A. Stark

K. Thomas

CW01502287

LEWIS'S PHARMACOLOGY

The previous editions of this book were dedicated to Charles and Dora Lewis, the parents of the original author. This edition is dedicated to the new author's family who have suffered much from his dedication to the book.

LEWIS'S PHARMACOLOGY

JAMES CROSSLAND

MA PhD FIBiol
Professor of Pharmacology
University of Nottingham

FIFTH EDITION

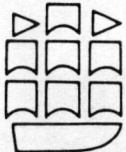

CHURCHILL LIVINGSTONE
EDINBURGH LONDON MELBOURNE AND NEW YORK 1980

CHURCHILL LIVINGSTONE
Medical Division of the Longman Group Limited

Distributed in the United States of America by
Churchill Livingstone Inc., 19 West 44th Street, New York,
N.Y. 10036, and by associated companies,
branches and representatives throughout
the world.

First Edition 1960 (J.J. Lewis)
Second Edition 1962 (J.J. Lewis)
Third Edition 1964 (J.J. Lewis)
Fourth Edition 1970 (revised by J. Crossland)
Fifth Edition 1980 (J. Crossland)

ISBN 0 443 02190 2
ISBN 0 443 01173 7 Pbk

British Library Cataloguing in Publication Data
Lewis, John Jacob
  Lewis's pharmacology. — 5th ed.
  1. Pharmacology
  I. Crossland, James   II. Pharmacology
  615'.1   RM300   80-40492

Printed and bound in Great Britain by
William Clowes (Beccles) Limited, Beccles and London

Preface to the Fifth Edition

The kind reception accorded to the Fourth Edition of *Lewis's Pharmacology* (the first under my authorship) has encouraged me to develop the book still further along the lines laid down in that edition. Although this has inevitably led to a considerable increase in the size of the book, I hope and believe that the style of writing, (which eschews unnecessary jargon, pays some attention to the niceties of English composition and assumes no previous knowledge of the subject on the part of the reader) will still make for easy and interesting reading that should be intelligible even to the most junior student who uses the book wisely. At the same time, the depth of treatment, combined with what I trust is a constructively critical approach to the subject, is intended to make the volume equally acceptable to the experienced pharmacologist. Several of the longer chapters are now substantial enough to be regarded as monographs in their own right.

Lewis's Pharmacology remains a single author text, a circumstance that ensures a uniformity of approach, style and outlook that is not always achieved by multiauthor projects. I hope that these substantial advantages are not completely offset by the obvious inability of a single author to achieve a total mastery of all the material with which he has to deal if he is to produce a comprehensive textbook of pharmacology. I leave my readers to adjudicate on this matter for themselves.

Nottingham, 1980
J.C.

Acknowledgements

The author of a textbook such as this receives his ideas, inspiration and information over a period of years from many sources. Some of this material becomes so integral a component of his total knowledge that he cannot always remember its origin and I must take this opportunity of apologizing to any writer who feels that his contribution to the subject of this book has been presented without due reference to its progenitor.

A large number of workers have generously supplied me with reprints of their own publications. These, particularly review articles, are of inestimable value and if I have not mentioned particular reviews in the text or bibliogrphy it is only because some restriction on coverage has to be imposed even in a book of this size.

I am indebted to authors and their publishers who have so readily given the permission to reproduce copyright material. More detailed acknowledgements are made at the appropriate points in the text but I would like to express my thanks to them as a group here.

A not inconsiderable number of those who perused the previous edition of this work have written to me with their suggestions for its improvement. Although pressure of work prevented my acknowledging all but a few of these letters, all the suggestions they contained were seriously considered and many of them have been adopted. I am most grateful to all those who took the trouble to write to me in this way and I hope that readers of the new edition will not hesitate to express their views on the book so that, with their help, it can be improved even further in future editions.

All the original diagrams in this (and the previous) edition of the book were drawn, or are based on drawings, by my son Mr. Paul G. Crossland whose artistic skills defy the laws of inheritance. I am most grateful to him for relieving me of the tedium of trying to draw them for myself.

My biggest debt of gratitude is owed, as always, to my wife, who converted my handwritten manuscript with its all but unintelligible instructions into a virtually perfect typescript that must have made the printer's task an easy one. She also corrected many of the proofs, checked the references and gave invaluable help in the formidable task of preparing the Index. The finished volume is almost as much her work as mine.

Finally I wish to place on record my appreciation of the efficiency, courtesy and never failing patience and understanding of all those members of the Churchill Livingstone organization who have been associated in any way with the production of this work.

Nottingham, 1980   J.C.

Extracts from the preface to the Fourth Edition

An *Introduction to Pharmacology* by J. J. Lewis first appeared in 1960. No comment concerning its value could be more telling than the fact that the Third Edition of the book was already on sale when Mr Lewis met his tragically premature death in 1965 and I felt more than flattered when the publishers invited me to undertake the preparation of a new edition.

My original intention was simply to bring the book up to date by adding new material where necessary, deleting that which had become outdated and altering the emphasis in certain chapters. It soon became clear that the results of such a patchy revision would have pleased neither my readers nor myself and the book which is now offered has been completely revised, rearranged and rewritten with the addition of a very considerable amount of entirely new matter.

The reader might justifiably enquire why I should wish—egocentricity apart—to make such drastic alterations in so conspicuously successful a book. The reason is twofold. Since the Third Edition of the book appeared a number of new and modestly-sized texts have been published. They also seek to fulfil the role of 'Introductions' to pharmacology and it seemed to me that the time was ripe for completing the conversion of 'Lewis' into the fully comprehensive textbook it was already becoming.

The other reason for redrafting the book so extensively was that emphases must change with authors and the times. For my part, I wish to stress the physiological and theoretical aspects of pharmacology at least as much as the chemical approach and I hope that in future editions it will be possible to complete the changes that have been initiated in this one. Nevertheless, I also hope that the spirit in which the original author approached his subject has not been lost and the retention of 'Lewis' in the title is much more than a formal gesture of respect to the book's creator.

The introductory chapter of previous editions has been expended into a series of eight chapters which examine several aspects of theoretical pharmacology and form Part I of the book. Part II discusses at some length the actions of a number of humoral substances and the nature of their involvement in fundamental physiological processes. Part III is concerned with the action of drugs on the various systems of the body. Chemotherapy is retained and forms Part IV of the book.

Although it is assumed that the reader will have completed at least an elementary course in physiology, some chapters and sections of chapters deal with topics in physiology. These topics are ones to which the pharmacologist has to make constant reference and particular attention has been paid to those that are often treated inadequately in elementary courses.

I hope that the detail provided is adequate for those who wish to study particular problems in some depth so that they can the more profitably read the review articles and original papers which no textbook can ever supplant. At the same time, the needs of those to whom pharmacology is a new subject have been kept constantly in mind. I have extended the practice, initiated by my predecessor, of explaining the origin and meaning of all the specialist terms used and I have provided a brief description of every clinical condition mentioned in the text. I hope that this will encourage the novice not to shun this work, for it is my belief that the beginner in any subject can benefit from a relatively large textbook. His teachers can tell him which parts he *must* study, but this enthusiasm is more likely to be kindled by his browsing, in however desultory a fashion, among those parts of the text that have not been categorized as prescribed reading.

Students new to pharmacology can have no immediate sense of its historical perspective nor of the soundness or shortcomings of the hypotheses by which it seeks to explain the facts of drug action. In this book, therefore, the major pharmacological topics have been approached, wherever possible, from the historical point of view and no attempt has been made to conceal the fact that not all the experimental findings are as reliable, nor the interpretations as valid, as they might at first sight appear. If some of these deficiencies are pointed out to the student, he may be encouraged to examine other pharmacological data with a critical eye and in this way he may come to realise that he, too, may be able to contribute something to the advancement of the subject.

This book contains the chemical formulae, therapeutic doses and proprietary names of all the drugs mentioned in the text. The multiplicity and the terminological ingenuities of pharmaceutical manufacturers defeat any effort to make lists of proprietary names complete; I hope that all the more common ones are given and that the reader may thus be spared the embarrassment so many of us have experienced when we have been made to appear ignorant of the nature of drugs with which we are perfectly familiar when they are identified by other names. As a further aid, the index incorporates a glossary of proprietary names with the corresponding approved names for quick or surreptitious reference. Although this work is in no sense a textbook of therapeutics, drug doses are included so that the reader may have some idea of the relative potencies and durations of action of different agents.

Pharmacology is a science in its own right and its practitioners, be they physiologists, physicians, pharmacists or pharmacologists proper, should speak the same language and be guided by the same pharmacological principles. Those who develop drugs, those who use them in their academic investigations, those who prescribe them and those who dispense them have much to gain by being made aware of each other's needs, problems and approaches and I trust that this volume may do something in the future, as its antecedents did in the past, to bring about this understanding.

Nottingham, 1969   J.C.

Contents

PART I

GENERAL PHARMACOLOGY

1. Introduction

'Pharmacology' means the 'science of drugs' but—even if we leave aside for a moment the question as to what constitutes a drug—this purely etymological definition is not a very satisfactory one. In one respect it is too broad, for there are several aspects of the 'science of drugs' which are of no interest to the pharmacologist as such. In other ways, however, the definition is far too narrow, for the scope of pharmacological research extends far beyond mere efforts to determine 'how drugs work'. In particular, the work of the pharmacologist has contributed much to our knowledge of fundamental physiological mechanisms. Equally, of course, many of the most important advances in pharmacology have come from the physiological laboratory. A rather more detailed consideration of this intimate and mutually rewarding interrelationship between physiology and pharmacology may serve to shed some light on the aims and status of pharmacology as a science in its own right.

The discovery, in 1889, that the removal of the pancreas from a dog led to the animal's drinking its own urine was a physiological observation which brought about the further discovery that carbohydrate metabolism is controlled by a hormone (insulin) liberated from specialised regions of the pancreas and that diabetes mellitus in the human subject is caused essentially by a deficiency of insulin. The use of insulin for the treatment of diabetes was prompted by these physiological observations: it is obviously a rational treatment since it represents an effort to restore normal physiological conditions by replacing the substance whose deficiency has led to the diseased state. When insulin is given to the diabetic subject, it is a drug in the layman's sense of the term—that is, it is a chemical substance given for therapeutic reasons—and the study of its actions in both the healthy and the diabetic subject clearly lies within the pharmacologist's province.

Relatively few drugs have been developed on the basis of a knowledge of the disturbances of physiological function which underlie specific disease processes but it is clear that this approach is an essential one if medicine is to be provided with an armoury of safe and effective drugs. Since all physiological responses involve, in the final analysis, the activity of chemical substances, the pharmacologist is vitally interested in efforts to determine the nature of these fundamental processes in the belief that he will be able to point the way to the development of other substances (drugs) which will potentiate, antagonize or otherwise modify these reactions. Thus progress in applied pharmacology and therapeutics is very much dependent on progress in physiology.

The discussion so far has emphasized the dependence of pharmacology on physiology but physiology in its turn owes much to pharmacology. However much we may hope and believe that the development of drugs in the future will be the result of advances in physiological knowledge, the fact remains that many of the most valuable therapeutic agents in use today were discovered (and are still being discovered!) as a result of purely empirical observations, some of them made in the very distant past. Pharmacologists seeking an explanation of the action of these drugs have not only discovered much that is important to the physiologist but on the basis of the knowledge they have acquired they have been able to provide him with useful tools to help unravel the complexities of physiological function. For instance, the experimental use of curare (the South American arrow poison which causes paralysis of skeletal muscle) was instrumental in elucidating the physiological processes involved in the initiation of muscle contraction by impulses in the motor nerve.

Another preoccupation of the pharmacologist is with the relationship between chemical structure and pharmacological action. This type of study has a twofold purpose. In the first place it aims to provide information for the chemist which will enable him to synthesize new compounds with special kinds of activity. In this connection, it should be noted that even when a disease process can be certainly attributed to deficiency of a known chemical substance, simple replacement therapy might not be the best, or even an adequate, treatment for the disease. The liberation of many of the body's regulatory substances fluctuates in response to the varying demands made upon them and after liberation they may be rapidly destroyed by enzymatic or other actions. Artificial administration of a substance of this type to a patient who cannot produce it from endogenous sources may only be able to reproduce the compound's physiological action if it is given more frequently than is convenient to the patient or according to a dose schedule too complex for him to understand. A synthetic or a semisynthetic derivative with a similar physiological action may well prove to be a more valuable therapeutic agent if, for instance, it is not susceptible to enzymatic inactivation or if it can be presented in a form enabling it to be slowly liberated into the blood stream.

Again it may sometimes be necessary to develop a drug, perhaps of a type that does not occur in the body, in order to counter the effect of a natural chemical such as a hormone which is causing disease because it is being liberated in abnormally large amounts. A detailed knowledge of the structure of the natural compound is clearly needed if a specific antagonist is to be produced. Thus chemistry is as important an adjunct to pharmacology as is physiology.

The other reason why studies of structure-action relationships are important is that they provide the sort of information that is required for the proper understanding of the chemical nature of the subcellular structures (the receptors, Chap. 8) through the medium of which many of the body's own chemical regulators exert their action.

The foregoing discussion may enable the reader to appreciate more clearly what is implicit in what is, to the author at least, the most acceptable definition of pharmacology—that it is the science which studies the mode of action of chemical substances on living tissues and organisms. It will be appreciated that the pharmacologist's definition of a drug (any chemical substance which has an action on living tissues) is considerably wider than that likely to be offered by the layman, the physician or the pharmacist.

A knowledge of pharmacology is required by students of several disciplines including medicine and dentistry, veterinary surgery, physiology and pharmacy but it is important to recognize that pharmacology is a science in its own right and that it can be studied as an independent subject. It is, in fact, both a pure and an applied science and it is this which makes its study a peculiarly fascinating and rewarding pursuit. The academic pharmacologist knows that his work may quite suddenly prove to have important therapeutic implications while the applied pharmacologist, actively seeking or testing new compounds of therapeutic interest, knows equally well that he may quite suddenly make a discovery of immediate theoretical and academic significance.

THE HISTORY OF PHARMACOLOGY

Sir John Gaddum (1900–1965) who was for many years a dominant figure in English pharmacology, once wrote that pharmacology began when man first used a plant extract to relieve the symptoms of disease. If we were to accept this view we would certainly have to place pharmacology among the oldest of the sciences for, since the dawn of his turbulent history, man has looked for substances that might ease his pain, lighten the burden of his illnesses, elevate his spirits and provide him with previews of a joyful after-life and with glorious visions of the gods who are to provide it. His unremitting search for these drugs, charms and potions grew out of his natural curiosity and was sustained by a belief in magic and by a faith in the superior power of beneficent gods (or of the one God when monotheism prevailed) who, though they might advertise their power by afflicting us with disease, also provided, for those who cared to look, the wherewithal to cure these very ills.

That pharmacology was originally a branch of magic is a fact that is enshrined in its very name for it is derived from the Greek *pharmakon,* a word which, according to Liddell and Scott, that famous pair of lexicographers, means 'a drug, whether healing or noxious; a healing remedy or medicine; an enchanted potion or philtre hence charm, spell; poison; a lye for laundry'. So we might perhaps be tempted to define pharmacology as the 'science of drugs, charms and magic'. It is a much more picturesque and romantic definition than the one we arrived at earlier and it is not without its merits: it is etymologically sound and it emphasises the inextricable mingling, throughout history, of medicine and magic, science and superstition and the activities of physicians and priests. The great literary figures of the past would certainly have accepted this definition. Thus Chaucer's 'perfect practising physician'

> ... watched his patient's favourable star
> and, by his Natural Magic, knew what are
> the lucky hours and planetary degrees
> for making charms and magic effigies,
> The cause of every malady you'd got
> he knew and whether dry, cold, moist or hot;
> he knew their seat, their humour and condition.

while Shakespeare put into Othello's mouth an explanation of how he won Desdemona. He will, he says

> ... a round unvarnished tale deliver
> of my whole course of love; what drugs, what
> charms, what conjuration and what mighty magic
> .... I won his daughter (with).

In this reputedly scientific age, remnants of our primitive beliefs persist: many of us well recall how, as children, we tried to alleviate the discomfort of nettle stings by rubbing dock leaves on to the insulted limb and how right it seemed to us that the nettles and the docks—the sword and the shield—should grow together side by side. As for belief in magic, this seems to be, in some respects, as compelling as it ever was. Many otherwise quite sophisticated people retain a touching faith in the ability of drugs to perform miracles of restorative healing and the course of many illnesses is favourably influenced by substances that have demonstrably no pharmacological action whatever (*placebos,* p. 143.)

In his search for anodynes and remedies, early man obviously had to make use of the materials he found around him and it was inevitable that among them he should fortuitously discover some substances of real and lasting value. It would be difficult to name a more valuable trio of drugs than opium, salicylates and digitalis but they (and many other therapeutic agents that find their place in this book) all made their appearance in the distant past, opium at least 7000 years ago. But those who stumbled across these early drugs were not scientists in any acceptable sense of that word because their outlook was still dominated by irrational, untenable and untestable beliefs in the power of magic and supernatural agencies. The first premonition of the change that was slowly to transform medicine into a branch of science came, fittingly enough, from Jean Fernel (1497–1558), the father of physiology. Fernel's greatest work *De Naturali Parte Medicinae* was first published in 1542 but the 1554 edition was retitled *Physiologia* and this marks—74 years before Harvey described the circulation of the blood—the first use of the word 'physiology' to describe the study of bodily functions. Fernel (who wrote treatises on pharmacy and on therapeutics as well as on physiology) had no use for magic: he could not believe, for instance, that epilepsy could be treated by administering spring water from the scalp of a man killed by fire. 'The scalp of any man soever enjoys the same powers and the manner of his death makes no difference to that'.

'Pharmacology' was not added to the language until 1693. In that year, Samuel Dale produced the first edition of his *Pharmacologia seu Manuductio ad Materiam Medicam*, a book that was dedicated to the then stripling Royal College of Physicians of London. Dale saw pharmacology as a purely descriptive science whose task was to systematize and catalogue existing knowledge of natural medicinal substances whether they were used in their native state or were modified by some preparative process. His book is a remarkable compilation of information and anyone who is prepared to devote the time and effort required to translate its 656 pages of scholarly Latin will be amply rewarded by the fascination of discovering the extraordinary range of naturally occurring materials (including water and earths from an astonishing variety of sources) that the physicians of the time had at their disposal.

Dale's book cannot be regarded as a textbook of pharmacology in the way that Fernel's masterpiece is even now recognised as a textbook of physiology. As a descriptive and organised catalogue of drugs it more closely resembles a pharmacopoiea and it is, indeed, referred to as such by its author. And for many years after Dale, the skill of the physician depended on his being able to recognise medicinally useful plants and to distinguish them from poisonous species. The relevance of this study is illustrated by the fact that several universities created combined chairs of botany and medicine but our physician-botanists for the most part made no ordered study of the properties of the plants they collected. Such rudiments of pharmacology that they managed to acquire became incorporated into 'materia medica', a name that lingered in the titles of textbooks and university departments long after the subject itself ceased to be dominated by identifying descriptions of medicinal plants.

If it is not too presumptuous to question Gaddum's dating we should surely say that pharmacology was born when man first conducted experiments to establish *why* his medicaments relieved the ills for which they were prescribed. This is a very recent activity: although experiments of an indubitably pharmacological nature were performed in the early years of the nineteenth century (notably by Magendie in France and by Christison in Scotland) the first laboratory actually to be called pharmacological and to be devoted exclusively to a study of this subject was set up, as recently as 1849, by Rudolf Buchheim in the German university of Dorpat in Estonia. In his later years Buchheim established another pharmacology laboratory, this time in Giessen. Buchheim investigated the actions of a wide range of drugs including purgatives, anthelminthics and the heavy metals but his chief claim to recognition by the modern pharmacologist is his insistence that the investigation of the mode of action of drugs could only be satisfactorily undertaken by properly trained pharmacologists. A brief quotation from his writings will indicate how closely the views of this pioneer pharmacologist accord with those of his modern counterpart.

The investigation of drugs, therefore, is a task for a pharmacologist and not for a chemist or pharmacist, who until now have been expected to do this ... The advantages which we expect to gain from a scientific development of pharmacology will benefit other medical sciences. Physiology can use drugs as tools for analysing the function of organs and certainly will repay handsomely for the service rendered by pharmacology. (Quoted in Holmstedt & Liljestrand, 1963).

Twenty years after Buchheim founded his laboratory, Carl Binz (1832–1913) instituted a pharmacology laboratory in Bonn. Binz demonstrated that quinine is lethal to a number of organisms including the malarial parasite but he is best known for his published lectures which were widely read both inside and outside Germany. The greatest of the early German pharmacologists, however, was undoubtedly Oswald Schmiedeberg who became professor of pharmacology at Strasbourg in 1872, where he remained until his death, at the age of 83, in 1921. Schmiedeberg's writings were as influential as those of Binz but his claim to fame rests on the very large numbers of enthusiastic workers he attracted to his laboratories. Many of these workers themselves became prominent pharmacologists who were then able to promote the subject in many countries of the world. Included among their number were the first occupants of chairs of pharmacology in the United States and England. John Jacob Abel (1857–1938) took up his appointment at Ann Arbor, Michigan in 1891 and Arthur Robertson Cushny (1866–1926) a Scotsman who had previously succeeded Abel at Ann Arbor, became professor of pharmacology at University College, London in 1905. The development of pharmacology in Britain was not quite so tardy as the latter date might suggest because Sir Thomas Brunton (1844–1916), influenced by what he had seen in Germany, established a pharmacology laboratory in a tiny room in St Bartholomew's Hospital in 1873 and twelve years later he published a voluminous textbook (*Textbook of Pharmacology, Therapeutics and Materia Medica*), much of which dealt with truly pharmacological topics. Even earlier than this, Robert Christison (1797–1882) who became professor of materia medica and therapeutics in Edinburgh in 1832 and Thomas Richard Fraser (1841–1920), his erstwhile assistant, who succeeded him in 1877, were experimental pharmacologists in all but name: some of their work preceded, by a few years, the setting up of Buchheim's laboratory. In this very first piece of pharmacological research, Christison examined an extract of calabar bean, the nut of Etu Esere, which had been used in Nigeria since time immemorial for the trial of witches by ordeal. If the accused could save her life by vomiting the poison she was deemed to be innocent. Christison studied the pharmacological actions of the extract in considerable detail and Fraser, who isolated its active principle (physostigmine, p. 213), was able to recommend its use, which it still enjoys, in the treatment of ophthalmological conditions—a far cry from the trial of witches! Perhaps, then, we should identify Edinburgh as the birthplace of pharmacology: birthplace or no, that university continued to attract pharmacologists. In 1918, Fraser was succeeded by Cushny, whose own chair at University College was filled by Alfred Joseph Clark (1885–1941) who in his turn went to Edinburgh when Cushny died in 1926. Clark was particularly interested in the general mechanisms of drug action and his hypothesis that in many instances drugs exert their action as a result of a unimolecular reaction with specific receptors in the tissues is the foundation of many present day ideas concerning the kinetics of drug action and the mechanisms of drug antagonisms. The recognition of pharmacology as an independent science was confirmed, in Britain, in 1931 when the British Pharmacological Society was formed by a small group of pharmacologically minded physiologists.

It has already been made clear that Germany was the cradle of pharmacology and the development of pharmacology in Britain and the United States was considerably helped by refugees from Hitler's Germany who, by their contributions to science, have repaid many times over any debt they owed to their host countries.

The work of contemporary pharmacologists is described in the main body of this book but the brief historical sketch just presented would not be complete without mention of Sir Henry Dale, the doyen of British pharmacologists. He was born in 1875 and died in 1968: his forebears were in no way related to Samuel Dale. Sir Henry's contributions to pharmacology (particularly in connection with histamine, the ergot alkaloids and the hypothesis of humoral transmission in the nervous system) were massive. His life and work are surveyed in an absorbing memoir by Feldberg (1970).

Space does not permit a discussion here of the development of pharmacology elsewhere than in Britain but a glance at the historical information presented in other chapters will make it clear that recent advances in pharmacology have come from many parts of the world and that the contributions made by some of the smaller nations such as Belgium, Switzerland and Scandinavia have been out of all proportion to the size of their countries.

Chemotherapy, like pharmacology itself, is of German origin. Much of Binz's work was of an essentially chemotherapeutic nature but the universally recognized father of chemotherapy is Paul Ehrlich (1854–1915) whose discovery of the value of the organic arsenicals in the treatment of syphilis ranks as one of the milestones of medicine. The development of chemotherapy since Ehrlich is fully discussed in Part IV of this book.

BIBLIOGRAPHY

Books, monographs and reviews

Feldberg, W.S. (1970) Henry Hallett Dale, 1875-1968. *Biog. Mems. Fellows Roy. Soc.* **16**, 77-174.

Holmstedt, B. and Liljestrand, G. (1963). *Readings in Pharmacology*. Oxford and London: Pergamon Press.

Marquardt, M. (1949) *Paul Ehrlich*. London: Heinemann.

Sherrington, Sir Charles (1946) *The Endeavour of Jean Fernel*. Cambridge: University Press.

Singer, C. and Underwood, E.A. (1962) *A Short History of Medicine*. Oxford: University Press.

2. Some aspects of cell structure and function

As more has become known about the effects of drugs on whole animals and isolated tissues there has developed a natural and laudable desire to discover the cellular and molecular changes that underlie the overt manifestations of drug action. It is no accident that this is the first of the several editions of this book to carry a chapter devoted to the cell, for it is only quite recently that advances in pharmacology and related sciences have demanded frequent mentions of cellular reactions in a variety of contexts. Every young student today (and even the television viewer who retains a modicum of what he sees) knows something about the finer details of cell structure but not all who read this book will be young students (or, it is to be hoped, ardent televiewers) and the information supplied in this chapter should provide a necessary, if skeletal, background for those with no previous knowledge of biology or with knowledge that was acquired in the days before 'The Double Helix' became compulsory nursery reading.

The idea that living organisms, however complex, are made up of discrete units can be said to have begun in 1665 when Robert Hooke first used the word 'cell' in a biological sense. Hooke had just invented the microscope and his new instrument was revealing details of plant structure that had never before been seen. When he studied 'an exceeding thin piece of wood' he noticed that it possessed a porous structure 'much like a honeycomb, but...these pores, or cells, were not very deep but consisted of a great many little boxes separated out of one continuous long pore by certain diaphragms'. He demonstrated similar structures in a variety of other plants but it is clear that he and his contemporaries thought of the cells as nothing more than empty chambers, analogous (hence their very name) to the small cells occupied by solitary monks or prisoners (Latin *cella*, a storeroom). Later biologists came to realize that the empty spaces described by Hooke were occupied, in living tissue, by a semi-liquid material (*protoplasm*) which is the real substance of living matter. Later still it became clear that all living organisms, animals as well as plants, consist of ordered agglomerates of cells and that the rigid cell walls that Hooke had described so vividly occur only in plant tissue where their sole function is to maintain the shape and form of the organism.

This unified cell theory is usually attributed to Schleiden and Schwann who in 1838 brought together the scattered observations and hypotheses that had appeared since the time of Hooke. Schleiden was a botanist and

Schwann was a zoologist whose name is perpetuated in the Schwann cells of peripheral nerves. They had been working independently and the most important fruit of their short lived collaboration (it is said to have begun and ended over the dinner table) was the recognition that the structures that Schwann had seen in animal tissues were cells with essentially the same form and structure as those that Schleiden and his predecessors had described in plants. Animals and plants, then, were assembled from the same kind of 'building blocks' but it was some time before the ubiquity of cells and the overriding importance of their activity was fully appreciated. At least twenty years were to elapse before biologists realized that new cells can only arise from other cells and that the birth of a new member of an animal species is preceded by the fusion of germ cells (ovum and spermatozoon) to form a parent cell from which the offspring develops by a process of repeated cell division and the growth of the daughter cells so produced. And it was not until 1871 that Waldeyer published his theory that the whole of the nervous system is made up of anatomically discrete (but functionally integrated) cells or neurones.

Among the biologists who were active between the times of Hooke and of Schleiden and Schwann and whose work tends for that reason to be overlooked, Purkinje merits special mention. Purkinje, a Bohemian physician, was born in 1787 and he failed by only one year to be alive a century later. His name is commemorated in the Purkinje fibres of the heart and the Purkinje cells of the cerebellum, he made a number of extremely valuable contributions to physiological and pharmacological knowledge and it was he who was responsible, about 1829, for the introduction of the word protoplasm to describe the semi-solid substance of cells. Purkinje had been educated by Piarist monks and he had himself been a monastic member of that order for a short time. His studies had made him familiar with the theological concept of protoplasm (literally the first flesh), a synonym for Adam, the prototype of us all. Purkinje's transfer of the theological term to biology displayed great perspicacity.

As we have seen, animal cells are not bounded by rigid cell walls. The overall volume of an individual organ is often maintained by a surrounding membranous capsule and its final shape is moulded and maintained by the pressure of neighbouring organs and other bodily structures. Many of the minute details of organ shape that are so carefully described in the older textbooks of anatomy disappear when an organ is removed from the living body: placed on a bench it tends to collapse into a shapeless mass. The form of the body as a whole, as opposed to that of its individual organs, is, of course, determined by its bony skeleton.

Some structural features of the animal cell

The optical microscope, which reached the peak of its development in the early 1940's, revealed some of the more gross features of the cell's anatomy but the finer structural details which are commonly pictured in even the most elementary of contemporary textbooks of biology remained hidden until the advent of the electron microscope some thirty years ago.

A simple and schematic sketch of the animal cell is presented in Fig. 2.1: the reader who wishes to acquire a more substantial knowledge of the appearance and structure of the several components of the cell is referred to the many excellent textbooks of cell biology now available including those listed in the bibliography appended to this chapter (p. 32). He will also profit from studying the splendid diagrams and photographs in *Gray's Anatomy* (Warwick and Williams, 1973).

The bodies found within most cells are commonly described as *organelles:* particular functions have been assigned to each species of organelle. Cells specialized in this fashion are known as *eucaryotes* (or eucaryotic cells) while those that carry little in the way of immediately evident inclusions are said to be *procaryotic.* The only procaryotes with which the pharmacologist is concerned, directly or indirectly, are the bacteria.

The paragraphs that follow provide very brief descriptions of the components of animal eucaryotes.

The nucleus

In any cell (save the mammalian erythrocyte, which is anucleate) the most prominent organelle is the nucleus. Because of its size, the nucleus was recognized as early as 1673 so that the major division of the cell's structure into nucleus and cytoplasm is of long standing.

The nucleus plays a dominent role in cell physiology, imposing its will, by way of its own inclusions (*chromatin* material and *nucleoli*), on the processes of reproduction, growth, development and repair. A cell without a nucleus—the most familiar example of such a cell is the mature red blood corpuscle—is indeed a very poor specimen of living matter, being denied so many of the activities permitted to nucleated cells and destined for early death.

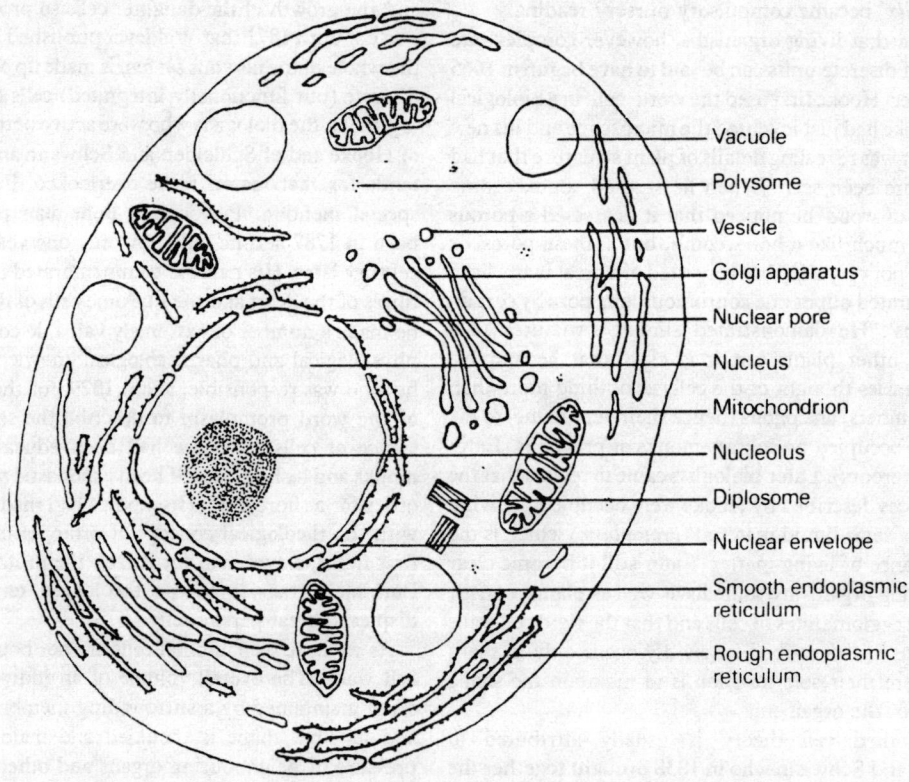

Vacuole
Polysome
Vesicle
Golgi apparatus
Nuclear pore
Nucleus
Mitochondrion
Nucleolus
Diplosome
Nuclear envelope
Smooth endoplasmic reticulum
Rough endoplasmic reticulum

Fig. 2.1 Principal features of the animal cell.

Most nuclei possess between one and four nucleoli. These are prominent, roughly spherical bodies made up largely of protein and ribonucleic acid (RNA). Chromatin, the material of the *chromosomes*, exists in both tightly coiled and relatively uncoiled states known as *heterochromatin* and *euchromatin* respectively. Chromatin is made up of strands of deoxyribonucleic acid (DNA). The nature and activity of the nucleolus and the chromosomes and of their constituent nucleotides are more fully described below.

The nucleus is surrounded by a narrow bag or sac (the *nuclear envelope*) which is continuous with and, indeed, forms a part of, the endoplasmic reticulum (p. 11) which permeates the whole of the cytoplasm (Fig. 2.1). In places, the two walls of the nuclear envelope are fused over a short distance and are here perforated by the *nuclear pores* which provide a two way channel of communication between the nucleus and the cytoplasmic matrix or *hyaloplasm*.

That part of the nucleus that does not consist of chromatin material is called *nuclear sap*: it contains dissolved material on its way from nucleus to cytoplasm together with fine particulate material of a so far unidentified structure and function.

The plasma membrane

We have already noted that, unlike those in plants and some bacteria, animal cells are not surrounded by a rigid cell wall. They are, however, bounded by an extremely delicate *plasma membrane* which provides an effective functional boundary between a cell and its neighbours or the extracellular fluid in which it is bathed. Knowledge of the differences between the extracellular and the intracellular fluids demanded the existence of just such a limiting membrane long before electron microscope studies demonstrated its physical reality.

Under the electron microscope the plasma membrane appears as two dense lines each about 2nm thick and separated by a less dense area, the overall thickness of the membrane amounting to some 8nm. Preparation of tissues for electron microscopy inevitably results in a degree of dehydration and in the living state plasma membranes probably have thicknesses of 9 or 10nm. The plasma membranes of adjacent cells are separated by a gel like substance that does not impede the free passage of anything but the larger protein molecules. In some regions the intercellular gap reaches a width of 50nm or so but in others it disappears completely, the plasma membranes of adjacent cells being fused together. The region of fused membranes is sometimes called the *junctional complex* and it appears to serve two purposes: it helps to bind the cells together and it also prevents the direct passage of material from the extracellular fluid into fine vessels or ducts (such as the bile canaliculi in the liver) that might be making their way through the intercellular space (Fig. 2.2a).

Although the gross chemical composition of the plasma membrane of several cell types is now reasonably well established, our knowledge of the way in which the individual constituents are disposed so as to provide a structure with the known properties of the membrane is much more controversial. Much of the work that has attempted to provide an answer to this problem has utilized red blood corpuscles. These cells are nothing more than plasma membrane bags filled with haemoglobin. When the corpuscles are haemolysed and washed, only plasma membranes ('ghosts') remain and this provides a simple way of obtaining the membranes in quantity and from known numbers of cells. It hardly needs to be said that conclusions based on studies of red cell ghosts are not necessarily (perhaps it should be 'necessarily not') applicable in their entirety to all other cells.

The plasma membrane of human erythrocytes is made up of protein (about 60 per cent of the dry weight of the membrane), cholesterol (about 9 per cent) and a number of phospholipids including sphingomyelin, phosphatidyl choline (lecithin), phosphatidyl ethanolamine and phosphatidyl serine. The membranes of the other cells that have been intensively studied have quantitatively, and to some extent qualitatively, different compositions: liver cells, for instance, contain more cholesterol (about 13 per cent) in their membranes with negligible amounts of phosphatidyl serine and phosphatidyl ethanolamine. Details of the composition of the plasma membranes of several cell types can be found in textbooks of cell biology such as that by Haggis (1974).

The chemical formulae of cholesterol, together with those of lecithin and sphingomyelin—these latter to illustrate structural features common to all the phospholipids—are displayed in Fig. 2.2b. The long hydrocarbon chains in all these molecules are strongly hydrophobic but the polar groups (hydroxyl in cholesterol and the charged nitrogen atoms and phosphate groups in the phospholipids) are hydrophilic. At an oil-water interface, molecules of this type dispose themselves in such a fashion that their hydrophobic ends lie in the oil while their hydrophilic ends enter the water.

Knowledge of the properties of their component molecules and of the actual mass of the membranes themselves led to the proposal that plasma membranes consist essentially of a double layer of the polar molecules arranged in such a way that the hydrophobic ends are directed towards the interior while the hydrophilic ends form the outer and inner boundaries of the membrane. The protein molecules are visualized as coating and interdigitating with the hydrophilic extremities of the double structure. To complete the picture, in accordance with the known facts of diffusion across the membrane (p. 39), perforations or 'pores' are added (Fig. 2.2c).

This concept of the nature of the plasma membrane (which was originally due to Danielli and his co-workers) is almost certainly an overly simple one. The reader should

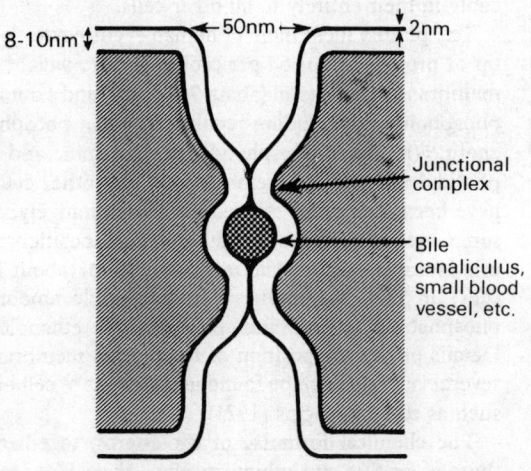

(a) Schematic representation of the plasma membrane

8-10nm   50nm   2nm

Junctional complex

Bile canaliculus, small blood vessel, etc.

Cholesterol

(b) Lipid components of the plasma membrane

phosphatidyl choline (lecithin)

sphingomyelin

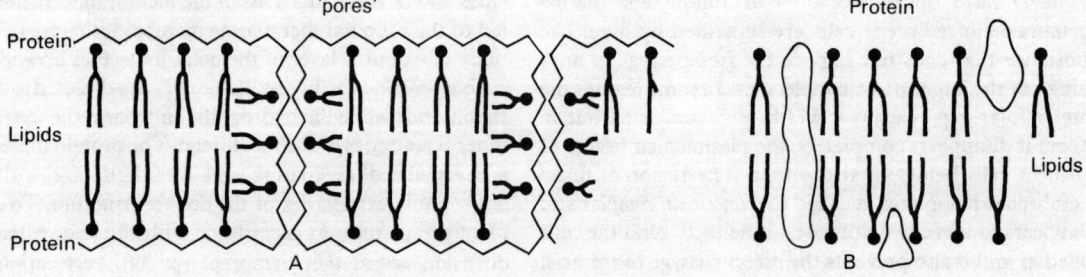

'pores'

Protein

Lipids

Protein

A

Protein

Lipids

B

(c)(i) The plasma membrane according to Danielli's concept. (ii) In the alternative Singer mosaic model the protein molecules are seen as being intermingled with and partially embedded in the double layer of lipid molecules.

Fig. 2.2 The structure of the plasma membrane.

be particularly careful not to assume that the two dark lines seen in electron micrographs of the membrane correspond to the hypothetical two rows of hydrophilic moieties of polar molecules with their associated proteins. Nevertheless, even if it is a caricature rather than an accurate representation of the real thing, the structure depicted in Fig. 2.2c should prove acceptable to most pharmacologists. From their point of view, cells certainly behave as if they were bounded by membranes of this type.

Endoplasmic reticulum

The electron microscope has revealed that the cytoplasm of almost all cells is permeated by a system of interconnected spaces that appear as flattened sacs (often known as *cisternae*) and tubules. The boundaries of these spaces, which together constitute the endoplasmic reticulum, consist essentially of phospholipid membranes. The endoplasmic reticulum usually communicates with the perinuclear space. Some parts of the reticulum are studded with ribosomes (see below) but other parts of the same system are free of ribosomes: the two forms are known, for obvious reasons, as rough (or granular) and smooth (or agranular) endoplasmic reticulum respectively. The relative amounts of the two forms varies with the cell type, the rough form being particularly prominent in cells that synthesize and secrete protein in quantity.

When cell homogenates are subjected to ultracentrifugation, the endoplasmic reticulum breaks up into spherical fragments. These fragments, with their associated ribosomes, constitute the *microsomes*. Surrounded by intact membranes, the microsomes retain the chemical activity of the parent structure. Microsomal enzymes are involved in both synthetic and catabolic processes.

The endoplasmic reticulum in muscle cells is known as the *sarcoplasmic reticulum*.

Ribosomes

The rough endoplasmic reticulum, as we have seen, carries ribosomes but these particles also occur independently in the cytoplasm either singly or in small groups (the *polysomes*) arranged as clusters or rosettes. In sections prepared for electron microscopy, ribosomes are some 15nm in diameter but they are presumably a little larger in fresh tissue.

Ribosomes consist of ribonucleic acid and protein and they are intimately involved in the process of protein synthesis. They are themselves manufactured in the nucleoli and are discussed in more detail later (p. 20).

The Golgi apparatus

This structure was first identified as long ago as 1898 by the famous neurohistologist whose name it bears and who is also eponymously commemorated in a number of neural structures and stains. For many years, the Golgi apparatus was the centre of controversy, many authorities averring

that it was nothing more than a histological artefact but electron microscopy and the development of a specific stain finally established the reality of its existence.

The Golgi apparatus is almost universally present in cells (the mammalian erythrocyte provides the usual exception) and it takes the form of 'stacks' of membrane-bound saccules, separated from one another by distances of approximately 25nm. These are associated with a number of vesicles and larger vacuoles, most of which are derived by budding from the saccules themselves. In the peripheral reaches of the saccules, the limiting membrane is punctured by a number of holes (*fenestrations*) analogous to those found in the nuclear membrane.

The number of saccules in a Golgi stack in the cells of animals and higher plants normally ranges from three to seven (there are five in the one represented in Fig. 2.1) though there are often more in the stacks of more elementary organisms. The Golgi apparatus is more widespread in neurones and gland cells than it is elsewhere but its general structure is everywhere the same.

The Golgi stack as a whole often takes on a curved configuration, the 'top' of the stack (the region nearer the apex of the cell) being convex and the 'bottom' being concave. The concentration of the saccular contents increases from the topmost to the lowest member of the stack as does the number of associated vesicles. It seems likely that saccules move progressively down their stacks, the lowest ones breaking up into vesicles as a new one is added at the top.

The products of secretory cells are elaborated by the conjoint activity of the endoplasmic reticulum and the Golgi apparatus. Enzyme proteins, for instance, are synthesized in the cisternae of the rough endoplasmic reticulum under the control of the associated ribosomes and are then passed into the Golgi saccules. The transfer is probably effected by *transport vesicles* which bud off from the cisternae in the immediate neighbourhood of a Golgi apparatus and are then taken into the topmost saccule of the stack. On their way down the stack the saccule contents are concentrated. They finally leave the apparatus as the granular contents of the vesicles and vacuoles.

Secretory cells also elaborate polysaccharides but these compounds are actually synthesized within the Golgi stacks. Glycoproteins are assembled in the Golgi apparatus from carbohydrate molecules collected there and protein synthesized by the rough endoplasmic reticulum.

Lysosomes

Unlike the other cellular inclusions, lysosomes are identified by their biochemical activities and not by their morphological characteristics. Their name was coined by de Duve to indicate that they are repositories of hydrolytic enzymes (*hydrolases*). Lysosomal enzymes are some forty in number and they include phosphatases, lipases, proteases including cathepsin, glycosidases, β-glucuronidase, sulphatases, ribonuclease and deoxyribonuclease. This formidable battery of enzymes is capable of handling every kind of large molecule normally encountered by the cell. A lysosome is properly defined as an intracellular structure that contains at least two of the known lysosomal enzymes.

Lysosomes are synthesized in the rough endoplasmic reticulum and the newly created molecules (*primary lysosomes*) first appear in the Golgi vesicles. *Secondary lysosomes* are lysosomes that have taken up material and are in the process of digesting it. Secondary lysosomes that have accumulated large quantities of undigested material are known as *residual bodies*.

Lysosomes, as would be expected, are particularly prominent in phagocytes but since most cells are continually engaged in digesting and replacing their components, lysosomes are found in virtually all cells. Structures that have reached the end of their useful life collect in *autophagic vacuoles* which then fuse with lysosomes. Polymorphonuclear leucocytes contain primary lysosomes that are released when the leucocytes congregate at sites of inflammatory activity and there destroy bacteria and other cells.

Lysosomes are bounded by resistant limiting membranes that protect the contents of the cell (other than those taken up by the lysosomes) from digestion.

Genetic abnormalities sometimes result in the production of lysosomes that are deficient in one or other enzyme. This gives rise to such *storage diseases* as Pompe's disease in which the liver, heart and muscles become engorged with undigested glycogen. The vital importance of the lysosomal enzymes is testified to by the fact that Pompe's disease is invariably fatal.

Peroxisomes

Peroxisomes are membrane limited vesicles reminiscent of lysosomes but of no more than 1μ in diameter. They contain oxidases (urate oxidase, α-hydroxyacid oxidase and D-aminoacid oxidase) that give rise to hydrogen peroxide and catalase, which destroys it. Some peroxisomes will, in addition, break down purines while many bacteria possess peroxisomes that contain the enzymes necessary to operate the glyoxalate cycle, a system that supplements and supports the citric acid cycle.

Mitochondria

As long ago as 1850, von Kölliker reported the presence of granular structures in striated muscle and some thirty years later Fleming found thread-like bodies in the cytoplasm of other cells. It eventually became clear that these two types of structure were different versions of the same organelle and Benda's naming of these bodies as mitochondria (from the Greek *mitos*, a thread and *chondros*, a grain) was most appropriate. This inspired nomenclature dates from the end of the last century.

Mitochondria most often appear as elongated bodies some $5-10\mu m$ long and one-tenth of that in diameter. They are present in all cells, except erythrocytes and bacteria, in numbers that range from one or two to more than a thousand. They are sites of energy production and cells with the highest rates of oxidative metabolism contain the most (and also the largest) mitochondria.

Under the electron microscope, the mitochondrion reveals itself as essentially a double walled sac. The outer wall is smooth and is separated by a distance of some 8nm from a much convoluted inner wall characterized by the presence of prominent projections (or *cristae*) some of which extend all the way across the organelle (Fig. 2.3). The cristae, which are formed by infoldings of the inner wall, greatly increase the internal surface of the organelle. It should be noted that, although a simple diagram inevitably conveys a different impression, the cristae are usually attached to the inner wall of the mitochondrion over only a short length of their circumference.

The mitochondrion is filled with a finely granular *matrix* which often contains a number of much denser granules which may reach diameters of 50nm.

The mitochondrial membranes or walls are made up of mixtures of proteins and lipid material held together by hydrophobic bonds. The general structure recalls that of the plasma membrane but some of the proteins in the inner wall and its cristae are enzymes.

As we shall discuss later (p. 27), oxidative metabolism involves the activity of the citric acid cycle and an electron

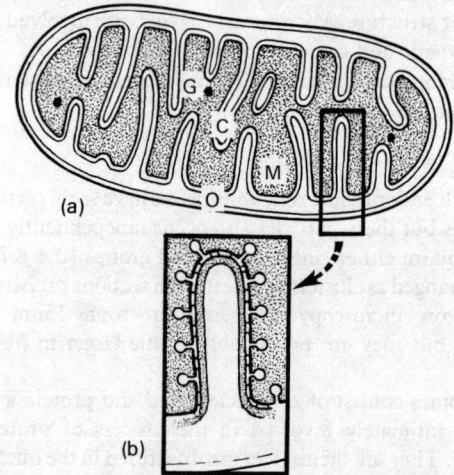

(a) General structure. *Reproduced by kind permission of the authors and publisher of Toner & Carr (1971).* M-matrix; C-crista; G-intramitochondrial granules; O-outer mitochondrial space. (b) To illustrate the position of the spheres containing ATPase

Fig. 2.3 The mitochondrion

transport chain and results in the formation of adenosine triphosphate (ATP). The enzymes of the citric acid cycle are dissolved in the matrix of the mitochondrion while those of the electron transport chain are in the cristae. ATPase, an enzyme required for the final step in ATP production is located on tiny projections with which the cristae are studded.

Mitochondria are unique among intracellular organelles in that they contain their own machinery for synthesizing some of their component proteins independently of any control by chromosomal genes. This circumstance has led some biologists to speculate that mitochondria have evolved from what were originally intracellular parasitic bacteria.

Centrioles
The centrioles are a pair of cylindrical structures some $0.5\mu m$ long and $0.2\mu m$ in diameter. They are found together near the nucleus and often in close association with the Golgi apparatus. Typically they are disposed with their long axes lying at right angles to one another. The two centrioles together are sometimes described as a *diplosome* and the diplosome and the immediate area of the cell in which it lies is sometimes called the *centrosome*.

Each centriole is invariably composed of nine flattened tubes (or they may possibly be solid rods) arranged in an imbricated fashion (that is to say they overlap one another slightly like the tiles on a roof) into a cylindrical form. The tubes spiral gently along the length of the centriole. Each of the component nine tubes is itself made up of a triplet of interconnected tubules or fibrils.

Small, dense cylindrical granules (the *centriolar satellites*) are often evident in the immediate vicinity of the centrioles.

The centrioles are involved in the processes of cell division: their behaviour during this activity is considered later (p. 17).

FRACTIONATION OF CELL COMPONENTS
The various subcellular organelles can be obtained for biochemical investigation by disrupting tissue samples and then subjecting them to repeated centrifugations at progressively increasing speeds (*differential centrifugation*). Because of their differing sizes, shapes and densities the individual components separate out at different stages of the centrifugation process (Fig. 2.4). The initial disruption of the cell is often brought about by gently homogenizing the tissue (liver is a rich source of intracellular inclusions) in 0.25M sucrose solution in a Potter type homogenizer, a device in which the tissue is trapped and broken up in a narrow annular space between a rotating cylindrical plunger (or pestle) and the walls of a matching cylindrical vessel containing the tissue and the homogenizing medium. Sucrose solution is used because it protects the integrity of the organelles and prevents their aggregating

together when they are separated from the cell. Other techniques including exposure to ultrasonic radiation, grinding with solid carbon dioxide or extrusion under pressure through a fine aperture can be used to produce a supply of disrupted cells which liberate intact organelles. The plasma membrane which completely encircles the cell and the endoplasmic reticulum which permeates it cannot, of course, escape fragmentation during this preliminary process. As we have already seen, fragments of endoplasmic reticulum constitute the so-called microsomes.

During centrifugation the mitochondria, the lysosomes and the peroxisomes separate out together (Fig. 2.4) but the microsomes can be separated from the other particles by suspending the precipitate in which they all appear in a tube containing sucrose solution in layers of progressively increasing density. On centrifuging the tube, the mitochondria on the one hand and the lysosomes and peroxisomes on the other will occupy the sucrose layer whose density matches their own. The lysosomes and peroxisomes which separate out together in a density gradient that is suitable for harvesting the less dense mitochondria can themselves be separated from one another by repeating the process of *density gradient centrifugation* in suitably chosen concentrations of sucrose. Density gradient centrifugation can also be used to separate fragments of rough endoplasmic reticulum from fragments of the smooth variety.

The homogeneity or otherwise of the fractions obtained by differential centrifugation has to be determined by electron microscopy.

THE CHROMOSOMES
It has been known for at least 150 years that small bodies with an affinity for aniline dyes make their appearance in the nuclei of cells that are in the process of dividing. Because of the ease with which they can be stained, these structures and the material of which they are composed soon became known as chromosomes (coloured bodies) and chromatin respectively. Chromosomes are readily discernible in the dividing cell because in that state lengths of chromatin are disposed in the form of very tight coils. At other times, they uncoil and become barely visible. As we have already noted (p. 9), the coiled and uncoiled forms of chromatin are called heterochromatin and euchromatin respectively.

At this stage of our discussion, chromosomes can be looked on as strings of *genes,* the structures that direct the development of the body's inherited characteristics. *Alleles* (or *allelomorphs*) is the term generally applied to different forms of the same gene.

All cells, apart from the mature gametes, in the normal members of a particular animal species carry the same number of chromosomes. This is the so-called *diploid number*. The gametes are provided with only one half of this complement of chromosomes—the *haploid number*. In

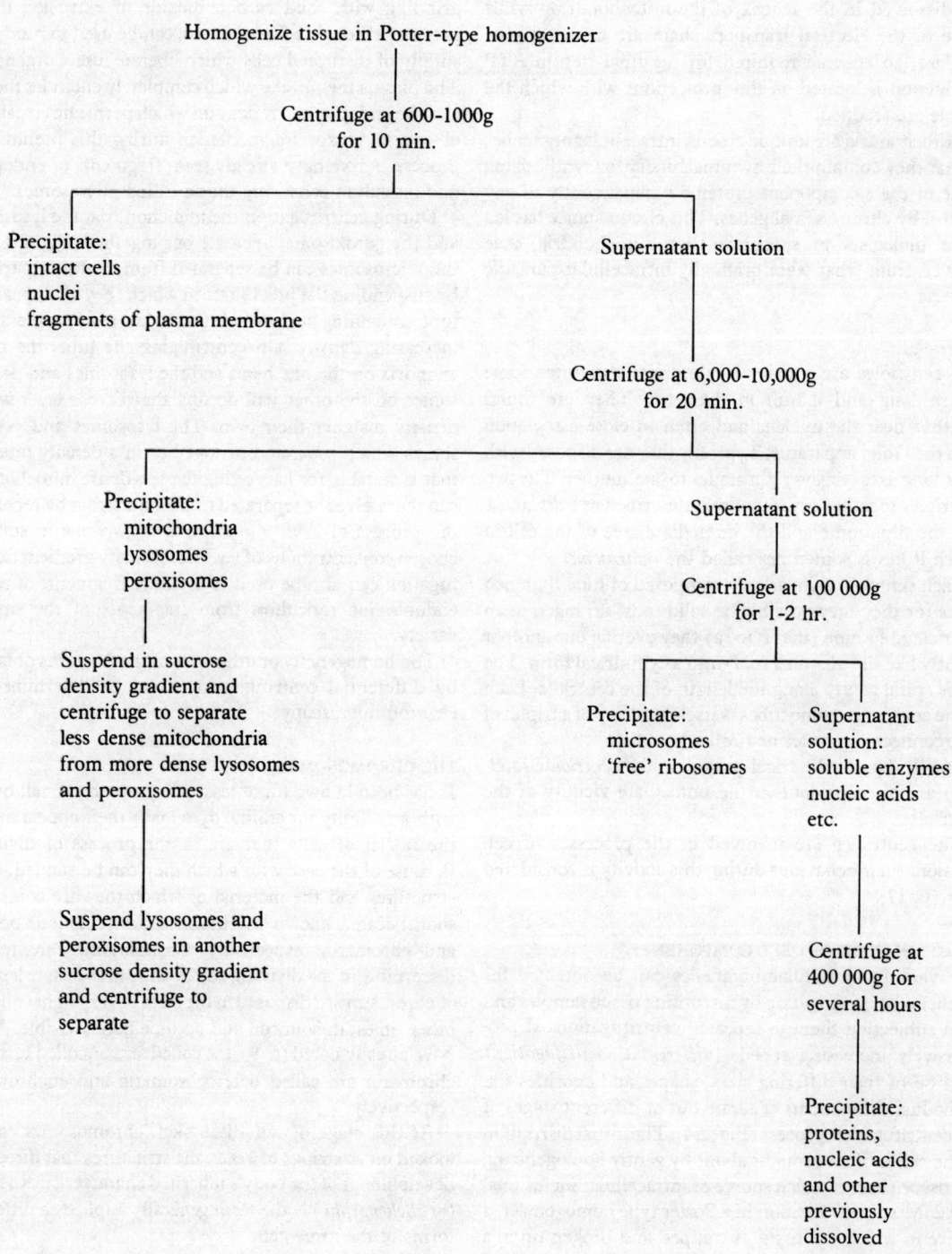

Homogenize tissue in Potter-type homogenizer

Centrifuge at 600–1000g
for 10 min.

Precipitate:
intact cells
nuclei
fragments of plasma membrane

Supernatant solution

Centrifuge at 6,000–10,000g
for 20 min.

Precipitate:
mitochondria
lysosomes
peroxisomes

Supernatant solution

Centrifuge at 100 000g
for 1–2 hr.

Suspend in sucrose
density gradient and
centrifuge to separate
less dense mitochondria
from more dense lysosomes
and peroxisomes

Precipitate:
microsomes
'free' ribosomes

Supernatant
solution:
soluble enzymes
nucleic acids
etc.

Suspend lysosomes and
peroxisomes in another
sucrose density gradient
and centrifuge to
separate

Centrifuge at
400 000g for
several hours

Precipitate:
proteins,
nucleic acids
and other
previously
dissolved
macromolecules

Fig. 2.4 Fractionation of cell components by differential centrifugation

the human being the haploid and diploid numbers are 23 and 46 respectively. Of the 46 chromosomes in human somatic cells, 44 (the *autosomes*) are present as homologous pairs. One member of each homologous pair was originally derived from the male and the other from the female parent but they are identical so far as their gene composition is concerned. The remaining two chromosomes are the sex chromosomes, so-called because they control the development of the primary and secondary sex characteristics. In females the sex chromosomes occur as a homologous pair (designated XX) but in males they form an unmatched pair, XY. The X chromosome comes from the mother and the Y chromosome from the father. Those who wish to deduce from the above that the female of the species is more complete and balanced than the male could assemble a formidable mass of collateral evidence from other sources. In fairness, though, it must be added that one of the female's X chromosomes soon becomes inactive, its chromatin becoming condensed into a minute button of material that takes up a position just inside the nuclear membrane.

Autosomes can be identified by numbering them from the longest (no.1) to the shortest (no.22) pair. They are sometimes further classified by segregating them into groups A to G. Group A consists of the autosomal pairs 1 to 3 and the other groups are as follows: B—4 and 5; C—6 to 12; D—13 to 15; E—16 to 18; F—19 and 20 and G—21 and 22. The sex chromosomes can be included within this classification. X is a member of group C while Y belongs to group G. The chromosome pattern for any individual or species is known as the *karyotype*.

Because of the essentially random nature of human breeding it will not infrequently happen that the allelomorphs of a particular gene will not be identical. Individuals carrying dissimilar allelomorphs are said to be *heterozygous* for the gene or for the characteristic it controls. They will be *homozygous* in respect of those of their genes with identical allelomorphs. Genes control such obvious physiological traits as body build, eye colour, hair type and so on but, as a result of spontaneous changes in their composition (*mutations*) they are sometimes responsible for effecting anomalies of structure and function that can give rise to recognizable disease. Whether or not a person who is heterozygous for a mutant gene of this type develops the disease depends on whether the mutant is *dominant* or *recessive* in type. A recessive allelomorph will exert no deleterious effect in a heterozygous individual because its influence will be countered by the activity of its normal allelomorph partner. Thus the mutant can be transmitted from generation to generation without manifesting its presence unless and until an offspring is born to parents both of whom by chance carry the mutant. When that happens there will be a one in four possibility (as readers can easily calculate for themselves) that the offspring will be homozygous for the mutant gene and that it will,

therefore, display the disease state that is the expression of the activity of that particular gene. Because of the restrictions that society places on unions between near relations this type of hereditary disease is relatively rare (it is most unlikely that identical mutations could arise spontaneously in two different individuals) except in those circles such as dynastic families where the consanguinity laws have customarily and perhaps necessarily been forgotten.

Some mutant genes are dominant so that they can cause disease or disorder even in heterozygous individuals. However, mutant genes are much more often recessive than dominant in type.

Although the X sex chromosome carries genes that are particularly concerned with the determination of sexual characteristics it also incorporates ones that control other activities. These genes can undergo mutations just as do those on autosomal chromosomes. The disorders produced by mutant genes on X chromosomes are said to be sex-linked. Since X chromosomes are paired in the female, a recessive sex-linked mutant will not normally be able to manifest its presence in the female offspring of a parent who carries this gene. Male offspring carrying the mutant will however, succumb to the disease because their X chromosomes are unpaired and there is thus no normal allelomorph to balance the influence of the mutant. Sex linked diseases, we can say, then, can be transmitted by females but, in the absence of breaches of the marriage laws, can only be suffered by males. We should also note that since a man gives his X chromosome only to his daughters he cannot pass on a sex-linked disease to his sons.

The best known examples of sex-linked disorders are haemophilia and disorders of colour vision.

There is no evidence that diseases are ever caused by mutant genes on Y chromosomes.

Abnormalities of chromosome number and structure

It occasionally happens that a pair of chromosomes fail to separate during meiosis (p. 17) so that the resulting gametes contain an unusual number of chromosomes. They are said to be *aneuploid:* one pair will carry 24 chromosomes and the other will have 22. These gametes can participate in fertilization processes in the usual way but the zygotes into which they become incorporated will carry 47 or 45 chromosomes instead of the usual 46. In the former instance the karyotype of the child that is eventually born will consist of 21 homologous pairs of chromosomes, one group of three homologous chromosomes and the usual pair of sex chromosomes. Its cells are said to be *trisomic*. In the latter instance the triplet of homologous chromosomes will be replaced by a single unmatched chromosome and the cells will be said to be *monosomic*. The most well known example of a disorder associated with aneuploidy is Down's syndrome (mongolism). In Down's syndrome, chromosome 21 occurs as a triplet and we can describe the condition as trisomy–21. In some other conditions in which physical and mental abnormalities are prominent features, single chromosomes in group D or group E display trisomy.

Abnormalities in the number of sex chromosomes are not very uncommon. Victims of Klinefelter's syndrome appear to be male but their male sex organs and functions are ill developed. They have abnormal numbers of sex chromosomes: most usually the pattern is XXY but others, even XXXY, have been reported. The analogous condition in females (Turner's syndrome) occurs in individuals whose karyotype includes only one X chromosome.

A variety of other sex chromosome patterns have been described. It includes XXYY and XYY.

Translocation and *deletion* are fates that not uncommonly befall chromosomes. In translocation, genes become transferred to unusual sites on the chromosomes and in deletion a gene or a group of genes becomes excluded from the chromosome with which it is usually associated.

In chronic myeloid leukaemia, autosomal chromosome 22 in blood cells derived from the bone marrow is very much smaller than it is in individuals free of leukaemia. The emasculated chromosome is sometimes known as the *Philadelphia chromosome*.

The cell cycle

Cells in the developing embryo and those in cancerous growths repeatedly reproduce themselves, the former in a controlled way, the latter in a most disorganized fashion. Two identical daughter cells are produced (by *mitosis*) from each parent cell and the offspring so created themselves grow and divide or, in the embryo, develop into highly specialized cells, such as neurones, that are incapable of reproducing themselves. Even in the adult animal some cells (spermatozoa, the cells of the liver and epidermis and the stem cells of the bone marrow, for example) retain an ability to replicate themselves and so can replace their discharged or effete fellows.

Mitosis, then, is the process of cell division. Cells which have just been formed by division of a parent cell are said to enter *interphase*, a state that is conventionally divided into the successive stages G_1, S and G_2. The letters G and S represent 'gap' and 'synthesis' respectively: the G_2 stage is also known as the premitotic interval since it heralds another mitosis. The complete *cell cycle* is schematically represented in Fig. 2.5.

Cells that no longer reproduce themselves can hardly be said to display a 'cycle' of change: once produced they enter what is described as the G_0 stage in which the only activity permitted to them is further differentiation into the specialized cells characteristic of mature animals.

The duration of the cell cycle varies from one cell type to another but the variability is largely attributable to variations in the duration of the G_1 stage. In cells in tissue

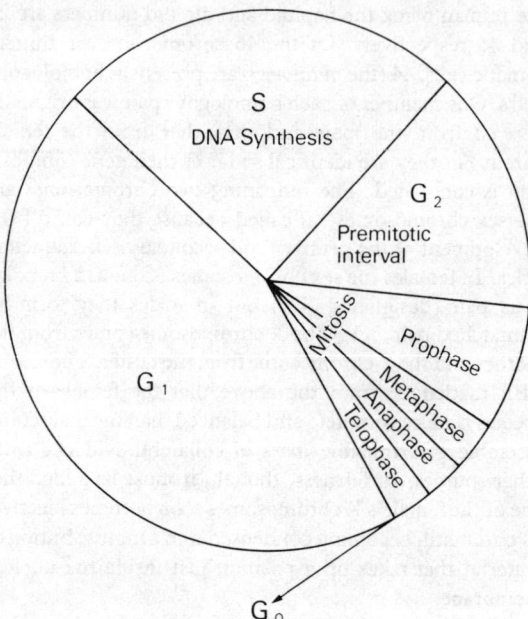

Fig. 2.5 The cell cycle.

culture the cell cycle typically occupies between 4 and 24 hours, mitosis taking up about one fifth of the cycle. The cell cycle is rather shorter in the living animal than it is in tissue culture.

Cells in the G_1 stage of their cycle are relatively quiescent and in this condition they are not very susceptible to the action of drugs that interfere with cell growth and reproduction. They are much more easily attacked in the S stage, when DNA is synthesized, and in the G_2 stage, which sees the synthesis of RNA and protein.

Cytotoxic substances are of potential value as antineoplastic agents (Chap. 61, p. 912): they are said to be *phase dependent* if they interfere more or less specifically with just one phase of the cell cycle or *cycle dependent* if they exert toxic actions throughout the cycle. Somewhat confusing alternatives to these terms are *cycle dependent* and *cycle independent* respectively.

MITOSIS

Mitosis can be described by reference to the changes that take place in cells maintained in tissue culture. The fibroblast has been extensively studied in this connection and Fig. 2.6 and the account which follows refers to this type of cell. The Figure is taken from Haggis (1974) and the description of mitosis to which it relates owes much to the same source.

Mitosis begins with *prophase*. In prophase, the cell takes on an almost spherical conformation and recognizable chromosomes appear. Each can be seen to be split longitudinally into two *chromatids* which are joined to one another at only one point, the *centromere* or *kinetochore*. The chromosomes become visible as a result of their being

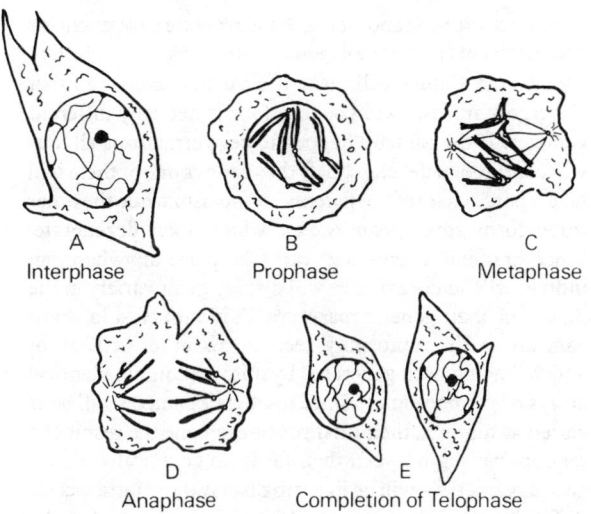

A	B	C
Interphase	Prophase	Metaphase

D	E
Anaphase	Completion of Telophase

Fig. 2.6 The stages of mitosis *taken from Haggis, 1974, by kind permission of the author and publisher.*

more tightly coiled than they were during interphase. The splitting of the chromosomes into chromatids occurs during interphase.

Other changes take place during prophase. The nuclear membrane fragments into vesicles too small to be seen under the light microscope and the nucleoli also disappear so that the distinction between nucleus and cytoplasm virtually vanishes. Another important process—*spindle formation*—is initiated during prophase. During the S period of interphase the diplosome (p. 13) has replicated itself. On electron microscopy, small microtubules are seen radiating from and between the two diplosomes giving the units a star like appearance. At this stage the diplosomes and their associated tubules are known, predictably, as *asters*. During prophase the asters (which are large enough to be visible under the optical microscope) migrate to opposite poles of the cell but they remain interconnected by a few microtubules.

In *metaphase* (Fig. 2.6C) the microtubules connecting the two asters multiply and become more well defined. They now constitute the definitive spindle which, with the virtual disappearance of the nucleus, can now take up a central position in the cell. As the name indicates, the spindle is broad at the equator and constricted at the polar regions of the cell. The spindle microtubules are sometimes described as fibres or threads. When the spindle is formed the chromatids move towards the equatorial region of the cell and there become attached, by their centromeres, to the spindle microtubules. Each centromere divides so that the previously conjoined chromatid pairs become completely separate.

During *anaphase* (Fig. 2.6D) the separated chromatids are pulled towards the opposite poles of the cell (the members of a chromatid pair moving to different poles)

apparently as a result of shortening of the spindle microtubules. In anaphase a furrow also appears in the cytoplasm.

In *telophase* (Fig. 2.6D) the chromatids unwind (and so become invisible again), associate with new nucleoli and become surrounded with a newly constituted nuclear membrane. Finally, the cytoplasm divides by a progressive deepening of the furrow that appeared during anaphase and the two daughter cells are now free to take on the form and function of mature fibroblasts.

Some authorities record the process of cytoplasm division as a distinct stage (*cytokinesis*) in the cell cycle, immediately following, but distinct from, telophase.

As is probably apparent from the foregoing description, prophase is the more prolonged of the several stages of the mitotic process. It occupies about one half of the time during which the cell is actively dividing.

MEIOSIS

When cells divide by mitosis, the longitudinal splitting of the chromosomes into chromatid pairs and the strict segregation of the members of each pair, one to each of the daughter cells, ensures that all the offspring of a particular cell shall be genetically identical. Moreover since all the cells in the body of a multicellular organism are derived from a single ancestor (the *zygote*) it is clear that this identity of genetic composition should extend to all the cells in an individual's body. The zygote itself is, however, produced by the union of a male and a female *gamete* (a spermatozoon and an ovum respectively) and if the gametes of a particular species themselves contained the same number of chromosomes as the generality of body cells in that species it is clear that the zygote (and hence all the cells derived from it in the new individual) would contain twice as many chromosomes as the parental cells. And, in their turn, cells in the next generation of offspring would possess twice the number of chromosomes carried by the cells of *their* parents. That this absurdly impossible situation does not develop is a consequence of the fact that mature gametes carry only half the number of chromosomes (the haploid number, p. 13) possessed by the other cells in the body of which they are a part. This arises because the developing gamete, after a number of normal mitoses, undergoes *meiosis* (Greek 'diminution', hence meiosis, an understatement) or reduction division. In meiosis a cell divides twice but its nuclear material divides only once.

We saw that in the anaphase of a normal mitosis, the paired chromatids separate and migrate to opposite poles of the dividing cell. We also noted that the chromatids were actually produced during the preceding interphase. Chromatids are similarly formed in gametes that are about to enter meiosis but they remain paired during the anaphase of the immediately succeeding cell division in which whole chromosomes, rather than their component chromatids, are segregated into the two daughter cells. The next cell division is essentially a normal mitosis (except, of course, that no chromatid formation and no nucleic acid synthesis is needed during the preceding interphase) with separation of chromatids during anaphase and the final production of mature gametes containing the haploid number of chromosomes.

Meiosis actually achieves much more than the mere reduction in the number of chromosomes in the gametes. The process is also associated with an exchange of genetic material between the members of homologous chromosome pairs. The way in which this is brought about is indicated schematically in Fig. 2.7.

In the prophase of the first meiotic division, the homologous pairs of chromosomes, already cleft into chromatids held together by centromeres in the usual way, come to lie close to one another in an accurate alignment that ensures that any gene in one member of the pair is immediately adjacent to the same gene in its fellow. Chromatids in each homologous pair of chromosomes approach and fuse with one another over short portions of their length (Fig. 2.7B). At the points of contact the chromatids appear to be actually crossing over one another and it is for this reason that the points of contact are often called *chiasmata*, the plural of *chiasma*, a crossing. At anaphase, the centromeres begin to migrate to opposite poles of the cell in the usual fashion and in so doing they break the chromatids at their points of fusion. The fragments so formed then recombine in such a way that the chromatids that had been

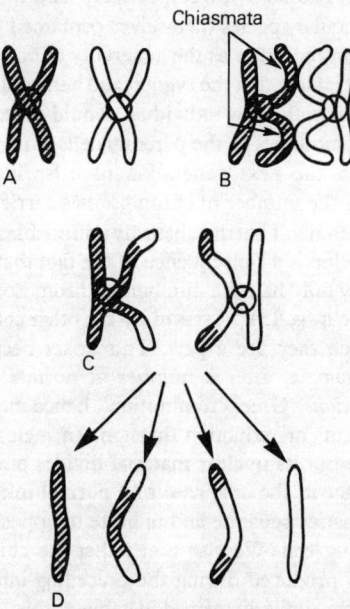

In the first meiotic division (A, B and C) the homologous chromosomes exchange material; in the second division (D) four different gametes are produced from the original homologous pair of chromosomes.

Fig. 2.7 Meiotic division

in contact with one another each incorporate a fragment, or fragments, of their homologous partner (Fig. 2.7C). Reference to the Figure will make it clear that every cell that undergoes meiosis will produce four genetically different gametes. If the gametes happen to be spermatozoa all four will continue to develop but if they are ova one of them will take a lion's share of the parental cytoplasm while the other three form small *polar bodies,* which soon degenerate. Since chromatid 'crossing' can take place anywhere, an individual's many gametes will display great variety in the details of their genetic make up. This variety is in sharp contrast to the uniformity seen in his other cells all of which, having been generated by mitosis, contain identical arrays of chromosomes. Since his mate's gametes will be as varied as his own, their offspring—each one the result of a random pairing between their far from genetically homogenous gametes—will be likely to display those intraspecies differences in appearance and behaviour that makes the living world so fascinating.

Some authorities use a special and somewhat erudite terminology to describe particular features of meiosis. These terms include *leptotene,* when the chromosomes have become sufficiently tightly coiled to be visible as discrete objects, *zygotene* when the individual chromosomes join their homologous mates, *pachytene* when complete alignment has been achieved, *diplotene* when the chromosomes coil even more tightly and *diakinesis* when the chiasmata are formed.

The nucleic acids

Chromosomes are composed of deoxyribonucleic acid (DNA) and smaller amounts of protein. Our attention will be focussed on the DNA component since little is known concerning the role of the protein.

The DNA molecule is an elongated structure consisting of two cross linked chains (or strands) that twist gently around one another in a helical fashion—the famous double helix. Each strand has an essentially simple structure since it is composed of a number of repeating units or *nucleotides.* The number of nucleotides in the cell is immense: the 46 chromosomes in every human cell represent a collection of some 10 000 million nucleotides. Each nucleotide is made up of a molecule of phosphoric acid attached to deoxyribose (a pentose sugar) which itself carries either a purine (adenine or guanine) or a pyrimidine (cytosine or thymidine) base. The nature of the phosphoric acid-pentose linking enables a distinction to be made between the two ends of the molecule for purposes of description: one extremity is the 3'-end and the other the 5'-end (Fig. 2.8*b*). The four bases occur in approximately equal numbers. The component strands of the DNA molecule are disposed in such a way that the phosphoric acid-deoxyribose skeletons lie on the outside of the double helix while the bases are directed inwards (Fig. 2.8*c*) and, united by hydrogen bonding, form the cross links that maintain the structural integrity of the whole molecule. The four bases units with one another according to a 'rule' which demands purine-pyrimidine pairing: adenine (A) must join thymine (T) and guanine (G) must join cytosine (C). This ensures that the products of chromosome replication shall be exact copies of the original. Chromosomes reproduce themselves, as we have seen (p.

16) in the S period of interphase: the two DNA strands of the chromatin separate and each then attaches itself, following the base pairing rule, to nucleotides manufactured in the nuclear sap (Fig. 2.8c). The newly attached nucleotides are then joined by enzyme action to give a new strand of DNA. Thus, when mitosis sets in, each chromosome in the parent cell is already replicated and a complete set of chromo-

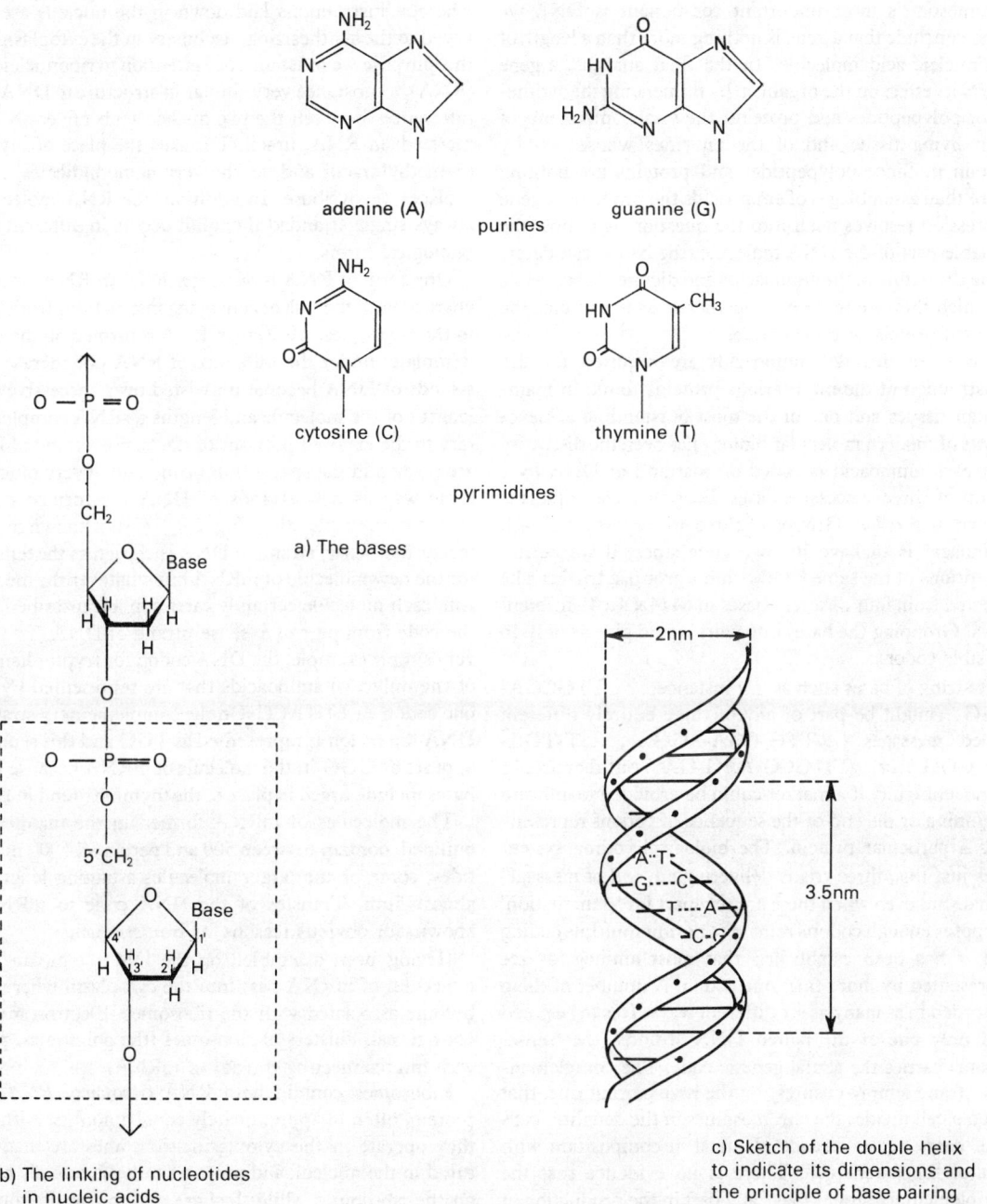

a) The bases

b) The linking of nucleotides in nucleic acids

c) Sketch of the double helix to indicate its dimensions and the principle of base pairing

Fig. 2.8 The structure of DNA.

somes will be available for each of the two daughter cells. In perhaps one in a million cell cycles, a nucleotide base, failing to recognize its proper partner, becomes attached to the 'wrong' one so that an inappropriate sequence of bases is introduced into the new DNA strand. Such an event constitutes a mutation.

In this simplistic account we can assume that chromosomes are simply strings of genes. Since we know that the chromosome's most important component is DNA we must conclude that a gene is nothing more than a length of the nucleic acid molecule. In the final analysis, a gene exerts its effect on the organism by influencing the synthesis of polypeptides and proteins, the vital components of both living tissue and of the enzymes whose activity sustain it. Since polypeptides and proteins are nothing more than assemblages of aminoacids the problem of gene expression resolves itself into the question as to how the variable part of the DNA molecule (the bases) can determine the nature of the aminoacids and dictate the sequence in which they are to be put together so as to produce the relevant protein or polypeptide.

No more than 20 aminoacids are required for the construction of the multifarious proteins found in mammalian tissues and one of the most outstanding achievements of modern molecular biology has been the discovery that each aminoacid is coded on a strand of DNA by a group of three successive bases. Each of these triplets is known as a *codon*. Groups of three are necessary if each aminoacid is to have its own code since, if we permit repetitions of the same base within a group, a triad can be selected from four different bases in 64 (4 x 4 x 4) different ways. Grouping the bases into pairs would give us only 16 possible codons.

A string of bases such as, for instance,. . . TTGCGA-AGG...might be part of any of three entirely different coded messages (...TTG-CGA-AGG..., ...T-TGC-GAA-GG...or...TT-GCG-AAG-G...) but there could be no ambiguity if a marker could be provided to indicate beginning or end of the sequence of codons representing a particular protein. The biological coding system does just this, three triads delivering an 'end of message' signal. But even when these are set apart for 'punctuation' purposes enough codons remain to permit multiple coding and it has been established that most aminoacids are represented by more than one codon. A number of them are coded in as many as six different ways. It is to be noted that only one of the paired DNA strands (the 'sense' strand) carries the actual genetic code. The complementary strand simply ensures, by the base pairing rule, that when a cell divides the chromosomes in the daughter cells shall carry 'sense' strands identical in composition with that of the parent cell. There is no evidence that the complementary strand plays any part in the production of messenger RNA (see below).

Proteins are synthesized on ribosomes in the cytoplasm.

Many ribosomes are attached, as we have seen, to the endoplasmic reticulum while others lie free in the cytoplasm. It has been suggested that the free ribosomes synthesize protein that will be used within the cell in which it is produced while those attached to the endoplasmic reticulum manufacture protein for use elsewhere. However, the processes of protein synthesis are identical at the two sites and we must now enquire into the mechanisms whereby instructions laid down in the nucleus are conveyed to the synthesizing machinery in the cytoplasm. For this purpose we must turn our attention to ribonucleic acid (RNA), a substance very similar in structure to DNA. The differences between the two nucleic acids are easily summarized: in RNA, uracil (U) takes the place of thymine (5–methyluracil) and, as the very name indicates, ribose replaces dexoyribose. In addition, the RNA molecule is always single stranded though it occurs in different morphological forms.

One form of RNA is *messenger RNA* (mRNA) which is charged with the task of conveying instructions from DNA to the ribosomes. Messenger RNA is formed on the DNA 'template' under the influence of RNA polymerase. The strands of DNA become untwisted over successive short lengths of the molecule and lengths of RNA complementary to the exposed portions of the 'sense' strand of DNA are formed in the spaces thus opened up in very much the same way as new strands of DNA are formed during chromosome replication (Fig. 2.9). It is not known by what means the 'sense' strand of DNA is chosen as the template for the new molecule of mRNA but whatever the mechanism, each molecule certainly carries in a transcribed form the code from part of a 'sense' strand of DNA. To take a very simple example, the DNA codon for tryptophan (one of the only two aminoacids that are represented by only one codon each) is ACC. On the complementary strand of DNA the codon is represented as TGG and this sequence appears as UGG in the molecule of mRNA because RNA bases include uracil in place of the thymine found in DNA.

The molecules of mRNA formed in the manner just outlined, contain between 500 and perhaps 10 000 nucleotides, some of the larger molecules attaining lengths of almost $5\mu m$. Transfer of the DNA code to mRNA is known, for obvious reasons, as *transcription*.

Having been assembled on the DNA 'template', the molecules of mRNA pass into the cytoplasm where they become associated with the ribosomes. Electron microscopy reveals clusters of ribosomes (the polysomes, p. 11) with interconnecting threads of mRNA.

Ribosomes contain both RNA (*ribosomal RNA*) and protein, often in approximately equal amounts. Although they operate in the cytoplasm, ribosomes are manufactured in the nucleoli and protein synthesis actually begins on the ribosomes while they are still in transit from the nuclear region to their stations in the cytoplasm. Each ribosome is composed of two components whose associa-

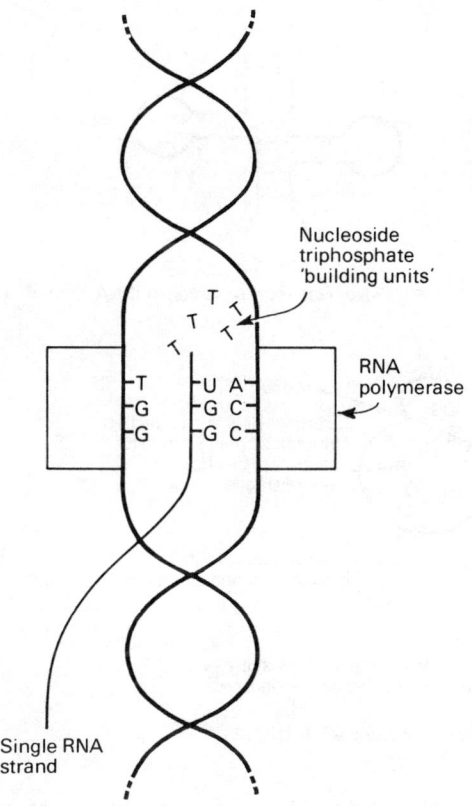

Fig. 2.9 To illustrate the synthesis of RNA on the DNA template under the influence of RNA polymerase. The codon for tryptophan has just been added to the molecule.

tion depends on the presence of magnesium ions. Intact ribosomes, which have molecular weights in the region of 5 million daltons have sedimentation coefficients of 80S. The two subunits have coefficients of about 60S and 40S respectively.

S, the Svedberg unit, measures the speed at which particles sediment. It depends, among several other factors, on the mass of the sedimenting particle.

The molecular weights of ribosomal RNA in the large and small ribosomal subunits are about 1.5 and 0.75 million daltons respectively. The precise functional significance of the ribosomal ribonucleic acids is not clear but it is known that the integrity of the ribosomal subunits depends upon their RNA component.

A ribosome that is about to synthesize a polypeptide chain attaches itself to the first codon on a strand of messenger RNA, other ribosomes attaching themselves at the same time to points further along the strand. This attachment is effected by the ribosome's momentarily dissociating into its component subunits, the smaller one of which unites with the molecule of mRNA before rejoining its larger partner. All is now ready for synthesis

to begin. The ribosome takes up from the surrounding cytoplasm the aminoacid that is represented by the particular codon at the point on the strand of mRNA at which the ribosome is temporarily attached. The ribosome then moves on to the next codon, selects the appropriate aminoacid from the cytoplasmic pool and links it to the aminoacid it has already taken up. This process of selecting aminoacids from the cytoplasm and of joining them in the order prescribed in the assembly instructions carried by the strand of mRNA continues until the ribosome has 'read' the whole of the strand (or the segment of strand) to which it is attached. When the ribosome encounters an 'end of sequence' code the now complete sequence of aminoacid residues is separated from the ribosomal machinery and synthesis of a new chain begins.

Aminoacids involved in polypeptide and protein assembly are taken to their ribosomal destinations by molecules of yet another form of ribonucleic acid. This is *transfer RNA* (tRNA), a compound sometimes also known as *soluble* (sRNA) or *acceptor RNA*. Each molecule of tRNA carries one molecule of aminoacid: there are specific forms of tRNA for each species of aminoacid but we remain in ignorance of the structural features that confer this specificity.

The molecule of tRNA is made up of about 75 to 80 nucleotides and it has a molecular weight of about 25 000 daltons. Notwithstanding the occurrence of different varieties of the nucleic acid for each aminoacid, the 3'-end of the molecule invariably terminates in the base sequence CCA. It is to the final adenine that all amino acids are attached. The common CCA sequence is added to the newly produced tRNA molecule (which has been assembled in the nucleus on the DNA template) by enzymatic action in the cytoplasm. The base at the 5'-end of the molecule of tRNA is always guanine.

Transfer RNA includes within its structure not only the four bases found in all types of RNA but also a considerable proportion of novel bases that do not appear in other varieties of ribonucleic acid. The most common of these bases are inosine, and pseudouracil (Fig. 2.10*a*) and they are probably produced by enzymatic transformation of the corresponding common bases after the tRNA molecule has been synthesized in a precursor form.

Although tRNA is, of course, single stranded in structure, the molecule is folded on itself in a fashion that permits base pairing of the type seen in DNA. Indeed, in those parts of the molecule where base pairing occurs, the double strand so formed adopts the double helix configuration. The twists and convolutions of the molecule of tRNA are often simplified for illustrative purposes into a 'clover leaf' form (Fig. 2.10*b*) but the ubiquity of the kind of structure implied by this type of representation is not completely established and a 'hairpin'-like caricature (Fig. 2.10*c*), which is certainly easier to fit into schematic diagrams, can also be utilized.

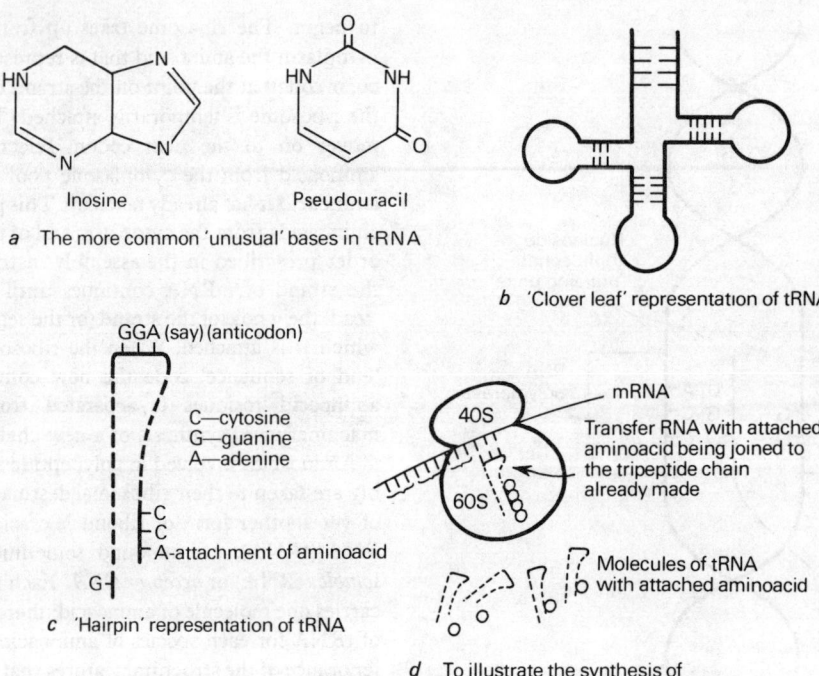

a   The more common 'unusual' bases in tRNA

b   'Clover leaf' representation of tRNA

GGA (say) (anticodon)

C—cytosine
G—guanine
A—adenine

C
C
A-attachment of aminoacid
G

c   'Hairpin' representation of tRNA

mRNA

Transfer RNA with attached
aminoacid being joined to
the tripeptide chain
already made

Molecules of tRNA
with attached aminoacid

d   To illustrate the synthesis of
protein molecules on the ribosome

Fig. 2.10 The structure and function of transfer RNA (tRNA)

When the common nucleotide bases lie opposite one another along the course of the apparently double stranded portion of the tRNA molecule, pairing occurs in the usual way but the intrusion of the unusual bases causes complications. Inosine is capable of forming hydrogen bonds with any of the common bases but none of the other members of the 'unusual' group can unite with any base opposite which they might find themselves. Thus some bases in the double stranded portions of the tRNA molecule are left exposed. This may provide the molecule with an opportunity for binding to the ribosome or to the enzyme that is required to effect the union between tRNA and its associated aminoacid. Whatever the true significance of the exposure that results from the presence of the unusual bases, there is no doubt that the disposition of these bases in the molecule is as rigidly determined as is that of any other element in the hereditary apparatus.

Approximately midway along the length of each molecule of tRNA there occurs a group of three bases that are complementary to one of the aminoacid codons found on mRNA. The bases are unpaired and they are directed 'outwards' (Fig. 2.10c). The triad is usually known, for obvious reasons, as the *anticodon* though some authorities with more ingenuity than wit refer to it as the *nodoc*. It is the anticodon which ensures that the molecule of tRNA with its attached aminoacid will only enter the polypeptide synthesizing system when the ribosome has itself moved to a point on the strand of mRNA that bears the appropriate

codon. The reader will recall that the twenty or so aminoacids are represented by no fewer than 61 codons and it follows that at least this number of forms of tRNA must be available. Molecules of tRNA differ from one another, however, in more respects than in the composition of their anticodons. A length of the molecule containing some 17 nucleotides and the CCA receptor region is of constant composition and it is presumably involved in the nonspecific attachment of the molecule to the ribosomes. The other end of the molecule, after guanine, includes a number of highly variable sequences and we must suppose that it contains within itself the means by which it can recognize (or be recognized by) both the aminoacid designated by its anticodon and the specific enzyme (one of the *aminoacyl–tRNA synthetases*) required to bring about the union of aminoacid and tRNA. This enzyme promotes a reaction between the specific aminoacid and ATP which results in the formation of a complex of the acid and AMP with the elimination of pyrophosphate. The enzyme, still associated with the acid-AMP complex, then attaches itself to the appropriate molecule of tRNA and effects a transfer of the aminoacid to the nucleic acid with the elimination of AMP. We can summarize these reactions simply as follows:

Aminoacid + ATP → Aminoacid-AMP + Pyrophosphate

Aminoacid-AMP + tRNA → Aminoacid-tRNA + AMP

The energy released in these reactions by the hydrolysis of ATP is utilized in the synthesis of the peptide bonds.

The synthesis of polypeptides on ribosomes is illustrated in a schematic fashion in Fig. 2.10d.

Cell metabolism

We saw in the preceding section that the energy required for the bonding of aminoacids into polypeptide chains is provided by the hydrolysis of ATP. Many other biologically important processes are equally dependent on the availability of this energy donor and ATP, which serves as both a store and a ready source of energy, has been well described as the body's metabolic currency (Edelstein, 1973). Its central position in the economy of the cell will become progressively more obvious with every increment in the reader's knowledge of biological processes.

Adenosine triphosphate (its full chemical formula will be found on p. 322) can be regarded as a complex of adenine, ribose and three phosphoric acid residues. Its resemblance to the component nucleotides of the nucleic acids (p. 19) will not be lost on the reader.

ATP is readily hydrolysed to the diphosphate (ADP) and inorganic phosphate (Pi). Hydrolysis is accompanied by the release of some 7000 cal (approximately 30500J) of energy per mole. In its turn, ADP can be converted to the monophosphate (AMP) with the release of the same amount of energy as that which accompanied the breaking of the first bond. Removal of the phosphate group from AMP occurs less readily and when it is achieved only 3000 cals (approximately 12500J) of energy per mole are released.

Most of the biological reactions that feature ATP necessitate only its conversion into ADP but in a few instances the two terminal phosphates are removed together (as pyrophosphate) to give AMP.

For obvious, if not entirely sound, reasons ATP and a number of other substances (these include, among others, acetyl coenzyme A, S-adenosylmethionine, creatine phosphate, acetyl phosphate and phosphoenol pyruvate) are known as high energy compounds. To indicate that energy is released when they are fractured, the bonds uniting the phosphate groups in ATP are commonly represented by a $\sim$ sign instead of the straight line that is otherwise employed to designate interatomic connections in the conventional representation of a chemical molecule. Phosphate groups are sometimes shown as $\textcircled{P}$ and the reader will probably encounter works in which ATP appears as adenosine $- \textcircled{P} \sim \textcircled{P} \sim \textcircled{P}$

Most of the other high energy compounds that occur in the body also include phosphate groups in their molecules but acetyl CoA and S-adenosylmethionine are sulphur containing compounds.

In physiological conditions, ATP exists largely in the tetraionic form:

$$\text{adenosine—O—P—O} \sim \text{P—O} \sim \text{P—O}^-$$

and the mutual repulsion between the negatively charged groups makes for instability in the molecule. Moreover ATP has fewer resonance forms than has ADP and this too makes ATP unstable because resonance energy confers stability on a molecule. This inherent instability allows easy splitting of ATP and the release of energy that inevitably occurs when a less stable changes into a more stable system.

The essential function of ATP, then, is to act as an intermediary between the reactions that produce energy and those that utilize it. Energy is supplied, of course, by the breakdown of the food we take and we now have to enquire, however briefly, into the mechanisms whereby this catabolic energy is captured and stored by the adenosine compounds. Before doing so, however, a few words concerning the nature of the coenzymes we shall meet may not be out of place.

All enzymes are protein in nature but many of them need to be associated with metal ions or with organic radicals if they are to exercise their function properly. These additional components sometimes form an integral and inseparable part of the molecule and cannot perform their duties independently of the rest of the enzyme. In this event they are usually known as *prosthetic groups*. On the other hand (and the dehydrogenases provide a particularly good example of this), some enzymes use co-factors that can exist independently of the enzyme itself. These separable co-factors are described, not surprisingly, as *coenzymes*. A particular coenzyme may serve a multiplicity of enzymes. Most coenzymes cannot be synthesized in the body from simple precursor molecules so that at least part of the molecule has to be provided in the diet in a preformed state. Essential regulatory substances that need to be obtained in this way are, by definition, vitamins and many coenzymes are, or are derived from, members of the B group of vitamins.

Two of the most important coenzymes are coenzyme I (nicotinamide adenine dinucleotide, NAD) and coenzyme II (nicotinamide adenine dinucleotide phosphate, NADP). Earlier names for these compounds were di- and triphosphopyridine nucleotide (DPN and TPN) respectively. When a compound undergoes dehydrogenation under the influence of an enzyme that utilizes NAD as its co-factor the hydrogen atoms that it loses are taken up by the oxidized form of NAD which thereby becomes reduced.

The structure of NAD is indicated in Fig. 2.11a. Nicotinamide is a derivative of nicotinic acid, the anti-pellagra member of the vitamin B complex. Looking at the Figure, the reader will realize that he is once again being

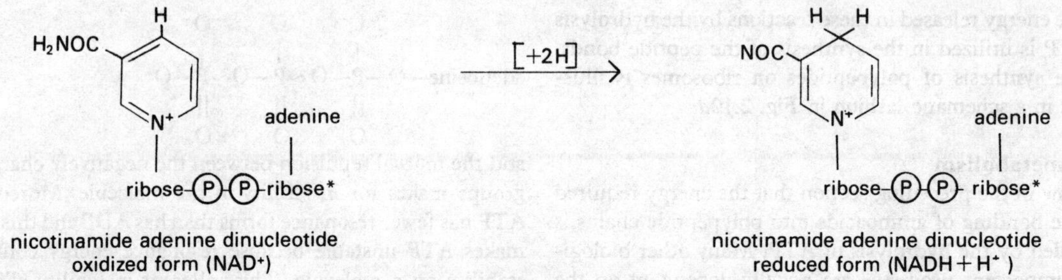

nicotinamide adenine dinucleotide
oxidized form (NAD⁺)

nicotinamide adenine dinucleotide
reduced form (NADH + H⁺)

In nicotinamide adenine dinucleotide phosphate (NADP), the hydroxyl group on carbon atom 2 of the indicated ribose molecule is phosphorylated.

(a)

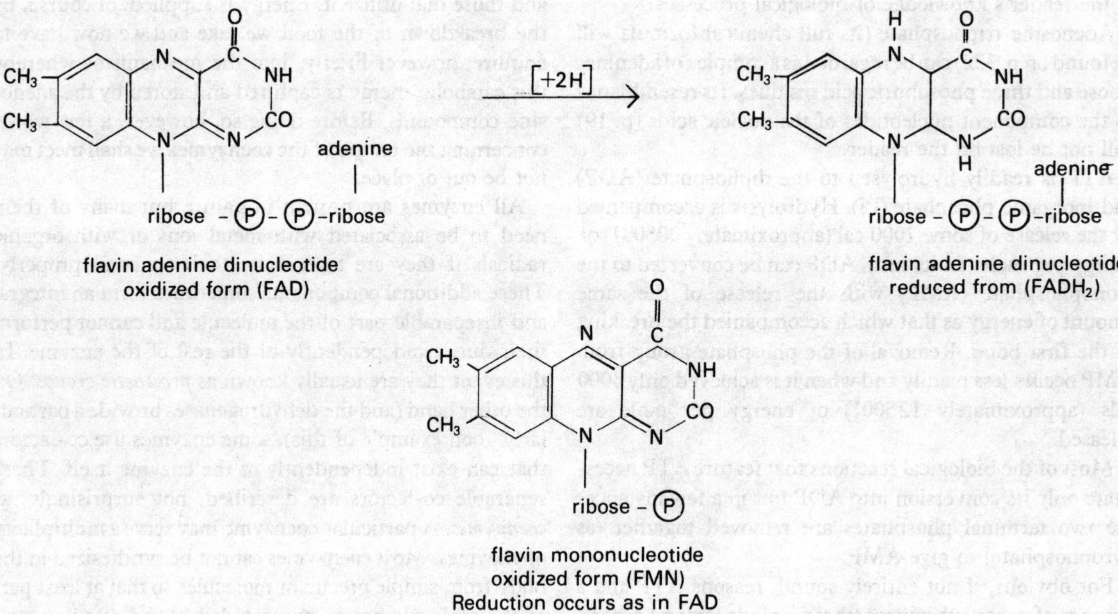

flavin adenine dinucleotide
oxidized form (FAD)

flavin adenine dinucleotide
reduced from (FADH₂)

flavin mononucleotide
oxidized form (FMN)
Reduction occurs as in FAD

(b)

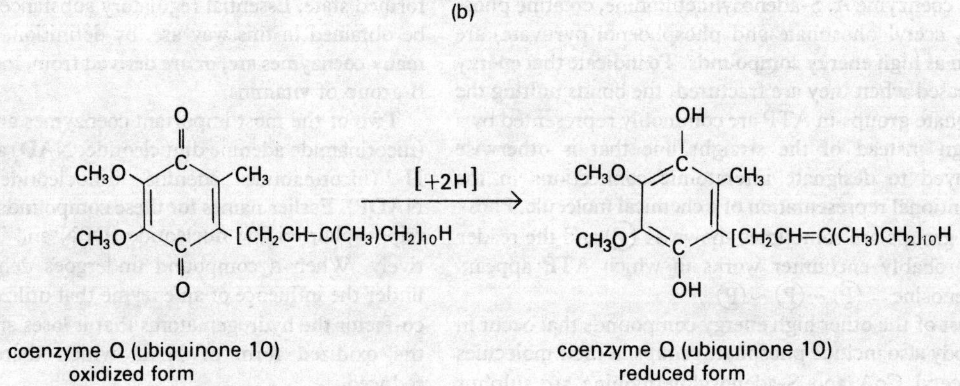

coenzyme Q (ubiquinone 10)
oxidized form

coenzyme Q (ubiquinone 10)
reduced form

(c)

Fig. 2.11 Some important coenzymes

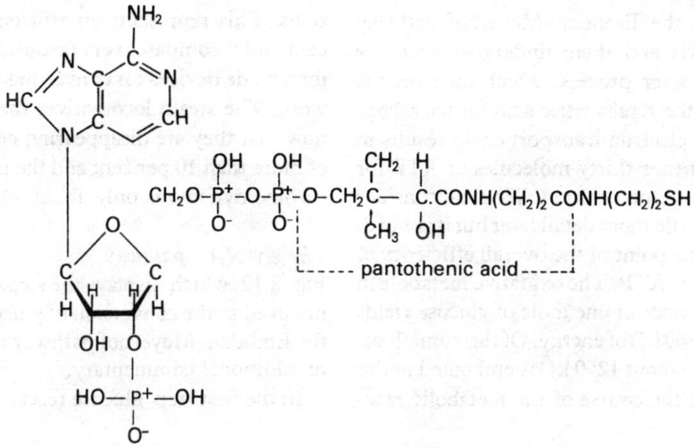

Coenzyme A
(d)

Fig. 12.11 (Contd)

confronted by a substance with the nucleotide structure that has featured so prominently in this chapter. He will also be able to see why the oxidized coenzyme is often (and in this author's opinion, preferably) represented as NAD^+. When the compound takes up two atoms of hydrogen the nicotinamide moiety of the molecule loses a double bond and its nitrogen atom loses its positive charge. This still leaves a hydrogen ion (proton) over and we can represent the whole reaction as

$$NAD^+ + 2H \rightarrow NADH + H^+$$

A precisely similar state of affairs obtains when the coenzyme is NADP.

Not all writers adopt the nomenclature adopted in the immediately preceding paragraph. Some prefer to represent the oxidized and reduced forms of coenzyme I as NAD and $NADH_2$. This avoids the clumsiness of $NADH + H^+$ as an expression for the reduced coenzyme but otherwise it has little to recommend it. Still other authors escape the embarrassing questions that are implicit in the other representations of the coenzyme by resorting to the simple NAD_{ox} and NAD_{red}.

Flavin mononucleotide (FMN), flavin adenine dinucleotide (FAD) and coenzyme A (CoA) also appear in Fig. 2.11, coenzyme A being given its complete structural formula. Both the flavin coenzymes incorporate vitamin B_2 (riboflavin, p. 790) in their molecules while coenzyme A is a derivative of pantothenic acid (p. 790), yet another member of the vitamin B complex.

The reduced form of flavin adenine dinucleotide is usually represented simply as $FADH_2$ since the coenzyme is essentially a hydrogen carrier, unlike $NADH + H^+$ which has to carry electrons as well. The biochemically reactive radical in coenzyme A is the sulphydryl (-SH) group and it is often convenient to refer to the molecule as CoA–SH.

Another coenzyme that will be encountered in the course of the following discussion is coenzyme Q or ubiquinone. It occurs in several forms. That present in mammalian tissues contains ten isoprene units (in other tissues the number is often lower than this) and it is for that reason that the mammalian coenzyme is sometimes referred to as ubiquinone-10.

Finally brief mention must be made of the cytochromes. At least four (designated a, a_3, b and c) take part in the oxidative metabolism of the cell's fuels and all of them except cytochrome c (which has been obtained in a pure form) are very tightly bound within the mitochondria. The cytochromes consist of porphyrin rings containing iron so that their structure is analogous to that of haemoglobin (p. 693). The iron can be readily and reversibly converted from the ferric (Fe^{3+}) to the ferrous (Fe^{2+}) form; this property allows the cytochromes to function as electron carriers.

We can now turn, somewhat belatedly, to our examination of the way in which the production of ATP is linked to the catabolism of foodstuffs by considering the metabolism of glucose.

Glucose undergoes anaerobic breakdown in the cytoplasm along the Embden-Meyerhof (glycolytic) pathway. The sequence of reactions involves both the utilization and the regeneration of ATP but the balance sheet shows a net production of eight molecules of the high energy compound for every molecule of glucose that joins the glycolytic pathway. The generation of ATP during anaerobic glycolysis is described as *substrate level phosphorylation*. In the presence of oxygen, the pyruvate that is the end product of activity in the Embden–Meyerhof pathway enters the mitochondria and there undergoes *oxidative phosphorylation*. This latter process, which involves the interlinked activity of the Krebs citric acid (or tricarboxylic acid) cycle and an electron transport chain results in the production of a further thirty molecules of ATP for every molecule of glucose metabolized. We shall consider all these reactions in a little more detail later but it is worth making a mention at this point of the overall efficiency of the system that generates ATP. The oxidative metabolism to carbon dioxide and water of one mole of glucose yields about 685 kcal (about 2860 kJ) of energy. Of this something of the order of 300 kcal (about 1250 kJ) is embodied in the ATP that is formed in the course of the metabolic reac-

tions. This represents an efficiency of more than 40 per cent and it compares very favourably with that achieved by man made devices for converting fuel energy into external work. The steam locomotives that so many of us cherish now that they are disappearing never attained efficiencies of more than 10 per cent and the more sophisticated steam turbine dynamo is only about 30 per cent efficient.

The glycolytic pathway
Fig. 2.12, which displays the steps and names the enzymes involved in the conversion of glucose to pyruvic acid along the Embden–Meyerhof pathway demands little in the way of additional commentary.

In the first step, glucose reacts with ATP to give glucose

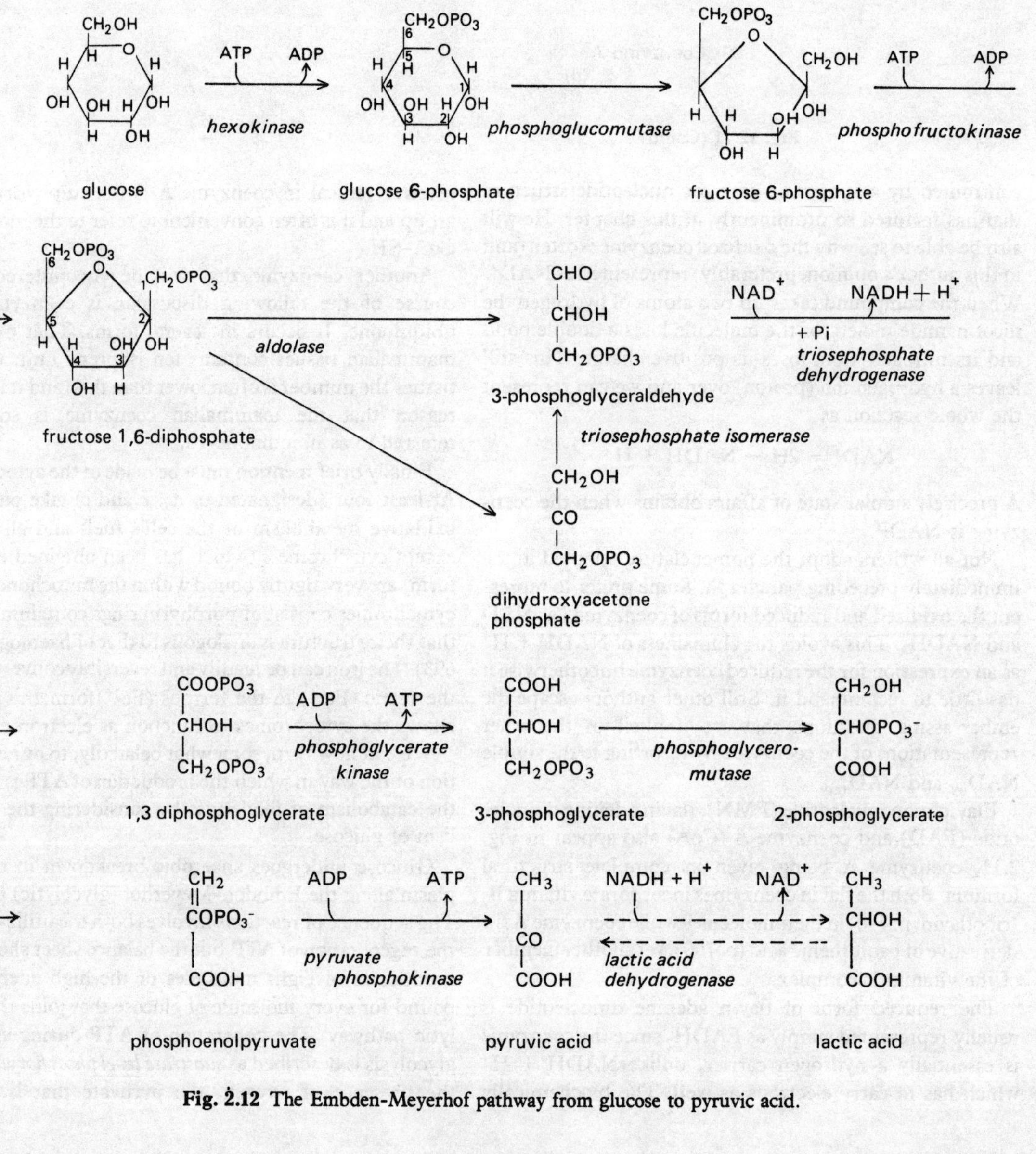

Fig. 2.12 The Embden-Meyerhof pathway from glucose to pyruvic acid.

6-phosphate and ADP, hexokinase catalysing the process. The glucose 6-phosphate then undergoes a simple molecular re-arrangement, under the aegis of phosphoglucomutase, to fructose 6-phosphate. The fructose phosphate reacts in its turn with ATP to give fructose 1,6 diphosphate, phosphofructokinase being the responsible enzyme. Aldolase cleaves the diphosphate into two three-carbon sugars namely 3-phosphoglyceraldehyde and dihydroxyacetone phosphate. The first named of these fragments is oxidized to 1,3-diphosphoglycerate with NAD^+ acting as co-factor to the triose phosphate dehydrogenase that supports this reaction. The phosphate required for this conversion comes from inorganic sources. As the reaction proceeds, more 3-phosphoglyceraldehyde is provided by hydrolysis of dihydroxyacetone phosphate. The next event is the conversion of 1,3-diphosphoglycerate and ADP into 3-phosphoglycerate and ATP. The remaining steps to pyruvic acid are easy to follow in Fig. 2.12. The reader should note that *each* of the two triose sugars derived from glucose gives rise to the production of two molecules of ATP. Taking into account the two molecules lost in the early stages of glycolysis we see that we have achieved a net gain of two molecules of ATP for every molecule of glucose that has been degraded as far as pyruvic acid. In addition, the two molecules of NAD^+ used in this reaction need to be regenerated. The regeneration of each molecule is associated, as we shall explain later, with the production of three molecules of ATP. Thus the origin of the eight molecules of ATP produced by substrate level phosphorylation and referred to earlier, is now clear.

In vigorous exercise the amount of oxygen that would be required for the complete oxidation of the fuel required by skeletal muscle outstrips the supply. Some of the pyruvic acid is converted into lactic acid. The hydrogen required for this reduction is carried by the reduced nicotinamide adenine dinucleotide that was formed when 3-phosphoglyceraldehyde was converted into 1,3-diphosphoglycerate earlier in the glycolytic process. This re-oxidation of the coenzyme, only limited supplies of which are available to the cell, ensures that glycolysis is not interrupted during a period in which demands for fuel are high. When the exercise is over the muscle repays its 'oxygen debt'—the lactic acid is re-oxidized to pyruvic acid, which rejoins the oxidative pathway it had to leave when oxygen supplies became inadequate.

Lactic acid can also be formed by the fermentation of glucose, another process in which anaerobic metabolism occurs.

In all animal tissues other than skeletal muscle the pyruvic acid that is produced by glycolysis immediately undergoes oxidative metabolism, none of it having to be delayed in the lactic 'lay by'. These stages in the conversion of glucose to carbon dioxide and water and the associated events that culminate in the production of further supplies of ATP all take place in mitochondria. Pyruvic acid reacts with coenzyme A to give acetyl coenzyme A (Fig. 2.13) and the last named compound then joins the Krebs citric acid (or the tricarboxylic acid) cycle which now has to be described. It should, perhaps, be noted at this stage, that at a physiological pH organic acids are completely ionized in solution. Consequently they are often named by their anions, so that pyruvic acid, for instance, becomes pyruvate. In this chapter we shall persist in designating them as acids. This practice is not without merit.

The citric acid cycle

The sequence of events that constitutes the citric acid cycle was elucidated by Krebs who received the Nobel prize for his discovery, as indeed did the pioneers who discovered most of the other fundamental cellular processes discussed in this chapter.

The acetate group in the acetyl coenzyme A derived from pyruvic acid, is transferred to oxaloacetic acid under the influence of citrate synthetase, so forming citric acid with the liberation of the coenzyme A which is thus made immediately available again for union with other molecules of pyruvic acid. A succession of chemical changes (molecular re-arrangements, dehydrogenations, decarboxylations, addition of water) then take place to produce a variety of intermediates, the last of which is oxaloacetic acid. The cycle has thus turned full circle and the oxaloacetic acid is ready for another circuit. A knowledge of the

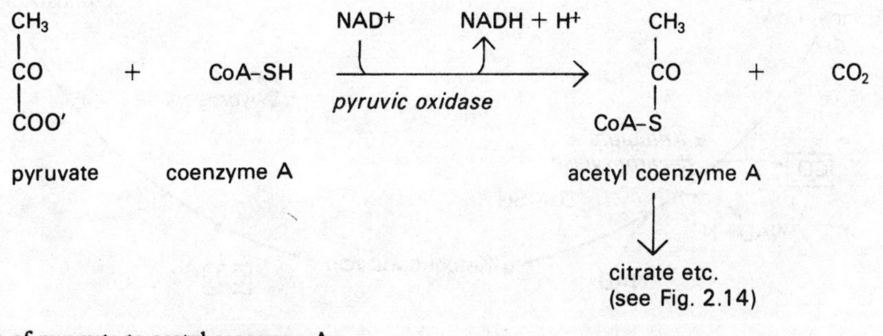

Fig. 2.13 Conversion of pyruvate to acetyl coenzyme A

precise details of the Krebs cycle operation is not to be regarded as being essential for the pharmacologist but the names of the compounds produced together with the enzymes and coenzymes involved in their formation are presented, for reference purposes, in Fig. 2.14. To provide further help for any reader who is (commendably) determined to see for himself the exact nature of the changes that take place, Fig. 2.15 supplies the chemical formulae of the cycle intermediates in the order in which they are generated.

Although a biochemist's knowledge of the Krebs cycle is not required, it is important to be aware of the results of its operation. In the first place, it will be noted that two molecules of carbon dioxide are evolved in every turn of the cycle. Remembering that another was produced during the formation of acetyl coenzyme A and that every mole-

cule of glucose produces two of pyruvic acid we can see that the six molecules of carbon dioxide demanded by the equation for glucose oxidation ($C_6H_{12}O_6 \rightarrow 6CO_2 + 6H_2O$) have duly made their appearance. It will be seen, though, that no oxygen has yet been used.

One molecule of ATP is generated in each turn of the cycle. More important than this, from the point of view of creating ATP, is the fact that two molecules of reduced nicotinamide adenine dinucleotide and one of reduced flavin adenine dinucleotide are also produced. Another molecule of the reduced nicotinamide coenzyme appeared when pyruvic acid was converted to acetyl coenzyme A to start the cycle. The re-oxidation of the reduced coenzymes is linked to ATP production during oxidative phosphorylation, the operation that completes the catabolic process.

It should be noted that the Krebs cycle is not the

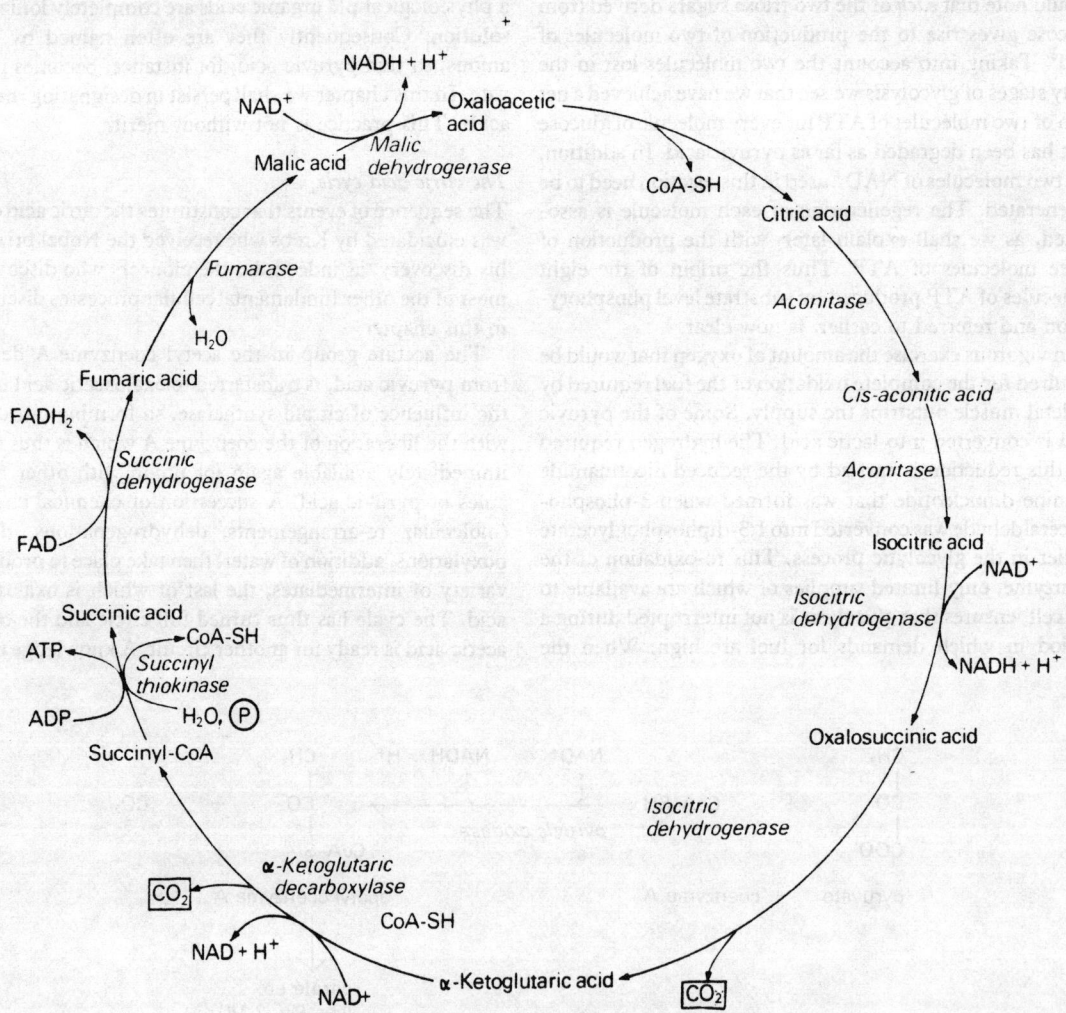

Fig. 2.14 The Krebs citric acid cycle (Enzymes are in *italics*).

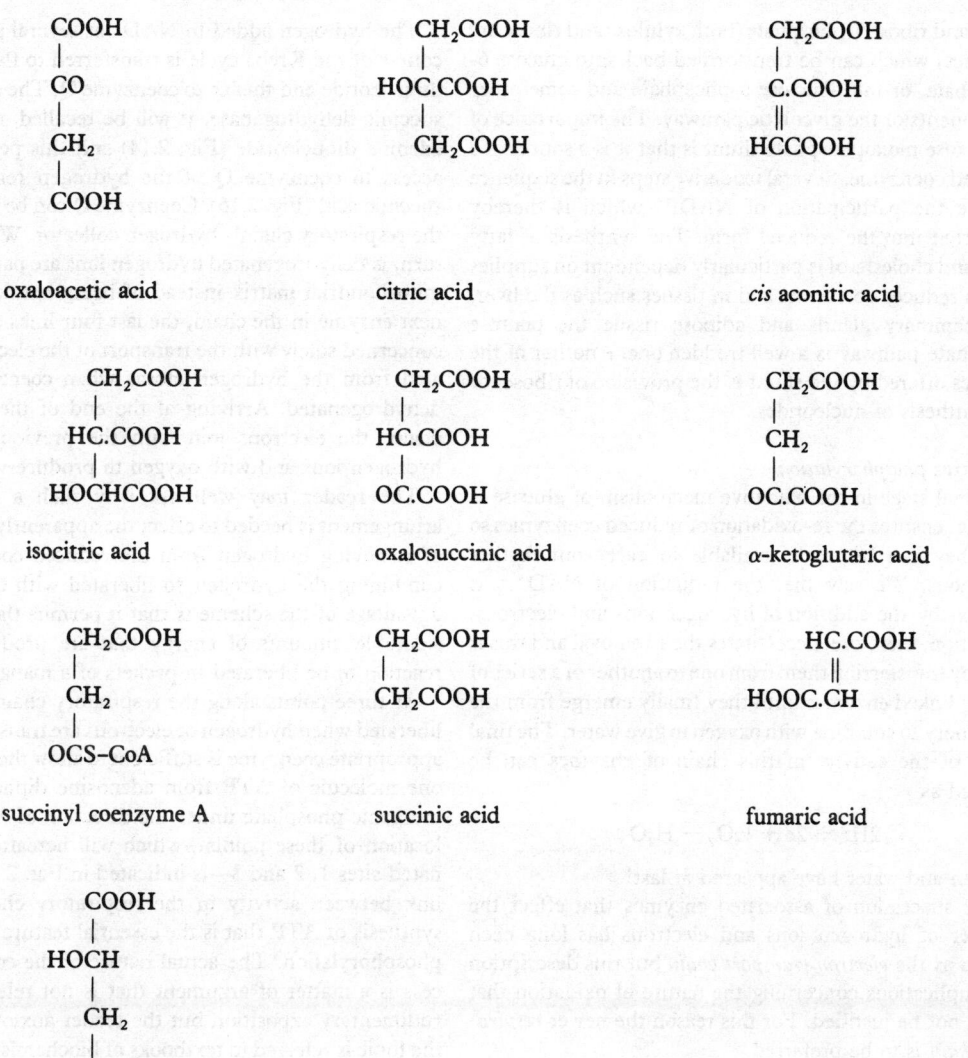

oxaloacetic acid   citric acid   *cis* aconitic acid

isocitric acid   oxalosuccinic acid   α-ketoglutaric acid

succinyl coenzyme A   succinic acid   fumaric acid

malic acid

Fig. 2.15 The Krebs cycle acids

completely closed and exclusive system that might appear from the foregoing discussion. A number of aminoacids are structurally related to some of the Krebs cycle intermediates, differing only in their possession of an amino group instead of the keto (–CO) group in the corresponding cycle intermediates. Aspartic acid, glutamic acid and alanine form *homologous pairs* in this sense with oxaloacetic, α-ketoglutaric and pyruvic acids respectively. The members of a homologous pair can be converted the one into the other by a *transamination* reaction. Transamination can also be effected between some other pairs of aminoacids that are not strictly homologous. This type of reaction allows the provision of aminoacids when these are needed.

Conversely, unwanted aminoacids that can undergo transamination can be used to provide additional material for the Krebs cycle.

It should be noted that not all the glucose utilized by the cell traverses the glycolytic and Krebs pathways. Some enters the pentose phosphate pathway, alternatively known as the hexose monophosphate shunt or, less commonly, the phosphogluconate pathway. The details of this complex metabolic sequence need not concern us here. Suffice it to say, by way of a summary, that glucose that is to be diverted into the shunt is first phosphorylated, in the usual way, to give glucose 6-phosphate. The glucose phosphate is subsequently converted into xylulose 5-phosphate and ribose 5-phosphate (both xylulose and ribose are pentoses) which can be transformed back into glucose 6-phosphate, or into fructose 6-phosphate and some other components of the glycolytic pathway. The importance of the hexose monophosphate shunt is that it is a source of a reduced coenzyme. Several oxidative steps in the sequence require the participation of $NADP^+$ which is thereby converted into the reduced form. The synthesis of fatty acids and cholesterol is particularly dependent on supplies of this reduced coenzyme and in tissues such as the liver, the mammary glands and adipose tissue the pentose phosphate pathway is a well trodden one. Another of the services offered by the shunt is the provision of ribose for the synthesis of nucleotides.

Oxidative phosphorylation

The final stage in the oxidative metabolism of glucose is one that ensures the re-oxidation of reduced coenzymes so that they can be made available to carry out further oxidations. We saw that the reduction of NAD^+ was effected by the addition of hydrogen ions and electrons. Oxidation, therefore, necessitates their removal and this is done by transferring them from one to another of a series of closely linked enzymes until they finally emerge from the machinery to combine with oxygen to give water. The final result of the activity of this chain of enzymes can be denoted as

$$2H^+ + 2e + \tfrac{1}{2}O_2 \rightarrow H_2O$$

Oxygen and water have appeared at last!

The succession of associated enzymes that effect the transfer of hydrogen ions and electrons has long been known as the *electron transport chain* but this description has implications concerning the nature of oxidation that might not be justified. For this reason the newer *respiratory chain* is to be preferred.

The respiratory chain is depicted in Fig. 2.16, which names the coenzymes but ignores the enzymes.

The hydrogen added to NAD^+ at several points in the course of the Krebs cycle is transferred to flavin adenine dinucleotide and thence to coenzyme Q. The coenzyme of succinic dehydrogenase, it will be recalled, is also flavin adenine dinucleotide (Fig. 2.14) and this permits direct access to coenzyme Q of the hydrogen removed from succinic acid (Fig. 2.16). Coenzyme Q can be looked on as the respiratory chain's hydrogen collector. When it, in its turn, is dehydrogenated hydrogen ions are passed into the mitochondrial matrix instead of being handed on to the next enzyme in the chain, the last four links of which are concerned solely with the transport of the electrons separated from the hydrogen atoms when coenzyme Q was dehydrogenated. Arriving at the end of the respiratory chain, the electrons join with the previously released hydrogen ions and with oxygen to produce water.

The reader may well ask why such a complicated arrangement is needed to effect the apparently simple task of removing hydrogen from the reduced coenzyme and combining the hydrogen so liberated with oxygen. The advantage of the scheme is that it permits the not inconsiderable amounts of energy that are produced in the reaction to be liberated in packets of a manageable size.

At three points along the respiratory chain the energy liberated when hydrogen or electrons are transferred to the appropriate coenzyme is sufficient to allow the synthesis of one molecule of ATP from adenosine diphosphate and inorganic phosphate under the direction of ATPase. The location of these points—which will hereafter be designated sites 1, 2 and 3—is indicated in Fig. 2.16. It is this link between activity in the respiratory chain and the synthesis of ATP that is the essential feature of oxidative phosphorylation. The actual nature of the coupling process is a matter of argument that is not relevant to this rudimentary exposition but the reader anxious to pursue the topic is referred to textbooks of biochemistry where he will find discussions concerning the relative merits of the rival 'chemical' and 'chemiosmotic' hypotheses. Some of

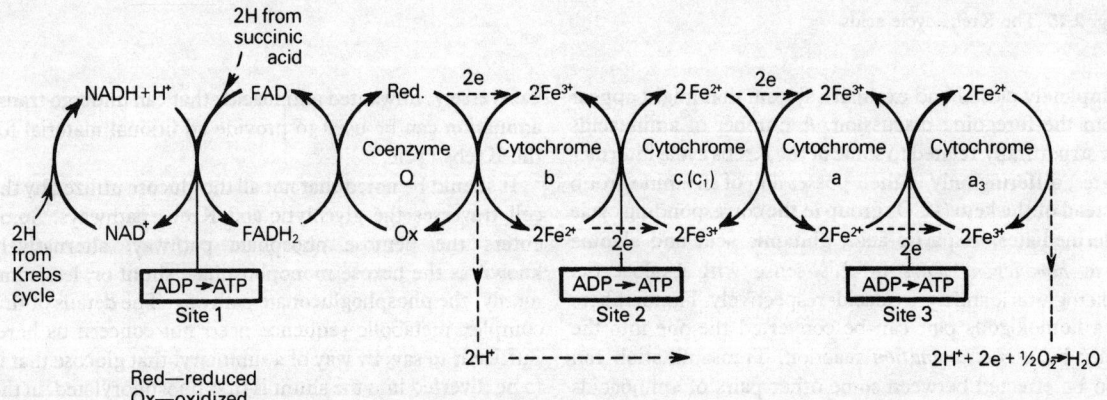

Fig. 2.16 The respiratory chain (For details, see text)

the many suitable textbooks are named in the bibliography appended to this chapter (p. 32).

The progress of hydrogen and electrons along the respiratory chain and their triggering of ATP synthesis en route is not the laboured procession that might have been implied by the foregoing descriptions. We saw earlier (p. 13) that ATPase and the components of the respiratory chain are very closely associated on the stalks of the mitochondrial cristae and we must try to visualize virtually instantaneous exchanges of hydrogen and electrons among the tightly knit enzymes and an immediate synthesis of ATP each time the initiating trigger is pulled by the successive bursts of metabolic energy.

We can see that for each atom of oxygen utilized by the respiratory chain, three molecules of ATP are produced provided that the hydrogen makes its entry into the system by way of reduced NAD. We say that the P : O ratio is 3. When hydrogen is introduced by the flavin adenine nucleotide route, however, the P : O ratio is only 2 because the route taken by hydrogen from the reduced coenzyme bypasses the first of the loci at which synthesis of ATP occurs. Noting these facts the reader should be able to satisfy himself that the oxidation of one molecule of pyruvic acid is associated with the production of 15 molecules of ATP and that, consequently, the two 3-carbon sugars produced from one molecule of glucose as it travels the glycolytic pathway will yield twice this amount of ATP. Added to the eight produced during glycolysis, this gives 38 as the grand total of molecules of ATP produced by the oxidation of one molecule of glucose.

A number of substances can inhibit oxidative phosphorylation by an action at one or other of the three sites at which ATP is formed. These substances include guanethidine, rotenone, chlorpromazine and barbiturates (inhibitors at site 1), antimycin, naphthaquinone and phenformin (site 2 inhibitors) and azide, cyanide and carbon monoxide (site 3 inhibitors). Some others (oligomycin provides a good example) act unspecifically at all three sites. Yet other substances break the link between respiratory chain activity and the synthesis of ATP. In the jargon of the business they 'uncouple oxidative phosphorylation'. Unlike the specific site inhibitors, uncouplers do not interrupt the oxidative reaction but because the synthesis of high energy phosphate is compromised the P : O ratio falls (to zero when uncoupling is complete) and the oxidative energy that can no longer be trapped by ATP appears as heat. In the laboratory, dinitrophenol is used as an uncoupling agent but pharmacologists have been more interested in the possibility that some drugs might owe their therapeutic or toxic properties to an uncoupling effect. However, most drugs that can be shown to uncouple oxidative phosphorylation in *in vitro* experiments do so only when they are present in concentrations they are unlikely to attain in the tissues of the living animal even when they are taken in toxic doses. An exception to this generalization is provided by the salicylates and this accounts for the surprising fact that aspirin, a drug with a well marked antipyretic action (p. 443) nevertheless induces fever, particularly in children, when it is taken by accident or suicidal intent in very large doses.

Up to this point, the provision of metabolic energy has been discussed entirely in terms of glucose but fats too are rich sources of energy. Neutral fats are hydrolysed into glycerol and fatty acids. Glycerol is converted into dihydroxyacetone phosphate and thereby gains admission to the Embden–Meyerhof pathway. The fatty acids are broken down into two-carbon fragments which become converted into acetyl coenzyme A which then, of course, is taken on board the Krebs cycle in the usual way. As an indication of the energy supplied by fatty acid metabolism it is worth noting that the complete oxidation of a single molecule of palmitic acid ($C_{15}H_{31}COOH$) is associated with the synthesis of no fewer than 130 molecules of ATP. Proteins are not normally thought of as suppliers of energy but they can serve this function. The aminoacids into which they are hydrolysed can be metabolized in a variety of ways: some, as we have seen, undergo transamination to give Krebs cycle intermediates, and are then either oxidized or converted into glucose. Others appear as acetyl coenzyme A but whatever their fate it is evident that, if they are not to be incorporated into new protein or polypeptide molecules, they will eventually have to join the system that handles the other types of foodstuff.

Microsomes, like the mitochondria, also possess an efficient oxidation system. It is based on enzymes linked with $NADP^+$ and flavoprotein coenzymes and its cytochrome component is called cytochrome P_{450}. The microsomal enzyme systems are considered in more detail later (p. 52).

BIBLIOGRAPHY

Books, monographs and reviews

Ambrose, E.J. and Easty, Dorothy M. (1977) *Cell Biology,* 2nd edn., Sunbury-on-Thames: Nelson.

Barker, G.R. (1968) *Understanding the Chemistry of the Cell.* London: Edward Arnold.

Edelstein, S.J. (1973) *Introductory Biochemistry,* San Francisco: Holden-Day.

Gillie, O. (1971) *The Living Cell,* London: Thames and Hudson.

Haggis, G.H. (1974) *Introduction to Molecular Biology,* 2nd edn, London: Longmans.

Hopkins, C.R. (1978) *Structure and Function of Cells,* London, Philadelphia and Toronto: W.B. Saunders Co.

Howland, J.L. (1973) *Cell Physiology,* New York: Macmillan.

Montgomery, R., Dryer, R. L., Conway, T. W. and Spector, A.A. (1977) *Biochemistry. A Case-Orientated Approach,* 2nd edn. Saint Louis: The C.V. Mosby Company.

Novikoff, A.B. and Holtzman, E. (1976) *Cells and Organelles,* 2nd edn, New York: Holt, Rinehart & Winston.

Routh, J.I. (1978) *Introduction to Biochemistry,* 2nd edn, Philadelphia, London and Toronto: W.B. Saunders Co.

Toner, Peter G. and Carr, Katherine E. (1971) *Cell Structure,* 2nd edn, Edinburgh and London: Churchill Livingstone.

Warwick, R. and Williams, P.L. (eds) (1973) *Gray's Anatomy,* 35th edn., Edinburgh: Longman.

Watson, J.D. (1968) *The Double Helix,* London: Wiedenfeld and Nicholson.

Wolfe, S.L. (1972) *Biology of the Cell,* Belmont, California: Wadsworth.

Yudkin, M. and Offord, R. (1973) *Comprehensible Biochemistry,* Edinburgh: Longman.

3. The administration of drugs

When a drug is being used for prophylactic, therapeutic or experimental purposes it must reach the site or sites at which an action is wanted and a sufficiently high concentration of the drug must be maintained there long enough for the desired effect to be achieved. Although these requirements are obvious they are not always fulfilled and many instances are known of drugs being ineffective as a result of their being administered by the wrong route or in accordance with an unsatisfactory dose schedule.

The concentration of a drug at its site of action is clearly determined by the balance between the rates of its arrival at and clearance from this site. The factors that promote and influence these processes will be discussed in detail later: in this chapter we shall be concerned only to describe the means by which drugs can be given to patients and laboratory animals and to compare, in purely practical terms, the relative advantages and disadvantages of these several modes of administration.

ROUTES OF ADMINISTRATION

ORAL AND RELATED ROUTES
Oral administration is the one most acceptable to the patient and it has a number of advantages. It is cheap, because sterilization and special purification procedures are not necessary. It is convenient because drugs can be given in the form of tablets or capsules which contain an exact dose. It is easy and the patient can take the drug without interrupting the activity in which he is engaged and without drawing attention to himself.

Drugs taken by mouth have to be absorbed (usually from the small intestine) before they can be transported to their site of action. Absorption may be slow, unpredictable and irregular because of the presence of variable amounts of food in different stages of digestion and to the varying degrees of acidity and alkalinity of the digestive juices (p. 41). Moreover, blood from the intestinal tract passes first to the liver: some drugs are metabolized in the liver and others may be stored there to be released only slowly. These considerations make it clear that oral administration is usually unsuitable in emergencies or on other occasions when a rapid effect is needed. On the other hand, it is sometimes an advantage to retard the absorption of an orally-administered drug so that a more prolonged action can be obtained. One method of doing this is to use a combination of the drug and an ion exchange resin.

Some substances are destroyed by the acid of the gastric juice but are immune to attack by alkali or the intestinal digestive enzymes. Some irritate the gastric mucosa and may cause nausea and vomiting. These drugs can still be given by mouth if they can be presented in a form which ensures that they are not released until they reach the intestine. They may, for instance, be placed in a capsule of gelatin or some other material which is not rapidly destroyed by gastric juice. If such capsules are swallowed on an empty stomach they pass very quickly to the intestine where they are digested, releasing their contained drug. Enteric coatings, which are immune to attack by gastric juice but which disintegrate readily in the small intestine, serve a similar purpose. Drugs which are attacked by gastric acid but which do not irritate the intestine are sometimes combined with a suitable alkali for oral administration.

It should hardly be necessary to add that no form of oral administration is practicable for drugs which irritate the intestine, which are destroyed by intestinal enzymes or which cannot be absorbed from the gastrointestinal tract.

A disadvantage of oral administration, apart from the uncertainties attendant on the irregular absorption, springs from its very convenience. Patients on a therapeutic regime that requires the regular taking of a drug may forget their drug on one occasion and may then attempt to compensate for their omission by taking a double dose on the next occasion. The dangers of such actions, though obvious, seem to be rarely appreciated by patients. The fidelity with which patients follow instructions is illustrated by the results of a study in which hospital outpatients were each given one hundred tablets of a drug, told to take four tablets a day for a week and return the rest to the hospital. The number returned ranged from none to ninety-seven!

In laboratory work on animals it is not usual to administer drugs by mouth since it is a more convenient and accurate procedure to give them by injection. However, when toxicity tests or exploratory studies are being undertaken on drugs which it is hoped to give by mouth to human beings it is advisable to administer them by this route also to the experimental animals. They can be given by capsule in the food, or by tube directly into the stomach. In the anaesthetized animal, they can be injected into the duodenum. In long term experiments it is sometimes possible to administer soluble and stable drugs in drinking water. In the author's laboratory, for instance, drugs such as alcohol and barbiturates have been given in this way over long periods. By noting the daily fluid intake it is possible to adjust the concentration of the drug in the drinking water so that a predetermined amount of drug is taken daily. The method is simple and it results in the maintenance of a steadier drug concentration in the tissues than is possible by injection methods. This is a valuable feature in experiments designed to study such problems as the development of drug tolerance (p. 83). The taste of bitter substances, such as barbiturates, can be disguised by saccharin or by sucrose.

Sublingual administration

A tablet containing the drug is placed under the tongue and is allowed to dissolve. The drug does not have to enter the intestine so it is absorbed rapidly and it reaches the general circulation without first passing through the liver. Substances that can be taken sublingually therefore act more rapidly and are likely to be effective in a lower dose than if they are swallowed. Sublingual tablets can be spat out as soon as relief is obtained and this can be a boon in situations that call for the rapid alleviation of distressing symptoms. The patient can take his drug without fearing, as he might if he had to swallow it, either that he will receive too little medicament to provide the relief he so urgently needs or that he will suffer the effects of an overdose. Sublingual tablets of glyceryl trinitrate and isoprenaline are available, for example, for the treatment of acute attacks of angina pectoris and asthma respectively. A further occasional use of the sublingual route is for the administration of drugs that would be destroyed in the gastrointestinal tract. Steroids sometimes have to be given over long periods of time to patients in whom a deficient output of endogenous steroid hormones demands supplementation from outside sources. Intramuscular injection and subcutaneous implants (p. 35) are usually made use of for this purpose but sublingual administration has also been employed with some success (Moffat, 1971). This provides an interesting contrast to the emergency situations that provide the other main indication for the use of sublingual preparations.

Inhalation

Substances in the gaseous form or in sprays and aerosols are readily absorbed through the pulmonary epithelium. Medicinal gases and volatile or gaseous anaesthetics such as ether and nitrous oxide have to be administered by inhalation. Bronchodilators are conveniently given from inhalers in aerosol form which brings the drugs into immediate contact with the structures on which they act. The development of inhalers which allow the supply of accurately metered doses of drug promises to extend the scope of this method of drug administration. It need not be restricted to drugs that act only on the lungs. Vaporizing drugs can be absorbed in smoke: nicotine is the most obvious example but smoke has also been used as a vehicle for atropine (in stramonium cigarettes), and, by addicts, for opium and other drugs.

Drugs can also be absorbed by the nasal mucous membrane if they are applied by *sprays* or taken by *insufflation*. In the last named method a fine powder or snuff is used. Pituitary snuff is administered by insufflation while cocaine and heroin are sometimes taken in this way by addicts.

Inhalation anaesthesia is employed in laboratory animals as it is in clinical practice. The administration of histamine or other bronchoconstrictor substances in an aerosol is a useful method of producing bronchoconstriction in guinea pigs when drugs are being screened for bronchodilator activity.

Rectal administration

Some drugs cause vomiting when they are given by mouth to sensitive subjects. If it is impracticable to administer them by capsule and if they are absorbed by the rectal mucous membrane they can be given *per rectum* in the form of suppositories. Ergotamine is presented in this form for the treatment of migraine when vomiting is present. The rectal route can be utilized in unconscious patients who cannot, of course, take drugs by mouth. Another form of preparation for rectal administration is the *enema*, a solution or suspension of the drug in water or some other vehicle. The anaesthetic bromethol is given by this route. Suppositories can also be used in the local treatment of rectal conditions: benzocaine is applied in this way to relieve pain and itching caused by haemorrhoids. Suppositories and enemas are less popular in Britain than they are in some European countries, a circumstance that should, perhaps, be passed over without further comment.

LOCAL ADMINISTRATION

The routes of administration so far discussed are used for drugs which are readily absorbed from the gastrointestinal or respiratory tracts into the general circulation. It is sometimes necessary, however, to restrict the action of drugs to the part of the body to which they are applied. The routes already mentioned can be used for local treatment. Thus, some gastrointestinal disorders can be treated by the oral or rectal administration of suitable drugs which are not absorbed from the intestine and bronchodilators can be given by inhalation. The methods of drug application described in this section, however, are used solely for local treatment.

Application to the skin

Drugs may be applied to the surface of the skin in the form of ointments, pastes, creams, liniments and lotions. A superficial action is usually sought but if suitable ointment bases or other vehicles are used some penetration into the subcutaneous tissues may take place. Absorption is by the sebaceous glands but it is slow and erratic. *Iontophoresis* consists of driving the substance in aqueous solution into the skin by means of a direct electric current. Though it was once popular, the therapeutic usefulness and applicability of iontophoresis is limited.

It should be remembered that although the healthy skin provides an impervious covering, its protective function may be lost if the skin is cut or damaged. In these circumstances, drugs intended to have a local action may be absorbed into the general circulation. Substances that are quite innocuous when applied to the skin may be highly toxic if they enter the circulation and care has to be exercised when prescribing drugs for dermatological conditions in cases where the skin is broken. Drugs suitable for local application to the skin are discussed elsewhere (p. 807).

Vaginal administration

The drug is presented in the form of a pessary or tablet or it may be used to impregnate a vaginal tampon. Although the method can be used for drugs which are absorbed through the vaginal mucous membrane into the circulation it is usually restricted to cases requiring the local treatment of vaginal conditions.

Drugs can also be applied locally to the *eye*. Rarely they are administered, by *urethral bougies,* directly to the urethra. In emergencies, adrenaline may be directly injected into the wall of the heart, providing a rather extreme example of the local application of a therapeutic agent.

Microinjection and microiontophoretic administration

These are the most refined forms of local administration yet devised for use in the laboratory. These techniques, which are more fully discussed elsewhere (p. 179) permit the application of minute quantities of drug directly to individual neurones in the central nervous system. They are of the utmost value to the laboratory worker. They have, of course, no clinical application.

Intraarterial, intrathecal and intraventricular injections are also, strictly, forms of local application but since they involve the introduction of the drug directly into the body fluids they are more conveniently classified with the other forms of parenteral administration.

PARENTERAL ADMINISTRATION

The term *parenteral* administration (par—beyond, enteral—intestinal) implies that the drug is given by a route which takes it directly into the body fluids, by-passing the preliminary process of transport through the intestinal wall or pulmonary alveoli which is necessary when drugs are ingested, inhaled or placed in the rectum. With all forms of parenteral administration, sterile precautions are necessary.

Subcutaneous administration

Provided that they do not cause irritation at the injection site, drugs in solution can be injected into the subcutaneous tissues from which absorption is slow but uniform. This method of administration is very useful for the treatment of conditions that demand the continued presence of the drug in the tissues over long periods. Diabetics take their insulin (which is destroyed by intestinal enzymes) by this route. When large volumes of a drug solution have to be given into the subcutaneous tissues (a technique which is sometimes rather splendidly called *hypodermoclysis*) it is helpful to add hyaluronidase to the mixture. Hyaluronidase (the spreading factor, page 420) reduces the degree of polymerization of the ground substance of connective tissue and so permits a more rapid and extensive spread of the injected material. The usefulness of the subcutaneous route is increased by the use of depot preparations from which the drug is released more slowly than it is from simple solution. Thus larger doses of drug can be given and the patient has to receive injections less frequently. Depot preparations are described in several places in this book. Examples include the long-acting insulins and some trypanocidal agents. A particular form of depot preparation is the *subcutaneous implant*. Instead of using the drug in solution a sterile compressed pellet is inserted into the subcutaneous tissues. The drug is liberated slowly and evenly and the drug effect is very prolonged. The method has a limited application but it is used to administer certain hormones such as testosterone and in the laboratory it has been used with success to provide a continuous supply of morphine to rats and mice and so to establish tolerance to the drug.

Intramuscular injection

Injection is made into a large muscle usually, in human subjects, the deltoid muscle in the shoulder or the gluteus muscle in the buttocks. The needle is inserted deeply and the injection may be painful. The advantages of intramuscular injection are that it results in uniform absorption and that it can be used for solutions too irritant for subcutaneous injection. The speed of absorption of drugs given by intramuscular injection depends on the vehicle in which they are dissolved: absorption is rapid from aqueous solutions and slow from oily ones.

Intraperitoneal injection

This is probably the most widely used route of drug administration in laboratory animals but since it necessitates the penetration of thick muscle layers and blind injection into the organ-filled and infection-prone abdominal cavity it is only very rarely employed in human beings. In experimental animals, intraperitoneal injection is easy and, provided that a sharp and sufficiently large needle is used, the animal suffers no discomfort. If the animal has been starved overnight it is unlikely that the needle will penetrate the intestines. After intraperitoneal injection, absorption of the drug is very rapid since the absorbing surface (the whole of the peritoneum) is very large.

Intravenous injection

Injection of the drug solution is made directly into a vein so that it is diluted in the venous blood, carried to the heart and circulated to the tissues. Since the total circulation time in man is of the order of fifteen seconds the onset of effect of intravenously injected drugs can be very rapid. This is a great advantage in emergency treatment and in the induction of anaesthesia. Another advantage of intravenous injection is that it can be used for the administration of drugs which cause irritation of the tissues when they are given by subcutaneous injection. When they are given intravenously they are rapidly diluted and carried away from the site of injection. Great care, however, has to be taken when administering irritant drugs to ensure that the vein is properly entered and that none of the drug escapes into the surrounding tissue. A disadvantage of the intravenous route is that, because of the rapidity with which the drug reaches the tissues, overdosage may have effects so immediate that it is impossible to reverse them. Strict sterile precautions are essential whenever a drug is given by the intravenous route to human beings since any infecting organisms introduced by the syringe would spread widely through the body.

In anaesthetized laboratory animals, intravenous injections are usually made by way of a cannula tied into the femoral, jugular or other suitable vein. The cannula is attached to a suitable reservoir of saline solution. If injections are made into the tubing connecting the cannula and the reservoir the drug can be washed into the vein by a constant volume of saline solution. Injection into the jugular vein carries the disadvantage that, if the cannula becomes accidentally dislodged, the negative intrathoracic pressure may draw large quantities of air into the venous system through the hole in the vein. The air passes directly to the heart which may stop since the froth produced by the admixture of air and blood provides too insubstantial a material for the heart to contract on. In addition, bubbles of air may form emboli in the pulmonary vessels. Air embolism is indeed a hazard theoretically attendant on any form of intravenous injection and it is prudent to exclude all air from the needle and syringe when giving drugs by the intravenous route. The dangers of injecting small quantities of air have, however, been rather exaggerated.

In conscious animals, intravenous injection is simpler in some species than in others. Drugs can be easily injected into the marginal ear vein of the completely unrestrained rabbit and into several superficial veins of dogs which have become accustomed to laboratory procedures. In rats and mice the tail veins are accessible, but injection failures are not uncommon and the animals usually have to be res-

trained in a suitable cage from which the tail projects. In the rat, the veins on the dorsum of the foot can also be used. It is a simple matter to make injections into the wing vein of young chicks.

A distinction should be made between intravenous injection and *intravenous infusion*. When a drug is injected it is given more or less rapidly over a short period of time. In infusions it is allowed to pass slowly into the vein over a period of hours or longer. In laboratory work the method is useful when it is desired to mimic the effect of substances that are continuously secreted in the normal animal. Infusions of appropriate agents can also be used for maintaining blood pressure, hydration and so on throughout a long experiment. In experimental work, infusions are conveniently given by mechanically-driven syringes. Similar devices are used in human surgery but in the ward continued intravenous administration is usually maintained by means of an intravenous drip, the drug solution being allowed to pass into the vein under the influence of gravity. The patient is not then dependent on the continued functioning of a mechanical device.

Intra-arterial injection

In human patients, this technique is limited to the injection of radio-opaque media for diagnostic purposes. In suspected cerebral tumours, for instance, the medium is injected into the carotid artery; for obvious reasons the technique is called *arteriography*. Arterial injection has a wider application in experimental work. In many circumstances it suffices to introduce the drug into the arterial circulation supplying the area of the body under investigation. Thus if the hind limbs are being studied the drug can be injected into the abdominal aorta. Sometimes, however, *close arterial injection* is needed. In this technique, steps are taken to restrict the area over which the drug exerts its effect. The solution is injected into a suitable artery at a point that is as close as possible to the desired site of action. Collateral arteries below the point of injection are tied off. The advantages associated with this method are that it sharply reduces the dilution of the drug by the blood and the time of contact with the blood enzymes. It also enables the drug to be applied almost exactly to the desired site of action so that there can be little doubt that any effect observed is due to an action at that site and is not a secondary response to an effect occurring elsewhere. Thus when drugs are given by close arterial injection into the spinal cord, effects on ventral root activity can be attributed to a direct action on anterior horn cells and not to reflex stimulation from some peripheral receptor. Close arterial injection, if given rapidly, can produce the effects of chemical mediators liberated by nerve impulses. The demonstration, by Dale and his colleagues, that the close arterial injection of acetylcholine into skeletal muscle produced a contraction similar to that following nerve stimulation provided an important argument for the view

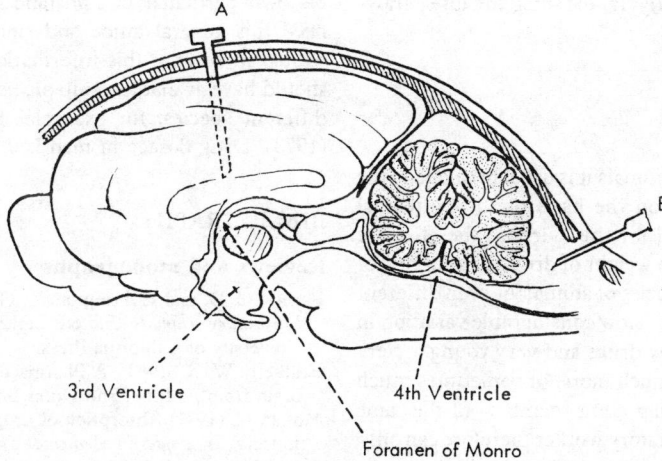

A

B

3rd Ventricle

4th Ventricle

Foramen of Monro

Fig. 3.1 Cross section of the mammalian brain to show at A, a Feldberg-Collision cannula permanently implanted in the skull and passing into the lateral ventricle which is lateral to the plane of the paper but communicates with the 3rd ventricle at the foramen of Monro. At B, a hypodermic needle passes through the skin, at a point located between the skull and the first vertebra, into the cisterna magna. The membranes which line the skull and cover the brain are omitted.

that the transmission of impulses from nerve to muscle is mediated by acetylcholine (p. 172).

Intrathecal and intraventricular injection

Injections can be made into the subarachnoid space (*intrathecal injection*) and the effects of the drug are then localized to the spinal nerves and meninges. This will be made clear by reference to Figure 28.1 on page 465. The intrathecal route is used to produce regional anaesthesia and to ensure that an injected drug reaches the central nervous system in a high concentration. In tuberculous meningitis, streptomycin may be given intrathecally.

Injection into the cerebrospinal fluid is a particularly important technique in experimental neuropharmacology. Because of the blood-brain barrier (which is described on page 47) many substances injected into the blood stream are excluded from the brain and in order to determine their effect on the nervous system it is necessary either to apply them directly to the exposed brain or to inject them into the cerebrospinal fluid. The latter method of application is often preferable since injection can be carried out on the completely unanaesthetized animal or on the animal anaesthetized just for the period of the injection.

Direct application to the brain is advisable even when studying the central action of substances which do pass the blood-brain barrier since, on intravenous injection, peripheral effects may completely overshadow the changes produced by the action on the central nervous system. This is particularly important when the substance under investigation is one which occurs in the central nervous system,

destroyed or otherwise inactivated before it can enter the general circulation.

for in the living animal the substance might be liberated in the course of normal cerebral activity. Its physiological actions will be restricted to nerve cells if, as is usual, it is

Cerebrospinal fluid covers the external surface of the brain and spinal cord and it also fills the cerebral ventricles in the interior of the brain. The walls of the ventricles, particularly the third ventricle include many important and sensitive structures and drugs very often have different actions according to whether they are applied to the surface or to the interior of the brain. In a thorough-going pharmacological analysis it is necessary to study the action of the drug at both sites. In many animals it is easy to inject material into the cisterna magna (Fig 3.1) and in mice the cerebrospinal fluid overlying the brain can be reached by a needle inserted between the eyes.

The best method of applying drugs to the ventricular fluids is by means of an indwelling cannula inserted at a previous operation. This method was developed and exploited by Feldberg whose monograph (Feldberg, 1963) discusses the method and gives details of the results obtained with its aid. Some of these may surprise the reader. Thus adrenaline, which many will think of as an 'excitatory' substance, produces a condition resembling light anaesthesia when it is placed in the ventricles while curare, which causes complete paralysis when it is given intravenously, produces convulsions on intraventricular injection. The dose of curare needed to cause convulsions is quite small since the drug is applied directly to nerve cells. The amounts of curare which pass into the general circulation are, consequently, far too small to cause paralysis.

DRUG DOSAGE

In experimental work on animals it is usual to calculate the required dose of a drug on the basis of the individual animal's body weight and for this purpose the effective dose is usually quoted as a weight of drug per kilogram of body weight. Different species of animal (or even different strains of the same species) show considerable variation in their susceptibility to many drugs and very young or very old animals may be very much more, or sometimes much less, susceptible than young adult members of the same strain or species. The laboratory worker therefore can only use published dosages as a general guide, relying on experience to teach him how to judge the dose required in his own particular circumstances. Nevertheless he does need this general guide and since a lot of time can be wasted in seeking this information in original papers he should have available a suitable manual of drug dosages in different species, for example, Barnes and Elthrington (1973). Drug dosage in man is discussed on page 70.

BIBLIOGRAPHY

Reviews and monographs

Barnes, C. D. and Elthrington, L. G. (1973). *Drug Dosage in Laboratory Animals.* 2nd ed. Berkeley and Los Angeles: University of California Press.
Feldberg, W. S. (1963). A Pharmacological Approach to the Brain from its Inner and Outer Surfaces. London: Arnold.
Moffat, C. (1971) Absorption of drugs through the oral mucosa. In *Topics in Medicinal Chemistry* Rabinowitz J.L. and Myerson, R.M. (eds) 4, pp. 1-26. New York: Wiley.

4. Transport across the cell membrane and the absorption of drugs

The ubiquity of the plasma membrane needs no emphasis. As we read in Chap. 2, living cells and many of their inclusions are surrounded and permeated by membranes across which there is a ceaseless movement of nutrients, metabolites and regulatory substances. This thunder of traffic does not end until life itself is extinguished (indeed we might say that the traffic *is* life) and the processes that permit, promote and direct the flow of molecules and ions across membranes lie at the root of many of the most fundamental physiological activites. Drugs and their metabolites passing into and out of the tissues participate in this criss-cross traffic but they can, of necessity, achieve this only by trespassing on the transport systems that have been evolved to subserve purely physiological processes. We must note, in addition, that some drugs exert their therapeutic or toxic effects because they modify physiological transport mechanisms. Thus membrane biology is as important a study for the applied pharmacologist as it is for the academic physiologist.

This chapter first considers, in a necessarily summary fashion, the several mechanisms and factors that control the passage of molecules and ions across biological membranes. It then examines the operation of these processes in the more immediately pharmacological situations represented by the absorption and distribution of drugs from the intestine and elsewhere and the excretion of drugs and their metabolites from the body. The more prudent reader will wish to acquire a more detailed and authoritative account of the basic mechanisms than can be provided here. He should consult one or more of the many monographs on membrane function that are now available. Some of the best (and their scope is often indicated by their titles) are included in the bibliography on page.

THE PASSAGE OF MOLECULES ACROSS BIOLOGICAL MEMBRANES

The basic processes we have to consider are those of simple diffusion, facilitated diffusion, active transport and filtration. We must also glance at phagocytosis and pinocytosis.

SIMPLE DIFFUSION
Water poured very carefully into a vessel that already contains a concentrated aqueous solution of, say, sucrose will form a layer on top of the more dense liquid. This separation is not permanent because thermal agitation permits the exchange of sucrose and water molecules so that a mixture of uniform composition is eventually produced. Diffusion of sucrose into the water layer would clearly still occur if a permeable membrane were situated at the interface of the two original solutions (although the time required for equilibration would be considerably lengthened by virtue of the barrier properties of the membrane) and we can begin our study of transport processes from this model, defining simple diffusion, at least provisionally, as the passage of a substance across a cell membrane from a solution of higher to one of lower concentration without involving the expenditure of metabolic energy on the part of the membrane.

When transfer is by simple diffusion, the rate of passage of a substance across a membrane permeable to it is directly proportional to the surface area of the membrane (A) and the concentration gradient across it. The latter is determined by the difference in the concentrations of the diffusing material on the two sides of the membrane ($C_a - C_b$, where C_a is greater than C_b) and the membrane thickness (x). The rate of passage is simply the amount of material that is transferred in unit time. If we represent this by T and introduce a constant (k) to convert the proportionality into an equality we can summarise the statements of the foregoing paragraph in the simple form:

$$T = k \, A \, \frac{(C_a - C_b)}{x}$$

The thickness of a particular membrane remains constant and we can therefore replace $\frac{k}{x}$ by another term which we can conveniently call the *permeability constant* of the membrane and represent by *P*. Hence

$$T = -P \, A \, (C_a - C_b)$$

which is essentially the same formula as that derived by Fick in 1885 and which is now usually known as Fick's law of diffusion. The minus sign has been introduced into the formula as a conventional indication that the material leaves the more concentrated and passes into the less concentrated solution. We can formally define *P*, the permeability constant, as the amount of substance that would cross unit area of the membrane in unit time if the concentration difference were maintained at unity. The magnitude of the constant will, it is clear, be influenced both by the nature of the membrane and the properties of the substance that is crossing it. The reader will appreciate that C_a and C_b (and hence the rate of transfer) will be changing all the time as material passes from one side of the membrane to the other. However, in the biological situation, the volumes of solution on the two sides of the membrane will often be large in comparison with the size of the membrane itself so that the concentrations will change only slowly and the simplified Fick formula as we have derived it provides a quite adequate background to a general discussion of the factors that influence diffusion.

It is customary to state, somewhat baldly, that two physical properties – *lipid solubility* and *molecular size* – determine the ease or otherwise with which a substance traverses a biological membrane and that high lipid solubility and low molecular volume favour penetration. Although this is essentially true, it is important to realise that the two factors do not operate in a regularly additive way and that their relative importance varies greatly among different groups of compounds.

We saw in Chapter 2 that the plasma membrane can be usefully thought of as a double layer of protein–lipid studded with water filled pores. We would expect lipid soluble substances to cross such a membrane by dissolving in, and diffusing through, the lipid layers. Material that could not dissolve in lipid would have to pass through the pores and these channels would obviously only be accessible to smaller molecules. These expectations are fulfilled in practice. We can use the oil-water partition coefficient as an approximate indication of the likely solubility of a substance in membrane lipid and it is found that the permeability of a membrane to the different members of a homologous series of lipid soluble compounds is directly proportional to their partition coefficients. The slowly increasing molecular weight as the series is ascended exerts a negligible effect. On the other hand, molecular size is all important with substances that dissolve in water but not in lipid and some small molecules of this type (urea is an example) traverse plasma membranes with ease.

The foregoing must not be taken to imply that molecular size is entirely without effect on the diffusion of lipid soluble compounds. The relationship between oil–water partition coefficients and the ability to cross biological membranes is not so precise for a mixed group of compounds as it is for the members of a homologous series and, in particular, many larger molecules diffuse less rapidly than might be expected. This may be a consequence of the fact that many large organic molecules are only slightly soluble in water and it is possible that, having dissolved in and crossed the lipid membrane they have difficulty in detaching themselves from it to re-enter an aqueous solution.

Diffusion of ions across membranes
Ions are not soluble in lipids but, like water soluble non polar molecules, they can diffuse across a membrane down a concentration gradient provided that they are not too big. However many biological membranes are polarized, one side being positively charged and the other being negatively charged. A positively charged ion (cation) in an aqueous solution in contact with the positively charged face of a polarized membrane will be driven through the membrane (Fig. 4.1) and the effectiveness of this process will depend on the degree of polarization of the membrane, that is on the potential gradient across it. Anions can, of course, pass with equal ease in the opposite direction. The transport of ions by this mechanism does not require there to be a difference in the concentration of the diffusing ion on the two sides of the membrane.

It should now be clear that the diffusion of ions can occur either in response to the establishment of a concentration difference between solutions separated by a permeable membrane or because there is an appropriately directed polarization across the membrane itself. One, the other or both of these factors will operate in individual situations and our original definition of simple diffusion ought properly to have referred to the passage of material down its *electrochemical concentration gradient,* a term that encompasses both the factors that influence the rate of passive diffusion. For non-electrolytes it is synonymous with concentration gradient as we have already used that term.

The potential difference across a biological membrane is itself the consequence of ion movements.

The influence of pH on the diffusion of lipid soluble substances
Many drugs are weak electrolytes, being only partly dissociated in solution. In general, the undissociated molecule is soluble in lipid but the ions are not. Indicating a weak acid as HA we can represent its reversible dissociation in solution as

$$HA \rightleftharpoons H^+ + A^-$$

Simple mass action considerations tell us that if the concentration of hydrogen ions in the system is increased—by adding acid to the solution, for instance— the equilibrium will be shifted to the left, so that the

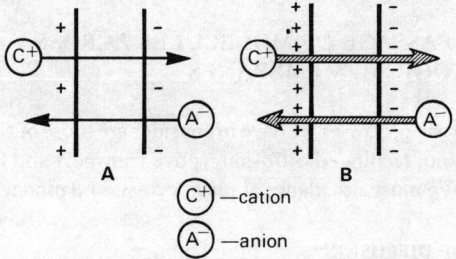

C^+ —cation
A^- —anion

Fig. 4.1 To illustrate the passage of ions across a polarized membrane. The membrane potential and the speed of passage is greater in (B) than in (A).

proportion of undissociated (and hence lipid soluble) molecules will increase. Thus, *the transfer of a weak acid across a membrane is favoured if it is presented in an acid medium.* Similarly the transfer of weak bases is increased if the pH of the solution is increased.

The effect of pH on ionization and hence on the transport of drugs across cell membranes was illustrated in a spectacular way by Travell (1940) who introduced strychnine in aqueous solution into the stomachs of a group of anaesthetized cats. He had previously tied off the pyloric end of each stomach so as to prevent passage of the strychnine into the intestine. The pH of the solutions he gave ranged, among the different animals, from 3 to 8. Strychnine is a weak base (so a high pH would favour its absorption) and a deadly poison and a cat that received the drug at pH 8 died within the half-hour. Death was progressively delayed in animals that were given solutions of increasing acidity and at pH 3 a strychnine solution was quite harmless. Calculations show that at pH 3 only 0.001 per cent of the strychnine would have been in the unionized form and that the fraction rose to 54 per cent at pH 8.

The rate of dissociation of an electrolyte is proportional to its concentration or, more properly, its activity. The difference between concentration and activity need not concern us here. Indicating concentration by square brackets and remembering that a proportionality can be converted into an equality by the use of an appropriate constant, the rate of dissociation of our acid can be represented as k_1 [HA]. The rate of re-association of its component ions is proportional to the product of their individual concentrations (or activities) and since, at equilibrium, the two reactions proceed at the same rate, we can say that

$$k_1 [HA] = k_2 [H^+] \times [A^-]$$
$$\text{or } [H^+] = \frac{k_1 [HA]}{k_2 [A^-]}$$

Let us now replace $\frac{k_1}{k_2}$ by a single constant which we will designate as K_a. Re-arranging our equation we obtain

$$\frac{1}{[H^+]} = \frac{1}{K_a} \frac{[A^-]}{[HA]}$$

If we now take logarithms and use the symbol pK_a in the same sense that pH is used we arrive at

$$pH = pK_a + \log \frac{[A^-]}{[HA]}$$

It is sometimes helpful to remember the last ratio as $\frac{\text{ionized acid}}{\text{unionized acid}}$. The reader will appreciate that the constant K_a is a measure of the net tendency of the acid to dissociate in solution. The weaker an acid the lower will be its K_a and the higher, therefore, its pK_a. Just as a highly

acid solution has a low pH so a highly acid substance has a low pK_a.

It was as long ago as 1908 that Henderson first established the relationship between the hydrogen ion concentration and the ratio of unionized to ionized acid. Because of his particular interests—he was a respiratory physiologist—Henderson expressed the equation in terms of carbonic acid and the bicarbonate ion but he could not use the symbols pH and pK_a because the 'potenz' notation was only introduced in 1909 by Sörensen. In 1917, Hasselbalch translated the Henderson equation into the new language, converting it into the version we have ourselves just derived. Ever since, it has been known as the Henderson-Hasselbalch equation. It appears in pharmacology and biochemistry in a number of guises and contexts since a variety of fundamental mechanisms depend on—or are assumed to depend on—simple unimolecular reactions.

It is to be hoped that the reader (unlike the authors of at least one half of the current textbooks of pharmacology and biochemistry) will have noticed the spelling of Hasselbalch.

The Henderson-Hasselbalch equation provides a quantitative expression of the relationship between the degree of dissociation of a weak acid and the pH of the solution in which it is dissolved. In particular, we can see (since the logarithm of 1 is zero) that the acid will be half ionized (i.e. $A^- = HA$) when the pH of the solution is the same as the acid's pK_a value. It is also evident that changes in acidity will have their most marked influence on the degree of ionization when the pH is near the pK_a value. Suppose, for instance, that the pK_a of a drug is 6. When it is in solution at this pH, 50 per cent of its molecules will be ionized. If the pH is now increased to 7, the ratio of ionized to unionized molecules will rise to 10 (log 10 = 1) so that approximately 91 per cent of its molecules will already be ionized ($\frac{91}{9} \simeq 10$). If the pH is adjusted by a further unit, to

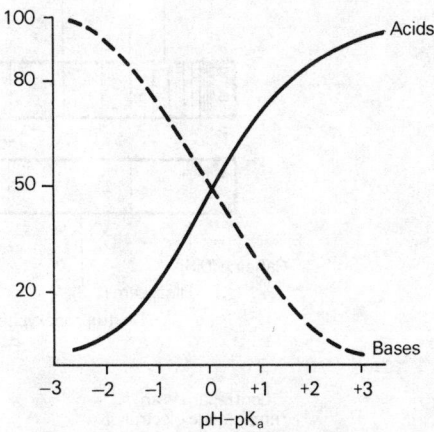

Fig. 4.2 The influence of pH on the dissociation of weak electrolytes.

8, the ionized: unionized ratio will rise to 100 (log 100 = 2) indicating that rather more than 99 per cent of the acid will be present in the ionized form. The change of pH from 7 to 8 has clearly resulted in a much smaller change in the number of ionized molecules than did that from 6 to 7. These changes are illustrated in Fig. 4.2.

An acid can be defined as a proton donor and this definition is implicit in our representation of an acid as HA which dissociates in solution to give H^+ and A^- ions. A base, correspondingly, can be defined as a proton acceptor and we can represent its behaviour in solution as

$$B + H^+ \rightleftharpoons BH^+$$

We can proceed from this simple relationship to derive the Henderson-Hasselbalch equation again. If we remember that k_1 refers to the reaction that supplies hydrogen ions, that k_2 is the constant for the reaction that mops them up again and that K_a is the ratio between the two, we shall arrive at the relationship:

$$pH = pK_a + \log \frac{[B]}{[BH^+]}$$

If we think of the last ratio as $\dfrac{\text{unionized base}}{\text{ionized base}}$, we can immediately see that the effect of changes in pH on the ionization of a base will be precisely the opposite to that on acids. Thus an increase in pH will bring about an increase in the unionized: ionized ratio (Fig. 4.2). Moreover, its K_a value (which measures a compound's nett ability to *donate* hydrogen ions) will be high and its pK_a value will be low.

Thus strong acids and weak bases are characterized by low pK_a ratios.

Some substances are amphoteric, behaving as both acids and bases. Not surprisingly, an amphoteric electrolyte has two pK_a values.

A knowledge of the pK_a of his drugs is evidently of some value to the pharmacologist. Those for a number of well known agents are displayed in Figure 4.3 but the chief purpose of this Figure is to underline some of the points that have been made in the text. A long list of pK_a values has been assembled by Smith and Rawlins (1973) *inter al* but their catalogue is not complete and the investigator who requires to know the pK_a of a particular drug may well have to reconcile himself to a tedious search in the original literature.

The effect of the acidity of the medium in which a weak acid finds itself is illustrated in Fig. 4.4 which is found in almost every contemporary textbook of pharmacology. Let us suppose that a weak acid with a pK_a of 4.4 is placed in a solution with a pH of 7.4 (this could, for instance, be blood plasma) which is separated by a typical cell membrane from a solution with a pH of 1.4 (this could be gastric juice). The undissociated acid will pass readily from one compartment to the other and at equilibrium it will attain the same concentration on both sides of the membrane. The Henderson-Hasselbalch equation tells us that, in the solution at pH 7.4, the logarithm of the ratio of the concentration of ionized to unionized acid must be 3 (pH − pK_a = 3) so that the ratio itself must be 1000 (log 1000 = 3). By a similar argument the ratio in the highly acid

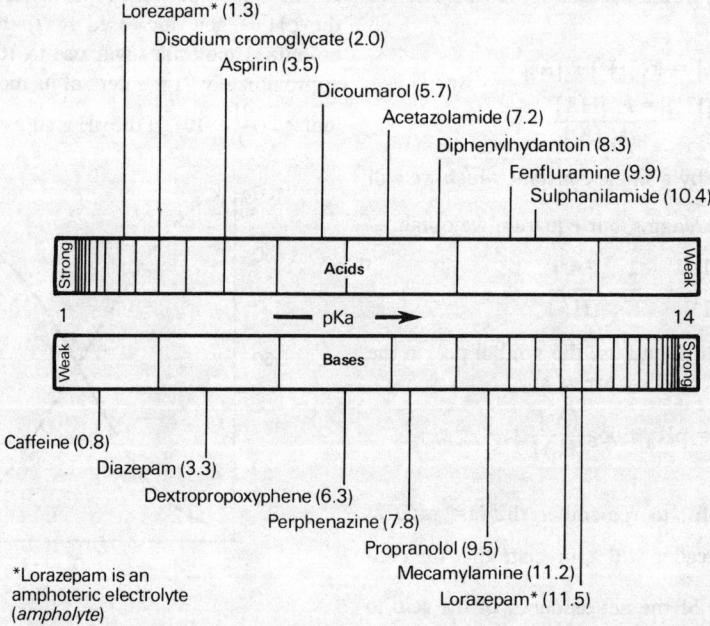

Fig. 4.3 The pKa values of some acidic (anionic) and basic (cationic) drugs.

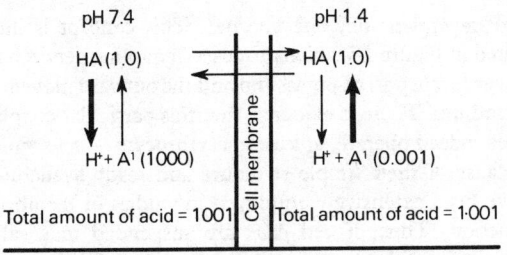

pH 7.4

HA (1.0)

H⁺ + A¹ (1000)

Total amount of acid = 1001

Cell membrane

pH 1.4

HA (1.0)

H⁺ + A¹ (0.001)

Total amount of acid = 1·001

Fig. 4.4 To illustrate the effect of pH on the distribution of a weak acid ($pKa = 4.4$) between a neutral (pH 7.4) and an acid (pH 1.4) solution. Figures in parentheses indicate relative concentrations of the two forms of the acid.

solution is 0.001 (pH ÷ pK_a = −3; log 0.001 = −3). The net result is the 'trapping' of ions in the solution at pH 7.4 and the production, without the expenditure of energy, of a large ion concentration gradient across the membrane. Ion trapping is made use of in the treatment of poisoning. Thus, alkalinization of the urine of a person who has taken an overdose of amphetamine, a weak base, will ensure that the drug is kept in the ionized form in the kidneys so that it is not reabsorbed into the blood. Recovery is consequently accelerated.

FACILITATED DIFFUSION
Some substances diffuse through some membranes more rapidly than would be predicted from a consideration of their lipid solubility or molecular size. Provided that this accelerated movement does not depend on energy generated in the membrane we can attribute it to facilitated diffusion. Like simple diffusion, this process can only carry molecules or ions down their electrochemical concentration gradients ('downhill') although sometimes, as we shall see (p. 45) facilitated diffusion brings in its train a secondary 'uphill' movement of material against a concentration gradient.

Facilitated diffusion confers a certain degree of selectivity on a membrane because substances carried by this means will be taken into or through cells more rapidly than those which, though possessing similar physical characteristics, can only move by simple diffusion.

Most authorities agree that facilitated diffusion is probably brought about by the activity of *carriers* that are attached to, or are incorporated within, the membrane and which oscillate back and forth across it. Some molecules or ions in a solution in contact with the membrane will, it is assumed, be able to form a loose complex with an appropriate carrier molecule. This will establish a concentration gradient for the complex which will cross the membrane at a rate determined by the diffusion characteristics of the carrier molecule. Arriving at the other side of the membrane, the carrier will discharge its passenger (the dissociation of the complex will be favoured by the low concentration of the transported material in the solution

into which it is carried) and will itself eventually return across the membrane as a simple result of its own thermal agitation.

The capacity of a ferry system of this type would clearly be limited (as any high season cross-Channel passenger will readily appreciate) by the number of available carriers and good evidence for its involvement in facilitated diffusion is provided by the observation that the amount of substance transferred by the process is proportional to the concentration gradient only up to a critical point. Beyond this, no further increase occurs. In addition, it is possible to demonstrate that the transport of one molecular species by facilitated diffusion can be impeded by the introduction of substances of similar molecular structure, a clear indication for the operation of competition for a scarce component of the transport system, presumably the carrier.

Many cells can transfer sugars, amino acids and ions by facilitated diffusion and this process certainly assists the absorption of sugars and amino acids by the intestine. It may also promote the absorption of a few drugs—tetracycline and quaternary ammonium compounds have been mentioned in this context (Levine, 1971)—but its importance for drug absorption generally would seem to be limited.

ACTIVE TRANSPORT
Some substances pass across biological membranes from less concentrated to more concentrated solutions. In other words, their direction of movement is the opposite to that which would be effected by simple or facilitated diffusion. This contrary movement is often (but by no means invariably) dependent on, and sustained by, energy that is supplied by the membrane itself and if this metabolism is inhibited, by cold or cyanide for instance, material that has been transported across the membrane drifts back again until it reaches the same concentration on both sides of the barrier. Active transport is fully defined as the process that enables substances to cross a membrane against their electrochemical concentration gradients and which depends on the utilization of energy supplied by the metabolic activity of the membrane. It is important to remember that we are only justified in diagnosing an active transport process if *both* the conditions mentioned in the definition have been fulfilled.

As we have seen, the composition of the fluid interior of the cell differs from that of the circumambient medium. As a particular example we may consider sodium and potassium: potassium is essentially an intracellular ion but sodium is found in only small amounts in the cell although it is present in quantity in the extracellular fluid. Cell membranes are permeable to both ionic species, so we can immediately rule out the possibility that sodium and potassium are distributed as they are simply because the membrane constitutes a barrier to their moving into or out of the cell. In fact, the separation of the ions is the result of active transport processes that bring about the extrusion of sodium from, and the transfer of potassium ions into, the cell. Both these movements occur against electrochemical concentration gradients and the mechanisms that bring these (and similar) movements about are often referred to as pumps. The reader will agree that this is an apt terminology for a device that keeps a cell clear of the sodium ions in which it is bathed just as a bilge pump keeps a boat clear of the water in which it floats.

The nature of the processes that bring about active transport still awaits clarification but there is some unanimity in the view that active transport, like facilitated diffusion, is mediated by carriers. It is easy to produce conceptual models of carrier mechanisms—some of these are entertainingly illustrated by Levin (1969)—and to visualize possible transport processes in general terms. We could suppose, for instance, that the substance to be transported formed a complex with a carrier molecule (we will designate this as C_A) which would diffuse across the membrane down its electrochemical concentration gradient. Arriving at the other side of the membrane, the complex would, we suppose, become involved in an energy consuming chemical reaction that converted the carrier into a new form (C_B) with liberation of the transported material. The new carrier would diffuse back across the membrane, undergo a spontaneous conversion to its original form (C_A) and thus make itself ready to accept another load for transport. The carrier C_B would not necessarily have to make its journey empty handed since it would be able to take back through the membrane any available material for which it had the necessary affinity. Thus the movements of two substances in opposite directions might be coupled with,

and dependent on, one another. This concept is illustrated in Figure 4.5 which proposes a coupling between the inward transport of potassium and the outward movement of sodium. There is evidence that this particular coupling does indeed operate, at least in erythrocytes—cells which, because of their simple structure and ready availability, have been extensively employed in studies of membrane function. Thus, if red cells are suspended in a saline solution containing no potassium there is a rapid ingress of sodium. This observation finds a ready explanation on the coupled transport hypothesis because if there is no potassium to be transported there will be no movement of the potassium-carrier complex across the membrane and hence no source of the sodium carrier C_B. The sodium that passes into the cell by diffusion from the surrounding saline solution is not expelled because the pump has failed.

The energy required for active transport is ultimately derived (probably in all instances) from the breakdown of adenosine triphosphate (ATP). So far as the transport of sodium and potassium is concerned, there is now a considerable body of evidence to support this conclusion and, further, to indicate that the hydrolysis of ATP is promoted by an enzyme that is itself activated by sodium and potassium. Complete activation requires both cations. The enzyme labours under the name sodium-potassium-activated adenosine triphosphatase but even this author must in this instance permit—and himself be driven to use—an abbreviation to sodium-potassium ATPase or even Na^+-K^+-ATPase. It was discovered in cell membranes by Skou in 1957 and has since been found to be an invariable component of the plasma membrane. The membranes of cells that retain high concentrations of potassium exhibit high enzyme activity and cells with only a limited concentrating power display a much lower activity. It has also been demonstrated that, in red cell 'ghosts', the enzyme is orientated in such a way that the portion of its molecule that reacts with sodium faces the inside of the cell while the part influenced by potassium is directed towards the outside. Erythrocyte ghosts are essentially red cells that have been emptied of their normal contents and then refilled with a simple solution containing ATP. The metabolic activity of 'ghosts' is similar to that of whole erythrocytes.

Much of the Na^+-K^+-ATPase can be inhibited by the cardiac glycosides (p. 691) and it is customary to refer to this as the ouabain-sensitive fraction since ouabain is the glycoside that is most often used in experimental work.

Apart from the cations we have been discussing, some other substances are concentrated within or expelled from cells by active transport processes. These substances (which include, inter al, sugars, amino acids, some vitamins, metabolites and some ions) are those whose absorption into, retention within, or excretion from the body is demanded by the necessity of maintaining physiological functions. It is perhaps not surprising that rela-

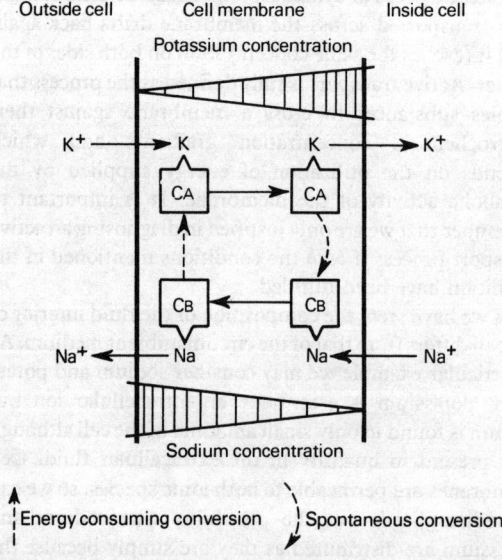

Fig. 4.5 Suggested mechanism for coupled potassium-sodium exchange against concentration gradients.

tively few drugs are carried by active transport. The pharmacologist is more interested in the fact that some drugs (like the cardiac glycosides we have already mentioned) interfere with active transport processes and thereby influence, for good or ill, the distribution of ions across cell membranes. This is particularly important in nerves and muscles whose normal functions are dependent on ordered changes in ion distribution across their plasma membranes.

Before leaving the subject of active transport we must refer again to a comment made earlier, in passing, that the movement of substances against their electrochemical concentration gradients does not invariably imply that active transport processes are at work. Consider, for example, the position indicated in Fig. 4.6 which represents two compartments, I and II, separated by a membrane incorporating a carrier which is capable of transporting each of the substances A and B but which has a greater affinity for A than for B. Let us further assume that, to begin with, there are equal numbers of B molecules (or ions) in the two compartments but that A is largely confined to compartment I.

Because of its higher affinity for this substance the carrier will form a complex with A rather than B and will then cross the membrane by facilitated diffusion. When it reaches the other side the carrier will give up its passenger (because of the low concentration of A in compartment II) but will now be open to occupation by molecules of B which here face no serious competition from A. Consequently, when the carrier drifts back across the membrane it takes some B with it. On arrival in compartment I, these B molecules will be rapidly displaced by A and the cycle will begin again. It can continue for as long as the concentration of A in compartment I exceeds that in compartment II and there is a supply of B in compartment II. This could be for an indefinite period if substances A and B were being added to or removed from the two compartments at appropriate rates. Thus the facilitated diffusion of A is linked with the transport of B against its concentration gradient. This is the process of *counter diffusion* and the energy for it is derived, not from catabolic processes in the membrane but from the 'downhill' flow of A. Counter diffusion must be distinguished from coupled transport (p. 44) which, as we have seen, also results in the transport of two substances in opposite directions but in this latter instance both substances travel against their respective concentration gradients, propelled by the energy derived from metabolic processes in the membrane.

The circumstances in which counter diffusion occurs are clearly rather unusual but they serve to emphasize the fact that the production and maintenance of an 'uphill' concentration gradient is not sufficient evidence that an active transport process is in operation. This lesson is further reinforced by the existence of other mechanisms that promote the flow of substances against their concentration gradients at no energy cost to the membrane. Ion trapping (p. 43) provides a good example of one such mechanism.

None of the foregoing must be taken to detract from the importance of active transport processes which play a vital role in the regulation of the most fundamental physiological processes.

FILTRATION

If mechanical (hydrostatic) pressure is applied to a solution contained in a vessel with pervious walls, water will ooze out of the container taking with it (by a process called *solvent drag*) those dissolved substances whose molecular size permits them ready passage through the holes in the walls. This constitutes the well-known phenomenon of filtration. The energy needed for filtration is derived entirely from the imposed hydrostatic pressure and biological membranes, so far as their properties as filters are concerned, are in no way different from the inanimate materials that constitute the familiar laboratory filters. Simple diffusion, the other process in which the membrane plays a purely passive role, also occurs across living and inanimate barriers alike but filtration can occur more rapidly than diffusion by virtue of the external energy that drives it. The rate of filtration increases with increase in driving pressure up to a limit that is determined by the maximum pressure that can be supplied to the system or that can be withstood by the filter whichever, of course, is the smaller.

There are, then, three possible mechanisms by which a substance can be passively transported across a membrane. These are:

a. diffusion down a concentration gradient
b. diffusion down a gradient of electric potential
c. solvent drag.

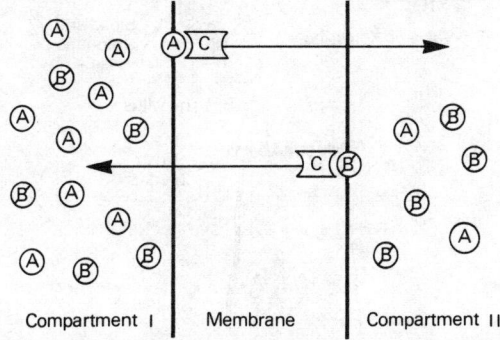

Compartment I   Membrane   Compartment II

Fig. 4.6 To illustrate that the facilitated diffusion of one substance (A) can lead to the transport of another (B) against its concentration gradient and without the expenditure of energy. For details see text.

With ions, all these processes may be operating simultaneously but solvent drag will be a dominant influence when the solution in contact with the membrane is under pressure. This occurs in the blood capillaries but not, for instance, in the gastrointestinal tract.

To these mechanisms for passive transfer we must, of course, add active transport to complete the list of processes that promote the passage of substances across membranes.

PHAGOCYTOSIS AND PINOCYTOSIS
Phagocytosis ('cell eating') is the term employed to describe the ingestion of macromolecules (such as proteins), bacteria, dye particles, etc. by cells. Pinocytosis ('cell drinking') is a similar process by which cells engulf droplets of extracellular fluid and substances dissolved in them.

THE ABSORPTION AND EXCRETION OF DRUGS

ABSORPTION FROM THE GASTROINTESTINAL TRACT
A few therapeutic substances, such as iron, aminoacids and fluorouracil, are related to dietary components that are absorbed by facilitated diffusion or active transport and they can therefore make use of specific transport systems to carry them across the intestinal wall. However, most of the drugs that are absorbed from the gastrointestinal tract cross the intestinal endothelium by simple diffusion and we can discuss the factors that regulate their passage into the blood stream in terms of the simple Fick equation we have already derived (p. 39).

$$T = -P \, A \, (C_a - C_b)$$

In the present context, C_a and C_b represent the concentrations of 'free' (diffusible) drug in the intestinal lumen and the draining capillary blood respectively.

From the point of view of comparing the absorptive capacities of the different segments of the gastrointestinal tract the most important term in the Fick equation is A, the area of the absorbing surface. It is much greater in the small intestine (duodenum, jejunum and ileum) than it is elsewhere and this more than counterbalances the effect of factors such as the pH of the intestinal contents that might be expected to hinder the absorption of particular substances. Thus, while weak acids are well absorbed and weak bases are not absorbed from the stomach (whose contents are strongly acid) both acids and bases are absorbed from the small intestine notwithstanding the neutral or slightly alkaline medium in which they find themselves and which would be expected not to favour the absorption of weak acids (p. 41). The low rate of passage of acid across unit area of the membrane is of little significance when the available area is so large.

The small intestine is, of course, a lengthy structure. By dint of careful packing, no fewer than five or six metres of this sinous tube are accommodated within the restricted confines of the abdominal cavity but the area of the outer surface of the tube is trivial in comparison with that of the absorptive surface that lines it. The mucous membrane is thrown into folds (these are sometimes called the valves of Kerckring, after their discoverer, a 17th century Dutch anatomist) and this has the effect of making its superficial area at least twice that of the outer surface of the small intestine. Further multiplication (this time by eight times) is achieved by the villi, the long, fingerlike processes that provide a dense feltwork like the pile of a carpet. Finally, electron microscope studies have revealed that the free border of the columnar epithelial cells that clothe the villi is itself crenellated and this still further augments the surface area. The total effect of these foldings and refoldings is to provide an absorbing area of some 4500 square metres. This is incomparably greater than the 55 square metres of surface provided by the pulmonary alveoli we were asked to marvel at when we were first introduced to human physiology. Those who crave for homely illustrations might like to think of the area available for intestinal absorption in terms of a carpet, one yard wide and nearly three and a quarter miles long!

The blood flow through the gut is vigorous and voluminous. This ensures that, when a drug is being absorbed, its concentration in plasma (C_b in the Fick equation) is kept low, to the advantage of the concentration gradient. Many drugs as they pass into the blood stream become bound to plasma proteins to a considerable extent. This further accentuates the concentration gradient which is determined only by the concentrations of freely diffusible

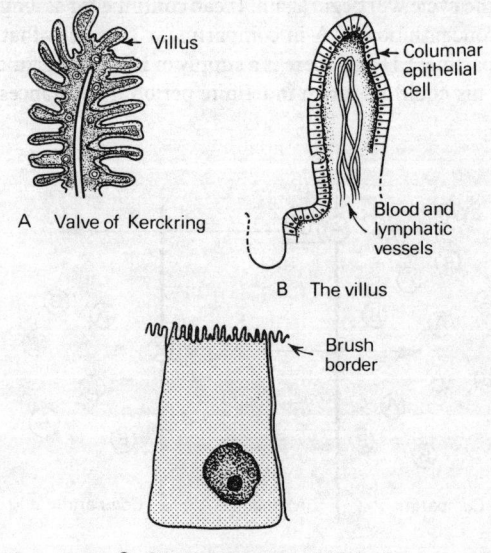

Fig. 4.7 To illustrate the enlargement of the intestinal absorption area achieved by the valves of Kerckring and the villi

(unbound) drug on the two sides of the membrane across which diffusion is taking place.

C_a, the drug concentration in the intestinal lumen, depends primarily on the amount ingested, the rate at which it is released from the dosage form in which it is presented and the volume of the gastrointestinal contents with which it is mixed. Preparations for oral administration are occasionally provided as multiple dose or slow release forms which are designed to release their contained medicament in small amounts over a period of a day or more so that they need to be taken only infrequently. It may happen, because of local conditions in the intestine, that the drug is released more quickly than had been intended. The resulting increase in the concentration of free drug may lead to its being absorbed in toxic amounts. The value of slow release preparations of drugs that can be taken by such a convenient route as the mouth is, in any event, questionable.

The term P in the Fick equation incorporates all the other factors that may influence drug absorption in a particular individual. These include the physical properties of the drug, the pH of the gastrointestinal contents and the condition of the intestine itself. Pathological conditions of the intestine may give rise to malabsorption syndromes.

Effect of gastrointestinal movements on drug absorption.
Movements of the stomach and intestines influence drug absorption in several ways but it is generally true to say that they facilitate absorption. Intestinal movements help to maintain the blood flow through the intestine and they also encourage the fragmentation and dissolution of drug tablets. Movements of the stomach ensure the more rapid passage of material into the upper intestine where, as we have seen, conditions for absorption are especially favourable. Drugs that inhibit gastric emptying (atropine, amphetamine and morphine are just three examples) may reduce the rate of absorption, and hence the effectiveness, of other drugs taken at the same time. Food in the stomach also inhibits gastric emptying and a voluminous meal will, in addition, have the effect of reducing the concentration of drug in the gastrointestinal tract. Generally, then, drugs should be taken on an empty stomach rather than immediately after a meal. An exception to this generalization is provided by drugs that irritate the gastric mucosa since food in the stomach provides a degree of protection to the mucosa.

Although a moderate amount of gastrointestinal activity clearly promotes drug absorption, a very rapid passage of material through the gut, such as might occur in diarrhoea, will hinder absorption if the drug is swept out of the body before it has had time to be taken up into the portal circulation.

TRANSFER OF DRUGS FROM BLOOD TO TISSUES
Protein free plasma is filtered from the capillaries into the tissue spaces. Solvent drag (p. 45) will ensure that any drug molecules dissolved in the plasma (but not bound to protein) will leave the capillaries with the tissue fluid. Filtration, as we have already seen (p. 45), is a very effective (but an unselective) process since the plasma is driven under pressure through pores or other breaches of continuity in or between the endothelial cells. Once in the tissue fluid, the molecules of many drugs are readily taken up by the cells.

The blood-brain barrier
Although small molecules generally pass with ease from the blood to the tissues, some blood borne substances do not pass readily into the substance of the brain. This is the result of the operation of metabolic and physical barriers (collectively known as the blood-brain barrier) and it explains why some drugs have to be administered by intrathecal injection (p. 37). It is best to think of the capillaries in the brain as having no pores so that they cannot act as filters; any material that leaves the vessels must do so by passing through the substance of the endothelial cells. As we have seen, this form of transfer is restricted to non polar (unionized) hydrophobic (lipid soluble) molecules. The consequence of this partial impermeability of the cerebral capillary endothelium is that the transfer of material into the brain is a far more selective process than it is for other tissues. The selectivity operates as well for substances passing from the brain into the blood stream as it does for those moving in the opposite direction. In other words, the barrier to free exchange helps to maintain stable conditions within the nervous system where homeostatic control has to be much tighter than it need be elsewhere in the body.

The brain is surrounded, and its ventricles are filled, by cerebrospinal fluid which is secreted into the ventricles by the chorioid capillary plexuses. Material in the cerebrospinal fluid passes readily into brain tissue and if a drug were secreted with the cerebrospinal fluid it would reach the brain cells as easily as if it had passed directly from the cerebral capillaries. In general, drugs that cannot leave the cerebral capillaries are also denied access to the cerebrospinal fluid and for the same reasons. Thus although we ought to recognise the separate existence of blood-cerebrospinal fluid and blood-extracellular fluid barriers, no harm is done by speaking simply of the blood-brain barrier with the implication that this term includes all the obstacles to the free passage of a substance from the blood stream to the cells of the brain.

Details of the blood-brain barrier are to be found in appropriate textbooks (such as that of Davson, 1967) but it is necessary to add here that caution has to be exercised when assessing the results of experiments in which the blood-brain barrier might have been operative. The barrier is not equally impenetrable in all parts of the central nervous system (it appears to be relatively permeable in the hypothalamic region and in the area postrema) and its effectiveness may vary with the experimental conditions and with the species of animal used. Some substances to which the barrier is normally impermeable may appear in the brain if they are given in large doses and when two substances are given together the presence of one may alter the ability of the other to penetrate into the brain. A thought-provoking review of the blood-brain barrier is that of Dobbing (1961), to which the reader is referred.

EXCRETION OF DRUGS

For the most part, drugs and their metabolites are eliminated from the body by the kidneys. In their passage from blood stream to bladder, drug molecules are carried across a number of cellular barriers by one or more of the transport systems—filtration, diffusion, secretion and active transport—that abound in the kidney to make this organ a repository of almost all the mechanisms we have discussed in this chapter. Kidney function is, however, more appropriately discussed elsewhere (Chap. 36).

Small amounts of drug may be excreted in the milk, saliva, sweat, tears, bile and faeces. Mention of these routes of excretion is made, as necessary, throughout the text.

THE DISTRIBUTION VOLUME OF DRUGS

Water makes up about 70 per cent of the adult body mass; in children the fraction is even higher. Of adult man's 50 litres of water, 25 litres (the *intracellular fluid*) are present within the cells. The remaining 25 litres (the *extracellular fluid*) are distributed between the blood plasma (five litres) and the *interstitial fluid* which amounts to about 15 litres. The five litres of extracellular fluid not accounted for in these figures are sequestered in bone and cannot participate in the exchanges of water that otherwise occur freely among the fluid compartments. It can be called *inaccessible water*. About 10 per cent of the extracellular fluid finds itself in the lumina of various tubular organs (the gastrointestinal tract, bronchi, glands and kidney), in the aqueous humour or in the cerebrospinal fluid. This small fraction of the interstitial fluid is sometimes identified as *transcellular water*.

Evans' Blue, a non-toxic dye, cannot pass through the capillary walls so that if we give an intravenous injection, say of *x* grams of the dye, it will be confined to the blood

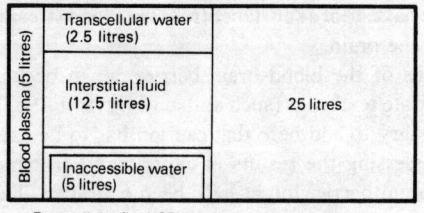

Fig. 4.8 The water compartments of the body.

plasma. If its concentration after thorough mixing in the blood stream is *a* grams per millilitre it is evident that the plasma volume will be given by $\frac{x}{a}$. This use of Evans' Blue is, of course, a recognised method for the determination of plasma volume. Similarly, a substance like inulin (which passes readily from plasma to the extracellular fluid but is excluded from cells) and antipyrine (an analgesic drug that distributes itself freely throughout the body water) are employed to measure the volumes of extracellular fluid and total body water respectively. The simple method of dividing the amount of marker by the plasma concentration is only applicable if the injected material can become evenly distributed throughout the appropriate fluid compartments before any of it is lost by excretion. It is not difficult, however, to derive a formula that will enable a fluid volume to be determined by taking measurements even after excretion has begun (see, for instance, Butler, 1971).

It should be self evident that the volume of interstitial fluid can only be obtained by subtracting plasma volume from that of the total extracellular fluid.

The physiologist may be interested in measuring the size of the fluid compartments *per se*, but the pharmacologist is more concerned to discover where his drugs have gone. He can calculate a drug's *apparent volume of distribution* either by simply dividing the amount administered by the concentration in the plasma at equilibrium or, if necessary, by utilizing a calculation that takes into account the fact that metabolism and excretion have set in before the drug has become completely distributed. In either event, he will normally expect to obtain a volume of distribution that corresponds at least approximately to that of one of the three fluid compartments and this may provide useful information concerning the fate of the drug after administration. On the other hand, the apparent volume of distribution may not correspond to that of any of the compartments and it will have to be concluded that the drug is not distributed evenly throughout the fluid to which it is localized. The example usually quoted in illustration of this is quinacrine (p. 867) whose apparent volume of distribution appears to be a thousand times greater than the volume of the body! The drug is heavily concentrated in the liver, so that at equilibrium the plasma concentration is extremely low. Concentration in any other organ or in a tissue such as body fat will be reflected in the same way. Binding of a drug to plasma protein reduces the amount of material that is available for diffusion into the extravascular compartments. Failure to appreciate the fact that protein binding has occurred will lead to completely distorted estimates of the volume of distribution and the distortion will be most serious for drugs that exhibit the highest degree of binding. If the method used for determining the amount of drug in the plasma is one that measures both free and bound drug the apparent volume will be lower than the true volume of distribution. The opposite situation will arise if only the amount of unbound drug is measured. A brief reflection is all that should be needed to convince the reader of the truth of these assertions.

Substances differ in the extent to which they can enter the several components of the transcellular water but the contribution made by this fluid to the total volume of the extracellular water is so small that we can, for pharmacological purposes, ignore the fact that the extent to which drugs enter it is highly variable.

BIBLIOGRAPHY

Books, monographs and reviews

Butler, T. (1971) The distribution of drugs. In: *Fundamentals of Drug Metabolism and Drug Distribution.* La Du, B. N., Mandel, H. G. and Way, E. L. (eds.) pp. 44-62. Baltimore: The Williams & Wilkins Co.

Davies, M. (1973) Functions of Biological Membranes. London: Chapman and Hall.

Davson, H. (1967) *The Physiology of the Cerebrospinal Fluid.* London: Churchill.

Dobbing, J. (1961) The blood-brain barrier. *Physiol. Rev.*, **41**, 130-188.

Dowben, R. M. (ed) (1969). *Biological Membranes.* Boston: Little, Brown and Co.

Finean, J. B., Coleman, R. and Michell, R. H. (1978). *Membranes and their Cellular Function,* 2nd edn. Oxford and London: Blackwell Scientific Publications.

Goldstein, A., Aronow, L. and Kalman, S. M. (1974). *Principles of Drug Action: The Basis of Pharmacology,* 2nd edn. New York and London: John Wiley.

Harrison, R. and Lunt, G. G. (1975) *Biological Membranes: their Structure and Function.* Glasgow and London: Blackie.

Jamieson, G. A. and Robinson, D. M. (eds.) (1977). *Mammalian Cell Membranes.* Vols. 1-5. London and Boston: Butterworths.

Levine, Ruth R. (1971). Intestinal absorption. In: *Topics in Medicinal Chemistry,* Vol. 4. Rabinowitz, J. L. and Myerson, R. M. (eds.) pp. 27-95. New York and London: Wiley-Interscience.

Neame, K. D. and Richards, T. G. (1972). *Elementary Kinetics of Membrane Transport.* Oxford and London: Blackwell Scientific Publications.

Nystrom, R. A. (1973). *Membrane Physiology.* Englewood Cliffs, N.J.: Prentice-Hall.

Rothfield, L. I. (ed) (1971). *Structure and Function of Biological Membranes.* New York and London: Academic Press.

Saunders, L. (1974). *The Absorption and Distribution of Drugs.* London: Ballière and Tindall.

Skou, J. C. (1969) The role of membrane ATPase in the active transport of ions. In: *The Molecular Basis of Membrane Function,* pp. 445-482. Ed. by D. C. Tosteson. Englewood Cliffs, N.J.: Prentice Hall.

Original papers

Skou, J. C. (1957). The influence of some cations on the adenosine triphosphatase from peripheral nerves. *Biochim. biophys. Acta.*, **23**, 394-401.

Travell, J. (1940). The influence of the hydrogen ion concentration on the absorption of alkaloids from the stomach. *J. Pharmac. exp. Ther.*, **69**, 21-33.

Williams, R. T., Millburn, P. and Smith, R. L. (1965). The influence of enterohepatic circulation on the toxicity of drugs. *Ann. N.Y. Acad. Sci.*, **123**, 110-124.

5. The disposal of drugs and toxic substances

In the course of their long evolution, complex living organisms have acquired a number of mechanisms that provide protection against material that might otherwise be harmful when taken into the body. This protection extends to essential regulatory substances, such as hormones and neurotransmitter substances which are produced in the body itself but which would disturb normal function if they were allowed to persist or accumulate in the tissues after their immediate tasks had been fulfilled. And it is also, of course, directed against the drugs we use, so that drug treatment resolves itself into a contest between the therapist who attempts to provide material that can be readily transferred to, and held at, its site of intended action and the patient's defences which are designed to defeat those very ends. The therapist usually wins the struggle but only because he can arrange for his drugs to arrive at the tissues more rapidly than the body can dispose of them. However, as we shall see, his victory is sometimes but short lived and even when it is longer lasting it may have to be purchased at the expense of exposing the patient to new hazards.

The most effective way of dealing with a foreign substance is to expel it from the body and urinary excretion is a very important component of the drug disposal system. Some drugs are excreted very rapidly but others cannot be eliminated so expeditiously and some way is therefore required for making a foreign substance less harmful—less effective if it is a therapeutic agent—while it remains in the body. To this end, the organism is equipped with a number of rather unspecific enzymes that break down, or otherwise modify, the drug. Usually these enzymatic changes produce molecules that are not only less active but are also more readily excreted than the parent compound.

Although it is of prime importance, the urinary excretion of drugs and their metabolites is not the only defence mechanism with which the body is armed and before turning to consider metabolic and excretory systems, we shall survey and briefly discuss the other means that are available for rendering drugs temporarily or permanently ineffective. It is important that the reader should appreciate from the outset that protein binding, drug sequestration, tolerance and some other processes that are so often treated in isolation from one another are, with metabolism and excretion, all parts of the same disposal system.

Let us look then at the possible fates of a drug that has been taken by mouth. If it is a therapeutic substance, it will have been provided in a form that permits ready absorption from the gastrointestinal tract. However, vomiting occasionally occurs and this will cause rejection of the drug. If this defence does not operate (or if it is outflanked by parenteral injection) the drug will enter the blood stream but some of it may find itself temporarily confined within the vascular system by becoming bound to plasma protein. That which remains free in the plasma is exposed to the risk of metabolic degradation in the liver. Indeed, some drugs suffer so considerable a degree of inactivation in their first passage through the liver (the so-called 'first pass' effect) that even if they are readily absorbed from the intestinal tract they are best given by a route (sublingual or parenteral) that permits them to enter the systemic circulation before their first visit to the liver.

The remnant of the original dose of drug that appears in the systemic circulation is available for general distribution: some of it will have to circulate through the liver, lungs and kidneys (and will there have to face the possibility of being metabolized or suffering expulsion into the glomerular filtrate) while some may be taken up and sequestered by the body fat, the bones and other tissues from which depots it will be released only slowly if at all. And some will reach its intended goal in the target tissues.

It should be possible to maintain a steady concentration of drug in the tissues by supplying it at a rate equal to that at which it is being lost but the organism's defence mechanisms can, in many instances, defeat this manoeuvre too. In the first place, the continued administration of certain drugs can lead to an increase in the activity of the mechanisms that destroy or otherwise exclude them from the tissues. Secondly, even if the concentration of drug at the target organ can be maintained, the tissue itself might become progressively less responsive. These two consequences of continued drug administration—*dispositional tolerance* and *cellular tolerance* respectively—are discussed in more detail in Chap. 7 (p. 83). In order to overcome these effects drug doses must be increased, sometimes to unacceptable levels.

We can now examine in turn each of the processes mentioned in the preceding paragraphs apart from those (vomiting, absorption from the intestine and tolerance) to which separate chapters (or part chapters) are devoted.

Binding to plasma proteins

Many substances that arrive in the blood stream become

more or less firmly bound to one or other of the plasma proteins. This binding is sometimes highly specific and subserves a particular physiological process. Thus transferrin (p. 660), a β globulin, provides a vehicle for the transport to the bone marrow of ferrous ions which are needed for haemoglobin formation but which would be toxic were they not bound to protein. At the other extreme, some ionized substances become loosely and quite unspecifically attached to plasma proteins by virtue of the fact that, at the pH of blood, the proteins carry a number of net positive or negative charges that permit union with appropriately charged ions. This type of binding is of no real importance since the coulombic forces provide only weak bonds and these are readily disrupted. There remains a third, and from our point of view, the most important category of binding. It occurs more particularly with plasma albumin and it involves the union of some of the chemical groups that are found in many types of drug with specific binding sites on the protein.

The specific binding sites are in every way analogous to drug receptor sites in the tissues and the reaction between a drug and its binding site yields to the same mathematical treatment as does that between a drug and its receptor or between a substrate and its enzyme. Thus we can depict the situation in plasma in terms of a simple equilibrium between 'free' drug (D), albumin (P) and the drug-protein complex (DP):

$$D + P \rightleftharpoons DP$$

Many substances have a high affinity for albumin so that at equilibrium the balance of the equation lies heavily to the right.

When small amounts of a drug with a high affinity for albumin are introduced into the plasma, the fraction that is bound will clearly be much higher than when there is more than enough drug fully to saturate the binding sites. Thus a statement to the effect that a particular drug is, say, 85 per cent bound to plasma protein, is not really very informative unless some additional information is provided or implied. In pharmacological and medical contexts it can be assumed that quoted binding figures relate to therapeutic doses.

Only unbound drug can pass through capillary walls to reach its intended target in the tissues. Of course, as supplies of 'free' drug become exhausted, the bound moiety will dissociate to release more of the 'free' form but this often takes place so slowly that an adequate supply to the tissues can only be maintained by taking in more drug. Sometimes, though, the rate of dissociation of the complex and the efficacy of the drug are such that a single dose combined with its binding protein provides a useful depot that can supply the patient's need over an extended period. Thus suramin, an antitrypanocidal drug, needs to be taken no more frequently than four times a year.

Slow breakdown of the albumin-drug complex usually results in slow excretion of the drug since only the free form can appear in the glomerular filtrate. However, some protein bound drugs are excreted very rapidly. A good example is provided by penicillin (p. 824) which is eliminated by secretion, still bound to protein, into the tubular fluid. An extreme example of the more usual state of affairs is the delayed excretion of iophenoxic acid, once a popular X-ray contrast medium. It is so slowly released into the glomerular filtrate from its combination with albumin that it has a plasma half life of more than two years.

Binding to plasma protein may facilitate drug absorption since, if many of the drug molecules become bound to plasma protein as soon as they have crossed the intestinal wall, the concentration of 'free' drug in the plasma is kept low and a high concentration gradient between intestine and blood (on which the rate of absorption depends) is thereby maintained. This effect probably explains why anticoagulant drugs of the coumarin type are so effective when taken by mouth. Their physicochemical properties are such as to indicate that they should be absorbed with difficulty from the alimentary tract but this disadvantage is offset by the very high degree of protein binding they undergo.

Clinically, the most important aspect of protein binding concerns the potentially dangerous consequences of the formation in the blood stream of depots of drugs that might have toxic effects if they were permitted to reach high concentrations in the body fluids. This can happen if plasma containing a protein bound drug is exposed to another agent that has a higher affinity for the binding sites than the original drug. In this circumstance the invader, by simple competition, displaces the original drug from its union with the albumin. This provides the basis of an important class of drug interactions (p. 78).

Sequestration in the tissues

Once in the interstitial fluid, some drugs are taken up avidly by particular tissues or tissue components. Those soluble in lipids can dissolve in body fat and this may immobilize considerable quantities of drug, particularly in obese individuals. The drug is gradually released from the fatty tissue but the process is often a very slow one and sequestration in fat undoubtedly provides some defence against toxic materials. Modern man is, for instance, continuously exposed to minute quantities of insecticides such as dieldrin and DDT which are successfully retained by fatty tissue so that, even after years of exposure, only minimal and innocuous amounts of the insecticides circulate in his body. It has even been argued that vigorous slimming should be avoided lest the breakdown of fatty tissue release perhaps toxic quantities of insecticides into the circulation. This argument should not be taken too seriously: the consequences of voluntary reduction in weight are overwhelmingly more beneficial than deleterious.

As a result of the slow release of the drugs, the action of some of the sex hormones may continue for some time after drug administration has ceased and this should be borne in mind when changes are made in hormone treatment schedules because the beneficial (or adverse) effects apparently attributable to the new treatment might be partly caused by the unsuspected persistence of the previous drug.

The therapeutic action, or the characteristic side effects of some drugs arise from their being taken up preferentially by particular tissues: iodine by the thyroid gland, mepacrine by collagen tissue in the skin and chloroquine by the liver and retina.

Finally, we must note that some substances are taken up so avidly and released by the sequestering tissues so reluctantly that they persist in the body for very long periods of time. These virtually permanent accumulations of material can produce local effects. Examples are *siderosis*—the deposition of iron in the tissues—and the accumulation of radioactive strontium in bone. Those zealots who cannot resist the temptation of using esoteric terms to describe simple phenomena rose to new heights when they coined the word *pharmacothesaurismosis* (from thesaurus, a treasury) to mean long term storage in the tissues.

Storage in hair and nails is mentioned later (p. 68).

Drug metabolism

As we have already noted (p. 50), the most effective weapon at the body's disposal for ridding itself of foreign substances is excretion in the urine. Metabolic processes (detoxication, biotransformation) convert these intruders into forms that are less toxic (and less effective) and more readily excreted than their parents.

Drugs are conveniently provided in the form of lipid soluble and non polar compounds that are readily absorbed into the body (p. 40). The same properties that encourage absorption from the intestine also favour the drugs' reabsorption from the kidney tubules and hence its retention in the tissues. Biotransformation processes are directed towards the production of metabolites that are less lipid soluble and more strongly ionized—and, consequently, less readily reabsorbed from the tubular fluid—than their parents. Moreover, some organic cations and anions appear in the urine partly or wholly as the result of their being secreted directly into the tubular fluid and this constitutes an additional reason why the more polar compounds are more promptly eliminated.

Metabolic processes, then, result in the production of molecules that are often less active and usually less lipid soluble and more strongly ionized than those from which they are derived. They are not, however, necessarily more soluble in water though water solubility clearly favours excretion in the body fluids. The solubility of a compound is often enhanced (and its activity may be still further reduced at the same time) by *conjugation* with glucuronic acid or one of a number of other substances that will be detailed later. Conjugation can only occur if the conjugating agent is presented with a compound with which it can readily unite by virtue of the latter's possessing (usually) an anionic grouping such as, for example, the hydroxyl radical. A few drugs meet this requirement and can be conjugated without further transformation but more often only their metabolites can participate in conjugation reactions. Some drugs or their metabolites are so water soluble that they can be rapidly excreted without the necessity for previous conjugation. The overall position is summarized in Fig. 5.1.

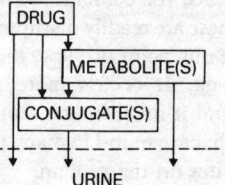

Fig. 5.1 Relationships between conjugation and metabolism

Metabolic and conjugation processes are sometimes designated as Phase I and Phase II reactions respectively.

Although metabolic and conjugation processes eventually produce substances that are less active than the parent compounds the initial stages of the transformation sometimes generate *more* active substances. Parathion, for instance, is a highly toxic substance as a result of its being converted, in vivo, into paraoxon (Fig. 5.2 vi) while the antidepressant action of imipramine is mediated through desmethylimipramine, its first metabolite (Fig. 5.2 vii). Drugs that rely on metabolic conversion into their active forms are often called 'pro-drugs'.

The major site of drug metabolism is, of course, the liver but some other tissues (including kidney, skin, lungs and blood) play a subsidiary (but sometimes a physiologically important) role in drug transformation processes.

Many of the enzymes that catalyse metabolic reactions are inseparably associated with the lipoprotein of the endoplasmic reticulum and they therefore appear in the microsomal fraction of tissue homogenates (p. 14). A few reactions depend on the activity of enzymes located elsewhere in the cell. Enzymes in intestinal microorganisms can effect metabolic transformations in drugs taken by mouth or excreted into the gastrointestinal tract in the bile or other secretions.

Drug metabolizing enzymes catalyse a large number of reactions but the resulting transformations can be conveniently segregated under three main heads: *oxidation, reduction* and *hydrolysis*. It is convenient to describe the reactions separately and to use a different drug to illustrate each one but it must be remembered that the breakdown of a single drug may involve the sequential or simultaneous operation of several metabolic processes. Since each of these processes may result in the production of substances each of which may be excreted in several conjugated forms it will be readily appreciated that one drug can give rise to a multiplicity of products in the urine—a figure of one hundred has been quoted for chlorpromazine. Not all animal species deal with an individual drug in the same way: the rabbit deaminates amphetamine but the dog hydroxylates it.

Oxidative reactions

Oxidation is the most common type of metabolic reaction. It takes many forms and most of the enzymes involved are of microsomal origin. A list of the oxidative reactions utilized in metabolic processes, with one example of each type, is provided in Fig. 5.2. Many other examples will be encountered in sections of this book that deal with the metabolism of individual drugs.

A. *Oxidations involving microsomal enzymes*

(i) aromatic hydroxylation

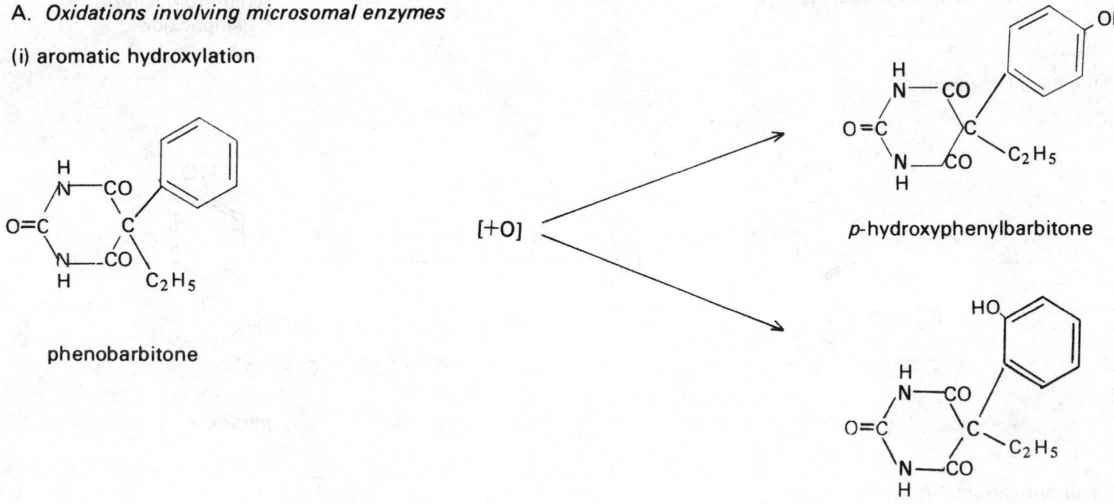

phenobarbitone

[+O]

p-hydroxyphenylbarbitone

o-hydroxyphenylbarbitone

(ii) aliphatic (side chain) hydrolylation

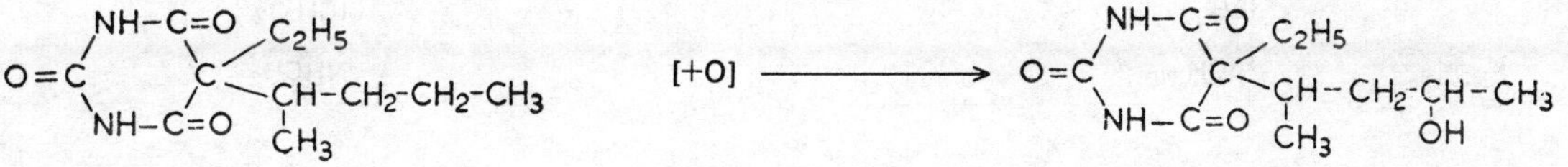

pentobarbitone

[+O]

5-ethyl-5(3-hydroxy-1-methylbutyl) barbituric acid

(iii) N-hydroxylation

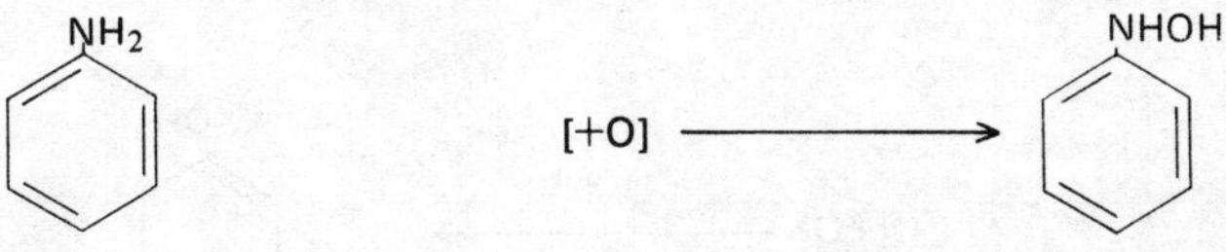

[+O]

(iv) N-oxidation

$(CH_3)_3N$ [+O] $\longrightarrow$ $(CH_3)_3NO$

trimethylamine

trimethylamine N oxide

Fig. 5.2 Metabolic oxidative reactions

(v) S-oxidation (sulphoxidation)

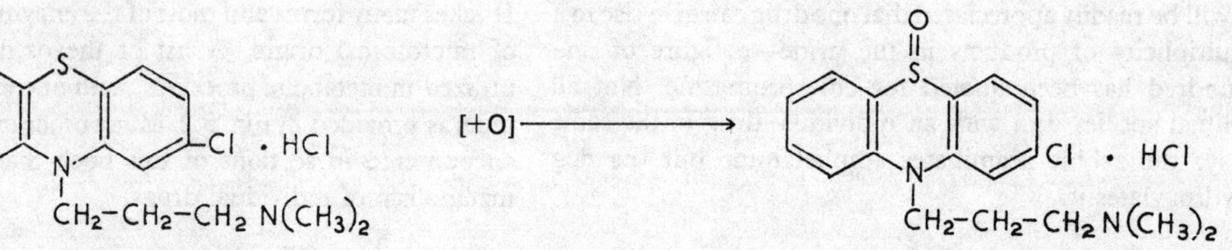

chlorpromazine

[+O] ⟶

chlorpromazine
sulphoxide

(vi) desulphuration

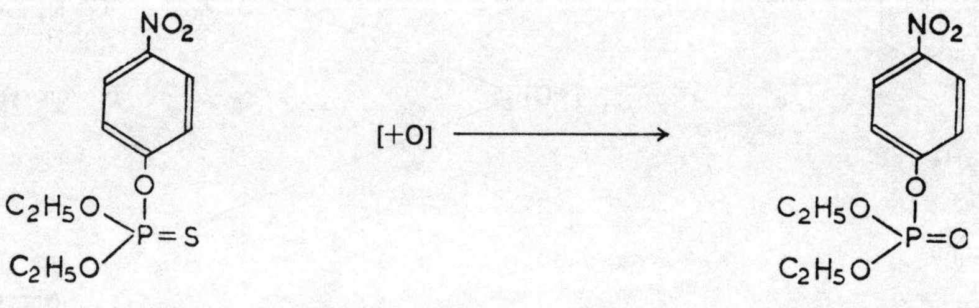

parathion

[+O] ⟶

paraoxon

(vii) N-dealkylation

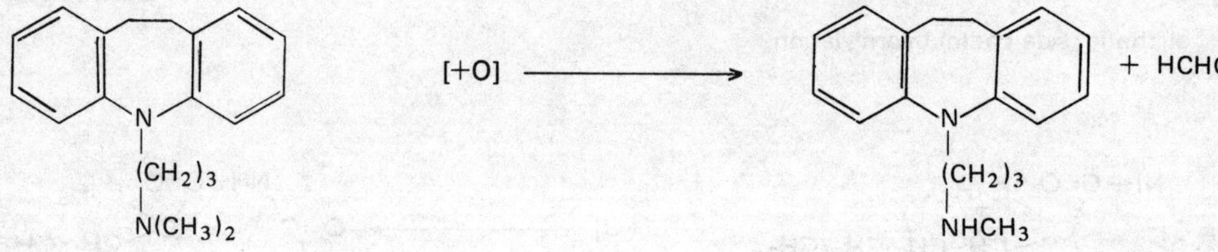

imipramine

[+O] ⟶

+ HCHO

desmonomethylimipramine
(desipramine)

(viii) O-dealkylation

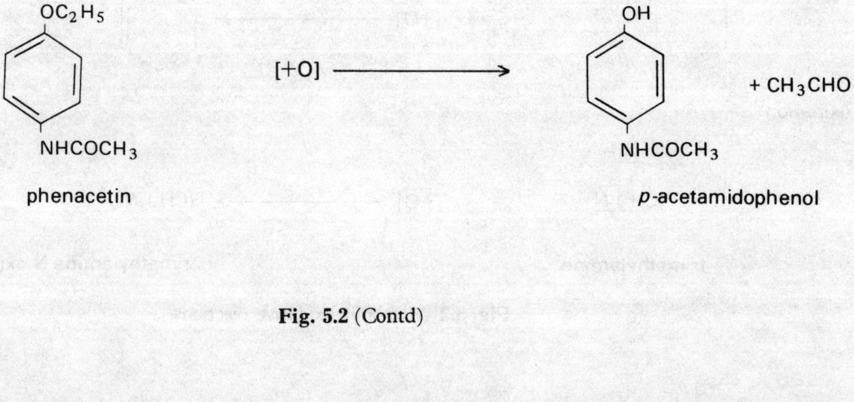

phenacetin

[+O] ⟶

+ CH_3CHO

p-acetamidophenol

Fig. 5.2 (Contd)

(ix) S-dealkylation

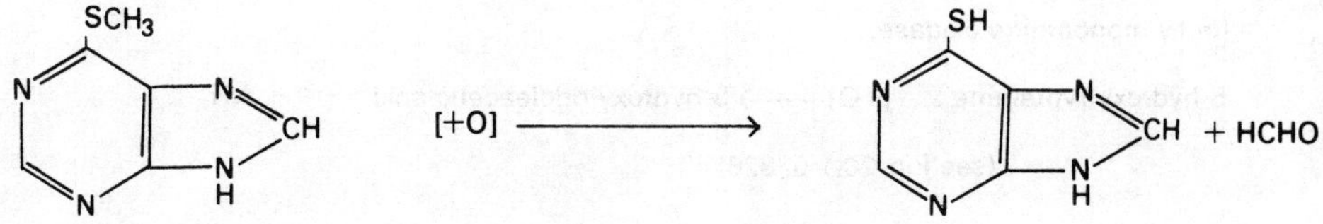

6-methylthiopurine   [+O] $\longrightarrow$ 6-mercaptopurine   + HCHO

(x) oxidative deamination

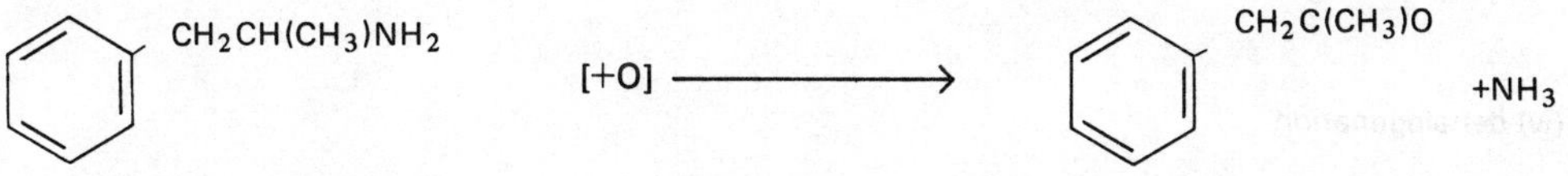

amphetamine   [+O] $\longrightarrow$ phenylacetone   +NH$_3$

(xi) epoxidation

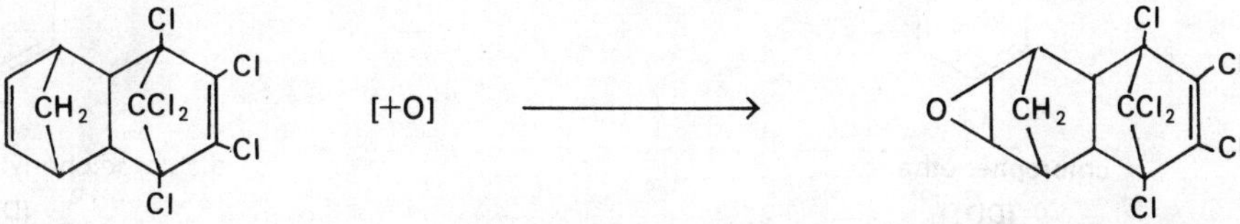

aldrin   [+O] $\longrightarrow$ dieldrin

B. *Oxidations involving enzymes not of microsomal origin*

(i) alcohol and aldehyde oxidation

$$C_2H_5OH \;\; [-H] \longrightarrow CH_3CHO \;\; [+O] \longrightarrow CH_3COOH$$

ethanol   acetaldehyde   acetic acid

(ii) aromatization

cyclohexane
carboxylic acid   [-H] $\longrightarrow$ benzoic acid

Fig. 5.2 (Contd)

(iii) deamination

(a) by monoamine oxidase

5-hydroxytryptamine $[+O] \longrightarrow$ 5-hydroxyindoleacetic acid $+ NH_3$

(see Fig. 20.1 p. 328)

(b) by diamine oxidase

Histamine $[+O] \longrightarrow$ imidazole acetaldehyde $+ NH_3$

(see Fig. 21.5 p. 340)

(iv) dehalogenation

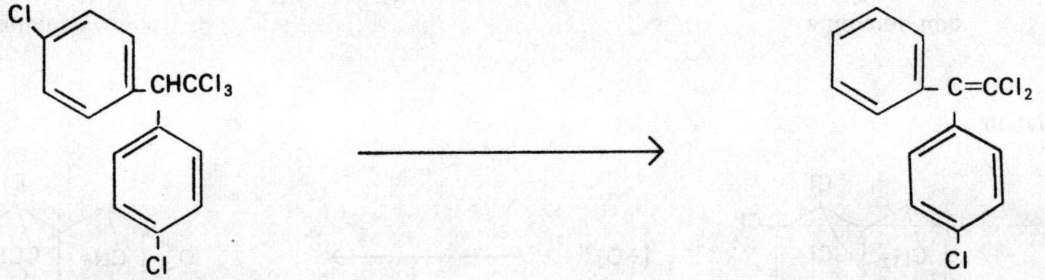

chlorophenothane
(DDT)

dichlorodiphenyldichloroethylene
(DDE)

(v) oxidation by xanthine oxidase

hypoxanthine $[+O] \longrightarrow$ xanthine $[+O] \longrightarrow$ uric acid

(see Fig. 27.10, p. 460)

Fig. 5.2 (Contd)

Reduction

Only a few drugs are inactivated by reduction. The enzymes involved are of both microsomal and non-microsomal origin; in addition some intestinal microorganisms elaborate reductive enzymes.

Compounds containing halogens can be reduced by a microsomal dehalogenating enzyme. Halothane, for instance, is reduced in this way to trifluoroethane. The last named compound then undergoes microsomal oxidation. A classical example of a reductive transformation which is still frequently referred to, although the drug has long been obsolete, is the conversion of Prontosil Red to sulphanilamide (p. 816). Prontosil Red has no antibacterial activity: it provides an early example of a pro-drug (p. 52).

Chloramphenicol is reduced to aminochloramphenicol by a microsomal enzyme and this provides an example of *nitroreduction*. Nitroreduction, azoreduction and dehalogenation constitute the three principal categories of reductive reactions encountered in biotransformation systems. An interesting feature of the enzymes that promote these reactions is that they are not confined to the liver. They are found in other tissues too in contrast to microsomal oxidative enzymes.

Some reductions are catalysed by non-microsomal enzymes. An interesting example is provided by chloral hydrate, which is reduced to trichloroethanol by alcohol dehydrogenase, an *oxidative* enzyme which in this instance is catalysing the reverse reaction to that in which it

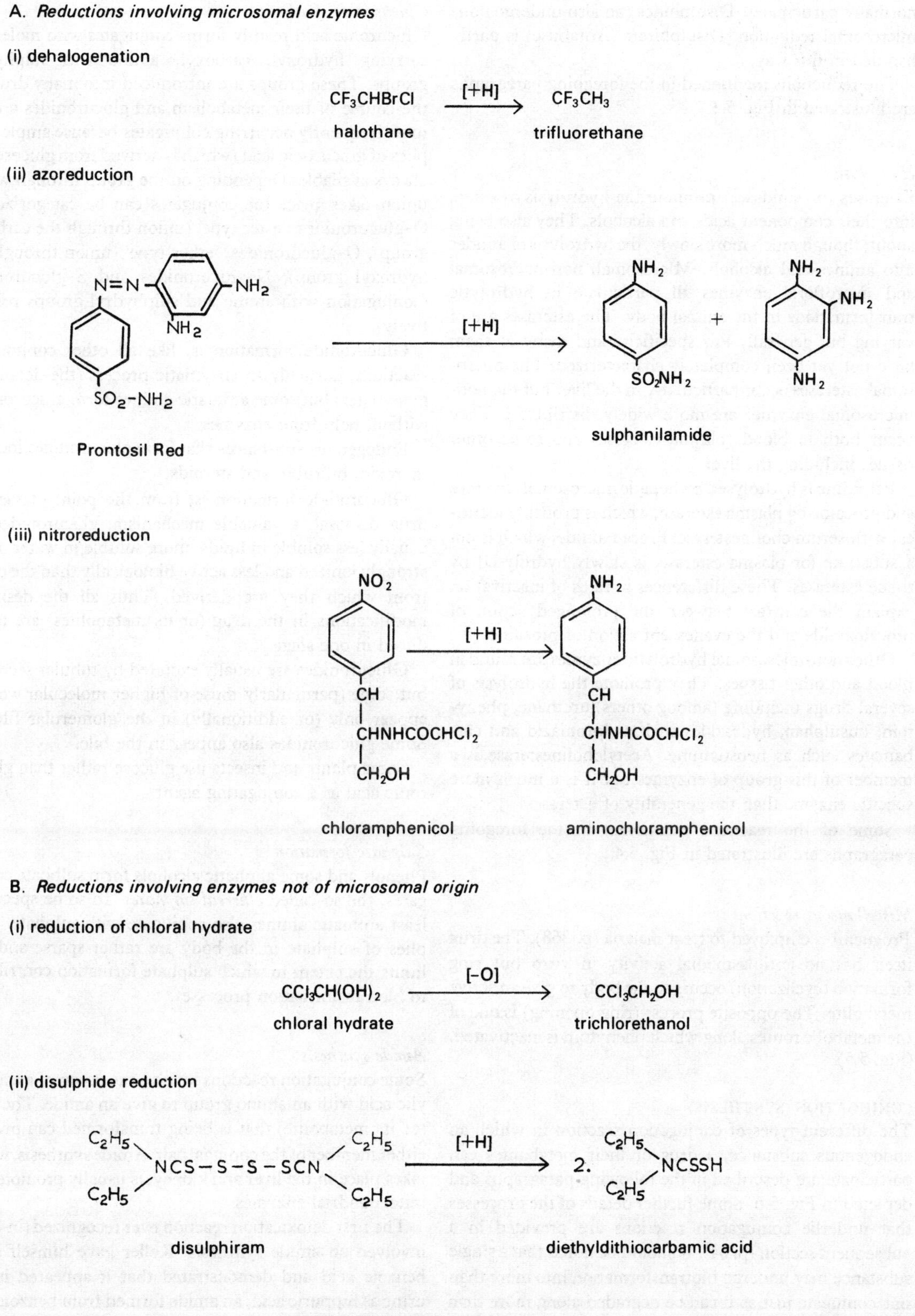
A. Reductions involving microsomal enzymes
(i) dehalogenation
CF3CHBrCl
[+H]
CF3CH3
halothane
trifluorethane
(ii) azoreduction
N=N
NH2
NH2
SO2–NH2
Prontosil Red
[+H]
NH2
SO2NH2
sulphanilamide
+
NH2
NH2
NH2
(iii) nitroreduction
NO2
CH
CHNHCOCHCl2
CH2OH
chloramphenicol
[+H]
NH2
CH
CHNHCOCHCl2
CH2OH
aminochloramphenicol
B. Reductions involving enzymes not of microsomal origin
(i) reduction of chloral hydrate
CCl3CH(OH)2
chloral hydrate
[-O]
CCl3CH2OH
trichlorethanol
(ii) disulphide reduction
C2H5
C2H5
NCS–S–S–SCN
C2H5
C2H5
disulphiram
[+H]
2.
C2H5
NCSSH
C2H5
diethyldithiocarbamic acid

Fig. 5.3 Metabolic reductive reactions

normally participates. Disulphides can also undergo non-microsomal reduction. Disulphiram (Antabuse) is partly handled in this way.

The reductions mentioned in the foregoing paragraphs are illustrated in Fig. 5.3.

Hydrolysis

Esterases (or amidases) promote the hydrolysis of esters into their component acids and alcohols. They also bring about, though much more slowly, the hydrolysis of amides into amines and alcohols. Microsomal, non-microsomal and microfloral enzymes all participate in hydrolytic transformations in the animal body. The esterases are of varying but generally low specificity and many of them have not yet been completely characterized. The microsomal esterases occur particularly in the liver but the non-microsomal enzymes are more widely distributed. They occur both in blood (plasma esterase) and some other tissues including the liver.

Pethidine is hydrolysed by hepatic microsomal enzymes and procaine by plasma esterase, which is probably identical with serum cholinesterase. Procainamide, which is not a substrate for plasma esterase, is slowly hydrolysed by tissue esterases. These differences in rates of inactivation explain the contrast between the prolonged action of procainamide and the evanescent action of procaine.

Other non-microsomal hydrolytic enzymes are found in blood and other tissues. They promote the hydrolysis of several drugs including (among others) urethane, phenytoin, busulphan, hydrazides such as iproniazid and carbamates such as neostigmine. Acetylcholinesterase is a member of this group of enzymes but it is a much more specific enzyme than the generality of esterases.

Some of the reactions mentioned in the foregoing paragraphs are illustrated in Fig. 5.4.

Miscellaneous reactions

Proguanil is employed to treat malaria (p. 868). The drug itself has no antiplasmodial activity in vitro but ring formation (cyclization) occurs in the body to give an active metabolite. The opposite process (ring opening) is one of the metabolic routes along which phenytoin is inactivated. (Fig. 5.5).

CONJUGATION (SYNTHESIS)

The different types of conjugation reaction in which an endogenous substance, a drug or their metabolites can participate are described in the following paragraphs and depicted in Fig. 5.6. Some further details of the processes that underlie conjugation reactions are provided in a subsequent section (p. 64). It should be noted that a single substance may undergo biotransformation into more than one conjugate just as it can be degraded along more than one metabolic pathway.

Glucuronide synthesis

Glucuronic acid readily forms conjugates with molecules carrying hydroxyl, carboxyl, amino and sulphydryl groups. These groups are introduced into many drugs in the course of their metabolism and glucuronides are the most frequently occurring conjugates because ample supplies of glucuronic acid (which is derived from glucose) are always available. Depending on the group through which union takes place the conjugates can be categorized as O–glucuronides, 'ester type' (union through the carboxyl group), O–glucuronides, 'ether type' (union through the hydroxyl group), N–glucuronides and S–glucuronides (conjugation with amino and sulphydryl groups respectively).

Glucuronide formation is, like all other conjugation reactions, normally an enzymatic process (the details are given later) but some aromatic amines form glucuronides without help from enzymes.

Endogenous substances that form glucuronides include thyroxin, bilirubin and steroids.

Glucuronide formation is, from the point of view of drug disposal, a valuable mechanism: glucuronides are usually less soluble in lipids, more soluble in water, more strongly ionized and less active biologically than the drugs from which they are derived. Thus all the desirable modifications in the drug (or its metabolites) are introduced in one stage.

Glucuronides are usually excreted by tubular secretion but some (particularly those of higher molecular weight) appear only (or additionally) in the glomerular filtrate. Some glucuronides also appear in the bile.

Some plants and insects use glucose rather than glucuronic acid as a conjugating agent.

Sulphate formation

Phenols and some aliphatic alcohols form sulphate conjugates, the so-called ethereal sulphates. In some species at least aromatic amines also conjugate with sulphate. Supplies of sulphate in the body are rather sparse and this limits the extent to which sulphate formation contributes to biotransformation processes.

Amide synthesis

Some conjugation reactions involve the union of a carboxylic acid with an amino group to give an amide. The drug (or its metabolite) that is being transformed can provide either member of the conjugal pair. Amide synthesis, which takes place in the liver and kidney, is usually promoted by mitochondrial enzymes.

The first detoxication reaction ever recognized (in 1842) involved an amide synthesis. Keller gave himself some benzoic acid and demonstrated that it appeared in the urine as hippuric acid, an amide formed from benzoic acid and glycine. The extent to which a dose of benzoic acid is

A *Hydrolyses involving microsomal enzymes*

(i) hydrolysis of esters

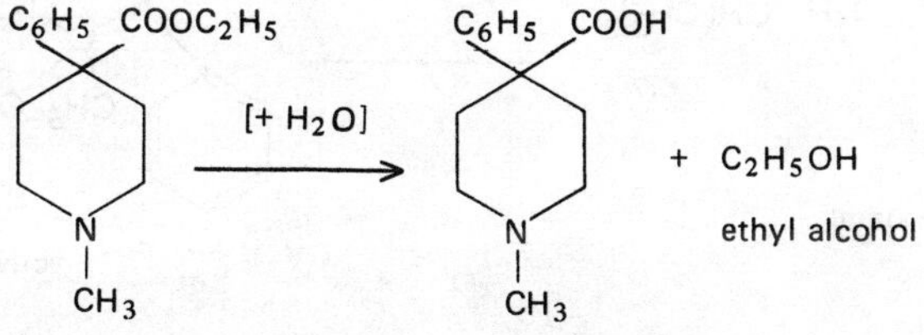

pethidine   meperidinic acid

B *Hydrolyses involving enzymes not of microsomal origin*

(i) hydrolysis of esters

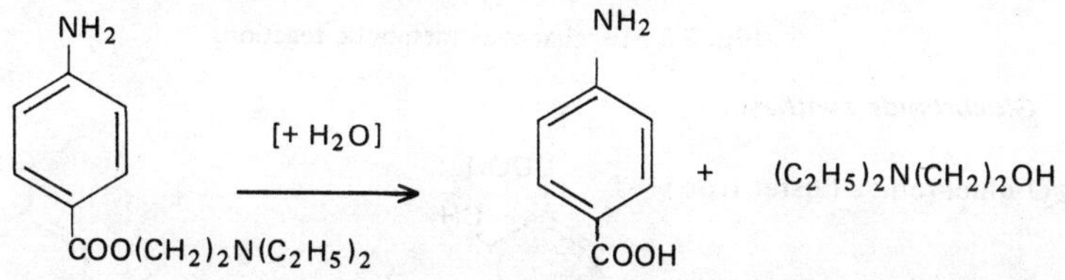

procaine   *p*-aminobenzoic acid   diethylaminoethanol

(ii) hydrolysis of amides

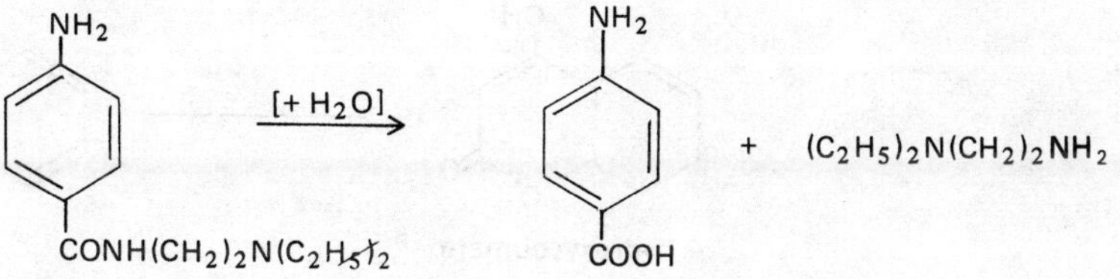

procainamide   *p*-aminobenzoic acid   diethylaminoethylamine

(iii) hydrolysis of hydrazides

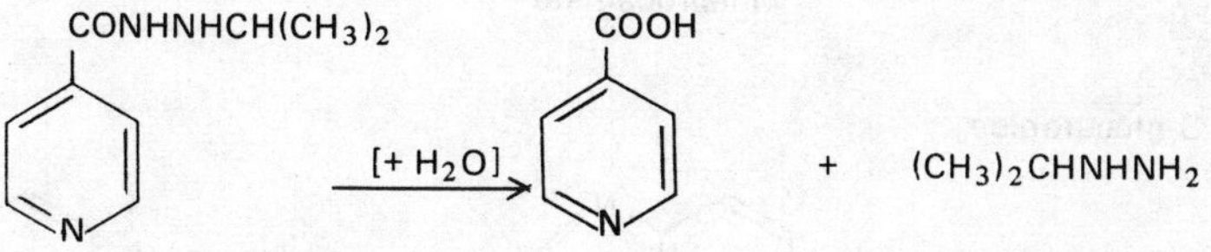

iproniazid   isonicotinic acid   isopropylhydrazine

Fig. 5.4 Metabolic hydrolytic reactions

Ring formation

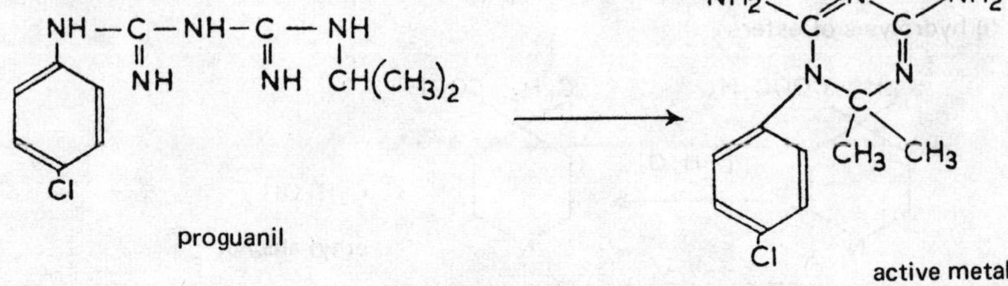

proguanil

active metabolite

Ring opening

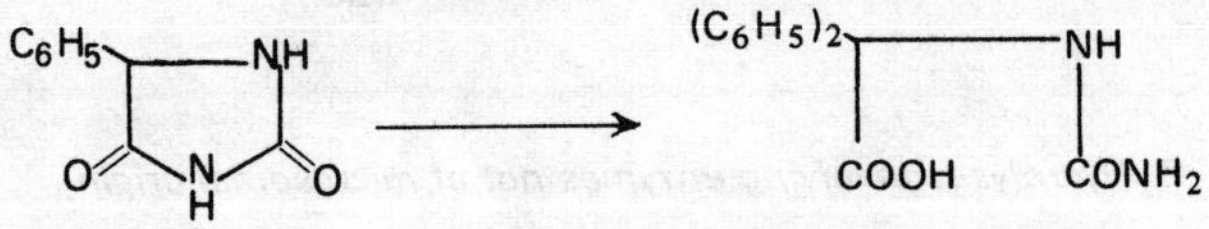

phenytoin

diphenylureidoacetic acid

Fig. 5.5 Miscellaneous metabolic reactions.

A. *Glucuronide synthesis*

(i) O-glucuronide ('ester type')

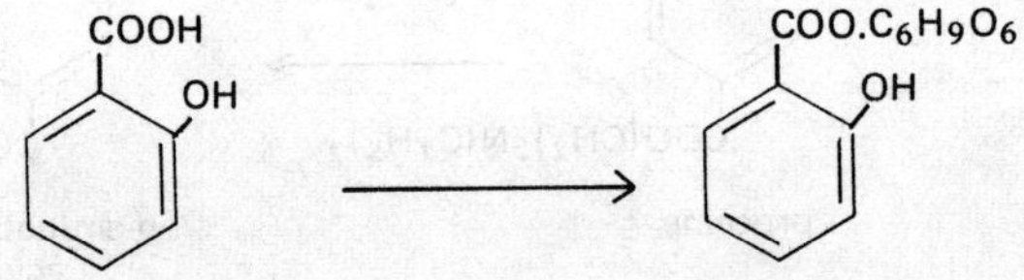

salicylic acid

(ii) O-glucuronide ('ether type')

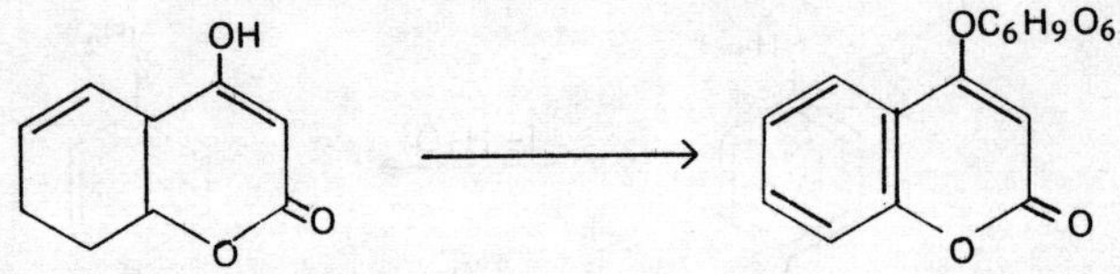

4-hydroxycoumarin

(iii) N-glucuronide

$$CH_2OCONH_2$$
$$|$$
$$C(CH_3)CH_2CH_2CH_3 \longrightarrow$$
$$|$$
$$CH_2OCONH_2$$

meprobamate

$$CH_2OCONHC_6H_9O_6$$
$$|$$
$$C(CH_3)CH_2CH_2CH_3$$
$$|$$
$$CH_2OCONHC_6H_9O_6$$

(iv) S-glucuronide

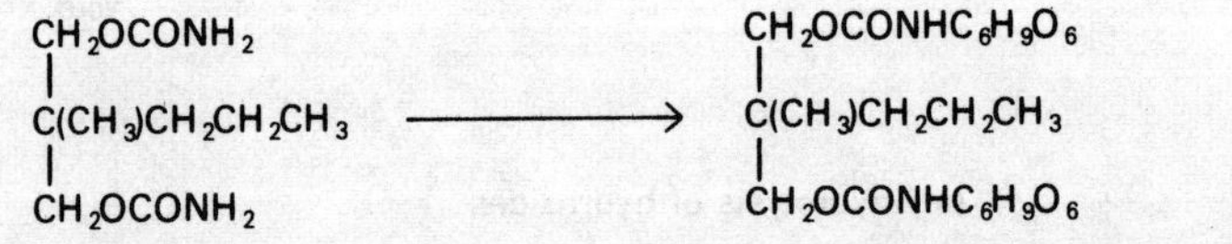

2-mercaptobenzothiazole

Fig. 5.6 Conjugation reactions operative in man.

B. *Ethereal sulphate synthesis*

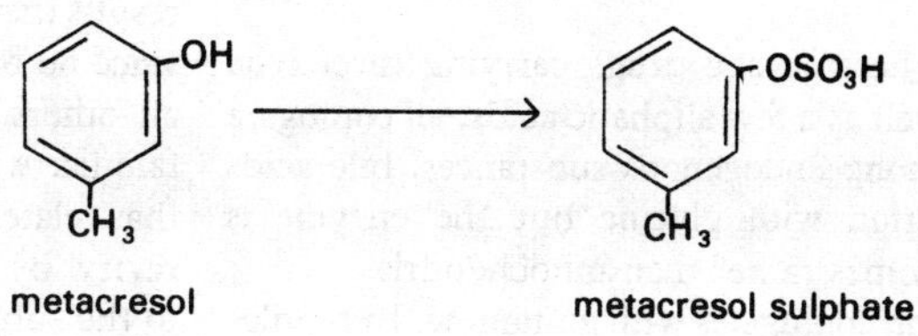
OH
CH3
OSO3H
CH3
metacresol
metacresol sulphate

C. *Amide synthesis*

(i) with amino conjugating agent (usually glycine)

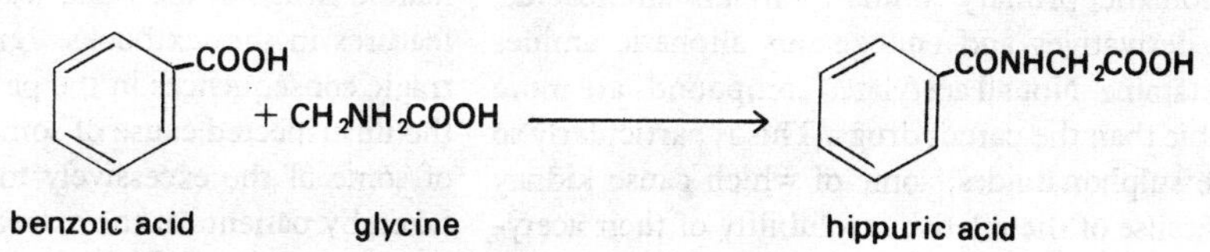
COOH
+ CH2NH2COOH
CONHCH2COOH
benzoic acid
glycine
hippuric acid

(ii) with carboxylic acid conjugating agent (usually acetic acid)

$$H_2NNH_2 \quad + \quad 2CH_3COOH \longrightarrow CH_3COHNNHCOCH_3$$

hydrazine acetic acid hydrazine conjugate

D. *Methylation*

(i) N-methylation

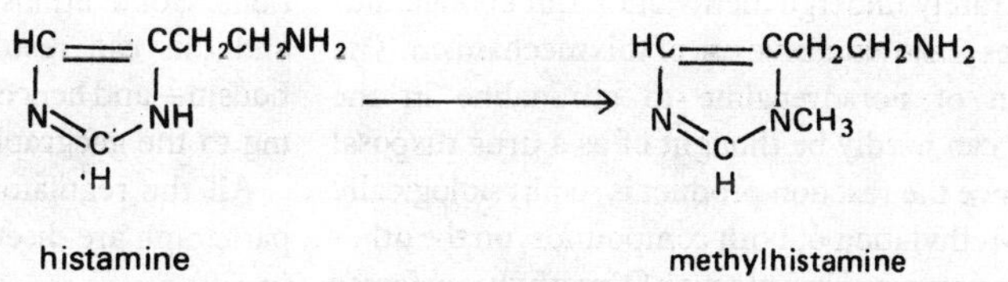
HC
CCH2CH2NH2
N
NH
C
H
NCH3
histamine
methylhistamine

(ii) O-methylation

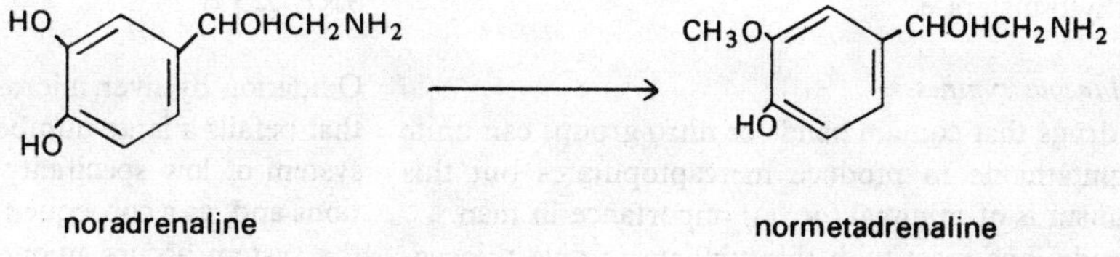
HO
CHOHCH2NH2
HO
CH3O
noradrenaline
normetadrenaline

(iii) S-methylation

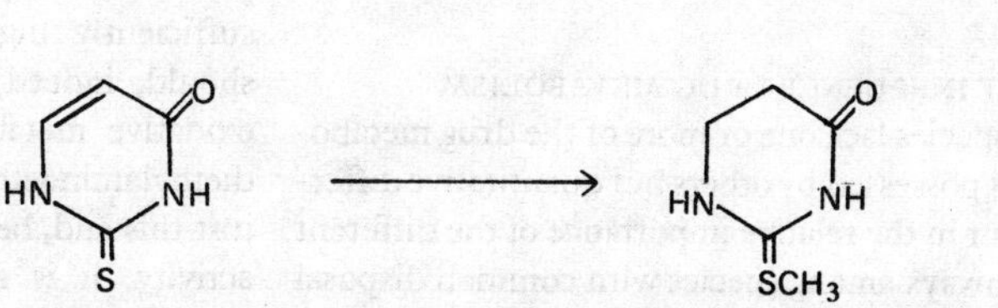
O
HN
NH
S
SCH3
thiouracil
5-methylthiouracil

Fig. 5.6 (Contd.)

converted into hippuric acid has been used as a test of liver function.

Aromatic and heterocyclic drugs carrying carboxylic acid groups, as well as a few aliphatic acids, all conjugate with glycine. Among endogenous substances, bile acids undergo conjugation with glycine but the enzyme is located in microsomes rather than mitochondria.

A few acids form conjugates with glutamine. In reptiles and a number of avian species, ornithine takes the place of glycine.

Acetic acid is the most usual acid component of the amides formed from drugs that carry amino groups. These include aromatic primary amines, foreign aminoacids, hydrazine derivatives and endogenous aliphatic amines such as histamine. Not all acetylated compounds are more water soluble than the parent drugs. This is particularly so among the sulphonamides, some of which cause kidney damage because of the relative insolubility of their acetylated derivatives.

Formylation reactions have also been reported.

Methylation

Methylation involves the introduction of methyl groups into primary aliphatic amines, phenols and compounds containing sulphur. The designations N-methylation, O-methylation and S-methylation indicate the atom to which the methyl group is attached. Drugs containing aliphatic amine groups rarely undergo methylation but endogenous primary amines make extensive use of this mechanism. The N-methylation of noradrenaline to adrenaline in the adrenal gland can hardly be thought of as a drug disposal mechanism since the reaction product is so physiologically valuable. O–Methylation of both compounds, on the other hand, which is promoted by catechol-O-methyltransferase (p. 260), constitutes an important step in their degradation. Histamine is methylated under the influence of imidazole N-methyltransferase.

Miscellaneous syntheses

Some drugs that contain halide or nitro groups can unite with glutathione to produce mercaptopurates but this mechanism is of minimal (or no) importance in man.

Cyanide ions react with thiosulphate to give thiocyanate.

FACTORS THAT INFLUENCE DRUG METABOLISM

Some animal species lack one or more of the drug metabolizing enzymes possessed by others but quantitative differences also occur in the relative importance of the different metabolic pathways among species with common disposal systems. The fact that different species may handle a particular drug in different ways is a matter of importance to the pharmacologist or toxicologist attempting to predict from animal experiments the likely effectiveness or safety of the drug in the human being. It is, unfortunately, not possible to declare that a particular animal will always yield results that will best predict responses in the human being since no one species resembles man more uniformly than all others. The laboratory worker should make himself familiar with those aspects of comparative pharmacology that relate to drug biotransformation systems. The short review by Williams (1971) provides a useful introduction to the subject.

Differences in the nature and effectiveness of the drug disposal systems also occur within species, including man and it is important that the physician be aware of these differences. The very young and the very old do not always handle drugs in the same way as the 'normal adult' who features in the textbooks. Ignorance of this fact has had tragic consequences in the past and it is undoubtedly still the unsuspected cause of some failures to respond to, and of some of the excessively toxic reactions against, drugs taken by patients at the extremes of their life spans. Some racial and genetic factors exert effects on patients of all ages. The best known of several genetic factors that influence drug metabolism is that which determines that some individuals are 'fast' acetylators of isoniazid (and some other substances) while others are 'slow' acetylators. Again, the ability of one drug to induce the production of microsomal enzymes in the liver that will promote not only its own degradation but also that of other substances constitutes one of the more usual causes of drug interactions. Some atmospheric pollutants have the same effect and this can result in differences in the rate of metabolism—and hence in the effective dose—of a drug according to the geographical locality in which it is used.

All the regulatory factors mentioned in the foregoing paragraph are discussed in more detail in the next chapter (p. 70).

SKF 525 A

Oxidation by liver microsomes, as we have seen, is a fate that befalls a large number of drugs. A single biochemical system of low specificity subserves most of these oxidations and, as a consequence, competition for possession of the system occurs among potential substrates if they are present in adequate concentrations. One substance with a sufficiently high affinity for the microsomal enzymes should, indeed, be capable of completely blocking the oxidative metabolism of many others. SKF 525 A (ß-diethylaminoethyl diphenylpropylacetate; Fig. 5.7) does just this and, because it is itself devoid of pharmacological activity, it is a useful laboratory tool. It inhibits the metabolism of all but a few of the compounds that are normally degraded by microsomal oxidation (and also, oddly enough, some of those that are broken down by enzymes not of microsomal origin) and with its aid it is possible to decide, for instance, whether the observed

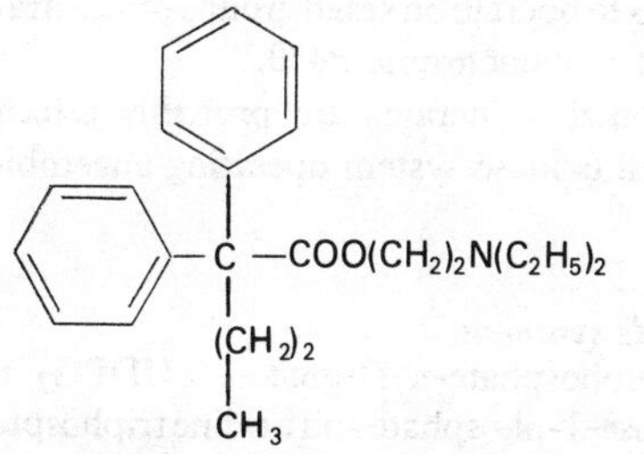

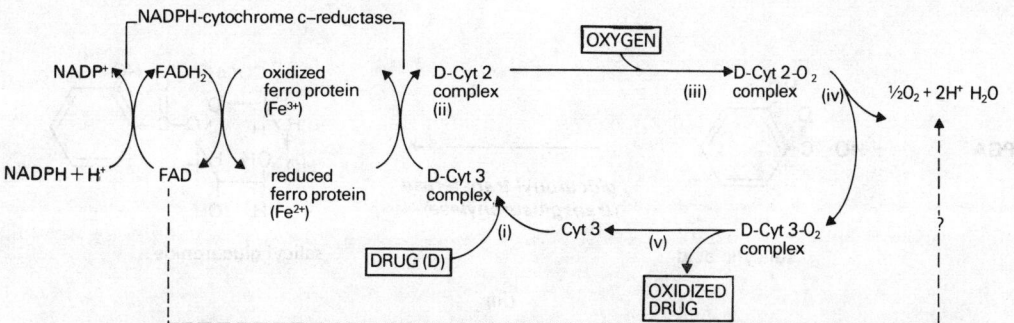

Fig. 5.7 SKF 525 A

actions of a drug are attributable to the drug itself or to an oxidation product.

Other inhibitors of metabolism

A large number of useful drugs operate by inhibiting the enzymatic breakdown of endogenous and sometimes of foreign substances. Disulphiram comes in the latter category: it prevents the conversion of acetaldehyde (derived from ethanol) into acetic acid and it finds application in the treatment of alcoholism. The many substances that intervene in the disposal of endogenous substances include monoamine oxidase inhibitors, anticholinesterase agents and drugs that inhibit xanthine oxidase. They are all described in detail elsewhere in this volume.

BIOCHEMICAL FEATURES OF THE DRUG METABOLIZING SYSTEMS

Having described the end results of the various metabolic reactions that are used by the body for drug disposal purposes, we can proceed to inspect a little more closely the nature of the biochemical mechanisms involved in these processes. The treatment will necessarily have to be superficial but the interested reader can obtain further details from biochemical texts or from appropriate monographs. Those listed in the bibliography on p. 69 can be recommended.

Microsomal oxidations

The key compound in these reactions is cytochrome P450, so labelled because it can unite with carbon monoxide (as

well as with atmospheric oxygen) to give a complex with an absorption peak at 450 nm. Cytochrome P450 is present in the microsomes of the liver and kidney (and in a few other tissues in which microsomal oxidations occur) but it is not found elsewhere in these tissues nor at all in those in which microsomal oxidations do not take place. Because of the low specificity of microsomal oxidative processes, cytochrome P450 is described as a *mixed function oxidase*.

Cytochrome P450 transfers atmospheric oxygen to the drug substrate. Only the reduced (Fe^{2+}) form of cytochrome P450 can collect oxygen for transfer in this way but in the course of its activity it is oxidized to the Fe^{3+} form. The transfer of electrons necessary to effect the change back to the reduced form and so maintain metabolic activity requires the nicotinamide adenine dinucleotide phosphate ($NADP/NADPH_2$) coenzyme system (p. 23). The whole process as so far elucidated, is shown in Fig. 5.8 and can be summarized as follows:

i. The drug forms a complex with oxidized (Fe^{3+}) cytochrome P450.

ii. $NADPH_2$ is oxidized to NADP under the influence of $NADPH_2$-cytochrome$c$ reductase. This name is a little misleading in the present context because cytochrome$c$ is not present in microsomes. A more appropriate (but rarely used) name is P450-reductase.

The reductase has two components—a flavoprotein (FAD, p. 24) and a ferroprotein. When $NADPH_2$ is oxidized, the flavoprotein becomes reduced to $FADH_2$. Electrons are then transferred to the ferroprotein (which thereby becomes reduced) from $FADH_2$ leaving protons (H^+) for use later in the cycle and returning the flavoprotein to its original oxidized state (FAD). Finally, an electron is passed to the oxidized cytochrome P450.

iii. The now reduced cytochrome, still complexed with drug, takes up a molecule of oxygen.

iv. The drug-cytochrome-oxygen combination loses an atom of oxygen. After transfer of electrons from the cytochrome (which thereby becomes converted

Fig. 5.8 Drug oxidation by microsomal enzymes. Cyt 2—reduced cytochrome P450 (Fe^{2+}) Cyt 3—oxidised cytochrome P450 (Fe^{3+}). For other abbreviations *see text*. Roman numerals relate to the similarly numbered paragraphs in the text

into the Fe^{3+} form again) to H^+ ions the latter react with the released oxygen to give water. The source of the proton (H^+) donor required for this stage of the process is not entirely clear but, as indicated in Fig. 5.8, it may well be that the protons are provided by the oxidation of $FADH_2$.

v. The oxidized cytochrome releases the oxidized drug and the cycle is complete.

It is to be noted that microsomal oxidations are not totally unspecific in nature. Cytochrome P450 is certainly the most abundant of the microsomal cytochromes and its activity accounts for most of the oxidative reactions effected by the microsomes. Small amounts of about six other cytochromes are, however, present in the liver and

each seems to operate on small groups of substrates that are indifferent to cytochrome P450.

Microsomal reductions are probably effected by the microsomal oxidase system operating anaerobically.

Glucuronide synthesis

Uridine diphosphate-α-D-glucose (UDPG) is formed from glucose-1-phosphate and uridine triphosphate (UTP) under the influence of uridyltransferase (pyrophosphory-lase). UDPG is then oxidized to the glucuronate (UDPGA). Nicotinamide adenine dinucleotide (NAD) and UDPG dehydrogenase are involved in this transformation. Finally, a glucuronide transferase catalyzes the transfer of glucuronide to the compound that is to be conjugated (Fig. 5.9).

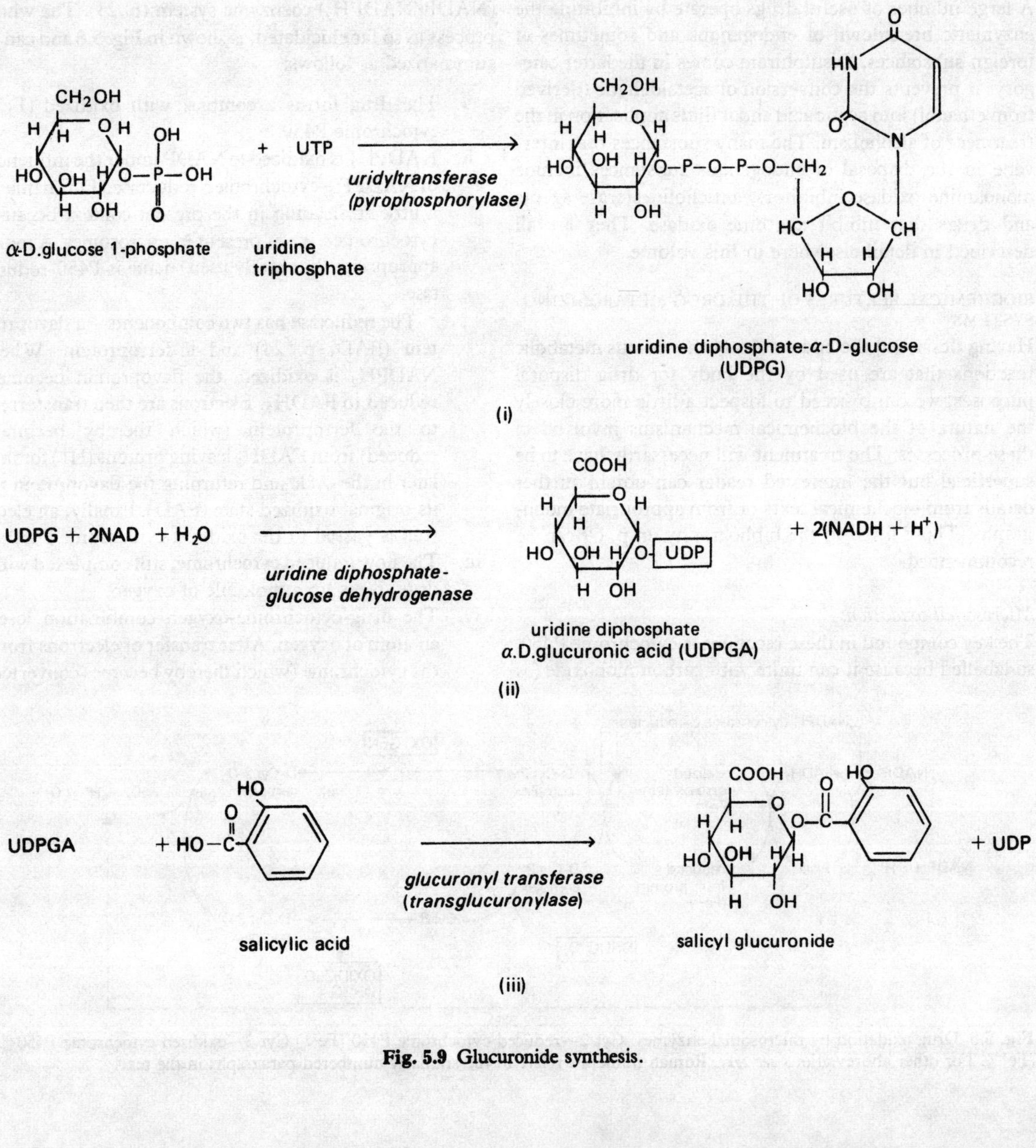

Fig. 5.9 Glucuronide synthesis.

As will be clear by reference to Fig. 5.9, the glucuronic acid-phosphate bond in UDPGA takes the α-configuration but the corresponding link in the conjugated compound adopts the β form. This change provides an example of the Walden inversion and it results in the conjugate's becoming susceptible to attack by β-glucuronidase, an enzyme found (among other sites) in the gastrointestinal tract and the urine. Although β-glucuronidase is not normally an important component of biotransformation systems, its action may sometimes have deleterious consequences. It is known, for instance, that naphthylamine (a substance that was used for many years in the dye industry) can cause carcinoma of the bladder and ureter in those exposed to it for a long time. Naphthylamine itself is not carcinogenic but its metabolites are. These metabolites are rendered innocuous by glucuronide conjugation in the liver but once in the urine the conjugates are exposed to enzyme attack so that the ureters and bladder are likely to be in contact, over a prolonged period, with small amounts of the carcinogenic metabolites.

Several glucuronyl transferases are known so that glucuronide synthesis exhibits a degree of specificity. The glucuronyl transferases are microsomal enzymes but those responsible for the initial formation of UDPGA are of cytoplasmic origin.

Sulphate formation

Sulphate ions must be activated before they can participate in conjugation reactions. Activation necessitates the formation, first of adenosine 5'-phosphosulphate (APS) and then of 3'-phosphoadenosine 5'-phosphosulphate (PAPS) under the aegis of ATP-sulphurylase and APS-kinase respectively. Adenosine triphosphate is needed in both these conversions. The final transfer of sulphate is promoted by a sulphotransferase. These reactions are shown in Fig. 5.10.

The sulphotransferases (which are of non-microsomal origin) are relatively specific, separate enzymes being available for each class of chemical compound that is susceptible to sulphate conjugation.

The enzyme systems involved in sulphate conjugation reactions also take part in the biosynthesis of sulphated polysaccharides such as heparin.

Amide formation

In this process the acid (irrespective of whether this is the conjugating agent or the molecule to be conjugated) is activated by union with coenzyme A (CoA). This occurs in two stages catalyzed by acyl synthetase and acyl thiokinase respectively. The first stage requires ATP. Transacylases bring about the final stage of the synthesis, promoting the union of amine and the activated acid with liberation of the coenzyme A. The sequence of reactions is indicated in Fig. 5.11.

Many endogenous fatty acids are activated by the system that prepares acids for conjugation into amides.

Methylation

Methylation can be accomplished by several biochemical systems but the most important one utilizes 5-adenosyl methionine. This compound is formed from methionine and ATP and the reaction is promoted by methionine adenosine transferase. A methyl transferase brings about the final transfer of the methyl group to the molecule that is to undergo conjugation. The reactions are shown in Fig. 5.12.

A large number of methyl transferases is known. Each of them can deal with only a limited number of substrates. They are found in a variety of tissues, some in the microsomes and others elsewhere.

Excretion of drugs

The principal medium in which drugs, metabolites and conjugates leave the body is, of course, the urine but almost every other secretion—bile, saliva, gastric juice and other gastrointestinal secretions, milk, sweat and genital secretions—can convey drugs out of the body. Particular aspects of drug carriage in all these vehicles are itemized in the following paragraphs.

Urine. The mechanisms that underlie urine formation are discussed in Chap. 36 (p. 617).

Bile. Some substances, particularly the glucuronide conjugates, are excreted into the duodenum in the bile. They reach the bile as a result of active secretory processes across the walls of the bile canaliculi. Separate transport systems apparently exist for organic acids, bases and unionized substances but the most favoured candidates for excretion in the bile are polar compounds with molecular weights of more than about 400 daltons.

Arriving in the duodenum, glucuronides are exposed to the action of β-glucuronidase and the previously conjugated drug or metabolite is released by the enzyme. It is reabsorbed into the portal circulation, enters the liver and again becomes enmeshed in the conjugation machinery. In this way a repeating cycle of release from conjugation, absorption and reconjugation is set up as the drug or metabolite repeatedly travels the *enterohepatic circulation*. With each turn of the cycle, some of the conjugate will, of course, escape hydrolysis in the intestine and some of the drug or metabolite will avoid reconjugation but some material (albeit in a progressively diminishing quantity) will remain trapped in the enterohepatic circulatory system for a considerable period of time.

Only a few drugs (as opposed to drug metabolites) form glucuronides that are excreted in the bile. The best known of those that do is stilboestrol.

It is possible that some substances that are excreted in the bile suffer enzymatic attack in the intestine and yield products that will be toxic if they are reabsorbed. It is not clear whether this mechanism is of any significance in the

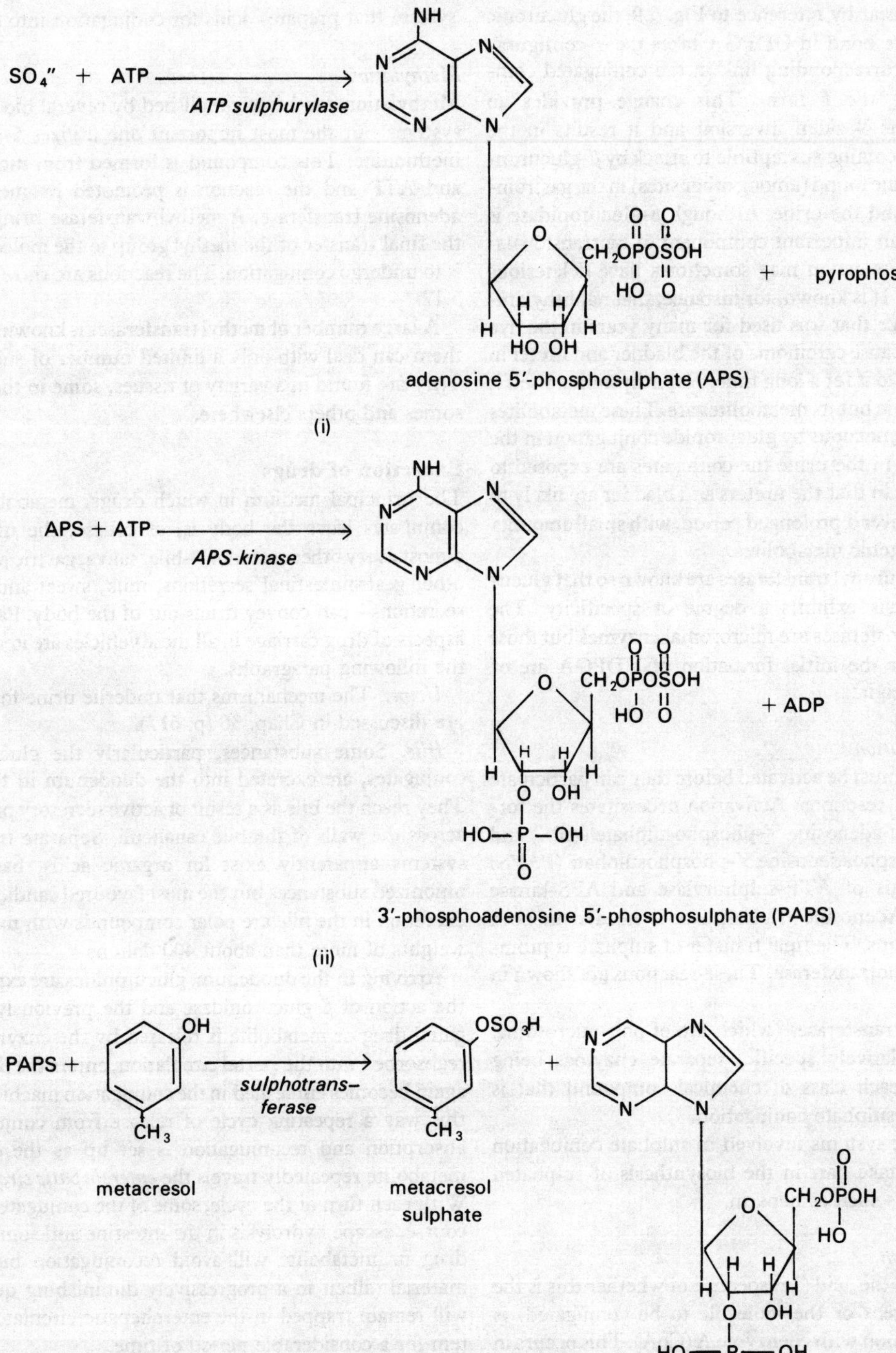

$$SO_4'' + ATP \xrightarrow{\textit{ATP sulphurylase}}$$

adenosine 5'-phosphosulphate (APS)   + pyrophosphate

(i)

$$APS + ATP \xrightarrow{\textit{APS-kinase}}$$

3'-phosphoadenosine 5'-phosphosulphate (PAPS)   + ADP

(ii)

$$PAPS + \xrightarrow{\textit{sulphotransferase}}$$

metacresol   metacresol sulphate   + 3'-phosphoadenosine 5-phosphate

Fig. 5.10 The synthesis of ethereal sulphate.

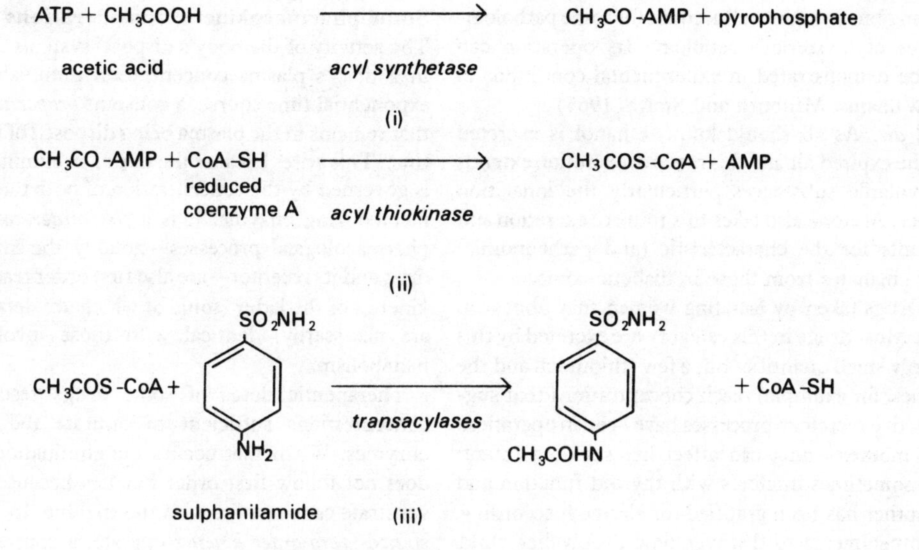

$$ATP + CH_3COOH \xrightarrow{} CH_3CO\text{-}AMP + \text{pyrophosphate}$$

acetic acid   *acyl synthetase*

(i)

$$CH_3CO\text{-}AMP + CoA\text{-}SH \xrightarrow{} CH_3COS\text{-}CoA + AMP$$

reduced
coenzyme A   *acyl thiokinase*

(ii)

$$CH_3COS\text{-}CoA + \quad \xrightarrow{\textit{transacylases}} \quad + CoA\text{-}SH$$

sulphanilamide   (iii)

Fig. 5.11 Acetylation of sulphanilamide to illustrate amide formation.

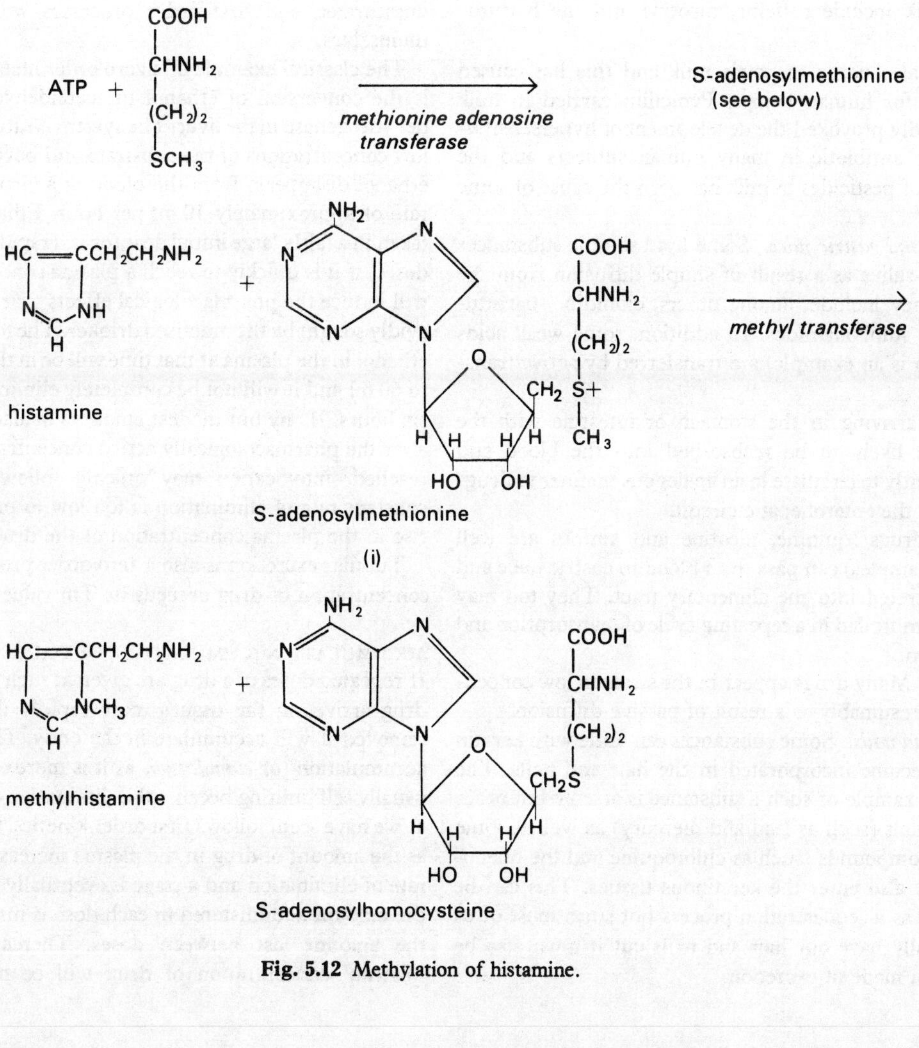

$$ATP + \begin{array}{c} COOH \\ | \\ CHNH_2 \\ | \\ (CH_2)_2 \\ | \\ SCH_3 \end{array} \xrightarrow[\textit{transferase}]{\textit{methionine adenosine}} \begin{array}{c} \text{S-adenosylmethionine} \\ \text{(see below)} \end{array}$$

methionine

histamine   +   S-adenosylmethionine $\xrightarrow{\textit{methyl transferase}}$

(i)

methylhistamine   +   S-adenosylhomocysteine

Fig. 5.12 Methylation of histamine.

human being but it might well account for some pathological changes of mysterious aetiology. Its operation can certainly be demonstrated in experimental conditions in animals (Williams, Millburn and Smith, 1965).

Expired air. As all should know, ethanol is excreted partly in the expired air and this mode of excretion extends to other volatile substances particularly the inhalation anaesthetics. Acetone also takes this route of excretion and this accounts for the characteristic (and pathognomic) smell that emanates from those in diabetic coma.

Milk. Drugs taken by lactating women may appear in their milk. Most drugs in this category are excreted by this route in only small quantities but a few (thiouracil and the tetracyclines, for example) reach concentrations that suggest that active secretory processes have been in operation. Drugs in mother's milk can affect her suckling infant: thiouracil sometimes inteferes with thyroid function and many a mother has been gratified (or alarmed, according to her temperament) to discover how deeply her child has slept after a feed taken after she herself has been indulging a taste for alcohol. Other common drugs that reach milk include caffeine, nicotine and the barbiturates.

Drugs also occur in cow's milk and this has caused problems for human beings. Penicillin carried in milk undoubtedly provoked the development of hypersensitivity to the antibiotic in many human subjects and the presence of pesticides in milk has been the cause of some concern.

Saliva and gastric juice. Some lipid soluble substances enter the saliva as a result of simple diffusion from the blood. They include, among others, clonidine, barbiturates and sulphonamides. In addition, some weak acids (penicillin is an example) are transferred by active transport.

Drugs arriving in the stomach or intestine with the saliva are likely to be reabsorbed into the blood and consequently to circulate in an analogous manner to drugs caught in the enterohepatic circuit.

Basic drugs (quinine, nicotine and amines are well known examples) can pass from blood to gastric juice and so be excreted into the alimentary tract. They too may become embroiled in a repeating cycle of reabsorption and resecretion.

Sweat. Many drugs appear in the sweat in low concentration, presumably as a result of passive diffusion.

Hair and nails. Some substances can unite with keratin and so become incorporated in the hair and nails. The classical example of such a substance is arsenic but other heavy metals (such as lead and mercury) as well as some organic compounds (such as chloroquine and the phenothiazines) also enter the keratinous tissues. This can be regarded as a sequestration process but since most of us occasionally have our hair and nails cut it must also be listed as a mode of excretion.

Some pharmacokinetic considerations

The activity of the body's disposal systems usually results in a drug's plasma concentration diminishing along an exponential time course, a constant *proportion* of the drug that remains in the plasma being disposed of in each unit of time. This arises because the rate of an elimination reaction is governed by the concentration of both the drug and the metabolizing enzyme: it is a *first order* reaction. Other pharmacological processes—notably the interaction of a drug and its receptor—are also first order reactions and the kinetics of the latter (some of which are detailed on p. 98) are necessarily identical with those involved in drug metabolism.

Therapeutic doses of some drugs result in plasma concentrations sufficient to saturate the metabolizing enzymes. When that occurs the elimination of the drug does not follow first order kinetics because some of the substrate cannot unite with the enzyme. In these circumstances *zero order kinetics* operate, a constant *amount* of drug being lost in unit time. Of course, as the concentration of the drug in the plasma falls the enzyme may become unsaturated and first order processes will then assert themselves.

The classical example of a zero order metabolic process is the conversion of ethanol to acetaldehyde by alcohol dehydrogenase in the liver. The system is saturated by very low concentrations of the substrate and beyond this point ethanol disappears from the blood at a virtually constant rate of approximately 10 ml per hour. Ethanol has to be taken in a fairly large initial dose (or in a rapid succession of doses) if it is quickly to reach a plasma concentration that will induce the pharmacological effects that seem to be so avidly sought by the practised drinker. The total amount of ethanol in the plasma at that time will be in the region of 50 to 60 ml and it will not be completely eliminated for some six hours. If any but modest amounts of alcohol are taken after the pharmacologically active concentration has been reached, intoxication may quickly follow because the constant rate of elimination is too low to prevent a rapid rise in the plasma concentration of the drug.

Tubular excretion is also a zero order process when the concentration of drug exceeds its Tm value (p. 619).

ACCUMULATION (CUMULATION) OF DRUGS
If repeated doses of a drug are given at such a rate that the drug arrives in the tissues more rapidly than it can be removed it will accumulate in the body. This process of accumulation (or *cumulation,* as it is more often called) is usually self limiting because the elimination of most drugs, as we have seen, follows first order kinetics. Consequently as the amount of drug in the plasma increases, so does its rate of elimination and a stage is eventually reached when the amount administered in each dose is just balanced by the amount lost between doses. Thereafter a steady 'plateau' concentration of drug will be maintained. A

moment's reflection will make it clear that the 'plateau' concentration is determined by the rate at which the drug is given. If the rate is too low the plateau concentration will fall short of that required to give the desired therapeutic effect while if the rate is too high the concentration may reach toxic levels before the steady state is achieved. In the latter instance, signs of toxicity will be delayed if the drug accumulates only slowly. Consequently, the absence of these signs in the early stages of drug administration cannot therefore be taken as evidence that toxic doses are not being given.

When a drug is given in repeated doses the same average concentration of drug in the tissues can be produced by a small dose given frequently or by a larger dose administered less often. The difference between the two administration programmes is seen in the resulting fluctuations of drug concentration between doses which will, clearly, be more marked when the drug is given infrequently. The number of doses into which the daily dose requirement is to be divided is determined partly by the rate at which the drug is disposed of and partly by the extent to which its effectiveness depends on the maintenance of a very stable concentration in the tissues. From the patient's point of view, the dose schedule should be arranged so that he needs to take, or be given, the drug as infrequently as is possible, consistent with the prevention of too wide fluctuations in the amount of drug in the plasma.

Although cumulation will permit the concentration of a drug to reach the desired level in the tissues after a number of doses have been given it is sometimes desirable to produce an immediately effective concentration. In these

instances, an initial *loading dose* of the drug is given. This creates an immediate effect which can then be prolonged by the administration of *maintenance doses*. The cardiac glycosides (p. 691) are given according to this type of schedule.

Cumulation has to be taken into account only when the drug under consideration is eliminated relatively slowly from the body.

Pharmacokinetic processes are discussed in formal detail in texts devoted wholly or partly to the subject. They include Curry (1974) and Goldstein *et al.* (1974).

BIBLIOGRAPHY

Books, monographs and reviews

Briggs, M. and Briggs, M. (1974). *The Chemistry and Metabolism of Drugs and Toxins.* London: Heinemann Medical Books.

Curry, S.H. (1974). *Drug Disposition and Pharmacokinetics.* Oxford, London, Edinburgh and Melbourne: Blackwell Scientific Publications.

Goldstein, A., Aronow, L. and Kalman, S.M. (1974). *Principles of Drug Action,* 2nd ed. New York, London, Sydney and Toronto: John Wiley

La Du, B.N., Mandel, H.G. and Way, E.L. (1971). *Fundamentals of Drug Metabolism and Drug Disposition.* Baltimore: The Williams and Wilkins Co.

Stowe, C.M. and Plaa, G.L. (1968). Extrarenal excretion of drugs and chemicals. *A. rev. Pharmac.,* **8**, 337-356.

Williams, R.T. (1959). *Detoxication Mechanisms,* 2nd ed. London: Chapman and Hall.

Williams, R.T., Millburn, P. and Smith, R.L. (1965). The influence of enterohepatic circulation on the toxicity of drugs. *Ann. N.Y. Acad. Sci.* **123**, 110-124.

6. Factors that influence the response to drugs

As we have already seen, the concentration of a drug in a particular tissue is determined by the balance between the drug's rate of arrival from the part of the body in which it is originally deposited and its rate of departure as a result of metabolic and other drug disposal processes. The individual components of these absorption and disposal mechanisms vary in their effectiveness from one individual to another so that it is impossible to know precisely how much of a drug dose will eventually reach its target tissue. If we also take into account the fact that the response of the tissue to the drug will itself be subject to this inherent biological variation we can readily appreciate why it is that a dose of drug that has a therapeutic effect in one individual might be useless (or, on the other hand, dangerously toxic) in another. Just two of the many examples quoted by Smith and Rawlings (1973) will serve to illustrate the influence of these random biological variations: the effective daily dose of phenindione (an anticoagulant) ranges from 25 to 200 mg and a standard intramuscular dose of atropine sulphate (0.02 mg per kilogram) given to 27 normal subjects had an effect on the heart rate ranging from a slowing of about five beats a minute to an acceleration of 60 beats a minute. It says much for the therapeutic ratio (p. 141) of modern drugs, the vigilance of physicians and, most of all, the effectiveness of the body's defences against pharmacological insult, that the frequency of seriously toxic drug reactions is so relatively low.

Up to this point we have mentioned only those variations in the response to drugs that are a simple consequence of the random variability that is inherent in all biological systems. However, other factors may intrude to superimpose their effects on these innate ones. In these circumstances, the responses to drug administration may be quite different (sometimes dramatically so) from those that were expected. Unlike the unexpected responses that may arise as a manifestation of biological variation, those that derive from the operation of these other factors should, in many cases, be predictable and therefore avoidable. In recent years, a considerable amount of attention has been directed towards *iatrogenic* disease. Iatrogenic means 'caused by physicians' and not a few cases of iatrogenic disorder (and, conversely, drug ineffectiveness) arise because the factors we are about to discuss are ignored or forgotten. They can conveniently be grouped as follows:

1. personal factors—age, weight, nutritional status
2. genetic and racial factors
3. environmental factors
4. immunological factors
5. pharmacological factors resulting from the concurrent administration of other drugs or the presence of other substances.

It is not always possible to ascribe an unexpected drug response to the exclusive operation of only one of these factors. Thus, one of the environmental effects we shall discuss is important only in the very young while immunological factors frequently have a genetic origin. Nevertheless, the classification provided here should assist the reader towards an understanding of factors that influence drug response even if the several categories are not mutually exclusive.

PERSONAL FACTORS

AGE

In the young child, drug disposal mechanisms have not reached the adult level of effectiveness. As a result, infants (particularly when premature) may suffer unexpectedly severe reactions to drugs that are quite innocuous to older children or adults. Two vivid illustrations of the consequences of this biochemical immaturity are commonly provided. Both relate to the comparative ineffectiveness of conjugation mechanisms in the very young.

Bilirubin is derived from the haemoglobin that is liberated from effete erythrocytes. Some bilirubin is slowly excreted in an unchanged form in the urine but most of it is converted into the glucuronide which is excreted quite rapidly. When the conjugation mechanisms are defective or (as with premature infants) incompletely established, bilirubin may appear in the blood more rapidly than it can be cleared from it. The excess is rendered harmless by being bound to plasma proteins. In the normal course of events bilirubin is gradually released from this combination as conjugating capacity becomes available. However, as we have seen (p. 51), compounds bound to plasma proteins are readily displaced by substances with a higher affinity of the binding sites and among the drugs that can displace bilirubin in this way are vitamin K and the sulphonamides. Given to premature infants (as they have been in the relatively recent past) these normally harmless drugs may release free bilirubin into the circulation. If drug administration is continued, access to the binding sites will be denied to the bilirubin that is still being formed and which will, therefore, be progressively deposited in the tissues. Deposition in the brain (*kernicterus*) may lead to rigidity, convulsions, coma, deafness, mental deficiency or death. As these sequelae indicate, the basal ganglia (p. 163) and the auditory nerve nuclei are particularly sensitive to bilirubin which depresses the oxidative metabolism of the nerve cells.

It should be mentioned in passing that deposition of bilirubin in the tissues can occur in the absence of drug administration if the rate of bilirubin production is so high that the storage capacity of the plasma proteins is exceeded. This is particularly likely to occur in the first few days of life when large numbers of foetal erythrocytes are being broken down. A slight degree of jaundice (a sign of bilirubin deposition in the skin) is indeed frequently seen even in the normal full-term infant and a fatal kernicterus may ensue if the rate of erythrocyte breakdown is abnormally high as it is in haemolytic disease of the newborn. Although these conditions are not directly relevant to the present discussion, which is concerned only to examine responses to drugs, they do serve to underline the importance of making sure that the bilirubin disposal system in the newborn is not impeded in any way since it is clearly operating, even in the normal infant, near to the limit of its capacity.

The other well publicized example of the vulnerability to drugs of infants who have not yet acquired an effective glucuronyl transferase system concerns chloramphenicol. Some fifteen years ago the practice arose in some quarters of giving chloramphenicol (p. 841) to premature infants in an attempt to protect them from infection in the immediately neonatal period. Many of the treated infants became cyanosed after they had received a few doses of the antibiotic and an alarming number—more than 60 per cent of one of the groups that were studied—died from circulatory failure. Because the afflicted infants became ashen grey in colour their condition was named the *grey syndrome*. Chloramphenicol is normally excreted as the glucuronide but since this mechanism of drug disposal was only partially operative in the premature infants the drug was not completely metabolized so that, after a few doses, unchanged drug had accumulated to a dangerously toxic concentration.

Factors other than immaturity of the conjugating systems also operate to produce unexpected reactions in the very young. Because of the instability of their homeostatic systems, young children often exhibit rapid and unpredictable swings in body temperature, blood glucose concentration, body water content and other components of the internal environment. All these changes may be associated with fluctuations in the response to drugs. In addition, absorption from the intestine is less effective than it is in older children and the circulation is less brisk so that drugs are not delivered so readily either to the target tissues or to the disposal systems. Finally, the actual responses to some drugs vary, quantitatively or qualitatively, with age. Thus, young children are more sensitive to morphine and less sensitive to atropine than are older members of the community, toxic doses of salicylates bring about acidosis in very young children but alkalosis in older children and adults (p. 442) and the barbiturates, which are classified as sedative drugs, not infrequently induce excitement in children. Unexpected reactions arising from the operation of the factors we have just enumerated are not confined to the immediately neonatal period (unlike those attributable to immaturity of the conjugation mechanisms) but they do tend to occur most frequently in the first year of life.

A final striking example can be quoted to illustrate the operation of some of the factors we have listed in the foregoing paragraphs. Some years ago, in the United States, a number of apparently healthy children, all under six months old, died from methaemoglobinaemia. They had not been given any drug that might itself have caused the production of methaemoglobin and the origin of the condition remained a mystery until it was realized that the infants had been given feeds made up in well water that contained a minute quantity of inorganic nitrate which was nevertheless fatally toxic by reason of three peculiarities of infant physiology: the acidity of the stomach contents is less than that in the older child and this permits the proliferation of bacteria that reduce nitrate; the nitrite thus produced oxidizes foetal haemoglobin (considerable amounts of which persist in infant blood) much more readily than it does the adult variety and the reductase that in older children would convert the methaemoglobin back to haemoglobin is deficient in the early months of life.

It is hardly necessary to add that drugs that might cause the production of methaemoglobin should only be given to very young children in cases of extreme necessity.

Drug doses in children

Children have, of course, a smaller body mass than adults and calculations of drug doses for them are sometimes based only on this fact. Assuming an adult mass of 65 kg, simple proportion suggests that the appropriate dose of drug for a child weighing x kg is obtained by multiplying the recommended adult dose by a factor of $\frac{x}{65}$. However— and particularly in this age of the obese child—this procedure is neither so logical nor so reliable as may at first appear and many would argue that the calculations should be based on age. It has been suggested that, for young children, the suitable fraction of the adult dose is given by $\frac{\text{age in years}}{\text{age} + 12}$ so that a child of three, for instance, would receive one-fifth of the recommended adult dose.

Some drug doses are now quoted as mg per square metre of body surface. The surface area can be obtained from the height and weight if a suitable nomogram is available but for children it is even easier to use the formula recommended by Catzel (1974)

Surface area (in square metres) = 0.07 × (Age + 6)

This formula implies that the surface area does not reach its adult value (1.7 m²) until age 18 but it is very satisfactory when applied to the age groups which require lower than adult drug doses. It should be clear, however, that no formula can be uniformly applicable to all drugs and all children since, as we have seen, children are more sensitive than adults to some drugs and less sensitive to others. A knowledge of the drugs is more important than a knowledge of formulae.

Drug responses in old age
Although the subject has not yet been extensively explored, it now seems clear that old people may react to drugs in a different way from younger adults not only because of regressive changes in their apparatus for drug absorption, metabolism and excretion (so that they revert in this as in other ways to the childhood condition) but also because changes in the functioning of the tissues cause drug responses to become qualitatively altered. The central nervous system is particularly likely to be affected in this way. The situation is likely to be aggravated by the fact that the aged brain loses much of its earlier ability to adjust to changes in the internal or external environment, minor disturbances of which may induce anxiety, confusion and disorientation. Care must be exercised therefore when psychotropic and other centrally acting drugs are prescribed for the elderly and the physician must be alert to the possibility that behaviour that appears to be a manifestation of senility in his patient may in fact be of iatrogenic origin, the result of his own injudicious prescribing.

BODY WEIGHT
The pharmacologist in his laboratory weighs his animals and calculates the dose of drug he is to give them from a knowledge of the mg per kilogram requirement. The same pharmacologist at the bedside will prescribe 'normal adult doses' of drugs for his human patients, usually without taking their body masses into account. At first glance, it may seem to provide a sad commentary on the relative values we attach to experimental animals and human patients but, in this instance at least, such cynicism would be misplaced. Animal doses relate to creatures whose adult body weights range from a few grams to several kilograms but the lean body masses of human adults of similar heights exhibit little variation. Differences in total body weights which may, of course, be considerable are referable almost entirely to differences in fat content. It would, therefore, be quite illogical to calculate, by reference to the total body weight, the required dose of a drug that is known to be distributed only among non fatty tissue. Such

a method of establishing the appropriate dose of a drug, applied blindly, is just as uncertain as is simple reliance on the 'normal adult dose'. At the same time, it must be remembered that the lean body mass of many people (particularly small and slender women) is considerably below that of the normal adult of the textbooks. For such individuals, the difference between the quoted adult dose and the toxic dose of a drug can become very small. If we further take into account the widespread predilection for overenthusiastic self medication and the popular if misbegotten belief that two doses of a drug will do more good than one, we can appreciate the extent of the hazards to which small persons are exposed and against which they should be warned.

There has been an increasing tendency in recent years to express drug doses, even for human beings, in terms of the total weight (or, sometimes, the surface area) of the body. This has been particularly applied to very potent substances. It should be evident, from what has already been said, that the practice has much to recommend it but its widespread adoption will not automatically ensure that all patients will receive optimum amounts of drug.

NUTRITIONAL STATUS
To the extent that the nutritional state is reflected in body weight and fat content, we have already partly considered its influence on drug responses but we now have to discuss the additional complications that follow in the train of serious undernourishment, a condition that is still, unfortunately, only too common in too many parts of the world.

The detoxication of drugs is impaired in seriously malnourished individuals because their inadequate diet does not provide the quantities of aminoacids that are needed to effect the conjugation processes that constitute so important a part of the detoxication mechanism. Blood pressure will be low and kidney circulation sluggish so that the excretion of unchanged drug will be slowed. Protein lack may lead to a serious deficit of plasma proteins and a much smaller fraction of the drug dose than usual will then be bound in a temporarily inactive form. Similarly there will be no possibility of any of the drug's being sequestered in fatty tissue. All these factors combine to produce abnormally high concentrations of drug in blood and tissues even if the amount originally given has been reduced in proportion to the reduction in lean body mass. Toxic reactions will, consequently, be more likely to occur and their impact may well be more than usually serious by virtue of their occurring in a patient whose debilitated state renders him ill fitted to resist them.

Vegetarians produce alkaline urine while those who take diets rich in animal protein produce acid urine. The rate of excretion of weak acids and bases is influenced by the acidity of the urine and unexpectedly severe reactions to normal doses of some drugs can sometimes be traced to the patient's having indulged in diets that hindered the excretion of the drug or its metabolites.

GENETIC AND RACIAL FACTORS

ENZYME ANOMALIES

As we reminded ourselves in the opening page of this chapter, the concentration of a drug in plasma or tissues at a particular moment is determined by a number of independently variable factors that control absorptive, metabolic and excretory processes. We know, therefore, that if we gave the same dose of a drug to a large number of people we would not find, some time later, that the concentration of drug in the plasma was the same in all our subjects. We would, instead, encounter a range of plasma concentrations and we would expect that, if we incorporated our findings in a graph that displayed the number of individuals (n) attaining each plasma concentration (x), the result would be a so-called normal curve of distribution with a mean of $\bar{x}$ and a form similar to that illustrated in Fig. 6.1(a) and discussed in detail in Chapter 9 (p. 114). This expectation is often realized in practice but some drugs do not give a normal distribution of plasma concentrations. In one of the by now classical investigations in this field (Evans, Manley and McKusick, 1960) a large group of normal subjects received the same dose (about 10 mg per kilogram) of isoniazid. Six hours later the concentrations of drug in the plasma were determined and a distribution curve was plotted. It assumed a bimodal form similar to that shown at Fig. 6.1(b), and consisting essentially of two conjoined normal distributions with mean concentrations (corresponding to $\bar{x}_a$ and $\bar{x}_b$ in the Figure) of about 1 μg per ml and 4.5 μg per ml respectively. The bimodal form emerged because, in addition to the multifactoral influences common to all the subjects, another factor that promoted the biotransformation of isoniazid was present in a majority of the subjects but was lacking in the minority. This additional feature was the ability to bring about the acetylation of isoniazid. Investigations into the families of 'slow' and 'rapid' inactivators have made it clear that acetylating ability (which resides in the hepatic enzyme N-acetyltransferase) is genetically determined and that it is inherited as a dominant characteristic. Studies such as this laid the foundations of the new specialty of *pharmacogenetics*, a discipline that concerns itself not only with the influence of genetic factors on the body's response to drugs but also with the effects of drugs on hereditary processes. The topic has stimulated much interest and the production of a number of monographs (Kalow, 1962; Meier, 1963; Szórády, 1973).

Sulphonamides are also disposed of partly by acetylation and slow inactivators of isoniazid handle sulphonamides in a similarly sluggish fashion.

A dose regime that would provide a satisfactory concentration of isoniazid in the tissues of those who inactivate the drug slowly might be quite inadequate in patients equipped with an acetylating mechanism. Hitherto, it has not been usual to determine the acetylator status of patients (although it is known that side effects occur more often in the slow inactivators) but recently the practice has arisen in some quarters of giving isoniazid and other antituberculosis drugs in large doses once or twice weekly instead of in smaller doses once or twice daily. These 'intermittent dose' regimens are therapeutically effective and convenient to the patient, but they do demand that the dose of drug to be given be very carefully determined: it is necessary to give enough to ensure that a therapeutically effective concentration of the drug is maintained in the tissues until the next dose is taken while ensuring that not enough is ingested to induce toxic reactions. In this situation, the rate at which the drug is metabolized becomes a critical factor and it would seem prudent to establish whether a patient who is to receive intermittent doses of isoniazid is a fast or a slow inactivator. Simple laboratory tests are available for this purpose (Russell, 1970; Ellard, Gammon and Tiitinen, 1973).

An individual who displays an unexpected and rare reaction to isoniazid by virtue of his being unable to acetylate the drug can be said to respond in an *idiosyncratic*

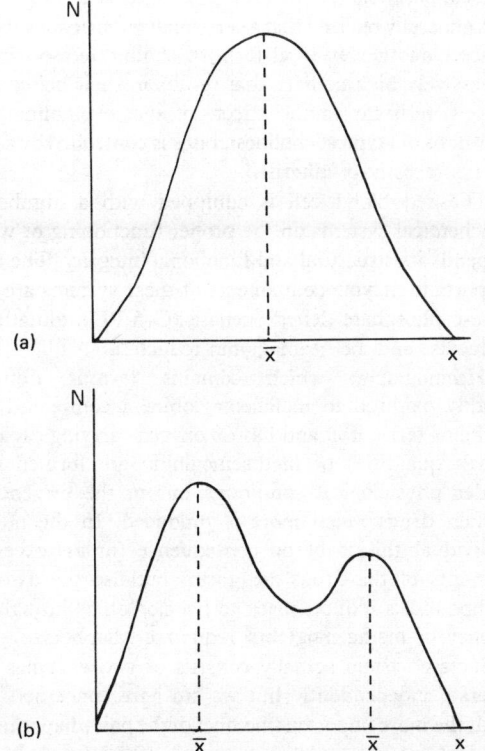

Fig. 6.1 Frequency distribution curves: (a) is the normal curve of distribution (see p. 115); (b) is a bimodal curve.

fashion. In the past it has been usual to categorize as idiosyncratic any unexpected reaction to a drug. Although this usage is semantically impeccable, the growing recognition of the importance of genetic factors had led some authorities to suggest that the adjective should be used only to describe reactions that are attributable to genetic peculiarities. There is much to be said for restricting in this way the use of a term that would lose its utility if it were permitted to embrace too large a variety of abnormal drug responses. Throughout this book, the word is used in the restricted sense.

The fine structure of enzymes, like that of all proteins, is apt to show slight variations from one species or individual to another and the acetylating enzyme is by no means the only one whose activity is critically influenced by genetic factors. It is well known that, as a result of peculiar features of their cholinesterase systems, some individuals experience idiosyncratic responses to succinylcholine. In most people, this muscle relaxing agent has a very fleeting action because it is very rapidly hydrolyzed by serum cholinesterase and the drug is employed in situations where just such an evanescent effect is required (p. 244). However, about 0.03 per cent of human subjects synthesize an atypical form of the cholinesterase with a very low affinity for some choline esters. If succinylcholine is given to a person whose cholinesterase is of the atypical variety, the resulting muscle paralysis will be both prolonged and severe. It is less generally realized that a very small minority of subjects possess another atypical form of cholinesterase with an excessively high activity that results in their being completely resistant to the effects of succinylcholine. The synthesis of atypical cholinesterases is controlled by a gene that is recessively inherited.

The red blood cell is equipped with a number of biochemical systems on the proper functioning of which depends its structural and functional integrity. The most important enzyme components of these systems are glucose-6-phosphate dehydrogenase (G-6-PD), glutathione reductase and methaemoglobin reductase.

Haemoglobin, which contains ferrous iron, is readily oxidized to methaemoglobin, a compound that contains ferric iron and has no oxygen carrying capacity. Small quantities of methaemoglobin are formed even under physiological conditions but in the presence of certain drugs much more is produced. In the normal individual this is of no consequence (unless excessive amounts of the drugs are given) because the oxidized compound is reduced back to haemoglobin through the agency of methaemoglobin reductase (diaphorase). The reductase system actually consists of two enzymes that operate independently but we are here concerned only with the more important member of the pair (diaphorase I, NADH–methaemoglobin reductase) which we shall, as is usual, simply refer to as methaemoglobin reductase.

Methaemoglobin reductase activity is genetically deter-mined and is subject to a considerable degree of variation. A few individuals lack the enzyme entirely so that they exhibit the signs of methaemoglobinaemia (predominantly an intense cyanosis) all the time since they cannot adequately handle even the small amounts of methaemoglobin that appear in the absence of drugs. A more usual condition, however, is associated with a relative deficiency of the enzyme which only becomes apparent after taking one of the drugs that can produce methaemoglobin. Among the commonly used compounds in this category are the sulphonamides, chloramphenicol, paracetamol, quinine, nitrofurantoin, primaquine, mepacrine, p-aminosalicyclic acid, sulphones, nitrates and nitrites. If the cyanosis that develops after drug taking is so deep that it indicates a gross deficiency of functional haemoglobin the methaemoglobin has to be reduced by intravenous injections to methylene blue.

A genetically determined deficiency of glucose-6-phosphate dehydrogenase is not uncommon but since it occurs predominantly in Negro and Mediterranean races it is probably better to classify it as a racial variation. A number of drugs that are innocuous when they are given in therapeutic doses may cause haemolytic anaemia and haemoglobinuria with associated nausea, vomiting and epigastric pain when they are given in excessive amounts. The erythrocyte's principal protection against haemolysis is provided by reduced glutathione, supplies of which are dependent on the activity of glucose-6-phosphate dehydrogenase. In the presence of adequate amounts of the enzyme, haemolysis does not occur unless the amount of drug that is given depletes the supplies of reduced glutathione quicker than they can be restored, but in those whose enzyme activity is deficient, haemolysis may occur, often in a very severe form, after quite small doses of the drug. This type of enzyme deficiency first came to light when it was noticed that Negro subjects sometimes reacted violently to normally therapeutic doses of primaquine (p. 867). The same deficiency also results in an increased sensitivity to nitrofurazone. This is a particularly unfortunate circumstance because nitrofurazone is a trypanocidal agent and those who are most in need of the drug will be members of coloured races. Other drugs that bring about haemolysis when glucose-6-phosphate dehydrogenase is lacking include nitrofurantoin, probenecid and a group of substances (some antipyretics, sulphonamides, sulphones and antimalarial agents) that have already been mentioned because they also cause methaemoglobinaemia.

Deficiency of glucose-6-phosphate dehydrogenase is determined by a gene carried on the X–chromosome. Because women have two such chromosomes per cell (only one of which is likely to bear the responsible gene) while men have only one, the enzyme deficiency is much more likely to appear in men than in women.

A congenital lack of glucose-6-phosphatase, the enzyme that catalyses the last step in the conversion of glycogen to glucose, occurs in (and is responsible for) von Gierke's form of glycogen storage disease. Because the glycogen cannot be broken down, it accumulates in large amounts in the liver and muscles and neither adrenaline nor glucagon is capable of exerting its normal effect of increasing the amount of glucose in the blood.

The subject of enzymes cannot be closed without at least a brief mention of acatalasia, the first genetically determined enzyme deficiency to be recognized as such. When hydrogen peroxide comes into contact with the tissues, it froths and bubbles because oxygen is released under the influence of catalase. About a quarter of a century ago, Takahara noticed that frothing did not occur when he was cleaning the wound of a particular patient with hydrogen peroxide (Takahara, 1952). He suggested, and later proved, that the patient's tissues lacked catalase and he demonstrated that acatalasia is a hereditary condition. All the cases of acatalasia so far reported have occurred in Japanese subjects but this is not to say that the condition will not appear elsewhere.

Among other effects of their condition, acatalasic subjects are hypersensitive to alcohol but if they should be tempted or driven to take methanol they will have to pay less dearly for their folly than if their enzyme system were complete. Catalase promotes the conversion of methanol to formaldehyde, the substance that causes blindness in methanol addicts. Thus the effects of a psychological weakness are blunted by a biochemical deficiency.

GENETIC DISEASES AND DRUG RESPONSES
Genetic factors can influence the body's response to drugs in a rather less direct fashion than do genetically determined enzyme abnormalities since certain diseases and abnormalities that are associated with abnormal responses to drugs have a genetic basis. Thus, in acute intermittent porphyria—a hereditary condition in which there are sporadic breakdowns of porphyrin synthesis—the metabolic disturbances consequent on the accumulation of porphyrin precursors and their metabolites produce a number of effects, the most dramatic of which are severe abdominal pain and psychotic episodes that may lead to misdiagnoses of peptic ulcer and schizophrenia respectively. The world's best known victim of intermittent porphyria, if the disputed diagnosis of Macalpine and Hunter (1969) is accepted, was George III whose well publicised madness would thus appear to have a metabolic origin. Patients who are subject to attacks of intermittent porphyria are extremely sensitive to some hypnotic drugs (especially the barbiturates), antipyretics and the sulphonamides all of which may aggravate or precipitate an attack of porphyria. These responses are truly abnormal in the sense that porphyria cannot be induced in normal subjects by these drugs in however high a dose they are given.

Porphyrins are the structural units of a number of important compounds, the best known of which are haemoglobin and the cytochromes.

Every textbook of pharmacology, including this one, issues a warning against the use of atropine, or other mydriatics, in patients with glaucoma. The thickening of the iris that accompanies pupillary dilatation may lead, it is pointed out, to an obstruction of the canal of Schlemm and hence to a further increase in intraocular pressure (p. 225). In fact, this effect occurs only in those in whom the anterior chamber of the eye is so narrow that the thickened iris can readily fill the irido-corneal angle. In this instance, drug action is modified by a genetically determined anatomical peculiarity.

OTHER RACIAL FACTORS INFLUENCING DRUG RESPONSES
The mydriatic action of atropine and of sympathomimetic amines such as cocaine is more pronounced in white than in Negro subjects. In the Chinese an intermediate degree of mydriasis is produced. It was once believed that this effect might have its origin in purely mechanical factors, the heavier deposits of pigment in the iris of Negroes restricting the contraction of the radial muscle. It is now clear that the actions of atropine elsewhere in the body are also less pronounced in Negroes and this may be related to differences in the rate with which different races dispose of the drug. In animals, too, different species show varying degrees of sensitivity to atropine. The rabbit can tolerate large doses of the drug because its tissues are rich in atropine esterase. Both the pharmacological actions and the toxic side effects of a number of other drugs differ among individuals from different races.

ENVIRONMENTAL FACTORS

Atmospheric pollution constitutes a threat to our health and well being and it has become one of the principal targets of conservationists and others who wish to save us from ourselves. This barrage of well intentioned propaganda was slow to evoke a response from pharmacologists but under the pressure of events a few are now beginning to see that atmospheric pollution can influence drug responses. Some of the pollutants are capable of inducing hepatic microsomal enzyme activity and this is probably the basis of the observation that pentazocine is disposed of more rapidly by those who breathe polluted city air than it is in country dwellers. The inducing agents are also present in tobacco smoke and their effects are additive with those of the industrial pollutants so that a heavy smoker living in a large city may well metabolize pentazocine—and, presumably a wide range of other drugs—considerably more rapidly than a non smoking countryman (Keeri-Szanto and Pomeroy, 1971).

The whole subject of the link between drug responses and environmental factors deserves a more intense study than it has so far been accorded. There are more factors than atmospheric hydrocarbons to be considered: insecticides such as DDT influence drug metabolism and we have already seen that in some circumstances our very drinking water can become lethal (p. 71).

IMMUNOLOGICAL FACTORS

For most people, penicillin is the most acceptable of drugs because it discriminates completely between infecting organisms, which it attacks, and their victim who is completely spared and who, consequently, escapes the unpleasant side effects that may occur during treatment with other drugs. A minority of patients, however, react violently to the administration of penicillin experiencing an anaphylactic shock which, in its most extreme form, may prove immediately fatal. Similarly unexpected (or 'allergic') responses of various kinds may, rarely, follow exposure to some other drugs. Allergy is certainly, therefore, one of the factors that can influence the organism's response to a drug but it is more appropriate to examine it in detail in the context of a general discussion of immunological phenomena and this is provided in Chapter 24 (p. 393).

PHARMACOLOGICAL FACTORS—DRUG INTERACTIONS

If two drugs are given together their combined effects may be greater than, the same as or smaller than the sum of the effects of the individual drugs. These three possible consequences are known as *potentiation* (or *synergism*), *addition* (or *summation*) and *antagonism* respectively. Some drug synergisms and antagonisms are well known, have been recognized for many years and are deliberately made use of for therapeutic purposes. Others may produce effects that are the reverse of beneficial and if the possibility that these interactions may occur is not taken into account when the drugs are prescribed, a dangerous potentiation or attenuation of the effect of one (or both) of the drugs might have dire consequences for the patient. The practice of giving two or more medicaments simultaneously is an old one and it is likely to become both more common and more potentially hazardous as therapeutic regimes become more sophisticated and drugs become more potent. It is undeniable that the physician needs a knowledge of drug interactions and their consequences but there is a real danger of the whole subject's attracting a disproportionate amount of attention at the expense of other equally important aspects of drug toxicity. The last few years have seen the compilation of vast catalogues of drug interactions and the uncritical or inexperienced reader can hardly be blamed if he assumes that almost any two drugs can exhibit mutual interactions, that all interactions are necessarily undesirable and that two drugs should never be given when one might serve. 'Polypharmacy', or pharmacomania as Prescott (1973) so delightfully dubs it, has almost become a term of abuse and much play has been made with the recent disclosure that in one, presumably typical, hospital, patients received an average of more than five drugs at the same time while some of them were given up to twenty different substances in the course of a single day. In the interests of acquiring a balanced outlook on the subject, the reader should bear in mind the following facts.

1. Pharmacologists should always advocate the giving of as few drugs as possible. There are indeed many conditions that require no drug treatment at all and when (as is usual) it is given it is most often merely a response to patient demand. Nevertheless, when an active intervention is needed, two drugs may well be better than one. Quite apart from the situation that arises when a patient needs to be treated for two conditions at once, there are many indications for multiple drug treatment. It may happen, for instance, that two agents have similar therapeutic actions but different side effects. Given together, they might be effective (because of summation of their therapeutic actions) at dose levels of each too small to produce side effects. Again, the successful treatment of hypertension and some other conditions is often achieved by using a number of drugs each with a different locus of action. Atropine can be used to antagonize the unwanted actions of the acetylcholine that accumulates in the body when anticholinesterases are given (p. 218) while inhibitors of dopa decarboxylase can be used to restrict the formation of dopamine to the area where it is needed by patients with Parkinson's disease receiving L-dopa (p. 590). The foregoing list could be extended almost indefinitely.

2. The fact that an interaction can occur between two drugs is not necessarily a contraindication to their use. Phenobarbitone and diphenylhydantoin given together provide a favoured treatment for grand mal epilepsy. There is an interaction between the drugs (p. 525) but, provided that the individual doses are periodically adjusted to take this into account, the utility of the combination is unimpaired.

3. Many articles on the subject of drug interactions open with a declaration of what their authors evidently believe is the self evident proposition that at least two drugs must be given before an interaction can occur. The implication that a therapeutic substance, given alone, cannot produce the interaction effect it may induce when it is a constituent of a mixture is incorrect because we all consume, or are exposed to, substances that are dealt with by the same disposal systems that rid us of drugs. Most physicians, and even some patients, are now aware that the actions of many drugs can be drastically altered by alcohol and some articles of diet but it is easy to ignore the effects of such apparently innocuous substances as laxatives, the alkali in the indigestion remedies or the iron in the 'tonics'

that are still taken by surprisingly large numbers of people whose urge to self medication ensures the continued affluence of the patent medicine manufacturer. We can go further than this because, as we have seen (p. 75), not only the tobacco smoke we can avoid but also the very air we breathe or the water we drink may be the source of potentially dangerous interactions. There is, finally, the apparently paradoxical situation that an untoward reaction may appear in a patient who, having been satisfactorily maintained on two drugs, reverts to a single drug regime (p. 81).

4. Not a few of the interactions reported in the literature are of doubtful significance. They may involve pairs of substances that are rarely, if ever, given together or the interaction effects may be so trivial that they can be disregarded. Moreover, an unexpected turn of clinical events in a patient receiving multiple drug therapy is not necessarily attributable to an interaction between some of the drugs. By the very nature of the situation it is often not practicable, desirable or permissible to carry out the further investigations that would be needed to establish the true origin of the incident which, in the absence of any other plausible explanation may enter the literature as a drug interaction effect.

5. Even when a drug interaction *can* occur this is not to say that it *will* occur in individual patients. There is a lamentable dearth of information concerning the incidence of particular reactions and of the factors that determine their appearance. It does seem, though, that interactions occur much less frequently than might be expected in view of the number of ways in which two drugs can, in theory at least, influence one another. However, as we shall see, it not infrequently happens that an interaction results in the production of two or more mutually antagonistic effects, the nett result of which is a minimal change in the effectiveness of either drug.

6. The enthusiasm of some writers may lead their more unwary readers to believe that drug interaction phenomena are invariably dramatic in onset and crippling in their impact. It is important to remember that this is not so and neither the patient nor his physician may be aware that an interaction is occurring. This is not to say that an interaction that does not announce itself is an unimportant one. On the contrary, it may take a form that results in a reduction in the amount of drug available in the tissues and the failure of a treatment that might have been successful had the physician been aware that the efficacy of his drugs had been impaired by their mutual interaction. Situations such as this will be largely avoided when we learn to regulate drug dosage by reference to measurements of the amount of drug actually present in the blood of the individual patient rather than by the blind administration of recommended doses.

Physicians and pharmacists presumably need to have access to compendia of drug interactions. They have plenty to choose from (some of the better ones are listed on p. 81) although it might be better if the information they contain were stored in accessible computers. The needs of the pharmacologist are different because he has to understand, and may have to investigate, the mechanisms of drug interactions. These are summarized in the following paragraphs. Only a few examples of the operation of each mechanism are given but they have been selected in such a way that they embrace the majority of the seriously adverse interactions that cause trouble in clinical practice. It may be that this modest list is not much less useful than the more ambitious compilations we have referred to. In this connection, the reader should be warned that manuals of drug interactions do not necessarily agree among themselves concerning either the occurrence or the effects of particular interactions. Some are not compiled or written as carefully as they might have been and in particular there is a tendency to imply, if not to declare, that all members of a group of drugs (the 'barbiturates', etc.) will interact in a fashion that has actually been established for only one or two individuals in the group. This may well be so, of course, and the wise man, warned of the potential danger attending the use, say, of one barbiturate will treat all barbiturates with circumspection. Nevertheless, a writer on a topic such as this must be as precise and accurate as possible and in the account that follows, groups of drugs will only be mentioned in a particular context if it is known that all (or at least a majority) of their members are equally suspect.

Some of the drugs that are featured in the interactions we shall examine will not yet be familiar to all readers but all of them are described, and can be located, elsewhere in this book.

Drug interactions can occur in infusion fluids, in syringes and even in prepared tablets and capsules. They are important but of no direct interest to the pharmacologist. Those who need information on the subject are referred elsewhere (see, for example, Griffin and D'Arcy, 1975).

We have seen (Chap. 5) that drug molecules are beset by many kinds of obstacles and menaced by many threats to their continued existence on the way to their site of action. Drug doses have to be large enough to ensure that a sufficient number of molecules survive these hazards and reach their targets. When one drug interacts with another it does so by influencing the effectiveness of one or more of the body's drug defence and disposal systems. We can consider them in turn.

INTERACTIONS IN THE GASTROINTESTINAL TRACT
Metal ions react with some organic compounds to form insoluble chelates (p. 796) which cannot, of course, be absorbed. Iron interferes with the absorption of tetracyclines in this way and the effectiveness of the antibiotics may be seriously impaired if iron salts are taken at the same

time. Many a patient takes iron in 'tonics' and other proprietary preparations without the knowledge of his physician whose tetracycline therapy may fail if he neglects to enquire into his patient's self medication habits.

The tetracyclines are likely to provoke gastrointestinal upsets and, unless forewarned, those who suffer in this way may seek to relieve their symptoms by taking milk or antacids. Unfortunately, the aluminium or magnesium in some antacids and the calcium in milk interfere with the absorption of tetracyclines just as does iron. A half pint of milk is sufficient to prevent almost completely the absorption of a normally therapeutic dose of a tetracycline.

While metal ions and the tetracyclines form insoluble complexes, ergotamine and caffeine form a complex that is more soluble and readily absorbed than ergotamine itself. The two drugs occur together in Cafergot.

Movements of the intestine, the acidity of its contents and pathological changes in its absorption mechanisms all influence drug absorption. These factors may themselves be modified or induced by drugs and this is the source of some other drug interactions. Thus, antacids affect the pH of the gut and self medication with sodium bicarbonate may inhibit the absorption of weakly acid substances such as salicylic acid. Atropine, morphine and their congeners delay gastric emptying and hence the absorption from the intestine of drugs taken by mouth.

p-Aminosalicylic acid, neomycin, colchicine and other drugs may give rise to malabsorption syndromes that may seriously impair the absorption of other substances. p-Aminosalicylic acid, for instance, may hinder in this way the absorption of rifampicin, an unfortunate circumstance because both drugs have antituberculosis activity and this interaction militates against their being used together as a therapeutic pair. Vitamin K is another substance whose absorption is affected in the malabsorption syndromes. Neomycin in addition prevents the endogenous production of vitamin K by reason of its lethal action on the intestinal organisms that synthesize the vitamin. A reduction of the amount of vitamin K that reaches the blood constitutes a hazard for the many people who need anticoagulant therapy because the deficiency may seriously potentiate the effect of the anticoagulants (vitamin K promotes coagulation, p. 673) in conditions where survival may depend on the maintenance of a critical degree of blood coagulability. The malabsorption syndrome produced by colchicine particularly affects the absorption of vitamin B_{12} while absorption of the fat soluble vitamins may be hampered by cholestyramine (which combines with bile salts) and liquid paraffin. Conversely, dietary components may have an effect on the absorption of drugs: a high fat diet promotes the absorption of fat soluble drugs such as griseofulvin and tetrachloroethylene. As far as the last named substance is concerned, this constitutes a disadvantage because the drug should be confined to the intestine.

INTERFERENCE WITH PROTEIN BINDING

We have seen in an earlier chapter (p. 51) that many drugs are extensively bound to plasma protein, that the bound portion of the dose cannot exert a pharmacological action and that a substance with a high affinity for the binding sites can competitively displace one with a lower affinity. Consequently, if a patient is receiving a potent drug that undergoes a high degree of binding to plasma protein and whose effectiveness had been secured by a careful dose adjustment, the intrusion of another drug might release some of the protein bound fraction of the original agent to provoke a dangerous increase in the amount of pharmacologically active material in the tissues. The danger, in theory at least, is greatest for drugs that are most extensively bound to the plasma proteins: some substances (warfarin, an anticoagulant drug, is an example) are bound to the extent of 98 per cent or more, so that a mere two per cent reduction in the quantity of bound drug would virtually double the amount of active material available for distribution. In practice, adverse reactions from this cause do not occur nearly as often as might be expected in the light of the high incidence of protein binding. This is partly because an increase in the amount of uncombined drug in the plasma will often be accompanied by an increased metabolism and urinary excretion by virtue of the fact that more drug is available for the enzymes and the glomerular filters and partly because the increase in the concentration of the free drug will not be very great if the distribution volume (p. 48) is large, as it is for many basic drugs. The relatively few adverse interactions attributable to drug displacement all relate to acidic substances with a restricted volume of distribution.

Anticoagulants of the coumarin type (particularly warfarin) can be displaced by antiinflammatory drugs such as phenylbutazone, oxyphenbutazone and the salicylates and by clofibrate. Any of these substances can dangerously reduce the coagulability of the blood if it is given to a patient whose intake of anticoagulant drug is not suitably adjusted. Chloral hydrate, the hypnotic, also displaces anticoagulants from the binding sites on the plasma proteins and this interaction is instructive on two counts. In the first place, it is to be noted that the actual displacing agent is trichloroacetic acid, a metabolite of the hypnotic. The second feature of this interaction is that, against all expectations, the taking of chloral hydrate may not affect, or may even increase, the coagulability of the blood of patients who are already receiving anticoagulant drugs. This appears to be the result of an enhanced metabolism and it underlines the point made earlier concerning the relative rarity of adverse drug reactions attributable to drug displacement.

The antiinflammatory agents mentioned in the preceding paragraph also displace tolbutamide and chlorpropamide (these are oral hypoglycaemic agents of the sulphonylurea group) from the binding sites and can induce a profound hypoglycaemia in mildly diabetic patients being maintained on these drugs. Some of the sulphonamides can also displace the sulphonylureas but not the anticoagulant drugs. On the contrary, the anticoagulants dislodge the sulphonamides. Salicylates also displace diphenylhydantoin and both they and the sulphonamides have a similar effect on methotrexate, an anticancer drug.

In another context, we have already mentioned the ability of vitamin K and the sulphonamides to displace bilirubin from its temporary union with plasma proteins with possibly fatal results in the newborn (p. 70). It should also be noted that one drug can dislodge another from binding sites in the tissues. Thus, among the antimalarial drugs, chloroquine and mepacrine can displace pamaquin from hepatic binding sites.

INTERACTION AT A COMMON RECEPTOR

'Drug interaction at receptor sites' could almost be offered as a definition of the field of study of pharmacologists. Many of our drugs operate at receptor sites where they antagonize or potentiate the effects of the endogenous substances that normally activate the receptor. Indeed, our hopes of developing rational treatments for the diseases that remain unconquered will in many instances have to wait on the discovery of more agents that will interact with physiological agonists at the appropriate receptor sites. On the other hand, the number of adverse and unexpected responses that can be attributed to this mechanism is very small. The best known instance concerns a group of antihypertensive drugs (bethanidine, debrisoquine and guanethidine) that are taken up into noradrenergic neurones by the mechanism that brings about the termination of transmitter action (p. 291). A number of psychotropic drugs including imipramine, chlorpromazine and amphetamine, are transported into the neurone in the same way and they can compete with the antihypertensive drugs (and with noradrenaline) for the receptor and the carrier. A patient whose hypertension has been stabilized with the aid of one of the drugs that are taken up by adrenergic neurones may suffer serious hypertension if he is then incautiously given one of the psychotropic drugs.

INTERACTIONS ON A COMMON PHYSIOLOGICAL SYSTEM

Drugs do not necessarily have to influence the same receptor in order to exert an effect on a physiological system (see, for example, the discussion on noncompetitive antagonism on p. 101) and some adverse interactions arise because drugs intervene at different points in a particular chain of functional control. Thus, thiazide diuretics bring about a reduction in the potassium content of the tissues and thereby increase the toxicity of the cardiac glucosides which may well be being given at the same time. Again, propranolol can be employed to correct disturbances of cardiac rhythm in unanaesthetized subjects but it has a depressant action on cardiac muscle which can become dangerously potentiated in patients anaesthetized with ether, an anaesthetic that itself depresses the myocardium. Propranolol also potentiates the hypoglycaemia induced by insulin because it prevents the production of glucose by the liver. Salicylates and the monoamine oxidase inhibitors exert a similar action.

As we discuss in detail elsewhere (p. 239), some general anaesthetics potentiate the action of neuromuscular blocking agents of the antidepolarizing variety. Since the two types of drug are frequently given together, it is important that the anaesthetist should be aware of the extent to which he should reduce the dose of the muscle relaxant when particular anaesthetics are to be given. The aminoglycoside antibiotics have a similar potentiating action.

The list of reactions of the type just mentioned could be extended almost indefinitely (as indeed it is in some publications) but many of the so-called 'interactions' that are commonly cited in this context hardly warrant inclusion in lists intended to draw attention to adverse reactions that might take an unwary practitioner by surprise. Thus, since both sedatives and, say, thiazide diuretics are well known as antihypertensive agents, it should be self evident that the blood pressure of a patient receiving treatment with the diuretic will be likely to fall still further if he is then given a sedative.

INTERFERENCE WITH DRUG METABOLISM

Those who have witnessed the development of the present interest in drug interactions will recall that it all began some twelve years ago with reports of the severe and sometimes fatal hypertensive crises that occurred in patients who partook of certain items of food or drink during treatment with monoamine oxidase inhibitors. The offending materials included such delicacies as cheese and Chianti wine as well as the more prosaic pickled herrings, yeast extracts (such as Marmite), Bovril and beer. They all contain small amounts of tyramine, a pressor amine. The eating of broad beans (which contain dopamine) or bananas (which contain 5-hydroxytryptamine) by those receiving monoamine oxidase inhibitors is fraught with the same danger as that which attends the ingestion of substances that contain tyramine. All three monoamines are normally destroyed by monoamine oxidase in the gut and liver but if the enzyme is inhibited they pass without hindrance to the tissues and so can exert a hypertensive action. The enzymatic inactivation of pethidine is also prevented by monoamine oxidase inhibitors and a normally harmless dose of the analgesic may become seriously toxic (even to the point of causing death) in patients who are also receiving a monoamine oxidase inhibitor.

Monoamine oxidase inhibitors also potentiate the action of indirectly acting sympathomimetic amines (which operate by releasing noradrenaline from neurones) such as amphetamine, ephedrine and many of the appetite suppressing drugs even though these substances are not substrates for monoamine oxidase. This is because the enzyme inhibitors, by preventing the intraneuronal destruction of noradrenaline, increase the amount of transmitter available for release. It is also known that they can unspecifically reduce the activity of a number of hepatic microsomal enzymes and this action might, theoretically at least, contribute to the interaction by retarding the inactivation and so prolonging the action of the sympathomimetic amines. The relevance of this last mentioned mechanism is difficult to assess because animal experiments indicate that it only begins to assume importance at dose levels far in excess of those used therapeutically. If the microsomal enzymes are affected in man at more modest dose levels than they are in the animal species that have so far been studied, monoamine oxidase inhibitors might (as some authors declare they do) potentiate the action of a large number of other drugs including alcohol, the coumarin type of anticoagulants and some of the antiacetylcholine agents employed in the treatment of Parkinson's disease.

Monoamine oxidase inhibitors are certainly the villains of this particular piece and seemingly endless lists of the adverse interactions in which they are said to participate can be found in the literature. It is, perhaps, fortunate (for all except those who have devoted so much energy to the compilation of these lists) that monoamine oxidase inhibitors now occupy a very insignificant place in the therapeutic armoury.

Other examples of drug interactions that can be attributed to one drug's inhibiting the metabolism of another include the potentiating effect of chloramphenicol, dicoumarol, diphenylhydantoin, phenylbutazone and sulphaphenazole on the hypoglycaemia induced by the oral hypoglycaemic agents, the potentiation of the tricyclic antidepressant drugs by perphenazine and the toxic responses to alcohol in patients taking metronidazole (p. 882).

An important group of drug interactions occurs because of the ability of some substances to stimulate the metabolic transformation of others. It is worth noting that the discovery of some of them considerably predated that of the interaction between foods and monoamine oxidase inhibitors.

If a drug that is partly or wholly metabolized by enzymes in the liver microsomes is taken repeatedly, it may induce the synthesis of more enzyme protein so that the drug is more rapidly inactivated and so less effective. This response provides a partial explanation for the phenomenon of tolerance (p. 83). However, the microsomal enzymes are far from specific and the enhanced metabolizing capacity extends to other substances that are degraded by the induced enzyme. Sometimes, both members of a pair of drugs induce enzyme activity so that each accelerates the breakdown of the other. The barbiturates, among which phenobarbitone is especially active, constitute the best known group of microsomal enzyme inducers. They hasten not only their own transformation but also that of a number of other drugs particularly the coumarin anticoagulants and diphenylhydantoin but including also the tricyclic antidepressant drugs, chlorpromazine and some steroids. In a similar fashion, glutethimide promotes the metabolism of warfarin and dipyrone while griseofulvin does the same for warfarin. Diphenylhydantoin stimulates the catabolism of metyrapone and some steroids while alcohol reduces the effectiveness of diphenylhydantoin and tolbutamide. It also accelerates the breakdown of barbiturates but nevertheless potentiates their action because of a similar depressant action on central nervous function.

A drug that simulates microsomal enzyme activity does not invariably accelerate the disappearance of other drugs that suffer degradation by the same mechanism. An illuminating example is provided by the fate of mixtures of phenytoin and phenobarbitone. Although each drug can stimulate the metabolism of the other, the amount of phenytoin in the blood of an individual who has been receiving only this drug may fall, rise or undergo no change if phenobarbitone is added to his medication. A fall (the 'expected' response) is the result of the increased activity of the hepatic microsomal enzymes induced by the barbiturate, a rise occurs if the phenobarbitone successfully competes with phenytoin for the available enzyme and no change takes place if the two other effects just counteract each other. The three possible responsers occur with equal frequency (p. 525).

We have seen already that chloral hydrate stimulates the disposal of dicoumarol and have mentioned that atmospheric pollutants, tobacco smoke and some pesticides are effective enzyme inducers.

Attempts have been made to turn to good therapeutic effect the enzyme inducing proclivity of the barbiturates (Wilson, 1972). Bilirubin is a potentially lethal substance in infants because of the immaturity of their conjugating mechanisms (p. 70). Provided that some enzyme activity is present in the first place, phenobarbitone will induce glucuronyl transferase activity and lead to a more effective clearance of bilirubin. The suggestion that premature infants should receive phenobarbitone for some days after birth has not been generally adopted (there are other ways of treating hyperbilirubinaemia and the barbiturates are not the safest of drugs) but the investigations have certainly served to underline the considerable potency of the barbiturates as enzyme inducers.

INTERACTION WITH EXCRETORY MECHANISMS

Acid and alkali conditions in the tubular fluid of the kidney favour the re-absorption (and thus the retention in the body) of weak acids and weak bases respectively, just as they do in the gastrointestinal tract. Thus, sodium bicarbonate taken in an attempt to quell the gastrointestinal upsets that so often accompany the ingestion of amphetamine will facilitate both the absorption of the drug and its retention in the body and so will enhance its effects. Conversely of course, acidification of the urine will hasten the drug's elimination and the manoeuvre of adjusting urinary acidity in the appropriate direction is one of the steps that can be taken to treat poisoning by weakly acid or weakly basic drugs. In this context, 'weak' can be taken to include substances with pK_a values (p. 41) of about 7.5 to 10.5 for bases and 3.0 to 7.5 for acids. It should hardly be necessary to add that tubular reabsorption is only a significant factor in prolonging a pharmacological effect if the material in the tubular fluid is either unchanged drug or an active metabolite.

A number of drugs enter the urine by secretion across the tubular wall and they can compete with one another for the available carrier. This competition is made use of when probenicid is given in association with penicillin in order to ensure a high tissue concentration of the antibiotic but it may also cause an adverse reaction if two (or more) drugs are given in ignorance of their tendency to compete in this way. Thus phenylbutazone can prevent the excretion of chlorpropamide and the active metabolite of acetohexamide and this can be the origin of an unexpectedly severe hypoglycaemia. Dicoumarol has a similar effect, at least on chlorpropamide excretion, while salicylates and sulphonamides hinder the disposal of methotrexate. The interaction between salicylates and uricosuric drugs constitutes a problem that is discussed on p. 459.

Before leaving this subject, two points need to be made. The first is the reiteration of the fact that drug interactions may make their presence felt when a patient reverts to taking one drug after a period of multiple drug therapy. Consider, for instance, the person who, after a myocardial infarction is taking an anticoagulant drug such as warfarin but who is also receiving a barbiturate either as a general sedative or as a means of securing a night of undisturbed sleep. As we have seen, the barbiturate will, after a time, accelerate the metabolism of warfarin but this is of no consequence because laboratory facilities will be available to monitor the effectiveness of the drug, the dose of which will in any event need occasional adjustment at first because of the operation of several factors of which the drug interaction is only one. Leaving hospital with his drug doses stabilized the patient, unless forewarned, may decide that he does not need to take the barbiturate now that he has exchanged the stress and disturbances of his hospital days for a life of domestic peace and tranquillity. If he does omit the barbiturate, the metabolism of his anticoagulant will slow and this may lead to a dangerous decrease in his blood's coagulability and to serious haemorrhages. The danger is greater by reason of the fact that a period of two to three weeks must elapse before the activity of the microsomal enzyme reverts to its pre-induction level. Since no untoward event will occur in the period

immediately following withdrawal of the barbiturate, our patient is likely to be lulled into the belief that no harm has been done by this unauthorized modification of his drug intake.

The other point concerns the multiplicity of drug interactions. If we are to judge by the compendia, the number that can occur is almost limitless but the reader will have noticed that only a few substances have featured in our descriptions of life-threatening interactions. He will also have seen that some drugs and drug groups have been referred to in several different contexts. While nothing absolves the practitioner from considering the potential hazards of any drug combination (or indeed of any single drug) that he is to prescribe, it may be useful to remind him that, while the price of safety is eternal vigilance, the patients most exposed to danger from adverse drug interactions are those who are receiving, among their other medicaments, anticoagulants, oral hypoglycaemic agents, cytotoxic drugs or cardiac glycosides (Prescott, 1973).

Some other interactions are more appropriately described in sections of this book that consider the actions of particular groups of drugs. The reader is referred particularly, in this connection, to discussions of interactions involving anticonvulsive agents (p. 525) and oral contraceptives (p. 750).

BIBLIOGRAPHY

Books, monographs and reviews

Catzel, P. (1974) *The Paediatric Prescriber.* 4th edn. Oxford: Blackwell.

Gant, B. R. and Waller, R. H. (1973 on.) *Drug Interaction Index.* Kelowna, Canada: Meditec Publications.

Garb, S. (1973) *Undesirable Drug Interactions.* London: Harvey Miller and Metcalf.

Gillette, J. R. and Mitchell, J. R. (eds.) (1975) *Concepts in Biochemical Pharmacology, Part III.* Berlin: Springer.

Griffin, J. P. and D'Arcy, P. F. (1975) *A Manual of Adverse Drug Interactions.* Bristol: Wright.

Hansten, P. D. (1973) *Drug Interactions,* 2nd ed. Philadelphia: Lea and Febiger.

Kalow, W. (1962) *Pharmacogenetics,* Philadelphia and London: Saunders.

Macalpine, Ida and Hunter, R. (1964) *George III and the Mad Business.* London: Allan Lane, the Penguin Press.

Meier, H. (1963) *Experimental Pharmacogenetics.* New York and London: Academic Press.

Prescott, L. F.(1973) Clinically important drug interactions. *Drugs,* **5,** 161–186.

Smith, S. E. and Rawlins, M. D. (1973) *Variability in Human Drug Responses.* London: Butterworths.

Stockley, I. H. (1973) *Drug Interactions and their Mechanisms.* London: Pharmaceutical Press.

Swidler, G. (1971) *Handbook of Drug Interactions.* New York: Wiley Interscience.

Szórády, I. (1973) *Pharmacogenetics—Principles and Paediatric Aspects.* Budapest: Hungarian Academy of Sciences.

Wilson, J. T. (1972) Developmental pharmacology: a review of its application to clinical and basic science. *A. Rev. Pharmac.* **12,** 423–450.

Original papers

Ellard, G. A. Gammon, Patricia and Tiitinen, Hilkka (1973) Determination of the acetylator phenotype from the ratio of the urinary excretion of acetylisoniazid to acid labile isoniazid: a study in Finnish Lapland. *Tubercle,* **54,** 201-210.

Evans, D. A. P., Manley, K. A. and McKusick, V. A. (1960) Genetic control of isoniazid metabolism in man. *Br. med. J.,* **ii,** 485-491.

Keeri-Szanto, M. and Pomeroy, J. R. (1971) Atmospheric pollution and pentazocine. *Lancet,* **i,** 947-949.

Prescott, L. R. (1969) Pharmacokinetic drug interactions. *Lancet,* **ii,** 1239-1243.

Russell, D. W. (1970) Simple method for determining isoniazid acetylator phenotype. *Br. Med. J.,* **3,** 324-325.

Takahara, S. (1952) Progressive oral gangrene probably due to lack of catalase in the blood (acatalazemia). *Lancet,* **ii,** 1101-1104.

7. Drug dependence and related conditions

In the not so distant past it was possible to speak of drug addiction and to define the condition in terms which would satisfy most pharmacologists. It was also possible, though with rather more difficulty, to define a condition of habituation and to differentiate it from addiction. With the recent increase in the range of drugs whose consumption for non-therapeutic purposes poses special social problems, it has become clear that the older definitions are no longer tenable and that to extend them to include all types of drug abuse would result in the formulation of definitions so vague and tortuous as to be quite useless. Recognizing this, the World Health Organization suggested in 1964 that the general term *drug dependence* should be used to include the conditions previously described as habituation and addiction. When drug dependence is referred to, its nature can be specified, if necessary, by reference to a known drug. Thus it might have to be said of a newly discovered analgesic that 'this drug produces dependence of the morphine type'.

In this chapter, some of the more easily defined consequences of repeated drug administration are discussed before consideration is given to the general problem of drug dependence. Some account is also given of the history of the term addiction.

TOLERANCE

It is a well known fact that if a drug is taken repeatedly it is likely to become progressively less effective so that the dose has to be increased if the drug's original action is to be maintained. This is the phenomenon of *tolerance*. Tolerance occurs to a large proportion—but by no means all—of the drugs taken by man and some examples will be familiar to the reader who recalls the effects produced by his first cigarette or first dose of alcohol. Tolerance will develop if the drug becomes more rapidly metabolized or excreted or less readily absorbed or if its distribution in the tissues changes. This form of tolerance can be called *dispositional tolerance*. Another major form of tolerance, that may occur independently of or in association with, a degree of dispositional tolerance, is *cellular tolerance*. This is the result of an actual change in the responsiveness of the tissues to the drug and it is a manifestation of an important property of living matter—that of *adaptation*. Living organisms tend in general to respond to changes in their environment rather than to the environment itself. If the environment is altered for a more or less lengthy period within immedi-

ately tolerable limits, the organism adapts itself so that it now responds to acute changes in this new environment. Touch receptors in the skin, for instance, very soon become adapted to the imposition of a steady pressure and a conscious sensation of touch is experienced only when this steady pressure changes. Again (though a different nervous mechanism is involved in this instance) if one sits in a bath of hot water the sensation of intense warmth soon disappears but it is immediately experienced again if a previously unimmersed limb is placed in the water. This type of adaptive response clearly has the same sort of survival value as has the development of tolerance to drugs. That it involves a different mechanism should occasion no surprise: adaptation is so vital a process and it demands a changed response to so wide a range of stimuli that it is only to be expected that the organism should have available a range of mechanisms to effect it.

Tolerance is clearly a form of *drug resistance*. It is induced by exposure of the individual to the drug in question. In some species, however, resistance to some drugs is inborn. Thus exposure of bacteria to sulphonamides or antibiotics may result in their being able to produce highly resistant strains of the organism. Another type of drug resistance is that exemplified by the rabbit, which is unaffected by doses of atropine which would be lethal in other species.

When tolerance develops it is not necessarily exhibited equally towards all the actions of the drug. Thus pethidine has analgesic and atropine like properties. Tolerance to the analgesic effect may develop even when sensitivity to the atropine like actions is unimpaired.

The tolerance that develops to some drugs also causes tolerance of drugs of the same pharmacological class. This is the phenomenon of *cross tolerance*. Cross tolerance may be specific or non-specific in type. Specific cross tolerance occurs between drugs with closely related pharmacological actions. A drug to which an individual has become tolerant may be replaced by one showing specific cross tolerance with the original drug and the state of tolerance will be completely maintained. Specific cross tolerance is exhibited between morphine and many morphine like analgesics. In non-specific cross tolerance, adaptation to the first drug causes only partial tolerance to others. Thus the person who has become tolerant to morphine is capable of taking somewhat larger doses of barbiturate before becoming heavily sedated than is the normal subject.

Attempts to elucidate the physiological and cellular reactions which underlie the development of tolerance are discussed below (p. 93).

TACHYPHYLAXIS

Tolerance to drugs usually develops over a more or less lengthy period in contrast to the rapid adaptation to touch, heat and other modalities of sensation. Rapid adaptation to the action of some drugs does, however, occur both in isolated preparations and, less frequently, in the whole animal. Thus, if 5-hydroxytryptamine is repeatedly added to, and washed out from, an organ bath in which is suspended a piece of guinea pig ileum, successive contractile responses are progressively reduced in amplitude. This rapidly developing tolerance is known as *tachyphylaxis*. The word means 'rapid protection' (*cf*. prophylaxis and anaphylaxis) and it clearly expresses the adaptive nature of the rapidly changing response. It should be noted that tachyphylaxis is much less commonly seen than is tolerance and it tends to be rather selective in its incidence. Thus, although the response of the guinea pig ileum to 5-hydroxytryptamine shows tachyphylaxis, the response to acetylcholine usually does not. Equally, the action of 5-hydroxytryptamine on the smooth muscle of some other organs does not display tachyphylaxis.

No single mechanism is responsible for the appearance of tachyphylaxis. In some instances it is caused by exhaustion of the stores of the agent which is ultimately responsible for the effect evoked by the drug. Thus, some of the sympathomimetic agents exert their pharmacological effects by causing the liberation of noradrenaline from tissue stores and the response to the drug will fall off if repeated doses deplete the stores more rapidly than they can be replenished. When tachyphylaxis is the result of the operation of this type of mechanism, related compounds will show cross tachyphylaxis.

Tachyphylaxis will also occur if the drug dissociates only slowly from its combination with the receptor so that a progressively increasing proportion of the receptor molecules is not accessible to successive doses of the drug. In the majority of instances, however, tachyphylaxis probably represents a truly adaptive response in the tissue. The nature of this adaptive response is still obscure.

SENSITIZATION

It sometimes happens that repeated doses of a drug cause a progressive increase in the response of the tissue or the organism. This is the phenomenon of *sensitization*. Sensitization is seen less often than tachyphylaxis. It should be distinguished from the sensitization which is produced in the whole animal by the administration of a foreign protein and which results in anaphylactic shock if another dose of protein is given (p. 402). In anaphylaxis the response of the animal to the second dose of protein is qualitatively different from the response to the first dose. In sensitization of the type discussed here, the response progressively increases in magnitude until a maximum is reached but the nature of the response does not alter.

Another type of sensitization occurs as a result of the interaction of two different drugs, the first of which acts as a sensitizing agent. Sensitizing drugs can operate in several ways: they may facilitate the absorption, prevent the destruction or inhibit the excretion of the second drug. On the other hand, the sensitizing drug may exert its effect at the receptor level by making receptors more accessible, by increasing the affinity of drug and receptor or by increasing the intrinsic activity (p. 98) of the second drug.

A particular form of sensitization is that shown by denervated structures which become supersensitive to the transmitter which, in the absence of denervation, would have been liberated from their nerves. Striated muscle, for instance, becomes much more sensitive to acetylcholine after its motor nerve supply has been cut. When the nerve degenerates, the muscle is no longer exposed to continued bombardment by molecules of acetylcholine. This seems to be the origin of the supersensitivity, for exactly the same result is achieved if the motor nerves are left intact and the animal is given botulinum toxin, a drug that prevents the release of acetylcholine from the nerves. The relationship between cessation of acetylcholine output and the development of increased receptor sensitivity is discussed elsewhere (p. 94).

PHYSICAL DEPENDENCE

In the majority of instances in which tolerance to a drug has developed, the adaptive changes that have taken place in the organism are such that no untoward reaction occurs if administration of the drug ceases. Some drugs, however—and they are all central nervous system depressants—produce more far-reaching adaptive changes and the metabolism of the nervous system is apparently affected to such an extent that normal functioning can only continue in the presence of the drug. A condition of *physical dependence* has been produced. If the drug is withheld after physical dependence has developed, withdrawal symptoms (*the abstinence syndrome*) occur since the brain is no longer being supplied with what has become an essential component of its environment. The withdrawal symptoms (which are described in more detail below) are always unpleasant, sometimes exceedingly so. It was this condition of physical dependence that was originally defined as *addiction*. There are still a few authorities who use the word in its original sense, insisting that the only drugs which can be truly called drugs of addiction are those which produce physical dependence. It is, however, misleading to place these drugs in a separate category from those that cause other types of dependence. To do so implies that drugs that cause physical dependence are somehow 'worse' than the rest, that when an individual takes one of these drugs he necessarily becomes dependent on it and that he continues to take it only because he fears the consequences of withdrawal. None of these supposi- tions is any more correct than the implicit corollary that the drug taker becomes less firmly 'hooked' to a drug that does not induce physical dependence than to those that do.

The drugs most likely to cause physical dependence are morphine and its congeners, alcohol, some barbiturates and a few of the so-called tranquillizers. As will be seen, the symptoms produced by withdrawal of these drugs from the dependent subject vary with the drug but they are all of an excitatory nature—that is, they affect the central nervous system in the opposite sense to that of the drugs themselves.

Physical dependence cannot occur without tolerance but tolerance does not of itself produce physical depen- dence. One or more of a variety of ill defined symptoms— drowsiness, restlessness, tremor, apprehension, a general sense of unease, etc.—commonly follows the abrupt with- drawal of almost any centrally acting drug that has been taken regularly over a period of time. There are those who would maintain that these changes constitute an absti- nence syndrome, albeit a mild one, and that, therefore, all habit forming drugs can induce a degree of physical dependence. To assert this, and to invoke the fact of these changes to justify the extension of the term 'addiction' (in the sense in which it was originally defined) to the state generated by all the drugs that are taken for nontherapeu- tic purposes is to misunderstand the true nature of a physical abstinence syndrome. Abstinence syndromes take forms that are quite specific to the particular type of drug that has been withdrawn. In other words, it should be possible by observing an individual in the throes of a withdrawal state to deduce from his behaviour the nature of the drug from which he has recently been separated.

In the interests of absolute accuracy it should be added here that we know of at least one drug that sometimes induces in those who take it a condition that can be properly described as physical dependence but which does not affect the central nervous system. The identity of this drug is revealed on page 630.

PSYCHIC (PSYCHOLOGICAL OR EMOTIONAL) DEPENDENCE

Even when the original definition of addiction was formu- lated, it was realized that there were some drugs that caused no physical dependence but once taken, resulted in their user's developing an overpowering compulsion to continue taking the drug. The best known example of this type of drug is cocaine. Cocaine takers acquire little or no tolerance to the drug—many, indeed, become partly sensitized to it—and physical dependence does not develop. Nevertheless the cocaine taker continues taking the drug because the euphoria and excitement which cocaine produces contrasts so vividly with the drabness of life without it. Thus he becomes as firmly 'hooked' to his drug as the opium eater is to his. For this reason, many

wished to include cocaine among the drugs of addiction and in order to achieve this while still making at least a token gesture of respect to the original definition, the term *psychic, psychological* or *emotional dependence* was intro- duced. A drug of addiction thus came to mean, for many, a drug that caused either physical or psychic dependence. This extension of the definition, however, brought its own difficulties because a large number of substances cause some degree of psychic dependence in the sense that the taker would be unhappy with them. Caffeine and tobacco are two very obvious examples of this. Millions of people throughout the world are emotionally dependent on caf- feine but no one wished to call caffeine a drug of addiction. Equally, tobacco was not classified as addictive, although there is overwhelming evidence that smoking is harmful to the individual's health and, as many people know only too well, it can be extremely difficult to break the tobacco habit. So yet another term had to be coined and caffeine, tobacco and other drugs that produce a more or less benign type of dependence (at least from the psychological point of view) were designated habit forming. The condition they produce was called *habituation*.

In order to make clear the differences between addiction and habituation and to enable such drugs as cocaine to be incorporated within the category of drugs of addiction, the World Health Organization formulated the following definitions in 1957. They are now moribund but it is worth reviving them at this stage in our story if only to demon- strate the impossibility of constraining the effects of a wide variety of drugs within rigid definitions.

'*Drug addiction* is a state of periodic or chronic intoxication produced by the repeated consumption of a drug (natural or synthetic). Its characteristics include:

1. an overpowering desire or need (compulsion) to continue taking the drug and to obtain it by any means
2. a tendency to increase the dose
3. a psychic (psychological) and, generally, a physical depen- dence on the effects of the drug
4. a detrimental effect on the individual and society.

Drug habituation (habit) is a condition resulting from the repeated consumption of a drug. Its characteristics include:

1. a desire (but not a compulsion) to continue taking the drug for the sense of improved well-being which it engenders
2. little or no tendency to increase the dose
3. some degree of psychic dependence on the effect of the drug but absence of physical dependence and hence of an abstinence syndrome
4. detrimental effects, if any, primarily on the individual.'

A careful examination of these definitions in the light of present day knowledge concerning drugs and drug takers will reveal their many weaknesses. The differences between 'desire' and 'compulsion' are tenuous, there is sometimes a tendency to increase the dose of drugs which would be otherwise described as habit forming rather than addictive and a definition of what is detrimental to society varies with the individual. None would deny that morphine is, in the original sense of the term, a drug of addiction yet it is difficult to see in what way the addict, taking the drug in the solitude of his room, is damaging society. On the other hand it might quite reasonably be asserted that the man who kills himself in his prime by an excessive consumption of tobacco damages society because he deprives it prematurely of the skills and talents he has acquired over the years. The word 'intoxication' is not well defined and there is not generally a physical dependence on drugs that otherwise fit the definition of addiction. Finally, the two definitions tend falsely to suggest that two entirely different conditions are being named and that one of them is necessarily less dangerous than the other. For these and other reasons, the more recent recommendations of the World Health Organization will be adopted here and the term dependence will be taken to include the conditions previously defined as addiction and habituation. 'Addict', however, need not be entirely eschewed: it is still a useful word if it is simply used to describe a person who has a strong desire to take a drug other than for therapeutic purposes. It can also, of course, be attached even more loosely to an individual with an obsessional adherence to some particular pursuit. Attempts to restrict it to one who takes a drug of addiction, as defined by the earlier formulations, should, however, be avoided.

For the purposes of description, it is convenient to divide drugs causing dependence into those that induce physical dependence (and hence an abstinence syndrome) and those that cause only psychological dependence.

Drugs that cause physical dependence

It has already been mentioned that all the drugs in this category are central nervous system depressants and that the abstinence syndrome produced on withdrawal is dominated by signs of central excitation. Broadly speaking, this excitation takes two forms: a generalized hyperirritability of the somatic and autonomic nervous systems characterizes withdrawal from morphine and related analgesics while psychotic behaviour and convulsions typify the abstinence syndrome produced by a number of sedative-hypnotic drugs and some tranquillizers.

MORPHINE AND RELATED COMPOUNDS

Morphine is the archetype of all the drugs that cause physical dependence. The traditional source is opium. It is smoked or taken by mouth in the form of opium pills or as laudanum (tincture of opium). More sophisticated addicts take morphine itself by hypodermic injection. Considerable tolerance develops towards morphine: De Quincey (whose book 'Confessions of an English Opium Eater', first published in 1821, provides a fascinating insight into the motivations and experiences of an opium addict) took more than 20 grams of opium daily. The maximum therapeutic dose is 20 mg. There is cross tolerance with the other morphine like analgesics.

Although tolerance develops towards the central depressant actions of morphine, there is less adaptation to the excitatory and peripheral actions and the morphine taker itches, has pinpoint pupils and suffers severe constipation.

The morphine dependent person tends to be a solitary, introverted individual: his sensibility is depressed and he becomes unconscious of his own miseries, a fact which explains why, in the past, some rulers have not discouraged opium taking by their subjects. The psychological characteristics of the morphine taker, as just enumerated, may be as much predisposing factors which precipitate his drug habit as consequences of it.

The regular taking of morphine is not necessarily incompatible with the maintenance of normal health and undiminished mental powers. Tolerance, after all, implies adaptation and the psychiatrically normal individual who remains in full control of himself and his drug taking behaviour can continue to live a productive life. The English Lakeland poets, to quote just one example, included a number of opium addicts among their number. The situation is entirely different when the drug taking reflects an abnormal mental state and is adopted in an effort to escape from the realities of life or to create a euphoric state of mind that enables those of inadequate personality to forget their deficiencies.

With but a few exceptions, all the other morphine like analgesics produce dependence. Special mention must be made of two of them—pethidine (meperidine) and heroin (diacetylmorphine).

Pethidine is an analgesic with minimal hypnotic properties so that it has been widely used, particularly in obstetrics. Its ability to produce dependence is not always fully appreciated but it is in fact a favourite drug among those addicts (such as hospital workers and medical practitioners) who have easy access to it.

There is an impression among both addicts and those who work among them that heroin gives rise to a much more intense euphoria than does morphine. It is by no means certain that this is so—the more rapid onset of heroin's action may be partly responsible for its popular reputation—but many drug users certainly believe that heroin provides the ultimate in drug induced states and those who have once adopted the drug tend to remain very firmly attached to it. It has been stated that the personality degenerates rapidly under the influence of heroin but it is difficult to know whether the personality changes are the consequence or the cause of the drug taking.

Heroin can be taken by mouth or as a snuff but the hardened drug taker prefers hypodermic ('skin pops' in the addict's jargon) or intravenous injection ('mainlining' or 'shooting up'). Among drug takers, syringes are sometimes difficult to come by, particularly in the United States, and they are sometimes loaned in exchange for doses of heroin. The possibly dire consequences of intravenous injections made by inexperienced operators using communal and often home made syringes need no elaboration here. The reasons why 'mainlining' is preferred and the immediate effects of a heroin injection, are described by a young heroin taker:

'When you snort heroin, you know, it got a bad bitter taste, like a taste that would turn your stomach inside out. It got some way-out taste…so I started shooting up. Shooting up you don't get the taste: all you get is a fast rush and a boss feeling…you're in your own world in other words. You ain't got no problems whatsoever…you got that boss feeling, man, like you're your own boss, there ain't nobody can tell you what to do in this world' (Rodriguez, 1964).

THE MORPHINE ABSTINENCE SYNDROME

All the morphine like analgesics produce identical abstinence syndromes. Restlessness appears first with coldness, increased nasal secretions and irregular respiration. As the syndrome develops there are painful abdominal cramps, vomiting, diarrhoea, profuse sweating, muscle pains and violent muscle twitching. The victim may threaten violence. Sleep may interrupt the development of the abstinence syndrome, but it does not reduce its severity for the symptoms recur with renewed intensity on waking. There may be cardiovascular collapse, sometimes fatal in the older patient. The initial coldness causes widespread 'gooseflesh' and this, together with the muscle twitching, explains the addict's description of the abstinence syndrome as 'kicking cold turkey'. The withdrawal symptoms reach their peak about three days after withdrawal of morphine or heroin but they may persist for up to two weeks. With pethidine the abstinence syndrome follows an accelerated time course, reaching its peak about six hours after withdrawal and lasting for up to six days.

Treatment of morphine dependence

It is a simple matter to wean an addict from his drug without disturbing him so much that he withdraws his cooperation before the process is completed. Unfortunately, unless the underlying cause of his habit is also tackled or unless he receives continuing psychological support he remains exposed to the risk of reverting to his earlier behaviour and becoming heavily dependent again. These remarks apply equally to the opiates and to many other drugs of dependence.

Methadone is the drug of choice in the treatment of dependence of the morphine type. Methadone is a morphine like analgesic and specific cross tolerance permits the replacement of the morphine like drugs of dependence by methadone: 1 mg. of methadone replaces 2 mg of heroin, 4 mg of morphine, or 20 mg of pethidine. The replacement can be brought about in two ways. In the first,

the drug of dependence is completely withdrawn and methadone, at the calculated dose level, is administered as soon as symptoms of the abstinence syndrome appear. The dose of methadone is itself gradually reduced over a period of about a week. In the second method of replacement, a 'tapering' procedure is adopted. The intake of morphine or the related drug is gradually reduced and methadone is given, in the doses indicated, to replace the withdrawn drug. Eventually the drug is completely replaced by methadone which is itself then gradually withdrawn as before.

Methadone itself causes physical dependence and a methadone abstinence syndrome inevitably occurs in patients who have been weaned from the morphine like drug with its aid. Though similar to the morphine abstinence syndrome, that following withdrawal from methadone is much less severe and the symptoms can be largely alleviated by the use of an anxiolytic drug. In the United States it is customary not to withdraw methadone on the principle that it is preferable to leave the patient dependent on a relatively benign opiate than to deprive him entirely of his previous solace and so run the risk of his returning to a more dangerous agent.

Cyclazocine, another morphine like analgesic (p. 433), has also been used in a similar fashion to methadone (Martin, Gorodetzky and McClane, 1966). Like the latter drug, cyclazocine produces a mild abstinence syndrome but no craving for the drug is engendered. In addition to its value in ensuring a smooth withdrawal from morphine like drugs, cyclazocine in twice daily oral doses of 0.5 to 1 mg. can be used to prevent restlessness and depression in the patient whose withdrawal from a morphine like drug has already been completed.

ALCOHOL DEPENDENCE

The difficulties inherent in any attempt to construct rigidly formal definitions of addiction and dependence are never better illustrated than when we are considering the problem of alcohol abuse. The habitual consumption of large quantities of alcoholic drinks induces a state of physical dependence which, in its fully developed form, can result in an abstinence syndrome as horrifying as any provoked by withdrawal of an opiate. Thus alcohol would have to be classified as a drug of addiction even if we were to adhere to the original and restricted definition of that word. But the problems posed by alcohol for both the individual and the community do not relate solely to the relatively few who become physically dependent on the drug. Millions of people throughout the world consume alcohol to such an extent that their physical health, mental wellbeing and overall efficiency are seriously impaired. It is usual nowadays to describe these individuals (together with those who are physically dependent on alcohol) as alcoholics. An alcoholic suffers from *alcoholism* but this condition is no more easy to describe than are the other terms that have to be employed in efforts to define the many essentially undefinable aspects of drug dependence. A much quoted definition of alcoholism—and it is the one that will be adopted for the purpose of the present discussion—is that offered by the American Medical Association. It goes as follows:

> Alcoholism is an illness characterized by preoccupation with alcohol and loss of control over its consumption such as to lead usually to intoxication if drinking is begun; by chronicity; by progression and by a tendency towards relapse. It is typically associated with physical disability and impaired emotional, occupational and/or social adjustments as a direct consequence of persistent and excessive use of alcohol.

The very length of this definition testifies to the difficulty of creating it but two of its features should be particularly noted. It describes alcoholism as a disease (largely, this author suspects, to take away some of the stigma that otherwise attaches to 'alcoholic' and so to encourage the victim to seek treatment) and it emphasizes the 'loss of control' that might indeed be regarded as a cardinal feature of many other forms of drug dependence. But the alcohol problem does not end with alcoholism as we have just defined it.

In most countries of the world, the consumption of alcohol is a perfectly legal activity and this has tended to obscure the fact that alcohol is a very dangerous drug. Another consequence of this general acceptance of alcohol has been a tendency to overstress the dangers and to overcondemn the use of intrinsically safer drugs such as marihuana while ignoring the greater threat posed by alcohol. Indeed many otherwise knowledgeable folk do not even think of alcohol as a drug while many of the more well informed divide the population into alcoholics and 'social drinkers'. The latter, by implication, have no alcohol problem and the description of alcoholism as a disease has helped to perpetuate this rather unfortunate tendency to create a 'them' and 'us' dichotomy. The situation is by no means as simple as this. Many apparently well controlled 'social drinkers' take more alcohol than is good for them (and, often without realizing it, they cannot reduce their intake) and they suffer minor degrees of psychological and physical ill health as a result. It has been estimated that a daily alcohol intake equivalent to two pints (about 1.2 litres) of an ordinary beer is sufficient to cause significant physical damage: in Great Britain the *average* consumption of alcohol among the adult population is already equivalent to about one pint of beer daily and this figure is rising. Finally, it has to be remembered that very modest amounts of alcohol can impair driving ability and so be the instrument that converts an apparently law abiding citizen into a criminal. Although this aspect of alcohol abuse is more properly considered elsewhere (p. 561) it should be said here that, from the point of view of the community at large, the car driver rendered careless by a modest dose of alcohol is much more dangerous than the true alcoholic

quietly drinking in his own home. The lesson that the circumstances in which a 'social drinker' takes his alcohol are no less important than the amount he takes, should not be lost on the reader. This generalization applies equally, of course, to many other drugs of dependence.

Western societies are so wedded to their alcohol that suspicion inevitably falls on those who campaign against its abuse and, in order to maintain any regard that his readers may have for his scientific objectivity, this author must declare that he does not himself abstain from alcohol. He still, however, reiterates his conviction that alcohol has been responsible for a greater total of human misery than any other drug that man has discovered.

It is not easy to be dogmatic about the incidence of alcoholism (as defined by the American Medical Association's criteria) since so many cases never come to light (many alcoholics are quite proficient in hiding the cause of their physical and mental disabilities) and many others dwell in the vague borderland between heavy drinking and alcoholism, but reliable and probably conservative estimates put the number of alcoholics in the United States and Great Britain as six millions and upwards of half a million respectively. The latter figure represents an incidence of something approaching one in fifty of the adult population, a huge figure by any epidemiological standard.

Tolerance to alcohol develops rapidly (and also recedes rapidly when drinking stops) as a result of the operation of both metabolic and cellular tolerance mechanisms but it never reaches the same degree as does that to morphine. The lethal dose of alcohol among alcoholic subjects is not greatly different from that among abstainers. Nevertheless it would be a mistake to assume that 'alcoholic' and 'drunkard' were synonymous terms and many alcoholic subjects are sufficiently tolerant of nonlethal doses of their drug to be able to present an apparently sober face to the world notwithstanding their frequent recourse to the bottle. The situation is complicated by the fact that some of the effects of alcoholism are nutritional in origin and are consequent on the alcoholic's inability or unwillingness to maintain an adequate intake of other nourishment. The well to do alcoholic who is aware of his condition finds it easier to disguise it than do the poor and the ignorant. This is not, of course, to deny that alcohol itself is responsible for causing serious physical damage and it is unfortunate that methyl alcohol, which is resorted to by those whose state has sunk so low that they cannot afford to buy ethanol, should be even more dangerous in this respect. The physical effects of alcoholism are considered in more detail in another chapter (p. 656).

Alcohol rids the drinker of feelings of depression, anxiety and incompetence. As Samuel Johnson put it, 'in the bottle, discontent seeks for comfort, cowardice for courage, shyness for confidence' and we can perhaps visualize the alcoholic as someone with a sense of inadequacy in the face of his and the world's problems that is only relieved by alcohol. As the effect of one drink wears off the depression returns and it can only be blunted by more alcohol. As tolerance develops, the prescription calls for increasing and more frequent doses of alcohol and the eventual development of a more or less serious degree of alcoholism. On this far too facile analysis we may suppose that those who are not psychologically predisposed to alcoholism drink alcohol simply for the sense of wellbeing and relaxation it brings but that they are under no compulsion to use it continuously in an effort to forget their normal state.

THE ALCOHOL ABSTINENCE SYNDROME

Although some authorities maintain that a simple 'hangover' of the type many of us have experienced on the morning after a single bout of drinking itself constitutes an abstinence syndrome it is generally agreed that a relatively prolonged period of alcohol consumption is necessary before abstinence can provoke noticeable physical changes. The most extreme form of the abstinence syndrome is *delirium tremens*. Shortly after the alcoholic stops drinking there is tremor, nausea, vomiting and profuse perspiration. Further drink will arrest the development of his condition but if he continues to abstain his tremor becomes much worse and he begins to experience visual hallucinations. These become more frequent and vivid and since they are frequently of a terrifying nature the subject becomes violently agitated and may develop delusions of persecution. There may also be auditory hallucinations, fever and epileptiform convulsions. The combination of violent tremors and the psychotic condition underline the aptness of the description of the abstinence syndrome as delirium tremens (originally tremulous delirium). The syndrome reaches its peak of severity about three days after the last drink. Thereafter it declines in intensity and the subject gradually recovers his normal condition. Death from cardiovascular collapse may occur at the height of the abstinence syndrome. Coloured animal shapes are a not uncommon feature of the visual hallucinations and the layman's description of the alcoholic state as 'seeing pink elephants' is more accurate than he may realise.

Delirium tremens of the most severe form only follows prolonged bouts of very heavy drinking and many of those who reach this condition have been taking the equivalent of one or two pints of whisky daily for several months. Less heavy drinking (say one pint of spirits daily for one or two weeks) produces a less violent abstinence syndrome characterized by tremors, nausea and vomiting, and a feeling of weakness and nervousness (the 'shakes' or 'jitters'). A night's sleep provides a sufficiently prolonged period of abstinence to precipitate the 'shakes' in an established alcoholic when he wakes in the morning. In order to make himself steady enough to shave and dress and to hide the telltale tremors from his workmates he will have to take alcohol on waking and on several occasions later in the day.

This state of affairs provides one of the very few instances of a drug dependent individual having to take his drug for fear of the consequences of withdrawal rather than from the pleasure he derives from the drug itself.

Treatment of alcohol dependence

If a patient is seen in the early stages of delirium tremens, it is necessary to prevent the further development of the condition. This can be done with alcohol, but longer acting depressant drugs (pentobarbitone, paraldehyde or chlordiazepoxide) are to be preferred. The dose of the chosen drug is determined by the seriousness of the condition when the patient is first seen, but once the withdrawal symptoms are controlled the dose can be progressively reduced at a rate that prevents the development of further symptoms. Obvious nutritional deficiencies and any dehydration resulting from alcoholic diuresis should be treated at the same time. It needs hardly to be added that, as with all the drugs which cause dependence, the mere withdrawal of the patient from his drug is insufficient. Unless attempts are made to discover the causes of his original attachment to the drug and to eliminate those causes by the appropriate psychiatric or physical treatment, relapse into alcoholism is almost inevitable.

A number of alcoholics who retain some insight into the seriousness of their condition ask for help in breaking their habit. Aversion therapy is sometimes useful in these cases. The patient is given a dose of emetine or apomorphine, together with pilocarpine. Immediately afterwards, he is given his favourite drink. The drugs cause violent nausea, vomiting and sweating which the patient associates with the taking of his drink. If this operation is repeated frequently enough, a conditioned aversion response is established, so that eventually the drink alone will produce vomiting.

A drug that appears to offer advantages over those just mentioned is tetraethylthiuram disulphide or disulphiram (Antabuse, Aversan, Refusal).

Disulphiram has been used for many years in the rubber industry and several workers who came into regular contact with the substance realized that they had become intolerant to alcohol. These observations led, in 1948, to the employment of disulphiram in the treatment of alcoholism.

Disulphiram is taken orally in doses of about 500 mg daily. It produces no untoward effects but when alcohol is taken disagreeable symptoms appear. They include flushing, sweating, nausea, violent headache, palpitations, hypotension and respiratory embarrassment. The dose mentioned is sufficient to maintain active levels of disulphiram in the blood throughout the day so that the ingestion of alcohol is inevitably followed by the symptoms described and it is not necessary to take the drug before every drink. Thus the patient is encouraged in his resolve to avoid alcohol. Nevertheless, successful treatment is still dependent on his continuing willingness to cooperate by taking disulphiram once a day and he can easily recapture the joys of drinking by the simple process of 'forgetting' his dose for a day or two. Depot preparations of disulphiram are now available. Once implanted they provide a sure guarantee against backsliding.

It is usually assumed that disulphiram inhibits aldehyde dehydrogenase in the liver, preventing the complete oxidation of alcohol and permitting the accumulation of acetaldehyde in the blood. While this is largely true it seems likely that disulphiram also inhibits a whole range of other enzymes. Its metabolic effects may therefore be more far reaching than was originally supected. Moreover, in some treated patients the response to alcohol is excessively severe. This is particularly likely to occur in those who are unusually sensitive to acetaldehyde some of whom have died as a result of their disulphiram treatment. It is always prudent to assess a patient's reaction to small doses of acetaldehyde before exposing him to disulphiram: not only is the treated hypersensitive individual likely to suffer a gross overreaction to any alcoholic drink he imbibes but he might also experience an unpleasant reaction to minute amounts of alcohol—such as that in after shave lotion—to which he quite innocently exposes himself.

It is said that a newer drug, citrated calcium carbimide (Abstem; Temposil) which has, apparently, the same mode of action as disulphiram, is less likely to cause serious reactions.

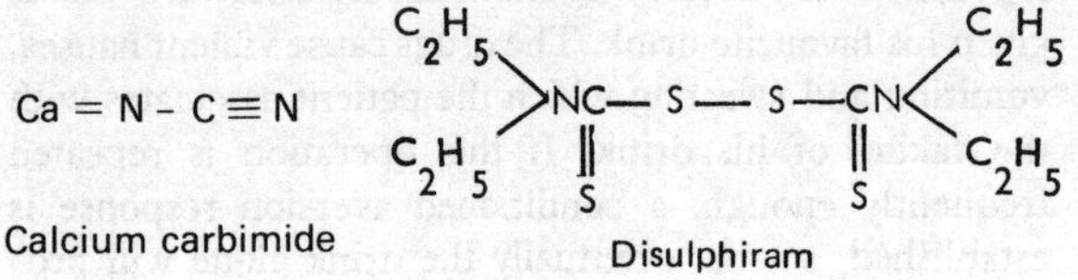

Calcium carbimide   Disulphiram

Fig. 7.1

Recent reports suggest that sodium valproate (p. 528) given before withdrawal of alcohol will considerably reduce the intensity of the abstinence syndrome.

DEPENDENCE ON BARBITURATES AND OTHER DEPRESSANT DRUGS
Although its occurrence was first reported in 1914, very early in the history of the drugs, many are still surprised to learn that barbiturates can cause physical dependence. In fact, this type of dependence is not uncommon, particularly in countries where barbiturates are prescribed almost routinely for large numbers of patients. Shorter-acting barbiturates are much more likely to cause physical dependence than are the compounds with a longer duration of action.

Many barbiturate takers develop their dependence as a result of having the drug prescribed for some minor nervous condition but others have actively sought out the drugs ('goof balls') for their alcohol like effects. The barbiturate addict behaves in many ways like the alcoholic with slurring of the speech, muscular incoordination and sluggishness of thought. He usually continues to take an adequate diet so the nutritional disorders that are so obvious a feature of the alcoholic and which contribute to his progressive deterioration, do not appear. Indeed studies of barbiturate dependence in the author's laboratory have shown that, in rats at least, the continued consumption of barbiturate leads to an acceleration of growth in young animals.

It is not surprising that other central depressant drugs produce a similar type of dependence to the barbiturates. Very early examples of this were chloral hydrate and paraldehyde and well authenticated cases of barbiturate like dependence on meprobamate, glutethimide, methyprylon, chlordiazepoxide and diazepam have now appeared. The tendency of the two last named drugs, and of their fellow benzodiazepines (p. 572), to induce serious dependence is, however, quite low.

THE BARBITURATE ABSTINENCE SYNDROME
The physiological actions of the barbiturates are similar to those of alcohol and a considerable degree of cross tolerance develops between alcohol, the barbiturates and the other compounds named in this section. Correspondingly, the abstinence syndromes to barbiturates and the other depressant drugs generally resemble delirium tremens. Major convulsions, however, are much more common after barbiturates than after alcohol.

TREATMENT OF BARBITURATE DEPENDENCE
It is important to prevent the development of the abstinence syndrome in alcoholics and in those dependent on barbiturates since the delirium which is likely to be precipitated by sudden abstinence may be difficult to suppress, even if the patient's drug intake is restored to pre-abstinence levels. In the treatment of barbiturate dependence, the short acting drug upon which the patient is likely to have become dependent should be withdrawn and replaced by a longer acting barbiturate which must be given in a sufficiently high dose to prevent the appearance of the abstinence syndrome. Pentobarbitone is a suitable substance to use, provided that the dose (200-400 mg) is repeated at six-hourly intervals. The dose of the substitute drug is then very slowly reduced until after about two weeks it has been completely withdrawn. If signs of an incipient abstinence syndrome (tremor or restlessness) appear at any time during the 'tapering' process, the patient is given an extra dose of barbiturate and the withdrawal process is continued at a slower rate than previously.

In cases of dependence on the non-barbiturate depressants, it is usually sufficient gradually to withdraw the drug itself.

After complete withdrawal of a depressant drug, it may be necessary to sedate the patient in order to prevent the restlessness which tends to occur however gradually withdrawal has been carried out. In view of the ease with which dependence develops, extreme care has to be taken to select a suitable drug.

Drugs that do not cause physical dependence

An extremely large number of drugs cause psychological but no physical dependence. They range from those such as cocaine which are as dangerous as the opiates to those such as caffeine which produce dependence of a very benign type.

COCAINE

The pharmacology of cocaine is discussed in full elsewhere (p. 466).

Cocaine is extracted from coca leaves which are chewed by many of the male members of several Peruvian and other South American communities. The cocaine improves muscle power and reduces the fatigue to which dwellers at very high altitudes are prone. Cocaine appears to produce no harmful effects in these natives, presumably because it is taken only to improve physical efficiency by individuals who are well adjusted to their social environment. The situation is entirely different in the addict who becomes dependent on cocaine because it provides an illusion of power and superiority which enables him to forget his inadequacies and the drabness of life without the drug.

The traditional way of taking cocaine ('snow', 'coke') is in the form of a snuff but it has become more common recently to use intravenous injection often in association with heroin. Cocaine sniffers develop ulceration of the nasal septum. Unlike opium takers, cocaine addicts tend to be gregarious and euphoric. They have widely dilated pupils which contrast with the pinpoint pupils of the morphine addict. They develop neither tolerance to, nor physical dependence on, cocaine.

The regular taking of cocaine causes a hyperexcitability of the nervous system with twitching or spasm of the muscles. It may also produce a psychotic state which includes a strong element of paranoia and the cocaine taker can become a very dangerous individual because his psychosis makes him see enemies everywhere while his cocaine induced excitement and energy provide him with the drive to attack them physically. Degenerative changes develop in the central nervous system after prolonged exposure to cocaine and there is rapid mental and physical deterioration. Although the pharmacological effects of the two drugs are virtually identical, a frankly schizophrenic psychosis is less often produced by cocaine than by amphetamine. Moreover, although the amphetamine taker becomes very tolerant of his drug the cocaine user, as we have seen, rarely does. Both these differences are probably attributable to differences in the duration of the drugs' action. Cocaine has a very short lived effect and even with

repeated intravenous injections the user cannot maintain a sufficiently high concentration of the drug in the brain to provide the necessary condition for the development of either tolerance or the complete psychosis.

Since there is no abstinence syndrome, cocaine can be completely withdrawn without having any immediate effect on the patient. Peruvian natives apparently find no difficulty at all in adapting to a cocaine free life if they take up occupations at lower altitudes. It is, however, very difficult to break the cocaine habit in the addict. Recollections of the euphoria and sense of wellbeing conferred by cocaine cause many relapses and as the degenerative changes in the nervous system progress, the patient may lose the will to change his ways so that his whole life is devoted to obtaining the drug. Nevertheless, some habitual sniffers of small amounts of cocaine preserve well integrated personalities and retain their intellectual powers. It is difficult to believe that Sherlock Holmes would have been a more successful detective if he had abstained from either his tobacco or his cocaine.

Cocaine, except when mixed with heroin has lost its earlier popularity among drug takers.

THE AMPHETAMINES

In the account that follows, references to 'the amphetamines' can be understood to apply equally to amphetamine and methylamphetamine. Both drugs are known colloquially as 'speed' (particularly in the United States) or, sometimes, as 'wakeamine'.

The effects of the amphetamines parallel those of cocaine, as might be expected from the fact that all the drugs have sympathomimetic actions. Before their sale was as rigidly controlled as it is today, the amphetamines were used to ward off fatigue, for instance by students preparing for examinations or by drivers faced with long overnight journeys. Because it was resorted to relatively infrequently and for the purpose of supplying a real physical need, this form of drug taking rarely if ever led to abuse—the student or driver was only too happy to stop taking his drug as soon as the examination or the journey was completed. The situation is entirely different when the amphetamines are taken in large doses for the deliberate purpose of providing a drug induced euphoria, particularly since, as with cocaine, it is usual for the drug to be taken in the company of others. Dangerous outbreaks of violence by groups of people under the influence of an amphetamine have been reported from time to time. A particularly striking example of this occurred in Japan immediately after the last war when thousands of people, humiliated by their nation's defeat, began taking methamphetamine. The two most obvious results of this were a great increase in crimes of violence and in admissions to mental hospitals. The psychosis produced by large doses of the amphetamines is so strongly reminiscent of schizophrenia that it can be used as a model for this disease. It may appear within two days of the ingestion of a large dose of an amphetamine. The psychosis usually disappears soon after the amphetamine is withdrawn but occasionally a permanently psychotic state is induced. Tolerance to amphetamine develops rapidly and the addict may take up to 1 gram of the drug daily. The therapeutic dose, by contrast, is of the order of 15 mg.

Although the amphetamines are usually taken by mouth, 'speed freaks' use the intravenous route, repeatedly injecting their drug in rapidly increasing doses in 'runs' that may last for periods of up to two weeks. Hallucinations and paranoid delusions, progressing to a fully blown amphetamine psychosis, are frequently experienced by 'speed freaks' during a 'run' as are patterns of repetitive behaviour (repeated cleaning of shoes or dismantling and reassembly of radios for example) that recall the stereotypy exhibited by rats given amphetamine (p.277).

The amphetamines are often taken with other drugs causing dependence. The person who has become dependent on barbiturates may, for instance, take an amphetamine as well, at first because the amphetamine enables him to remain alert during working hours. Later, he finds that the combination of drugs provides more satisfaction than either drug alone. The notorious 'purple hearts' (Drinamyl tablets) contain both dexamphetamine (5 mg) and amylobarbitone (30 mg). The barbiturate diminishes the fear and anxiety that might otherwise be produced by amphetamine but it does not reduce the euphoria and excitement. This enables larger doses of amphetamine to be taken. Drinamyl is often taken in circumstances in which alcohol is also available to add its own euphoriant effect to that of the other drugs.

HALLUCINOGENS

The powerful hallucinogens such as mescaline, psilocybin and lysergic acid diethylamide provide a temptation for many who hope by their aid to increase the depths and sensitivity of their perception. Unfortunately, the drugs are just as likely to produce prolonged periods of depression or psychotic reactions. Subjects under the influence of the hallucinogens, particularly lysergic acid diethylamide, may also develop bizarre or grandiose beliefs (such as, for instance, that they have the power to stop all traffic simply by stepping out into the street) that expose them to danger. The hallucinations produced are not always pleasant and they sometimes induce extreme terror. These effects justify the strict controls to which the distribution of the drugs is now subjected but dependence on the hallucinogens as irrevocable as that produced by drugs such as heroin does not occur. A considerable degree of cross tolerance develops between the different hallucinogenic drugs notwithstanding the differences in their chemical structure.

CANNABIS (MARIHUANA)

Although cannabis, in large doses at least, is a hallucinogen, it is appropriate to consider it separately since it is so much more widely used than the other hallucinogenic drugs.

Cannabis has been used since time immemorial. It is an exudate from the top of the female hemp plant (Cannabis sativa, C. indica, etc.) and it is known by a variety of other names including hashish, charas and dagga. Bhang is the name given to the upper leaves of the hemp plant. They contain relatively small amounts of the active principle. For the purpose of general description, all forms of the drug whether in the form of the resin or leaf extracts, can be called marihuana.

The active principle of marihuana is now known to be tetrahydrocannabinol.

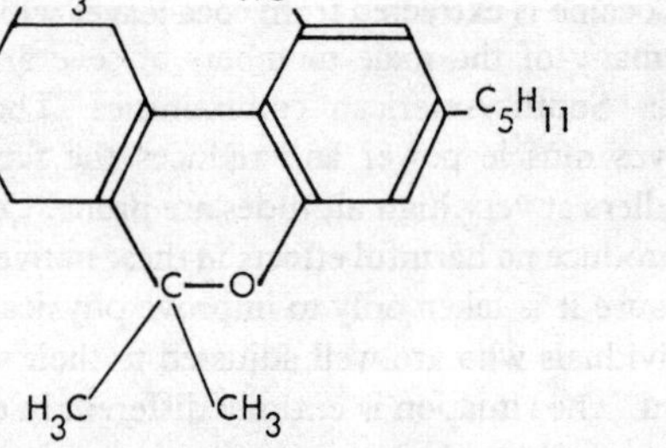

Fig. 7.2 Tetrohydrocannabinol

Marihuana is often taken in the form of cigarettes ('reefers', 'joints') but it is also effective by mouth and it is sometimes taken in drinks or in sweets. Among devotees of the drug, marihuana is called 'pot'.

In the relatively small amounts in which it is usually taken, marihuana causes euphoria and a feeling of elation. An individual in an elated ('high') condition due to marihuana is easily amused and readily breaks into song or silly laughter. His mood, however, may suddenly change to one less pleasant. His appreciation of time and space may be distorted so that objects take on a different identity and long periods of time may seem to be mere minutes or minutes become hours. Like cocaine, marihuana tends to be taken by those of a gregarious nature, for the garrulousness it produces feeds on that of others in a similar condition. The lone marihuana taker tends to be more often depressed than elated. Sometimes the drug causes aggressiveness and some workers maintain that there is an association between the taking of marihuana and outbreaks of violent crime. There is no real evidence of a causal connection between the two events.

There are considerable differences of opinion concerning the dangers of marihuana. Most authorities now agree that it causes little deterioration of personality and no physical harm and that it is not difficult to break the marihuana habit. In this respect, it is a considerably less dangerous substance than alcohol. On the other hand, those who oppose greater permissiveness in the use of the drug maintain that marihuana takers are likely to graduate to the more dangerous drugs of dependence, particularly heroin. While it is true that almost all heroin addicts began their career by taking marihuana, it seems that only a small proportion of marihuana takers turn to the 'harder' drugs. The most dangerous aspect of the situation is certainly the fact that those who supply marihuana usually have other (and higher priced) drugs available with which to tempt their customers, who are often young and impressionable.

TOBACCO

It is a remarkable fact that, although the subjective sensations produced by cannabis smoking—according to those best qualified by experience to pronounce on this subject—are more immediately pleasurable than those evoked by tobacco, the tobacco smoker is likely to be much more firmly 'hooked' to his drug than is the cannabis user. This intriguing fact is perhaps related to the cigarette smoker's ability to regulate at will the excitability of his nervous system in response to his needs as we discuss in more detail on p. 207. Unfortunately, to be 'hooked' to tobacco (particularly when it is in the form of cigarettes) is to be attached to a very dangerous substance indeed and tobacco should most certainly appear on any list of the drugs of dependence. That it so rarely does so reflects rather badly on the validity of most of our attempts to define dependence. Or perhaps it constitutes another manifestation of the all too human predilection to divide the population into 'them' (who in this instance take 'drugs' and are therefore to be censored) and 'us' who are innocent because we only take alcohol and tobacco.

GLUE, CLEANSING FLUIDS, AEROSOL PROPELLANTS, ETC.

Some twentyfive or so years ago, young adolescents (and not a few adults) in the United States found that they could achieve a satisfying 'high' with attendant euphoria and hallucinations by inhaling the vapours of organic liquids. Petroleum spirit seems to have been the first substance to have been so used and there exists at least one report of lead poisoning following the continued inhalation of the vapour of leaded petrol (Law, 1968). It was not long before the early 'sniffers' found other types of material and the cement provided in plastic model construction kits soon established itself as a firm favourite. Commonly the contents of several tubes were evacuated into a paper or a polythene bag from which the solvent vapour (usually benzene) could be inhaled. Stories abound of dustbins (garbage cans) being found full to the brim with model kits intact except for their tubes of cement that had constituted the whole reason for their purchase of the first place. Some cases of glue sniffing were reported from Britain but these were relatively few in number perhaps because the British youngster derived more satisfaction from assembling the model than from sniffing its glue. Another form of sniffing

involved the inhalation of carbon tetrachloride from clothes cleansing fluids.

Both benzene and carbon tetrachloride are very toxic substances and the advent of sniffing led to their being excluded from plastic cements and cleansing fluids. Toluene, a much less dangerous substance, replaced benzene in the former and, to make assurance double sure, American model manufacturers began to add allyl isothiocyanate (oil of mustard) to the glues supplied in their kits. This compound provided an effective deterrent to the potential 'sniffer': when inhaled it causes a severe irritation of the nasal mucous membrane.

Other substances that have enjoyed a vogue as sniffing agents (with the culprit solvent indicated in parentheses) include cigarette lighter fuel (naphtha), nail varnish remover (acetone), paint thinner (toluene), aerosol propellants (fluorinated hydrocarbons) and the newer cleansing fluids (trichloroethylene).

The 'sniffing' habit seems to be soon shed and it can hardly be indicated as a major cause of physical or psychological ill health.

MISCELLANEOUS DRUGS OF DEPENDENCE

There is hardly a drug with an action on the central nervous system that has not been reported to cause dependence. Aping adolescent sniffers, anaesthetists have been known to become dependent on inhalation anaesthetics, particularly ether and nitrous oxide, and some patients have taken to phenacetin, a drug that is apparently capable of producing a degree of physical dependence. A condition similar to that aroused by marihuana follows the ingestion of large amounts of grated nutmeg and some enthusiasts claim—on a basis, it seems, of a fervid imagination rather than of sober fact—to have obtained satisfying amounts of hallucinogens from banana skins.

THE PHARMACOLOGICAL BASIS OF DRUG DEPENDENCE

Not all aspects of drug dependence can be expected to yield easily to a pharmacological analysis and it would be premature (although a tentative speculation is offered later) to seek an explanation on other than psychological or sociological grounds as to why human beings begin to take drugs in the first place. On the other hand, the phenomena of tolerance and physical dependence clearly involve changes of a type that should be susceptible to an explanation in pharmacological terms. A number of hypotheses have been advanced along these lines but none is yet supported by completely persuasive experimental evidence.

Collier (1966) formulated a theory which attempted to explain tolerance and physical dependence in terms of modern concepts of receptor action. Tissues may contain two types of receptor for particular drugs. Receptors of the first type ('pharmacological receptors') cause a pharmacological response when the drug comes into contact with them. Receptors of the second type ('silent receptors') elicit no response. Collier suggests that tolerance involves the production of a change in the relative numbers of the two types of receptor, the pharmacological receptors decreasing and the silent receptors increasing in number. Thus the response to a previously effective dose of the drug is reduced. There is nothing inherently impossible in this explanation, since there is evidence that this type of adaptation occurs in some experimental situations. For instance, the increased sensitivity to acetylcholine produced by motor denervation or the administration of botulinum toxin is best explained by assuming that the number of pharmacological receptors has increased (Thesleff, 1960). There is, however, no direct evidence that the number of pharmacological receptors in the brain decreases in response to the administration of drugs like morphine.

In order to explain the development of physical dependence, Collier proposed a different mechanism. This is justifiable since tolerance may occur without causing physical dependence and it is not unreasonable to assume that different mechanisms might subserve the two conditions. Collier suggested that drugs that cause physical dependence produce tolerance by reducing the supply of an excitatory transmitter, with a consequent increase in the number of pharmacological receptors. After withdrawal of the drug, the amount of available transmitter returns to its normal level more rapidly than the extra receptors return to their 'silent' state. As an alternative, it is suggested that the drug increases the supply of inhibitory transmitter. In a variant of this latter hypothesis, Collier proposed that the pharmacological receptors increase in number because the depressant drug occupies receptors for an excitatory transmitter substance and that the abstinence syndrome arises because the drug molecules leave the receptors before the original number of silent receptors has been restored. Normal amounts of transmitter impinging on neurones bearing an abnormal proportion of pharmacological receptors would be expected to produce the exaggerated responses so characteristic of abstinence syndromes.

Hypotheses that invoke changes in the receptor population are not as readily susceptible to direct experimental testing as are those that focus attention on the transmitters rather than on their receptors. Among those who have favoured transmitter hypotheses, Crossland has considered the possibility that adaptation to a depressant drug simply involves an increase in the amount of available excitatory transmitter (or a decrease in the amount of inhibitory transmitter) sufficient to overcome the depressed condition of the nerve cells. When the drug is withdrawn, hyperexcitability might be expected to occur if the condition of the nerve cells returned to normal more

rapidly than did the supplies of transmitter Indirect evidence for this view came from the observation (Wulff, 1959) that among patients dependent on barbiturates, withdrawal convulsions occur more readily in those dependent on the short acting drugs. The longer acting barbiturates are eliminated more slowly and the nerve cells will therefore return more slowly to their normal condition.

While it is true that this observation can be just as readily explained by Collier's hypothesis there is other evidence in favour of the view that changes in transmitter release underlie the development of tolerance and the precipitation of the abstinence syndrome in at least one group of drugs.

It has long been known that morphine and its congeners inhibit the release of acetylcholine from both the intestine and the brain. Crossland and his colleagues have adduced evidence that as rats become tolerant to morphine, the initially depressed release of acetylcholine returns to that characteristic of unmedicated animals but that when an abstinence syndrome is initiated by the administration of nalorphine or naloxone there is a massive release of acetylcholine which seems to be responsible for the major part of the syndrome (Crossland, 1972; Crossland, Ali and Jepson, 1976). Experiments by Knoll and his colleagues have led to an essentially similar conclusion (Fürst, Vizi and Knoll, 1976) but in mice it seems that serotonin plays a more important part than acetylcholine (Way, 1972).

Although morphine certainly influences the amounts of acetylcholine and serotonin in the brain, recent studies have emphasized the importance of the enkephalins (p. 437). In rats, tolerance appears to be associated with the accumulation of enkephalins in the brain (indicating perhaps that the release of the enkephalins from their neurones is depressed) while the opposite change takes place when tolerant animals are made abruptly abstinent (Simantov and Snyder, 1976). The changes in enkephalin content provoked by abstinence are not as dramatic as the increases in acetylcholine release but it is not impossible that both substances play a part in mediating the responses to the opiates.

There is no evidence that cholinergic (or serotoninergic) mechanisms are involved in the development of tolerance to the barbiturates or to the alcohols or in the genesis of the abstinence syndromes to these drugs. Some very recent work in the author's laboratory has revealed a very sharp rise in the amount of 5–methyltetrahydrofolic acid in the brains of rats withdrawn from barbiturates. It seems that this change is a necessary antecedent to the development of abstinence convulsions. These observations further support the conclusion that no single mechanism is uniquely involved in the production of all types of abstinence syndrome.

The enkephalins and the endorphins have analgesic properties and it seems likely that they exert euphoriant actions too. The possibility that we produce our own pleasure substances tempts this author at least to speculate on the possibility that some forms of drug taking are indulged in as an unconscious attempt to compensate for a deficiency of endogenous euphoriants.

THE TESTING OF DRUGS LIKELY TO CAUSE PHYSICAL DEPENDENCE

If it is suspected that a drug might induce physical dependence, it may be possible to confirm this suspicion in the laboratory. The drug is given to the experimental animals over a period of time, progressively increasing the dose as tolerance develops. Dosage is then stopped and the animals are watched for unusual symptoms such as restlessness, muscular weakness, rigidity, vomiting or convulsions. Rats that do not show spontaneous convulsions on drug withdrawal may become hypersensitive to sound and convulsions may then be precipitated by the noise made by shaking a bunch of keys or by sounding a door bell near the cage. These sound induced convulsions arise in similar circumstances to the spontaneous convulsions seen after withdrawal of some drugs from dogs, cats or man.

The time over which drug administration should be continued before withdrawal depends on the drug under test and the species of animal being used. Thus, whereas barbiturates must be given to cats and dogs for several months before the animals become physically dependent on the drugs, dependence can be produced in rats by four weeks of drug administration (Crossland & Leonard, 1963).

If the drug being tested is derived from, or has similar properties to, a drug known to cause physical dependence, the test just described can be usefully modified. The animals are first made dependent on the known drug, which is then replaced by the drug under investigation. If no abstinence syndrome develops, it is clear that the second drug is able to maintain the state of physical dependence induced by the first. Confirmation that the second drug is itself capable of producing physical dependence can be obtained by continuing its administration for three or four weeks and then withdrawing the drug. An abstinence syndrome should develop. It should be noted that the second drug will only replace the first if the two drugs exhibit cross dependence. This is to be expected if they are structurally similar. If they are not cross dependent, an abstinence syndrome will develop when the second drug is given but this does not necessarily mean this drug is incapable of producing *any* kind of physical dependence. This can only be determined by a separate experiment in which animals are given progressively increasing doses of the drug in the way already described.

In a quantitative version of the replacement test, a dose of the second drug is found which will just prevent an abstinence syndrome to the first. This enables an estimate to be made of the relative doses of the two drugs required to produce the same degree of physical dependence.

It is sometimes possible to carry out tests on man. Morphine addicts who are receiving the normal supply of morphine can be used when a new morphine like analgesic is being tested. The new drug is gradually substituted for the morphine and its ability to prevent the appearance of an abstinence syndrome is assessed. If no sign of morphine withdrawal appears, it can be concluded that the new drug produces the same kind of physical dependence as morphine itself.

Finally it should be noted that drugs that are capable of inducing physical dependence will only do so in practice if their other properties are such that individuals are tempted to take them—and then to continue to take them—for non medical reasons in the first place.

BIBLIOGRAPHY

Books, monographs and reviews

Collier, H. O. J. (1966). Tolerance, physical dependence and receptors. In *Advances in Drug Research*, Vol. 3, pp. 171-188. Ed. Harper, N. J. and Simmonds, Alma B. New York: Academic Press.

Deneau, G. A. and Seevers, M. H. (1964). Pharmacological aspects of drug dependence. In *Advances in Pharmacology*, Vol. 3, pp. 267-284. Ed. Garattini, S. & Shore, P. A. New York: Academic Press.

Edwards, G. and Grant, M. (eds) (1977). *Alcoholism—New Knowledge and New Responses*. London: Croom Helm.

Hofmann, F. G. (1975). *A Handbook on Drug and Alcohol Abuse*. New York, London and Toronto: Oxford University Press.

Seevers, M. H. (1962). Medical perspectives on habituation and addiction. *J. Am. med. Ass.*, **181**, 112-118.

Seevers, M. H. and Deneau, G. A. (1963). Physiological Aspects of Tolerance and Physical Dependence. In *Physiological Pharmacology*, Vol. 1, pp. 565-640. Ed. Root, W. S. & Hofmann, F. G. New York: Academic Press.

Wulff, M. H. (1959). *The Barbiturate Withdrawal Syndrome*. Copenhagen: Munksgaard.

Original papers

Crossland, J. (1972) Acetylcholine and morphine dependence. In: *Agonist and Antagonist Actions of Narcotic Analgesic Drugs*, pp. 232-234. London and Basingstoke: Macmillan.

Crossland, J., Ali, T. A. J. and Jepson, P. (1976). Morphine dependence and transmitter release. In: *Symposium on Analgesics*, pp. 97-102. ed. Knoll, J. and Vizi, E. S. Budapest: Akadémiai Kiadó.

Crossland, J. and Leonard, B. E. (1963). Barbiturate withdrawal convulsions in the rat. *Biochem. Pharmac.*, **12** (Suppl.), 103 (Abstract).

Fürst, Susanna, Vizi, E. S. and Knoll, J. (1976). Azidomorphines and acetylcholine release. In: *Symposium on Analgesics*, pp. 103-112, ed. Knoll, J. and Vizi, E. S. Budapest: Akadémiai Kiadó.

Law, W. R. (1968). Gasoline sniffing by an adult (lead encephalopathy). *J. Am. med. Assoc.* **204**, 1002-1004.

Le Friend, D. (1967). Accidental therapeutic drug addition. *Clin. Pharmac. Ther.*, **7**, 832-834.

Martin, W. R., Gorodetsky, C. W. and McClane, T. K. (1966). An experimental study in the treatment of narcotic addicts with cyclazocine. *Clin. Pharmac. Ther.*, **7**, 455-465.

Rodriguez, H. (1964). In: *The Addict in the Street*, pp. 25-34. Ed. Larner, J. and Tefferteller, R. New York: Grove Press Inc. and Harmondworth, Middlesex: Penguin Books.

Simantov, R. and Snyder, S. H. (1976). Elevated levels in morphine-dependent rats. *Nature*, **262**, 505-507.

Thesleff, S. (1960). Supersensitivity of skeletal muscle produced by botulinum toxin. *J. Physiol.*, **151**, 598-607.

Way, E. L. (1972). Reassessment of brain 5-hydroxytryptamine in morphine tolerance and physical dependence. In: *Agonist and Antagonist Actions of Narcotic Analgesic Drugs* pp. 153-163. London and Basingstoke: Macmillan.

8. Receptors

Histamine, 5-hydroxytryptamine, acetylcholine and some other choline esters all cause contraction of the isolated ileum of the guinea pig. The effect of the choline esters is prevented by doses of atropine which do not antagonize the action of histamine or 5-hydroxytryptamine. Other antagonists are as specific for each of these last named substances as is atropine for the choline esters and observations such as this can be repeated in many fields of pharmacology. A structural resemblance between the active substance (the *agonist*) and its antagonist is often evident. Sometimes the resemblance is very close. Again, in many instances a maximal pharmacological response can be elicited by minute quantities of agonist. Findings such as these are best explained on the assumption that agonists exert their action by becoming attached to specialized portions (the *receptors*) of the excitable cell and that the receptors for a particular agonist occupy only a tiny part of the cell surface. The receptor theory is generally accepted by pharmacologists and in recent years much interest has been aroused by attempts to derive quantitative descriptions of drug action based on acceptable assumptions concerning the relationship of drugs to their receptors. It is not to be concluded that all drugs operate through receptor mechanisms. Some, notably the general anaesthetics, show no structural specificity and these drugs presumably owe their action to a more general effect on the cell membrane or cellular processes. The mode of action of structurally non-specific drugs is discussed elsewhere (p. 493).

The existence of what we now know as receptors seems to have been clearly visualized by J. N. Langley, one of Britain's pioneer physiologists. Writing in 1878, in the very first volume of the *Journal of Physiology*, Langley described experiments in which he had studied the mutual antagonism of pilocarpine and atropine as exemplified by their effects on salivary secretion in the cat and he went on to say

> '....we may, I think, without much rashness, assume that there is some substance or substances in the nerve endings or gland cells with which both atropin and pilocarpin are capable of forming compounds. On this assumption then the atropin or pilocarpin compounds are formed according to some law of which their relative mass and chemical affinity for the substances are factors'.

This is a clear statement of what we shall later define as competitive antagonism and if the quotation were modified by replacing 'substances' by 'receptors' it could easily be passed off as an extract from a modern textbook of pharmacology. Even before Langley, other workers such as Luchsinger and Heidenhain had also described antagonisms of the pilocarpine-atropine type in terms of a competition between the two agents but neither they nor Langley found it necessary to identify, as a specialized region of the cell, the point at which the competition occurred. It was left to Paul Ehrlich actually to express, as late as 1900, the receptor concept in formal terms. Langley, indeed, never felt impelled to speak of receptors as such even though he survived until 1925.

Ehrlich was the father of chemotherapy and it was his work in this field which led him to the conclusion that specialized regions of microorganisms, the receptors, were vital in the organism's function inasmuch as they were the means by which it attached itself to nutrient molecules. Substances which poisoned the cell did so, Ehrlich surmised, because they could attach themselves to the receptors thereby depriving the organism of its means of obtaining nourishment. The toxicity of the substance would be considerably increased if, as well as being able to attach itself to the cell, it possessed another chemical grouping (the toxophoric group) capable of actively injuring the cell. Ehrlich later extended his concepts so as to embrace the more general case of drug action on excitable tissues. Like Langley, Ehrlich took as his model the antagonism of atropine and pilocarpine: he assumed that both compounds would, by means of 'anchoring groups', attach themselves to the receptors of the tissue cells. The fact that atropine, in contrast to pilocarpine, has no excitatory action on the tissues, was seen as being due to the different activities of the active groups (analogous to the toxophoric groups) in the two substances. Ehrlich's views are epitomized in his phrase '*Corpora non agunt nisi fixata*' (substances do not act unless fixed)— the only Latin tag which finds a place in modern textbooks on pharmacology and itself derived from the chemists' rather more famous '*Corpora non agunt nisi liquida*'. Ehrlich likened the relationship of drugs and their receptors to a lock and its matching key, just as Emil Fischer had pictured enzymes and their substrates.

Receptor theory is one of the few theoretical and unifying concepts in pharmacology. It stands in relation to the science in much the same way that atomic theory does to the physical sciences. Just as he knows that atoms can no longer be regarded as solid and immutable objects, the reader should appreciate that receptors are not fixed and rigid groups of atoms. 'Drug-receptor interaction must be seen as a mutual moulding of drug and receptor. There is mutual adaptation as far as shape and charge distribution is concerned. This adaptation plays an important role in the activation of drug and receptor and therefore is essential to drug action' (Ariëns and Simonis, 1964).

The first attempt to incorporate the receptor concept into some quantitative generalizations was made by A. J. Clark in 1937. Clark assumed that the response of a tissue was dependent on the number of receptors which were occupied by the drug and that the interaction between drug and receptor was a simple unimolecular reversible process. Clark's equation, which is discussed later, provides the basis of many of the mathematical formulations of drug action in use today. His treatment has, however, been modified in one important respect. As Ehrlich—and Clark himself—had clearly recognized, attachment to a receptor is a necessary but not a sufficient prerequisite for pharmacological activity. A compound may have a high affinity for a receptor but it will elicit no visible response unless it is also capable of setting into motion the train of events which culminates in an overt response of the tissue. The ability to do this is referred to as the *efficacy* (Stephenson, 1956) or the *intrinsic activity* (Ariëns, 1954; van Rossum and Ariëns, 1962). The current definition of intrinsic activity makes it virtually identical with efficacy and the two terms may be used interchangeably. In the present discussion 'intrinsic activity' is used in recognition of the extensive contributions made by Ariëns and his colleagues to receptor theory. It should already be clear that a drug with a low affinity but a high intrinsic activity can produce the same pharmacological response as one with a high affinity but a low intrinsic activity.

QUANTITATIVE ASPECTS OF DRUG-RECEPTOR INTERACTIONS

Throughout this section, the approach and nomenclature which is adopted is essentially that of Ariëns.

Intrinsic activity, affinity and dose-response curves

In order to establish the basic relationships between intrinsic activity, affinity and the response of a tissue, it is convenient and reasonable to assume that when a drug is present in a concentration sufficient to enable it to exert its maximum effect it will be occupying all the available receptors. This assumption will have to be modified later (p. 104) but the conclusions reached by accepting it in its present form will not have to be radically altered.

If a number of drugs which act on the same receptor system elicit quantitatively different maximal responses, it is clear that their intrinsic activities must differ. If there is a linear relationship between the intrinsic activity of a drug which is occupying all the available receptors and the pharmacological response it evokes, it becomes a simple matter to compare intrinsic activities. When a number of related agonists is compared in this way, it is usual to assign an intrinsic activity of unity to the most active member of the group. The intrinsic activities of the other compounds then receive appropriate fractional values calculated in terms of the size of the maximal responses they evoke in relation to that produced by the most active compound. The assumption that the pharmacological response is directly related to intrinsic activity does not, of course, necessarily represent the true state of affairs but it is one which permits a simple and productive mathematical treatment and there is no substantial evidence of any alternative relationship which would more adequately explain the experimental data.

It is important to note that comparisons of intrinsic activities only have meaning within groups of substances which act on the same receptor system: it would, for instance, be pointless to attempt to compare the intrinsic activities of acetylcholine and histamine by reference to their actions on the guinea pig ileum.

The intrinsic activity may be represented in mathematical formulations as α. When it is necessary to distinguish, in the same expression, between different agonists, appropriate indices or subscripts may be added. The intrinsic activity of antagonists can be denoted by the letter β.

The affinity of a drug for its receptors is treated in the way originally proposed by Clark. The concentration of the agonist is represented by [A] and the concentration of receptors not already occupied by drugs is given by [R]. It can be assumed that the number of molecules of A which become attached to the receptors is small in relation to the total number available so that the interaction between drug and receptor will not sensibly affect [A]. The rate of combination of drug and receptor can therefore be expressed, following simple mass action principles, as

$$k_1 [R] \times [A]$$

where k_1 is a constant (the association constant), the magnitude of which is determined by the avidity with which the drug becomes associated with the receptor. Similarly, the rate of dissociation of the drug-receptor complex is given by the expression

$$k_2[RA]$$

where k_2 (the dissociation constant) reflects the tendency of the drug to leave the receptor. [RA] is the concentration of receptors occupied by the drug.

At equilibrium—that is, when the drug is exerting the maximum effect of which it is capable in the dose in which it has been administered—

$$k_1[R] \times [A] = k_2[RA]$$

This relationship can be expressed in a more useful way by taking account of the fact that $[R] + [RA]$ is equal to $[r]$, the total concentration of receptors.

Thus,

$$k_1[A]([r] - [RA]) = k_2[RA]$$

$$\text{or} \quad \frac{[RA]}{[r]} = \frac{k_1[A]}{k_1[A] + k_2}$$

$$= \frac{1}{1 + \frac{k_2}{k_1[A]}}$$

$\frac{k_2}{k_1}$ can be replaced by K_A, the equilibrium constant. K_A measures the balance of the tendencies of the drug to dissociate from, and to become associated with, the receptors: it is the reciprocal of the drug's affinity for the receptors. The term $\frac{[RA]}{[r]}$ represents the fraction of the total number of receptors occupied by the drug. If it is multiplied by α, the intrinsic activity, it provides a measure of the response of the preparation, expressed as a fraction of that elicited by maximal doses of a drug with maximal intrinsic activity (unity) on the receptor system.

Thus,

$$\text{Relative response} = \frac{[RA]}{[r]} \; \alpha = \frac{\alpha}{1 + \frac{K_A}{[A]}} \quad \text{---} \quad (1)$$

When $[RA] = [r]$ all the receptors are occupied and the response is thus proportional to α. This is the relationship which has already been established. Reference to the equation shows that when the concentration of the drug $[A]$ equals K_A, the response will be one half of the maximum (α) obtainable. This provides us with the means of comparing the affinities of different drugs. The affinities are proportional to the reciprocals of the concentrations required to produce one half of the maximal effect obtainable with the drugs. For obvious reasons, the concentrations are expressed in molar terms. Fig. 8.1(a) illustrates the type of dose-response curve obtained with drugs with different intrinsic activities but the same affinity. The drugs whose dose-response curves are shown in Fig. 8. 1(b) have the same intrinsic activity but different affinities.

Equation (1) is the basic formulation on which Ariëns and his colleagues have built a sophisticated theoretical structure supported by a vast amount of experimental data. The interested reader is referred to the book by the Ariëns group (Ariëns, 1964): even a casual glance at the volume will indicate the extent of the contribution it makes to the subject. Equation (1) arises from simple mass action considerations. It is formally—and inevitably—the same as that derived for a number of unimolecular physiological reactions including, for instance, the combination of muscle haemoglobin with oxygen, the dissociation of carbonic acid and, of course, the reaction of an enzyme with its substrate to form the enzyme-substrate complex. The affinity of a drug for its receptor is qualitatively and quantitatively analogous to the affinity constant (the Michaelis constant) of an enzyme for its substrate. The Michaelis constant is the substrate concentration necessary to enable an enzyme reaction to proceed at half its maximum velocity.

The Ariëns equation predicts that the dose-response curve should be a rectangular hyperbola and that the log (dose)-response curve (the form in which the relationship is usually constructed) should take a sigmoid (S-shaped)

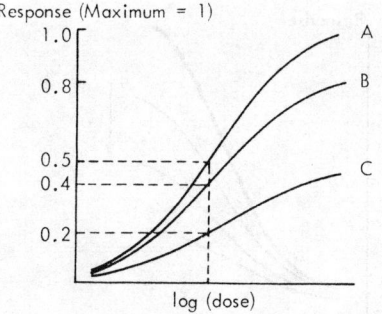

Intrinsic activity: Compound A—1, Compound B—0·8, Compound C—0·4. The three compounds have the same affinity.

(a)

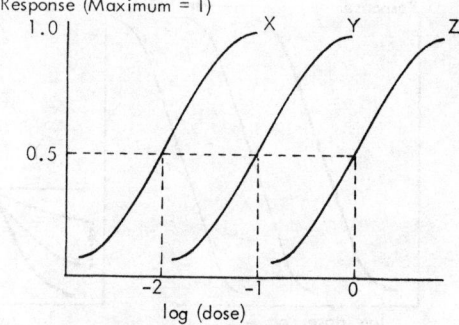

The affinities of compounds X, Y and Z stand in the ratio 100:10:1. The three compounds have the same intrinsic activity.

(b)

Fig. 8.1 Assessment of intrinsic activity and of affinity.

configuration. In general this prediction is borne out although, for reasons which will be discussed later, (p. 104), the slope of the sigmoid curve is frequently steeper than that predicted. The derivation of equation (1) involved the making of a number of assumptions, some of which have already been mentioned. In addition, it has been assumed that intrinsic activity and affinity are completely independent variables though it is clear that this may not be so. Nevertheless, the agreement between theoretical prediction and many of the experimental findings is remarkably close. It provides convincing evidence of the essential validity of the Clark-Ariëns treatment.

If the reciprocals of the dose and the response are plotted against one another, a straight line should be obtained. This is analogous to the Lineweaver-Burk line plotted by enzyme biochemists but it is rarely employed in pharmacological work.

DRUG ANTAGONISTS

A drug whose intrinsic activity is zero will produce no overt response in a preparation to which it is applied, however high its affinity for the receptors. However, it will hinder the access of other molecules to the receptors and in this way it may completely or partially block the response to the agonist. The extent to which the response is interfered with is determined by the relative concentrations and

affinities of the agonist and antagonist, each being able to displace the other if its concentration is sufficiently increased. For this reason, the blocking agent is known as a *competitive antagonist*. In the presence of doses of antagonist insufficient to cause a complete blockade of agonist activity, the dose-response curve of the agonist is moved to the right exactly as if its affinity for the receptors had been reduced. This, in effect, is what has happened. The situation is shown diagrammatically in Fig. 8.2(a).

Thus, a competitive antagonist has an intrinsic activity of zero, it shifts the dose-response curve to the right and the inhibition it causes can be removed by increasing the concentration of agonist.

A compound with a high affinity and a low or moderate intrinsic activity will also be capable of reducing the effect of an agonist. The inhibition will again be removed by increasing the concentration of the agonist but the antagonist will itself be capable of producing a response in the preparation. Such a compound is consequently described as a *partial agonist*. It is also sometimes known as a *dualist* because it behaves as both an agonist and an antagonist. The effect of a partial agonist on the dose-response curves of an agonist is illustrated in Fig. 8.2(b). The form of the curves is simply explained, at least qualitatively. In the presence of very small doses of the agonist, the response obtained is determined almost entirely by the partial

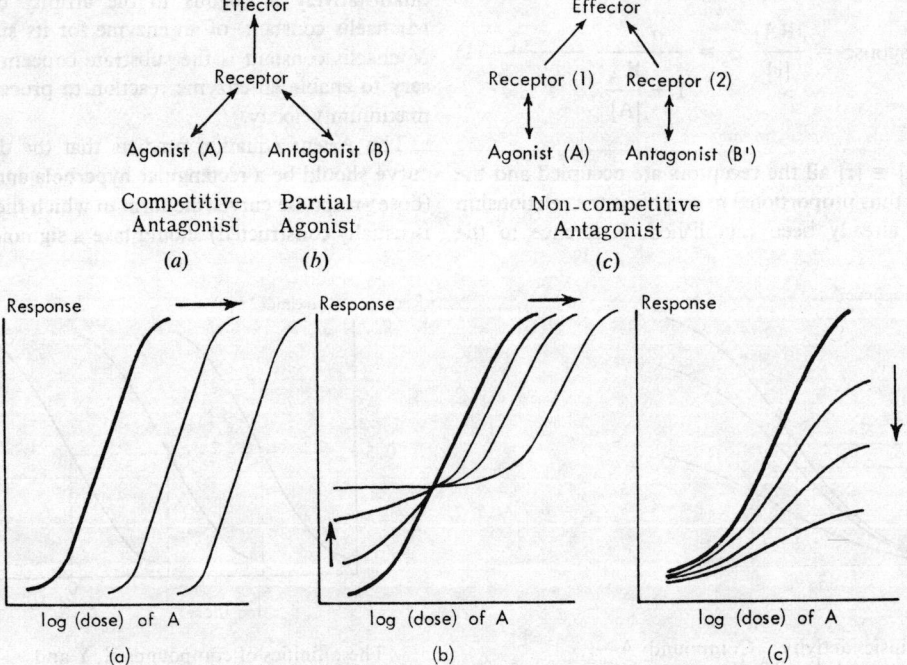

In all the diagrams the dose-response curve of the agonist in the absence of antagonist is represented by the bolder line and the arrow indicates the direction of increasing concentration of the antagonist.

Fig. 8.2 Dose-response curves of an agonist in the presence of different types of antagonist.

agonist. This response will increase as the concentration of the partial agonist is increased until it is exerting its maximum effect which is determined, of course, by its intrinsic activity. As the concentration of agonist is increased in the presence of a constant concentration of the partial agonist, its effects become progressively more dominant and the dose-response curve takes on the form characteristic of that of the agonist although, because of the continuing presence of the partial agonist, the curve is displaced to the right. It will be seen that in the presence of high doses of the partial agonist the response of the preparation remains constant over a range of concentrations of the agonist. This is a reflection of the fact that under these conditions the agonist is ineffective until it is present in a concentration sufficiently high to enable it to free some of the receptors by displacement of the antagonist. It can also be shown that there is one dose of agonist which will always produce the same response, irrespective of the concentration of partial agonist. This response is equal to the latter's intrinsic activity. This explains why the dose-response curves in Fig. 8.2(b) have a common point of intersection.

Using the convention adopted in equation (1) and adding the terms [B], K_B and β to characterize the antagonist, the effect of an agonist in the presence of an antagonist active on the same receptor system can be expressed by the equations

$$\text{Response} = \frac{[RA]}{[r]}\alpha + \frac{[RB]}{[r]}\beta$$

$$= \frac{\alpha}{1 + \left(1 + \frac{[B]}{K_B}\right)\frac{K_A}{[A]}} + \frac{\beta}{1 + \left(1 + \frac{[A]}{K_A}\right)\frac{K_B}{[B]}} \quad (2)$$

As before, the response is expressed as a fraction of the maximum effect obtainable from the receptor system. For a purely competitive antagonist, $\beta = 0$ and the second terms in equations (2) disappear. The expression which remains is identical with that relating to the agonist alone except that the affinity has been in effect decreased by a factor determined by the concentration and the affinity of the antagonist. This explains the shift to the right of the dose-response curve, to which reference has already been made. For the partial agonist, $\beta > 0$, and the equations (2) express the form of the curves in Fig. 8.2(b).

Some substances are capable of combining irreversibly with drug receptors. They reduce the number of receptors available to the agonist and they cannot be displaced by high concentrations of the latter. The equations (2) do not, of course, apply to irreversible antagonists, which behave rather in the fashion of the non-competitive antagonists discussed below.

A *non-competitive antagonist* is one which operates on a different population of receptors from those activated by the agonist but which can nevertheless alter the response of the effector system. A non-competitive antagonist depresses the response to the agonist to an extent dependent on the concentration of antagonist. Because the agonist and antagonist affect different receptor systems, the inhibitory effect of the antagonist is independent of the concentration of agonist and no amount of the latter, however great, will overcome the inhibition. To put it in another way, the agonist is incapable of evoking the maximum response it is capable of when no antagonist is present—in effect, its intrinsic activity has been reduced. In quantitative terms, a non-competitive antagonist reduces the effect of any dose of agonist by a factor of

$$1 - \frac{\beta'}{1 + \frac{K'_B}{[B]}} \quad (3)$$

In this expression the superscripts indicate that the antagonist B reacts with its own receptor system and not with that activated by the agonist. Dose-response curves in the presence of a non-competitive antagonist are illustrated in Fig. 8.2(c).

Some non-competitive drugs increase the response of a tissue to the agonist. They are *sensitizers* rather than inhibitors. Their effect on the response to the agonist is represented by expression (3), modified by changing the minus to a plus sign.

Both non-competitive antagonists and those that combine irreversibly with drug receptors are sometimes categorized, following Gaddum, as *unsurmountable* antagonists.

It should be added that the three types of agonist-antagonist relationship discussed above, though the most important, do not by any means exhaust the possible ways in which two or more drugs may act on the same effector system. Other types of interaction and the appropriate mathematical treatments can be found in the book by Ariëns and his colleagues already referred to.

The pA_x, pD_x and pD'_x scales

Competitive antagonists can be quantitatively compared on the basis of their pA_x values, an index of activity devised by Schild (1947). It is usual to measure the pA_2 value, which is the negative logarithm of the molar concentration of the antagonist which results in the dose of agonist having to be doubled in order to produce the effect it had in the absence of the antagonist. The pA_{10} and, more rarely, other pA_x values may have to be calculated and pA_x can be generally and succinctly defined as the negative logarithm of the molar concentration of the antagonist required to reduce the effect of a multiple dose (x) of the agonist to that of a single dose. The more active an antagonist is the smaller will be the dose required to reduce the effect of the agonist and the larger, therefore, its pA_x values. The pA_x

scale was introduced on purely empirical grounds as a convenient index of antagonistic activity but it fits very well into the framework of modern receptor theory.

Competitive antagonists, as has been seen, in effect reduce the affinity of an agonist for its receptor and it can be shown that the pA_2 value is proportional to the affinity of the antagonist for the common receptors.

Measurement of the pA_x values can be put to practical use in several ways.

a. Dose-response curves obtained in the presence of different concentrations of a competitive antagonist are parallel with one another and with the curve obtained in the absence of the antagonist. Consequently pA_x values will be independent of the concentration of agonist used in their calculation, provided that the antagonism is truly competitive. If, in a particular instance, a pA_x value is found to increase with the dose of agonist, it must be concluded that the antagonism is not competitive in type.

b. Theory predicts (p. 104) that pA_2-pA_{10} will be 0.95 for any competitive antagonist. This relationship can be used to establish whether a particular agent is acting as a competitive antagonist. For a number of practical and theoretical reasons, a consistently close agreement with the predicted figure cannot be expected but if pA_2-pA_{10} is the order of 0.5 or less, it can be concluded that competitive antagonism is not being measured. Some indubitably competitive antagonists exert a measure of non-competitive block at high concentrations. For this reason, the amount of drug which is required to bring about a tenfold reduction of the effect of the agonist is rather smaller than would be expected. Consequently, pA_{10} is larger and pA_2-pA_{10} is smaller than that required by theory. The intervention of non-competitive antagonism into the action of a competitive antagonist can be suspected if its pA_2-pA_{10} value, though greater than 0.5, is appreciably less than 0.95. In this event, tests for non-competitive antagonism should be applied with the antagonist present in a high concentration.

c. An agonist may act on a number of different tissues, on each of which it may be inhibited by the same competitive antagonist. The pA_x value for the antagonist should be the same for all tissues bearing the same type of receptor. An actual example will illustrate this. The pA_{10} values for atropine against acetylcholine on a number of tissues were found to be 8.1 (guinea pig ileum), 7.6 (guinea pig lung), 8.1 (rat intestine), 8.3 (frog atrium) and 4.2 (frog rectus) (Arunlakshana and Schild, 1959). These results provide a clear indication that the receptors in the frog rectus muscle differ from those in the other tissues and that the latter are identical one with another. In this particular instance, it was, of course, already known that this was so (the receptors in the rectus muscle are nicotinic in type while the other tissues carry muscarinic receptors) but measurement of pA_x values might well throw light on the nature of

receptors whose identity has been less certainly delineated than those of the acetylcholine system.

d. A number of substances may all evoke a response in a particular preparation. In order to determine which of these are operating through a common receptor system, a competitive antagonist active against all the agonists is sought and a pA_x value against them all is calculated. This should be the same for each agonist-antagonist combination which affects the same receptor type.

The activities of non-competitive antagonists are measured on the pD'_x scale. The pD'_x value is the negative logarithm of the molar concentration of the antagonist which is required to reduce the maximum effect of the agonist to $\frac{1}{x}$ of that which it exerts in the absence of the antagonist. The pD'_x value is analogous to the pD_x value which is applied to agonists and which is defined as the negative logarithm of the molar concentration of the agonist which produces an effect equal to $\frac{1}{x}$ that of the maximum response. As in the case of the pA_x scale, theoretical and practical considerations indicate that the pD'_2 and pD_2 values are the measures of choice. It will be recalled that the concentration of agonist required to produce half its maximum effect is inversely related to the drug's affinity (p. 99). From this relation it will be clear that the pD_2 value is directly proportional to the logarithm of the affinity of an agonist and the pD'_2 value is similarly related to the affinity of the non-competitive antagonist for its particular receptors. This can be seen by putting $\beta' = 1$ and $K'_B = [B]$ in the expression (3) on p. 101. The pD'_2 is a logical measure of antagonistic activity because the more avidly the drug seeks its own receptors the greater will be its action on the common effector system and the greater the hindrance offered to the action of an agonist on that system.

Like the pA_x value, the pD'_x value should be independent of the dose of agonist used in its measurement, provided that the antagonist is acting in a truly non-competitive way. If it is found in an individual case that pD'_x falls as the dose of agonist increases, it must be concluded that the antagonist is behaving wholly or partly in a competitive way, the higher dose of agonist partially reversing the inhibition imposed by the antagonist. The effect of agonist concentration on pA_x and pD'_x values is summarized in Table 8.1.

The pD'_x values of non-competitive antagonists can be put to the same kind of practical use as pA_x values. Thus papaverine is a non-competitive antagonist and atropine a competitive antagonist of a number of agents which cause

Table 8.1 The effect of increasing the dose of agonist on pA_x and pD'_x values

	pA_x	pD'_x
Competitive Antagonist	No effect	Decreases
Non-competitive Antagonist	Increases	No effect

Table 8.2 The effect of antagonists on the response of the isolated guinea pig ileum (after Ariëns, 1964)

	Agonist		
	Barium Chloride	Histamine	Acetylcholine Analogue
pA$_2$ of atropine	3.2	6.5	8.1
pD$'_2$ of papaverine	5.0	4.9	5.3

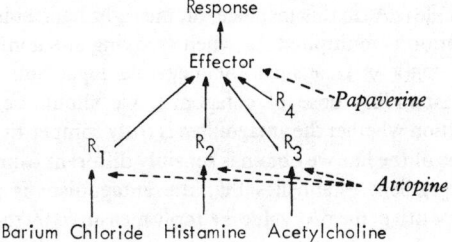

Fig. 8.3 Analysis of the sites of action of agonists and antagonists deduced from the data of Table 8.2.

contraction of the guinea pig ileum. The pA$_2$ and pD$'_2$ values of atropine and papaverine respectively against three agonists (barium chloride, histamine and an acetylcholine analogue) are displayed in Table 8.2. The pD$'_2$ values for papaverine are approximately the same against all three agents but the pA$_2$ values differ. It can be concluded that the receptors for barium chloride, histamine and acetylcholine are dissimilar but that they all operate through a final common mechanism which is inhibited by papaverine. Results such as these, incidentally, illustrate how inaccurate it is to speak of specific antagonists: atropine has some action, albeit a small one, on the histamine and barium receptors as well as those which respond to acetylcholine.

CALCULATION OF pA$_x$

We can now examine a little more formally the basis of some of the assertions concerning competitive antagonism made in the course of the foregoing paragraphs. In so doing we shall discover how to measure pA$_x$ values.

Let us suppose that a dose [A] of agonist, acting alone, provokes the same response in a tissue preparation as does the higher dose [A$_1$] in the presence of a dose [B] of a competitive blocking agent. We can express this situation in terms of equation (2) on p. 101 when we shall see that

$$\frac{\alpha}{1 + \dfrac{K_A}{[A]}} = \frac{\alpha}{1 + \left(1 + \dfrac{[B]}{K}\right)\dfrac{K_A}{[A_1]}}$$

It is a very simple matter to show, as the reader can do for himself by suitable manipulation of the terms, that this reduces to

$$\frac{1}{[A]} = \frac{1}{[A_1]} + \frac{[B]}{K_B[A_1]}$$

or

$$\frac{[A_1]}{[A]} = 1 + \frac{[B]}{K_B}$$

$\dfrac{[A_1]}{[A]}$, the ratio of the higher to the lower dose of agonist, can be conveniently replaced by the single term x. When this is done it becomes clear that we have defined the conditions for measuring pA$_x$ since [B] is the concentration of anta-

gonist required to reduce the effect of a multiple dose, x, of the agonist to that of a single dose.

We noted on p. 99 that the terms K$_A$ and K$_B$ as employed in the Ariëns equations refer to the *reciprocals* of the affinity constants of the agonist and antagonist respectively. We can, therefore, replace K$_B$ by the affinity constant which we shall have to represent as k_B. Thus

$$(x - 1) = k_B \cdot [B]$$

Taking logarithms and remembering that, by definition, pA$_x$ = $-$log[B] we reach the final form of our equation

$$\log(x - 1) = \log k_B - pA_x \quad\quad\quad (4)$$

It is important to remember that this equation is valid only in cases of simple and strictly competitive antagonism, that is in conditions where $\beta = 0$ and when only one molecule of antagonist attaches itself to an individual receptor.

The following points, some of which have already been mentioned in passing, emerge from a consideration of equation (4).

(a) The equation is that of a straight line with a gradient of -1. The gradient of a line is the constant by which the

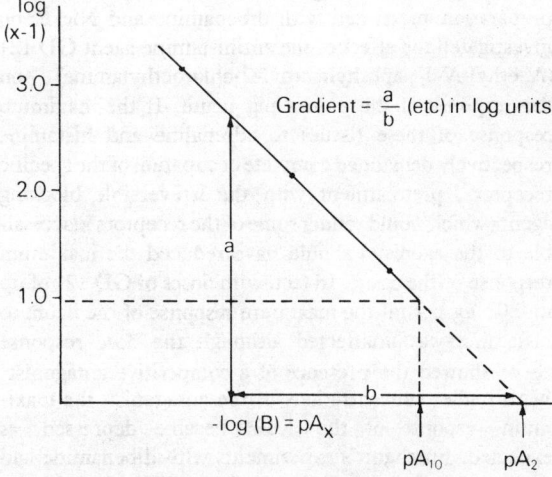

Fig. 8.4 To illustrate the relationship between dose ratio (x) and pA$_x$.

variable (pA_x in this instance) on the right hand side of the equation is multiplied. If, when studying antagonists, we plot $\log(x - 1)$ against the negative logarithm of the corresponding dose of antagonist, we should seriously question whether the antagonism is truly competitive if the shape of the line we obtain is sensibly different from −1. If the gradient establishes that the antagonism is indeed competitive, the pA_2 value is simply measured by the point where the line cuts the abscissa because $\log(x - 1)$ is 0 when x is 2 (Fig. 8.4). Any other pA_x value can, of course, be read from the graph. In practice, the several values of x required to construct the graph are obtained from dose-response curves of the agonist in the presence of different amounts of antagonist.

(b) We can see from the equation that $pA_2 = \log k_B$, a formal version of the statement already made (p. 102) that the pA_2 value is a measure of the affinity of the antagonist for the common receptor. We can also confirm the assertion that pA_x values are independent of the doses of agonist used in their calculation: neither of the variables [A] and [A_1] appear in equation (4).

(c) If we replace $\log k_B$ by pA_2 we have, for x = 10,

$$\log 9 = 0.95 = pA_2 - pA_{10}$$

another relation we have discussed (p. 102) without previously offering a formal proof of its validity.

Modifications of the basic theory

SPARE RECEPTORS

So far it has been assumed that a maximum response of an effector system is obtained only when all available receptors have been occupied. Furchgott (1954) and Nickerson (1957), who studied the effects of irreversible blocking agents, were the first to show that this assumption is not always justified. Furchgott used the rabbit aortic strip preparation pretreated with dibenamine and Nickerson investigated the effect of the antihistamine agent GD 121 (N-ethyl-N-1-naphthylmethyl-2-chloroethylamine) on the response of the guinea pig ileum. If the maximum response of these tissues to adrenaline and histamine respectively demanded complete occupation of the specific receptors, pretreatment with the irreversible blocking agent (which would render some of the receptors inaccessible to the agonists) should have reduced the maximum response of the tissue. In fact, with doses of GD 121 of up to 0.01 μg per ml the maximum response of the ileum to histamine was unaffected although the dose response curve showed the presence of a competitive antagonist. With higher concentrations of the antagonist, the maximum response of the ileum became depressed, as expected. Furchgott's experiments with dibenamine had produced essentially similar results to those on the ileum except that in this instance the maximum response began to fall off at much lower concentrations of the antagonist.

The fact that the response to histamine was less easily depressed than that to adrenaline indicated that a much smaller proportion of the ileal receptors had been occupied in order to obtain a maximum effect. The dose required to produce a given response had to be increased one hundred fold before the maximum response began to fall off. This implies that only one per cent of the ileal receptors have to be occupied in order to elicit the maximum response of which the tissue is capable. The remaining 99 per cent are *spare* or *reserve receptors*. The spare receptors are in no way different from those whose occupation has produced the maximum response. The interaction of an agonist with any of the receptors can evoke a response but the maximum effect is produced as soon as the appropriate number of receptors have delivered their stimulus to the effector organ. We have already seen that not all drugs which become associated with a particular receptor system have an intrinsic activity of unity and it should be obvious that there can be no spare receptors when such partial agonists are exerting the maximum effect of which they are capable. Thus not all agonists operate with a receptor reserve and those that do (compare adrenaline and histamine in the examples quoted) do so with reserves of greatly differing sizes. A practical point to be noted is that mechanical factors in a pharmacological preparation may prevent the tissue from developing the maximum response of which it should be capable. This can have the effect of indicating a larger receptor reserve than would be disclosed if a more suitable arrangement were employed.

The existence of spare receptors adds a complication to the simple quantitative treatment of drug-receptor interaction summarized in equation (1) on page 99. Receptor occupation can still be thought of as being determined by the concentration and the affinity of the agonist. The response of the tissue, however, is only proportional to the number of occupied receptors until the maximum response of which the receptor system is capable has been reached. Thereafter, the response will increase no more. The effect of this is to shorten the dose range over which the response changes from zero to the maximum. In other words, the dose-response curve will be steeper for some agonists than is predicted by theory. Another circumstance which is not allowed for in the simple theory is that some agonists elicit no response at all until their concentration exceeds a particular threshold value. This also will make the dose-response curve steeper than it would be if any dose of agonist, however small, produced some response. In fact, as has already been mentioned (p. 100) dose-response curves obtained in the laboratory are not infrequently steeper than predicted. In a somewhat negative way, this serves to confirm the essential validity of the Ariëns treatment.

SILENT RECEPTORS

Silent receptors must be distinguished from spare receptors. A silent receptor is one to which the agonist may become attached but which is incapable of producing a pharmacological response. Different authorities have applied the term 'silent' to what would seem to be two essentially different types of receptor systems. It is a well known fact that many drugs are adsorbed on to plasma protein molecules. This has the effect of reducing the immediate effect of the drug because fewer molecules reach the 'pharmacological' receptors in the tissues but it also prolongs the action of the drug, which is slowly released from the plasma proteins. Drugs adsorbed on to the proteins in this way may be displaced by other drugs (this is the origin of one of the types of drug interaction enumerated on p. 76) and the adsorption sites are often described as silent receptors. Even in isolated preparations, the possibility exists that a drug may be taken up by nonactive adsorption sites of this type. The term silent receptor has, however, also been applied (and in the writer's view this is a more acceptable use of the term) to sites on the reactive tissue itself. Silent receptors envisaged in this way can be regarded as moieties of the tissue protein. If striated muscle is denervated, there is an increase in the number of pharmacological receptors at the end plate (Axelsson and Thesleff, 1959; Thesleff, 1960) and it may well be that these new receptors are produced from previously silent receptors. As we discuss elsewhere (p. 94) one of the hypotheses which seeks to explain the development of physical dependence on drugs is founded on the view that silent receptors in the brain can be readily transformed into pharmacological receptors and back again under the influence of a changing chemical environment.

Both types of silent receptor will have the effect of reducing the amount of drug available to the pharmacological receptors and this will tend to flatten the dose-response curve thus partly offsetting the effect of the spare receptors and the threshold.

THE RATE THEORY OF DRUG ACTION

Of the several variations of the Clark-Ariëns hypothesis which have been proposed from time to time, that put forward in 1961 by Paton is the most interesting and challenging. Paton supposes that the most important factor determining drug action is the *rate* at which drug-receptor combinations take place (Paton, 1961; Paton & Rang, 1965). The basic formulations of the rate theory can be easily developed from the relationships assembled in the earlier sections of this chapter where it was seen (p. 99) that the rates of forward and backward drug-receptor interactions could be represented as $k_1[A]([r]-[RA])$ and $k_2[RA]$ respectively. At equilibrium, the two reactions proceed at the same rate and the rate of receptor occupation is then given by

$$\frac{k_1[A]([r] - [RA])}{[r]} = \frac{k_2[RA]}{[r]}$$

By simple mathematical manipulation similar to that exercised earlier it can be shown that

$$\text{Rate of receptor occupation} = \frac{k_2}{1 + \dfrac{K_A}{[A]}} \quad\text{——— (5)}$$

If the response is proportional to the rate of receptor occupation rather than to the proportion of receptors occupied, equation (5) must replace equation (1) on page 99 as the basic expression of receptor function. The only difference between the two formulations is that the intrinsic activity, α, of the occupation theory is replaced by k_2, the dissociation constant of the drug-receptor complex. Paton believes that each time a drug molecule comes into apposition with a receptor site a 'quantum' of excitation is transmitted to the effector system. The dissociation constant takes the place of the intrinsic activity in all the other expressions previously discussed. Thus, on the rate theory, agonists, partial agonists and competitive antagonists are characterized by the possession of high, moderate and low dissociation constants respectively. The principal arguments for and against the rate theory are summarized in the succeeding paragraphs.

a. The rate theory is basically much more simple than the occupation theory since it avoids the awkward concept of intrinsic activity. Association and dissociation constants are more readily acceptable parameters. Many antagonists have a characteristically slow onset of action and this is completely in accord with the rate theory requirement that an antagonist should leave the receptors only slowly. Moreover, Paton has been able to demonstrate, in some series of compounds, that the predicted inverse relationship between dissociation constants and antagonistic potency does indeed exist. In these experiments (Paton, 1961), the kinetic constants were calculated from the speed of onset and disappearance of the drug's action. Against the rate theory must be cited the not inconsiderable objection that, in order to account for the behaviour of both agonists and antagonists, the theory has to postulate a range of rates of association and dissociation far outside any of those actually known to occur in other chemical reactions.

b. When a drug is first applied to a preparation, the rate at which it becomes associated with the receptors is high. Thereafter, the rate falls until equilibrium is reached. The *number* of receptors occupied increases progressively (at first rapidly and then more slowly) until equilibrium is reached. According to the rate theory, therefore, the response of the tissue should rise rapidly to a peak and then fall to a steady value (the phenomenon of *fade*) while occupation theory predicts that the response will increase progressively until a steady state is attained (Fig. 8.5). Thus, the time course of development of drug action should provide decisive evidence in support of one or other

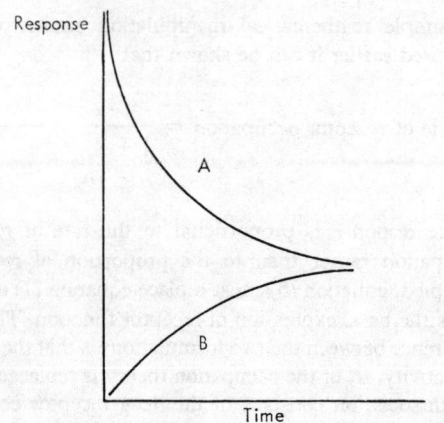

Fig. 8.5 Time course of development of a pharmacological response as predicted by rate theory (A) and occupation theory (B).

of the theories. Many a beautiful theory has been slain by a cruel fact but in this particular instance, the facts leave both theories unscathed. It is true that fade can be demonstrated with a number of agonists (including acetylcholine and histamine) and when it does appear the time course of the response corresponds closely to that predicted. Moreover, and again as predicted, the extent and the rate of development of fade increase as the dose of agonist is increased. Fade cannot always be demonstrated. When it cannot, it may be that some other circumstance (the existence of a diffusion barrier, for example) retards the rate of drug-receptor association and so prevents the appearance of the expected large initial response. However, in one much-quoted experiment (Higman, Podleski & Bartels, 1963), fade could not be demonstrated and its absence could not be attributed to any hindrance of drug access. In this experiment, a single electroplax cell of the electric eel was exposed to carbamyl choline. Different concentrations of the drug brought about differing degrees of partial depolarization but in each instance the time course of the response reproduced that predicted by the occupation theory. Finally, it should be added that some workers have suggested that the whole phenomenon of fade is an artefact consequent on the mechanical arrangements used for recording the contractions of the isolated tissues traditionally used for studying drug-receptor interactions. Up to now, then, experiments designed to demonstrate the occurrence or otherwise of fade have given equivocal rather than the decisive results hoped for.

   c. If the initial rate of drug-receptor interaction is high, even an antagonist should produce some degree of receptor activation when it is first applied. Some drugs do in fact behave in this way (see particularly the discussion of neuromuscular blocking agents in Chap. 16 but it is not yet possible to say whether all antagonists would behave in this manner if they were tested in situations free of physical obstructions to drug-receptor association.

The evidence summarized in the preceding paragraphs does not permit a firm decision to be made concerning the validity of the rate theory. The theory certainly explains many phenomena in quantitative terms as well as—and sometimes better than—the occupation theory but it is in some respects more restrictive, requiring a consistency of behaviour on the part of a variety of drug types which is rarely seen in practice. In many ways, of course, the modifications it imposes on the occupation theory are of no more than minor importance: the concept of spare receptors, for instance, is replaced by 'spare capacity for more rapid association' and measurements such as pA_x and pD'_x retain their quantitative validity. Perhaps the best conclusion that can be reached at this stage is that of Ariëns who believes that the dissociation constant of the drug-receptor complex, which figures so prominently in the rate theory, is only one of several factors which together constitute the intrinsic activity. This is an ingenious suggestion and it lends itself, in the present writer's view, to experimental testing. Thus, for drugs in whose action fade can readily be demonstrated, the dissociation constant is presumably a more than usually important determinant of intrinsic activity and the behaviour of these drugs ought to be more accurately described by rate theory formulations than is that of drugs which do not exhibit fade.

THE NATURE OF RECEPTORS

Most of the experimental investigations into the quantitative aspects of drug-receptor interaction have made use of isolated preparations, such as the guinea pig ileum, which are simple to set up and whose responses can be measured with ease and accuracy. Drugs, however, do more than cause the contraction of muscle and the concepts and relationships discussed in the preceding sections of this chapter are of more general application than might be suggested by the limited number of preparations to which reference is customarily made in text book treatments of receptor theory. To take but one example, the antivitamins (p. 795) are competitive antagonists of the vitamins and they have as much claim to be so categorized as has atropine in its relationship with acetylcholine.

   At least since Ehrlich's time, drugs have been visualized as molecules whose shape enables them to become closely associated with specialized regions of the cell. A similar 'lock and key' congruency has been regarded, and properly so, as the crucial relationship between an enzyme and its substrate although recent views indicate that both lock and key should be thought of as being made of some material which permits each to induce some conformational change in the other. Although the association between a substrate and its enzyme may lead to a different type of end result from that initiated by the association of a drug with its receptor, it is clear that there must be an essential similarity (if not an identity) in the chemical and physical changes which determine and accompany the binding of drugs and substrates to their respective sites. It is, therefore, not unreasonable to look to enzymes and other active macromolecules for clues to the structure and activity of drug receptors. Some drugs receptors *are* enzymes (see for instance the discussion on adrenaline β receptors in Chap. 18) but others are not. Acetylcholine must clearly have close structural affinities with active groups on both cholinesterase and receptor molecules but, it is difficult to sustain the view that enzyme and receptor are identical.

We have already noted that recent studies of enzyme structure suggest that substrates are capable of inducing conformational changes in enzyme molecules and a similar change may well take place when a drug molecule meets its receptor. This has led Mautner (1967) to suggest that two specialized regions of the drug molecule should be distinguished. One enables the compound to become attached to the receptor molecule and it is responsible for the drug's affinity. The other portion of the molecule, which induces a configurational change in the receptor (and hence initiates the pharmacological response) determines the drug's intrinsic activity. An antagonist is incapable of bringing about this change (it has zero intrinsic activity) and a partial antagonist has only a limited ability to do so. It will be realized that this hypothesis, the best we have, echoes that of Ehrlich which was propounded so long ago. This is at once a tribute to the latter's prescience and a confession of our own inability to penetrate to the heart of the structural unit of pharmacological activity.

There can be little doubt that receptors exist as actual entities. If a suitable tissue is exposed to a radioactively labelled drug, the sites at which the drug is bound can be revealed by autoradiography. Using this technique, Waser demonstrated, as long ago as 1957 (see Waser, 1966) that tubocurarine, a competitive antagonist of acetylcholine, accumulated at the end plates of the muscle fibres in a mouse diaphragm. He calculated that 1.4×10^6 molecules of tubocurarine were bound at each end plate. This presumably reflects the number of acetylcholine receptors in each muscle cell: it is quite surprisingly close to the figure (1.6×10^5 receptor molecules per cell) calculated for the longitudinal muscle of guinea pig ileum by Paton and Rang (1965). The final confirmation of the reality of receptors has been provided in very recent years by the isolation in milligram quantities of the purified acetylcholine receptor protein from the electroplaques of electric fish.

It should be possible, by studying the structure of agonists to deduce the chemical features of at least part of the corresponding receptor system. Studies of structure-action relationships pursued with this (and other) ends in view are discussed in some detail in the appropriate chapters of this book but it must be said that the knowledge of receptor structure so gained is hardly commensurate with the amount of effort which has been expended. The obstacle to rapid progress in this field probably arises from the fact that many of the crucial features in the relationship of drug and receptor are too subtle to be represented by conventional chemical formulae which give no precise indication of the disposition of the intramolecular and intra-atomic forces which govern chemical reactivity.

BIBLIOGRAPHY

Books, monographs and reviews

Ariëns, E. J. (Ed.) (1964). *Molecular Pharmacology*. New York and London: Academic Press.

Ariëns, E. J. and Simonis, A. M. (1964). A molecular basis for drug action. *J. Pharm. Pharmac.*, **16**, 137-157 and 289-312.

Ciba Foundation Symposium (1962). *Enzymes and Drug Action*, Ed. Mougar, J. L. and de Reuck, A. V. and London: Churchill.

Clark, A. J. (1937). General Pharmacology. In *Handbuch der Experimentellen Phaarmakologie*, Vol. 4. Ed. Heffter, A. Berlin: Springer-Verlag.

Cohen, J. B. and Changeux, J.-P. (1975). The cholinergic receptor protein in its membrane environment. *A. Rev. Pharmac.*, **15**, 83-103.

Danielli, J. F., Moran, J. F. and Triggle, D. J. (1970). *Fundamental Concepts in Drug-Receptor Interactions*. New York: Academic Press.

Furchgott, R. F. (1964). Receptor mechanisms. *A Rev. Pharmac.*, **4**, 21-50.

Goldstein, A., Aronow, L. and Kalman, S. M. (1974). *Principles of Drug Action*, 2nd edn., New York: John Wiley.

Mautner, H. G. (1967). The molecular basis of drug action. *Pharmac. Rev.* **19**, 107-144.

Paton, W. D. M. (1961). A theory of drug action based on the rate of drug-receptor combination. *Proc. R. Soc. B.*, 21-69.

Paton, W. D. M. and Rang, H. P. (1966). A kinetic approach to the mechanism of drug action. *Adv. Drug Res.*, **3**, 57-80.

Porter, Ruth and O'Conner, Maeve (Eds) (1970). *Molecular Properties of Drug Receptors*. London: Churchill.

Rang, H. P. (Ed) (1973). *Drug Receptors: A Symposium*. London: Macmillan.

Thesleff, S. (1960). Effects of motor innervation on the chemical sensitivity of skeletal muscle. *Physiol. Rev.*, 40, 734-752.

Triggle, D. J. (1965). *Chemical Aspects of the Autonomic Nervous System*. New York and London: Academic Press.

Waser, P. G. (1966). Autoradiographic investigations of cholinergic and other receptors in the motor end plate. *Adv. Drug Res.*, **3**, 81-120.

Waud, D. R. (1968). Pharmacological receptors. *Pharmac. Rev.*, **20**, 49-88.

Original papers

Ariëns, E. J. (1954). Affinity and intrinsic activity in the theory of competitive inhibition. Part I (1954). *Archs int. Pharmacodyn. Thér.*, **99**, 32-49.

Arunlakshana, O. and Schild, H. O. (1959). Some quantitative uses of drug antagonists. *Br. J. Pharmac. Chemother.*, **14**, 48-68.

Axelsson, J. and Thesleff, S. (1959). A study of supersensitivity in denervated mammalian skeletal muscle. *J. Physiol.*, **149**, 178-193.

Furchgott, R. F. (1954). Dibenamine blockade in strips of rabbit aorta and its use in differentiating receptors. *J. Pharmac. exp. Ther.*, **111**, 265-284.

Higman, H. B., Podleski, T. R. and Bartels, E. (1963). Apparent dissociation constant between carbamylcholine, *d*-tubocurarine and the receptor. *Biochim. Biophys. Acta*, **75**, 187-193.

Langley, J. N. (1878). On the mutual antagonism of atropin and pilocarpin, having especial reference to their relations in the sub-maxillary gland of the cat. *J. Physiol.*, **1**, 339-369.

Nickerson, M. (1956). Receptor occupancy and tissue response. *Nature, Lond.*, **178**, 697-698.

Paton, W. D. M. and Rang, H. P. (1965). The uptake of atropine and related drugs by intestinal smooth muscle of the guinea pig in relation to acetylcholine receptors. *Proc. R. Soc. B.*, **163**, 1-44.

Schild, H. O. (1947). pA, a new scale for the measurement of drug antagonism. *Br. J. Pharmac. Chemother.*, **2**, 189-206.

Stephenson, R. P. (1956). A modification of receptor theory. *Br. J. Pharmac. Chemother.*, **11**, 379-393.

van Rossum, J. M. and Ariëns, E. J. (1962). Receptor-reserve and threshold phenomena. *Archs int. Pharmacodyn. Thér.*, **136**, 385-413.

9. Statistics in pharmacology

Statistical methods provide the pharmacologist with a very powerful tool for the control and quantitative analysis of his experimental work. Statistical techniques are now highly developed and it is impossible in a brief chapter such as this to do more than indicate the situations in which their application is useful or necessary and to sound a few warnings concerning the pitfalls which await those who apply the techniques uncritically or inappropriately. Readers who wish to acquire a more detailed knowledge of the theoretical foundations and the biological applications of this interesting branch of mathematics are referred to the volumes listed in the bibliography appended to this chapter.

Everybody knows that statistics is concerned with the collecting of numerical data but few realise that the word *statist* (the original form of 'statistician') means a statesman. Rulers have always been anxious to know the numbers of their subjects (and hence the potential size of their armies) and the numerical data they thus amassed became known as statistics. It is only in the last century or so that statistics has become a preoccupation of scientists, sociologists and industrialists and modern statistical methods have been developed in response to demands from these workers for more sophisticated information than simple numerical totals of men capable of bearing arms or paying taxes.

So far as their scientific applications are concerned, statistical methods were originally developed as a means of providing summary descriptions of the behaviour of very large numbers of objects—the molecules in a volume of gas, for instance. The pharmacologist, however, usually has to work with small numbers of animal or human subjects and statisticians have been called upon to provide methods of analysis which will enable him to assert with a stated degree of confidence whether or not the results obtained on a small sample of a particular population (young rats, victims of a certain disease, etc.) are applicable to the population as a whole.

Why are statistical methods necessary? If, for instance, a pharmacologist finds that the growth rate of a group of rats is accelerated by the administration of a particular drug, why cannot he assume, without further ado or statistical analysis, that he has discovered an incontrovertible fact about the drug and that its administration to any other group of rats will cause their growth rate to increase? He cannot do so because rats grow at different rates and it may

have happened that, when he divided his rats into two groups, he by chance (or unconscious design) selected for drug treatment animals whose average increase in weight would in any event, drug treatment or no, have been greater than those chosen to receive no drug. The purpose of statistical analysis is to determine whether the observed differences between the treated and the untreated animals could have arisen by chance. There is, however, another important point to be considered. Even if, in our imaginary experiments, the average growth rate of the animals chosen to receive the drug has no inherent tendency to be greater than that of the untreated animals, it is possible that growth might be stimulated, not by the drug itself, but by circumstances attendant on the fact of the drug's administration. Thus, if the drug is to be given by injection several times daily, the treated animals might be handled more frequently or more gently than the untreated animals so that, as contented animals will, they eat more food. The intervention of influences such as these (which occur more frequently than might be supposed) cannot be detected by the mere application of statistical formulae to the results obtained at the end of the experiment. They must be foreseen at the outset and steps must be taken to design the experiment in such a way that their effect is neutralized: in the present instance, of course, the untreated animals should be given injections of a 'dummy' substance whenever their fellows receive the drug. It is not always so easy to detect possible complicating factors nor to devise means of eliminating or neutralizing their effects. The important principle, which cannot be repeated too often, is that the *design* of an experiment is as much a part of the statistical process as is the analysis of the results. An investigation is worthless, however elaborate the statistical analysis of the experimental results, if the experiments themselves have been badly designed. Excellent counsel, which is often quoted but so rarely heeded, is that any research worker who needs statistical advice should seek it *before* he embarks on his experiment.

Some aspects of experimental design are discussed elsewhere in this chapter and in Chap. 10 but every investigation presents its own problems of design and hard and fast rules to fit any occasion cannot be laid down. Because of this and because the modern pharmacologist needs to be acquainted with many methods of statistical analysis (if only to enable him to appraise the work of others) most teachers and textbooks (including this one) devote most of their available time and space to a discussion of the techniques of analysis. This should not blind the reader, particularly if he is a laboratory worker, to the overwhelming importance of good experimental design.

It might be useful to end these introductory paragraphs with a definition of statistics. Statistics is the technique used to design the strategy for collecting, and then to analyse, numerical data which are affected by a multiplicity of causes and to assess the relative importance of these various causes.

SOME BASIC STATISTICAL TERMS AND CONCEPTS

Probability, statistical significance and the null hypothesis

The idea of probability is a familiar one. In statistics, the probability of an occurrence is expressed on a scale ranging from zero (for an impossibility) to 1 (for a certainty). Thus, the probability that a tossed coin will come down as a 'head' is 0.5 (1 in 2), the probability that a shaken die will expose a '6' is 0.17 (1 in 6) and so on.

Many statistical calculations have the aim of establishing whether observed differences between two groups of measurements can have arisen by chance. If the calculations indicate a low probability of a chance occurrence, the observed differences are said to be *statistically significant*. Thus, to take the example quoted earlier, if the difference between the mean weights of the two groups of animals are shown to be statistically significant, it has to be concluded that the difference has arisen because one group of animals has received the drug. It is usual to regard a probability of 1 in 20 ($P = 0.05$) as being sufficient to establish statistical significance. If P falls to 0.01 or less, the results are said to be 'highly significant'.

It is important to remember that the figure of 0.05 which is chosen as the criterion of statistical significance is a purely arbitrary one and that statistical significance does not necessarily parallel pharmacological or clinical significance. A particular experimental manoeuvre or drug treatment may cause an effect which, though statistically highly significant, is quantitatively trivial and pharmacologically unimportant. Conversely, because of difficulties in measurement, or some other circumstance, a very important response may reveal itself in results of only marginal statistical significance. Statistical probabilities must not be looked on as magic tokens, signals to despair if they rise above 0.05 or to elation if they fall below that figure. They must always be interpreted in the light of the actual experimental results to which they refer.

Statistical calculations which assess the probability that a particular difference has arisen by chance are in effect testing a *null hypothesis*—that is, the hypothesis that the experimental treatment has no effect on the parameter being measured. A low value of P indicates that the null hypothesis is unlikely to be correct.

Degrees of freedom

Many statistical calculations have to take into account the number of degrees of freedom in the system being studied. This concept has the same connotation that it has in chemistry. Thus, if a series of n variables has a mean value of x, $(n-1)$ of those variables can theoretically take any value but the value of the remaining item is then fixed if the mean of x is to be maintained. The series is said to have $(n-1)$ degrees of freedom. Similarly, if we are comparing two series of variables containing respectively n_1 and n_2 items, the total number of degrees of freedom will be (n_1+n_2-2).

'Controls'

In assessing the effect of a particular experimental treatment, it is usual to divide the experimental material into two or more groups, one of which, the so-called 'control' or normal group, does not receive the experimental treatment. It serves to provide baseline values against which the effects of the treatment can be gauged. Statistical analysis then assesses the significance of any difference found between the 'control' and treated groups. The selection and handling of the animals or subjects which are to form the 'control' group is one of the most important features of an experimental design but it is frequently performed in so uncritical a manner as to cast grave doubts on the validity of the results of the investigation, however 'significant' they may appear to be on statistical analysis.

Let us reconsider the simple case of studying the effect of drug administration on the growth rate of rats. It is clear that, in a situation like this, it is not sufficient to give the drug to one group of animals and to leave the members of the control group untouched. Most investigators would readily see the necessity of treating these animals in a similar fashion to those receiving the drug. Thus, if the drug is to be given by a thrice daily intraperitoneal injection, the untreated animals should receive thrice daily injections of the vehicle in which the drug is dissolved or suspended. However, a properly designed experiment should go much further than this. The animals to be used in the investigation should be allocated by some random process to 'control' and 'experimental' groups. One way of doing this is to determine the fate of each animal in turn by tossing a coin. Alternatively, the animals may be divided into pairs, the members of the individual pairs being matched for weight, sex, docility, etc. One member of each pair is then selected, by the toss of a coin, to receive the drug: the other will receive vehicle only. Ideally, the animals should then be housed individually (unless the nature of the experiment requires that the effects of group interaction should be allowed to operate) and the cages should be arranged in a random order and labelled by some disinterested person in such a way as to make it impossible for the experimenter himself to know or to suspect which animals are receiving the drug and which are not. The same disinterested person should supply the experimenter with syringes, one for each cage, containing the appropriate amount of drug or vehicle whose appearance should not, of course, enable them to be distinguished from one another. The experimenter administers the drug but it may not always be appropriate to allow him to record the weights of his animals. Not until the experiment is complete should he be permitted to know which animals had formed the experimental group. Very few laboratory investigations are conducted under conditions as rigid as those prescribed here. This is unfortunate, because poor experimental design may lead to results of dubious pharmacological significance. Much time, money and material has then to be wasted in efforts to confirm results which would not have needed confirmation had they been obtained from properly designed experiments. Those who work with animals should remember that the life of no animal should be sacrificed in vain. It *is* a vain sacrifice if the animal is included in an experiment which yields unreliable results.

It will be appreciated that a proper experimental design may result in the investigator's being partially deprived of participation in his own experiment. This is inevitable but it may lead to difficulties, particularly when the subjects are human patients and the investigator is the physician who is responsible for their welfare. This problem is mentioned again in Chap. 10 (p. 137).

It should be added that the design outlined for the simple experiment just discussed is not flawless. It is, for example, difficult for a disinterested person who becomes involved in a project to remain totally disinterested and his own unconscious desire that the experiment should succeed (or fail) may influence the results. This possibility looms large in the conduct of clinical trials; it is referred to again in the next chapter.

Difficulties of another type can be illustrated by reference to a specific example. Suppose that it is required to determine what effect removal of the adrenal medulla has on pharmacological responses in conscious animals. The operation itself is simple to perform in the rat but it involves the excision of a considerable amount of the adrenal cortex, the tissue whose hormonal secretion enables the animal to resist the stress of surgery. It is conceivable, therefore, that rats which have undergone this operation suffer some permanent change which might affect their subsequent behaviour quite independently of their having lost their adrenal medullae. It is difficult to prepare satisfactory 'control' animals for an operation like this: it is usual to produce them by subjecting some animals to a 'sham' operation in which the adrenals are exposed and handled but are not interfered with surgically. This procedure obviously does not produce animals which

differ from the experimental group only in their possession of adrenal medullae. Situations in which it is impossible to establish a true 'control' group are by no means uncommon in pharmacology.

In setting up or assessing experimental work, the reader should always ask himself whether every possible step has been taken to design the study in a fashion which will ensure that the results are influenced only by the treatment or manoeuvres under investigation.

Retrospective and prospective studies

Investigations involving human beings can rarely be carried out under the same rigid conditions as those that can and should be applied to experiments in the animal laboratory. We could hardly, for instance, take a group of healthy young people, divide them into carefully matched pairs and then proceed to study the effects of cigarette smoking on the lungs by requiring that one member of each pair should smoke heavily for twenty years while the corresponding 'control' subject abstained completely. If we were interested in the relationship between smoking and the development of pathological changes in the lungs we would have to institute a *retrospective* survey. We would enquire about the smoking habits of a group of patients with pulmonary disease and compare them with those of a group of patients (or normal subjects) whose lung function was unimpaired. Retrospective investigations of this kind are sometimes known as *case-control* studies, a description that implies comparisons between patients and appropriate control subjects.

Not all clinical investigations are subject to restraints that demand retrospective studies. If, for instance, we wished to compare the therapeutic effectiveness of two similar drugs we could plan an experiment that incorporated all the refinements of design that are customarily demanded in animal experiments. Investigations that can be planned in this way are of a *prospective* nature. *Cohort* surveys involve a carefully selected group (or cohort) of subjects: these surveys are usually prospective in nature although they may include retrospective elements.

Attributes and variables

An *attribute* is a character or a quality. Thus a patient may have a particular disease, a person has eyes of a restricted number of colours and so on. The essential feature of an attribute is that it enables experimental results to be classified into a number of categories or 'cells'. A *variable*, on the other hand, is a measurement—such as the height of a patient, the weight of an animal, the amount of histamine in a tissue extract—which can take any one of a large and undefined number of numerical values. It is possible, if the need arises, to convert variables into attributes and thus to use the statistics of attributes to analyse variables. Consider, as an example, an investigation which involves measuring the heights of a group of people. The results obtained are variables but they can be converted into attributes by categorizing all those whose height exceeds an arbitrary value as 'tall' and all those below that height as 'short'. The converse process-the conversion of attributes into variables—cannot be carried out.

THE STATISTICS OF ATTRIBUTES

The χ^2 (chi-squared) test

It is not possible, within the limitations imposed by the necessity of treating the subject of this chapter as succinctly as possible, to explain or discuss the theoretical basis of the χ^2 test which is, incidentally, pronounced *kye* square (or squared). Fortunately, ignorance of its origin need not preclude its successful application, unlike the situation with some other tests that will be considered later.

We can begin our inspection of the test with a very simple example. Suppose that a coin is tossed 100 times: it comes down showing 'heads' on 60 occasions and 'tails' on the remaining 40. We require to know whether these figures supply evidence that the coin is biassed. Our null hypothesis is that the coin is not biassed so that we should have expected to see 50 'heads' and 50 'tails'. In order to assess the likelihood that the difference between the observed and expected figures has arisen by chance, we make use of the formula

$$\chi^2 = \Sigma \frac{(\text{actual-expected})^2}{\text{expected}}$$

Σ represents 'the sum of' and in the present instance χ^2 is very simply calculated as $\frac{(60-50)^2}{50} + \frac{(40-50)^2}{50} = 4$. Since there are only two possible responses in this experiment ('heads' and 'tails') there is only one degree of freedom. Some indication of the χ^2 values for the number of levels of P and various degrees of freedom (d.f.) is provided by the figures presented in Table 9.1. Complete tables of χ^2 can be found in textbooks of statistics but the fragment given in Table 9.1 is sufficient to indicate that the possibility that the observed difference from expectation has arisen by chance is just less than 0.05 ($P < 0.05$). Thus our null hypothesis is falsified and we conclude that the coin may be biassed.

Table 9.1 Some χ^2 values

P	df 1	5	10
0.10	2.71	9.24	15.99
0.05	3.84	11.07	18.31
0.01	6.64	15.09	23.21
0.001	10.83	20.51	29.59

A rather more complicated example is illustrated in Table 9.2 which purports to display the relationships between eye and hair colour. The figures, incidentally, are completely fictitious. The 'expected' values are given in brackets and are calculated as follows: of the 165 subjects included in the imaginary study, 80 (48.5 per cent) have blue eyes, 55 (33.3 per cent) have grey eyes and the remaining 18 per cent have brown eyes. The null hypothesis (that hair colour and eye colour are not associated) requires that a similar distribution should be evident among the individuals in the separate 'hair colour' categories - 48.5 per cent of the 50 subjects with light hair should have blue eyes and so on. The χ^2 calculation involves the addition of the nine terms

$$\frac{(14-24)^2}{24} + \frac{(30-17)^2}{17} \cdots\cdots + \frac{(9-7)^2}{7}$$

Table 9.2 A 3 $\times$ 3 contingency table

	Blue		Eye colour Grey		Brown	
Light hair	14	[24]	30	[17]	6	[9]
Dark hair	43	[36]	17	[26]	15	[13]
Ginger hair	23	[20]	8	[13]	9	[7]

There are four degrees of freedom—if the totals of each row and each column are to be maintained, no more than four of the component figures can be independently varied—and this exemplifies the general rule that a table with p columns and q rows (a $p \times q$ *contingency table*) permits $(p - 1) \times (q - 1)$ degrees of freedom.

The 2 $\times$ 2 contingency table. Although contingency tables may contain any number of cells, the 2 $\times$ 2 form is that which is most frequently encountered in practice. This is because so many investigations involve simple double dichotomies—for instance, into patients with or without a disease who have or have not received a particular treatment. We must therefore examine the analysis of a 2 $\times$ 2 contingency table in rather more detail and we can do this with the aid of the data set out in Table 9.3(a) which compares the incidence of an illness in 50 inoculated children with that in a group of 60 children who had not received inoculations. It is evident that a higher proportion of the uninoculated children (40 per cent as against 22 per cent of the inoculated group) have succumbed to the disease but we wish to know how likely it is that this difference could have arisen by chance. We have, in other words, to test the validity of the null hypothesis that inoculation does *not* provide protection against the disease. Now, if the null hypothesis is valid, the incidence of illness in the inoculated group of children will be just as reliable a guide as the disease's infectivity as is the incidence in the uninoculated group and we must take this into account when we compute the 'expected' values for our χ^2 determi-

Table 9.3(a) A 2×2 contingency table

	Inoculated	Uninoculated	Totals
With disease	11	24	35
Without disease	39	36	75
Totals	50	60	110

Table 9.3(b) 'Expected' values calculated for the observations in Table 9.3(a)

	Inoculated	Uninoculated	Totals
With disease	16	19	35
Without disease	34	41	75
Totals	50	60	110

nation. Thus, 35 of the total of 110 patients included in the study succumbed to the disease and the null hypothesis requires that this proportion should be maintained in both the inoculated and uninoculated groups: $\frac{35}{110}$ of 50 and of 60, rounded up to the nearest whole number, give 16 and 19 respectively and these are the values that appear in Table 9.3(b). The other two figures in that table are derived in an analogous manner—or by simple subtraction—and our χ^2 value is calculated as the sum of $\frac{(11-16)^2}{16}$, $\frac{(24-19)^2}{19}$, $\frac{(39-34)^2}{34}$ and $\frac{(36-41)^2}{41}$. This is 4.22; the significance of this result will be discussed shortly.

In practice, it is not necessary actually to calculate the 'expected' values when our data are disposed in a 2 x 2 contingency table. Instead, we substitute the observed values in the formula:

$$\chi^2 = \frac{n(ad-bc)^2}{(a+b)\,(c+d)\,(a+c)\,(b+d)}$$

where the terms have the meanings indicated in Table 9.4. The formula is a very easy one to remember; applied to the figures of Table 9.3(a) it gives

$$\chi^2 = \frac{110[(11 \times 36) - (24 \times 39)]^2}{35 \times 75 \times 50 \times 60}$$

$$= 4.07$$

This estimate differs slightly from our earlier one but this is merely the consequence of our having 'rounded off' figures when calculating for Table 9.3(b) the values to be expected if the null hypothesis holds.

χ^2 values obtained when the number of observations is rather small (as in the present example) often give spuriously high estimates of statistical significance and a better estimate is obtained by applying a formula that incorporates a correction introduced by Yates. The Yates formula is

$$\chi^2 = \frac{n\left[|ad - bc| - \dfrac{n}{2}\right]^2}{(a+b)\,(c+d)\,(a+c)\,(b+d)}$$

The symbol | | (the *modulus*) indicates that the sign of the difference between *ad* and *bc* is disregarded, a positive quantity being entered. Although it is not always necessary to apply the Yates' correction to the figures in a 2 x 2 contingency table, no harm is done if the formula is used in cases where the simple χ^2 formula would have sufficed.

The reader will see that the Yates correction involves no more than the subtraction of half the total number of observations from the difference between *ad* and *bc* before proceeding to treat the figures in the same way as when applying the uncorrected formula. The 'corrected' χ^2 value for the data we are discussing is given by

$$\chi^2 = \frac{110 \,[|(11 \times 36) - (24 \times 39)| - 55]^2}{35 \times 75 \times 50 \times 60}$$

$$= 3.29$$

Thus the χ^2 value obtained by this method is lower than that arrived at by applying the uncorrected formula. Indeed, according to Table 9.1, a χ^2 of 3.29 with one degree of freedom will occur with differences between 'observed' and 'expected' quantities that have rather more than a 1 in 20 (0.05) probability of having arisen by chance and which are, therefore, not statistically significant. We have, however, to take another factor into consideration. The χ^2 values in Table 9.1 are taken from a 'two-tailed' table which sets out the values that must be attained in order to establish the statistical significance of deviations from expected values that can occur in either the positive or negative direction. To illustrate this, let us suppose that we were evaluating the performance of a new scientific instrument by using it to measure a series of quantities which had already been accurately determined by an older instrument of established reliability. The new instrument would give results that were sometimes larger and sometimes smaller than those obtained with the older instrument and it would be appropriate to appeal to the two-tailed table if we were applying the χ^2 test to see whether the differences between the readings given by the two instruments could have arisen by chance. The situation is quite different when we consider our inoculation data, because the figures themselves and collateral evidence from other sources (as well as plain common sense!) make it clear that the

Table 9.4 The generalized 2×2 contingency table

	Observed values		Totals
	a	b	a + b
	c	d	c + d
Totals	a + c	b + d	a + b + c + d $= n$

treatment we are studying can only possibly operate in one direction—if it has any effect at all, it will reduce the incidence of disease. We therefore have to convert our 'two-tailed' into a 'one-tailed' table to enable us to assess the significance of departures from 'expected' values in the one direction only. The rule for doing this is simple: the 'one-tailed' χ^2 value required for a degree of statistical significance P is the same as that for a two-tailed value at a probability level of $2P$. Thus for one degree of freedom and a probability level of 0.05, χ^2 must reach 3.84 if deviations in both directions are possible but only 2.71 (see Table 9.1) if it is known that the effect of the experimental treatment will be exerted in only one direction. In the present example, therefore, we can say that an *association* between inoculation and freedom from the disease has been established and that the level of statistical significance lies between 0.05 and 0.025 ($0.025 < P < 0.05$). As we shall see, some other statistical tables can relate to either a two-tailed or a one-tailed situation and care may have to be exercised, first to decide which table to use in a particular analysis and then to ensure that the correct version is being referred to.

It is extremely important to realise that the establishment of an association does not by itself imply that the two attributes are causally related. They may both be determined by a third factor. Thus, if our inoculation data were acquired in the course of a retrospective survey, it could be argued that the group of inoculated children was not representative of the population at risk by virtue of the fact that the more conscientious parents would be the more disposed to seek protection for their children. Consequently the children's relative freedom from the disease might be a manifestation of some other effect of parental care such as attention to diet or to the physical environment. In order to determine whether there is indeed a causal relationship between two associated attributes, additional studies have to be undertaken.

The χ^2 test should not be applied if any cell in a contingency table indicates an *expected* value smaller than 5. When small values do occur, it may be possible to eliminate them—if the table has dimensions greater than 2 x 2—by incorporating the rows or columns that contain them into neighbouring cells. The distorting effect of small values in a 2 x 2 contingency table can be countered by making an 'exact' computation of χ^2 (see Bailey, 1959 *inter al*) but the method is fairly laborious. In any event, too much importance should not be attached to results of marginal significance obtained from a small number of observations.

The χ^2 test is widely used both by pharmacologists and by those who pursue research in the clinical field: the association between cigarette smoking and lung cancer was first demonstrated by the use of this statistic. It is suitable for analysing the result of any experimental investigation in which the observations can be set out in 'cells' and it may also be employed to determine the 'goodness of fit' of an observed set of quantitative values to a theoretical distribution.

THE STATISTICS OF VARIABLES

The normal curve

Suppose that we measure the heights of a large number of randomly-chosen adult males. Most of them would have a height within a few inches of the average of the group as a whole, some would differ from the average height by a larger margin and a few would be very short or very tall. If we constructed a frequency diagram showing the number of individuals (p) attaining particular heights, a curve similar to that shown as A in Fig. 9.1 would be obtained. This is the so-called *normal curve*, which was originally known as the normal curve of error because it describes the distribution of the errors made in physical measurements. Thus, if a large number of people each measure the weight of the same object, most of them will arrive at a value within a few grams of the true weight and a few will return weights markedly different from this.

The normal curve was first described, as long ago as 1733, by De Moivre (whose theorem plagued so many of us at school) but it was also discovered quite independently by Gauss, one of the greatest mathematicians of all time. For this reason, the normal distribution is sometimes described as Gaussian. Gauss was not, however, born until 1777 and the use of his name in this way provides an illustration of the well recognized fact that eponymous descriptions do not always bestow credit on those who most deserve it.

Some considerable time elapsed after the discovery of the normal curve before it became apparent that it describes the distribution of many phenomena, particularly biological ones. The ubiquity of the distribution is surprising—the cross section of a pile of dry sand takes this form!—and many of the statistical tests commonly used in biological work are based on the assumption that the variables being measured are normally distributed. This assumption is often justified and many variables which do not follow a perfectly Gaussian distribution are only

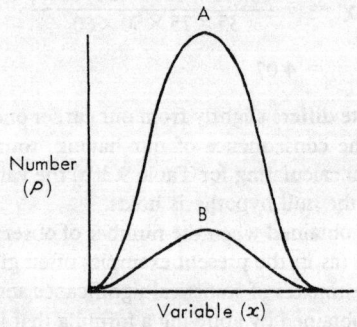

Fig. 9.1 The normal curve.

slightly assymmetrical (or *skew*) so that no great error is introduced if they are examined by statistical techniques designed for perfectly symmetrical distributions. Nevertheless the possibility that variables may not be normally distributed must always be borne in mind.

The curves labelled A and B in Fig. 9.1 both illustrate normal distributions. They differ only in that the variables whose distribution is portrayed by curve A are more closely concentrated about the mean than are those of curve B, which are more evenly spread.

The equation for the normal curve is given by:

$$p = \frac{n}{\sigma\sqrt{2\pi}} \, e^{\frac{-x^2}{2\sigma^2}}$$

where p represents the frequency of occurrence of the variable x and n is the total number of observations. The symbol σ (sigma) locates the points at which the gradient of the curve is steepest. In mathematical terms these are the *points of inflection,* where the convexity of the middle part of the curve changes into the concavities of its extremities. Because of the symmetry of the normal curve the two points of inflection occur equidistantly on both sides of the mean, $\bar{x}$ (Fig. 9.2). The quantity σ is the *standard deviation.* The way in which it is calculated is described later but it should be noted now that the standard deviation provides some important quantitative information. The range of values of x from $(\bar{x}-\sigma)$ to $(\bar{x}+\sigma)$ embraces 68.2 per cent of the total number of observations. The spans $(\bar{x}-2\sigma)$ to $(\bar{x}+2\sigma)$ and $(\bar{x}-3\sigma)$ to $(\bar{x}+3\sigma)$ include, respectively, 95.5 and 99.78 per cent of the total. Another relationship, which is convenient to remember because reference to it will be made frequently in the following pages, is that the range $(\bar{x}-1.96\sigma)$ to $(\bar{x}+1.96\sigma)$ includes 95 per cent of the observations.

The standard deviation provides a very succinct way of summarizing a large number of observations. Thus the statement that the body temperature of a group of normal young adult males was 98.1 $\pm$ SD 0.4°F (150) tells us that 150 subjects were studied, that their average body temperature was 98.1°F and that 102 (68.2 per cent of 150) had a body temperature in the range 97.7 to 98.5°; similarly 143 had temperatures in the range 97.3 to 98.9°F. It should also be noted that the standard deviation offers a prediction as well as a description. Taking the present example, we can say that there is a 95.5 per cent chance that the body temperature of *any* young adult male will fall between 97.3 and 98.9°F.

The meaninglessness of the term 'normal'. The reader should pause at this point to reflect that the figures just quoted for body temperature (they are taken from an actual study) falsify the commonly held notion that there is a single 'normal' body temperature which is maintained by all healthy people. It is true that the mean body temperature (98.1°F in our example) is the most common in the sense that more individuals exhibit this than any other

particular temperature. Nevertheless, subjects with a body temperature other than the mean value far outnumber those with it. A similar situation occurs with other physiological measures and statements about 'normal' values only have meaning if standard deviations are quoted so that it is possible to estimate the ranges of values within which known proportions of the samples lie.

Calculation of the standard deviation. We shall first inspect and apply a method of calculating the standard deviation which, though tedious, does have the merit of providing a clear idea of the nature and properties of the parameter and of some of the important quantities related to it.

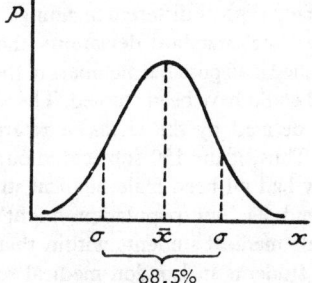

Fig. 9.2 To show the relationship of the mean ($\bar{x}$) and standard deviation (σ).

Let us represent the n members of a series of measurements as x_1, x_2, x_3 and so on to x_n. We obtain the arithmetic mean ($\bar{x}$) of the group and then find the difference between each individual measurement and the group mean. The n quantities so derived—$(x_1 - \bar{x})$, $(x_2 - \bar{x})$......$(x_n - \bar{x})$—are squared and added together, a process represented by $\Sigma\,(x - \bar{x})^2$ and often symbolised as s^2. This gives us the *sum of squares,* a statistic which ought properly to be (but never is) called the sum of squares of deviations from the mean and which, as we shall see, often appears in statistical analyses. The sum of squares is divided by n (this gives the *variance*) and we arrive finally at the standard deviation (SD) by taking the square root of this quotient, remembering that the square root of a positive number can be either positive or negative. We can summarise these manipulations in the formula

$$SD = \pm \sqrt{\frac{\Sigma\,(x-\bar{x})^2}{n}}$$

In biological work in general, and in pharmacological investigations in particular, conclusions have often to be based on results obtained from very small samples and in these circumstances the standard deviation of the sample is likely to be rather different from that of the population from which the sample was taken. Mathematical analysis shows that an acceptable correction to the sample standard deviation can be made by a simple modification of the formula just derived. The 'corrected' formula is

$$SD = \pm \sqrt{\frac{\Sigma (x - \bar{x})^2}{n - 1}}$$

As n increases, the difference between the standard deviation obtained by dividing the sum of squares by $(n - 1)$ and that obtained by dividing by n becomes progressively smaller and the laboratory worker does not have to decide whether he has a sufficiently large number of observations to justify his dividing by n. The use of the 'corrected' formula is, therefore, always appropriate.

The observant reader will have noticed that in the course of the last few pages the symbol for the standard deviation has been slyly changed from σ to SD. The two abbreviations have, in fact, slightly different meanings. The letter σ represents the 'true' standard deviation—the value that would be obtained if all possible members of the *population* being sampled could have been studied. The nature of the population is defined by the terms of reference of the investigation. Thus, if the 150 subjects in our body temperature study had all been male medical students aged between 18 and 23, our population might have been defined as male medical students within that age range, male medical students in London medical schools, etc., depending on the point the study was intending to establish. The abbreviation SD is the value of the standard deviation calculated from the sample actually studied. If the number of items in the sample is large, the calculated SD will be virtually identical with σ.

Before we proceed to an actual calculation it will be helpful, for future reference, to bring together some of the relationships that have appeared in the preceding paragraphs and to add one or two new ones. So far we have

$$\text{variance} = \frac{\text{sum of squares } (s^2)}{n - 1}$$

$$\text{standard deviation (SD)} = \pm \sqrt{\text{variance}}$$

A very important statistic, to which we shall devote some attention later, is the standard error of the mean (SEM) which is more often simply called the standard error and is arrived at by dividing the standard deviation by the square root of n. Hence

$$SEM = \frac{SD}{\sqrt{n}} = \sqrt{\left(\frac{\text{sum of squares}}{n(n - 1)}\right)} \text{ or } \sqrt{\frac{\Sigma (x - \bar{x})^2}{n(n - 1)}}$$

Finally we must mention the *coefficient of variation*. The standard deviation tells us something about the scatter of the observations it refers to, but if we wish to assess the breadth of the scatter we have to take into account the magnitude of the standard deviation relative to that of the mean with which it is associated. A standard deviation of 1°C attached to a series of readings that have a mean of 5°C clearly reflects a wider relative spread of observations than would the same standard deviation if the average tempera-

ture were 100°C. The coefficient of variation (CV) enables us to compare the standard deviations of samples that have different means. It is given by

$$CV = \frac{100 \times SD}{\text{mean}} \%$$

Thus for the temperature readings just referred to, the coefficients of variation are $\frac{(100 \times 1)}{5} = 20$ and $\frac{(100 \times 1)}{100}$ = 1 per cent respectively. In practice the coefficient finds few applications.

A moment's reflection on the formula for the standard deviation should make it clear that it represents an average (the *root mean square*) of the variations about the mean. The root mean square (often identified simply as r.m.s.) is a familiar average measure in other fields: in electricity, for instance, the root mean square of the voltage of an alternating current gives the magnitude of the steady voltage in a direct current supply that would provide the same amount of electrical energy.

We can now proceed to make an actual calculation of the standard deviation and this is done in Table 9.5 which illustrates the application of the formula we have already discussed to a relatively small group of nine observations. Squaring the differences eliminates the minus quantities that appear in the $(x - \bar{x})$ column but the signs should always be entered particularly if the calculation is being performed without the assistance provided by a calculating machine. They provide a useful check on the arithmetic because the sum total of the negative differences will be the same as that of the positive ones if no arithmetical error has been made.

Although they are arithmetically simple, the calculations involved in finding the standard deviation can become extremely tedious when they are applied to a

Table 9.5 Calculation of the standard deviation of the mean of a series of blood sugar estimations by direct calculation of the sum of squares

Blood sugar in mg/100 ml (x)	$x - \bar{x}$	$(x - \bar{x})^2$
98	12.56	157.7536
90	4.56	20.7936
78	- 7.44	55.3536
80	- 5.44	29.5936
90	4.56	20.7936
75	-10.44	108.9936
66	-19.44	377.9136
79	- 6.44	41.4736
113	27.56	759.5536
TOTAL	Sum of squares (s^2)	1572.2224
(T) 769	Variance ($\frac{s^2}{n-1}$)	196.5278
n 9		
Mean	S.D.	$\pm\sqrt{196.5278}$
($\bar{x}$) 85.44		$= \pm$ 14.02

group of more than a very few variables. Fortunately there is a simple algebraic manipulation that leads to a more acceptable method of calculation because $\sum (x - \bar{x})^2$, the sum of squares, can be expressed in the form $\sum x^2 - \dfrac{(\sum x)^2}{n}$. The reader who is disposed to do so, can confirm the validity of this relationship for himself by applying the elementary rules of algebra and recalling that $(x - \bar{x})^2$ gives $x^2 + \bar{x}^2 - 2x\bar{x}$.

The term $(\sum x)^2$ in our new formula is called the *correction factor:* it is arrived at, quite simply, by adding all the observations together (a process that will already have been performed when the arithmetic mean was calculated), squaring this sum and dividing it by the number of items in the group. The correction factor can be expressed in the form $\dfrac{T^2}{n}$, where T is the sum total of all the observations. This version is, indeed, preferable because it avoids reference to $(\sum x)^2$, a term that can easily be confused with $\sum x^2$ by those who apply statistical methods only infrequently.

All we have to do, then, to obtain the sum of squares is to square and add the individual values ($\sum x^2$) and to subtract the correction factor from this total. The calculation is worked in Table 9.6 for the same set of variables that were examined previously. Most of the advantages of this method of calculation are obvious but it can be even easier to apply than may appear at first sight because many electronic calculators will yield both the sum, and the sum of the squares, of a series of numbers in a single operation. Moreover, this method is intrinsically more accurate than the 'direct' method of calculation which usually involves a rounding up or down of the mean. The small inaccuracy thus introduced finds its way into every one of the differences $(x - \bar{x})$ and thence into the sum of squares.

Standard error of the mean.

We have seen that the standard deviation provides information concerning the scatter of *individual* values about the mean. The standard error of the mean (SEM), which we have already defined (p. 116) gives similar information concerning the scatter of *means*. To take once again the example of the mean body temperature, the standard error of the mean of the 150 observations is $\pm\dfrac{0.4}{\sqrt{150}} = \pm 0.03$ and it enables us to say that, if another sample of 150 young adult males was taken the mean body temperature of the group as a whole would have a 68.2 per cent chance of falling between 98.07°F and 98.13°F and a 95 per cent chance of coming within the range 98.04°F to 98.16°F. The last quoted values (which represent, of course, the mean $\pm$ 1.96 SEM) are known, for obvious reasons, as the 95 per cent *confidence* (or *fiducial*) limits (or *intervals*) and they enable us to declare the degree of reliability that can be placed on the estimated means. Other fiducial limits (the 99 per cent or the 99.9 per cent limits) can be calculated if the need arises. Although the descriptions 'confidence' and 'fiducial' are frequently used interchangeably, there is a distinction between the two, but this need not concern the general reader.

If, as is usual in pharmacology, we calculate means from only a few items, we cannot be sure that the range, mean $\pm$ 1.96 SEM, will give us the 95 per cent fiducial limits. The smaller the sample size, the more scattered will be the values obtained on repeated determinations of the mean and the wider, therefore, will be the fiducial limits. In order to determine *how* wide the limits should be, we make use of the statistic t which indicates the distance (in terms of the number of standard errors) from the mean at which we must place our boundaries in order to be certain of including 95 per cent (or other fractions) of the total population of means. When the samples are 'infinitely' large (in practice this means that they must contain more than 20 items), the 95 per cent confidence limits are represented, as we have seen, by the mean $\pm$ 1.96 SEM but when they contain only six items (that is, when the number of degrees of freedom is 5) the 95 per cent limits stretch from 2.6 SEM below, to 2.6 SEM above, the mean (Table 9.7). Reference to the table shows also that the 99 per cent limits for 5 degrees of freedom extend to 4 standard errors on each side of the mean.

The 95 per cent fiducial limits indicate the bounds within which 95 per cent of a series of grouped observa-

Table 9.6 Calculation of the standard deviation for the data of Table 9.5 using the formula:

Sum of squares $= \sum x^2 - \dfrac{T^2}{n}$

Blood sugar in mg/100 ml (x)	x^2
98	9604
90	8100
78	6084
80	6400
90	8100
75	5625
66	4356
79	6241
113	12769

TOTAL
(T) 769   Total ($\sum x^2$) 67279

n 9   Sum of squares (s²) 67279 − 65706.7777
= 1572.2223

Mean ($\bar{x}$) 85.44

Correction factor $\left(\dfrac{T^2}{n}\right)$ $\dfrac{591361}{9}$

The variance and standard deviation are calculated as before

= 65706.7777

Table 9.7 Some values of 't' (two-tailed test)

n	P 0.05	0.01
2	4.2	9.9
5	2.6	4.0
10	2.2	3.2

tions are likely to lie. There is thus a 5 per cent likelihood ($P = 0.05$) that an estimate will fall *outside* these limits and that is the reason for indicating probabilities in the t table which is widely used, not only for calculating fiducial limits, but also for assessing the statistical significance of the differences between series of variables.

Fiducial limits often need to be quoted in the presentation of information concerning the potency of one drug relative to others or to known standards. The reader will encounter several methods of calculation of the limits, each appropriate to particular experimental situations.

Student's t-test of significance

Gosset, a statistician who wrote in the early years of this century, sometimes called himself 'Student' and it was over this pseudonym that he first published details of the t test. In the event the eponym proved to be extremely apt, for research students (and, indeed, many of their elders) seem to be particularly attracted by this particular test which they use more widely (and wildly) than any other statistical method.

One use of the ratio t has already been mentioned and it is easy to understand the principal whereby it is used to assess the statistical significance of the difference between the means of two series of variables. Suppose that we have been investigating the action of a drug on a particular variable and that the mean value of this variable in a group of animals given the drug is x_1 with a standard error of ϵ_1. Let the corresponding values in a group of untreated animals ('controls') be x_2 and ϵ_2. Suppose further that these parameters are such that the distributions to which they refer are located in the position shown in figure 9.3— that is, that they intersect at a point located at a distance of 1.96 standard errors away from the respective means. Now we know that 5 per cent of the observations represented by

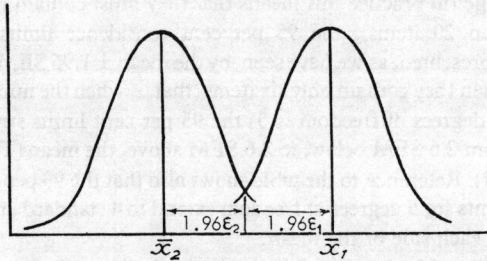

Fig. 9.3 To illustrate the basis of Student's t-test.

the curves will fall outside the range spanned by points that lie 1.96 standard errors below and above the mean and it is self-evident that these 5 per cent will be equally divided between the two extremes of the distribution. Consequently we can say that the difference between the means x_1 and x_2 in our example is statistically significant at the 0.025 level of probability because if repeated samples of the variable x_1 (or x_2) are taken they will by chance come within the distribution of x_2 (or x_1) no more than 2.5 times in a hundred. The condition for the 0.025 level of probability is therefore

$$\bar{x}_1 - \bar{x}_2 = 1.96\,(\epsilon_1 + \epsilon_2)$$

or

$$\frac{\bar{x}_1 - \bar{x}_2}{\epsilon_1 + \epsilon_2} = 1.96$$

For mathematical reasons, this condition is expressed in the quantitatively different but conceptually similar form

$$\frac{x_1 - x_2}{\sqrt{(\epsilon_1^2 + \epsilon_2^2)}} = 1.96$$

Now the argument presented above is only valid if the number of items in our samples is sufficiently large to ensure that the interval, mean $\pm$ 1.96 SEM, really does include 95 per cent of the total possible population of means. When samples are small the ratio given above must reach the t value corresponding to the appropriate number of degrees of freedom if it is to indicate a probability level of 0.025. Other values of t, of course, signal other degrees of probability.

The formula actually employed for calculating t is

$$t = \frac{\bar{x}_1 - \bar{x}_2}{s}\sqrt{\frac{n_1 n_2}{n_1 + n_2}}$$

where

$$s^2 = \frac{1}{n_1 + n_2 - 2}\left\{\Sigma\,(x_1 - \bar{x}_1)^2 + \Sigma_n(x_2 - \bar{x}_2)^2\right\}$$

n_1 and n_2 are the number of items in the two series; the number of degrees of freedom in the system is $n_1 + n_2 - 2$.

The argument in the preceding paragraphs has led us to the conclusion that a t of 1.96, when derived from a reasonably large number of observations, indicates that the difference between the means is statistically significant at the 0.025 level of probability. However, reference to Fig. 9.3 will make it clear that this conclusion is only justified if we know that the effect we are investigating can operate in one direction only—in the type of experiment illustrated in Fig. 9.3 for instance, we must be quite sure that the only possible effect that the drug can have, if it has any at all, is to increase the value of the variable x. This is the 'one-tailed' condition we encountered when discussing the χ^2-test but when we apply the t-test, particularly in pharmacology, it only rarely happens that we can have solid grounds for believing that the manoeuvre we are testing really can operate in one direction only, though we might have a strong suspicion that it does so. Usually, then, we have to take both tails of the distributions into account and we do this by applying (this time in the opposite direction) the very simple rule we have already used (p. 114), doubling the P value for a one-tailed distribution in order to meet the two-tailed situation. Our t of 1.96, therefore, when derived from values that require a two-tailed test, indicates a statistical significance at only the threshold 0.05 level of probability. Tables that set out the probability level of different t-values usually give the two-tailed probability because, as we have seen, t-values are also used to determine confidence limits and these are essentially two-tailed since they are placed on both sides of the mean. The user can always check his t-tables by noting whether a t of about 1.96 indicates, for the highest number of degrees of freedom, a probability of 0.05 or of 0.025. Rarely, he will encounter t-tables in their original form in which probabilities are displayed as numbers that have to be subtracted from unity to obtain the one-tailed values.

It is important to note (and this point is frequently ignored) that the t-test is only valid if there is no significant difference between the variances of the two series. The method of checking that this is so is indicated later.

The application of the t-test in a typical two-tailed situation is illustrated in Table 9.8 which shows the effect of the drug bulbocapnine on the glycogen content of rat brain (Crossland and Rogers, 1968).

By referring to Table 9.7 it can be seen that the value of t indicates a statistically significant difference at almost the 0.01 level of probability. Before accepting this value we must satisfy ourselves that there is no significant difference between the variances of the two samples. This is done by calculating F, the ratio of the larger to the smaller variance. In the present example, the variance of the series x_1 is $\frac{0.40}{5}$ = 0.08 and that of x_2 is $\frac{0.68}{5}$ = 0.14. F, which is known as the *variance ratio* (or sometimes *Snedecor's ratio*) is there-

fore $\frac{0.14}{0.08}$ or 1.8. From two-tailed tables it can be found that, with the number of degrees of freedom in the present example (5 in each series), F must exceed 5.05 before the difference between the variances can be considered significant at the 0.05 level of probability. The use of the t test is therefore justified in the present case. Methods are available for comparing the means of small samples whose variances do differ significantly from each other (Bailey, 1959). Alternatively, a non-parametric assessment (p. 128) may be used.

As was pointed out earlier (p. 110), pharmacological investigations sometimes make use of a 'paired sample' design. Animals are grouped into carefully matched pairs and one member of each pair receives the treatment under investigation, while the other serves as the 'control'. A series of differences between treated and untreated animals is thus obtained. The null hypothesis requires that the mean value of these differences should be zero and in this situation the t test resolves itself into a comparison of the actual differences and a series of zeros. The formula for the determination of t is thereby simplified into

$$t = \frac{\bar{x}}{\text{SD}}\sqrt{(n-1)}$$

where $\bar{x}$ is the mean, SD is the standard deviation of the observed differences and n is the number of matched pairs. The number of degrees of freedom is, of course, $n - 1$.

Analysis of variance

This technique, whose development is due largely to R. A. Fisher, provides the pharmacologist with one of his most powerful statistical tools. It is an invaluable procedure for the analysis of properly designed experiments and it underlies many bioassays. It is unfortunate that it is not possible, within the compass of a single chapter, to give more than a brief and inadequate account of the technique

Table 9.8 Calculation of student's 't'

	Untreated animals (x_1)			Treated animals (x_2)		
x_1	$(x_1 - \bar{x}_1)$	$(x_1 - \bar{x}_1)^2$		x_2	$(x_2 - \bar{x}_2)$	$(x_2 - \bar{x}_2)^2$
3.6	-0.3	0.09		3.6	0.3	0.09
3.7	-0.2	0.04		3.8	0.5	0.25
4.4	0.5	0.25		3.0	-0.3	0.29
4.0	0.1	0.01		2.9	-0.4	0.16
3.9	0.0	0.00		3.6	0.3	0.09
4.0	0.1	0.01		3.0	-0.3	0.09
23.6		$\sum (x_1 - \bar{x}_1)^2$ 0.40		19.9		$\sum (x_2 - \bar{x}_2)^2$ 0.68
$\bar{x}_1$ 3.9				$\bar{x}_2$ 3.3		
n_1 6				n_2 6		

$$t = \frac{3.9 - 3.3}{\sqrt{\frac{1}{10}(0.40 + 0.68)}} \times \sqrt{\frac{36}{12}} = \frac{0.60}{0.33} \times 1.7 = 3.1$$

The figures relate to the glycogen content (expresses as μ moles of glucose per gram) of rat brain.

Table 9.9 Data for an analysis of variance

SAMPLE			SAMPLE			SAMPLE		
A	*B*	*C*	*A*	*B*	*C*	*A*	*B*	*C*
4(0)	5(1)	6(2)	3(1)	5(1)	4(0)	1	0	2
4(0)	6(2)	2(2)	3(1)	5(1)	4(0)	1	1	2
2(2)	4(0)	7(3)	3(1)	5(1)	4(0)	1	2	3
2(2)	7(3)	3(1)	3(1)	5(1)	4(0)	1	2	1
3(1)	3(1)	2(2)	3(1)	5(1)	4(0)	0	2	2

	15	25	20
Means	3	5	4

Individual values with differences from overall mean (4) in parentheses.

(a)

Calculation of variation *between* samples. Individual values have been replaced by the appropriate sample mean. Differences from the *overall* mean are in parentheses.

(b)

Calculation of variation *within* sample. The figures indicate the difference of the individual values in Table 6. 8(a) from their sample mean (3, 5, & 4 respectively).

(c)

and its potentialities but an attempt will be made to describe it in terms that will enable readers to understand the analyses of variance they will encounter in many of the scientific papers they will (or ought to) read. Some may be encouraged to delve deeper into the applications of the method while others, whether they like it or not, will have to employ it in the course of their professional duties. These groups of readers will have to progress to sources of more detailed information such as the monographs listed in the bibliography to this chapter. The writer himself found that he set about the task of understanding variance analysis with rather more enthusiasm when he found it described as *anovar* (Campbell, 1969), a euphonious and gently seductive term that deserves a wider currency than it presently enjoys.

'Student's' *t* test is a form of variance analysis but it is only applicable to data which are grouped into two series. In its more generalized form, the analysis of variance is used for the examination of multiple groups of variables. Suppose, to take first a very simple example, that we are to perform an experiment involving measurements on a group of 15 animals and that these animals have to be obtained from three sources. We wish to know whether, notwithstanding their different origins, the animals form a homogeneous group in respect of the variable we are to measure. To simplify the analysis so that the reader may follow the arithmetic involved, let us assume that the variable has the small and simple values indicated in Table 9.9(a).

The mean value of the variable, calculated from all 15 animals, is 4 and the deviation of the individual values from this overall mean are shown in parentheses in Table 9.9(a). These differences are squared and added: the 'sum of squares' so obtained is 46 with 14 degrees of freedom. Now the variation represented by this overall sum of squares arises from two sources: there is a difference *between* the means of the three samples and the individual values *within* each sample also differ. In order to obtain the

sum of squares relating to the first mentioned source of variation, we eliminate the differences within each sample by replacing the individual values by the sample mean, as shown in Table 9.9(b). The difference of each value from the overall mean is 1, 1 and 0 respectively in the three samples: the differences are squared and added. The result is 10 and there are 2 degrees of freedom in the system. We now need to calculate the sum of squares due to variation *within* the samples. We obtain the difference of each value from its sample mean. The figures, which are displayed in Table 9.9(c) are squared and added. As the reader can easily calculate, the result of this operation gives 36 with 12 degrees of freedom. The results of our computations are summarized in Table 9.10 which is the usual form in which an analysis of variance is displayed. The 'within sample' sum of squares and degrees of freedom could of course have been obtained by subtracting the 'between sample' figures from the corresponding totals but by making separate calculations for the two sources of variation we have provided a useful check on the accuracy of the arithmetic.

The analysis is completed by calculating F as before. It is $\frac{5}{3} = 1.67$. The number of degrees of freedom (n_1) in the system responsible for the larger variance is 2 and that (n_2) for the smaller variance is 12. Tables show that the value of F required to establish a significant difference at the 5 per

Table 9.10 Analysis of variance for the data of Table 9.9

Source of variation	Sum of squares	Degrees of freedom	Mean square	Variance ratio (F)
Between samples	10	2	$\frac{10}{2} = 5$	1.67
Within samples	36	12	$\frac{36}{12} = 3$	1.00
Totals	46	14		

cent level with these degrees of freedom is 3.89 and we can conclude that the differences between the means of our three samples has arisen purely by chance and that the 15 animals can be treated as a homogeneous group.

Before passing on to discuss a more complicated anovar we must draw attention to the fact that, in the simple analysis just described, the smaller variance arose from the 'within-sample' figures and this is what we would expect since each supplier would strive to produce as uniform a strain of animal as possible. The 'within-sample' parameter in our example measures the 'residual' variance, a term that appears in all anovars. It is the variance that remains after the effects of all the imposed sources of variation have been taken into account and it reflects the inevitable and irreducible variability that is inherent in any group of experimental results. It is attributable to the random operation of a number of factors such as unavoidable experimental and observer error as well as to the natural innate variations in biological samples however carefully they are chosen.

We can now proceed to discuss a rather more complex analysis of variance. It has been selected almost arbitrarily from among the very many that could have been taken from the recent literature and it is therefore representative of those that the pharmacologist will repeatedly encounter. The interested reader should, ideally, work the whole calculation for himself the better to appreciate the meaning of the various quantities that are derived from the experimental results and the nature of the arithmetical manipulations that produce them. This is important because scientific papers themselves never discuss, as we are about to do, the calculations that transform their masses of numerical information into succinct analyses of variance since it is assumed that their readers will be familiar with the technique.

Our sample study (Williams *et al.*, 1974) concerned itself with the effect of diphenhydramine (an antihistamine drug) and of pH on the absorption of methaqualone (a hypnotic agent) from the mouth. The reasons for studying the buccal absorption of this drug need not be entered into here.

Seven volunteer subjects were given solutions of methaqualone (1 mg per ml) containing three different concentrations of diphenhydramine (0, 0.1 and 0.2 mg per ml) and each mixture was presented at two different acidities (pH 5 and pH 8). All the subjects took, in turn, all six mixtures each of which was held in the mouth for five minutes and then spat out. The amount of methaqualone in the expectorate (together with that in an appropriate buffer solution with which the mouth was washed out after each test) was measured in order to determine the amount of drug that had been absorbed. The 42 results are assembled in Table 9.11 and are analysed in Table 9.12 which, like our earlier table, takes the form that is now invariably adopted for the display of analyses of variance.

The values in Table 9.12 are derived as follows.

We first of all compute the total sum of squares (ss) for all 42 results using the formula with which we are already familiar –

$$ss = \sum x^2 - \frac{T^2}{n}$$

The 42 individual values in Table 9.11 are squared and added (19321.44) and from this total we subtract $\frac{T^2}{n}$ which, as we have seen, is also known as the correction factor (CF). In the present instance it amounts to 16602.35 (the sum total of the 42 values is squared and divided by 42) so that the total sum of squares is 2719.09. The number of degrees of freedom in the calculation for the total sum of squares is clearly 41.

We now have to assess the contributions to the total sum

Table 9.11 The effect of diphenhydramine and of pH on the absorption of methaqualone from the buccal cavity (figures from Williams *et al*, 1974)

		Amount of methaqualone absorbed (per cent of administered dose)				
		Methaqualone 1 mg/ml		Methaqualone 1 mg/ml + Diphenhydramine 0.1 mg/ml		Methaqualone 1 mg/ml + Diphenhydramine 0.2 mg/ml	
Subject		pH5 (1)	pH8 (2)	pH5 (3)	pH8 (4)	pH5 (5)	pH8 (6)
	1	23.58	22.60	15.75	20.38	15.52	18.60
	2	11.38	26.37	10.84	14.35	8.86	10.35
	3	11.31	16.88	20.52	22.20	17.33	18.84
	4	33.08	34.31	22.31	19.22	13.11	13.58
	5	19.80	31.49	18.55	27.56	11.42	17.81
	6	30.03	33.43	26.04	21.78	10.10	14.76
	7	33.52	39.84	22.15	21.41	5.04	9.04
Means		23.243	29.274	19.451	20.986	11.626	14.711

Table 9.12 Analysis of variance for the figures in Table 9.11

Source of variation	Sum of squares	Degrees of freedom	Mean square	Variance ratio (F)
Main effects				
pH	132.37	1	132.37	20.21*
dose	1201.82	2	600.91	91.74*
subjects	379.62	6	63.27	9.66*
Interactions				
pH × dose	36.48	2	18.24	2.78
pH × subjects	95.12	6	15.85	2.42
dose × subjects	795.12	12	66.26	10.12*
Residual				
pH × dose × subjects	78.56	12	6.55	—
				* P < 0.001
Totals	2719.09	41		

of squares that are made by the three imposed sources of variation—pH, dose of diphenhydramine and the subjects themselves. We proceed in precisely the same manner as we did when we worked our simple example. Taking pH, for instance, we imagine that each of the 21 values appearing in the three pH 5 columns has been replaced by the overall mean of the 21 figures (18.107). In a similar fashion we replace the 21 values in the pH 8 column by their overall mean (21.657). The sum of squares attributable to the pH is then given by

$$[21 \times (18.107)^2 + 21 \times (21.657)^2] - CF$$

This gives us 132.37 with a mean square (variance) of the same magnitude since there is only one degree of freedom.

Analogous calculations provide the sums of squares due to the changing dose of diphenhydramine (all values in columns 1 and 2, 3 and 4, 5 and 6 are replaced by their respective means; two degrees of freedom) and to inter-subject variation (all six values for each subject replaced by the subject mean; six degrees of freedom) and these sums of squares and the corresponding mean squares are inserted in the table.

If we add together the sums of squares relating to pH, diphenhydramine dose and subjects we shall find that their total falls considerably short of the overall sum of squares we originally calculated. The deficiency cannot yet be defined as the residual sum of squares because we still have to take into account the effect of possible *interactions* between the experimental variables. It has been implicit in our discussions so far that if, for instance, pH and diphenhydramine both influence the absorption of methaqualone they will do so quite independently of each other. This however is not necessarily so because the effect of pH may alter as the dose of diphenhydramine is varied. Analogous interactions might occur between pH and subjects (different subjects responding in quantitatively different ways to alterations in the pH of the mixture they take) and between subjects and the dose of diphenhydramine.

In order to calculate, and to assess the significance of, the variance attributable to interaction between pH and the diphenhydramine dose we have first to compute the sum of squares for the two factors taken together. We do this by replacing the individual values in each of the six columns of Table 9.11 by the appropriate column mean. What we do, in effect, is to eliminate the variation that arises from the third variable (the subjects), a source which is not relevant to our immediate calculation. The sum of squares we need is given by:

$$7[(23.243)^2 + (29.274)^2 + (19.452)^2 + (20.986)^2 + (11.626)^2 + (14.711)^2] - CF$$

Our ubiquitous correction factor is 16602.35 as before and the combined sum of squares for pH and dose becomes 1370.67. From the latter figure we subtract the sums of squares that relate to the two separate factors and these amount, as we know, to 132.37 for pH and to 1201.82 for dose (Table 9.12). The remainder (36.48) is the sum of squares relating to the interaction of the two factors. The number of degrees of freedom (1×2) is the product of those for the two separate components.

For the interaction between dose and subject $(2 \times 6$ degrees of freedom) we exclude the effect of pH by replacing, for each subject at each of the three dose levels, the methaqualone absorption at pH 5 and pH 8 by the mean of these two values so that the six entries for each subject are reduced to three (23.09, 18.07 and 17.06 respectively for subject 1 and so on) and the sum of squares calculation is

$$2[(23.09)^2 + (18.07)^2 + \ldots\ldots (7.04)^2] - CF$$

A total of 21 terms will appear within the square brackets. We arrive at 2376.56 for the joint sum of squares and we must subtract those relating to dose (1201.82) and subjects (379.62) to obtain the sum of squares for the dose × subject interaction. It is 795.12.

The last interaction we have to calculate is that between pH and subject (1 x 6 degrees of freedom) and for this purpose we have to eliminate the influence of the varying dose of diphenhydramine by replacing the six values for each subject by the two obtained by taking, respectively, the means of the three values at pH 5 and the three at pH 8. Thus for the first subject in Table 9.11, we have 18.28 (the mean of 23.58, 15.75 and 15.52) and 20.53 and the sum of squares is given by

$$3[(18.28)^2 + (20.53)^2 + \ldots\ldots (23.43)^2] - CF$$

There will be 14 terms inside the square brackets and the interaction sum of squares is arrived at by a process that should now be familiar to the reader.

We can now, at last, calculate the residual variation. It can be regarded as equivalent to the pH x dose x subject interaction and consequently it has 12 (1 x 2 x 6) degrees of freedom. It is computed quite simply by adding together the six sums of squares for the individual factors and their interactions and subtracting this aggregate from the total sum of squares we originally calculated. We note that the degrees of freedom for the seven sources of variation total 41, as they should.

The variance ratios are calculated as before and we discover their statistical significance by reference to the appropriate tables. To take the pH effect as an example, the tables tell us that if a variance ratio has been arrived at as a result of dividing a variance with one degree of freedom by one with 12 degrees of freedom it must reach 4.75, 9.33 or 18.64 to establish statistical significance at the 0.05, 0.01 or 0.001 levels of probability respectively. Since the variance ratio we obtain for pH is rather larger than 18.64 we can assert that changing the pH of the administered mixture caused changes in methaqualone absorption greater than those that could be accounted for by experimental error or simple biological variation and that the probability that this result arose by chance is less than one in a thousand ($P < 0.001$). Inspection of Table 9.11 will make it clear that the influence of pH is such that absorption is encouraged by a rise of pH. Three of the other variance ratios are also significantly greater than unity (the value that would be expected if the factor being analysed had no effect on absorption), all of them at a probability level of less than 0.001. The remaining two ratios are not significantly different from unity.

Thus our analysis of variance (read in conjunction with the data on which it is based) informs us that the absorption of methaqualone from the mouth is significantly depressed, in a dose-dependent manner, by diphenhydramine but that it is encouraged by increasing the pH of the solution in which it is presented and that subjects differ significantly one from another in the readiness with which they can absorb the drug and in the extent to which the absorption is impeded by diphenhydramine. On the other hand, the response to a change in pH does not vary from subject to subject and it is unaffected by the presence of diphenhydramine.

The reader who is new to statistical methods will now be in a position to appreciate the force of the remarks made earlier (p. 119) concerning the value of variance analysis in pharmacology.

The anovar we have described in such detail can be classified as a three-way analysis because three main sources of variation had to be taken into account. In a more involved experimental situation there would be more than three imposed sources of variance and the analysis would be·correspondingly more involved. For instance, in a four-way analysis we would have to consider the variance attributable to the four sources themselves (let us call them a, b, c and d) and to interactions both between pairs ($a \times b$, $a \times c$, $a \times d$, $b \times c$, $b \times d$, $c \times d$) and among triplets ($a \times b \times c$, $a \times b \times d$, $a \times c \times d$ and $b \times c \times d$). Fortunately, modern statistical calculators relieve their operators of

much of the tedious arithmetic that statical analysis once demanded: some need to be provided with nothing more than the raw data and an instruction to produce, say, the sum of squares. The arrival of these instruments in our laboratories does not however absolve us from the duty of becoming familiar with the principles of the calculations we order them to perform.

Correlation and regression

If we measured the height and weight of a number of individuals, we could display our results in the form of a *scatter diagram*, similar to that illustrated in Fig. 9.4 in which there is one point, giving the value of the variables x and y, for each individual in the sample. Because some short people are very fat and some tall people are very thin, we would expect the points to exhibit a degree of scatter, but at the same time we would also expect to notice a tendency for high values of x to be associated with high values of y. We would, in other words, expect x and y to show some degree of *correlation*. Statistical methods permit correlations of this type to be detected and quantitatively assessed.

The reader will appreciate that in respect of variables, correlation has much the same meaning as has association in respect of attributes. As with an association, the establishment of a correlation between two variables must not be taken as an indication that a causative relationship has necessarily been established.

For the examination of correlation we can derive one or both of two measures—the *correlation coefficient* and the *regression lines*.

The correlation coefficient This statistic, always represented by r, measures the closeness of the correlation between x and y. Suppose that the points in Fig. 9.4 had fallen on a perfectly straight line instead of being scattered. We could then have said that there was a perfect correlation between the two variables and that no change in x could occur without a predictable and proportionate change in y. The correlation coefficient is such that a perfect correlation is represented by a coefficient of $+1$ or -1. The positive sign is appropriate to cases in which y increases as x increases; a negative coefficient indicates that y decreases as x increases.

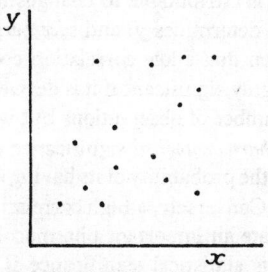

Fig. 9.4 A scatter diagram.

The formula to be given for the calculation of the coefficient of correlation assumes that the variables x and y are representative samples of normally distributed populations. If they are not, the coefficient loses much of its quantitative significance but regression line analysis (see below) is still permissible.

The correlation coefficient is given by

$$r = \frac{\frac{1}{n-1} \Sigma (x - \bar{x})(y - \bar{y})}{(SD)x \times (SD)y}$$

where the terms have the meanings they have held throughout this chapter; $(SD)x$ and $(SD)y$ refer to the standard deviations of the x and y variables respectively. A word is necessary concerning the quantity $(x - \bar{x})(y - \bar{y})$. The difference of each 'x' from $\bar{x}$, the mean of the series, is multiplied by the difference of the corresponding 'y' from $\bar{y}$ and the n products are then added together. Now, the individual terms of the $(x - \bar{x})$ and the $(y - \bar{y})$ series—and therefore their products—may be either positive or negative quantities. The signs must be taken into account when computing $\Sigma (x - \bar{x})(y - \bar{y})$.

Having determined the correlation coefficient, which must lie somewhere between -1 and $+1$, we have to decide whether a statistically significant relationship has been established or whether the particular r could have arisen by chance. To do this, we make use of Student's t yet again, using the formula

$$t = r \sqrt{\frac{(n-2)}{1-r^2}}$$

There is, in fact, no need to calculate t because tables are available which show the value of r which must be attained before the coefficient can be regarded as statistically significant. Thus, if we have 12 comparisons (11 degrees of freedom), r must exceed 0.55 to establish significance at the 5 per cent level of probability. With one hundred degrees of freedom, an r of as little as 0.16 reaches statistical significance at the 5 per cent level.

The correlation coefficient provides useful information concerning the extent to which changes in one variable are linked with changes in the other. This information is obtained by multiplying r by 10 and then squaring. Thus, if r is 0.7 it is possible to estimate that 49 per cent of the variation in x is attributable to changes in y (or to some process which determines y) and vice versa.

We have seen that a low correlation coefficient can be statistically highly significant if it is derived from a sufficiently large number of observations but we must remember that the pharmacological significance of a low r is the same whether the probability of its having arisen by chance 0.01 or 0.001. Conversely, a high correlation coefficient is likely to indicate an important pharmacological relationship even if its statistical significance is marginal. This distinction between pharamcological or clinical signifi-

cance and statistical significance is an extremely important one that should be borne in mind whenever experimental findings are being analysed, irrespective of the statistical technique that is used.

Regression lines. A regression line is the line (or its equation) which most accurately describes the relationship between x and y. It enables us to predict the value of x (or y) corresponding to any value of y (or x).

It is normally assumed that the relationship between x and y can best be represented by a straight line. This assumption is not always justified but the mathematics of curvilinear relationships is too formidable for the amateur mathematician and the pharmacologist usually has to restrict his analysis to situations in which a straight line provides the best fit to the experimental data. Fortunately, these conditions are often fulfilled.

'Regression' was introduced into the statistician's vocabulary by Sir Francis Galton towards the end of the nineteenth century. He pointed out that although very tall men are likely to father tall sons, these children will deviate from the normal height by a smaller amount than their fathers. A similar generalization applies to the offspring of abnormally short men and to the magnitude of other inherited qualities. Galton described this phenomenon as 'the regression to mediocrity' and he illustrated it with graphs he called regression lines. The name has become attached to all lines which display the relationship between linked variables although the lines rarely describe regressions in the sense used by Galton. Galton's findings incidentally did not establish any fundamental principle of heredity: a real Victorian, he had ignored the fact that sons have mothers as well as fathers.

If we were asked to fit by eye a straight line to the points in Fig. 9.4, we would obviously try to draw it in such a position that the average distance of the individual points from the line reached a minimum. This is virtually what is done when the line is fitted mathematically except that the computation gives the line from which the squares of the distances of the points reaches a minimum value. This is called the method of least squares. In fact, mathematical analysis gives two straight lines. The reason for this will emerge from a consideration of the two parts of Fig. 9.5.

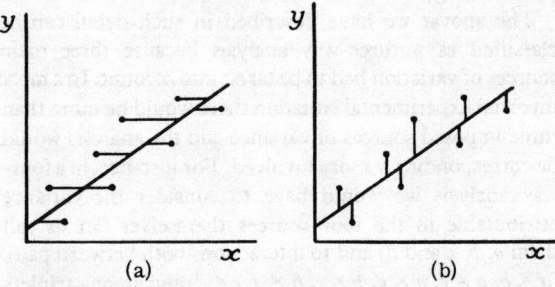

Fig. 9.5 To illustrate the method of deriving the equation for the regression of y on x (a) and of x on y (b).

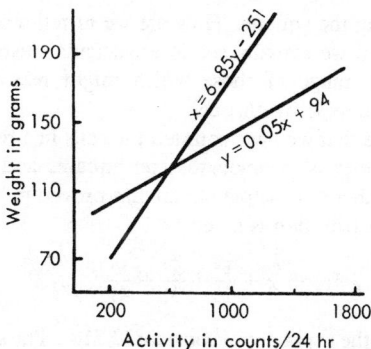

The regression line in Fig. 9.5(a) is fixed so that the deviations from it along the x axis reach a minimum. It (or its equation) enables y to be predicted from x. The line in Fig. 9.5(b) shows that in which deviations along the y axis reach a minimum. It shows the regression of x on y; it enables x to be calculated if y is given. If r is 1 the two regression lines coincide. The further the correlation coefficient falls short of unity, the further the lines diverge from one another. It is usual to insert both lines on the scatter diagram (Fig. 9.6).

Straight lines are represented by the equations $y=mx+c$ (for the regression of y on x) and $x=m'y+c'$ (for the regression of x on y).

If the regression lines are to be calculated from variables for which it will also be necessary to calculate the correlation coefficient, the equations for the regression lines can be obtained from the relationships:

$$y = r\left(\frac{SDy}{SDx}\right)(x-\bar{x})+y$$

and

$$x = r\left(\frac{SDx}{SDy}\right)(y-\bar{y})+\bar{x}$$

The appropriate values of r, $\bar{x}$, $\bar{y}$, SDx and SDy are substituted to give two simple expressions (of the form, $y=mx+c$) in x and y. Two arbitrary values of x are then chosen and the corresponding values of y are calculated from the first of these expressions. The two points thus found enable us to draw the regression line on the scatter diagram. The regression line of x on y is fitted in a similar fashion using the second expression. The equations of the lines may of course be used, instead of the lines themselves, if it is necessary to predict the values of y (or x) corresponding to values of x (or y) other than those used for the construction of the scatter diagram.

If r is not to be calculated, we make use of the general equation for the straight line and calculate the constants m and c from:

$$m = \frac{\Sigma(x-\bar{x})\,(y-\bar{y})}{\Sigma(x-\bar{x})^2}; \quad c = \bar{y}-mx$$

The constants for the regression line of x on y are calculated similarly, replacing $\Sigma(x-\bar{x})^2$ by $\Sigma(y-\bar{y})^2$ etc. The quantity $\Sigma(x-x)(y-\bar{y})$ is calculated in the manner described for the calculation of r.

It is often useful to be able to quote confidence limits for the regression line. The standard error of m is given by

$$SEM = \frac{s}{\sqrt{(x-\bar{x})^2}}$$

where $s^2 = \dfrac{1}{n-2}\left\{\Sigma(y-\bar{y})^2 - \dfrac{[\Sigma(x-\bar{x})\,(y-\bar{y}]^2}{\Sigma(x-\bar{x})^2}\right\}$

If the number of the observations is large, the lines obtained using $m\pm1.96$ SEM and the appropriately adjusted value of c (calculated from $c = y - mx$) will lie on

Fig. 9.6 Relationship between locomotor activity and body weight.

either side of the regression line and will indicate the boundaries of the 95 per cent confidence limits. If n is small the SEM will have to be multiplied by the appropriate value of t to give the limits.

Some of the points discussed in the preceding paragraphs may be clarified by reference to Fig. 9.6, which shows the relationship between locomotor activity and body mass in young rats (Crossland and Turnbull, 1972). Locomotor activity (x) is measured in terms of the number of times the animal crosses a light beam in 24 hours. The mass of the animals (y) is in grams and the equations of the two regression lines are shown, as is usual, on the lines themselves. For the sake of clarity, the actual points of the scatter diagram are omitted. In this particular investigation the value of r was $+0.60$ ($P<0.001$), indicating that 36 per cent of the variation in locomotor activity among different animals in the group was attributable to differences in the animals' weights.

The Poisson distribution

Not all variables exhibit a normal distribution. One of the non-Gaussian distributions which may be encountered in pharmacological work is that first described by Poisson in 1837. It can be illustrated by reference to the problem of counting red blood cells in an ordinary haemocytometer. The reader will recall that a drop of diluted blood is placed on a microscope slide on which is engraved a grid of small squares. When the cover slip is properly in position, a precise volume of the diluted blood overlies each marked square. The number of erythrocytes in each of a block of squares is counted and from this the number of cells in the blood which yielded the diluted sample can be computed. Similar methods are available for the counting of white cells, the number of bacteria in a liquid suspension and so on.

It is highly unlikely that every square of the haemocytometer will contain the same number of cells. At the same time, mistakes in preparing the diluted sample or in placing the cover slip will cause an uneven distribution of cells among the squares. How are we to tell whether the distribution we actually see in a particular instance falls within the range of those which might reasonably be expected to arise by chance?

Suppose that we have counted the cells in a reasonably large number of haemocytometer squares and that the mean number of cells per square has proved to be x. The Poisson distribution is given by

$$e^{-x}(1 + \bar{x} + \frac{\bar{x}^2}{2!} + \frac{\bar{x}^3}{3!} + \frac{\bar{x}^4}{4!} \dots\dots)$$

where e is the exponential constant (2.718). The symbol $n!$ is read as 'factorial n': 3! indicates the product 3x2x1, and so on for the other factorial products. The terms within the brackets of the Poisson distribution give successively the proportion of the total number of squares which will contain 0, 1, 2, 3, 4 .... red cells. In order to calculate the absolute number of squares we expect to be so occupied, we multiply the individual fractional values by n, the total number of squares examined.

The 'expected' distribution given by the Poisson distribution can be compared with that actually obtained if we use the χ^2 test, the result of which will indicate whether the observed distribution differs significantly from that which would be expected to arise by chance.

Many discontinuous variables are distributed in the Poisson fashion. One example which is frequently quoted in text books is that described by Bortkewitch. It relates to the number of cavalrymen in the Prussian army who suffered death in successive years from horse kicks!

Measures of average
Asked to calculate the 'average' of a series of n variables, most of us would add the individual values together and divide the resulting total by n, computing in this way the *arithmetic mean* which is a logical and readily understood concept. Indeed it is so well known and understood, even by those with no pretension to numeracy, that we did not feel any compulsion to define or explain the term when it first entered our discussions earlier in this chapter. The arithmetic mean is a very useful parameter too, because it can form, in a way that is denied to other measures of average, the basis of analyses that provide much additional information about the series of observations from which it has been derived. The reader will realise that all the calculations relating to normally distributed variables that he has so far encountered in this chapter have centred on the arithmetic mean.

The arithmetic mean is not, however, the only way we have of expressing an average value nor is it always the most appropriate and we must now devote some attention to the *median*. To obtain the median of a number of variables we simply arrange them in ascending order of magnitude. The value that then occupies the middle place in the order is the median. Thus, in the group 1, 2, 5, 6, 9,

the median is 5: two values are smaller than 5 and two are greater. For groups made up of an odd number of values the median is immediately identifiable; the median of an even number of variables is taken as the arithmetic mean of the two central values. By this convention the median of the sequence 1, 2, 5, 8, 9, 11 is 6.5, the mean of 5 and 8. No modification of either of the described procedures is required when a value occurs more than once: the median of the series 1, 2, 5, 6, 6, 6, 9 is 6, the number that occupies what we might perhaps call the 'geometrical' midpoint of the order. Special, but simple, techniques are required for assembling and finding the median value of a large group of variables but they need not concern us here.

We see that the median is obtained without our having to subject the individual items to any arithmetical treatment beyond the calculation, when appropriate, of the mean of the two central values. All we have to do is to locate the midpoint of an ordered sequence of numbers.

Quantities that are arranged in ascending order of their magnitudes can be said to be disposed in ranking order and, in later pages, we shall have to look at some other statistics that can be derived from a consideration of the rank order of collections of variables.

It should be evident, from what has already been said, that the median, unlike the arithmetic mean, will not be influenced by the intrusion of a few extreme values into a group of otherwise similar variables and it is in this property that the one real strength of the median lies. To illustrate this, and to indicate the way in which the median can be employed in descriptive statistics, let us consider an imaginary group of five pharmacologists with individual annual incomes of £3500, £3800, £4200, £4700 and £20 000 respectively. The arithmetic mean of the salaries is £7240 but the median is only £4200. It is clear that the median provides a more realistic idea of the income level of the group as a whole than does the arithmetic mean which gives a distorted impression because of the impact of the one extreme value. If an increase in salary were denied to the group on the grounds that the average income of its members was £7240, four of the five would be condemned to continuing penury but if an increase were granted on the grounds that the average income was but £4200, only one member of the group would receive an unwarranted increment. Thus the use of the median would ensure justice for the majority but the arithmetic mean would secure it only for the minority.

It would not, of course, be necessary in a real life situation to invoke either the median or the arithmetic mean if we were discussing the salary levels of a group of only five people since the precise circumstances of each individual could be comprehended at a glance. However, the principle enunciated in our simple example is a valid one, because arguments do have to be based on summary values when large groups of supplicants are involved and the median is frequently appealed to when salary structures are being erected or modified. It is particularly applicable to groups of individuals such as architects, actors, barristers—and authors!—a very few of whose members enjoy incomes that are substantially higher than those of their fellows while a few others may live in at least temporary poverty. The utility of the median in this context can be widened by dividing the range of salaries (arranged, of course, in rank order) into four equal parts or *quartiles* and quoting the medians of the first (the lowest) and the fourth (the highest) quartiles as well as the overall median. This provides a more realistic view of the rewards offered by a particular occupation because it brings into focus not only the general level of renumeration but also the earnings of the least well paid members and those of the giants of the profession.

A number of other variables, particularly in the biometric field, exhibit the same sort of fluctuations as do salary levels and, in these instances too, the median may provide a more realistic summary of the mass of data then would the arithmetic mean. In addition, and as we shall see later, a comparison of medians forms the basis of statistical tests that can be applied to sets of variables taken from populations that do not show a normal distribution and which, in consequence, cannot be analysed by the usual parametric methods.

The median salary of our imaginary group of pharmacologists was considerably below the mean salary. This arose because the individual salaries were very unevenly distributed around the central value. If they had been more evenly spread, the arithmetic mean and the median would have been closer together and if the distribution had been perfectly symmetrical the two measures would have been coincident. The reader can readily confirm the truth of this last assertion for himself by calculating the arithmetic mean and locating the median of the numbers 1, 3, 7, 11, 13. It is a general property of any statistically normal distribution that its mean and median coincide: an inspection of Fig. 9.2 should make it quite clear that $\bar{x}$, the arithmetic mean, is also the median, because the same number of values exceed $\bar{x}$ as fall short of it.

Another way of expressing the average value which is, however, of only limited utility, is to use the *mode*, the most 'fashionable' member (cf. *à la mode*) of a group. Thus, in the sequence 1, 3, 3, 4, 6, 6, 6, 7 the modal value is 6 because it appears more often than any other value. In a normal distribution the mode, like the median, coincides with the mean. An empirical and approximate relationship links the mode, the mean and the median of a series of variables taken from a population whose distribution is no more than moderately skew (p. 115). It is:

$$\text{Mode} \simeq \text{Mean} - 3(\text{Mean} - \text{Median})$$

Finally, we must refer to the *geometric* and *harmonic* means. To illustrate the application and calculation of the geometric mean, let us suppose that we wish to estimate the likely size in 1965 of a community that numbered 50 000 in 1955 and 90 000 in 1975. The larger a population becomes, the greater will be the number of children born into it each year so that its growth rate progressively increases. Our community will, therefore, have grown more rapidly in the later than in the earlier part of the twenty years period. Consequently, although the arithmetic mean of the two population figures would yield the midpoint (70 000) of the population range, this would overestimate the size of the community at the midpoint of the period. The geometric mean provides a better estimate. It is obtained, for our particular example, by multiplying together the figures for 1955 and 1975 and taking the square root of the product. This is 67 082 and we can accept this as the best available estimate of the 1965 population.

The geometric mean (G) can be calculated for any number of variables. The general formula, assuming n variables $(x_1, x_2\ldots\ldots x_n)$ is:

$$G = \sqrt[n]{(x_1 \times x_2 \times \ldots\ldots x_n)}$$

Apart from its use for estimating the average of a group of variables whose rate of change depends on the size of the variable itself (as in our example), the geometric mean can be applied to the calculation of the averages of groups of values that increase by a constant multiplying factor, as in the sequence 3, 6, 12, 24, 48. Variables of this kind are encountered in serological work: when sera are assayed their activity is expressed in terms of the dilution (*titre*) at which a required end point is reached. The different dilutions are related to one another by a constant multiplying factor (usually 2) and it is a matter of empirical observation that, when a number of assays of the same serum are made, the geometric mean of the several determinations approaches the true value more closely than does their arithmetic mean. The geometric mean is also employed for averaging quantities like price indexes that are expressed as fractions of a fixed reference or base value.

Speeds (rates of reaction etc.) are averaged by taking the harmonic mean (H) which is calculated for our n variables $(x_1, x_2\ldots\ldots x_n)$ from the formula

$$\frac{1}{H} = \frac{1}{n}\left(\frac{1}{x_1} + \frac{1}{x_2} + \ldots\ldots\frac{1}{x_n}\right)$$

or, more succinctly,

$$H = \frac{n}{\Sigma \frac{1}{x}}$$

We can illustrate the application of the harmonic mean by referring to the old problem of the optimistic motorist who, calculating the arithmetic mean, believes that he averages 45 mph if he covers half his journey at 30 mph and the other half at 60 mph. He should use the harmonic mean to compute his average speed. In this example it is given by $\frac{1}{2}(\frac{1}{30} + \frac{1}{60})$ or 40 mph.

For the same set of figures, the harmonic mean is smaller than the geometric mean which is, in its turn, smaller than the arithmetic mean.

NON-PARAMETRIC STATISTICS

Non-parametric methods have earned no more than a dubious reputation for themselves for while some professional statisticians are attracted to them, others (probably, it would seem, the majority) either abhor them or ignore them altogether. This author's unenthusiastic (but unauthoritative) view is that non-parametric statistics do have a place, but a severely limited one, in pharmacology.

In non-parametric statistics, the absolute value of the variables is not taken into account. Instead, the values are arranged in a ranking order of magnitude and the statistical manipulations are performed on the ranking positions so obtained. The arithmetic involved in making non-parametric calculations is very simple because the variables, however large or complex, are reduced to a series of simple integers. However, a good deal of valuable information is lost by this manoeuvre and, except when the techniques are used merely to obtain a preliminary estimate of the significance of results which are to be more thoroughly investigated later, non-parametric methods should not be applied to variables which can be analysed by parametric methods. They are required when the variables to be analysed are not derived from a normally distributed population or when they do not have a precise quantitative meaning. It is, for instance, possible to grade subjective responses such as pain on numerical scales (0 for no pain, 1 for slight pain, etc.) which, though useful for comparative purposes, yield figures which cannot be handled in the same way as normally distributed variables.

A number of non-parametric tests are available; the one used in a particular case is determined by the nature of the investigation. Rümke and de Jonge (1964) gives a useful summary of seven experimental designs and the non-parametric tests appropriate to each design. More complete details of the methods are to be found in those textbooks of statistics that deign to mention them or those (such as Siegel, 1956) devoted entirely to the subject. Three non-parametric tests are described here so that the reader who has no occasion to use them may have at least some idea of the manipulations involved.

The Mann-Whitney test
The statistic (U) calculated in this test was developed in 1947 from one derived by Wilcoxon some two years earlier.

It is used for estimating the significance of the difference between two groups of values and it might therefore be regarded as a non-parametric equivalent of the t-test.

For the purpose of illustration we will take some figures from the results of an experiment designed to study the effect of drug pretreatment on the severity of the abstinence syndrome produced by the sudden withdrawal of morphine from rats that had become tolerant to the drug and were consuming it in large quantities daily. The nature of the morphine abstinence syndrome is discussed in detail elsewhere (p. 87); all that need be said here is that in our experiments its severity was recorded by a scoring system that depended to some extent on the subjective judgment of the observer. The scoring schedule permitted scores ranging from zero (no abstinence sign) to ten.

The severity of the abstinence syndrome in five animals that had not been given any other drug before withdrawal of morphine was represented by scores that ranged from 2.1 to 3.3: the individual scores, labelled x_1 to x_5, are arranged in ascending order of magnitude in Table 9.13. In five rats that had been given physostigmine immediately before the abstinence syndrome had been precipitated the scores ranged from 2.5 to 5.1. They are also ranked in ascending order of magnitude in Table 9.13 and are labelled y_1 to y_5. We require to know whether pretreatment with physostigmine significantly affected the animals' reaction to morphine withdrawal.

To determine U, we arrange all ten scores in a single rank order. If we identify the scores simply by their code letters we can see the overall order is:

$$x_1 \; y_1 \; x_2 \; y_2 \; x_3 \; x_4 \; x_5 \; y_3 \; y_4 \; y_5$$

We now proceed to calculate the statistic U_1. To do this, we count the number of y values that rank below each of the x values taken in turn. Thus, there is no y lower than x_1 and only one is smaller than x_2. Two values of y come below each of x_3, x_4 and x_5. The sum of these numbers (0, 1, 2, 2, 2) gives us U_1 which is 7. We repeat the process for y, counting and adding the number of x values that rank below each y to obtain U_2 which is clearly $18 (1 + 2 + 5 + 5 + 5)$. U, the statistic we need, is always taken as the smaller of U_1 and U_2 so that for our series of values it is 7.

When there are more than a few values to be processed it is more convenient to calculate U from a formula. The values are arranged in overall rank order as before and the

Table 9.13 The effect of physostigmine on the morphine abstinence syndrome

	Untreated rats (x)			Rats given physostigmine (y)		
No.	Score	Overall rank		No.	Score	Overall rank
x_1	2.1	1		y_1	2.5	2
x_2	2.6	3		y_2	2.7	4
x_3	2.8	5		y_3	3.4	8
x_4	3.0	6		y_4	4.5	9
x_5	3.3	7		y_5	5.1	10
$n_x = 5$		$R_x = 22$		$n_y = 5$		$R_y = 33$

numerical position of each value is noted. These overall rank order positions have been inserted in Table 9.13. The positions of all the x values are totalled to give the quantity Rx and a similar addition of the y positions yields Ry. In our example these rank totals are 22 and 33 respectively. The formulae for calculating U_1 and U_2 are

$$U_1 = n_x n_y \times \tfrac{1}{2} n_y (n_y + 1) - Ry$$
$$U_2 = n_x n_y \times \tfrac{1}{2} n_x (n_x + 1) - Rx$$

where n_x and n_y are the number of observations in the x and y series respectively. For our figures U_1 becomes $25 + 15 - 33 = 7$ and U_2 is $25 + 15 - 22 = 18$ as before.

It frequently happens that a particular value appears more than once in the groups of figures we are analysing so that there might, for instance, be two candidates for position 4 in the rank order. In that event, both would be allocated position 4.5 and the next member of the series would take position 6.

The appropriate tables show that when $n_x = n_y = 5$, the value of U must not exceed 4 to establish significance at the 0.05 level of probability. We can say therefore that the figures in Table 9.12 do not establish any effect of physostigmine on the intensity of the morphine abstinence syndrome. The reader who inspects the figures closely will probably suspect that the lack of statistical significance is largely a consequence of the fact that, for the sake of simplicity, two very small series of values were analysed. He might like to confirm for himself that if the groups in Table 9.12 were increased by adding 2.0 and 2.9 to the x column and 3.5 and 4.9 to the y column, the value of U would be 9, which is sufficiently low when n_x (and n_y) is 7 to establish statistical significance.

The Spearman test
The Spearman rank correlation test is employed when it is necessary to determine whether two variables are independent or are in any way correlated with one another. The

Table 9.15 Some values of R (Spearman Test)

n \ P	Positive Correlation			Negative Correlation		
	0.05	0.01	0.001	0.05	0.01	0.001
5	0			40		
10	58	34	16	272	296	314
15	226	175	97	854	945	1023

method of performing the test is shown in Table 9.14, which compares the marks obtained by ten students in an essay type ('subjective') examination with those scored in an examination in which the correct answer to a number of questions had to be selected from a list provided ('objective' examination). The actual marks in column 2 are converted into rank positions in column 3: student 8 is given position 1, student 7, who scored the lowest mark, occupies position 10. A similar transformation of the marks in the objective examination (column 4) is shown in column 5. The differences (column 6) between the ranks for individual students are squared (column 7) and added to give the statistic R which in this instance is 44. The reader will appreciate the simplicity of the arithmetic.

A moment's reflection will make it clear that, if two variables exhibit a perfect positive correlation, each subject in an experiment will receive the same rank number for both variables. Consequently R will be zero. Conversely, if the two variables show a perfect negative correlation, R will be very large. In the present instance, where we have 10 subjects, the maximum possible value is 330; generally it is given by $\tfrac{1}{3}n(n^2-1)$.

The values of R required to establish a positive or negative correlation at a particular level of significance are obtained from the appropriate table, a fragment of which appears in Table 9.15.

The value of R obtained from the data of Table 9.15

Table 9.14 Calculation of the Spearman coefficient

Student	'Subjective' Examination		'Objective' Examination		Rank Difference	(Difference)^2
	Marks	Rank	Marks	Rank		
1	50	8	45	4	4	16
2	60	4	35	6	-2	4
3	53	7	34	7	0	0
4	72	2	60	2	0	0
5	54	6	47	3	3	9
6	58	5	33	8	-3	9
7	42	10	32	9	1	1
8	73	1	61	1	0	0
9	62	3	42	5	-2	4
10	48	9	31	10	-1	1
						$R = 44$
(1)	(2)	(3)	(4)	(5)	(6)	(7)

indicates a positive correlation at a probability level between 0.01 and 0.05.

The statistic R can be manipulated to provide a rank correlation coefficient (r_s) which, like the correlation coefficient r discussed earlier, has a range of -1 to $+1$. It is calculated as $1 - \dfrac{6R}{n^3 - n}$, an appropriate sign being attached. For the figures of Table 9.14, r_s is 0.73.

The Friedman test

Friedman was the originator of non-parametric statistics. The test which bears his name may be applied to the analysis of experiments designed to compare the mode of action of a number of different drugs or procedures in circumstances in which it is possible to administer each in turn to all subjects used in the experiment. It goes almost without saying that the order in which the treatments are given to the individual subjects must be randomized.

Table 9.16 shows the effect of two drugs, A and B, on the heart rates of six human subjects. The rate, in beats per minute, was calculated from observations made over a suitable period after administration of the drug. The ranking orders of the three different treatments are entered, for each patient, in the table. Thus, for subject 1 the rate after drug B is higher than it is after no drug but it is higher still after drug A. If we give a rank of 1 to the lowest heart rate, the ranking order of treatment for subject 1 becomes 1–3–2. In subject 6 none of the treatments affects the heart rate and the arithmetic sum of the rank numbers (1+2+3) is divided equally among the three treatments. Similarly, if the heart rate after drug A had been the same as after drug B but higher than that in the untreated subject, the rank order would have been entered as 1–2.5–2.5. These rules are of general application in determining ranks in all types of non-parametric tests.

Our null hypothesis is that neither drug affects heart rate. Thus, we would have expected the rank order for each

Table 9.17 The Friedman Test

No. of Subjects	No. of Treatments		
	3	6	12
5	32	183	1210
10	62	388	2558
15	90	582	3837

Values of M required for $P = 0.05$

subject to have been 2–2–2 and the totals in each of the ranking order columns would have been 12. The differences between the actual and expected totals are squared and added to give the statistic M which, in the present instance, amounts to 14. Reference to Table 9.17 shows that the value of M is not high enough to enable us to reject the null hypothesis. It is interesting to note that exactly the same value for M would have been obtained however great the absolute changes in heart rate, if the ranking orders had remained the same. If the value of M had been such as to lead to a rejection of the null hypothesis, it would then have been necessary, by inspection of the results and perhaps by the application of other tests, to determine which of the drugs was exerting a statistically significant effect on the heart rate.

SEQUENTIAL ANALYSIS

Sequential analysis is a statistical technique that was originally developed for use by the Armed Forces of the United States and their advisers but which was then applied to industrial problems and now has some place (albeit a controversial one) in the analysis of drug trials in man (Chap. 10).

The problems encountered by those who have to decide whether to permit full scale production of a new weapon are not dissimilar to those faced by the drug manufacturer.

Table 9.16 The application of the Friedman Test

Subject	Heart Rate After			Ranking Order		
	No Drug	Drug A	Drug B			
1	70	110	79	1	3	2
2	72	70	92	2	1	3
3	93	106	89	2	3	1
4	57	70	62	1	3	2
5	72	82	106	1	2	3
6	80	80	80	2	2	2
Totals				9	14	13
Totals expected on null hypothesis				12	12	12
Differences				−3	+2	+1
(Differences)²				9	4	1
TOTAL					14	

The production of new weapons and drugs are both expensive processes which cannot be justified unless the new agent is demonstrably more effective than an established one. On the other hand, if it *is* more effective, it is essential that this should become known as soon as possible so that production can begin with the minimum of delay, if rivals are to be outwitted. The essential feature of sequential analysis is that the results are collected as they become available (hence the description 'sequential') and the investigation is stopped, and a decision concerning further action is taken, as soon as the accumulated results indicate that a statement can be made at a predetermined level of significance concerning the effectiveness of the new agent. Sequential analysis is particularly useful when the drug under test is to be used in the treatment of a rare condition. As patients become available they are exposed to the drug and the effectiveness of the new treatment is compared with that of the old. Accumulated results are entered on a chart similar to that illustrated in Fig. 9.7. Thus, at stage A, six patients have been given the drug and four of them have shown a favourable response. The instruction is to 'continue testing'. More patients are sought and studied and the findings are added to those previously obtained. The process is continued until the point indicating the accumulated results crosses the 'accept' line (as at C) or the 'reject' line (as at D). The trials are then terminated. Some drugs may, of course, continue to give equivocal results (as at B) over many trials.

Instructions for the construction of the 'accept' and 'reject' lines corresponding to different levels of probability are given in some textbooks of statistics (see, for instance, Moroney, 1956) and it is also possible to purchase suitable analysis charts on which individual results can be marked as they are obtained.

BIOLOGICAL ASSAY

Finney, one of the leading workers in the field, defines biological assay (or *bioassay*) as 'the estimation of the nature, constitution or potency of a material (or of a process) by means of the reaction that follows its application to living matter'. This is rather a wide definition—it does not exclude, for example, purely qualitative observations of the effect of drugs on living matter—and, in the context of the present chapter, it is permissible to confine attention to quantitative assays. These may be conveniently grouped under three heads, although a particular assay method may be applicable to more than one of the three categories of assay.

(*a*) The potency of drugs may be expressed in terms of the dose required to produce a therapeutic, pharmacological or toxic response. It is usual to calculate the dose which will be required to produce the effect in 50 per cent of the test population. If the response is death, this dose is called the LD_{50} (LD=lethal dose); otherwise it is usually described as the ED_{50} (ED=effective dose) although it may sometimes be necessary to resort to other symbols, the meanings of which are usually clear from the context of the reports in which they appear. Dose levels other than that expected to produce the response in 50 per cent of the animals, may also have to be calculated. In that event the subscript is appropriately altered.

(*b*) Drugs which cannot be obtained in a chemically pure form have to be standardized by comparing their activity with that of preparations whose activity has been defined in terms of internationally agreed units. International standards are available for a number of hormone and vitamin preparations, for some antibiotics or antisera, for digitalis (but not for the individual alkaloids, which can be prepared in the pure form) and for heparin. Prescribed methods of standardizing drugs against the international standards are laid down in national pharmacopoeiae.

(*c*) It is often necessary to estimate the amount of active material (such as acetylcholine, histamine or 5-hydroxytryptamine) in a tissue extract, a body fluid or a perfusate. Notwithstanding the recent development of sensitive chemical methods, these estimations have frequently to be performed with the aid of a biological preparation such as the isolated intestine. The effect of the extract is compared with that of known amounts of the substance whose content in the tissue extract is to be determined.

Because of the inherent variability in the responses of living tissues, quantitative bioassay procedures only give reliable results if they are subjected to a tight statistical control and those who undertake a substantial amount of bioassay work should explore, as far as they can, the statistical basis of the methods they use. Far too many laboratory workers are satisfied to apply, blindly, formulae they have been told are suitable for the assays upon which they are engaged. Exhaustive treatments of the statistical principles of bioassay can be found in the texts by Burn, Finney and Goodwin (1950), Emmens (1948) and Finney (1964) to which the interested reader is referred.

The data on which bioassays are based may be either *quantal* or *graded* in nature. A quantal response is mea-

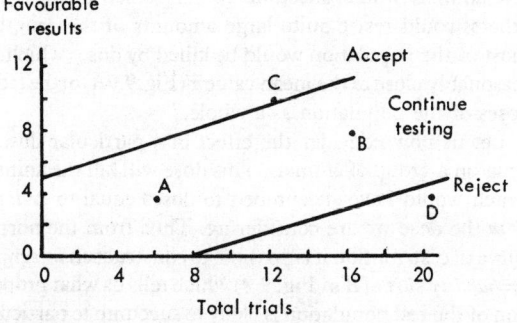

Fig. 9.7 Chart for sequential analysis.

sured by the proportion of the test population which exhibits a particular 'all-or-none' effect. Thus, if we are interested in calculating the LD_{50} of a drug, we may administer. it in different doses to groups of animals and record the number of deaths in each group. Death is obviously an all or none, ungraded response: an animal is either dead or it is not. Methods used for the calculation of the LD_{50} are, of course, applicable to the assessment of other types of quantal response. Graded responses are those which are measured by continuous variables such as weight, body temperature, the extent to which an isolated preparation contracts, etc.

Both quantal and graded assays depend ultimately on our plotting, or making assumptions concerning the form of, dose-response curves. The assay process is considerably simplified if this relationship can be expressed in the form of a straight line. This will be clear from the simple example illustrated in Fig. 9.8. Suppose that we wish to determine the amount of a pharmacologically active substance in t ml of a tissue extract. The responses (S_1 and S_2 respectively) of doses (s_1 and s_2 ml) of a standard solution of the active substance will be sufficient to establish the position of the dose-response curve it it takes the form of a straight line. The effect of the test dose (t ml) of the tissue extract is recorded (T, Fig. 9.8). The amount of active material in this dose is determined by simple interpolation. In the example of Fig. 9.8 it is equivalent to the activity of x ml of the standard solution.

As we discussed in the preceding chapter, log (dose)-response curves are usually sigmoid in form, the middle part of the curve being virtually a straight line. Outside this region the dose-response relationship is a curvilinear one. Moreover, as can be seen by referring to the illustrations in Chapt. 8 the curve becomes more horizontal at low and high dose levels, an appreciable increase in dose being reflected by only trivial changes in response. It is obviously desirable, for the purposes of bioassay, to use the test preparation over a dose range which corresponds to the steepest part of the log (dose)-response curve for it is here that the preparation exhibits its maximum ability to discriminate between doses of different sizes. The steepest part of the curve is also the straightest and it thus becomes a cardinal principle of bioassay that calculations should be based on responses which avoid the extremities of the dose-response curve.

A terminological detail should be noted at this point. Measurements such as responses and doses are called *parameters*. When the raw data are expressed in a form different from that in which they were collected (for instance, when we make use of the logarithms of doses rather than the doses themselves) the transformed parameters are called *metameters*.

The details of experimental design in bioassay work vary with the nature of the assay technique which has been adopted as well as with the preparation to which it is

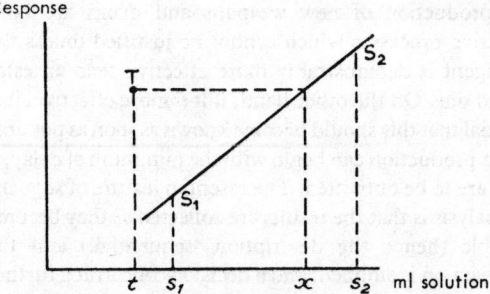

Fig. 9.8 A 3-point assay.

applied. If, however, the response can be measured on intact animals which will not suffer long term effects from the drug administration, it is always advisable to incorporate a *crossover* feature in the overall design. This is illustrated by the method of assaying insulin by reference to its effect on the glucose content of the blood of rabbits. Two doses (S_1 and S_2) of the insulin standard and two of the preparation to be standardized (T_1 and T_2) are used. Rabbits are randomly divided into four groups. On the first day of the experiment each group receives one of the doses of the standard or 'unknown' preparation. The effect of these doses on the blood sugar is measured. On the next day the group which had previously received the lower dose of standard (S_1) is given the higher dose of 'unknown' (T_2) and corresponding crossover arrangements are adopted with the other three groups of animals. In this way, inaccuracies in the assay arising from variations among individual animals are reduced. Crossover tests can sometimes be used in therapeutic trials. Examples will be found in several places in this book, among the chapter sections which are concerned with the laboratory and clinical evaluation of individual drugs.

Calculation of LD_{50} and ED_{50}. In the calculation of these quantities it is convenient to make use of the probit transformation. The transformation is easy to understand from the following considerations. If we knew the precise lethal or effective dose for each animal of a large population we would expect to find that the doses (or more generally the logarithms of the doses) were normally distributed: a few animals would succumb to very small doses, a few others would resist quite large amounts of the drug but most of the population would be killed by doses which lay reasonably close to the mean value $\overline{x}$ (Fig. 9.9A) of the lethal doses of the population as a whole.

Let us now consider the effect of a particular dose of drug on a group of animals. This dose will kill the animals which would have succumbed to doses equal to *or lower than* the dose we are considering. Thus from the normal curve of distribution it is possible to construct an *integrated probability curve* (B in Fig. 9.9) which tells us what proportion of the test population is likely to succumb to particular doses of the drug. The integrated probability curve is

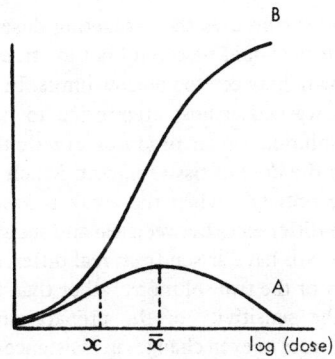

Fig. 9.9 Conversion of the normal curve into the integrated probability curve.

sometimes known as the *cumulative frequency curve*. It is, of course, applicable to any variable which is distributed normally.

The integrated probability curve is, quite clearly, the dose-response curve and the number of deaths corresponding to $\bar{x}$ is the LD_{50}. It will only take the form shown in Fig. 9.9 if the frequency-dose curve from which it is constructed indicates a normal distribution. In pharmacological practice it is found that this is more likely to occur if the scale of the abscissa is logarithmic rather than linear. If it happens that a plot of the actual doses against the response gives a normal distribution, a similar distribution will emerge if the logarithms of the doses are used in the graph. Thus there is no disadvantage in basing calculations on the logarithms of doses even in situations in which the doses themselves could have been used.

To bring about the probit transformation we have to introduce a new metameter, the *normal equivalent deviation*. This quantity is defined, for any value of the log (dose) as $\frac{x-\bar{x}}{\sigma}$: in other words, it represents the distance, in multiples of the standard deviation, of the point x from the mean $\bar{x}$. For values of x less than $\bar{x}$, the normal equivalent deviation is a negative quantity and for arithmetical convenience we eliminate negative values of the deviation by adding 5 to the normal equivalent deviation. This gives the *probit* (a contraction of *probability unit*). The quantity 5 is chosen because it brings the zero of the probit scale to a point located five standard deviations below the mean. It will be clear, from what has already been said about the normal distribution, that this zero point is farther from the mean than we shall ever need to go: it will be recalled that only 0.25 per cent of our population will be expected to respond to a dose of the drug located only 3 standard deviations below the mean.

Probits are related to doses in a linear fashion. If, therefore, we take two groups of animals and expose the members of one group to one dose of the drug and those of the other group to another dose, we shall be able to calculate the percentage mortality (or other quantal response) in each group. The probits corresponding to the two percentages enable us to fix the line relating mortality probits to the logarithm of the dose. From this line we can read off the logarithm of the dose corresponding to a probit of 5. This gives us the LD_{50} because a probit of 5 implies a normal equivalent deviation of zero, *i.e.* $x=\bar{x}$.

Tables are available which enable percentages to be converted directly into probits. Alternatively, it is possible to use a special graph paper in which the ordinate is ruled on a probit scale and the abscissa on a logarithmic scale. However, the concept of probits may be clarified for the reader if he attempts to derive some probits for himself in the fashion illustrated by the following examples. Consider the point x in Fig. 9.9 which, we will assume, is situated one standard deviation away from the mean. Its normal equivalent deviation is therefore –1 and its probit (–1+5) is 4. Now, we know that the range of values from the (mean–SD) to the (mean+SD) includes 68.2 per cent of the population. Thus 31.8 per cent of the population falls outside this range, one half (15.9 per cent) below the (mean–SD) point and the other half above the (mean+SD) point. If therefore we give a dose of drug whose logarithm is one standard deviation less than the logarithm of the mean, we should expect 15.9 per cent of the animals to die. In other words, a percentage response of 15.9 corresponds to a probit of 4. Similarly, if we take a value of x which equals the (mean+1.96SD) we have a probit of 6.96. Now the dose range (mean–1.96SD) to (mean+1.96SD) includes 95 per cent of the population so that, if we administer a dose of (mean+1.96SD) we would expect 97.5 per cent of our sample to die because one half of the 5 per cent falling outside the range we are considering would be killed by doses which fell below the (mean–1.96SD) point. Thus we conclude that a mortality of 2.5 per cent corresponds to a probit of 6.96. Reference to tables shows that this is so.

It should be noted that probits are related to mortality in the same way as are the doses (or the logarithms of the doses) themselves. It is for this reason that the relationship between probits and doses is a straight line.

Several other methods are available for calculating LD_{50} or ED_{50}. Some (for instance that of Weil, 1952) are useful if only small numbers of animals are available. All the methods are based on considerations similar to those discussed in the preceding paragraphs.

Threshold dose assays

All-or-none responses sometimes form the end point of biological standardization procedures. Although it is theoretically possible to perform these assays by measuring the ED_{50} of the 'standard' and the 'unknown' preparations it is often simpler and more economical to measure the threshold dose on individual animals. Thus the standardization of digitalis involves determining the dose which causes death (due to cardiac arrest) in the anaesthetized guinea pig. The preparation is given by slow intravenous infusion and the mean volume of the standard solution required to kill a group of animals is compared with the mean volume of the test solution required to produce the same end point.

The assay methods about to be described for the assessment of graded responses may also be applicable to quantal responses.

Bracketing dose assays

Suppose that we wish to determine the amount of acetylcholine in a tissue extract and that we are to use for this purpose the isolated frog rectus muscle (p. 208). We add a dose of the extract to the organ bath and record the contraction (T_1) which is produced. After washing out the bath we add a known amount (s μg) of the authentic acetylcholine. Suppose that the contraction produced (S_1) is greater than T_1. This can mean either that the extract contains fewer than s μg of acetylcholine or that the sensitivity of the muscle has increased between the addition of the test and standard solutions. The same dose of extract is added to the bath once more. If the contraction produced (T_2) is again less than S_1, it is permissible to conclude that the dose of extract contains fewer than s μg of acetylcholine. We now find a dose of acetylcholine (s' μg.) which produces a smaller contraction than our dose of extract. The amount of acetylcholine in the extract is thus 'bracketed' between s and s' μg. If s and s' are not very close together and if sufficient tissue extract remains, the extremes of the bracket can be brought closer together. The final assessment of the acetylcholine content of the extract is the mean of the values which provide the closest bracket.

The bracketing dose assay is very useful if the amount of material available for assay is not very large and if the sensitivity of the preparation is not very steady. It will be appreciated that the assay result is in no way dependent on the making of actual measurements. All that we have to decide is whether a particular contraction is greater or smaller than the dose between which it lies. Thus, in the sequence of contractions T_1-S_1-T_2 just described, our conclusion that the extract contained fewer than s μg of acetylcholine would not be affected if, because of changes in the sensitivity of the preparation, T_1 and T_2 were not identical in size, provided that *both* were smaller than S_1.

Quite accurate assays of the pharmacological activity of a tissue extract can be achieved by this method, even if the amount of material available only permits the determination of a 'wide' bracket. It is surprising how often a preliminary assay based on the mid point of the first bracket gives a result very close to that obtained by bracketing the test solution between two doses of standard whose separation is close to the limits of resolution of the preparation.

The reader who uses the bracketing dose technique in the laboratory should be careful not to attempt to bracket his 'unknown' between too narrow limits. In particular, he should be warned against attempting to find a dose of standard solution which produces *exactly* the same contraction as the dose of tissue extract. Much more reliable results are obtained when the assay is based on clearly observable differences between test and standard solutions since these will have arisen from real differences between the activity of the two solutions rather than from fluctuations in the sensitivity of the preparations, timing or pipetting errors or even changes in resistance offered to the movement of the recording lever by local variations in the thickness of the soot deposited on the kymograph drum.

In all bioassay preparations which make use of isolated tissues, care has to be taken to ensure that the standard solution is present in a form similar to that in which it is present in the tissue extract. In particular, when the acetylcholine content of a brain extract is being assayed on a frog rectus muscle, the standard acetylcholine has to be added to a portion of brain extract from which acetylcholine has previously been removed by boiling the extract in alkaline solution. This point is discussed in detail elsewhere (p. 208).

So far as the general design of bracketing dose assays is concerned, the most important point is to put in standard and 'unknown' solutions in a sequence (usually a strict alternation) that will permit the effects of changes in the sensitivity of the preparation to be minimized.

If the preparation is likely to give stable responses and if ample material is available, the amount of pharmacologically active substance in extracts, perfusates and other solutions can be more accurately determined by the more formal assays described in the next section.

Four-point and other assays

The method of a four-point assay can be illustrated by reference to the problem considered in the preceding section—the determination of the amount of pharmacologically active material in a tissue extract. Let us assume that we have recorded the responses (S_1 and S_2) given by two volumes (x_1 and x_2) of the standard solution and by the same two volumes of the 'unknown' solution. These contractions are represented as T_1 and T_2 respectively. Assuming that we have chosen a logarithmic scale for the abscissa and that the response of the assay preparation lies in the middle of its range, the four points will be sufficient to fix the two dose-response lines shown in Fig. 9.10. If all the pharmacological activity of the extract is caused by the material present in the standard solution, the two lines will be parallel although they will not coincide unless the concentration of the active material in the standard solution has been chosen so that, by an unlikely coincidence, it is the same as that in the extract. In the situation illustrated in Fig. 9.10 the test solution is clearly more active than the

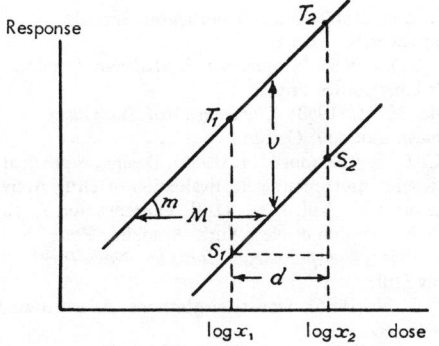

Fig. 9.10 Data for a 4-point assay.

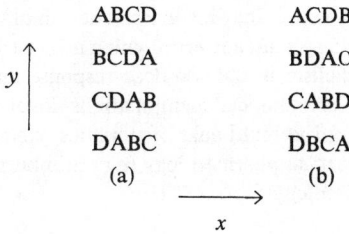

ABCD	ACDB
BCDA	BDAC
CDAB	CABD
DABC	DBCA
(a)	(b)

Fig 9.11 Some Latin squares.

standard. The horizontal separation, M, of the two curves represents the logarithm of the ratio of the concentration of active material in the test and standard solutions. The assay, therefore, reduces to a calculation of the distance M. This could, of course, be done by direct measurement from the actual curves. In practice, however, the experimentally determined points S_1, S_2, T_1 and T_2 of the four-point assay will rarely fall on two perfectly parallel lines. A large number of lines could thus be fitted by eye and it is better to calculate M. This is done as follows.

If the slope of the two lines is represented by m, we have the simple relationship

$$M = \frac{v}{m}$$

where v is the vertical separation of the two curves. v clearly equals $T_1 - S_1$ which should be the same as $T_2 - S_2$. The best estimate of v is obtained by taking the mean of these two values. Thus $v = \frac{1}{2}(T_1 - S_1 + T_2 - S_2)$. The slope of the curve m is given by $\frac{S_2 - S_1}{d}$ where d is $\log x_2 - \log x_1$, that is, the logarithm of the ratio of the two volumes x_2 and x_1. The slope is also given by $\frac{T_2 - T_1}{d}$ and, as in the case of v, the best estimate is given by $\frac{S_2 - S_1 + T_2 - T_1}{2d}$.

$$\text{Therefore } M = \frac{(T_1 - S_1 + T_2 - S_2)d}{S_2 - S_1 + T_2 - T_1}$$

The volume of test and standard solutions used in four-point assays need not, in fact, be the same although it is usual and convenient to arrange that the ratio of the larger to the smaller dose of the test solution is the same as that of the standard solution. In other words, if we call the doses of standard solution s_1 and s_2 and those of the test solution t_1 and t_2, it is usual to arrange that $\frac{s_2}{s_1} = \frac{t_2}{t_1}$. It is also convenient to arrange that this is a simple ratio (such as 2) since its logarithm (d) has to be used in the calculation.

If the volumes of test and standard solutions are not the same, the calculation for M given above must be modified

by multiplying the term on the right by $\frac{s_1}{t_1}$ (or $\frac{s_2}{t_2}$ which is the same).

In order to reduce the effects of irregular fluctuations in the sensitivity of the pharmacological preparation, several values of T_1, T_2, S_1 and S_2 are obtained and the mean (or total) values are used in the final calculation. An important point in the assay design is that the order in which the four solutions are added to the preparation should be changed in successive cycles. For this purpose it is usual to employ the so-called *Latin square* design. This design was originally developed for agricultural work. Suppose that we wished to discover which of four varieties of corn, A, B, C and D, would grow best in a particular soil. The area available for our experiment could be divided into sixteen equal squares and these could be planted with the crops in one of the orders shown in Fig. 9.11. The effect of any regular fluctuations in the fertility of the soil in either of the directions x or y would be annulled by this arrangement. Thus if the yield from all the squares planted with variety A were higher than that from the other squares, it would be reasonable to assert that this variety of corn would be most suitable for the type of soil in the experimental plot. There are 24 different ways of arranging the letters ABCD and if we had another plot divided into 16 areas we could use the alternative planting arrangement shown in Fig. 9.11 or one of the other two possibilities which the reader can work out for himself.

Returning to the four-point assay, the arrangement of the letters in Fig. 9.11 can be used to indicate the order in which test and standard solutions might be added to the bath (A=s_1, B=t_1, etc.).

The assay just described is called a four-point (or a 2×2) assay for obvious reasons. Other assay designs are possible—thus the very simple assay illustrated in Fig. 9.8 is a three-point (or a 1×2) assay and six-point (3×3) assays sometimes have to be used. The four-point assay is, however, of general utility. Indeed, in some circumstances, the four-point assay gives more reliable results than a six-point assay.

The four-point assay method lends itself to performance in automatic apparatus since the Latin square order of addition of the standard and test solutions can be set up in the instrument's programme.

Methods are available for calculating the fiducial limits

of a four-point assay. They involve an analysis of variance which takes into account any error which might arise from a lack of parallelism in the two dose-response lines. For details of the arithmetical manipulations involved, the reader is referred to text books of statistics (*e.g.* Finney, 1964) or of practical pharmacology (*e.g.* Edinburgh University Pharmacology Staff, 1971).

BIBLIOGRAPHY

Books, monographs & reviews

Bailey, N. T. J. (1959). *Statistical Methods in Biology.* London: English Universities Press.
Burn, J. H., Finney, D. J. & Goodwin, L. G. (1950). *Biological Standardization.* London: Oxford University Press
Campbell, R. C. (1974). *Statistics for Biologists,* 2nd edn. Cambridge: University Press.
Cox, D. R. (1958). *Planning of Experiments.* New York: Wiley.
Edinburgh University Pharmacology Staff (1968. *Pharmacological Experiments on Isolated Preparations.* Edinburgh: Livingstone.
Emmens, C. W. (1948). *Principles of Biological Assay.* London: Chapman & Hall.
Finney, D. J. (1964). *Statistical Method in Biological Assay.* London: Charles Griffin.
Galton, F. (1869). *Hereditary Genius.* London: Macmillan.
Kendall, M. G. (1948). *Rank Correlation Methods.* London: Griffin.
Mainland, D. (1963). *Elementary Medical Statistics.* 2nd edn. Philadelphia: Saunders.

Moroney, M. J. (1960). *Facts from Figures,* 3rd edn. Harmondsworth: Pelican.
Oldham, P. D. (1968). *Measurement in Medicine.* London: English Universities Press.
Quenouille, M. H. (1953). *The Design and Analysis of Experiment.* London: Griffin.
Rümke, C. L. and de Jonge, H. (1964). Design, Statistical Analysis and Interpretation in Evaluation of Drug Activities: Pharmacometrics, Vol. 1 (ed. D. R. Laurence and A. L. Bacharach). London & New York: Academic Press.
Siegel, S. (1956). *Non-parametric Statistics.* New York: McGraw Hill.
Snedecor, G. N. (1956). Statistical Methods. Ames: Iowa State College Press.
Stewart, G. A. and Young, P. A. (1963). Statistics as applied to pharmacological and toxicological screening. *Progr. med. Chem.,* **3,** 187-260.
Yule, G. U. and Kendall, M. G. (1964). *An Introduction to the Theory of Statistics,* 14th edn. London: Griffin.

Original papers

Crossland, J. and Rogers, K. J. (1968). Glycogen, glucose and lactic acid content of the brain in experimental catatonia. *Biochem. pharmac.,* **17,** 1637-1645.
Turnbull, M. J. (1966). *Nature and Neurochemical Correlates of Barbiturate Withdrawal Convulsions in the Rat.* PhD. Thesis, University of Nottingham.
Weil, Carrol S. (1952). Tables for convenient calculation of median effective dose (LD_{50} or ED_{50}) and instructions in their use. *Biometrics,* **8,** 249-255.
Williams, M. E., Kendal, M. J., Mitchard, M., Davis, S. S. and Poxon, R. (1974). Availability of methaqualone from commercial preparations *in vitro* and *in vivo* studies in man. *Br. J. clin. Pharmac.,* **1,** 99-105.

10. The screening and testing of drugs

A chemical compound becomes a useful drug if it possesses relevant pharmacological and therapeutic activity, if it is free of short or long term toxicity and if it is superior in any way to existing medicaments. The means by which the possession of each of these qualities is established is the subject of the present chapter.

SCREENING FOR PHARMACOLOGICAL ACTIVITY

Although supervisors of undergraduate pharmacology classes often like to pretend otherwise, the pharmacologist in an industrial laboratory does not spend all his time in endeavours to characterize the activity of compounds of whose chemical structure and likely actions he is totally ignorant. The substances he is called upon to test have not infrequently been synthesized (or extracted from plant or animal tissues) with a definite aim in mind. The likely origins of new compounds and the pharmacologist's approach to them may be summarized as follows:

a. The new compound may have been produced by effecting a simple modification of the structure of a substance of proved therapeutic value. This may have been undertaken in an attempt to increase the drug's stability, to improve its physical properties or pharmacological activity, to reduce its toxicity or simply to produce an alternative to a commercial rival's successful product. Whatever the motive for producing the drug, a particular type of activity will be expected of it and the pharmacologist's first task is to see whether the chemist's expectations are fulfilled.

b. A few new drugs (and it is devoutly to be hoped that their numbers will increase) are produced on rational biochemical or pharmacological grounds. Thus benzonatate (p. 609) was developed with the deliberate intention of combining local anaesthetic activity with an inhibitory action on stretch receptors in the lungs. This particular combination of actions was sought because physiological considerations indicated that it would provide a rational way of suppressing cough. Again, the pharmacologists who tested this compound had to ensure first of all that the new drug was indeed capable of abolishing cough. In this category of 'rational' drugs must also be included those that are related to substances—such as hormones, enzymes and neurotransmitters—which occur naturally in the body.

c. There remain many compounds that are produced with no particular therapeutic end in view. The ingenuity of organic chemists leads to the development of whole new series of compounds which have to be tested for possible pharmacological activity. In addition, it is only prudent to investigate the properties of intermediates and side products of synthetic processes which may not originally have been directed towards the production of substances of medicinal interest.

When a compound of this type comes into the hands of the pharmacologist, it has to be subjected to a series of simple tests designed to reveal the nature of any pharmacological activity it does possess and thus to indicate the direction to be taken by more detailed investigations if these seem to be justified. For obvious reasons, the application of this battery of simple tests is described as *blind screening*. The technique is, incidentally, also used by the academic pharmacologist who wishes to examine the pharmacological activity of a 'new' substance he has detected in tissue extracts.

In practice, the overall strategies which are adopted for the pharmacological investigation of new compounds do not differ greatly from one another. Thus, if a substance has been produced for the purpose of obtaining a particular type of activity, it will still be necessary, when the presence of the primary activity has been confirmed, to apply tests for other pharmacological effects. Conversely, if pharmacological activity of a particular kind is discovered in the course of a blind screening programme, it will be necessary to investigate it in more detail by one of the methods employed for the study of that particular activity.

For every new drug that is found to be suitable for clinical trial, at least one thousand others have been tested in the laboratory and found wanting (Smith, 1961). This statistic may give some idea of the volume of work which has to be undertaken in industrial pharmacology laboratories and it is essential that preliminary (or 'primary') screening tests shall be quick, simple and inexpensive to perform. The word 'screen' implies that the substances under test are exposed to a process which will hold back substances of potential value and let through the rest. In order to achieve this satisfactorily, the 'mesh' of the screen should be small enough to retain all compounds of interest, even if some have to be rejected when they are subjected to the more rigorous procedures which constitute the secondary screening tests.

Tests suitable for detecting particular types of pharmacological activity are described in the chapters of this book that discuss the properties of individual groups of drugs. A number of textbooks (which are listed in the bibliography on p. 146) are devoted exclusively to the subject of screening tests.

It should be mentioned here that screening tests vary in the extent to which they indicate the therapeutic potentiality, as opposed to the pharmacological activity, of new compounds. At one extreme, substances synthesized for possible use as antibacterial agents or as trypanocides etc. are tested by injecting them into animals infected with the appropriate organism. The activity of the drug is measured in terms of its ability to prolong the survival of the infected animals, to reduce the number of pathogens in their tissues or to prevent tissue damage. The activity so measured bears a direct relationship to the desired therapeutic action. At the other extreme have to be placed tests designed to discover suitable drugs for the treatment of mental illness (*psychotropic* drugs). Mental illness cannot be produced in experimental animals and tests for possible psychotropic activity are purely empirical in form. They are developed by observing the effect on animal behaviour of a number of drugs of proved therapeutic value. A battery of these tests (p. 593) is employed when new compounds are being tested. A weighty criticism of these screening tests is that the observed behavioural effects in normal animals may not be caused by the operation of those actions on the nervous system upon which the drugs' therapeutic activity depends. It is difficult to see how entirely new *types* of psychotropic drugs can be discovered by these screening procedures. The tests only permit the detection of psychotropic activity similar to that exhibited by the major groups of established psychotropic agents. The latter were themselves developed from drugs which, used for the treatment of other kinds of disorder, had been observed to evoke pronounced changes of mood in patients who took them.

Most screening procedures involve the detection of activity whose relationship to the drugs' potential therapeutic actions lies somewhere between the two extremes just discussed. It is important to note that many tests give rather less indication of a new compound's therapeutic potentiality than might at first sight be supposed. An example, which is discussed in some detail on p. 702 concerns drugs used in the treatment of angina of effort (angina pectoris), a condition which is due to a restriction of blood flow through the coronary arteries. The drug traditionally used for the relief of anginal pain is amyl nitrite and it is easy to demonstrate that this substance causes dilatation of the coronary arteries, an action which

clearly is related to its therapeutic effect. Screening tests for antianginal activity would therefore reasonably be expected, as they do, to involve the detection of coronary vasodilator activity. Yet dilatation of the coronary arteries is not of itself a sufficient condition for the relief of anginal pain: some substances dilate the arteries as a result of, or coincidentally with, actions which demand a greater output of energy by the heart. Such drugs are at best useless and may be dangerous.

The foregoing discussion should make it plain that drug screening is not merely a routine process, the mechanical application of which will invariably give unequivocal answers to questions concerning the therapeutic possibilities of new compounds. Pharmacologists in screening laboratories have real opportunities of contributing to the advance of medical science by the development of new tests and by critical appraisal of the old.

Blind screening

It is not possible to devise a scheme of testing which will infallibly reveal all the different types of potentially useful pharmacological activity which may be possessed by a particular substance. The person in charge of a screening programme must decide on the precise procedure which is to be adopted in individual cases but a few general points may be made here.

Much can be learnt by making simple observations on the effect of the compound on the behaviour of conscious animals. One of the best known methods (and that favoured by this author) of obtaining the maximum amount of information from these simple tests is that designed some years ago by Irwin. Mice are given intraperitoneal injections of the substance under test and its effects are assessed by systematic observation of the animals' subsequent behaviour and responses. The observations to be made are itemized in Table 10.1; they enable an activity 'profile' to be built up so that the actions of the compound being tested can be compared with that of reference drugs of known activity. Most of the observations listed in Table 10.1 are simple enough to understand though it should perhaps be mentioned that 'visual placing' is related to the animal's ability to re-orientate itself, without falling over, if it is placed in an unusual position. 'Stereotypy' is the continuous repetition of a particular movement; the 'passivity' score reflects the animal's reaction to being held in a vertical position by the loose skin on the scruff of its neck; the 'Straub tail' response is a phenomenon referred to elsewhere (p. 427). The presence of a 'startle response' is adjudged by exposing the animal to a loud noise.

When a drug's 'profile' is being drawn by the application of Irwin's method, small groups of mice are given the drug at a number of dose levels—a useful range is 1, 3, 10, 30 and 100 mg per 100 grams of body weight but with very active substances it may be necessary to establish thresh-

Table 10.1 Items examined in the Irwin primary tests for pharmacological activity

BEHAVIOURAL RESPONSES

Awareness	*Mood*	*Motor Activity*
Alertness (4)	Grooming (4)	Reactivity (4)
Visual Placing (4)	Vocalization (0)	Spontaneous Activity (4)
Passivity (0)	Restlessness (0)	Touch Response (4)
Stereotypy (0)	Irritability (0)	Pain Response (4)
	Fearfulness (0)	

NEUROLOGICAL RESPONSES

Motor Incoordination	*Muscle Tone*	*Posture*
Staggering Gait (0)	Limb Tone (4)	Body Posture (4)
Abnormal Gait (0)	Grip Strength (4)	Limb Posture (4)
Righting Reflex (4)	Body Sag (0)	
	Body Tone (4)	
	Abdominal Tone (4)	

Reflexes	*Central Nervous System Excitation*
Pinna (4)	Startle Response (0)
Corneal (4)	Straub Tail (0)
Ipsilateral Flexor (4)	Tremors (0)
	Twitching (0)
	Convulsions (0)

AUTONOMIC RESPONSES

Writhing (0)	Piloerection (0)
Pupil Size (4)	Hypothermia (0)
Palpebral Opening (4)	Skin Colour (4)
Exophthalmos (0)	Heart Rate (4)
Urination (0)	Respiratory Rate (4)
Salivation (0)	

The peak effect of the drug on each of the responses listed is assessed in a scale ranging from 0 to 8. Numbers in parentheses indicate the score which is given to untreated mice.

olds of activity by reducing the dose in progressive steps below the level of 1 mg per 100 grams of body weight. Practical details concerning the conduct of these tests are given by Irwin himself in the textbook edited by Nodine and Siegler (1964).

This preliminary screening procedure is particularly useful for detecting psychotropic and some other forms of nervous and neuromuscular activity and the method is also of value when the acute toxicity of new drugs is being assessed. Pharmacological activity detected by these simple tests must of course be thoroughly investigated by the methods discussed in the relevant chapters of this book. Some actions on the central and peripheral nervous systems—local anaesthesia and anticonvulsive activity, for instance—do not manifest themselves in tests based on simple observation of a normal animal's response to drug administration but the appopriate tests can be added to the schedule of screening tests if this is thought desirable.

Many forms of pharmacological activity are attributable to effects exerted on the autonomic nervous system or its transmitters or on the specialized receptors found in blood vessels, viscera and skeletal muscles. Relevant information concerning these actions can be obtained by analysing any action that the new drug has on the blood pressure and respiration of intact anaesthetized animals, usually the rat and the cat. When the last named species is examined in

this way, it is useful to record also the effect of the drug on the contractions of the nictitating membrane evoked by stimulation of the cervical sympathetic chain (p. 257). Isolated preparations, especially that of the guinea pig ileum, may be used to determine whether the drug mimics or antagonizes the actions of such fundamentally important substances as acetylcholine, histamine, noradrenaline or 5-hydroxytryptamine. The use of the ileum in this way is discussed in some detail elsewhere (p. 652); the properties it reveals will indicate the form which should be taken by later tests.

Some potentially useful properties may escape detection in ordinary screening tests. Unless these forms of activity are being actually sought, it is, for instance, unusual to subject drugs to tests for antiemetic, antitussive or chemotherapeutic potentiality.

TOXICITY TESTING

No drug is absolutely safe and some of the most valuable are, by their very nature, the most dangerous. The toxicity of a newly discovered drug has to be assessed in the light of the purpose for which it might be used, the period over which it will have to be administered, the effective dose and the potency and toxicity of older drugs. Vomiting, for instance, is a toxic effect which would disqualify a drug intended for the treatment of a trivial complaint. Yet this same toxic effect might be quite acceptable in a drug which promised to arrest the growth of a malignant tumour. Again, a toxic effect which developed only after a long continued administration would be of no importance in a drug intended for the treatment of an acute condition or for only occasional administration.

Two rather different aspects of drug action are included within the phrase 'drug toxicity'. There are, first of all, the untoward responses that may follow the taking of an overdose of the drug and that represent an exaggeration of the effect on which the drug's therapeutic action depends. Thus, the barbiturates, which depress the central nervous system, constitute a group of valuable sedatives, hypnotics and anaesthetics but, taken in excessive doses, they depress the central nervous system to the point of respiratory paralysis and each year they are responsible for many thousands of suicide and accidental deaths. This type of toxic response is inseparable from the drug's therapeutic actions and it is important to have some idea of the drug's margin of safety—that is, the difference between the toxic or the lethal dose and that required to produce a therapeutic effect.

The other group of toxic effects are those included in the general category of *side effects*: they are not related to a drug's therapeutic action and their occurrence may place limitations on the use of what might otherwise be valuable medicinal agents. The aim of those who develop new drugs must be to provide effective agents with the least possible tendency to produce side effects of this type.

Toxicity testing must, inevitably, be performed largely on laboratory animals. It is advisable to use at least two phylogenetically different species for this purpose. The rat and the dog (especially the beagle) are most commonly used but particular effects may have to be examined on a wider variety of animals. In addition, other suitably sensitive species may be required for investigating special aspects of drug toxicity such as carcinogenicity, teratogenicity, a tendency to evoke hypersensitivity reactions or to produce dependence.

The preliminary and routine testing of new drugs can be performed on rats, which can be housed and handled in large numbers. The results of these preliminary investigations should enable the tests on dogs to be planned so as to abstract the maximum amount of information from the necessarily less extensive studies which will be undertaken on this species. The reactions of the dog are often surprisingly similar to those exhibited by man but it is known that some drugs (amphetamine is an example) are metabolized along different routes in man and dog. A drug of this type may not reproduce in man the effects recorded in the dog and care has to be taken when the potentiality of a new drug is being assessed not to assume too close a parallelism between the reactions of the two species.

Toxicity testing, however carefully it is performed, cannot be expected to reveal all the adverse effects that might possibly follow the administration of a new drug to man. Quite apart from the difficulty of predicting the responses of human beings from the results of animal experiments, there is the fact that some toxic effects appear in only a tiny minority of patients. The antibiotics, for instance, are among the safest of drugs yet, very rarely, penicillin precipitates a fatal anaphylactic reaction and chloramphenicol may cause aplastic anaemia. Side effects as rare as these are unlikely to manifest themselves until tens of thousands of patients have received the drug. Even if they occur with the same frequency in laboratory animals, it is clearly impracticable to test thousands of animals in the hope of detecting a rare toxic action. And even if these very unusual reactions were detected in laboratory experiments it would not necessarily be advisable to abandon a drug that was otherwise full of therapeutic promise: the number of fatalities attributable to the administration of antibiotics, for instance, is miniscule in comparison with those that would occur if the drugs were withheld. The purpose of toxicity tests is to make a realistic assessment of the potential hazards of a new form of drug therapy in relation to the benefits likely to follow its adoption. In the final analysis it is impossible to make this assessment with any assurance until the drug has been in actual use for many years and every person who observes the effect on a patient of any drug (however well established) is an experimental toxicologist who, by his observations, adds to our store of information about the drug. The mere addition of a few more individuals to the list of those who have shown no adverse reactions (and this is the form that the new information so frequently takes) improves the reliability of the statistics on which the ultimate judgment of the drug's value will be made.

It should not be necessary to add that nothing written in the foregoing paragraph absolves the laboratory worker from exerting himself to the utmost to ensure that a potentially useful drug can be offered for clinical trial with a reasonable chance that it will do no harm to the patient. Just what is meant by 'a reasonable chance' depends, as has been hinted earlier, on the likely value of the new drug. In the nature of the situation, most new drugs offer no more than a slight advantage over well established medicaments and it follows that they must be as completely beyond suspicion as it is possible to go.

Those responsible for the organization of toxicity tests must be aware of the existence of toxic responses which are particularly difficult to predict on the basis of ordinary laboratory experiments. These side effects include those which arise from an interaction between the drug and particular items of human diet, hypersensitivity reactions, polyneuritis and subjective feelings such as headache and nausea.

It is impossible to lay down rigid 'programmes' for the

guidance of toxicologists. Each new drug has to be tested according to a plan determined by a knowledge of its pharmacological actions and the circumstances in which it will be administered. 'No fool-proof prescription for tests to determine the toxicity of drugs can be prescribed, but no fool should be testing drugs for this or any other property' (Paget and Barnes, 1964).

Acute toxicity tests
The purpose of an acute toxicity test is to determine the nature and extent of the untoward reactions which might follow the administration of a single dose (or an overdose) of the drug. A quantitative aspect of acute toxicity testing is the determination of the drug's lethal dose. This is usually expressed as the LD_{50} (p. 131). Standing alone, it conveys less information than does the ratio of the lethal to the effective doses ($LD_{50} : ED_{50}$), a quantity which is often known as the *therapeutic index*. The greater a drug's therapeutic index, the less likely is it that fatalities will follow an accidental overdosage. The formula just quoted for the index is not entirely satisfactory and some authorities recommend, instead, the use of the ratio of the maximum therapeutic dose to the minimum lethal dose. It is usual to calculate the lethal dose after administration of the drug by several routes, but most attention will, naturally, be directed towards the effects caused by the mode of administration which most nearly approaches that by which the drug will be given if it is introduced into clinical practice.

Determination of the LD_{50} demands the use of a relatively large number of animals (but see p. 133) and it is customary to make an accurate determination on one species (the rat or mouse) only. The dose thus arrived at is then administered to a few members of other laboratory species and the lethal dose is calculated only for those species whose response is appreciably different from that expected.

An advantage of determining the LD_{50} at an early stage in the investigation of a new drug is that the doses used to establish the drug's spectrum of pharmacological activity can be related to its lethal dose.

The LD_{50}, and the incidence of toxic responses, should be separately determined for male and female animals.

Many of the immediately toxic effects of new drugs come to light during the initial screening procedures but the formal programme of toxicity testing enables these to be investigated in more detail. In particular, it is necessary to determine whether lethal doses of the drug cause death by an exaggeration of the pharmacological action upon which their therapeutic potentiality depends or whether death is the result of the operation of completely independent side effects.

Animals that die soon after a single dose of drug rarely exhibit changes extreme enough to alter the histological appearance of the tissues. Nevertheless, post mortem examinations should be carried out on at least a sample of the animals that receive lethal doses of drug. Histological examination may be revealing if death has been delayed beyond about six hours after administration of the drug.

The administration of a sub-lethal dose of the compound under test may provide evidence to suggest that such side effects as vomiting, muscle tremors, catatonia (p. 594) or changes in autonomic function are likely to occur if the drug is given in comparable doses to human beings. It is often pointed out (and rightly so) that dogs vomit on the slightest provocation—even the sight of a person who has previously given them an emetic drug—but their vomiting in response to the administration of a new drug must never be lightly dismissed. A vomiting response may be the result of direct stimulation of the vomiting centre (p. 599) and, as such, may indicate an unwelcome propensity on the part of the drug to stimulate other parts of the central nervous system.

Longer term toxicity tests
If the results of the acute toxicity tests prove satisfactory, the new drug has to be administered to experimental animals over a more prolonged period. Only if no adverse change follows this more extended contact is it permissible to test the drug on human patients. The duration of these longer term tests is determined by the period over which the drug will be taken if it is finally accepted for clinical use. It is usually suggested that animals should receive the drug for at least twice as long (up to a limit of two years) as human patients will require it. There is a twofold reason for placing an upper limit of about two years on the duration of chronic toxicity tests: this period represents almost the complete life span of the most commonly used experimental animal (the rat) and it is unlikely that toxic effects which have not been seen after a two years' administration of drug will make their appearance later. The one possible exception to this generalization is the development of tumours (see below).

In chronic toxicity tests, the drug is given in amounts several times greater than the pharmacologically active dose and frequently enough to ensure that a high plasma concentration is maintained throughout the period of testing. It is usual to divide the experimental animals into a number of groups that receive different doses of the drug. Throughout the test, the general appearance and condition of the animals, their weights and their food intakes are noted. Regular haematological examinations, including at least the determination of red and white cell counts and the haemoglobin content of the blood, must be undertaken. Many drugs produce blood dyscrasias as undesirable, and sometimes serious, side effects and any abnormality, however slight, which appears in the blood picture during chronic toxicity testing should be taken as a signal that a thorough going haematological investigation is needed. Biochemical tests for liver and kidney function and for the state of the electrolyte balance are also performed. Another duty of the biochemist at this stage of the investigation is the determination of the drug's mode of absorption and excretion and the elucidation, if possible, of the pathways of its metabolic degradation *in vivo*. Important though all these tests are, however, a detailed pathological examination of the treated animals remains the sheet anchor of successful long term toxicity testing. Groups of animals are killed after different periods of exposure to the drug. Their internal organs are weighed and subjected to macroscopic examination before they are prepared for histological study. Examination of the slides is a time consuming process and because it is worthless if it is not performed with the utmost care and detail, it is usual to restrict the complete histological study of the body tissues to those animals which have received the highest dose of drug. If a pathological change is detected in a particular organ or tissue, the relevant slides from animals which have received lower doses of the drug are then examined.

In addition to the general pathological examination just referred to, a number of special tests may have to be performed as described in the following paragraphs.

Teratogenicity.   Everybody now knows that thalidomide, an apparently safe sedative, caused some of the pregnant women who had received it to give birth to grossly deformed infants. The production of foetal abnormalities by drugs was not an unknown phenomenon: the real tragedy of the thalidomide disaster was that the abnormalities, gross though they were, were not incompatible with continued intra-uterine life. Consequently, the affected foetuses grew and were born alive. It is now mandatory to subject all new drugs to tests which will ensure, as far as possible, that substances with teratogenic activity (*teras* is the Greek for 'monster') are never again administered to human patients.

Because of the ease with which foetal abnormalities can be induced in this species, the rabbit is the animal of choice for teratogenicity testing but parallel tests should also be performed on at least one other species. The rat is generally used for this purpose but some workers also inoculate fertilized hens' eggs with the drug under test.

It is usually true to say that a toxic effect that does not appear after the administration of a large dose of drug will not be produced by smaller doses. This statement is not valid so far as teratogenic activity is concerned because a drug which produces foetal abnormalities in small doses may cause foetal death followed by abortion in larger amounts. For this reason, it is essential to conduct teratogenicity tests with several groups of animals which receive different doses of drug.

Foetal abnormalities are only produced if the active drug is administered at the time when development is proceeding most rapidly and, for the purpose of detecting teratogenic activity, drug administration should commence as early in the animals' pregnancy as possible.

Groups of pregnant animals, then, are given the drug at different dose levels. Some of the mothers should be killed at different stages of pregnancy so that the uterine contents can be examined for dead or deformed foetuses. Others are allowed to deliver their litters which are then carefully inspected. This examination should include a study of the internal organs as well as the external appearance. Some apparently normal litters should be permitted to survive so that they can be examined throughout their life. This will reveal whether the drug has caused a developmental abnormality which manifests itself only by causing illness, sterility or premature death in the older animal. If the drug causes the death and abortion of foetuses, a strong suspicion should be entertained that it has teratogenic activity even if the expelled foetuses appear to be anatomically normal. Drugs which cause foetal death in some species or dose levels often induce foetal abnormalities in other circumstances.

Some rabbits produce deformed foetuses even if they have received no drugs at all, while others are relatively insusceptible to known teratogenic agents. Teratogenicity tests must therefore be performed under adequately controlled conditions. It is useful to include some animals which are given normally teratogenic doses of thalidomide. In this way the possibility that the test drug has produced no foetal abnormality simply because the animals are resistant to its effects can be properly allowed for. The incidence of spontaneously developing abnormalities can be assessed by including some animals that receive neither thalidomide nor the test drug.

If foetal abnormalities do occur, the dose of drug required to produce them should be noted so that its relation to the normal therapeutic dose can be assessed.

Carcinogenicity.   Many chemical substances are capable of producing malignant tumours in animals and man. These *carcinogenic* substances are often particularly dangerous if they are taken in small doses over a long period of time. Modern pharmacology is producing more and more compounds (oral contraceptives, other hormonal preparations and psychotropic drugs are examples) which are taken in just this way and it is essential that every effort should be made to establish their innocence before they are released for general use.

Tumours may appear in animals subjected to two-year toxicity tests but the absence of tumours cannot be taken as absolute evidence that the drug will not induce tumour formation in man: the experimental species may be one that is resistant to the carcinogenic action of the drug under test or the drug may be one that only produces tumours after administration over a longer period of time than can be achieved within the lifetime of an animal such as the rat. In some laboratories, substances that have been demonstrated to be otherwise innocuous are tested for carcinogenic activity by being given to dogs over a period of at least seven years. No manufacturer can be expected to withhold a new drug for this length of time and, commercial considerations apart, a delay of seven years would be quite unacceptable if the drug had a potentially high therapeutic value. However, if the drug survives the two-year test, there is no good reason why it should not be released for clinical trial provided that it is withdrawn from use if continuing toxicity tests in animals give the slightest cause for suspicion that, in the doses and duration of its likely administration to human beings, the drug is not entirely safe. Careful examination of experimental animals should result in the detection of a malignant change before irreversible damage is done to human beings.

Special care has to be taken to examine a drug for carcinogenic activity if its structure is related to that of known carcinogens. It may be that the known carcinogen only produces tumours in animals if it is administered in a particular way, such as by skin painting. If this is so, the new drug should be applied in a similar fashion, even if this is entirely different from the intended route of administration to human beings.

The choice of species for carcinogenicity testing is difficult unless there is some reason for believing (on the basis of the activity of compounds of similar structure, for instance) that a particular species will be especially sensitive to any carcinogenic action the drug may possess. In the absence of any such information, the rat and mouse are probably the animals of choice for tests of short duration. For more prolonged tests, the dog is the only really suitable species.

Drug dependence. Drugs with an action on the central nervous system may cause dependence ('addiction') in human beings. Tests which may reveal the tendency of a drug to produce withdrawal symptoms after protracted use are discussed elsewhere (p. 95) but the possibility that a psychological dependence may be induced can only be assessed on the basis of what is known about the drug's central nervous actions. Thus a stimulant of the central nervous system may produce euphoria, a condition which predisposes to abuse of the drug. A substance which causes hallucinations or other disorders of perception is also potentially dangerous but no test which makes use of experimental animals is capable of revealing whether a drug will be hallucinogenic in man.

CLINICAL TRIALS

Clinical trials of a new drug may begin when toxicity tests on experimental animals and on healthy volunteers have established that the administration of potentially therapeutic doses of the drug to patients is unlikely to be attended by untoward effects. In Britain, drugs have first to be cleared by the Committee on Safety of Drugs but this body is solely concerned with drug safety. It does not pronounce on the clinical effectiveness of drugs—indeed, it cannot do so, since it has to make its adjudications before the drug is ever given to patients. Consequently, the clinical trial is an important stage in the overall assessment of the drug's potentialities and no more than one in twenty of those subjected to trial justifies itself sufficiently to merit commercial production.

A clinical trial needs to be planned and executed and its results interpreted with the same care as any laboratory experiment. And, like laboratory experiments, not all clinical trials can follow the same design. The drug to be tested may be intended for self administration by ambulant patients in their own homes. In these circumstances the conduct of the trial may have to be entrusted to the family physician who will usually have no means of ensuring that his instructions are followed. As a class, patients are notoriously unable or unwilling to follow simple instructions. Joyce (1968) reports the instance of a group of 37 patients who were given supplies of one of four analgesics (aspirin, phenylbutazone, flufenamic and mefenamic acids) for the treatment of rheumatic conditions. On their periodic visits to the clinic, the patients were examined: urine analysis revealed that, on an average of one in three visits, all had failed to take the prescribed drug during the preceding 48 hours. Some of the patients had taken other analgesics in addition to the one prescribed. It is clear that clinical trials carried out under these conditions pose questions of method and interpretation which are not encountered when a ward full of supervised patients is available. Again, the disease to be treated might be a rare one, so that it may not be possible to obtain more than one or two patients for study at any one time. Information concerning the effectiveness of the drug has therefore to be accumulated slowly and the conditions under which the different small groups of patients have to be studied are likely to show considerable variation. Further complications arise if the clinical condition is short lived, if it is likely to exhibit spontaneous remissions or if the drug is to be given in order to prevent an occurrence, such as vomiting, which occurs irregularly and unpredictably. For the purpose of the immediate discussion, it will be assumed that the drug is to be tested on hospitalized patients suffering from a non-acute condition. It will be further assumed that there is a sufficient number of patients available to enable at least a tentative conclusion to be drawn from the results of one trial. The manoeuvres that have to be adopted when these conditions are not fulfilled are mentioned later in this chapter and in those sections of other chapters that are concerned with the testing of individual drugs.

It is common knowledge that the clinical condition of a patient who has been told that he is receiving a new drug is likely to show a temporary improvement quite irrespective of whether the new drug exerts a relevant pharmacological effect—irrespective, indeed, of whether he has in fact been given a drug different from that he had been previously receiving. This is the *placebo* response: its effect in a particular situation can be gauged by giving the patients a completely inert substance such as lactose (but see below,) in a form which resembles as closely as possible the drug being investigated. Although an awareness of the placebo effect is widespread, few who have not studied it realise just how powerful an influence it may exert. Nor is it generally appreciated that the placebo effect is as likely to influence the physician's judgement, or even the 'objective' readings he makes, as it is to affect the patient's subjective symptoms. If a physician believes that the drug he is giving is a highly effective one, his patients may well recover more rapidly than those who receive the same drug from an unenthusiastic prescriber.

It will be obvious that placebo responses are particularly likely to occur when drugs are being used for the relief of symptoms which, though real, are ill-defined, vaguely localized or not susceptible of objective measurement: pain, feelings of nausea, malaise or depression and similar symptoms all fall into this category. Placebo effects are also very likely to appear during the treatment of the many disorders (peptic ulceration and essential hypertension are examples) in whose make up there is a strong psychosomatic element. However, these effects are by no means unknown in the response to diseases which would not be expected to be much influenced by psychological factors. Almost all drugs have their greatest successes when they are first introduced into clinical use, a testimony to the universality of the placebo response.

> 'Those who have been disillusioned are inclined to sum up their experience by claiming that the best way to cure any disease is to announce a clinical trial of remedies for it. For example, the illegitimate birth rate in one London borough is rumoured to have fallen almost to zero since the medical officer of health announced his intention to carry out a comparative trial of oral contraceptives in the local authority clinics' (Joyce, 1968).

The part played by placebo effects in the actions, attitudes and assessments of those actually involved in the control of the trial must not be underestimated. The mere act of participating in an investigation of any type is likely to influence the participant, however disinterested and unbiassed he may be before the study begins. Participation inevitably leads to involvement and the investigation must be protected as much from the enthusiasms, conscious or otherwise, of the research workers as from the expectations of the patient.

With these points in mind, it is possible to devise what at first sight might appear to be an almost flawless design for a clinical trial. When this has been set out, the possible deficiencies in such a design and some of the difficulties which may beset attempts to implement it in the ward will be discussed.

The patients are randomly divided into two groups. One group will receive the drug. Patients in the other group will be given a placebo except when it is felt necessary to compare the effectiveness of a new drug with that of an established medicament. In these circumstances, the second group of patients will receive (or continue to receive) the established drug instead of placebo. The patients will be aware that they are subjects in a clinical trial and it is essential that neither the individual patients nor their attendants should know who is receiving the new drug. Thus, if the new drug is to be taken in the form of tablets, the placebo (or the other drug) must be incorporated into tablets whose size, shape, colour, texture and taste are such as to render them indistinguishable from those of the new drug. If suitable placebo tablets are not supplied by the drug's manufacturers, they will have to be produced in the hospital and it may then be convenient for the pharmacist who produces them to allocate the patients to the 'treated' or 'control' groups and to send drug or placebo to the ward in identical containers labelled for individual patients. If he does this, he should not be permitted to take any further part in the investigation since he (and ideally it should be he alone) will know the make up of the two groups. Care has to be taken that the allocation of patients is a truly random process (a coin may be tossed or tables of random numbers may be used) but if it is felt desirable to know how the effectiveness of the drug is influenced by factors such as the age, sex or clinical condition of the patients, it is permissible to divide the patients into a number of suitable groups (male and female, young and old, etc.) and then to allocate treatments randomly within the selected groups.

When the drug has been given for a suitable period, it may be possible and desirable to interchange the treatments so that those who previously received drug now receive placebo and *vice versa*. Not until the treatment programme has been completed and the patients' progress has been finally assessed should the identity of those who received the drug in each half of the trial be revealed.

This type of trial has a *double blind* character (neither patients nor physician knowing who has received a drug) with a *cross over* design if drug and placebo groups are interchanged in the middle of the trial. Its possible shortcomings may now be discussed.

The placebo. Too often the placebo is given as a mere gesture to statistical design without any real appreciation of the function of control groups. An inert substance such as lactose (the traditional 'dummy' drug) provides a completely inadequate control substance if the active drug produces side effects (such as a dry mouth, gastrointestinal upsets, increased cardiac activity, etc.) that completely defeat the purpose of the double blind technique by making it clear to both the patient and his physician that he is a member of the treated group. Attempts have been made to develop placebos with side effects similar to those produced by active drugs and it is important that this approach should be more generally adopted, particularly when psychotropic drugs are being studied. There is more than a suspicion that the beneficial effects exerted by some of the most successful of these drugs owe more to their peripheral side effects than to any direct action on the brain. Of course, the perfect placebo (like the perfect control animal in a laboratory experiment) does not exist, because the only substance that can properly reproduce all the side effects of a particular drug is the drug itself. The impossibility of producing a perfect placebo does not absolve the designer of a clinical trial from recognizing that different drugs demand different placebos and that a placebo which does not successfully disguise from the patient the fact that he is not receiving the active drug is worse than none at all.

Operation of the cross over design may itself provide a hint as to when the active drug has been given to a particular patient, though this might not have been evident if the design of the investigation had not involved a change in treatment.

Studies on normal subjects and on patients have established that some individuals (the placebo reactors) exhibit more marked placebo responses than others. Some investigators attempt to identify placebo reactors among volunteers for clinical trials and to exclude them from the study. This, however, should not be necessary if the trial is properly designed. Some, indeed, might ask whether the conditions of the 'ideal' clinical trial are not unrealistically artificial, since placebo effects contribute to a large number of successful medical treatments. However, the point of a clinical trial is to establish whether a new drug has any direct effect on the disease process or its symptoms: the magic can be added later.

The ethics.   What is scientifically desirable may not always be ethically acceptable. It is axiomatic that the comfort, health and safety of the patient take precedence over all other considerations, even if a promising clinical trial has to be abandoned, or its design made less rigid, in order to secure them. However undesirable it may be from a scientific point of view for the physician in charge of the patients in the trial to be given precise details about the likely immediate side effects of the new drug, he has an inalienable right to be given, at any time, all the information he asks for should he feel that lack of it is prejudicial to the welfare of his patients. Extreme diligence is needed to ensure that humanity does not leave the ward when science enters it. Again, it is resonable to ask whether, in the interests of obtaining 'control' subjects, it is justifiable to withhold from an ill patient a drug which might promote or hasten his recovery. In practice, the situation rarely arises in the extreme form in which it is posed here. A new

drug which promised a dramatic cure for diseases from which no relief had hitherto been available would hardly need to be subjected to a rigorously controlled therapeutic trial: it could be given openly to all who needed it. Miracle drugs are, however, rare and most new medicaments offer no more than slight improvements over existing drugs. It is these drugs which require the most careful assessment but fortunately they can usually be subjected to a rigorous trial since no harm will be done to any patient by withholding the new drug in favour of a placebo, or an established medication, during the trial.

The subjects.   All patients who take part in a controlled therapeutic trial should be volunteers. It may be that the motives which impel them to volunteer indicate that they, and their response to drugs, are not representative of the population as a whole. It is difficult to imagine that this factor will significantly affect the prognostic value of a therapeutic trial. Nevertheless, the possibility that it may do so should be kept in mind by those who design the trial.

The results.   The results of clinical trials are statistical in nature since the assessment of the potential value of the drug must be based on the average responses of groups of patients. A few individuals may derive considerable benefit from an agent which has little effect on the condition of most of the participants in the trial. Consequently a drug may sometimes, in carefully selected cases, be of greater therapeutic value than is indicated by the results of early clinical trials. Equally, of course, a drug of apparently proved effectiveness may prove to be useless in a minority of patients.

Analysis of the results of clinical trials
The statistical methods appropriate to a particular trial will be determined by the nature of the measurements made and the conditions under which the trial has to be conducted. Usually the statistician who controls the investigation will be able to say how many patients should be needed to establish the worth of the drug and it is desirable that they should all be included in the same trial. If only a very few patients are available at any one time, a method of assessment such as sequential analysis (p. 130) will have to be adopted. This enables the results to be assessed as they are gradually accumulated and the end point of the trial comes when the analysis shows a statistically significant result.

Quantitative results can be assessed by traditional statistical techniques but nonparametric methods (p. 128) will have to be adopted if the responses of the patient cannot be expressed in a suitable numerical form.

The data collected in a clinical trial should be sufficiently precise and sensitive to detect the effects of the drug. If there is any doubt concerning the adequacy of the assessment, it can be checked by collecting comparable data from patients given a drug of known effectiveness whose action is similar to that of the drug under trial. This information will of course be available if the design of the trial requires the inclusion of such patients for other reasons.

There is a widespread but erroneous belief that 'objective' measurements on the patient are *necessarily* more reliable and informative than reports by the patient himself. It is possible to devise methods by which the patient can indicate fluctuations in the intensity of his symptoms and these methods, properly used, are often as reliable as measurements made by an external observer. An indication on a meter provides an objective measure but it has always to be remembered that the meter has to be read, and the readings recorded by, a human being.

BIBLIOGRAPHY

Books, monographs and reviews

Burger, A. (ed.) (1968) *Selected Pharmacological Testing Methods*, vols. 1-3. London: Edward Arnold and New York: Marcel Dekker.

Casarett, L. J. and Doull, J. (1975) *Toxicology: The Basic Science of Poisons*. New York: Macmillan.

Good, C. S. (ed.) (1976) *The Principles and Practice of Clinical Trials*. Edinburgh, London and New York: Churchill Livingstone.

Jouhar, A. J. and Grayson, M. F. (eds.) (1973) *International Aspects of Drug Evaluation and Usage*. Edinburgh and London: Churchill Livingstone.

Joyce, C. R. B. (1968) Psychological factors in the controlled evaluation of therapy. *In* Joyce, C. R. B. (ed.) *Psychopharmacology: Dimensions and Perspectives*. London: Tavistock Publications.

Loomis, T. A. (1970) *Essentials of Toxicology*. Philadelphia: Lea and Febiger.

Laurence, D. R. and Bacharach, A. L. (eds.) (1964) *Evaluation of Drug Activities: Pharmacometrics*, vols. 1 and 2. London and New York: Academic Press.

Nodine, J. H. and Siegler, P. E. (eds.) (1964) *Animal and Clinical Pharmacologic Techniques in Drug Evaluation*. Chicago: Year Book Publishers.

Paget, G. E. and Barnes, J. M. (1964) Toxicity tests. *In* Laurence, D. R. and Bacharach, A. L. (eds.) (1964)—*see above*—Vol. 1, pp. 135-166.

Smith, W. G. (1961) Pharmacological screening tests. *In* Ellis, G. P. and West, G. B. (eds.) *Progress in Medicinal Chemistry*, Vol. 1. London: Butterworths.

Turner, R. A. (1965) *Screening Methods in Pharmacology*. New York and London: Academic Press.

11. Some aspects of experimental pharmacology

This chapter is not offered as a practical guide for the laboratory worker. Its purpose is to indicate for the benefit, particularly, of the nonspecialist reader a few of the possibilities and limitations inherent in the experimental techniques to which he will find the most frequent reference during his perusal of this and other books and papers. Practical details may be found, by those who need them, in manuals of experimental pharmacology (Burn, 1952; Edinburgh University Pharmacology Staff, 1970a and b), in the specialized texts dealing with laboratory screening methods (Chap. 10) and in the original papers referred to in this chapter and elsewhere in this book.

Elaborate apparatus is now as commonplace in the pharmacology laboratory as it is in any other, but a considerable amount of work, including much that is fundamental, is still successfully undertaken with equipment of surprising simplicity. Foremost in this category is the traditional isolated organ bath in which a fragment of intestine, a uterine horn or some other tissue is suspended

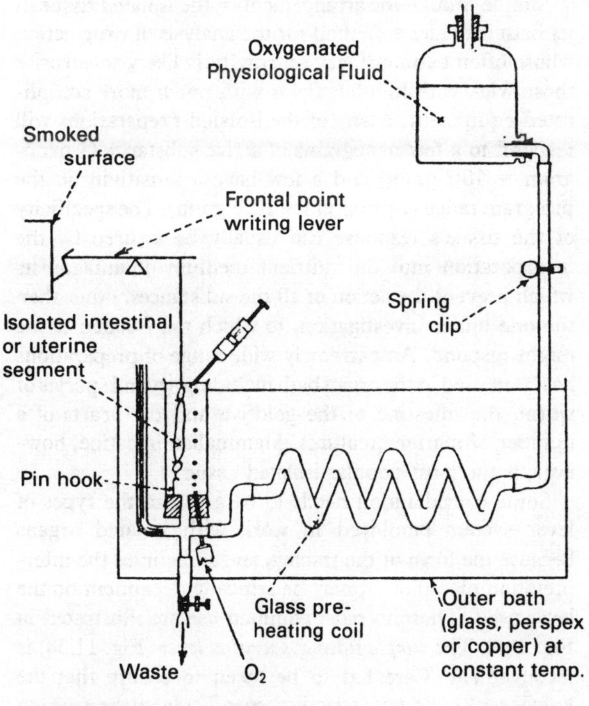

Fig.11.1 Isolated organ bath.

in a suitable nutrient medium maintained at a steady temperature. One end of the tissue is fixed and the other is attached to an almost counterbalanced lever carrying a point which impinges lightly on the surface of a piece of sooted paper. The paper encircles the slowly rotating cylinder of a kymograph and the response of the tissue to a drug added to the bath can thus be followed as the pointer, scraping soot from the paper, produces a tracing of the response. A schematic diagram of the apparatus usually employed is presented in Fig. 11.1. If the tissues of a poikilothermic animal such as a frog, a fish or an invertebrate are being examined, the outer bath can usually be dispensed with. In some experiments provision has to be made for the accommodation of suitable electrodes for stimulation of the tissue or its attached nerve.

The nutrient solution used in the organ bath is one of a number of modifications of the solution unwittingly discovered (ca. 1890) by Sydney Ringer's lazy technician who brought fame to his master by making up sodium chloride in tap water (and so adding some other ions) because he was not inclined to walk the extra distance involved in obtaining distilled water. The composition of some of the more commonly used variants of Ringer's solution is indicated, for reference purposes, in Table 11.1. The choice of solution and of the temperature at which it is held in a particular experiment is governed by the nature of the tissue and of the response which is being examined and also, to some extent, by personal preference.

The apparatus supplied commercially is usually provided with a relatively large bath (25 or 50 ml capacity) but except for the simpler class experiments it is more convenient in practice to use the smaller bath, similar to that illustrated in Fig. 11.1, which is easily made from glass tubing and need have a capacity of no more than 1 to 2 ml. The use of a small bath is essential when only small amounts of material (such as the extract of a few milligrams of tissue) are available. In special circumstances the microbath designed by Gaddum (1965) may be called for. The microbath has a capacity of less than 0.05 ml. An alternative manoeuvre when only tiny quantities of active material are available is to use the technique of *superfusion* (Fig. 11.2). In this method the nutrient solution and its added drug is permitted to flow slowly over the isolated preparation. The superfusion method was another of the ingenious devices invented by Gaddum (Chap. 1) who was a pioneer in the development of techniques for the extraction and

Table 11.1 Composition of solutions more commonly used in pharmacological preparations

	Ringer's (Frog)	Ringer-Locke's	Tyrode's	De Jalon's	Krebs'
	%	%	%	%	%
Sodium chloride	0.6	0.9	0.8	0.9	0.69
Potassium chloride	0.0075	0.042	0.2	0.042	0.035
Magnesium chloride			0.01		
Magnesium sulphate 7H$_2$O					0.029
Sodium bicarbonate	0.01	0.05	0.1	0.05	0.21
Calcium chloride	0.01	0.024	0.02	0.006	0.028
Glucose		0.1	0.1	0.05	0.2
Typical uses	Frog tissues	Cardiac muscle	Intestine	Uterus	Skeletal muscle (diaphragm, etc.)

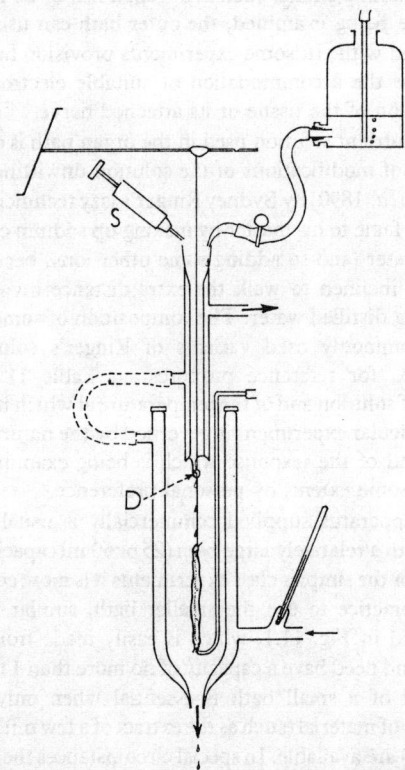

Fig 11.2 *Superfusion Apparatus* Water from a thermostat is circulated through the apparatus as indicated (W). Aerated physiological salt solution from the reservoir is warmed as it passes through the upper jacketed tube. It drips on to the thread at D and hence over the tissue. Doses of drug or tissue extract are added from the syringe S. *Reproduced by kind permission of the authors from Pharmacological Experiments on Isolated Preparations* (Edinburgh University Pharmacology Staff, 1968).

quantitative assay of pharmacologically active substances in tissue extracts. It is possible to arrange for a solution that contains pharmacologically active material to superfuse in succession a number of different isolated preparations. This is a particularly valuable arrangement when the solution contains two or more closely related substances that have to be individually assayed by the technique of differential bioassay (p. 210). The use of such a cascade of preparations to assay a mixture of prostaglandins is described later (p. 389).

Simple though the arrangement is, the isolated tissue in its bath provides a method for the analysis of drug action whose often extraordinary sensitivity is likely to surprise those who work in other fields with much more complicated equipment. Many of the isolated preparations will respond to a few nanograms of active substance (1 nanogram = 10^{-9} gram) and a few have a sensitivity in the picogram range (1 picogram = 10^{-12} gram). The specificity of the tissue's response can usually be assured by the incorporation into the nutrient medium of antagonists which prevent the action of all the substances, other than the one under investigation, to which the isolated tissue might respond. An extremely wide range of preparations has been used in the organ bath including several species of worm, the intestine of the goldfish and the hearts of a number of marine creatures. Mammalian intestine, however, is the most popular isolated tissue.

Some consideration needs to be given to the types of lever system employed in work with isolated organs because the form of the tracing, and sometimes the interpretation placed on it, may be critically dependent on the lever used. Those in most common use are illustrated in Fig. 11.3. The *simple sideways writing lever* (Fig. 11.3a) is inconvenient. Care has to be taken to ensure that the kymograph cylinder is strictly perpendicular to the working bench and that the lever moves in the same vertical plane.

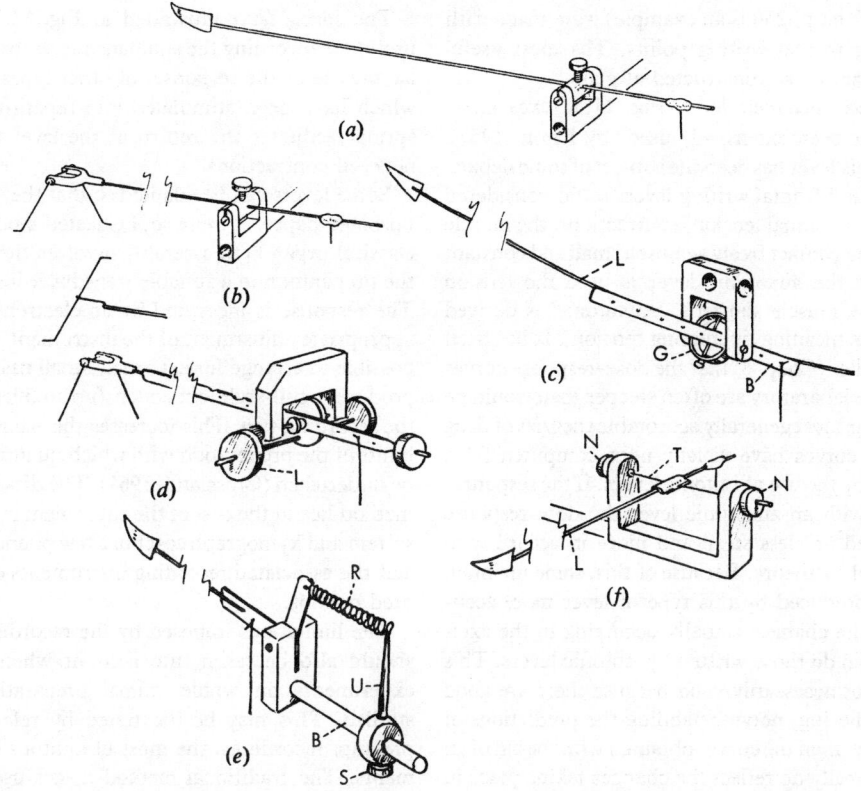

Fig. 11.3 *Some levers used in pharmacology*   (a) Side-ways writing lever. (b) Frontal-writing
lever. The point is hinged and the distribution of its weight is such that its lower tip falls
against the paper. The lower picture shows an alternative and better type of point. It is made of
glass and the hinge of paper. (c) Gimbal lever. (d) Pendulum auxotonic lever. As the
preparation contracts, the load L moves further out from the fulcrum and so exerts a greater
effect. Loads of different sizes may be fitted as required. (e) Sprung (or Spring) lever. The
tension of the spring R can be set as required by altering the position of the upright U.
(f) Torsion (Isometric) lever. The lever is mounted on a nylon thread, T, or a fine metal strip
whose tension can be adjusted by the nuts N. *Reproduced by kind permission of the authors from
Pharmacological Experiments on Isolated Preparations* (Edinburgh University Pharmacological
Staff, 1968).

If this is not done the lever will either leave the paper at
some point in its excursion or it will press more heavily at
some points on the paper and the increased friction will
retard or distort its movements. This may introduce errors
when the preparation is used in quantitative work such as
the construction of dose-response curves or the assay of
active material in tissue extracts. These disadvantages are
avoided if a *gimbal lever* (Fig. 11.3c) is used. This type of
lever has a sideways writing action but because the writing
arm is mounted in gimbals it always falls on to the paper.
Changes in frictional resistance—apart from any occasioned by localized accumulations of soot due to heavy
smoking of the paper—are thus avoided and the adjustment of the kymograph and the positioning of the organ
bath in relation to it is made easier. Both the simple and the
gimbal forms of the sideways writing lever trace curved
lines in response to a linear pull. Consequently the vertical

distance travelled by the lever from the base line is not
directly proportional to the degree of shortening of the
preparation. With large excursions of the lever, distortion
may introduce serious errors into any quantitative work
that necessitates actual measurements of the contraction of
the preparation. It is a less important source of error in
'bracketing dose' assays (p. 132), in which it is only
necessary to decide whether a particular response is greater
or smaller than those which immediately precede and
follow it. The effects of arc distortion can be minimized by
reducing the magnification imparted by the lever or they
can be eliminated completely if recourse is had to a frontal
writing lever (Fig. 11.3b). This type of lever has much to
recommend it: it writes with a constant friction, its writing
point falls lightly against the paper like that of a gimbal
lever and it traces linear contractions as straight lines
instead of arcs. Many of the tracings reproduced in this

book (Fig. 16.7 on p. 256 is an example) were made with levers carrying frontal writing points. Ths most useful frontal points are those constructed of glass.

The *pendulum auxotonic lever* (Fig. 11.3*d*) was introduced, and has been extensively used, by Paton (1957). The value of this lever has been the subject of some debate. The sideways and frontal writing levers so far considered record isotonic (= equal tension) contractions, the muscle being allowed to contact freely against a small and constant tension. When the auxotonic lever is used the tension increases as the muscle shortens. 'Auxotonic' is derived from the Greek meaning 'increasing tension'. It has been mentioned earlier (Chap. 8) that the dose-response curves obtained in the laboratory are often steeper than would be predicted by the most generally acceptable theories of drug action. These curves have usually been computed from data obtained by the use of isotonic levers. If the responses are recorded with an auxotonic lever the dose-response curves obtained are less steep and more in accord with those predicted by theory. Because of this, some maintain that tracings produced by this type of lever more accurately reflect the changes actually occurring in the excitable tissue than do those written by isotonic levers. This argument is not necessarily valid because there are good reasons for believing, notwithstanding the predictions of receptor theory, than the curves obtained with the aid of an isotonic lever really do reflect the changes taking place in the preparation. This point is discussed in Chapter 8 (p. 106). The status of the auxotonic lever as a recording instrument needs clarification in another connection. Using the lever, Paton has adduced evidence for the occurrence of 'fade' in pharmacological responses (Chap. 8). This finding is in accordance with the predictions of Paton's own 'rate theory' of drug action but the principal rival theory predicts a different type of response (see Fig. 8.5, p. 106). It might appear, therefore, that the experimental results lend support to Paton's theory but some believe that the fade is an artefact introduced by the auxotonic lever, the load leading to a rapid readjustment of internal tensions in the muscle.

The discussion in the preceding paragraph should serve to emphasize a point to which attention is not sufficiently often paid—the possibility that the recording apparatus may itself distort the response of sensitive and delicate tissues.

The pendulum auxotonic lever imposes a certain restraint on the contraction of the isolated preparation. Shortening is almost completely prevented by a properly adjusted *isometric* or *torsion lever* (Fig. 11.3*f*). Thus muscle contraction occurs under virtually isometric (= equal length) conditions. A very long lever is required in order to magnify the very slight shortening response. It is unusual to make isometric recordings from isolated preparations but it is useful to be able to record the development of isometric tension in the skeletal muscle of whole animal preparations.

The *spring lever* illustrated in Fig. 11.3*e* is especially useful for recording the spontaneous contractions of cardiac muscle or the responses of other types of preparation which have been stimulated into repetitive activity: the spring facilitates the return of the lever to the baseline between contractions.

Some levers can be adapted so that they write in ink on unsooted paper. A more sophisticated modification of the classical organ bath assembly involves the attachment of the preparation to a suitable transducer instead of a lever. The response is measured by an electronic recorder. By appropriate adjustment of the instrument's amplifier, it is possible to arrange for extremely small tissue responses to produce a full-scale deflection (up to 30cm. or more) of the recording pen. This increases the accuracy within the limits of the preparation with which quantitative work can be undertaken (Crossland, 1961). The disadvantage of this method lies in the cost of the equipment required. A lever system and kymograph cost but a few pounds; a transducer and the associated recording instruments cost a few hundred pounds.

The limitations imposed by the recording instruments should also be taken into account when the results of experiments on whole animal preparations are being studied. This may be illustrated by reference to blood pressure recordings, the most ubiquitous of all measurements. The traditional method makes use of a mercury manometer connected to a cannula inserted into a suitable artery—the common carotid and the femoral arteries are most commonly used. The simple manometer illustrated in Figure 11.4*a* can be used for dogs, cats and rabbits. It should be clear to the reader that the movement of the pointer in millimetres indicates a blood pressure change of twice that number of millimetres of mercury. For small animals, such as rats, the Condon manometer (Fig. 11.4*b*) is required: because the long arm of this manometer has only a small bore, very little blood passes into the manometer system when the animal experiences even a considerable rise of blood pressure. The haemodynamic disturbances that might occur if the larger manometer were used are thereby avoided. An incidental advantage of Condon's instrument is the fact that the level of mercury in the wide bulb that constitutes the short arm of the manometer remains virtually unaltered however much the height of the column in the recording limb fluctuates. Consequently, a change of blood pressure of, say, 20 mm of mercury will cause a vertical shift of 20 mm in the kymograph tracing instead of the 10 mm that would occur with the larger manometer with its more conventional form of U-tube. Unfortunately the columns of mercury in both forms of the apparatus have a considerable inertia and the fluctuations of blood pressure between systolic and diastolic are considerably damped, particularly when the heart rate is high. Consequently, the effects of a drug which differentially affects the two pressures are not clearly seen,

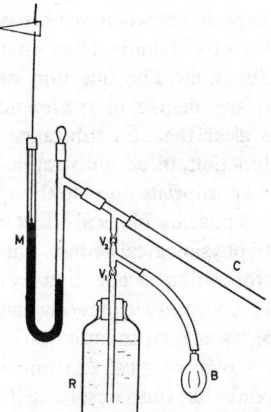

Fig. 11.4 (a) *Mercury manometer:* A useful form of the conventional mercury manometer. When the bulb B is pressed and released, anticoagulant fluid is drawn from the reservoir R. When the bulb is again pressed, the fluid is either forced, *via* the valve V_2 through the rubber tube (c) going to the arterial cannula if this is open or into the mercury manometer (M) if C is closed. In using the apparatus, the system is filled with fluid and the pressure in the manometer is set at a level which will ensure that there is no appreciable loss of blood into the system when the cannula is in open connection with the manometer. *Reproduced by kind permission of the author from Experimental Physiology, 7th edn. by B.L. Andrew).*

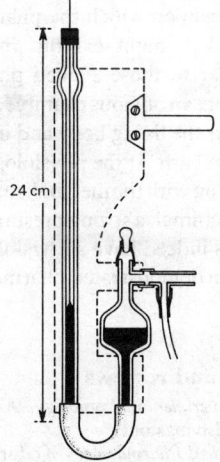

24 cm

(b) *The Condon version of the mercury manometer. Reproduced by kind permission of the authors from Pharmacological Experiments on intact preparations* (Edinburgh University Pharmacology Staff and L.J. McLeod, 1971).

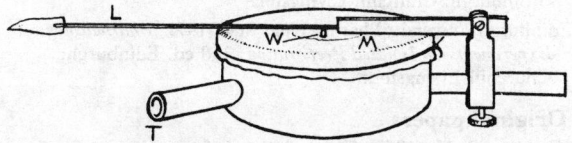

(c) *Membrane manometer:* The arterial cannula is connected by pressure tubing to the tube T which leads into the cylinder covered by the stretched elastic membrane M. The lever (L) is supported on the membrane by the wedge W.

the trace indicating what is essentially the mean pressure. Another form of pressure recording, which is used less frequently than it ought to be, is the membrane manometer. A small cylinder, the top of which is covered by a stretched elastic membrane is attached by pressure tubing directly to the arterial cannula (Fig. 11.4c). Blood enters the system, stretching the membrane whose tension increases until it is sufficient to oppose any further entry of blood. The inertia of the system is low and rapid fluctuations of pressure are followed by the membrane, whose movements are recorded by the lever which is supported on it. Membrane manometers are available in several sizes. A disadvantage of the system is that there is no simple relation between the excursions of the lever and the blood pressure change and the response becomes less sensitive as the pressure falls. There is an increasing tendency to use transducers and oscilloscopes or pen writing oscillographs for the purpose of recording physiological events in the whole animal. The blood pressure transducers commonly used for this purpose provide low inertia systems which not only show fluctuations between systolic and diastolic pressures but also reveal, when an oscilloscope is used, the minor fluctuations of pressure which occur during the cardiac cycle. It should be remembered that an oscilloscope beam has no inertia and it will demonstrate small and rapid changes which cannot be followed by heavy recording pens. A minor disadvantage of blood pressure transducers is that their response is not related in a linear fashion to the blood pressure and each one has to be calibrated before use by applying a series of known pressures to the instrument and noting the response produced in the record.

The amount of information supplied by a respiration record is also dependent on the method of recording used. This is discussed in Chapter 35 (p. 613).

Another question that should be asked when a record is being inspected is whether the response shown is really caused by the action claimed. For instance, the myographic method of recording the effects of drugs on spinal reflexes involves the recording of muscle activity by an isometric lever and the initiation of reflex responses by electrical stimulation of a peripheral nerve or by mechanical stimulation of the patellar tendon. A changed response is not necessarily the result of an action of the drug on the reflex centres. It may have arisen from some systemic effect such as a fall of blood pressure, from an effect on the processes of neuromuscular transmission or from some other action. When the equipment is available, this type of problem is much better attacked by electrophysiological methods. One or more of the dorsal roots is stimulated electrically and the action potentials transmitted along the appropriate ventral roots are recorded. The drug is administered by close arterial injection into the spinal cord. It is possible to distinguish the ventral root responses which have been conducted over a monosynaptic pathway from those which have taken the more circuitous polysynaptic route and thus to be able to say whether the drug affects monosynaptic or polysynaptic responses. Some of the traditional methods retain their value, as has been seen, but the pharmacologist should not spurn the new techniques made available to him by advances in other fields.

Modern laboratories are beginning to provide even their most junior undergraduates with electronic recording equipment and transducers instead of the traditional kymograph. Admirable though this trend is, it is not without its small disadvantages. Apart from the cost, to which reference has already been made, the traces obtained from most recorders can have a maximum amplitude of only 5 cm and even enthusiasts for the new system—like this writer—have to admit to some sense of loss now that they can no longer encourage their students to produce the elegant and distinctive kymograph tracings that were the reward for diligence, delicacy of touch and attention to detail in the laboratory.

Dose-response curves

It was pointed out in Chapter 8, that much of the evidence that has been adduced to support modern hypotheses concerning the mode of interaction of drugs and their receptors rests on the construction of dose-response curves for such simple actions as that of histamine or acetylcholine on the guinea pig ileum. It is obvious that dose-response curves may be constructed by recording the effect of a number of different doses of the drug, washing out each dose after its effect has been exerted and not adding another until the preparation has returned to its baseline condition. Another less obvious method, and this is the one favoured by Ariëns and his colleagues because it gives more regular and reproducible curves, is to produce a *cumulative dose-response curve*. The effect of a dose of the drug is recorded and another dose is then added, the first being retained in the bath. After the second dose has exerted its action, the total change from baseline (which is, of course, the summed effect of both doses of the drug) is measured. A third dose is now added to those already in the bath and the procedure is continued until a suitable range of values has been obtained.

Pharmacological actions

Before concluding this chapter, it is appropriate to consider briefly the relationship between physiological and pharmacological actions. The pharmacological actions of a substance are those produced when the substance is applied to an isolated tissue preparation or administered to the intact animal. Many of the compounds given in this way do not occur naturally in the body of the animal which provides the preparation. The interpretation of the actions of drugs of this type demands no further discussion in the context of this secretion. When the substance given does occur naturally, the question often arises whether the observed pharmacological response has any relevance to the physiological action of the substance. Indeed, on many occasions, the experiment will have been performed for the precise purpose of obtaining clues in the compound's physiological function. The question cannot always be answered with any degree of confidence. As a general principle, it is clear that if a substance has a particular physiological function, its administration by an appropriate route, in an appropriate dose, to the appropriate organ should result in a pharmacological effect which is at least a caricature of its physiological action. The converse of this self evident proposition is not, however, necessarily or invariably true. An observed pharmacological effect cannot, of itself, be taken as an unequivocal indication that the substance has a physiological function in the organ on which the response has been observed. This is an important principle which is not always paid the respect it merits. Some indication as to the extent to which the observed response presages a physiological function may sometimes be gleaned from the circumstances attendant on the experiment. If, for instance, the compound has a pharmacological action in very small doses on a tissue which is known to synthesize and retain it, the chances of its having a physiological function in that tissue are considerably enhanced. Collateral evidence must, however, be assembled before it is justifiable to conclude that the pharmacological experiment signals physiological function. Satisfactory collateral evidence may, for instance, take the following form. The organ on which the pharmacological effect has been recorded might exhibit, in its normal activity, changes similar to those evoked pharmacologically. Peristalsis, to quote an obvious example, occurs both in the intact intestine in the living body and in a fragment of intestine in the organ bath. If the physiological activity is disturbed by interfering with the metabolism of the active substance in the intact animal, a strong presumption exists that the substance does indeed have a physiological function related to the action demonstrated pharmacologically.

BIBLIOGRAPHY

Books, monographs and reviews
Andrew, B. L. (1972) *Experimental Physiology*. 9th ed. Edinburgh: Churchill Livingstone.
Burn, J. H. (1952). *Practical Pharmacology*. Oxford: Blackwell.
Crossland, J. (1961). Biological estimation of acetylcholine. In *Methods in Medical Research*, Vol. 9. Ed. Quastel, J. H. New York: Year Book Medical Publishers.
Edinburgh University Pharmacology staff and McLeod, L. J. (1971) *Pharmacological Experiments on Intact Preparations*. Edinburgh: Churchill Livingstone.
Edinburgh University Pharmacology Staff(1971).*Pharmacological Experiments on Isolated Preparations* 2nd ed. Edinburgh: Churchill Livingstone

Original papers
Gaddum, J. H. (1953). The technique of superfusion. *Br. J. Pharmac. Chemother.*, **8**, 321-326.
Gaddum, J. H. (1965). An improved microbath. *Br. J. Pharmac. Chemother.*, **23**, 613-619.
Paton, W. D. M. (1957). A pendulum auxotonic lever. *J. Physiol.*, **137**, 35-36P.

PART II

HUMORAL SUBSTANCES AND MECHANISMS

12. Some aspects of the physiology of the nervous system

A large number of pharmacologically active substances affect nervous function and many drugs owe their usefulness (or their side effects) to an action on one or other division of the nervous system. A knowledge of neurophysiology is therefore of some importance to the pharmacologist but he does not always receive, in elementary physiology courses, information concerning those aspects of the subject which are most relevant to his particular speciality. The purpose of this chapter is simply to point out to the reader the topics with which he should make, or renew, acquaintance if he is to appreciate fully the intricacies of neuropharmacological action. Limitations of space preclude more than a superficial treatment of the selected topics and those who feel the need to acquire a more detailed knowledge are referred to standard text-books of neurophysiology. Some discussion of other specialized areas of neurophysiology will be found elsewhere in this book in connection with the actions of drugs that influence particular types of nervous activity.

THE NERVE IMPULSE

Impulses travelling along nerve fibres provide the only means by which information can be transmitted to, from or within the central nervous system.

A nerve fibre consists of a core of semi-fluid gelatinous material (the *axoplasm*) which is bounded by a membrane (the *axolemma*) so thin that it can only be seen with the electron microscope. In the thinnest mammalian nerve fibres the axon with its axolemma is surrounded only by the *neurilemma* (the sheath of Schwann) a very fine lipoprotein membrane. In the larger fibres (the myelinated or medullated fibres) a myelin (or medullary) sheath intervenes between the axolemma and the neurilemma. This sheath is interrupted at regular intervals along its length at the *nodes of Ranvier*. As a matter of fact, the myelin sheath is derived from the neurilemma which wraps itself, jam roll fashion, up to twenty times around the axon.

From the physiological point of view the most important structure is the axolemma because it represents the boundary between the axoplasm and the extracellular fluid. A potential difference (the *demarcation potential*) exists across the axolemma of unstimulated nerve. It should be noted that similar, but smaller, demarcation potentials exist across all other cellular boundaries that separate solutions of different compositions. As far as nerve is concerned, the membrane potential arises as follows.

An energy consuming process (the sodium pump) extrudes sodium ions across the axolemma so that the concentration of these ions in the axoplasm is lower than it is outside. An inevitable result of this state of affairs is that predicted by the Gibbs-Donnan equations: the *freely diffusible* ions (largely potassium and chloride in this instance) distribute themselves on the two sides of the membrane in such a way that the concentration of potassium ions in the axoplasm is greater than that in the surrounding extracellular fluid. An opposite distribution is established for the chloride ions. Diffusible ions disposed in this way would tend to diffuse along their concentration gradients but this tendency is offset by the fact that positively charged ions align themselves immediately outside the axolemma and negative ions take up a corresponding position on the inside of the membrane. The potential difference thus established is just sufficient to prevent the diffusion of the ions. Thus the distribution imposed by the Gibbs-Donnan effect is maintained in the face of conditions which tend to destroy it.

It should be clear that the size of the membrane potential is determined by the extent of the disparity between the concentrations of potassium (or chloride) on the two sides of the axolemma. This disparity, in its turn, is dependent on the extent to which sodium has been extruded from the axoplasm. The membrane potential (E) can be calculated as

$$E = 58 \log_{10} \frac{[K^+] \text{ inside}}{[K^+] \text{ outside}} = 58 \log_{10} \frac{[Cl'] \text{ outside}}{[Cl'] \text{ inside}}$$

In mammalian nerves the resting potential lies between 60 and 90 millivolts.

The resting potential is preserved until the nerve is stimulated. An effective stimulus produces a patch of reversed polarization, the inside of the nerve, at the point where the stimulus is applied, becoming positive with respect to the outside. As a result, local action currents are set up (Fig. 12. 1) which have the effect of transferring the area of reversed polarization to an adjoining region of the nerve while normal resting conditions are re-established in the stimulated region. In this way the patch of reversed polarization (which is the nerve impulse) is transmitted along the nerve.

In unmyelinated nerve fibres, transmission of the nerve impulse is continuous, the region of reversed polarization

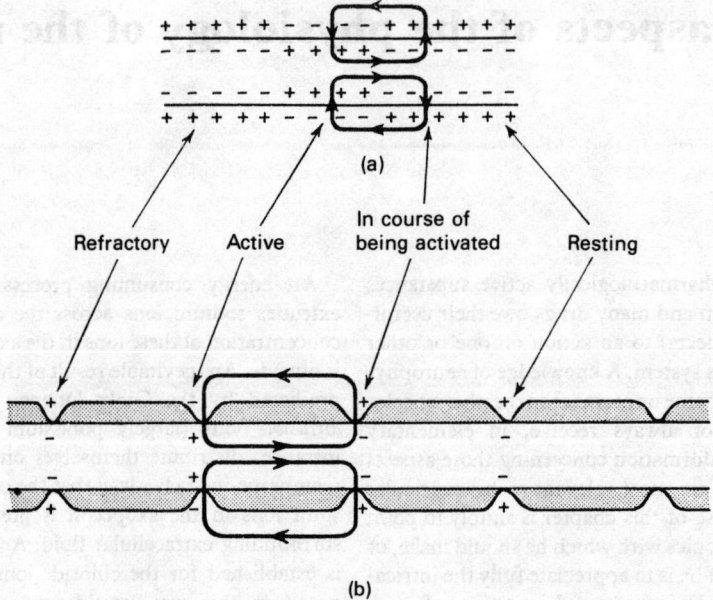

Fig. 12.1 The conduction of a nerve impulse along an unmyelinated (a) and a myelinated (b) nerve fibre. The action currents generated by the active region lead to the development of activity in a neighbouring region of nerve and to the re-establishment of the resting state in the originally active area.

being conducted, in the way described, to an immediately adjacent region of the nerve membrane. The process is continued until the whole length of the nerve has been visited by the impulse. In myelinated fibres, on the other hand, the stimulus initiates the membrane change at a node of Ranvier and this is then transferred from node to node. The nerve impulse, in other words, 'jumps' from node to node—the process of *saltatory conduction*. This type of impulse transmission has clear advantages. The impulse travels more rapidly by saltatory than by continuous conduction and saltatory conduction is a more economical process because the energy which is expended in restoring the membrane after the passage of an impulse is localized to restricted regions of the nerve.

Nodes of Ranvier are spaced more widely in nerves of large diameter than they are in thinner fibres. Consequently, conduction velocity is highest in the largest fibres.

If a nerve fibre is stimulated in the middle of its length, impulses pass in both directions from the point of stimulation. However, when the stimulus is applied at one end of the nerve fibre (as it is under most physiological circumstances) the impulse is conducted along the nerve with no tendency at any stage for new impulses to be fired back to the starting point. This is because the region of a nerve over which an impulse has just passed is refractory to further stimulation for a period of about one millisecond. By the time that the refractoriness has disappeared the impulse has moved so far away that the action currents it generates do not reach the now excitable region of nerve in sufficient intensity to cause re-excitation.

It remains to discuss the origin of the condition of reversed polarization.

Stimulation of the nerve electrically, mechanically or by a natural stimulus (such as that from a receptor or from action currents engendered by an activated area of the nerve) results in an increase in the permeability of the axolemma to sodium which therefore passes into the nerve notwithstanding the continuing activity of the sodium pump. Following the theory outlined above (p. 155), it would be expected that the ingress of sodium would be accompanied by an efflux of potassium. In fact, a delay intervenes between the movements of sodium and potassium ions probably because the potassium ions need, for their own transport, the carriers that take sodium into the nerve. The result is that for a brief period, both ionic species are present in the axoplasm. The inside of the nerve is now positive with respect to the outside and the development of this reversed potential (which reaches a magnitude of 90 to 120 millivolts) constitutes the rising phase of the action potential (Fig. 12.2). As potassium leaves the nerve the potential difference reverts to its original state. During the recovery period which follows the passage of the nerve impulse, the pump mechanism returns the sodium to the extracellular fluid, potassium re-enters the nerve and the resting state is restored.

The foregoing oversimplified account needs to be elaborated in one important respect if the reader is properly to appreciate modern ideas concerning the mode of action of a number of drugs including particularly the local anaesthetics and a range of cardioactive agents. Ion movements

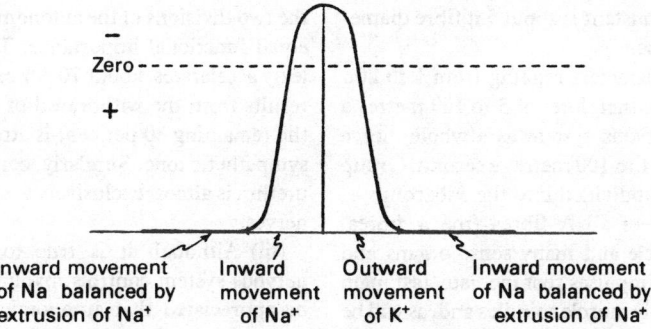

Inward movement of Na balanced by extrusion of Na⁺ | Inward movement of Na⁺ | Outward movement of K⁺ | Inward movement of Na balanced by extrusion of Na⁺

Fig. 12.2

across the membrane of cardiac muscle cells duplicate those that occur in nerve fibres and the following account is applicable to both tissues.

In a series of elegant and careful experiments, Hodgkin and Huxley (1952) made a detailed quantitative analysis of the membrane currents and associated ion movements that occur during the several phases of the nerve action potential and they were able to derive a series of mathematical equations that describe these events.

We have seen that the essential first stage in the generation of a propagated nerve (or muscle) action potential is the rapid ingress of sodium ions. The conductance of the membrane for sodium ions (C_{Na}) during this process is given by the Hodgkin and Huxley equations as

$$\bar{C}_{Na} = \bar{C}_{Na} \times m^3 h$$

where $\bar{C}_{Na}$ represents the maximal possible sodium conductance and m and h are variables that refer to factors that, respectively, promote and hinder the ingress of sodium ions (Hodgkin & Huxley, 1952). Although this is a purely mathematical formulation, the m and h functions are seen as representing the activity of molecules located respectively on the inside and outside of the membrane. It is customary to picture these molecules as gates. The cubic function implies the existence of a group of three 'm' gates that are opened or closed in series as suggested in Fig. 12.3.

The increased permeability of the membrane to sodium produced by application of an electrical, mechanical or a physiological stimulus is described mathematically in terms of a progressive increase in the value of m ('the m gates are opened') and by a fall in h ('the h gate, initially wide open, is gradually closed') that eventually leads to a cutting off of the sodium inflow. The h gate remains closed until the membrane is partially repolarized. The period of complete closure of the h gate corresponds to the absolute refractory period. Thereafter the h gate opens and the m gates are progressively closed until the nerve is restored to its initial state.

TYPES OF NERVE FIBRE

Nerve fibres are divided into three groups, designated A, B

and C. The fibres of groups A and B are myelinated, those of group C are unmyelinated. Group C fibres have the smallest diameter (about 1μ) and they conduct nerve impulses at the rate of 1 to 2 metres a second. In unmyelinated fibres generally, conduction velocity is proportional to the square root of the fibre diameter. Postganglionic nerves in the autonomic nervous system are made up predominantly of C fibres. C fibres also carry nerve impulses which subserve 'slow' pain.

For reasons already explained, myelinated fibres conduct nerve impulses more rapidly than do unmyelinated fibres of the same diameter: among myelinated fibres conduction velocity is directly proportional to the diame-

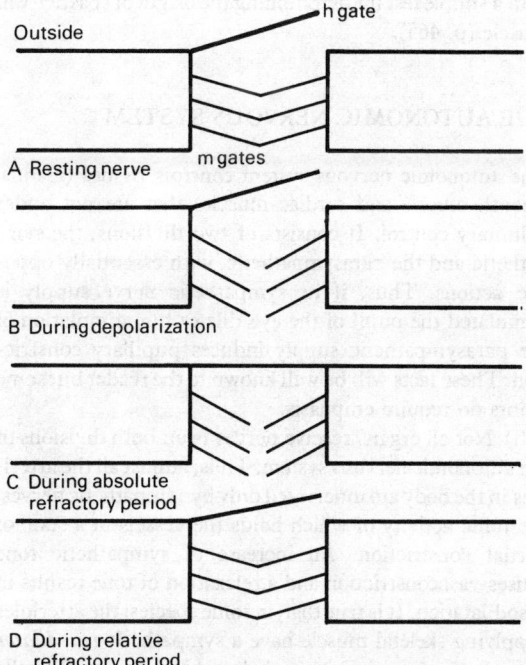

Fig. 12.3 Schematic diagram to show the position of the m and h 'gates' before, during and after the passage of a nerve impulse.

ter. The proportionality constant is about 5 if fibre diameter is measured in microns.

Group A fibres have diameters ranging from 1 to 20μ and conduction velocities, therefore, of 5 to 100 metres a second. Thus, in the nervous system as a whole, nerve impulses travel at rates of 1 to 100 metres a second. Group A fibres are themselves subdivided into the subgroups α, ß, γ and δ. The largest of all A fibres (the α fibres) innervate voluntary muscle and many sense organs and they also carry the nerve impulses that mediate 'fast' pain (p. 417). The γ fibres supply muscle spindles and, as will be seen, the γ-motor system (the γ fibres and the muscle spindles) is of considerable importance in the control of muscle tone.

The nerve fibres of Group B are restricted in diameter to 2-3μ (conduction velocity 10-15 metres a second). They can be distinguished from A fibres of the same diameter by the direction and magnitude of the potential changes which immediately succeed the propagated action potential. Group A fibres exhibit both negative and positive after potentials, but B fibres develop only large positive after potentials. Preganglionic nerves in both divisions of the autonomic nervous system are made up of B fibres.

The smaller a nerve fibre, the greater is its sensitivity to local anaesthetics and some other drugs. Thus 'slow' pain is easily suppressed by local anaesthetics but 'fast' pain may be only partly blunted. Similarly γ-motor fibres are more susceptible than α fibres and this has been made use of in a simple test for determining the origin of spasticity in muscle (p. 465).

THE AUTONOMIC NERVOUS SYSTEM

The autonomic nervous system controls tissues (glands, smooth muscle and cardiac muscle) that are not under voluntary control. It consists of two divisions, the sympathetic and the parasympathetic, with essentially opposite actions. Thus, if its sympathetic nerve supply is stimulated the pupil of the eye dilates but stimulation of the parasympathetic supply induces pupillary constriction. These facts will be well known to the reader but some points do require emphasis.

(i) Not all organs receive nerves from both divisions of the autonomic nervous system. Thus, almost all the arterioles in the body are innervated only by sympathetic nerves, the tonic activity of which holds the vessels in a state of partial constriction. An increase of sympathetic tone causes vasoconstriction and a relaxation of tone results in vasodilatation. It is true that, in some species, the arterioles supplying skeletal muscle have a sympathetic *vasodilator* (as well as a constrictor) supply but this does not affect the general validity of the assertions that have been made in this paragraph.

(ii) Even in organs which do receive a dual innervation, the two divisions of the autonomic system are not always of equal functional importance. Thus, if the heart rate reflexly accelerates, about 70 per cent of the observed change results from the withdrawal of parasympathetic tone and the remaining 30 per cent is attributable to an increase of sympathetic tone. Similarly, control of the bladder and the urethra is almost exclusively vested in the parasympathetic nerves.

(iii) Although it is true to say that the autonomic nervous system controls involuntary movements, it must be appreciated that autonomic activity may accompany events initiated in the cerebral cortex. Thus, voluntary motor activity is accompanied by an increased blood flow in the contracting muscles and when muscles are paralysed as a consequence of a cerebral haemorrhage, their blood supply is also disturbed.

(iv) Postganglionic fibres of the sympathetic nervous system bring about their effects by the liberation of noradrenaline. Parasympathetic fibres liberate acetylcholine. Acetylcholine is also the transmitter substance at all autonomic ganglia, sympathetic and parasympathetic alike. The actions of these transmitter substances are discussed in detail in later chapters.

General effects of autonomic stimulation. Stimulation of the sympathetic nervous system causes dilatation of the pupils, acceleration of the heart, vasoconstriction (particularly in the skin and viscera), the liberation of glucose from glycogen in the liver and muscles, inhibition of intestinal motility and of gastrointestinal secretory activity and constriction of the sphincters. The bronchi dilate, the fur of animals becomes ruffled, the hairs of men are erected (giving the appearance of goose flesh), the spleen contracts (in those species of animal that possess a contractile splenic capsule) and micturition is inhibited. Stimulation of the sympathetic nervous system also evokes the liberation of adrenaline from the adrenal medulla. The effects of adrenaline augment and complement those of sympathetic nerve stimulation although on a few organs the action of adrenaline is not the same as that of sympathetic stimulation. The significance of these differences between the effects of adrenaline action and of sympathetic stimulation is discussed elsewhere (p. 262).

The activity of the sympathetic nervous system reaches its peak in strenuous exercise and in extreme emotion. This led Cannon to formulate his now famous aphorism that the sympathetic-adrenal system prepared the body for 'flight or fight'. It is certainly true that the changes brought about by stimulation of the sympathetic nervous system all facilitate the production of energy, the exchange of respiratory gases and the circulatory adjustments appropriate to intense physical activity. On the other hand, the sympathetic nervous system comes into play in less extreme circumstances than those envisaged in Cannon's dictum— when a recumbent subject stands up, for instance. Moreover, some degree of sympathetic tone is applied to many organs (the heart and blood vessels, for instance) even in the completely relaxed subject. It is probably more accurate simply to say that sympathetic nervous activity is increased whenever there is any increase, however trivial, in the body's activity so that its energy output is increased. In other words, sympathetic nervous activity is associated with catabolic conditions. By the same token, the parasympathetic system is associated with anabolic conditions, its activity being increased when energy is being taken in, as during the digestion of a meal, or conserved, as in rest or sleep.

Stimulation of the parasympathetic nervous system induces constriction of the pupils and bronchi, slowing of the heart and an increase in the activity of the digestive system—salivary and gastro-intestinal secretions are promoted, the motility of the intestine is increased, the sphincters relax and the gall bladder contracts. The bladder also contracts and the urethral sphincters relax in response to stimulation of their parasympathetic supply. Defaecation and micturition do not, of course, necessarily occur in the intact animal since these functions are to some extent under voluntary control.

Although it is generally supposed that emotional states are associated with activity of the sympathetic nervous system, it should be noted that this demarcation of the physiological function is not so clear cut as is sometimes believed. Some people who receive bad news suffer bradycardia, a fall in blood pressure and collapse; an angry man is as likely to be flushed (indicating inhibition of sympathetic activity) as pale, and defaecation or micturition sometimes accompany feelings of intense fear or pleasure. All these events are of parasympathetic rather than sympathetic origin.

The organization of the autonomic nervous system

It is assumed that most readers will be familiar with the details of the structural organization of the autonomic nervous system so that only the main features need to be stressed here.

It is important to remember that the autonomic nervous system is essentially a *motor* system. Sensory fibres from the viscera certainly travel in the autonomic nerves and many pass through the ganglia. However, they pass into the dorsal roots without synaptic interruption. Thereafter they take the same course as do somatic sensory impulses.

In both divisions of the autonomic nervous system, the nerve fibres that leave the brain or spinal cord (the *preganglionic* fibres) are interrupted in ganglia, where synaptic contacts are made with the cells that give rise to the *postganglionic* fibres. In the parasympathetic system the ganglia are located very close to, or on, the innervated organs. Thus the ciliary ganglion within the orbit gives rise to the postganglionic fibres that cause constriction of the pupil and accommodation of the lens for near vision. The preganglionic fibres to the ciliary ganglion are conveyed in the oculomotor nerve.

The parasympathetic nerve supply to all but the pelvic organs travels with some of the cranial nerves—the 3rd (oculomotor), the 7th (facial), the 9th (glossopharyngeal)

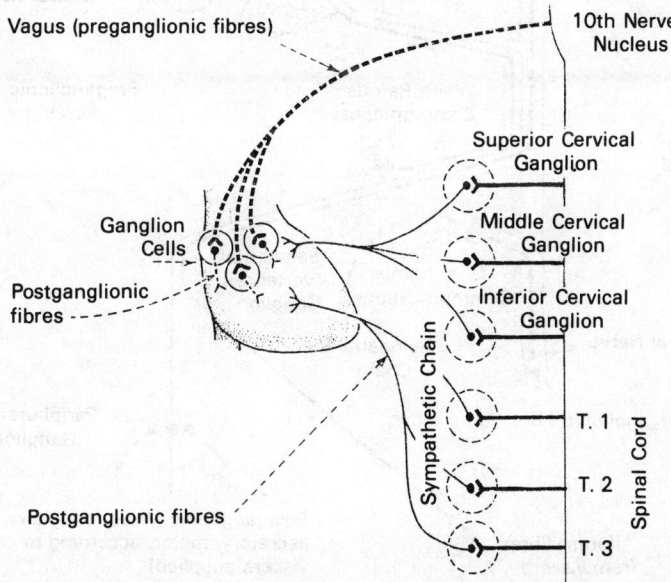

Fig. 12.4 Innervation of the heart. Preganglionic parasympathetic fibres (cholinergic) are shown as thick, broken lines, preganglionic sympathetic fibres (cholinergic) as thick lines, postganglionic sympathetic fibres (adrenergic) as thin lines and postganglionic parasympathetic fibres (cholinergic) as thin, broken lines.

and the 10th (vagus). Of these nerves, the vagus has much the widest distribution (the word vagus itself means wanderer) supplying, as it does, all the involuntary musculature in thoracic and abdominal organs. Pelvic organs (the uterus, the terminal portions of the colon, the rectum, the bladder and the external genitalia) receive their supply from the second, third and fourth sacral segments of the cord. Because of its anatomical origins the parasympathetic nervous system is sometimes called the cranio-sacral division of the autonomic nervous system.

Sympathetic ganglia are located some distance from the autonomically innervated organs so that, in contrast with the situation that obtains in the parasympathetic division, preganglionic sympathetic fibres are short and postganglionic fibres are long. This can be seen from an inspection of figure 12. 4 which illustrates the innervation of the heart.

Sympathetic ganglia are found in two locations in the body. A few unpaired ganglia (the coeliac, the superior and the inferior mesenteric ganglia) together with the hypogastric plexus (which is similar to a ganglion proper) lie in the abdominal cavity. The others, linked together by nerve fibres whose function will be mentioned later, form two *sympathetic chains*, which extend from the base of the skull

to the coccyx. They are situated, one on each side of the midline, close to the muscles that clothe the vertebrae (the prevertebral muscles).

In the early stages of development, one pair of sympathetic ganglia is laid down for each segment of the spinal cord but some fusion then takes place in the cervical region which retains only three pairs of ganglia (the superior, middle and inferior cervical ganglia) although the cervical cord has eight segments. Because the superior cervical ganglia are each formed from the fused rudiments of four ganglia (the other cervical ganglia are each derived from two rudiments) they are much larger than those elsewhere along the sympathetic chain and they provide very useful preparations for the study of ganglionic transmission processes (p. 175). In the thoracic, lumbar and sacral regions, one pair of ganglia is found for each segment of the cord so that the total number of ganglia in each chain is 26 (3 cervical, 12 thoracic, 5 lumbar, 5 sacral and 1 coccygeal) except in the dog. In this species, the upper four thoracic ganglia on each side are fused to form the large *stellate ganglia*.

Although there is a ganglion corresponding to each spinal segment, the preganglionic fibres themselves are

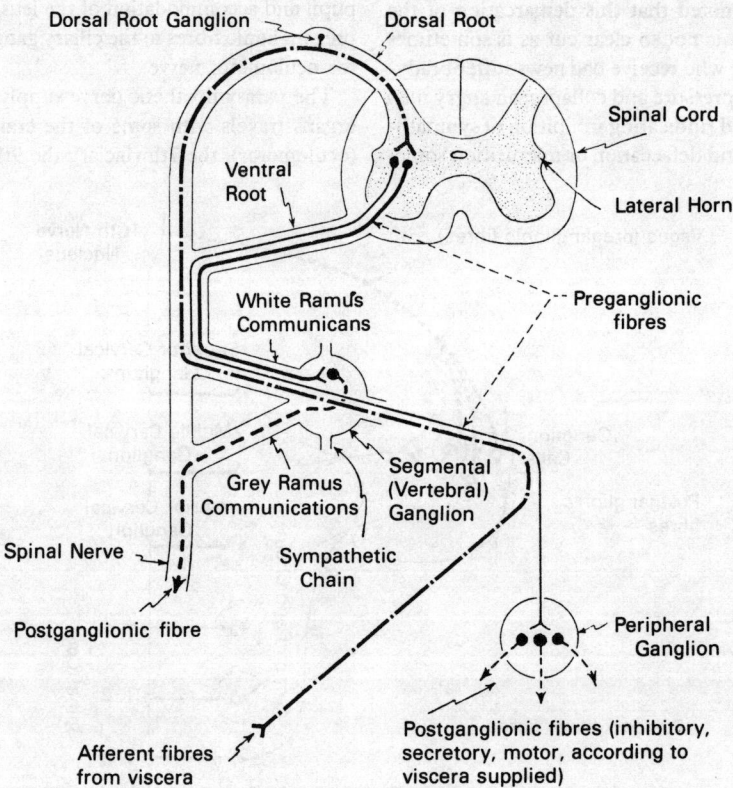

Fig. 12.5 Origin of sympathetic fibres from neurones in the lateral horn of the spinal cord. Preganglionic fibres (cholinergic) are shown as unbroken lines and postganglionic fibres (adrenergic) fibres as broken lines. Afferent fibres from the viscera are shown thus —·—·—. Note that the spinal nerves also contain afferent and efferent somatic nerve fibres.

derived only from cells in the grey matter of the thoracic region of the spinal cord and from the upper two lumbar segments. The sympathetic nerves are, for this reason sometimes described as forming the thoracolumbar division of the autonomic nervous system.

The preganglionic fibres leave the spinal cord with the anterior roots from which they pass to the corresponding sympathetic ganglia in the *white rami communicantes* (Fig. 12. 5). Thereafter they take one of several possible courses.

(i) Many preganglionic fibres terminate in their own ganglia and there make synaptic contact with secondary neurones whose axons, the *grey rami communicantes* pass back to the somatic nerve and are thereby distributed to the autonomically innervated structures in the area of distribution of the nerve. Postganglionic fibres, as was mentioned earlier (p. 157) are unmyelinated C fibres and they thus appear grey in colour. Preganglionic fibres are myelinated B fibres and they take on a white appearance. This is the origin of the designation 'grey' and 'white' for the two types of ramus.

(ii) Some of the preganglionic fibres which leave the cord at thoracic segments 5 to 12 and the first two lumbar segments pass straight through the ganglia and into the abdominal cavity (Figs. 12. 5 and 12. 6). There they form the splanchnic nerves which terminate in the abdominal ganglia already referred to (p. 160). Post-ganglionic fibres pass to various parts of the intestine where they meet vagal or pelvic parasympathetic fibres to form the autonomous plexuses which control the movements of the intestine and which are more fully discussed in a later chapter (p. 652). The origin of the preganglionic supply to the individual abdominal ganglia is indicated in Figure 12. 6. Some fibres of the splanchnic nerves traverse the coeliac ganglion without synaptic interruption and terminate in the adrenal medulla whose chromaffin (adrenaline secreting) cells thus behave as postganglionic elements.

(iii) Some preganglionic fibres branch as they enter the ganglion. One branch terminates in the ganglion in the fashion already described. The other branch turns upwards or downwards in the sympathetic chain, passing through a number of ganglia, to which it gives branches which themselves make synaptic contact with postgangli-

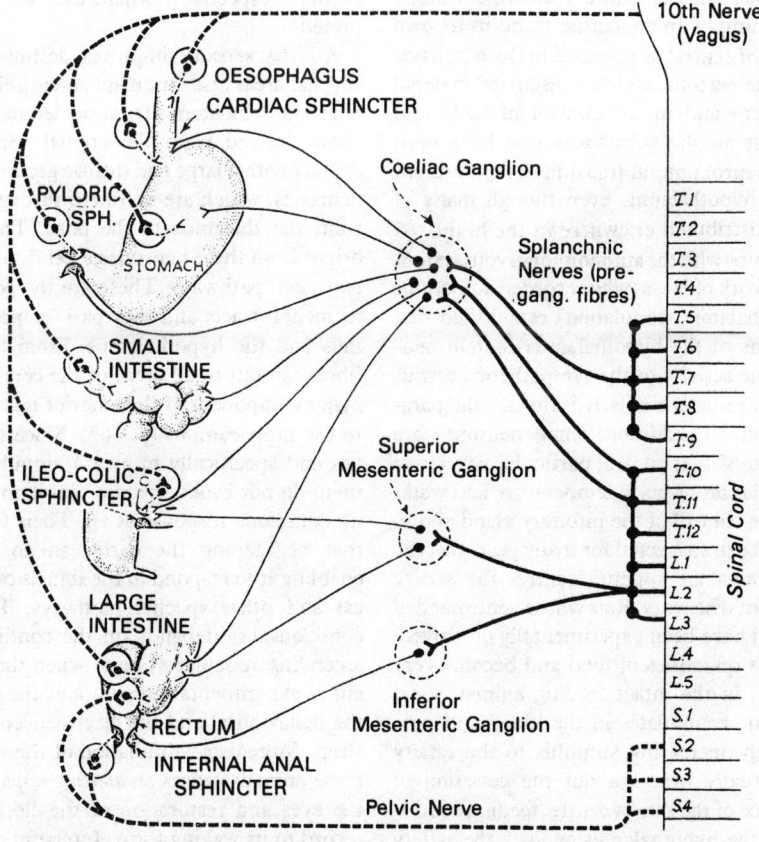

Fig. 12.6 Innervation of the gastrointestinal tract. Note that in this instance the preganglionic sympathetic fibres pass *through* the paravertebral ganglia, T5 to L3, without synaptic interruption. Nerves are represented according to the convention adopted in Figure 12.4.

onic neurones. The cervical, the lower lumbar and the sacral ganglia receive their preganglionic supply from the thoracic and the upper lumbar outflow, respectively, in this way but some of the thoracic ganglia which receive preganglionic fibres directly from the corresponding segments of the cord also receive some of their supply from more distant rami.

The fibres which pass upwards or downwards in the way described form the longitudinal strands which connect the sympathetic ganglia together to form the chains.

It will be seen that impulses passing along a single white ramus may activate ganglia over a considerable length of the sympathetic chain and thereby exert an influence over a wide region of the body.

THE HYPOTHALAMUS

The hypothalamus (Fig. 12. 9) though small in size is one of the most important and fascinating regions of the nervous system. It is in functional connection on the one hand with the autonomic nervous system and on the other hand with the frontal lobes and the highest centres of the brain. It supervises the activity of the pituitary gland and thus has an influence on the entire endocrine system. Indeed, it is something of an endocrine gland in its own right (p. 770). It is of central importance in the regulation of the emotional state—a topic which is discussed in detail later in this chapter—and in the control of sleep and wakefulness. Almost all the substances that have been named as possible neurohumoral transmitters are present in quantity in the hypothalamus even though many of them are sparsely distributed elsewhere in the brain.

So far as relationships with the autonomic nervous system are concerned, the work of Hess (who recorded autonomic responses to hypothalamic stimulation) established that the posterior regions of the hypothalamus contain neurones that control the activity of the sympathetic nervous system while anterior nuclei similarly influence the parasympathetic division. In addition, some neurones are organized into 'centres' that control particular vegetative activities—the regulation of body temperature and water balance, feeding, the control of the pituitary gland and so on. Although it has been suspected for many years that the hypothalamus contains an appetite centre, the *satiety centre* is a more recent discovery. Rats whose ventromedial hypothalamic nuclei have been experimentally destroyed, eat abnormally large quantities of food and become very fat. It is clear that, in the intact feeding animal, some product of digestion accumulates in the blood and provides a progressively increasing stimulus to the satiety centre which eventually brings about the cessation of eating. In the absence of the satiety centre, feeding continues. Its location in the hypothalamus exposes the satiety centre to emotional influences and this may partly explain the gross overeating or extreme anorexia that may accompany psychological disturbances. It is also possible that

nicotine (p. 205) stimulates the satiety centre and this may explain why those who give up smoking tend to put on weight.

THE ASCENDING RETICULAR SYSTEM

Sensory nerve impulses destined to reach consciousness travel from the periphery to the brain by well defined pathways in the spinal cord. These include the lateral and anterior spinothalamic tracts and the dorsal white columns. These several tracts come together in the medulla and continue as the *lemnisci* to the thalamus, whence they are relayed by way of the internal capsule, to the sensory cortex (Area 3) in the parietal lobe of the hemisphere. Sensory impulses in the cranial nerves also travel to the thalamus and the parietal cortex. The information transmitted along these routes is interpreted in terms of specific sensations well localized in consciousness to the part of the body from which they originate. In addition, the organs of special sense—the eye and the ear—give rise to impulses which reach the temporal and occipital cortices respectively where they are appropriately interpreted.

All the sensory impulses destined for these specific cortical areas also stimulate an entirely separate system of neurones. Collaterals from the lemniscal fibres (and from those derived from the cranial nerves) make synaptic contact with a large and diffuse group of cells, the reticular neurones, which are scattered throughout the brain stem from the thalamus to the pons. The fibres which take origin from these neurones ascend the nervous system by two main pathways. These are the posterior and anterior tegmental tracts and they pass, respectively, to the thalamus and the hypothalamus. From the latter structures, fibres fan out to all areas of the cerebral cortex. Another major component of the anterior tegmental system passes to the hippocampus (p. 167). Since the cortical fibres do not end specifically in area 3, impulses conducted along them do not evoke specific sensations: indeed, they elicit no conscious response at all. Their function seems to be that of keeping the cortex in an 'alerted' condition, enabling it to respond to the signals carried by the lemniscal and other specific pathways. The maintenance of consciousness depends on the continued activity of the ascending reticular system: when the reticular fibres are cut in experimental preparations the animal exhibits both the behavioural and the electroencephalographic signs of sleep. Moreover, stimulation of the reticular neurones in these animals causes an *alerting response*, with opening of the eyes and restoration of the electroencephalographic record to its waking form. Interruption of impulses in the direct sensory pathway has no effect on the level of consciousness. Thus, although impulses which travel to the cortex by way of the reticular system are not themselves appreciated in consciousness, the conscious appreciation of impulses travelling by the specific routes is impossible in the absence of activity in the reticular system.

The sleep and waking centres of the hypothalamus are connected with the ascending reticular system and diseases which affect the hypothalamus, or the structures that impinge upon it, may be associated with disturbances of the sleep rhythm.

The multiplicity of synapses in the reticular system makes it particularly susceptible to chemical influences and a large number of drugs is capable of modifying its activity, thus producing changes in the level of consciousness, alertness and behavioural responsiveness. Acetylcholine, noradrenaline, 5-hydroxytryptamine and dopamine are particularly important transmitter substances at these synapses.

The *cerveau isolé* preparation has been widely used to investigate the action of drugs on the reticular activating system. The animal is anaesthetized only during the operative procedure. A section is made across the brain stem at the midbrain (mid-collicular) level but care is taken not to interrupt the circulation above this level. The brain therefore remains viable but, because the reticular fibres have been severed, the electroencephalographic record is dominated by long bursts of regular waves of high amplitude separated by periods of quiescence. This highly synchronized pattern is typical of that seen in sleep or anaesthesia. Drugs that stimulate the reticular system have a desynchronizing effect, changing the electroencephalographic pattern to one dominated by fast, low amplitude waves. The animal may show overt signs of being alerted.

The *encéphale isolé* is a similar preparation except that the section is made between the medulla and the first cervical segment of the cord. In this preparation, the animal has to be artificially respired.

For obvious reasons, the ascending reticular system is sometimes called the reticular activating (or alerting) system. The reticular system also has an important descending component, the physiological significance of which is discussed in the next section.

Sleep and the drugs that influence it are discussed in more detail in Chapter 29 (p. 478).

THE CONTROL OF MUSCLE TONE AND OF VOLUNTARY MOVEMENTS

Voluntary movements are initiated in area 4 of the cerebral cortex and the impulses which arise there are transmitted to the anterior horn cells in the spinal cord by way of the pyramidal tract. However, if this were the only mechanism involved, voluntary motor activity would be clumsy, incoordinated and imprecise. Muscle movements are smoothed and controlled, and resting muscle tone is

regulated, by means of the *extrapyramidal system* which is best thought of as comprising all those nerve fibres, save those of the pyramidal tract itself, that carry impulses from supraspinal regions of the central nervous system to the anterior horn cells. Although there is some overlap of function, it is broadly true to say that extrapyramidal activity that influences voluntary movement is controlled by the cerebellum while that controlling muscle tone comes from the basal ganglia. Both the cerebellum and the basal ganglia exert their effects on the anterior horn cells by way of fibres that have their origin in nuclei of the reticular system.

The descending tracts of the reticular system are of two types, facilitatory and inhibitory. Facilitatory neurones predominate but their activity is restrained by impulses derived from the suppressor areas of the cortex and from the basal ganglia. Decerebration (which involves destruction of the brain above the level of the midbrain) releases this restraint and causes decerebrate rigidity. In the intact animal, inhibitory and facilitatory effects balance one another so as to maintain normal muscle tone.

During the execution of voluntary movements the cerebellum receives nerve impulses from proprioceptors in the joints, muscles and tendons and also from the motor cortex. It is thus in possession of information concerning the nature of the intended voluntary movement and it is able to adjust the tone and activity of the contracting muscles in the light of the information it receives from the proprioceptors so that the intended movement is smoothly and accurately executed.

The basal ganglia are nuclear masses at the base of the brain. For the purpose of the present discussion it is sufficient to enumerate the basal ganglia and to provide a general description of their disposition: the interested reader who requires details of their precise location and of their interconnections should refer to standard textbooks of anatomy.

The principal basal ganglia are the caudate nucleus, the putamen and the globus pallidus. These three nuclei are collectively described as the corpus striatum; the putamen and globus pallidus are together called the lentiform nucleus. These structures lie just deep to the thalamus which itself forms a major part of the wall of the third ventricle. The anterior part of the caudate nucleus is enlarged to form the 'head'. The 'body' and 'tail' complete the nucleus whose general shape is reminiscent of a question mark. Closely associated with the 'tail' of the caudate nucleus is the almost spherical amygdaloid nucleus—the 'point' in the question mark—which is actually located within the temporal lobe (Fig. 12. 8). Another important component of the basal ganglia is the substantia nigra, a midbrain structure.

The caudate nucleus receives fibres from the suppressor motor areas and sends fibres to the descending reticular system and to the other components of the basal ganglia.

Among the latter can be traced a circuit of fibres which links the caudate nucleus, by way of the putamen, globus pallidus and thalamus, to area 4 of the cortex, thus providing a route (albeit a circuitous one) whereby the suppressor area 4s can influence the activity of the immediately adjacent area 4 at the cortical as well as at spinal cord level.

Lesions of the basal ganglia give rise to a variety of diseases, all of which are characterized by a symptomatology which includes varying degrees of athetosis (involuntary writhing movements of the limbs and facial muscles), rigidity and tremor. The diseases include cerebral palsy, torsion spasm, Huntington's chorea (St. Vitus' dance), ballismus (in which the involuntary muscle movements are of a violent, flinging nature) and two disorders—Wilson's disease and Parkinson's disease—which are of particular interest to the neuropharmacologist.

Wilson's disease (hepatolenticular degeneration) results from an inborn error of metabolism which deposits protein bound copper in the liver and brain, particularly in the thalamus and—as the name suggests—the lentiform nucleus. Large quantities of free amino acids are excreted in the urine. Extrapyramidal symptoms and intellectual deterioration are severe. In Parkinsons's disease (paralysis agitans) the muscles are rigid and a characteristic tremor is intensified during emotional stress. It may take the form of a 'pill rolling' movement of the thumb and index finger. The facial muscles are immobile and the gait is festinant (hurrying).

The existence of many different forms of extrapyramidal disease is a reflection of the complexity of the basal ganglia and their interconnections. We have already noted that the extrapyramidal system exerts its major effects by way of the descending component of the reticular system

and that the cells of origin of the reticular tracts are particularly susceptible to chemical influence by reason of the multisynaptic nature of the routes along which excitatory and inhibitory impulses reach them. This explains why extrapyramidal effects ranging from slight rigidity to a fully blown Parkinson's syndrome are frequently seen during psychotropic drug therapy. Parkinsonism is further discussed later (p. 588).

THE GAMMA MOTOR SYSTEM

The motor nerves which supply skeletal muscle contain both α fibres and γ fibres. The α fibres innervate the muscle fibres proper and the γ fibres control the muscle spindles. The spindles form part of an extremely interesting mechanism for the maintenance of posture and muscle tone. If the γ fibres are stimulated the spindles shorten and this elicits a reflex contraction of the muscle fibres mediated by the α fibres (Fig. 12. 7). Exactly the same final result could, of course, be obtained by direct stimulation of the α neurones and it seems likely that the pyramidal and the extrapyramidal system exert their influences on both types of neurones. Which system is responsible for the production of a particular type of motor activity—or, indeed, whether the γ system is ever solely responsible for initiating activity—is still a matter of dispute but it is obvious that the direct pathway along the rapidly conducting α fibres will offer distinct advantages when rapid voluntary movements have to be executed. On the other hand, activity such as the maintenance of a fixed posture, which does not depend on rapidly changing muscle contractions, can probably be adequately performed through the γ system with the advantage that the voluntary effort need be exerted only on the muscle spindles, the contraction of the rest of the muscle being reflexly and accurately

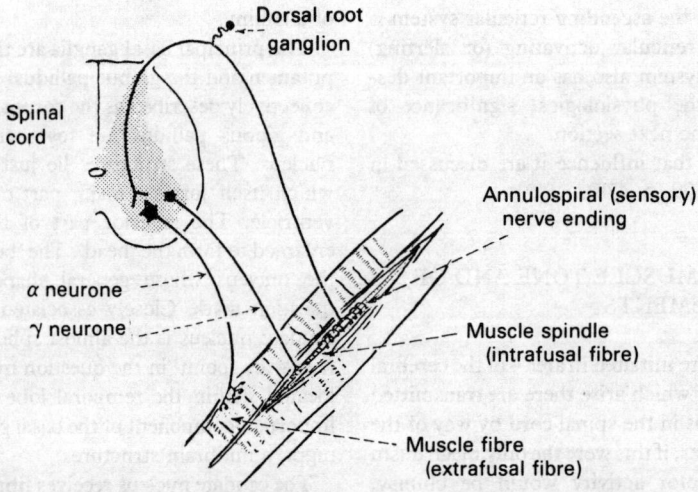

Fig. 12.7 The production of muscle contraction by the direct and by the γ-neurone mediated activation of α-neurones.

maintained so that the muscle takes up the same length as the spindles themselves. It should be noted that the spindles are delicate structures which form only a very small part of the total muscle mass and when they contract they do not themselves produce any direct shortening of the muscles.

Lesions of the basal ganglia or of the extrapyramidal system may produce disturbances of muscle tone as a result of interference with the activity of the γ motor system. Thus, some forms of spasticity result from the withdrawal of the restraint that is normally exerted on the γ neurones in the anterior horn of the spinal cord by the inhibitory component of the descending reticular system. In other conditions, spasticity is caused by the withdrawal of reticular inhibitory influences from the α cells.

THE NEUROLOGICAL BASIS OF EMOTION

Disturbances of mood or *affect* (which may take such forms as anger, anxiety, depression, fear or unbridled elation) are responsible for much unhappiness and mental ill health and the demand for their relief is the reason why vast quantities of some psychotropic drugs are consumed in the world's more affluent communities. Controlled emotions, on the other hand, form the basis of human happiness and satisfaction.

Emotion, as every reader will recognize, has both a sensory and a motor component. It is, in other words, both a way of feeling and a way of acting. Normally, a particular kind of overt activity is associated with a particular kind of subjective feeling: when we see someone weeping we know (or believe we know) how he feels and if a person behaves in a calm and 'unemotional' way, we assume that his mood is placid. In fact, the two aspects of emotion do sometimes become dissociated. The patient with Parkinson's disease may feel intense emotion although his face remains expressionless. Conversely, victims of some other types of nervous disorder may dissolve into floods of tears or explode into bursts of laughter while remaining subjectively unmoved.

It is clearly impossible to provide a complete and satisfactory explanation of the origin of so complex and almost infinitely variable a state as 'emotion' in terms of simple and unequivocally established nervous pathways. Emotional changes probably involve modifications in the activity of the brain as a whole. Nevertheless some structures are of particular importance in the generation of these changes. They will be briefly discussed here.

THE HYPOTHALAMUS

The 'motor' component of an emotional change particularly affects structures controlled by the autonomic nervous system. Much—but not all—of the associated activity in the somatic nervous system (striking an opponent in anger, for instance) is essentially a voluntary response to the emotional state and can, in theory at least, be suppressed, but an individual who is exercising complete restraint in this respect usually betrays his state by autonomic signs. Pallor or flushing, changes in cardiac rate or output, dilated pupils, involuntary micturition or defaecation, gooseflesh, erection of the hairs on the scalp (and ruffling of the fur in animals), weeping and dryness of the mouth, are all events that indicate a heightened emotional state.

Electrical stimulation of the posterior hypothalamus in conscious animals carrying implanted electrodes, produces a rage-like outburst of autonomic and somatic motor activity. The activity of the somatic musculature presumably arises as a result of impulses ascending from the hypothalamus to the cortex. A similar type of response appears in animals whose brain has been severed headwards of the thalamus. This response is called 'sham rage' because it is evoked by trivial stimuli which would not disturb an intact animal. Stimulation of some other hypothalamic sites seems to evoke pleasurable sensations in animals, while human subjects, similarly stimulated, may report feelings of ecstatic joy of an intensity never experienced in real life situations. The clear implication is that, like 'sham rage', this emotional response too is normally curbed by the restraining influence of the higher centres of the brain.

These two examples illustrate the important fact that one of the primary functions of the higher centres of the brain is to moderate the activity generated in the lower reaches of the central nervous system. This inhibitory activity extends to more areas than the hypothalamus and related structures—indeed it influences responses initiated even in the spinal cord—and it embraces more than obviously emotional ('affective') responses. Thus an animal from which the cerebral hemispheres and the associated brain stem have been excised exhibits a considerable increase in muscle tone that particularly affects the extensor (anti-gravity) musculature. This is the condition of *decerebrate rigidity*.

Man is characterized by his possession of a brain whose frontal lobes are, in relative terms, much larger than they are in other primates, an anatomical feature that is witnessed to by his high forehead. The parts of the frontal lobes that are situated forward of the areas concerned with the initiation of voluntary motor activity were for long known as the 'silent areas' of the brain because no overt response follows their electrical stimulation. Since they are obviously related to man's unique status in the animal kingdom they were at first assumed to be the loci of rational and creative thought but it is now recognized that they represent the seat of civilized and intellectual activity only insofar as they are the principal site of origin of the inhibitory influences that suppress the more extreme emotions and wilder instincts that would otherwise result in his being an ungovernably aggressive victim of his own basic drives. In such a state, man could hardly be described as civilized, nor could he ever indulge in the quiet contemplation that is essential to constructive thought. There must be many who would wish that man's inhibitory processes were not even more strongly developed.

An inhibitory area in the motor cortex is the suppressor area, to which reference has already been made (p. 163). Removal of its influence precipitates decerebrate rigidity.

An accident that most dramatically demonstrated the influence of the prefrontal areas at a time when knowledge of their function was still fragmentary occurred, in 1848, to one Phineas Gage, who as the foreman of one of the teams engaged in the construction of the then new Rutland and Burlington Railroad, was charged with the duty of instructing young apprentices in the technique of rock blasting. A hole, drilled in the rock, was filled with explosive and sealed with a clay stopper. A long fuse passed into the explosive through the stopper. Before the charge was fired it had to be compressed by hammer blows on a cylindrical tamping iron—the one used by Gage was some 42 inches long and over one inch in diameter—applied to the clay cap. On the day of the accident some of the apprentices had drilled the hole, filled it with charge and inserted the fuse. They had, unfortunately, forgotten to seal the hole with the regulation clay stopper. This circumstance was unknown to Gage when he decided that he himself should wield the tamping iron. The inevitable happened: when he hammered the iron it struck a spark from the rock. The unprotected charge was ignited and the force of the resulting explosion drove the tamping iron through Gage's upper jaw and brain, finally emerging through the cranial vault. Miraculously the luckless Gage escaped death. He survived for some years but when the post mortem examination was made it was found that the destruction caused by the passage of the tamping iron and by the huge abscess that resulted from the inevitable infection had destroyed a large part of the prefrontal areas although the motor areas of the brain were completely spared (Fig. 12. 8).

In the years remaining to him, Phineas Gage suffered epileptic attacks attributable to cerebral irritation from scar tissue but the most overtly remarkable change was in his character. Before his accident he had been a considerate, neat, conscientious, well organized, pious and quiet individual. After the accident he became aggressive, coarse, obstinate, quarrelsome, loud mouthed, blasphemous, untidy and careless.

In the permanent character changes induced in Phineas Gage, the reader will no doubt recognise some of the temporary ones seen in some drunks, for alcohol produces a depression of central nervous activity that affects the frontal lobes first of all. He may also realise that the tamping iron had effected a crude and primitive form of leucotomy. In the days when that operation was a popular technique for eradicating pathologically excessive inhibitory activity, injudiciously sited incisions in the frontal lobe occasionally produced individuals who displayed over-violent emotional reactions.

Although the overall effect of the removal of the control exercised by the higher centres is clearly excitatory not all areas of the central nervous system exert restraint on the

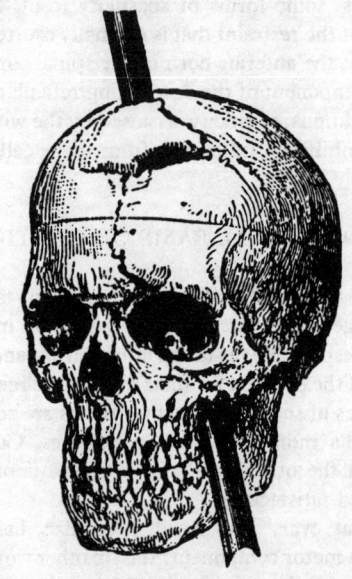

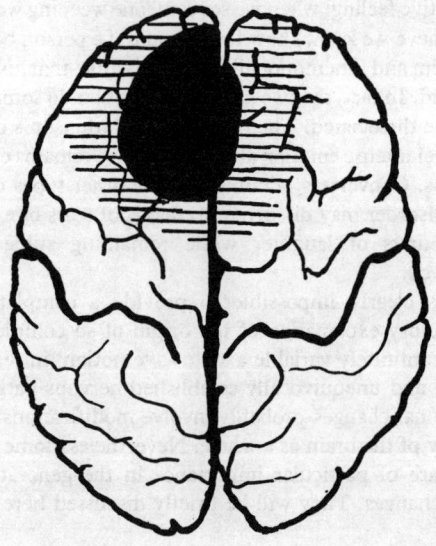

Fig. 12. 8 Phineas Gage's skull and brain showing the path taken by the tamping iron and the extent of the destruction and damage caused to the brain. Note that the motor areas of the brain were completely spared. Reproduced by permission of the author and publishers from Cobb (1946).

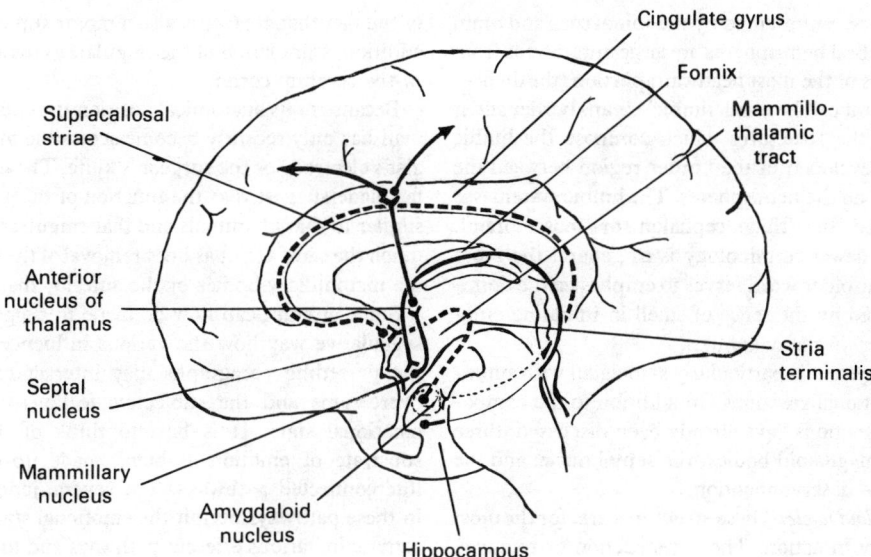

Fig. 12.9 This diagram illustrates the interconnections of some of the structures involved in the initiation and modification of emotional (affective) changes. Note the two pathways: (a) hippocampus, via the fornix, to the mammilary nuclei of the hypothalamus → anterior nucleus of the thalamus via the mammillothalamic tract (the tract of Vicq d'Azyr) → cingulate gyrus → cerebral cortex; (b) amygdaloid nucleus via the stria terminalis to the septal nuclei → hippocampus via the supracallosal striae.

hypothalamus. Some areas stimulate it. This, after all, is to be expected since it is highly unlikely that the visceral component of all grades of emotional response could be generated in the hypothalamus itself simply by modifying the degree of inhibitory tone. The suppression of violent reactions by the higher centres permits other excitatory impulses to be brought to bear on the hypothalamic and other centres. The nature and origin of these excitatory effects will now be briefly discussed.

THE TEMPORAL LOBES
More than forty years ago, Klüver and Bucy removed the temporal lobes of monkeys and produced a condition they described as 'psychic blindness'. After the operation, the animals no longer displayed fear, aggression or affection towards monkeys which had previously aroused these emotions: they behaved, indeed, as though they could no longer see other members of their community although their vision as such was not affected by removal of the temporal lobes. Similarly, articles of food that had previously been seized upon with avid delight and those which had previously evoked disgust were taken with equal equanimity, their identity being discovered only by actual sampling. Sexual activity, on the other hand, was usually intensified but the animals were quite indiscriminate in their choice of objects, animate or inanimate, upon which to direct their sexual energies.

Disorders of temporal lobe function in man are often associated with disturbances of perception and of emotional response. Outbursts of activity in temporal foci may coincide with episodes of fear, depression or aggressive behaviour in patients with temporal lobe epilepsy.

The hippocampal area of the temporal lobe has neuronal connections with the hypothalamus. Bilateral excision of the hippocampus in man causes loss of immediate memory but this may be because of the abolition of the affective response which is inseparably associated with the successful recall of a fact or an event. If this affective response— the sense of recognition—is absent, it is impossible to differentiate a correct from an incorrect recall.

THE LIMBIC SYSTEM
The limbic system is a collection of interconnected nuclei and nerve tracts, the complexity of whose anatomical interrelations defies simple description. Of the structures mentioned or illustrated (Fig. 12. 9) in this chapter, the hippocampus, parts of the amygdaloid nucleus, the fornix, the mamillary bodies of the hypothalamus and the anterior nucleus of the thalamus form one circuit (the phylogenetically older one) of the limbic system. Other portions of the amygdaloid nuclei, the septal nuclei and the cingulate gyrus constitute the phylogenetically newer parts of the system. The amygdaloid and the septal nuclei are connected by way of the stria terminalis and impulses conducted along this pathway pass along the supracallosal striae to the hippocampus. The cingulate gyrus is in direct communication with the anterior nucleus of the thalamus. Thus the two parts of the limbic system are closely interconnected.

The central nervous system consists essentially of an

almost solid tube, represented by the spinal cord and brain stem. The cerebral hemispheres are large outgrowths from the lateral walls of the most headward portion (the diencephalon) of the tube. The word 'limbic' means border and it indicates that the structures which compose the limbic system have developed in the border region between the diencephalon and the hemispheres. The limbic system was formerly called the rhinencephalon or 'nose brain'. Although the newer terminology is in general the more satisfactory, the older word serves to emphasize the dominant role played by the sense of smell in initiating emotional responses in many animals.

The limbic system is particularly associated with autonomic and emotional reactions. In addition to the components whose functions have already been discussed, three others—the amygdaloid bodies, the septal nuclei and the cingulate gyri—deserve mention.

The amygdaloid nuclei These structures are, for the most part, excitatory in action. Their destruction or removal, performed in such a way as to leave the rest of the hemispheres intact, produces an animal of extraordinary calmness and docility. Even animals as wild as the lynx have been rendered tame by this procedure. The reader may be confused if he has read reports of some of the earlier work, according to which amygdalectomy led to extreme ferocity. This may have been due to incomplete destruction of the nuclei or to damage to surrounding inhibitory structures.

Some investigators have stimulated the amygdaloid nuclei in conscious human subjects, who reported uncontrollable feelings of fear or rage during the periods of stimulation. In similar experiments on animals, amygdalar stimulation evoked a number of coordinated responses (such as chewing, clawing, snarling and crying) of the type normally associated with emotional states.

The septal nuclei Stimulation or removal of the septal nuclei has consequences that are the opposite of those provoked by similar manipulations of the amygdaloid nuclei. The pacifying effect of septal stimulation was, perhaps, most dramatically illustrated by Delgado, an American neurophysiologist, who devised a system whereby electrodes implanted in the brains of his experimental animals could be activated by radio signals. Untamed bulls so equipped became as docile as lambs whenever the radio signal was directed towards them.

The fact that our affective 'tone' is under the control, *inter alia*, of opposing drives from the amygdaloid and septal nuclei presumably ensures a refinement of regulation analogous to that provided in organs such as the heart that are subjected to both sympathetic and parasympathetic influences.

The cingulate gyrus Stimulation of the anterior cingulate gyrus (area 24) produces activation of the sympathetic nervous system, vocalization and relaxation of existing muscle tone. The last mentioned effect is a manifestation

of the fact that area 24 is also a motor suppressor area. In addition, stimulation of the cingulate gyrus affects all areas of the cerebral cortex.

Because of its anatomical position the cingulate gyrus in man has only recently become accessible to the physiologist's electrode or the surgeon's knife. The observations so far made suggest that the function of the gyrus in man is similar to that of animals and that cingulectomy produces much the same effect as does removal of the hippocampus, the mammillary bodies or the anterior thalamic nuclei.

Some attempt can now be made to suggest in a rather speculative way how the various influences discussed in the preceding paragraphs may interact to produce the overt signs and the subjective feelings of a particular emotional state. It is best to think of the anatomical substrate of emotion as being made up of a series of interconnected pathways. The several junctional regions in these pathways permit the emotional state to influence activity in various efferent pathways and to be influenced itself by afferent impulses from the periphery.

The emotional state is initiated in the first place by events which are consciously experienced—the sight of an enemy or of a loved one, the sound of music and so on. The nervous responses evoked in the appropriate areas of the cerebral cortex by these events are funnelled into the temporal lobe which in some way 'sets' the emotional state. Impulses are then transmitted along the hippocampus—fornix—hypothalamus (mammillary body)—anterior thalamus pathway and the amygdaloid—septal nuclei—hippocampus link (Fig. 12. 9). On arrival at the hypothalamus the nerve impulses send out appropriate signals to the autonomic nerves and at hypothalamic and thalamic levels they are themselves influenced by impulses from the periphery. Impulses from the thalamus pass to the cerebral cortex and these may be responsible for eliciting the subjective symptoms of the emotional condition as well as the voluntary somatic responses to it. It must also be remembered that the hypothalamus is an important relay station on the ascending reticular pathway so that the 'alerting' response may itself be influenced by the emotional state.

It will be clear from Fig. 12.9 that activity arising in the amygdaloid and septal nuclei (modified, of course, by afferent impulses from many sources) will itself be transmitted to the temporal lobes.

The anterior thalamus is connected by way of the cingulate gyrus (which adds its own contribution to the autonomic and somatic response) to all areas of the cerebral cortex which thereby 'colour' the incoming sensory information according to the nature of the prevailing emotional condition: when we are happy the ugliest object may arouse feelings of pleasure but when we are sad the most beautiful sight may leave us unmoved.

An important point to appreciate is that the final response to a particular situation depends not only on the information being passed along the pathways just described, but also on the overall degree of alertness of the cortex, which is determined by impulses passing up the ascending reticular system. Thus an emotional response may be modified by drugs that act at points along the specific 'emotion' pathway or equally by those that depress the arousal response.

THE BLOOD-BRAIN BARRIER

Some blood borne substances do not pass readily into the substance of the brain. This is because of the operation of metabolic and physical barriers (collectively known as the blood-brain barrier) and it explains why some drugs have to be administered by intrathecal injection (p. 37).

Details of the blood-brain barrier are to be found in appropriate textbooks (such as that of Davson, 1967) but it is necessary to add here that caution has to be exercised when assessing the results of experiments in which the blood-brain barrier might have been operative. The barrier is not equally impenetrable in all parts of the central nervous system (it appears to be relatively permeable in the hypothalamic region and in the area postrema) and its effectiveness may vary with the experimental conditions and with the species of animal used. Some substances to which the barrier is normally impermeable may appear in the brain if they are given in large doses and when two substances are given together the presence of one may alter the ability of the other to penetrate into the brain. A thought-provoking review of the blood-brain barrier is that of Dobbing (1961), to which the reader is referred.

BIBLIOGRAPHY

Books, monographs and reviews

Blakemore, C. (1977). *Mechanics of the Mind.* Cambridge and London: Cambridge University Press.

Boyd, I. A., Eyzaguirre, C., Matthews, P. B. C. and Rushworth, G. (1964). *The Role of the Gamma System in Movement and Posture.* New York: Association for the Aid of Crippled Children.

Brain, Lord (1962). *Recent Advances in Neurology and Neuropsychiatry,* 7th Ed. London: Churchill.

Campbell, H. J. (1966). *Correlative Physiology of the Nervous System,* New York and London: Academic Press.

Davson, H. (1967). *The Physiology of the Cerebrospinal Fluid.* London: Churchill.

Dobbing, J. (1961). The blood-brain barrier. *Physiol. Rev.,* **41,** 130-188.

Eliasson, S. G., Prensky, A. L. and Harden, W. B. (Jr.) (eds) (1974). New York, London and Toronto: Oxford University Press.

Noback, C. R. and Demarest, R. J. (1976). *The Nervous System,* 2nd Ed. New York: McGraw-Hill Book Co.

Mitchell, G. A. G. (1953). *Anatomy of the Autonomic Nervous System.* Edinburgh: Livingstone.

Patton, H. D., Sundsten, J. W. and Sunanson, P. D. (1976). *Introduction to Basic Neurology.* Philadelphia, London and Toronto: W. B. Sauders Co.

Paul, D. H. (1975). *The Physiology of Nerve Cells.* Oxford, London and Edinburgh: Blackwell Scientific Publications.

Pincus, J. H. and Tucker G. (1974). Behavioural Neurology. New York. London and Toronto: Oxford University Press.

Read, Cynthia (1978). *A Primer of Human Neuroanatomy.* London: Lloyd-Luke.

Ruch, T. C. and Fulton, J. F. (1960). *Medical Physiology and Biophysics,* Chaps. 1-22, Philadelphia and London: Saunders.

Simon, A., Herbert, C. C. and Strauss, R. (Eds.) (1961). *The Physiology of Emotions.* Springfield: Thomas.

Strongman, K. T. (1973). *The Psychology of Emotion.* London: John Wiley and Sons.

Walsh, E. G. (1957). Physiology of the Nervous System. London. New York and Toronto: Longmans. Green and Co.

Original papers

Granit, R., Holmgren, B. and Merton, P. A. (1955). The two routes for the excitation of muscle and their subservience to the cerebellum. *J. Physiol.,* **130,** 213-224.

Hodgkin, A. L. and Huxley, A. F. (1952). A quantitative description of membrane current and its application to conduction and excitation in nerve. *J. Physiol.,* **117,** 500-544.

13. Neurohumoral transmission

The nerve impulse is essentially an 'electrical' event since it consists of the movement of ions across the nerve membrane (p. 155). It is, however, generally agreed that the impulse transmits its effects to other cells by a chemical or *humoral* process. As each nerve impulse reaches the end of the nerve fibre it liberates a small amount of a *transmitter substance* which passes across the synapse or the neuroeffector junction to initiate activity in another neurone or in a muscle or a gland cell.

This chapter considers the development of contemporary ideas concerning neurohumoral transmission mechanisms and discusses the evidence that supports the claims of various substances to be considered as transmitter agents. Those new to pharmacology may need to refer, while reading this chapter, to other parts of this book in order to familiarize themselves with relevant aspects of the chemistry, metabolism and elementary pharmacology of some of the established and putative transmitter substances that are featured in this chapter.

Neurohumoral transmission has been extensively investigated and it is very well documented. Readers who wish to study it further are referred to the reviews listed in the bibliography to this chapter.

The idea that a nerve transmits its effects by liberating a chemical substance must have been discussed for many years before it was ever put forward formally, for humoral theories of physiological function are of very ancient origin. Du Bois-Reymond certainly suggested, as early as 1877, that nerves exert their excitatory action on muscle by liberating a chemical substance, but the neurohumoral hypothesis, as we know it today, is usually regarded as having its origin in the observations of T. R. Elliott, made in 1904. Elliott was impressed by the similarities between the effects of sympathetic stimulation and of adrenaline injection and he suggested that sympathetic nerves might bring about their actions by liberating adrenaline. This view was expressed in a brief preliminary communication concerning the innervation of the bladder and urethra (Elliott, 1904). In the full paper, which was published in the following year, no mention was made of the possibility of chemical mediation of the effects of sympathetic stimulation and Elliott never again referred, in print, to his hypothesis. Nevertheless, the honour of being the first to visualize the nature of junctional transmission is undoubtedly his, not least because he planted the idea in Dale's mind, as the latter readily and repeatedly

acknowledged in his writings. Dale himself did more than any other individual to establish the universality of chemical transmission processes.

In 1906, Dixon followed up Elliott's suggestion by proposing that the transmission of impulses from parasympathetic nerves might also be chemically mediated and he obtained some experimental evidence which indicated that the transmitter substance might be related to choline. These experiments made little impact at the time and physiologists were remarkably slow to follow the lead given by Elliott and Dixon. It was not until 1921 that Otto Loewi published the first of a series of papers that were destined to become landmarks in the history of pharmacology. They are described in the next section.

TRANSMISSION AT AUTONOMIC NEUROEFFECTOR JUNCTIONS

In his first experiments, Loewi took an isolated frog heart to which the vagus and the acceleratory (sympathetic) nerves were left attached. The heart was filled with Ringer's solution from a cannula attached to it. The solution in the heart could be transferred to a second isolated heart. Both hearts beat spontaneously; in the absence of nerve stimulation, the Ringer's solution in the first heart did not affect the spontaneous activity of second when transferred to it. Vagus stimulation brought about the expected reduction in the rate and strength of cardiac contraction and the fluid contained in the heart during the period of stimulation acquired the ability to induce similar effects when it was passed into the second heart. In a similar fashion, stimulation of the sympathetic nerve accelerated the heart and the Ringer's solution in it at that time caused acceleration of the second heart on transfer to it. On the basis of this and similar experiments, Loewi concluded that stimulation of the two nerves led to the liberation of substances which he provisionally called 'Vagusstoff' and 'Acceleransstoff'. That the two substances had separate chemical identities was indicated by the fact that the fluid collected during stimulation of the vagus did not affect recipient hearts pretreated with atropine although the acceleratory effect of fluid collected during sympathetic stimulation was still demonstrable. Ergotamine, on the other hand, was able to prevent the action of Acceleransstoff without affecting the inhibitory action of Vagusstoff. The results so far described established, in Loewi's later words, that 'nerves do not influence the heart directly but liberate from their terminals specific chemical substances which, in their turn, cause the well-known modifications of the function of the heart characteristic of the stimulation of its nerves' (Loewi, 1960).

Loewi at first believed that Vagusstoff was choline. He knew that choline inhibited the heart and that this action was prevented by atropine. He was able to isolate choline from Ringer's solution which had been contained in an isolated heart and he showed that it appeared at a faster rate during vagus stimulation. However, he also found that the amount of choline which was liberated by even a prolonged period of nerve stimulation was far too small to have any effect on the heart. It was not until five years and ten papers later that he realised that the active material was probably acetylcholine. With the benefit of hindsight, it is easy to be surprised at this delay: Reid Hunt and Taveau had described the properties of acetylcholine as early as 1906 and they had shown that, so far as actions on the cardiovascular system were concerned, acetylcholine was 100,000 times more potent than choline. Loewi was well aware of this. Indeed, in order to measure the amount of choline in the Ringer's solution contained in his isolated hearts, he converted it into acetylcholine and used the frog heart as a bioassay preparation!

In the paper which recorded the close similarity between the properties of acetylcholine and Vagusstoff (Loewi and Navratil, 1926), the authors also demonstrated that the action of both substances was potentiated by physostigmine (p. 213) and they suggested, correctly of course, that this sensitization was the result of physostigmine's ability to inhibit the enzymatic inactivation of acetycholine.

Thus, by 1926, it was established that acetylcholine (or something closely akin to it) was liberated by vagus stimulation and all the evidence suggested that the ester was itself responsible for transmitting the effects of nerve stimulation to the heart. It proved rather more difficult to demonstrate the liberation of acetylcholine from the mammalian vagus nerve but this was finally achieved by Feldberg and Krayer in 1933. Subsequent work resulted in the demonstration that an acetylcholine-like substance was liberated from other parasympathetic nerves and in 1934, Dale and Feldberg, using the method of differential bioassay (p. 210), were able to establish without any doubt that the parasympathetic transmitter substance liberated by stimulation of vagal fibres to the stomach (and hence, presumably, by other parasympathetic nerves) was indeed acetylcholine.

Many years were to elapse before Acceleransstoff was identified, notwithstanding the long-known fact that adrenaline mimics the effects of sympathetic nervous stimulation. The difficulty arose because although chemical examination of Acceleransstoff (or *sympathin,* as it became called) indicated that it might be adrenaline, pharmacological experiments revealed differences which made it difficult to accept the view that the two substances were identical. The nature of these discrepancies can be illustrated by reference to one of the experiments of Cannon and Rosenblueth, the most prolific workers in this field in the years immediately before the second World War. They used anaesthetized cats whose nictitating membrane had been denervated some time before the experiment. This operation conferred an increased sensitivity on the membrane, which was even further sensitized by giving the animals cocaine at the time of the experiment. The cocaine treatment also increased the sensitivity of other sympathetically innervated organs which could therefore be used to indicate the liberation of sympathin into the circulation. Contraction of the nictitating membrane and relaxation of the uterus revealed excitatory and inhibitory sympathomimetic effects respectively. When the nerve supply to the liver was stimulated the nictitating membrane contracted but the uterus was not affected. Adrenaline, on the other hand, produced a response in both organs. Cannon and Rosenblueth were enthusiastic protagonists of the view that the sympathetic transmitter substance was adrenaline. In this they were supported by Loewi. They explained their result by supposing that the adrenaline liberated by sympathetic nerves combined with a receptor substance loosely attached to the surface of innervated organs. Two receptor substances were postulated: combination of adrenaline with one of them would give rise to a substance (sympathin E) with excitatory effects while combination with the other would give sympathin I, a substance with inhibitory effects. Thus, to return to the example quoted, it was supposed that when the hepatic nerve was stimulated, sympathin E was formed. It exerted a vasoconstrictor action on the hepatic vessels and escaped into the general circulation in minute quantities where its presence was betrayed by the response of the nictitating membrane. The uterus would only be affected by sympathin I and it would not, therefore, respond to circulating sympathin E. Adrenaline, on the other hand, would form sympathin I with the uterine receptor substance and would thereby induce uterine relaxation. Equally, of course, it would form sympathin E at the nictitating membrane.

The 'two sympathins' hypothesis, though never entirely satisfactory, was the only one which went any distance at all to supplying an adequate explanation of these perplexing experimental facts. It remained the only acceptable hypothesis until 1946, when von Euler demonstrated that extracts of sympathetically-innervated organs contained more noradrenaline than adrenaline. The properties of noradrenaline parallel those of sympathin more closely than do those of adrenaline and by 1950 or so it was generally accepted that noradrenaline was the transmitter substance at the sympathetic neuroeffector junction. The idea of the two sympathins was then abandoned. The reason why the uterus did not respond to the noradrenaline liberated when the hepatic nerves were stimulated in the experiment referred to, is simply that the organ is not very sensitive to noradrenaline, even after cocaine treatment. It is, however, sensitive to adrenaline which affixes itself to different receptors from those occupied by noradrenaline.

Although nearly thirty years elapsed between the discovery of Acceleransstoff and its identification as noradrenaline, it is interesting to note that Barger and Dale had pointed out that noradrenaline more closely mimicked the effects of sympathetic stimulation than did adrenaline no fewer than ten years *before* Loewi announced the discovery of Acceleransstoff! (Barger and Dale, 1910).

The chemistry and the pharmacological properties of noradrenaline are described in Chapter 17 (p. 258). Here it is only necessary to add that it differs from adrenaline in lacking a methyl group on its terminal carbon atom.

Nerves that exert their action by liberating acetylcholine or noradrenaline are said to be *cholinergic* or *adrenergic* respectively. There has been an unfortunate tendency in recent years to use the terms loosely and in a much wider (and more inaccurate) sense than Dale intended when he introduced them. They should be restricted to a description of *nerves* that liberate acetylcholine or noradrenaline as transmitter substances. It is, for instance, entirely incorrect to speak of a substance that has similar actions to acetylcholine as a 'cholinergic' drug. It is a pity that so few workers have heeded Sir Henry Dale's caution that we should 'resist any impulse to widen the application of [the terms] by allusion or "transference of epithet". This can be attractive in a poem, no doubt, but for a scientific term it is destructive of its only value, precision' (Dale, 1953). Pharmacologists of all people should be careful to avoid this kind of poetic licence in their utterances. Our science is imprecise enough as it is and the condition should not be aggravated by avoidable semantic waywardness.

NEUROMUSCULAR TRANSMISSION

The idea that impulses in postganglionic autonomic fibres transmitted their effects by liberating a chemical mediator was immediately accepted, but attempts to extend the hypothesis to include events at other junctional regions met with vigorous opposition even after a considerable amount of experimental evidence in favour of this extension had been accumulated. Many physiologists, although they were prepared to accept the idea of chemical control of the viscera, felt that the flash of nerve impulses through the complex mesh of synapses in the central nervous system and the control of muscles capable, for instance, of moving fingers at the rate achieved by a competent pianist or typist required something with a more evanescent

existence and a more circumscribed area of activity that could be provided by a chemical substance. They regarded chemical mediation as a primitive mechanism, superseded in most parts of the body (even in the ganglia of the autonomic system) by an altogether faster, 'electrical' transmission system in which the action currents generated in a nerve were the direct means of stimulating neighbouring muscle or nerve cells. It is interesting to note that Loewi himself did not believe that humoral mechanisms were capable of effecting junctional transmission at other than autonomic postganglionic sites.

The first extension of the chemical hypothesis was made by Dale and his fellow workers who sought evidence for humoral transmission at the junction of motor nerve and striated muscle fibres. This region is known as the *neuromuscular junction,* a term which should be understood to exclude the less specialized junctional region between autonomic nerve and smooth (or cardiac) muscle fibres.

Dale and his colleagues showed that stimulation of the motor nerve to a perfused voluntary muscle led to the appearance of acetylcholine in the eserinized perfusate (Dale, Feldberg and Vogt, 1936). The muscles studied included the tongue of the cat, the gastrocnemius of the dog and the hind limb musculature of the frog. It was shown that the acetylcholine came from the motor nerves themselves: autonomic and sensory nerve fibres and the contracting muscles were excluded as possible sources. These experiments were followed by others in which acetylcholine was rapidly injected into muscles under conditions designed to reproduce as far as possible those under which it would arrive if it were liberated from a motor nerve. The technique of 'close arterial injection' was used for this purpose: the artery supplying a muscle was temporarily emptied of blood and the acetylcholine was injected rapidly and at a point as close as possible to the vessel's point of entry into the muscle (Brown, Dale, and Feldberg, 1936). Small amounts of acetylcholine (1-5 μg.) given in this way produced a contraction which resembled a muscle twitch in form but which occurred at only half the speed of twitches elicited by stimulation of the motor nerve. Later, it was found that the acetylcholine-induced 'twitch' was in fact a brief tetanus but, when account is taken of the fact that, even after close arterial injection, there remained several impediments to the rapid access of acetylcholine to its site of action, the similarities between the contractions produced by acetylcholine and those resulting from motor nerve stimulation are striking. Finally, the effects of anticholinesterase agents (p. 219) on neuromuscular transmission were shown to be consistent with the assumption that these substances permitted the accumulation of acetylcholine liberated from motor nerves in the course of their normal physiological activity. Bacq and Brown (1937) emphasized the parallel that exists between anticholinesterase activity and the ability to potentiate the response of a muscle to nerve stimulation.

Dale and his colleagues believed that the evidence they had assembled was sufficient to establish the fact of cholinergic transmission at the neuromuscular junction, but some other investigators, particularly Eccles, were unwilling to accept this conclusion. They proposed, instead, the electrical hypothesis of junctional transmission to which a brief allusion has already been made (p. 172). Other interested physiologists found themselves taking sides in this controversy, and the sharp division of opinion thus engendered enlivened meetings of the Physiological Society in Britain for a decade.

Although they are no longer relevant, Eccles's objections to the chemical hypothesis of neuromuscular transmission were weighty and, in the state of knowledge which existed in 1936, unanswerable by direct experiment. To take just one point, Eccles pointed out the wide disparity, in Dale's experiments, between the amount of acetylcholine released into the perfusion fluid by motor nerve stimulation and the minimum amount required to stimulate muscle. He argued, that is, that the observed effects of acetylcholine were pharmacological ones, unrelated to the physiological process of neuromuscular transmission. As is emphasized in several other places throughout this book, this kind of argument has to be taken very seriously. Dale and his colleagues countered it by pointing out that the dose of acetylcholine needed to evoke a muscle contraction became progressively smaller, as the point of injection was moved nearer and nearer to the muscle. They therefore maintained that the loss of acetylcholine by enzymatic destruction and by diversion to sites other than the excitable membrane was sufficient to explain the observed discrepancy between the amount liberated into the perfusion fluid and that required to stimulate muscle. However, it was impossible to provide direct evidence that this was so and Eccles's electrical hypothesis retained its appeal for the many who found it more acceptable on quantitative grounds.

The overall weight of Eccles's objections at that time to the chemical hypothesis can be judged by referring to his formidable review of the subject (Eccles, 1936).

The deadlock between the two opposing views of the mechanism of neuromuscular transmission was not finally broken until 1949 but the experimental investigations that were to lead up to this event were initiated much earlier.

Curare, a drug which causes muscle paralysis, is known to produce its effect by interfering with transmission processes at the neuromuscular junction (p. 237). In the curarized animal, stimulation of a motor nerve gives rise to a non-propagated change in electrical potential at the motor end plate. The end plate is a specialized region of the muscle with which the terminal ramifications of the motor nerve fibres are associated. This *end plate potential* became the object of a series of experiments by Eccles and his associates. They showed that it became progressively bigger as the effects of a dose of curare began to wear off.

Ultimately a stage was reached when the end plate potential gave rise to a propagated muscle action potential—that is, nerve stimulation once again produced an obvious muscle twitch (Eccles, Katz and Kuffler, 1941). These experiments made it clear that the end plate potential was the essential intermediary between propagated action potentials in nerve and muscle. The problem of neuromuscular transmission was thus reduced to that of discovering the origin of the end plate potential. Kuffler was always of the opinion that the potential was of chemical origin and he obtained some impressive experimental evidence that this was so (Kuffler, 1942). Eccles, however, still maintained that the change was brought about entirely by the action of local currents set up directly by the arrival of the nerve impulse at the motor nerve terminals. He continued to hold this view for some years, but in 1949 he published the results of an investigation into the effects of anticholinesterases on the end plate potential of frog muscle (Eccles and MacFarlane, 1949). He examined seven drugs, all of which intensified and prolonged the end plate potential, indicating that they were potentiating transmitter action. Since the one common property of these substances was that of being able to prevent destruction of acetylcholine, it was evident that the agent whose action was potentiated could only be acetylcholine. Thus the validity of the chemical hypothesis of neuromusclar transmission was finally established by the person who had been most active in drawing attention to its deficiencies.

During recent years it has been possible to study neuromuscular transmission in some detail and it is now possible to sketch a more complete outline of the process, as follows.

Acetylcholine is synthesized within the motor nerve terminals under the control of choline acetyltransferase. The choline required is conveyed into the nerve from the plasma by a process of active transport. The acetylcholine is stored in tiny vesicles immediately inside the limiting membrane of the nerve terminals. In the absence of motor nerve stimulation a succession of these vesicles approach and unite with the membrane of the nerve terminals. They then undergo spontaneous rupture and release their contained acetylcholine ino the junctional space. These spontaneous movements and rupture of the synaptic vesicles are probably the results of thermal agitation on the part of the molecular components of the nerve membrane. It has been calculated that on rupture each synaptic vesicle releases some 5000 molecules of acetylcholine. Subsequently it re-forms and takes up another complement of transmitter molecules.

The small amounts of acetylcholine released by the spontaneous rupture of single vesicles produce tiny areas of depolarization which appear as very small ('miniature') end plate potentials, none of which is large enough to generate a propagated muscle contraction. When a nerve impulse invades the nerve terminal, a large number of vesicles rupture simultaneously and sufficient acetylcholine is released to produce a full-sized end plate potential which initiates contraction of the muscle fibre. The surface of the end plate is richly supplied with cholinesterase which hydrolyses the acetylcholine as soon as it has exerted its depolarizing action. The end plate returns to its resting condition until another nerve impulse arrives to trigger off another depolarization-repolarization cycle.

The release of acetylcholine is the result of the ingress of calcium ions consequent on the depolarization of the nerve terminals by the arriving nerve impulse. That calcium is necessary for transmitter release is evident from the fact that acetylcholine does not appear in the absence of external calcium.

Each nerve impulse promotes the release of about one million molecules of acetylcholine (the contents, that is, of about 2000 vesicles) on to an end plate studded with about twenty times that number of acetylcholine receptors. Acetylcholinesterase binding sites are present in a density that approximates to that of the receptors. Four calcium ions are taken up for each molecule of acetylcholine released. It has been calculated that the amount of acetylcholine stored in a motor nerve terminal would be exhausted, in the absence of replenishment, after rather less than five minutes of normal activity. The function of the motor system is maintained even in the face of vigorous neuromuscular traffic by reason of the high concentration of choline acetyltransferase in motor nerves (p. 182). This ensures that synthesis proceeds briskly so that the very modest reserve of acetylcholine is never less than full.

Liberated into the neuromuscular space, acetylcholine depolarizes the muscle membrane. Contraction of the underlying muscle follows but this event is not the immediate consequence of the depolarization as is shown by the fact that stimulation of the myofibrils by electric currents that mimic the effects of a physiological depolarization does not result in contraction. The link between excitation of the muscle membrane and contraction of the muscle substance is provided by calcium ions. Concentrations of this ion as low as 10^{-6} mol/l are sufficient to initiate contraction and it is important that this critical concentration is not reached in the absence of motor nerve stimulation. It is here that the sarcoplasmic reticulum plays its part, active transport mechanisms enabling it to act as a reservoir from which calcium can be mobilized or into which it can be taken up.

As we have seen, the sarcoplasmic reticulum corresponds to the smooth endoplasmic reticulum in other cells (p. 11). It is disposed around the myofibrils (the subcellular muscle fibres) in the form of irregular cisternae which abut on a system of transverse tubules (the T-system) at right angles to the cisternae (Fig. 13.1). There is no continuity between the lumina of the cisternae and those of the tubules but the two elements are closely related to one another, both anatomically and functionally.

The tubules are generally found at fixed positions in the muscle cell, usually at the A-I junction but sometimes at the Z-lines and their lateral extremities which are slightly enlarged to form the *lateral sacs* impinge on (and indeed in some species are continuous with) those parts of the muscle's limiting membrane that are capable of generating depolarizing currents. Depolarization permits the entry of extracellular calcium ions into the tubules. In their turn these ions cause the release of intracellular calcium from its bound form within the sarcoplasmic cisternae and this presumably creates the conditions for the splitting of ATP that initiates muscle contraction. When the signal from the tubules ends the intracellular calcium ions are taken back into their bound state within the cisternae and the muscle relaxes. That extracellular calcium is the vital link in excitation-contraction coupling is evident from the fact that muscle contraction does not occur in the absence of external calcium ions even though depolarization of the muscle membrane is not affected in these circumstances.

THE NORADRENERGIC NEURONE

The reader who has perused the foregoing account can hardly fail to be impressed by the progress that has been made in our understanding of neuromuscular transmission since the first tentative formulation of the acetylcholine hypothesis little more than forty years ago. Almost as spectacular a progress has been recorded by those who chose to study the physiology of transmission processes initiated by noradrenaline, the other of the two mediators that were revealed to the early investigators.

Noradrenergic transmission is discussed in its several aspects in some other parts of this chapter and elsewhere in the book, but some aspects of the process need to be mentioned briefly here in order to increase the reader's appreciation of events that occur at synaptic junctions operated by some other transmitter substances. Most of the information given here has been derived from experimental studies of postganglionic sympathetic nerve fibres but there is no reason to believe that it is not, for the most part, equally applicable to noradrenergic neurones in the central nervous system.

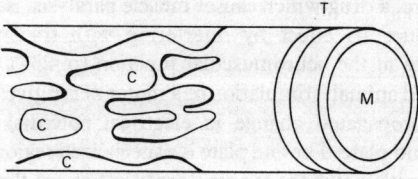

Fig. 13.1 Schematic illustration of the sarcoplasmic reticulum surrounding a myofibril (M). To show the irregular cysternae (C) and the transverse tubule (T). Note the lack of cisternae in the immediate vicinity of the transverse tubule.

The release of noradrenaline from nerve terminals in response to the arrival of a nerve impulse is dependent on an influx of calcium ions just as is the release of acetylcholine from somatic motor nerve terminals. Indeed, it seems likely that all neurotransmitter substances rely on the entry of calcium ions to bring about their release from the vesicles in which they are contained.

After release, noradrenaline becomes associated with the appropriate receptor but unlike acetylcholine at the somatic neuromuscular junction its subsequent inactivation is not affected by enzymes located on the postjunctional membrane. Transmitter action is terminated by a number of processes. Some of the noradrenaline diffuses from its site of action into the circumambient tissue fluids and blood and is there destroyed by catechol O-methyl transferase (p. 260). Another portion is probably taken up into the effector cell itself ('uptake 2') but the major part of the transmitter is returned into the postganglionic nerve fibre by a high affinity uptake process, usually designated 'uptake 1'. Back in the neurone the transmitter is re-incorporated in the vesicle granules whence it came, but on its way to this haven it is exposed to the possibility of hydrolysis by the monoamine oxidase (p. 260) present in mitochondria that are concentrated at the nerve terminals. The molecules of noradrenaline that successfully run this gauntlet are available for re-use once they are sequestered in the granules and the whole process clearly constitutes a valuable conservation mechanism.

The cholinergic link hypothesis
Until recently, a great deal of interest was centred on the hypothesis, originally formulated by Burn and Rand in 1959, that in postganglionic sympathetic nerve fibres the release of noradrenaline is triggered by acetylcholine. The main planks of the argument were that stimulation of postganglionic sympathetic fibres is accompanied by the liberation of acetylcholine as well as noradrenaline, that acetylcholine can bring about the liberation of noradrenaline from adrenergic nerves and that substances that prevent the synthesis or release of acetylcholine block the effects of sympathetic stimulation. The supporting evidence was discussed in some detail in the previous edition of this book and in the 1968 reviews by Burn that are cited in the bibliography to this chapter. The cholinergic link hypothesis does not enjoy the popularity and publicity that was once its lot and a substantial body of experimental evidence casts doubt on its validity. A simple but formidable objection to the hypothesis comes from the observation that sympathetic nerve fibres have a very limited ability to synthesize acetylcholine. Pending its possible revival the hypothesis can be noted but it does not now demand discussion in detail. Its apparent demise is a matter of regret at least to this author: by conferring on acetylcholine the role of universal transmitter substance in the peripheral nervous system it resolved the anomaly

that acetylcholine appears to be involved in transmission processes everywhere in the periphery except at some neuroeffector junctions in the sympathetic nervous system, for it is accepted that the sympathetic nerves to the sweat glands and the sympathetic vasodilator nerves to skeletal muscle bring about their effects by liberating acetylcholine. It also made the sympathetic postganglionic fibres even more analogous to the adrenal medulla for in this organ the release of adrenaline is also effected by acetylcholine liberated in this instance from what are essentially preganglionic fibres.

SYNAPTIC TRANSMISSION AT AUTONOMIC GANGLIA

At the time when Dale and his colleagues were first studying the neuromuscular junction, some members of the group also performed parallel experiments on sympathetic ganglia. The results were quite analogous to those obtained at the neuromuscular junction. Thus, stimulation of preganglionic fibres led to the appearance of acetylcholine in an eserinized solution perfusing the superior cervical ganglion, acetylcholine stimulated the cells of the ganglion and anticholinesterase agents modified the effects of pre-ganglionic stimulation in the way that would be expected if acetylcholine were a transmitter substance. Ganglionic transmission, like that at the neuromuscular junction was blocked by curare (Brown and Feldberg, 1936). These results convinced pharmacologists that acetylcholine was responsible for synaptic transmission at the ganglia but Eccles was able to marshal even more evidence against this conclusion than he did against the proposal that neuromuscular transmission was cholinergic in nature (Eccles, 1936). The dispute between the chemical and electrical hypotheses was resolved in the same way as it was in the case of the neuromuscular junction. Pre-ganglionic stimulation in curarized animals evokes a non-propagated potential change (the postsynaptic potential) in the ganglion cells. In normal animals the postsynaptic potential develops into the propagated action potential so that, like the end plate potential, it is an essential intermediary between action potentials in the pre- and post-junctional elements. Eccles was able to show that the ganglionic postsynaptic potential was affected by anticholinesterases and by curare in a fashion consistent with its owing its origin to acetylcholine.

Although the experiments just discussed made it clear that acetylcholine is the chemical mediator of synaptic transmission at autonomic ganglia as it is at the neuromuscular junction, it soon became clear that there are some considerable differences between the transmission processes at the two sites. These differences, which are detailed below, should be noted, because they illustrate the important fact that it is not possible to describe the events at one type of junction by analogy with what happens at others even when, as in this instance, the chemical mediators are the same.

The first point of difference concerns the localization of cholinesterase. At the neuromuscular junction, most of the enzyme is concentrated at the end plate where it is well placed to hydrolyse acetylcholine after the latter has iniated the muscle twitch. At autonomic ganglia, however, the cholinesterase is present in the preganglionic fibre and little is found in the ganglion cells. It must be concluded that enzymatic hydrolysis is not an important mechanism for terminating transmitter action in ganglia. At first sight, the position is not dissimilar to that which obtains in the noradrenergic neurone but there is no evidence of a high affinity uptake system for acetylcholine in the preganglionic terminals and an alternative mode of bringing acetylcholine's action to an end must be sought. Years before reuptake into the presynaptic fibres had become recognized as a mode of transmitter inactivation, Ogston showed that diffusion of acetylcholine from its site of liberation in autonomic ganglia would be sufficiently rapid to ensure expeditious curtailment of its action at the postsynaptic receptor (Ogston, 1955) and it seems that this is indeed the inactivation mechanism that is utilized at these sites.

The second point of difference concerns the nature and origin of the postsynaptic potential. The end plate potential, as we have seen, is a simple partial depolarization arising from the action of acetylcholine on typically nicotinic receptors. The ganglionic postsynaptic potential is more complex; an early negative wave (depolarization) gives way to a positive wave which is succeeded in its turn by a late negative phase of activity (Fig. 13.2). The first negative wave is depressed by curare, tetraethylammonium and hexamethonium and it is potentiated by nicotine, tetramethylammonium and acetylcholine. These observations make it clear that this initial phase of activity arises from the action of acetylcholine on nicotinic receptors (p. 201). The early negative phase is normally responsible for initiating activity in the postganglionic fibres so that it is broadly true to describe transmission at autonomic ganglia as a process mediated by acetylcholine and involving nicotinic receptors.

The late negative phase of the ganglion potential appears to result from the action of acetylcholine on muscarinic receptors; it is abolished by atropine but not by curare and it is potentiated by acetylcholine, muscarine and acetyl-β-methylcholine (p. 200). There is no doubt that the late negative phase is a physiological event in the sense that it develops in response to acetylcholine liberated from the preganglionic nerves (Volle, 1966a and b) but its physiological significance has not been unequivocally established. It may, perhaps, modulate the transmission effected by the earlier stimulation of nicotinic receptors. It is also possible that it might assume a greater significance under particular conditions. Thus until quite recently it was a common practice to treat hypertensive patients with ganglion blocking agents. These drugs (hexamethonium, which has already been mentioned, is one) reduce blood pressure by causing blockade of nicotinic receptors in the ganglia and they were often given over long periods of time. It sometimes happened that the blood pressure eventually escaped from their action, beginning to rise again even though drug administration continued. This may have been because transmission began to be effected through the medium of the muscarinic receptors.

It was at first believed that the positive wave of the ganglion potential was the result of adrenaline release from chromaffin tissue in the ganglia. It had been known for many years that adrenaline, as well as acetylcholine, was liberated when preganglionic fibres were stimulated and the fact that dibenamine (p. 299) depressed the positive wave lent added weight to the idea that adrenaline was involved. However it is now known that it is dopamine, liberated from small interneurones, that gives rise to this element of the postsynaptic potential. These interneurones belong to the 'small intensely fluorescent' (SIF) category of dopaminergic neurones. The interneurones themselves are activated by acetylcholine. The receptors involved are muscarinic in type.

The physiological significance of the positive wave of the ganglion potential is obscure but it may serve as a device to limit ganglion stimulation.

The action of dopamine is mediated by way of cyclic AMP formation while the muscarinic actions of acetylcho-

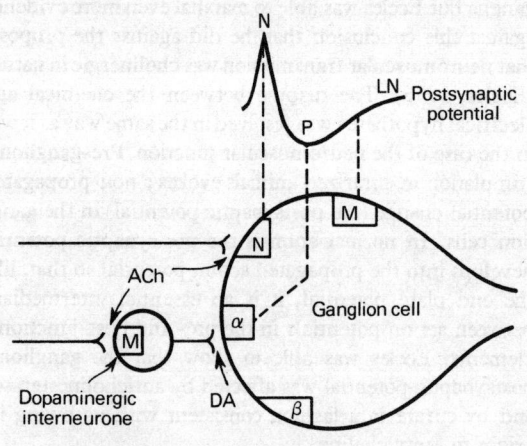

ACh=acetylcholine
DA=dopamine
N and M=nicotinic and muscarinic receptors
α and β =adrenaline receptors
N, P and LN=negative, positive and late negative phases of potential

Fig. 13.2 Possible origin of the several phases of the postsynaptic potentials in autonomic ganglia (based on Eccles and Libet, 1961; Greengard and others, 1976).

line in the ganglia are dependent on the formation of cyclic GMP.

Isoprenaline (p. 272) facilitates transmission through autonomic ganglia, suggesting that the ganglion cells also possess adrenaline β receptors. This may explain why, in some experimental circumstances, adrenaline has been reported to facilitate transmission through ganglia.

5-Hydroxytryptamine and histamine also affect transmission in ganglia. The physiological significance of these observations is obscure.

We must now return briefly to consider the significance of the fact that acetylcholinesterase is present in preganglionic autonomic fibres. Koelle has suggested that the nerve impulse arriving at the termination of the preganglionic nerve liberates a minute amount of acetylcholine which then brings about the release of more acetylcholine from the nerve terminals. This second wave of acetylcholine diffuses to and depolarizes the ganglion while the acetylcholinesterase hydrolyses the acetylcholine remaining in the neighbourhood of the preganglionic terminals and thus prevents the further release of transmitter. Koelle's hypothesis provides an ingenious explanation for the apparently anomalous location of ganglionic acetylcholinesterase. It also brings the preganglionic fibre neatly into line with the postganglionic sympathetic fibre: acetylcholine releases acetylcholine in one situation and noradrenaline in the other. No one has yet suggested, however, that an analogous state of affairs exists at the parasympathetic neuroeffector junction: the evidence would indicate that here a simple release of acetylcholine is sufficient to effect transmission. Some experimental evidence in support of his hypothesis is provided by Koelle (1962), but it has to be added that, in the absence of more recent experimental evidence, few authorities are disposed to embrace the Koelle view, ingenious though it is.

SYNAPTIC TRANSMISSION IN THE CENTRAL NERVOUS SYSTEM

At the time when Dale and his associates were canvassing the idea that junctional and synaptic transmission everywhere involved the liberation of chemical mediators, some of those who supported this hypothesis were attempting to obtain evidence for chemical transmission in the central nervous system. They naturally focussed their attention on acetylcholine but the experimental results, though very interesting in themselves, were not sufficiently direct to provide convincing evidence (except to those already converted to the concept) that cholinergic transmission occurred in the central nervous system. Eccles, on the other hand, was able to adduce what appeared at the time to be decisive evidence against the hypothesis of chemical transmission (Eccles, 1947). He took the longitudinally-sectioned spinal cord of the frog and recorded the electrical

activity produced in the anterior root fibres by stimulation of the posterior roots. By soaking the cord in a solution containing sodium pentobarbitone (p. 484), he was able to abolish all activity in internucial neurones so that the record he obtained reflected potential changes in the motor neurone arising in response to its direct stimulation along a monosynaptic pathway. Eccles found that neither anticholinesterases nor acetylcholine itself had any effect on the activation of the motor neurones by impulses in the sensory roots. The only valid interpretation of these results is that acetylcholine is not involved in the transmission of impulses across the synapse of a monosynaptic reflex but because acetylcholine was, at that time, the only substance with any claim to be considered as a transmitter substance between neurones, Eccles believed that his findings negatived the whole concept of chemical transmission in the spinal cord and, by implication, in the rest of the central nervous system.

Shortly after he had completed the experiments just described, Eccles succeeded in demonstrating the reality of chemical transmission at the neuromuscular junction. This led him to reconsider the problem of transmission in the central nervous system and in 1952 his group, using microelectrodes to study individual neurones, were able to demonstrate that synaptic transmission in the spinal cord required the intervention of a chemical mediator (Brock, Coombs and Eccles, 1952). The essence of their experiment was the demonstration that the excitatory postsynaptic potential (which generates the impulse in the neurone) does not arise until the action potential in the presynaptic nerve ending has died away and the action potential has no detectable direct action on neurones with which the fibre is in synaptic relationship. If the action currents themselves cannot excite neurones directly, they must do so indirectly, and the only conceivable mechanism whereby this can be brought about is by the liberation by the presynaptic fibres of chemical substances which then activate the postsynaptic sites in the central nervous system and they provided sufficient evidence to convince the majority of physiologists of the universality of chemical transmission. Later, additional support came from Grundfest (1957) who assembled a formidable mass of evidence, derived from his own work and that of others, which indicated that the synaptic regions of neurones in the central nervous system are not excitable by electrical means. If this is universally so, there can be no possibility of anything but chemical transmission throughout the nervous system. It must, however, be remembered that the results of the Eccles experiment which indicated that acetylcholine was not involved in the transmission of impulses in the monosynaptic reflex are still valid.

The recognition that specific chemical substances mediate the most fundamental of central nervous processes encouraged the belief that mental illness might have its origin in disturbances of the processes involved in the synthesis, storage, release or inactivation of these transmitter substances. The possibility of remedying these disturbances or of counteracting their effects by the administration of appropriate drugs makes the problem of chemical transmission one of considerable interest to psychiatrists and pharmacologists alike.

The known and putative transmitter substances will now be considered in turn but before this is done it is necessary to discuss some points of more general relevance.

Some general features of central synaptic transmission

The central nervous system evidently makes use of a number of different chemical transmitter substances. The actual number can only be guessed at but many (perhaps too many) of the pharmacologically active compounds known to be present in nerve tissue have been put forward as likely transmitter agents. The critical reader cannot fail to be less than impressed by the support that can be mustered for some of these substances and he should not be too ready to admit these marginal candidates to the roll of transmitter substances unless and until their claims have been more fully substantiated.

Those who wish to claim transmitter status for a particular substance often set down a list of generally accepted criteria that must be satisfied before any compound can be classified as a transmitter substance. They then proceed to demonstrate that, in their view, the substance they are championing meets the specified requirements. This exercise does no harm and it can serve a useful purpose if the items of experimental evidence on which it is based are critically examined in the light of the points they are intended to establish. Unfortunately, the evidence is sometimes interpreted rather uncritically and this may lead to the experimental results being accorded a greater significance than they warrant.

The criteria for transmitter potentiality are, inevitably, based on what is known concerning the behaviour of established transmitters such as acetylcholine. It is not to be expected that all mediators will behave in this way. On the other hand, all neurones serve but one purpose (the initiation and transmission of nerve impulses) and synaptic transmission processes are presumably broadly similar throughout the nervous system. It is reasonable to expect that other chemical mediators will bear *some* resemblances to acetylcholine and the reader should look with suspicion at claims made on behalf of substances whose behaviour is very different from that of the established transmitter agents.

With the reservations already outlined in mind, the properties required of transmitter substances can be listed and examined (Werman, 1966; Crossland, 1967; Davidson, 1976.). Some of the principal methods available to determine the possession or otherwise of these properties

by putative transmitter substances are also mentioned in the following paragraphs.

1. *Transmitter substances must be present in nerve fibres—particularly the presynaptic terminals—and must be released therefrom on stimulation.* —The presence of a substance in localized areas of the central nervous system is often taken as presumptive evidence that the substance has a humoral function in those areas, particularly in relation to the physiological activity of the regions in which it is found. This may well be so, but the function exerted is not necessarily a transmitter one. Indeed, the distribution of many of the substances that have been considered as possible mediators of transmission provides something of an argument against their being able to fulful this role.

Acetylcholine is quite widely distributed in the central nervous system. It is not present in quantity in all nerve fibres and tracts—this circumstance, indeed, provided one of the most convincing of the early arguments for the existence of non-cholinergic transmission—but its distribution is not obviously related to any one *functional* system. There seems to be no reason why other transmitters should not be equally widespread but some of the current candidates have a restricted distribution. Moreover, some areas of the brain such as the hypothalamus and some parts of the extrapyramidal system contain relatively large amounts of a multiplicity of humoral substances while others, such as the cerebellum, contain only very small amounts of a few compounds. The distribution of active substances in the central nervous system should be examined critically.

A substance that is present in the brain or spinal cord is not necessarily located in neurones. Non-neuronal elements (the *neuroglia*) outnumber neurones at least tenfold and may well contain pharmacologically active material. Again, the mere fact that an active substance is liberated from the central nervous system on stimulation (often under grossly unphysiological conditions) does not of itself provide very substantial support for its postulated transmitter status. Its transmitter function becomes more likely if it can be shown that the amount released by stimulation at an intensity encountered under physiological conditions is adequate to stimulate or inhibit neighbouring neurones.

Histochemistry is the most specific and sensitive technique at present available for determining the presence of endogenous chemical substances in the tissues. It has been applied to studies of the distribution of monoamines and of glutamic acid decarboxylase (p. 189) within the central nervous system and the information thus obtained has done much to confirm the respective claims of the monoamines and γ-aminobutyric acid to transmitter status. Unfortunately, histochemical methods can, as yet, be applied to only a very few of the humoral substances in which we are interested and for the rest, recourse has to be made to other techniques for assessing their distribution within the central nervous system. Most often these consist of measuring the amount of the substance under investigation, or of the activity of the enzyme that synthesizes it, by pharmacological or biochemical assays on extracts of discrete brain areas or nerve tracts. This approach is, clearly, limited by the sensitivity of the assay method and by the accuracy and fineness of the original dissection.

Corroborative evidence of the physiological importance of a presumed transmitter substance will be provided if it can be shown, by biochemical or pharmacological examination of subcellular fractions, that the material is concentrated in nerve terminals. Such a localization clearly ensures that a reservoir of transmitter is always available to meet the demands of nerve activity. Similar support for the candidature of a substance for transmitter status will be seen in demonstrations that it, or its precursors, can be actively taken up into neurones against a concentration gradient. Such high affinity uptake processes are involved in both the provision of neuronal supplies of transmitter and in the termination of the action of at least some released transmitters.

The reader should appreciate that the criteria enumerated in the foregoing paragraphs are neither sufficient nor always necessary to establish transmitter action. Some authorities, for instance, have suggested that prostaglandins might act as neurohumoral transmitter substances. If they did, they would presumably have to be synthesized in response to the arrival of impulses at the relevant nerve endings since tissues cannot store prostaglandins. Many of the criteria relating to the presence and the interneuronal and intraneuronal distribution of transmitter substances would not, of course, apply in these circumstances.

2. *Application of the presumed transmitter substance to a neurone must produce changes in the neurone characteristic of those that occur when it is excited or inhibited by physiological stimuli.* Electrophysiological investigations, largely those of Eccles and his colleagues, have revealed the nature of the changes that occur in the subsynaptic membrane of neurones in the spinal cord during excitation and inhibition. Excitatory transmission involves a local depolarization of the affected neurone and an increase in its permeability to all ions. Inhibition is rather more complex as two types of inhibitory process have been described. In *postsynaptic inhibition,* the transmitter causes an increased permeability of the neuronal membrane to potassium or chloride ions. This results in an increase in the resting potential of the cell (hyperpolarization) which thereby becomes stabilized so that it is unable to fire impulses. In *presynaptic inhibition,* impulses in the inhibitory fibres interrupt the arrival of impulses in the fine terminals of excitatory fibres. Thus, in one form of inhibition, the excitability of the neurones is depressed and in the other there is a reduction in the excitatory bombardment of the neurone. Eccles has provided a useful pharmacological test for differentiating between the two types of inhibition:

presynaptic inhibition is blocked by picrotoxin and postsynaptic inhibition by strychnine. In other parts of the central nervous system, excitation involves processes identical with that described for spinal cord neurones. Inhibition is usually of the postsynaptic variety and is associated with hyperpolarization but in the brain stem and the cerebral cortex the inhibitory process is not antagonized by strychnine.

The multibarrelled micropipette enables substances to be deposited in the immediate vicinity of neurones. One of the barrels serves as a recording electrode so that the neuronal responses can be measured; the multiplicity (five or more) of barrels permits several substances to be applied simultaneously or successively to the neurone. In this way it is possible to study the interactions of humoral substances with presumed antagonists or other material. Many nerve cells in the central nervous system exhibit spontaneous activity and the response of these cells (an increase or decrease in firing rate) can be readily detected. Cells that are not spontaneously active and are not excited by the humoral substance being studied, can be stimulated into activity by glutamate delivered through one of the barrels of the pipette. This manoeuvre may lead to complications of interpretation since it is not yet known how closely glutamate excitation mimics that evoked by nerve impulses.

Single barrelled electrodes, small enough to penetrate the neurone without destroying the integrity of the surface membrane, can be employed for the direct recording of membrane potentials.

Substances that are ionized in solution can be delivered to the neurones from the micropipette by means of a small electric current whose direction is determined by the charge on the ion that is to be deposited. A current in the opposite direction (the *backing current*) prevents the egress of the ion until the micropipette is in place. Any effect of the expelling current itself can be assessed by placing a pharmarcologically inactive substance in one barrel of the pipette and passing a current through it.

As an alternative to *microiontophoresis,* mechanical methods of ejecting substances into the immediate environment of a neurone are available.

It seemed reasonable to believe that microelectrode studies would provide information which, in the light of the newer knowledge concerning the membrane changes accompanying excitation and inhibition, would lead to a speedy identification of transmitter substances. This hope has not been completely realized, for it has become clear that neurones can show excitatory or inhibitory responses to a wide variety of compounds, many of which are demonstrably not transmitter substances at the neurones on which they act. It may also happen that a substance plays a physiological role at some of the neurones it affects on iontophoretic application but not at others.

Another fact that should be noted is that not all forms of nerve activity produce immediate effects on neuronal membranes. It sometimes happens that their effects are mediated through one of the cyclic nucleotides. Transmitters that evoke the production of these substances may not therefore display any activity on iontophoretic application. Recognizing this dichotomy of transmitter action, Eccles and his colleagues have divided the mediators into those with *ionotropic* and those with *metabotropic* actions (McGeer, Eccles & McGeer, 1978). Some transmitter substances (acetylcholine is a case in point) are ionotropic at some sites and metabotropic at others.

3. *The pharmacological actions of the putative transmitter and of substances that interact with it must be consistent with its presumed transmitter function.* The validity of this assertion will emerge from the discussion in the following pages. Here, it is sufficient to point out to the reader that compounds that interfere with the synthesis, release or disposal of the presumed transmitter substances (acetylcholine apart) not infrequently produce effects that are inconsistent with the humoral agent's postulated functions. The arguments advanced to explain these discrepancies should be carefully scrutinized since the experimental findings may sometimes be more satisfactorily explained by assigning a non-transmitter role to the substance in question.

Modulators of transmission

A problem which has been largely ignored concerns the function of those neurohumoral substances to which no transmitter action can be ascribed. They are usually thought of as *modulators* of transmission—substances that modify but do not initiate the processes of synaptic transmission. It is easy to suggest ways in which neuromodulator activity might be effected but experimental evidence for the existence of chemically mediated modulator activity in the central nervous system is almost completely lacking. The properties and likely modes of action of modulator substances are so ill-defined that it is impossible to enunciate criteria by which they might be recognized. The reader is advised to keep an open mind on the subject and, in the absence of adequate supporting evidence, to treat with caution claims that a particular substance serves in this capacity in the brain. It does seem however that the prostaglandins certainly behave as modulators not only of some forms of central and peripheral nervous activity but also of some other processes in the body (p. 389).

THE DALE PRINCIPLE

It is a mark of his amazing prescience that, long before most physiologists were prepared to accept even the idea that acetylcholine could act as a mediator of neuromuscular and synaptic transmission, Dale had already moved on to the next stage and was thinking of experiments that might reveal the identity of the chemical mediators that operate at synapses in the central nervous system that do not make use of acetylcholine. He pointed out that a branching nerve fibre would be likely to liberate the same transmitter substance at both (or all) of its branches. The strength of this now perhaps self-evident proposition (which has since become known as 'the Dale principle') lay in the experimental studies it suggested. In particular it provided the impetus for some early attempts to identify the transmitter substance liberated at central synapses by sensory nerve fibres entering the spinal cord. Many sensory fibres en route from the skin to the cord give off collateral branches which end in association with arterioles in the subcutaneous tissues. When the sensory fibres are activated by cutaneous stimuli, the nerve impulses passing into the cord also give rise to impulses that pass back along these collaterals (the so-called antidromic impulses) to cause dilatation of the arterioles (Fig. 21.3, p. 338). Dale's principle would suggest that the substance that causes the vasodilatation is the same as that liberated in the spinal cord and the search for the latter (the transmitter substance at the first synapse in the sensory pathway) would resolve itself into the much easier task of finding a suitable vasodilator substance in extracts of sensory nerve fibres. Three such substances were found: substance P, histamine and adenosine triphosphate (ATP) though the work of Holton and her colleagues indicated that the actions of the latter substance most closely reproduced the effects of antidromic stimulation (Holton and Holton, 1954). In his earlier writings the present author (and some of his contemporaries) discussed this work and its implications in some detail (see, for instance, Crossland, 1957) but in more recent years he has ignored it, largely because very little additional evidence seemed to be forthcoming to support the idea that one or more of the vasodilator substances might be neurotransmitter agents. It is a sign of the times that all three substances now find a place once again in reviews of the chemical mediation of synaptic transmission (including this one), largely because there is an increased readiness to believe that almost any type of active substance found in the central nervous system might serve a transmitter function. This willingness to consider everything might, of course, reflect a partial disenchantment with some of the substances that have attracted support in recent years but whatever opinion the reader forms of the claims now lodged on behalf of histamine, substance P and ATP he should remember that attention was originally focussed on the possible transmitter status of these substances by the application of a principle that was formulated so long ago by the father of the whole subject.

Among the claimants to transmitter status are substances as simple as glycine and others as complex as the prostaglandins. Some occur in the brain in nanogram quantities and others are found to the extent of hundreds of micrograms. It is difficult to believe that substances as disparate as this can subserve the same type of function but at the present state of our knowledge the claims of all of them must be considered.

Much of the experimental work that has sought to establish the transmitter function of particular substances has been of an indirect nature, involving the making of rather simple observations on animals receiving drugs that are believed to interfere with the action or metabolism of the putative transmitter substance. Many of these experiments are, by their very nature, unsatisfactory—most drugs have a number of actions other than that for which they have been administered and little precise information can be gained by casual observation of behavioural effects in intact animals—and those who wish to assess the situation objectively should pay most attention to the results of experiments that involve the substance itself (rather than drugs related to it) and those that permit the making of observations directly related to neuronal responses. The substances that might act as mediators of transmission in the central nervous system will now be discussed in turn. They are grouped, as far as possible, into particular chemical classes and they are led, naturally enough, by acetylcholine.

Acetylcholine

It is fitting that the first substance to be unequivocally established as a mediator of central synaptic transmission was acetylcholine. Throughout the length of the anterior horns of the spinal cord are located the Renshaw cells which are so called in commemoration of the neurophysiologist who first described their properties. These neurones exert an inhibitory influence on neighbouring motoneurones. The physiological stimulus to the Renshaw cells comes from the motor nerves: branches leave the motor fibres within the spinal cord and make synaptic contact with the Renshaw cells (Fig. 13.3). Impulses in the motor nerves thus have the effect of inhibiting activity in the very neurones which have given rise to these impulses. The system presumably operates as a feed back device that prevents excessive stimulation of muscle. It might, for instance, provide valuable protection during convulsive activity. Since motor nerves liberate acetylcholine at their peripheral terminals, it seemed reasonable to assume, in accordance with the Dale principle, that the collateral fibres to the Renshaw cells would do the same and that the transmission process between these elements would be cholinergic in nature. Experiments by Eccles and his colleagues confirmed that this is so (Eccles, Fatt and Koketsu, 1954). Minute amounts of acetylcholine, applied by microiontophoresis, depolarize Renshaw cells and this depolarization, as well as that which accompanies physiological activation of the cells, is blocked by curare and by dihydro-ß-erythroidine, specific antagonists of acetylcholine at nicotinic receptors. Anticholinesterases prolong

activity in the Renshaw cells whether this is evoked by acetylcholine or by stimulation of the motoneurones. Like the cells of autonomic ganglia, Renshaw cells are stimulated by tetramethylammonium and by nicotine. In the intact animal, acetylcholine, administered by intra-arterial injection into the spinal cord, inhibits reflex activity. Thus the pharmacological action of acetylcholine is consistent with the results obtained from microelectrode studies on single cells.

More recent studies have established that the course of events following the liberation of acetylcholine from the motor nerve collaterals is rather more complicated than was at first realized. A single electric shock to the nerve causes an immediate depolarization of the Renshaw cells which respond with a brief burst of repetitive activity lasting for about 50 msec. The cells then repolarize but immediately thereafter a slow depolarization sets in and the cells resume their discharge at a slow and gradually decreasing rate for some five seconds.

Whereas the first phase of Renshaw cell activity is the result of stimulation of nicotinic receptors as the Eccles group showed so long ago, the later less explosive response comes from stimulation of muscarinic receptors and is, accordingly, blocked by atropine.

The reader can hardly fail to be struck by the close parallel that exists between the events that take place following physiological stimulation of Renshaw cells and those that occur at autonomic ganglia. The difference between the two lies in the fact that whereas a phase of activity attributable to catecholamine release intervenes between the two negative phases of the postganglionic potential, the corresponding pause during Renshaw cell activation does not involve this mechanism. It seems, instead, to be the result of some form of mutual inhibition operating among the activated cells.

Spinal neurones other than the Renshaw cells are not depolarized by acetylcholine. This observation not only underlines the physiological significance of Renshaw cell stimulation by acetylcholine but it also indicates that the latter is not the transmitter substance at all synapes in the spinal cord. The three synaptic junctions illustrated in Figure 13.3 all utilize different mediators: one junction is cholinergic, one is operated by an inhibitory transmitter substance (probably glycine) whose effect is prevented by strychnine and the motoneurone is activated by an excitatory transmitter from the pyramidal tract whose identity has yet to be established.

As far as the other neurones in the central nervous system are concerned, some of the many that respond to acetylcholine do so as a result of stimulation of nicotine receptors and they give a typically 'sharp' response. Most of them, however, are activated through muscarine receptors (it has been estimated that there are a hundred times as many muscarine as nicotine receptors in the brain) and give either an inhibitory or an excitatory response with the typically slow time course already seen in the Renshaw cells.

Neurones that respond to acetylcholine (they can be described as *cholinoceptive*) are widely distributed throughout the brain. They have been found in the brain stem (including cells of the reticular system), in the thalamus, hypothalamus and basal ganglia, in the cerebellum and in the cerebral cortex (for references see Crossland, 1967, Bradley, 1968 and Phillis, 1970). In the caudate nucleus no fewer than 80 per cent of the tested cells responded to acetylcholine and in the cerebellum 75 per cent of the Purkinje cells were affected. In other regions of the brain between 30 and 60 per cent of the neurones appear to be cholinoceptive. In the cerebral cortex and cerebellum, acetylcholine almost invariably produces excitatory responses but in the medulla and pons, inhibition is produced almost as frequently as is excitation.

Neurones bearing nicotine receptors are found in the medulla, the diencephalon, the cerebellum and, sparsely, in the cortex. Those with muscarine receptors occur throughout the brain. Only stimulation of nicotine receptors produces the decrease in membrane resistance resulting from the opening up of ionic channels that follows the direct depolarization of neurones. It seems likely that the effects of stimulation of the muscarine receptors are mediated through cyclic guanosine monophosphate (p. 324).

It should be added that, in addition to stimulating its neuronal receptors, nicotine brings about the release of acetylcholine from the brain. This is the basis of some of the pharmacological effects of nicotine in tobacco smoke.

It should not be assumed that all the cholinoceptive neurones in the brain are necessarily activated by cholinergic fibres. At a cholinergic synapse, the postsynaptic element must, obviously, be cholinoceptive, but cholinoceptive neurones are not necessarily components of cholinergic synapses. In order to establish that they are, it is necessary to demonstrate that the nerve fibres that activate them contain, and can release, acetylcholine. It is not known what proportion of cholinoceptive neurones are so situated but it seems clear that not all are. The cerebellum, for instance, and many of the fibres that enter it, contain little acetylcholine but the proportion of cholinoceptive neurones in this part of the brain is quite high. On the other hand, all the pharmacological evidence (some of which is summarized below), as well as that provided by the work of Feldberg and Vogt, is consistent with the view that cholinergic synapses are widespread.

Motor nerves, autonomic preganglionic fibres and post-ganglionic parasympathetic fibres all transmit information by liberating acetylcholine and in all three types of nerve fibre the activity of choline acetyltransferase is high. Conversely, the enzyme activity is low in sensory nerve fibres and in those of the pyramidal tract; transmission from these fibres is demonstrably noncholinergic in

nature. It may therefore be assumed that the distribution of choline acetyltransferase activity mirrors that of cholinergic fibres. This point was first made by Feldberg and Vogt (1948) who studied the activity of the enzyme in a large number of nerve tracts and nuclei long before modern histochemical techniques made possible the direct demonstration of particular types of neurone. Their results revealed that, in some nerve pathways, there is a tendency for presumed cholinergic fibres to alternate with noncholinergic fibres. To take an example: in the sensory pathway, the connection between the periphery and the spinal cord is by way of the noncholinergic posterior root fibre, that from the spinal cord to the thalamus may constitute a cholinergic link and the final neurone, between the thalamus and the cortex is again noncholinergic in type. This alternation of cholinergic and noncholinergic fibres is by no means an invariable finding and indeed the work of Feldberg and Vogt is now rarely referred to. It did, however, serve to emphasize the wide distribution of probably cholinergic neurones. It also made clear the fact that fibres with a high choline acetyltransferase activity are not confined to particular functional systems.

In recent years it has proved possible to demonstrate the presence of choline acetyltransferase in individual neurones by immunohistochemistry (p. 184) using a method based on a technique originally developed by Sternberger *et al.* (1970). These studies have demonstrated that in some areas of the brain, such as the basal ganglia, that contain a variety of established or putative transmitter substances, cholinergic neurones are quite distinct from those that contain the other substances. They have shown too that the nerve tract that brings the septal nucleus into communication with the hippocampus is cholinergic in nature. This

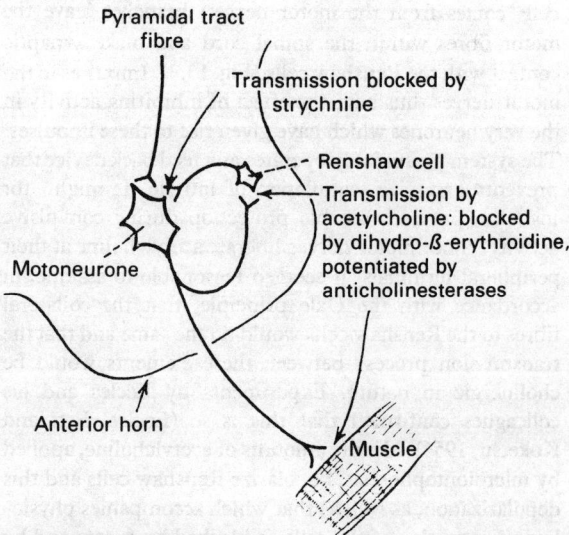

Fig. 13.3 Activation of a motoneurone by a pyramidal tract fibre and inhibition by a Renshaw cell fibre.

tract is an important component of the limbic system (p. 167) and its content of cholinergic neurones should give us pause for thought on occasions when we are tempted to interpret the activity of this system and of the psychotropic drugs that act on it exclusively in terms of monoamine transmitter systems.

Acetylcholine is unique among the postulated transmitter substances in that pharmacological experiments produce results that are almost invariably consistent with the view that acetycholine is a central transmitter substance. Thus, anaesthesia increases the acetylcholine content of all areas of the brain while convulsive activity lowers it (Richter and Crossland, 1949). These changes, which have been repeatedly confirmed, are assumed to be the consequence of a decreased liberation of transmitter during anaesthesia and of an increased release during the heightened central activity of the convulsive state. Evidence that acetylcholine release from the brain is affected in this way is provided by the experiments of several groups of workers who have measured the release of acetylcholine into Ringer's solution placed in contact with the exposed cortex of anaesthetized animals. As anaesthesia deepened, the rate of appearance of acetylcholine fell. The rate increased again when anaesthesia was lightened or when the cortex was stimulated into activity (Mitchell, 1963; Celesia and Jasper, 1966). Many other experiments of this type have produced equally consistent results: the fact that these results have frequently been obtained by analysis of whole brain extracts emphasizes the wide distribution of cholinergic neurones.

About 60 per cent. of the acetylcholine and choline acetyltransferase in a cholinergic neurone is concentrated in synaptosomal vesicles at the nerve endings. The rest of the transmitter is free in the cytoplasm. The neurones operate a high affinity uptake system for choline which ensures a continuing supply of material for the intraneuronal synthesis of transmitter. The acetyl moiety is provided by acetylcoenzyme A derived from the metabolism of glucose (p. 27). The choline uptake system may also constitute a regulatory system permitting the synthesis of acetylcholine to fluctuate in response to its rate of release.

Experiments using radioactive choline have established that cholinergic neurone activity normally liberates acetylcholine that has just been synthesized. A reserve supply of transmitter is stored in a separate compartment.

There is general agreement that, whatever we may think of the qualifications of the other contenders, acetylcholine is a transmitter substance at central synapses. Much (but not all) of the evidence in support of this view is circumstantial but it is overwhelmingly convincing in its consistency.

Monoamines

Since noradrenaline shares transmission duties with acetylcholine in the peripheral reaches of the autonomic nervous system, the catecholamine was an early and obvious candidate for consideration as a chemical mediator of transmission at central synapses and most authorities are now prepared to accord it that status. Much of the early evidence that was invoked to support noradrenaline's role was pharmacological in nature and the position was complicated by the fact that substances such as reserpine, iproniazid and their many psychotropic successors affect both noradrenaline and 5-hydroxytryptamine in the brain. This is a consequence of the fact that two enzymes, aromatic-L-aminoacid decarboxylase and monoamine oxidase are involved in the synthesis and catabolism, respectively, of both substances. A further complication arose when it became clear that dopamine, hitherto regarded as merely a precursor of noradrenaline and adrenaline, had transmitter properties in its own right. The roles of the individual monoamines have now been delineated to a large extent and it will be possible to consider them separately in the following account although cross references from one to another will still be necessary.

A discussion concerning the transmitter potentialities of the monoamines cannot be allowed to ignore adrenaline and a brief consideration of this substance's possible role in the central nervous system is appended to our discussion of the catecholamines.

NORADRENALINE

Noradrenaline has a patchy distribution in the central nervous system. The largest concentrations (which amount to about 1 μg per gram of tissue) are found in the hypothalamus and in the area postrema of the fourth ventricle while the grey matter of the medulla and mid brain contains about one third of this quantity. Smaller amounts of noradrenaline are widely distributed in other parts of the nervous system. Noradrenaline, like acetylcholine, is found in the presynaptic vesicles and fluorescence microscopy has revealed that noradrenaline is contained in different fibres from those that contain dopamine or 5-hydroxytryptamine.

Attempts to determine the distribution in the brain of neurones that contain noradrenaline have been greatly facilitated by the application of histochemical techniques. One of the seminal discoveries in this field was made by Eranko (1955) who found that slices of the adrenal medulla fixed in formaldehyde exhibited a bright yellow fluorescence. The Falck and Hillarp technique represents an extension of this procedure to the nervous system (Falck et al., 1962), cells that contain catecholamines and 5-hydroxytryptamine giving an apple green and a bright yellow fluorescence respectively. The substances responsible for the fluorescence are shown in Fig. 13.4.

One disadvantage of the histofluorescence method is that it does not readily pick out neurones that contain only small amounts of the monoamines. Another is that it does

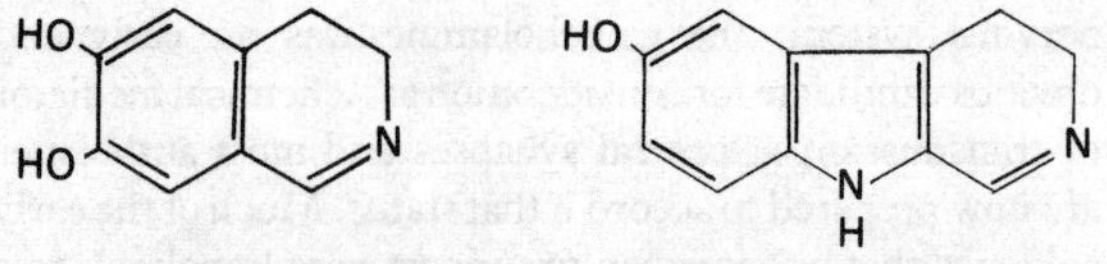

Green fluorescing
material derived from
the catecholamines
(a 3,4-dihydroisoquinoline)

Yellow fluorescing
material derived from
5-hydroxytryptamine
(a 3,4-dihydro-ß-carboline)

Fig. 13.4 Fluorescent substances derived from monoamines

not differentiate between noradrenaline and dopamine. A number of pharmacological and other manoeuvres have been adopted to overcome these drawbacks. The administration of compounds such as monoamine oxidase inhibitors to animals whose brains will later be examined will lead to the accumulation of endogenous monoamines to a point at which they will become more visible when the postmortem tissue is subjected to examination by fluorescent microscopy.

α-Methyldopa is one of the several agents that have been employed to distinguish between neurones that contain noradrenaline and those that synthesize only dopamine. The compound is converted into α-methylnoradrenaline in noradrenergic neurones. When reserpine is given to animals that have previously received α-methyldopa, the α-methylnoradrenaline, being much more resistant to the depleting action of reserpine, remains in the noradrenergic cells which can thus be identified by fluorescence histochemistry. Using techniques such as this, Dahlström and Fuxe (1965a and b) were able to plot the course of many of the noradrenaline-containing fibres in the brain. The diagrams that illustrate their findings feature in many of the texts and monographs the reader will encounter.

Two recent developments have led to improvements in the histochemical techniques employed to detect neurones that contain noradrenaline. Glyoxylic acid has replaced formaldehyde vapour in the preparation of tissues for fluorescent microscopy (Lindvall & Bjorklund, 1974) and an immunohistological method has been developed for the detection of dopamine ß-hydroxylase (Swanson & Hartmann, 1975). This enzyme is found in association with noradrenaline in the intraneuronal storage granules, a device that presumably prevents the accumulation of dopamine, the 'wrong' transmitter, in noradrenergic nerves.

Immunohistochemical techniques can be applied to the detection of any cell component against which an antibody can be prepared. The antibody is attached to a suitable marker and is applied to the tissue that is being examined. It becomes firmly and specifically attached to the appropriate antigen whose position is announced by the stain or other type of marker with which the antibody is associated.

The application of these new techniques has partly, but not entirely, confirmed earlier findings concerning the distribution of presumably noradrenergic neurones. The following outline of the disposition of these neurones is therefore necessarily tentative in some respects.

Groups of neurones containing catecholamines are found throughout the length of the brain stem. Their fibres ramify widely but in small numbers. These groups of neurones were labelled A1 to A14 by Dahlström and Fuxe: groups A1 to A4 are located in the medulla, A5 to A7 in the pons, A8 to A10 in the midbrain and A11 to A14 in the diencephalon. The cells in groups A1 to A10 contain noradrenaline while those of the most rostral groups (A12 to A14) contain dopamine. Some of the neurones in group 11 contain dopamine while the others synthesize noradrenaline. Important groups of noradrenaline-containing neurones are those labelled A4 and A6. These neurones constitute the *locus coeruleus*.

An important tract of fibres rising in the *locus coeruleus* projects dorsally to the cerebellum, the diencephalon, the limbic system and the cerebral cortex particularly the cingulate gyrus (p. 168). Descending fibres pass from the *locus coeruleus* to nuclei in the lower brain stem and from cell groups A1 and A2 to the anterior horn cells in the cord as well as to cells in the lateral horn of the cord from which the preganglionic fibres of the sympathetic nervous system take origin.

Earlier work indicated that cells in groups A1, A2, A5 and A7 gave rise to fibres that travelled, in close association with the ascending reticular system, to destinations in the lower brain stem, the mid brain and the diencephalon but recent work has questioned the reality of these connections.

Attempts to assess the nature of the responses evoked in the brain by noradrenaline administration in the intact animal may be complicated by indirect effects caused by the drug's affecting peripheral structures (particularly the blood vessels), stimuli from which might themselves affect cerebral activity. However, in some carefully designed experiments, blood pressure compensators were used and in these circumstances noradrenaline (and adrenaline, too) certainly had an 'alerting' action (p. 162), particularly in the sleeping animal (Rothballer, 1959). Since noradrenaline neurones occur in those parts of the brain that contain a large number of reticular synapses, this finding of an alerting effect provides a hint that transmission processes in the reticular system might be mediated or influenced by noradrenaline. It must, however, be added that it has not yet proved possible to demonstrate the liberation of noradrenaline during stimulation of the ascending reticular system.

The idea that noradrenaline and adrenaline are essentially excitatory substances is a familiar one, but both catecholamines often have depressant actions. Even on the reticular system, 'deactivation' as well as the alerting reaction has been observed in response to noradrenaline in the course of the same experiment and the injection of small amounts of adrenaline or noradrenaline into the cerebral ventricles causes a condition indistinguishable from light anaesthesia. Again, Marrazzi showed many years ago that adrenaline and noradrenaline inhibit the potential changes evoked in one occipital cortex by stimulation of a corresponding point in the cortex of the opposite side.

Several groups of workers have demonstrated that noradrenaline has a predominantly depressant action when it is applied by microiontophoresis to neurones in several regions of the central nervous system. This depressant effect is seen both on spontaneously firing neurones and on those that have been excited by glutamate. In the brain stem, however, both excitatory and inhibitory effects appear. The evidence suggests that 80 per cent. of neurones in this region are susceptible to noradrenaline. About one in four of these cells are excited and the rest are depressed (Bradley, 1968; 1973). These findings are in agreement, qualitatively at least, with the observation that, in the intact animal, noradrenaline exerts both alerting and deactivating actions on the ascending reticular system and inhibitory effects elsewhere. Some of the inhibitory effects caused by the iontophoretic application of noradrenaline are of rapid onset and short duration while others are more prolonged. It is likely that the latter type of response, at least, is mediated by cyclic AMP. It is certainly prolonged by substances that preserve the nucleotide by inhibiting the phosphodiesterase that would otherwise destroy it (p. 321).

The physiological significance of these neuronal responses to noradrenaline cannot yet be fully evaluated. The neuronal membrane is not very selective in its response to substances placed on it and, in most of the areas so far investigated, none of the agents that block noradrenaline receptors in peripheral tissues influence neuronal responses to noradrenaline. This suggests either that most central neurones do not carry specific noradrenaline receptors or that, if they do, their nature is very different from that at peripheral sites. The first possibility seems to be the more likely one because in one situation in the brain (the mitral cells of the olfactory bulb) the response to noradrenaline is partially inhibited by two substances (phentolamine and dibenamine, pp. 299–300) that are known to prevent the access of noradrenaline to its receptors in peripheral structures.

Chlorpromazine, the best known of the so-called major tranquillizers (p. 548), depresses activity in the reticular system. Bradley and his associates have shown (Bradley et al., 1966; Bradley, 1973) that chlorpromazine depresses those cells in the brain stem that respond to noradrenaline. It antagonizes the excitatory actions of noradrenaline and reproduces the inhibitory actions but it is without effect on neurones that are not affected by noradrenaline. Chlorpromazine does not modify the effects of acetylcholine, 5-hydroxytryptamine or histamine on brain stem neurones

although it is known to exhibit some antagonism towards the action of these substances on smooth muscle preparations. These results are not inconsistent with the idea that noradrenaline may be the chemical mediator of excitatory impulses in the reticular alerting system.

It may well be that the actions of noradrenaline, as revealed by iontophoretic studies, reflect its physiological function in some areas (such as the olfactory bulb and the neurones of the ascending reticular system) but not in others. If this is so, it may be that noradrenaline functions more often as an excitatory than as an inhibitory transmitter substance even though its pharmacological actions in the central nervous system are predominantly of an inhibitory type. It must, however, be emphasized that this hypothesis is not yet based on very substantial evidence and it is clearly not entirely satisfactory to have to attribute an excitatory function to a substance with such widespread inhibitory actions. On the other hand, it is difficult to sustain the alternative notion that the role of noradrenaline is essentially an inhibitory one.

The assumption that noradrenaline is involved, as mediator or modulator, in excitatory transmission processes is not inconsistent with the actions of a number of drugs. Indeed, analysis of the mode of action of these drugs together with investigations into the possibly biochemical aetiology of mental illness, provides the pharmacologist (if not the physiologist) with his most powerful reasons for believing that noradrenaline plays a leading role in the control of central nervous activity. The reader who wishes to savour the enthusiasm that these studies engender in the neuropharmacologist is referred to the sections of this book that discuss the mode of action of antidepressant drugs, the origin of the affective psychoses and the hallucinogenic agents.

DOPAMINE

A relatively recent addition to the assembly of putative transmitter substances, dopamine has rapidly established itself in the favour of pharmacologists. The secret of its success lies in the ease with which the actions of a not inconsiderable number of drugs can be explained on the basis of their influencing the activity of identified dopamine neurones.

It was in 1958 that Carlsson suggested that dopamine, as well as being a precursor of noradrenaline and adrenaline (p. 258), might also function independently as a neuroregulator in its own right (Carlsson, 1959). Carlsson was impressed by the fact that the distribution of dopamine in the brain did not correspond to that of noradrenaline as would have presumably been so if dopamine served merely as a precursor of the other catecholamines.

The basal ganglia are important components of the so-called extrapyramidal system and they are thereby involved in the control of muscle tone. The presence of high concentrations of dopamine in some of the basal ganglia, particularly the caudate nucleus and putamen (the corpus striatum) suggested to Carlsson that the catecholamine might be a mediator of activity in this control system, a possibility that was strengthened by the observation that reserpine, which depletes the basal ganglia of their contained dopamine, induces signs of extrapyramidal dysfunction reminiscent of those seen in Parkinson's disease. It was not long before evidence came to light of a deficiency of dopamine in the caudate nucleus of patients with idiopathic Parkinsonism (p. 588). The involvement of dopamine in the activity of the extrapyramidal system is now one of the most widely known facts of our science and the veriest tyro among contemporary pharmacology students finds no difficulty in discussing 'the rational treatment of Parkinson's disease'. This particular topic is discussed in more detail elsewhere in this book (p. 589).

Dopamine can be measured in extracts of nervous tissue by spectrophotofluorimetry. In all mammals so far studied (these include man), the highest concentrations of dopamine have been found in the thalamus, the hypothalamus and some of the basal ganglia. The overall brain content (about 0.5 μg per gram of brain tissue) and the maximum local concentration (5 to 8 μg per gram in the caudate nucleus and putamen) show little variation among different mammalian species. It is interesting that dopamine is absent from the brains of birds and amphibians, species in which extrapyramidal control is only poorly developed.

Dopamine fibres in the central nervous system were first plotted by Dahlström and Fuxe by the method of fluorescence histochemistry they employed for the identification of noradrenaline neurones. Their findings were later refined by the application of the glyoxylic acid method (Lindvall & Bjorklund, 1974 b) but no immunohistochemical technique for the localization of dopamine neurones is yet available.

We have already noted that the most headward of the catecholamine neurones contain dopamine. Those labelled A9 in the Dahlstöm and Fuxe classification are located in the substantia nigra and they project to the corpus striatum as the nigrostriatal pathway whose existence and dopaminergic nature are totally consistent with the known facts relating to the pathology of Parkinson's disease and its response to drugs that influence activity mediated by dopaminergic neurones.

A remarkable feature of the nigrostriatal neurones is the extent to which they branch. It has been estimated that each of them makes nearly 500 contacts with neurones in the corpus striatum.

Cell bodies of the A10 group of neurones lie just medial to those of the A9 group. Their axons proceed rostrally in company with the nigrostriatal fibres but they continue beyond the corpus striatum into some of the nuclei of the limbic system and into associated areas of the cerebral cortex. There is convincing evidence that many of the drugs employed in the treatment of schizophrenia owe

their effectiveness to an antidopamine action (p. 542). The destination of the terminal ramifications of the A10 group of neurones would indicate that it is here particularly that the antipsychosis drugs exert their therapeutic actions. Their antidopamine actions at the terminations of the A9 and A12 neurones account, on the other hand, for many of their side effects. This topic is discussed in more detail later (p. 551).

The cells in group A12 give rise to some of the nerve fibre tracts that effect communication between the hypothalamus and the pituitary gland. The secretion of the prolactin inhibitory factor is one of the activities that comes under the control of these dopaminergic fibres and this explains why the mammary glands of both sexes are sometimes spurred into activity by the antipsychosis drugs (p. 549). Dopaminergic neurones are also involved in the inhibition of ovulation and the stimulation of growth hormone secretion.

On microiontophoretic application to cortical, brain stem and spinal cord neurones, dopamine usually has a depressant action, particularly on cells that have been excited by glutamate. The action of dopamine on neurones in the caudate nucleus is not uniformly inhibitory. About one in four of the cells are excited and the rest are depressed.

Although dopamine produces hyperpolarization in most of the neurones that respond to it and might therefore be considered to behave in much the same fashion as γ-aminobutyric acid and glycine, there is convincing evidence that, in addition, it activates a specific dopamine-sensitive adenylyl cyclase and thus produces 'metabotropic' actions by way of cyclic AMP just like noradrenaline. These actions are rather prolonged and it may be that they serve to modulate the activity of other neurones, particularly those of the cholinergic system. The extensive ramifications of the dopaminergic fibres, to which attention has already been drawn, gives some additional weight to this supposition.

Although some (perhaps even the major part) of the dopaminergic system has been clearly brought to light by currently available histochemical methods, there can be little doubt that more remains to be discovered, originating perhaps from smaller (or smaller groups of) neurones. The extent to which dopamine-sensitive neurones occur in the central nervous system can be at least guessed at by considering the response of the whole animal to agents that affect the dopamine system. Dopamine agonists (whose properties are discussed elsewhere in this volume) include apomorphine, piribedil and bromocriptine. The best known inhibitors of dopamine activity are the antipsychosis drugs.

It is unusual to find so complete a convergence of physiological, pharmacological, pathological and therapeutic opinions as we have noted in respect of dopamine. Although the evidence is far from complete we can assert with confidence that of all the putative synaptic transmitter—or modulator—substances, dopamine is already one of the most firmly established.

ADRENALINE

Surprisingly enough, it is only recently that any serious attention has been paid to the possibility that adrenaline, like its two precursors, might have a claim to be considered as a putative transmitter substance.

The conversion of noradrenaline to adrenaline requires the intervention of phenylethanolamine-N-methyltransferase (p. 258) and neurones bearing this enzyme have been detected in the brain by an immunohistochemical method (Hokfelt *et al.*, 1974). They are aggregated in two main groups labelled C1 and C2 which are closely associated with the corresponding groups of noradrenaline neurones, A1 and A2. These cells project, by way of the reticular system, to the thalamus and the hypothalamus. They also send axons into the pons and the medulla and into the spinal cord. Whether central 'adrenergic' neurones will be discovered in greater numbers when methods for their detection become more refined and in what ways, if any, the central actions and presumed functions of adrenaline differ from those of noradrenaline are questions yet to be answered. It is possible, indeed, that the immunohistochemical method used to detect the adrenaline-synthesizing enzyme is not entirely specific for phenylethanolamine-N-methyltransferase and that the neurones picked out by the method do not contain adrenaline after all. It must, however, be admitted, in the latter connection, that purely biochemical determinations of the amount of enzyme in brain tissue have indicated its presence in those areas in which it had been detected by immunohistochemistry (Lew *et al.*, 1977).

It is to be hoped that more extensive information will shortly be forthcoming to enable adrenaline's claims to be more reliably assessed.

5-HYDROXYTRYPTAMINE (SEROTONIN)

The observation by Gaddum in 1954 that lysergic acid diethylamide, the well known hallucinogen, was a 5-hydroxytryptamine antagonist did much to stimulate interest in the then novel idea that psychotic illnesses might have their origin in disturbances of transmitter metabolism or action. It led to the flourish of activity in this field that resulted in the recognition of the catecholamines and some aminoacids as important regulators or mediators of synaptic transmission. But it did very little, ironically enough, to clarify the position of serotonin itself.

The suggestions that this brain monoamine is involved in sleep, in the generation of depressive and other 'affective' states, in the production of hallucinatory activity and in the control of body temperature are all fully discussed elsewhere in this text as is the unique place that serotonin occupies in pineal metabolism. Observations relating to these topics cannot, however, be incorporated into any scheme based on the known central actions of serotonin or of the disposition of neurones that carry it.

A large proportion of the voluminous experimental work that has been referred to has been indirect in the sense that it has been concerned with analysing the effects of drugs that are thought to interfere with the storage, release, action or inactivation of 5-hydroxytryptamine. The difficulties that arise in the interpretation of the results of this kind of study have already been alluded to and the reader is counselled to pay more regard to those investigations that study the actions of the amine itself, uncomplicated by the presence of other substances.

So far as the brain (excepting the pineal gland) is concerned, the highest concentrations of serotonin are found in the thalamus, the hypothalamus and the midbrain. The amounts found in these areas vary, with the investigator and with the species studied, within the range of 0.4 to about 2.5 μg. per gram of tissue. The amine content of whole rat brain is of the order of 0.5 μg. per gram. The distribution of 5-hydroxytryptamine recalls that of noradrenaline although as has been seen, the two amines are found in separate fibres. Fluorescence microscopy reveals that 5-hydroxytryptamine (like, indeed, all the other substances that have been mentioned in this chapter) is concentrated in the presynaptic terminals.

Neurones that contain serotonin can be detected by fluorescence microscopy and the same general methods as are applied to the detection of noradrenaline and dopamine. The relatively fleeting appearance of the fluorescence that signals the presence of serotonin constitutes something of a disadvantage.

Dahlström and Fuxe were able to distinguish nine groups of serotonin-containing neurones in preparations of rat brain. Located in the brain stem, the neurone groups, numbered *seriatum* from medulla to midbrain, are designated B1 to B9. Groups B3 and B9 are in the reticular formation but the others (which seem to be involved in the generation of sleep) are members of the raphe system (p. 481).

The axons of the most caudal group of neurones (B1 and B2) proceed to the lateral and anterior horns of the spinal cord and those form the most rostral group (B7) pass directly to the cerebellum. Cell groups B7 and B8 (together with small contributions from B5 and B6) give rise to a tract of fibres that passes to the hypothalamus and the septal nuclei. Axons from other members of the same cell groups pass to the cingulate gyrus and hippocampus while those from group B9 project directly to the corpus striatum.

Serotonin neurones are relatively few in number and they project to relatively few destinations. They do, however, ramify richly in the destinations they do reach.

On iontophoretic application, 5-hydroxytryptamine usually depresses neurones in the central nervous system but under the appropriate experimental conditions a minority of cells is excited. Thus about 80 per cent. of a sample of cortical neurones and 90 per cent. of brain stem neurones will respond to 5-hydroxytryptamine. About 40 per cent. of these cells will be excited (Bradley and Wolstencroft, 1965; Roberts and Straughan, 1966). 5-Hydroxytryptamine inhibits evoked potentials in the visual cortex. In this type of experiment, it has a more powerful inhibitory action than either noradrenaline or dopamine. It also has a general inhibitory action on the spontaneous electrical activity of the cerebral cortex with some tendency to cause excitation at higher dose levels. Excitatory activity can also be evoked, at all dose levels, in some subcortical structures.

Although the neuropharmacological effects of serotonin are thus predominantly depressant in type, there is some evidence that the less common excitatory responses may more closely mirror its physiological actions. The excitatory responses to microiontophoretic application of 5-hydroxytryptamine are blocked by specific antagonists such as lysergic acid diethylamide and methysergide (p. 334) but the inhibitory responses are unaffected, suggesting that the neurones may carry specific 5-hydroxytryptamine receptors through which neuronal excitation may be affected. Thus, if 5-hydroxytryptamine is a transmitter substance at all, it may be a mediator of excitatory impulses at least at some sites. It is important to emphasize that the fact that a cell bears 5-hydroxytryptamine receptors does not mean that excitation in that neurone is necessarily mediated by 5-hydroxytryptamine: the liberation of the amine on to the cell from fibres impinging upon it has also to be demonstrated. This has not yet been achieved. This point is underlined by the observation that the lateral geniculate body possesses some neurones that are inhibited and others that are excited by 5-hydroxytryptamine. The latter, like similar neurones elsewhere in the central nervous system, can be blocked by lysergic acid diethylamide but the fibres of the optic nerve—which forms the principal inflow into the lateral geniculate body—contain no 5-hydroxytryptamine. Moreover, many neurones respond equally well to acetylcholine, to noradrenaline and to 5-hydroxytryptamine.

The dietary precursor of 5-hydroxytryptamine is tryptophan (p. 327). Boullin (1963) fed rats on a diet that lacked tryptophan. In this way he produced animals whose brains contained no more than one fifth of the amount of 5-hydroxytryptamine found in pair-fed control animals. Some of the deficient animals exhibited behavioural changes that included tremor, ataxia and convulsions. 5-hydroxytryptamine does not readily pass the blood-brain barrier but the effects of administering it can be reproduced by giving 5-hydroxytryptophan, its immediate precursor. Small doses of 5-hydroxytryptophan cause sedation but larger amounts lead to an excited form of behaviour characterized by an apparently purposeless increase in locomotor activity. The treated animals seem to be unaware of the presence of obstacles in their path which they make no attempt to avoid.

5-Hydroxytryptamine synthesis can be inhibited in vivo by the administration of p-chlorophenylalanine (p. 327). Daily doses of the order of 300 mg per kilogram of body weight reduce the 5-hydroxytryptamine content of brain within a few days to 5 per cent. or less of its normal level and this condition can be maintained indefinitely by continued adminstration of the drug. Koe and Weissman (1968) found that the behaviour of rats, dogs and squirrel monkeys, suffering from severe degrees of cerebral serotonin deficiency produced in this way, differed remarkably little from that of normal animals. Some of the rats showed an increased irritability on handling and some of the dogs exhibited tremors, ataxia and an increase in muscle tone. In rats there was some reduction in the threshold for electroshock seizures. Some earlier workers had shown that p-chlorophenylalanine produced a condition of permanent wakefulness in cats but the few human beings who have been given the compound have not complained of sleeplessness.

The effects of p-chlorophenylalanine adminstration are consistent with those produced by the aministration of 5-hydroxytryptophan and the deprivation of tryptophan. They indicate that, so far as the brain is concerned, 5-hydroxytryptamine is usually depressant in its actions. This finding that 5-hydroxytryptamine is generally depressant in its actions is, unfortunately, not consistent with the tentative conclusion reached earlier, that the physiological receptors for 5-hydroxytryptamine may be those that give rise to excitatory responses.

There is convincing evidence that 5-hydroxytryptamine is a transmitter substance in some invertebrate species and it also seems to play an important role (though perhaps only as a precursor of melatonin) in the mammalian pineal gland (p. 332).

Brain monoamines and body temperature

In 1964, Feldberg and Myers found that the intraventricular injection of 5-hydroxytryptamine increased the body temperature of conscious cats while adrenaline and noradrenaline depressed it. Later experiments showed that dogs and monkeys respond in the same way as cats. On the other hand, 5-hydroxytryptamine has a hypothermic action on the goat, ox, rat and mouse. Less regularly it also reduces the body temperature of rabbits and sheep. Noradrenaline has a hyperthermic action in rabbits and sheep and does not affect the temperature of the ox or goat. In the rat and mouse, noradrenaline has a bivalent effect, small doses producing some degree of hyperthermia and larger doses having a more pronounced hypothermic action. Some of the drugs that influence the monoamine content of brain affect the body temperature and Feldberg has marshalled some persuasive arguments in support of his hypothesis that the regulation of body temperature depends on the co-ordinated release of the monoamines from hypothalamic structures (Feldberg, 1968). However, Feldberg's experiments, interesting though they are, are not immediately relevant to the question as to whether 5-hydroxytryptamine is a transmitter substance, particularly since a number of other naturally occurring substances can also influence body temperature in this way.

OTHER MONOAMINES

A number of other amines that are known to occur, or could theoretically be present, in brain tissue have been nominated as possible transmitter substances in the mammalian brain. They include octopamine (p. 259), a substance for which a transmitter role in crustacea has almost been established (Axelrod & Saavedra, 1977) and tyramine (p. 274) while among compounds related to serotonin, acetylserotonin (p. 328), 5 methoxytryptamine, tryptamine and hallucinogenic agents such as dimethyltryptamine and N-methyltryptamine all have, or have had, their champions. Although some evidence for transmitter action can be found for all these substances it does not, at the time of writing, amount to anything significant.

Aminoacids

Interest in the neurotransmitter roles of free aminoacids dates from 1953 and the discovery of clues pointing for the first time to the existence of a specifically inhibitory transmitter substance, soon to be identified as γ-aminobutyric acid (GABA). At almost the same time it became clear that glutamic acid had properties that were consistent with its having an excitatory transmitter function and since then a number of other aminoacids have been able to stake claims, with varying degrees of conviction, for inclusion in the list of recognized mediators, excitatory or inhibitory.

γ-AMINOBUTYRIC ACID

In 1953, Florey reported that extracts of mammalian brain contained a substance which he called Factor I, pending its chemical identification. Crude preparations of Factor I displayed a number of inhibitory actions: they blocked the discharge of impulses from crayfish stretch receptors, they antagonized the excitatory actions of acetylcholine on several pharmacological preparations, they depressed the stretch reflex when they were applied directly to the spinal cord of the cat and they protected mice against the convulsive action of strychnine. This last observation—which proved impossible to repeat—was particularly interesting at a time when the antagonism between strychnine and the chemical mediator of inhibition in the spinal cord had just been demonstrated and no inhibitory transmitter had been identified. The inhibitory action of Factor I on crayfish stretch receptors was made the basis of an elegantly simple method for assaying the Factor I content of tissue extracts.

Four years after Florey's first report, Factor I was identified as γ-aminobutyric acid. At the time when interest became thus focussed on γ-aminobutyric acid, it was not appreciated, as it is now, that many substances could depress central neurones and γ-aminobutyric acid was the obvious candidate for the role of inhibitory transmitter substance.

It had been known since 1950 that γ-aminobutyric acid was present in brain. In vertebrates, it does not occur elsewhere, an interesting finding in view of the fact that inhibitory processes are confined to the central nervous system. It has a wide and relatively even distribution in the brain, its concentration ranging from about 200 μg. per gram (about 2.0 μM) of cortical tissue to about 550 μg. per gram (about 5.3 μM) in the midbrain.

γ-Aminobutyric acid is formed from glutamic acid by an essentially irreversible reaction that requires the enzyme glutamic acid decarboxylase (GAD) with pyridoxal phosphate (vitamin B_6) as a cofactor. It also undergoes a transamination reaction with α-ketoglutaric acid (Fig. 13.5). Though reversible, this reaction normally serves as a catabolic pathway for γ-aminobutyric acid. It results in the production of succinic semialdehyde which can itself be enzymatically oxidized to succinic acid. The transaminase (GABA-T) also requires vitamin B_6 as a cofactor.

αKetoglutaric and succinic acids are both intermediates in the tricarboxylic acid cycle (p. 28) and the reactions just described provide an irreversible shunt that permits the continuing metabolism of α-ketoglutaric acid independently of the α-ketoglutaric oxidase system. Thus γ-aminobutyric acid occupies a unique position in the metabolic system of the brain and it is this, presumably, that explains its high concentration in central nervous tissue. There is, of course, no reason why γ-aminobutyric acid should not also subserve a transmitter function, a purpose which would presumably require only a small fraction of the available material.

In invertebrates, inhibition does not arise exclusively within the central nervous system and it was soon established that γ-aminobutyric acid is an inhibitory transmitter at peripheral sites in at least some invertebrate species. It was found that γ-aminobutyric acid and, particularly, glutamic acid decarboxylase were present in much higher concentrations (the enzyme by up to a hundred fold) in the inhibitory than in the excitatory fibres of crustacea and that the aminoacid was released from inhibitory nerve fibres when these were stimulated. Moreover in the crayfish stretch receptor, γ-aminobutyric acid perfectly reproduces the effects of stimulation of the inhibitory nerve fibres, bringing about an increase in the permeability of the membrane to potassium and chloride ions.

The situation in the vertebrate nervous system proved to be more difficult to determine and opinions concerning the role of γ-aminobutyric acid underwent some marked oscillations before general agreement was reached concerning its probable status. Those (including this author) who were at first not persuaded that γ-aminobutyric acid

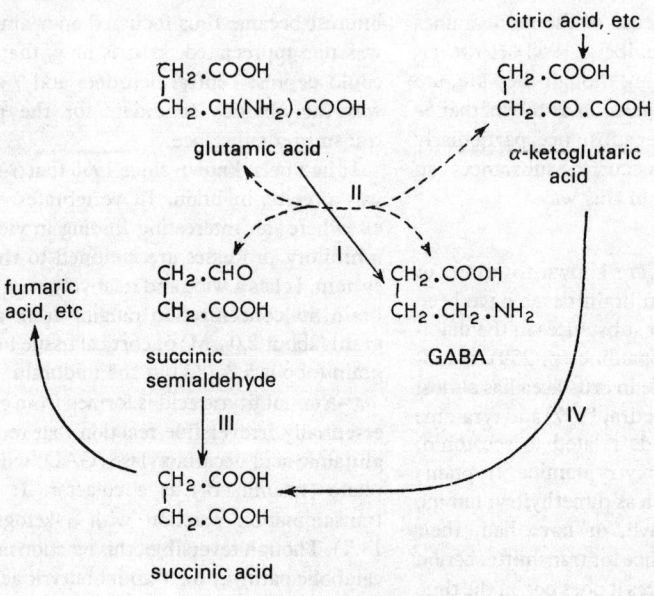

I – glutamic decarboxylase GAD + Vit B_6
II – GABA-α-ketoglutaric transaminase (GABA-T)
III – succinic semialdehyde dehydrogenase + NAD
IV – α-ketoglutaric oxidase

Fig. 13.5 The relationship of γ-aminobutyric acid to the tricarboxylic acid cycle. From Crossland (1967), by kind permission of Messrs. Butterworths.

had the properties to be expected of a transmitter substance found their doubts reinforced by the work of Curtis and his colleagues (Curtis, Phillis & Watkins, 1959) who applied γ-aminobutyric acid, by microiontophoresis, to spinal cord neurones. They found that all postsynaptic responses, excitatory and inhibitory alike, were depressed by γ-aminobutyric acid. This appeared to be the result of an increase in the permeability of the neurone membrane to all types of ion. This effect was seen in all types of nerve cell including the motoneurone. Here at least it was known that postsynaptic inhibition involves a hyperpolarization of the cell and a *selective* increase in its permeability (p. 179). Moreover, the development of the inhibitory postsynaptic potential on the motoneurone membrane is prevented by strychnine, a drug that did not affect the actions of γ-aminobutyric acid on spinal neurones.

The situation changed dramatically when attention was switched from the spinal cord to the cerebral cortex. Krnjević and his colleagues (Krnjević, Randić & Straughan, 1966; Krnjević & Schwarz, 1966) made a detailed study of inhibitory processes in the cerebral cortex, using both extracellular multibarrelled electrodes for recording the effects of drug application and single barrelled microelectrodes for intracellular recordings. They found that stimulation of the cortex of cats, monkeys and rabbits produced inhibitory responses in neurones in other cortical areas. These responses were particularly evident in cells

that had been made to fire by the microiontophoretic application of acetylcholine or L-glutamate. The inhibition was demonstrably postsynaptic in type, was associated with hyperpolarization of the neuronal membrane and was unaffected by strychnine and a range of other agents, including, in particular, antagonists of noradrenaline and acetylcholine. γ-Aminobutyric acid could abolish excitatory and inhibitory postsynaptic potentials in the cortex in exactly the same way that it was known to do in the spinal cord. In addition, however, it also produced a hyperpolarization whose characteristics were remarkably similar to those of the hyperpolarization induced in the same cells by the arrival of inhibitory impulses along cortical pathways.

Experiments performed on the cerebellum by Obata and his colleagues yielded evidence of an even more impressive nature. The Purkinje cells in this organ exert inhibitory actions of the hyperpolarizing type on the cells of Deiter's and other cerebellar nuclei. The Obata group demonstrated that when γ-aminobutyric acid was applied to neurones in the cerebellar nuclei it reproduced exactly the effects of Purkinje cell stimulation (Obata *et al.*, 1967). They went on further to demonstrate that γ-aminobutyric acid was released when Purkinje cells were stimulated (Obata & Takeda, 1969). Some time later, Roberts and his coworkers developed an immunohistochemical method for locating glutamic acid decarboxylase and with its aid they demonstrated that the enzyme was concentrated in the terminal reaches of the Purkinje axons (McLaughlin *et al.*, 1974). Not since we discussed the activation of Renshaw cells have we encountered such overwhelming evidence that a particular substance exerts a transmitter function at an identified junction.

γ-Aminobutyric acid is widely distributed in substantial amounts throughout the central nervous system. Information derived from the application of histochemical and immunohistochemical methodology coupled with corroborative evidence such as the finding of high affinity uptake systems in particular groups of neurones has led to the identification of tracts of fibres and groups of neurones that almost certainly employ γ-aminobutyric acid as a vehicle for transmitting the effects of their activation to other neurones. We shall have to steel ourselves against the horror of their becoming almost universally referred to as GABAnergic neurones. These neurones occur, among other locations, in the basal ganglia (those passing from the corpus striatum to the substantia nigra are referred to again on p. 589), the cerebral cortex, the retina, the hippocampus, and the posterior horns of the spinal cord. In the last mentioned location γ-aminobutyric acid probably acts as the mediator of presynaptic inhibition.

The loss of neurones of the γ-aminobutyric acid system linking the corpus striatum to the substantia nigra underlies at least some of the pathological changes seen in Huntington's chorea just as degeneration or inactivation of the dopamine neurones travelling in the opposite direction is associated with the development of Parkinson's disease. Another clinical aspect of γ-aminobutyric acid activity is the fact that the benzodiazepine group of drugs appears to operate by facilitating the action of the transmitter (p. 575).

γ-Aminobutyric acid is synthesized within nerve terminals but after release it is taken up not only by the presynaptic and postsynaptic elements by processes analogous to the 'uptake 1' and 'uptake 2' mechanisms that operate in noradrenergic neurones but also into neighbouring glial cells. Back in the presynaptic terminals the transmitter may be broken down by the transaminase (Fig. 13.5) but in that event the glutamic acid so formed can undergo decarboxylation to re-form the γ-aminobutyric acid. It seems that glutamic acid formed in the glial cells from the γ-aminobutyric acid that has been taken up is converted into glutamine by the action of glutamine synthetase. The glutamine can be taken back into the nerve terminals where, exposed to the action of glutaminase, it will be reconverted into glutamic acid. These reactions emphasize again the metabolic relationships between γ-aminobutyric acid and glutamic acid and the readiness with which they are converted the one into the other.

· Picrotoxin (p. 514) and bicuculline are both powerful convulsive agents and they have been shown to be specific antagonists of γ-aminobutyric acid. Their pharmacological actions on whole animals are, therefore, quite consist-

ent with the notion that γ-aminobutyric acid is an inhibitory transmitter in the brain. Other substances that cause convulsions may also operate by antagonizing γ-aminobutyric acid. Indeed, observations on the mode of action of the hydrazides (see below) provided a considerable encouragement to those who were attempting to establish an inhibitory role for γ-aminobutyric acid in the days before the definitive experiments on the cerebellar Purkinje cells had established this role beyond reasonable doubt. It must, however, not be assumed that all convulsions of cerebral origin are the result of interference with inhibitory mechanisms mediated by γ-aminobutyric acid. In particular, the reader should guard against a too ready acceptance, sodium valproate (p. 528) notwithstanding, of the view that grand mal epilepsy has its roots in this mechanism.

γ-Aminobutyric acid is present in the brain in what would appear to be quantities far in excess of those needed for maintaining synaptic activity even over so wide an area as that in which it seems to operate. This circumstance, coupled with the unique relationship between γ-aminobutyric and glutamic acids might suggest that, in addition to serving as the inhibitory transmitter substance it undoubtedly is, γ-aminobutyric acid also influences the overall excitability of the nervous system by some sort of modulating or metabolic action the intensity of which is determined by the relative amounts of the two aminoacids. A hypothesis such as this (for which there is no real experimental evidence) might go some way to explaining some of the anomalies, such as those recorded below, that sometimes arise when attempts are made to explain the pharmacological actions of drugs that are apparently related to γ-aminobutyric acid.

The convulsant hydrazides (among which are included isonicotinic acid hydrazide, thiosemicarbazide and thiocarbohydrazide) cause spontaneous convulsions, or an increased susceptibility to sound—or photically—induced seizures in experimental animals. Convulsions have also been reported in tuberculous patients who have received therapeutic doses of isonicotinic hydrazide (p. 846) over

bicuculline

long periods. The convulsant hydrazides cause a loss of pyridoxine from the body and hydrazide convulsions in experimental animals are associated with a large reduction in the amount of γ-aminobutyric acid in the brain. The convulsions can be prevented by pyridoxine and also by hydroxylamine, which inhibits γ-aminobutyric acid—α-ketoglutaric acid transaminase and thus prevents the reconversion of γ-aminobutyric acid into glutamic acid and the operation of the shunt mechanism (Fig. 13.5). Some other compounds that cause pyridoxine deficiency also produce convulsions and hydroxylamine will protect animals against some convulsant drugs such as leptazol that do not themselves bring about a reduction in the amount of γ-aminobutyric acid content of brain.

On superficial examination the results just quoted seem to indicate a relationship between deficiency of γ-aminobutyric acid and seizure susceptibility as direct as that revealed by picrotoxin or bicuculline. The relationship is, in fact, less simple that at first appears. Animals given both thiosemicarbazide and hydroxylamine, for instance, may show susceptibility to seizures at a time when the amount of γ-aminobutyric acid in the brain is elevated above normal levels. Again, amino-oxyacetic acid brings about an increase in the γ-aminobutyric acid content of brain and it also inhibits the convulsions that follow the withdrawal of barbiturates from dependent animals (p. 95). However, there is a dissociation between the prophylactic activity of amino-oxyacetic acid and its effect on the γ-aminobutyric acid system: convulsions can occur in the presence of increased amounts of γ-aminobutyric acid in the brain and at no time during the development of seizure susceptibility is there any change in the amount of this substance that can be extracted from brain tissue (Crossland & Turnbull, 1972).

Perhaps one of the conclusions we should draw from these results is that pharmacological experiments that require the analysis of material from large parts of the brain or which involve the administration of a number of drugs none of which is entirely specific in its action, cannot be expected to yield the clear cut information that comes from an examination of individual neurones or groups of neurones by today's elegant physiological techniques.

GLYCINE

We saw earlier that some of the early investigations that sought to establish an inhibitory transmitter role for γ-aminobutyric acid foundered because the experiments were performed on the spinal cord. The effect of γ-aminobutyric acid on spinal motoneurones did not mimic those of the natural transmitter in respect both of effects on the permeability of the neuronal membrane and of inhibition by strychnine. The later triumphant demonstration that γ-aminobutyric acid is an inhibitory mediator of inhibitory processes in higher reaches of the nervous system made it evident that inhibition of spinal motoneurones is dependent on a mediator other than γ-aminobutyric acid. The evidence suggests that glycine might be that mediator.

The first inkling that glycine might have a transmitter function came from the work of Aprison and Werman and their respective colleagues (Davidoff et al., 1967; Werman et al., 1968). They found evidence that this simplest of amino acids is associated with small internuncial neurones of the type that subserve inhibitory processes in the cord (Fig. 13.3). Thus it is present in the grey matter and, in an experiment in which degeneration of the small neurones but not of the motoneurones was induced by obstructing the blood supply to the spinal cord, almost one-third was lost. When glycine was applied to motoneurones by iontophoresis, it produced hyperpolarization, reduced the excitability of quiescent cells and inhibited the discharge rate of spontaneously firing cells. The inhibitory postsynaptic potential which is normally produced when inhibitory fibres are stimulated failed to develop in cells hyperpolarized by glycine. Finally, and perhaps most interesting of all, the action of glycine on spinal neurones was found to be antagonized by strychnine.

Glycine is found in all tissues of the body and throughout the nervous system, but it certainly occurs in about a threefold higher concentrations in the spinal cord, medulla and pons than in the rest of the central nervous system. Its concentration is highest of all (about 500 μg. per gram) in the anterior horn of the cord, a region that receives the nerve endings from the inhibitory internuncial neurones (Aprison, Davidoff & Werman, 1970). Perhaps even more impressive is the fact that a high affinity uptake system for glycine operates only in the spinal cord, medulla and pons (Neal, 1971). The glycine is taken up into synaptic vesicles and these have a morphology that has for some time been thought to be characteristic of inhibitory neurones. There is also evidence, consistent with the presence of the glycine uptake system in the brain stem, that glycine mediates inhibitory processes that influence activity in some of the cranial nerves that have their origin in this region. Many workers have demonstrated that glycine is released from slices of the mammalian spinal cord and that the rate of release is accelerated by electrical stimulation of the tissue (Davidson, 1976).

The available evidence suggests that glycine in the brain is synthesized in situ and is not derived to any extent from the preformed glycine that is certainly available in quantity from dietary sources. Synthesis is from serine (itself derived from glucose metabolism) under the influence of serine hydroxymethyltransferase.

All these observations indicate that glycine is uniquely capable, among the substances so far investigated, of mimicking the effects produced by stimulation of inhibitory nerves and that it is present in the terminals of these nerves. Its claim for serious consideration as a mediator of inhibitory processes in the spinal cord and brain stem is a powerful one.

The most serious bar to a complete and immediate acceptance of glycine's claim to transmitter status is that there is no evidence that any drug with a locus of action on the cord interferes in any way with the release or re-uptake of glycine. Moreover, metabolic disorders that result in the accumulation of glycine in the blood are not associated with any change that suggests that motoneurones are being exposed to abnormal amounts of inhibitory transmitter. But the physiological evidence for glycine's involvement in inhibitory processes is extremely convincing.

GLUTAMIC ACID

A number of naturally occurring amino acids and some related derivatives that do not occur naturally excite central neurones. Among the naturally occurring substances, glutamic acid is particularly active. Applied by microiontophoresis in molar concentrations as low as 10^{-15}, glutamate stimulates cells throughout the central nervous system, increasing membrane permeability in the same way as does an excitatory nerve impulse. Although its action is not entirely unselective—the Betz cells of the cerebral cortex have a high threshold and neurones of the olfactory bulb appear to be quite unresponsive —glutamate excites virtually all the cells to which it is applied. The response is typically 'sharp': neurones only discharge during the actual application of the amino acid but a continuous release produces continuous firing. Thus the neurone responds to glutamate in much the same way that it would be expected to respond to a physiological excitatory substance and many physiologists have been persuaded that glutamic acid is a major excitatory transmitter substance. Many of those who normally regard the uneven distribution and high concentration of glutamic acid in the nervous system as important pointers to its probable transmitter status do not regard the relatively even distribution and high concentration of glutamic acid in the nervous system as in any way weakening its claim to be a mediator of excitatory transmission. They argue, with reason, that the other roles that it is called upon to perform (it is, for

instance, a component of proteins and some coenzymes including folic acid, it is involved in fatty acid synthesis and in the regulation of ammonia concentration) demand that glutamic acid shall be everywhere available and that the amount required for synaptic transmission is so small that it makes no impact on the total amount present in any area of the brain. As evidence of its transmitter function they prefer to rely, instead, on the fact that a high affinity uptake system, specific for glutamic acid, exists in central neurones.

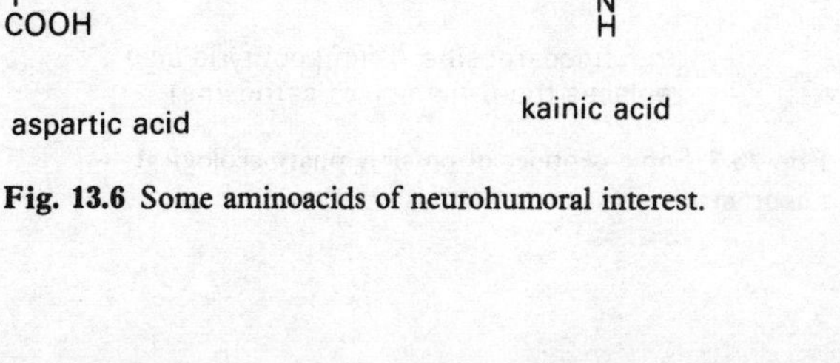

Neurones that possess this system are widely distributed. They include fibres that pass from the cortex to the corpus striatum, from the retina to the superior colliculus, some cerebellar cells and some internuncial neurones in the spinal cord.

Glutamic acid exhibits in an extreme fashion a state of affairs that was mentioned in connection with the putative transmitter function of glycine: it reproduces perfectly the effects of physiological stimulation of the neurones that are thought to contain it but there is virtually no drug whose action can be in any way attributed to an interference with glutamic acid metabolism or action in any way. Kainic acid (Fig. 13.6) is an agonist at glutamate receptors but it is a powerful neurotoxic substance and its actions can hardly be taken as indicative only of a receptor stimulation.

Glutamic acid occurs in brain tissue to the extent of approximately 1400 to 1800 μg per gram of tissue. The concentration in white matter is about two-thirds of that in grey matter.

Reference has already been made to the possibility that glutamic acid and γ-aminobutyric acid might be involved together in the regulation of cerebral excitability.

It is not easy to understand the widespread enthusiasm among physiologists for the idea that glutamic acid is a neurotransmitter in view of the critical assessment to which other candidates are rightly subjected.

OTHER AMINOACIDS

Those who believe that glutamic acid is a mediator of excitatory synaptic transmission are almost compelled to support the notion that *aspartic acid* enjoys a similar role. The molar concentration of aspartic acid in the brain is less than one third of that of glutamic acid but about 4 μmol per gram of tissue it is certainly enough to fill the 'pool' in the nerve endings which segregates the aminoacid used in connection with nervous function from that with more general metabolic actions elsewhere in the body. Aspartic acid excites a wide variety of neurones and its potency in this respect is comparable to that of glutamic acid. Like glutamic acid, aspartic acid is found throughout the nervous system but there is some evidence that in some locations, the two aminoacids are differentially distributed. In the spinal cord, for instance, glutamic acid tends to be more concentrated in the posterior than in the anterior nerve roots while the reverse is true for aspartic acid.

Fig. 13.6 Some aminoacids of neurohumoral interest.

Aspartic acid is taken up into synaptosomes by a high affinity uptake system indistinguishable from that utilized by glutamic acid while calcium ions release both substances from brain slices.

Taurine is the next most abundant aminoacid in the nervous system where it occurs in amounts comparable to those shown by γ-aminobutyric acid and glycine. Applied by iotophoresis to nerve cells in the spinal cord, taurine has powerfully depressant actions that are blocked by strychnine but not by bicuculline. In the cortex it has only a weak depressant action though there is evidence that when depression does occur it is blocked by bicuculline but not by strychnine. These observations suggest, perhaps, that taurine can modulate the actions of both glycine and γ-aminobutyric acid or alternatively that it may actually be the chemical transmitter at some of the sites that are currently assumed to be operated by the recognized aminoacid inhibitory transmitters. Taurine is taken up into nerves by a high affinity uptake system and is released by electrical stimulation of brain slices in vitro. Many more investigations are needed, however, before any transmitter or modulator function can be confidently assigned to it.

The place of taurine in biochemistry and physiology generally has been recently reviewed (Huxtable and Barbeau, 1976).

Polypeptides

Relatively simple polypeptides appear in many roles in the body particularly as hormones, systemic or local. In these guises they make frequent appearances elsewhere in this book but in the present context we need to notice only a few members of the group.

SUBSTANCE P

This substance was discovered in extracts of intestine and brain in 1931 (p. 357) but it was not until 1948 that it came under scrutiny as a possible noncholinergic transmitter substance when it was recognized as a possible (but apparently unlikely) mediator of antidromic vasodilatation (p. 180). Interest in the implication of this possibly faded rather quickly and substance P suffered a temporary eclipse, only emerging again in the early 1970s, when Leeman and her colleagues found that extracts of mammalian hypothalamus evoked salivary secretion in experimental animals. It eventually transpired that the active sialogogue in the extracts was substance P (Leeman and Mroz, 1974).

Substance P is an undecapeptide (Fig. 13.7). When it is attached to γ-globulin it develops antigenic properties and this permits its localization and concentration in tissues to be determined by immunohistochemical and radioimmunoassay methods.

In the central nervous system, substance P is found in highest concentration in the basal ganglia (especially the substantia nigra), the nucleus of the trigeminal nerve, the posterior horns of the spinal cord, the medial and middle hypothalamus and the interpenduncular nucleus. Within the neurones themselves, substance P is concentrated at the nerve endings, probably in dense-core vesicles. The amount of the peptide in the substantia nigra is reduced in patients with Huntington's chorea (p. 164), an observation that is consistent with the presence of fibres containing substance P in the strionigral tract, for the disease is associated with a loss of striatal neurones.

The high concentration of substance P in the posterior spinal roots and the posterior horns of the cord suggest the possibility that substance P might act as a transmitter substance from the first sensory neurone, a possibility that had, of course, been mooted many years before recent experiments revived the idea. The fact that some other, perhaps better qualified, substances have also been nominated as transmitters at the first synapse in the sensory system does not of itself constitute a reason for excluding substance P since it is not unreasonable to assume that sensory fibres are not chemically homogeneous. They may, for instance, be differentiated to some extent according to the sense modality they convey.

Mechanisms for the synthesis of substance P have not yet been defined but rat brain contains a neutral endopeptidase capable of cleaving the substance P molecule at the points indicated in Fig. 13.7 (Benuck and Marks, 1975).

On microiontophoretic application to cerebral and cord neurones, substance P often causes a slowly developing but long lasting excitation quite dissimilar from that evoked by

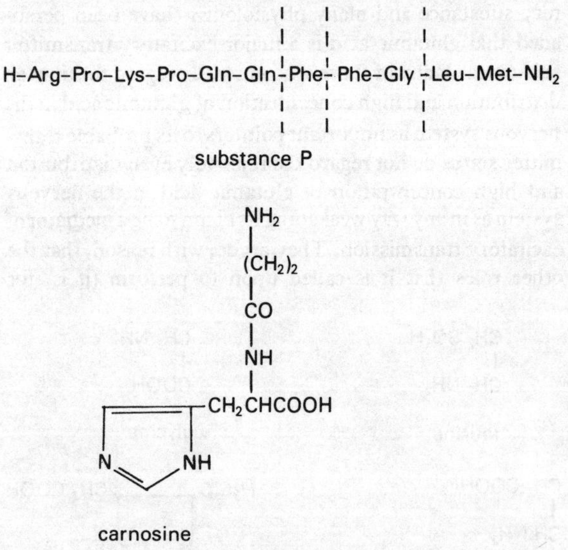

H–Arg–Pro–Lys–Pro–Gln–Gln¦Phe¦Phe–Gly¦Leu–Met–NH₂

substance P

NH₂
|
(CH₂)₂
|
CO
|
NH
|
CH₂ CHCOOH

N   NH

carnosine

(In homocarnosine, γ-aminobutyric acid replaces the ß-alanine of carnosine)

Fig. 13.7 Some peptides of possible pharmacological importance.

the excitatory aminoacids and perhaps indicative of a 'metabotropic' action of some kind. Pharmacological experiments have proved even less encouraging: no antagonist of substance P is known and, to the author's knowledge, no centrally acting drug exerts any effect on the turnover of the peptide in the brain.

Substance P has a long way to go before it can be recognized as a transmitter substance.

THE ENKEPHALINS AND THE ENDORPHINS

The possibility that the endogenous opiates might be involved in transmission processes, particularly in some sensory pathways, is fully discussed elsewhere in this volume (p. 438).

OTHER PEPTIDES

Most of the other active pepides found in living tissue probably exert local regulatory actions. They include angiotensin, carnosine and several hypothalamic hormones and releasing factors. However, a few of them also occur in the central nervous system and these need to be a little more closely examined in the present context in order to assess the possibility that further investigations might reveal that the mediation of synaptic transmission is to be included among their regulatory functions. *Carnosine* is a dipeptide (ß-alanylhistidine) which, as its name implies, occurs in quantity in skeletal muscle. Its properties and possible physiological significance were investigated many years ago but apart from the fact that it proved to bring about a sharp fall in blood pressure, nothing very exciting emerged from these studies and carnosine is rarely mentioned in contemporary textbooks of physiology. A flicker of interest has been rekindled by recent observations that carnosine is present in mammalian brain and that its concentration in the thalamus is appreciably greater and in the olfactory considerably greater than it is in the rest of the brain (Margolis, 1974). Denervation of the nerve fibres that pass from the nasal mucosa to the olfactory bulb is accompanied by an almost complete loss of carnosine from the bulb (Ferriero and Margolis, 1975) and a similar fate befalls the enzyme (carnosine synthetase) that synthesizes the dipeptide. Although these findings are not inconsistent with the idea that carnosine might prove to be the mediator of synaptic transmission from primary olfactory neurones it is difficult to believe in the existence of mediators with so restricted an area of transmitter activity and much more evidence must be forthcoming before carnosine can be added to the roll of established transmitter substances. These remarks apply even more forcibly to the related homocarnosine (γ-aminobutyrylhistidine) the subject of a few other recent investigations. Angiotensins I and II and the converting enzyme (p. 357) occur in the central nervous system, particularly and perhaps not surprisingly in the hypothalamus but there is little evidence that it performs a transmitter function in the usually accepted sense of that word. *Neurotensin*, a hypothalamic trideca-peptide with a variety of regulatory actions, also occurs in some other areas of the brain and spinal cord. Its distribution hints at a possible transmitter function but little other evidence is yet available to provide further support for the idea.

Miscellaneous substances

A large miscellany of compounds that display one or more of the postulated attributes of transmitter substances has been detected in the tissues of the central nervous system. Although none of these substances needs detailed consideration they merit at least a mention in this chapter, since during the lifetime of this textbook any one of them might spring into prominence as a regulator of central nervous activity. Some of them have received their mention in the sections of the chapter that deal with the particular groups of chemical compounds to which they belong but a few of them cannot be segregated in this way and they are, therefore, gathered together in this final section of this chapter.

HISTAMINE

Elsewhere in this book (p. 336) histamine is described as the enigma of pharmacology since it has, so far, proved impossible to attribute to it any physiological function commensurate with its wide distribution in the body and its by no means negligible pharmacological properties. Because histamine is present in the nervous system where it shows the patchy distribution that is often believed to presage a transmitter function, many investigators (including this author) have been attracted by the idea that it is at least partly in this sphere of activity that histamine will find its destiny. This belief received some encouragement from the experiments already referred to that suggested that histamine might be a mediator of antidromic vasodilatation and hence of synaptic transmission at the first synapse on the sensory pathway. This hypothesis had soon to be abandoned and we must look elsewhere for any evidence that histamine has a role in the central nervous system.

Histamine is present in highest concentration in sensory fibres, in the optic nerves (which, like spinal sensory nerves, are incapable of synthesizing acetylcholine), in the pineal body and in the hypothalamus. In these areas it reaches concentrations of up to several micrograms per gram of tissue. In the anterior nucleus of the thalamus, the substantia nigra, the periaqueductal grey matter and the raphé nuclei, histamine concentrations are of the order of 0.3 μg per gram. It is fairly evenly distributed among the other areas of mammalian brain but its overall concentration in the central nervous system does not exceed 0.05 to 0.1 μg per gram of tissue. It has proved impossible to confirm early reports (Kwiatkowski, 1943) that histamine reaches a higher concentration (1 to 2 μg per gram) in the cerebellum than elsewhere in the brain. In postganglionic fibres of the sympathetic nervous system, large quantities of histamine (up to 100 μg per gram) are found. Contrary to earlier reports, mast cells do occur in the nervous system. Like similar cells elsewhere (p. 405) they contain histamine. It has been estimated that about 50 per cent. of the brain's histamine is contained in the mast cells which are associated with non-nervous elements. The results of experiments designed to detect possible changes in the turnover of neuronal histamine will be difficult to interpret in ignorance of the relative contribution made by each of the histamine fractions to any change that takes place.

In the cerebral cortex of the anaesthetized cat, histamine depressed more than 65 per cent. of the neurones to which it was applied by microiontophoresis (Phillis, Tebēcis and York, 1968). This depression affected spontaneously firing cells as well as those that had been excited by acetylcholine, glutamate or hypothalamic stimulation. When the driving current was increased so that more histamine was deposited on the cells, excitatory effects were observed. Other workers have reported that cells elsewhere in the central nervous system are either inhibited or not affected by histamine. There is some evidence that nerve endings in the cortex may contain small amounts of histamine (Kataoka and De Robertis, 1967) but it is not yet known whether this histamine is liberated in the course of normal neuronal activity.

The pharmacological actions of histamine and antihistamines in the intact animal do not fit in very closely with those seen in single cortical neurones. It is well known, for instance, that H_1-histamine antagonists (p. 351) exert a sedative action. Yet in single cortical neurones these antihistamines often uncover excitatory responses because the depressant action of iontophoretically applied histamine is more easily prevented by these drugs than are the excitatory effects. Moreover, many authorities believe that the sedative effects of histamine antagonists are not directly attributable to an action at histamine receptors. It is true that there is some evidence that histamine stimulates the central nervous system of the whole animal: it certainly intensifies the electrical activity of the cerebellum, it stimulates the hypothalamus and it provokes vomiting by a direct action on the vomiting centre (p. 603). It also stimulates the superior cervical ganglion. These suggestions that histamine has excitatory actions on the central nervous system conflict with the picture of an essentially inhibitory substance evoked by the experiments on single cortical cells. Like the monoamines, histamine stimulates the formation of cyclic AMP by brain slices from some mammalian species. It is interesting to note that, in the chick at least, this action is antagonized by histamine H_2 receptor antagonists but not by those that block H_1 receptors (Nahorski, Rogers and Smith 1977).

Calcutt (1976) has marshalled the biochemical evidence in support of the view that histamine plays an important role in the brain but this evidence is not yet strong enough to be convincing.

Much still needs to be done before we can make a definite pronouncement concerning the part, if any, that histamine plays in synaptic transmission. A recent statement by Eccles and some of his colleagues that 'the evidence for histamine as a neurotransmitter in the mammalian brain is rather convincing' (McGeer, Eccles and McGeer, 1978) seems strangely premature.

ATP

Of the substances found in extracts of sensory nerves, ATP seemed at one time to be the one most likely to function as the mediator of antidromic vasodilatation and therefore, perhaps, as the transmitter at the central terminations of sensory nerve fibres (p. 180). The evidence that ATP had actions on the nervous system consistent with a transmitter function was, however, never very strong and interest in the possibility of its having neurohumoral activity soon flagged. In more recent years Burnstock has produced evidence for the existence of 'purinergic' nerve fibres in the postganglionic fibres of the autonomic nervous system (Burnstock, 1972). Although the idea of purinergic nerves has not, by any means, been taken to the heart of all pharmacologists, the possibility of their existence should be borne in mind and it may well be that in the near future the question of ATP's participation in transmission processes in the central nervous system will be re-opened.

PIPERIDINE

Piperidine is a simple compound (in the pure state it is a volatile liquid) that is certainly present in the mammalian brain and spinal cord. It is unevenly distributed, reaching its highest concentrations in the olfactory bulb, the cerebellum and the spinal cord. Piperidine is actively taken up by the brain in which tissue it is concentrated in the synaptosomes. Brain tissue can also convert pipecolic acid (2-carboxypiperidine) into piperidine *in vitro*. In its turn, pipecolic acid may be produced from lysine.

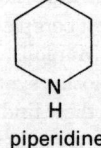

piperidine

In physiological experiments, piperidine mimics some of the synaptic actions of acetylcholine. Like acetylcholine too (p. 183) the amount of piperidine in brain increases during sleep. Further information concerning the pharmacology of piperidine can be found in the papers by Tasher *et al.* (1959) and by Kase *et al.* (1969).

CONCLUSION

It is impossible to say with certainty which substances, other than acetylcholine, mediate transmission processes in the central nervous system. The most important contenders fall into two disparate groups—the aminoacids and the monoamines. The aminoacids, which are widely distributed in quite high concentrations throughout the central nervous system, reproduce remarkably well the effects of stimulation of excitatory and inhibitory nerves and on these grounds their claims to transmitter status are very strong. Yet few of the drugs that affect central nervous function influence the release, metabolism, action or storage of these aminoacids (apart perhaps from γ-aminobutyric acid) in any regular way. The monoamines, by contrast, are present only in localized areas of the nervous system and in relatively minute amounts, there is a good deal of evidence that many of the more effective psychotropic drugs owe their effectiveness to interventions in the activity of 'monoaminergic' neurones and that some forms of mental illness have their origins in a disturbed physiology of these same neurones. On the other hand, the evidence for transmitter action gleaned from electrophysiological studies on single neurones are not nearly as convincing for the monoamines as they are for the aminoacids. This might be partly the result of the monoamines' exerting, in Eccles's terminology, a 'metabotropic' rather than an 'ionotropic' transmitter action.

The identity of any other transmitter substance remains as big a mystery as it has always done. Various arguments and counter arguments can be marshalled in favour of and against a large and an ever growing number of more or less likely candidates. As we have seen, these arguments are not always as consistent or as well thought out as they might be and much remains to be done to establish the precise status of the many substances referred to in the course of this chapter. Even when we have decided which of them are of physiological importance there remains the task of deciding, for each successful candidate, whether it is a transmitter substance, a modulator rather than an initiator of synaptic events or a regulatory substance of some other kind.

A particular task for the pharmacologist is to develop more agents that block specific forms of nervous activity in the central nervous system in the fashion that strychnine, to take an example, blocks postsynaptic inhibitory processes in the spinal cord. When this is done it should be possible to determine whether the actions of a putative transmitter substance are blocked in the same way as are the effects of nerve stimulation and so to decide whether the substance is indeed a transmitter or whether its excitatory or inhibitory action on the neurone is merely a pharmacological event.

One thing of which we can be sure is that the next few years will witness developments in this field as important as any that have gone before. The wise reader, recognizing this, will be ever vigilant for reviews of the topic that appear after the publication date of this book.

BIBLIOGRAPHY

Books, monographs and reviews

Aprison, M.H., Davidoff, R.A. and Werman, R. (1970) Glycine: its metabolic and possible roles in nervous tissue. In *Handbook of Neurochemistry*, Vol.3, pp.381-397. Lajtha, A. (ed.) New York: Plenum Press.

Burn, J.H. (1968a). *The Autonomic Nervous System*, 3rd edn. Oxford and Edinburgh: Blackwell.

Burn, J.H. (1968b). Catecholamines: (a) Pharmacology. In *Recent Advances in Pharmacology*, 4th edn., Robson, J.M. and Stacey, R.S. (eds.), pp.155-177. London: Churchill.

Burnstock, G. (1972) Purinergic nerves. *Pharmac. Rev.*, **24**, 509-581.

Calcutt, C.R. (1976) Mini-review: The role of histamine in the brain. *Gen. Pharmac.*, **7**, 15-25.

Crossland, J. (1957) The problem of non-cholinergic transmission in the central nervous system. In: *Metabolism of the Nervous System*, Richter, D. (ed.) pp.523-541. London: Pergamon.

Crossland, J. (1967) Psychotropic drugs and neurohumoral substances in the central nervous system. In: *Progress in Medicinal Chemistry*, Vol.5, Ellis, G.P. and West, G.B. (eds) pp.251-319. London: Butterworths.

Curtis, D.R. and Watkins, J.C. (1960) The excitation and depression of spinal neurones by structurally related amino acids. *J. Neurochem.*, **6**, 117-141.

Dale, Sir Henry H. (1953) *Adventures in Physiology*. London: Pergamon.

Davidson, N. (1976) *Neurotransmitter Amino Acids*. London, New York and San Francisco: Academic Press.

Eccles, J.C. (1936) Synaptic and neuro-muscular transmission. *Ergebn. Physiol.*, **38**, 339-444.

Eccles, J.C. (1964) *The Physiology of Synapses*. Berlin: Springer.

von Euler, U.S. and Pernow, B. (1977) *Substance P*. New York: Raven Press.

Feldberg, W. (1968) The monoamines of the hypothalamus as mediators of temperature responses. In: *Recent Advances in Pharmacology*, 4th ed., Robson, J.M. and Stacey, R.S., pp.349-398. London: Churchill.

Grundfest, H. (1957) Electrical inexcitability of synapses and some consequences in the central nervous system. *Pharmac. Rev.*, **37**, 377.

Huxtable, R. and Barbeau, A. (1975) (eds.) *Taurine*. New York: Raven Press.

Krnjević, K. (1974) Chemical nature of synaptic transmission in vertebrates. *Physiol. Rev.*, **54**, 418-540.

Loewi, O. (1960) An autobiographical sketch. *Perspect. Biol. Med.*, **4**, 3-25.

McGeer, P.L., Eccles, J.C. and McGeer, Edith G. (1978) *Molecular Neurobiology of the Mammalian Brain*. New York: Plenum Press.

Phillis, J.W. (1970) *The Pharmacology of Synapses*. Oxford: Pergamon Press.

Rothballer, A.B. (1959) The effects of catecholamines on the central nervous system. *Pharmac. Rev.*, **11**, 494-547.

Tebēcis, A.K. (1974) *Transmitters and Identified Neurons in the Mammalian Central Nervous System*. Bristol: Scientechnica.

Toner, P.G. and Carr, Katharine E. (1971) *Cell Structure*, Edinburgh and London: Churchill Livingstone.

Werman, R. (1966) A review—criteria for identification of a central nervous system transmitter. *Comp. Biochem. Physiol.*, **18**, 765-766.

Original papers

Axelrod, J. and Saavedra, J.M. (1977) Octopamine. *Nature, Lond.*, **265**, 501-504.

Bacq, Z.M. and Brown, G.L. (1937) Pharmacological experiments on mammalian voluntary muscle in relation to the theory of chemical transmission. *J. Physiol.*, **89**, 45-60.

Barger, G. and Dale, H.H. (1910). Chemical structure and sympathomimetic action of amines. *J. Physiol.*, **41**, 19-59.

Benuck, M. and Marks, N. (1975) Enzymatic inactivation of substance P by a partially purified enzyme from rat brain. *Biochem. Biophys. Res. Commun.*, **65**, 153-160.

Boullin, D.J. (1963) Behaviour of rats depleted of 5-hydroxytryptamine by feeding a diet free of tryptophan. *Psychopharmacologia*, **5**, 28-38.

Bradley, P.B. (1973) Excitatory effects of catecholamines in the central nervous system. In *Frontiers in Catecholamine Research*, pp.653-656 Usdin, E. and Snyder, S.H. (eds.) London and New York: Pergamon Press.

Bradley, P.B. and Wolstencroft, J.H. (1965) Actions of drugs on single neurones in the brain stem. *Br. med. Bull.*, **20**, 15-18.

Bradley, P.B., Wolstencroft, J.H., Hosli, L. and Avanzino, G.L. (1966). Neuronal basis for the central action of chlorpromazine. *Nature, Lond.*, **212**, 1425-1427.

Brock, L.G., Coombs, J.S. and Eccles, J.C. (1952) The recording of potentials from motoneurones with an intracellular electrode. *J. Physiol.*, **117**, 431-460.

Brown, G.L., Dale, H.H. and Feldberg, W. (1936) Reactions of the normal mammalian muscle to acetylcholine and to eserine. *J. Physiol.*, **87**, 394-424.

Brown, G.L. and Feldberg, W. (1936) The acetylcholine metabolism of a sympathetic ganglion. *J. Physiol.*, **88**, 265-283.

Celesia, G.G. and Jasper, H.H. (1966) Acetylcholine released from cerebral cortex in relation to state of activation. *Neurology*, **16**, 1053-1064.

Crossland, J. and Turnbull, M.J. (1972) γ-Aminobutyric acid and the barbiturate abstinence syndrome in rats. *Neuropharmac.*, **11**, 733-738.

Curtis, D.R., Phillis, J.W. and Watkins, J.C. (1959) The depression of spinal neurones by γ-amino-*n*-butyric acid and *ß*-alanine. *J. Physiol.*, **150**, 656-682.

Dahlström, A. and Fuxe, K. (1965a) Evidence for the existence of monoamine neurons in the central nervous system. 1. Demonstration of monoamines in the cell bodies of brainstem neurons. *Acta Physiol. Scand.*, Supp.**232**, 62.

Dahlström, A. and Fuxe, K. (1965b) Evidence for the existence of monoamine neurons in the central nervous system. IV. Distribution of monoamine nerve terminals in the central nervous system. *Acta Physiol. Scand.*, Supp.**247**, 64.

Dale, H.H. and Feldberg, W. (1934) The chemical transmitter of vagus effects to the stomach. *J. Physiol.*, **81**, 320-334.

Dale, H.H., Feldberg, W. and Vogt, Marthe (1936) Release of acetylcholine at voluntary motor nerve endings. *J. Physiol.*, **86**, 353-380.

Davidoff, R.A., Shank, R.P., Graham, L.T., Aprison, M.H. and Werman, R. (1967) Association of glycine with spinal interneurones. *Nature*, **214**, 680-681.

Eccles, J.C. (1947) Acetylcholine and synaptic transmission in the spinal cord. *J. Neurophysiol.*, **10**, 197-204.

Eccles, J.C., Fatt, P. and Koketsu, K. (1954) Cholinergic and inhibitory synapses in a pathway from motor-axon collaterals to motoneurones. *J. Physiol.*, **126**, 524-562.

Eccles, J.C., Katz, B. and Kuffler, S.W. (1941) Nature of the end-plate potential in curarized muscle. *J. Neurophysiol.*, **4**, 362-387.

Eccles, J.C. and MacFarlane, W.V. (1949) Actions of anticholinesterases on end plate potential of frog muscle. *J. Neurophysiol.*, **12**, 59-79.

Eccles, Rosamond M. and Libet, B. (1961) Origin and blockade of the synaptic responses of curarized sympathetic ganglia. *J. Physiol.*, **157**, 484-503.

Elliott, T.R. (1904) On the action of adrenalin. *J. Physiol.*, **31**, xx-xxi.

Eranko, O. (1955) Histochemistry of noradrenaline in the adrenal medulla of rats and mice. *Endocrinology*, **57**, 363-368.

Falck, B., Hillarp, N.A., Thieme, G. and Torp, A. (1962) Fluorescence of catecholamines and related compounds condensed with formaldehyde. *J. Histochem. Cytochem.*, **10**, 348-354.

Feldberg, W. and Vogt, M. (1948) Acetylcholine synthesis in different regions of the central nervous system. *J. Physiol.*, **107**, 372-381.

Ferriero, D. and Margolis, F.L. (1975) Denervation in the primary olfactory pathway of mice—II. Effects on carnosine and other amine compounds. *Brain Res.*, **94**, 75-86.

Greengard, P. (1976) Possible role for cyclic nucleotides and phosphorylated membrane proteins in postsynaptic actions of neurotransmitters. *Nature, Lond.*, **260**, 101-108.

Hokfelt, T., Fuxe, K., Goldstein, M. and Johansson, O. (1974) Immunohistochemical evidence for the existence of adrenaline neurones in rat brain. *Brain Res.*, **66**, 235-251.

Kase, Y., Miyata, T., Kamikawa, Y. and Kataoka, M. (1969) Pharmacological studies on alicyclic amines—II. Central actions of piperidine, pyrrolidine and piperazine. *Jap. J. Pharmac.*, **19**, 300-314.

Kataoka, K. and De Robertis, E. (1967) Histamine in isolated small nerve endings and synaptic vesicles of rat brain cortex. *J. Pharmac. exp. Ther.*, **156**, 114-125.

Kelly, J.S. and Krnjević, K. (1968) Effects of γ-aminobutyric acid and glycine on cortical neurones. *Nature*, **219**, 1380-81.

Koe, B.K. and Weissman, A. (1968) The pharmacology of p. cholorophenylalanine, a selective depletor of serotonin stores. In: *Advances in Pharmacology*, vol 6B, Garattini, S. and Shore, P.A. (eds.) 29-47.

Krnjević, K. and Schwartz, S. (1966) The action of gamma-aminobutyric acid on cortical neurones. *Exp. Brain Res.*, **3**, 320-336.

Krnjević, K., Randić, Marjana and Straughan, D.W. (1966) Pharmacology of cortical inhibition. *J. Physiol.*, **184**, 78-105.

Kuffler, S.W. (1942) Electric potential changes at an isolated nerve-muscle junction. *J. Neurophysiol.*, **5**, 18-26.

Kwiatkowski, H. (1943) Histamine in nervous tissue. *J. Physiol.*, **102**, 32-41.

Leeman, S.E. and Mroz, E.A. (1974) Substance P. *Life Sci.*, **15**, 2033-2044.

Lew, J.Y., Matsumoto, Y., Pearson, J., Goldstein, M., Hokfelt, T. and Fuxe, K. (1977) Localization and characterization of phenylethanolamine-N-methyltransferase in the brain of various mammalian species. *Brain Res.*, **119**, 199-210.

Lindvall, O. and Bjorklund, A. (1974a) The glyoxylic acid fluorescence histochemical method: A detailed account of the methodology for the visualization of central catecholamine neurons. *Histochemistry*, **39**, 97-127.

Lindvall, O. and Bjorklund, A (1974b) The organization of the ascending catecholamine neuron system in the rat brain. *Acta Physiol. Scand.*, **412**, supp.1-48.

Loewi, O. and Navrath, E. (1962) Über humorale Übertragbarkeit der Herznervenwirkung. XI. Mitteilung. Über den Mechanismus der Vaguswirkung von Physostigmin und Ergotamin. *Pflügers Arch.ges Physiol.*, **214**, 689-696.

McLaughlin, B.J., Wood, J.G., Saito, K., Barber, R., Vaughan, J.E., Roberts, E. and Wu, J.Y. (1974) The fine structural localization of glutamate decarboxylase in synaptic terminals of rodent cerebellum. *Brain Res.*, **76**, 377-391.

Margolis, F.L. (1974) Carnosine in the primary olfactory pathway. *Science*, **184**, 909-911.

Mitchell, J.F. (1963) The spontaneous and evoked release of acetylcholine from the cerebral cortex. *J. Physiol.*, **165**, 98-116.

Nahorski, S.R., Rogers, K.J. and Smith, B.M. (1977) Stimulation of cyclic adenosine 3',5'-monophosphate in chick cerebral hemisphere slices: Effects of H_1 and H_2 histaminergic agonists and antagonists. *Brain Res.*, **126**, 387-390.

Neal, M.J. (1971) The uptake of ^{14}C glycine by slices of mammalian spinal cord. *J. Physiol.*, **215**, 103-117.

Obata, K., Ito, M., Ochi, R. and Sato, N. (1967) Pharmacological properties of the postsynaptic inhibition of Purkinje cell axons and the actions of γ-aminobutyric acid on Deiter's neurones. *Exp. Brain Res.*, **4**, 43-57.

Obata, K. and Takeda, K. (1969) Release of GABA into the fourth ventricle induced by stimulation of the cat cerebellum. *J. Neurochem.*, **16**, 1043-1047.

Ogston, A.G. (1955) Removal of acetylcholine from a limited volume by diffusion. *J. Physiol.*, **128**, 222-223.

Phillis, J.W., Tebecis, A.K. and York, D.H. (1968) Histamine and some antihistamines: their actions on cerebral cortical neurones. *Brit. J. Pharmac. Chemother.*, **33**, 426-440.

Richter, D. and Crossland, J. (1949) Variation in acetylcholine content of brain with physiological state. *Am. J. Physiol.*, **159**, 247-255.

Roberts, M.H.T. and Straughan, D.W. (1967) Excitation and depression of cortical neurones by 5-hydroxytryptamine. *J. Physiol.*, **193**, 269-294.

Sternberger, L.A., Hardy, P.H., Cuculis, J.J. and Myer, H.G. (1970). The unlabelled antibody enzyme method by immunohistochemistry: Preparation and properties of soluble antigen-antibody complex (horseradish peroxidase-antiperoxidase) and its use in identification of spirochetes. *J. Histochem. Cytochem.*, **18**, 315-333.

Swanson, L.W. and Hartmann, B.K. (1975) The central adrenergic system. An immunofluorescence study of the location of cell bodies and their efferent connections in the rat utilizing dopamine-ß-hydroxylase as a marker. *J. comp. Neurol.*, **163**, 467-506.

Tasher, D.C., Abood, L.G., Gibbs, F.A. and Gibbs, E.L. (1959). Introduction of a new type of psychotropic drugs: Cyclopentimine. *J. Neuropsychiat.*, **1**, 266-273.

Werman, R., Davidoff, R.A. and Aprison, M.H. (1968) Inhibitory action of glycine on spinal neurons in the cat. *J. Neurophysiol.*, **31**, 81-93.

14. The choline esters and the cholinesterases

Acetylcholine is one of the most important and most widely distributed of all tissue constituents; it is referred to repeatedly and in a variety of contexts throughout this book as it is in all textbooks of pharmacology. It is certainly the most venerable of humoral substances, its properties having been first investigated in the opening years of this century. Although acetylcholine functions primarily as a synaptic and neuromuscular transmitter substance, it is also found in non-nervous tissue where it may control functions such as inherent cardiac rhythmicity, smooth muscle activity and ciliary movement, which can occur independently of nervous action. Acetylcholine occurs in animals, both vertebrate and invertebrate, and in plants. The nettle sting contains acetylcholine, the head of the common fly is capable of synthesizing large quantities of the ester and the motility of parasitic worms depends on its presence.

The position occupied by acetylcholine as a transmitter substance is fully discussed in Chapter 13.

GENERAL PROPERTIES OF ACETYLCHOLINE

Acetylcholine, the acetyl ester of choline, is a quaternary ammonium compound. The molecule possesses a cationic (positively charged) head joined by a chain of two carbon atoms to an ester grouping. Acetylcholine is stable in acid solution but it is very unstable in alkali. In the body it is combined with protein until it is liberated to exert its physiological action. Free acetylcholine, liberated in this way or injected into the blood stream, is rapidly destroyed by cholinesterase (p. 211). Acetylcholine is synthesized in the tissues by choline acetyltransferase (choline acetylase), an enzyme that promotes the transfer of the acetyl group from acetylcoenzyme A to choline. Acetylcoenzyme A itself is a product of normal glycolysis. It is formed by an energy consuming reaction from pyruvic acid and coenzyme A under the influence of pyruvic dehydrogenase.

The muscarinic and nicotinic actions of acetylcholine

MUSCARINIC ACTIONS

It was observed many years ago that muscarine, an alkaloid extracted from a poisonous fungus *Amanita muscaria*, produced effects in experimental animals similar to those resulting from stimulation of the parasympathetic division of the autonomic nervous system. Acetylcholine has similar effects since it mediates the transmission of impulses from the postganglionic terminations of the parasympathetic nerves to the effector organs. Thus all the actions of muscarine can be reproduced by acetylcholine but acetylcholine has other effects not shown by muscarine. Although muscarine does not occur in animal tissues, it is convenient to speak of the muscarinic actions of acetylcholine as a separate pharmacological entity. These actions have several features in common—they are all, for instance, blocked by atropine—and the evidence suggests that specific muscarinic receptors exist in the tissues.

Although it is true to say that muscarine mimics the effects of parasympathetic stimulation, its actions (and the corresponding actions of acetylcholine) go beyond this in several respects. In general, the peripheral blood vessels are innervated only by the sympathetic division of the autonomic nervous system and vasodilatation, insofar as it

Muscarine

is due to nervous influences, is the consequence of relaxation of sympathetic constrictor tone. Stimulation of parasympathetic nerves therefore has little effect on blood vessels (except those in some glands) but muscarine and acetylcholine cause vasodilatation. Moreover, muscarinic receptors are found in the central nervous system and in autonomic ganglia (Chap. 13).

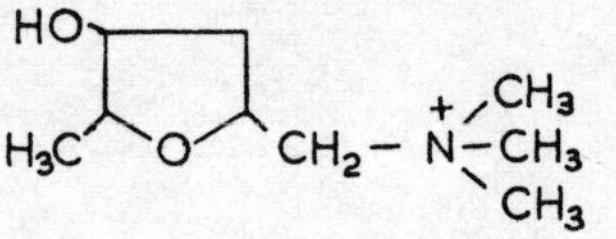

With these points in mind, the muscarinic actions of acetylcholine may be enumerated as follows:

1. Stimulation of sweat, salivary and tear glands and stimulation of the secretory activity of the stomach, intestines and pancreas.

2. Stimulation of the smooth muscle of the bronchi, the gastrointestinal tract, the gall bladder, bile duct, urinary bladder and ureters.

3. Relaxation of sphincters in the gastrointestinal, biliary and urinary tracts.

4. Vasodilatation and, in slightly higher doses, slowing of the heart.

5. Constriction of the pupil (*miosis*) and accommodation of the lens for near vision.

6. Actions on the central nervous system and autonomic ganglia. These are discussed in Chapter 13.

NICOTINIC ACTIONS

Nicotine has pharmacological actions different from those of muscarine and it happens that those actions of acetylcholine that are not mimicked by muscarine are reproduced by nicotine. Thus acetylcholine acts on both muscarinic and nicotinic receptors. The pharmacological actions of nicotine are considered in more detail later (p. 205) but they can be summarized as follows:

1. Stimulation of skeletal muscle.

2. Stimulation of autonomic ganglia (both sympathetic and para-sympathetic) and stimulation of the adrenal medulla. The latter structure is supplied by preganglionic sympathetic fibres and embryologically and functionally the medullary cells resemble post-ganglionic sympathetic elements. Reference has already been made to the occurrence of muscarinic receptors in ganglia but the nicotinic receptors are more important and, from the elementary point of view, the *pharmacological* action of acetylcholine at autonomic ganglia can be regarded as being exclusively nicotinic in type.

3. Actions on the central nervous system that are discussed elsewhere (Chap. 13 and below, p. 205). For the present it is sufficient to note that the central nervous system appears to possess both muscarinic and nicotinic receptors.

The actions of nicotine and muscarine differ from one another in an important general respect. The effects of muscarine increase progressively with the dose but high doses of nicotine inhibit structures that are stimulated by lower doses of the drug. Acetylcholine itself behaves in the same way: at muscarinic sites, high doses always have greater effects than low doses but at nicotinic sites where small doses of acetylcholine have a stimulant effect, larger doses cause receptor blockade. Thus, acetylcholine may prevent the operation of transmission mechanisms that are themselves due to acetylcholine.

The actions of acetylcholine on the blood pressure can be utilized to provide a convenient demonstration of muscarinic and nicotinic effects. A small dose of acetylcholine (2 to 20 μg.) given by intravenous injection to the anaesthetized cat causes vasodilatation (together with bradycardia with the higher doses in the range) and thus a fall in blood pressure. Because of the rapidity with which the acetylcholine is hydrolysed, the depressor effect is only short lived. It is a muscarinic action and it is no longer seen if acetylcholine is given after the animal has received atropine. If the cat is now given a large dose of acetylcholine (this may have to be of the order of 500 to 1 000 times as large as that required to demonstrate the muscarinic effect), the blood pressure rises sharply. In the absence of atropine, this amount of acetylcholine would have caused a fatal hypotension; in its presence the effects of acetylcholine on the heart and blood vessels are prevented and the stimulant actions on the ganglia are permitted to express themselves. Stimulation of the sympathetic ganglia and the release of adrenaline cause cardioacceleration and widespread vasoconstriction and this is responsible for the observed hypertensive response. The parasympathetic ganglia are also stimulated but the presence of atropine prevents the appearance of signs of parasympathetic stimulation. Some fibrillation (twitching of groups of fibres) may be seen in the muscles after the administration of doses of acetylcholine (or of equivalent quantities of nicotine) sufficient to cause nicotinic effects.

The amount of acetylcholine which can be safely given by intravenous injection to the unatropinized animal is such that any ganglion stimulant action it can exert is very small indeed and it is in any event overwhelmed by the concurrent muscarinic effects on the effector organs. The fact that large doses of acetylcholine are necessary before its nicotinic actions can be demonstrated is in large part due to the enzymatic and other barriers which hinder its penetration into the ganglia from the blood stream.

It should be added that, among common laboratory animals, the muscarinic and nicotinic actions of acetylcholine on the cardiovascular system can only be readily demonstrated on the cat.

Many of the disorders suffered by man involve disturbances of autonomic, neuromuscular or central nervous function and drugs that potentiate or antagonize the actions of acetylcholine would therefore be expected to have a wide range of therapeutic applications. It has already been mentioned that the muscarinic effects of acetylcholine are antagonized by atropine. The nicotinic effects are blocked by curare (Chap. 16). Both these drugs are unselective in their effects and a great deal of effort has been expended in attempts to produce drugs with a more restricted range of action. These attempts have been only partially successful. It has proved possible to develop drugs which selectively block transmission at either the neuromuscular junction or at ganglia and this is related to morphological differences in the nicotinic receptors at the two sites. On the other hand, all ganglia, whether sympathetic or parasympathetic, are morphologically and functionally similar so that selective blockade of sympathetic or parasympathetic ganglia has not yet been achieved. Among the atropine-like drugs some show relatively more activity against the secretory, the motor or the ophthalmological effects of autonomic activation but this slight degree of selectivity is probably due to the fact that the drugs have actions other than their ability to block muscarinic receptors.

Drugs that antagonize the muscarinic and nicotinic actions of acetylcholine are discussed in greater detail in Chapters 15 and 16 respectively.

OTHER COMPOUNDS WITH ACETYLCHOLINE-LIKE ACTIVITY

It is possible to make a few generalizations concerning the types of pharmacological activity exhibited by other choline esters (Fig. 14. 1). They may differ from acetylcholine in one or more of three ways: in their muscarinic activity, in their nicotinic activity or in their chemical stability, including their resistance to enzymatic hydrolysis. An increased chemical stability may cause prolongation of both nicotinic and muscarinic actions and may thus give a false impression of increased potency.

Muscarinic potency falls if the acetyl group is replaced, but some substituents produce compounds that resist enzymatic hydrolysis. Carbachol (in which the acetyl group is replaced by carbamyl) provides an example of this. Nicotinic activity is increased if acetyl is replaced by propionyl. Thus propionylcholine has powerful nicotinic actions and weak muscarinic actions. The nicotine actions become progressively less marked as the size of the terminal group increases so that many choline esters have neither muscarinic nor nicotinic activity. Some (tropylcholine and benzilylcholine are examples) actually have atropine-like antimuscarinic activity.

Changes in the alkyl chain separating the cationic head from the ester grouping of acetylcholine generally result in a reduction of muscarinic activity and an increase in chemical stability. Nicotinic activity is retained, eliminated or, very occasionally, increased. There is no clear relationship between changes in the two types of activity. Thus, acetyl-α-methylcholine has about the same degree of nicotinic activity as acetylcholine but its muscarinic potency is only one-twentieth of that of acetylcholine. Acetyl-β-methylcholine, on the other hand, has no nicotinic actions but its muscarinic activity is one-half that of acetylcholine.

We must now leave the choline esters to glance briefly at compounds produced by modifying the anionic head of the acetylcholine molecule. If one or more of the methyl groups on the quaternary nitrogen atom is replaced by a hydrogen atom or by an ethyl group, both muscarinic and nicotinic potencies are reduced. At least two methyl

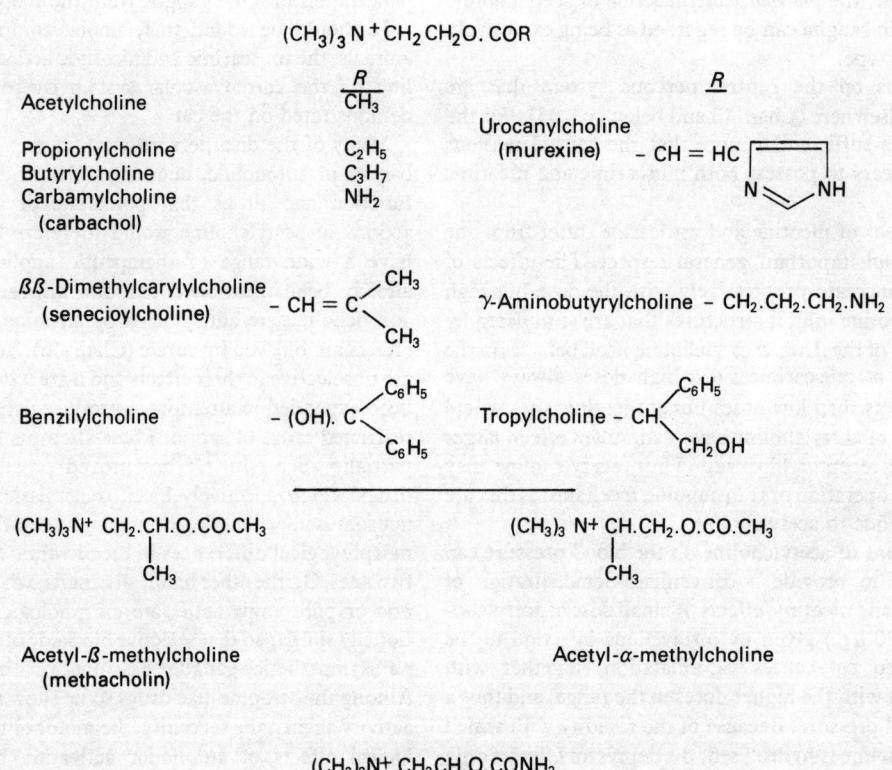

Fig. 14. 1 Some choline esters.

groups must be present for significant activity of either type. Barlow (1955) suggests that the two methyl groups on the anionic head are necessary to enable the head to fit into the cavity presumed to exist at the cationic site of the receptor protein (Chap. 17). If all three methyl groups are replaced by ethyl groups, antagonism to acetylcholine appears. This effect can be seen in quite simple compounds: tetramethylammonium, for instance, has a nicotine-like stimulant action on autonomic ganglion cells but tetraethylammonium is an acetylcholine antagonist at these sites. Acetylcholine, indeed, can be regarded as a more active derivation of tetramethylammonium.

The quaternary nitrogen atom itself may be replaced by arsenic, antimony, phosphorus or sulphur without loss of all acetylcholine-like activity. Nicotine itself (p. 205) does not possess a quaternary nitrogen atom, but at a physiological pH, it may be present as the quaternary nicotinium ion.

Ing (1949) suggested that, in compounds chemically related to acetylcholine, maximal muscarinic activity occurs when a chain of five atoms (usually carbon or oxygen but not hydrogen) is linked to the quaternary atom. This is the so-called 'five atom rule'.

Individual compounds

PROPIONYLCHOLINE
Propionylcholine is the only choline ester, other than acetylcholine, to have been unequivocally detected in mammalian tissues. Appreciable amounts are found, together with acetylcholine, in extracts of ox spleen (Banister, Whittaker and Wijesundera, 1953). It is possible that a careful examination of other tissue extracts might reveal its presence (or that of other choline esters) elsewhere. This point is taken up again below (p. 210).

UROCANYLCHOLINE (MUREXINE)
Urocanylcholine is another naturally occurring choline ester. It occurs in the hypobranchial body of *Murex trunculus*, the Mediterranean whelk, and in some related species. Urocanylcholine has no muscarinic activity but it has potent nicotinic actions. Small doses of urocanylcholine cause contraction of striated muscle but, as with other nicotine-like substances (p. 237) larger amounts bring about a neuromuscular blockade of a depolarizing type, a property which the whelk utilizes as a means of defence and for the purpose of obtaining food.

ββ-DIMETHYLACRYLYLCHOLINE (SENECIOYLCHOLINE)
This choline ester occurs in the hypobranchial glands of *Thais lapillus* (the dog whelk) and *T. floridana floridana* (the Southern oyster drill). These glands contain very large amounts of the ester. Expressed in terms of acetylcholine, the biological activity of extracts of these glands reaches 4000 μg per gram of tissue (Keyl, Michaelson and Whittaker, 1957). This figure should be compared with that for mammalian brain which contains about 4 μg of acetylcholine per gram. Senecioylcholine presumably serves the same function as does urocanylcholine. Some gastropods and the lobster contain acetylcholine itself.

γ-AMINOBUTYRYLCHOLINE
Some years ago it was believed that γ-aminobutyrylcholine might be an inhibitory transmitter in the central nervous system but there is now doubt concerning its presence in brain and γ-aminobutyrylcholine no longer claims the attention of neuropharmacologists.

CARBACHOL
Carbachol (carbamylcholine chloride, Carcholin, Doryl is a stable ester of choline which is not hydrolysed by cholinesterases. It possesses both the muscarinic and the nicotinic actions of acetylcholine but the muscarinic effects predominate. The effects of carbachol, which are both prolonged and intense, include, as would be expected, vasodilatation with increased skin blood flow and temperature and a subjective sensation of heat. There is increased secretion of saliva, sweat, tears and mucus; organs which contain smooth muscle (particularly the gastrointestinal tract, the ureters and the bladder) are stimulated. The last named actions may result in abdominal pain, diarrhoea and a persistent desire to urinate.

The therapeutic uses of carbachol and other choline esters are limited, since their actions can be more conveniently reproduced by anticholinesterase drugs (p. 219). Carbachol is sometimes employed to relieve urinary retention. For this purpose it is given by mouth (0.5 to 1 mg. two or three times daily) or by subcutaneous injection. By the last named route the dose is 0.25 to 0.5 mg. It is also occasionally used, alone or with an anticholinesterase, in the treatment of glaucoma (p. 225). For this purpose it is applied locally as a 1 to 1.5 per cent solution.

METHACHOLINE
Methacholine (acetyl-β-methylcholine, Amechol, Mecholyl) has the muscarinic activity of acetylcholine but it is almost devoid of nicotinic activity. It is slowly hydrolysed by acetylcholinesterase. The pharmacological effects of methacholine are those that would be expected of a compound with the properties of muscarine, but the cardiovascular effects (bradycardia and peripheral vasodilatation) are more pronounced than are the other signs of parasympathomimetic activity. Methacholine not only causes a more pronounced increase of peripheral blood flow than does carbachol but it may also cause cardiac arrhythmias—particularly heart block and atrial fibrillation—or cardiac arrest. These responses to methacholine are true muscarinic effects since they are prevented or abolished by atropine. Cardiac arrhythmias are particu-

larly likely to occur if methacholine is given to patients with thyrotoxicosis. Careful experiments reveal that methacholine has some ability to stimulate autonomic ganglia. This effect results from an action on the ganglionic muscarine receptors to which reference has already been made.

In the past, methacholine was used for the treatment of paroxysmal tachycardia but it is now only rarely employed for this purpose. Patients can often arrest attacks of paroxysmal tachycardia by manoeuvres, such as pressing on the carotid sinus, that increase vagal activity. Methacholine has the same effect as vagal stimulation and this is the basis of its antiarrhythmic action. However, as has been seen, the drug may itself produce cardiac arrhythmias and many better agents and procedures are now available.

Methacholine is still occasionally used to supplement the effect of anticholinesterases in the treatment of glaucoma. It also finds occasional application as a diagnostic agent. It causes the liberation of catecholamines from chromaffin tissue by an action analogous to that on sympathetic ganglia. In the normal subject the consequences of this are negligible but if a phaeochromocytoma (p. 274) is present there will be a sharp rise of blood pressure which overshadows and outlasts the hypotensive response. Methacholine has also been applied to the diagnosis of atropine poisoning. In this condition, injections of methacholine do not produce the parasympathomimetic effects which are otherwise so prominent. For diagnostic purposes methacholine is given, by subcutaneous injection, in doses of 20 mg.

BETHANECHOL

Bethanechol (ß-methylcholine carbamate) is a stable ester which is not hydrolysed by cholinesterase. It exerts a prolonged muscarinic action without evoking nicotine-like responses. Its properties, actions and uses are similar to those of carbachol, to which it is now preferred. Thus, it is used in the treatment of urinary retention and abdominal distension following surgery and in constipation arising as a consequence of vagotomy performed for the relief of peptic ulcer. The maximum oral dose is 30 mg., the subcutaneous dose is 5 mg. It is never given by intravenous injection.

PILOCARPINE

Pilocarpine is a liquid alkaloid obtained from the leaves (jaborandi leaves) of various species of *Pilocarpus*, a genus of trees and shrubs found in South and Central America and the West Indies. The natives of these countries have for long chewed the leaves to increase the flow of saliva.

Pilocarpine has a direct muscarine-like action on effector cells of the parasympathetic system. It does not possess significant nicotinic activity, but like methacholine, it causes some ganglionic stimulation by virtue of its action on the muscarine receptors in the ganglia. This effect is of little practical significance.

The most marked effects of pilocarpine are exerted on

Pilocarpine

the eye and on the exocrine glands. It causes profuse sweating and a copious secretion of saliva, bronchial mucus and gastric acid. In the last named respect it is as effective as histamine and the action may be partly a reflection of pilocarpine's chemical relationship with histamine. However, it shares none of the other actions of histamine.

Pilocarpine was formerly used as a *sialogogue* (an agent that promotes salivation) and a *diaphoretic* (an agent that promotes sweating) but the end sought by these means (the removal of oedema fluid) is now more effectively and comfortably achieved by diuretic agents (Chap. 36). The diaphoretic action of pilocarpine has, however, an interesting theoretical aspect. Denervation of a muscle or gland usually results in an increase in its sensitivity to the neurohumoral agent that activates it. This supersensitivity extends to related substances. Denervated sweat glands provide an exception to the general rule, for they lose their sensitivity to acetylcholine and to pilocarpine.

For therapeutic purposes, the use of pilocarpine is restricted to ophthalmological practice. The nitrate is employed as a 0.25 to 2.0 per cent. solution or as lamellae for application to the eye. It is a potent miotic with a prolonged action. It is used (usually in conjunction with an anticholinesterase) to reduce intraocular pressure in glaucoma and to abolish the mydriatic and cycloplegic actions of atropine and the ganglion blocking agents.

ARECOLINE

Arecoline is an alkaloid obtained from the areca or betel nut, the seed of *Areca catechu*. Like jaborandi leaves, betel nuts (which contain other active substances in addition to arecoline) are extensively chewed in the East to promote salivary secretion and to aid digestion.

Arecoline

Arecoline has muscarinic and weaker nicotinic properties. It has no therapeutic application in man but it is used as a vermifuge for dogs.

DEANOL

Deanol (2-dimethylaminoethanol; Deaner, Elevan) has been administered to schizophrenic patients with the aim of increasing the acetylcholine content of brain. It is reported to produce mild euphoria, central nervous system stimulation and a reduction of fatigue (Murphree, Jenney and Pfeiffer, 1959). These effects are reminiscent of those produced by amphetamine (Chap. 18). It has also been employed to treat mild mental depression. There is no evidence that deanol has any effect on the acetylcholine content of brain nor that the conditions for which deanol has been used are in any way due to acetylcholine deficiency. The essentially empirical nature of this treatment is underlined by the fact that, as a treatment for schizophrenia, atropine (which would be expected to have opposite central effects to deanol) has also had its adherents.

$$(CH_3)_2N.CH_2.CH_2.OH$$
Deanol

NICOTINE AND THE PHARMACOLOGY OF TOBACCO SMOKING

It will be clear from what has already been said that nicotine could claim classification as a ganglion or neuromuscular blocking agent, but the extent and intensity of the stimulant actions it produces in low doses justify its separate consideration as an acetylcholine-like excitatory substance.

Nicotine

Nicotine is a very poisonous alkaloid obtained from tobacco. The free base is a liquid but the alkaloid is usually met with as the hydrogen tartrate or sulphate. Pure nicotine is odourless but it decomposes on keeping, becoming dark brown in colour and taking on the characteristic smell of tobacco. As can be seen by reference to its formula, nicotine, a tertiary base, is a combination of pyridine and methylpyrrolidine.

Pharmacological properties
Although many of the actions of nicotine are explicable on the basis of its first stimulating and then depressing acetylcholine receptors in ganglia, striated muscle and the central nervous system, it has some other actions which necessitate a rather more detailed discussion of its pharmacology. It should be noted that, in the whole animal, the stimulant rather than the depressant effects of nicotine are most often in evidence. Even lethal doses of nicotine usually cause convulsions although these could arise (to use the neuropharmacologist's favourite escape route) from an inhibition of inhibitory systems. On the other hand, animals given nicotine sometimes collapse with complete muscle and respiratory paralysis.

Effects on the cardiovascular system
The effects of nicotine on the cardiovascular system are the resultant of a number of actions on the several components of the system, some mediated by the nervous system and some due to a direct action of nicotine.

Sympathetic and vagal ganglia are both stimulated. Since the vagus nerve generally exerts the greater control over the heart rate, the result of concurrent stimulation of both types of ganglia is normally cardiac slowing and nicotine would invariably cause bradycardia (or tachycardia when it reached a paralyzing concentration) if its cardiac effects were determined solely by its effects on autonomic ganglia, particularly since it also has a direct stimulant action on the vagus centre. Although nicotine does often cause bradycardia, tachycardia may occur as a result of the operation of other factors such as adrenaline release and a direct excitatory action of nicotine on cardiac muscle.

Stimulation of the sympathetic ganglia causes a widespread vasoconstriction which is augmented by adrenaline release and by the direct action of nicotine on the blood vessels and the vasomotor centre. Nicotine also stimulates the chemoreceptors of the carotid and aortic bodies. Although the effect of this stimulation is exerted primarily on respiration which is thereby stimulated, some stimulation of the cardioacceleratory and vasomotor centres also occurs. All these influences together cause the blood pressure to rise sharply.

Effects on the central nervous system
The stimulant action of nicotine on two medullary centres has already been mentioned. In addition, nicotine stimulates (and then paralyses) the respiratory centre, the vomiting centre and several hypothalamic centres. The nausea and autonomic distrubances which reward the young boy's first attempt to smoke a cigarette are manifestations of his autonomic responses to nicotine. Among the hypothalamic centres that are stimulated by nicotine is the supraoptic nucleus, stimulation of which causes the liberation of the antidiuretic hormone from the posterior lobe of the pituitary gland. This effect can readily be demonstrated if two subjects drink a large volume of water and one of them (preferably a non-smoker) also smokes a cigarette. The time at which maximum diuresis occurs will be found to be considerably later in the subject who has smoked. It is also possible that nicotine stimulates the satiety centre (p. 162) and this may explain why those who give up smoking tend to put on weight. This is not to suggest that smoking should be used as a way of arresting the development of obesity since this would simply involve the exchange of one suicide weapon for another.

It is important to appreciate the fact that nicotine does not exert its effects on the brain entirely as a result of stimulating nicotine receptors although these structures certainly exist in the central nervous system. Nicotine releases acetylcholine from cholinergic neurones and the released transmitter will, of course, be able to stimulate both muscarinic and nicotinic receptors. Consequently the apparently anomalous situation can arise of some of the central actions of nicotine being blocked by atropine. Some authorities maintain that all the effects of nicotine on the brain are the result of acetylcholine release.

Nicotine is a powerful convulsant agent. In experimental animals, the intraperitoneal injection of doses of nicotine of the order of 15 mg per kilogram rapidly produces powerful and generalized convulsions.

Effects on the neuromuscular system
It has already been pointed out that injections of nicotine (or of large doses of acetylcholine in atropinized animals) cause fibrillatory twitching of muscles. Larger doses may cause paralysis. When respiratory failure occurs as a direct result of nicotine administration, this is due partly to inhibition of the respiratory centre and partly to blockade at the neuromuscular junctions of the respiratory muscles.

Other effects
In the gut, stimulation of the intramural intestinal parasympathetic ganglia causes a marked increase in muscle tone and in peristaltic movements. Nicotine also causes contractions of the smooth muscle of the bladder and the uterus, probably because of stimulation of parasympathetic ganglia. Nicotine increases the secretion of saliva, sweat and bronchial mucus. The pupil is constricted, due partly to a direct action of nicotine on the constrictor muscle. All these effects are reversed by higher doses of the drug.

USES OF NICOTINE
Nicotine stimulates acetylcholine receptors on subsynaptic membranes but it has no action on other parts of the neurone. The application of nicotine to a ganglion containing synapses will therefore be followed by stimulation of structures innervated by nerves proceeding from the ganglion. If the ganglion (like those of the dorsal roots) is one which contains no synapses, the application of nicotine will have no effect on the structures with which the ganglion is connected. Langley made use of these facts as long ago as 1889 in his classical work that mapped the positions of autonomic ganglia in the body.

Nicotine is used as an insecticide and its convulsant action makes it a useful laboratory tool for investigating the mechanisms and sequelae of convulsive activity.

The extent to which nicotine is responsible for the subjective effects of tobacco smoking is discussed below.

The pharmacology of tobacco smoking
Smoking is one of the most ancient and widespread of man's activities, although Europeans had to discover America before they could savour the delights of tobacco.

Nornicotine

Lobeline

Many governments have capitalized on the attractions of tobacco by subjecting it to heavy taxation but neither the expense nor the certain knowledge that smoking is a major hazard to health prevents more than a relatively small number of people from succumbing to the smoking habit.

The fact that smoking is so compulsive suggests that tobacco, like alcohol and caffeine, satisfies a real need in many people. Some of the pleasure derived from smoking is due to the soothing effect of sucking a cigar, a cigarette or a pipe stem, to the ritual associated with selecting and lighting one's smoke and to the sight and smell of the smoke itself. However, there can now be little doubt that it is the nicotine in tobacco which is responsible for the major part of the immediate effects of smoking: injections of nicotine will still the longing for tobacco in heavy smokers deprived of their cigarettes and those who cannot, or do not wish to, smoke may chew tobacco or take it in the form of snuff. That man's craving is for a nicotine-like substance rather than for tobacco itself is further indicated by the fact that Australian aborigines learned long ago to chew the leaves of the pituri plant which contains nornicotine. Indian 'tobacco' (*Lobelia inflata*) contains lobeline, a compound which has nicotine-like properties. It was used in the past as a respiratory stimulant; because it is likely to cause nausea and vomiting it has also been used in attempts to produce a conditioned aversion to tobacco.

Animal experiments (Armitage, Hall and Morrison, 1968) have shed some light on the way in which smoking may bring about its psychological effects in man. In these experiments it was demonstrated that the intravenous injection of small doses of nicotine caused a marked stimulation of lever pressing activity in thirsty rats that had been trained to press the lever in order to obtain water. The dose of nicotine used (2 μg. per kilogram every 30 seconds for 20 minutes) was similar to that obtained by a man who slowly smokes two cigarettes in succession. The period of stimulation outlasted the period of nicotine administration by about an hour. When the same total dose of nicotine was given according to a different time schedule—4 μg. per kilogram every 60 seconds or 1 μg. per kilogram every 15 seconds—there was a tendency for the lever pressing activity to be reduced. These latter dose schedules reproduce the effects of smoking a cigarette by large deep inhalations or by the short sharp puffs of the nervous smoker. Experiments on cats produced even more striking results. In lightly anaesthetized animals, nicotine, given according to the dose schedule that produced stimulation in rats, caused activation of the electroencephalogram. At the same time the release of acetylcholine from the cortex was increased. As in the rat experiments, when the individual doses of nicotine were increased there was a tendency for the cortical activity and acetylcholine output to be reduced.

People sometimes smoke in order to stimulate mental activity; on other occasions they may wish to reduce nervous tension. The work just described indicates a possible way by which nicotine may bring about both these effects; taken in a number of small doses, as in the quiet smoking of the student or writer, it may have an essentially stimulant action, particularly if the prevailing circumstances (lateness of the hour, quiet surroundings, etc.) are otherwise such as to tend to cause drowsiness. On the other hand, if the cigarette is smoked quickly or if deep inhalations are taken, the nicotine may have a tranquillizing effect, particularly if the circumstances (an impending examination or interview) are otherwise such as to tend to stimulate nervous activity. Armitage, Hall and Morrison point out that the cigarette is an ideal device for delivering nicotine in doses which can be varied as required: 'It is worth noting that someone smoking a cigarette has literally finger tip control of how much nicotine he takes into his mouth; by reducing the puff volume or inhaling less frequently, he absorbs less nicotine.' Fine control of this type is not so readily produced in pipes and this may explain why pipes make little appeal to those who need tobacco to 'calm their nerves'. Pipes are attractive to the placid and contented individual who may need only the slight mental stimulation induced by the small amounts of nicotine gained by the contemplative puffing of a slowly burning bowl of fragrant tobacco mixture.

Kersbaum (1968) has pointed out that the nicotine absorbed from tobacco smoke is sufficient to augment the secretion of adrenocorticotrophic hormone (ACTH) by some 50 per cent. over its resting level and he suggests that because of this, smoking in times of stress increases the ability of the organism to adapt to the abnormal situation. This does not seem to provide a very adequate reason for the wide adoption of the smoking habit since it seems to assume that ACTH can calm the anxious mind and that, in the absence of nicotine, its secretion is not accurately geared to the intensity of the stress.

Although considerations such as the foregoing may serve to show that tobacco smoking helps to maintain and regulate central nervous activity, it has to be remembered that, however beneficial it might be to the mind, tobacco is certainly poison for the body. Present day emphasis on the now established relationship between cigarette smoking and carcinoma of the lung may tend to obscure the fact that tobacco has other toxic actions. It may cause bronchitis and the cardiovascular system is also very vulnerable. Smoking may cause cardiac extrasystoles (Chap. 40) or anginal pains. More serious effects may be seen in the blood vessels. The vasoconstriction produced by the continued inhalation of nicotine imposes an additional load on the heart and smoking should be avoided by those with coronary arterial disease, heart failure or peripheral vascular disorders. It seems probable, indeed, that the taking of nicotine actually encourages the development of cardiovascular disease. Those who are already predisposed to these conditions by reason of other circumstances (such as a sedentary occupation, obesity and occupational stress) should limit or abandon their smoking.

Tobacco amblyopia is a condition of partial or total blindness which arises from atrophy of optic nerve fibres. It occurs among those who smoke heavily for a long period of time. Early warning signs of the condition include dimness of vision and defects of accommodation.

A considerable degree of tolerance to the effects of tobacco occurs in the regular smoker. Those not accustomed to smoking may find that it causes nausea, vomiting, giddiness, tremors, sweating and disturbances of cardiac rhythm. The same symptoms are sometimes experienced by tobacco workers but they disappear rapidly when exposure to tobacco ceases.

Some of the toxic effects of tobacco (particularly those affecting the cardiovascular and nervous systems) are probably due to nicotine. Others (notably carcinoma of the lung, which seems to constitute a hazard only for cigarette smokers) are not.

THE DETECTION AND ESTIMATION OF ACETYLCHOLINE

Many investigations demand estimations of the acetylcholine content of tissue extracts, exudates, perfusates or incubates. A number of biological preparations are available for this purpose. Those which do not respond selectively to acetylcholine may be made insensitive to other substances by appropriate antagonists, or the extracts can be made in such a way as to exclude substances that might otherwise interfere with the determination. In general, these manoeuvres do not exclude or annul the effects of other choline esters but it is usually assumed that all the acetylcholine-like activity that is being assayed is in fact caused by acetylcholine. The extent to which this assumption is justified is discussed below.

The most suitable biological preparations for the quantitative estimation of acetylcholine are as follows. Practical details can be found in reviews (Lewis and Waton, 1958; Crossland, 1961) and in the original papers referred to there and in the following paragraphs.

Leech muscle
The isolated, physostigminized longitudinal dorsal muscle of the medicinal leech (*Hirudo medicinalis*) is one of the oldest established preparations. If the muscle is used in a

microbath of the type developed by Gaddum (Chap. 11) it can be used to estimate as little as 25 to 100 picograms (1 pg.= 10^{-12} gram) of acetylcholine (Szerb, 1961).

The frog rectus preparation

The isolated physostigminized rectus abdominis muscle of the frog is less sensitive than the leech but it is a very suitable preparation if the sample being assayed provides at least 1 μg of acetylcholine. A properly sensitized rectus muscle in a bath of 4 ml capacity will usually respond to doses of acetylcholine as small as 0.05 μg.

The rectus abdominis is a striated muscle but it responds to acetylcholine with a slow and dose dependent contraction (a *contracture*) and not by a twitch. Contractures are usually only obtained from chronically denervated muscles; the rectus muscle of the frog is the only muscle which responds in this way without previous denervation.

The rectus muscle (and in some circumstances the leech muscle, too) is affected by material present in some tissue extracts. This material does not itself cause the rectus to contract but it sensitizes the muscle to acetylcholine. Thus a tissue extract which contains acetylcholine may cause a bigger contraction of the muscle than will the same amount of acetylcholine in the absence of extract. Consequently, if attempts are made to assay the acetylcholine content of one extract by comparing its effects on the rectus with those produced by standard solutions of acetylcholine, too high an estimate of the acetylcholine content may be obtained. Brain extracts may contain large amounts of sensitizing material which, if ignored, may result in the acetylcholine content of the extracts being overestimated to the extent of 50 to 60 per cent. It is usual to counter the effect of the sensitizing substances by means of a manoeuvre suggested originally by Feldberg. The extract to be assayed is divided into two portions. The acetylcholine in one of the two portions is destroyed by brief boiling in alkali. It is assumed that this treatment does not affect the activity of the sensitizing material. In conducting the assay, the contractions produced by suitable amounts of the tissue extract are compared with those produced by known doses of acetylcholine to which have been added amounts of acetylcholine-free extract equivalent to those in the acetylcholine-containing samples being added to the bath for assay. A disadvantage of having to correct in the way described for the presence of sensitizing substances is that half the extract has to be used in the preparation of the acetylcholine-free solution.

The possibility of sensitizing material affecting other assay preparations should always be borne in mind when acetylcholine assays are being performed, particularly if the extract has been obtained from an unusual source, if it has been prepared by an unusual method or if the assay preparation is a novel one.

Isolated mollusc heart

The isolated heart of the bivalve mollusc *Venus mercenaria* (the clam) is sensitive to acetylcholine which inhibits the cardiac contractions. This provides the basis of a cheap and easily handled bioassay preparation. Other marine invertebrates have been used in the same way.

The guinea pig ileum

The methods so far described measure the nicotinic actions of acetylcholine. The remaining methods assay the acetylcholine by measuring its muscarinic actions. Acetylcholine causes contraction of the longitudinal muscle of the guinea pig ileum and this effect can be made the basis of a bioassay procedure. It has the advantage of being a cheap, convenient and simple preparation which is familiar (sometimes too familiar) to all pharmacologists. It is not selective in its response but the effect of other substances in the extracts can be eliminated. Treatment of the preparation with mepyramine maleate and tryptamine will render it insensitive to histamine and 5-hydroxytryptamine respectively. Some tissues contain substance P (Chap. 22). This is removed from the extracts before assay by incubation with chymotrypsin (Toru and Aprison, 1966). It is a sensible precaution when using this method to confirm, by demonstrating its abolition by atropine, that all the biological activity which has been measured is in fact due to acetylcholine—or, to be more precise (see below), to a substance with muscarine-like activity.

Some workers have been able to detect as little as one picogram of acetylcholine by using the guinea pig ileum.

Blood pressure

The hypotensive action of acetylcholine can be used as a bioassay method. If the anaesthetized cat is used, the animal should ideally be eviscerated, sympathectomized and adrenalectomized. By these means the blood pressure is stabilized, the preparation becomes more sensitive and reproducible responses are obtained. The operative procedures required for producing this highly sensitive preparation may prove formidable to the inexperienced. More recently, the rat blood pressure has replaced that of the cat (Straughan, 1958).

Chemical methods of assay

It is often said that bioassays are tedious, time consuming, unspecific and inferior to chemical methods which, it is thereby implied, are simple, speedy and specific. This is certainly so for some substances (histamine and the monoamines for instance) but chemical methods for the assay of acetylcholine still leave something to be desired and the reader should not be too ready to assume that all the methods that are available offer all the advantages that are sanguinely expected of chemical assays in general. Many of them demand the use of very costly apparatus, some do not have the sensitivity of the best bioassay methods, the chemical manipulations that are needed to convert acetyl-choline into an assayable product may be critically dependent on the maintenance of rigorous—and not always clearly defined—experimental conditions and there is always the danger that active material may be lost (or contaminants introduced) during one or more of the several steps of the conversion process. It should also be remembered that a method which is perfectly satisfactory for the determination of acetylcholine in simple solution may be far from adequate when it is applied to such a chemically complex mixture as a brain extract. The foregoing must not be taken as a blanket condemnation of chemical methods of acetylcholine assay. It is intended simply as a warning that, imperfect though bioassays may be, chemical methods have their drawbacks too. Those who have mastered bioassay techniques for acetylcholine should pause before moving from the pharmacology to the chemistry laboratory.

As long ago as 1949, Hestrin developed a chemical method for assaying acetylcholine. It was based on the fact that the ester reacts with hydroxylamine to give acetylhy-droxamic acid which can be converted by ferric chloride into a compound that Hestrin measured colorimetrically. In its original form, the method was too insensitive to attract widespread popularity but recent modifications have made it more acceptable. In the version developed by Maslova, the excess iron left after the coloured complex has been formed is estimated by polarographic analysis while Schumacher and Ehl isolate the acetylcholine by paper chromatography, develop the paper with hydroxyl-amine and ferric chloride and measure the amount of colour by densitometric analysis. Fluorimetric techniques have also been used: the fluorimetric compound produced in Fellman's method is acetylhydrazyl salicylhydrazone while O'Neill and Sakamato make use of reduced nicotin-amide adenine dinucleotide measuring the amount that is produced in a system in which acetate (derived from the acetylcholine that is to be assayed) is converted into acetylcoenzyme A under the influence of acetylcoenzyme A synthetase in the presence of (among other substances) the oxidised dinucleotide which is, of course, reduced in the process. Other workers prefer to combine enzymatic with radioassay methods: Reid & Haubrich employ cho-line kinase to produce radioactive phosphorylcholine from labelled ATP and choline derived from the acetylcholine that is to be assayed. Alternatively the choline can be converted into labelled acetylcholine by incubation with choline acetyltransferase and labelled acetylcoenzyme A

Acetylhydrazyl
salicylhydrazone

according to the method of Aprison. Gas chromatography has given some very encouraging results and several groups of workers have developed assay methods based on this technique. The acetylcholine has necessarily to be converted into a volatile derivative and one of the most popular is that produced by removing one of the methyl groups from the quaternary nitrogen atom of acetylcho-line. Jenden employs benzenethiolate for this purpose but an alternative method is that developed by Green and his colleagues in which demethylation is achieved by pyrolysis at a temperature of 450°. This last method has considerable promise.

In a recent laboratory manual (Hanin, 1974) to which the interested reader is referred, a number of authors (including all those mentioned in the foregoing paragraph) critically assess the chemical assay methods they recommend or have developed and they provide detailed instructions for carrying them out.

The origin of the acetylcholine-like activity of tissue extracts

It is an easy matter to demonstrate that the biological activity revealed by bioassay preparations of the type described is due to a substance, or substances, with acetyl-choline-like properties. Suitably treated, the test tissues respond selectively to substances which act on acetylcho-line receptors and confirmation of the nature of the active material in tissue extracts can be obtained by demonstrating its destruction by cholinesterase (p. 211) and the abolition of its effect when the test preparation is treated with curare or atropine, whichever is appropriate. Moreover, there is no doubt at all that many tissues do contain acetylcholine since it can be isolated and identified in a chemically pure form. It is less easy to be certain that no substance other than acetylcholine contributes to the total acetylcholine-like activity in tissue extracts.

Chang and Gaddum (1933) reported the occurrence of acetylcholine-like activity in extracts of a number of organs including the brain, blood, spleen, placenta, heart and intestine. Using the technique of parallel assay which is described below, they provided evidence that the activity of intestinal extracts was probably due only to acetylcho-line and it has been rather generally assumed by later workers that this conclusion extends to extracts of other tissues. Although this conclusion is clearly not necessarily valid, it was not seriously questioned even after the clear demonstration that propionylcholine is present in extracts of ox spleen (p. 210). Until recently the only other attempt to establish the identity of acetylcholine was that of Dale and Feldberg (1934) who showed that the material liberated in the heart of a dog during stimulation of the vagus was certainly acetylcholine. Some workers, however, notably Hosein and his collaborators (see, for instance, Hosein et al., 1965) attempted to demonstrate, by chemical means, the existence of acetylcholine-like material in addition to acetylcholine itself in tissue extracts. A more careful inspection of the pharmacological properties of tissue extracts was therefore indicated and a number of workers applied themselves to this problem, with particular reference to nervous tissue.

The method of pharmacological analysis used is best understood by considering a simple example. Propionylcholine, it will be recalled, has powerful nicotinic activity but relatively little muscarinic activity. Let us suppose that a hypothetical tissue extract contained only propionylcholine. An investigator, assuming that the biological activity was due, in fact, to acetylcholine could determine the 'acetylcholine' content of the extract by assaying it against acetylcholine, using any of the available methods. If he chose the frog rectus preparation, he would conclude that the acetylcholine content of the extract was quite high. If he used the guinea pig ileum, he would conclude that the acetylcholine content of the extract was very low. If he examined the extract by both methods, he would be able to assert that the extract contained active material other than, or in addition to, acetylcholine. As a generalization, then, it can be said that if the same estimate of the acetylcholine content of a tissue extract is given when it is assayed on two, or preferably more, preparations it is reasonable to conclude that the activity is indeed due to acetylcholine. It is possible that an individual compound may have the same activity as acetylcholine on more than one preparation and in order to avoid the possibility that the preparations chosen for the parallel assays might be incapable of distinguishing between acetylcholine and some other substance it is clearly desirable to examine the extracts on as many preparations as possible.

The method just described considered the case of a tissue extract containing only one substance but it will also detect the presence of material other than acetylcholine, even when considerable quantities of acetylcholine are also present. This is illustrated by the figures given in Table 14.1 which are taken from the results of an experiment performed in the author's laboratory.

The examples so far quoted have considered the situation when propionylcholine is present. In practice, propionylcholine would be detected quite readily because the relative intensity of its nicotinic and muscarinic activities is so different from that of acetylcholine that the frog rectus and the ileum preparations differentiate easily between the two esters. The detection of material with a spectrum of pharmacological activity closer to that of acetylcholine would be more difficult, particularly if it were present in small quantities. It is also important to note that the method of parallel assay as described does not in itself permit the identification of the material present in a tissue extract : it only reveals whether or not it is all acetylcholine. Identification of any other substance whose presence is so revealed constitutes another problem. It may be possible to isolate the individual active components by chromatography or by other separation techniques and then to examine each component by appropriate pharmacological and chemical methods but the tactics to be used depend on the circumstances and they cannot be discussed in detail here. It should, however, be added that, once the components of the mixture are identified, each can be quantitatively determined by assaying the mixture against standard solutions of the identified components on a number of preparations. This technique of *differential bioassay* was adopted by Banister, Whittaker and Wijesundera (1953) for the determination of acetylcholine and propionylcholine in extracts of spleen.

Table 14.1 Detection of propionylcholine in the presence of acetylcholine

Percentage of Propionylcholine	Rectus Assay Ileum Assay
0	1.00
5	1.05
10	1.13
20	1.30
50	2.28

Mixtures of acetylcholine and propionylcholine were assayed against acetylcholine. The figures show a disparity between the rectus and ileum assay when propionylcholine formed more than about 10 per cent of the mixture

Studies which involved parallel bioassays (Szerb, 1963; Crossland and Redfern, 1963) indicated that the acetylcholine-like activity of brain extracts is caused, after all, entirely by acetylcholine notwithstanding the neglect of earlier workers to establish this point and the contrary evidence adduced by Hosein. The conclusion reached from the biological studies received confirmation from a chemical investigation. Using a combined gas chromatography and mass spectrometry technique, Holmstedt and his colleagues (Hammar et al., 1968) were able to demonstrate that the only choline ester present in extracts of fresh rat brain was acetylcholine. The presence of propionylcholine and butyrylcholine was positively excluded. These findings not only disposed of an argument that had persisted for a decade but they also established the fact that brain extracts contain neither of the substances which might interfere with the fluorimetric determination of acetylcholine.

The situation in peripheral nerve is less clear. Carlini and Green (1963) obtained evidence that material other than acetylcholine was present in extracts of sciatic nerve but Crossland and Slater reached the opposite conclusion.

The results of none of the experiments described in the foregoing paragraphs absolves the pharmacologist from making a careful study of his own tissue extracts (particularly if they come from an unusual source) before he asserts that they contain only acetylcholine.

Table 14.2 Characterization of the cholinesterases

	Erythrocyte Cholinesterase e-cholinesterase	Serum Cholinesterase s-cholinesterase
Other Names	Cholinesterase I 'True' cholinesterase Acetylcholinesterase Acetocholinesterase Specific cholinesterase	Cholinesterase II 'Pseudo' cholinesterase Butyrocholinesterase ('Unspecified' or 'unspecific' cholinesterase)
Substrate specificity	Generally most active against acetate esters	Generally most active against butyrate esters
Activity against: acetylcholine	+	+
acetyl-ß-methylcholine	+	–
benzoylcholine	–	+
Present in high concentration in:	Brain	Cardiac and smooth muscle
	Striated muscle Erythrocytes	Glands: pancreas, mammary glands and (some species) salivary glands Skin Serum

CHOLINESTERASES

The observation that the pharmacological actions of acetylcholine are very short lived led Dale to suggest, as long ago as 1914, that acetylcholine was destroyed in the blood and other tissues by an enzyme. Ample evidence was forthcoming to support Dale's proposition and the name cholinesterase was given to what was at that time thought to be a single enzyme. However, in 1940 Alles and Hawkes found that the cholinesterase of erythrocytes differed from that in serum. The two enzymes were called e (for erythrocyte)-cholinesterase and s (for serum)-cholinesterase. Since then the actions of the enzymes have been studied in considerable detail and a number of other names (Table 14.2) have become attached to them.

The cholinesterase of erythrocytes was found to be very active against low concentrations (up to 0.003M) of acetylcholine and to be inhibited at higher substrate concentrations. The rate of hydrolysis of small amounts of acetylcholine by serum cholinesterase is, on the other hand, very low but it increases progressively as the substrate concentration is increased. Serum cholinesterase hydrolyses propionylcholine and butyrylcholine more rapidly than it inactivates acetylcholine. For this reason, serum cholinesterase became known as 'pseudo' cholinesterase and the erythrocyte enzyme as 'true' cholinesterase. This nomenclature was unfortunate (it is now obsolescent)

since, whatever its physiological substrate may be, 'pseudo' cholinesterase is as real an enzyme as any other and it is capable of destroying choline esters.

The cholinesterases are not very selective enzymes: both types hydrolyse a large number of esters both of choline and of other carboxylic acids. Erythrocyte cholinesterase is particularly active towards acetate esters (especially acetylcholine itself) while serum cholinesterase preferentially hydrolyses butyrate esters. This has led to the proposal that the enzymes should be named acetylcholinesterase and butyrocholinesterase respectively and this terminology is employed in this book. 'Cholinesterase', standing alone, is used when a property or an action common to both types of enzyme is under discussion. Acetylcholinesterase hydrolyses acetylcholine and acetyl-ß-methylcholine but not benzoylcholine. Butyrocholinesterase hydrolyses acetylcholine and benzoylcholine but not acetyl-ß-methylcholine. The use of these three substrates enables the enzymes to be identified, particularized and quantitatively estimated in tissue extracts.

The cholinesterases in different species, and even in different members of the same species, are not necessarily identical. This is particularly so among the butyrocholinesterases, individual variations in which account for abnormally prolonged (or unusually brief) responses to succinylcholine, a muscle relaxant (p. 243). Among animals, an esterase in guinea pig liver and kidney hydrolyses benzoylcholine but not acetylcholine and pig serum contains an enzyme that hydrolyses acetylcholine but not benzoylcholine. Rabbit plasma contains a benzoylcholinesterase which is probably identical with atropine esterase (p. 228), an enzyme unique to this species.

A number of other serum esterases share some of the properties of the cholinesterases. The aliesterases, which hydrolyse alkyl esters (but not choline esters) are, like the cholinesterases, inhibited by organophosphorus compounds but they are not affected by other types of cholinesterase inhibitors. The arylesterases are not inhibited by any of the anticholinesterase agents.

The functions of the cholinesterases are not yet completely understood although there seems to be no doubt that the physiological substrate of acetylcholinesterase is acetylcholine itself. The role of the enzyme in transmission is fully discussed in Chapter 13. It is not clear what is the usual substrate for butyrocholinesterase. In some situations it is likely to be acetylcholine. The rhythmical contractions of smooth and cardiac muscle, for instance, which can occur independently of their nerve supply, are probably maintained by acetylcholine but the enzyme at these sites is butyrocholinesterase. There is a general tendency, too, for butyrocholinesterase to be located in tissues innervated by the parasympathetic nervous system. At the same time, it will be recalled that propionylcholine occurs in the spleen of some mammalian species. If the function of the ester in that organ involves its own destruction, this is presumably effected by butyrocholinesterase.

Cholinesterases occur in some situations (the red cell membrane, the placenta, etc.) where it is difficult to relate their function to the destruction of acetylcholine or other choline esters and they may have quite independent actions. Possibilities which have been suggested include the control of membrane permeability and of the blood level of fatty substances such as cholesterol.

Figure 14.2 attempts to summarize the most generally accepted current views concerning the nature of cholinesterase and the mechanism of acetylcholine hydrolysis. The enzyme has two binding sites: an anionic site to which the cationic head of acetylcholine can be attached and a site which accepts the ester group of the molecule. The last named site itself carries both basic (anionic) and acidic (cationic) groups that bind the carbon and the carbonyl atoms respectively. So far as activity at the esteratic site is concerned, binding to the basic area seems to be the primary event.

Consideration of the structure and physico-chemical properties of a large number of substrates and inhibitors suggests that the separations between the anionic site and the anionic and cationic heads of the esteratic site are about 0.25 nm and 0.5 nm respectively. Some authorites believe that acetylcholinesterase may carry two anionic sites for each esteratic site and that butyrocholinesterase possesses the two sites in equal numbers. An alternative proposition

$$H_3C-\overset{\overset{\displaystyle CH_3}{|}}{\underset{\underset{\displaystyle CH_2-CH_2-O-C=O}{}}{C}}-\overset{\displaystyle CH_3}{}$$

γ,γ -dimethyl butyl acetate

is that the non-esteratic site is different in nature from the anionic site of acetylcholinesterase.

Some progress has been made towards an elucidation of the molecular structure of cholinesterase and there is good evidence that, at the esteratic site, the hydroxyl group of serine and the imidazole nitrogen of histidine provide the required basic area while the cationic spots may be contributed by the hydroxyl groups of tyrosine. The negative charges at the anionic site proper may come from glutamic or another dicarboxylic acid.

It seems that the esteratic site is the portion of the cholinesterase molecule that is primarily concerned with acetylcholine hydrolysis since γ,γ. dimethyl butyl acetate, a compound in which the quaternary nitrogen atom of acetylcholine has been replaced by carbon, is as rapidly hydrolysed by cholinesterase as is acetylcholine itself.

When the enzyme-substrate complex (Fig. 14.2) has been formed the acetylcholine molecule is 'pulled apart', perhaps because the distance between the binding sites on the enzyme is somewhat greater than the corresponding distance in the acetylcholine molecule. Choline is liberated first so that for a brief period of time the enzyme is acetylated. Liberation of acetic acid restores the enzyme to its active form.

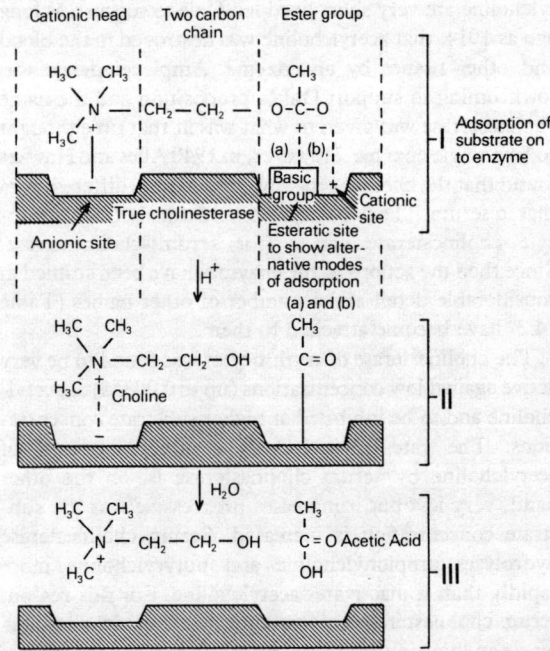

Fig. 14.2. Hydrolysis of acetylcholine by acetylcholinesterase.

ANTICHOLINESTERASES

The anticholinesterases inhibit the enzymatic hydrolysis of acetylcholine which consequently accumulates in the body so that its actions at effector sites are prolonged and intensified. It is convenient to classify the anticholinesterases into those such as physostigmine (eserine) and its analogues which interact reversibly with cholinesterase and the so-called 'irreversible inhibitors' such as the organophosphorus compounds which form a much more stable combination with the enzyme. Many anticholinesterase agents are themselves broken down by the enzyme so their inhibitory effect slowly declines even in the absence of other factors that might promote the reactivation of the enzyme. Esters such as neostigmine and physostigmine are particularly susceptible to hydrolysis in this way. Some authorities prefer to include among the irreversible inhibitors all those compounds that undergo hydrolysis by cholinesterase. On this basis the carbamates (physostigmine and related compounds, see below) would have to be classified with the organophosphorus compounds although the two groups of compounds are broken down at very different rates. Only a few compounds (edrophonium for one) would then be left in the reversible category. Except to a chemical purist, this change of terminology has little to recommend it and there are several sound reasons for adhering to the old terminology.

Anticholinesterases may react with the anionic site, the esteratic site or both sites of the enzyme. Thus, the quaternary ammonium salts are adsorbed on to the anionic site, the organophosphorus compounds are adsorbed on to the esteratic site and neostigmine and physostigmine interact with both sites.

The pharmacological actions of the anticholinesterase compounds as a group are discussed after the individual compounds have been catalogued.

Reversible inhibitors of cholinesterase

PHYSOSTIGMINE (ESERINE)

The first anticholinesterase to be recognized, identified and used clinically was physostigmine. Some aspects of its history are mentioned in Chapter 1 where reference is made to the work of Christison and of Fraser, Britain's pioneer pharmacologists, and to their work with the calabar bean. Christison has left a vivid account of the effects produced in himself by ingestion of the bean (in 1855) and Fraser isolated and purified the active principle of the bean in 1870. Jobst and Hesse had achieved its isolation some years earlier but Fraser was apparently unaware of their work. The name physostigmine (from the botanical name of the calabar bean, *Physostigma venenosum*) was given to the active principle by Jobst and Hesse; the alternative name, eserine, owes its origin to the fact that the calabar bean was also known as the bean (or nut) of Etu

Esére. The structure of physostigmine (Fig. 14.3) was elucidated by Stedman and Barger in 1925. Stedman believed that the anticholinesterase activity of physostigmine was attributable to the presence of the phenyl carbamate residue and not to the two nitrogen-containing (pyrollidine) rings.

It is now known that the possession of the phenyl carbamate moiety is not a necessary prerequisite for anticholinesterase activity, which can be demonstrated in simple tetra-alkylammonium salts, in compounds like hexamethonium and decamethonium (Chap. 16) and in some other compounds. Nevertheless, Stedman's hypothesis proved to be most fruitful for it led to the production of the first two synthetic anticholinesterases. These were neostigmine (Prostigmine) and miotine. Their chemical formulae (which should be compared with that of physostigmine) are displayed in Figure 14.3.

A large number of neostigmine derivatives and analogues with anticholinesterase activity have also been prepared. The names and formulae of some of them are given in Figure 14.3.

The presence of a quaternary nitrogen atom, while not essential for anticholinesterase activity, does confer increased potency on the molecule. Thus neostigmine, which has a quaternary nitrogen atom, is a more powerful anticholinesterase agent than either physostigmine or miotine, both of which are tertiary bases. The size and nature of the groups on the quaternary or tertiary atom are important.

A number of bisneostigmines also exhibit anticholinesterase activity. The examples shown in Figure 14.3 illustrate the fact, in partial vindication of the original Stedman hypothesis, that, in some compounds at least, the possession of a phenyl carbamate moiety increases anticholinesterase activity. The compound 3113CT is more than a hundred times as active as neostigmine itself. Demecarium is an interesting member of this group. It has a long-lasting action and finds some application in ophthalmology.

The bisneostigmines are bisquaternary compounds and some other substances of this type also possess anticholinesterase activity. Examples are given in Figure 14.3. An interesting feature of benzoquinonium and the oxamides (ambenonium and methoxyambenonium) is that they show both curare-like and neuromuscular facilitatory as well an anticholinesterase activity. Benzoquinonium indeed has been employed clinically as a neuromuscular blocking agent but it is no longer used in this way, largely because of the complications introduced by its other properties.

Many of the compounds so far discussed are active against both acetyl- and butyrocholinesterase. However, the bisquaternary compounds tend to be much more active against acetylcholinesterase. This is particularly so in the case of the oxamides, supporting the view that acetylcholinesterase may have two anionic sites separated by a

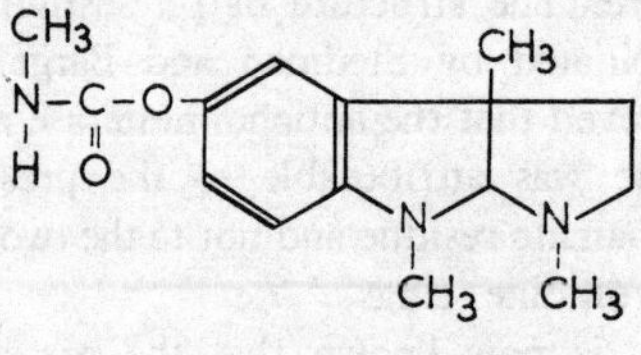

Physostigmine (eserine)

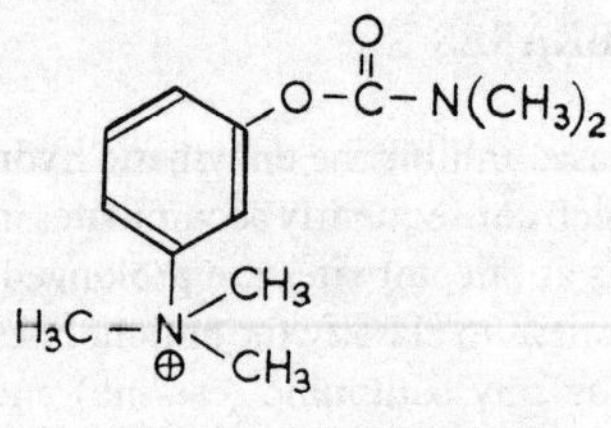

Neostigmine (Prostigmin)

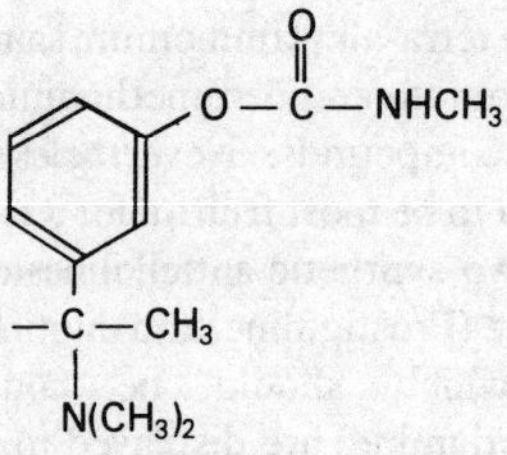

Miotine

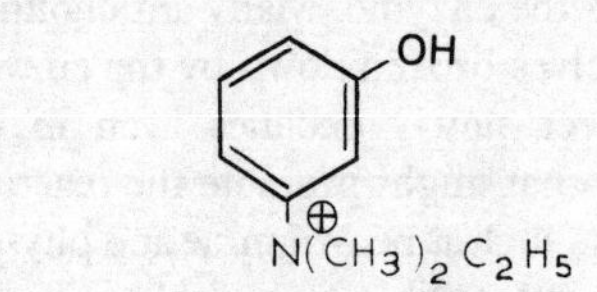

Edrophonium (Tensilion)

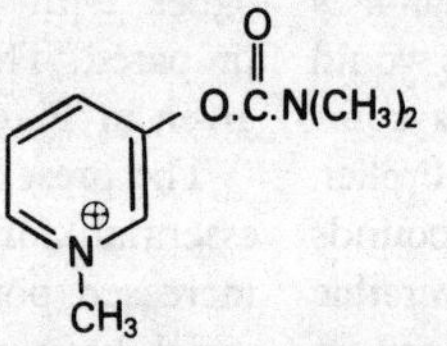

Pyridostigmine (Mestinon)

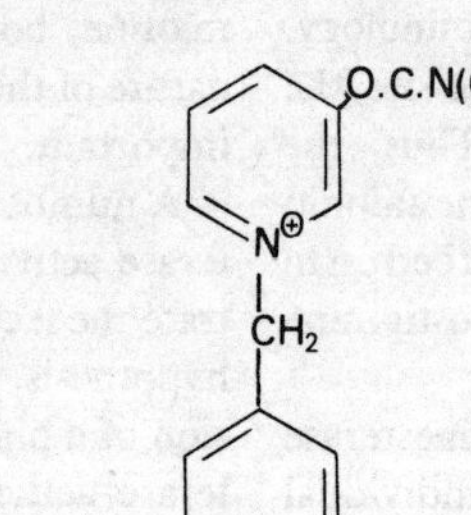

Benzpyrinium (Stigmonene)

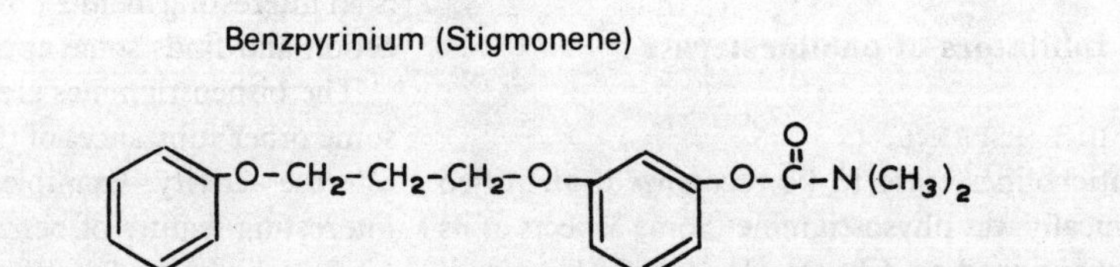

Potency = 10⁸

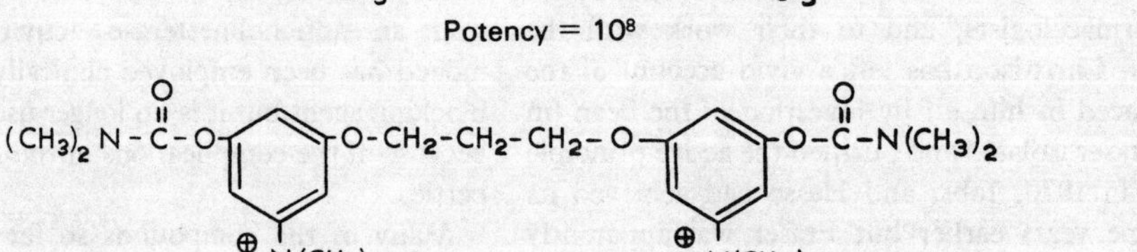

Potency = 10⁶
3113 CT

Fig. 14.3 Some reversible inhibitors of cholinesterase.

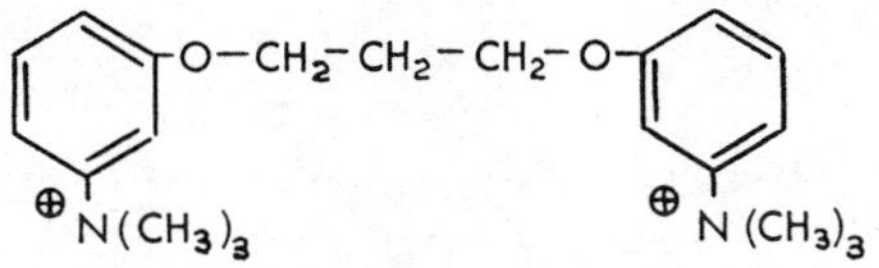

Potency = 1

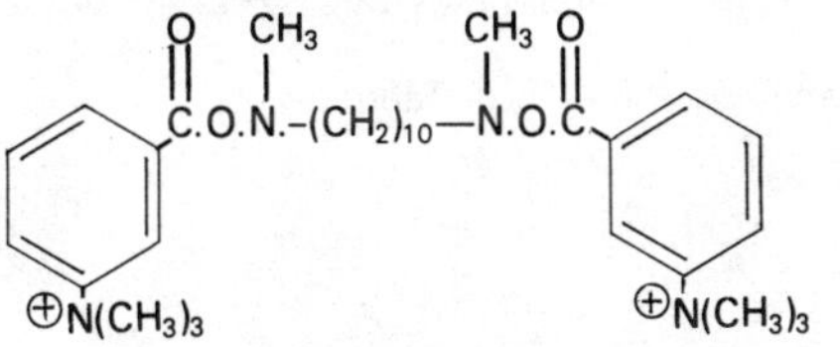

Demecarium (Humorsol)

Bisneostigmines

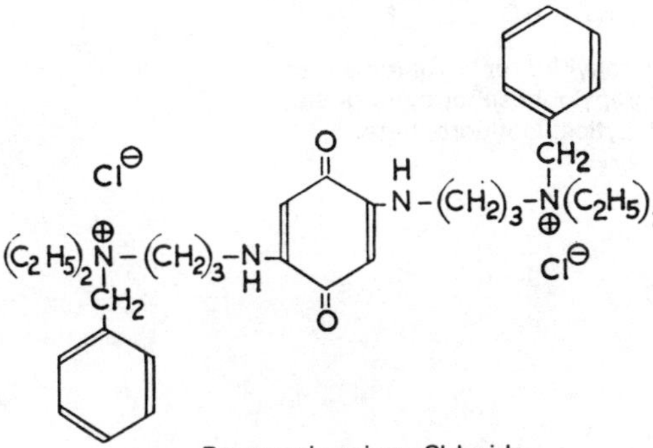

Benzoquinonium Chloride

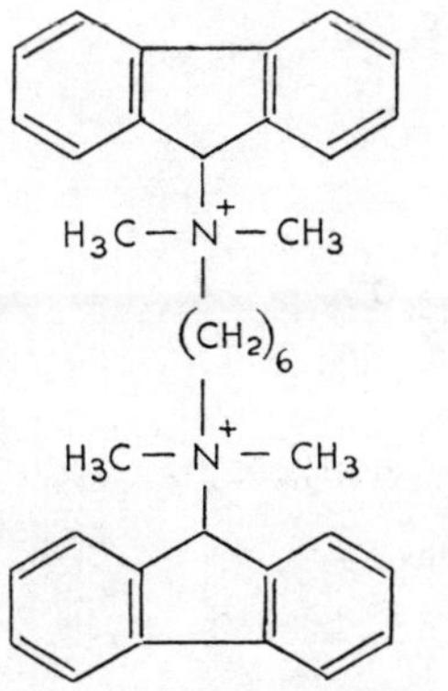

Hexafluorenium (Mylaxen)

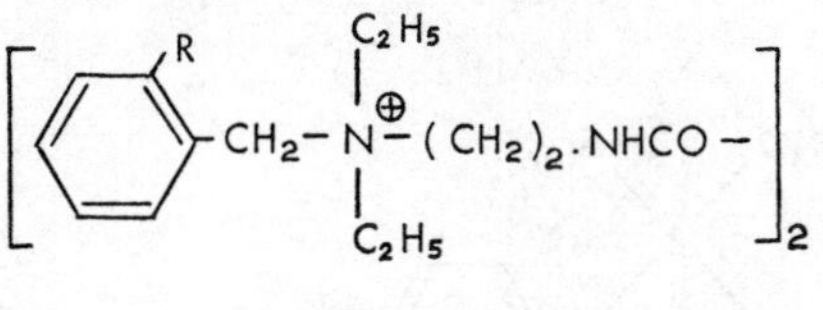

R = Cl   Ambenonium (Mytelase)
R = OCH₃ Methoxyambenonium

Fig. 14.3 (Contd)

distance of 1.4nm. Butyrocholinesterase presumably has only one anionic site although against this conclusion must be set the fact that hexafluorenium (Mylaxen, Fig. 14.3) specifically inhibits butyrocholinesterase.

Neostigmine has some acetylcholine-like properties, as is shown by the fact that it will partially remove a curare block (as acetylcholine would) in preparations in which the cholinesterase is already completely inhibited by another anticholinesterase. This observation led to the synthesis of a number of related compounds, of which the best known member is edrophonium, a compound used clinically as an anticurare. The anticurare action of neostigmine and edrophonium, though due primarily to their ability to inhibit cholinesterase, is therefore partially attributable to their possessing some nicotinic activity. Neostigmine does not readily cross the blood-brain barrier and this is an obvious advantage when the drug is taken other than locally since it restricts the anticholinesterase activity of the drug to the peripheral sites of action where it is needed.

Irreversible inhibitors of cholinesterase—The organophosphorus compounds

Organic esters of phosphoric acids have been known for very many years—tetraethylpyrophosphate was first synthesized in 1850—but their anticholinesterase activity was not recognized until 1943. They were used first as insecticides but their high degree of toxicity led to their development as war gases ('nerve gases') at first in Germany and then in Britain and elsewhere. A large number of organophosphorus anticholinesterases have been produced. The names and formulae of some of them are given in Figure 14.4 which adopts the classification proposed by Holmstedt (1959).

Inhibition of cholinesterase by organophosphorus compounds appears to be a two-stage process. In the first stage, the enzyme combines reversibly with the inhibitor to form a readily dissociable complex. In the second stage, a stable linkage is formed between the enzyme protein and the phosphorus. Cholinesterase activity disappears until the enzyme-phosphorus link is hydrolysed.

As we have already noted, phosphorylation occurs at the esteratic site of the enzyme and the phosphorus compounds attach themselves to the active centre of the enzyme in the same way as does the ester group of acetylcholine (Fig. 14.5) The enzyme phosphate, unlike the enzyme acetate, is very stable and the final stage of hydrolysis proceeds extremely slowly.

In the usual sense of that term, it is not strictly correct to speak of the organophosphorus compounds as 'irreversible' inhibitors since they are eventually hydrolysed with release of the enzyme. On the other hand, according to the alternative definition (p. 213) the organophosphorus compounds fall unreservedly into the category of irreversible inhibitors.

The organophosphorus compounds are not specific

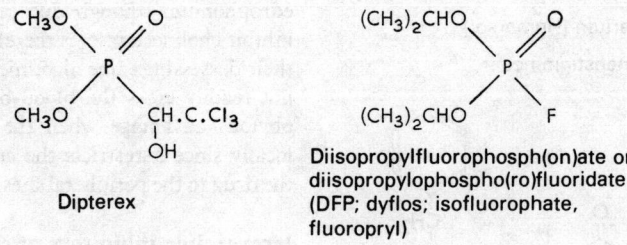

Alkoxy Compounds

Sarin

Soman

Tabun

Dialkoxy and Dialkyl Compounds

Dipterex

Paraoxon (See p. 54)

Diisopropylfluorophosph(on)ate or
diisopropylophospho(ro)fluoridate
(DFP; dyflos; isofluorophate,
fluoropryl)

Mipafox

Thiol Compounds

Demeton-S (Systox)

Isosystox

Thiono Compounds

Parathion (See p. 54)

Methyl Parathion

Fig. 14.4 Some organophosphorus compounds.

Thio-Thiono Compounds

Malathion (see p. 902)

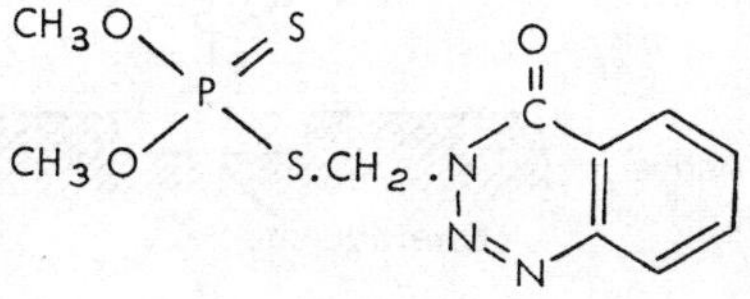

Guthion

Pyro- and Thionopyrophosphates

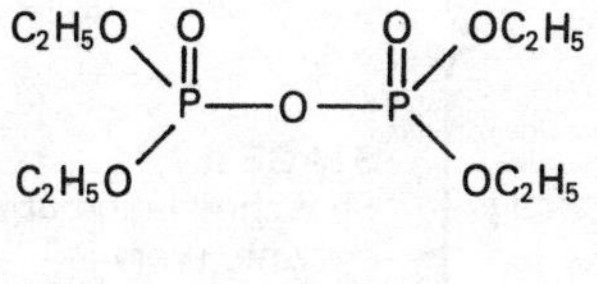

Tetraethylpyrophosphate (TEPP)

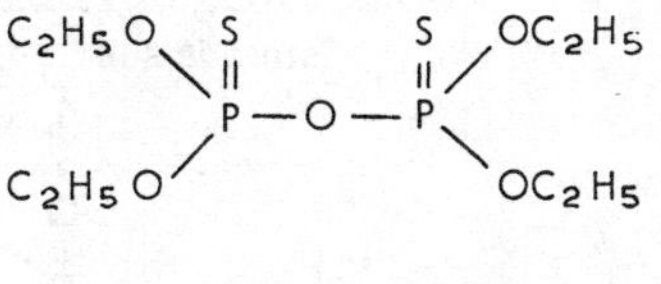

Tetraethylmonothionopyrophosphate

Phosphorylcholines   (Quaternary Compounds)

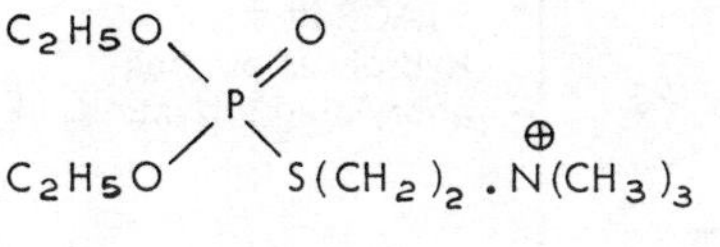

Echothiophate (Phospholine)

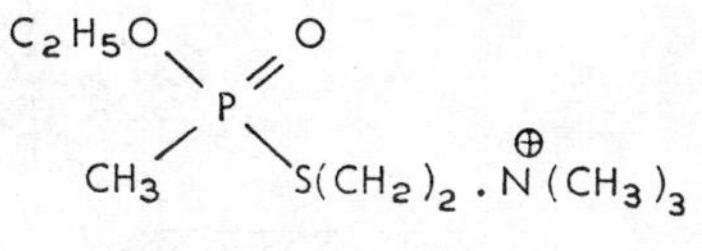

Ethoxymethylphosphorylthiocholine

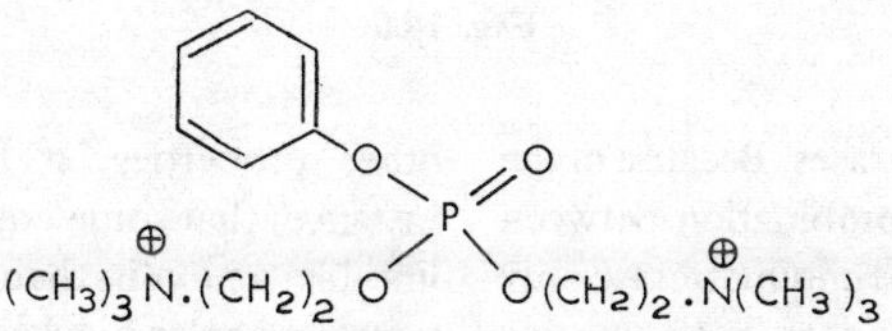

Phenoxyphosphoryl dicholine

Fig. 14.4 (Contd)

inhibitors of cholinesterases, since they also inhibit the whole group of carboxylic esterases which includes such enzymes as trypsin, chymotrypsin and the lipases. All but a few of the inhibitors are equally effective against both types of cholinesterase. The exceptions are provided by some (but not all) of the phosphorylcholines which preferentially inhibit acetylcholinesterase and by DFP, OMPA and mipafox which are rather more active against butyrocholinesterase.

Some generalizations can be made concerning the relationship between the structure of the organophosphorus compounds and their ability to inhibit cholinesterase. In the alkoxy series, compounds which contain fluorine are more active than those containing iodine or other radicals. The symmetrical dialkoxy compounds such as DFP are rather less potent than compounds like sarin, the British

nerve gas, which contain only one alkoxy group in their molecule. The quaternary organophosphorus compounds are the most powerful members of this group of anticholinesterases. Like neostigmine they also have some acetylcholine-like activity which contributes to their overall pharmacological effects.

It has already been mentioned that the organophosphorus compounds are slowly hydrolysed by cholinesterase. They are also susceptible to attack by a number of enzymes present in the liver, the kidney and other tissues. Some of these enzymes are relatively specific—some animal tissues, for instance, contain a malathionase and a DFPase—and this may be a factor that influences the toxicity of organophosphorus insecticides in man and domestic animals. The other enzymes which attack the organophosphorus compounds are less specific. The most important of these

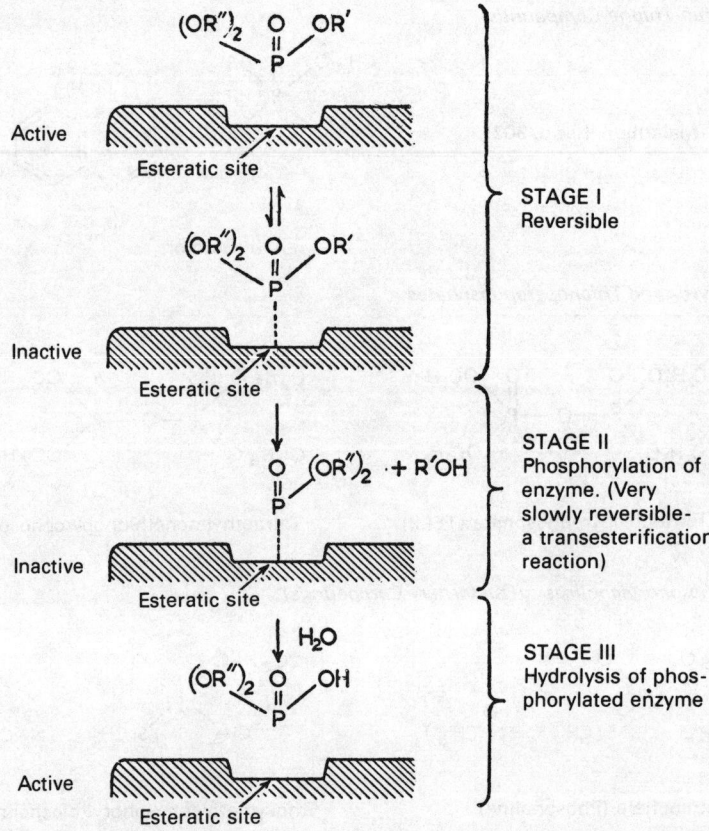

Fig. 14.5

enzymes are the plasma and tissue esterases. Because of the virtually irreversible nature of the combination between the organophosphorus compounds and cholinesterase only a small fraction of an administered dose need survive destruction in order to ensure inhibition of cholinesterase activity.

Some organophosphorus compounds become more toxic as a result of being altered by enzymatic changes in the body. Thus parathion, which itself has no anticholinesterase activity, is oxidised to paraoxon. Paraoxon is an anticholinesterase agent but some sulphur-containing organophosphorus compounds are converted into toxic substances (sulphones and sulphoxides) with no anticholinesterase activity.

Pharmacological properties of the anticholinesterases

The pharmacological effects of anticholinesterase administration are due primarily to the fact that the acetylcholine released in the course of normal physiological activity is not destroyed. It therefore accumulates in the body where it exerts both muscarinic and nicotinic actions. The effects of individual anticholinesterases may be modified by their other properties; it has already been mentioned, for instance, that some anticholinesterases have an acetylcholine-like action in their own right, while others may cause neuromuscular blockade. The effects of some compounds are complicated by the production in vivo of other toxic substances. Lipid soluble substances, such as the organophosphorus derivatives, penetrate easily into the central nervous system and their central effects are therefore more pronounced than those produced by anticholinesterases of lower lipid solubility. Finally, some of the anticholinesterases have additional actions which arise neither from their relationship to acetylcholine or cholinesterase nor to their metabolic transformation into toxic substances. While these possible sources of variation in pharmacological activity should be borne in mind, the major actions of all the anticholinesterases can nevertheless be summarized as follows:

1. Muscarinic effects

These include (a) effects on smooth muscle—increased peristalsis, relaxed sphincters, bronchoconstriction, vasodilatation, miosis and cycloplegia, (b) effects on cardiac muscle—bradycardia which, together with the vasodilatation, produces a fall in arterial pressure, (c) effects on exocrine glands—lachrymation, salivation and sweating. In the rat, chromodacryorhesis (Chap. 15) occurs. All these effects can be attenuated or abolished by atropine.

2. Nicotinic effects

These effects include generalized muscle twitching followed by muscle weakness. In addition, ganglion stimulation may accentuate or modify the muscarinic effects (see the discussion of nicotine, p. 205).

3. Central effects

The central effects vary in severity according to the drug used (see above) but they include restlessness, dizziness, tremor, aphasia, disorientation and hallucinations. In cases of severe poisoning coma, convulsions and death may occur.

Uses of the anticholinesterases

LABORATORY USES

Because free acetylcholine is so rapidly destroyed in the body, experiments designed to demonstrate its release during normal physiological activity are only successful when cholinesterase is inhibited. The use of an anticholinesterase for this purpose led to the discovery that acetylcholine was liberated from stimulated motor and preganglionic nerves. The further observation that anticholinesterases prolonged and intensified the end plate potential finally established that the latter—and hence the process of neuromuscular transmission—was due to acetylcholine. These and other crucial findings, without which the validity of the humoral theory of synaptic and neuromuscular transmission could never have been established, are described in more detail in Chapter 13. In general, it may be said that the modification of a physiological process by means of an anticholinesterase agent provides presumptive evidence that the process is in some way dependent on acetylcholine. Some care is needed in the application of this principle by virtue of the fact that the anticholinesterase used may have other properties. At least one hypothesis (that the propagation of an impulse along a nerve fibre is due to acetylcholine liberation) founded on the results of experiments which involved the use of anticholinesterases, is almost certainly erroneous.

The sensitivity to acetylcholine of the isolated frog rectus muscle, the dorsal muscle of the leech and the guinea pig ileum is considerably increased if the preparations are bathed in a solution containing an anticholinesterase agent. This increases their value as bioassay preparations.

OPHTHALMOLOGICAL USES

The earliest reported clinical use of an anticholinesterase was by Argyll Robertson, the famous ophthalmic surgeon, who introduced it into clinical practice in 1863 following the pioneer work of Christison and Fraser (p. 6). Anticholinesterases are used in the treatment of glaucoma, a condition of increased intraocular pressure due to impaired drainage (or excessive secretion) of aqueous humour. It is a potentially dangerous condition since if untreated it may lead to blindness. Anticholinesterases cause miosis and, as a result of the thinning of the ciliary body so produced, they open up the canal of Schlemm and so encourage drainage of the aqueous humour (Fig. 15.1). Physostigmine is most commonly used for the treatment of glaucoma. It is applied locally as a 0.25 to 1 per cent. solution. A muscarine-like drug such as pilocarpine (2 to 4 per cent.) is often added to the anticholinesterase solution: some authorities recommend the use of pilocarpine alone. Physostigmine is particularly useful for the treatment of acute attacks of glaucoma when the reduction of intraocular pressure is a matter of urgency. In chronic glaucoma, physostigmine is rather less useful since its relatively brief duration of action necessitates its application to the eye up to four times daily. Longer acting anticholinesterases such as decamarium, DFP, echothiophate, TEEP and paraoxon have all been used instead of physostigmine. They are applied once or twice weekly in solutions containing the anticholinesterase in a concentration of 0.1 to 0.25 per cent. It is usual to combine treatment with anticholinesterases with the administration of acetazolamide (Chap. 36) which reduces the secretion of aqueous humour.

Anticholinesterases increase the permeability of the blood-aqueous humour barrier and this of course tends to increase the rate of secretion of the aqueous humour. This is rarely sufficient to offset the effects of increased drainage but sometimes the application of the anticholinesterase induces a transient increase in intraocular pressure.

The repeated application to the eye of atropine followed by physostigmine will cause alternating dilatation and constriction of the pupil with associated changes in the ciliary body. This manoeuvre is sometimes employed in order to break down intraocular adhesions.

THE TREATMENT AND DIAGNOSIS OF MYASTHENIA GRAVIS

Myasthenia gravis is discussed in Chapter 16 where it is pointed out that this condition of muscle weakness is due to the lack of an effective concentration of acetylcholine at the motor end plates. The rational treatment of the disease therefore is to increase the amount of available acetylcholine and this is achieved by the administration of an anticholinesterase. Physostigmine was used at first for this purpose but it was soon replaced by neostigmine which has remained a drug of choice notwithstanding the large number of other cholinesterase inhibitors which have been discovered during the intervening 30 years. The acetylcholine-like properties of neostigmine augment its anticholinesterase activity and the fact that it is excluded from the central nervous system (p. 215) constitutes another advantage. Except in severe cases, or in myasthenic crises, the disease can usually be controlled by oral doses of neostigmine. The total daily dose and the frequency of administration have to be arrived at empirically by intelligent co-operation between physician and patient. Mild cases of the disease may be controlled by 10 to 15 mg of neostigmine daily, but severely afflicted patients may need up to 350 mg. In crises, where respiratory paralysis threatens, neostigmine is given (as the methylsulphate) by frequent subcutaneous or intramuscular injections or by intravenous infusion. Parenteral administration is sometimes used to supplement oral therapy at times when the patient needs additional muscular strength for swallowing or for other necessary exertions. The muscarinic effects of the accumulating acetylcholine may trouble some patients, particularly those who are receiving large doses of neostigmine parenterally. They serve no useful purpose but they can be antagonized by atropine.

Ephedrine (Chap. 18) may be given in oral doses of 25-30 mg thrice daily to potentiate the action of neostigmine. This effect of ephedrine was discovered accidentally by Mary Walker, one of the pioneers in the field of myasthenia treatment and herself a sufferer from the condition. Sympathomimetic substances potentiate the action of acetylcholine at the neuromuscular junction and this is presumably the basis of the beneficial effect of ephedrine treatment.

Neostigmine has a short duration of action and it often has to be given, or taken, at quite frequent intervals round the clock. Attempts to use longer acting anticholinesterase agents have not been very successful. The longest acting of all—the organophosphorus compounds—are unsuitable, partly because of their central actions and partly because their prolonged action prevents the adjustment of dose to fluctuating needs during the day. Pyridostigmine (Fig. 14.3), which has a somewhat longer lasting action than neostigmine, is preferred by some. Pyridostigmine is available as an injection and in tablets suitable for oral administration. A tablet containing 60 mg of the drug has an anticholinesterase activity equal to that of 15 mg of neostigmine.

Anticholinesterase agents are also used for diagnosis. If the condition of a patient complaining of muscle weakness is improved by an anticholinesterase, it is highly likely that he is suffering from myasthenia gravis. For diagnostic purposes, it is usual to use edrophonium (Tensilon), a drug with a very brief action: 2 mg are injected intravenously. If the response to this dose is equivocal, a second injection of 8 mg is given 30 seconds after the first. Edrophonium can also be employed to determine whether a patient maintained on neostigmine is receiving an adequate dose. If it produces a transient increase in muscle power in such a patient, the maintenance dose of neostigmine should be increased.

An overdose of neostigmine produces a condition of muscle weakness not dissimilar to myasthenia gravis itself and it may sometimes be difficult to determine whether extreme weakness in a myasthenic patient is due to his having taken too much or too little drug. Edrophonium can be used to provide an answer to this question, for it will improve the condition of a patient who has taken insufficient anticholinesterase and it will cause an even more pronounced weakness in those suffering from anticholinesterase overdosage.

Neostigmine and atropine are employed to reverse the effect of curare-like neuromuscular blocking agents (Chap. 16). The rationale of their use for this purpose is the same as that for the treatment of myasthenia gravis.

THE TREATMENT OF PARALYTIC ILEUS AND RELATED CONDITIONS

Paralytic ileus is a condition, often a sequel to abdominal surgery, in which lack of tone (*atony*) of the intestinal muscle leads to abdominal distension and retention of flatus and faeces. A similar state of atony may affect the bladder, leading to retention of urine and difficulty in micturition. These conditions are treated by anticholinesterases, a subcutaneous dose of 1 mg of neostigmine methylsulphate being usually sufficient. For preventitive treatment, smaller doses of neostigmine (0.25 mg) are given three or four times daily, beginning immediately after the operation and continuing for about three days. Some of the more recently discovered anticholinesterases—particularly DFP and benzpyrinium—have also been employed for the prevention and treatment of postoperative intestinal and bladder atony but they offer no particular advantage over neostigmine.

INSECTICIDES

Some of the organophosphorus compounds have found wide application as insecticides. Their use for this purpose is discussed in Chapter 59.

WAR GASES

Primitive man used an anticholinesterase as an ordeal poison, civilized man has adopted anticholinesterases as war gases. These include the alkoxy organophosphorus compounds sarin, soman and tabun (Fig. 14.4) which hold the doubtful distinction of being the most lethal substances ever synthesized by man for use against his fellows. Their toxic actions can be referred to the muscarinic and nicotinic actions of acetylcholine; the central nervous system is particularly susceptible and for this reason these anticholinesterase agents are also known as nerve gases. They are not, strictly speaking, gases but they can be distributed as aerosols. They are rapidly fatal in high doses and lower doses may cause prolonged incapacity due to effects on the eyes.

PROTECTIVE ACTION AGAINST OTHER CHOLINESTERASES

Koster demonstrated some considerable time ago that the

toxicity of DFP in cats was considerably reduced if the animals were first given a small dose of physostigmine (Koster, 1946). This observation has been confirmed and extended on many occasions since and it is clear that most of the easily reversible cholinesterase inhibitors confer a degree of protection against organophosphorus compounds given immediately afterwards.

An enzyme molecule to which an anticholinesterase is attached is immune from further attack and, because cholinesterase is present in the body in excess of normal requirements, a significant amount can be protected in this way before there is any gross interference with normal bodily mechanisms. An organophosphorus inhibitor given to an animal that has just been given another anticholinesterase will therefore only be able to react with those molecules of enzyme that have not already been inhibited and as soon as the protected cholinesterase becomes functional again it will provide a pool of enzyme sufficiently large to maintain life even though the rest of the organism's cholinesterase will remain inactivated for a long time. It should be possible to provide this sort of protection for human beings faced with the possibility of an inescapable exposure to an organophosphorus anticholinesterase. It will, however, be clear that prophylaxis will only be achieved if the period of exposure to the organophosphorus compound is shorter than the time required to reactivate the protected enzyme. For this reason, anticholinesterases like edrophonium, whose action is rapidly reversed, offer no protection against the organophosphorus inhibitors.

POISONING BY ORGANOPHOSPHORUS COMPOUNDS

Acute poisoning, qualitatively similar to that which would follow exposure to a nerve gas, may occur after accidental exposure to the organophosphorus compounds used as insecticides, but prolonged contact with low concentrations of the compounds may result in demyelination of nerves in the central nervous system and damage to anterior horn cells in the spinal cord. The consequences of this—a peripheral neuritis followed by motor incoordination and paralysis—may be serious.

The organophosphorus compound which has caused most cases of accidental poisoning is triorthocresylphosphate which was implicated in the outbreak of paralysis ('Ginger Jake paralysis') which occurred in the United States of America in 1930 and which affected about 15 000 people, some of whom died whilst others suffered permanent injury. The outbreak was due to an alcoholic beverage made illegally from ginger during Prohibition. It contained about 2 per cent. of triorthocresylphosphate. More recently a widespread outbreak of poisoning in North Africa was caused by the use for culinary purposes of an oil which contained organophosphorus compounds. Triorthocresylphosphate has little anticholinesterase activity but the neurological effects it produces are similar to those

which complicate some cases of poisoning by the organophosphorus anticholinesterase agents. It is not known why the organophosphorus compounds are neurotoxic but presumably they phosphorylate an enzyme or protein on which the integrity of the neurone depends (Aldridge, Barnes and Johnson, 1969). This is certainly not cholinesterase but, as we have seen (p. 217), the organophosphorus inhibitors are far from specific in their action.

In acute poisoning by an organophosphorus anticholinesterase agent, the muscarinic effects of the accumulated acetylcholine can be prevented or reversed by atropine. Doses large enough to exert an effect on the central nervous system have to be given. The nicotinic actions can in theory be antagonized by curare-like substances but it may be necessary to apply artificial respiration in order to counter paralysis of the respiratory muscles, the most serious consequence of the accumulation of acetylcholine to paralysing levels. It was pointed out earlier (p. 215) that some anticholinesterase agents also exhibit curariform and neuromuscular facilitatory activity. These properties are sufficiently pronounced to confer on these drugs the ability partially to reverse the neuromuscular block produced by toxic doses of the organophosphorous anticholinesterases.

A number of compounds are capable of reactivating cholinesterase that has been inactivated by the organophosphorus inhibitors. A representative selection of reactivators is shown in Figure 14.6; they are all oximes but some hydroxamic acids have some degree of effectiveness.

The reactivating oximes combine with the organophosphorus inhibitor which, it will be recalled, is attached to the esteratic site of the enzyme. However, in order to be effective, the reactivators must also fit into the unoccupied anionic site of the enzyme. When this occurs the reactivator-inhibitor complex 'lifts off' the enzyme. The reader will appreciate, therefore, why the most potent reactivators are quaternary ammonium compounds and why there is a critical length of molecule for maximum effectiveness.

The effectiveness of the oximes as antidotes is appar-

Triorthocresyl phosphate
(TOCP)

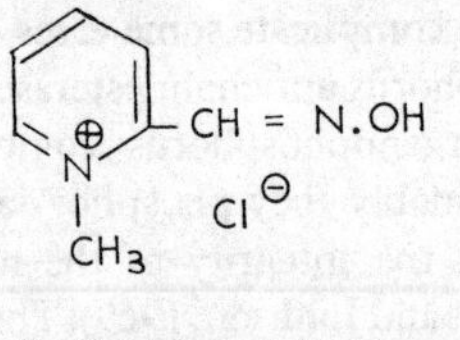

Pralidoxime chloride
2-PAM pyridine-2-aldoxime
methiodide)

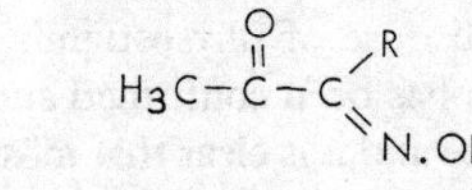

Diacetylmonoxime (DAM) R = CH$_3$

Pyruvaldoxime
(monoisonitrosoacetone;
MINA)   R = H

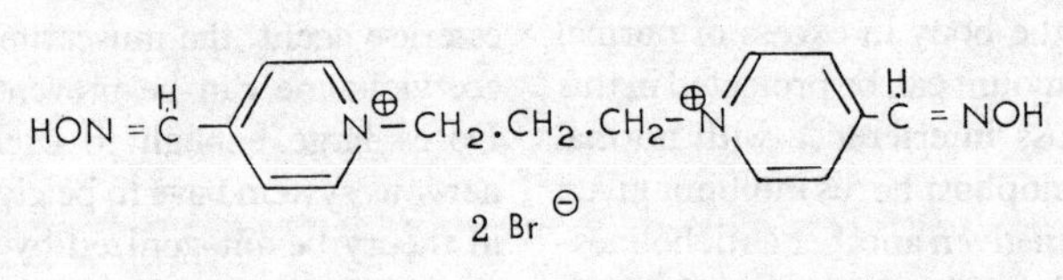

1,3 Bis(pyridinium-4-alloxime) propane dibromide
(TMB-4)

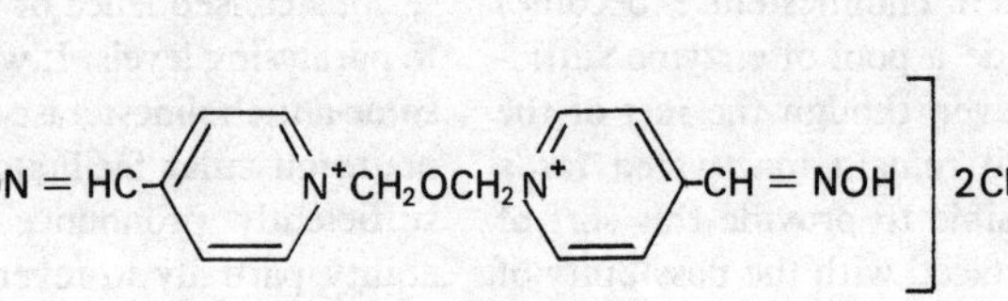

obidoxine chloride (Toxogonin)

Fig. 14.6 Some reactivators of cholinesterase.

ently not entirely attributable to their reactivating action. They may also alter the distribution of the inhibitor, diverting more to the liver as well as exerting a curare-like action sufficient to effect a partial relief of the neuromuscular blockade that is so potentially serious a consequence of cholinesterase deficiency.

The reactivators are only effective if they are given immediately before or soon after exposure to the inhibitor. The phosphorylated enzyme undergoes a fairly rapid process of 'ageing' (which probably involves the loss of an alkyl of alkoxyl group) as a result of which it becomes resistant to the action of the reactivating agent. 'Ageing' is, perhaps, something of a misnomer since it occurs within five minutes of phosphorylation. Even before ageing has occurred, the reactivators are not very successful in restoring cholinesterase activity in the central nervous system. Yet another limitation on their usefulness lies in the fact that they are not effective against all organophosphorus compounds the toxicity of a few of which is actually increased by the oximes.

Pralidoxime has been used clinically and toxogonin also shows promise. The intravenous dose of pralidoxime which might have to be repeated, is 1-2 grams. Given with atropine, it can also be administered prophylactically to those who expect to be exposed to a highly toxic organophosphorus compound. A useful degree of protection can only be assured if pralidoxime is given no earlier than fifteen minutes before exposure and even then it will not be effective against oxime-resistant inhibitors such as soman.

For protection against this type of compound, reversible anticholinesterases may prove to be useful (p. 221).

Sodium hypochlorite can be applied to destroy any of the anticholinesterase that comes into contact with the body.

BIBLIOGRAPHY

Books, monographs and reviews

Barlow, R. B. (1955). *An Introduction to Chemical Pharmacology.* London: Methuen.

Brimblecombe, R. W. (1974) *Drug Actions on Cholinergic Systems.* London: Macmillan.

Crossland, J. (1961). Biologic Estimation of Acetylcholine. In, Quastel, J. H. (Ed.), *Methods in Medical Research,* Vol. 9, 125-129. New York: Year Book Medical Publishers, Inc.

Hanin, I. (1974). *Choline and Acetylcholine: Handbook of Chemical Assay Methods.* New York: Raven Press.

Holmstedt, B. (1959). Pharmacology of organophosphorus cholinesterase inhibitors. *Pharmac. Rev.,* **11**, 567-688.

Karczmar, A. G. (1967). Pharmacologic, Toxicologic and Therapeutic Properties of Anticholinesterase Agents. In, *Physiological Pharmacology* (Root, W. S and Hofmann, F. G., eds.). New York and London: Academic Press. pp. 163-322.

Karczmar, A.G. (ed.) (1970). *International Encyclopedia of Pharmacology and Therapeutics. Section 13-Anticholinesterase Agents.* Oxford: Pergamon Press.

Koelle, G. B. (ed.) (1963). Cholinesterase and Anticholesterase Agents. In *Handbuch der Experimentellen Pharmakologie,* Vol. 15. Berlin: Springer.

Lewis, J. J. and Waton, N. G. (1958). The estimation of physiologically active, naturally occurring substances in the tissues and body fluids. Parts VII and VIII. *Lab. Practice,* **1**, 416-469.

Original papers

Aldrige, W. N., Barnes, J. M. and Johnson, M. K. (1969). Studies on delayed neurotoxicity produced by organophosphorus compounds. *Ann. N. Y. Acad. Sci.,* **140**, 314-322.

Armitage, A. K., Hall, G. H. and Morrison, Cathleen F. (1968). Pharmacological basis for the tobacco smoking habit. *Nature,* **217**, 331-334.

Banister, Jean, Whittaker, V. P. and Wijesundera, A. (1953). The occurrence of homolgues of acetylcholine in ox spleen. J. *Physiol.,* **121**, 55-71.

Carlini, E. A. and Green, J. P. (1963). Acetylcholine activity in the sciatic nerve. *Biochem. Pharmac.,* **12**, 1367-1376.

Chang, H. C. and Gaddum, J. H. (1933). Choline esters in tissue extracts. *J. Physiol.,* **79**, 255-285.

Crossland, J. and Redfern, P.H. (1963). Chromatographic behaviour of acetylcholine in brain extracts. *Life Sci.,* **10**, 711-716.

Dale, H. H. and Feldberg, W. (1934). The chemical transmitter of vagus effects to the stomach. *J. Physiol.,* **81**, 320-334.

Fellman, J. H. (1969). A chemical method for the determination of acetylcholine: its application to a study of presynaptic release and a choline acetyltransferase assay. *J. Neurochem.,* **16**, 135-143.

Hammar, C-G., Hanin, I., Holmstedt, B., Kitz, R. J., Jenden, D. J. and Karlen, B. (1968). Identification of acetylcholine in fresh rat brain by combined gas chromatography—mass spectrometry. *Nature, Lond.,* **220**, 915-917.

Hestrin, S. (1949). The reaction of acetylcholine and other carboxylic acid derivatives with hydroxylamine and its analytical application. *J.biol.Chem.,* **180**, 249-261.

Hosein, E. A., Rambaut, P., Chabrol, J. G. and Orzeck, A. (1965). Studies on the partition coefficient of 'bound' acetylcholine from rat brain and comparisons on the colorimetric and bioassay methods of determining its acetylcholine content. *Arch. Biochem. Biophys.,* **111**, 540-549.

Ing, H. R. (1949). The structure-action relationships of the choline group. *Science,* **109**, 264-266.

Kersbaum, A. (1968). Smoking, nicotine and adrenocortical secretion. *J. Amer. med. Ass.,* **203**, 275-279.

Keyl, M. J., Michaelson, I. A. and Whittaker, V. P. (1957). Physiologically active choline esters in certain marine gastropods and other invertebrates. *J. Physiol.,* **139**, 434-454.

Koster, R. (1946). Synergisms and antagonisms between physostigmine and diisopropylflurophosphate in cats. *J. Pharmac. exp. Ther.,* **88**, 39-46.

Murphree, H. B., Jenney, E. H. and Pfeiffer, C. C. (1959). *The Effect of Pharmacologic Agents on the Nervous System.* Baltimore: Williams and Wilkins.

Straughan, D. W. (1958). Assay of acetylcholine on the rat blood pressure. *J. Pharm. Pharmac.,* **10**, 783-4.

Stockley, I. H. (1969). The influence of ATP in brain extracts on the estimation of acetylcholine assayed on the frog rectus muscle, *J. Pharm. Pharmac.,* **21**, 302-308.

Szerb, J. C. (1961). The estimation of acetylcholine using leech muscle in a microbath. *J. Physiol.,* **158**, 8-9P.

Szerb, J. C. (1963). Nature of acetylcholine-like activity released from brain *in vivo. Nature, Lond.,* **197** 1016-1017.

Toru, M. and Aprison, M. H. (1966). Brain acetylcholine studies: a new extraction procedure. *J. Neurochem.,* **13**, 1533-1544.

Župančič, A. O. (1953). The mode of action of acetylcholine. A theory extended to a hypothesis on the mode of other biologically active substances. *Acta. physiol. Scand.,* **29**, 63-71.

15. Atropine and atropine-like drugs

Centuries ago, Italian women applied decoctions of the deadly nightshade to their eyes, causing dilatation of the pupils and giving themselves a lustrous, wide-eyed and—they hoped—alluring appearance. For this reason, and as early as the 16th century, the name *belladonna* (beautiful lady) was applied to the plant. The Italian ladies were also aware of less innocent use for the deadly nightshade which was popular as a poison. Its modern botanical name, *Atropa belladonna* commemorates both these ancient uses. Atropa comes from Atropos, the oldest of the Fates, who cuts the thread of life. The pharmacologically-active alkaloid obtained from belladonna became known as atropine and its constituent base as tropine.

Atropine occurs in a number of other plants in the family *Solanaceae*. It has also been synthesized. It is a racemic mixture of (+) and (—)-hyoscyamine; the pharmacologically-active component is (—)-hyoscyamine. Atropine, the tropic acid ester of tropine, is usually obtained by the racemization of (—)-hyoscyamine extracted from belladonna or from other solanaceous plants. Atropine was first isolated in a pure form in 1831.

Atropine

Atropine has widespread actions and it has been used in the treatment of a large number of clinical conditions. In attempts to obtain atropine-like drugs with a greater selectivity, with a different duration of action or with fewer side effects, a large number of related synthetic or semi-synthetic drugs has been introduced. In this chapter the pharmacology of atropine itself is first considered in detail. Related compounds are then catalogued and their principal properties are briefly discussed.

PHARMACOLOGICAL PROPERTIES OF ATROPINE

Atropine antagonizes the muscarinic actions of acetylcholine. This antagonism (which is competitive in nature) is the basis of most, but not all, of its pharmacological actions. Atropine is as effective in antagonizing the muscarinic effects of acetylcholine accumulating after the administration of an anticholinesterase as it is in preventing the actions of exogenous acetylcholine. It also blocks the muscarinic actions of other choline esters and the response to stimulation of parasympathetic nerves. When atropine is given alone to the intact animal or human subject, its anti-muscarinic effects are largely restricted to blocking the responses to acetycholine liberated in the course of normal nervous activity. Although it is true that muscarine mimics the effect of parasympathetic stimulation it is important to remember that muscarinic receptors are also present in some tissues (particularly blood vessels and central neurones) which are not supplied by parasympathetic nerves. The effects of muscarine—and of acetylcholine acting on muscarinic receptors—therefore include more than an imitation of parasympathetic activity and the actions of atropine similarly involve more than a simple blocking of parasympathetic nervous activity.

It is convenient to consider the pharmacological properties of atropine under four heads:
  (i) parasympathetic blockade
  (ii) other peripheral anti-muscarinic actions
  (iii) actions on the central nervous system
  (iv) peripheral actions not due to block of muscarine receptors

Parasympathetic blockade

The effect of atropine on structures innervated by the parasympathetic nervous system depends on the degree of parasympathetic tone that exists at the time of drug administration. This will vary not only from one species and individual to another but also among different organs in the same individual.

It should be clear from what has been said earlier that atropine does not prevent the liberation of acetylcholine from parasympathetic nerves. It simply prevents the access of acetylcholine to muscarine receptors.

THE EYE.
The muscle which causes constriction of the pupil—*the constrictor pupillae*—is supplied by parasympathetic fibres in the oculomotor (3rd cranial) nerve. Under normal circumstances these fibres exhibit considerable tonic activity and atropine therefore causes pupillary dilatation (*mydriasis*) since it leaves the pupil under the unopposed influence of its sympathetic (dilatatory) nerve supply.

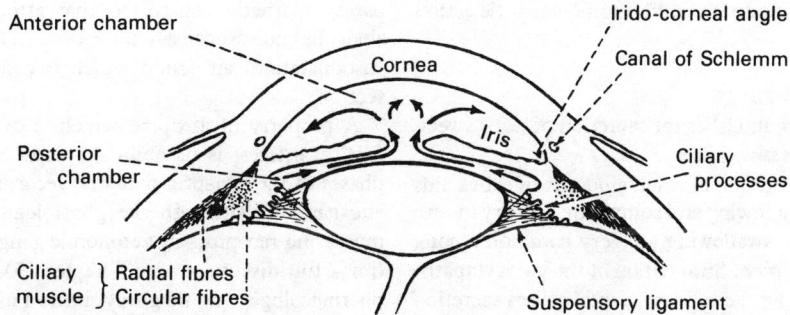

Fig. 15.1 Structures involved in ocular accommodation and the formation and drainage of aqueous humour. The arrows indicate the circulatory pathway taken by the aqueous humour.

Atropine administration also abolishes constrictor reflexes, such as that provoked by shining a light in the eye.

The oculomotor nerve also supplies the ciliary muscle. Contraction of this muscle slackens the suspensory ligament (Fig. 15.1) reducing tension on the lens and allowing it to become more convex. Accommodation for near vision is dependent on the ciliary muscle's ability to contract. Atropine prevents this contraction and causes paralysis of accommodation (*cycloplegia*): distant vision remains good but near vision is indistinct.

Atropine causes the intraocular pressure to rise. Intraocular fluid is secreted by the ciliary processes in the posterior chamber of the eye. It passes through the pupil into the anterior chamber from which it drains into the venous system *via* the canal of Schlemm which is situated at the irido-corneal angle (Fig. 15.1). Pupillary dilatation causes thickening of the peripheral part of the iris with a consequent narrowing of the irido-corneal angle. This restricts the drainage of the aqueous humour though secretion continues and the pressure therefore rises. Though this rarely does harm to the normal eye, it may create a dangerous situation in those already suffering from raised intraocular pressure (*glaucoma*).

It will be appreciated that the pressure-raising effect of atropine is a simple mechanical consequence of pupillary dilatation and that any mydriatic drug, whatever its mode of action, will aggravate glaucoma. Atropine, however, is particularly dangerous because of its prolonged action. Some nasal decongestants and other proprietary preparations contain atropine; people with increased intraocular pressure should be warned of the possible consequences of too enthusiastic self-medication with these preparations. It is pointed out elsewhere (p. 75) that, because of genetically determined differences in the geometry of the irido-corneal angle, atropine is more likely to bring about a dangerous increase in intraocular pressure in the members of some ethnic groups than it is in others.

CARDIOVASCULAR SYSTEM
Atropine removes the restraining influence normally exerted by the vagus on the heart rate. Parasympathetic tone in the cardiac branches of the vagus—and hence the cardioacceleratory effect of atropine—varies considerably: it is high in the cat and dog but low in the rabbit. In man, vagal tone is higher in the trained athlete than in the untrained individual. It is also higher in young people. Atropine also reduces or abolishes cardioinhibitory reflexes, though some reflex cardiac slowing, due to the reduction of sympathetic tone, can occur in the atropinized animal. Soon after its administration, atropine sometimes causes a transient slowing of the heart. This is the result of a stimulant action on the cardioinhibitory centre in the medulla and it disappears as soon as the peripheral action of atropine is fully established.

RESPIRATORY SYSTEM
The bronchi are normally exposed to the effect of tonic activity in the parasympathetic nerves which supply them and atropine consequently causes bronchodilatation. The larger vital capacity so produced implies an increased ventilatory exchange and respiration appears to be stimulated though atropine itself has no direct effect on respiration which is controlled by somatic and not by autonomic nerves. Atropine also inhibits secretion of the bronchial glands.

SMOOTH MUSCLE OF THE GASTROINTESTINAL TRACT
Gastrointestinal movements and the tone of intestinal muscle are under a predominant parasympathetic control. Even in the normal individual, therefore, atropine inhibits intestinal tone and motility. In experimental preparations it does not always entirely abolish the effects of vagal stimulation on gut motility though the responses to acetylcholine are completely blocked.

The origin of this apparently anomalous behaviour is not entirely clear, though it suggests the possibility that vagal stimulation causes the release of small amounts of an atropine-resistant transmitter as well as larger quantities of acetylcholine.

The bladder has a complex but predominantly parasympathetic innervation and atropine reduces its tone and spontaneous motor activity. The parasympathetic supply to the uterus is unimportant and atropine has little action on that organ.

GLANDULAR SECRETIONS

Atropine reduces or abolishes the secretion of tears, sweat, saliva, and the digestive juices.

The continual secretion of small amounts of saliva aids articulation and swallowing and complaints of a dry mouth and of difficulty in swallowing are very common among patients taking atropine. Stimulation of the parasympathetic nerves supplying the salivary glands causes secretion of saliva and an increased blood flow through the glands. It has been known for many years that in some species atropine does not abolish this vasodilator response, even when salivary secretion has been completely inhibited. It is usual to explain this as being due to the production by the stimulated gland of an enzyme which liberates plasma kinins but this explanation is not entirely acceptable (p. 639) and it is possible that the vasodilatation is due to acetylcholine's acting on atropine-resistant receptors. Variations in atropine sensitivity among different organs and different species are well known (Ambache, 1955).

The inhibitory action of atropine on sweat secretion explains the pyrexia and the hot dry skin seen in atropine poisoning.

Atropine depresses the resting secretion of gastric juice, reducing both the volume and the acidity. Although there is a very considerable hormonal component in the process of acid gastric secretion, the action of the hormone (gastrin) is inhibited by atropine just as is the secretion due to vagal stimulation. Atropine does not, however, completely abolish the secretion of gastric acid.

By suppressing the secretion of tears, atropine causes drying of the conjunctiva and exposes the eye to a greater risk of superficial injuries from dust and other particles in the atmosphere. The rat is unique in that it possesses Harderian glands as well as tear glands of the usual type. These glands secrete porphyrins and are very susceptible to circulating acetylcholine which causes *chromodacryorrhesis* ('bloody tears'). Chromodacryorrhesis occurs after administration of anticholinesterase drugs or during the tonic phase of convulsive activity when acetylcholine enters the bloodstream: it is prevented by atropine.

Other peripheral antimuscarinic actions

Acetylcholine causes dilatation of peripheral blood vessels. This is a muscarinic action and atropine will therefore antagonize the vasodilatation produced by acetycholine and other choline esters. Indeed this action forms the basis of the classical experiment to demonstrate the muscarinic and nicotinic actions of acetylcholine (p. 201). Similarly, atropine will counter the vasodilatation produced by anticholinesterase drugs and it has a valuable place in the treatment of poisoning by these compounds. However, most of the blood vessels in the body are not subject to parasympathetic control so that atropine, when given alone, has no vasoconstrictor action. In fact, it causes some vasodilatation, an action which is considered in a later section.

A property of atropine which is of considerable theoretical interest is its ability to abolish two of the three phases of the synaptic potential recorded from sympathetic ganglia. Although the physiological significance of muscarine receptors in autonomic ganglia is not yet clear (for a full discussion, see Chapter 13), the experimental pharmacologist should always bear in mind the possibility that the atropine he has administered may, in some circumstances, be affecting ganglionic transmission.

Central actions of atropine

Cholinergic synapses are widely distributed in the central nervous system and normal nervous activity is dependent on the continual release of acetylcholine. The experimental evidence suggests that a large proportion of the central acetylcholine receptors are muscarinic in type (Krnjević and Phillis, 1963, a and b) and since they are found in both excitatory and inhibitory systems it is not surprising that atropine has both inhibitory and excitatory properties. In addition to its specifically antimuscarine action, atropine also has a non-specific effect, stabilizing the neuronal membrane and depressing its response to such excitatory substances as amino acids (Curtis and Phillis, 1960). Although relatively large doses of atropine are required to demonstrate this effect in experimental preparations, it may well contribute to the drug's central actions in man, particularly, of course, when high doses have been taken.

In human subjects, excitation due to atropine is particularly evident after toxic doses of the drug. They cause increased respiration, restlessness, excitement and irritability. With very large doses, delirium and convulsions occur, followed by coma. As has already been pointed out, therapeutic doses of atropine sometimes cause medullary stimulation, made evident by transient bradycardia.

Notwithstanding these excitatory actions, the central effects of atropine are predominantly inhibitory while many atropine-like compounds only have inhibitory properties. It is because of their inhibitory action that atropine and related drugs are employed in the treatment of motion sickness and Parkinson's disease. In experimental animals, widespread inhibition can be demonstrated even when atropine is causing behavioural excitation (Wikler, 1952; Longo, 1956, 1962). Inhibition is shown in the electroencephalogram, which exhibits the slow, high-amplitude waves characteristic of depression. The arousal response to sciatic nerve stimulation is also blocked. The occurrence of behavioural excitation in the face of electroencephalographic signs of inhibition is presumably due to the inhibition of excitatory synapses in areas of the brain which normally restrain the activity of the lower centres.

Atropine administration produces a fall in the acetylcholine content of brain. The most likely explanation is that some of the acetycholine liberated in the course of normal central nervous activity is reincorporated into the nerve terminals and that the receptors for this incorporation are blocked by atropine. Support for this view is provided by the observation that atropine increases the amount of acetylcholine diffusing from the brain into saline-filled cups placed on the cortex. The progressive fall in the amount of acetycholine in the brain presumably reduces the efficiency of cholinergic synaptic transmission and may well contribute to the inhibitory actions of atropine. An alternative explanation, favoured by some, is that the activity of many central neurones is normally restrained by inhibitory impulses arriving along cholinergic nerves. If the appropriate receptors are of the muscarine variety, the administration of atropine will remove this restraint and the resulting increased activity of the central nervous system (some of which, of course, will involve cholinergic neurones) will lead both to an increased release of acetylcholine from the brain and to a depletion of the organ's store of transmitter. Thus the observed effect of atropine on the acetylcholine content of brain finds an explanation in two hypotheses, one linked with the fact that the drug has inhibitory actions and the other dependent on the equally valid observation that it has excitatory effects. This indicates yet again, if further illustration were needed, how tenuous, tentative and untested are many of the hypotheses that are profferred in explanation of the effects on the nervous system of simple and common drugs.

Peripheral actions of atropine not caused by block of muscarine receptors

Atropine has a quinidine-like action on the heart, prolonging the refractory period; it dilates peripheral blood vessels and it behaves as a local anaesthetic with about one-half the activity of procaine. It has some antihistamine activity and weak curariform properties. It also inhibits ciliary movement in the trachea and oesophagus of a number of animal species. None of these actions is due to its blocking specific muscarine receptors. Procaine also has quinidine-like, vasodilator and curariform properties, while quinidine has local anaesthetic and curariform actions. The fact that these drugs of different pharmacological classes have a number of properties in common has fascinating implications for those interested in the chemical nature of receptor molecules. These and other examples of common properties among different groups of drugs have been fully discussed by Burn (1958) and are mentioned elsewhere in this book (p. 473).

The vasodilator action of atropine is exerted, like that of papaverine (p. 705) directly on the smooth muscle cells of the blood vessels, though it can also interfere with the constrictor action of noradrenaline. The local anaesthetic action is another manifestation of atropine's ability to stabilize the nerve membrane unselectively against a range of excitatory substances. Ciliary movement appears to be maintained by the local production and liberation of acetylcholine in the epithelial cells though the receptors involved are not muscarinic in type since ciliary movement is inhibited as easily by D-tubocurarine as by atropine.

Although the properties of atropine mentioned in this section are primarily of theoretical importance, some of them may contribute to its therapeutic actions. The laboratory worker too should realize that they may add complications to his experimental system and may lead to misleading conclusions or to apparently irreconcilable discrepancies. It is, for instance, important to remember the antihistamine properties of atropine when studying systems in which both acetylcholine and histamine are involved. Again, the local anaesthetic action of atropine may cause inhibition of a response mediated by nerves and this may give rise to the erroneous conclusion that the mechanism initiating the response involves the stimulation of muscarine receptors. Many of these minor actions of atropine are only evident at higher dose levels and the complicating effects just mentioned are less likely to arise if careful attention is paid to the atropine dosage used in experimental work.

USES OF ATROPINE AND RELATED COMPOUNDS

The clinical uses of atropine are easily appreciated in the light of the pharmacological properties which have just been discussed. The many atropine substitutes which have been introduced into clinical practice have essentially the same actions and uses as atropine itself. Their peculiar advantages are summarized later in this chapter.

(i) In ophthalmology, atropine is used as a mydriatic to aid in the examination of the retina and for the treatment of inflammatory states such as acute iritis and keratitis (inflammation of the cornea). Daily application to the eye of a one per cent solution of atropine is usually employed. In diagnostic work it is usual to employ homatropine since the mydriasis and cycloplegia produced by a single dose of atropine may persist for three to seven days, which is far too long for the comfort of the patient. In iritis, however, prolonged mydriasis is useful, presumably because of the enforced relaxation of the iris. Moreover, the patient soon realizes that he cannot focus for near vision and he abandons his efforts at accommodation and thus 'rests' his eyes. For a similar reason, atropine is useful in the treatment of some forms of squint. The cycloplegia prevents accommodation and the extrinsic muscles of the eye which were previously causing excessive convergence will relax for a sufficiently long time to permit the carrying out of re-educative exercises.

(ii) Atropine is a valuable drug for pre-anaesthetic

medication. Some inhalation anaesthetics stimulate bronchial secretion. This can be prevented by atropine, which thus facilitates the work of the anaesthetist and the surgeon and it diminishes the risk of bronchial obstruction, pulmonary collapse and postoperative pneumonia. Atropine has the further advantage that it prevents the cardiac inhibition which might otherwise occur as a result of reflex stimulation of the vagus from intra-abdominal stimuli, such as traction on the intestine, occurring during the operation.

(iii) Because they reduce the tone of smooth muscle, atropine and atropine-like drugs find application as *antispasmodic* or *spasmolytic* agents. They are used in a variety of conditions characterized by smooth muscle spasm. These include biliary, intestinal and renal colic and constipation due to spasm of the large intestine. In peptic ulcer patients, atropine reduces gastric motility and acid secretion and as a result it effectively prevents the nocturnal pain which is a frequent and disturbing occurrence in this condition. It thus provides favourable conditions for healing. Atropine is a constituent of some preparations used in the treatment of asthma, for which its bronchodilator and antisecretory actions are both useful. It is used in conjunction with morphine to prevent the biliary or intestinal colic which is likely to occur if morphine is given alone.

(iv) The inhibitory action of atropine on central synapses is made use of in the treatment of Parkinson's disease (p. 590) and motion sickness (p. 603).

(v) Atropine is a valuable and specific antidote in poisoning by anticholinesterases such as the organophosphorus insecticides. It is also used, in conjunction with anticholinesterase drugs, in the treatment of myasthenia gravis if there is a danger of acetylcholine's accumulating to such an extent that its muscarinic actions (bradycardia, hypotension, bronchoconstriction and intestinal spasm) might threaten the life or comfort of the patient. The beneficial nicotinic actions of the acetylcholine on skeletal muscle are not impaired by atropine.

(iv) Atropine has been used to prevent excessive sweating (*hyperhydrosis*) particularly that occurring in pulmonary tuberculosis.

(vii) Very large doses of atropine were occasionally employed in the past to produce prolonged coma in the treatment of schizophrenia though the value of this heroic treatment was never established.

In experimental pharmacology, atropine is used in the whole animal and in isolated tissue preparations when it is necessary to prevent the muscarinic actions of acetylcholine as, for instance, in the analysis of a tissue extract containing more than one active substance. It is also used to confirm that the activity of a tissue extract is due to acetylcholine. Doses of tissue extract and equivalent doses of acetylcholine are added alternately to the test preparation after the latter has been in contact with atropine. As

the effect of atropine fades, the responses to the tissue extract and to acetylcholine should recover at identical rates. If they do not do so, doubt will be cast on the conclusion that the activity of the tissue extract is entirely due to acetylcholine.

Atropine resistance, atropine poisoning and atropine sensitivity

The usual therapeutic dose of atropine is 0.25 to 1 mg of the sulphate, the form in which it is most often prescribed. It can be taken by mouth or administered by subcutaneous injection. It is usually assumed that higher doses than this are dangerous but the fatal dose of atropine is not precisely known. It is known, however, that people have survived the ingestion of as much as 1000 mg and the dose suggested for the treatment of schizophrenia was 200 mg on alternate days for several weeks. It is, perhaps, surprising that such doses can be tolerated, in view of the deadly nightshade's long established reputation as a killer.

It is generally agreed that many animals are much more resistant than man to atropine. In the cat, the dose required just to block the muscarinic action of acetylcholine is 2 mg per kilogram or about 150 times the therapeutic dose in man. The lethal dose of atropine is very high in many mammals, the astronomical figure of 700 mg per kilogram having been quoted for the rat. In some animals, particularly the herbivores, atropine resistance is due to the presence in the blood of an atropinase which presumably protects the animal against the toxic action of solanaceous plants encountered in its foraging.

Atropine poisoning

Cases of atropine poisoning have occurred in children who have eaten the berries of the deadly nightshade, the bitter sweet or the black nightshade. In atropine poisoning there is dry mouth, difficulty in swallowing and hoarseness. Nausea and vomiting may occur and swallowing and talking become difficult. Although the victim is very thirsty, he cannot swallow fluid. The pupils are widely dilated, vision is blurred and there is photophobia. The skin is hot, flushed and dry and there may be a skin rash. There is fever and body temperatures as high as 43° C. (109° F.) have been reported in children poisoned with atropine. The increased body temperature is due partly to the inhibition of sweating and partly to a central action of atropine. As a consequence of the increased body temperature, respiration is rapid. There is restlessness, excitement and confusion and the patient may be very talkative. Hallucinations, mania, delirium and convulsions may occur. When very large amounts of atropine have been taken, the excitement gives way to severe depression and coma.

Atropine poisoning is treated by washing out the stomach to remove any unabsorbed drug. Neostigmine or pilocarpine are given to overcome the antimuscarinic effects and sedatives are administered to reduce the excitement and delirium.

Atropine sensitivity

Although, as we have seen, many people seem to be able to tolerate surprisingly high doses of atropine, some others display an abnormally high sensitivity to the drug and its congeners and may suffer unwelcome and prolonged side effects even after taking only a recommended therapeutic dose. Excitement, sometimes to the point of a wild delirium, has been reported in these circumstances but a more common response is confusion, disorientation and a patchy amnesia, some recent events being remembered clearly while others are forgotten. A person in this condition will obviously feel quite 'lost' and may behave in what appears to an uninformed onlooker to be a completely irrational or irresponsible fashion. The attendant thirst may impel an atropine sensitive individual to take more alcohol than he normally allows himself and this will not only aggravate his other symptoms but it may also lead to misinterpretation of his condition so that he finds himself receiving the attention of the law rather than the succour of a physician. In view of the popularity and easy availability of atropine-like compounds (particularly hyoscine) as motion sickness remedies, the existence of atropine sensitivity and an awareness of its consequences should always be kept in mind by both prescribers and imbibers of these drugs.

OTHER COMPOUNDS WITH ATROPINE-LIKE PROPERTIES

HYOSCINE (SCOPOLAMINE) AND HYOSCINE METHYL NITRATE (SKOPOLATE, SKOPYL)

The peripheral actions of hyoscine are very similar to those of atropine, but it has stronger actions on the eye and the exocrine glands. It is a more rapidly acting mydriatic and

stimulant activity. Its sedative property is made use of when it is combined with morphine or a barbiturate in preanaesthetic medication. In small doses, hyoscine causes amnesia and it has been used in obstetrics, in combination with morphine, to produce 'twilight sleep'. Hyoscine is also an effective motion-sickness preventive: a popular preparation is Sereen. Hyoscine is more potent than atropine in reducing the rigidity of Parkinson's disease. An overdose of hyoscine produces toxic symptoms that resemble those following atropine except that excitement and mania are less common. In sensitive individuals, therapeutic doses of hyoscine may precipitate the syndrome of confusion, disorientation and amnesia that has already been described. The therapeutic dose range is from 0.3 to 0.6 mg.

When the nitrogen atom of hyoscine is methylated to form the quaternary derivative, hyoscine methyl nitrate is obtained. This compound resembles atropine rather than hyoscine. It has a powerful peripheral antimuscarine activity and small doses can apparently produce complete achlorhydria in man. It is used as an antispasmodic to treat hypertropic pyloric stenosis in children and peptic ulcer in adults. The bromide (hyoscine methobromide) is also used.

HYOSCINE BUTYL BROMIDE (BUSCOPAN)

This is another quaternary derivative of hyoscine. In therapeutic doses it has no atropine-like action on the eye, circulation, sweat and salivary glands. There is only a slight decrease in acid gastric secretion, but peristalsis is inhibited and there is a reduction in the tone of intestinal smooth muscle. Hyoscine butyl bromide is used as an antispasmodic in treating peptic ulcer, gastritis and various disorders of the gastrointestinal tract which are characterized by spasm. It has also found employment for the relief of spasmodic conditions of the bile duct and urinary tract and for the treatment of dysmenorrhoea. The dose is 20 mg four times daily.

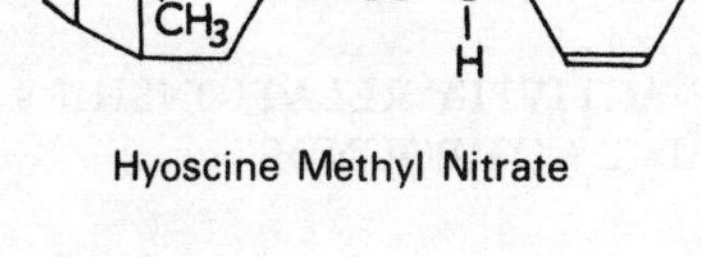

Hyoscine Methyl Nitrate

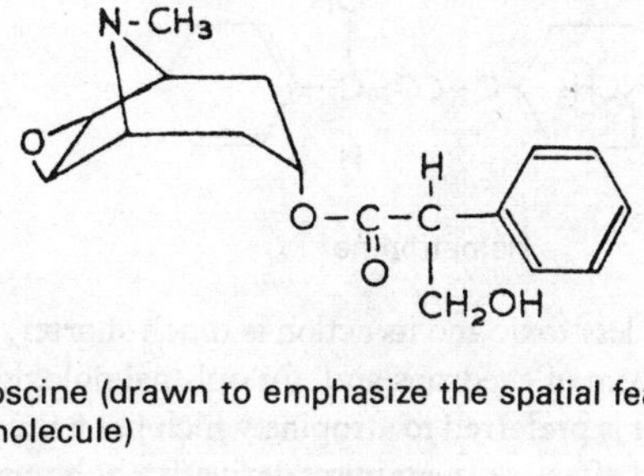

1-Hyoscine (drawn to emphasize the spatial features of the molecule)

cycloplegic than atropine but its effects pass off more rapidly. The most important qualitative differences between atropine and hyoscine are seen in their effects upon the central nervous system. Hyoscine is a sedative and hypnotic, though it is not entirely without central

ATROPINE METHONITRATE

Atropine methonitrate is the quaternary derivative of atropine analogous to the corresponding hyoscine derivative. It has peripheral antiacetylcholine actions similar to those of atropine itself but it is more potent. Because it cannot penetrate the blood barrier, atropine methonitrate has no action on the central nervous system. Its main therapeutic uses are in eye drops (a one per cent solution is used) and in the treatment of hypertrophic pyloric stenosis in infants. It is administered just before the infant is fed but it is not easy to see why the drug is efficacious in this condition since the gastric and intestinal sphincters are relaxed by *stimulation* of muscarine receptors: the promotion of gastrointestinal movements by parasympathetic nervous activity is compounded of an increased activity in the propulsive muscles and an associated relaxation of the sphincters. Atropine would therefore be expected either to increase sphincter tone or (in the absence of parasympathetic activity) to have no effect.

Atropine methonitrate is of particular value in experimental work as a consequence of its lack of central actions. If, for instance, a drug exerts effects on the nervous system which are blocked by atropine but not by atropine methonitrate, it is reasonable to conclude that the central effects arise in the brain itself and are not secondary to stimulation of peripheral structures. It is important to remember however that all the quaternary derivatives of atropine and hyoscine can effect a degree of neuromuscular and ganglion blockade. While this activity rarely manifests itself when the drugs are employed therapeutically it may appear in the less restricted conditions of the animal laboratory where it may introduce perplexing complications (such as respiratory depression) into the experimental results of those who think of the quaternary compounds only as substances with an atropine-like action limited to peripheral sites. Atropine methonitrate has been supplied under a number of proprietary names. These include Eumydrin, Metanite, Metropine and Pylostropin.

HOMATROPINE
Homatropine is the mandelic acid ester of tropine. It resembles atropine in its pharmacological properties but is

Homatropine

less potent and less toxic and its action is much shorter. It is used in the form of eyedrops and, for ophthalmological examinations, it is preferred to atropine which has a much more prolonged effect. A quaternary derivative of homatropine, homatropine methyl bromide, has similar properties to homatropine and it has been used as an antispasmodic agent in peptic ulcer. Proprietary names include Methatropin, Homapin, Malcotran, Mesopin and Novatrin.

OTHER COMPOUNDS
A very large number of compounds with atropine-like activity has been synthesized. The names, formulae and special properties of some of them are displayed, for reference purposes, in Table 15 1. Compounds whose central actions make them particularly useful in the treatment of Parkinson's disease are not included in Table 15 1; they are fully discussed in Chapter 32.

All the compounds shown in Table 15.1 have properties generally similar to those of atropine but several of them have more pronounced papaverine-like activity and their antispasmodic effects are therefore more obvious than their antisecretory or central nervous actions. Local anaesthetic activity is another feature of some of these compounds: those which combine marked papaverine-like and local anaesthetic actions should theoretically be more useful than atropine itself in the treatment of gastrointestinal conditions associated with pain and spasm.

Some of the compounds have well marked antispasmodic properties with little mydriatic action, while other substances have more pronounced mydriatic actions. As we have seen, these differences are in some instances largely or partly attributable to the drugs' possessing more than a simple antimuscarine action but there remains a number of purely antimuscarine substances that differ in their relative antispasmodic and mydriatic potencies. Attempts have been made to discern the structural features underlying these two types of action but they have not been very successful and there is little evidence to suggest that mydriatic and antispasmodic actions involve different types of receptor or different types of drug-receptor interaction. It is more likely that the variations in mydriatic and antispasmodic actions shown by the different compounds arise because of differences in the ease with which they gain access to the receptors. The relative potencies of the different drugs depend very much on the species of animal on which they are tested as well as the route of administration. Thus, on local application in the cat, atropine methonitrate is no more potent a mydriatic agent than atropine but when it is given to the mouse by intraperitoneal injection, it is over twice as potent as atropine (Ing, Dawes and Wajda, 1945).

Some antihistamines have atropine-like actions. These are discussed in Chapter 21.

STRUCTURE-ACTIVITY RELATIONSHIPS IN ATROPINE-LIKE COMPOUNDS

Atropine and hyoscine are both tertiary bases and are respectively the tropic acid esters of tropine and of a derivative of tropine, 6,7-epoxytropine. They are very potent muscarine antagonists and many synthetic compounds have been modelled upon them. On the other hand, many compounds which bear little or no chemical

Table 15.1 Some atropine-like compounds

Approved name	Formula	Proprietary name(s)	Remarks
Adiphenine R = Adiphenine–6H R =	 $CH.CO.O(CH_2)_2 N(C_2H_5)_2$	Trasentine Trasentine-6H	Papaverine-like action on smooth muscle. Local anaesthetic action. Little action on eye, heart or glands
Amptrotropine		Syntropan	Similar properties and uses to adiphenine
Carbofluorene aminoester hydrochloride Carbatrine		Pavatrine	Similar to adiphenine
Dibutoline		Dibuline	Powerful atropine-like actions but short lasting
Dicyclomine hydrochloride		Bentyl, Merbentyl Wyovin	Papaverine-like and local anaesthetic properties. Antispasmodic
Mepenzolate methylbromide		Cantil	Antispasmodic effect, particularly marked on colon
Piperidolate hydrochloride		Dactil	Some local anaesthetic activity. Used in treatment of gastro-intestinal spasm

Table 15.1 (contd)

Approved name	Formula	Proprietary name(s)	Remarks
Eucatropine		Euphthalamine	Very short acting mydriatic
Hexocyclium methylsulphate		Tral	Atropine-like action mainly exerted on gastro-intestinal tract
Lachesine bromide			Short acting mydriatic and anti-spasmodic. Sedative action. Useful in homatropine-sensitive patients.
Methantheline bromide		Banthine	Atropine-like properties. Ganglion and some neuromuscular blocking action. Used in treatment of peptic ulcer
Oxyphenonium bromide		Antrenyl Spastrex	Atropine-like properties
Penthienate bromide		Monodral	Atropine-like properties
Pipenzolate		Piptal	Antispasmodic

Table 15.1 (contd)

Approved name	Formula	Proprietary name(s)	Remarks
Poldine		Nacton	Antispasmodic
Propantheline bromide		Pro-Banthine	Similar properties and use to meth-antheline. More potent, less toxic
Sestron		Antispasmin Profenil	Papaverine-like actions. Anti-spasmodic
Tricyclamol methylsulphate		Elorine Lergine Tricoloid	Atropine-like properties

relationship to atropine or to hyoscine possess significant antiacetylcholine activity.

In homatropine, mandelic acid replaces the tropic acid of atropine. Other aromatic and aliphatic acids have been used in place of mandelic and tropic acids but of the compounds made, only homatropine has been widely used. Pyman suggested that the acid part of the molecule should contain an aromatic ring, an asymmetric carbon atom and an alcoholic hydroxyl group. Later work has only partly borne out this view.

The complex, bridged seven-membered tropine ring can be replaced by simpler structures. In eucatropine it has been replaced by 1,2,2,6-tetramethyl piperidinol and amptrotropine, tropic acid is esterified with 3-diethylam-ino-2,2-dimethyl-propanol. Benzilic acid has been used to

replace tropic acid, and a number of potent mydriatics contain a benzilic acid residue. The view has been put forward that tropic acid derivatives are predominantly antispasmodic and those of benzilic acid predominantly mydriatic, yet atropine and hyoscine, both tropic acid derivatives, are potent mydriatics.

Since atropine antagonizes the muscarinic actions of acetylcholine, it was natural to look for atropine-like activity among compounds related to acetylcholine. Acetylcholine is the ester of a fatty acid (acetic acid) with an amino alcohol (choline). Laschesine, which has potent atropine-like activity, is the ester of benzilic acid with an amino alcohol (choline). Lachesine, which has potent pavatrine and caramiphen are all esters of diethylamino-ethanol and heavily substituted derivatives of acetic acid.

In these compounds there is a tertiary nitrogen atom but lachesine is a quaternary base, as are oxyphenonium and methantheline. Oxyphenonium and methantheline are the methobromides of diethylaminoethanol esterified with heavily substituted derivatives of acetic acid. It is very difficult to draw any general conclusions as to the chemical structure necessary for a compound to possess atropine-like activity. Tertiary bases do not appear to possess any very marked advantages over the quarternary ones. The tropine ring system is not essential, nor is tropic acid. Many atropine-like compounds bear some relationship to acetylcholine but this is often rather difficult to see. The most that can be said is that many atropine-like compounds are esters of an amino alcohol with a substituted acetic acid. A generalized formula for atropine-like compounds is indicated in Figure 15.2 but many substances that do not display the structural features in the formula nevertheless possess atropine-like activity.

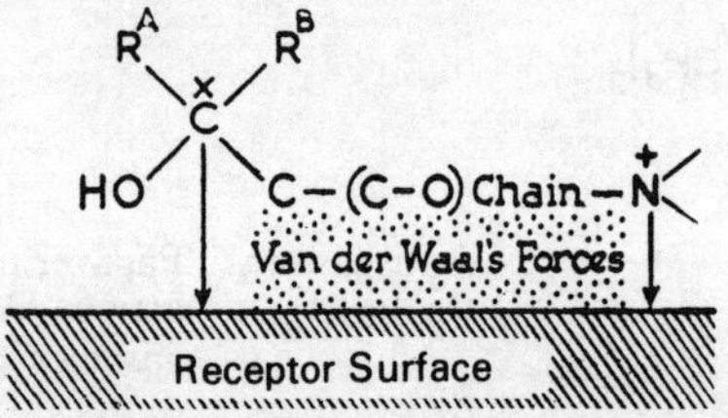

Fig. 15.2 Structural features associated with atropine-like anticholinergic activity.

The hypothetical compound contains a quaternary carbon atom (C^X) which bears an alcoholic hydroxyl group, a ring system (R^A) and (at R^B) an aromatic or aliphatic group or a hydrogen atom. The quaternary carbon atom is separated from a tertiary nitrogen atom (N^+) by a short (four or five membered) carbon or carbon-oxygen chain. The molecule is firmly held on to the receptor surface at the two points C^X and N^+. At the former, dipole bond formation may take place while at the latter the bond formed is ionic. Van der Waal's forces may assist in the binding to the receptor surface at points between these centres. The function of the hydroxyl group is not very clear but it may assist in fixing the molecule firmly to the cell surface.

BIBLIOGRAPHY

Books, monographs and reviews

Ambache N. (1955). The use and limitations of atropine for pharmacological studies on autonomic effectors. *Pharmac. Rev.*, **7**, 467-494.

Burn, J. H. (1958). *Functions of Autonomic Transmitters*, pp. 137-161. Baltimore: Williams and Wilkins.

Cavallito, C.J. and Gray, A.P. (1960). Chemical nature and pharmacological actions of quaternary ammonium salts. *Prog. Drug Res.*, **2**, 135-226.

Grant, W. M. (1955). Physiological and pharmacological influences upon intraocular pressure. *Pharmac. Rev.*, **7**, 143-182.

Original papers

Curtis, D. R. and Phillis, J. W. (1960). The action of procaine and atropine on spinal neurones. *J. Physiol.* **153**, 17-34.

Ing, H. R., Dawes, G. S. and Wajda, I. (1945). Synthetic substitutes for atropine. *J. Pharmac. exp. Ther.*, **85**, 85-102.

Krnjevic, K. and Phillis, J. W. (1963a). Acetylcholine-sensitive cells in the cerebral cortex. *J. Physiol.*, **166**, 296-327.

Krnjevic, K. and Phillis, J. W. (1963b). Pharmacological properties of acetylcholine-sensitive cells in the cerebral cortex. *J. Physiol.*, **166**, 328-350.

Longo, V. G. (1956). Action of atropine and scopolamine on the EEG and behavioural reactions due to hypothalamic stimulation. *J. Pharmac. exp. Ther.*, **116**, 198-208.

Longo, V. G. (1962). *Electroencephalographic Atlas for Pharmacological Research.* pp. 39-43. Amsterdam: Elsevier.

Wikler, A. (1952). Pharmacologic dissociation of behaviour and EEG 'sleep patterns' in dogs: morphine, N-allylnormophine and atropine. *Proc. Soc. exp. Biol.*, **79**, 261-265.

16. Drugs that block neuromuscular or ganglionic transmission

The processes involved in the transmission of impulses across the neuromuscular junction have been described in Chapter 13. Interruption of any of these processes will lead to paralysis of voluntary muscle and it is convenient to classify neuromuscular blocking agents by reference to the stage in the transmission sequence at which they exert their effects. The classes of drug thus categorized are:

I. *Drugs that Depress Acetylcholine Output*
   (a) by inhibition of synthesis or storage
   (b) by inhibition of release

II. *Drugs that Prevent the Action of Released Acetylcholine*
   (a) by depolarizing the muscle end plate
   (b) by preventing the depolarizing action of acetylcholine
   (c) by a mixed action

As yet, only drugs in the second of the two major categories have found clinical application.

Some drugs bring about relaxation of the skeletal musculature by an action on neurones in the spinal cord. They are not neuro-muscular blocking agents in the strict sense of the term but it is convenient to consider them in the context of the present chapter.

It will be clear that it will also be possible, theoretically at least, for drugs to facilitate neuromuscular transmission by increasing the output of acetylcholine or by potentiating its action after release. One such substance is guanidine, which potentiates the release of acetylcholine from motor nerves and which has been used sporadically in the treatment of botulism (p. 236) and myasthenia gravis. Although its champions have been pressing its claims for attention for nearly forty years, guanidine is still only used rarely. It is not very effective as an adjunct to other forms of treatment and it is prone to produce severe gastrointestinal upsets and tremulousness if the dose is not very carefully adjusted: on the rare occasions when it is used it is given in daily oral doses of 20 to 50 mg per kilogram.

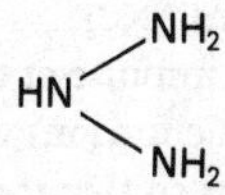

DRUGS THAT DEPRESS ACETYLCHOLINE OUTPUT

As yet no substance is known which can prevent acetylcholine synthesis by inhibiting the activity of choline acetyltransferase. However, a group of compounds (triethycholine and the hemicholiniums) inhibit synthesis

Guanidine

apparently by competing with choline for occupation of the intracellular transport mechanism to the site of synthesis. In accord with this hypothesis is the fact that their inhibitory action is reversed by choline.

HEMICHOLINIUMS

These compounds, which were first synthesized in 1955 by Schueler, have two choline moieties in the molecules. The best known member of the group is that named HC-3. As would be expected it also impairs the production of acetylcholine in other cholinergic nerves and in brain tissue. The block of neuromuscular transmission produced by the hemicholiniums develops only slowly. This is because the preformed stores of acetylcholine have to be depleted before transmission can be affected. For this reason, transmission failure occurs most rapidly at those junctions where activity is greatest. The hemicholiniums also depress the sensitivity of the motor end plate to acetylcholine but this effect is only apparent at dose levels

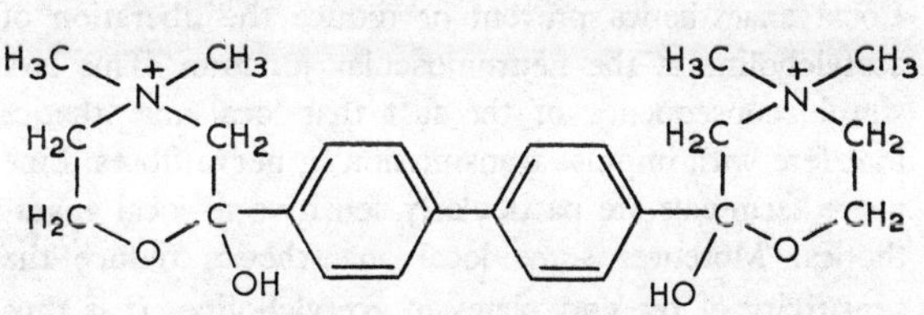

The hemicholinium,   HC-3

higher than those which can produce complete neuromuscular block by preventing acetylcholine synthesis.

TRIETHYLCHOLINE.

Triethylcholine behaves in every way like HC-3. The hemicholiniums and triethylcholine have not been used

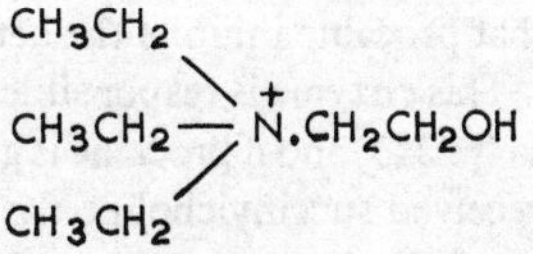

Triethylcholine

clinically. Since they produce transmission block most easily at junctions where activity is high, it was suggested (Bowman, Hemsworth and Rand, 1962) that they might find a use in conditions such as tetanus in which painful muscle spasms are due to over-activity of motor nerves but this expectation has not materialized.

Inhibitors of release

CHANGES IN IONIC BALANCE
The arrival of a nerve impulse at the motor nerve terminal permits the entry of calcium ions which alter the properties of the synaptic vesicles so that they liberate acetylcholine. There is a direct relationship between the concentration of calcium ions in the tissue fluid and the amount of acetylcholine which is liberated. Consequently any reduction in the amount of calcium in the plasma will be attended by some degree of neuromuscular block. Magnesium ions have the opposite effect and the actions of magnesium and calcium are mutually antagonistic except at high ionic concentrations when both species depress the excitability of the muscle by a direct action on the muscle membrane. Potassium ions facilitate transmission by increasing acetylcholine release.

ANTIBIOTICS
Kanamycin, neomycin and streptomycin produce neuromuscular block by a mechanism similar to that caused by calcium lack. They are also capable of causing an antidepolarizing blockade of muscle (p. 237) and some reports suggest that they inhibit acetylcholines synthesis.

LOCAL ANAESTHETICS
Local anaesthetics prevent or reduce the liberation of acetylcholine at the neuromuscular junction. This is a simple consequence of the fact that local anaesthetics interfere with impulse transmission in nerve fibres. Fine nerve terminals are particularly sensitive to local anaesthetics. Moreover some local anaesthetics reduce the sensitivity of the end plates to acetylcholine. It is thus relatively easy to produce muscle paralysis by injecting a local anaesthetic in the neighbourhood of the motor nerve terminals but the circumstances under which the anaesthetics are administered do not normally lead to any significant degree of neuromuscular blockade. However, care should be exercised when local anaesthetics are given to patients with myasthenia gravis for in this condition the muscles are extremely sensitive to any reduction in the amount of available acetylcholine (p. 245). It must also be remembered that procaine inhibits the activity of butyrocholinesterase. This enzyme is responsible for inactivating succinylcholine (p. 243) and if procaine is given to a patient who has just received succinylcholine the neuromuscular blocking effect of the latter drug may be unexpectedly prolonged.

Substances that interfer with the sodium pump mechanism (cardiac glycosides, uncoupling agents, etc.) will have the same action as a local anaesthetic.

BOTULINUM TOXIN
The anaerobic organism *Clostridium botulinum* may infect foods, particularly meat (*botulus* means sausage) and vegetables. If contaminated foods are canned without adequate sterilization the organism may multiply during storage of the food. It produces a toxin which, if the food is eaten in an uncooked form, is likely to give rise to the condition of *botulism*. Although botulism is a relatively rare condition, sporadic outbreaks still occur particularly among people who eat much prepared food or who are given to preparing preserves and bottled foods in their own homes. In botulism, skeletal muscles (including the muscles of respiration) are paralysed and parasympathetic nervous activity is inhibited so that, in addition to muscle weakness, there is paralysis of accommodation, dilated pupils, impairment of gastrointestinal activity and urinary retention. The toxin does not interfere with the transmission of impulses along the nerve terminals nor does it modify the response of the muscles to acetylcholine. It prevents the release of acetylcholine, perhaps by obstructing the exits by which the transmitter leaves the nerve terminals after its release from the synaptic vesicles. The only effective treatment in cases of the severe poisoning is artificial ventilation: there is no antidote to the toxin and such procedures as increasing the plasma calcium concentration have little ameliorative effect, since in botulism there is interference only with the final stage of the train of events which leads to the release of acetylcholine. The effects of the toxin are very long lasting and artificial respiration may have to be continued for several days or perhaps weeks. The toxin is extremely potent, as little as one microgram being sufficient to cause fatal poisoning in man.

The facts that botulinum toxin is potent, lethal and cheap to produce in quantity provide an irresistible temptation to those charged with their nations' defence and it has been the subject of study in biological warfare laboratories throughout the world.

OTHER TOXINS
Muscle paralysis is a feature of some other diseases notably diphtheria, the toxin of which inhibits the conduction of nerve impulses in the motor nerve and may also inhibit acetylcholine synthesis. Some parasitic ticks paralyse farm animals by a similar action.

DRUGS THAT PREVENT THE ACTION OF RELEASED ACETYLCHOLINE

Under normal circumstances acetylcholine, the physiological mediator of neuromuscular transmission, is rapidly destroyed by cholinesterase and this permits end-plate depolarizations (and hence muscle contractions) to follow rapidly upon one another when the motor nerve is repetitively stimulated. However, if depolarization is brought about by cholinesterase the end plate will be held in its depolarized state and the muscle will no longer respond to motor nerve stimulation. Substances that lead to muscle paralysis in this way are called, for obvious reasons, *depolarizing blocking agents*. It will be clear that, in appropriate circumstances, acetylcholine itself may produce a depolarization blockade. Thus, if cholinesterase is inhibited by an anticholinesterase agent or if the enzyme is overwhelmed by the injection of a large dose of acetylcholine, the motor end plate will suffer a more or less prolonged depolarization and it will be incapable of responding to motor nerve stimulation (or to depolarizing drugs) until the block is removed. The intra-arterial injection of small amounts of acetylcholine in the normal human subject causes a transient paralysis of the muscles supplied by that artery.

Muscle contraction can also be prevented by drugs that compete with acetylcholine for the receptors at the end plate but do not themselves cause depolarization. These agents do not cause muscle contraction but since they prevent the access of acetylcholine to its receptors they prevent—or in smaller doses reduce—muscle contraction in response to motor nerve stimulation or to the injection of depolarizing drugs. This type of blocking agent is described as *antidepolarizing, non-depolarizing* or *competitive*. All three terms are used interchangeably but the first is probably the most satisfactory if not the most generally popular. The best known antidepolarizing drug is tubocurarine: others are quoted later. Since these drugs compete with acetylcholine (and with other depolarizing

Table 16.1 Comparison between depolarizing and antidepolarizing blocking agents

	Depolarizing Blocking Agents	Antidepolarizing (Non-depolarizing or Competitive) Blocking Agents
1. *Effects of blocking agents on muscle tone*		
a) block preceded by increased muscle activity	Yes	No
b) agent causes contraction of isolated frog rectus muscle	Yes	No
c) type of paralysis in chick	Spastic	Flaccid
2. *Effects of blocking agents on the depolarizing action of acetylcholine and on the tension developed during and after a tetanus*		
a) depolarizing action of acetylcholine	Unaffected	Reduced
b) muscle responses, in presence of the agent, to a train of impulses	All responses reduced to the same extent	Progressive decline in responses
c) blocking action partially reversed by a tetanus	No	Yes
3. *Effect of applied electric currents on block*		
a) anodal current	Block reduced	Block intensified
b) cathodal current	Block intensified	Block reduced
4. *Effect of ether anaesthesia on block*	Block unaffected or reduced	Block potentiated and prolonged
5. *Sensitivity of myasthenic patients to blocking agents*	Normal or decreased	Very much more sensitive than normal subjects
6. *Block reversed by*	Antidepolarizing agents but block difficult to reverse	Anticholinesterases; Depolarizing agents; Potassium ions; Adrenaline; Ephedrine

agents) it follows that the depolarizing and the antidepolarizing blocking agents have mutually antagonistic actions.

Some compounds behave as simple depolarizing agents in some species but in others they may have a mixed action, producing a condition that exhibits some of the characteristics of both a depolarization and an antidepolarization blockade. 'Mixed' block is discussed after the features of the pure types have been considered in more detail.

Although the antidepolarizing agents are competitive antagonists of acetylcholine, the depolarizing drugs are *not* non-competitive antagonists in the sense in which that term is properly defined (p. 101) since they affect the same receptors as do acetylcholine and the competitive blocking agents. They are in fact partial agonists.

Table 16.1 summarises the principal characteristics of the depolarizing and the antidepolarizing drugs. Some of these features require further explanation and elaboration as follows.

1. Effects on muscle tone

Depolarization of the end plate initiates a propagated action potential in the muscle membrane and this provides the stimulus for contraction. A prolonged depolarization of the end plate might therefore be expected to cause muscle spasm: as the membrane recovered from its refractoriness another action potential would be generated by the still depolarized end plate and muscle contractions would follow one another at least as rapidly as they do in a complete tetanus. In fact this does not occur in mammals, which respond to depolarizing blocking agents by a few muscle twitches followed by a flaccid paralysis. This is because the depolarizing agents soon cause a persistent

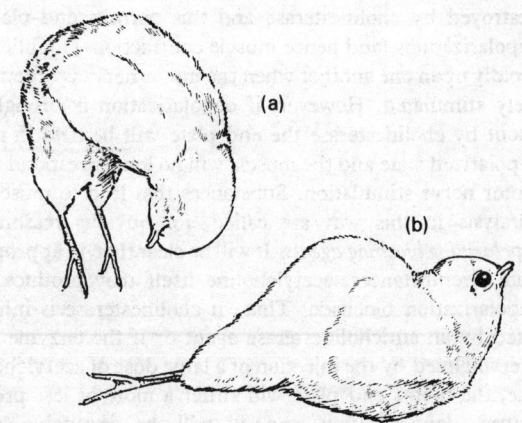

Fig. 16.1 The effects of neuromuscular blocking agents on the chick. (a) Flaccid paralysis produced by an antidepolarizing agent (D-tubocurarine). (b) Spastic paralysis produced by a depolarizing agent (decamethonium).

depolarization in the muscle membrane immediately adjacent to the end plate. This effectively prevents the propagation of further action potentials. Antidepolarizing blocking agents also produce a flaccid paralysis but this is not preceded by muscle twitching. In some avian species, depolarizing agents do produce a prolonged increase in muscle activity and a marked difference between the effects of the two types of blocking agent can be strikingly demonstrated if they are given by intravenous injection to the young conscious chick. Depolarizing agents cause a spastic paralysis, the chick's legs becoming forcibly extended and the head being thrust back. Antidepolarizing blocking agents produce a flaccid paralysis, the muscles becoming limp and lifeless (Fig. 16.1). The same differ-

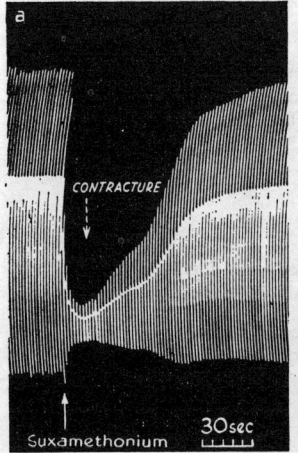
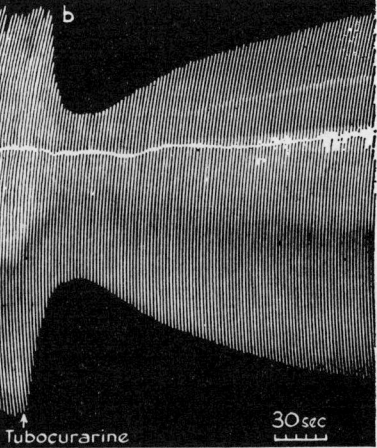

Fig. 16.2 (a) *Left-hand tracing*. Contracture of the hen gastrocnemius muscle induced by intravenous injection of suxamethonium. Note that not only is the twitch-height reduced, but the muscle is shortened. (b) *Right-hand tracing*. Partial neuromuscular blockade of the same preparation with tubocurarine. Twitch-height is reduced but there is no contracture. The muscle was stimulated indirectly *via* the sciatic nerve. (Reproduced by permission of the editor of the *Journal of Pharmacy and Pharmacology*).

ence can be seen in the contractions of avian muscles in response to motor nerve stimulation in the presence of the blocking agents. Both cause a reduction in twitch size but depolarizing drugs also produce an increase in muscle tone, because of the continued generation of action potentials (Fig 16.2).

2. Effects on the depolarizing action of acetylcholine and on the tension developed during a tetanus.

The extent by which a small dose of acetylcholine reduces the resting end plate potential is not affected by the presence of a depolarizing agent. A competitive blocking agent, on the other hand, prevents the access of acetylcholine to the receptors and reduces its depolarizing effect. The extent of this interference with the action of acetylcholine depends on the relative concentrations of acetylcholine and the blocking agent. These facts explain the changes in muscle tension which are seen when a motor nerve is repetitively stimulated at a fast rate in an animal which has received a blocking agent. During a tetanus the amount of acetylcholine released by each nerve impulse decreases as stimulation proceeds. In the normal animal this has no effect on muscle tension since the amount of transmitter liberated by even the later stimuli of the tetanus is more than sufficient to effect depolarization of all the end plates. In the presence of the depolarizing type of blocking agent the tension is even more easily maintained: because of the persisting state of partial depolarization the amount of acetylcholine required to produce complete depolarization is less than that in the untreated animals. A different state of affairs exists in animals which have been given a blocking agent of the competitive type, for as the amount of available acetylcholine falls off the effect of the blocking drug becomes more pronounced and the tension reduces as more and more end plates receive insufficient transmitter for adequate depolarization. The different effects of depolarizing and antidepolarizing agents on the tension developed during a tetanus are illustrated in Figure 16.3.

Post-tetanic facilitation is a response exhibited by muscles partially paralysed by blocking agents of the competitive type. If a motor nerve is subjected to slow repetitive stimulation, the corresponding muscle will respond with contractions of a constant size. If the repetitive stimulation is interrupted by a brief tetanus and the slow stimulation is resumed at the earlier rate, the response to the first of these renewed stimuli will be larger than those which immediately preceded the tetanus. It is this increased response which constitutes the phenomenon of post-tetanic facilitation and it is due to the fact that the first post-tetanic stimulus liberates an increased amount of acetylcholine (Hutter, 1952). This partially overcomes the blocking action of the competitive drug. Post-tetanic facilitation does not occur in animals which have received a blocking agent of the depolarizing type because acetylcholine does

not reverse the action of these drugs. Thus, if a neuromuscular block can be partially reversed by a tetanus it is a certain indication that the blockade is due to a drug of the competitive type.

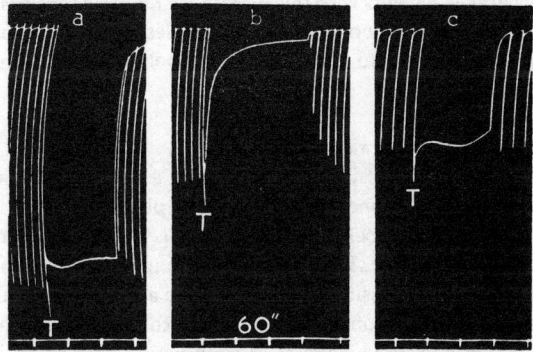

Fig. 16.3 (a) Tetanization of a non-curarized muscle. (b) Tetanization of a muscle partly paralysed with tubocurarine. (c) Tetanization of a muscle partly paralysed with decamethonium. The tracings were obtained from the gastrocnemius muscle of the cat stimulated indirectly *via* the sciatic nerve. Downstrokes represent muscle contractions in response to each electrical stimulus. Tetanic stimulation was commenced at T.

3. Effects of cathodal and anodal currents

A cathodal current (one which passes from the inside to the outside of the end plate) has a depolarizing action and therefore has the same action as acetylcholine. Consequently it will intensify blockade due to a depolarizing drug and antagonize that produced by an antidepolarizing drug. Anodal currents have the opposite effects.

4. Effects of anaesthetics

Ether and some other general anaesthetics (chloroform, cyclopropane and halothane) prolong and intensify the neuromuscular blockade produced by the antidepolarizing drugs. This is because the anaesthetics stabilize the end plate membrane and so oppose its depolarization. Ether is much the most active anaesthetic in this respect and tubocurarine is particularly sensitive to its potentiating action. The blocking action of the depolarizing drugs is usually unaffected by ether, though in some species (but not in man) the blockade is partially reversed. In general, the barbiturates intensify the relaxation produced by both types of blocking agent. The possibility that the degree of muscle relaxation produced by a relaxant drug may be modified by the anaesthetic used has obviously to be taken into account when the drugs are used in surgery. It has been suggested that when ether is used as the anaesthetic, antidepolarizing relaxants should be given in one-third to one-half of the dose which would provide the required degree of relaxation in the absence of an anaesthetic (Foldes, 1960).

5. *Effects of myasthenia gravis*

Muscles affected by myasthenia gravis (p. 245) are several times more sensitive than are normal muscles to the paralysing action of antidepolarizing drugs. This effect is sometimes made the basis of a diagnostic test for myasthenia gravis. Patients with this disease are no more sensitive, and they are sometimes considerably less sensitive, than normal subjects to the action of depolarizing blocking agents.

6. *Reversal of blockade*

Anticholinesterases, which bring about a rapid accumulation of acetylcholine at the motor end plates, reverse the neuromuscular blockade produced by agents that compete with acetylcholine. Depolarizing blocking agents have the same effect. Potassium ions, adrenaline and ephedrine all potentiate the action of acetylcholine at the neuromuscular junction and, used alone or in conjunction with an anticholinesterase, they antagonize the effect of antidepolarizing drugs.

Although the depolarizing and the antidepolarizing agents exert mutually antagonistic effects, the lifting of a depolarization block by an antidepolarizing agent is much less easily accomplished than is the reverse process.

Dual (mixed) block

Many of the investigations which have sought to establish the mode of action of neuromuscular blocking agents have made use of the tibialis anterior muscle of the cat. In this preparation, decamethonium behaves in every way as a depolarizing blocking agent. In man, too, decamethonium in most circumstances produces block by depolarization. However, in many other mammalian species, including, among others, the dog, monkey, guinea pig and rabbit, decamethonium always produces a dual or mixed type of block. When the drug is first injected, the muscles twitch and become depolarized as would be expected, but when the block is fully established it can be antagonized by an anticholinesterase or by a tetanus and prolonged by tubocurarine. These last features are all indicative of the presence of an antidepolarizing blockade. Similar effects are seen with other depolarizing agents. It has already been pointed out that depolarization and antidepolarization blocks are mutually antagonistic. Consequently, muscles which respond to depolarizing agents by developing a dual block rapidly become insensitive to the action of the drug. This provides an indication of yet another way in which tachyphylaxis (p. 84) may arise.

It is now clear that dual blocks may develop, under appropriate circumstances, in all species including those which have hitherto been assumed to develop only a pure depolarization block in response to the administration of depolarizing agents. The soleus muscle of the cat readily develops a dual block and among human subjects this type of blockade is often seen in the muscles of patients with

myasthenia gravis. This explains why myasthenic patients are sometimes very insensitive to depolarizing agents.

The possibility that an antidepolarization block may develop after administration of a depolarizing agent is of more than academic interest to the anaesthetist who uses blocking agents. The management of a patient who has been given a depolarizing drug will have to be altered, particularly in an emergency, if a substantial degree of antidepolarization blockade develops. Yet in general it will not be possible to predict that the patient is likely to develop a dual block and the transition from one type of blockade to the other, if and when it occurs, cannot be detected by superficial examination. One possible method for detecting the presence of antidepolarization blockade has been suggested by Churchill-Davidson and Christie (1959). It involves the rapid stimulation of an accessible motor nerve. If an antidepolarization block is present the resulting tetanus should lighten the paralysis. However, not all the muscles may be responding in the same way and the information obtained by stimulation of the nerves to a single muscle may not give a true indication of the state of affairs in the rest of the musculature, particularly that of the respiratory system, the preservation of whose function is the most vital requirement. Another way in which the diagnosis of a mixed block might theoretically be made consists of the administration of a small dose of neostigmine which should antagonize the antidepolarization phase of the blockade. However, as Bowman (1962) points out, this manoeuvre may lead to a misdiagnosis. Under conditions of light anaesthesia, the blocking agent may bring about a reduction in the amount of acetylcholine liberated by impulses in the motor nerves. An anticholinesterase may, by partially remedying this deficiency, cause a reduction of the paralysis by permitting the development of an increased tension in muscle fibres which have completely recovered from the effects of the drug. Thus, the partial reversal of a neuromuscular blockade by an anticholinesterase agent is not, in these circumstances, indicative of the presence of an antidepolarizing agent. When this factor is taken into account, it seems likely that, in the non-myasthenic patient, dual block is, after all, a relatively rare occurrence. In animal experiments, too, the uncritical interpretation of the results of experiments that involve the administration of neostigmine may lead to an erroneous conclusion that a dual blockade has occurred.

Individual blocking agents

The chemical formulae of the substances discussed below are displayed in Figures 16.4 (antidepolarizing agents) and 16.5 (depolarizing agents).

ANTIDEPOLARIZING AGENTS

TUBOCURARINE

For hundreds of years, the natives of South America tipped their arrows with plant extracts which paralysed the

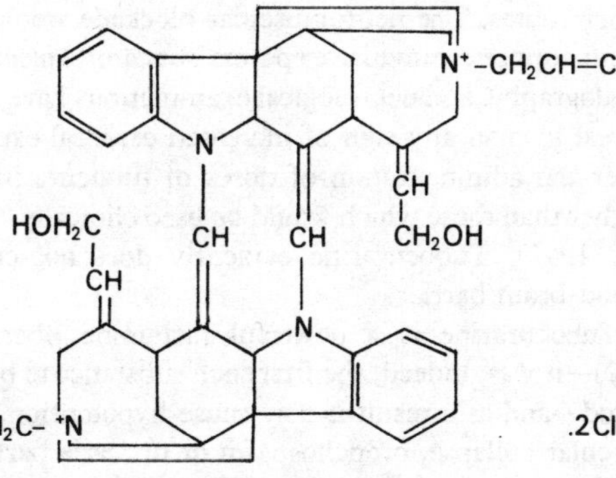

Alcuronium chloride

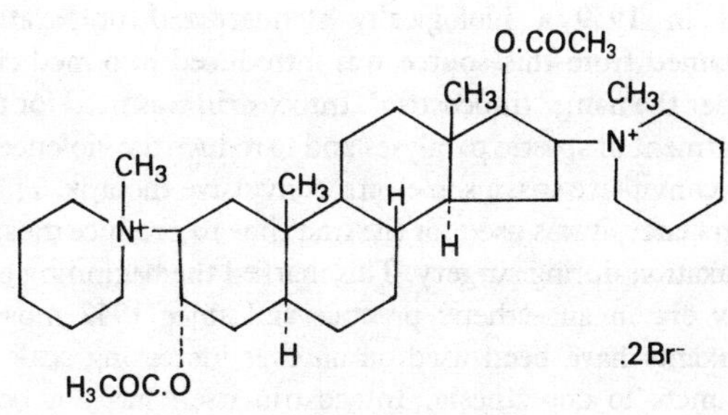

Pancuronium bromide

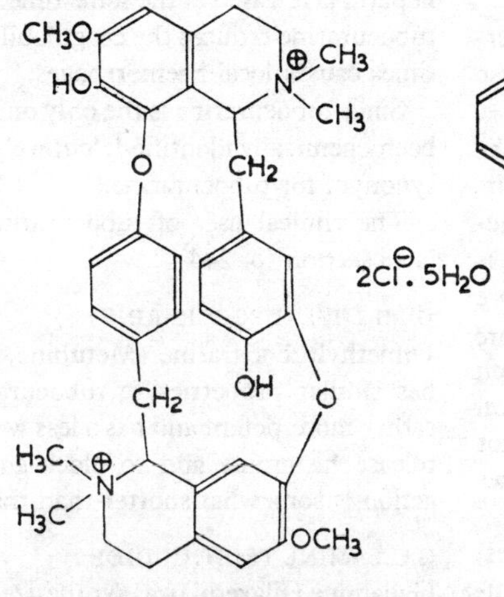

Tubocurarine chloride
(In dimethyltubocurarine the two –OH groups are replaced by –OCH_3)

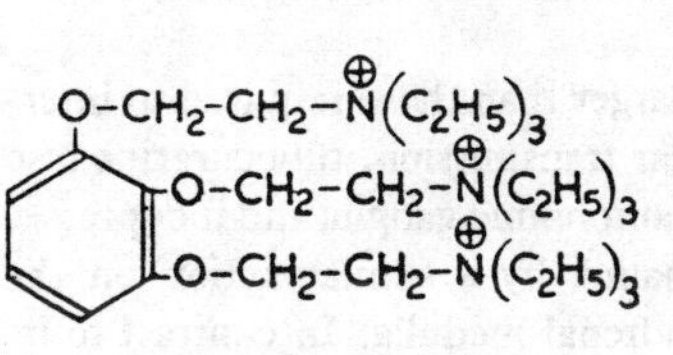

Gallamine triethiodide

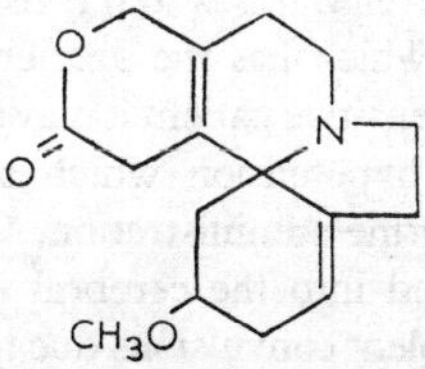

Dihydro-ß-erythroidine

Laudexium methylsulphate

Fig. 16.4 Some antidepolarizing (competitive) neuromuscular blocking agents.

game animals into which they were shot. These arrow poisons were known collectively as woorara, urari or curare: different tribes obtained their curare from a number of different plant species and prepared it in several types of vessels, including pots, calabashes and bamboo tubes. The precise chemical nature of many of the varieties of this ancient poison will probably never be elucidated but one form of tube curare has been available outside South America for many years. In 1935, King isolated the principal active constituent of this material and he established its structure and dextrorotatory optical activity. For obvious reasons, the active principle was called D-tubocurarine. Subsequently the same material was identified in extracts of the plant *Chondrodendron tomentosum* and in 1939 a biologically standardized preparation obtained from this source was introduced into medicine under the name 'Intocostrin'. Intocostrin was used for the treatment of spastic paralyses and to reduce the violence of the convulsive spasms in electroconvulsive therapy. Three years later, it was used for the first time to produce muscle relaxation during surgery. This marked the beginning of a new era in anaesthetic practice and since 1942 muscle relaxants have been used on an ever-increasing scale as adjuncts to anaesthesia. Intocostrin itself has not been used since tubocurarine and its dimethyl ether (dimethyl tubocurarine) have become available in quantity in the pure form.

In doses somewhat larger than those required to interfere with neuromuscular transmission, tubocurarine also blocks transmission in autonomic ganglia and it depresses the secretion of adrenaline by a similar action on the secretory cells of the adrenal medulla. In contrast to its action at the neuromuscular junction, tubocurarine sometimes stimulates the ganglia before depressing them. It is sometimes said that parasympathetic ganglia are more sensitive to the depressant action of tubocurarine than are sympathetic ganglia but, even if this is so it is the effect on the sympathetic ganglia which has the greater practical significance, since in the sensitive patient it may be a factor that contributes to the hypotension which sometimes develops during tubocurarine administration.

When it is administered into the cerebral ventricles, tubocurarine produces violent convulsions due to a stimulant action on structures in the neighbourhood of the ventricles. Excitation of the central nervous system does not, however, occur when tubocurarine is administered by other routes. The neuromuscular blockade would in any event suppress convulsive spasms but careful electroencephalographic and neurological examinations have failed to reveal in man any sign of increased cerebral excitability after the administration of doses of tubocurarine much higher than those which would be used clinically (Smith *et al.*, 1947). Tubocurarine evidently does not cross the blood-brain barrier.

Tubocurarine is a powerful histamine liberator (p. 342)—it was, indeed, the first such substance to be recognized—and as a result it may cause hypotension, cardiovascular collapse, bronchospasm or urticaria particularly in patients who suffer attacks of asthma or other allergic conditions. Histamine is liberated from mast cells and heparin is released at the same time. This may explain why tubocurarine reduces the coagulability of blood and sometimes causes local haemorrhages.

Since tubocurarine is the only one of the curares to have been chemically identified, 'curare' is sometimes used as a synonym for tubocurarine.

The clinical uses of tubocurarine are considered in a later section (p. 244).

DIMETHYLTUBOCURARINE

Dimethyltubocurarine (Metubine, Mecostrin; Fig. 16.4) has similar properties to tubocurarine except that it is rather more potent and has a less well marked tendency to release histamine and to block ganglia. Its duration of action is somewhat shorter than that of tubocurarine.

GALLAMINE TRIETHIODIDE.

Gallamine (Flaxedil) was synthesized in 1946 by Bovet and his colleagues as part of a programme aiming at the production of synthetic compounds which, while based on the tubocurarine molecule, would have a simpler struc-

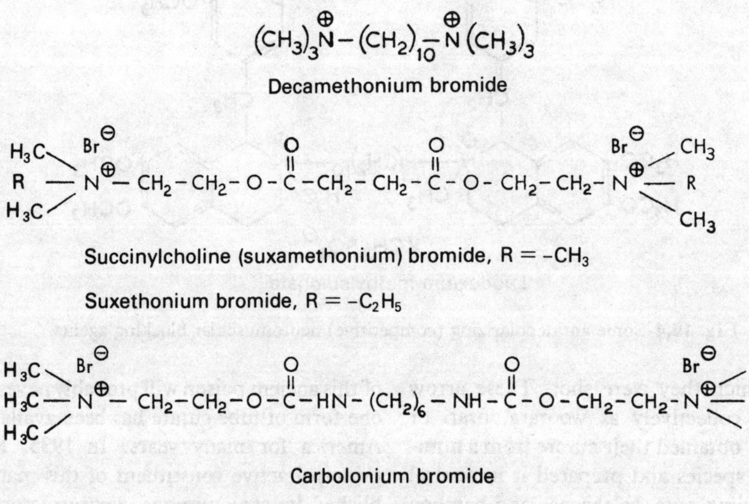

$$Br^{\ominus} \qquad Br^{\ominus}$$
$$(CH_3)_3\overset{\oplus}{N} - (CH_2)_{10} \overset{\oplus}{N} (CH_3)_3$$

Decamethonium bromide

$$H_3C, \quad Br^{\ominus} \qquad\qquad O \qquad\qquad O \qquad\qquad Br^{\ominus} \quad CH_3$$
$$R - \overset{\oplus}{N} - CH_2 - CH_2 - O - \overset{\|}{C} - CH_2 - CH_2 - \overset{\|}{C} - O - CH_2 - CH_2 - \overset{\oplus}{N} - R$$
$$H_3C \qquad\qquad\qquad\qquad\qquad\qquad\qquad\qquad\qquad\qquad\qquad CH_3$$

Succinylcholine (suxamethonium) bromide, R = –CH₃

Suxethonium bromide, R = –C₂H₅

$$H_3C, \quad Br^{\ominus} \qquad\qquad O \qquad\qquad\qquad O \qquad\qquad Br^{\ominus} \quad CH_3$$
$$H_3C - \overset{\oplus}{N} - CH_2 - CH_2 - O - \overset{\|}{C} - HN - (CH_2)_6 - NH - \overset{\|}{C} - O - CH_2 - CH_2 - \overset{\oplus}{N} - CH_3$$
$$H_3C \qquad\qquad\qquad\qquad\qquad\qquad\qquad\qquad\qquad\qquad\qquad CH_3$$

Carbolonium bromide

Fig. 16.5 Some depolarizing blocking agents.

ture. It was the first and is still the best of the synthetic antidepolarizing blocking agents. Its mode of action is similar to that of tubocurarine but it has little tendency to release histamine or to cause blockade of autonomic ganglia. It does, however, exert an atropine-like action on the cardiac branches of the vagus (but not on other parasympathetic nerves) and thereby causes an increase in heart rate and blood pressure. Its effect on the blood pressure is therefore the opposite of that exerted by tubocurarine and it is less suitable than the latter drug for use in hypertensive or thyrotoxic patients.

DIHYDRO-β-ERYTHROIDINE.

Some plants are known to contain substances with a curare-like action but they were never used as sources of arrow posion by natives who had access to them. Among these plants are the trees and bushes of the *Erythrina* genus, from one species of which—E. *americana*—have been isolated the isomeric alkaloids α- and β-erythroidine. Derivatives of β-erythroidine have been prepared; dihydro-β-erythroidine seemed to be the most potentially useful of these compounds and it has been subjected to an intensive study including clinical trials. Erythroidine and its derivatives, have, unlike tubocurarine, some activity when taken by mouth and this may explain why extracts of plants containing erythroidine were never used as arrow poisons: an animal which has had even large amounts of tubocurarine shot into it can be eaten with impunity. Although it has not found clinical application, dihydro-β-erythroidine is used in the laboratory (see, for instance, Fig. 13.3, p. 182).

ALCURONIUM

Alcuronium (Alloferin) is one of the newer antidepolarizing agents. It is a synthetic derivative of a calabash curare. Its properties and uses are similar to those of tubocurarine but it is a less potent histamine liberator and its hypotensive action is not so pronounced. The muscle paralyzing effect of alcuronium is potentiated by halothane. Alcuronium is an example *par excellence* of a pachycurare (p. 247)

PANCURONIUM

As can be seen by reference to its chemical formula, pancuronium (Pavulon) consists essentially of a steroid to which an acetylcholine grouping has been attached but it displays no steroid activity. It does not bring about histamine release of ganglion blockade and it is devoid of activity on the cardiovascular and central nervous systems. Like alcuronium its principal value is as an adjunct to anaesthesia. Muscle relaxation appears within two minutes of its intravenous injection. The neuromuscular activity of pancuronium is potentiated by ether.

OTHER DRUGS

The formula of laudexium methylsulphate (Laudolissin) is included for reference purposes in Figure 16.4. That of benzoquinonium (Mytolon) which has anticholinesterase

as well as neuromuscular blocking activity will be found on p. 215. The drugs are not discussed further here since neither is now used clinically for inducing neuromuscular blockade.

DEPOLARIZING DRUGS

DECAMETHONIUM

The only depolarizing agent that is commonly used is succinylcholine but decamethonium is an interesting drug that merits at least a passing mention. Decamethonium (C10; Syncurine), which is prepared as the bromide or iodide, is a member of a series of compounds (the methonium series) in which two quaternary nitrogen atoms are joined by a polymethylene chain. Neuromuscular blocking activity is maximal in compounds with ten methylene groups, as in decamethonium, when the distance between the quaternary nitrogen atoms is about 1.4 nm. The quaternary nitrogen atoms in tubocurarine are separated by a similar distance. It is believed that this corresponds to the separation between adjacent acetylcholine receptors at the end plate. The molecules of compounds like tubocurarine and decamethonium will therefore be able to occupy all the receptor sites more readily than those of other substances.

In man and the cat, decamethonium normally produces a 'pure' depolarization blockade but, as has been pointed out previously, it produces a dual block in most other species. In the cat, doses of the drug which relax the limb muscles are less likely than tubocurarine to cause paralysis of the respiratory musculature but this advantage is not retained in man. In ordinary doses, decamethonium does not release histamine or block ganglia. It has a slightly shorter duration of action than has tubocurarine but no generally effective method is available for terminating its action and this has led to its falling into disuse.

SUCCINYLCHOLINE

Succinylcholine (suxamethonium, succinyldicholine Anectine, Scoline) was, like gallamine, introduced (in 1949) by Bovet and his colleagues. It has a similar mode of action to decamethonium but the blockade it produces is very short lived: the effect of a single intravenous dose usually persists for no more than five minutes. This is an advantage in a compound whose blocking action is otherwise difficult to reverse for in the circumstances in which the drug is used it is not inconvenient to have to administer it by intravenous drip. Muscle relaxation is maintained for only as long as the drip operates.

The fact that the blocking action of succinylcholine is so evanescent is due to its rapid hydrolysis by butyrocholinesterase. The hydrolysis takes place, in plasma and in liver, in two stages: in the first succinylmonocholine and choline are produced; in the second stage, succinylmonocholine is more slowly hydrolysed to give succinic acid and choline. Succinylmonocholine itself has a weak neuromuscular blocking action. In patients with liver disease, hydrolysis may be slowed and this may result in succinylcholine's having a much more prolonged and intense effect than it has in the normal subject. A similar state of affairs arises in the not insubstantial group of subjects whose plasma and liver butyrocholinesterase is of an atypical form which is incapable of hydrolysing succinylcholine. Very rarely the opposite situation may arise and it proves impossible to establish a neuromuscular block because a highly active cholinesterase disposes of the succinylcholine before it can reach its target.

Procaine and some other local anaesthetics (Chap. 28) inhibit butyrocholinesterase and extreme care has to be exercised if, for any reason, succinylcholine and one of these local anaesthetics have to be given together. On the other hand, the judicious administration of an anticholinesterase agent may sometimes be resorted to if it is necessary to prolong the action of a single dose of succinylcholine. Hexafluorenium (p. 215) is a useful agent for this purpose.

Succinylcholine does not liberate histamine but it stimulates antonomic ganglia and it therefore tends to cause a rise in blood pressure. It causes muscle twitching before the musculature becomes completely relaxed. This stimulant effect is more marked with succinylcholine than it is with other depolarizing blocking agents (perhaps because the drug is commonly injected rapidly) and it may cause some actual damage, trivial but widespread, to the muscle fibres resulting in post-operative soreness in muscles throughout the body. Sometimes the pain produced in this way is very severe.

Succinylcholine is used as the chloride or bromide. Its clinical applications are discussed below.

SUXETHONIUM

The actions of this compound are qualitatively similar to those of succinylcholine. It is hydrolyzed even more rapidly than succinylcholine and it is said to be less likely to cause post-operative muscle pain.

CARBOLONIUM

This drug, which has anticholinesterase and some atropine-like activity (these two properties tend to offset one another) is no longer used clinically.

CLINICAL USES OF THE NEUROMUSCULAR BLOCKING AGENTS

The neuromuscular blocking agents find their principal use in surgery. They promote complete muscle relaxation and permit major abdominal surgery to be carried out on patients who are only lightly anaesthetized and who are therefore spared the hazards of deep anaesthesia. They are also of value in orthopaedic surgery, enabling corrective manipulations to be carried out with ease. A single dose of a short-acting agent such as succinylcholine will facilitate the passage of instruments into the larynx, oesophagus or

bronchi of the lightly anaesthetized patient. When blocking agents are employed in surgery they are not given until the patient is anaesthetized. Remedial measures can then be instituted without delay should the patient prove to be unusually sensitive to the drug.

The painful muscle spasms of tetanus can be reduced in intensity by neuromuscular blocking agents. The drugs have also been used in the treatment of status epilepticus and for attenuating the violent seizures which otherwise accompany electroconvulsive therapy. In these conditions it is useful to administer the muscle relaxant in conjunction with an appropriate anaesthetic.

Tubocurarine is sometimes used in diagnosis. The muscles of myasthenic patients are particularly sensitive to antidepolarizing agents and in cases where the diagnosis is in doubt the production of a severe paralysis by a small dose of tubocurarine (0.1 to 0.3 mg.) will make it plain that the condition is indeed myasthenia gravis. Tubocurarine may also be of assistance in the diagnosis of conditions characterized by immobility of joints. If the joints themselves are affected, the administration of tubocurarine will not make them more mobile, but if muscle spasm contributes to their immobility the drug will free them.

The contribution made by the blocking agents to the elucidation of the part played by acetylcholine in neuromuscular, genglionic and central synaptic transmission is detailed in Chapter 13.

Factors that influence the dosage requirements of neuromuscular blocking agents.

Some indication of the effective doses of the neuromuscular blocking agents is given in Table 16.2, but it is important to recognize that these doses can be no more than approximate. The administration of these drugs—particularly when they are to serve as adjuncts to anaesthesia—should be entrusted only to those with experience of their use. The anaesthetist will adjust the dose by taking into account the circumstances of the case in the light of his previous experience and a knowledge of the factors which

Table 16.2 Doses and duration of action of the neuromuscular blocking agents in current clinical use

	Mean Muscle Relaxing Dose mg./kg	Duration of Action min
Antidepolarizing Agents		
Alcuronium	0.2	15
D-Tubocurarine chloride	0.2	30
Dimethyltubocurarine	0.08	22
Gallamine triethiodide	1.0	25
Pancuronium	0.08	35
Depolarizing Agents		
Decamethonium bromide	0.04	20
Succinylcholine bromide	0.5	3
Suxethonium bromide	0.7	1

are known to influence the effect achieved by different blocking agents. Most of these factors have already been mentioned: they are summarized here for convenience and some additional ones are added:

The nature of the anaesthetic (p. 239).

The temperature of the patient.
If surgery is to be undertaken in a patient who has been rendered hypothermic, it has to be remembered that his sensitivity to depolarizing blocking drugs will be increased but his sensitivity to antidepolarizing agents will be reduced.

The condition of the patient.
Patients with myasthenia gravis and some other forms of muscle disease may exhibit an increased sensitivity to antidepolarizing drugs and a decreased sensitivity to the depolarizing agents (p. 240). Deficiency of butyrocholinesterase potentiates and prolongs the blocking action of succinylcholine. Tubocurarine should be avoided in patients with an allergic diathesis.

The age of the patient
Newborn infants are much less sensitive to depolarization blocking agents than are older children and adults, but they may be more sensitive to tubocurarine. Aged patients tend to be more sensitive than younger adults to both types of blocking agent.

Disturbances of potassium metabolism
Hyperkalaemia causes an increased sensitivity to depolarizing agents and a decreased sensitivity to antidepolarizing drugs. Hypokalaemia has the opposite consequences.

Concurrent administration of other drugs.
As we have seen (p. 236) a number of antibiotics potentiate the action of tubocurarine and other antidepolarizing agents. Antibiotics are sometimes placed in the peritoneal cavity in the closing stages of abdominal surgery. If this is done while the patient is still under the influence of an antidepolarizing agent, there may be a sudden deepening of the paralysis with arrest of respiratory movements. The effects of local anaesthetics on neuromuscular function are discussed on page 236.

Toxic effects
Muscles like those of the eye and digits, that are called upon to perform delicate and finely regulated movements receive a rich motor nerve supply and they are highly susceptible to paralysis by the neuromuscular blocking agents. The least sensitive are the muscles of respiration, particularly the diaphragm. This is a fortunate circumstance but the respiratory muscles are not immune to blockade and unexpected respiratory paralysis is the most potentially dangerous hazard attending the use of the blocking agents. Paralysis of the diaphragm carries an additional risk for it can lead to regurgitation of stomach contents and their aspiration into the lungs of the supine patient if the trachea has not been intubated. In thoracic surgery it may be necessary deliberately to produce respiratory paralysis but in these circumstances the dose will be carefully adjusted and the cessation of respiration will not assume the dimensions of an emergency. Cardiovascular collapse, bronchoconstriction or less serious manifestations of histamine release may occur when tubocurarine is used.

Respiratory paralysis demands the immediate institution of artificial respiration. In many cases no further treatment will be necessary but if spontaneous respiration is slow to return, more positive steps may have to be taken to reverse the action of the blocking agent. Before this is done, it is necessary, as Grob (1967) has emphasized, to be sure that the respiratory arrest is really due to persistent blocking agent and not to some other circumstance.

If an antidepolarizing drug has been given, treatment with atropine and an anticholinesterase agent should lighten the paralysis. Atropine is given in an intravenous dose of 0.5 to 1 mg. This is followed by the anticholinesterase—neostigmine, 0.5 to 1.5 mg or edrophonium, 10 to 20 mg are the drugs of choice. Edrophonium has a short duration of action and the dose may have to be repeated several times if the patient's respiration is to be maintained. Neostigmine is the better drug to use but it is essential to keep the patient fully atropinized throughout the period of neostigmine action if serious muscarinic effects (bronchoconstriction, excessive bronchial secretion, cardiac arrest, etc.) are to be avoided. The risk of administering an overdose of the anticholinesterase must always be borne in mind.

Some patients do not respond to anticholinesterase administration as rapidly as they should. In these cases, potassium chloride, adrenaline or both substances may be used to potentiate the action of the accumulating acetylcholine. Antihistamines may be useful to counter the effects of mild degrees of histamine release.

Reversal of the paralysis produced by a depolarizing agent is more difficult. The actions of decamethonium can sometimes be antagonized by hexamethonium (p. 253) but the attendant hypotension due to ganglion blockade is a disadvantage. Attempts to reverse the paralysis by tubocurarine administration, though theoretically a valid procedure, are usually no more than partially successful and it is probably best to rely on artificial respiration to bring about the restoration of normal breathing.

MYASTHENIA GRAVIS

The story of myasthenia gravis, particularly the instalments that are unfolding as these very words are being written is, to this author at least, one of the most fascinating in medicine.

Myasthenia gravis is a disease that causes its victims' muscles to become weak and easily fatigued. The disability may be trivial and restricted to the eye muscles which become more than normally fatigued at the end of the day. More commonly, the muscle weakness is more severe and widespread: it typically begins in the face and neck and then spreads progressively to involve the upper limbs, the abdomen and the muscles of respiration. The course of the disease may be punctuated by periods of more or less complete remission and by periods during which the muscle weakness becomes more marked. If untreated, the condition not infrequently has a fatal outcome.

As long ago as 1895, Jolly pointed out that the behaviour of myasthenic muscles resembled that of muscles poisoned with curare. This early observation has been amply substantiated. The careful reader will have already realized that the muscles most frequently affected in myasthenia gravis are those that are most susceptible to the action of curare. The similarity between myasthenic and curarized muscle that is obvious on superficial examination does not break down when the behaviour of the muscle is analyzed in the detail permitted by modern myographic techniques. Finally it is to be noted that, whatever other treatment is employed in myasthenia gravis, the mainstay is a combination of drugs—an anticholinesterase, atropine and ephedrine—that would the most effectively relieve neuromuscular blockade produced by an antidepolarizing agent.

That there is a link between myasthenia gravis and pathological conditions in the thymus has been suspected for many years. In 1911, Sauerbach removed the thymus from a young lady who had both thyrotoxicosis and myasthenia gravis. He had hoped that the operation would lead to an amelioration of the thyrotoxic state but in the event it was the myasthenia that responded to the surgery (see Goldstein and Mackay, 1969). In the years that followed and despite the reservations of sceptics, thymectomy became slowly established as a method of treating myasthenia gravis particularly in patients unresponsive to anticholinesterase therapy. Several recent surveys agree that between 60 and 70 per cent of those who have undergone thymectomy have enjoyed either a complete recovery from their illness or a considerable improvement in their clinical state.

The first report of the occurrence of a thymic tumour (*thymoma*) in a patient with myasthenia gravis appeared in 1901 but thymomas are not found in more than 10 per cent of myasthenia victims. On the other hand, it has recently become clear that the thymus glands of more than 70 per cent of myasthenia patients exhibit histological evidence of what Goldstein believes is a chronic inflammatory condition or *thymitis* (Castleman, 1966; Goldstein and Mackay, 1969). Since a thymoma will also cause thymitis we can see

that fewer than 20 per cent of patients with myasthenia gravis will be free of obvious thymitis.

We must now enquire into the nature of the association between thymitis and the characteristic disturbances of neuromuscular function in myasthenia gravis.

Even in the days when obvious pathological changes in the thymus had been detected in only a small proportion of patients with myasthenia gravis, the similarities between myasthenic and curarized muscle prompted the notion that myasthenia gravis is the result of the liberation into the blood stream of a curare like substance elaborated by the thymus. This attractive hypothesis explained not only the features of the disease to which we have already drawn attention but also the fact that the infants of myasthenic mothers not infrequently display signs of myasthenia gravis during their first days of life as they might be expected to do if the disorder were caused by the activity of a blood borne blocking agent easily transferred from mother to foetus. Some of the experimental evidence adduced in support of this hypothesis was very persuasive. Thus, Wilson and his colleagues reported that extracts of the thymus glands of myasthenic patients produced a curare like block of neuromuscular transmission in laboratory preparations such as the rat's isolated phrenic nerve-diaphragm. Extracts of normal thymus were without effect (Wilson *et al.*, 1953). If these results could have been regularly confirmed they would have provided powerful support for the idea that the thymus gland can elaborate and secrete a substance with curare like properties. Unfortunately, other workers (see, for instance, Parkes and McKinna, 1967) were unable to confirm these findings and the simple 'humoral' hypothesis became less popular. It suffered an almost total eclipse when it became clear that myasthenia gravis is an autoimmune disease (p. 395) and the idea gained currency that the neuromuscular blocking agent in myasthenia would prove to be an antibody to the acetylcholine receptor at the end plate. The thymus also carries acetylcholine receptors. They are located on the myoepithelial elements that form an integral part of the organ's structure and if autoantibodies developed against these receptors, moved on to the end plates the involvement of the thymus in myasthenia gravis would be very neatly explained. Acetylcholine antibodies can certainly be demonstrated in the blood of patients with myasthenia gravis but opinion is divided on the crucial question as to whether they are capable of combining with end plate receptors. There are other objections to the idea that receptor antibodies are the cause of the muscle weakness: they can sometimes be detected in the blood of newborn infants whose neuromuscular function is perfectly normal and it is difficult, since antibodies would not be expected to disappear rapidly, to explain the immediate effect of thymectomy in myasthenia gravis.

An alternative hypothesis, and one which in this writer's opinion has much to recommend it, is that of Goldstein

(Goldstein, 1968, Goldstein and Schlesinger, 1975) who maintains that the thymitis which is so regular a finding in myasthenia gravis is the result of an autoimmune reaction in the thymus itself and that this leads to the overproduction of the gland's normal secretion. Goldstein at first gave the name *thymin* to the active material presumably secreted by the thymus and he showed that simple extracts of normal bovine thymus, injected daily for ten days into guinea pigs, caused changes in muscle histology and function similar to those seen in myasthenia gravis. More recently he has been able to establish both the structure of thymin (it is a polypeptide with 49 aminoacid residues) and its likely physiological function (it seems to control the differentiation of lymphocytes) and he had renamed it *thymopoietin*. Experiments with synthesized material have established that the neuromuscular blocking activity of thymopoietin resides in a 13 residue fragment of the complete molecule. Single intraperitoneal injections in mice of microgram quantities of the synthesized fragment ('thymopoietin 29-41') are followed by an impairment of neuromuscular transmission that is reversed by neostigmine.

The reader will appreciate that Goldstein has resuscitated the original humoral theory and has established the status of the thymus as an endocrine gland and of myasthenia gravis as an endocrine disease. He has brought into sharp focus the similar origin of thyrotoxicosis and myasthenia gravis both of which are seen as the result of excessive hormonal secretion of autoimmune origin and which not infrequently occur together. To emphasize the affinities between the two conditions, Goldstein has coined the word *thymotoxicosis* to describe the condition in the thymus. This is a particularly apt and happy neologism which will deserve to be generally adopted if more detailed studies establish the validity of Goldstein's still tentative hypothesis.

That plasma of patients with myasthenia gravis contains *something*, be it antibody or humoral factor, that makes the end plate receptors inaccessible to acetylcholine has been recently demonstrated by Bender and his colleagues. α-Bungarotoxin is a snake venom that combines specifically and irreversibly with the nicotinic acetylcholine receptor. Plasma from myasthenic patients (but not that from individuals with other forms of muscle disease) blocked the binding of α-bungarotoxin to the acetylcholine receptors on the end plates of normal muscle (Bender *et al.*, 1975).

Whatever is the true aetiology of myasthenia gravis, the main features of the disease, and the rationale of the methods used to treat it, can be readily understood for most purposes if it is remembered that the muscles of myasthenic patients behave *as if* they were exposed to curare.

STRUCTURE-ACTION RELATIONS IN THE NEUROMUSCULAR BLOCKING AGENTS.

The neuromuscular blocking agents have been studied more intensively and for a longer period of time than any other group of substances by those interested in establishing relations between chemical structure and pharmacological activity. As in so many other instances in this field, few completely valid generalizations have emerged from this protracted study.

Bovet (1951) pointed out that from the standpoint of their chemical structure the neuromuscular blocking agents fall into two groups. Some (the *pachycurares*) have thick, fat and rigid molecules, others (the *leptocurares*) have long slender molecules. He also drew attention to the fact that, in general, the pachycurares (tubocurarine, for example) are antidepolarizing agents while the leptocurares (decamethonium, for example) are depolarizing drugs. Reference to Figures 16.4 and 16.5 will make it evident that Bovet's generalizations have some validity, though exceptions can be found and it is, of course, impossible to accommodate compounds with mixed activity into a simple dichotomous classification of the type proposed.

Most quaternary ammonium compounds have neuromuscular blocking activity and nitrogen-containing compounds with little activity in their original state often develop a well marked ability to produce neuromuscular blockade if their nitrogen atoms are converted into the quaternary form. Atropine and strychnine provide good examples of substances whose properties can be altered in this way. However, although the possession of a quaternary nitrogen atom tends to confer neuromuscular blocking activity, not all of the established blocking agents are quaternary compounds. A particularly interesting example is provided by β-erythroidine and its dihydro derivative. Not only do these compounds not contain quaternary nitrogen but their activity is very considerably reduced if their nitrogen is quaternized.

The functional importance of the quaternary nitrogen atom is presumably related to the necessity of binding the molecule to the acetylcholine receptor if it is to exert its characteristic action. It is easy to see that electrostatic bonds could be readily established between the quaternary atom and the anionic sites in the receptor (p. 212) Substances that contain quaternary atoms of other kinds—antimony, arsenic, iodine, phosphorus and sulphur—may also have neuromuscular blocking activity. Other pieces of evidence which indicate the importance of electrostatic binding between the blocking agent and anionic sites include the fact that if one of the quaternary nitrogen atoms and its attached methyl groups in decamethonium is replaced by a primary amine, there is a considerable loss of neuromuscular blocking activity. A similar consequence follows the replacement of the methyl groups by ethyl or other groups that reduce the charge on the nitrogen atom. The ease with which the compound is attached to the receptor is not, of course, determined solely by the intensity of the charge on the quaternary atom. A large substituent which did not affect the actual charge on the atom might nevertheless reduce the mutual attraction between the blocking agent and the receptor if, because of its size, it prevented the molecule from approaching the receptor surface. Moreover, other forms of bonding are certainly involved and such factors as lipid solubility which determine the ease with which the compound can approach the muscle membrane in the first place will also influence the activity of the compounds.

It was mentioned earlier that the distance between the two nitrogen atoms in the methonium series reaches its optimum so far as the ability to induce neuromuscular blockade is concerned, in decamethonium and it is generally assumed that this distance (1.2 to 1.4 nm) represents that which separates adjacent receptor sites at the muscle end plate. This same interatomic distance is found in other blocking agents, among them tubocurarine and succinylcholine, but it is not a necessary requirement for blocking activity. It is easy to see that two 'short' molecules (say of acetylcholine or nicotine) would fit the receptors as easily as would one molecule of decamethonium. The situation is different when longer molecules are involved. In these the distance separating the quaternary or other 'binding' atoms becomes of more critical importance.

INTERNEURONAL BLOCKING AGENTS.

These compounds produce muscle relaxation by an action on the central nervous system. Doses which produce relaxation of tension do not markedly impair voluntary motor activity. The first member of the group to be used clinically was mephenesin: some of the compounds developed from it have proved to be of more value as psychotropic drugs than as muscle relaxants. Conversely muscle relaxation is often best achieved by giving a so-called 'anxiolytic' drug such as diazepam. The relationship between emotional and physical tension is discussed elsewhere (p. 563). The actions of mephenesin, the most intensively studied member of this group of blocking agents can be taken as typical of them all.

Mephenesin

Mephenesin (Myanesin, Lissephen, Tolserol) is the most potent member of a series of glycerol ethers studied by Berger and Bradley (1946). Mephenesin produces a flaccid paralysis superficially similar to that seen after the administration of tubocurarine but it can easily be demonstrated that, except in massive doses, mephenesin has no action on neuromuscular transmission. The muscles of respiration are the last to be paralysed by both mephenesin and the neuromuscular blocking agents, but mephenesin offers a wider margin of safety between the dose which causes paralysis of the muscles of respiration and that which paralyses the rest of the skeletal musculature. Unfortu-

nately, the anaesthetist is prevented from taking advantage of this valuable property because the action of mephenesin is very short lived and intravenous injection carries the risk of haemolysis, haemoglobinuria and phlebothrombosis.

By the intravenous route, mephenesin brings about a sharp fall in blood pressure in experimental animals. This is due partly to a direct action on the heart, whose output is reduced and partly to a reflexly induced vasodilatation in response to stimulation of chemoreceptors in the right atrium and lungs (the Bezold-Jarisch reflex). The hypotensive action of mephenesin in human beings presumably has a similar origin.

Mephenesin inhibits polysynapic reflexes such as the flexor reflex but it has no effect on the knee jerk, a typical monosynaptic reflex. On the other hand, it does inhibit both the facilitation and the inhibition of the knee jerk produced by stimulation of the appropriate divisions of the reticular system and of some other brain centres. These observations led to the conclusion that mephenesin preferentially inhibits activity in internuncial neurones (interneurones) so that polysynaptic pathways are blocked while monosynaptic ones are spared. There is, however, no clear evidence that all the forms of muscle spasm and tension which are relieved by mephenesin necessarily arise from activity in polysynaptic pathways. A characteristic feature of interneurones is that their activity is repetitive and it has been suggested that the selectivity of mephenesin might have a functional rather than an anatomical basis, the drug being capable of inhibiting activity in any repetitively firing neurone whatever its location. Thus, the sudden brief discharge of motoneurone such as occurs in response to sharp blow on the patellar tendon would not be affected but if the same neurone were discharging repetitively its activity would be inhibited by mephenesin. This hypothesis (for which there is some experimental evidence) explains why small doses of mephenesin will reduce muscle spasm while leaving voluntary movements relatively unimpaired. Larger doses cause a more generalized depression of the neurones involved in the control and maintenance of muscle tone and movements.

Mephenesin prolongs barbiturate sleeping time in mice, and patients given the drug not uncommonly complain of drowsiness, though this may in part be a feeling induced by the muscle relaxation. Mephenesin has local anaesthetic activity and there are some reports that it has analgesic properties. Even when all these effects are taken into consideration, however, it is clear that mephenesin has relatively little effect on systems other than those concerned with the regulation of motor activity. Sedative or tranquillizing effects are more evident in some of the mephenesin congeners mentioned below. The actions of mephenesin on the central nervous system are fully discussed by Smith (1965).

Mephenesin reduces both tremors and increased reflex activity. It causes muscle relaxation, reduces decerebrate rigidity and abolishes or reduces the intensity of strychnine and electroshock convulsions and those due to tetanus toxin. It is rather less effective in convulsions produced by leptazol and it has virtually no effect on the autonomic nervous system. Its therapeutic applications are limited by the undesirability of administering it by the intravenous route. It is active when taken by mouth in large doses (2 to 3 grams). By this route its action is considerably more prolonged and a continued effect can be obtained by three or four daily doses of this size. Mephenesin has been used in this way for the treatment of various conditions in which there is spasticity or involuntary movements of the limbs and it is sometimes of some service for the reduction of muscle tone as a preparation for physiotherapeutic or orthopaedic manipulations. In attempts to increase its usefulness, mephenesin has been used in combination with other drugs: mephenesin and quinalbarbitone have been used to treat anxiety and tension states and a combination of mephenesin and salicylamide was introduced for the relief of painful conditions associated with muscle spasm. *Mephenesin carbamate* (Solseran) has similar properties to mephenesin itself but it has a more prolonged action. It has been used, again with only limited success, in low back pain, in anxiety states, to control the tremors of acute alcoholism and in tetanus. It is given by mouth in doses of 500 mg. four times daily.

Other compounds with a mephenesin-like action

When mephesin was first put to clinical use it seemed likely that it would be a much more useful substance than it has since proved to be and a large number of new compounds was produced in the hope of finding (and profiting from) drugs that would retain all the advantages but none of the disadvantages of mephenesin. The first generation of new drugs were derivatives of glycerol (like mephenesin itself) or of butanediol and many of them found their way into textbooks and pharmacies. They failed to fulfil their early promise and the few survivors (their names and formulae are displayed in Figure 16.6) are of limited utility.

We have already noted that some psychotropic drugs possess the ability to relax skeletal muscle but it is more appropriate to discuss their properties in the context of psychotropic drugs as a whole and this is done on pp. 563-564.

METHOCARBAMOL

Methocarbamol (Robaxin) has pharmacological properties very similar to those of mephenesin although it is said to be a more effective inhibitor of electroshock convulsions. It has some sedative action and may cause hypothermia. It appears to be incapable of promoting muscle relaxation in the dog although it is active in other species. It has been used to treat pain due to muscle spasm following strains and fractures and that of fibromyositis. Methocarbamol

can be given by very slow intravenous injection (maximum dose one gram) as it is less likely than mephenesin to cause haemolysis or phlebitis. It may also be taken by mouth in thrice daily doses of one or two grams.

MEPROBAMATE.

Although meprobamate has muscle relaxant properties similar to, but less marked than, those of mephensin, interest in the drug is now entirely centred in its sedative actions which have led to its being extensively used for the treatment of tension and anxiety states (p. 563).

CARISOPRODOL

Carisoprodol (Rela, Carisoma) has clear structural affinities with meprobamate (Fig. 16.6) but its pharmacological activities are rather different. It is a more potent muscle relaxant and a less potent sedative. Unlike mephenesin and most of its congeners, including meprobamate, carisoprodol inhibits monosynaptic as well as polysynaptic reflexes. It depresses the facilitatory effect of reticular formation stimulation more readily than the inhibitory effect. In illustration of this selective action may be cited the fact that carisoprodol suppresses decerebrate rigidity in laboratory animals more effectively than does mephenesin or meprobamate. It antagonizes convulsions due to strychnine but it is very much less effective than mephenesin in this respect.

Carisprodol is a mild analgesic. This effect is apparently independent of its muscle relaxing properties: other muscle relaxants only produce analgesia when they are given in doses large enough to induce a pronounced ataxia.

Carisprodol can be employed for the relief of pain in muscles, joints and bones especially when this is associated with spasm. Suggested therapeutic indications are muscular rheumatism, lumbago, sprains and dislocations. The oral dose of carisoprodol is 350 mg which may be taken up to four times daily.

PHENYRAMIDOL

Phenyramidol (Analexin) resembles carisoprodol in its properties but it is a more powerful analgesic.

OTHER COMPOUNDS.

The remainder of the compounds displayed in Figure 16.6 need only a brief mention. Styramate (Sinaxar), chlorzoxazone (Paraflex) and chlormezanone (Trancopal) are employed primarily as muscle relaxants (though chlormezanone has also found limited favour as an 'anxiolytic' drug) but some reports indicate that they have no more than a placebo action. Chlorzoxazone is chemically similar to zoxazolamine, a compound so toxic that it has now been withdrawn from general use. Chlorzoxazone is less toxic than zoxazolamine but headache, depression and, sometimes, hypersensitivity reactions may attend its use and there can be few occasions when it is necessary to use the drug in preference to less toxic agents. Chlormezanone has some analgesic properties and styramate is long acting. Since chlormezanone possesses muscle relaxing, analgesic

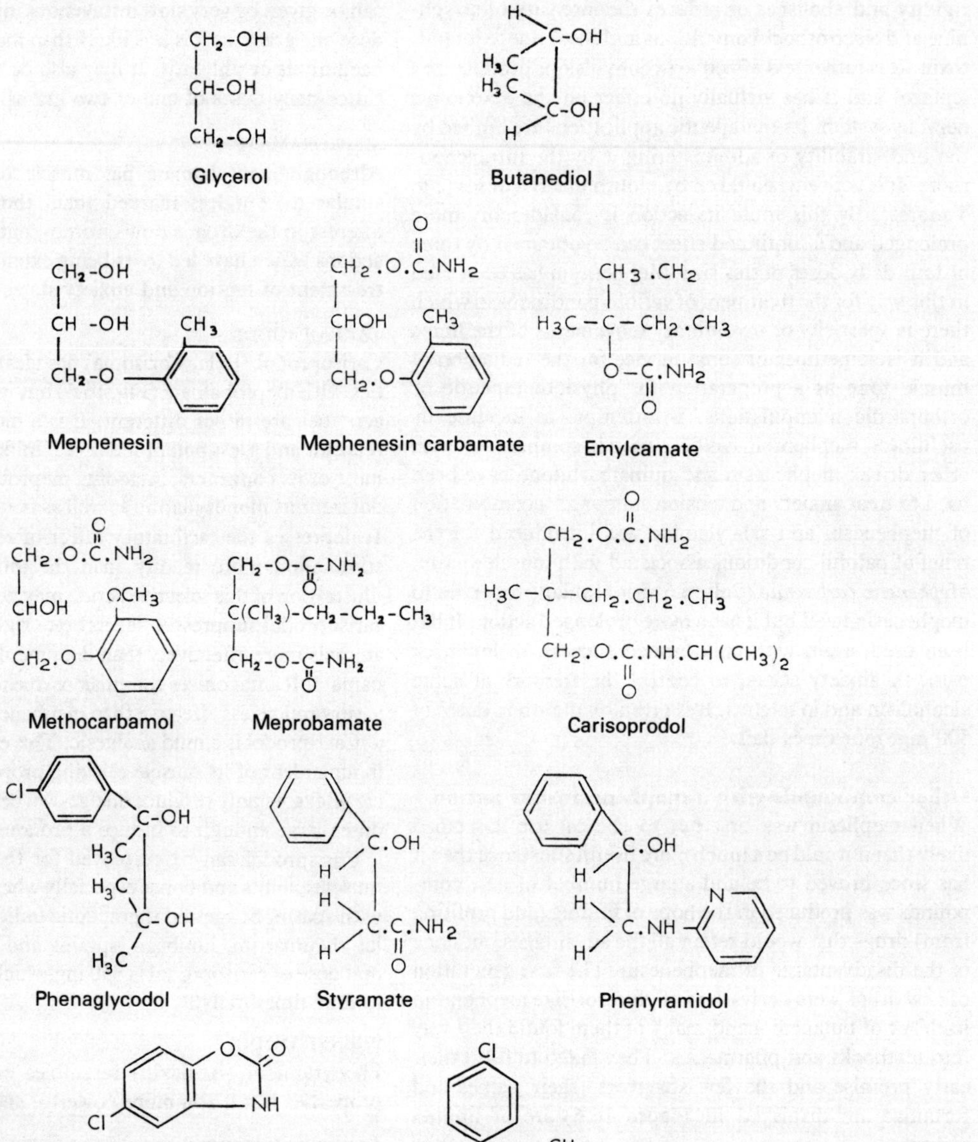

Glycerol

Butanediol

Mephenesin

Mephenesin carbamate

Emylcamate

Methocarbamol

Meprobamate

Carisoprodol

Phenaglycodol

Styramate

Phenyramidol

Chlorozoxazone

Chlormezanone

Fig. 16.6 Mephenesin and some related muscle relaxants.

and a mildly sedative action it is sometimes prescribed in combination with paracetamol for the relief of dysmenorrhoea. The combined preparation is known as Lobak.

On the very rare occasions when they are used, emylcamate (Nuncital, Striatran) is given with the hope of relieving anxiety or muscle spasm while phenaglycocol, by virtue of its central depressant activity, supplements antiepileptic medication.

BACLOFEN

Baclofen (Lioresal) is a newly introduced compound which has found application in the treatment of muscle spasm associated with multiple sclerosis and other disorders that affect the spinal cord. Chemically, baclofen is γ-amino-β-p-chlorophenyl butyric acid and this makes it a substance of particular interest to the pharmacologist

$H_2N.CH_2.CH.CH_2COOH$

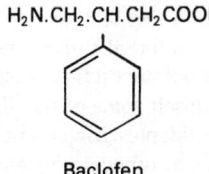

Baclofen

because it is closely related to γ-aminobutyric acid, a presumed inhibitor of synaptic activity in the central nervous system (p. 189). The initial daily dose of baclofen (given in three instalments) is 15 mg which can be slowly increased to about 50 mg.

THE LABORATORY TESTING OF MUSCLE RELAXANTS

The screening of compounds for interneuronal or neuromuscular blocking activity is not one that can be adequately achieved by the use of simple tests. Rats and mice, the screening laboratory's principal stock-in-trade, are relatively insensitive to both types of blocking agent so that—although used in some tests—they are not really suitable species on which to conduct screening procedures. When a compound has been shown to possess some form of muscle relaxing activity, the elucidation of its locus of action necessitates the setting up of quite elaborate preparations.

When muscle relaxing activity has been detected by preliminary observations on a variety of animals, it is necessary first to decide (if this is not already evident from the history of the drug's development) whether its site of action is at the periphery or in the central nervous system. A suitable animal for this purpose is the rabbit. In general, drugs that act centrally produce relatively little impairment of respiratory movements when they are given in doses sufficient to induce muscular relaxation. High doses do not cause the complete flaccidity seen with neuromuscular blocking agents. On the other hand, righting reflexes are lost when muscle tone is only moderately reduced. In the rabbit, the intravenous injection of neuromuscular blocking agents causes 'head drop', the animal being unable to hold its head in the usual position. Centrally acting muscle relaxants are less likely to cause head drop in small doses but they readily inhibit the polysynaptic pinna reflex—the withdrawal or shaking of the head produced by gently touching the centre of the ear. It was mentioned earlier that mephenesin elevates the threshold for electroshock and strychnine convulsions and the discovery of this property in a compound may provide a hint of interneuronal blocking activity. Mice can be used for this test, the value of which can be augmented by making additional observations (of motor activity, muscle co-ordination, etc.) of the effect of the drug in these animals (Bastian, 1961). At the same time, it must be emphasized that anticonvulsant activity is not necessarily associated

with the possession of mephenesin-like properties: diphenylhydantoin (p. 523) the anticonvulsant drug *par excellence* has no useful muscle relaxant action. The further investigation of the two classes of drug is described below.

INTERNEURONAL BLOCKING AGENTS.

The ability to inhibit the activity of internuncial neurones and hence to produce some degree of muscle relaxation is one which is shared by a number of compounds which are not primarily muscle relaxants. The barbiturates and the phenothiazine 'tranquillizers' are good examples of drugs in this category. What is needed in a centrally acting muscle relaxant is a mephenesin-like ability selectively to depress the motor system. Ideally, the compound should be active on both α and γ mechanisms (p. 164). When compounds are being screened for potential use as muscle relaxants, an attempt should therefore be made to assess the extent to which muscle relaxation is accompanied by depression of systems other than those that directly control muscle activity. In particular, sedative or hypnotic effects should be looked for.

Interneuronal blocking activity is most convincingly established by demonstrating a differential effect on monosynaptic and polysynaptic reflexes. Myographic methods should not be used for this purpose because they cannot exclude the possibility that the drug is exerting its effects by influencing neuromuscular transmission. Instead, action potentials in a ventral spinal root should be recorded. In response to stimulation of the appropriate dorsal root, the ventral root produces a large spike potential (due to transmission through the monosynaptic pathway) followed by a series of smaller responses, the result of activity in a number of polysynaptic pathways. An interneuronal blocking drug should abolish the polysynaptic responses at a dose level which has no effect on the monosynaptic spike.

In order to assess the potential utility of a newly discovered interneuronal blocking drug, its ability to reduce abnormal muscle tension should be examined. A useful approach is to use the decerebrate cat. Decerebration can be brought about either by sectioning the brainstem or by ligating the arterial supply to the higher centres of the brain. Both methods should be used, because the rigidity produced by section of the brain stem arises from overactivity in the γ-motoneurones while that which follows arterial ligation arises from α motoneurones (p. 165) and a useful drug will inhibit both forms of activity. Spasticity can be produced by simpler, if less useful, methods including the administration of tetanus toxin or the production of asphyxia by occluding the arterial supply to the spinal cord.

NEUROMUSCULAR BLOCKING AGENTS

Not all species are equally sensitive to neuromuscular blocking agents and drugs that are pure depolarizing agents in some species may produce a mixed neuromuscular blockade in others. For the detailed examination of blocking drugs it is therefore important to use a preparation whose responses resemble those seen in man. The chloralosed cat best meets these requirements and, except when other species are mentioned, it may be assumed that the procedures described in the succeeding paragraphs relate to this preparation. It is usual to record the responses of the tibialis anterior muscle in response to stimulation of the sciatic nerve. Contractions of the soleus muscle should also be recorded as this may reveal the production of dual blockade by substances that have a purely depolarizing effect on the tibialis anterior muscle. As a preliminary screening test, however, substances may usefully be given by intravenous injection to the young conscious chick: a depolarizing agent will cause a spastic paralysis while other types of paralysing drug produce a flaccid condition (Fig 16.1). An indication of depolarizing activity may indeed already have appeared if the drug has been administered to sensitive mammals, because depolarizing agents cause twitching of mammalian muscle before paralysis sets in.

In order to be able to conclude that a drug operates only on junctional mechanisms, it is necessary to establish that activity in the nerve trunk or in the muscle is not directly affected. This is easily tested by recording action potentials in the stimulated motor nerve and the response of the muscle to direct stimulation. Neither should be affected if the drug acts only at the neuromuscular junction.

A drug that causes a flaccid paralysis may do so because it prevents the synthesis or release of acetylcholine. If it inhibits acetylcholine synthesis, it will bring about a gradual but progressive reduction in the muscle tension generated in response to a *rapid* stimulation of the motor nerve. The muscle response to a close intra-arterial injection of 5 to 10 μg. of acetylcholine will not be reduced unless the drug also has, like hemicholinium or triethylcholine, some degree of depolarizing activity. In that event, the response to injected acetylcholine will be partially depressed. The administration of choline will result in a gradual restoration of neuromuscular function. Substances that prevent the release of acetylcholine cause a much more rapid development of neuromuscular blockade than do inhibitors of acetylcholine synthesis and their action cannot be reversed by choline. In general, they will not have the structural affinity with choline which is a feature of all the inhibitors of acetylcholine synthesis so far discovered. Consequently, they are unlikely to have any depolarizing action and they will not even partially depress the response to acetylcholine.

If the blocking agent under test abolishes or substantially reduces the response to injected acetylcholine, it is reasonable to conclude that it affects the reactivity of the end plate region of muscle. In order to determine the type of blockade it produces, experimental tests based on some of the known differences between depolarizing and anti-depolarizing agents (Table 16.1) are applied. For practical details the reader is referred to Bowman (1964).

In the teaching laboratory it is possible for the student to demonstrate for himself some of the differences between depolarizing and antidepolarizing agents by making use of such familiar agents as tubocurarine and decamethonium and such preparations as the frog rectus muscle and the isolated phrenic nerve-diaphragm of the rat. These simple isolated preparations, though useful for demonstration purposes, are not recommended for the identification of the pharmacological activity of new compounds in the research laboratory because their response to individual drugs may be very different from that of muscles in the intact human being.

GANGLION BLOCKING AGENTS

It has been known for many years that tubocurarine blocks the transmission of impulses across autonomic ganglia as well as neuromuscular junctions. In 1949, however, Acheson and his colleagues reported that tetraethylammonium blocked the ganglia at dose levels which did not affect neuromuscular transmission. In the same year, Paton and Zaimis discovered that hexamethonium and pentamethonium were more powerful, longer acting and even more selective in their action than tetraethylammonium. Since then a large number of other ganglion blocking agents has been discovered. The names and formulae of the more important members of the group are presented in Table 16.3.

Because they reduce the level of sympathetic activity, the ganglion blocking drugs cause a diminution of vascular tone with a consequent fall in blood pressure and for some years after their discovery they were extensively used as antihypertensive agents. Their popularity is now declining with the advent of drugs that selectively block activity in the adrenergic neurones themselves. The mechanism of synaptic transmission is the same in all autonomic ganglia and the blocking agents therefore interrupt both sympathetic and parasympathetic processes, a fact that partly explains their eclipse by drugs which selectively influence postganglionic sympathetic fibres.

Like the neuromuscular blocking agents, substances with an action on ganglia may occupy receptors on the postsynaptic membrane by simple competition with acetylcholine or they may produce persistent depolarization. All the compounds that are conventionally classified as ganglion blocking agents belong to the first group but substances like tetramethylammonium, nicotine and lobeline are ganglion depolarizing agents. There is a clear difference between the behaviour of depolarizing substances at the motor end plates and at ganglion cells. It will be recalled that, at the mammalian neuromuscular junction, depolarizing agents have only a momentary stimulant

Table 16.3 Some ganglion blocking agents

Official name	Proprietary name(s)	Chemical formula	Remarks
Hexamethonium chloride (or bromide, iodide, bitartrate)	C_6; Vegolysen T	CH_3–$\overset{\oplus}{N}(CH_3)_2$–$CH_2$-$CH_2$-$CH_2$-$CH_2$-$CH_2$-$CH_2$–$\overset{\oplus}{N}(CH_3)_2$–$CH_3$ $2Cl^{\ominus}$	Poorly absorbed when given by mouth. Now rarely used. Initial dose 1.5-2.5 mg Final daily dose: Up to 400 mg.
Pentamethonium chloride		$(CH_3)_3\overset{\oplus}{N}$–$(CH_2)_5$–$\overset{\oplus}{N}(CH_3)_3$ $2Cl^{\ominus}$	Rarely used
Pentolinium bitartrate	Ansolysen	[pyrrolidinium] $\overset{\oplus}{N}$–$CH_2CH_2CH_2CH_2CH_2$–$\overset{\oplus}{N}$ [pyrrolidinium] $\cdot 2C_4H_5O_6^{\ominus}$	Well absorbed after oral administration. Has been used in the treatment of hypertension and for producing controlled hypotension. Initial dose: 2.5-3 mg. Final daily dose: 30-60 mg or more.
Azamethonium		H_5C_2–$\overset{\oplus}{N}(CH_3)_2$–$(CH_2)_2$–N($CH_3$)–$(CH_2)_2$–$\overset{\oplus}{N}(CH_3)$–$C_2H_5$ $2Br^{\ominus}$	Similar to hexamethonium
Mecamylamine	Inversine; Mevasine	[bicyclic structure with NH-CH₃ and CH₃ groups] $\cdot$ HCl	Some central side effects (malaise, tremor and psychotic symptoms). May have a constrictor effect on blood vessels. Initial dose: 2.5-3 mg. May be increased at 48 hr. intervals to a final total dose of 10 mg. three times daily.
Pempidine	Perolysen; Tenormal	[piperidine ring with H_3C, CH_3 substituents and N-CH_3]	Potent agent with prolonged action. Large doses stimulate central nervous system and have curare-like action. Initial dose: 2.5-3 mg. Final daily dose: Up to 80 mg.

Table 16.3 (contd)

Official name	Proprietary name(s)	Chemical formula	Remarks
Trimetaphan camphorsulphonate (camsylate)	Arfonad		Short acting. Also has direct action on blood vessels. Causes histamine release. May be given by infusion for producing controlled hypotension.
Trimethidinium	Ostensin		For oral use. Initial dose: 20 mg twice daily. Final daily dose: Up to 450 mg.

action so that the muscles only exhibit a few fasciculations before they pass into a condition of flaccid paralysis. At the ganglia, small doses of depolarizing agents produce prolonged repetitive stimulation of the postganglionic elements with no blockade, while the blockade induced by larger doses is preceded by a considerable degree of stimulation. Substances that depolarize the ganglion thus act both as stimulants and as blocking agents. This precludes their being employed for the production of ganglion blockade for clinical purposes. Many other substances display variable degrees of ganglion blocking activity as a side effect of their main actions.

Substances that prevent the synthesis or release of acetylcholine by motor nerves (triethylcholine, the hemicholiniums, botulinum toxin, etc.) have a similar effect on preganglionic fibres of the autonomic ganglia and lead to ganglion blockade. Potassium and adrenaline facilitate synaptic transmission in the ganglion as they do at the neuromuscular junction. This is to be expected in view of the similarity of the neurohumoral transmission processes at the two sites. However, as a result of the existence of a number of subsidiary mechanisms, ganglionic transmission is modified by some substances which do not influence neuromuscular transmission. These substances—whose actions are not immediately relevant to the production of ganglion blockade—are discussed elsewhere (p. 176). Another point of difference between the neuromuscular junction and the ganglion synapse concerns the response to anticholinesterases. At the former site, these

drugs exert a profound effect on transmission processes and they may also be employed to reverse the paralysis produced by antidepolarizing substances. They are much less effective at the ganglion synapse where the transmitter action of acetylcholine is terminated by diffusion away from the receptor sites or by other processes which do not involve its hydrolysis by cholinesterase (p. 176).

Clinically useful ganglion-blocking agents should prevent the stimulant action of depolarizing agents or of preganglionic stimulation without themselves having any stimulant action either on the ganglion cells or on the structures innervated by the postganglionic nerves. A 'pure' blocking agent will not inhibit the release of acetylcholine by the preganglionic nerves though the possession of this action will not of itself reduce the drug's potential usefulness unless the effect is sufficiently well marked to influence neuromuscular transmission. There is evidence that pempidine may, in large doses, bring about a reduction in the release of acetylcholine from preganglionic nerves (Corne and Edge, 1958). On the other hand, tetraethylammonium increases the rate of release of acetylcholine though this is insufficient to overcome the ganglion blockade produced by this compound (Matthews and Quilliam, 1964).

Pharmacological properties of ganglion blocking drugs
The most obvious effects of ganglion blockade are seen in the cardiovascular system. The blood vessels are normally

in a partially constricted state due to the tonic activity of their sympathetic nerve supply. Ganglion blockade causes vasodilatation. The increased blood flow so produced results in an increased skin temperature and a deepening of the skin's usual pink colour. The removal of vasoconstrictor tone from the resistance vessels (the peripheral arterioles) brings about a sharp fall of blood pressure. The vasodilation also affects the veins so that they accommodate more blood. The rate of return of blood to the heart and consequently the cardiac output, is thus reduced. This effect contributes to the overall hypotensive response. In congestive cardiac failure the venous dilatation produced by ganglion blockade may result in an increased cardiac output instead of the usual reduction since cardiac performance improves if a failing heart becomes less distended (p. 693). Ganglion blocking agents often increase the power of contraction of an isolated perfused heart and this provides additional evidence that their influence on the output of the healthy heart in vivo is not to be attributed to a direct action on cardiac muscle. So far as the heart rate is concerned, the response to the blocking agents is dependent on the prevailing degree of vagal tone. Usually, vagal tone is high and ganglion blockade produces cardiac acceleration. Less often, the vagus is exerting a smaller degree of tone than the sympathetic nerves. In these circumstances ganglion blockade results in bradycardia.

An unfortunate consequence of the blockade of the sympathetic ganglia is the loss of the regulatory mechanisms that normally permit the circulation to adjust itself to changes in the position of the body. When a change is made from the recumbent to the erect position, there is a tendency for the blood flow through the vessels of the head and neck to be reduced. This is a simple result of the fact that, under the influence of gravity, blood 'pools' in the lower limbs and abdomen. In normal circumstances the consequent fall of blood pressure in the carotid sinus reflexly stimulates the cardioaccelerator and vasomotor centres. The heart accelerates and the blood vessels constrict so that the blood pressure rises, some blood is diverted from the lower parts of the body and normal blood flow through the head is restored. This compensatory response is mediated through the sympathetic nervous system and it is therefore ineffective after ganglion blockade. Patients under treatment with ganglion blocking agents may faint or feel dizzy—the result of the *postural hypotension*—when they change from a reclining to a more erect position. Almost every reader will occasionally have experienced mild symptoms of postural hypotension even with an alert sympathetic system and should therefore be able to appreciate the more serious discomfort and embarrassment felt by those whose postural compensatory mechanisms are inoperative.

Blockade of the parasympathetic ganglia, which is an inevitable concomitant of sympathetic blockade, has its own consequences. These are inconvenient and therapeutically valueless in the hypertensive patient. Smooth muscle is relaxed, but the sphincters may be closed so that stomach emptying is delayed and there is constipation and retention of urine. The secretion of saliva and of gastric and intestinal juices is arrested. The pupil dilates and the vision may be blurred due to paralysis of accommodation.

The individual drugs are listed in Table 16.3. It will be seen that most of them are quaternary nitrogen compounds. It is possible that the others are quaternized at the site of action. A few of the compounds (mecamylamine, pempidine, trimetaphan camphorsulphonate and phenacyl homatropinium sulphate) have some side effects, detailed in the Table, which are not attributable to blockade of autonomic ganglia. Central side effects are more likely to occur with compounds that lack a quaternary nitrogen atom and which can therefore pass easily into the brain.

Clinical uses of the ganglion blocking agents
The ganglion blocking agents have now passed the peak of their popularity and their therapeutic use is limited.
Reduction of blood pressure. Blockade of sympathetic ganglia results in a fall of blood pressure in hypertensive and in normal subjects. The blocking drugs may therefore be used, in theory at least, both for the treatment of hypertension and for the production of controlled hypotension in surgery. The treatment of hypertension is discussed in detail elsewhere (p. 315). For the production of a hypotensive state during surgery, trimetaphan is useful. A one in a thousand solution of the drug is infused at a rate which will maintain the patient's systolic blood pressure at about 70 mm of mercury. The part of the body on which surgery is to be performed is raised above the level of the rest of the patient and the blood supply to the operation area is thus considerably diminished. This reduces the extent of bleeding and helps to provide the surgeon with a clear operating field. This is a valuable aid to the successful completion of complex neurosurgical or cardiovascular procedures. Because trimetaphan has a short duration of action, the blood pressure can be restored to its normal level within a few minutes of stopping the infusion.

Diseases of the gastrointestinal tract
Blockade of the parasympathetic ganglia, which is the origin of some tiresome side effects in those who are taking ganglion blocking drugs for their effect on sympathetic ganglia, has occasionally been turned to good effect in those with some disorders of gastrointestinal function, particularly duodenal ulcer. In their turn, however, patients being so treated suffer as side effects the results of sympathetic blockade and blocking agents are now rarely used for the inhibition of parasympathetic activity.

The administration of ganglion blocking agents is not to be undertaken lightly or by those not experienced in their use. When the drugs are employed to produce a controlled hypotension, the infusion must be regulated with the greatest of care to prevent too precipitous and perhaps irreversible falls of blood pressure. The possibility that a patient may respond in a violent fashion to histamine liberated by trimetaphan must always be borne in mind. When the drugs are given by mouth the initial dose must be quite low (Table 16.3). It is then cautiously increased at intervals dictated by the speed with which the drug is eliminated from the body, until the desired level of blood pressure is reached. It is usual to give the daily requirement as divided doses which are repeated at four to six hour intervals. Because they also inhibit gastrointestinal activity, ganglion blocking drugs may be retained for considerable periods in the stomach. This may give the impression that the patient is receiving inadequate amounts of the drug and the dose may be inadvisably increased. When this is eventually absorbed, a dangerously excessive hypotensive effect may be produced. This danger is reduced if the dose is only increased slowly and at reasonably long intervals.

When hypertensive patients take ganglion blocking drugs over long periods, tolerance is likely to develop and the dose has to be increased if the hypotensive response is to be maintained. This type of tolerance may arise because alternative ganglionic transmission mechanisms which do not involve activation of nicotinic receptors and which normally play only a subsidiary role may be capable of partially re-establishing the transmission of impulses across the ganglia. On the other hand some hypertensive patients, particularly if they are receiving other drugs, are unexpectedly sensitive to ganglion blocking agents.

Not all ganglia are equally influenced by the ganglion blocking agents but attempts to develop substances with an action restricted to either the sympathetic or the parasympathetic ganglia (or to functional groups of ganglia within these major subdivisions) have not been successful.

LABORATORY TESTING OF DRUGS THAT AFFECT AUTONOMIC GANGLIA.

Some of the available methods for distinguishing between drugs that block transmission in sympathetic ganglia and those that inhibit activity in the postganglionic fibres are mentioned elsewhere (p. 307). The ganglion blocking agents arrest transmission in the parasympathetic ganglia as well as in those belonging to the sympathetic system. Evidence of parasympathetic ganglion blockade is provided if a drug, known from other tests to be devoid of atropine-like properties, causes dilatation of pupil in undisturbed animals. The mydriatic effect will, of course, be more evident if the animal is observed in bright light so that the pupils are initially well constricted. Mice may be used in this test; rats are unsuitable. Blockade of parasympathetic ganglia also leads to inhibition of the peristaltic

reflex. This reflex can be easily evoked in the isolated intestine by distending the lumen with a saline solution. The changes in volume accompanying the waves of peristalsis are recorded. The effect of a ganglion blocking drug on this system (the Trendelenburg preparation) is illustrated in Figure 16.7. It is also possible to record action potentials in pre-and postganglionic fibres in response to preganglionic stimulation and thus to confirm that the drug under test abolishes activity in the postganglionic fibres without affecting transmission of impulses in the preganglionic elements.

One of the most useful methods for investigating in closer detail the mode of action of drugs that modify

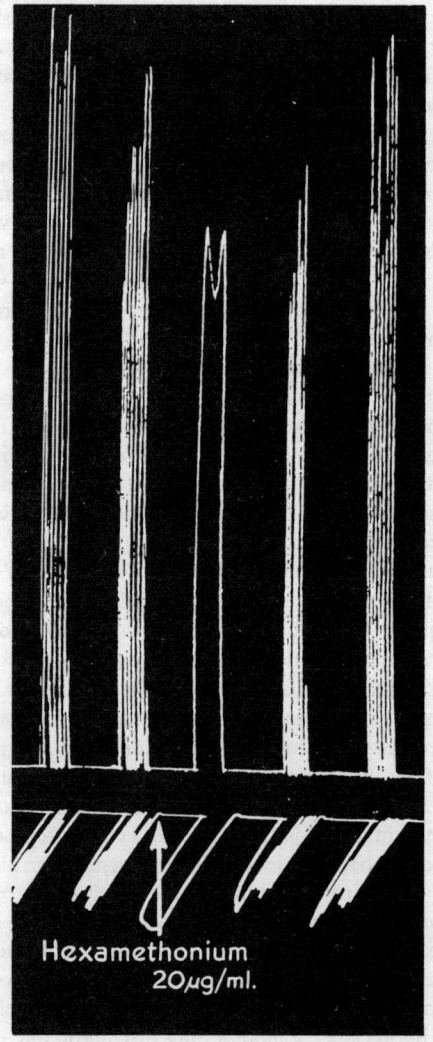

Fig. 16.7 Effect of hexamethonium upon peristalsis (lower record) and longitudinal muscular contractions (upper record) in response to repeated distensions of the guinea-pig ileum. Note that after drug addition, peristaltic activity ceased. This effect is believed to be due to blockade of synaptic transmission in the intramural intestinal ganglia.

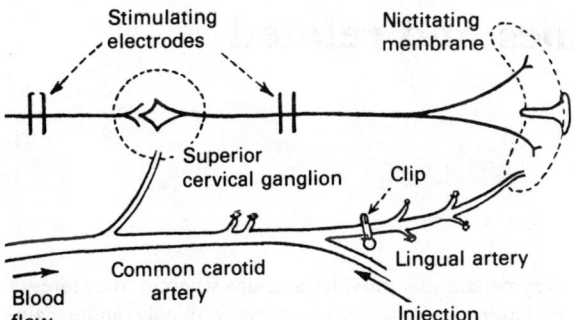

Fig. 16.8 Arrangement used for locating the point of action of drugs that influence autonomic activity.

ganglionic transmission or influence processes in the postganglionic fibres is illustrated in Figure 16.8. The contractions of the nictitating membrane in response to stimulation of both pre- and postganglionic nerves are recorded. Drugs are injected into the lingual artery close to its junction with the external carotid artery. Closure of the clip on the latter vessel ensures that the drug passes only to the ganglion; if the clip is open, the arterial blood flow sweeps the drug to the nictitating membrane. By this technique it is easy to locate with precision the point or points at which the drug acts.

For the measurement of acetylcholine release from stimulated preganglionic fibres, a perfusion technique similar to that originally described by Kibjakow is used.

BIBLIOGRAPHY

Books, monographs and reviews

Bovet, D. (1951). Some aspects of the relationship between chemical constitution and curare-like activity. *Ann. N.Y. Acad. Sci.*, **54**, 407-437.

Bowman, W. C. (1962). Mechanism of neuromuscular blockade. In Ellis, G. P. and West, G. B. (Eds.) *Progress in Medicinal Chemistry*, Vol. **2**, 88-131. London: Butterworths

Bowman W. C. (1964). Neuromuscular blocking agents. In, Laurence D. R. and Bacharach, A. L. (eds.) *Evaluation of Drug Activities: Pharmacometrics*, Vol. **1**. 325-352. London and New York: Academic Press.

Foldes, F. F. (1960). The pharmacology of neuromuscular blocking agents in man. *Clin. pharmac. Therap.*, **1**. 345-395.

Goldstein, G. and MacKay, I. R. (1969) *The Human Thymus:* London: Heinemann.

Green, A. F. and Boura, A. L. A. (1964). Depressants of peripheral sympathetic nerve function. In, Laurence, D. R. and Bacharach, A. L. (eds.) *Evaluation of Drug Activities: Pharmacometrics.* Vol. **1**. 369-430.

Grob, D. (1963). Therapy of myasthenia gravis. In Koelle, G. B. (ed.) *Cholinesterases and Anticholinesterase Agents* (Handbuch der exptl. Pharmak., Erganzungswerk 15). 1028-1050. Berlin: Springer.

Grob D. (1967). Neuromuscular blocking drugs. In, Root. W. S. and Hofmann, F. G. (eds.) *Physiological Pharmacology.* Vol. **3**, 389-460. New York and London: Academic Press.

Original papers

Bastian, J. W. (1961). Classifications of CNS drugs by a mouse screening battery. *Arch. int. Pharmacodyn.*, **133**, 347-364.

Bender, A. N., Engel, W. K., Ringel, S. P., Daniels M. P. and Vogel, Z. (1975). Myasthenia gravis: a serum factor blocking acetylcholine receptors of the human neuromuscular junction. *Lancet* (i) 607-608.

Berger, F. M. and Bradley, W. (1946). The pharmacological properties of α:ß-dihydroxy-γ-(2-methylphenoxy)-propane (myanesin). *Br. J. Pharmac. Chemother.*, **1**. 265-272.

Bowman, W. C., Hemsworth, B. A. and Rand, M J. (1962). Triethylcholine compared with other substances affecting neuromuscular transmission. *Br. J. Pharmac. Chemother,* **19**. 198-218

Castleman, B. (1966). The pathology of the thymus gland in myasthenia gravis. *Ann. N. Y. Acad. Sci.,* **135**, 496-503

Churchill-Davidson, H. C. and Christie, T. H. (1959). The diagnosis of neuromuscular block in man. *Br. J. Anaesth.,* **31**, 290-301

Corne, S. J. and Edge, N. D. (1958). Pharmacological properties of pempidine, a new ganglion blocking compound. *Br. J. Pharmac. Chemother,* **13**, 339-349

Goldstein, G. (1968). The thymus and neuromuscular function. *Lancet,* **ii,** 119-122.

Goldstein, G and Schlesinger, D. H. (1975). Thymopoietin and myasthenia gravis: neostigmine-responsive neuromuscular block produced in mice by a synthetic peptide fragment of thymopoietin. *Lancet* (**ii**). 256-259.

Hutter, O. F. (1952). Post-tetanic restoration of neuromuscular transmission blocked by D-tubocurine. *J. Physiol.,* **118**, 216-227.

Matthews, E K. and Quilliam, J. P. (1964). Effects of central depressant drugs upon acetylcholine release. *Br. J. Pharmac. Chemother.,* **22**. 415-440.

Parkes, J. D. and McKinna, J. A (1967). Effects of thymic extract on the neuromuscular junction. *Nature, Lond.,* **214**. 1116-1117.

Smith, S. M., Brown, H. O., Toman J. E. P and Goodman, L. S. (1947). Lack of cerebral effects of D-tubocurarine. *Anaesthesiology,* **8,** 1-14

Wilson A., Obrist, A. R. and Wilson, H. (1953). Some effects of extracts of thymus glands removed from patients with myasthenia gravis. *Lancet,* ii, 368-371.

17. Sympathomimetic amines and related substances

Dopamine, noradrenaline and adrenaline are naturally occurring (*biogenic*) catecholamines—that is they contain the catechol (3,4-dihydroxyphenyl) nucleus. Their status as humoral transmitter substances is fully discussed in Chapter 13 (p. 170). This chapter is concerned with more general aspects of the pharmacology and metabolism of these and some related compounds.

The metabolism of the catecholamines

BIOSYNTHESIS

It is now well established that the naturally occurring catecholamines arise from phenylalanine and tyrosine by way of the pathway shown in Fig. 17.1. The reaction sequence is a simple one but it is necessary to add a few notes on the enzymes involved in the biosynthetic process.

(*a*) Phenylalanine hydroxylase appears to consist of two enzymes. They have been found to occur together in the liver.

(*b*) The activity of the tyrosine hydroxylase is low and the conversion of tyrosine to DOPA is the rate-limiting step in the formation of adrenaline and its precursors.

Activity in sympathetic nerves influences tyrosine hydroxylase, and hence the synthesis of noradrenaline, in two ways. In the first place, noradrenaline inhibits the enzyme and this provides a means whereby the stores of noradrenaline in adrenergic nerve terminals can be maintained in the face of fluctuating demands. Increased sympathetic activity, or exposure to drugs that evoke noradrenaline release, will tend to deplete the terminal vesicles of their immediately available stores of noradrenaline (p. 288) but the resulting release of the noradrenaline brake will permit a more rapid synthesis of transmitter. As the noradrenaline stores refill, the brake is reapplied.

The second regulatory mechanism governs noradrenaline synthesis in the nerve cell bodies rather than in the terminals. If preganglionic fibres are stimulated, more tyrosine hydroxylase is induced transsynaptically in the postganglionic elements so that noradrenaline synthesis is enhanced. In contrast to the inhibition of tyrosine hydroxylase by noradrenaline, this mechanism operates sluggishly, a noticeable increase in enzyme activity becoming evident only after several hours of increased sympathetic activity, while the peak effect needs days to develop. The existence of this mechanism serves to explain why it is that noradrenaline synthesis proceeds more vigorously in sympathetic nerves that are continuously active than in those that exhibit only sporadic bursts of activity.

The two mechanisms just discussed constitute the fast and slow components respectively of a negative feedback

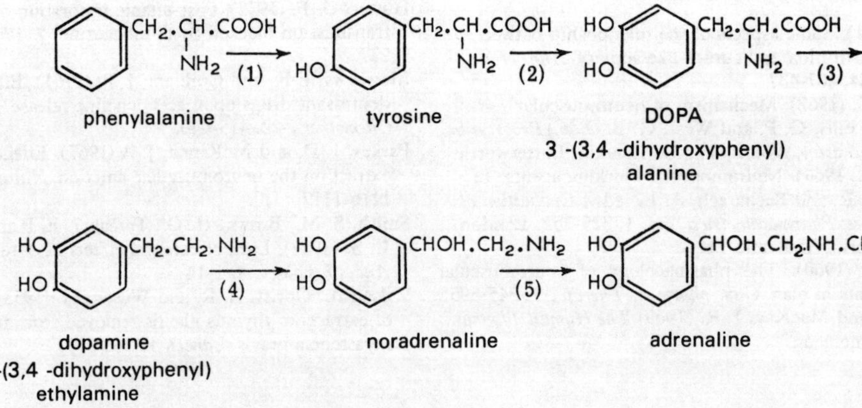

Enzymes (1) phenylalanine hydroxylase
          (2) tyrosine hydroxylase
          (3) DOPA-decarboxylase (aromatic-L-amino acid decarboxylase)
          (4) dopamine-β-oxidase (dopamine-β-hydroxylase)
          (5) phenylethanolamine N-methyltransferase

Fig. 17.1 The principal biosynthetic pathway for dopamine, noradrenaline and adrenaline.

system that controls the synthesis of noradrenaline. The reader should note that other feedback systems regulate the *release* of noradrenaline in response to the prevailing degree of sympathetic activity. These systems, which involve the prostaglandins, are discussed elsewhere (p.383). α-Methyl-*p*-tyrosine inhibits tyrosine hydroxylase *in vivo:* when it is given to experimental animals it arrests synthesis of the catecholamines. The actions and laboratory uses of α-methyl-*p*-tyrosine are discussed in more detail in Chapters 13 and 18.

(*c*) The remaining enzymes are of generally low specificity. That converting DOPA to dopamine is still sometimes known as DOPA decarboxylase although it has been known for many years that it, or an enzyme closely akin to it, is also responsible for the conversion of 5-hydroxytryptophan to 5-hydroxytryptamine. It also promotes the decarboxylation of some other aromatic aminoacids so that it is better to designate it 'aromatic-L-aminoacid decarboxylase', a descriptive, if not a very euphonious, name.

Dopamine-β-oxidase can catalyse the β-hydroxylation of a number of tyramine derivatives while phenylethanolamine *N*-methyltransferase is equally unselective in the noradrenaline derivatives it *N*-methylates. This lack of specificity among the biosynthetic enzymes raises the possibility that alternative pathways for the formation of adrenaline and its precursors may exist. Some of the possibilities are indicated in Fig. 17.2. Octopamine, a substance found in quantity in the octopus, occupies a prominent position in this scheme. It occurs in small amounts in many tissues that contain adrenaline or noradrenaline and some of the putative changes illustrated can undoubtedly occur *in vivo* in the sense that if the presumed precursor is administered in quantity the expected transformation occurs. Cardiac tissue, for instance, readily converts tyramine to octopamine. This type of experimental result cannot be taken as an indication that any of the alternative pathways is used in physiological conditions and the consensus of informed opinion is that the route of synthesis of virtually all of the body's adrenaline, noradrenaline and dopamine is that traced in Fig. 17.1. Nevertheless, the possibility that an alternative pathway might be opened up in abnormal conditions has clearly to be considered. Thus, monoamine oxidase inhibitors prevent the oxidative deamination of dietary tyrosine the metabolism of which is then diverted along the tyramine-octopamine route. The octopamine formed in this way can be taken up by adrenergic nerve terminals to become a false transmitter (p. 288). It is possible that this provides an explanation of the surprising fact that some monoamine oxidase inhibitors can be used as antihypertensive agents (p. 319).

Long continued stimulation of preganglionic sympathetic fibres promotes the activity of dopamine-β-hydroxylase as well as that of tyrosine hydroxylase (see above).

Adrenaline is the hormone of the adrenal medulla. In this tissue, noradrenaline is simply a precursor of the active substance: it is not liberated from the gland in any but small amounts and its physiological effects, so far as medullary activity is concerned, are negligible. In sympathetic nerves, however, synthesis proceeds no further than noradrenaline which exists in these nerves as a transmitter substance in its own right. Noradrenaline is also present in the brain but dopamine, its immediate precursor, also has transmitter functions in the central nervous system. The unique situation thus arises that two of the natural precursors of a humoral substance have humoral functions in their own right.

Dopaminergic neurones lack dopamine-β-hydroxylase and this preserves their chemical specificity by preventing the formation of noradrenaline.

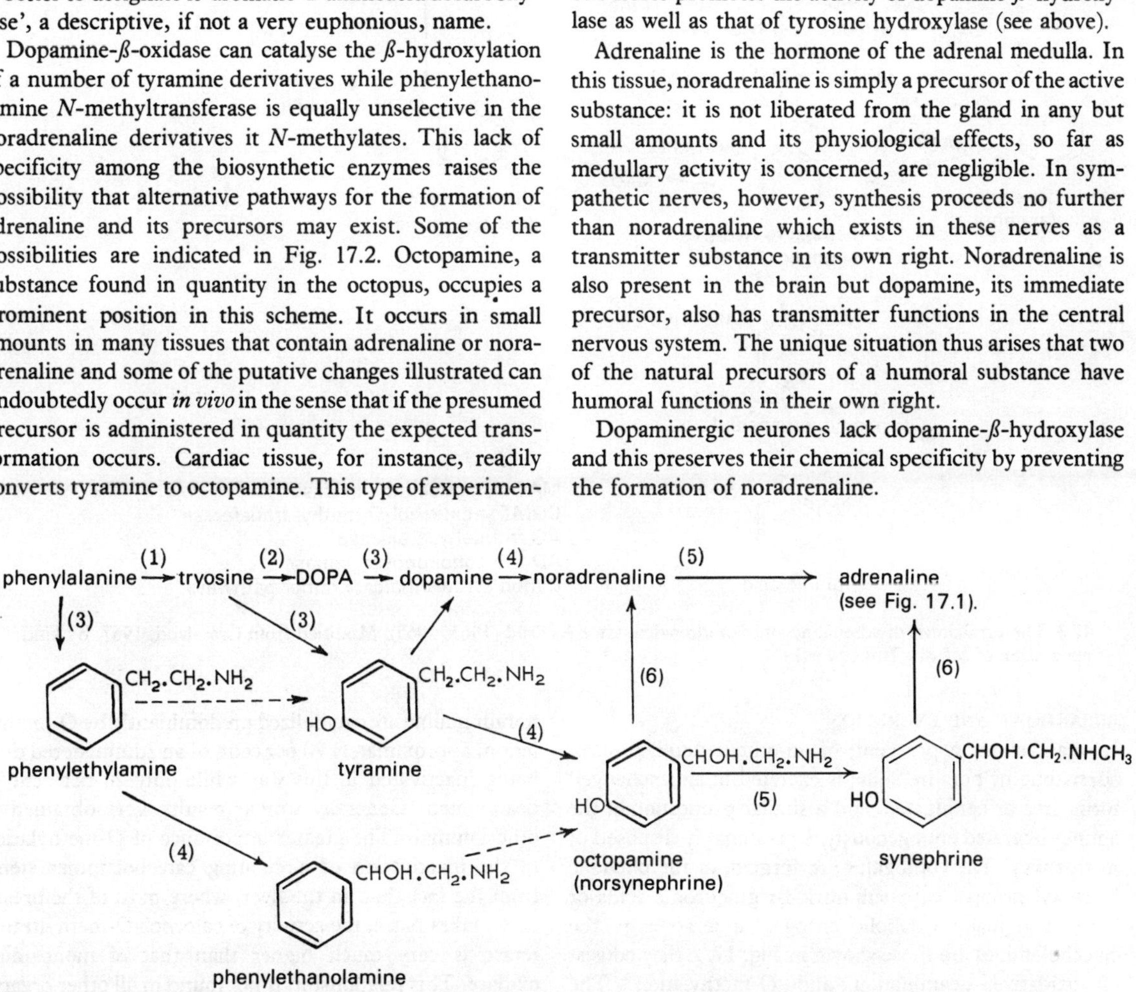

Fig. 17.2 Possible minor pathways for the biosynthesis of dopamine, noradrenaline and adrenaline. The enzymes involved are indicated, when known, by the numbers used in Fig. 17.1 and by (6) which is a mixed function oxidase. Reactions which have not been demonstrated *in vivo* are designated by dotted lines.

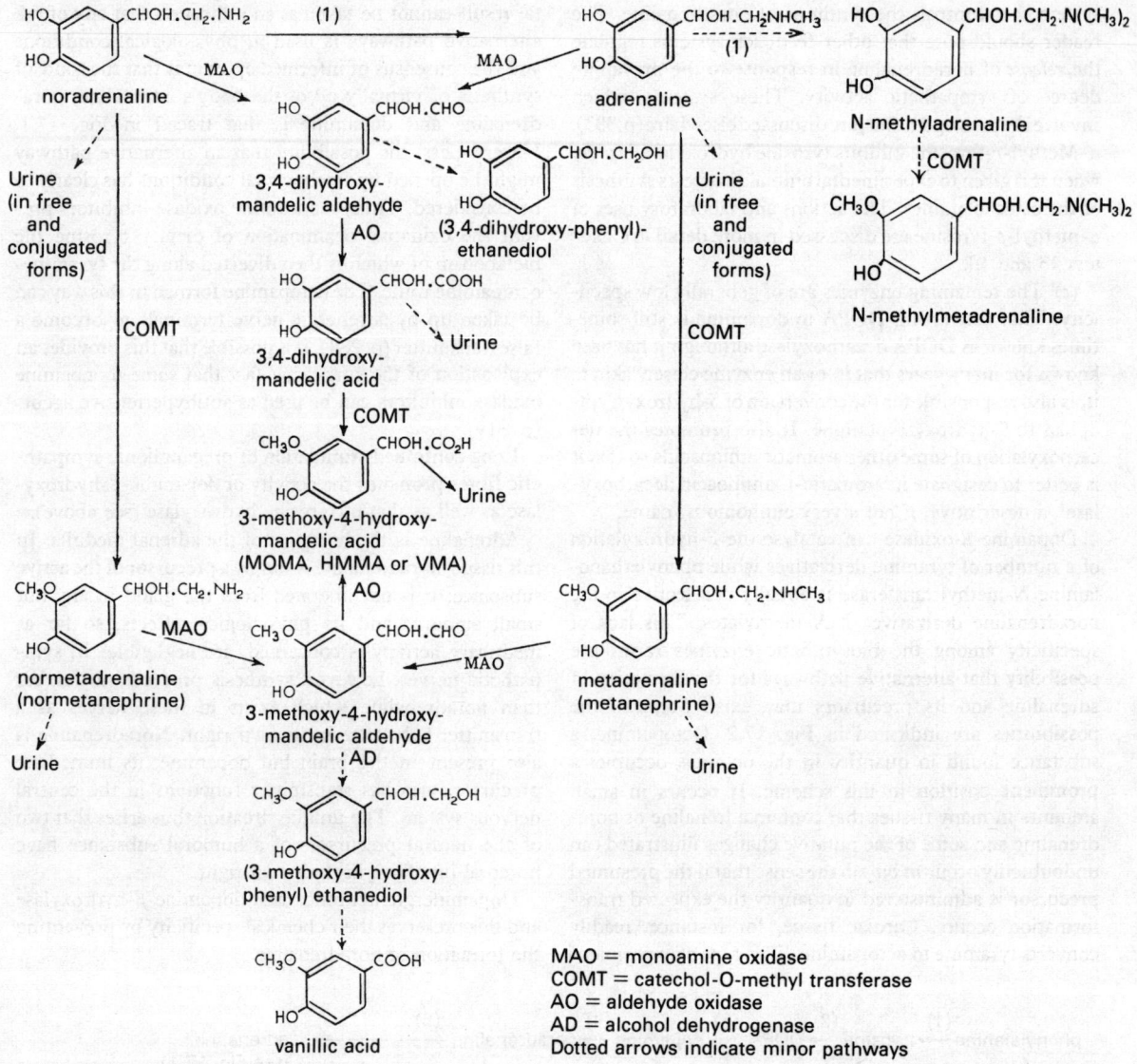

17.3 The breakdown of adrenaline and noradrenaline after Axelrod (1963, 1965). Modified from Crossland, 1967, by kind permission of Messrs. Butterworths.

BREAKDOWN AND EXCRETION

In man, about 6 per cent. of an administered dose of adrenaline or noradrenaline is excreted in an unchanged form, free or conjugated, and a similar proportion of the amines liberated endogenously is presumably disposed of in this way. The conjugates are formed, at the phenolic hydroxyl groups, with sulphuric or glucuronic acids or both. The major catabolic changes undergone by the catecholamines are those shown in Fig. 17.3: they consist of oxidative deamination and O-methylation. The enzymes involved are monoamine oxidase and catechol O-methyltransferase respectively.

Axelrod showed that, in man, circulating adrenaline and

noradrenaline are catabolized predominantly by O-methylation, approximately 70 per cent. of an administered dose being inactivated in this way while only 20 per cent. is deaminated. Generally similar results were obtained in other animals. The greater importance of O-methylation in the inactivation of circulating catecholamines stems from the fact that, in the liver, where most of the breakdown takes place, the activity of catechol-O-methyltransferase is very much higher than that of monoamine oxidase. This relationship is not found in all other organs: in the heart, for instance, monoamine oxidase is about five times more active than catechol-O-methyltransferase. The destruction of free noradrenaline in the cytoplasm of adrenergic neurones is also brought about by monoamine oxidase (p. 175).

In the presence of monoamine oxidase, the final product of catechol-O-methyltransferase activity is 3-methoxy-4-hydroxymandelic acid (Fig. 17.3) but much of the adrenaline or noradrenaline degraded by this enzyme is excreted as the simple methylated compounds metadrenaline (metanephrine) and normetadrenaline (normetanephrine) respectively. These substances appear in the urine mostly as conjugates but small amounts are present in the free form. A small proportion (probably no more than 10 per cent.) of the material catabolized by catechol-O-methyltransferase takes the alternative route shown in Fig. 17.3 and it appears in the urine as the glycol, (3-methoxy-4-hydroxyphenyl) ethanediol.

Reference to Fig. 17.3 will make it clear that catechol-O-methyltransferase can break down the products of monoamine oxidase activity and only very small amounts of 3,4-dihydroxymandelic acid appear in the urine. Thus we can conclude that the urine's content of 3-methoxy-4-hydroxymandelic acid (vanillyl-mandelic acid, MOMA, HMAA or VMA) is an index of catecholamine breakdown by both routes.

The points made in the foregoing discussion are underlined by the information presented in Table 17.1 which is taken from a paper by Axelrod and his colleagues (La Brosse, et al., 1961) and which indicates the relative importance of the different pathways shown in Fig. 17.3 for the breakdown of an administered dose of adrenaline in man. Much of our knowledge concerning the metabolism of adrenaline and noradrenaline, and most of the information concerning this topic to be found in this (and other) books comes from the writings of Axelrod, to whose reviews (Axelrod, 1963, 1965, 1966) the interested reader is directed for further discussion of the problem. More recent work has only confirmed the essential accuracy of the pioneer work of Axelrod.

It has been mentioned that phenylethanolamine N-methyltransferase is an enzyme of low specificity. It is capable of bringing about the N-methylation of adrenaline and the N-methyladrenaline so formed is susceptible to O-methylation by catechol-O-methyltransferase. It is possible that these reactions constitute a minor pathway for adrenaline inactivation in vivo. The possibility that adrenaline can be converted into adrenochrome and adrenolutin and that these compounds are responsible for producing schizophrenia is now discounted.

THE CATABOLISM OF DOPAMINE

Precursor dopamine is, of course, converted into noradrenaline but an alternative method of disposal is presumably required if the compound is to exercise an independent role. This is probably brought about through the agency of catechol-O-methyltransferase and monoamine oxidase which convert dopamine into homovanillic acid according to the scheme shown in Fig. 17.4.

MONOAMINE OXIDASE INHIBITORS

Although monoamine oxidase appears to take relatively little part in the metabolism of the endogenous catecholamines, compounds which inhibit the activity of the enzyme do exert marked pharmacological effects particularly on the central nervous system. The origin of this apparent contradiction is threefold: monoamine oxidase participates in intraneuronal processes concerned with the regulation of noradrenaline stores, it is very much involved in the catabolism of 5-hydroxytryptamine and the inhibitors may have independent actions not directly related to their ability to interfere with monoamine oxidase activity. Monoamine oxidase is also responsible for inactivating some exogenous sympathomimetic amines such as tyramine (which is ingested in a number of foodstuffs) and inhibition of the enzyme can also produce dramatic effects on this account. Monoamine oxidase inhibitors are discussed in detail in Chapter 32 (p. 578).

SUBSTANCES THAT INHIBIT THE ACTIVITY OF CATECHOL-O-METHYLTRANSFERASE

Inhibition of catechol-O-methyltransferase activity has remarkably few pharmacological consequences other than prolonging the actions of released or injected adrenaline and, to a lesser extent, those of noradrenaline. Interest in the inhibitors is centred on the light they cast on the nature

Table 17.1 The products of adrenaline metabolism in man (La Brosse, Axelrod, Kopin & Kety, 1961)

Free and conjugated adrenaline	6.5%
Metanephrine	
(a) free	5.0%
(b) conjugated	33.7%
3-Methoxy-4-hydroxymandelic acid (MOMA or VMA)	39.2%
(3-Methoxy-4-hydroxyphenyl) ethanediol	6.8%
3,4-Dihydroxymandelic acid + (3,4-dihydroxyphenyl) ethanediol	
(a) free	0.85%
(b) conjugated	0.75%

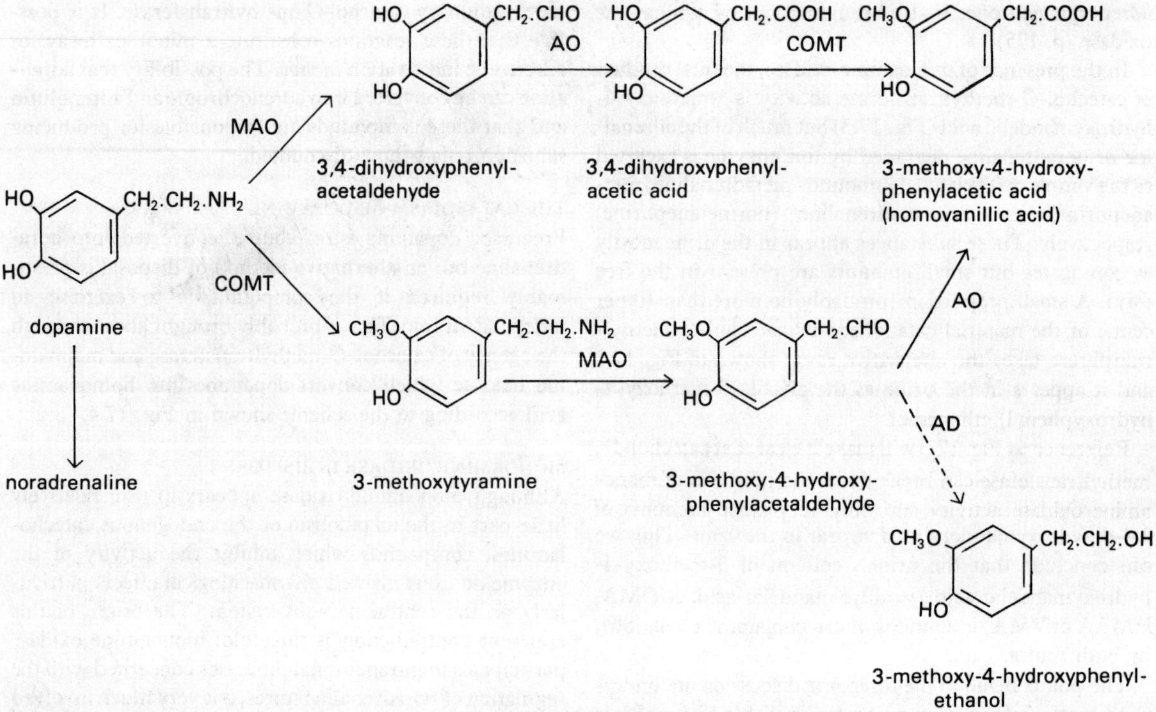

HO—CH₂.CHO

$CH_2.CHO$ → AO → $CH_2.COOH$ → COMT → $CH_2.COOH$

3,4-dihydroxyphenyl-acetaldehyde   3,4-dihydroxyphenyl-acetic acid   3-methoxy-4-hydroxy-phenylacetic acid (homovanillic acid)

MAO

dopamine $CH_2.CH_2.NH_2$

COMT

noradrenaline

CH_3O—$CH_2.CH_2.NH_2$ MAO → CH_3O—$CH_2.CHO$

3-methoxytyramine

3-methoxy-4-hydroxy-phenylacetaldehyde

AO

AD

CH_3O—$CH_2.CH_2.OH$

3-methoxy-4-hydroxyphenyl-ethanol

Abbreviations as in Fig. 17.3

Fig. 17.4 The catabolism of dopamine

of the adrenaline receptor (p. 280) rather than on their pharmacological actions or therapeutic potentialities. Substances that inhibit the activity of catechol-O-methyl-transferase include pyrogallol and the tropolones (Fig. 17.5).

The physiological and pharmacological properties of adrenaline and noradrenaline

It is customary to regard the sympathetic nervous system and the adrenal medulla as components of a single system, the secretions of the gland potentiating, prolonging or otherwise supporting the effects of the nervous activity. To some degree this is true and it is not surprising that in many respects the pharmacological actions of adrenaline, the hormone, are similar or complementary to those of noradrenaline, the neurohumour. In a few ways, however, the actions of the two substances are qualitatively different and this will serve to confer some flexibility on the system if, as seems likely, the hormonal and the nervous components are involved to different proportionate extents in their response to situations which activate them. Thus, it seems that in physical exercise the adrenal medulla is particularly active whereas the corrective response to a sudden haemorrhage involves a relatively greater participation of the sympathetic nerves.

The actions of adrenaline and noradrenaline on the major systems of the body will now be considered.

Cardiovascular system
The primary action of *adrenaline* on the heart is to increase its force of contraction. As a result, the heart empties more completely and adrenaline increases cardiac output even in the absence of any increase in venous return. Its ability to

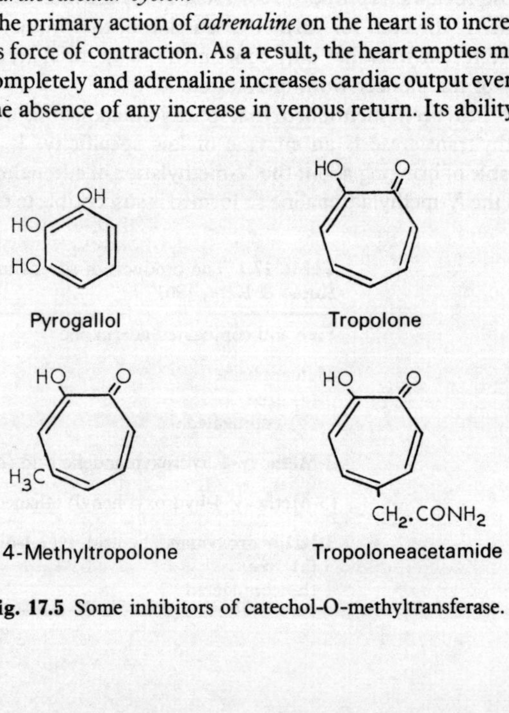

Pyrogallol

Tropolone

4-Methyltropolone

Tropoloneacetamide

Fig. 17.5 Some inhibitors of catechol-O-methyltransferase.

do this explains the marked rise in cardiac output which occurs at the very beginning of a period of physical exercise. The increase in the force of cardiac contraction is sometimes called, for no very good reason, a *positive inotropic* action. One of the first experiments performed by many students of pharmacology involves the application of adrenaline to the sinus venosus of a frog. The heart accelerates (a *positive chronotropic* effect) and this result, coupled with the popular belief that the heart beats more rapidly in conditions of emotional stress, often leads to the firm but mistaken conviction that the most prominent cardiac action of adrenaline is to increase the rate of beat. In the grossly unphysiological preparation represented by the pithed, and often bloodless, frog cardiac acceleration is certainly the most obvious response to adrenaline application. In the intact animal, however, this effect contributes little to adrenaline's overall action on the circulation, particularly since the elevated blood pressure resulting from the increased cardiac output leads to a reflex inhibition of the heart rate which partly offsets the stimulant action on the pacemaker. The subjective sensation experienced in acute emotional stress is caused by the increased force of cardiac contraction which gives the impression of an acceleration simply because in normal circumstances the beat of the heart is not felt at all. As well as increasing the cardiac output, adrenaline increases the irritability of the myocardium and increased concentrations of adrenaline may precipitate cardiac arrhythmias (p. 689).

Adrenaline constricts the blood vessels of the skin and viscera but dilates those in skeletal muscle. As a result of these changes the peripheral resistance—and hence the diastolic pressure—undergoes little alteration. It rises or falls slightly depending upon the extent of the vasodilatation produced in the muscles. The systolic blood pressure is determined largely by the cardiac output and so the overall effect of adrenaline injection or release is to increase the systolic pressure while inducing little change in the diastolic pressure.

Adrenaline increases the blood flow through the heart and brain but it must not be assumed that this is the result of a direct action on the blood vessels. Adrenaline certainly has some dilatatory effect in the coronary vessels but it actually causes some constriction of isolated cerebral vessels. The origin of the increased blood flow is mechanical rather than pharmacological. The coronary arteries leave the aorta immediately beyond its valve and the brain also is fed by vessels which receive the full force of the blood ejected on cardiac systole. Blood flow through heart and brain is thus determined by the systolic pressure and the increase in pressure produced by adrenaline is sufficient in itself to account for the increased flow. Another, and perhaps more important factor, operates in the coronary vessels because adrenaline's stimulant action on the myocardium causes the appearance of vasodilator metabolites such as adenosine.

Noradrenaline is primarily a vasoconstrictor agent. It reduces blood flow in skeletal muscle as well as that in the skin and viscera and thus brings about a sharp rise in diastolic pressure. It increases both the force and the rate of contraction of the isolated heart but it is much less potent than adrenaline in these respects. In the intact animal, however, noradrenaline brings about a reduction in heart rate with a consequent fall in cardiac output and oxygen consumption. The bradycardia arises because noradrenaline brings about a larger increase in mean blood pressure than does adrenaline so that it evokes a more powerful reflex cardioinhibitory response. The cardioinhibitory reflex (Marey's reflex) arises in response to stimulation of pressure receptors in the carotid sinus and aortic arch.

Respiratory system

Adrenaline causes relaxation of the bronchial musculature with a consequent increase in vital capacity. *Noradrenaline* does not relax the bronchi: it sometimes brings about some bronchoconstriction.

Following a large intravenous dose of adrenaline or noradrenaline there is a period of apnoea. This is a reflex response to stimulation of the carotid and aortic pressure receptors. Smaller doses of adrenaline stimulate pulmonary ventilation, perhaps by direct action on the respiratory centre. Noradrenaline is much less effective.

Other smooth muscle

Adrenaline relaxes the smooth muscle but stimulates the sphincters of the gastrointestinal tract unless sphincter tone is high, in which event adrenaline relaxes the sphincter too. The spleen of some animal species is surrounded by a contractile capsule. Adrenaline causes the capsule to contact and stored erythrocyte rich blood is added to the circulating volume. This effect is not of great significance in man.

The responses of the uterus to adrenaline vary with the species and other circumstances. The isolated rabbit uterus contracts, as does the pregnant uterus of the cat. On the other hand, adrenaline relaxes the uterus of the rat and the non-pregnant cat. The response of the human uterus depends on the dose of adrenaline and other factors (pregnancy, etc.) but it is worth remembering that, in the human female during late pregnancy and labour, uterine contractions are invariably inhibited by adrenaline. Adrenaline also causes contraction of the isolated seminal vesicles of the rat and guinea-pig.

Everybody knows that fear and other emotional responses are signalled by physical changes, prominent among which are the dilated pupils that result from contraction of the dilator pupillae. This muscle is controlled by sympathetic nerves and it also responds to circulating adrenaline. However, neither noradrenaline nor adrenaline is capable of causing pupillary dilatation when it is instilled into the conjunctival sac of healthy subjects unless the dilator pupillae has been previously denervated. Dilatation is also likely to occur in those suffering from one of a number of systemic diseases such as serious diabetes mellitus, thyrotoxicosis and pancreatitis.

Unlike adrenaline, some other sympathomimetic agents such as ephedrine and phenylephrine do cause dilatation of the pupil if they are given locally. They differ from mydriatic agents of the atropine type in that their use is not contraindicated in patients with glaucoma (p. 225). Indeed they actually bring about some reduction of intraocular pressure by restricting the blood supply to the ciliary processes and so reducing the rate of formation of aqueous humour and they have been used clinically for this purpose. They have the advantage of interfering only minimally with ocular accommodation. Adrenaline itself is also sometimes employed in the treatment of glaucoma, and it may be that its action in this respect, unlike that of the other agents we have mentioned, is not entirely attributable to its vasoconstrictor action: salbutamol (p. 272), a sympathomimetic amine with no constrictor effect, also brings about a reduction in intraocular pressure on local application to the eye.

The effects of *noradrenaline* on the organs listed in this section are qualitatively similar to, but quantitatively smaller than, those of adrenaline.

The central nervous system

It is a matter of common experience that the quantities of adrenaline liberated from the adrenal medulla in emergency situations cause sensations of fear and anxiety with shaking, weakness and tremor of the limbs. It must not be assumed that these effects are manifestations of a direct action of adrenaline on the central nervous system. Adrenaline does not readily pass the blood-brain barrier and many of the subjective effects it evokes represent responses to changes taking place in peripheral tissues. The forcibly beating heart, for instance, will remind a person of the circumstances attendant on other occasions when a similar sensation was experienced and this will add to his apprehensiveness and to his generally disturbed behaviour. Adrenaline does have pharmacological actions if it gains access to the central nervous system. In the laboratory it is easy to avoid the blood-brain barrier by injecting directly into the cisterna magna or into the cerebral ventricles (p. 37) and under these circumstances very small amounts of active material are often sufficient to evoke responses in the brain which are not complicated by the effect of nervous stimuli arriving from peripheral organs as is likely to happen if the drug is given by intravascular injection. Introduced directly into the brain in this way, adrenaline induces drowsiness or light anaesthesia, a surprising response to an agent that is popularly associated with alerting responses and emotional upheavals. It also causes

changes in body temperature (usually a depression) and, sometimes, vomiting.

Noradrenaline is much less likely to cause anxiety, fear and tension. Released in the brain by the activity of adrenergic neurones, noradrenaline has transmitter actions that are discussed in detail elsewhere (p. 183).

Exocrine glands

Adrenaline stimulates the secretion of sweat and saliva but inhibits the secretion of other glands. *Noradrenaline* can also stimulate the secretion of sweat but it has little effect on the other glands.

Metabolism

Adrenaline stimulates the breakdown of glycogen (*glycogenolysis*) in liver and muscle and brings about an increase in the concentration of glucose and lactic acid in the blood. This very old observation provided the stimulus for many of the biochemical studies that were undertaken during the earlier years of the present century and which contributed so much to our knowledge of carbohydrate metabolism. The glycogenolytic action of adrenaline provides an increased supply of energy-yielding nutrients to the tissues and this is clearly in accord with the simple view that the function of adrenaline is to bring about changes which permit the organism to respond to acute emergencies. *Noradrenaline* stimulates glycogenolysis to a much smaller extent than does adrenaline and there is evidence that when the blood glucose concentration falls, the resulting activation of the sympatho-adrenal system involves the adrenal component to a greater extent than when the situation is one, such as a haemorrhage, in which the necessary corrective is an overall vasoconstriction such as is provided by noradrenaline.

Adrenaline also affects fat metabolism. This action is shared by noradrenaline. Adipose tissue is broken down to release free fatty acids and glycerol. The reincorporation of the free fatty acids into adipose tissue is stimulated by glucose. Adrenaline, as has been seen, is a much more potent hyperglycaemic agent than is noradrenaline and this explains why noradrenaline produces an increase in the concentration of free fatty acids in the plasma which is of the same order as that induced by adrenaline.

The glycogenolytic and lipolytic actions of the catecholamines are set in motion by the activation of phosphorylase and lipase, respectively, through the adenyl cyclase-cyclic AMP link. This linking mechanism (the 'second messenger' system) mediates the action of so many hormones and other humoral substances that it demands a separate discussion and this is provided in Chapter 19 (p. 321). In the meantime, it is worth pointing out that the system's march to its present pre-eminent status began with the discovery of the part it plays in adrenaline induced glycogenolysis.

Adrenaline receptors

It was pointed out that, although Loewi had established the principle of chemical transmission in the autonomic nervous system and had identified the post ganglionic parasympathetic transmitter as acetylcholine, it proved surprisingly difficult to determine the nature of the sympathetic transmitter notwithstanding the long established fact that a known hormone, adrenaline, reproduced the effects of sympathetic stimulation. The difficulties lay partly in the fact that the properties of the transmitter, though generally similar to, were in a few ways perplexingly different from, those of adrenaline. Another problem was posed by the fact that sympathetic stimulation produced both excitatory and inhibitory effects. It could hardly be maintained that excitation and inhibition were mediated by different transmitter substances because adrenaline itself, a single substance, also produced both types of effect. However, antagonists such as ergotoxine (p. 295) were known to be incapable of blocking all the actions of adrenaline, inhibitory responses such as vasodilatation being, in general, unaffected. It was therefore concluded that some factor residing in the effector cell determined whether the sympathetic transmitter produced an excitatory or an inhibitory response. The possibility that the dual response might be caused by the presence of two kinds of receptor was dismissed because Cannon and Rosenbleuth, the most prominent workers in this field in the 1930's, had produced some evidence that when an organ gave an excitatory response to stimulation of its sympathetic supply an excitatory substance 'overflowed' into the blood. Similarly an inhibitory response was associated with the appearance of an inhibitory substance. The only hypothesis which could encompass an explanation of all these facts was that a single transmitter (perhaps adrenaline, perhaps some related substance) was released by stimulation of the sympathetic nerves and that this transmitter (M) combined with one of two 'receptive substances' E or I in the effector cell. The substance so produced, ME or MI (sympathin E or sympathin I) evoked an exitatory or an inhibitory response respectively. There the matter rested until 1948.

α- AND β-RECEPTORS

The concept of two sympathins, formed in the effector cell from a common precursor, was always a difficult one to accept fully and in 1948 Ahlquist provided evidence for the existence of at least two different kinds of adrenaline receptor. For reasons that are discussed elsewhere (p. 172), these structures should *not* be called adrenergic or adrenotropic receptors. Ahlquist studied the actions of five sympathomimetic substances on a number of pharmacological responses in both intact animals and isolated tissues.

The sympathomimetic agents Ahlquist used were adrenaline, noradrenaline, α-methylnoradrenaline, α-methyladrenaline and isoprenaline and he found that he could divide the pharmacological responses into two clear groups on the basis of their relative sensitivities to the five agonists. One group of responses consisted of vasoconstriction, contraction of the uterus, ureter and dilator pupillae muscle and relaxation of the intestine. Adrenaline and noradrenaline proved to be the most potent effectors of all six responses with isoprenaline the least so. The other three responses were vasodilatation, relaxation of the uterus and increased rate and force of the heart beat. For the evocation of all these responses, isoprenaline and adrenaline were the most effective and noradrenaline was least so. Ahlquist's findings are summarized in Table 17.2.

Ahlquist concluded (and his experimental results clearly made this conclusion eminently reasonable) that the tissues he examined carried two kinds of adrenaline receptor. He proposed that they be designated α and β receptors and this nomenclature has been universally accepted. On this classification our first group of six responses involves the activation of α receptors while the remaining three responses result from stimulation of β receptors. It is also clear from Ahlquist's data that adrenaline strongly stimulated both α and β receptors, that noradrenaline is more active on α than on β receptors and that isoprenaline is more active on β receptors. It is to be noted that noradrenaline is not entirely devoid of an action on β receptors—after all, stimulation of the sympathetic nerves to the heart causes the liberation of noradrenaline and a consequent cardioacceleration. On the other hand, noradrenaline has little effect on β receptors in tissues other than the heart. Isoprenaline has minimal actions on α receptors. Noradrenaline and adrenaline occur naturally in the animal body and it would have provided a satisfyingly neat and symmetrical situation if isoprenaline, the 'specialist' β stimulant, also occurred in the body. Indeed it is possible to argue that the evolution of an 'isoprenalinergic' nerve supply to a few tissues would have been a boon and considerable interest was aroused some years ago by reports that isoprenaline had been detected in some sympathetic nerves. Unfortunately it has proved impossible to confirm these findings. Ahlquist was careful not to assert that α and β receptors mediated exclusively excitatory and

Table 17.2 The Ahlquist experiment

Group 1 responses [mediated by α-receptors]	Group 2 responsers [mediated by β-receptors]
Vasoconstriction	Vasodilatation
Contraction of uterus	Relaxation of uterus
Contraction of ureters	Increased rate and force
Contraction of dilator pupillae	of heart beat
Relaxation of the intestine	
Order of Potency	*Order of potency*
Adrenaline > noradrenaline > α-methylnoradrenaline > α-methyladrenaline > isoprenaline	Isoprenaline > adrenaline > α-methyladrenaline > α-methylnoradrenaline > noradrenaline

inhibitory effects respectively. Nevertheless, five of the six responses classified as resulting from stimulation of α receptors involved stimulation of muscle. The one inhibitory response in the group was inhibition of gut motility but more recent work has indicated that intestinal receptors are predominantly of the β type. Of the three β responses, two (vasodilatation and inhibition of uterine activity) were inhibitory and the third (myocardial contraction) was excitatory in nature.

When Ahlquist first put forward his hypothesis, the sympathetic transmitter had not been identified. He himself thought that it was probably adrenaline and he believed that his two-receptor concept did no more than provide a simple and acceptable alternative explanation to the one then available for the origin of the excitatory and inhibitory responses to sympathetic stimulation and adrenaline injection. In so doing, he had (justifiably, as it later transpired) to ignore some of the findings of Cannon and Rosenblueth and at the time there was no substantial body of evidence to suggest that his two-receptor hypothesis corresponded more closely to the facts than did the rival two-sympathin hypothesis. A short time later, it became clear that noradrenaline was the sympathetic transmitter and the realization that the effects of sympatho-adrenal stimulation were mediated by both noradrenaline and adrenaline made Ahlquist's notion of two receptor types more generally acceptable. Its final vindication came with the discovery of separate and specific antagonists for α and β receptors. The pharmacology of these antagonists is discussed in the next chapter. It is worth pointing out that Ahlquist's hypothesis has found its most impressive support in experiments which became available long after the hypothesis was originally formulated. This provides strong evidence of its essential validity: so many hypotheses propounded to explain a particular series of experimental results become less, rather than more, tenable in the light of later discoveries.

β_1 and β_2 receptors

The conclusions that can be drawn from pharmacological experiments on simple preparations are rarely as unequivocally clear cut as textbook commentaries tend to imply. Among the factors that lead to confusion is the lack of complete specificity in agonist and antagonist molecules and some of those who followed Ahlquist reported findings that, superficially at least, were difficult to interpret on the simple assumption that tissues carry no more than two types of adrenaline receptor. Furchgott, for instance, found it necessary to postulate for a time the existence of four types of receptor which he designated as α (for the contraction of smooth muscle), β (for the relaxation of smooth muscle other than that of the intestine), γ (for metabolic actions) and δ (for relaxation of intestinal smooth muscle). Neither Furchgott's analysis nor others that rested on a postulate of more than two adrenoceptors

stood the test of time or of the rigorous examination permitted by the advent of new agents and a growing knowledge of the distribution of α and β receptors. Not, that is, until 1967 when Lands and his coworkers and, close on their heels, a group headed by Arnold, provided evidence that β receptors are of two types (Lands, Luduena and Buzzo, 1967; Arnold and McAuliff, 1968).

The approach adopted by Lands and his collaborators was not very dissimilar to that favoured by Ahlquist twenty years earlier. They took a number of β-agonists (in some experiments, fifteen were used) including adrenaline, noradrenaline and their derivatives and they measured the relative potency, in relation to that of isoprenaline, of all these agents on a number of β-mediated pharmacological responses. These included rate and force of heart beat, intestinal and uterine relaxation, vasodilatation, bronchodilatation and lipolysis. Taking the responses in pairs, Lands then calculated the extent to which the relative potencies of the agonists on one response correlated with those on the other member of the pair. When looked at in this way, the responses fell into two sharply differentiated sets. There was a very high degree of correlation between the relative potencies of the different agonists on any pair of responses that came from the same set but a very low degree of correlation if the pair came from different sets. Specific examples should make the procedure clear. Taking as a pair of responses the power of cardiac contraction and the rate of heart beat, the correlation coefficient (p. 123) between the relative potencies of twelve β stimulants on the two preparations was 0.923. Similarly, for vasodilatation and bronchodilatation, the correlation coefficient was 0.957. However, for power of cardiac contraction and vasodilatation, the coefficient was only 0.312. These results clearly indicate that the receptors involved in the production of changes in heart rate have the same characteristics as those that mediate changes in the force of cardiac contraction and that these differ from those that initiate vasodilatation and bronchodilatation. In their turn, the receptors mediating the last two responses are, on this analysis, identical or very closely similar. Examination of the other responses studied by Lands and by Arnold confirm that all of them can be allocated to one or other of the two sets. The first set of responses is initiated by what, following Lands, we now call β_1 receptors. They consist of cardiac effects, lipolysis and intestinal relaxation (though there is some dispute concerning the allocation of the last named response to the β_1 set) while β_2 receptors are associated with glycogenolysis and relaxation of blood vessels, bronchi, ureters and the uterus. It will be noted that both types of β receptor are involved in the metabolic responses to adrenaline. This last conclusion comes largely from Arnold's work. A succinct discussion of both Lands' and Arnold's studies is provided by Furchgott (1972).

This early work on the subdivision of β receptors did not entirely escape criticism on both methodological and

Table 17.3 The probable nature of the adrenaline receptors in the principal tissues containing them

Tissue	Nature of receptor	Response	Remarks
Heart	β_1	Increase in heart rate, in myocardial contractility and in conduction though conducting tissue	—
Blood vessels skeletal muscle liver	α, β_2 α, β_2	α—vasoconstriction β_2—vasodilatation	In skeletal muscle β receptors predominate over α
other viscera skin brain mucous membranes	α α α α	Vasoconstriction	
Stomach and Intestine sphincters other muscle	α α, β_1	Constriction α—relaxation of rhythmicity and tone β_1—relaxation of rhythmicity and tone	
Bronchi	β_2	Relaxation	Bronchi also carry a few α receptors
Eye radial muscle of iris (Dilator pupillae)	α	Contraction (pupil dilates)	
ciliary muscles	β_2	Paralysis of accommodation	
nictitating membrane	α, β	α—contraction β—relaxation	Effect not very strong; α receptors predominate; β receptors presumably of β_2 variety
Skin pilomotor muscle sweat glands	α α	Hair 'stands on end' Secretion	Sweating limited to parts of body which show 'emotional sweating'—palms of hands and axillae
Splenic capsule	α	Contraction	Not all species have spleens with contractile capsules
Bladder detrusor muscle sphincters	β_2 α	Relaxation Constriction	
Vas deferens Uterus	α, β_2 α, β_2	α—contraction β_2—relaxation α—contraction (rabbit and human; possibly relaxation in rat and cat) β_2—relaxation	Nature of response to stimulation of both receptors (e.g. by adrenaline) depends on species, stage of menstrual or ovarian cycle, stage of pregnancy, hormonal factors. etc.
Metabolic effects	β	β_1 lipolysis β_2 glycogenolysis	

Noradrenaline stimulates α receptors and β_1 receptors in the heart; isoprenaline stimulates β receptors, adrenaline stimulates both. Note that α responses are *predominantly* excitatory in nature, while β responses are excitatory in the heart and inhibitory elsewhere.

interpretative grounds but the advent of relatively specific β_2 (p. 305) and β_1 antagonists (p. 304) has established the idea as firmly as earlier events vindicated the original Ahlquist classification.

It is not impossible that more sophisticated experiments and analyses will reveal differences within each group of adrenoceptors (some minor ones indeed are already appearing) and that we shall be confronted with demands that we subdivide α, β_1 and β_2 receptors still further. On the other hand, it may equally well be that we have reached the limit of useful resolution. Indeed, as Furchgott (1972) points out, even β_1 and β_2 receptors are not necessarily structurally different from one another. It may be that, in any one species, they 'are identical molecules ....(whose)....properties are influenced by their interactions with surrounding molecules in the macromolecular structures such as cell membranes in which they are located or "embedded"'. Whatever may be the ultimate future of the receptors the present division is sharp enough for therapeutic purposes.

We have seen that noradrenaline has some action on β_1 receptors in the heart. Since cardiac β_1 effects are essentially excitatory as are almost all responses to stimulation of α receptors, it is permissible to look upon noradrenaline as having almost exclusively excitatory actions, at least in the periphery. The brain presents a more complex situation.

The nature of the adrenaline receptors present in a representative selection of tissues is indicated in Table 17.3. This information has been gleaned from a study of the effects of noradrenaline, adrenaline, isoprenaline and specific blocking agents on the tissues, together with analyses of the Lands' type. Reference to the Table will make clear the origin of the differences between the pharmacological actions of noradrenaline and adrenaline. To take one example, the blood vessels in skeletal muscle carry both α and β_2 receptors, stimulation of which causes vasoconstriction and vasodilatation respectively. The β_2 receptors outnumber the α receptors so that adrenaline, stimulating both kinds of receptor, will cause vasodilatation but noradrenaline, with no action on β_2 receptors, will cause vasoconstriction. Isoprenaline, of course, is a more powerful vasodilator agent than adrenaline because it does not influence the α receptors.

The reader should note that the alimentary tract carries both α and β receptors, both mediating relaxation.

SYMPATHOMIMETIC AMINES

Adrenaline, noradrenaline and a number of synthetic amines structurally related to the naturally occurring compounds are designated *sympathomimetic*, the adjective implying that they mimic the effects produced by stimulation of the sympathetic nerves. In fact this is not a very accurate description: stimulation of a sympathetic nerve

never results, for instance, in an exclusive activation of β receptors but isoprenaline, a substance which elicits only β responses is justly classified as a sympathomimetic amine. It is best to think of a sympathomimetic amine, semantics notwithstanding, as one that produces a pharmacological effect as a result of a direct or indirect stimulation of α or β receptors or both.

It is usual to adopt a three-way classification of the sympathomimetic amines into those that have *direct*, *indirect* and *mixed* actions respectively.

Directly acting sympathomimetic amines produce pharmacological responses by agonist actions on the adrenoceptors. The indirectly acting compounds do not themselves directly influence the receptors but they do cause the liberation of noradrenaline from noradrenergic nerve terminals. Not surprisingly, none of them has any action on the adrenal medulla (its physiological activator is acetylcholine) so that none operates through the medium of adrenaline release. Mixed action sympathomimetic amines operate both directly and indirectly.

Some of the indirectly acting and mixed action amines pass the blood-brain barrier and exert central actions that are the result of dopamine liberation from dopaminergic neurones as well as the expected noradrenaline release.

MODE OF ACTION OF THE INDIRECTLY-ACTING SYMPATHOMIMETIC AMINES

Gaddum and Kwiatkowski (1938) suggested that compounds such as tyramine and ephedrine might owe part of their pharmacological activity to an ability to prevent the enzymatic destruction of the sympathetic transmitter. Blaschko, Richter and Schlossman (1937) had earlier suggested that a similar action might explain the effects of amphetamine. We now know that enzyme activity is not an important factor in bringing about the termination of sympathetic transmitter action (p. 175) and there is general agreement that indirectly-acting sympathomimetic amines operate by causing the release of noradrenaline from nerve terminals in sympathetically innervated organs. The evidence which supports this conclusion can be summarized as follows:

(*a*) Indirectly-acting sympathomimetic amines increase the concentration of noradrenaline in the venous blood draining sympathetically innervated organs. This has now been demonstrated for a large number of amines and organs. (Iversen, 1967).

(*b*) Tyramine and amphetamine (the only indirectly-acting amines so far studied in this way) reduce the noradrenaline content of tissues.

(*c*) Reserpine treatment leads to a loss of noradrenaline from adrenergic neurones and indirectly-acting sympathomimetic agents have little or no action in reserpinized animals unless a noradrenaline infusion is first given to bring about a partial replenishment of the stores of transmitter (Burn and Rand, 1958).

The indirectly-acting sympathomimetic amines probably liberate noradrenaline by displacing it from its storage sites. It seems that they are carried to the intracellular sites by the transport mechanism which normally permits the accumulation of noradrenaline and which is responsible for bringing about the reincorporation into the neurones of noradrenaline liberated in the course of adrenergic nerve activity. Thus the amines not only liberate transmitter but they also potentiate its effects by ensuring its persistence at the receptors. This part of the mechanism is essentially the same as that envisaged by the early workers in this field except that blockade of re-uptake takes the place of inhibition of catabolic enzyme activity.

It has been suggested that the indirectly-acting sympathomimetic amines might be converted into their β-hydroxylated derivatives within the nerve terminals and that the derivatives have a greater affinity for the storage sites than has noradrenaline itself.

Identification of directly- and indirectly-acting sympathomimetic amines

Cocaine increases the sensitivity of sympathetically innervated organs to directly-acting sympathomimetic amines but reduces or abolishes the response to indirectly-acting substances. Like the latter themselves, cocaine prevents the uptake of noradrenaline by the nerve terminals and this is the basis of its ability to increase the sensitivity of organs to noradrenaline. Presumably it has an even greater affinity for the transport mechanism than have the indirectly-acting amines. This would explain why the actions of the latter are blocked. Cocaine does not greatly influence the activity of sympathomimetic amines with a mixed action.

Denervation of sympathetically innervated organs leads to an increase in their sensitivity to noradrenaline and other directly acting amines. Responses to indirectly acting amines are depressed or abolished. The action of compounds with a mixed action is unaffected.

Reserpine can also be used to distinguish the various classes of sympathomimetic amine. It is usual to examine the effect of reserpinization on the dose response curve of the compound under investigation. Reserpine does not alter the dose response curves of compounds that act directly on adrenoceptors but it moves to the right, and depresses the maxima of, those derived from indirectly-acting sympathomimetic substances. The curves of compounds with a mixed action are moved to the right but their maxima are not affected. This method of identification is particularly useful for determining the classification of substances whose actions have proved difficult to characterize.

Individual sympathomimetic amines

Tables 17.4, 17.5 and 17.6 list the names and formulae of

sympathomimetic amines with direct, indirect and mixed actions respectively. The catalogue of directly-acting compounds is subdivided according to the type of receptor involved in the drugs' action. Typical members of each of the subgroups so recognized are adrenaline (which acts on α, β_1 and β_2 receptors), noradrenaline (a predominantly α antagonist), isoprenaline (predominantly β_1 and β_2) and salbutamol (predominantly β_2). The reader will note the absence of compounds that act exclusively on β_1 receptors. That such substances are not available probably reflects a lack of demand rather than chemical incompetence. The indirectly-acting amines liberate only noradrenaline peripherally and to this extent their actions are referable to α receptor stimulation. However, as we have seen, many indirectly-acting substances pass into the brain with ease and have pronounced central actions. Even those actions that are attributable to noradrenaline stimulation of α receptors add extra features to the drugs' spectrum of activity which are not exhibited by noradrenaline itself, which does not penetrate the blood-brain barrier. Actions on other types of central dopaminergic and other neurones may still further complicate the pharmacological picture. Amphetamine will be taken as a typical representative of the group of indirectly-acting sympathomimetic amines. Finally, compounds with a mixed action stimulate either or both types of receptor and may also have a central action. Ephedrine is the most widely used mixed-action amine. The following paragraphs provide additional information concerning some of the substances that appear in Tables 17.4 to 17.6

ADRENALINE

The pharmacology of adrenaline has been considered in detail in earlier pages and it only remains to discuss its therapeutic actions. It has been extensively used for the treatment of acute attacks of asthma. By its action on β_2 receptors, adrenaline relieves bronchospasm and the vasoconstriction it produces through the medium of α receptor stimulation reduces congestion of the bronchial mucous membrane. It seems that adrenaline also has some ability to prevent the release of bronchoconstrictor substances resulting from antigen-antibody unions (Assem and Schild, 1969). In this respect it resembles, although it is much less active than, sodium cromoglycate (p. 410). This effect is probably mediated through β_2 receptors and it obviously contributes to the effectiveness of adrenaline and its congeners in the treatment of asthma (p. 408) Adrenaline can be given by subcutaneous injection (in doses of up to 0.5 mg) or taken by inhalation of a one per cent solution delivered in a fine spray from a nebulizer operated by the patient. In the emergency situation presented by severe anaphylactic shock, adrenaline may have to be given by *slow* intravenous injection. This route of administration is so hazardous that its use is only justified in life threatening emergencies.

Table 17.4 Substances that act directly on adrenaline receptors

Approved name(s)	Proprietary name(s)	Formula	Remarks
Substances that act on both α and β receptors			
Adrenaline Epinephrine Suprarenin			see text
α-Methyladrenaline Dihydroxyephedrine Epinine	—	HO—⬡—$CHOH.CH.NH.CH_3$ $\mid$ CH_3 with HO	—
Dopamine	Intropin	see text	see text
Substances that act predominantly on α receptors			
Noradrenaline Norepinephrine Levarterenol	Levophed	see text	see text
α-Methylnoradrenaline Nordefrin Corbasil; Corbefrine		HO—⬡—$CHOH.CH.NH_2$ $\mid$ CH_3 with HO	Used as a vaso-constrictor agent with local anaesthetics
Phenylephrine Neo-Synephrine	Isophrin	⬡—$CH.CH_2.NHCH_3$ $\mid$ OH with OH	Used as a nasal decongestant and for maintaining blood pressure in shock and spinal anaesthesia
Oxedrine; Synephrine	Sympatol	HO—⬡—$CH.CH_2.NHCH_3$ $\mid$ OH	Used as a nasal decongestant and for maintaining blood pressure in shock and spinal anaesthesia
Norphenylephrine	—	⬡—$CHOH.CH_2.NH_2$ with OH	—
Methoxamine	Vasoxyl Vasylox	OCH_3 ⬡—$CHOH.CH.NH_2$ $\mid$ CH_3 with OCH_3	Used to treat the hypotension of shock and spinal anaesthesia; antagonizes the metabolic actions of adrenaline
Substances that act predominantly on β receptors (both types)			
Isopropylnoradrenaline Isoprenaline Isoproterenol	Aludrine; Isuprel; Neo-epinine; Norisodrine; Saventrine; Suscardia	see text	see text
α-Ethylnoradrenaline	Bronkephrine	HO—⬡—$CHOH.CH.NH_2$ $\mid$ C_2H_5 with HO	Has been used in the treatment of asthma
Orciprenaline Metaproterenol	Alupent; Metaprel	see text	Some preference for β_2 receptors

Table 17.4 (contd)

Approved name(s)	Proprietary name(s)	Formula	Remarks
Methoxyphenamine	Orthoxine		Has been used in asthma
Protochylol Protokylol	Ventaire		Has been used in the treatment of asthma
Nylidrin	Arlidin		Used (not very successfully) in the treatment of dysmenorrhoea and intermittent claudication
Isoxsuprine	Vasodilan Vasotran		As for nylidrin

Substances that act selectively on β_2 **receptors**

Approved name(s)	Proprietary name(s)	Formula	Remarks
Isoetharine	Dilabron Bronchilator	see text	see text
Salbutamol Albutamol Albuterol	Ventolin	see text	see text
Hexoprenaline	Etoscol; Ipradol	see text	see text
Rimiterol	Pulmadil		See text
Terbutaline	Bricanyl Filair		Uses as for salbutamol
Fenoterol	Berotec		Uses as for salbutamol
Ritodrine	Prepar Yutopar		Uses as for salbutamol
Soterenol			

Adrenaline is applied locally to produce vasoconstriction in surgical procedures on the ear, nose and throat. It shrinks the mucous membrane and permits better visualization of the operative field as well as reducing capillary oozing. A pledget of cotton wool soaked in adrenaline and inserted into the nostril may be needed to arrest troublesome nose bleeding. Some local anaesthetics cause vasodilatation. The addition of adrenaline to the anaesthetic localizes and prolongs the anaesthetic action. All these vasoconstrictor actions result from α receptor stimulation and it might be thought that noradrenaline or some other compound which acted exclusively on the α receptors would be as useful an agent. Some compounds of this type are, indeed, now used as nasal decongestants (Tables 17.4 to 17.6) but when localized vasoconstriction is required for other purposes it is still usual to employ adrenaline, which is a very effective constrictor of superficial vessels and is of proven worth.

Adrenaline administration by systemic routes is not without its dangers. Palpitations, tremors and a sensation of intense fear are not uncommon, even after subcutaneous injections. More serious side effects (which sometimes prove fatal) include cardiac arrhythmias, attacks of anginal pain and a rise of blood pressure which may precipitate cerebral or subarachnoid haemorrhages. These accidents are particularly likely to occur if an injection intended for the subcutaneous tissues enters a vein or if an intravenous injection is given too rapidly.

ISOPRENALINE

Isoprenaline (isopropylnoradrenaline, isoproterenol) stimulates only β receptors and thereby brings about vasodilatation, bronchodilatation and an increase in cardiac output. It is employed for the relief of asthmatic attacks for which purpose it is taken in sublingual tablets in a dose of 5 to 20 mg. (racemic form). The dose of the (—) form is 5 to 15 mg.

Isoprenaline is also available in inhalers that provide metered doses as a pressurized aerosol. Each 'puff' of vapour provides 0.1 or 0.15 mg. of isoprenaline and up to three doses can be taken at any one time to relieve bronchospasm. Low doses are effective by this route because the drug penetrates deeply into the lung and directly to its target. Unfortunately, patients whose asthma attack does not yield to the recommended dose may be tempted to take more and some years ago an alarming number of fatalities was recorded, particularly in Britain, among users of the then novel isoprenaline aerosol inhalers. The cause of death lay in the heart. Isoprenaline increases the power of cardiac contraction and hence that organ's oxygen demands but the concurrent vasodilatation brings about a fall in blood pressure that may deprive the heart of the increased oxygen supply it needs. The possibility cannot be entirely excluded that the aerosol propellant itself has some toxic effect on the heart.

By the intravenous route, isoprenaline is sometimes applied to the treatment of shock.

Side effects sometimes accompany even modest doses of isoprenaline by whichever route they are taken. They are, for the most part, confined to the heart and they are similar to those produced by adrenaline. Peripheral vasodilatation may cause flushing but hypertensive episodes, such as may be caused by adrenaline, do not, of course, occur. Patients with heart disease, thyrotoxicosis, diabetes mellitus and disorders of the liver and kidney are particularly likely to suffer adverse side effects as are those with an inborn hypersensitivity to sympathomimetic amines: they should be warned of the dangers.

The effect of a dose of isoprenaline persists for no more than half an hour, the drug being completely inactivated during that period. When it arrives in the bloodstream from the lungs, sublingual vessels or a syringe, it is exposed to the action of catechol-O-methyltransferase and it is metabolized to 3-O-methylisoprenaline, a compound that has, interestingly enough, some ability to block β receptors and so partly to offset the beneficial effect of its parent. This might well explain why some patients become tolerant to the drug. Isoprenaline is also inactivated by conversion to the ethereal sulphate in the intestinal wall and liver and this militates against its administration by the oral route.

In addition to being metabolized, isoprenaline is also taken up into tissues by the uptake-2 mechanism for catecholamines (p. 175) and this further accelerates the inactivation of therapeutic doses. There are, indeed, those who maintain that this constitutes the most important route of isoprenaline disposal.

COMPOUNDS WITH A SELECTIVE ACTION ON β_2 RECEPTORS

In an attempt to design a bronchodilator drug that would spare the heart and also have a reasonably prolonged action, the isoprenaline molecule was systematically modified and this led to the discovery, first, of orciprenaline (metaproterenol, Alupent) and isoetharine (Dilabron). It was in the course of this work, it should be observed, that Lands conceived the notion of β_1 and β_2 receptors.

Orciprenaline is not a catecholamine since its two phenolic hydroxy groups occupy meta positions relative to one another (Fig. 17.6). Consequently it is immune to attack by catechol-O-methyltransferase (and, presumably, to tissue uptake) and so has a satisfactorily prolonged action. On the other hand, it has agonist activity at both β_1 and β_2 receptors though the β_1 type are less sensitive to the drug than the β_2 type. Contrariwise, isoetharine operates rather selectively on β_2 receptors and so does not affect the heart but it is a catecholamine and so has only a short lived action. A more successful outcome of the chemist's manipulative skill was the emergence, in 1968, of salbutamol.

Salbutamol (albutamol, Ventolin) couples the selectiv-

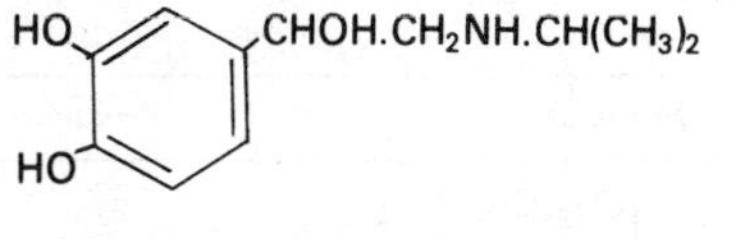

HO— / \ —CHOH.CH₂NH.CH(CH₃)₂   (with HO)

HO ... $CHOH.CH_2NH.CH(CH_3)_2$

Isoprenaline

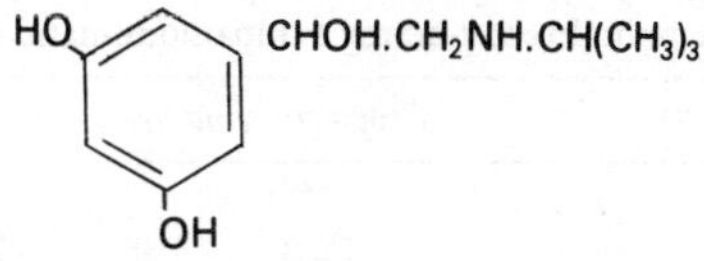

HO ... $CHOH.CH_2NH.CH(CH_3)_3$ ... OH

Orciprenaline

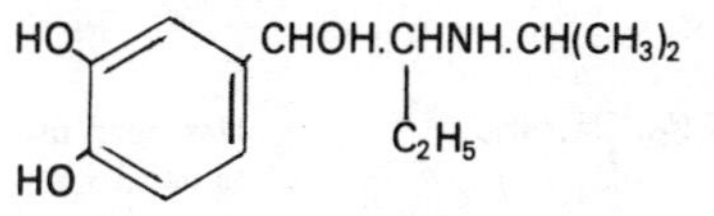

HO ... $CHOH.CHNH.CH(CH_3)_2$ ... C_2H_5 ... HO

Isoetharine

HOH_2C ... $CHOH.CH_2NH.C(CH_3)_3$ ... HO

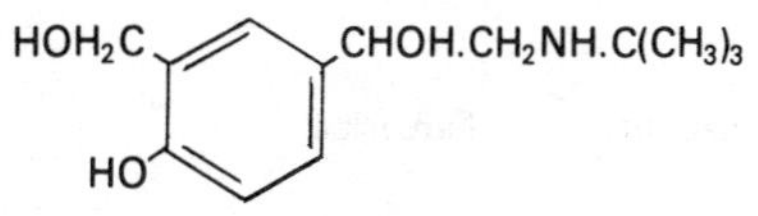

Salbutamol

Fig. 17.6 Isoprenaline and some of its derivatives.

ity of isoetharine with the prolonged action of orciprenaline. The formulae of the three compounds are displayed, for comparison, in Fig. 17.6.

For the relief of asthma and of attacks of bronchospasm from other causes, salbutamol is supplied in inhalers that provide metered doses of 0.1 mg in an aerosol. Unlike isoprenaline, salbutamol is readily absorbed from the gut in an unchanged form and several oral preparations, including some of the prolonged release variety, are available for clinical use. The oral dose of salbutamol is 2 to 4 mg three or four times daily. Like other β_2 agonists, salbutamol inhibits the contractions of uterine muscle and it can be given, by intravenous injection, to ward off threats of premature labour.

An aerosol dose of salbutamol is effective for up to four hours. It is eventually excreted in the urine, partly unchanged and partly as an O-phenylglucuronide.

Salbutamol has virtually no action at all on β_1 receptors and its use carries with it no danger of death from cardiac arrest. It does, however, exert a metabolic action that may, in its turn, lead to tachycardia particularly in those with hyperthyroidism who should be circumspect in their use of the drug.

The success of salbutamol naturally inspired a search for other long acting drugs with β_2 selectivity. Not surprisingly, some were found but none seems to offer any real advantage over salbutamol. A few are listed in the appropriate section of Table 17.4: some, it will be seen, are relatively simple derivatives of isoprenaline but others are possessed of novel structures, a particularly interesting example being provided by hexoprenaline, the most recent (1970) addition to the list.

Hexoprenaline (Ipradol, Etoscol) consists of two noradrenaline molecules united by a hexamethylene chain. Notwithstanding the noradrenaline moieties in its molecule, hexoprenaline is at least as selective a β_2 agonist and as long acting a drug as salbutamol. Its prolonged action is attributable to the fact that, although it is a substrate for

catechol-O-methyltransferase, it is metabolized quite slowly. Moreover, its metabolites (the mono- and di-3-O-methylhexoprenalines) are also β_2 agonists.

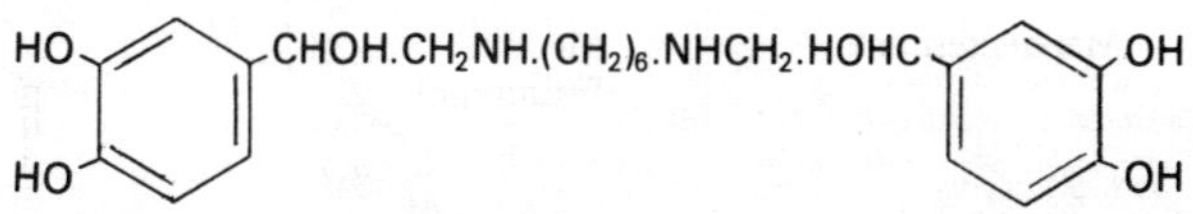

HO ... $CHOH.CH_2NH.(CH_2)_6.NHCH_2.HOHC$ ... OH ... HO ... OH

Hexoprenaline

Hexoprenaline, like salbutamol, can be taken by mouth or as an inhalant and can be given intravenously. When incorporated in an aerosol, the metered dose is 200 μg. A double dose can be taken if necessary. The oral dose is 0.5 to 1 mg, three or four times daily. The indications for hexoprenaline and the precautions to be taken in its use are precisely the same as those that apply to salbutamol. The drug is described in detail by Pinder, et al., (1977).

Rimiterol (Pulmadil). Rimiterol is a selective β_2 agonist that retains a catechol structure and so is inactivated by catechol-O-methyltransferase: its total duration of action after inhalation is, not surprisingly, similar to that of isoprenaline (1 to 3 hours) but shorter than that of salbutamol and terbutaline. This feature reduces the risk of cumulation of the drug if doses are taken with injudicious frequency. Rimiterol is taken by inhalation in doses of 0.2 to 0.6 mg but it can also be given by intravenous infusion (in doses of up to 0.2 μg per kilogram of body mass per minute) in cases of severe asthma. Although the drug is described as a 'selective' agonist it does, of course, have some actions on β_1 receptors and an increase in heart rate during the course of treatment should be taken as evidence that overdosing has occurred. Other signs of overdosage include, as might be expected, tremor, dizziness and feelings of anxiety. It is contraindicated in pregnancy.

NORADRENALINE
Interest in noradrenaline is centred largely on its function as a transmitter substance in the sympathetic and central

Table 17.5 Some indirectly-acting sympathomimetic amines

Approved name(s)	Proprietary name(s)	Formula	Remarks
p-Tyramine		$CH_2.CH_2.NH_2$ benzene ring with HO	
Amphetamines	Benzedrine ; Dexedrine; Desoxyn; Didrex; Pervitin	see text	see text
Hydroxyamphetamine	Paredrine	benzene ring with HO, $CH_2.CH.NH_2$ with CH_3	Has been used as nasal decongestant
β-Phenylethylamine derivatives used as anorexigenic drugs. See Fig. 17.9 (p. 279)			
Pholedrine	Parendrinol Veritol	benzene ring with HO, $CH_2.CH.NH.CH_3$ with CH_3	Used to maintain blood pressure in shock and spinal anaesthesia
Mephentermine	Mephine Wyamin(e)	benzene ring, $CH_2-\overset{CH_3}{\underset{CH_3}{C}}-NHCH_3$	Was used as nasal decongestant and to maintain blood pressure

nervous systems. Its therapeutic uses are limited. An intravenous infusion may have to be given during the excision of a phaeochromocytoma (an adrenaline-secreting tumour of the adrenal medulla) to prevent the catastrophic fall in blood pressure which might otherwise occur immediately after the tumour's removal from the body. Noradrenaline is better for this purpose than is adrenaline, partly because it maintains a better degree of overall vasoconstriction and partly because it has less action on the heart. A noradrenaline infusion is sometimes useful for maintaining blood pressure in experimental animals but the use of vasoconstrictor agents for the treatment of shock in human beings is no longer popular (see also p. 299).

DOPAMINE

Although its physiological actions are exerted predominantly, if not exclusively, on the central nervous system, dopamine has some pharmacological actions on the cardiovascular system and these have been put to therapeutic use (Goldberg, 1972, 1974; Anonymous, 1977). Dopamine causes dilatation of the renal and mesenteric arteries, it increases cardiac contractility and (in higher doses than are necessary to evoke the other two responses) it constricts the peripheral blood vessels. These changes are the result of stimulating dopamine, adrenaline β_1 and adrenaline α receptors respectively and their nett effect is to increase cardiac performance, blood pressure and blood flow through the kidney.

Dopamine is available as a preparation for intravenous infusion (Intropin) in patients with acute or chronic heart failure or for those in severe shock. The initial dose is 0.5 to 1.0 μg per kilogram and minute; it can be increased, with careful monitoring of the responses, up to a maximum of about 15 μg per kilogram and minute.

Given by the intravenous route, dopamine does not readily enter the brain (in order to produce dopamine effects in the central nervous system, L-DOPA must be given; see page 590) but it may, nevertheless, cause vomiting, the result presumably of a stimulation of the dopamine sensitive neurones of the vomiting centre.

AMPHETAMINES

The best known indirectly acting sympathomimetic amines are members of the amphetamine family. Until quite recently they (particularly methylamphetamine) were numbered among the physician's favourite prescriptions for a variety of conditions that are detailed below. Because of the danger of amphetamine abuse their use is now severely restricted in many parts of the world. The danger of permitting the unfettered prescribing and distribution of amphetamines lies as much in the opportunities that the well stocked pharmacy offers to the drug thief as in the temptation placed in the way of patients who receive the drugs legitimately. Amphetamine abuse, the amphetamine psychosis and drug dependence in general are discussed in full elsewhere (p. 83). Here it is only necessary to point out, particularly to the younger reader, the extraordinary change which has taken place recently in the views which are held concerning the dangers of the amphetamines. Not more than twenty years ago a famous pharmacologist was able to say in his widely read text book: 'Addiction to the amphetamines is uncommon and easily overcome' (Gaddum, 1959). Today many psychiatrists believe that the amphetamines are more dangerous than heroin.

Even though they are now rarely used clinically, the amphetamines are still of the utmost interest to pharmacologists. Studies utilizing these drugs have contributed much towards our present fund of knowledge concerning the activity of 'monoaminergic' neurones in the brain and there is little doubt that they still have much to offer. They have also done much to bolster current postulates of the chemical origin of mental illness (p. 544).

The clinical uses to which the amphetamines have been put illustrate the therapeutic potential of the indirectly acting sympathomimetic amines. It seems that, for most purposes, amphetamine substitutes will have to be drawn from those members of this class of compounds that are not likely to be abused.

Amphetamine base (Fig. 17.7) is a colourless volatile liquid but it, and its congeners, are most often used as the solid sulphates. Amphetamine itself is a racemic mixture of optically active isomers of which only the dextro (+) form has significant pharmacological activity. The active isomer is dexamphetamine (Dexedrine). Dexamphetamine, as would be expected, is about twice as active, gram for gram, as amphetamine itself.

The description of the amphetamines which follows applies, except where it is stated otherwise, to all the drugs shown in Fig. 17.7

The volatile amphetamine base was originally used as a local vasoconstrictor agent. Incorporated into a suitable absorbent, it was the active agent in Benzedrine inhalers. These were inserted briefly into the nostrils. The heat of the hand was sufficient to release a vasoconstrictor amount of amphetamine which provided a welcome relief of nasal congestion in colds, sinusitis and hay fever. Some amphetamine was also absorbed into the circulation and exerted a central stimulant action which was not unwelcome in view of the mental depression which so frequently accompanies the common cold. Benzedrine inhalers provided a ready source of the drug and their manufacture has now ceased.

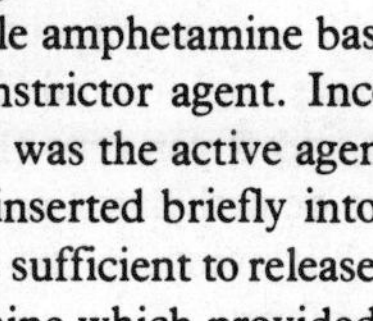

Amphetamine (Benzedrine)
Dexamphetamine (Dexedrine) $\Big\}$ R = NH_2

Methylamphetamine (Desoxyn Pervitin) R = $NH.CH_3$
Benz(yl)amphatamine (Didrex) R = $N(CH_3)CH_2$

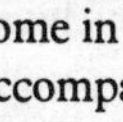

Fig. 17.7 The amphetamines.

The amphetamines are powerful stimulants of the central nervous system and this is the basis of many of their therapeutic uses.

(a) *Narcolepsy* is a condition in which the victim periodically succumbs, wherever he might be, to a quite irresistible desire to sleep. A related state is *cataplexy*. The victim of cataplexy suffers attacks of extreme muscular weakness so that he falls helplessly to the ground, unable to utter a sound. The factor that precipitates a cataplectic attack is invariably an emotional response—very often the laughter occasioned by a joke or an amusing situation. Consciousness is not lost during these episodes, which are not, therefore, epileptic in nature. Narcolepsy and cataplexy may be the result of encephalitis but they often have no obvious aetiology. Both conditions are treated with dexamphetamine or methamphetamine in doses of 5 to 10 mg or 2.5 to 10 mg respectively, given three or four times daily. It is a well attested fact that in post-encephalitic conditions the patient may exhibit a decreased susceptibility to the effects of the amphetamines and daily doses of up to 60 mg or more may have to be given. As an alternative to an amphetamine, ephedrine (p. 277) or methylphenidate (Ritalin) may be tried.

Narcolepsy and cataplexy are probably the only two conditions for the treatment of which the use of the amphetamines is still justified. Other sympathomimetic amines with a smaller addictive liability should, however, be tried first. Ephedrine seems to have been very successful in some patients but since both narcolepsy and cataplexy are very rare conditions, extensive clinical experience with drugs other than amphetamine is lacking.

(b) Amphetamine has been successfully used to control children who exhibit an abnormal degree of restlessness and general motor activity (*hyperkinesis*). This apparently paradoxical effect of an essentially stimulant drug has its explanation in the fact that true hyperkinesis is but one element in the 'minimal brain dysfuction' syndrome, other aspects of which include lack of ability to concentrate, impairment of memory and other manifestations of depressed intellectual function. Amphetamine, by its general alerting effect, arouses the sleeping intellect (hyperkinetic children are not mentally backward) and the child calms down when he has something to occupy his mind. We all know that restlessness is often a symptom of boredom.

Amphetamine has now been largely and successfully superseded by other less dangerous drugs, particularly methylphenidate.

The minimal brain dysfunction syndrome and its treatment is extensively discussed by Kornetsky (1976) to whom the interested reader is referred.

(c) Amphetamine is an *anorexigenic*—more commonly but less accurately *anorectic*—drug (that is, it reduces the appetite) and this is the basis of its use in the treatment of obesity. The anorexigenic effect is probably the resultant of a number of pharmacological actions. The most important of these is a stimulation of the pathways that are physiologically activated to cause cessation of feeding when sufficient nourishment has been taken and whose sensitivity is probably depressed in the obese. In addition, the amphetamines inhibit gastric motility and secretions and may reduce the acuity of the sense of smell and taste. Finally, the elevation of mood they produce may tempt the patient away from the table to an indulgence in less introvert pleasures.

There is evidence that while the effects of the systems that cause cessation of eating utilize dopamine and serotonin as their neurotransmitters, those that underlie the appetite, by reinstating the urge to eat in response to the appropriate chemical stimulus, are operated by noradrenaline. Amphetamine promotes the release of both noradrenaline and dopamine and hence, presumably, the activation of both the satiety and appetite mechanisms. We must, perhaps, conclude that, when both operate simultaneously, the satiety control exerts dominance over the appetite regulator just as, for instance, extensor muscles overwhelm flexor muscles when their motor nerves are simultaneously and maximally stimulated.

The treatment by amphetamines of a condition such as obesity is a hazardous practice because obese patients may suffer from disturbances of mood which render them particularly likely to become dependent on the drugs.

Obesity and the drugs used in its treatment are discussed in more detail later (p. 281).

(d) The amphetamines have been rather extensively used for the treatment of depression too mild and fleeting to warrant attention by a psychiatrist. The benefits conferred by the drugs seems to be determined more by the physician's optimism than by any relevant pharmacological action. The position of amphetamine in relation to that of other antidepressant drugs is discussed in more detail elsewhere (p. 586).

(e) Amphetamine, like so many other drugs, once had a small place in the treatment of epilepsy, particularly the petit mal variety. The rationale of this measure appears to reside in the fact that drugs which increase cerebral activity may interfere with the march of the epileptic disturbance across the brain. Amphetamine has also been used in patients with grand mal epilepsy to offset the drowsiness induced by the barbiturate that so often features in their treatment schedules. There is little justification for using amphetamine in either epilepsy.

(f) There is no doubt that the amphetamines not only promote a degree of euphoria but that they also delay the onset of fatigue in the normal subject. These facts were common knowledge to students, car rally drivers, night workers and aviators in the days when the amphetamines were more easily available than they are today. They also became known to competitors in cycle races and other endurance events: they led to at least one widely publicized

fatality and to a prohibition of their use by athletes, whose urine is now tested as frequently as that of racehorses in order to check that their sporting spirit has been strong enough to keep them to the rules.

Toxic effects of amphetamine administration. For the most part, the amphetamines produce toxic side effects that are readily predictable from a knowledge of the drugs' principal pharmacological actions. They are, that is to say, merely manifestations of overdosage and they include (among many other responses) tremor, restlessness, euphoria, garrulity, headache, irritability, insomnia, cardiac arrhythmias, palpitations, anxiety and increased libido. Some of these effects are actively sought by those who take amphetamines for nontherapeutic purposes but, at the dose levels they prefer, aggressiveness, feelings of superabundant power and energy and a sense of being persecuted tend to dominate the picture so that the amphetamine taker, like the cocaine addict, is likely to become socially dangerous. It is but a short step from the state just described to the full blown amphetamine psychosis, a schizophrenia like consequence of amphetamine abuse that is fully discussed, together with other aspects of amphetamine dependence, in Chapter 7 (p. 83).

The metabolism of the amphetamines. Amphetamine itself is excreted in the urine partly unchanged and partly as the conjugates of a number of metabolites appearing as the result of hydroxylation and deamination processes (Fig. 17.8).

The relative importance of these several routes of amphetamine disposal varies with the species. In man, the approximate fractions of an amphetamine dose that are excreted unchanged, as deaminated and as hydroxylated metabolites are 34, 24 and 3 per cent respectively. For the rat, the corresponding figures are 14, 2 and 60 per cent and for the guinea pig 4, 62 and 0 per cent (Estler, 1975). Methamphetamine can be demethylated and then set on the amphetamine route but some of the drug is also excreted in the unchanged form.

Some amphetamine metabolites have pharmacological actions in their own right and may be responsible for producing or prolonging some of the effects usually attributed to amphetamine itself. p-Hydroxyamphetamine, a powerful vasoconstrictor agent devoid of central nervous activity, has been used as a nasal decongestant.

In man, as we have seen, a substantial fraction of a dose of amphetamine is eliminated in an unchanged form. This excretion is favoured if the urine is acid but those who use amphetamine not infrequently generate an alkaline urine as a consequence of their indulgence in sodium bicarbonate taken in an effort to quell the gastric discomforts that so commonly follow amphetamine ingestion. Unexpectedly severe toxic reactions to the amphetamines can sometimes be traced to this cause.

Mode of action of the amphetamines. Amphetamine is an indirectly acting sympathomimetic amine and many of its

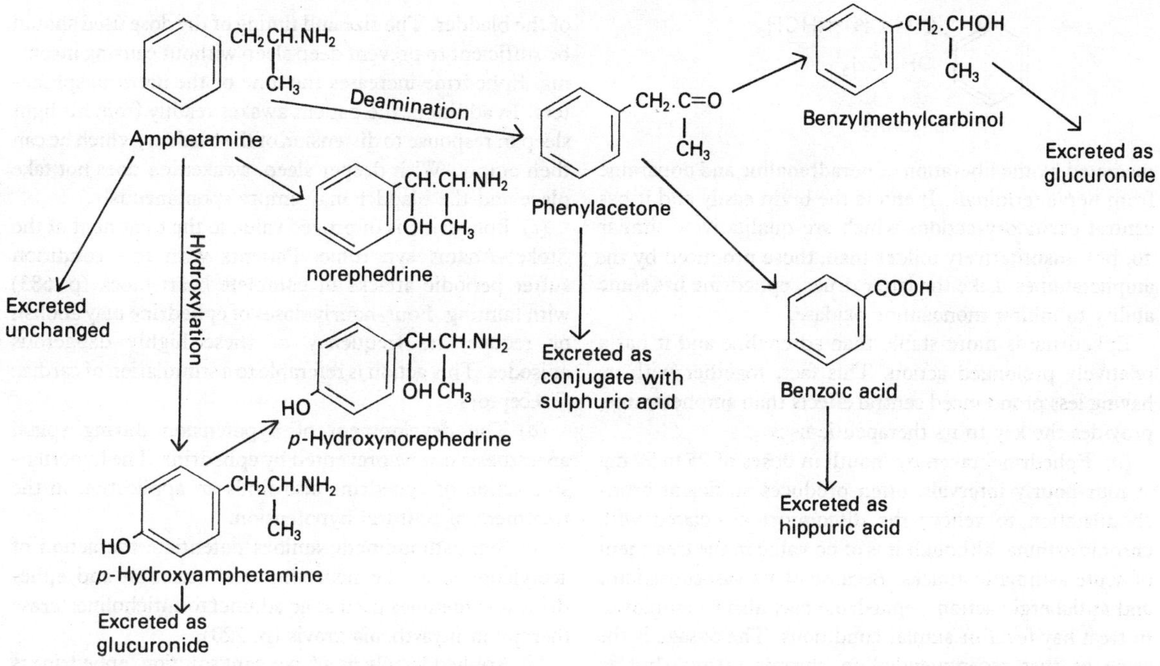

Fig. 17.8 Pathways of amphetamine metabolism

actions are mediated by the release of noradrenaline and dopamine from neurones that contain them. Some progress has been made towards the delineation of the contribution made by each catecholamine to the overall picture of amphetamine action. Thus, in rats, amphetamine brings about a general increase in locomotor activity together with the appearance of repetitive and apparently purposeless movements (such as licking, sniffing and gnawing) that are collectively described as *stereotypy*. It seems that noradrenaline release in the brain accounts for the increased locomotor activity while the stereotypy is the result of dopamine release from elements of the extrapyramidal system (p. 163). Although stereotypy is often thought to indicate exploratory activity it may well be the rodent equivalent of aggressive behaviour in man. If this is so, it provides an explanation of some aspects of the amphetamine psychosis syndrome and it strengthens the case for the involvement of dopamine as an aetiological factor in mental illness. Noradrenaline release is evoked by lower doses of amphetamine than are required for the release of dopamine and this may well explain why the psychotic sequelae of amphetamine ingestion appear only with higher doses.

Although catecholamine release is accepted as the principal one, several other mechanisms have been invoked to account for the actions of amphetamine. The literature overflows with reports of experiments, frequently leading to contradictory conclusions and not all well designed, intended to provide evidence for the operation of these additional mechanisms. One of the better authenticated of these is an inhibition of the uptake-1 process whereby the catecholamines, after release, are reincorporated into their neurones. The effect of this action, of course, is further to add to the amount of transmitter at the synapse, already increased by the releasing action of the amphetamine.

There is evidence that the amphetamines have some inhibitory action on monoamine oxidase, thus recalling the hypothesis originally proffered to explain their action. They may also cause the release of transmitter from serotoninergic neurones but there is little authority for the view that this is of more than minimal importance.

There are those who claim that the amphetamines exert direct actions on both α and β receptors so that the drugs should be included among the mixed action sympathomimetic amines. This, however, is an unlikely conclusion. Some effect on β_1 receptors is to be expected by virtue of noradrenaline's ability to stimulate them but glycogenolytic effects that might argue for some β_2 agonist activity are probably the indirect consequence of the generally increased level of central nervous activity.

EPHEDRINE

Ephedrine is an extremely ancient drug. It formed the active constituent of the plant extracts used, under the name of 'Ma-huang', by the ancient Chinese. Its introduction into Western medicine dates from 1925.

Ephedrine has an adrenaline-like action, stimulating both α and β receptors. In addition, it has indirect actions,

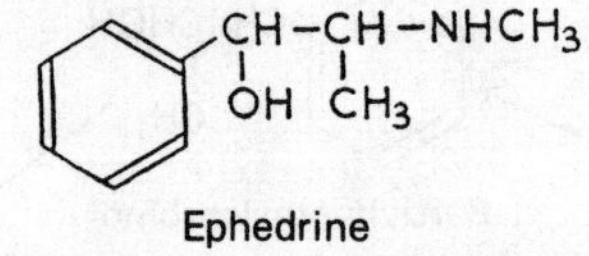

$$CH-CH-NHCH_3$$
$$\quad | \quad\quad |$$
$$\quad OH \quad CH_3$$

Ephedrine

mediated by the liberation of noradrenaline and dopamine from nerve terminals. It enters the brain easily and it has central excitatory actions which are qualitatively similar to, but quantitatively milder than, those produced by the amphetamines. Like the latter drugs, ephedrine has some ability to inhibit monoamine oxidase.

Ephedrine is more stable than adrenaline and it has a relatively prolonged action. This fact, together with its having less pronounced central effects than amphetamine, provides the key to its therapeutic uses.

(a) Ephedrine, taken by mouth in doses of 25 to 50 mg at four-hourly intervals, often produces sufficient bronchodilatation to relieve the discomfort associated with chronic asthma, although it is of no value in the treatment of acute asthmatic attacks. Because of its vasoconstrictor and antiallergic actions, ephedrine may also be employed to treat hay fever or similar conditions. The dosage is the same as that recommended in chronic asthma but in conditions in which nasal congestion is the only symptom demanding relief, ephedrine may be applied directly to the nostrils in the form of a one per cent solution in isotonic saline. In this way the systemic effects of ephedrine are minimized. When ephedrine is taken by mouth, the central excitatory effects sometimes prove disturbing. Some individuals, however, welcome the slight elevation of mood induced by ephedrine because it counteracts the feelings of depression and impaired efficiency so often associated with hay fever.

(b) Ephedrine is used in efforts to prevent bed-wetting in children and in patients with impaired nervous control of the bladder. The size and timing of the dose used should be sufficient to prevent deep sleep without causing insomnia. Ephedrine increases the tone of the urethral sphincters. In addition, the patient awakes readily from his light sleep in response to distension of the bladder, which he can then empty. With deeper sleep, awakening does not take place and the bladder may empty spontaneously.

(c) Ephedrine is of proved value in the treatment of the Stokes-Adams syndrome. Patients with this condition suffer periodic attacks of complete heart block (p. 683) with fainting. Four-hourly doses of ephedrine may abolish or reduce the frequency of these highly dangerous episodes. This action is referable to a stimulation of cardiac β receptors.

(d) The development of hypotension during spinal anaesthesia can be prevented by ephedrine. The hypertensive action of ephedrine also finds an application in the treatment of postural hypotension.

(e) Sympathomimetic amines potentiate the action of acetylcholine at the neuromuscular junction and ephedrine is sometimes used as an adjunct to anticholinesterase therapy in myasthenia gravis (p. 220).

(f) Applied locally as a 5 per cent solution, ephedrine is a useful mydriatic agent with no tendency to cause glaucoma. In the past the central actions of ephedrine led to its being employed in a number of conditions for which the amphetamines were later used. The recognition of the dangers associated with amphetamine may well lead to ephedrine's being restored to favour. However, ephedrine itself is not without abuse potential and prudence would dictate that the drug should not be made widely available.

Side-effects of ephedrine administration. These include palpitation, insomnia, nervousness, irritability and a feeling of weakness. Ephedrine may also cause headache, nausea and vomiting.

Table 17.6 Sympathomimetic amines with a mixed action

Approved name(s)	Proprietary name(s)	Formula	Remarks
Ephedrine			see text
Pseudoephedrine Isoephedrine	Sudafed	Isomer of ephedrine with similar uses	
Metaraminol	Aramine	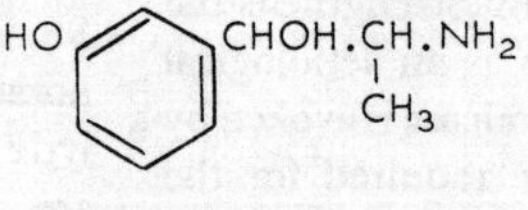 $HO-C_6H_3(OH)-CHOH.CH.NH_2$ with CH_3	Used in the treatment of hypotension from many causes
Phenylpropanolamine Norephedrine	Propadrine	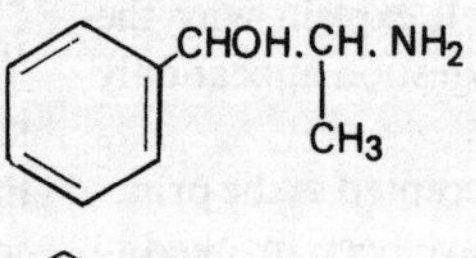 $C_6H_5-CHOH.CH.NH_2$ with CH_3	Used as a nasal decongestant
m-Tyramine		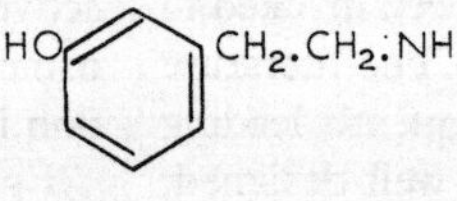 $HO-C_6H_4-CH_2.CH_2.NH_2$	

Structure-action relationships in the sympathomimetic amines

The laevorotatory (—) isomers of adrenaline and noradrenaline are much more active than the dextrorotatory compounds. Epinine (Table 17.4), a compound which differs from adrenaline only by the absence of an OH group in the side chain, is about as potent a sympathomimetic agent as D-adrenaline. Similarly, dopamine has the same activity as D-noradrenaline. Again, L-corbasil (α-methoxynoradrenaline, Table 17.4) exhibits a much higher sympathomimetic potency than does the D-isomer which itself shows about the same activity as α-methyldopamine. These examples could be multiplied: they indicate that the greater activity of the laevorotatory isomers is determined by the orientation of the hydroxyl group on the β-carbon atom of side chain (Fig. 17.10). This fact has to be taken into account when the nature of the sympathetic receptor is being considered and it is important to note that the greater activity of the L-isomers applies equally to compounds which act on β receptors as to those which affect α receptors.

In most instances the effect of the hydroxyl group is simply to increase the affinity of the compound for the receptors but the orientation of the group also plays some part in determining the nature of the pharmacological response: isopropyldopamine and D-isoprenaline, for instance, cause blockade of α receptors. Dextrorotatory substituents on the α carbon atom produce compounds with more pronounced central excitatory activity than the corresponding laevorotatory isomer. Thus D-amphetamine is a more powerful stimulant than L-amphetamine.

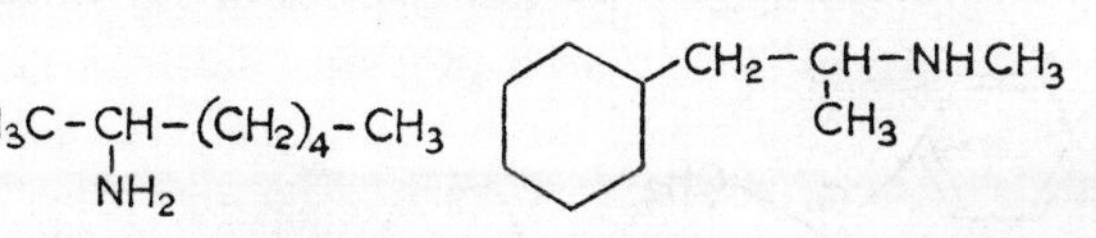

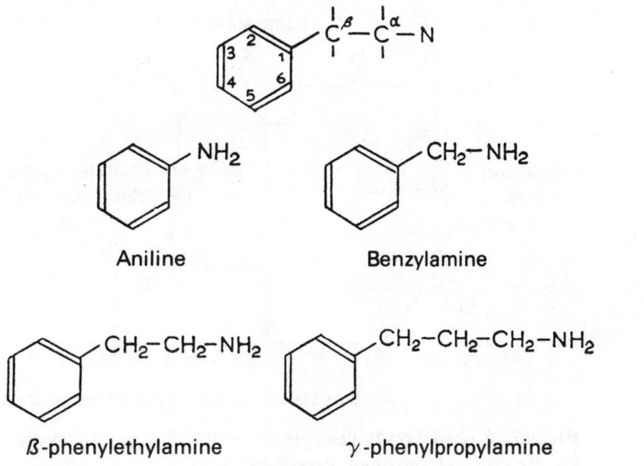

Fig. 17.9 Some phenylamines

Aniline

Benzylamine

β-phenylethylamine

γ-phenylpropylamine

H₃C–CH–(CH₂)₄–CH₃
      |
      NH₂

2-Aminoheptane

CH₂–CH–NHCH₃
     |
     CH₃

Propylhexedrine

Some aliphatic and alicyclic compounds possess a degree of sympathomimetic activity: 2-aminoheptane (Tuamine), 2-methylamino heptane (Octin) and propylhexedrine all have vasoconstrictor and pressor activity. They are much less active on β receptors and have minimal central excitatory actions. They have been used as nasal decongestants or to prevent falls in blood pressure during spinal anaesthesia. Propylhexedrine (Benzedrex) is the most active of these compounds. The sympathomimetic amines proper can be regarded as derivatives of β-phenylethylamine.

β-Phenylethylamine itself has some pressor activity but aniline, benzylamine and γ-phenylpropylamine are almost completely inactive in this respect. Thus the separation between the ring and the peripheral amino group provided by the –C–C–NH₂ linkage would appear to be optimal for the α type of activity. Sympathomimetic activity is still evident in compounds in which the carbon atoms are

replaced by oxygen or sulphur. The presence of hydroxyl groups on the benzene ring is not an absolute requirement for activity but the most potent directly-acting sympathomimetic compounds are catecholamines—compounds in which the benzene ring of β-phenylethylamine has hydroxyl substituents in positions 3 and 4. Compounds in which the hydroxyl groups occupy *para* positions, or which lack one or both of the hydroxyl groups, retain some α-sympathomimetic activity but they have virtually no action on β receptors. Salbutamol, which lacks a hydroxyl group but which is a powerful stimulant of β_2 receptors provides an important exception to this generalization. When hydroxyl groups are in the *meta* relationship (occupation of positions 3 and 5) the compounds will stimulate β_2 receptors if the substituent on the terminal nitrogen is bulky enough.

The most active α sympathomimetic agent is noradrenaline. The more bulky the substituents on the nitrogen atom the smaller is the α activity. Thus isoprenaline has only a small degree of α-type activity and butylnoradrenaline has none. On the other hand, within the series noradrenaline-adrenaline-isoprenaline, the affinity for β receptors increases as the bulk of the substituents increases. It should be added that the reduction in the affinity for the α receptor induced by increasing the bulk of the substituent is partly offset if a hydroxyl group in the *laevo* orientation is also present. Thus, L-isoprenaline still has *some* α-sympathomimetic activity but D-isoprenaline blocks α receptors.

With these points in mind, it is possible to theorize on the nature of the α and β receptors. The most profitable speculations along these lines have been those of Belleau and much of what is discussed below is based on his work (see Belleau, 1963).

It can be concluded from what has already been said that the α adrenaline receptor probably carries at least two binding sites. The more important will be that which binds

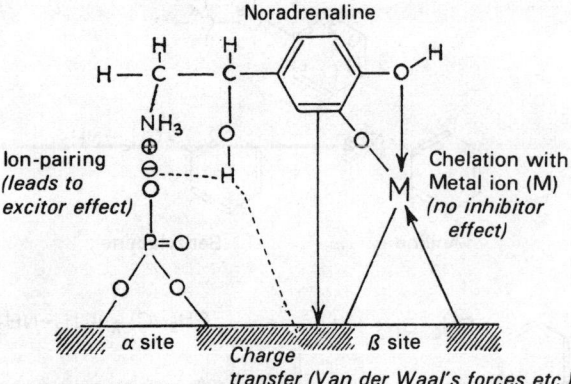

Fig. 17.10 (Based on Belleau (1963) by the kind permission of Dr. Belleau and Pergamon Press Ltd.)

the amino nitrogen of sympathomimetic amines; the secondary site will be related to the ring structure. Belleau in fact visualized the latter as the β receptor site (Fig. 17.10). On this view, a compound such as isoprenaline is bound predominantly to the β site, attachment to the α site being hindered by the bulky nature of the isopropyl group. Adrenaline might be attached to both sites and this is consistent with its possessing both α and β effects. A difficulty arises when noradrenaline is considered, for it should have the same affinity as adrenaline or isoprenaline for the β site. The fact that it has predominantly α effects has to be explained by assuming that its high affinity for the α site ensures that it is first attached to that portion of the conjoint receptor and that α effects are thus initiated before occupation of the β site can take place. This subsidiary hypothesis is not entirely satisfactory and it is probably better to think of α and β receptors as separate structural entities. On this alternative view, the primary binding site of the α receptor is related to the amino nitrogen of the sympathomimetic substances and is identical with Belleau's α site. The secondary site, which accounts for the increased sympathomimetic activity of compounds containing the hydroxylated benzene ring, is equivalent to Belleau's β site. If this hypothesis is accepted, it is possible to propose for the β receptor proper a structure or mechanism quite distinct from that of the α receptor and there is much to recommend this view.

Whatever may ultimately emerge as the most acceptable represensation of the adrenaline receptor, there is unanimity that the most acceptable concept of the process by which the amino nitrogen is bound to the receptor site is that due to Belleau. He noted that dibenamine, an agent that blocks adrenaline α receptors, exerts its pharmacological action through an ethyleneimmonium intermediate which becomes attached to the receptor. The ethyleneimmonium ion possesses a carbon atom ($C^\star$ in Fig. 17.11) with a carbonium character—that is, it carries a partial positive charge. This is induced by the neighbouring positively

charged nitrogen atom. The charged carbon atom has the same steric relationships as the nitrogen atom in the cations formed at physiological pH values by noradrenaline, β-phenylethylamine and other compounds that are known to stimulate α receptors. Thus the α receptor should carry a negatively charged group which will react with the cations formed by sympathomimetic amines and with the induced carbonium ion of debenamine and like compounds. The most likely group to carry a partial negative charge is phosphate and the reaction at the α site can be visualized as an ion pairing between the phosphate ion at the receptor site and the cation formed by the drug. Bulky substituents on the amino nitrogen would hinder the approach of cation and anion and α-sympathomimetic activity would be reduced. Moreover, the presence of these large groupings would serve to prevent the access of the transmitter to the α site by forming a mechanical barrier and this may partly explain why compounds with bulky substituents cause some degree of α receptor blockade. Belleau's views are summarized in Fig. 17.10 which also indicates how the presence of the hydroxyl grouping in the side chain may facilitate binding to the receptor site.

There is rather less unanimity concerning the nature of the β receptor or of the β site of the conjoint α-β receptor. Phenylethylamine derivatives readily form metal chelates (p. 796) and it is known that the first step in the inactivation of catecholamines by catechol-O-methyltransferase is the chelation of the magnesium ions which are an essential cofactor in the enzyme's activity (Fig. 17.12). The tropolones (p. 262) inhibit the enzyme. They chelate divalent metal ions and they also antagonize the actions of isopren-

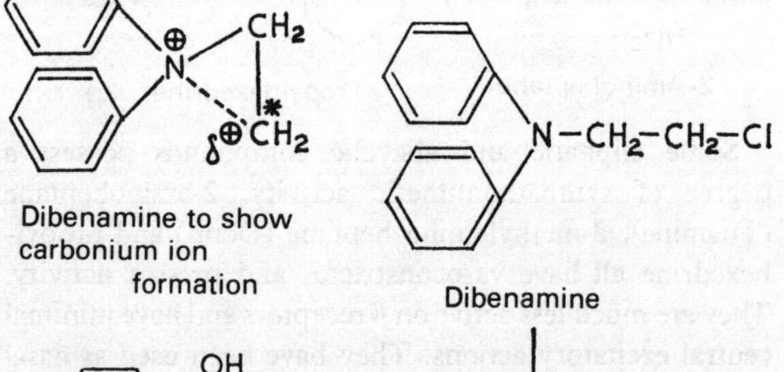

Fig. 17.11 Dibenamine and its ethyleneimmonium derivative.

aline. On these grounds Belleau suggested that the β site bears a resemblance to the prosthetic group of catechol-*O*-methyltransferase and that the binding to it of isoprenaline and other agents with β-sympathomimetic activity also involves a chelation process (Fig. 17.10). It is possible that this mechanism is responsible for bringing about the binding of the benzene nucleus to the secondary α site but not to the β receptor proper if the latter is a separate entity. It must be emphasized that these representations of adrenaline receptors (like those of so many other subcellular structures) are hypothetical and over-simplified. Any finally acceptable conceptualization of the structural features of the β site must be able to accommodate facts that are not explained by the models discussed here. These include the observation that the *laevo* orientation of the hydroxyl group on the side chain plays as important a part in determining the affinity for β receptors of isoprenaline and related compounds as it does that of substances which stimulate only α receptors.

The relationsip of β receptors to cyclic AMP is discussed in Chapter 19 (p. 321).

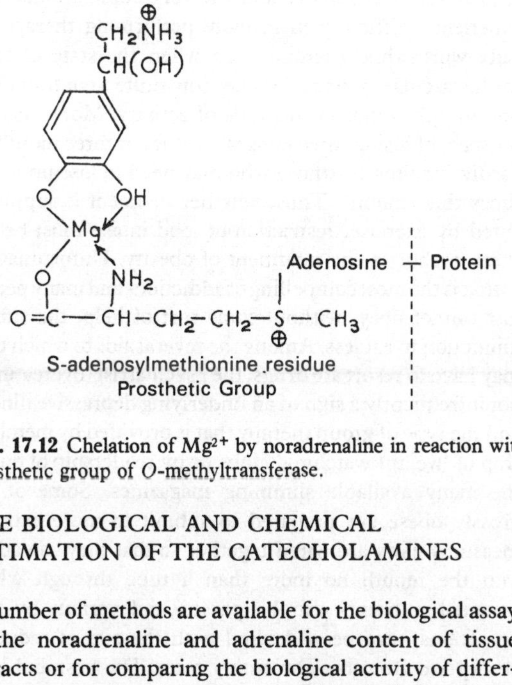

Fig. 17.12 Chelation of Mg^{2+} by noradrenaline in reaction with prosthetic group of *O*-methyltransferase.

THE BIOLOGICAL AND CHEMICAL ESTIMATION OF THE CATECHOLAMINES

A number of methods are available for the biological assay of the noradrenaline and adrenaline content of tissue extracts or for comparing the biological activity of different sympathomimetic substances. Biological assay methods are sensitive and (in the proper hands) accurate but they are time-consuming and they demand a degree of pharmacological skill and delicacy of touch that few seem disposed to acquire. Moreover none of the methods is suitable for the assay of dopamine, a substance that cannot be ignored by those who wish to examine catecholamines, particularly those in extracts of nervous tissue. For all these reasons, chemical methods of assay now rule in the catecholamine laboratory.

Bioassay preparations include the pithed rat, the fowl's rectal caecum, the rabbit duodenum and the rat uterus. The pithed rat gives a pressor response. All the isolated preparations respond to the catecholamines by relaxation but when the rat uterus is used it is preferable to adopt de Jalon's method of assay. A virgin rat is pretreated with stilboestrol and the uterus is supended in de Jalon's solution (p. 148) at a relatively low temperature (31 °C) so that any spontaneous movements cease. Small doses of carbachol are added to the bath every 1.5 to 2 minutes. Each dose is allowed to remain in contact with the tissue for 30 seconds before it is washed out. In this way, regular and repeated responses are obtained. Adrenaline, noradrenaline or a portion of the solution to be assayed is added to the bath 30 seconds before a dose of carbachol and the extent to which the induced contraction is inhibited measures the response to the catecholamine. The regularly repeated dosing with carbachol is not interrupted: when the evoked uterine responses have returned to their initial height another dose of the standard or 'unknown' catecholamine solution can be added to the bath.

Some of the available biological assay methods are particularly sensitive to one or other of the catecholamines (Table 17.7) and they can be employed to estimate the amount of adrenaline or noradrenaline in the presence of appropriately small quantities of the other. If appreciable quantities of both substances are present, they must first be separated by column or paper chromatography. Alternatively, a differential assay method, (Burn, Hutcheon and Parker, 1950) can be tried but the method is only suitable if the total concentration of the two amines is not less than 10 µg per ml. Under these circumstances chemical estimation is much more simple and far less tedious. In all the biological methods, care has to be taken, by the use of suitable antagonists or by other means, to ensure that the recorded responses arise only as a result of stimulation of adrenaline receptors.

Satisfactory fluorimetric methods for the determination of adrenaline and noradrenaline are now available (Anton and Sayre, 1962, 1964, 1972). Fluorimetric methods are convenient, quick and accurate. They have the additional advantage of being applicable to the assay of dopamine and of catecholamine metabolites. The measurement of metabolites is nowadays assuming the same importance as assay of the catecholamines themselves.

Other newly developed methods of catecholamine determination include gas liquid chromatography and radioenzymatic methods. They are reviewed briefly by Butt (1976) and more extensively by Nagatsu (1973).

OBESITY

Obesity is the most common and most serious nutritional disorder in the affluent half of the world. Almost 50 per

Table 17.7 Some suitable preparations for the biological estimation of adrenaline and noradrenaline

Preparation	Response	Sensitivity to:	
		Noradrenaline	*Adrenaline*
Blood pressure of pithed rat	Increase	1 ng	10 ng
Isolated duodenum of rabbit	Inhibition of tone	3-30 ng/ml	3-30 ng/ml
Isolated rectal cae-cum of fowl	Inhibition of tone	50 ng/ml	1.5 ng/ml
Isolated rat uterus	Inhibition of carbachol-induced contractions	150 ng/ml	1.5 ng/ml

cent of Britons (60 per cent or more of the 40 to 60 age group) weigh more than they should, if we adopt as a criterion of ideal weight that which is known, from actuarial studies, to be associated with lower than average morbidity and mortality rates (Montegriffo, 1971).

It is hardly necessary to define obesity, but some formal definitions do appear in the literature. The most apt of these, in this author's opinion, is the one offered by McMullan (1959) to the effect that 'obesity is a condition in which the body contours are distorted by a diffuse accumulation of adipose tissue'. Those who wish to judge for themselves both the force of this definition and the prevalence of obesity need only glance at the profiles presented for their inspection in bars, bathing beaches, common rooms and mirrors. They can assess the extent of their own departure from the ideal state by calculating their Ponderal index (Seltzer, 1966). This is the ratio of the height in inches to the cube root of the weight in pounds. A value below 13 indicates a departure in the wrong direction from the ideal weight.

Obesity is to be deplored on more than aesthetic grounds. Superfluous fat is a useless burden that has to be carried everywhere to the detriment of its owner's cardiovascular system. A number of metabolic disorders such as diabetes mellitus, cirrhosis of the liver and gallstones lie in wait for the obese. Obesity is often an enemy of successful surgery and tranquil anaesthesia and, among the elderly, falls leading to fatal fractures are more often the lot of the obese than of their leaner brethren. 'The longer the belt, the shorter the life'.

If energy intake in the form of food falls below energy expenditure, reserves of body fat are called on to supply the deficit and body weight falls. Thus, however varied and complex the origins of obesity, its cure is simple: food intake must be reduced or energy output must be increased. The only practicable way of increasing energy expenditure is by taking exercise. Too much is not to be expected from physical exertion. The addition of an hour's walking to the daily routine of an individual in a sedentary occupation will result in the loss of 3 to 4 kg of body mass in three months—total abstention from food would achieve

the same loss in under two weeks—provided that the extra energy expenditure during walking is not partly offset, either by an increased food intake consequent on the increased appetite engendered by the exericse or by too long a period of self congratulatory relaxation after the daily exercise has been completed. Unfortunately, many people can find neither the time nor the opportunity for regular physical activity and the very obese are likely to experience difficulty in actually performing therapeutically worthwhile exercise even when the state of their cardiovascular systems does not constitute a contraindication to indulgence in this type of activity. Moreover, the prospect of losing three kilograms of fat in three months is hardly dazzling for those who may need to lose up to ten times this amount. Thus, whether or not it is supplemented by exercise, restriction of food intake must be the sheet anchor in the treatment of obesity. Unfortunately, eating is the most compelling of addictions and many people just cannot obey, without some sort of help, the simple injunction to eat less. Among the several aids to which they may have to resort are drugs, the psychiatrist (overeating is not infrequently a sign of an underlying depressive illness) and the type of group therapy that is provided by membership of 'weight watching' clubs or by readership of one of the many available slimming magazines. Some of the grossly obese are prepared to submit to more extreme measures: jaws are wired together so that they can admit into the mouth no more than a tube through which essential nutrients can be passed and various by-pass operations have been devised with the aim of reducing absorption from the alimentary tract. The best and least dangerous of these involves anastomosis of the jejunum to the ileum at points that lead to the exclusion of about half a metre of the small intestine.

Even the most successful and energetically pursued dietary regime cannot spirit away overnight the huge and repulsive masses of adipose tissue that will have accumulated in the excessively obese and, as a preliminary to the institution of other measures, the surgical removal of subcutaneous fat (and sometimes of the omental apron) followed by cosmetic plastic surgery has something to recommend it on medical, psychological and aesthetic grounds.

Drugs used in the treatment of obesity

Pharmacologists are, of course, primarily concerned with the use of drugs but it must not be forgotten that, in the control of obesity, drugs can serve as no more than aids to the reduction of food intake. Those that have, from time to time, found favour can be grouped as follows:

1. Drugs that influence carbohydrate metabolism: biguanides and glucagon
2. Metabolic stimulants
3. Bulk forming agents and purgatives
4. Anorectic (anorexigenic) drugs.

Only those in the last mentioned category merit more than superficial attention.

The possibility that suitable prostaglandin antagonists may eventually find a place in this list of antiobesity drugs is discussed on p. 386.

DRUGS THAT INFLUENCE CARBOHYDRATE METABOLISM

In patients with maturity onset diabetes, phenformin and metformin (p. 728) stimulate glucose utilization, inhibit gluconeogenesis and interfere with the absorption of glucose and some other nutrients from the gut. All these actions encourage the loss of fat and biguanides are sometimes given to obese nondiabetic subjects as aids to weight loss. Objective assessments have made it clear that, except possibly in those with a family background of diabetes, these drugs have no more than a placebo effect. Evidently, the nature of the metabolic disturbance in maturity onset diabetes is such as to render glycolytic and other systems abnormally responsive to the biguanides.

Glucagon (p. 722) promotes the mobilization of glucose and so banishes hunger. The long term use of glucagon in the obese would, however, be impracticable even if it were desirable. The drug has to be given by injection and its action is not free of side effects.

METABOLIC STIMULANTS

A drug that stimulated tissue metabolism would be expected to be as therapeutically effective as gentle exercise and it would carry the added recommendation that it would allow energy expenditure to be boosted round the clock instead of only during the relatively short time that can be devoted to exercise before the onset of fatigue or the call of duty brings it to an end.

The thyroid hormones stimulate metabolism but they are only effective in euthyroid subjects at dose levels that cause thyrotoxicosis. When there is evidence of depressed thyroid activity in obese patients, judiciously chosen doses of triiodothyronine or thyroxine can be safely given and they may bring about an agreeable loss of weight.

BULK FORMING AGENTS AND PURGATIVES

On the assumption that a distended stomach induces feelings of satiety, methyl cellulose and other bulk forming agents (p. 648) have been added to frugal repasts in the hope of converting them into meals voluminous enough to satisfy the appetite. They have proved to be singularly useless, for hunger returns as soon as the mass leaves the stomach.

Bulk forming agents exert another supposedly beneficial effect in obese subjects because they stimulate intestinal movements and so hurry the contents of the alimentary tract past their absorption sites. This brings about the elimination of material that would otherwise be absorbed. All purgative drugs have this action and some proprietary slimming preparations number a purgative among their components. There is no evidence that it contributes in any way to the effectiveness of the preparations.

ANORECTIC DRUGS

Drugs that blunt the appetite are the only ones that offer any real help to the obese. They do so by providing pharmacological props to the resolve to eat less.

We have already excluded glucagon and bulk forming substances from the list of useful anorexigenic agents on the grounds of inconvenience and ineffectiveness respectively. Arguments began a quarter of a century ago concerning the anorectic activity of chorionic gonadotrophin. They continue: reports that purport to demonstrate the drug's effectiveness appear at the same rate as those that maintain either that it is no better than placebo or that in some subjects it actually sharpens the appetite. In any event, chorionic gonadotrophin has to be given parenterally and it seems that it will have to take its place alongside glucagon as a failed hope.

The first really effective anorectic drug to appear on the scene was amphetamine. For many years it enjoyed, among physicians and patients alike, a wide, if not entirely justified reputation, as an aid to weight loss. Amphetamine is a phenylethylamine derivative and some other drugs based on this structure also won clinical recognition (Fig. 17.13). With the advent in the late 1960's of stricter controls on its use, amphetamine had to be abandoned as a routine anorectic drug. Some of the other phenylethylamine derivatives found themselves under the same cloud as amphetamine itself and the only healthy survivors are diethylpropion and fenfluramine with phentermine and chlorphentermine retaining a minor place in the list of favoured drugs. The newest anorectic agent (mazindol) is not related to phenylethylamine.

The mode of action of amphetamine has already been discussed in some detail (p. 276).

Diethylpropion

The mechanism of this drug's anorectic action is similar to that of amphetamine but it is much less prone to cause cerebral excitation and the likelihood of its being abused is, consequently, low. Nevertheless a few cases of diethyl-

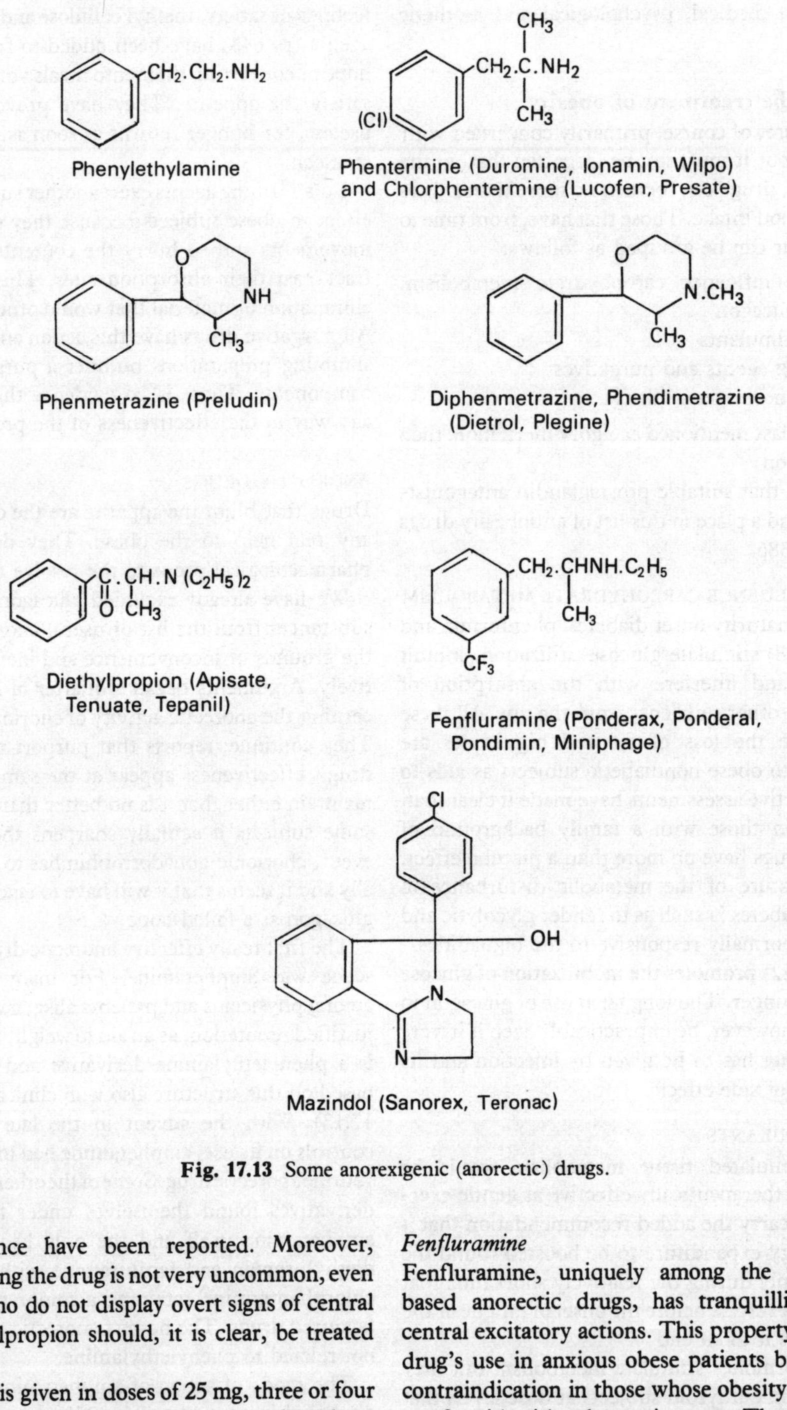

Fig. 17.13 Some anorexigenic (anorectic) drugs.

propion dependence have been reported. Moreover, insomnia after taking the drug is not very uncommon, even among patients who do not display overt signs of central excitation. Diethylpropion should, it is clear, be treated with respect.

Diethylpropion is given in doses of 25 mg, three or four times daily. For obvious reasons, the last dose should not be taken later than the early evening. Sustained action preparations are also available. They permit the taking of a single 100 mg dose of diethylpropion each morning. The drug seems to yield the best results if it is taken intermittently, one-month periods of treatment alternating with drug free periods of similar duration.

Fenfluramine

Fenfluramine, uniquely among the phenylethylamine based anorectic drugs, has tranquillizing rather than central excitatory actions. This property recommends the drug's use in anxious obese patients but it constitutes a contraindication in those whose obesity is associated (as it so often is) with a depressive state. The unusual combination of depressant and anorectic activity is probably a consequence of the fact that the major targets for fenfluramine's actions are neurones that contain serotonin whereas the other anorectic drugs operate predominantly on neural mechanisms that utilize dopamine or noradrenaline. It will be recalled that serotonin, like the catecholamines, is involved in both feeding and affective (p. 188) processes.

Fenfluramine exerts a number of metabolic actions. In particular it promotes the mobilization and metabolism of fat and the uptake of glucose by muscle. For some time it was believed that these mechanisms might operate to increase energy expenditure in those who took the drug and so provide a partial realization of the fat man's dream of a drug that will cause him to lose weight without demanding any dietary sacrifice on his part. It is now clear that any action that fenfluramine has on tissue metabolism is too small to cause any weight loss. Like all the other drugs listed in Fig. 17.13 fenfluramine is useful simply because it moderates the appetite.

Fenfluramine is said to be the drug of choice for the treatment of the obesity that sometimes develops in patients who are taking drugs of the phenothiazine type (p. 548), in obese diabetic subjects, in those with hypertension and in children. It is taken in twice daily doses of 20 to 80 mg. The smallest dose is tried first but this can be cautiously increased if side effects are not troublesome until an optimum dose is found. The most common side effects are drowsiness and gastrointestinal disturbances (particularly diarrhoea and abdominal pain), but dizziness and headache are also seen. Cases of serious overdosage show pyrexia, mental confusion and convulsions, a picture that is very similar to that seen in atropine poisoning. Even the mydriasis is there! In view of the postulated mode of action of fenfluramine, it is interesting that the signs of toxic overdosage can be reversed by serotonin antagonists.

When fenfluramine treatment has to be interrupted, the drug should be withdrawn gradually over a period of days, the dose being steadily reduced during this period. Abrupt withdrawal of fenfluramine may, surprisingly enough, precipitate a mental depression that is likely to persist for some days.

Fenfluramine only rarely causes dependence, though some cases of deliberate abuse have been reported.

Mazindol

Although mazindol is an indole compound, the most recent investigations (Kruk and Zarrindast, 1976) indicate that in its mode of anorectic action it resembles amphetamine much more closely than do some of the phenylethylamine derivatives (particularly fenfluramine) notwithstanding the latter's structural affinities with amphetamine.

It appears that mazindol increases the availability of dopamine at the synapses partly by blocking the reuptake of the catecholamine and partly by promoting its release. Although the results of some earlier studies had pointed to the participation of noradrenaline in the responses evoked by the drug, it now seems unlikely that this mediator plays no more than an insignificant role. Thus, in rats, the anorexia induced by mazindol is antagonized by pimozide

(a specific dopamine antagonist) but not by agents that oppose the actions of noradrenaline or serotonin.

Mazindol is a new and relatively untried drug but, on present evidence, it seems to be effective in doses of 1 mg taken thrice daily. The fact that its neuropharmacological actions are so similar to those of amphetamine should, however, give pause for thought among those who are concerned with the abuse potential of anorexigenic drugs.

Phenylpropanolamine

Phenylpropanolamine is a mixed action sympathomimetic amine (Table 17.6, p. 278) that is used as a nasal decongestant. It also causes a degree of anorexia. At first sight this should occasion no surprise because the drug is a β-phenylethylamine derivative like so many other anorexigenic drugs. What is surprising is the fact that its mode of action may differ from that of the other drugs that suppress appetite: it appears to stimulate peripheral glucose receptors that signal satiety so that it should be classed with glucagon (p. 722) rather than with the other β-phenylethylamine derivatives. Its use for the treatment of obesity is not recommended.

BIBLIOGRAPHY

Books, monographs and reviews

Anton, A.H, and Sayre, D.F. (1972) In: *Methods in Investigative and Diagnostic Endocrinology*, Vol. 1. ed. Kopin, I.J. pp.398-436 Amsterdam: North-Holland Publishing Co.

Axelrod J. (1965) In: Varley and Gowenlock (eds.) *The Clinical Chemistry of the Monoamines*, London and New York: Elsevier.

Axelrod, J. (1965). The metabolism, storage and release of catecholamines. *Recent Prog. Horm. Res.*, **21**, 597-622.

Axelrod, J (1966). Methylation reactions in the formation and metabolism of catecholamines and other biogenic amines. *Pharmac. Rev.*, **18**: 95-113

Belleau, B. (1963) An analysis of drug receptor interactions. In: *Modern Concepts in the Relationship between Structure and Pharmacological Activity, Proceedings of the First International Pharmacological Meeting*, 1961, vol. **7** 75-99, London: Pergamon Press.

Blaschko, H. and Muscholl, E. (1972) (eds) *Catecholamines* (Handbook of Experimental Pharmacology, Vol. 33). Berlin: Springer-Verlag.

Butt, W.R. (1976) *Hormone Chemistry* 2nd edn. pp. 217-242. Chichester: Ellis Horwood.

Craddock, D. (1973) *Obesity and its Management* 2nd edn., Edinburgh and London: Churchill Livingstone.

Crossland. J. (1967) Psychotropic drugs and neurohumoral substances in the central nervous system. In: Ellis, G.P. and West, G. B. (eds) Vol. 5 pp. 251-319 London: Butterworths.

Estler, C.-J. (1975). Effect of amphetamine-type psychostimulants on brain metabolism. *Adv. Pharmac. Chemother.* **13**, 305-357

Gaddum, J.H. (1959) *Pharmacology*, 5th ed. Oxford: University Press.

Goldberg, L.I. (1972) Cardiovascular and renal actions of dopamine: potential clinical applications. *Pharmac. Rev.*, **24**, 1-29

Hoebel, B.G. (1977). Pharmacologic control of feeding. *A. rev. Pharmac. Toxicol.* **17**, 605-621.

Iversen, L.L. (1967). *The Uptake and Storage of Noradrenaline in Sympathetic Nerves*. Cambridge: The University Press.

Kornetsky, C. (1976). *Pharmacology. Drugs affecting Behaviour*. pp. 223-252. New York: John Wiley.

Nagatsu, T. (1973). *Biochemistry of Catecholamines*. pp.209-273. Baltimore: University Park Press.

Pinder, R.M., Brogden, R.N., Sawyer, Phyllis R., Speight, T.M. and Avery, G.S. (1975) Fenfluramine: a review of its pharmacological properties and therapuetic efficacy in obesity. *Drugs* **10**: 241-323.

Pinder, R.M., Brogden, R.N., Speight, T.M. and Avery, G.S. (1977) Hexoprenaline: a review of its pharmacological properties and therapeutic efficacy with particular reference to asthma. *Drugs*, **14**, 1-28

Root, W.S. and Hoffmann, F.G. (eds.) (1967). *Physiological Pharmacology*. Vol. IV. New York and London: Academic Press.

Silverstone, T. (1975). *Obesity: its Pathogenesis and Management*. Lancaster, England: Medical and Technical Publishing Co.

Symposium (1971). Salbutamol. *Postgrad. med. J.* **47**: (Jan. supp.) 1-112.

Trendelenburg, U. (1963). Supersensitivity and subsensitivity to sympathomimetic amines. *Pharmac. Rev.* **15**: 225-276

Udenfriend, S. (1966). Tyrosine hydroxylase. *Pharmac. Rev.*, **18**, 43-52.

Original papers

Ahlquist, R.P. (1948). A study of the adrenotropic receptors. *Amer. J Physiol.*, **153**: 586-600.

Anonymous (1977). Intravenous dopamine. *Lancet* (ii) 231-232.

Anton. A.H. and Sayre, D.F. (1962). A study of the factors affecting the aluminium oxide trihydroxy-indole procedure for the analysis of catecholamines. *J. Pharmac. exp. Ther.*, **138**: 360-375.

Anton. A.H. and Sayre, D.F. (1964) The distribution of dopamine and dopa in various animals and a method for their determination in diverse biological material. *J. Pharmac. exp. Ther.*, **145**, 326-336.

Assem, E.S.K. and Schild, H.O. (1964). Inhibition by sympathomimetic amines of histamine release induced by antigen in passively sensitized human lung. *Nature (Lond.)*, **224**, 1028-1029.

Blaschko, H., Richter, D. and Schlossman, H. (1937). The oxidation of adrenaline and other amines. *Biochem. J.*, **31**, 2187-2196.

Burn, J.H., Hutcheon, D.E. and Parker, R.H.O. (1950). Estimation of adrenaline-noradrenaline mixtures. *Brit. J. Pharmac. Chemother.*, **5**: 142-146.

Burn, J.H. and Rand, M.J. (1958). The action of sympathomimetic amines in animals treated with reserpine. *J. Physiol.*, **144**, 314-346.

Gaddum, J.H. and Kwiatkowski, H. (1938). The action of ephedrine. *J. Physiol.*, **94**, 87-100.

Goldberg, L.I. (1974). Dopamine—clinical uses of an endogenous catecholamine. *New Eng. J. Med.*, **291**, 707-710.

Kruk, Z.L. and Zarrindast, M.R. (1976). Mazindol anorexia is mediated by activation of dopaminergic mechanisms. *Br. J. Pharmac.*, **58**, 367-372.

La Brosse, E.H., Axelrod, J., Kopin, I.J. and Kety, S.S. (1961). Metabolism of 7-H^3-epinephrine-α-bitartrate in normal young men. *J. clin. Invest.*, **40**: 253-260.

McMullan, J.J. (1959). Obesity and body weight in general practice. *The Practitioner*, **182**: 222-227.

Montegriffo, V.M.E. (1971). A survey of the incidence of obesity in the United Kingdom. *Postgrad. med J.*, **47**: (June supp.) 418-422.

Seltzer, C.C. (1966). Some re-evaluations of the build and blood pressure study, 1959, as related to Ponderal Index, Somatotype and Mortality. *New Eng. J. Med.*, **274**, 254-259.

18. Antagonists of adrenergic neurone activity

All the substances described in this chapter interfere, to a greater or lesser extent, with the activity of the sympathetic nervous system. Those that pass the blood brain barrier also have central actions but in this chapter we are concerned primarily with drug effects on peripheral structures. The antagonists fall into two distinct groups. The first group includes drugs that inhibit the synthesis, storage or release of the catecholamines. They therefore remove the influence of the sympathetic system from its effector organs and they also prevent the action of the indirectly acting sympathomimetic drugs. It is clear that they will not prevent the action of noradrenaline, adrenaline or other directly acting substances which reach the circulation from exogenous sources. The second group of agents acts on the receptors themselves. They block the effects both of sympathetic nervous activity and of circulating sympathomimetic substances but most of them are selective in the sense that individual drugs block either the α or the β receptors.

It will be appreciated that, so far as their action on systems which are predominantly under sympathetic control is concerned, both groups of drugs have some of the actions of ganglion blocking agents. Thus many of them reduce blood pressure and may cause postural hypotension. Side effects such as blurred vision, dry mouth and so on, which are attributable to block of the parasympathetic system, do not, of course, occur except with those drugs which have some ganglion blocking activity independently of their action on the adrenergic neurone or its receptors.

The substances discussed in this chapter are sometimes collectively known as the adrenergic blocking agents. However, the term 'adrenergic' should be applied only to nerves: to extend it to drugs and receptors is incorrect and may be misleading. This topic is discussed in more detail elsewhere (p. 172). Here it is only necessary to repeat that 'adrenaline receptor' is as easy to say and to write as 'adrenergic receptor' and it should be equally acceptable to the etymologist, the historian and the scientist who believes that his terms should be rigidly defined.

DRUGS THAT PREVENT THE ACTION OF THE ADRENERGIC NEURONE

Substances that prevent the liberation of noradrenaline

from the adrenergic neurone can be classified as follows:

(i) substances that prevent the *storage* of catecholamines—reserpine and related compounds,

(ii) substances that prevent the *synthesis* of catecholamines—α-methylDOPA, α-methyl-*m*-tyrosine, α-methyl-*p*-tyrosine,

(iii) substances that prevent the *release* of catecholamines—xylocholine, bretylium, guanethidine,

(iv) substances that destroy sympathetic nerves—6-hydroxydopamine, antiserum to nerve growth factor.

Substances that prevent storage of catecholamines

RESERPINE

Reserpine has both central and peripheral actions and its effects in the brain are complicated by the fact that it affects 5-hydroxtryptamine, dopamine and other substances as well as noradrenaline. It is therefore more appropriate to discuss the general properties and uses of the drug elsewhere and this is done in Chapter 32 (p. 557). Here attention is confined to a discussion of the pharmacological action of reserpine on the peripheral adrenergic neurone; its use as an antihypersentive drug is considered below (p. 288).

When reserpine is administered to experimental animals, it causes a slow but progressive reduction in the catecholamine content of the tissues. Within twenty-four hours, a single dose of the order of 1 mg per kg produces an almost complete depletion of catecholamine stores. The tissues do not regain their normal complement of catecholamine for at least a week. Reserpinization can also be produced by giving very small doses (5 μg per kg) of reserpine on several successive days.

Kopin and Gordon (1963) administered tritium-labelled noradrenaline to rats. They waited until the tissues had accumulated the labelled compound and then gave the animals a small dose of reserpine. During the next 12 hours there was only a small increase in the urinary excretion of labelled noradrenaline and normetadrenaline but the excretion of deaminated metabolites increased more than three-fold. Tyramine, on the other hand, which is known to cause the release of noradrenaline from adrenergic nerves, caused a three-fold increase in the urinary excretion of labelled noradrenaline and normetadrenaline but it had virtually no effect on the excretion of deaminated metabolites. These results indicate that reserpine does not promote the liberation of noradrenaline as such from sympathetic nerves. This explains why it is that, except in large doses, reserpine does not cause signs of sympathetic stimulation during the period when the noradrenaline is being lost from the adrenergic neurones.

It has already been pointed out (p. 175) that much of the noradrenaline liberated from nerve fibres is reincorporated into the fibres. This represents an important channel of inactivation after the noradrenaline has exerted its physiological action. Experiments with tritum-labelled noradrenaline have made it clear that reserpine does not influence the rate of reuptake of noradrenaline (Kopin, Hertling and Gordon, 1962; Gillespie and Kirpekar, 1965) but the noradrenaline which is taken up is immediately metabolized, as is evidenced by the accumulation of deaminated metabolites in the tissues. The most likely explanation of these findings is that reserpine prevents the passage of noradrenaline into the nerve storage vesicles.

Reserpine disrupts the function of the storage vesicles to such an extent that they cannot retain the newly synthesized noradrenaline (the last stage in the synthesis takes place within the vesicles themselves) any more effectively than that which arrives by reuptake processes. Noradrenaline that is left in, or allowed to escape into, the cytoplasm is promptly destroyed by monoamine oxidase. Consequently reserpine rids neurones of their noradrenaline even though it does not interfere with catecholamine synthesis.

It might be asked why, if reserpine prevents the uptake of noradrenaline into the storage vesicles, adrenergic function can be temporarily and partially restored in reserpinized animals by an infusion of noradrenaline. The explanation appears to be that the infused material enters the small 'pool' of noradrenaline from which the transmitter is released by nerve impulses and entry to which is not prohibited by reserpine. This pool is normally replenished from a larger reservoir of storage vesicles but which is empty, for reasons we have already discussed, in reserpinized animals. In these circumstances the small pool can only be filled from extraneous sources and adrenergic activity ceases again when the infusion is stopped.

Reserpine also removes serotonin and dopamine from nerves that contain these transmitters.

Reserpine and the treatment of hypertension. Once popular as an antihypertensive agent, reserpine is still favoured by some physicians. Provided that the daily dose of reserpine is kept below 0.25 mg serious mental depression (p. 558) should not occur. The mode of action of reserpine is still not clear. It certainly depletes the postganglionic terminals of their contained noradrenaline but it seems to cause arteriolar dilatation in doses which do not completely inhibit the activity of the sympathetic nerves. It may be that the noradrenaline associated with the nerve terminals is capable of exerting a tonic constriction in the absence of activity in the sympathetic nerves and that this effect disappears at a time when suffficient noradrenaline

remains to enable the continued functioning of the sympathetic nerves. The tranquillizing action of reserpine may contribute to its antihypertensive effect although resperine has little effect on the discharge of impulses from the sympathetic centres in the hypothalamus.

Reserpine and psychiatric illness. This topic is considered in the chapter that discusses psychotropic drugs (p. 558).

Substances that prevent the synthesis of catecholamines

α-METHYLDOPA AND α-METHYL-M-TRYOSINE

It is pointed out elsewhere (pp. 258 and 327) that DOPA decarboxylase (L-amino acid decarboxylase) is involved in the biosynthesis of dopamine, noradrenaline and 5-hydroxytryptamine. When it was discovered (Sourkes, 1954) that α-methylDOPA inhibited this enzyme *in vitro*, it seemed reasonable to suppose that its administration to animals would lead to impairment of amine synthesis. This view was strengthened when it was found that α-methyl-DOPA does indeed cause a very marked reduction in the noradrenaline content of animal tissues. Dopamine and 5-hydroxytryptamine are affected to a smaller extent. In 1960, α-methylDOPA (Aldomet) was introduced into clinical practice for the treatment of hypertension on the assumption that it would prevent the synthesis and hence the release, of noradrenaline by the sympathetic fibres. α-MethylDOPA has proved to be a most popular and effective drug but it is now clear that the premiss on which it found its way into therapeutics was a false one and that its mode of action is a good deal more complex than was originally believed.

The depletion of noradrenaline produced by α-methyl-DOPA considerably outlasts the period of enzyme inhibition. So far as its effect on noradrenaline is concerned, it seems that the most important effects of α-methylDOPA result from its ability to compete with DOPA as a substrate for DOPA decarboxylase. As a result of this, α-methylnoradrenaline (Fig. 18.1) instead of noradrenaline is produced in the neurone. The enzymes involved in this conversion are the same as those which form noradrenaline from DOPA and it will be evident that α-methylnoradrenaline cannot be formed at its maximal rate until the DOPA decarboxylase has recovered from its initial inhibition. There is doubt, in fact, whether the enzyme is inhibited at all by doses of α-methylDOPA which cause depletion of noradrenaline. Some powerful *in vitro* inhibitors of DOPA decarboxylase do not affect the noradrenaline content of adrenergic neurones.

Stimulation of sympathetic nerves causes the release of α-methylnoradrenaline in animals which have been given α-methylDOPA (Muscholl & Maître, 1963) and α-methylnoradrenaline is therefore said to be a *false transmitter*. If the sympathomimetic activity of the false transmitter was much less than that of noradrenaline itself,

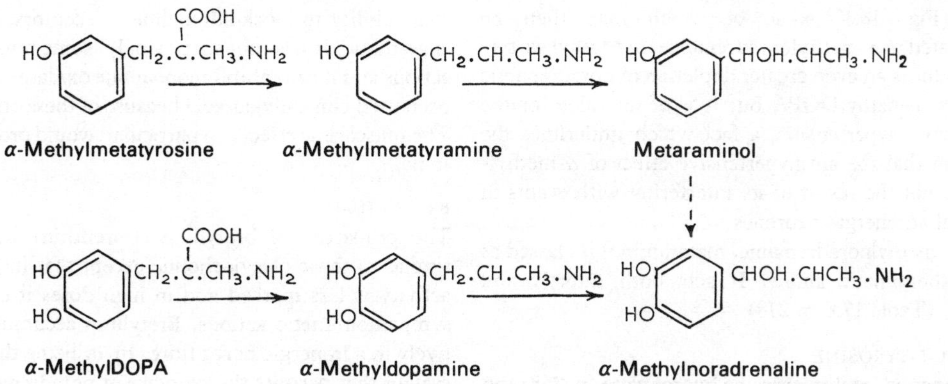

Fig. 18.1 α-Methylated derivatives of the catecholamines

α-methylDOPA would lead to a reduction in the effects of sympathetic nervous activity and this would explain the drug's antihypertensive activity. It is, however, clear that the sympathomimetic activity of α-methylnoradrenaline is not so uniformly less than that of noradrenaline as was at first believed. Indeed it is itself used clinically as a vaso-constrictor drug (Table 17.4, p. 270). Moreover the replacement of noradrenaline by α-methylnoradrenaline is accompanied by an increased sensitivity to noradrenaline of the sympathetic effector organs (Haefely, Hurlimann & Thoenen, 1966). It appears that α-methylDOPA does not noticeably affect sympathetic nervous activity and the origin of its antihypertensive action must be sought elsewhere. Day, Roach and Whiting (1973) noted that the antihypertensive action of α-methylDOPA was prevented by inhibitors of DOPA decarboxylase that penetrate into the central nervous system but not by those whose action is restricted to peripheral sites. They also found that the antihypertensive effect was annulled by inhibitors of dopamine-β-hydroxylase. Taken together, these observations indicate that α-methylDOPA has a locus of action in the central nervous system, that the drug must be decarboxylated before it can exert its therapeutic effect and that the active product is α-methylnoradrenaline and not α-methyldopamine. The reader will not have failed to notice that the action of a substance that was originally introduced into medicine because of its ability to inhibit an enzyme actually depends for its effectiveness on the continuing activity of that very enzyme!

α-MethylDOPA, then, influences sympathetic nervous activity by reducing the outflow into the nerves from central sources. This effect is abolished by phentolamine (an α-receptor blocking agent, p. 300), indicating that α-methylnoradrenaline is a false transmitter, usurping the role of noradrenaline in the mediation of the depressor influences of the vasomotor centres. If this is the correct interpretation of the situation we must conclude that, contrary to that in peripheral arterioles, α-methylnoradrenaline is a substantially more effective activator than noradrenaline of α-receptors on some central neurones. α-MethylDOPA also has a sedative action (which is presumably mediated through α-methylnoradrenaline) and this will form part of its overall effect on sympathetic outflow. There is also some evidence that it is not entirely devoid of peripheral actions, though these may prove to be clinically insignificant. It may be, for instance, that α-methylnoradrenaline, though generally no less active a vasoconstrictor substance than noradrenaline, is less so in some special regions (such as the renal vasculature) that are particularly important in the regulation of blood pressure.

The daily dose of α-methylDOPA for hypertensive patients can reach 2 grams, divided into four instalments, but amounts as low as 750 mg are sometimes adequate. The effects of the drug appear only slowly (it may be 48 hours before the maximum response to the first oral dose is seen) so that care has to be exercised when attempts are being made to determine the maximally effective dose for an individual patient. The drug may cause drowsiness, nasal stuffiness (a common occurrence with agents that inhibit sympathetic outflow) and, occasionally, impotence. Infrequently, it causes gastrointestinal upsets and jaundice, and a few cases of agranulocytosis (completely reversible by withdrawal of the drug) have been reported. α-MethylDOPA does not produce more than a slight degree of postural hypotension. This may be related to the finding that, in animals treated with the drug, the effects of a low rate of stimulation of the sympathetic nerves disappear more readily than do those of a high rate of stimulation.

α-MethylDOPA has been used with some slight success in the treatment of malignant carcinoid (p. 329). In this condition, it may be that the drug does act as an enzyme inhibitor, preventing the synthesis of 5-hydroxytryptamine. Its use for the relief of symptoms caused by phaeochromocytomas has also been explored.

α-Methyl-m-tyrosine behaves in a similar fashion to α-methylDOPA. The false transmitter it produces is metaraminol (Fig. 18.1) some of which may then be hydroxylated to α-methylnoradrenaline. α-Methyl-*m*-tyrosine produces an even greater depletion of noradrenaline than does α-methylDOPA but it is of no value for the treatment of hypertension, a fact which underlines the conclusion that the antihypertensive effect of α-methylDOPA is not the result of its interfering with events in peripheral adrenergic neurones.

Like α-methylnoradrenaline, metaraminol is classed as a sympathomimetic amine. It acts both directly and indirectly (Table 17.6 p. 278).

α-METHYL-*P*-TYROSINE

This compound inhibits tyrosine hydroxylase (p. 258) and prevents the synthesis of noradrenaline without affecting the production of 5-hydroxytryptamine. The compound has no therapeutic use but it can be a useful pharmacological tool, particularly in studies on the brain.

Substances that prevent the release of catecholamines

XYLOCHOLINE

Xylocholine (TM. 10) was the first compound recognized as being capable of blocking the effects of stimulation of sympathetic nerve fibres. Both inhibitory and excitatory effects are prevented. It has been suggested that xylocholine may interfere with the biosynthesis of noradrenaline from dopamine and that this is the basis of its sympathetic blocking action. Among other explanations is one based on the hypothesis that acetylcholine liberation in sympathetic nerves is a necessary preliminary to noradrenaline liberation. Xylocholine can be shown to block ganglionic and neuromuscular transmission and it might therefore equally well block the action of acetylcholine at the sympathetic nerve terminals. Support for this idea comes from from the observation that in the atropinized heart, acetylcholine has sympathomimetic actions because it liberates noradrenaline from the sympathetic nerve endings. This action is blocked by xylocholine (Huković, 1960). The structure of xylocholine lends some credence to the view that it may intervene in actions mediated by acetylcholine. However, the view that the release of noradrenaline at sympathetic nerve endings is mediated by acetylcholine is not generally accepted and it may well be that xylocholine and bretylium (see below) share a common mode of action.

Xylocholine has a number of other actions, though these are evident only at dose levels slightly higher than those which cause sympathetic nerve blockade. Thus, it causes some liberation of catecholamines from the tissues, it has some ability to block adrenaline α receptors, it is a local anaesthetic, it has (not surprisingly) some muscarine-like actions and it can inhibit monoamine oxidase. It has never been used clinically, largely because of these other actions. The muscarinic effects, in particular, would prove troublesome.

BRETYLIUM

The properties of bretylium (Darenthin) are generally similar to those of xylocholine except that its muscarinic activity is less marked and in high doses it exerts some sympathomimetic actions. Bretylium accumulates selectively in adrenergic nerve fibres by utilizing the transport system that permits the reuptake of noradrenaline by the nerves. Once in the nerves, bretylium prevents the release of noradrenaline in response to nerve impulses. It is possible that this is the result of a local anaesthetic action. However, it can be shown that the release of noradrenaline can be prevented by doses of bretylium too small to prevent conduction of nerve impulses. It may, of course, be that these small doses of bretylium are sufficient to halt the action potentials in the fine sensitive terminals of the nerves without affecting impulse propagation in the main trunk but there is no direct evidence that this is so. Moreover, guanethidine (see below) which is a more effective adrenergic nerve blocking agent than bretylium is a much less powerful local anaesthetic. A more likely explanation may be that bretylium, by competition with calcium, interferes with excitation-secretion processes in the nerve terminals.

The sympathomimetic activity of bretylium (which might seem to be something of an anomaly in a drug that inhibits the release of noradrenaline) to which reference has already been made, appears transiently soon after the drug is given. It arises partly because bretylium causes an initial release of noradrenaline from the nerves and partly because it enforces the retention at the neuroeffector junction of some of the transmitter that is liberated before nerve block is established. It does this by virtue of its competition with the catecholamine for the available uptake capacity.

Although bretylium initially liberates noradrenaline from adrenergic nerves it does not bring about any detectable decrease in the catecholamine content of sympathetically innervated tissues. This is because it is a monoamine oxidase inhibitor so that it prevents the destruction of noradrenaline released from the storage granules into the cytoplasm. Only that escaping into the neuroeffector spaces is lost.

$$H_3C - \overset{\overset{\displaystyle CH_3}{|}}{\underset{\underset{\displaystyle CH_3}{|}}{N^+}} - CH_2 - CH_2 - O - \text{(xylyl)}$$

Xylocholine

$$\text{(bromophenyl)} - CH_2 - \overset{\overset{\displaystyle CH_3}{|}}{\underset{\underset{\displaystyle CH_3}{|}}{N^{\oplus}}} - CH_2 - CH_3 \quad Br^-$$

Bretylium bromide

Drugs, such as amphetamine and imipramine, that prevent the reuptake of noradrenaline reverse or antagonize the actions of bretylium.

Bretylium (which was first used in 1960) enjoyed a brief spell of popularity as an antihypertensive drug. However, tolerance develops very rapidly and bretylium causes some uncomfortable side effects. The most characteristic of these is pain in the parotid gland but nasal stuffiness, breathlessness on exertion, diarrhoea, postural hypotension, muscular weakness and even mental changes have been reported. The drug is not used as an antihypertensive agent but it still finds a minor place in the treatment of cardiac arrhythmias (p. 690). The rationale of its use in these conditions is the fact that, by preventing noradrenaline release, it reduces cardiac irritability.

GUANETHIDINE

Guanethidine (Ismelin) has qualitatively similar properties to bretylium. It is widely used as an antihypertensive drug. It has more marked reserpine-like actions than either xylocholine or bretylium but it does not deplete the brain or the adrenal glands of their contained catecholamines. The lack of effect on the brain is presumably due to the drug's inability to cross the blood barrier. It is not known why it has no action on the adrenal glands. Unlike xylocholine and bretylium, guanethidine does not inhibit monoamine oxidase so that the noradrenaline content of sympathetically innervated structures falls to a very low level after guanethidine treatment.

The reserpine-like action of guanethidine together with its ability to prevent the release of noradrenaline in response to activity in the sympathetic nerves result in a very sharp decline in the liberation of sympathetic transmitter and explains its hypotensive effect. It is to be noted that guanethidine exerts its antihypertensive effect before the nerves are seriously depleted of noradrenaline. This indicates that the drug's ability to prevent transmitter release (the mechanism of this action is probably identical with that made use of by bretylium) is of more significance than its reserpine-like proclivity. Like bretylium guanethidine has some sympathomimetic actions and when it is first given it may, as a result, cause a transient increase in blood pressure. After repeated administration, guanethidine causes a considerable increase in the sensitivity of adrenaline receptors but this does not offset the drug's antihypertensive action since noradrenaline output is so low. It has already been mentioned that guanethidine is a less powerful local anaesthetic than xylocholine or bretylium.

The side effects of guanethidine are similar to those produced by bretylium except that tolerance does not develop so rapidly and parotid pain is rare. Diarrhoea may be troublesome and there may be impairment of ejaculatory ability in the male. The diarrhoea may be caused by 5-hydroxytryptamine liberated in the intestine as a result of the reserpine-like action of guanethidine. Imipramine and other tricyclic antidepressant drugs antagonize guanethidine. Conversely, guanethidine potentiates the effects of sympathomimetic agents by reason of the increased sensitivity of the adrenaline receptors and the reduced uptake of some of these agents into the nerves. Hypertensive crises have been recorded among patients taking guanethidine who have had recourse to cold cures containing sympathomimetic substances.

Guanethidine is extensively bound to plasma proteins. With a plasma half life of five days it has a prolonged duration of action. Because of this and of the fact that its effects develop only slowly, some time is usually required before a suitable dose is arrived at for the individual patient. The usual daily dose ranges from 10 to 300 mg.

BETHANIDINE

Bethanidine (Esbatal) has similar properties and uses to, but has some advantages over, guanethidine. It has a more rapid onset of action and this enables a satisfactory dose to be found quickly. Bethanidine is rather less likely than guanethidine to cause diarrhoea and because its effects are rapidly reversed and re-established it is permissible for the patient periodically to abstain from the drug so that he may enjoy a normal sex life. He begins to take the drug again

Bethanidine

immediately after successful intercourse; during the day or so during which the drug has been withheld, his blood pressure is kept in check by appropriate adjustment of the doses of the other drugs he will be taking. The dose of bethanidine is 5 to 50 mg twice daily.

DEBRISOQUINE

The properties, uses and dosage of debrisoquine (Declinax) are similar to those of bethanidine. Its antihypertensive action, like that of bethanidine, is seen within four hours of its oral administration and the effect of a single dose lasts for 12 to 24 hours. Debrisoquine may cause diarrhoea, though it does so less often than guanethidine. Minor degrees of postural hypotension have been

Guanethidine

Debrisoquine

reported, as they have with all drugs which impair the activity of sympathetic nerve fibres but they are never so severe as that experienced with the ganglion blocking agents.

Substances that destroy sympathetic nerves

Substances in this category are clearly unsuitable as therapeutic agents but they are of continuing value in the laboratory where they are helping to unravel the complexities of noradrenergic and dopaminergic function.

6-HYDROXYDOPAMINE

Some ten years ago, Tranzer and Thoenon (1967) discovered that 6-hydroxydopamine selectively destroyed the fine terminals of the postganglionic adrenergic nerves to produce what has been aptly described as a chemical sympathectomy. When injected directly into the brain, 6-hydroxydopamine prevents synaptic transmission from fibres that utilize either noradrenaline or dopamine. With high doses, nerve terminals that contain 5-hydroxytryptamine are also affected.

The selectivity of 6-hydroxydopamine is attributable to the fact that it is carried into nerve fibres by the transport system that subserves the reuptake of catecholamines (the uptake-1 process, p. 175) by their parent nerves. Once in the nerves, it behaves at first as a false transmitter but as it begins to destroy the nerve endings (this may occur within one hour of the drug's injection) it causes the release of noradrenaline from damaged storage vesicles and its effects now resemble those of a very active, indirectly acting sympathomimetic amine. As the destructive process progresses, all activity in the affected nerves ceases. The changes are usually reversible, new terminal fibres replacing the lost ones within some weeks or months by the usual processes of nerve regeneration. In the newly born, neurone degeneration is more extensive than it is in older animals and it is sometimes so complete that regeneration does not occur.

6-Hydroxydopamine

6-Hydroxydopamine is probably most useful when it is injected into localized regions of the central nervous system. Thus, when it was injected into the lateral hypothalamus it brought about degeneration of noradrenergic fibres that course past the hypothalamus. The experimental animals became aphagic and adipsic, clearly indicating that the system whose integrity had been breached is involved in the control of food and water intake. Other examples of the use of chemical sympathectomy are provided elsewhere.

6-Hydroxydopamine is reviewed by Malmfors and Thoenen (1971) and by Kostrzema and Jacobwitz (1974).

COMPOUNDS RELATED TO 6-HYDROXYDOPAMINE

6-HydroxyDOPA is converted in the body into 6-hydroxydopamine and so has similar actions. Unlike 6-hydroxydopamine, however, the parent compound can pass through the blood-brain barrier. 6-Aminodopamine, α-methyl-hydroxydopamine and α-methyl-6-aminodopamine are similar in their actions to, but are only about half as potent as 6-hydroxydopamine.

5,7-Dihydroxytryptamine selectively destroys neurones that contain 5-hydroxytryptamine.

IMMUNOSYMPATHECTOMY

A nerve-growth factor, protein in nature, is essential for the growth and survival of sympathetic neurones. A specific antiserum to this protein permanently destroys paravertebral and prevertebral sympathetic ganglia (Levi-Montalcini and Booker, 1960). The effects are more widespread in mice than in rats and other laboratory animals and immature animals are more extensively affected than adults. The ganglia of immature mice that have received the antiserum retain no more than two per cent of their original complement of cells but in immature rats the surviving cells may reach 15 per cent of the original total. Moreover, the cells in outlying ganglia such as those of the pelvic plexuses escape the destructive action of the antiserum. The antiserum does not cross the blood-brain barrier.

Immunosympathectomy is reviewed by Levi-Montalcini and Angeletti (1966). It is clearly not as useful an investigative tool as 6-hydroxydopamine.

DRUGS THAT BLOCK ADRENALINE RECEPTORS

Substances that prevent the effects both of sympathetic stimulation and of adrenaline injection have been known for many years. When they were first studied, neither the idea of chemical transmission of the effects of nerve stimulation nor the existence of more than one type of adrenaline receptor was recognized. Nevertheless, it was realized at an early date that the substances then available prevented the excitatory effects of sympathetic nerve stimulation and spared the inhibitory actions. Dale emphasized this as early as 1906, when he wrote that preparations of ergot caused 'a specific paralysis of the motor elements in the structures, associated with sympathetic innervation, which adrenaline stimulates; the inhibitor elements retaining their normal function...' We would now say, of course, that substances which antagonize the effects of sympathetic nerve stimulation in this way selectively block adrenaline α receptors. Until 1958 (ten years after Ahlquist had formulated the hypothesis of α and β receptors) the only blocking agents known were of this type. Many such drugs were known by then and it seems strange that no substances had appeared with an action that could be attributed to selective blockade of the β receptors. However, the general acceptance of the idea of α and β receptors stimulated a search for β receptor blocking agents and several have now been discovered. The selectivity of the blocking agents is rather surprising. All of them have actions other than receptor blockade yet most of them are incapable of effectively blocking more than one type of adrenaline receptor. The exception to this generalization is provided by labetalol, a new drug (p. 306) that blocks both α and β receptors.

Substances that cause blockade of alpha receptors

It is important to appreciate that, so far as their blocking action on adrenaline receptors is concerned, all the α receptor blocking agents have identical effects. Differences in their overall pharmacological actions in the intact animal are the result of their affecting a variety of other systems. It will also be realised that, when given alone, the extent of the effect produced by any of these drugs will depend upon the degree of sympathetic tone which prevails.

Before the individual blocking agents are discussed in detail, the properties common to them all will be briefly reviewed. Although the reader should have no difficulty in working out, in general terms, the effects which would be expected to result from blockade of α receptors, he should note that, in the account which follows, some apparently anomalous effects are mentioned. These have sometimes led to hasty and unjustified conclusions concerning the nature of the receptors present in individual organs.

HEART

Adrenaline receptors in cardiac muscle are of the β type. Nevertheless, in pharmacological experiments, drugs that block α receptors sometimes produce alterations in the rate or force of the heart beat. These effects are sometimes the result of reflex stimulation of the heart following blockade of peripheral receptors: a fall in blood pressure produces reflex tachycardia. In addition some of the blocking agents have a direct action on the heart. Tolazoline, for instance, produces a marked increase in cardiac output but this is simply a manifestation of its sympathomimetic action which is exerted independently of its blocking effect on α receptors (p. 300).

As is discussed later, agents that block β receptors will restore normal rhythms in irregularly beating hearts. A number of drugs that block α receptors also possess this property. This might suggest either that the heart possesses α receptors or that some α blocking drugs can cause blockade of β receptors. In fact, there is no evidence that either of these conclusions is correct. The α blocking agents cause a reduction of the blood pressure and this itself exerts a beneficial effect in cardiac arrhythmias. In addition, many of the blocking agents exert a quinidine-like depressant action on the myocardium. The relative intensities of this action among different agents bears no relationship to their receptor blocking activity and some blocking agents do not depress the myocardium at all.

BLOOD VESSELS

One of the best known effects of the α receptor blocking agents is their ability to reverse the pressor action of adrenaline. In the absence of blocking agents, adrenaline and noradrenaline both cause the blood pressure to rise. After the α receptors have been blocked, the pressor effect of noradrenaline is reduced or abolished while adrenaline brings about a fall in blood pressure. The explanation is simple: adrenaline stimulates both α and β receptors in the blood vessels but noradrenaline only stimulates α receptors. After blockade of the latter, only the β receptors can be stimulated and adrenaline causes a transient increase in blood pressure (the result of cardiac stimulation) which is soon overcome by the extensive dilatation of the muscle blood vessels. The reversal of the blood pressure response to adrenaline can be produced by doses of an α receptor blocking agent which do not completely eliminate the effect of noradrenaline and in these circumstances the adrenaline response can be 're-reversed' to a pressor effect by administration of a drug which blocks the adrenaline β receptors.

The extent of the depressor response to adrenaline after α receptor blockade varies with the species and with the depth of anaesthesia. The blood vessels in the muscles of some animals such as the rabbit are but poorly supplied with adrenaline β receptors. Cats and dogs, on the other hand, give a good depressor response provided that they are not too deeply anaesthetized. Deep anaesthesia causes a maximal dilatation of blood vessels and depressor responses can therefore not be demonstrated. For the same reason a hypotensive response to adrenaline cannot be elicited in spinal animals.

In cats and dogs whose α receptors have been blocked, stimulation of the sympathetic nerves sometimes causes a fall in blood pressure. This is not an effect of stimulation of β receptors, since the sympathetic nerves liberate only noradrenaline. The response represents an unmasking of the effects of sympathetic vasodilator fibres. These fibres are cholinergic in type. Like the adrenaline β receptors in muscle arterioles, these cholinergic fibres are plentiful only in those species (including man) which can undertake vigorous physical activity.

Blockade of the α receptors in the conscious animal which has received no other drug will cause a fall of blood pressure to an extent dependent on the prevailing degree of sympathetic tone. However, with some drugs, this effect is overwhelmed by direct actions on the blood vessels. The naturally occurring ergot alkaloids, for instance, have a direct vasoconstrictor action.

Compensatory pressor reflexes, such as those that

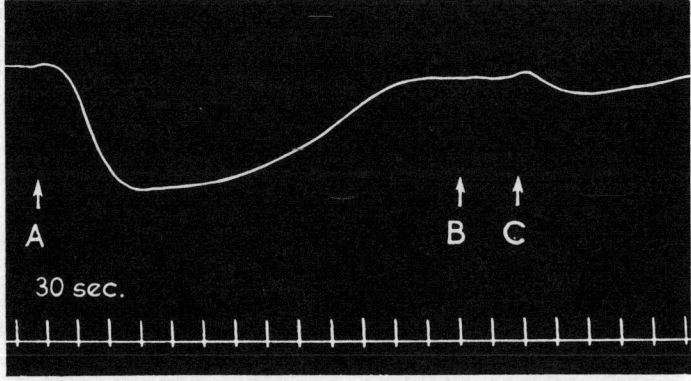

Fig. 18.2 Inhibition by phentolamine of the vasoconstrictor action of adrenaline on the blood vessels of the rats hindquarters. Injections were made into the injection cannula as follows: A 1 μg of adrenaline; B 0.5 μg of phentolamine, C 1 μg of adrenaline. The apparatus used to obtain the record is shown in Fig. 40.9, p. 707.

prevent postural hypotension are mediated by way of sympathetic nerves. They cannot occur in animals given full doses of α receptor blocking drugs. The pressor effect of nicotine is also prevented by blockade of α receptors.

The effect of an α receptor blocking drug on the vasoconstrictor action of adrenaline in the rat hind quarters is illustrated in Fig. 18.2.

OTHER SMOOTH MUSCLE

In the resting state, both the parasympathetic and sympathetic nerves to the iris exhibit some tone. Administration of an α receptor blocking agents therefore causes some pupillary constriction. The fact that the responses to parasympathetic stimulation remain unaffected allows some pupillary responses (constriction in bright light, for instance) to be partially retained.

In the cat, contractions of the nictitating membrane is inhibited by blockade of α receptors (Fig. 18.3) Adrenaline receptors in intestinal muscle are of both types (p. 267) and α receptor blocking agents only partially antagonize the inhibitory actions of adrenaline or noradrenaline. Some of the blocking drugs have motor or inhibitory effects independently of their ability to block the receptors.

Both types of blocking agent inhibit the reuptake of noradrenaline by adrenergic nerve endings. This inhibition of uptake has the curious consequence that the administration of one type of blocking agent increases the response to stimulation of the other type of receptor. Thus phenoxybenzamine, an α blocking agent, increases the effect of noradrenaline on the rate of spontaneous contraction of isolated rabbit atria (Stafford, 1963).

The central nervous system. Interpretation of the actions of these drugs on the central nervous system is complicated by uncertainties concerning the nature and distribution of adrenaline receptors in the central nervous system, and the

permeability of the blood brain barrier to the drugs. The central effects of individual drugs are mentioned when the drug itself is discussed in the succeeding sections.

Drugs that block adrenaline α receptors fall into the following classes:

   i) the ergot alkaloids
   ii) the 2-haloalkylamines
   iii) the imidazolines
   iv) the benzodioxans
   v) the dibenzapepines
   vi) other compounds

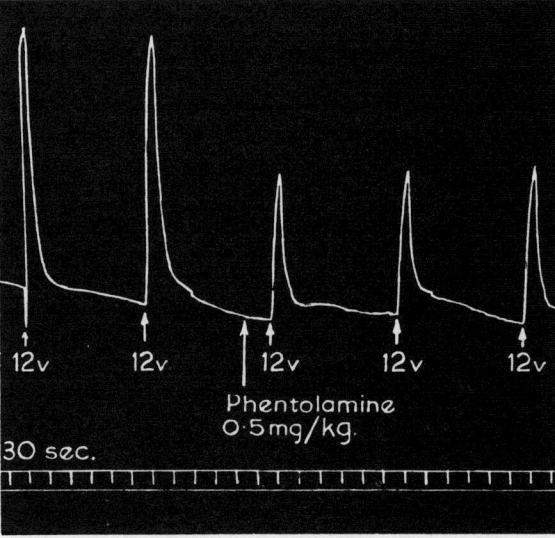

Fig. 18.3 The effect of intravenous phentolamine on the response of the nictitating membrane of the cat to electrical stimulation of preganglionic fibres of the cervical sympathetic. The vertical arrows indicate the points at which stimulation began. The stimulus intensity was 12 volts.

THE ERGOT ALKALOIDS

Ergot is a fungus (*Claviceps purpurea*) to which rye is particularly susceptible. The fungal growths on the rye are of a purple colour. The eating of bread made from contaminated rye was responsible in the past for many outbreaks of *ergotism* in those parts of the world where the grain was extensively cultivated. The knowledge that it is dangerous to eat infected rye and the relative ease with which the fungus can be recognized, have served almost to eliminate ergotism but sporadic outbreaks still occur—there was one in France as recently as 1951.

The effects of ergotism are alarming and explain why the disease was once regarded with superstitious dread. The most usual symptom of ergotism was gangrene which was a consequence of vasoconstriction and which resulted in fingers, toes or whole limbs becoming dried, shrivelled and black so that they sometimes fell off. The nerves to the limbs also suffered lack of nourishment because of the inadequacy of the circulation (and perhaps also to a concomitant vitamin deficiency) with the result that the victim experienced sensations of tingling and intense burning in the extremities. It was for this reason (and perhaps also because the blackened limbs appeared to have been charred by fire) that ergotism was popularly known as St Anthony's fire. St Anthony's name was attached because it was believed that pilgrims to his shrine would be cured of their affliction. This promise did not go entirely unfulfilled, for the act of pilgrimage ensured that the victim left the area in which the infected rye was growing.

Ergotism is also associated with the occurrence of spontaneous abortions and with disturbances of central nervous function, including convulsions and acute mania.

The relative intensity of the three major manifestations of ergotism—gangrene, abortion and mania—varied from one outbreak to another. The most recent one, to which reference has already been made, occurred in the small French town of Pont St Esprit in the Rhone valley and many of its victims suffered terrifying hallucinations or bizarre disturbances of thought which drove them to reckless or pointless acts of a type they would never contemplate when in their right minds. A detailed account of their sufferings and of the events that led up to and followed the outbreak is provided by Fuller (1968). Although it is the work of a layman, Fuller's book paints a vivid picture of the impact made by a powerful hallucinogenic agent on the minds of a population that was completely unprepared for, and largely ignorant of the likely effects of, an attack by hallucinogens of the type found in ergot. It must be remembered that the vast majority of those who take hallucinogenic agents do so on an experimental basis and the reports they present of the effects of the substances they have taken (and even, perhaps, their actual experiences) are inevitably coloured by their own previous knowledge and expectations.

Ergot is one of the most remarkable of all organisms. A wide range of pharmacologically active substances including several whose actions are of the greatest interest to the academic pharmacologist, can be extracted from this unpleasant little fungus.

The constituents of ergot with pharmacological interest can be divided into two main groups. The first group is composed of substances which are not specific to ergot and it includes acetylcholine, histamine, tyramine, isoamylamine, ergothioneine, ergosterone and a miscellaneous collection of other compounds of less immediate interest. The compounds in the second group are peculiar to ergot. They are all derivatives of lysergic acid (the name of this substance indicates its origin) and they are known collectively as the ergot alkaloids. In the context of the present chapter, the importance of the ergot alkaloids lies in the fact that nearly all of them cause blockade of adrenaline α receptors. They have a number of other actions which are dissociated from their ability to block the receptors but all their actions are considered together here. This is not only convenient but it also helps to emphasize the fact, which is sometimes forgotten, that it is not correct simply to classify the ergot alkaloids as α receptor blocking agents.

In 1906, Barger and Carr isolated a crystalline substance from ergot. Believing that they had obtained a single substance and that it was responsible for the symptoms of ergotism they called it ergotoxine. It later became clear that ergotoxine was a mixture of alkaloids but before the individual components of this mixture were identified, three other alkaloids were extracted from ergot. They were all shown to be single substances. The first, isolated by Stoll in 1920, was called *ergotamine*. The second alkaloid was isolated independently and almost simultaneously in several laboratories in 1936. It received a number of names—ergometrine, ergosterine, ergobasine and ergotocine. Of these names, only *ergometrine* is now used but in the United States the compound is known officially as ergonovine. The next alkaloid to be isolated and identified was *ergosine*. The constituents of ergotoxine were identified in 1943 by Stoll and Hofmann as *ergocristine, ergocryptine* and *ergocornine*.

The ergot alkaloids are optically active, the L isomer being the pharmacologically active form. The D isomers, which have no biological activity, are named by adding the suffix -ine: thus ergotaminine is D-ergotamine. The laevorotatory compounds are not very stable and they are readily converted into the inactive form in solution.

The chemical formulae of the ergot alkaloids are set out in Figure 18.4. It will be seen that ergometrine is an amide of lysergic acid while the other five naturally occurring compounds are amino acid alkaloids of lysergic acid.

The range of ergot alkaloids has been extended by the production of a number of semi-synthetic derivatives. These are of two types. In one, the double bond indicated in Figure 18.4 in the lysergic acid moiety of the molecule, is saturated to produce dihydrogenated compounds, the

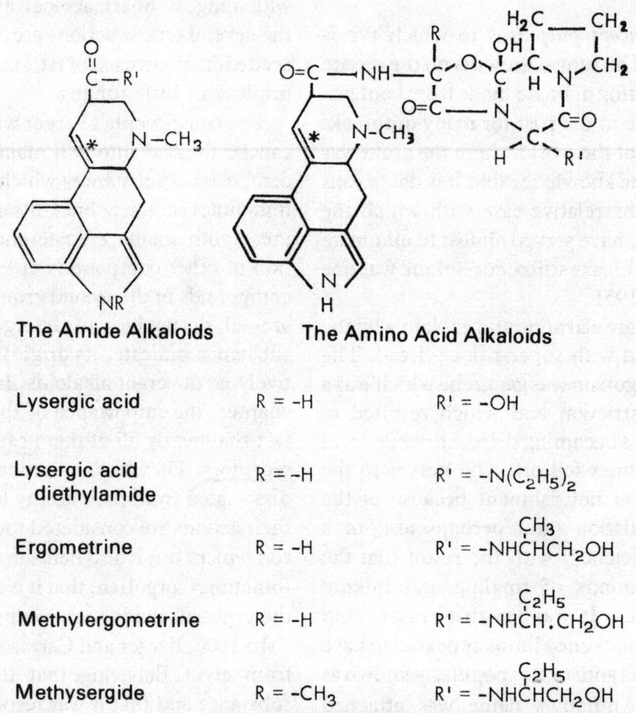

The Amide Alkaloids

The Amino Acid Alkaloids

Lysergic acid	R = –H	R' = –OH
Lysergic acid diethylamide	R = –H	R' = –N(C$_2$H$_5$)$_2$
Ergometrine	R = –H	R' = –NHCHCH$_2$OH (CH$_3$)
Methylergometrine	R = –H	R' = –NHCH.CH$_2$OH (C$_2$H$_5$)
Methysergide	R = –CH$_3$	R' = –NHCHCH$_2$OH (C$_2$H$_5$)

The Amide Alkaloids

Ergotamine,	R = –CH$_3$,	R' = –CH$_2$⬡
Ergocornine,	R = –CH(CH$_3$)$_2$,	R' = –CH(CH$_3$)$_2$.
Ergocristine,	R = –CH(CH$_3$)$_2$,	R' = –CH$_2$⬡
Ergocryptine,	R = –CH(CH$_3$)$_2$,	R' = –CH$_2$–CH(CH$_3$)$_2$.
Ergosine,	R = –CH$_3$	R' = –CH$_2$–CH(CH$_3$)$_2$.

The Amino Acid Alkaloids

Fig. 18.4 The ergot alkaloids. The double bond marked with an asterisk* is the one which is saturated in the dihydro derivatives.

names of which are obtained by adding the prefix 'dihydro-' to that of the corresponding alkaloids. Dihydrogenated derivatives of all the naturally occurring ergot alkaloids have been prepared. The second type of semisynthetic compound is obtained by combining lysergic acid with an amine. They are thus analogous to ergometrine. They include lysergic acid diethylamide, methylergometrine (methylergonovine) and methysergide.

It is possible to provide a brief summary of the main properties of all the ergot alkaloids by dividing them into three groups as follows:

(a) the naturally occurring amino acid alkaloids. They are powerful constrictor agents and they also cause a powerful but delayed contraction of the uterus. They block adrenaline α receptors

(b) the dihydrogenated derivatives of the amino acid alkaloids are much less active vasoconstrictor and oxytocic agents but they are more effective blockers of adrenaline receptors

(c) the amide alkaloids, both natural and semisynthetic, cause an immediate and powerful contraction of the uterus but they have little action on blood vessels and none on adrenaline receptors.

Mention should also be made here of bromocriptine, a derivative of ergocryptine, with interesting therapeutic possibilities. The drug is discussed in full on p. 777.

All the ergot alkaloids antagonize the action of 5-hydroxytryptamine and in some instances (lysergic acid diethylamide and methysergide, for example) the pharmacological activity is dominated by this effect.

ERGOTAMINE AND DIHYDROERGOTAMINE

Ergotamine is the most extensively used member of the group of amino acid alkaloids. It is a powerful vasoconstrictor agent and it finds its chief use, usually as the tartrate, in the treatment of migraine (p. 418). Ergotamine is poorly absorbed from the gastrointestinal tract and it is most effective when it is given by subcutaneous injection in doses of 0.25 to 0.50 mg or more depending on the severity of the attack. Subcutaneous injection is not, however, a convenient route for self medication and ergotamine can be taken sublingually or by mouth. The oral dosage is 2 to 4 mg followed, if necessary, by 2 mg doses every hour until relief is obtained or until a total of 10 mg of the drug has been taken. Ergotamine is also available in rectal suppositories, which provide a convenient preparation for patients whose migraine is associated with severe vomiting. Caffeine increases the effectiveness of ergotamine in migraine, partly because of its own constrictor action on the cerebral vessels and partly because it promotes the absorption of ergotamine from the alimentary tract. A proprietary preparation (Cafergot) combines ergotamine tartrate (1 mg.) and caffeine (100 mg.) in the same tablet. Proprietary preparations of ergotamine tartrate without caffeine include Femergin, Gyneran, Gynergen and Lingraine. Histamine H_1 antagonists are sometimes added to ergotamine and caffeine in an attempt still further to improve the effectiveness of the mixture. Proprietary preparations of this type include Ergodryl and Migril which contain diphenhydramine and cyclizine respectively.

The gangrene of ergotism is due largely to ergotamine which, as well as causing vasoconstriction, can produce actual damage to the capillaries and to the tunica intima of small arteries and arterioles. The use of ergotamine is therefore contraindicated in patients with degenerative disease of the arteries. The generalized vasoconstrictor action of ergotamine also renders it unsuitable for use in those with evidence of coronary disease. Ergotamine treatment should be discontinued if it causes anginal pain even in subjects who have not previously exhibited symptoms of cardiac insufficiency. Gangrene is essentially the result of a nutritional defect in the tissues and it occurs most readily in patients with metabolic disorders such as diabetes mellitus or in those with kidney or liver disease. The occurrence of any of these conditions should therefore also be regarded as constituting a bar to the use of ergotamine.

The amino acid alkaloids cause contraction of the uterus and ergotamine should be withheld in pregnancy even though large doses can normally be taken before the uterus is affected.

Nausea and vomiting occur in a substantial minority of those who take ergotamine. This is an unfortunate circumstance in view of the frequency with which vomiting ushers in or accompanies an attack of migraine. It is mentioned elsewhere (p. 601) that the ergot alkaloids stimulate the chemoceptor trigger zone of the vomiting centre so that there is a risk of ergotamine's causing vomiting after administration by any route. Metoclopramide (p. 645) can be given to counter the nausea and vomiting associated with ergotamine use.

Because of the many limitations on the use of ergotamine, the effect of other ergot alkaloids on migrainous headaches was investigated and dihydroergotamine was found to be almost as effective as ergotamine itself. Dihydroergotamine has no action on the uterus and it is a much less powerful vasoconstrictor agent. It is given at half-hourly intervals in oral doses of up to a total of 6 mg. By subcutaneous or intramuscular injection, the dose is 1 to 2 mg repeated if necessary in two hours' time. Methysergide (Sansert) has also been used with considerable success (p. 334). Methylergometrine (Methergine) is effective in some patients and clonidine (p. 310) enjoys some popularity among migraine sufferers.

Dihydroergotamine, methysergide and methylergometrine are all less powerful vasoconstrictor agents than ergotamine while clonidine has vasodilator activity, and it has been suggested by some that drugs which relieve the pain of migraine do not, as is usually supposed, do so entirely by virtue of their vasoconstrictor action. Nevertheless, there is much to support the view that the underlying cause of migraine is extracranial vasodilatation (p. 418). All the ergot alkaloids antagonize the action of 5-hydroxytryptamine and it may well be that those which do not have vasoconstrictor activity on their own account antagonize vasodilatation or the pain caused by 5-hydroxytryptamine or other substances whose liberation is responsible for the migrainous attack.

Symptoms of a mild ergotism (such as a feeling of coldness or tingling in the extremities) are not uncommon in patients treated with ergotamine but, except in the circumstances enumerated earlier, these provide no occasion for undue alarm. Muscle pains may also be experienced. If the peripheral circulation is seriously interfered with, the drug must be withdrawn and it may be necessary to administer a vasodilator drug such as phenoxybenzamine (p. 299).

The effects of ergotamine on adrenaline receptors cannot be put to any therapeutic use since the consequence of blockade of the receptors in blood vessels is completely overcome by the direct vasoconstrictor action. Ergotamine can be used to provide an interesting laboratory demonstration. It has already been mentioned that agents that block α receptors convert the pressor action of adrenaline into a depressor response. Ergotamine, however, is capable of converting the depressor action of isoprenaline into a pressor response. In its presence, isoprenaline stimulates the cardiac β receptors but cannot cause vasodilatation because of the constriction imposed by the ergotamine.

HYDERGINE

A mixture of the methanesulphonates of the dihydrogenated derivatives of the alkaloids found in ergotoxine has been marketed under the name of Hydergine. Hydergine does not have the direct vasoconstrictor action of ergotamine nor, of course, does it stimulate the uterus. Its actions are largely the result of its blocking adrenaline α receptors and it has been used therapeutically in this capacity, as a vasodilator and antihypertensive agent. Claims that it improves cerebral blood flow and mental function in senile patients are not widely supported and the therapeutic value of the drug seems to be no more than minimal.

ERGOMETRINE

Ergometrine (ergonovine) is an amine alkaloid and its major action is on the uterus. It is virtually devoid of agonist activity on adrenaline receptors. Ergometrine is responsible for the abortions seen in ergotism but it is a less toxic substance than ergotamine since it has little effect on blood vessels.

The sensitivity of the uterus to ergometrine varies according to the physiological state of the organ. The non-pregnant uterus is fairly sensitive but, after a period of quite low sensitivity, the gravid uterus responds very readily late in pregnancy. Sensitivity reaches its maximum just before full term and is retained during the immediately post-partum period. In obstetric practice, ergometrine is most often used after the placenta has been expelled, although it may also be given immediately after the child has been delivered if it is felt necessary to hasten delivery of the placenta. Ergometrine arrests and prevents post-partum haemorrhage. It is also valuable for promoting involution of the uterus if this is delayed.

Ergometrine is given in doses of 0.2 mg. by intravenous or intramuscular injection. It can also be taken by mouth and this provides a convenient route of administration when the drug is used to promote uterine involution in an otherwise fit patient. The oral dose is 0.2 mg thrice daily: treatment may have to be continued for up to 12 weeks. Even under normal circumstances, involution of the uterus is not complete until about two months after parturition.

Methylergometrine (methylergonovine, Methergine) has actions and uses similar to those of ergometrine.

LYSERGIC ACID DIETHYLAMIDE

Lysergic acid diethylamide is a psychotomimetic drug and its properties and uses are discussed in detail elsewhere (p. 542) It does not occur as such in ergot but the fact that a simple derivative of lysergic acid has such striking effects on mental processes indicates the likely origin of the psychic disturbances that may occur in ergotism.

The 2-haloalkylamines

Among this group of compounds (of which more than 1,500 have been synthesized) are to be found substances that cause a more complete and long-lasting blockade of the adrenaline α receptors than any of the other blocking agents so far discovered. Dibenamine and phenoxybenzamine are the best known haloalkylamines but before the individual drugs are described it is convenient to consider the group as a whole.

The availability of so large a number of compounds of one type provides a unique opportunity for studying structure-action relationships and on the basis of such a study Nickersen (1949) concluded that only those compounds which met a few rigidly defined criteria were capable of blocking adrenaline receptors. Subsequent studies have substantially confirmed Nickersen's earlier conclusions. The criteria are as follows:

(1) The compound must have a halogen (other than fluorine) or an aklyl- or aryl-sulphonate group in the β position of the alkyl group of the alkylamine. This confers sufficient reactivity on the molecule to permit the formation of an ethyleneimmonium compound upon which depends the blocking activity of the parent substance (Fig. 18.5). Iodine and bromine provide more active compounds than does chlorine but compounds containing chlorine lose less activity during absorption from the gastrointestinal tract. The 2-haloalkylamines have a similar structure to the nitrogen mustards (p. 913) whose cytotoxic action is also attributable to the formation of ethyleneimmonium compounds. The 2-haloalkylamines have no cytotoxic action but the nitrogen mustards have some ability to antagonize the effects of adrenaline.

(ii) The compound must possess at least one unsaturated ring attached to the nitrogen atom. This increases the stability of the ethyleneimmonium intermediate. The unsaturated ring must satisfy certain steric requirements. In particular, any substituents in the ring must lie in the same plane as the ring itself. Thus compounds in which the ring substituents are groups such as isopropyl are inactive while those that contain methyl or methoxy groups are active. Substitution of a phenoxy for a benzyl group increases potency so that phenoxybenzamine is more active than dibenamine.

(iii) Most, but not all, of the series of compounds included in the 2-haloalkylamine group require a tertiary nitrogen atom as a prerequisite for blocking activity.

The blocking action of the haloalkylamines takes some considerable time (up to 2 hours) to manifest itself after the

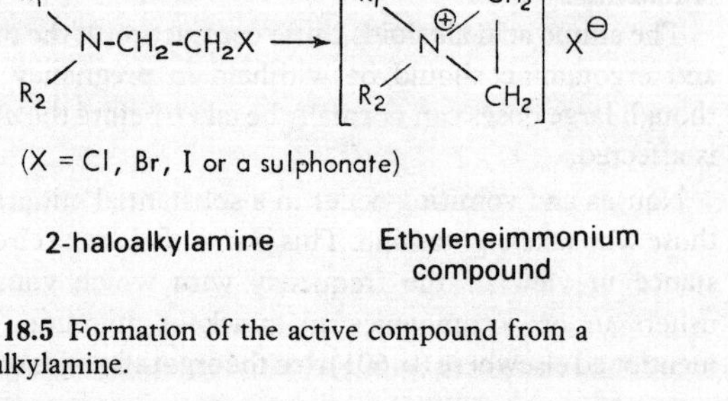

(X = Cl, Br, I or a sulphonate)

2-haloalkylamine   Ethyleneimmonium compound

Fig. 18.5 Formation of the active compound from a haloalkylamine.

drug has been administered, but once established it persists for several days. The long latency of the drug's action is attributable to the slow production of the active ethyleneimmonium compound. The long duration of action is partly the result of the compound's firm attachment to the adrenaline receptors. This firm attachment prevents displacement of the blocking agent by large doses of adrenaline or noradrenaline. Thus the receptor blockade produced by the haloalkylamines is essentially non-competitive although the features of a competitive antagonism can be recognized before blockade is fully established. The haloalkylamines are lipid soluble and the production of reservoirs of the drugs in body fat contributes to the prolongation of their action.

The haloalkylamines are not completely specific in their action. They have actions on the central nervous system which are not caused by blockade of adrenaline receptors and they all block histamine and 5-hydroxytryptamine receptors. Large doses prevent the muscarinic actions of acetylcholine. Although the haloalkylamines vary in their ability to cause blockade of these other receptors, some are quite potent: phenoxybenzamine, for instance, is a powerful an antihistamine as are many of the compounds classified as antihistamine drugs. On the other hand, so far as their action on sympathetically innervated structures is concerned, the haloalkylamines are highly specific in the sense that their action is almost entirely attributable to their preventing the access of sympathomimetic amines to the α receptors. One exception to this generalization is provided by the observation that some of them cause catecholamine release and hence a transient increase in blood pressure.

DIBENAMINE

Although dibenamine has little action on receptors other than the adrenaline α receptors, it is not used clinically. It causes local tissue damage if it is injected and it is virtually

Dibenamine

inactive when taken by mouth. In addition, it stimulates the central nervous system and may cause restlessness, nausea and vomiting. High doses have caused convulsions in experimental animals.

PHENOXYBENZAMINE

Phenoxybenzamine (Dibenyline, Dibenzyline) is a much more potent blocking agent than dibenamine. It can be given by mouth without causing gastric upsets, nausea or vomiting. Phenoxybenzamine has been used with some success in the treatment of Raynaud's disease, Buerger's

disease, intermittent claudication, frost bite and in other conditions in which blood flow through the limbs is restricted by spasm or obstruction of the arteries. The oral doses used for this purpose are of the order of 50-100 mg daily but treatment should be initiated with lower doses. Phenoxybenzamine has been used for the diagnosis of phaeochromocytoma (p. 274) but compounds with a less prolonged action are to be preferred for this purpose. On the other hand, phenoxybenzamine is valuable for the treatment of patients with inoperable phaeochromocytomas, for the pre-operative treatment of those who are awaiting operation and for the prevention of hypertensive crises that might otherwise occur as a result of catecholamine release caused by manipulation of the tumour during surgery.

Phenoxybenzamine
hydrochloride

Since drugs that block α receptors should theoretically have the same effect on sympathetic activity as ganglion blocking agents, it seemed likely that phenoxybenzamine, with its prolonged action, would be a useful antihypertensive drug. This hope has not been generally realized because phenoxybenzamine does not affect β receptors and its antihypertensive effect is offset by a compensatory reflex stimulation of the sympathetic nervous system which restores the blood pressure by its stimulant action on the heart. Nevertheless, phenoxybenzamine is not entirely useless in all hypertensive states. In small doses, it has been applied to the treatment of hypertensive patients who have become resistant to the usual antihypertensive drugs by reason of their arterioles having become hypersensitive to noradrenaline. It has also been given to terminate hypertensive crises in patients who have been injediciously withdrawn from clonidine (p. 311) or who have been unwise enough to eat forbidden food while taking monoamine oxidase inhibitors (p. 579).

Phenoxybenzamine has been used for the treatment of severely shocked patients. The idea that shock should be treated by producing vasodilatation represents a complete reversal of earlier practice. However, shock is characterized by excessive sympathetic vasoconstrictor activity and if vasodilatation is induced it encourages the restoration of blood flow to the tissues, hastens the removal of toxic metabolites from the cells, reduces the passage of water from blood to the extracellular fluid and promotes urine flow. At the same time, the action of the heart is not interfered with. For the treatment of shock, phenoxybenzamine is given by intravenous injection in doses of about 1 mg per kg.

It has already been mentioned (p. 293) that some of the drugs which block adrenaline α receptors can restore normal heart beat in patients showing cardiac irregularities and phenoxybenzamine has been used to suppress extrasystoles in patients under deep cyclopropane anaesthesia.

Side effects of phenoxybenzamine treatment include orthostatic hypotension, dizziness and failure of ejaculation. In contrast to debenamine, phenoxybenzamine has a depressant action on the central nervous system.

In view of its long lived action and the possibility of its storage in fat depots, the possibility that phenoxybenzamine may accumulate in the body must always be kept in mind.

The imidazolines

A large number of imidazolines have been synthesized and tested. They are remarkable for the large number of pharmacological activities they show. To varying extents they have histamine-like, sympathomimetic and parasympathomimetic activity, they inhibit monoamine oxidase, diamine oxidase and cholinesterase and they cause blockade of adrenaline α receptors. In addition, they may have other actions unrelated to these effects. Although not all of the compounds exhibit all these properties, it is equally true that none of them has only one type of pharmacological activity. Consequently, care has to be exercised when attempts are made to explain the actions of these agents and this is particularly so when they are being used in the laboratory to analyse the actions of drugs on adrenaline receptors. The best known imidazolines are tolazoline and phentolamine. Tolazoline has been the more thoroughly investigated. The blockade of α receptors produced by the imidazolines is short lived and easily antagonized by large doses of noradrenaline. Thus the block, unlike that due to the haloalkylamines, is truly competitive in nature.

TOLAZOLINE

Tolazoline (Priscol, Priscoline) is chemically related to histamine, to antazoline (an H_1-antihistamine), to naphazoline (a sympathomimetic drug) and to pilocarpine. In its properties, it is one of the most protean of the imidazolines and its ability to block adrenaline α receptors was only noticed some years after its other pharmacological properties were first described.

Tolazoline is a powerful vasodilator agent. This is only partly the result of its antagonizing the effects of sympathetic nervous activity since the drug causes vasodilatation in doses that are too small to prevent the vasoconstrictor action of noradrenaline. Moreover, it also causes vasodilatation in sympathectomized limbs. In the rabbit, tolazoline, like histamine in this species (p. 336) causes arteriolar constriction and a rise of blood pressure. These findings suggest, but do not unequivocally establish, that the direct

Tolazoline hydrochloride

vascular actions of tolazoline involve stimulation of histamine receptors. Tolazoline has other histamine-like actions: it stimulates the secretion of gastric juice and it produces an atropine-resistant contraction of the isolated intestine and uterus of several mammalian species. In the intact animal, however, movements of the intestinal tract brought about by tolazoline can be prevented by atropine and it must be concluded that under these conditions the drug is exerting a parasympathomimetic action. Among its other cholinomimetic actions, tolazoline stimulates the secretion of mucus, of saliva and of pancreatic juice, it causes bradycardia in the rabbit and it potentiates the action of acetylcholine on many preparations including some, such as autonomic ganglia and the frog rectus muscle, in which the actions of acetylcholine are nicotinic in type. Sympathomimetic actions of tolazoline include the production of tachycardia (in most species), an increased cardiac stroke volume and coronary vasodilatation.

Tolazoline is used primarily as a vasodilator drug in the same sort of conditions as those for which phenoxybenzamine is useful. It has also been used for testing the ability of the stomach to secrete gastric acid. It is employed for this purpose in the same way as histamine. (p. 641).

Because a direct vasodilator action is allied to the ability to block adrenaline α receptors, tolazoline is a much more powerful vasodilator than is phenoxybenzamine, but, as might be expected, it also causes many more troublesome side effects. These include flushing, shivering, 'gooseflesh', hypertension, tachycardia, anginal pain, headache, abdominal pains, nausea, vomiting and diarrhoea. Tolazoline is contraindicated in patients with peptic ulcer and in those with coronary arterial disease.

The usual dose of tolazoline is of the order of 50 mg, taken thrice daily by mouth.

PHENTOLAMINE

Phentolamine (Rogitine, Regitine) is a more powerful blocking agent than tolazoline but its other actions are less well marked. It does not stimulate the secretion of gastric juice.

Phentolamine finds its chief use in the diagnosis of

Phentolamine

phaeochromocytoma (p. 274). For this purpose a 5 mg dose of phentolamine is administered intravenously during a phase of hypertension. A sharp, though temporary, fall in blood pressure occurring within two minutes of injection is taken as a positive response and it suggests that a phaeochromocytoma is present. Phentolamine sometimes reveals the existence of a phaeochromocytoma in this way when other blocking agents give negative results. False positive and false negative responses are not uncommon and the patient should be subjected to other tests before a final diagnosis is made. In particular, the urinary excretion of catecholamines must be measured. Phentolamine is also useful for controlling the patient's blood pressure during the removal of a phaeochromocytoma.

The benzodioxans

A number of aminoalkyl derivatives of benzodioxan are powerful α receptor blocking agents. The names and formulae of the more important members of the group are presented in Fig. 18.6. The benzodioxans are short acting drugs which cause competitive block of the α receptors. In addition to their action on the receptors, they also have a direct action on smooth muscle. They stimulate the uterus, intestine, bronchi, blood vessels and nictitating membrane and they cause contraction of the coronary blood vessels. On the other hand, they cause a direct depression of the myocardium. The benzodioxans have a complex action on the central nervous system. They cause stimulation of the lower brain stem and hypothalamus and this accounts for the bradycardia (caused by stimulation of the vagus centre) which the drugs produce. Hypothalamic stimulation results in antidiuresis and hyperglycaemia. The benzodioxans also cause depression of the central nervous system and large doses may produce hypotension, analgesia and some degree of anaesthesia.

Like other drugs which block adrenaline receptors, the benzodioxans antagonize the effects of circulating catecholamines more effectively than the effects of sympathetic stimulation. Piperoxane (Benodaine), however, shows this difference to a much greater degree than do other blocking agents and it was this which led to the extensive use of piperoxane for the diagnosis of phaeochromocytoma. The fact that its stimulant action on the blood vessels produces a hypertensive response in the patient with essential hypertension contributed to its usefulness as a diagnostic agent, since blocking agents that do not have this action on the vessels, or which antagonize activity in sympathetic nerves more effectively than piperoxane, are likely to produce a false diagnosis of phaeochromocytoma in patients who are in fact suffering from hypertension. Unfortunately, piperoxane sometimes precipitated serious hypertensive crises in patients with essential hypertension and it has now been almost completely replaced as a diagnostic agent by phentolamine. Toxic side effects also preclude its use as a therapeutic agent.

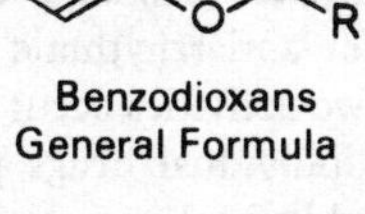

The side effects of piperoxane treatment include headache, hypertension, anginal pain, tachycardia, nausea and vomiting.

Dibenzapepines

The most active dibenzapepine derivative is azapetine (Ilidar). Its properties are similar to those of tolazoline. Thus it causes vasodilatation and stimulates gastrointestinal motility. Its histamine-like actions are less pronounced than those of tolazoline.

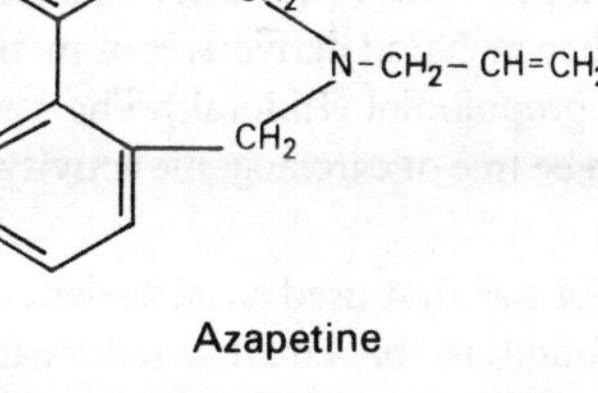

Azapetine

Other compounds

YOHIMBINE

Yohimbine produces a short lived blockade of the α-receptors and it also causes blockade of receptors for 5-hydroxytryptamine. If yohimbine is given to an experimental animal it blocks the response of the nictitating membrane both to sympathetic nerve stimulation and to injected adrenaline. As the effect of the yohimbine passes off, the nictitating membrane passes through a stage of hypersensitivity to the effects of nerve stimulation at a time when its response to adrenaline is still blocked. The explanation for this effect is probably that acetylcholine is liberated from the sympathetic nerve (p. 175) and that yohimbine temporarily increases the sensitivity of the nictitating membrane to acetylcholine.

**Benzodioxans
General Formula**

Prosympal (883F) $R = -CH_2-N(C_2H_5)_2$

Piperoxane $R = -CH_2-N$ 〈 〉

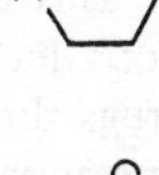

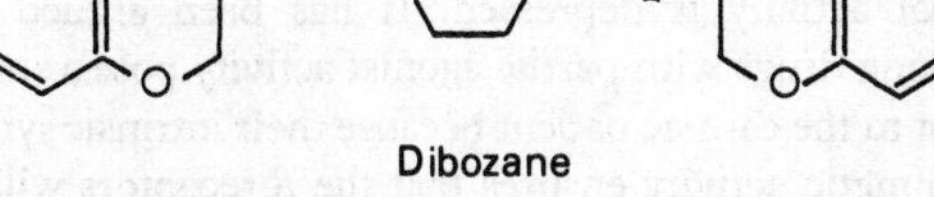

Dibozane

Fig. 18.6 Some benzodioxans

Yohimbine

Yohimbine has something of a reputation as an aphrodisiac. If this reputation if founded on any basis more substantial than optimistic faith, it is presumably attributable to stimulation of the central nervous system, to vasodilatation in the genitalia or both.

Yohimbine has an obvious chemical similarity to reserpine (p. 557).

CHLORPROMAZINE
Among its actions (p. 549), chlorpromazine has some degree of α receptor blocking activity.

Substances that cause blockade of adrenaline β receptors

The first β receptor blocking agent to be discovered was dichloroisoprenaline (dichoroisoproterenol) whose properties were first described in 1958 by Powell and Slater. In 1962, pronethalol (nethalide, Alderlin) became available. It underwent extensive clinical trials and was used therapeutically for a short time until it was withdrawn following the observation that it produced tumours of the thymus in mice. Two years later, other agents became available. They included derivatives of methane sulphanilamide and propranolol (Inderal.) The last named drug was found to be free of carcinogenic activity in experimental animals.

Propranolol was first used as an antianginal drug but it was soon found to be equally serviceable in cardiac arrhythmias. On the heels of these two successes, other uses (some of them, as we shall see, rather surprising) were found for the drug and β blockade soon established itself as a major therapeutic technique, a fate strikingly different from that which befell α blockade.

Propranolol's overnight success led, it need hardly be said, to a flourish of activity in the laboratories and to the emergence of a steady procession of new blocking agents some of which feature in Table 18.1. Reference to their formulae will make it clear that all the drugs have structural affinities with isoprenaline, the archetypical β receptor agonist.

Propranolol sometimes precipitates acute attacks of bronchospasm in sensitive subjects. This is presumably the consequence of blockade of the bronchial (β_2) receptors and hence the removal of tonic bronchodilator impulses. Because of this, attempts were made to find substances that would effectively block cardiac (β_1) receptors while sparing β_2 receptors. The first successful outcome of this search was the discovery, reported in 1968, of practolol. Practolol enjoyed wide popularity for some years until reports of its toxicity began to appear. These soon became too clamorous to be ignored and the drug had to be hurriedly withdrawn. The list of alarming conditions caused by practolol includes corneal damage associated with reactions in the skin and oral mucous membrane (the oculomucocutaneous syndrome), deafness, sclerosing retroperitoneal fibrosis (which gives rise to symptoms of peritonitis) and a state resembling disseminated lupus erythematosus. All these reactions are of immune origin. Fortunately other and (one hopes) safer cardioselective blocking agents (see Table 18.1) were waiting to step into the breach created by the loss of practolol.

It is to be noted that the so-called cardioselective drugs are not wholly specific. They are up to one hundred times more effective on β_1 than on β_2 receptors but it is by no means unknown for them to cause bronchospasm in sensitive patients. Nevertheless, the selective drugs are still to be preferred when β blockade is required in asthma-prone subjects because if bronchospasm does occur it can be readily relieved by a β agonist by virtue of the blocking agent's low affinity for the bronchial receptors. Propranolol and the other less selective drugs cannot be so easily displaced from the receptor sites.

Butoxamine has a greater affinity for β_2 than for β_1 receptors but it has not been used clinically because there is no known condition that responds to blockade of the β_2 receptors alone. Labetalol is unique in its ability to block α and both types of β receptor. Its properties and uses are dealt with later (p. 318).

Partial agonist and membrane stabilizing actions of β blocking agents. Table 18.1 draws attention to the fact that some of the drugs that block β receptors exert a degree of isoprenaline-like (or 'intrinsic sympathomimetic') activity and so qualify as partial agonists (p. 100) while some have membrane stabilizing effects that might be expected to confer antiarrhythmic and local anaesthetic properties. The two activities occur independently of one another so that individual drugs possess one, both or neither of these additional characteristics.

By its tonic activity, the sympathetic nervous system exerts an important control over the rate and force of the heart beat. This drive is particularly important in the diseased heart for without it the organ might fail completely. Drugs that suppress activity at β receptors are, therefore, potentially dangerous in patients whose myocardial activity is depressed. It has been argued that blocking drugs with partial agonist activity pose a smaller threat to the cardiac patient because their intrinsic sympathomimetic activity ensures that the β receptors will not suffer complete blockade. The argument is not a good one

Table 18.1 Drugs that block adrenaline β receptors

Approved name(s)	Proprietary name(s)	Formula or R in general formula: $R\text{-CH(OH)CH}_2\text{NHCH}\begin{smallmatrix}CH_3\\CH_3\end{smallmatrix}$	Partial agonist activity	Membrane stabilizing effect	Potency relative to propranolol	Plasma half-life (hr) after oral dose
		The early (now obsolete) compounds				
Dichloro-isoprenaline	—					
MJ 1999	—					
Pronethanol Nethalide	Alderlin					
		Drugs that block both β_1 and β_2 receptors				
Propranolol	Inderal Avlocardyl		0	++	1	3–5.5
Alprenolol	Aptin(e) Betacard Betaptin		++	+	0.3	2–3
Bunolol		$OCH_2.CH(OH)CH_2NH.C(CH_3)_3$				
Oxprenolol	Trasicor		++	+		2

Table 18.1 (contd)

Approved name(s)	Proprietary name(s)	Formula or R in general formula: $R\text{-CH(OH)CH}_2\text{NHCH}$ CH_3 CH_3	Partial agonist activity	Membrane stabilizing effect	Potency relative to propranolol	Plasma half-life (hr) after oral dose
		Drugs that block both B_1 and B_2 receptors				
Pindolol	Visken	OCH_2-	++	+	6	3-4
Sotalol	Beta-Cardone Sotacor	CH_3SO_2HN-	0	0	0.3	6-12
Timolol	Blockadren	OCH_2	0	0	6	
		Drugs that act predominantly of β_1 receptors				
Practolol	Eraldin	CH_3CONH- $O-$	++	0	0.3	6
Acebutolol	Sectral	OCH_2- H_7CONH- $COCH_3$	+	+	0.3	6-8
Atenolol	Tenormin	OCH_2- H_2NCOCH_2-	0	0	1	6-8
Metoprolol	Betaloc Lopresor Seloken	OCH_2- $CH_3OCH_2CH_3-$	0	0	1	3-4
Tolamol(ol)		$OCH_2.CH(OH).CH_2NH.CH_2CH_2O$ CH_3 $CONH_2$ (full formula)	0		1	

Table 18.1 (contd)

Approved name(s)	Proprietary name(s)	Formula or R in general formula: $R-CH(OH)CH_2NHCH\begin{smallmatrix}CH_3\\CH_3\end{smallmatrix}$	Partial agonist activity	Membrane stabilizing effect	Potency relative to propranolol	Plasma half-life (hr) after oral dose
Drug that acts prediminantly on β_2 receptors						
Butoxamine		OCH$_3$ ... CH(OH)CH(CH$_3$)NHC(CH$_3$)$_3$ CH$_3$O ... (full formula)	—	—	—	—
Drug that acts on both α and β receptors						
Labetalol		H$_2$NOC ... CH(OH).CH$_2$.NHCH ... CH$_3$ CH$_2$.CH$_2$ ... HO ... (full formula)	0	+	0.3	4–6

and clinical experience has certainly failed to supply any evidence to sustain it. The wise physician who wishes to establish β-blockade in those with depressed cardiac function will not rely on intrinsic activity to protect his patients. He will use digitalis to maintain the heart's action.

In some circumstances the intrusion of partial agonist activity constitutes a positive disadvantage: in high doses, partial agonists may partly offset the antihypertensive and antithyroid consequences of β blockade and so reduce the drug's therapeutic effectiveness.

Drugs with instrinsic sympathomimetic activity will also stimulate β_2 receptors and the situation here is clearer than it is in the case of β_1 receptors for there seems to be little doubt that drugs of this type exert a useful degree of bronchodilator activity in bronchosensitive patients. On paper at least, the β-blocking drug of choice for asthmatic patients would combine cardioselectivity with intrinsic sympathomimetic activity. Atenolol possesses these qualifications but it has not yet been widely used.

The membrane stabilizing effect of β receptor blocking agents is of no clinical significance since it only appears with doses many times in excess of those used therapeutically. To quote a leader in this field: 'The membrane stabilizing action is only important because of the confusion that it has caused' (Prichard, 1977).

The ability to cause blockade of β receptors is invested in *laevo* rotatory isomers but membrane stabilizing effects are inhibited equally by *laevo* and *dextro* isomers.

Metabolism and pharmacokinetics. Aspects of the metabolism and pharmacokinetics of the β blocking agents that might to some extent determine the choice of drugs for particular purposes can be enumerated as follows:

a. Some of the drugs (propranolol, alprenolol, metroprolol, oxprenolol) are disposed of almost entirely by hepatic enzyme activity and, except in those with liver disease, they have a fairly short survival time in the plasma (Table 18.1). Others (practolol and sotalol) are removed from the body almost entirely by glomerular filtration and they have a much longer half life, particularly in the presence of serious kidney disease. The remaining drugs utilize both mechanisms and their half lives are influenced by the extent to which one or other mode of elimination is dominant. The plasma half lives of all the drugs are prolonged in elderly patients.

b. The bioavailability of modest oral doses of the drugs that are metabolized in the liver is low because the drugs are taken up from the portal vein and suffer 'first pass' elimination by the liver (p. 33). When larger doses are taken, progressively more of the drug reaches the systemic circulation.

c. Propranolol and alprenolol have a higher solubility in lipid than have the other agents and they therefore cross the blood brain barrier the more readily. This property may constitute a recommendation when central nervous effects are being deliberately sought for therapeutic reasons but a contraindication when actions on the nervous system might be the cause of unwelcome and unnecessary side effects.

d. All the ß blocking drugs are absorbed from the alimentary tract (some more effectively than others) and so can be taken by mouth. Intravenous injection is permissible in appropriate circumstances.

e. Some of the metabolites of propranolol and alprenolol (but not, apparently, those of the other agents that are disposed of by the liver) retain pharmacological activity and this may lead to some prolongation of the drugs' action.

Pharmacological actions of the blocking agents. Apart from their influence on membrane stability, the ß blocking agents exert few effects that cannot be attributed to their interaction with ß receptors. In the normal resting animal, there is little activation of ß receptors other than those in the heart. The pharmacological actions of drugs that block ß receptors are, consequently, unimpressive. The drugs come into their own when the receptors are pathologically stimulated.

Therapeutic uses of the ß blocking drugs. As we have already noted, more and more therapeutic uses have been found for these drugs in the course of the past few years. The impressive tally of conditions that have yielded more or less successfully to ß blockade follows with an indication of the pages in which the treatment is more fully discussed:

(i)   angina pectoris and myocardial infarction (p. 702).
(ii) cardiac arrhythmias (dysrhythmias) (p. 689).
(iii) hypertension (p. 318).
(iv) phaeochromocytoma
(v)   obstructive cardiomyopathy and dissecting aneurysm of the aorta
(vi) thyrotoxicosis (p. 717).
(vii) anxiety states (p. 569).
(viii) migraine
(ix) schizophrenia (p. 571).
(x)   drug withdrawal syndromes (p. 571).

Toxicity and side effects of drugs that block ß receptors. The alarming sequelae of practolol administration, to which reference has already been made, are apparently unique to that drug and need not be considered here. This account relates particularly to propranolol, the most widely used of the drugs that cause ß blockade, but the side effects of the other members of the group differ only quantitatively, when they differ at all, from those provoked by propranolol. All the side effects are referable to actions on ß receptors.

a. The possibility that attacks of bronchospasm will occur in sensitive individuals has already been discussed. The likelihood of this complication is least with cardioselective drugs that have intrinsic sympathomimetic activity.

b. ß Blockade can induce heart failure in patients with myocardial insufficiency who have not been protected against this eventuality by prior digitalization.

c. Other cardiac side effects include excessive slowing of the heart, impairment of conduction through the atrioventricular bundle and hypertension after large doses of blocking agents that are also partial agonists.

d. Skeletal muscles are equipped with blood vessels that carry ß as well as the more usual α receptors. Stimulation of these receptors by circulating adrenaline partly offsets the vasoconstriction that results from tonic sympathetic activity. In some individuals, the vasoconstrictor tone that remains after blockade of the ß receptors is sufficient to cause a serious reduction in limb blood flow and this gives rise to cold extremities, chilblains or even Raynaud's disease (p. 702). Unlike cardiac side effects, excessive constriction of the peripheral vessels is less likely to occur with blocking agents that possess intrinsic sympathomimetic activity.

e. Some patients taking ß blocking agents complain of vivid dreams, hallucinations or nightmares. Others suffer bouts of depression. Propranolol, which penetrates readily into the central nervous system (p. 305), is particularly likely to produce these side effects but they are not uncommonly induced also by pindolol.

f. Side effects attributable to the blockade of metabolic processes mediated through ß receptors are unusual but a few—disturbances of carbohydrate metabolism (appearing as either hypoglycaemia or hyperglycaemia) and potassium retention—have been reported.

g. Muscle weakness and cramps have occasionally been noted in patients receiving ß blocking agents.

LABETALOL
Labetalol which first appeared in 1971 is, at the time of writing, the only compound in clinical use that is a competitive antagonist at all types of adrenaline receptor.

Labetalol is more active against ß than it is against α receptors and it shows some preference for cardiac ($ß_1$) receptors (Symposium, 1976). Like some other ß receptor antagonists it has membrane stabilizing properties at high dose levels but it is devoid of partial agonist activity. Labetalol does not exhibit the additional pharmacological activity that is characteristic of so many other drugs that effect blockade of α receptors but it does prevent the reuptake of noradrenaline into sympathetic nerve terminals. In this respect it resembles all the other α receptor antagonists save prazosin (p. 312).

Labetalol is readily absorbed from the gastrointestinal tract. It is bound to plasma protein to the extent of about 50 per cent and has a plasma half life of some four to six hours. About two thirds of an administered dose appears in the urine largely as conjugates. One such conjugate is the O-phenylglucuronide but the major conjugate in man has yet to be identified. Metabolism to hydroxylabetalol occurs in some animals but only to a trivial extent in man. Drug that does not appear in the urine is excreted in the faeces after passage into the bile. Uptake into, and conjugation by, the liver is associated with a considerable first pass elimination of labetalol.

Because it prevents the effects of sympathetic stimulation on the blood vessels, labetalol has a hypotensive action that cannot be counteracted by cardiac reflexes because the β receptors, through which the reflexes would be mediated, are also inaccessible. For this reason, labetalol has been applied to the treatment of hypertension. Its status as an antihypertensive agent (which is discussed on p. 318) is the subject of current controversy.

Laboratory uses of the β receptor blocking drugs. Provided that the results are interpreted with caution, the β blocking agents can be used in the laboratory to determine the distribution of α and β receptors. It has already been pointed out that the presence of α receptors in the bronchi has been established in this way and other interesting examples are provided by the intestine and the uterus. Adrenaline causes relaxation of both these organs and its action on the uterus can be completely inhibited by drugs that block β receptors. For complete inhibition of the intestinal effect, however, it is necessary to apply both an α and a β blocking agent. Thus, it may be concluded that the inhibitory action of adrenaline on the uterus involves only β receptors while the intestine can be inhibited by stimulation of either α or β receptors.

A further pharmacological use for the β receptor blocking agents is in the analysis of drug action. Thus, both 5-hydroxytryptamine and histamine increase the force of contraction of isolated atria (Trendelenburg, 1960). The action of 5-hydroxytryptamine but not that of histamine is blocked by dichloroisoprenaline. It can therefore be concluded that 5-hydroxytryptamine operates by causing noradrenaline release while histamine does not.

THE SCREENING OF DRUGS THAT ANTAGONIZE ACTIVITY IN ADRENERGIC NEURONES

Since the activity of the sympathetic nervous system can be interfered with by drugs which act at many different points along the route from the central nervous system to the adrenaline receptor, the detection of substances that antagonize activity in the adrenergic neurone and the identification of their locus of action is not easy. It must be remembered that many of the drugs discussed in this chapter have more than one action so that, to take an example, a direct vasoconstrictor action of a substance which also blocks adrenaline α receptors may result in the drug's having a pressor rather than the expected depressor effect. It is impossible to summarize here all the experimental methods that are available for screening these

drugs and for determining the range of their actions but a comprehensive review of the subject is provided by Boura and Green (1964).

The nictitating membrane of the unanaesthetized cat provides a useful means of distinguishing ganglion blocking agents from drugs that act on adrenergic neurones or their receptors. A ganglion blocking agent causes relaxation of the nictitating membrane and dilatation of the pupil. Substances that block the receptors or inhibit activity in the postganglionic sympathetic fibres cause relaxation of the nictitating membrane without affecting pupillary size which is maintained by activity in the parasympathetic nerve. It will be recalled that the action of reserpine-like drugs appears only slowly and it may be necessary to administer the drug on several successive days in order to detect this kind of response. It will also be recalled that many of the drugs that block adrenaline α receptors are not very effective against noradrenaline released from sympathetic nerves and they may escape detection in this simple test.

Another useful preparation is the anaesthetized cat from which are taken records of the blood pressure, the heart rate and contractions of the nictitating membrane. Substances that prevent the liberation of noradrenaline will inhibit the response of the nictitating membrane to stimulation of the cervical sympathetic nerve. Unlike the ganglion blocking agents, they will be equally effective against both preganglionic and postganglionic stimulation. Drugs that cause blockade of the adrenaline receptors will also inhibit the response of the membrane but they are likely to be more effective against injected catecholamines. Drugs that act only on the nerves will of course have no effect on the latter response. Provided that the anaesthesia is not too deep and that the substance has little or no direct vasoconstrictor action, a drug which causes blockade of adrenaline α receptors will cause reversal of the pressor action of adrenaline but it will have no action on the heart beyond that which can be accounted for by reflex responses to the blood pressure changes. Drugs that block adrenaline β receptors will reduce or abolish the hypotensive action of isoprenaline. The action of isoprenaline on the heart will also be prevented. Ethylnoradreanline is another useful agent for detecting drugs that block β receptors. Ethylnoradrenaline acts on both α and β receptors but its action on the β receptors is predominant. It therefore causes a fall in blood pressure even though it stimulates the rate and force of the heart. After administration of a drug that blocks the β receptors, ethylnoradrenaline has a pressor effect and no longer stimulates the heart.

The conclusions reached by experiments on intact animals can be confirmed and extended by the use of isolated preparations exposed to the action of the appropriate catecholamines. Among such preparations are the perfused heart, the isolated atria, the perfused hind quarters of the rat, the perfused rabbit ear, isolated strips of arterial muscle, the isolated vas deferens and such conventional preparations as the guinea pig ileum and the rabbit uterus.

A very useful preparation for distinguishing between drugs that act on the adrenergic neurone and those that cause blockade of the receptors is the Finkleman preparation. It is particularly valuable for demonstration purposes. A piece of small intestine with its attached mesentery is removed from a rabbit and is set up in an organ bath. A piece of the mesentery containing a branch of the mesenteric artery and its accompanying nerves is placed between the jaws of a conventional electrode. Spontaneous movements of the intestine and their inhibition by nerve stimulation or adrenaline are recorded. A compound that prevents the action both of nerve stimulation and of added adrenaline is likely to be acting on the receptors. One that only inhibits the effect of nerve stimulation is exerting its action on the adrenergic neurone.

DRUGS THAT REDUCE ARTERIOLAR TONE

It is convenient at this stage to summarize the mechanisms that control the calibre of the resistance vessels (the arterioles), to consider the ways in which drugs can influence these mechanisms and to follow this with a discussion of the management of hypertension. Many of the substances which have to be mentioned are treated in detail in the earlier parts of this chapter or elsewhere; those which cannot be so allocated are described below (pp. 309-314). It should be emphasized that the first part of the present discussion relates to *all* the mechanisms that may cause relaxation of arterioles: it is not suggested that they are all necessarily capable of being exploited to produce potentially useful antihypertensive agents. On the other hand, the laboratory worker seeking the origin of an observed hypotensive effect must remember that it might have arisen by the operation of any one of these mechanisms.

The blood vessels are normally held in a state of tonic constriction by the activity of the sympathetic nervous system and changes in this activity are responsible for many of the fluctuations of vascular tone that occur in response to physiological demands. The activity of the sympathetic vasoconstrictor nerves is under the control of the vasomotor centre which is located in the fourth ventricle near the junction of the medulla and pons and in close anatomical and functional association with the cardiac and respiratory centres. The vasomotor centre receives and acts on information supplied from a number of sources. It is sensitive to the carbon dioxide and oxygen content of the blood passing through it and it is influenced by nerve impulses originating from other parts of the central nervous system (the other medullary centres, the hypothalamus and the higher reaches of the brain) and from the periphery. From the point of view of the physiological control of the blood vessels, the most important peripheral sources of information are the pressor receptors of the carotid sinus and the aortic arch. The corresponding chemoreceptors (in the carotid and aortic bodies) are also linked with the vasomotor centre but they are more important in respiratory than in vasomotor control.

A number of substances are capable of stimulating receptors located in the ventricles (particularly in the coronary artery bed), the atria and the lungs. Stimulation of these receptors results in bradycardia and vasodilatation. This reflex was first described by von Bezold and Hirt in 1867 but it was more completely studied by Jarisch and Richter in 1939. It is now generally known as the Bezold-Jarisch reflex. It is of much more interest to the pharmacologist than it is to the physiologist for it is not evoked by any of the known naturally-occurring blood-borne substances on which cardiovascular control normally depends. It seems likely that the receptors involved are proprioceptive in nature, signalling information concerning the pressure in the chambers of the heart and perhaps in the coronary and pulmonary circulations. Their stimulation by drugs therefore constitutes a purely pharmacological effect, albeit an important one, for many substances can be shown in the laboratory to activate the reflex and thus to produce some degree of bradycardia and hypotension. Some of them do so in therapeutic doses. When a drug produces a fall in blood pressure either as its main or as a side effect, the possibility that it is doing so by way of the Bezold-Jarisch reflex must always be considered.

It is now possible to enumerate the possible loci and modes of action of drugs that increase the calibre of the arterioles as follows (see also Fig. 18.7).

1 and 2. Depression of the hypothalamus and higher centres of the brain. Any depressant drug is likely to cause some relaxation of sympathetic outflow by an action on the hypothalamus or the higher centres. Many sedative drugs have this action and many antihypertensive agents have sedative properties.

3. Action on the vasomotor centre The vasomotor centre is sensitive to oxygen lack and carbon dioxide excess and a number of drugs modify vasopressor or vasodepressor reflexes that operate through the centre. α-Methylnoradrenaline (p. 289) and clonidine (p. 310) have this action.

4. Initiation of the Bezold-Jarisch reflex. The veratrum alkaloids (p. 309) provide the classical example of drugs that produce a hypotensive response through the medium of the Bezold-Jarisch reflex. This effect is sufficiently marked to have made the alkaloids once popular as antihypertensive agents. They are not now used for this purpose and none of the drugs currently favoured for the treatment of hypertension operates through this mechanism. Drugs

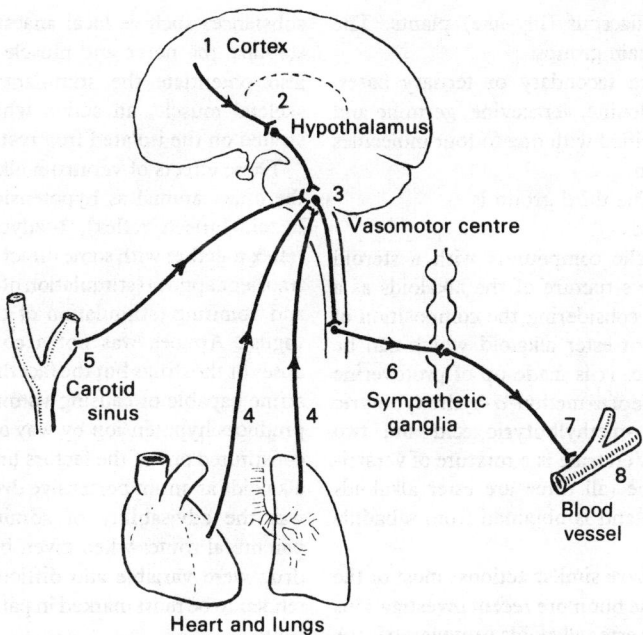

Fig. 18.7 Possible sites of action of drugs which cause relaxation of arteriolar tone. The numbers refer to those used in the text (p. 308-309)

which do evoke the reflex independently of their main action include thiourea (p. 716) and mephenesin (p. 248) the latter in therapeutic doses.

5. Stimulation of receptors in the carotid and aortic sinuses and bodies. The primary function of the baroreceptor mechanism of the carotid and aortic sinuses is to restore the blood pressure to its normal level by adjusting sympathetic outflow in the appropriate direction when the blood flow through the sinuses alters as a result of a temporary change in the local or general blood pressure. The veratrum alkaloids may stimulate the receptors as they do those in the heart but none of the drugs in current use noticeably affect the sensitivity of the pressor receptors, nor do they stimulate, to any significant degree, the chemoreceptors in the carotid or aortic bodies.

6. Inhibition of transmission processes in sympathetic ganglia. A number of substances inhibit activity in the sympathetic ganglia. They may do this

a. by preventing the synthesis or release of acetylcholine by the preganglionic nerve fibres. Triethylcholine, the hemicholiniums and botulinum toxin (p. 236) act in this way. These drugs have no therapeutic importance in the management of hypertension,

b. by preventing the access of acetylcholine to its receptors in the ganglion—the ganglion blocking agents (p. 252).

7. Inhibition of activity in the adrenergic neurone. These drugs have already been classified in the present chapter into

a. those which prevent the storage of noradrenaline—reserpine and its congeners,

b. those which prevent the synthesis of noradrenaline—α-methylDOPA, etc.

c. those which prevent the release of noradrenaline—xylocholine, bretylium, guanethidine, etc.

8. Direct action on the blood vessels. Substances in this category may cause arteriolar dilatation either

a. by preventing the access of noradrenaline to adrenaline α-receptors—phenoxybenzamine, prazosin, labetalol, etc.

b. by a direct action on vascular smooth muscle—nitrites (p. 699), papaverine (p. 705), hydrallazine (p. 311), diazoxide (p. 313), minoxidil (p. 312) etc.

It should be noted that a number of antihypertensive drugs owe their effectiveness to actions at more than one of the sites listed above.

Miscellaneous drugs

THE VERATRUM ALKALOIDS

Although the veratrum alkaloids are now outdated as therapeutic agents, they still seem to have a peculiar fascination for pharmacologists. It is true that the use of these agents has helped to unravel the nature of a number of cardiac and respiratory mechanisms, including the Bezold-Jarisch reflex, but this hardly justifies the excessive attention still lavished upon them by the writers of many textbooks.

The veratrum alkaloids are derived from members of a

number of genera of liliaceous (lily-like) plants. The alkaloids fall into three main groups:

a alkamines, which are secondary or tertiary bases. Some of the latter (zygadenine, veracevine, germine and protoverine) may be esterified with one to four molecules of an organic acid to form

b the ester alkaloids. The third group is

c the glycosidic alkaloids

The bases are polycyclic compounds with a steroid structure. An idea of the structure of the alkaloids as a whole can be gleaned by considering the composition of protoveratrine A, a potent ester alkaloid which can be obtained in the pure state. It is made up of protoverine esterfied with one molecule of α-methyl-α-hydroxybutyric acid, one molecule of α-methylbutyric acid and two molecules of acetic acid. Veratrine is a mixture of veratridine, cevine and cevadine (all three are ester alkaloids derived from veracevine) and is obtained from sabadilla seeds.

All the ester alkaloids have similar actions: most of the early studies used veratrine but more recent investigations have made use of the pure ester alkaloids protoveratrine A and B. Unlike the tertiary alkamines and their derivatives, the secondary alkamines do not lower the blood pressure but one of them, veratramine, is of some pharmacological interest because it antagonizes the increased heart rate produced by adrenaline or by stimulation of the sympathetic nervous system. It seems that this effect of veratramine is attributable to an action on the cardiac pacemaker.

The veratrum alkaloids stimulate or sensitize a variety of receptors and nerve cells outside the central nervous system, so that the cells discharge repetitively in response to stimuli that are ordinarily of subthreshold intensity. They have an analogous effect on striated muscle. It appears likely that they do this by increasing the sodium conductivity of the nerve and muscle membrane: as a result there is an associated loss of potassium from, as well as an increased entry of sodium into, the nerve and muscle. Consonant with this explanation of the action of the alkaloids is the observation that it is antagonized by substances such as local anaesthetics and calcium which stabilize the nerve and muscle membrane. The alkaloids also potentiate the stimulant action of potassium on skeletal muscle, an action which can be easily demonstrated on the isolated frog rectus abdominis preparation.

These effects of veratrum alkaloids show themselves in the intact animal as hypotension (from activation of the Bezold-Jarisch reflex), bradycardia (the Bezold-Jarisch reflex together with some direct action on the vagus nerve), transient apnoea (stimulation of vagal endings in the lungs) and vomiting (stimulation of the nodose ganglion of the vagus). Apnoea was not a complication of therapeutic doses of the drugs but the fact that the amount of protoveratrine capable of causing vomiting is close to that which produces hypotension by way of the Bezold-Jarisch reflex constituted one of the factors limiting the usefulness of the alkaloids as antihypertensive drugs. Another disadvantage was the advisability of administering the drugs by a parenteral route: when given by mouth the effects of the drug were variable and difficult to predict. Side effects tended to be most marked in patients given the drug by this route.

The amount of the veratrum alkaloids required to cause repetitive contraction of muscle is larger than that which will stimulate peripheral receptors. The effects on muscle can be simply demonstrated on the frog sciatic nerve-gastrocnemius preparation. If the muscle is treated with the alkaloids, stimulation of the nerve gives rise to a normal muscle twitch followed in succession by a partial relaxation, a secondary sustained contraction (the *veratrinic contracture*) and a slow relaxation. If the dose of alkaloid is large the initial partial relaxation is not seen, the myogram is smooth and the muscles do not relax for a considerable time. The description 'contracture' in connection with this phenomenon is in fact a misnomer. As has already been suggested, the sustained muscle contraction produced by the veratrum alkaloids is a tetanus.

Those interested in the veratrum alkaloids are referred to an authoritative review by Benforado (1967).

CLONIDINE

Clonidine (Catapres, Dixarit) is an imidazoline compound with structural similarities to tolazoline (a drug that blocks α adrenaline receptors but also has a direct vasodilator action), naphazoline (a sympathomimetic agent) and antazoline, an antagonist of histamine at H_1 receptors. It is hardly surprising that clonidine enjoys a wide range of pharmacological activities.

Immediately following an intravenous injection of clonidine there is a short lived increase in blood pressure. The view that this is the consequence of a direct stimulation of α receptors is corroborated by the concurrent appearance of other signs of sympathetic stimulation. In the cat, for instance, the nictitating membrane contracts.

The pressor response soon gives way to a more pro-

Protoveratrine A

Clonidine (hydrochloride)

longed fall in blood pressure. This may be partly the result of a blockade of presynaptic α receptors but a central action probably provides a much more important contribution to the depressor response. Doses of clonidine too small to have any vascular action when they are introduced into the general circulation produce a prompt fall in blood pressure when they are injected into the brain by way of the vertebral arteries. This hypotensive response is accompanied by a measurable reduction in the sympathetic outflow along the splanchnic nerves. It is abolished by guanethidine, section of the spinal cord and by blockade of central α neurones. An inescapable conclusion is that clonidine inhibits activity in the sympathetic nerves by *stimulating* central adrenergic (or perhaps dopaminergic) neurones. These neurones are located in the vasomotor centre and perhaps also in the hypothalamus.

The reduction in sympathetic activity is accompanied by a corresponding increase in parasympathetic tone. These reciprocal changes account for the bradycardia that is so prominent a response to clonidine.

When clonidine is taken by mouth the initial pressor response is not seen.

At high dose levels, clonidine has a guanethidine-like action but this is hardly likely to contribute to the antihypertensive effect of therapeutic doses of the drug.

Although the cardiovascular responses to single doses of clonidine can be adequately explained on the basis of the mechanisms that have just been discussed, it is by no means certain that the long term effects of the drug in hypertensive patients are entirely explicable in this way. An additional—or alternative—mechanism that might come into operation in these circumstances is a reduction in the response of the arterioles to sympathomimetic influences and substances (Zaimis and Hanington, 1969).

Clonidine has a number of chlorpromazine-like actions. Thus it causes sedation and hypothermia and it inhibits conditioned avoidance responses in experimental animals. It has, however, no useful psychotropic activity in man.

Clonidine inhibits salivary secretion by a central action. This is a rather surprising effect in view of the drug's ability to enhance parasympathetic nervous activity.

Clonidine is applied to the treatment of hypertension. Its effectiveness in this respect approximates to that of α-methylDOPA, the two drugs having similar modes of action. Postural hypotension is not a troublesome side effect because, with the modest doses usually employed, sympathetic activity is not suppressed so firmly that it cannot be aroused by afferent impulses from the barore-

ceptors. Side effects that can prove troublesome include sedation, dry mouth, allergic skin reactions and (less often) constipation and impotence. Although clonidine is said to reduce the output of renin by virtue of its effect on sympathetic activity, it not infrequently causes retention of sodium and water but this is easily countered by the contrary action of the diuretic agent in association with which clonidine is almost invariably given.

A particular hazard in clonidine therapy is the occurrence of a rebound hypertensive response, sometimes accompanied by nausea, vomiting and cerebral irritability, if the drug is withdrawn. Drugs such as phentolamine, which protect the α-receptors, should be given, if a hypertensive crisis of this type threatens.

Tricyclic antidepressant agents reverse the actions of clonidine and the two types of drug should not be taken together.

Clonidine attains peak plasma levels some 2 to 4 hr after oral administration. Its half life is about 12 hr. The usual dose is 0.1 to 0.6 mg three or four times daily.

Clonidine has also found favour in the treatment of migraine.

DRUGS WITH A DIRECT ACTION ON VASCULAR SMOOTH MUSCLE.
Some of the drugs that are employed exclusively or predominantly as antihypertensive agents are effective because they induce relaxation of the resistance vessels by a direct action on the vascular musculature. It is convenient to discuss these drugs here so that they can be separated in the reader's mind from substances such as the nitrites, papaverine and aminophylline whose direct action on the smooth muscle of blood vessels (and other organs) is exploited for other therapeutic ends. This latter group of drugs is considered separately (pp. 705-707).

Hydrallazine and Dihydrallazine These compounds have had rather a chequered history. Some years ago both were widely used in Europe and hydrallazine was popular in the United states but neither drug found favour in Britain. More recently, hydrallazine has lost some of its popularity in the United States but it has gained many advocates in Britain. It cannot be used alone because the dose needed to control the blood pressure over long periods is likely to give rise to the toxic side effects detailed below. In small non-toxic doses, however, it can usefully add to the antihypertensive effect of other drugs. Hydral-

Hydrallazine
hydrochloride

Dihydrallazine
dihydrochloride

lazine and dihydrallazine have essentially the same pharmacological actions but hydrallazine (Apresoline, Lopress) has been the more widely used in clinical practice. The American spelling of hydrallazine omits an '1'.

The mode of action of the phthalazine compounds is not well understood but it appears that they have a direct action on the blood vessels: they have been shown to cause relaxation of isolated artery strips and to antagonize the contractions produced in this preparation by adrenaline and noradrenaline. It may be that they chelate the trace metals on which the contraction of smooth muscle seems to depend. The drugs increase heart rate and stroke volume. This is partly a reflex response to the reduced blood pressure but the change in cardiac output is greater than might be expected from the extent of the fall in blood pressure and a stimulant effect on the medullary centres cannot be excluded as a possible contributory factor to the overall cardiac response. The increased cardiac activity partly offsets the depressor effect of the vasodilatation and it can precipitate anginal attacks in susceptible patients but this should cause no problem when (as often will be the case) a β blocking agent is given at the same time. Although single doses of hydrallazine increase renal blood flow out of proportion to the increased flow to other organs, this effect disappears with repeated dosing and hydrallazine is of no particular advantage in patients with advanced renal disease.

The phthalazines can cause nausea and vomiting, headache, tachycardia and nasal congestion. Plasma renin activity is elevated, with retention of sodium and water and a hypertensive response that partly offsets the antihypertensive effect of the vasodilator drug. This disadvantage does not appear if a diuretic drug is also given.

Chronic effects are more serious and include conditions that resemble acute rheumatism and disseminated lupus erythematosus. The incidence of rheumatism in patients taking the phthalazines reaches 10 per cent.

The reader will have noted that hydrallazine can only exert its full therapeutic effect when it is given in association with a β blocking drug and a diuretic agent. Analogous situations arise with some other antihypertensive drugs. Polypharmacy is evidently more to be desired than decried in this field.

Hydrallazine is readily absorbed from the alimentary tract and is bound to plasma protetins to the extent of some 90 per cent. It is rapidly excreted in the urine and has a serum half life of some three hours. Acetylation constitutes the principal mode of inactivation (some actually occurs in the intestinal mucosa during absorption) and it is a wise precaution to determine the acetylator status (p. 73) of those who are to receive the drug.

The initial dose of hydrallazine is 25 mg, given two to four times daily. This can be slowly increased, if necessary, until a maximum dose of 75 mg is reached.

Prazosin

Prazosin (Hypovase, Minipress, Peripress, Sinetens) is a new drug with unique properties. It occludes α receptors but, unlike most other agents of this type, it has no other pharmacological action. Extensive experiments have failed to demonstrate any direct effect on vascular muscle, on central neurones, on ganglia or on peripheral receptors other than α adrenoceptors. The specificity of prazosin extends even further than this because its blocking action is restricted to the postsynaptic receptors. The presynaptic α receptors are spared so that the feedback inhibition of noradrenaline release (p. 384) is not compromised as it is when any other α blocking agent is given. It is partly for this reason that the administration of prazosin is not attended by tachycardia and renin release to the extent seen with drugs that occupy the presynaptic receptors.

The vasodilatatory effect of prazosin is focussed predominantly on the arterioles.

Prazosin is readily absorbed from the gastrointestinal tract. Peak plasma levels are reached some two hours after administration and the plasma half life is about three hours. The drug is extensively metabolized by the liver, O-dealkylation and glucuronide formation providing the principal routes of inactivation.

Prazosin

The therapeutic action of prazosin reaches its peak some 4 to 5 hr after administration and it is maintained for up to ten hours. These times are considerably longer than might have been expected from a consideration of the drug's half life. The discrepancy is probably a reflection of the fact that prazosin has a predilection for blood vessels which retain it longer than do other tissues.

Prazosin is used instead of, or in addition to, β blocking drugs in the management of hypertension. The dose, given two or three times daily, ranges from 0.5 to 10 mg. Orthostatic hypotension sometimes occurs in the early stages of treatment but this usually becomes less troublesome as treatment proceeds. A few patients suffer a profound cardiovascular collapse after their first dose of prazosin. This so-called *first dose effect* can be avoided or minimized by initiating treatment with the lowest practicable dose and by giving the first dose at bed time. Other side effects include drowsiness, palpitations and, rarely, acute parotid pain. Although prazosin does not provoke renin release it does occasionally cause fluid retention.

Minoxidil

Minoxidil is so new a drug that it has not yet acquired a

Minoxidil

proprietary name. It is the most powerful of the directly acting vasodilators currently made use of in hypertensive therapy. Its principal seat of action, like prazosin's, is the arterioles. The arteries and veins are affected only minimally. The profound arteriolar dilatation evokes a reflex increase in cardiac output and the liberation of renin. If unopposed by concurrent diuretic therapy, fluid retention, sometimes of gross proportions, may follow.

Minoxidil has a plasma half life of no more than three hours but the effect of a single dose persists for more than twenty four hours presumably because—again like prazosin—the drug is retained in the arteriolar wall.

Minoxidil is employed only for the treatment of severely hypertensive patients who have failed to respond to the more usual antihypertensive measures. In these circumstances it can be most useful. It retains its effectiveness in the presence of renal failure. The therapeutic dose, taken once daily, is 10 to 40 mg.

Apart from the fluid retention already referred to, unwanted sequelae of minoxidil include gastrointestinal symptoms and hirsutism that can reach embarrassing proportions. Haemorrhagic lesions have been produced by minoxidil in the hearts of experimental animals and there is a suspicion that human patients may occasionally suffer in a similar fashion.

Diazoxide

As can be seen, diazoxide (Eudemine, Hyperstat) has close structural similarities with chlorothiazide (p. 632) but it is devoid of diuretic activity. Indeed, like the other powerfully vasodilator drugs, it induces sodium and water rentention and it has usually to be given in partnership with a loop diuretic such as frusemide.

Like minoxidil, diazoxide causes relaxation of arteriolar smooth muscle. The haemodynamic consequences (increased cardiac output and renin release) are similar and it seems likely that hydrallazine, minoxidil and diazoxide have a common mode of action related to their ability to interfere with the action of calcium or of other trace metals that play a vital role in smooth muscle physiology.

Diazoxide finds its therapeutic role in hypertensive crises in which life is threatened by an otherwise uncon-

Diazoxide

trollable rise in blood pressure. For this purpose, it is given by rapid intravenous injection. The response is immediate and the recommended adult dose of 300 mg can be repeated, if necessary, within half an hour. Once the blood pressure has returned to a manageable level, the effect of a successful dose will be maintained for up to twenty four hours. Rapid injection is mandatory if combination of diazoxide with plasma proteins is to be minimized.

Diazoxide should, ideally, be avoided in patients with an impaired blood supply to the heart or brain lest the sharp fall of blood pressure should result in a complete denial of blood to these organs. For these patients, sodium nitroprusside is to be preferred.

Sodium nitroprusside

Like diazoxide, sodium nitroprusside (Nipride)—$Na_2Fe(CN)_5NO,2H_2O$—is given intravenously to control the blood pressure in hypertensive crises. Its powerful action on arteriolar smooth muscle extends to the veins and this operates to the advantage of the drug since the increased capacity of the venous system reduces the return of blood to the heart. The resulting fall in cardiac output contributes to the antihypertensive effect of sodium nitroprusside which is, in consequence, the most powerfully depressant of all the drugs available for the restoration of normal blood pressure. Many other vasodilator agents, as we have seen, induce a reflex increase in cardiac output that partly neutralizes their antihypertensive effect.

Sodium nitroprusside owes its vascular properties to the nitroso group in its molecule. Its action is evanescent—the action of a single dose persists for no more than two minutes—so that it must be administered by intravenous infusion. Although this circumstance demands a continuous monitoring, it does make for easy regulation of the blood pressure and it is for this reason that sodium nitroprusside is to be preferred to diazoxide in patients with coronary or cerebral vascular insufficiency.

Sodium nitroprusside is decomposed into thiocyanate when it is exposed to light. Infusion bottles and syringes containing the drug must be covered with aluminium foil or some other light excluding material. Conversion to thiocyanate occurs also in the liver (after a preliminary transformation into cyanogen by the erythrocytes) and if nitroprusside infusion is continued for more than a day or two, the amount of thiocyanate in the plasma should be measured regularly. Because the drug is usually given in intensive care units with full laboratory support, this requirement can easily be met and there is no reason why toxic reactions should be permitted to manifest themselves. A concentration of more than 12 mg per cent of thiocyanate in the plasma constitutes a warning that the danger level is being reached.

The signs of thiocyanate poisoning include delirium and psychotic reactions. Less severe reactions—nausea, skin rashes, headache and feelings of anxiety and apprehension—are usually the consequence of too precipitate a fall of blood pressure and they can be remedied by reducing the infusion rate.

Angiotensin antagonists

Some forms of hypertension are associated with abnormally high concentrations of renin—and hence of angiotensin II—in the plasma. A number of substances that prevent the production or annul the effects of angiotensin II have recently become available although they have not yet acquired therapeutic significance. One such substance is a nonapeptide isolated from the venom of the pit viper. Known only as compound SQ20881, it inhibits the enzyme that converts angiotensin I into angiotensin II, the active form of the compound. Another is saralasin, an analogue of angiotensin II in which the aspartic and phenylalanine residues at the two extremities of the latter molecule (p. 358) have been replaced by sarcosine and alanine respectively. Saralasin occupies the receptor sites for angiotensin in vascular muscle and the adrenal cortex but it is itself devoid of agonist activity. Thus it antagonizes the action of angiotension II by competitive inhibition.

Saralasin is only effective when it is administered by parenteral routes and it is, therefore, unsuitable for long term use. It is, however, important as the potential parent of more useful drugs. Moreover it can itself be employed in a diagnostic capacity to determine whether a case of hypertension is angiotensin dependent.

HYPERTENSION AND ITS TREATMENT

Because stimulation of sympathetic nerves leads to vasoconstriction and a consequent increase in blood pressure, much of the effort devoted to the discovery of means of treating hypertension has centred on the development of drugs that will reduce sympathetic activity. The logic of this procedure is open to discussion but it is worth stressing at the outset that some of the most widely used of all antihypertensive drugs (the diuretics) have no direct action at all on the sympathetic nervous system.

Hypertension can be of primary or secondary origin. Secondary hypertension is a condition of elevated arterial pressure arising as a consequence of a recognizable pathological lesion. Among its more important causes are renovascular disease, diabetes mellitus, phaeochromocytoma and Cushing's syndrome. An increased secretion of aldosterone (aldosteronism) from any cause, enzyme deficiencies leading to an impaired production of cortisol (and hence to an increased secretion of adrenocorticotrophic hormone), tumours invading the juxtaglomerular apparatus in the kidney and pregnancy toxaemia are other conditions that can cause secondary hypertension. The continued taking of diuretic drugs (particularly those of

the benzothiadiazine variety) and of oral contraceptives can also provoke hypertension. Nevertheless, most cases of hypertension are of primary origin (essential hypertension), the arterioles becoming constricted as a result of the operation of as yet unidentified factors.

In some circumstances, secondary hypertension yields to the appropriate surgical treatment but in the majority of cases (when, for instance, both kidneys are affected by disease) specific forms of treatment are not available. In this event, secondary hypertension is treated in the same way as the primary condition except that, in the presence of kidney disease the physician must consider whether any of the drugs he intends to use may cause a further embarrassment of renal function.

In hypertension the calibre of the arterioles throughout the body is reduced, causing an increased peripheral resistance and an increase of diastolic blood pressure. The heart, having to operate against a permanently increased load, is exposed to conditions which, if uncorrected, may lead to cardiac failure. Organs such as the brain, the kidney and the eye, whose normal function depends on the maintenance of a copious blood supply, are also likely to suffer irreparable damage.

In some hypertensive individuals the amount of renin (and hence of angiotensin II) in the blood is abnormally high while in others it falls within or below normal limits. In many cases of secondary hypertension the origin of this difference is easily explained: tumours of the juxtaglomerular apparatus increase and hyperaldosteronism suppresses renin secretion. So far as essential hypertension is concerned, dispute still surrounds the questions whether the high plasma renin variety of hypertension differs fundamentally from the low renin type and whether the difference has therapeutic implications.

Four grades of hypertension are conventionally recognized. The approximate blood pressure corresponding to each of these grades are set out in Table 18.2

Malignant hypertension is a condition of gross and progressive hypertension associated with serious heart, brain or kidney damage. In almost all cases of malignant hypertension plasma renin activity is very high.

The diastolic pressure is of greater diagnostic significance than is systolic pressure. If the diastolic pressure is high, the systolic pressure must also be high but the systolic pressure may be temporarily increased in the absence of changes in the diastolic pressure. Systolic pressure is very susceptible to changes in cardiac output, which may undergo frequent and rapid fluctuations throughout the course of a normal day. The stress of a medical examination can cause a considerable increase in the cardiac output and hence in systolic pressure. Of itself, this rise of pressure is of no serious import, for as soon as the patient relaxes, his systolic pressure falls. Sometimes, however, the systolic pressure is permanently increased by an amount that is out of porportion to the elevation in

Table 18.2 Grades of hypertension

Grade of hyper-tension	Approximate upper limit of diastolic pressure	Likely systolic pressure	Retinal findings
	mm.Hg.	mm.Hg.	
Mild (borderline)	105	150–190	Arteries narrowed. Veins distended
Moderate	115	180–200	Thickened arteries compress veins at crossing points.
Severe	130	200–220	Flame shaped haemorrhages. Some exudation giving 'cotton wool' patches.
Gross	> 130	> 220	Above signs + papilloedema (oedema of the head of the optic nerve).

In SI units, pressure is measured in pascals (newtons per square metre) but clinicians still generally express blood pressure as millimetres of mercury, the units in which their sphygmomanometers are calibrated. One kilopascal is approximately equivalent to 7.5 mm Hg

diastolic pressure. This condition is of clinical significance and has implications for treatment.

Diastolic pressure is a measure of the pressure which has to be developed to enable blood flow to be maintained against the resistance offered by the arterioles. Diastolic pressure reflects the calibre of the arterioles: if these vessels are permanently narrowed, as they are in untreated hypertension, the heart will have to work against an abnormally high load all the time, even during sleep.

It is for this reason that discussions concerning hypertension and its treatment usually centre on the diastolic pressure.

The only part of the body in which arterioles are visible is the retina and the ophthalmoscopic signs which serve to confirm the grades of hypertension diagnosed by the sphygmomanometer are shown in Table 18.2. Papilloedema is diagnosed when the edges of the head of the optic nerve appear indistinct and by the finding that, when the nerve is in focus, the rest of the retina is blurred. Papilloedema is a consequence of increased vascular or extravascular pressure and it may arise in the course of several conditions (such as raised intracranial pressure caused by a tumour) other than hypertension itself: in hypertension papilloedema is associated with the other retinal signs noted in Table 18.2

It will be appreciated that the boundaries between the several grades of hypertension are drawn in a somewhat arbitrary fashion and that at the lower end of the scale it is impossible to delineate a frontier between 'normal' and 'abnormal' blood pressure: the blood pressure readings of a whole population form a continuum from the lowest to the highest. The appropriate treatment in an individual case cannot be determined in a mechanical fashion simply by assigning it, on the basis of blood pressure readings, to one of the categories of hypertension. Each case must be considered on its merits.

The treatment of hypertension

In the majority of cases, hypertension is symptomless and the condition is usually discovered by chance in the course of medical examinations for other purposes. It is not possible, therefore, to make completely accurate statements concerning the incidence of the disease, particularly since we cannot draw a firm line of demarcation between normotensive and hypertensive pressures. Reliable estimates, based on the results of well planned screening programmes and surveys indicate that, in developed countries at least, something like 15 per cent of the adult population have diastolic blood pressures greater than 95 mmHg. Whatever the true figure, it is evident that hypertension is one of the scourges of our time and almost every recent volume of every contemporary medical or pharmacological journal contains at least an article if not a symposium on the subject. It is not surprising, either, that a legion of drugs parade their attractions before the physician. None is entirely satisfactory if only because it is difficult to persuade patients to adhere to a regime that involves the life long taking of drugs, often with annoying side effects, for a condition that itself so often causes no symptoms at all. The physician has therefore to decide whether to treat the symptomless case of essential hypertension and, if so, which therapeutic measures he should adopt.

The question as to when hypertension should be treated is outside the remit of this book. Suffice it to say that the factors that have to be taken into account are the height of the blood pressure (the higher it is the more necessary it is to bring it down), the sex, age and race of the patient (males are more likely to succumb to the effects of untreated hypertension than are females even though blood pressures often reach higher levels in women; those under 50 are more vulnerable than older people; coloured races are more susceptible than white races) and the presence or otherwise of diseases of the heart, kidney or brain consequential on the hypertensive state. There is now general agreement that a successful reduction in the blood pressure of those with untreated diastolic pressures greater than 110 to 115 mm of mercury is rewarded with a reduced risk of illness or death from cerebrovascular accidents, renal disease and heart failure. The value of treating less severe grades of hypertension is still a matter of dispute.

It is inevitable, in a situation where a multiplicity of drugs is available for the treatment of a disease of varied and debatable aetiology, that opinions concerning treatment should differ. Nevertheless, the general statements concerning antihypertensive therapy that follow do represent a reasonably unanimous view. The reader needs to be reminded again of the importance of treating each case on its merits and that the choice of particular drug from a group of agents of equivalent efficacies is determined by such individual factors as the nature of any other condition from which the patient suffers, his relative susceptibility to the side effects of the different available drugs and the judgment and predilection of his physician.

Contemporary strategies in antihypertensive therapy involve beginning with the simplest form of treatment and progressively adding more potent drugs in the light of the responses obtained by the simpler regimes.

A number of reviews and monographs concerned with the treatment of hypertension and the mode of action of antihypertensive drugs are available. Among those to be recommended are included Berglund, Hansson and Werko (1975), Davies and Reid (1975), Prichard and Tuckman (1977) and Wollam, Gifford and Tarazi (1977).

1. First of all, the general measures detailed below (p. 317) are instituted. In some cases of mild hypertension, this suffices of itself to bring the blood pressure back to acceptable levels.

2. If a further reduction of blood pressure is sought, diuretic drugs are also given. Some authorities recommend β blocking instead of diuretic drugs at this stage, particularly for younger patients, but in this writer's opinion the higher incidence of side effects with drugs that cause blockade of β receptors leaves the advantage with the diuretics.

It has been estimated that one half of all hypertensive patients with a diastolic pressure of no more than 115 mm of mercury can be satisfactorily controlled by diuretic therapy and general measures alone.

3. If the blood pressure is still too high, the combined effect of the measures already described needs to be augmented by the addition to the programme of another moderately antihypertensive drug. The choice here is embarrassingly large but a β blocking agent emerges as the clear current favourite. α-MethylDOPA, clonidine, hydrallazine or prazosin can be employed instead, while even reserpine still finds a few advocates. Reserpine apart, no one of these alternative drugs can be preferred to another on the grounds of either clinical efficacy or relative freedom from side effects. Reserpine is (rightly) less popular than it was some years ago.

In the midst of current enthusiasms for β blocking agents the reader should recall the long list of possible side effects (p. 306) that may be experienced by those who take the drugs. Remembering the fate of practolol he should not be too surprised if, with the passage of time, these drugs lose some of their present reputation.

4. The drugs that have just been named as alternatives to drugs that cause blockade of β receptors can also be used further to augment the therapeutic effect achieved by the general measures + diuretic drug + blocking agent programme. Hydrallazine and prazosin seem to be particularly useful when paired with propranolol or one of its relatives.

If one member of this group of drugs has been given in the earlier programme in preference to a blocking agent, another can be added as a supplement at this stage. When this is done, the optimal response will be obtained if an agent that interferes with activity in the sympathetic nervous system (α-methylDOPA, clonidine) is paired with one (hydrallazine, prazosin) that has a direct action on the vascular musculature.

5. The programme just outlined may well prove ineffective in cases of severe or gross hypertension. In that event, recourse will have to be made to one of the more powerful drugs such as guanethidine, bethanidine, debrisoquine or minoxidil. Ganglion blocking agents (p. 252) were once popular in severe hypertension but they are now obsolete.

6. Hypertensive crises demand the institution of emergency treatment directed towards an immediate reduction of blood pressure. Suitable drugs for this purpose include diazoxide, sodium nitroprusside, phentolamine and phenoxybenzamine.

The possible uses of labetalol and pargyline are discussed separately later (pp. 318, 319).

It will be clear that some hypertensive patients will require treatment with a number of drugs. As we have already seen (p. 76) this form of polypharmacy is not necessarily to be deplored—diuretic drugs antagonize the fluid retaining proclivities of hydrallazine, diazoxide and minoxidil while β blocking agents prevent the reflex cardiac acceleration that might otherwise be produced by depressor drugs—but care must be taken to keep the treatment programme as simple as possible if the patient is to be encouraged to keep to it. It will be appreciated that it is foolish to adhere to a complicated programme of drug taking that just develops as a result of adding one agent after another to the programme without stopping to enquire at any stage whether any drug can be removed from it.

The modes of action of many antihypertensive drugs and procedures have already been discussed in detail in this and other chapters of this book. The following paragraphs fill in the gaps that remain.

GENERAL MEASURES

In all forms of cardiovascular disease, obesity is to be avoided: fat adds useless extra weight which has to be carried at the cost of an additional energy output by an already overworked heart. Particularly in cases of mild hypertension, a reduction of weight to a figure below that regarded as normal for individuals of the sex, age and height of the patient may have a more valuable therapeutic effect than any form of drug treatment. For reasons discussed below, it is often useful to restrict the intake of sodium but not to the point of making food unpalatable. Excessive indulgence in alcohol and tobacco should be discouraged. The patient should try to avoid situations in which he is likely to be exposed to continuous stress; a sedative may help to reduce over-activity of the sympathetic nervous system. At the same time, it is important that the patient should not be made too conscious of the state of his blood pressure. Cardiovascular disease is prone to precipitate a hypochondriacal state in its victims. The neurotic condition itself produces symptoms which the patient believes are indicative of a damaged cardiovascular system and he may rapidly develop into a permanent invalid, incapable of performing any useful work at a time when his physical condition really requires that he does no more than avoid dietary indiscretions or extremes of physical effort.

DIURETIC DRUGS

Diuretics are used alone or as adjuncts to other antihypertensive drugs. For most patients the diuretic agent of choice is one of the benzothiadiazine group of diuretic agents (p. 631); chlorothiazide, bendrofluazide and cyclopenthiazide given twice daily are equally effective. Alternatively, one of the longer acting members of the group, such as polythiazide, can be used. It is often advisable to initiate treatment with a low dose which is increased gradually.

In cases of renal failure, it may be necessary to prescribe one of the powerful 'loop diuretics', particularly frusemide (p. 629) and this drug may also be required in patients taking antihypertensive drugs that induce massive fluid retention (see above, p. 312) In those in whom it is important to avoid potassium loss, a potassium sparing agent such as spironolactone, amiloride or triamterene can be employed but the antihypertensive effect of this type of drug is so weak that it needs boosting by the concurrent administration of a benzothiadiazine.

The origin of the antihypertensive action of diuretic agents is obscure. It was at first believed that the reduction in blood pressure was a simple consequence of a diminished volume of circulating blood. This is unlikely to be the explanation: the blood volume and cardiac output do fall in the early stages of treatment but they soon return to almost their initial levels though there is no concomitant return of the blood pressure. Moreover, if the plasma volume of a patient who is being successfully treated with chlorothiazide is increased by an infusion of dextran, there is no marked increase in blood pressure.

It is known that sodium is involved in the control of blood pressure. In conditions associated with depletion of the body's sodium, the blood pressure falls and the renin-angiotensin mechanism for the maintenance of blood pressure operates at least in part by regulating sodium retention by the kidney. The benzothiadiazine diuretics cause an initial loss of sodium but, like the blood volume, the sodium content of the blood fluids soon returns towards its normal level. Nevertheless, careful measurements indicate that there is a permanent, if small, sodium deficit in patients receiving that thiazide diuretics. It is also known that the antihypertensive effect of these agents is nullified if sodium chloride is given. Taken in conjunction with the well-established fact they hypertensive patients benefit from a low salt diet, this evidence would suggest that thiazide diuretics owe their antihypertensive action to a promotion of sodium release (Tobian, 1967; Tarazi, 1973). It may be that the loss of sodium from the arterial and arteriolar walls is out of proportion to the loss from other tissues and that this results in the vessels losing some of their sensitivity to noradrenaline and perhaps other endogenous vasoconstrictor agents.

DRUGS THAT INHIBIT SYMPATHETIC NERVOUS ACTIVITY

Many of the drugs that have hitherto been used in the treatment of hypertension inhibit activity in the sympathetic nervous system. There is no evidence that essential hypertension is attributable to overactivity of this division of the autonomic nervous system or that the arterioles are excessively sensitive to the action of the sympathetic transmitter. However, blood vessels are usually in a state of tone caused by the activity of the sympathetic nervous system and it is not unreasonable to suppose that removal of this tone would permit some degree of relaxation even of blood vessels which were also under the influence of another constrictor agent. The validity of this argument rests on the assumption that sympathetic nervous activity continues unabated in the hypertensive subject and it might well be asked why the increased blood pressure, operating through the carotid sinus mechanism, should not reflexly inhibit all activity in the sympathetic vasoconstrictor nerves so tending to restore blood pressure to more normal levels. There is, in fact, no evidence that this occurs: it appears that in hypertension the carotid sinus mechanism is 'set' at a higher level so that blood pressure adjustments operate to a base line higher than that in normotensive subjects. It may be that this resetting of the base line is a simple adaptive response to the changed conditions: in other words, if the primary aetiological event takes place in the blood vessels, elevation of the blood pressure is necessary if the circulation is to continue normally. Thus, if the carotid sinus is to continue to subserve a regulatory function it must operate to a higher base line. On the other hand, there is at least a possibility that the 'resetting' of the carotid sinus is the primary event and that the cause of essential hypertension should be sought in the activity of the vascular pressor receptors. Whatever the basic disturbance may be, it is clear that there is some point in attemtping to induce vascular relaxation by inhibiting sympathetic nervous activity.

The modes of action of most of the drugs that oppose the influence of the sympathetic nervous system have already been considered. Only the β receptor blocking agents, labetalol and pargyline remain for discussion.

β Blocking agents

Although there were, apparently, sound theoretical reasons for believing that propranolol would be useless for the control of blood pressure, clinical experience has confounded that view. Since Prichard (1968) first used the drug, propranolol and other members of its family have grown steadily in importance and popularity.

Because it causes blockade of β receptors, propranolol reduces the cardiac output and it was at first believed that this action provided the key to its antihypertensive action. Those who took this point of view maintained that propranolol was effective only in hypertensive patients whose condition was characterized, and perhaps caused, by an increased cardiac output. There is, however, no evidence either that the drug's usefulness is limited in this way or that hypertension ever arises elsewhere than in the resistance vessels. This hypothesis was succeeded by the inherently more reasonable one that propranolol, by rendering β receptors inaccessible to adrenaline prevented the liberation of renin. It is generally accepted that this event is at least partly mediated by way of β receptors. Propranolol does indeed depress plasma renin concentrations but some related drugs such as pindolol and atenolol whose antihypertensive efficacy is in no way inferior to that of propranolol leave unaffected the amount of renin in the plasma. Moreover, propranolol is not noticeably more effective in patients with high renin hypertension than it is in those who fall into the low renin category. Finally, doses of

propranolol just sufficient to normalize plasma renin activity are often below the threshold for antihypertensive activity.

More recently a cause for the antihypertensive effect of propranolol has been sought in the central nervous system. Propranolol has useful sedative and 'anxiolytic' properties (p. 569) and this must at least make a contribution to its therapeutic effect. That it cannot provide the whole explanation is evident from the fact that practolol and sotalol, which cannot surmount the blood brain barrier are nevertheless effective antihypertensive agents.

The full antihypertensive effect of propranolol and its congeners does not appear until treatment has been kept up for some weeks and it has been suggested that during this period the baroreceptors are being 'reset' at a lower level. The implication is that the blood pressure is reduced during the early stages of treatment by one of the mechanisms already discussed (or by a different one) and that this is later maintained and intensified by reason of the fact that the baroreceptors have adapted to the lower pressure and are no longer capable of evoking corrective pressor responses to depressor events. If this hypothesis were to be substantiated, propranolol's mode of action would be neatly explained as the antithesis of the hypothesis that essential hypertension arises because the baroreceptors are set at a higher than normal level (see above). There are, unfortunately, physiological arguments to be set against this otherwise attractive hypothesis and the mode of antihypertensive action of drugs that effect β blockade has still to be numbered among the mysteries of pharmacology.

In the treatment of hypertension, propranolol is given twice or four times daily in doses of 40 to 240 mg. The dose of other β blocking agents is determined by their potencies relative to propranolol (Table 18.1, p. 303).

Labetalol

Labetalol is a new drug which is fully described earlier in this chapter (p. 306). It combines α and β blocking activities and it has already been made use of (in daily doses of 300 mg to 4 grams) to treat all grades of hypertension but its therapeutic value is questionable. Combined antihypertensive therapy with agents that separately occlude α and β receptors has not been very successful largely because of the postural hypotension that is an inevitable accompaniment of α receptor blockade and there is no reason to believe that the combination of the two properites in a single molecule will prove to be any more so. Indeed it is likely to be less so because labetalol denies the user the opportunity of adjusting the relative degree of α and β blockade.

Prazosin, the reader will recall, escapes the criticisms that can be levelled against the more conventional α blocking agents and it is difficult to believe that labetalol will be able to gain ascendancy over combined therapy with prazosin and propranolol or a congener.

Labetalol has been given by intravenous injection to resolve hypertensive crises. It brings about an immediate and abrupt fall of blood pressure but the operation is not without hazard since the β blockade removes from the heart its ability to compensate for too precipitous a fall in blood pressure.

Pargyline
Hypertensive crises constitute a recognized and much publicized side effect of therapy with monoamine oxidase inhibitors unless care is taken to avoid the ingestion of tyramine (p. 79) and it must come as something of a surprise to many people when they discover that one of these enzyme inhibitors (pargyline) has enjoyed a brief reputation as an antihypertensive drug.

Many of the drugs that are employed to control the blood pressure exert a depressant effect on the central nervous system (indeed this action contributes to their efficacy) but pargyline is an antidepressant substance and it should therefore be particularly useful in depressed hypertensive patients who would certainly not relish the thought that treatment of their high blood pressure could only be bought at the expense of a deepening of their depression. It was for this type of patient that pargyline was used for a time but the drug has come under the cloud that has darkened the reputation of all monoamine oxidase inhibitors and it has been superseded by antihypertensive agents that do not depress mood.

A number of equally unsatisfactory hypotheses have been formulated to explain pargyline's mode of antihypertensive action. It might, for instance, prevent the synthesis of noradrenaline in sympathetic nerves and its well documented ability to prevent the release of noradrenaline in response to stimulation of preganglionic nerves in experimental animals might reflect a similar action in the human subject which would obviously contribute to an antihypertensive action. Another possibility is that inhibition of monoamine oxidase, by preventing the degradation of dopamine would cause the accumulation of this amine and possibly of octopamine (p. 259) which might displace noradrenaline from noradrenergic nerves and act as a false transmitter with less sympathomimetic activity than noradrenaline itself.

DRUGS WITH A DIRECT ACTION ON THE BLOOD VESSELS All these antihypertensive agents are fully discussed elsewhere in this chapter (pp. 311-314).

BIBLIOGRAPHY

Books, monographes and reviews

Benforado, J. M. (1967). The Veratrum Alkaloids. In: Root, W.C. and Hofmann, F.G. (eds.) *Physiological Pharmacology*, Vol.IV. New York and London: Academic Press.

Berglund, G. Hansson L, and Werko, L. (eds) (1975). *Pathophysiology and Management Arterial Hypertension*. Stockholm: Lingdren and Soner.

Boura, A.L.A. and Green A.F. (1964). Depressants of Peripheral Sympathetic Nerve Function. In: *Evaluation of Drug Activities: Pharmacometrics*, pp. 369-430 Ed. Laurence, D.R. and Bacharach, A.L. New York: Academic Press.

Conference, *Ann. New York Acad. of Sciences* (1967), **139**, 541-1009. New Adrenergic Blocking Drugs, their Pharmacological, Biochemical and Clinical Actions.

Conolly, M.E.(1970) (ed) *Catapres in Hypertension*. London: Butterworths.

Davies, D.S.and Reid, J.L. (eds) (1975) *Central Actions of Drugs in Blood Pressure Regulation*. Baltimore: University Park Press.

Fuller, J.G. (1968) *The Day of St Anthony's Fire*, London: Hutchinson.

Graham, J.D.P. (1962) 2-Halogenoalkylamines. *Progr. Med. Chem.*, **2**, 132-175.

Iversen, L. L. (1967) *The Uptake and Storage of Noradrenaline in Sympathetic Nerves*. Cambridge: The University Press.

Julian, D. G. (1977) (ed) *Angina Pectoris*, Edinburgh, London and New York: Churchill Livingstone.

Kostrzewa, P. M. and Jacobwitz, D. M. (1974). Pharmacological actions of 6-hydroxydopamine. *Pharmac. Rev.*, **26**, 200-288.

Levi-Montalcini, Rita and Angeletti, P.U. (1966). Immunosympathectomy. *Pharmac. Rev.* **18**, 619-628.

McDevitt, D. G. (1977) The assessment of β-adrenoceptor blocking drugs in man. *Br. J. clin. Pharmac.*, **4**, 413-426.

Malmfors, T. and Thoenen, H. (1971). *6-Hydroxydopamine and Catecholamine Neurons*. Amsterdam and London: North-Holland Publishing Co.

Nickersen, M, and Hollenberg, N. K. (1967). Blockade of α adrenergic receptors. In: *Physiological Pharmacology*, pp. 243-306. Ed. Root, W. S. and Hofmann, F. G. New York: Academic Press.

Prichard, B. N. C. (1977). Beta-adrenoceptor blocking drugs. *Practitioner* **219**, 501-508.

Prichard, B. N. C. and Tuckman, J. (1977). Treatment of hypertension. In: *Recent Advances in Cardiology*, Vol. 7, ed. Hamer, J. Ch. 9. Edinburgh and London: Churchill Livingstone.

Symposium (1976). Labetalol. *Br. J. clin. Pharmac.*, **3**, 681-824.

Tarazi, R. C. (1973). Diuretic drugs: mechanisms of antihypertensive action. In: Onesti, G., Kim, KE. and Moyer, J. H. (eds) Hypertension: *Mechanisms and Management*, New York: Grune & Stratton.

Tobian, L. (1967). Why do thiazide diuretics lower blood pressure in essential hypertension? *A. Rev. Pharmac.*, **7**, 399-408.

Waal-Manning, Hendrika J. (1976). Hypertension: which beta-blocker? *Drugs*, **12**, 412-441.

Wang, H. H. (1967). Blockade of β adrenergic receptors. In: *Physiological Pharmacology*, pp. 307-329. Ed. Root, W. S. & Hofmann, F. G. New York: Academic Press.

Wollam, G. L., Gifford, R. W. and Tarazi, R. C. (1977). Antihypertensive drugs: clinical pharmacology and therapeutic use. *Drugs* **14**, 420-460.

Zaimis, E. and Hanington, E. (1969). A possible pharmacological approach to migraine. *Lancet* (ii), 298-300.

Original papers.

Barger, G. and Carr, F. H. (1906). Note on ergot alkaloids. *Chem. News*, **94**, 89.

Dale, H. H. (1906). On some physiological actions of ergot. *J. Physiol.*, **34**, 163-206.

Day, M, D., Roach, A G. and Whiting, R. L. (1973). The mechanism of the antihypertensive action of α-methylDOPA in hypertensive rats. *Eur. J. Pharmac.*, **21**, 271-280.

Dunlop, D. and Shanks, R. G. (1968). Selective blockade of adrenoceptive beta receptors in the heart, *Br. J. Pharmac. Chemother.*, **32**, 201-218.

Gillespie, J. S. and Kirpekar, S. M. (1965). The inactivation of infused noradrenaline by the cat spleen. *J. Physiol., Lond.*, **176**, 205-227.

Haefely, W., Hürlimann, A. and Thoenen, H. (1966). The effect of stimulation of sympathetic nerves in the cat treated with reserpine, α-methyldopa and α-methylmetatyrosine, *Br. J. Pharmac. Chemother.*, **26**, 172-185.

Hukovic, S. (1960). The action of sympathetic blocking agents on isolated and innervated atria and vessels. *Br. J. Pharmac, Chemother.*, **15**, 117-121.

Kopin, I. J. and Gordon, E. K. (1963). Metabolism of administered and drug release norepinephrine-7-^{3}H in the rat. *J. Pharmac. exp. Ther.* **140**, 207-216.

Kopin, I. J, Hertting, G. and Gordon, E. K. (1962). Fate of norephinephrine-H^3 in the isolated perfused rat heart. *J. Pharmac, exp. Ther.*, **138**, 34-40.

Levy, B and Ahlquist, R. F. (1961). An analysis of adrenergic blocking activity, *J. Pharmac, exp. Ther.*, **133**, 202-210.

Levy, B. (1966). Dimethylisopropyl methoxamine: a selective β receptor blocking agent. *Br. J. Pharmac. Chemother.*, **27**, 277-285

Levi-Montalcini, Rita and Booker. B. (1960). Destruction of the sympathetic ganglia by an antiserum to a nerve growth protein. *Proc. natn. Acad. Sci. USA*, **46**, 324-331.

Muscholl, E and Maître, L. (1963). Release by sympathetic stimulation of α-methyl noradrenaline stored in the heart after administration of α-methyl dopa. *Experimentia*, **19**, 658-659.

Nickerson, M. (1949). The pharmacology of adrenergic blockade. *Pharmac, Rev.*, **1**, 27-101.

Powell, C. E. and Slater, I. H. (1958). Blocking of inhibitory adrenergic receptors by a dichloro analog of isoproterenol. *J. Pharmac, exp. Ther.*, **122**, 480-488.

Prichard, B. N. C. (1968). Hypotensive drugs. *Practitioner*, **200**, 30-39.

Sourkes, T. L. (1954). Inhibition of dihydroxyphenlalanine decarboxylase by derivatives of phenylalanine. *Archs Biochem. Biophys.*, **51**, 444-456.

Stafford, A. (1963). Potentiation of some catechol amines by phenoxybenzamine, guanethidine and cocaine. *Br. J. Pharmac. Chemother.*, **21**, 361-367.

Stjärne, L. (1961). Tyramine effects on catechol amine release from spleen and adrenals in the cat. *Acta physiol. scand.*, **51**, 224-229.

Trendelenburg, U. (1960). The action of histamine and 5-hydroxytryptamine on isolated mammalian atria. *J. Pharmac, exp. Ther.*, **130**, 450-460.

19. The cyclic nucleotides

New drugs are introduced into medicine more often than old ones are discarded. Each provides the physician with yet another means of treating his patients and the medical scientist with yet another means of testing old or formulating new hypotheses of drug action. The information that accumulates as a result of this clinical and laboratory experience has to be added to the large stock of existing information that is still too valuable to lose. And so textbooks of pharmacology and therapeutics grow ever bulkier. In these circumstances it is only too easy to overlook the fact that, from this tangled jungle of detail some broad general principles are beginning to emerge. The intervention of the prostaglandins in a large variety of disparate physiological processes provides one example of a unifying principle of this type. In a similar fashion, cyclic nucleotide formation constitutes a common link in the action of many endogenous compounds, particularly hormones and transmitter agents and of substances that mimic them. This chapter surveys general aspects of cyclic nucleotide action. More specific points are dealt with in those sections of this volume that discuss individual physiological systems in which the nucleotides intervene. The location of these additional mentions can be found by referring to the Index.

It is historically appropriate that we should initiate our discussion by considering the actions of adrenaline and, in particular, that hormone's ability to bring about the conversion of glycogen to glucose in both liver and muscle. The liver was investigated first.

The first and rate limiting step in hepatic glycogenolysis is the production of glucose-1-phosphate (p. 323). The enzyme involved is a phosphorylase and adrenaline activates this enzyme. The mechanism whereby this activation is effected was elucidated by Sutherland and his colleagues in a series of experiments that culminated, in 1956, in the discovery of cyclic AMP (Fig. 19.1), the immediate activator of phosphorylase. The chain of events that leads to this activation is illustrated in Fig. 19.1 and can be itemized as follows:

1. Adrenaline activates adenyl cyclase, an enzyme more often known today as adenylate cyclase or, most recently, as adenylyl cyclase. Glucagon (p. 722) has a similar action.

2. Adenylate cyclase promotes the conversion of adenosine triphosphate (ATP) to adenosine 3',5' monophosphate (cyclic AMP or cAMP). The accumulation of cyclic AMP is limited by the activity of a specific phosphodies-terase (cyclic adenosine 3',5' monophosphate phosphodies-terase) which is widely distributed in the tissues and which converts cyclic AMP into the noncyclical form of the nucleotide (Fig. 19.1). The activity of this enzyme (which, like adenylate cyclase, requires magnesium ion for its activation) is inhibited by methylxanthines such as theophylline and caffeine and by diazoxide, puromycin and papaverine. Imidazole stimulates the enzyme.

3. Cyclic AMP in association with ATP activates a specific protein kinase that activates, in its turn a phosphorylase kinase. It does this by catalyzing the transfer of the terminal phosphate of ATP to the unactivated form of the enzyme.

4. The activated phosphorylase kinase, again in association with ATP, phosphorylates and thereby activates the phosphorylase with which our discussion began.

Similar reactions to those just outlined underlie the induction of glycogenolysis by adrenaline in skeletal muscle. In this tissue, the inactive and active forms of phosphorylase are labelled *b* and *a* respectively as indicated in Fig. 19.2. In addition, it seems that cyclic AMP also activates phosphofructokinase, the enzyme that converts fructose 6-phosphate into fructose 1,6-diphosphate en route to the production of lactic acid.

In the sequence of reactions that culminate in glycogenolysis, each activated enzyme activates the next in the line. This provides yet another example of a cascade system of the type that features in so many physiological regulatory processes and that permit the rapid amplification of the effects of an initially trivial change. Other examples of cascade processes include the coagulation of blood, the production of plasma kinins and the activation of complement.

It is usually assumed that adrenaline brings about glycogenolysis by way of its action on β receptors and it was natural to enquire whether other manifestations of β receptor stimulation also involved the intervention of adenylate cyclase and cyclic AMP. This was a particularly important matter at the time when cyclic AMP was first discovered for many authorities were still unwilling to concede that the receptors involved in initiating such 'mechanical' responses as an increased power of cardiac contraction could be the same as those that brought about 'chemical' events such as the mobilization of glycogen. Experimental evidence sufficient to still their doubts was soon forthcoming. Thus cardiac muscle contains adenylate

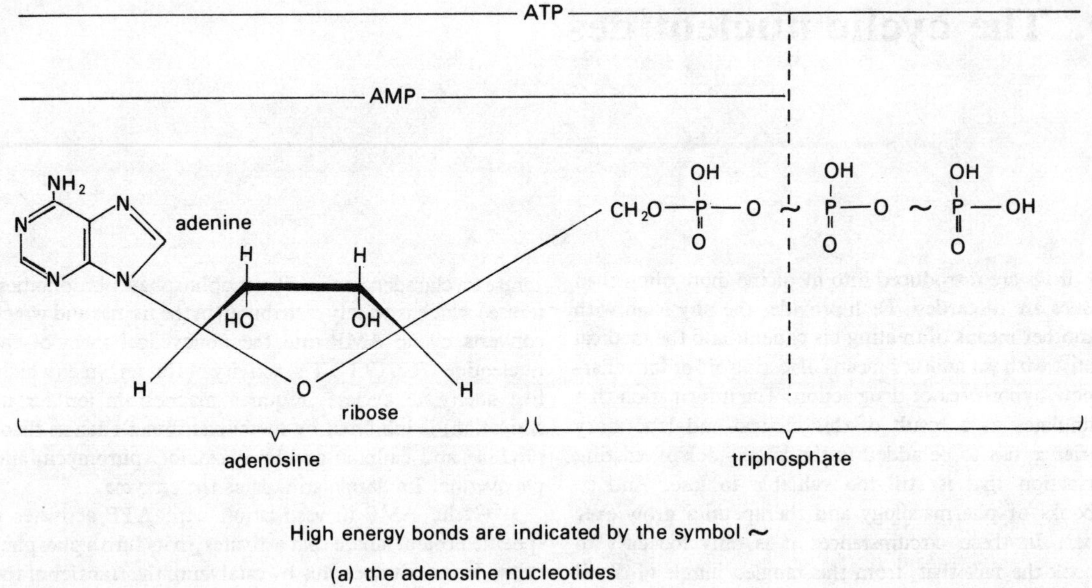

High energy bonds are indicated by the symbol ~

(a) the adenosine nucleotides

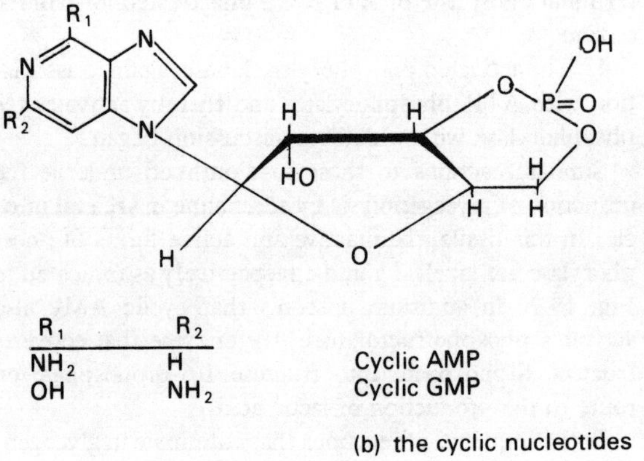

R_1	R_2	
NH_2	H	Cyclic AMP
OH	NH_2	Cyclic GMP

(b) the cyclic nucleotides

Fig. 19.1 The adenosine and the cyclic nucleotides

cyclase, phosphoroylase and phosphodiesterase and the first of these enzymes is activated by substances that stimulate β receptors. Moreover, when appropriate measures are taken to prevent uptake of the drugs by the cardiac nerves, a close parallelism can be demonstrated between the ability of a sympathomimetic amine to induce cardiac responses and its ability to activate adenylate cyclase. The overt cardiac responses and the enzyme activation are equally susceptible to the effects of β blockade; cyclic AMP formation and phosphorylase activation follow in the wake of adenylate cyclase activation and the effects of adrenaline on the rate and power of cardiac contraction are potentiated by the methylxanthines. Analogous lines of argument establish the role of adenylate cyclase in other processes dependent on stimulation of β receptors.

Stimulation of β receptors, then, results in an increased formation of cyclic AMP. On the other hand, there is a fall in the concentration of the nucleotide in tissues whose α receptors are stimulated.

Following the pioneer work with adrenaline, it soon became clear that other hormones also operated by way of the cyclic AMP mechanism. No useful purpose would be served by detailing them all at this point but hormonal functions that depend on an increased formation of cyclic AMP include the actions of glucagon on the liver and the pancreas; of the respective pituitary trophic hormones on the adrenal cortex, ovary, testis and frog melanocytes; of thyrotrophin releasing hormone and thyroid stimulating hormone on the anterior pituitary and thyroid glands respectively and of vasopressin on the kidney tubules. On the other hand the actions of prostaglandins on adipose tissue, of melatonin on frog skin and of insulin on the liver and on fatty tissue all involve inhibition of cyclic AMP formation.

The traditional interpretation of the word 'hormone' is 'chemical messenger' and the recognition that cyclic AMP participates in so many hormonal activities has led to its being described as a 'second messenger'. However its actions are by no means confined to the mediation of conventional hormonal actions. There is, for instance, clear evidence that dopamine exerts its action on some (but not all) of the central neurones that respond to it by activating adenylate cyclase (Kebabian, 1978) and the same mechanism may well explain the action of some other central neurotransmitter agents.

It is necessary now to enquire how a common mechanism can underlie a wide variety of seemingly specific reactions. Adenylate cyclase is incorporated into all membranes and it seems that it must be associated with specific

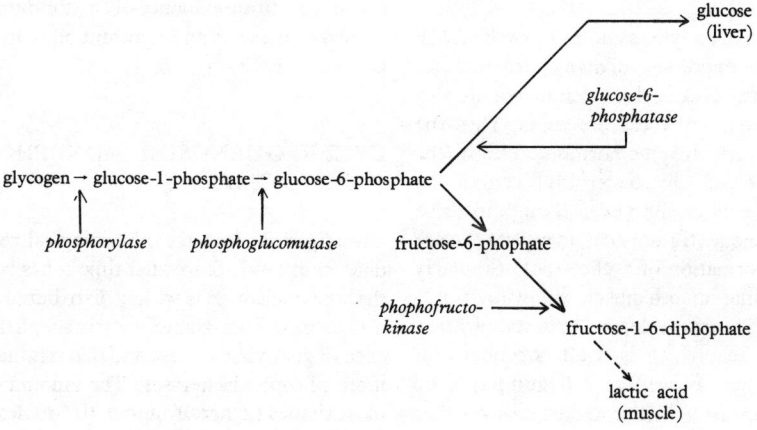

(a) Reactions involved in glycogenolysis (outline)

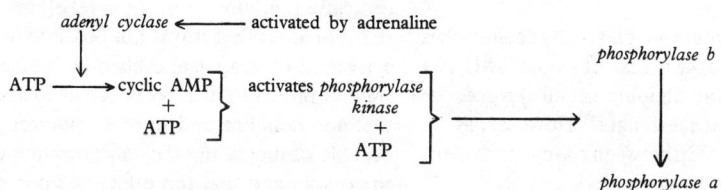

(b) Sequence of reactions involved in activation of phosphorylase by adrenaline

Fig. 19.2 Reactions and substances involved in the metabolic actions of adrenaline. (Enzymes are indicated in *italics*.)

receptors that determine the nature of the agonists that will activate it in any particular cell. It was believed until recently that these receptors formed an integral part of the enzyme molecule but it now seems that, though closely associated, the two structures enjoy separate identities. In an impressively ingenious experiment Orly and Schramm (1976) were able to culture two cell lines. One of the lines carried an adrenaline β receptor but no adenylate cyclase while the other possessed the enzyme but no β receptor. Fusion of the two lines produced hybrid cells with adenylate cyclase that responded to adrenaline. Other workers have succeeded in separating receptor and enzyme by chemical means (Limbird & Lefkowitz, 1977).

In some cells the adenylate cyclase is influenced by more than one hormone and we must assume, therefore, that the enzyme can be associated with more than one receptor in the same cell.

The nature of the reaction set in motion by the activated cyclase is governed by the particular sort of biochemical machinery that is available to it. It seems that in many (if not all) instances the primary event is the activation of a protein kinase. The system as a whole is schematically indicated in Fig. 19.3.

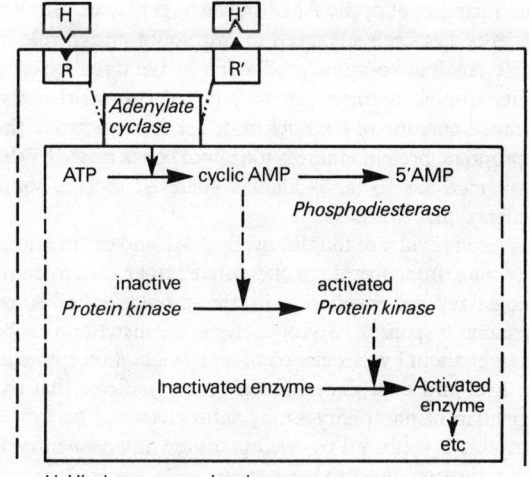

H, H'—hormone molecules;
R, R'—hormone receptors;
enzymes are indicated in *italics*;
broken arrows indicate 'activation'

Fig. 19.3 Schematic representation of the cyclic AMP system.

CYCLIC AMP AND CALCIUM

Although the activation of enzyme systems by cyclic AMP plays a central role in the expression of many hormonal and some transmitter effects it is clear that calcium ions are also critically involved in many of these processes. Thus the final effect of adrenocorticotrophic hormone release (the synthesis and release of corticosteroids) cannot be achieved in the absence of calcium even though in these circumstances the hormone still activates adenylate cyclase and so promotes the formation of cyclic AMP. Similarly the relaxation of intestinal smooth muscle following stimulation of its β receptors seems to depend on a stabilization of the muscle membrane which is itself dependent on calcium. It may be that, as well as activating specific biochemical systems, cyclic AMP promotes changes that result in an increase or a decrease in the amount of available calcium that permits completion of the hormone's action.

An appreciation of the vital role played by calcium has led several authorities to suggest that, if cyclic AMP is a second messenger, calcium should, in all justice, be assigned the status of 'third messenger'. However, as we shall note later, the relationship between the cyclic nucleotides and calcium is by no means settled.

HOW ESSENTIAL IS CYCLIC AMP?

Although there is wide agreement that cyclic AMP operates as a second messenger in many hormonal and humoral systems, the idea that it is the unique intermediary in these systems has not escaped criticism. It has recently been demonstrated by several groups of workers that ACTH can stimulate hormone production by the adrenal cortex in doses that are too small to induce detectable changes in the concentration of cyclic AMP in the target tissue. Similar evidence has been advanced to cast doubt on the role of cyclic AMP in hormone production by the testis exposed to its trophic hormone. It may be, of course, that the minimal quantity of the nucleotide needed to activate the appropriate protein kinase is too low to be estimated by the assay methods so far available. There is, indeed, some evidence that this is so.

There is evidence too that cyclic AMP and calcium ions may sometimes operate as alternative rather than as complementary intermediaries in the promotion of some hormone responses. Glycogenolysis, for instance, can be brought about by stimulation of α as well as β receptors in the liver and some experimental results indicate that the activation of phosphorylase by substances that occupy α receptors is mediated by calcium release independently of any activation of adenylate cyclase.

Experiments of the type mentioned in the two foregoing paragraphs are more thoroughly discussed by Earp and Steiner (1978). They should serve to prevent too uncritical an acceptance of assertions that the cyclic AMP mechanism is both unique and universal in its operation but they do not constitute evidence of any fundamental defect in the view that it exerts an important regulatory function in the animal body.

CYCLIC GUANOSINE MONOPHOSPHATE (CYCLIC GMP)

Investigations into the physiological role of cyclic GMP date from 1960. Since that time it has become established that the nucleotide is widely distributed in the tissues, that it is formed from guanosine triphosphate under the influence of guanylate cyclase and that it is inactivated by one or more phosphodiesterases. The amount of cyclic GMP in most tissues (generally about 10^{-8} moles per kilogram wet weight of tissue) is considerably smaller than that of cyclic AMP (about 10^{-7}M) but much higher than average concentrations are found in the cerebellum and, particularly, the retina. At first it was not possible to demonstrate any activation of guanylate cyclase by biologically active substances but in 1970 reports began to appear to the effect that acetylcholine and some substances related to it were capable of increasing the concentration of cyclic GMP in the tissues and that this effect was prevented by atropine (Ferrendelli et al., 1970; George et al., 1970) Among the actions of acetylcholine that seem to be mediated in this way are those on the heart, the vas deferens and intestinal smooth muscle. Both the cyclic nucleotides have also been implicated in the regulation of polymorphonuclear leucocyte migration in response to chemotactic factors secreted by bacteria. Acetylcholine and other muscarinic drugs, substances that stimulate adrenaline α receptors, some of the prostaglandins and a number of other agents accelerate this migration and increase the amount of cyclic GMP in the infected tissues. Migration is decreased, on the other hand, by substances that stimulate adrenaline β or histamine H_2 receptors, by some other prostaglandins and by a number of other substances including cholera toxin. All these agents increase the amount of cyclic AMP in the tissues. Opposing actions of the two cyclic nucleotides are also seen in the sensitized mast cell exposed to the appropriate antigen. Adrenaline acting on its β receptors increases the concentration of cyclic AMP in the cell and inhibits the release of the mediators of anaphylaxis while acetylcholine increases the concentration of cyclic GMP and promotes mediator release.

It would be easy to guess, from the foregoing, that cyclic AMP and cyclic GMP might operate as a duo, respectively mediating mutually opposing reactions. This hypothesis has its attractions in the light of the undoubted and important fact that many physiological responses are the result of reciprocal alterations in the activity of balanced systems. The sympathetic and parasympathetic divisions of the autonomic nervous system and the excitatory and inhibitory components of the extrapyramidal motor system provide just two examples of such systems. The ancient Chinese, lacking modern knowledge of the anatomical and physiological organization of the animal body, nevertheless placed this principle of control by opposing systems at the very hub of their medical philosophy. They called it the 'Yin-Yang' principle and in recent years the term has been used by Goldberg in a vigorous advocacy of his proposal that the reactions mediated by cyclic AMP and cyclic GMP respectively are indeed opposed to one another (Goldberg *et al.*, 1975). This view, intellectually attractive though it is, should not be too enthusiastically embraced until a number of other factors has been considered. In the first place, it must be noted that it has not been possible to demonstrate the intervention of cyclic GMP in more than a small number of hormonally or humorally mediated reactions and some of those in which it is evidentially involved are similar to, rather than the opposite of, those mediated by cyclic AMP. Again it must not be too readily assumed that the role of cyclic GMP is completely analogous to that of cyclic AMP. In some cells for instance, the production of cyclic GMP requires that guanyl cyclase (which is located in the cytoplasm) be activated by the influx of calcium into the cells. In these cells we should, perhaps, designate calcium as the second messenger and cyclic GMP as the third.

Not all the reactions promoted by cyclic GMP require stimulation of acetylcholine receptors. Oestrogen effects on the uterus (contraction, lysosome release and glycogen deposition) are facilitated by cyclic GMP and are suppressed by cyclic AMP and there is evidence that oestrogens can increase the amount of cyclic GMP in the uterus. The actions of oxytocin, serotonin and prostaglandin $PGF_{2\alpha}$ on the uterus and those of serotonin and histamine on the intestine may also involve the production of the nucleotide. The release of growth hormone and the actions of calcitonin also fall into the category of those possibly mediated by cyclic GMP.

We have already noted that higher than average amounts of cyclic GMP are found in the retina and the cerebellum. In the nervous system generally three separate guanylate cyclase—cyclic GMP systems have been identified (Ferrendelli, 1978). One of them has already been mentioned: the enzyme is associated with the cytosol and it is activated by calcium influx as might happen on nerve depolarization. Another system involves a particle bound form of guanylate cyclase which is not activated by calcium and has not yet been fully investigated. Finally the retina contains yet another particulate form of guanylate cyclase which is actually inhibited by calcium ions. The most interesting aspect of the retinal system, however, is that the cyclic GMP formed by it is destroyed by a light sensitive phosphodiesterase and it is difficult to escape the conclusion that the nucleotide is involved in the regulation of fundamental visual responses.

A number of drugs induce quite large changes in the amount of cyclic GMP in the cerebellum. Morphine and the benzodiazepines among other drugs can deplete it by up to 50 per cent while apomorphine and isoniazid produce even greater changes in the opposite direction. These alterations in the cyclic GMP content of the cerebellum seem to result, in many instances at least, from activation of neurones that utilize γ-aminobutyric acid as their transmitter substances (Guidotti, 1978).

Investigations into the actions and physiological significance of cyclic GMP are still in their infancy but progress in the field is rapid—the annual Advances in Cyclic Nucleotide Reasearch is always a volume of substantial proportions—and the reader should be alert to the likelihood that some of the tentative hypotheses presented or hinted at in the foregoing paragraphs will have been completely demolished or triumphantly vindicated by the time that this chapter sees the light of day.

RELATIONSHIPS BETWEEN THE PROSTAGLANDINS AND THE CYCLIC NUCLEOTIDES

This topic is discussed elsewhere (p. 387).

BIBLIOGRAPHY

Books, monographs and reviews

Breckenridge, B. M. (1970). Cyclic AMP and drug action. *A. rev. Pharmac.*, **10**, 19034.

Earp, H. S. and Steiner, A. L. (1978). Compartmentalization of cyclic nucleotide-mediated hormone action. *A rev. Pharmac.*, **18**, 431-458.

Ferrendelli, J. A. (1978). Distribution and regulation of cyclic GMP in the central nervous system. *Adv. cyclic Nucleotide Res.*, **9**, 453-464.

Goldber, N. D., O'Dea, R. F. and Haddox, Mari K. (1973). Cyclic GMP. *Adv. cyclic Nucleotide Res.*, **3**, 155-223.

Greengard, P., McAlfee, D. A. and Kebabian, J. W. (1972). On the mechanism of action of cyclic AMP and its role in synaptic transmission. *Adv. cyclic Nucleotide Res.*, **1**, 337-355.

Rabin, B. and Freedman, R. (eds) (1972). *The Effect of Drugs on Cellular Control Mechanisms*. London: Macmillan.

Rall, T. W. (1972). Role of adenosine 3',5'-monophosphate (cyclic AMP) in actions of catecholamines. *Pharmac. Rev.*, **24**, 399-410.

Rall, T. W. and Gilman, A. G. (eds) (1970). The role of cyclic AMP in the nervous system. *Neurosci. Res. Prog. Bull.*, **8**, 221-323.

Robison, G. A., Butcher, R. W. and Sutherland, E. W. (1971). *Cyclic AMP*. New York and London: Academic Press.

Sutherland, E. W. and Robison, G. A. (1966). The role of cyclic 3':5'-AMP in response to cathecholamines and other hormones. *Pharmac. Rev.*, **18**, 145-161.

Vollicer, L. (1977). *Clinical Aspects of Cyclic Nucleotides*. New York: Spectrum Publications.

Original papers

Ferrendelli, J. A., Steiner, A. L., McDougal, D. B. and Kipnis, D. M. (1970). The effect of oxotremorine and atropine on cGMP and cAMP levels in the mouse cerebral cortex and cerebellum. *Biochem. biophys. Res. Commun.*, **41**, 1061-1067.

George, W. J., Polson, J. B., O'Toole, A. B. and Goldberg, N. D. (1970). Evaluation of guanosine 3',5'-cyclic phosphate in rat heart after perfusion with acetylcholine. *Proc. natn. Acad. Sci. USA.* **66**, 398-403.

Goldberg, N. D., Haddox, Mari K., Nicol, S. E., Glass, D. B., Sandford, C. H., Kuehl, F. A., Jr. and Estensen, R. (1975). Biological regulation through opposing influences of cyclic GMP and cyclic AMP: the Yin Yang hypothesis.

Adv. cyclic Nucleotide Res., **5**, 307-330.

Guidotti, A. (1978). Synaptic mechanisms in the actions of benzodiazepines. In: *Psychopharmacology: A Generation of Progress*, pp. 1349-1357. eds. Lipton, M. A., DiMascio, A. and Killam, K. F. New York: Raven Press.

Limbird, L. E. and Lefkowitz, R. J. (1977). Resolution of β-adrenergic receptor binding and adenylate cyclase activity by gel exclusion chromatography. *J. biol. Chem.*, **252**, 799-802.

Orly, J. and Schramm, M. (1976). Coupling of catecholamine receptor from one cell with adenylate cyclase from another cell by cell fusion. *Proc. natn. Acad. Sci. USA*, **73**, 4410-4414.

20. 5-Hydroxytryptamine (serotonin)

As long ago as the middle of the nineteenth century, physiologists were aware that blood serum contained a vasoconstrictor material which they named, for obvious reasons, 'vasotonin' or 'serotonin'. The substance attracted little attention, however, and no mention of it will be found in text books published before 1950. In 1948, Rapport isolated serotonin in the pure form and in the following year he was able to report that he had identified it as 5-hydroxytryptamine.

Some 20 years before Rapport announced the identity of serotonin, Erspamer had detected a pharmacologically active material in acetone extracts of the intestine. Believing it to be an amine, Erspamer called his substance Enteramine. When he learned of Rapport's work, Erspamer realized that Enteramine might be 5-hydroxytryptamine. In 1952 he confirmed that this was indeed so.

The investigations by Rapport and Erspamer provoked an interest in 5-hydroxytryptamine which grew at an ever accelerating pace as it became clear that the substance was widely distributed in nature and that it had a variety of interesting pharmacological properties. The simplicity of its structure, the ease with which it can be estimated in tissue extracts and the conviction that it plays a fundamental role in physiological processes combined to produce the extraordinary interest in 5-hydroxytryptamine which has characterized the past two decades. This rush of interest has only recently been stemmed and then only by the arrival on the scene of rivals (the prostaglandins) that are even more siren like in their ability to seduce, fascinate and dominate the minds of pharmacologists.

Much of the interest shown in 5-hydroxytamine stems from the belief that it plays a fundamental part in transmission processes in the central nervous system. This possibility is discussed in detail elsewhere (Chap. 13). In this chapter, attention is directed to the metabolism of 5-hydroxytryptamine, to its general pharmacological actions and to a consideration of its possible functions outside the central nervous system.

It is usual to abbreviate 5-hydroxytryptamine to 5-HT or simply HT. Some, like the author, try to resist the tendency to corrupt their native language into a succession of esoteric and discordant symbols. For this reason, 'serotonin', an inoffensive and euphonious trivial name, which is quite acceptable on historical grounds, will be used throughout this chapter when an alternative is needed to the clumsy 5-hydroxytryptamine.

THE FORMATION AND METABOLISM OF 5-HYDROXYTRYPTAMINE

5-Hydroxytryptamine is formed from tryptophan by way of 5-hydroxytryptophan (Fig. 20.1). The enzymes involved are tryptophan-5-hydroxylase and 5-hydroxytryptophan decarboxylase. The last named enzyme is probably identical with DOPA decarboxylase (aromatic *l*-amino acid decarboxylase; p. 259). Except in the pineal gland, the rate limiting step in the biosynthesis of serotonin is the hydroxylation of tryptophan and *p*-chlorophenylalanine interferes with this process. It does this partly by acting as a competitive inhibitor of, and partly by actually inactivating, tryptophan-5-hydroxylase. In addition, in nervous tissue *p*-chlorophenylalanine prevents the transport of tryptophan to the sites of serotonin synthesis (the synaptosomes).

Although *p*-chlorophenylalanine is not entirely specific in its actions (it inhibits phenylalanine hydroxylase as well as tryptophan-5-hydroxylase) it can be used to deplete an animal's tissues of serotonin without markedly influencing the synthesis of other humoral substances such as noradrenaline. It has occasionally been used clinically, under its proprietary name (Fenclonine) in attempts to reduce serotonin synthesis and hence the troublesome diarrhoea in carcinoid patients (p. 329). In the laboratory, *p*-chlorophenylalanine is given in daily doses of 80-100 mg per kilogram until the required degree of serotonin depletion has been achieved. In human beings the daily dose is about 1 gram.

Serotonin synthesis can also be prevented in experimental animals by giving them a tryptophan-free diet. The physiological responses of animals whose tissues lack serotonin are referred to elsewhere in this chapter and in Chapter 13.

Tissues that contain 5-hydroxytryptamine usually contain both tryptophan-5-hydroxylase and 5-hydroxytryptophan decarboxylase but in some instances there is no close relationship between the serotonin content and the hydroxylase and decarboxylase activities of individual tissues. Thus, notwithstanding its high serotonin content, the intestine appears to have little hydroxylase activity and the blood platelets have virtually no ability to decarboxy-

p-Chlorophenylalanine

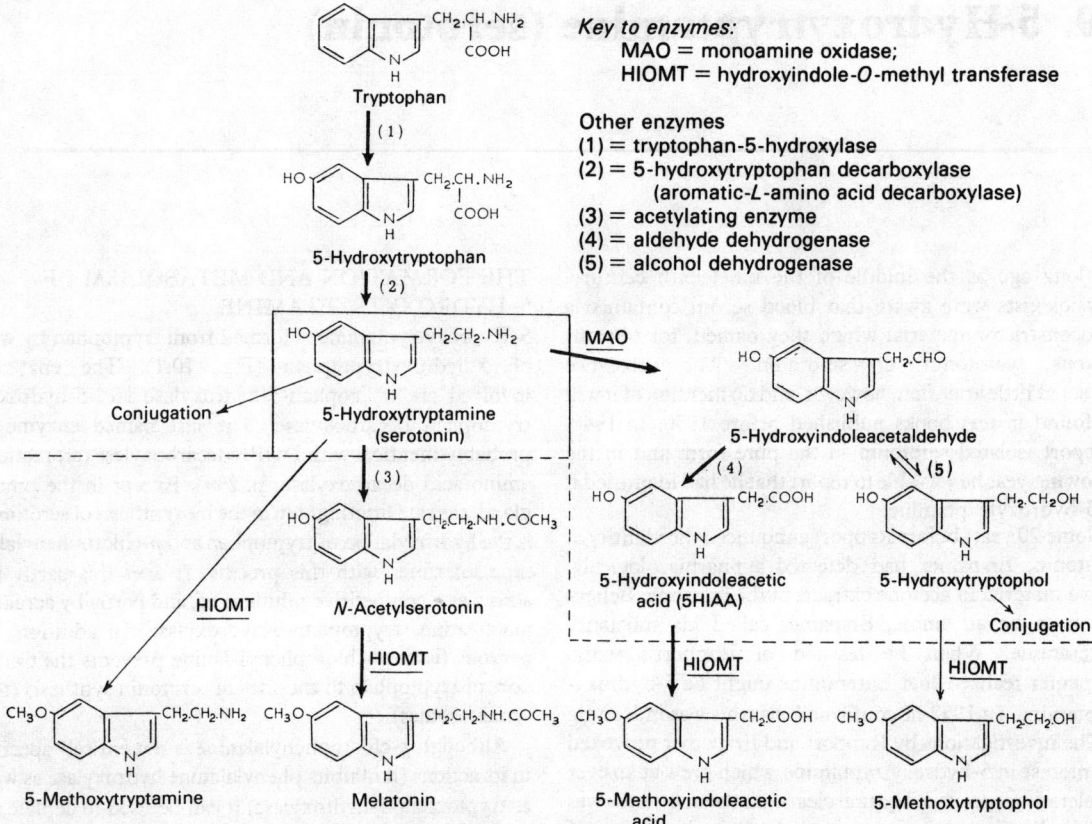

Fig. 20.1 The principal pathways of serotonin synthesis and metabolism. The reactions enclosed by the dotted line occur only within the pineal gland. Bold arrows indicate the more important reactions.

late 5-hydroxytryptophan. It may be that the turnover of serotonin in the intestine proceeds only slowly and it is known that the platelets obtain most of their serotonin by taking up the preformed amine during their circulation through the tissues. In the platelets, serotonin is bound to storage granules similar to those in which it is stored in nerve endings.

It is theoretically possible for tissues to obtain their serotonin by taking up the preformed amine, by decarboxylating 5-hydroxytryptophan produced in and provided by another tissue or by themselves synthesizing serotonin from tryptophan. There is little doubt that, except in platelets, the last named source is the most important.

The formation of 5-hydroxytryptamine could, in theory, proceed by way of tryptamine but there is no substantial evidence that this occurs in living tissues.

THE METABOLISM OF SEROTONIN
Serotonin metabolism follows a different course in the pineal gland from that in other mammalian tissues. The generality of tissues will be considered first.

Serotonin can be broken down or otherwise inactivated by a number of routes but the most important involves

degradation by monoamine oxidase, which promotes the formation of 5-hydroxyindoleacetaldehyde (Fig. 20.1). Most of this compound is oxidised, through the agency of an aldehyde dehydrogenase, into 5-hydroxyindoleacetic acid (the principal urinary metabolite of serotonin) but, at least in some tissues, a little is reduced to 5-hydroxytryptophol, under the influence of an alcohol dehydrogenase. The reduction is reversible but conjugation of the 5-hydroxytryptophol with glucuronic and sulphuric acids minimizes its reconversion to the aldehyde.

A little serotonin is also excreted as conjugates and still smaller amounts appear in the urine in the free form.

The pineal gland is unique among mammalian tissues in containing hydroxyindole-*O*-methyltransferase (HIOMT), an enzyme that is more widely distributed in the central nervous system of the lower vertebrates. The enzyme converts 5-hydroxyindoles into the corresponding methylated compounds so that in the pineal gland the metabolites of serotonin include 5-methoxytryptamine, 5-methoxyindoleacetic acid and 5-methoxytryptophol (Fig. 20.1). In addition, the pineal gland is capable of converting serotonin into *N*-acetylserotonin and thence, through the agency of hydroxyindole-*O*-methyltransferase, into *N*-

acetyl-5-methoxytryptamine (melatonin). Some of the melatonin formed in the pineal gland is released into the circulation. Part of this is taken up by other tissues (p. 332) and the rest is subjected to 6-hydroxylation by a liver enzyme. The 6-hydroxylated compound is excreted as the conjugated form.

The serotonin acetylating enzyme is found throughout the brain but only trivial amounts of N-acetylserotonin are found elsewhere than in the pineal gland, presumably because the further conversion to melatonin cannot take place.

Even in the pineal gland, the 5-hydroxyindoleacetaldehyde pathway provides the principal route of serotonin breakdown but the production of melatonin is of greater physiological interest. Its possible significance is discussed later (p. 332).

The widespread distribution of hydroxyindole-O-methyltransferase in sub-mammalian species suggests that methylation reactions constitute a primitive means of inactivating serotonin. The reader will have noticed the analogy between hydroxyindole-O-methyltransferase and catechol-O-methyltransferase.

DISTRIBUTION OF 5-HYDROXYTRYPTAMINE

Serotonin is very widely distributed in nature. It is found in some plants and fruits, including the avocado pear, the banana, the tomato and the Australian (but not the South African) pineapple. Among these fruits, banana skin has the highest amount of serotonin, the concentration reaching 150 μg per gram. It is a common constituent of plant and animal stings and venoms, the wasp sting apparatus containing about 300 μg per gram. It is strange that serotonin should be present in appreciable quantities both in delectable fruits and in poisonous stings.

In mammalian tissues, serotonin reaches its highest concentration in the pineal gland where it is present to the extent of 60 to 80 μg per gram. It is approximately equally distributed between the gland cells proper (the pinealocytes) and the plexuses of sympathetic nerve terminals that form a prominent feature of pineal structure. These nerve endings are unique among sympathetic nerves in containing serotonin instead of noradrenaline. However, if noradrenaline is infused into the pineal gland, it replaced serotonin in the nerves.

Most of the body's serotonin is contained, though at a lower concentration than in the pineal gland, in the intestine, where it is particularly associated with the argentaffin (so called because they can be detected with the aid of silver stains) or enterochromaffin cells. In the intestine, the highest concentration of serotonin is found in the mucous layer but the absolute amount varies both with the species and with the part of the gastrointestinal tract from which the sample is taken: the range of concentration is from 1 to 10μg per gram of mucosa.

In blood, serotonin is found predominantly, if not exclusively, in the platelets. As a result, appreciable amounts can also be obtained from extracts of the spleen. The serotonin content ranges from about 0.4 μg per 10^9 platelets in the rat to 7.5 μg in the rabbit. In human platelets, the value is about 0.7 μg per 10^9 platelets. In the rat and mouse (but not in other species) serotonin is present in mast cells and consequently in the skin.

Small amounts of serotonin are present in the liver, lung and kidney but the concentrations in these organs rarely exceed 0.5 μg per gram of tissue.

In view of the attention which has been directed towards the possible function of serotonin in the brain, it is worth mentioning here that even in those parts of the brain which are richest in the amine (the thalamus, the hypothalamus and the midbrain) the concentration is only of the order of 1 to 1.5 μg per gram. However, the functional importance of a substance is not necessarily proportional to its concentration in particular tissues and the sensitivity of nerve cells is different from that of muscle.

For a more detailed account of the distribution of serotonin, the reader is referred to the comprehensive tables in the monograph by Garattini and Valzelli (1965).

PHARMACOLOGICAL ACTIONS AND PHYSIOLOGICAL FUNCTIONS OF 5-HYDROXYTRYPTAMINE

Throughout this book, we repeatedly emphasize that although the physiological actions of a naturally occurring substance should be mirrored (if only in a distorted form) by its pharmacological effects, not all of the latter are necessarily reflections of physiological function. It is particularly necessary to emphasize this point in any discussion of the possible physiological functions of serotonin, since, although its pharmacological actions are varied, its physiological functions are not yet clearly defined. In this section, the actions of serotonin on various systems are outlined and an attempt is made to assess the relevance of these actions to physiological function. Reference will also be made to disturbances of function seen in patients suffering from tumours of the argentaffin cells of the intestinal mucosa—the so-called argentaffinomas or malignant carcinoids. These tumours secrete large quantities of serotonin (and other substances) and carcinoid patients thus provide some information concerning the pharmacological responses of the human subject to continuous serotonin release.

GASTROINTESTINAL TRACT
Serotonin stimulates the smooth muscle of the gastrointestinal tract. Different species and different parts of the tract vary in their sensitivity to serotonin but the rat is particularly sensitive and the isolated terminal colon and strips of

isolated stomach fundus from this species have been used for the bioassay of serotonin in tissue extracts.

When serotonin is applied to the mucosal surface of the isolated intestine, it stimulates peristalsis but it is without effect if it is applied to the serosal side of the preparation. It has also been demonstrated that serotonin is released from the intestine during peristaltic activity while diarrhoea is frequently complained of by carcinoid patients. These observations have led to the suggestion that serotonin is involved as a local hormone in the control of peristaltic activity. It is assumed that an increase in pressure in the intestine causes the liberation of serotonin which then stimulates intestinal movements. Against this hypothesis, however, must be set the fact that peristaltic activity is in no way impaired in rats whose intestines have been almost completely depleted of serotonin as a result of the animals' having been fed a tryptophan-free diet. This more recent work indicates that serotonin probably plays but a minor role in the control of intestinal activity.

Large doses of serotonin produce peptic ulcers in rats. Reserpine (p. 557) has a similar action and this may well be due to the drug's ability to release serotonin. The ulcerogenic action of serotonin is potentiated by adrenalectomy and inhibited by vagotomy, atropine and hexamethonium. There is a high incidence of peptic ulcer among patients with carcinoid tumours. On the other hand, disturbances of serotonin metabolism are not common in patients with peptic ulcer. It may be that serotonin is involved in some way in the regulation of the secretory and motor activity of the stomach. If this is so, large doses of serotonin might be expected to have the effects actually observed, even if peptic ulceration is not itself attributable to disorders of serotonin metabolism. There is certainly some evidence (p. 645) that acetylcholine is not the only transmitter substance influencing gastric activity.

Gaddum and Picarelli (1957) showed that the action of serotonin on the smooth muscle of the intestine was partially antagonized by dibenzyline (p. 299) but that, whatever the concentration of the blocking agent, the inhibition was never complete. Morphine also partially inhibited contractions produced by serotonin. Dibenzyline and morphine together, however, completely blocked the response. In the light of these observations, Gaddum concluded that the intestine carries two types of serotonin receptor and he named these 'D' and 'M' receptors to indicate their susceptibility to blockade by dibenzyline and morphine respectively. The D receptors are also blocked by lysergic acid diethylamide and the M receptors by atropine and cocaine. These findings suggest that the M receptors are associated with nervous elements in the intestine, while the D receptors are more closely related to the muscle. The isolated uterus contains few nerve elements and it is consonant with Gaddum's views concerning the location of the M receptors that the action of serotonin on the uterus, though completely inhibited by

lysergic acid diethylamide, is not antagonized at all by morphine, atropine or cocaine.

Gaddum's conclusions were at first criticized on the ground that the inhibitors he used were far from specific and had a number of actions unrelated to their ability to occupy serotonin receptors. However, later work established that his conclusions were essentially correct. Drakontides and Gershon (1968) demonstrated that the nerve receptors (M receptors in the original terminology) were blocked by phenylbiguanide and the muscle receptors (D) by methysergide (p. 334). Tryptamine also stimulates the intestine. It appears to do this by way of the muscle receptors because its action is antagonized by methysergide but is unaffected by phenylbiguanide.

Phenylbiguanide

If smooth muscle from the stomach or uterus is incubated with neuraminidase it loses its ability to respond to serotonin but it can be resensitized by exposure to compounds containing sialic acid (Woolley and Gommi, 1964; Wesemann and Zilliken, 1967). It is therefore suggested that sialic (N-acetylneuraminic) acid is an integral part of the serotonin receptor. This substance is a component of all gangliosides, which are themselves complex lipids found in the membranes of cells, particularly neurones. Gangliosides that can specifically bind serotonin have been isolated.

N-acetylneuraminic acid

CARDIOVASCULAR SYSTEM

Although serotonin has a vasoconstrictor action on isolated preparations, its effect on the blood pressure of the intact animal is not uniformly pressor. In rats, serotonin causes a brief fall followed by a short-lived rise and finally a prolonged fall in blood pressure. This has been called an *amphibaric* (literally 'both pressures') response. In cats, dogs and rabbits, serotonin often has a hypotensive action. In man, it usually causes the blood pressure to rise. The reason for these variable and often unpredictable effects is that serotonin has a variety of actions in the intact animal, the relative intensities of which vary with the species, the initial blood pressure, the dose of serotonin and the anaesthetic used. The individual effects which may contribute to the final blood pressure response are as follows:

(i) peripheral vasoconstriction due to a direct action on the blood vessels;

(ii) a reflex bradycardia and vasodilatation due to reflexes mediated by way of the vagus nerve and initiated by stimulation of chemoreceptors in the right atrium (the Bezold reflex) and the carotid and aortic bodies;

(iii) transient ganglion blockade;

(iv) inhibition of activity in the postganglionic sympathetic fibres when the sympathetic tone is high. This inhibition is brought about either by an action on the fibres themselves or by noradrenaline antagonism;

(v) a direct stimulant action on the vagus centre;

(vi) a direct stimulant action on cardiac muscle, causing tachycardia and an increased stroke volume. In the rabbit (but not, probably, in other species) this action is mediated by the liberation of noradrenaline;

(vii) constriction of the pulmonary artery;

(viii) release of histamine and adrenaline.

For an extended discussion of these mechanisms the reader is referred to the review by Page (1958) and by Garattini and Valzelli (1965).

It is only possible to hazard informed guesses concerning the function of serotonin in the physiological control of the human cardiovascular system. Carcinoid patients are often hypertensive and display a degree of pulmonary stenosis and this may certainly be a consequence of serotonin liberation. On the other hand, most authorities now believe that the peripheral dilatation and deep flushes experienced by these patients arise because of the liberation of plasma kinins so that we cannot take the occurrence of these vascular phenomena as evidence that serotonin may have a vasodilator action in the human subject. The evidence from migraine prophylaxis is no more helpful: migraine is associated with dilatation of the extracranial blood vessels and methysergide, a serotonin antagonist, prevents migraine attacks in some susceptible subjects. However, and as we shall see (p. 334), we must avoid the too facile conclusion that serotonin acts as a vasodilator substance in migraine. The consensus of evidence and opinion suggests that serotonin is, if anything, a local regulator of vasoconstrictor tone.

Like histamine (p. 336), serotonin dilates the capillaries and increases their permeability. These responses are probably only of importance in rats and mice. In these species, serotonin and histamine occur together in the mast cells and both substances participate in the mediation of cutaneous anaphylactic and anaphylactoid responses (p. 407). In other mammalian species, mast cells contain no serotonin.

RESPIRATORY SYSTEM

Serotonin is a powerful bronchoconstrictor agent and guinea pigs exposed to an aerosol containing serotonin suffer an anaphylactic-like shock similar to that produced by histamine. In addition to its direct action on the bronchioles, serotonin influences respiration by way of the respiratory components of the cardiovascular reflexes initiated by chemoreceptor stimulation. Like the cardiovascular responses, the respiratory changes are species dependent: in cats, apnoea is followed by a short-lived hyperpnoea, in dogs and man there is hyperpnoea and in rabbits dyspnoea occurs. The cardiorespiratory reflexes also affect bronchiolar tone independently of the direct action of serotonin.

Paroxysms of dyspnoea, similar to those seen in asthma are common in carcinoid patients. The evidence suggests, however, that if serotonin is involved at all in the production of asthmatic attacks in non-carcinoid patients, its role is only a minor one.

BLOOD

Serotonin is released from platelets when blood clots: the released amine presumably has a vasoconstrictor action and it may give rise to reflex cardiovascular and respiratory responses. Bleeding time (which is a measure of the ability of injured capillaries to produce haemostasis by vasoconstriction) is reduced by serotonin but there is no substantial evidence that any form of haemorrhagic disease is due to the platelets being deficient in serotonin or incapable of releasing the amine.

A fascinating recent hypothesis is that the platelets behave in the same way as do central neurones as far as the uptake and retention of serotinin is concerned so that events in the platelets might provide a clue to activity in the neurones. To take one example, the concentration of total 5-hydroxyindoles (predominately serotonin) in the blood of a group of children with Down's syndrome ('mongolism') averaged 49 ng per ml. In a comparable group of mentally normal children the concentration was 124 ng per ml (see Coleman, 1973). The implication that Down's syndrome is associated with a deficient uptake or retention of serotonin by central neurones led directly to the use of 5-hydroxytryptophan as a treatment for the condition though not yet, it must be confessed, to any great advantage to the treated patients. The analogy between platelets and neurones must not be pressed too hard—the platelet receptor seems, for instance, to be of the D variety (Michael, 1969).

THE KIDNEY

Serotonin has an antidiuretic action. This is brought about by a decrease in glomerular filtration rate consequent on constriction of the afferent arterioles. In some species, serotonin also acts on the tubules, causing an increase in water reabsorption. The antidiuretic action of serotonin can be produced by doses as low as 4 μg per kilogram in the rat. Blood serum and urine contain an antidiuretic substance distinguishable from the antidiuretic hormone. This material (the 'stable antidiuretic substance' of Ginsburg and Heller, 1953) has been identified as serotonin. All these observations have led some to suggest that serotonin may act as a local hormone in the kidney, being liberated from platelets as they pass through the kidneys in amounts determined by the state of the body's water content. There is little evidence to support this hypothesis and in patients with carcinoid tumours renal function is usually normal.

THE PERIPHERAL NERVOUS SYSTEM

The pain producing properties of serotonin and its effect on transmission processes in autonomic ganglia are mentioned on pages 417, and 177 respectively. Many of the peripheral actions of serotonin are similar to those of histamine and the nature of the interrelationships of these two substances in the production of allergic and anaphylactic reactions provides a problem of considerable interest. In the central nervous system the actions of serotonin parallel those of noradrenaline and raise questions concerning the significance of this parallelism which are as fascinating as those concerning the relationship between serotonin and histamine.

From the foregoing discussion, it will be clear that we are still quite ignorant of the physiological function of serotonin outside the central nervous system. It may act as a local hormone, regulating blood flow in localized regions in response to the body's needs but the evidence which supports this view is not very strong. Its central nervous functions are discussed elsewhere (p. 187).

SEROTONIN AND THE PINEAL GLAND

It has already been pointed out that serotonin and tryptophan-5-hydroxylase attain their highest concentrations in the pineal gland and that the gland's possession of hydroxyindole-O-methltransferase renders it unique among mammalian tissues. Work by Axelrod and his colleagues (Wurtman and Axelrod, 1968; Axelrod and Wurtman, 1968; Wurtman, Kelly and Axelrod, 1969) has raised fascinating possibilities concerning the physiological significance of these observations. These hinge particularly on the pharmacological properties of melatonin and on the factors that regulate its production in the mammalian pineal gland.

Although some have suggested that its appearance in pineal extracts is an extraction artefact, most authorities are satisfied that melatonin does occur in the pineal gland. This would certainly be the view of Lerner and his colleagues who had to use the pooled pineal extracts from no fewer than 250 000 cattle in order to obtain melatonin in sufficient quantity to permit its chemical identification.

The pineal gland is the only mammalian tissue capable of synthesizing melatonin but a few others (peripheral nerves, sympathetic ganglia, the ovary and the pituitary gland) take it up from the blood following its release from the pineal gland.

Melatonin lightens the skin of frogs and it prevents the skin-darkening action of the melanocyte stimulating hormone (p. 771). It has no direct action on mammalian skin.

In mammals, melatonin inhibits smooth muscle, including that of the gastrointestinal tract, the bronchi and the uterus. When small quantities are implanted in the hypothalamus, melatonin induces sleep. However, its most interesting actions are those which it exerts on the endocrine system. If melatonin is injected daily into immature rats, sexual maturation is delayed and when it does occur the growth rate of the ovaries is depressed and the dioestrus phase occupies a longer fraction of the sexual cycle that it does in untreated animals. In male animals, the development of the seminal vesicles is retarded.

Melatonin suppresses the secretion of luteinizing hormone and the melanocyte stimulating hormone of the pituitary gland and it depresses the activity of the thyroid and the parathyroid glands.

Methoxytryptophol (Fig. 20.1) behaves like melatonin. Both substances exert their effects on the pituitary gland as a result of a direct action on hypothalamic nuclei.

The real interest of these pharmacological observations lies in the fact that rats exposed to conditions of continuous darkness suffer endocrine changes similar to those produced by daily injections of melatonin. Exposure to continuous light produces the opposite effects—for instance, the oestrus phase of the oestrus cycle is prolonged. Moreover, the hydroxyindole-O-methyltransferase activity of the pineal glands of animals exposed to continuous light is no more than 40 per cent of that of rats living in darkness. Continuous darkness affects the actual synthesis of the enzyme: in animals given puromycin, an inhibitor of protein synthesis, darkness does not bring about the usual increase in enzyme activity.

The activity of 5-hydroxytryptophan decarboxylase is also influenced by environmental conditions, being almost twice as great in animals exposed to continuous light as in those kept in the dark.

The interesting possibility arises that the diurnal alternation of day and night and seasonal variations in their relative duration might bring about fluctuations in the synthesis and release of melatonin which in their turn induce cyclic and coordinated changes in the activity of the sex and other endocrine glands. Melatonin, in fact, may be one of the regulators of the 'biological clock'.

The effects of light and darkness on the activity of the pineal enzymes are certainly initiated in the eye. Impulses generated in the retina in the usual way pass along the optic nerve and then traverse a tract of fibres—the medial forebrain bundle—to the hypothalamus. They pass to the pineal gland in sympathetic fibres that are relayed in the superior cervical ganglion: cervical sympathectomy abolishes the effect of light and darkness on pineal enzymes.

The serotonin content of the pineal gland exhibits diurnal variations reaching a maximum value (under natural lighting conditions) during the early afternoon and minimum values near midnight. Neither blinding nor exposure to continuous darkness abolishes these fluctuations in serotonin content. On the other hand, exposure to continuous light does abolish them and the times of maximum and minimum content can be interchanged by reversing the lighting conditions. These findings are best explained on the assumption that the changes in the serotonin content are determined by an endogenous rhythm which is not dependent on, but can be modified by, light.

Changes in the rate of release of serotonin from its 'bound' form appear to underlie diurnal fluctuations in the amount of amine present in the pineal gland, since 'free' serotonin is rapidly metabolized.

The experimental pharmacologist should bear in mind the possibility of diurnal variations whenever he is investigating neurohumoral, endocrinological or other regulatory systems. It is advisable to expose experimental animals to a regular rhythm of darkness and artificial light and, as far as possible, to take measurements and prepare tissue extracts at the same time each day.

THE ESTIMATION OF
5-HYDROXYTRYPTAMINE IN TISSUE
EXTRACTS

Most investigators now estimate serotonin by the spectro-photofluorimetric method which is sensitive and specific. The tissue is homogenized with a protein precipitant (perchloric acid is very suitable for this purpose) and the serotonin in the alkalinized supernatant solution is treated with a mixture of borate buffer, sodium chloride and butanol. The organic phase is then shaken with a sodium chloride-saturated buffer and then with a phosphate buffer (pH7) and heptane. After centrifugation and removal of the organic phase, an appropriate volume of the aqueous solution is treated with ninhydrin. The fluorescence thus produced permits the serotonin to be determined. In tissues containing much serotonin, advantage can also be taken of its natural fluorescence. For further details of the ninhydrin method, the reader is referred to the paper by Snyder, Axelrod and Zweig (1965).

More recently, another fluorescence method has been developed, for the assay of serotonin, melatonin, and some other serotonin metabolites. The method involves condensation of the individual indolealkylamines with O-phthalaldehyde and it can be applied to the determination of both serotonin and noradrenaline in the same sample of brain

tissue, which need weigh no more than 50 mg (Maickel et al., 1968).

Because serotonin affects a variety of isolated tissues, a number of methods for its biological assay are available. These include the isolated atropinized oestrous uterus of the rat, the terminal colon of the rat, the blood vessels of the perfused rabbit ear, the isolated heart of the clam (Venus mercenaria) and the fundus of the rat stomach.

When the serotonin content of a tissue is to be determined by bioassay, it is usual to prepare the tissue extract with acetone in which serotonin is highly soluble. After evaporating off the solvent, fatty material is removed with petroleum ether. The residue is dissolved in an appropriate saline solution before bioassay. The presence of substance P (p. 194) in brain extracts may interfere with the assay of serotonin on some preparations, particularly the rat uterus. It can be removed by incubating the extract with chymotrypsin.

5-HYDROXYTRYPTAMINE ANTAGONISTS

A large number of substances antagonize the action of serotonin. Some are antagonists only in the sense that their actions are the opposite of those of serotonin or that they interfere with a mechanism (such as the depressor reflex) which is set in motion by serotonin. There remain many substances which are true antagonists and which block the action of serotonin on isolated preparations. Many of them have actions on the intact animal but it must not be too readily assumed that all the effects seen in the whole animal are necessarily due to serotonin antagonism. This is particularly important in connection with their actions on the central nervous system.

Notwithstanding the widespread occurrence and varied actions of serotonin, its antagonists have only a very limited use in clinical medicine.

The alkaloids of ergot (p. 295) all exhibit antiserotonin activity. Many of them have other pharmacological actions in addition but lysergic acid diethylamide (LSD) and compounds related to it are powerful and relatively specific antagonists. It was the ability of lysergic acid diethylamide to cause hallucinations in man which first led to the suggestion that serotonin plays a part in the regulation of nervous activity in the brain. A number of other compounds with a structural resemblance to serotonin are also effective antagonists. Those which are hallucinogenic are discussed as a group in Chapter 32 where their chemical formulae will also be found. Those without hallucinogenic activity are mentioned below.

Since all the serotonin antagonists mentioned here and in Chapter 32 bear a structural resemblance to serotonin itself, it is not surprising that many are competitive antagonists of serotonin.

Many psychotropic drugs have some degree of antiserotonin activity but the extent to which this explains their actions on the brain is disputed.

2-BROMO-LYSERGIC ACID DIETHYLAMIDE

This compound (often known as BOL) is as active a serotonin antagonist as lysergic acid itself when it is tested on isolated preparations but it is devoid of hallucinogenic activity. It is used in the laboratory when it is desired to identify the active material in tissue extracts: that part of the pharmacological response which is blocked by BOL can be attributed to serotonin. As when atropine or mepyramine are being used to block the actions of acetylcholine or histamine respectively, this test is only valid if it can be shown that, after removal of BOL from the bath, the responses to authentic serotonin and to the tissue extract recover at the same rate.

METHYSERGIDE

Methysergide (Deseril, Sansert), like BOL, antagonizes serotonin on isolated preparations but has no hallucinogenic activity. Its chief claim to attention is provided by its undoubted value in the prevention of migraine attacks in some susceptible subjects although it will not cut short an established headache. As a prophylactic, it is taken in doses of 1 to 2 mg four times daily.

The mode of action of methysergide in migraine is not known but it is unlikely to be a direct result of its serotonin antagonism. It is true that, in some patients, the urinary excretion of 5-hydroxyindoleacetic acid is sharply increased during migraine attacks and this may indicate a loss of serotonin from the body and hence the loss of a humoral factor that has been helping to maintain a degree of vasoconstrictor control on the extracranial blood vessels. But there is no evidence that methysergide is only of utility in those whose hydroxyindole metabolism is disturbed in this way and serotonin does not seem to be critically involved in the aetiology of more than a minority of cases of migraine. In any event, it is difficult to understand how a serotonin antagonist could correct a condition attributable to a deficiency of the agonist.

As we repeat in many places in this book, drug antagonists not infrequently display some agonist activity and it is theoretically possible that, in some circumstances, methysergide acts as a vasoconstrictor substance in its own right. However, it has to be admitted that laboratory experiments provide no evidence for such direct vasoconstrictor activity and a vasoconstrictor agent should be able to relieve, as well as to prevent, headache. A more tenable explanation may be that, in migrainous subjects, methysergide is capable of potentiating the action of a natural vasoconstrictor substance such as noradrenaline. An alternative view is that its protective effect derives from a central action on vascular reflexes. The problem of migraine, its aetiology and treatment is further discussed on p. 418.

Methysergide has also been employed—in these cases

certainly because of its antiserotonin properties—in the management of carcinoid patients and, very occasionally, to control mania.

Methysergide is not an entirely innocuous substance. Prolonged use carries with it the risk of retroperitoneal

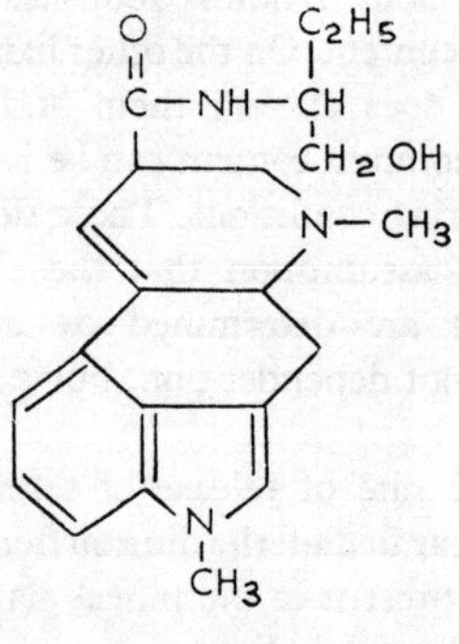

Methysergide

inflammatory fibrosis or of pulmonary fibrosis with valvular heart disease. Less serious complications include gastrointestinal upsets and symptoms of central nervous origin such as ataxia, dizziness, paraesthesiae and insomnia.

The dose of methysergide is 2 mg four times daily.

CYPROHEPTADINE

Cyproheptadine is a powerful antagonist of both histamine and serotonin. Its formula recalls that of two groups of psychotropic drugs—the phenothiazine tranquillizers and the imipramine-like antidepressants—which also possess the ability to antagonize the amines though to a lesser degree.

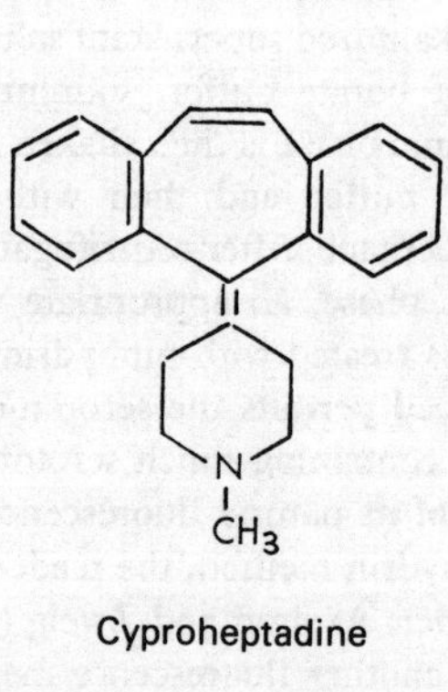

Cyproheptadine

By virtue of its antihistamine activity, cyproheptadine (Periactin, Perideca, Antegan) has been used in the treatment of allergic conditions. The dose is 4 mg taken four times daily.

BIBLIOGRAPHY

Books, monographs and reviews

Coleman, Mary (1973). *Serotonin in Down's Syndrome.* Amsterdam, London and New York: North Holland-American Elsevier.

Cummings, J.N. (ed.) (1973) *Background to Migraine.* London: Heinemann.

Garattini, S. and Shore, P.A. (eds.) (1968). Biological role of indolealkylamine derivatives. *Advances in Pharmacology,* Vols. 6A and 6B. New York and London: Academic Press.

Garattini, S. and Valzelli, L. (1965). *Serotonin.* Amsterdam, London and New York: Elsevier.

Lewis, G.P. (1958). *5-Hydroxtryptamine.* London: Pergamon Press.

Offermeier, J. and Ariëns, E.J. (1966). Serotonin, *Arch. int. Pharmacodyn.* **164** 192-245.

Page, I.H. (1954). Serotonin (5-hydroxytryptamine). *Physiol. Rev.,* **34,** 563-588.

Page, I.H. (1958). Serotonin (5-hydroxytryptamine); the last four years. *Physiol. Rev.,* **38** 277-335.

Wurtman, R.J., Kelly D.E. and Axelrod, J. (1969). *The Pineal,* New York and London: Academic Press.

Original papers

Axelrod, J. and Wurtman, R.J. (1968). Photic and neural control of indoleamine metabolism in the rat pineal gland. In, Garattini, S. and Shore, P.A. (1968)—see above—pages 157-169.

Drakontides, A.B. and Gershon, M.D. (1968). 5-Hydroxy-tryptamine receptors in the mouse duodenum. *Br. J. Pharmac. Chemother.,* **33,** 480-492.

Gaddum, J.H. and Picarelli, Z.P. (1957). Two kinds of tryptamine receptor. *Br. J. Pharmac. Chemother.,* **12,** 323-328.

Ginsburg, M. and Heller, H. (1953). Antidiuretic activity in blood obtained from various parts of the cardiovascular system. *J. endocrin.,* **9,** 274-282.

Makkel, R.P., Cox, R.H., Saillant, J. and Miller, F.P. (1968). A method for the determination of serotonin and norepinephrine in discrete areas of rat brain. *Inter. J. Neuropharmac.,* **7,** 275-283.

Michael, F. (1969). D-receptor for serotonin on blood platelets. *Nature,* **221,** 1253-1254.

Snyder, S.H., Axelrod, J. and Zweig, M. (1965). A sensitive and specific fluorescence assay for tissue serotonin. *Biochem. Pharmac.,* **14,** 831-835.

Wesemann, W. and Zilliken, F. (1967). Receptors of neurotransmitters—II. Sialic acid metabolism and the serotonin induced contraction of smooth muscle. *Biochem. Pharmac.* **16,** 1773-1779.

Woolley, D. W. and Gommi, B. W. (1966). Serotonin receptors VI—methods for the direct measurement of isolated receptors. *Arch. int. Pharmacodyn,* **159,** 8-17.

Wurtman, R.J. and Axelrod, J. (1968). The formation, metabolism and physiologic effects of melatonin. In, Garattini, S. and Shore, P.A. (1968) see above—pages 141-151.

21. Histamine and its antagonists

Histamine is widely distributed in plant and animal tissues. It was first synthesized in 1907 and in 1910 Barger and Dale showed that, like so many other substances of intense pharmacological interest, it was present in ergot. During the next few years, Dale and his colleagues investigated the properties of histamine. Much of our knowledge concerning its main pharmacological actions comes from these early papers which provoked an interest in histamine which is still intense and which still provides the major impetus to research in a number of laboratories throughout the world. It is, however, not yet possible to state with any certainty what are the physiological functions of this ubiquitous but puzzling substance whose most obvious action in the living animal is to cause untoward reactions when it is liberated from the cells that contain it. Histamine, indeed, is the enigma of pharmacology.

The word histamine means 'tissue amine' and it is an appropriate name for an amine which is so widely distributed. In the early years of its history, histamine went by its chemical name—β-iminazolylethylamine—because, as Sir Henry Dale (1953) explained in a later annotation to his and Laidlaw's classic paper of 1910, he had been asked not to use the word histamine (which he had already coined) because of the possibility of its being confused with a proprietary preparation with a vaguely similar name. Others were less sensitive to the rights of holders of trade marks and 'histamine' crept in, gaining general currency in about 1916.

$$HC \!\!=\!\! C.CH_2.CH_2.NH_2$$

(ring positions: 4, 5, N 3, 2, 1 NH, C, H)

Histamine

Histamine readily forms salts: the acid phosphate and the dihydrochloride are commonly used in the laboratory though the base is stable. A remarkable property of histamine is its stability towards acid. In a normal solution of hydrochloric acid, histamine can be boiled for up to two hours with no detectable loss of activity.

All pharmacologists should read at least some of the early papers on histamine. A selection of them is included, with their senior authors' later comments, in Dale's *Adventures in Physiology* (1953).

Pharmacological properties of histamine

The principal pharmacological actions of histamine can be summarized in a sentence. It causes contraction of smooth muscle, dilatation of capillaries and secretion of hydrochloric acid by the stomach. The relative intensity of these effects and the extent to which smooth muscle in different parts of the body is affected by histamine varies considerably with the species. Thus, in the cat, histamine causes widespread capillary dilatation which results in a profound fall of blood pressure notwithstanding a slight constriction of the arterioles resulting from stimulation of the vascular smooth muscle. Lethal doses of histamine cause so large a pooling of blood in these vessels that the return of blood to the heart is reduced to such an extent that the heart fails. The cat has, so to say, died of a haemorrhage into its own capillaries. In the rabbit, on the other hand, histamine causes constriction of the pulmonary artery and the blood flow through the lungs is restricted. With large doses of histamine this will be sufficient to cause death from asphyxia, but with non-lethal doses, the pulmonary arterial constriction together with some contraction of the smooth muscle in the arterioles of the splanchnic region causes a rise in blood pressure. The contrasting effects of histamine on the blood pressure of the cat and the rabbit are illustrated in Figures 21.1 and 21.2. It will be noticed that considerably larger doses of histamine must be given to the rabbit than the the cat in order to produce a vascular response. Rabbit tissues generally are relatively insensitive to histamine. Guinea pigs are extremely sensitive and in this species histamine causes an intense bronchoconstriction which may cause death from asphyxia. Finally, in the dog the hepatic sphincter (which controls the hepatic vein where it leaves the liver) is tightly constricted. The liver becomes engorged with blood which accumulates in the splanchnic vessels so that the blood pressure falls because of the reduced venous return.

With these general points in mind, the pharmacological actions of histamine can be considered in more detail.

(i) In the living animal, as has already been indicated, the actions of histamine on smooth muscle are most clearly seen in the blood vessels and bronchi. In isolated preparations, it can also be shown that the smooth muscle of the uterus and the intestine responds to histamine. The isolated terminal ileum of the guinea pig, indeed, is the most widely used preparation for the bioassay of histamine in tissue extracts and in Dale's early work the isolated uterus

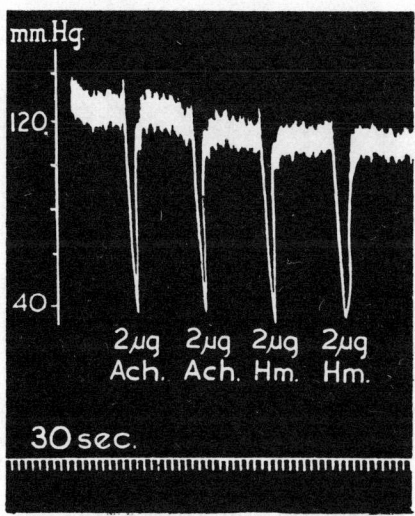

Fig. 21.1 The depressor effects of acetylcholine (ACh) and histamine (Hm) on the anaesthetized cat.

was employed to demonstrate the liberation of histamine in anaphylactic reactions (p. 405).

(ii) When it is injected into the blood stream, histamine produces effects that depend on the relative intensity of the constrictor and dilator actions on the arterioles and capillaries respectively. When histamine is injected into, or liberated from, the skin, however, it produces dilatation of both the capillaries and the neighbouring arterioles. Dilatation of the capillaries is associated with an increased permeability of these vessels and the increased exudation of tissue fluid gives rise to a weal. These three effects—dilatation of capillaries, formation of weals and dilatation

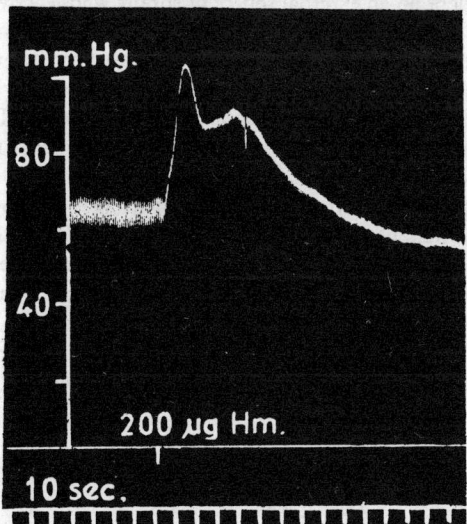

Fig. 21.2 The pressor effect of histamine (Hm) on the anaesthetized rabbit.

of the arterioles—constitute the well known *triple response* which can be very easily demonstrated in the human subject if a needle prick is made into the skin through a drop of histamine. The triple response can also be demonstrated in sensitive subjects without the necessity of actually injecting histamine. An object such as a ruler or the end of a pencil is drawn firmly several times over an area of the skin of the forearm or back. There is first of all a transient pallor which is no part of the triple response and is due simply to the fact that the blood has been pushed out of the superficial vessels. The pallor soon gives way to redness which accurately marks out the track of the object drawn over the skin. The accuracy of this delineation indicates that it is due to capillary dilatation. Weal formation develops in the area of capillary dilatation and at the same time an irregular area of redness appears. It covers a larger area than that due to capillary dilatation. This spreading *flare* is caused by arteriolar dilatation. Arterioles supply relatively large areas of the skin and when an arteriole in the path of the moving object dilates, it produces an area of cutaneous hyperaemia which spreads in an irregular fashion over the boundaries of the path.

Two components of the triple response (the capillary dilatation and the weal) are the direct result of histamine's being injected into the skin or liberated by the mechanical trauma. The arteriolar dilatation is an indirect effect caused by the operation of the *axon reflex*, the mechanism of which can be understood by reference to Figure 21.3. It can be seen that the sensory nerve fibre has two branches, one from an area of skin and the other from the neighbouring arteriole. Histamine stimulates the cutaneous branch of the sensory fibre and sends nerve impulses to the central nervous system in the usual way. However, when the impulses meet the junction with the branch from the arterioles, they send other impulses along that branch *towards* the vessel. When they reach it, vasodilatation occurs. Since the impulses pass along the branch in the 'wrong' direction (impulses in sensory fibres normally pass towards the central nervous system) they are said to be *antidromic*. There is nothing particularly unusual in the phenomenon of antidromic conduction since if a stimulus is applied to the middle of a length of any nerve, impulses will pass in both directions from the point of stimulation until they reach a synapse. Electrical stimulation of sensory nerve fibres will also cause dilatation of arterioles in the area from which the fibres arise. It should be added that although the arteriolar dilatation in response to histamine is said to be caused by an axon reflex, the mechanism is not a reflex in the usual physiological sense of that term, since it occurs independently of the central nervous system and no synapse intervenes in the 'reflex' pathway. Axon reflexes can still be elicited if the sensory fibre is cut between the cord and the bifurcation of the fibre. They are, however, reflexes in a literal sense, the

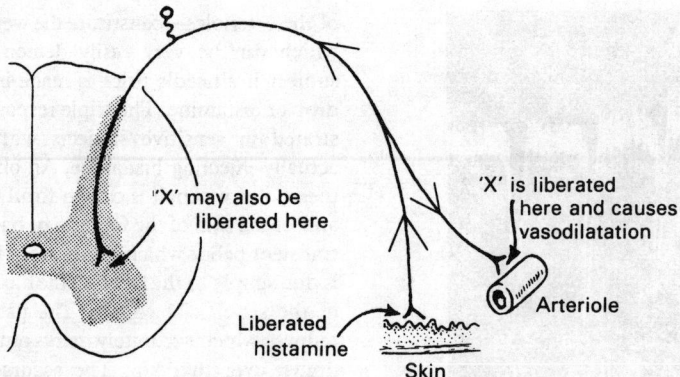

Fig. 21.3 The production of arteriolar dilatation by histamine liberation from the skin

nerve impulses being 'reflected' when they reach the junction.

The triple response in human skin was first investigated by Sir Thomas Lewis (1927). Lewis pioneered experimental work in the human being and by means of quite simple experiments he was able to illustrate differences and similarities between the human and the animal subject. He recognised that the triple response to mechanical stimulation was mediated by a histamine-like substance but with characteristic caution he suggested that it should be given the noncommittal name 'H-substance'. However, the presence of histamine in the skin, the action of histamine antagonists and the similarity of the triple responses produced by mechanical stimulation to that evoked by histamine, combine to make it clear that Lewis's 'H-substance' is indeed histamine.

The appearance of the skin after the injection of histamine is similar to that seen after a nettle sting. Histamine is one of the constituents of the fluid in nettle stings.

(iii) It has already been seen that histamine stimulates sensory nerves in the skin and thereby initiates an axon reflex. These same sensory impulses continue into the central nervous system and if of sufficient intensity they give rise to the sensation of itching or, less often, pain. The actions of histamine on other parts of the nervous system are less well defined. However, histamine will usually stimulate autonomic ganglia (Trendelenburg, 1954), and the adrenal medulla (Burn and Dale, 1926). This latter effect is responsible for the increase in blood pressure which often follows the hypotensive action of histamine in the cat. Histamine also augments the electrical activity of the cerebellum either directly or by way of an action on midbrain neurones.

(iv) Histamine causes the secretion of hydrochloric acid by the stomach. This action is discussed elsewhere (p. 641)

(v) In the human subject, histamine causes an intense headache, the result of dilating the intracranial blood vessels.

FORMATION, DISTRIBUTION AND METABOLISM OF HISTAMINE

Formation of histamine

Histamine is produced in the tissues from histidine under the influence of histidine decarboxylase. Some of the bacterial inhabitants of the intestinal tract also contain this enzyme and it was believed until recently that a proportion of the histamine in tissues (particularly those of carnivores) arrived there by uptake from the bloodstream of material that had been formed in the gut by bacterial decarboxylation of dietary histidine. It now seems clear that the tissues do not rely on exogenous sources for their supplies of histamine and that the activity of the endogenous enzyme is controlled by biochemical feedback mechanisms that ensure that tissue stores can be maintained at a more steady level than would be possible if they were even partly dependent on an external source of supply whose activity might well vary capriciously. It is true that many tissues can take up histamine but this facility is used to clear the bloodstream of excessive amounts of histamine appearing as a result, for instance, of an anaphylactic process. The material taken up in this way is slowly released to the metabolizing and excretory systems.

Histidine decarboxylase is widely distributed in animal tissues often, however, at a low level of activity. It is highly specific and utilizes pyridoxal phosphate as a coenzyme. A number of factors, including catecholamines and stimuli that provoke inflammation, promote the formation of histidine decarboxylase and hence that of histamine.

Histidine decarboxylase is inhibited by a number of

$$HC = C.CH_2.CH.NH_2$$

with the ring $N = C$ (H) — NH and COOH substituents

Histidine

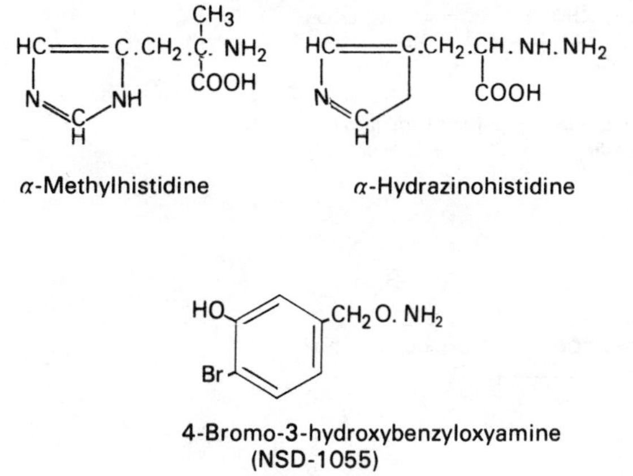

α-Methylhistidine

α-Hydrazinohistidine

4-Bromo-3-hydroxybenzyloxyamine
(NSD-1055)

Fig. 21.4 Inhibitors of histidine carboxylase

substances including α-methylhistidine. The last named serves to differentiate the enzyme from aromatic-L-amino-acid decarboxylase (DOPA decarboxylase, p. 259), an unspecific enzyme which is also capable of bringing about the decarboxylation of histidine. For its part, this enzyme is inhibited by α-methylDOPA (p. 288), neatly completing the parallel with histidine decarboxylase.

Other useful inhibitors of histidine decarboxylase include α-hydrazinohistidine and 4-bromo-3-hydroxy-benzyloxyamine (NSD-1055) (Fig. 21.4).

Distribution of histamine in the tissues

Although histamine is widely distributed, the relative amounts in different tissues vary with the species. Thus while amounts of up to 40 μg per gram are found in the livers of dogs and rabbits, the concentration in rat and guinea pig liver rarely exceeds 5 μg per gram. Guinea pig lung, on the other hand, has a histamine content of the order of 50 μg per gram, whereas that of the rabbit is less than 10 μg per gram of tissue.

The histamine content of brain is much lower than is often quoted but there is general agreement that the hypothalamus and the optic nerves contain more than the rest of the brain. Although the absolute amount of histamine in the central nervous system is very small in comparison with that in an organ such as the liver or lung, it is not small in relation to the amount of some other neurohumoral substances such as the monoamines (p. 183). Among different species, the histamine content of brain is much more uniform (the overall concentration being about 50 ng per gram) than that of other organs. Nonmyelinated nerve fibres are rich in histamine which thus seems to be associated with nervous tissue proper and not with the material of the sheath. These considerations all suggest that histamine may play a part in the regulation of nervous activity though the nature of this regulatory activity is, as yet, completely unknown.

In the gastrointestinal tract, the histamine content is high in the stomach (except the pyloric region) and the duodenum. Beyond the small intestine, there is a progressive fall in the histamine content of the gut, although even the colon contains appreciable amounts of the amine (Douglas, Feldberg, Paton and Schachter, 1951). In the stomach, a particularly high concentration of histamine is found in the parietal cells. This finding underlines the importance of histamine in the regulation of acid secretion.

In many tissues, histamine is bound with heparin within the mast cells which are themselves capable of slowly synthesizing the amine. Mast cells are contained in the connective tissue and are characterized by the presence of cytoplasmic granules which stain with basic dyes. The basophil leucocytes of the blood have similar characteristics and they are sometimes known as the mast leucocytes. The mast cells of the rat and mouse (but not those of other species) contain 5-hydroxytryptamine as well as histamine and heparin. There is a broad correlation between the mast cell and the histamine content of a tissue. It is important to note, however, that not all of the body's histamine is stored in mast cells. The brain, for instance, is virtually devoid of mast cells and in the stomach the histamine the parietal cell region does not appear to be associated with mast cells. It is tempting to offer the generalization that the histamine sequestered within the mast cells does not normally perform any physiological function while that which is free of the cells does have a physiological role. Certainly there is little experimental evidence to suggest that mast cell histamine is ever released in an orderly fashion in response to recognizably physiological stimuli.

Metabolism of histamine

Histamine can be metabolized along several pathways, some of which are of little importance in the mammal, although they may be of more significance in bacterial metabolism. In studying these and other metabolic systems, it is usual to give radioactive histamine to the animal and to determine the nature of the labelled metabolites which appear in the blood and urine. It is assumed that the metabolic processes involved in the degradation of this added or exogenous histamine are the same as those that break down tissue (endogenous) histamine. This is not necessarily so and some caution is needed in interpretation of the results of this type of experiment. The position is complicated by the fact that the path by which exogenous histamine is metabolized is to some extent dependent on the route by which it is administered.

Up to 80 per cent of the histamine administered to the mammal is metabolized along the two pathways shown in Fig. 21.5. The relative importance of the two major catabolic pathways varies with the species. The oxidative pathway to imidazoleacetic acid and its conjugated products is very important in the female rat but in the dog, cat, mouse, male rat and man, ring N-methylation accounts for most of the histamine loss. In other animals the two

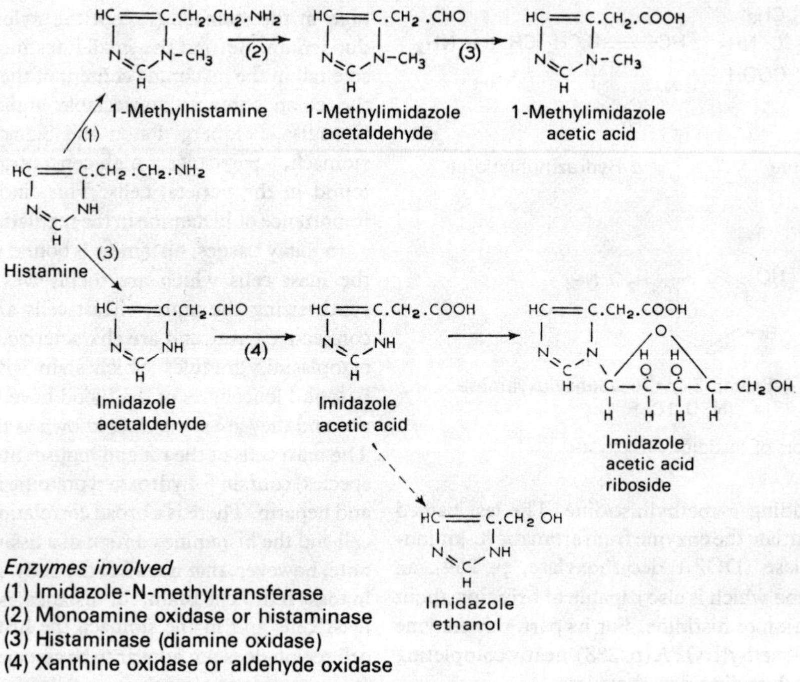
1-Methylhistamine
1-Methylimidazole acetaldehyde
1-Methylimidazole acetic acid
Histamine
Imidazole acetaldehyde
Imidazole acetic acid
Imidazole acetic acid riboside
Imidazole ethanol
Enzymes involved
(1) Imidazole-N-methyltransferase
(2) Monoamine oxidase or histaminase
(3) Histaminase (diamine oxidase)
(4) Xanthine oxidase or aldehyde oxidase

Fig.21.5 Major pathways of histamine metabolism (minor pathways are discussed in the text)

pathways contribute approximately equally to the breakdown of histamine.

Although oxidative deamination provides a relatively unimportant catabolic pathway for histamine in many species, it would be unwise to disregard histaminase completely. The activity of this enzyme in human blood increases during pregnancy and this is associated with (though it is by no means necessarily the cause of) a more effective disposal of exogenous histamine. The additional enzyme is of placental origin. Heparin injections also bring about an increase in the histaminase activity of plasma. Moreover, histaminase is present in high concentration in the intestine, kidney, liver (in some species) and thoracic duct lymph even in those mammals whose endogenous histamine does not apparently tread the path of oxidative deamination to destruction. This observation was originally made by Carlston (1950) using dogs, cats and rabbits. Later workers have reported similar findings in other species.

The thoracic duct opens directly into the venous system but, except in pregnancy, the histaminase activity of the blood is normally very low. It is still not known by what mechanism thoracic duct lymph so promptly loses its enzyme activity when it passes into the blood stream. The mystery is further confounded by the fact that both hypophysectomy and adrenalectomy bring about very large increases in the histaminase activity of thoracic duct lymph at the expense of that in the intestine and kidney. Again none of the enzyme apears in the plasma. This effect of interrupting the pituitary-adrenal axis can be reversed by giving an intravenous infusion of cortisone. The functional significance of these changes in histaminase activity in species that normally inactivate histamine largely by methylation cannot yet be discerned. It may be that the physiological substrate for histaminase is some substance other than histamine. The specificity of the enzyme is not high.

As long ago as 1938, Zeller showed that an extract of pig kidney that had histaminase activity was also capable of bringing about the deamination of other diamines such as putrescine and cadaverine (Table 21.1) and for this reason he proposed that the enzyme should be called 'diamine oxidase' instead of histaminase. The pig kidney enzyme has now been obtained in a purified state and it retains both histaminase and diamine oxidase activity. A similar remark applies to a purified enzyme preparation obtained from the human placenta. Moreover, both types of enzyme

Table 21.1 Some diamines and polyamines of physiological interest

$H_2N.(CH_2)_4.NH_2$	Putrescine
$H_2N.(CH_2)_5.NH_2$	Cadaverine
$H_2N.(CH_2)_3.NH.(CH_2)_4.NH_2$	Spermidine
$H_2N.(CH_2)_5.NH.(CH_2)_4.NH(CH_2)_3.NH_2$	Spermine

activity in these preparations are inhibited by aminoguanidine. For these reasons the terms 'histaminase' and 'diamine oxidase' are used interchangeably in the present account but the reader should remain alive to the possibility that some tissues may yield enzymes that act only on histamine or only on other diamines or whose action on these substances is not inhibited by aminoguanidine.

The nature of the enzyme that converts 1-methylhistamine into 1-methylimidazole acetic acid is not yet clearly established. The conversion can be brought about *in vitro* by diamine oxidase but in *in vivo* experiments it has been shown that aminoguanidine does not prevent the oxidative deamination of 1-methylhistamine. Iproniazid—which inhibits both monoamine oxidase and diamine oxidase—does prevent the conversion. This suggests that a monoamine oxidase is involved in the breakdown of 1-methylhistamine but it is not necessarily the same enzyme as that which is concerned in the metabolism of the catecholamines and 5-hydroxytryptamine.

In all species except the rat, the major route of metabolism of histamine added to the brain is by ring N-methylation. In rat brain *in vivo*, added histamine is converted largely to imidazoleacetic acid (Snyder, Glowinski and Axelrod, 1966). There is some evidence (White, 1960; Jonson and White, 1966) that, in the brain, endogenous histamine is less susceptible than exogenous histamine to enzymatic attack. The same conclusion has been reached by the present author and his colleagues in independent experiments of a different type.

Minor pathways of histamine metabolism include the following:

(i) Acetylation to acetylhistamine. This pathway is important in bacteria;

(ii) The nitrogen in the amino group of histamine can be methylated to give N-methylhistamine and N-dimethylhistamine. Both of these compounds have been detected in human urine but they could be of bacterial origin. A similar remark applies to imidazole ethanol (Fig. 21.4), which has also been found in human urine.

(iii) When large quantities of histamine are administered to animals, 1,5-dimethylhistamine (and the corresponding acetaldehyde and acetic acid) appear in the urine. Although these are abnormal metabolites in the sense that they only appear after large doses of histamine, it is possible that they may be formed when large amounts of histamine are liberated locally in allergic and anaphylactic reactions. However, the experimental evidence so far available indicates only that there is an increased urinary excretion of free histamine during anaphylaxis.

Further details concerning the metabolism of histamine can be found in reviews (Schayer, 1959, 1966; Buffoni, 1966; Kahlson and Rosengren, 1971) on which the above discussion is largely based.

Histaminase inhibitors

In the laboratory, aminoguanidine is a very useful and specific inhibitor of tissue histaminase activity. Guanidine itself, diguanidines such as Synthalin A (p. 730) and diamidines also inhibit histaminase. Diamidines have, in addition, histamine liberating properties (p. 342). Several other histamine liberators inhibit histaminase activity but there is no regular association between these two types of action. The diamidines and the diguanidines also inhibit monoamine oxidase to some degree. Similarly, those monoamine oxidase inhibitors that are hydrazide or hydrazine derivatives also inhibit the histaminase activity of tissues, as does semicarbazide, better known as an inhibitor of glutamic dehydrogenase (p. 191). Of the many other substances known to inhibit this enzyme, mention should be made of the hallucinogen, mescaline, the antispasmodic drug, papaverine and the vitamin, thiamine. A detailed survey of histaminase inhibitors is provided by Zeller (1963).

Substances that release histamine

Tissue histamine may be released, in a physiologically active form, in a variety of circumstances. The effects produced depend on the amount and site of histamine release: they range from a trivial itching to fatal anaphylactic shock. The nature and mode of action of substances that

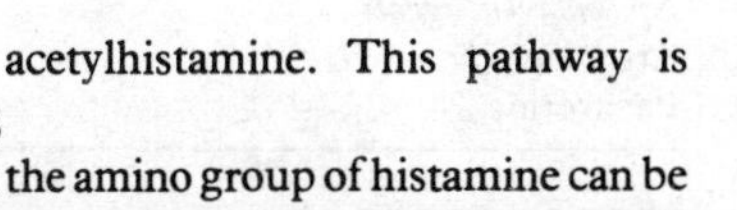

$$HC \!=\!=\! C.CH_2.CH_2.NH.COCH_3$$

Acetylhistamine

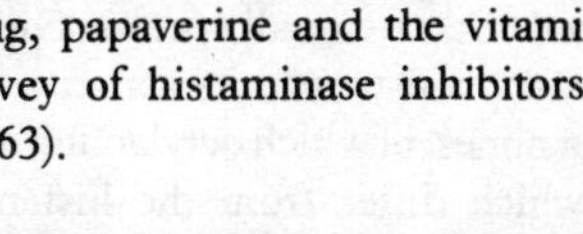

$$HC \!=\!=\! C.CH_2.CH_2.NH.CH_3$$

N-methylhistamine

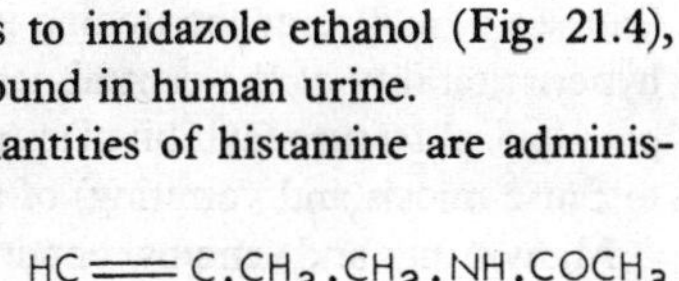

$$HC \!=\!=\! C.CH_2.CH_2.N(CH_3)_2$$

N-dimethylhistamine

$$HC \!=\!=\! C.CH_2.CH_2.NH_2$$

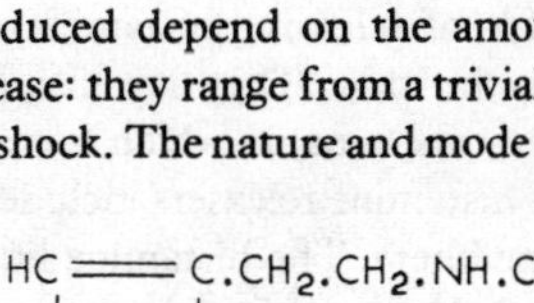

1,5 dimethylhistamine

Fig. 21.6 Some histamine metabolites

release histamine were reviewed in a well known paper by Paton (1957) and the classification of histamine releasing agents which follows is that adopted by Paton.

Histamine releasers fall into seven groups:

1. Antigens and simpler substances which can combine with proteins to form antigens. Under the appropriate circumstances, which are fully discussed elsewhere, antigens combine with antibodies and the combination is followed by the release of histamine and other substances.

2. Mechanical trauma and substances such as stings and venoms which damage the skin. As has already been discussed (p. 337) very mild mechanical stimulation is sufficient to cause histamine liberation in sensitive individuals.

3. Proteolytic enzymes.

4. Surface active agents such as detergents, bile salts and lysolecithin. The detergent, Tween 20 produces urticaria and other signs of histamine release in the dog but not in the rat. Some detergents, including Triton X-100 bring about the release of enzymes, ATP and potassium as well as histamine. This suggests that they cause actual damage to the mast cell membrane. Most of the other releasers are more specific in their effects, liberating mainly histamine.

5. High molecular weight compounds such as dextrans and polyvinylpryrrolidine. These substances, too, exhibit a degree of special specificity: dextrans are active in the rat and polyvinylpyrrolidine in the dog. A histamine releaser much used in the laboratory is compound 48/80, a polymer of p-methoxy-N-methyl phenyl ethylamine. Although compound 48/80 is a powerful and specific histamine releaser it is not effective in all species. Guinea pig tissues, for example, are resistant to its action.

6. A number of monoamines, of which octylamine is the best known example, which differ from the histamine liberators described below, in that they release potassium as well as histamine and their action is more prolonged.

7. Histamine liberators. A number of chemically unrelated substances are capable of releasing histamine very rapidly, particularly from the skin. They are classified together as histamine liberators, a name which serves to distinguish them from the histamine releasers included in the other six categories listed here. The histamine liberators are listed in Table 21.2. Many of them happen to be useful drugs, though their therapeutic actions are in no way related to their ability to release histamine. The histamine liberators are also capable, at least in some species, of releasing heparin and (at a high dose level) some of the other mediators of anaphylaxis.

Although small doses of antihistamines (H₁ antagonists) can prevent the histamine releasing action of compound 48/80, larger amounts promote histamine release.

It will be appreciated that a drug may cause histamine release by one of two mechanisms. It may be a histamine liberator of the type which has just been discussed or it may, in sensitive individuals, act as an antigen or as a part-antigen and so provoke an allergic response. In either instance the release of histamine (and associated substances) may be the cause of an unwelcome side effect of the drug's therapeutic action. The histamine liberators characteristically release histamine in a sudden 'explosive' manner from the skin and they are less likely to produce troublesome symptoms than drugs that give rise to allergic responses in which the release of the responsible agents is more prolonged and may be more widespread. Nevertheless, the intense itching that accompanies pentamidine treatment (p. 878) seems to be certainly attributable to histamine release. It is also usually assumed that the itching produced by morphine is the result of histamine release. In this instance, however, a rather more compli-

Table 21.2 The histamine liberators

Chemotherapeutic agents	Sympathomimetic agents
Chlortetracycline	Amphetamine
Pentamidine	Phenylethylamine
Phenamidine	Tyramine
Propamidine	
Quinapyramine	Vasodilator agents
Stilbamidine	Hydrallazine
	Tolazoline
Centrally-acting drugs	Trimetaphan
Apomorphine	
Codeine	Quaternary neuromuscular
Morphine	blocking agents
Pethidine	Benzoquinonium
Thebaine	Laudexium
Strychnine	d-Tubocurarine
Spasmolytic agents	
Atropine	
Papaverine	

cated mechanism may be involved since the itching outlasts the likely period of histamine release. It is possible (but see p. 428) that the itching is a manifestation of the hyperirritability of the central nervous system which is a paradoxical feature (exhibited also by the drug's tendency to cause miosis and vomiting) of morphine action.

Many stings and venoms contain histamine or histamine liberators. This point is discussed in detail elsewhere (p. 420).

The reader should note that most of the substances that evoke histamine release are basic in nature.

Physiological significance of histamine and histaminase

Histamine has dramatic effects when it is liberated into the tissues during allergic or anaphylactic reactions and it might be thought that these effects are merely exaggerated forms of the responses produced by smaller quantities of histamine liberated in the course of normal physiological activity. There is no evidence that this is so: there has, for instance, been no suggestion that bronchial or vasomotor tone is in any way regulated by histamine.

There is general agreement that histamine is a physiological regulator of gastric acid secretion but it would be surprising if that were the only function of so widespread a substance. Nevertheless, we are still quite ignorant of histamine's other physiological functions.

Perhaps the most interesting problem concerns the possible role of histamine in the central nervous system. It is discussed elsewhere (p. 195); here it is sufficient to say that, notwithstanding some suggestive evidence, we have no clear idea what part histamine plays in the regulation of nervous activity. The fact that histamine is present in the lungs, the intestinal tract and the skin—parts of the body that are in contact with the external environment—has led some authorities to suggest that histamine is involved in the defence of the organism against attack by external agents. The nature of histamine's participation in such activity is not specified.

Under normal conditions much of the body's store of histamine remains bound in an inactive form within the tissues so that little breakdown of the endogenous amine occurs. It is, however, worth enquiring a little more closely into the possible significance of the histamine catabolizing enzymes.

Histaminase activity is found in the gastrointestinal tract of animals that can produce histamine in the gut by bacterial decarboxylation of histidine and it may be that the enzyme serves to limit the absorption of histamine. In this connection, it is interesting to note that when the intestine of rats was sterilized by adding a sulphonamide to the diet for several weeks, the intestinal histaminase activity was reduced by almost one third (Abdel-Aziz and Boullin, 1964). Again, in some animals histaminase is absent from the gastric mucosa where free histamine must be liberated to regulate the secretion of acid. Presumably the lack of histaminase helps to maintain the histamine at the required concentration. Placental histaminase may serve to prevent the passage of histamine from foetus to mother or alternatively to protect the mother against histamine liberated in her own uterus, since sex hormone activity tends to cause disruption of mast cells. Finally, it is to be remembered that histaminase is not specific and its physiological activity may be exerted on substances other than histamine.

The histaminases of blood are also not specific. Benzylamine, the preferred substrate of plasma histaminase, is not a normal constituent of the animal body and the enzyme may serve to destroy any benzylamine absorbed from articles of diet. The benzylamine oxidase of human plasma also has diamine oxidase activity and the possibility that the enzyme has a protective function is suggested by the fact that the amount in plasma increases during pregnancy, a condition which is associated with increased plasma concentrations of histamine, putrescine and cadaverine.

The quantitative estimation of histamine

A number of methods has been used in the past for the determination of histamine but only two of these—one biological and one chemical—merit the serious attention of the modern pharmacologist.

BIOLOGICAL DETERMINATION

The isolated atropinized terminal ileum of the guinea pig provides a sensitive method for the assay of histamine. When tissue extracts are studied it is essential to free them from other substances that might cause the ileum to contract or otherwise influence its activity. The best available method is still that of Barsoum and Gaddum which was developed more than 40 years ago. In outline, the procedure involves homogenization of the tissue in trichloroacetic acid, washing the supernatant solution with ether and boiling the washed material with hydrochloric acid for at least 90 minutes. The boiled solution is evaporated to dryness and taken up in ethanol. The final solution is itself evaporated to dryness in which state it can be stored almost indefinitely in the cold. It is dissolved in water and neutralized on the day of assay. Details of the procedure are given by Crossland (1961). It should be noted that none of the steps in the procedure can be omitted or curtailed. Failure to observe this precaution may lead to the retention of active material other than histamine and to an exaggerated estimate of the amount of histamine present in the extract. It is usual to confirm that the biological activity of each extract tested is indeed attributable to histamine. This is done with the aid of a suitable antihistamine drug, as described on page 352.

This method of histamine determination suffers from the disadvatage of tediousness, since both the extraction and the assay processes are time consuming. On the other hand, the method is extremely reliable and it can be used to assess the accuracy of the chemical method.

It is a wise precaution when embarking on a new project in which it is intended to estimate histamine by a chemical method, to perform preliminary experiments in which the histamine content of the relevant tissue is determined by the biological as well as the chemical method. A coincidence of the results obtained by the two methods provide an assurance that the chemical method is suitable for that particular investigation. If the two methods do not agree it is prudent to use bioassay instead of the chemical method.

CHEMICAL DETERMINATION

In 1959, Shore, Burkhalter and Cohn introduced a fluorimetric assay for histamine. The method involves the taking up of histamine into butanol from a perchloric acid homogenate of the tissue. It is condensed with o-phthalaldehyde to give a strongly fluorescent solution whose intensity is compared with that produced in standard solutions of histamine taken through the same procedure. The original paper gives details of the several precautions which must be taken if reliable and reproducible results are to be obtained.

The fluorescence method in its original form is adequate when tissues rich in histamine are being examined. As several groups of workers have shown, it is, however, unsuitable for brain tissue which contains little histamine but considerable quantities of substances that are not eliminated in the extraction process and which themselves form fluorescent products with o-phthalaldehyde. The most important of these substances is spermidine (Kremzner and Pfeiffer, 1966). As a result of their presence, the unmodified fluorescence method consistently produces falsely high estimates of brain histamine content, as can be readily demonstrated by comparing these estimates with those obtained by application of the biological method (Crossland, Woodruff and Woodruff, 1966). Recently a method has been developed in which brain extracts are adsorbed on to an ion exchange column from which histamine, spermine and spermidine can be eluted and separately estimated (Shaw, 1968). This technique has the advantage not only of producing reliable assays of the brain histamine content but also of permitting the determination on the same extract of both spermine and spermidine, substances that are of interest in their own right.

HISTAMINE ANTAGONISTS

There are three types of substance that might, on theoretical grounds, be expected to counteract the actions of free histamine:

(i) those that accelerate its destruction or inactivation;

(ii) those whose pharmacological actions are the opposite of those of histamine itself;

(iii) those that prevent the access of histamine to its receptors.

Useful substances of the first type are as yet not available, since it is impracticable to administer sufficient quantities of a purified enzyme to the intact animal. Several compounds fall into the second category and some of them find clinical application. Adrenaline, isoprenaline, aminophylline and atropine-like compounds, for instance, all counteract bronchoconstriction provoked by histamine and they have all been used in the treatment of asthma. Substances of the third type, which more or less specifically antagonize the actions of histamine, form the subject of the following paragraphs.

The development of histamine antagonists progressed along a remarkably similar course to that followed by antiadrenaline agents. The reader will recall that, over a period of many years, a large number of compounds capable of blocking adrenaline receptors were introduced into the laboratory and clinic. All those that appeared before 1958 had additional pharmacological effects but

none of them was able to antagonize all the known actions of adrenaline (p. 292). With the general acceptance of Ahlquist's hypothesis that adrenaline receptors are of two types, it became clear that this first group of antagonists blocked α receptors but spared those of the β variety. This led to the quest for specific β blocking agents. Since β blocking activity had not emerged in any of the α antagonists, notwithstanding the variety of chemical structures they displayed, it was evident that a new approach would have to be adopted if a β receptor antagonist was to be found. Success followed a decision to examine the pharmacological activity of substances derived from isoprenaline, the prototypical agonist at β receptors. The first β blocking agent appeared in 1958; it has been followed by a deluge of similar substances. All members of the group are much more specific in their actions than are those that occupy only α receptors.

The first histamine antagonist appeared in 1937 and it triggered a positively explosive development of agents of this type. All of these so-called *antihistamines* exhibited a variety of other pharmacological actions but, as with the early adrenaline antagonists, none was capable of preventing all the actions of the agent it was meant to oppose. In particular none could antagonize histamine's ability to provoke the secretion of gastric acid. Over the years, several explanations were proffered for this deficiency but the general climate of pharmacological opinion eventually veered to favour the idea that the action of histamine on gastric secretion involved different receptors (the H_2 receptors) from those (the H_1 receptors) blocked by the antihistamines.

A positive search for antagonists of H_2 receptors then began. Structural modifications were made to the histamine molecule, analogous to those that, in the case of isoprenaline, changed an agonist into an antagonist and after a somewhat protracted labour, the first H_2 antagonist was born. Two others followed: all three compounds specifically block H_2 receptors but, like those that block β receptors, they have few other pharmacological actions.

Although only one H_2 receptor antagonist (cimetidine) is currently in clinical use, others will inevitably make an appearance and a range of therapeutic applications, greater than can presently be visualized, will no doubt be found for them because it is clear that H_2 receptors are much more widely distributed than was at first thought. It is possible that H_2 blocking agents will become at least as important as those that occupy H_1 receptors and the present dichotomy into 'antihistamines' and H_2 'receptor antagonists' will offend against both common sense and semantics. It is better to speak of histamine H_1 antagonists and histamine H_2 antagonists and to reserve 'antihistamine' as a generic term that relates to histamine antagonists in general. As far as possible, this nomenclature is adhered to throughout this book, although slight modifications of terminology

(H$_1$ antagonists, H$_2$ blocking agents, H$_1$ antihistamines) will appear in the interests of literary elegance.

Substances that cause blockade of histamine H$_1$ receptors (the antihistamines)

In 1937, Bovet in France was able to announce the discovery of thymoxyethyldiethylamine (929F), the first antihistamine. During the war years, Bovet and his group pursued their study of compounds of this type intensively and they discovered many active compounds. Their work stimulated research in other countries and a vast number of substances with antihistamine activity was discovered. Antergan (Table 21.3) was the first histamine antagonist to be introduced into clinical practice but it was soon followed by many more. At the time when the H$_1$ antagonists were being actively developed, it was generally believed that all the symptoms of allergic and anaphylactic conditions were the result of histamine release and it was hoped that the new drugs would bring considerable therapeutic benefits. Although they have proved useful in a number of conditions and sales have reached a high level, the early hopes have not been completely fulfilled.

The names, chemical formulae and recommended doses of some of the drugs that block histamine H$_1$ receptors are given in Table 21.3. No useful purpose would be served by attempts to memorize the information given in this Table, which is provided for reference and for illustrating some of the general features of antihistamine structure.

In Fig. 21.6 (p. 341) the formula of histamine is compared with those of β-2-pyridyl ethylamine and β-3-pyrazole ethylamine. Both of these last named compounds mimic the action of histamine but blocking activity appears when alkyl groups replace the hydrogen atoms on the nitrogen of the ethylamine chain. Almost all of the many hundreds of H$_1$ antagonists that have been synthesized are substituted ethylamines—compounds, that is, that contain the –CH$_2$.CH$_2$.N= chain. This is illustrated by the examples given in Fig. 21.6 and the many more displayed in Table 21.3. In some compounds (promethazine, for instance) one of the carbon atoms in the ethylamine residue, as well as the nitrogen, bears an alkyl substituent. It is reasonable to conclude that it is the presence of the substituted ethylamino group which confers antagonist activity. It should be noted that a similar transition from mimetic to antagonistic activity as a result of substitution of small by larger radicals occurs in other classes of compound—those related to acetylcholine and noradrenaline, for instance. In some of the H$_1$ antagonists, part of the ethylamine is incorporated within a ring structure.

Substituted ethylamino groups appear in a variety of compounds and the ability to exert a degree of H$_1$ antagonism activity is a not uncommon feature of many drugs whose principal actions are exerted on other systems. Phenoxybenzamine (p. 299), which is classified as an adrenaline blocking agent, is as potent an antihistamine as mepyramine and many local anaesthetics, tranquillizers and atropine-like drugs have some antihistamine activity.

Structural features in the drugs that occupy histamine H$_2$ receptors are discussed later (p. 353).

Several chemical classifications of the drugs that block histamine H$_1$ receptors are possible. None has any special advantage since it is not possible to relate particular facets of the action of different antihistamine drugs to their chemical structures. The classification in Table 21.3, though not the most popular, was chosen in order to emphasize the occurrence of types of compound that are also encountered among other groups of drugs. Many phenothiazines, for instance, are used as tranquillizers and diphenylmethane derivatives are found among the atropine-like drugs and the anti-Parkinsonian agents. An alternative, and apparently more rigidly chemical, classification groups the drugs according to the nature of the atom or group that connects the ethylamine residue to the rest of the molecule. This gives us the ethanolamines (in which the connecting link is provided by an oxygen atom), the alkylamines (carbon link) and the ethylenediamines (nitrogen link) together with piperazines and phenothiazines. However, even this classification still leaves a residue of 'other drugs' that cannot be allocated to any of the major categories and it is not always easy to divine the logic that has determined the place of some of those that are included in the major categories.

Pharmacological properties of drugs that cause blockade of histamine H$_1$ receptors

Some of the effects produced by this group of drugs clearly spring from their ability to antagonize the actions of histamine while others are equally clearly the result of properties that are independent of their antihistamine activity. There remain a number of actions which cannot readily be assigned to either of the other two categories.

The histamine antagonizing actions can be demonstrated both on isolated preparations and in the intact animal. Thus, the H$_1$ antagonists inhibit histamine-induced contractions of the intestine, uterus, bronchioles and arterioles. They also prevent the capillary dilatation and weal formation which otherwise occurs when histamine is injected into, or liberated from, the skin. It can be shown on isolated preparations that they are competitive antagonists of histamine; they do not prevent histamine liberation.

Thymoxyethyldiethylamine (929F)

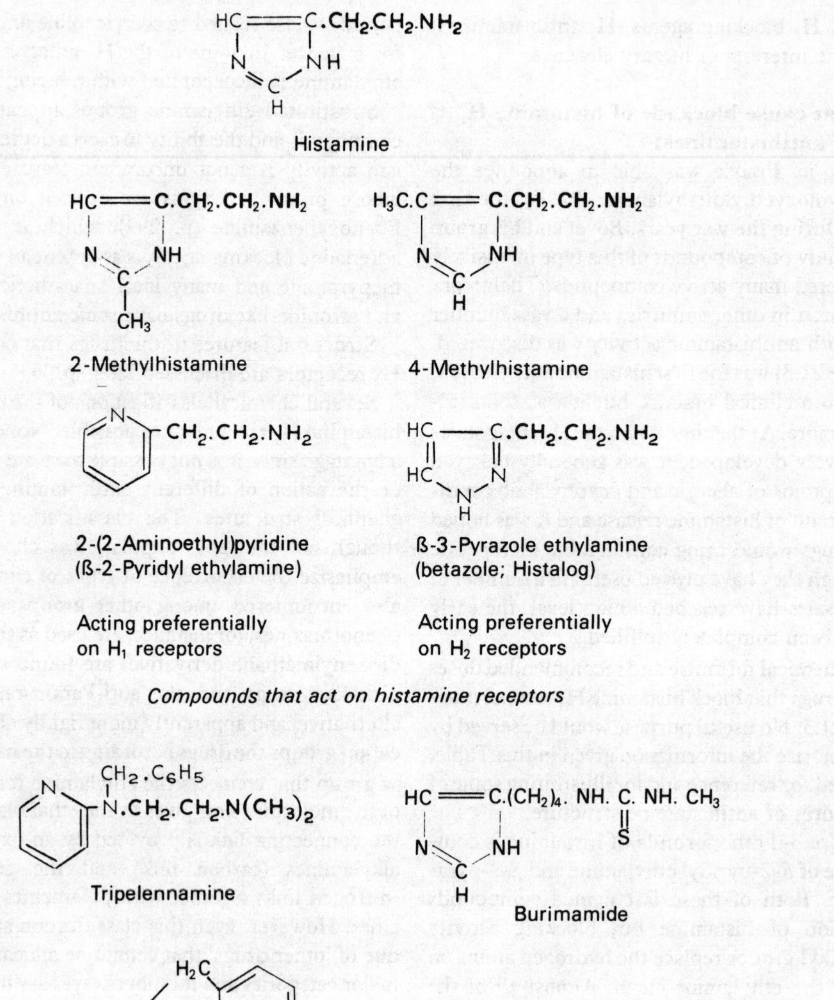

HC══C.CH₂.CH₂.NH₂

Histamine

HC══C.CH₂.CH₂.NH₂

2-Methylhistamine

H₃C.C══C.CH₂.CH₂.NH₂

4-Methylhistamine

CH₂.CH₂.NH₂

2-(2-Aminoethyl)pyridine
(ß-2-Pyridyl ethylamine)

Acting preferentially
on H₁ receptors

HC══C.CH₂.CH₂.NH₂

ß-3-Pyrazole ethylamine
(betazole; Histalog)

Acting preferentially
on H₂ receptors

Compounds that act on histamine receptors

CH₂.C₆H₅

N.CH₂.CH₂.N(CH₃)₂

Tripelennamine

HC══C.(CH₂)₄. NH. C. NH. CH₃

Burimamide

H₂C

N

CH₂.CH₂.N(CH₃)₂

Antergan

H₃C. C══C.CH₂. S(CH₂)₄. NH. C. NH. CH₃

Metiamide

H──C──N   N.CH₃

Cyclizine

H₁ antagonists

H₃C. C══C.CH₂. S(CH₂)₂. NH. C. NH. CH₃

Cimetidine

H₂ antagonists

Antihistamines

Fig. 21.7 To illustrate the structural relationships among histamine agonists and antagonists

Table 21.3 Some drugs that block histamine H_1 receptors
The form in which the drug is normally supplied is indicated in parentheses

1. ANILINE DERIVATIVES

Approved name(s)	Proprietary name(s)	R_1	R_2	Dose and remarks
Antergan		(phenyl)	$-CH_2.CH_2.N(CH_3)_2$	The earliest 'antihistamine'. Not now used
Antazoline (hydrochloride, mesylate, phosphate)	Antistin	(phenyl)	$-CH_2-$ (imidazoline)	50–100 mg 4 times daily
Methaphenilene (hydrochloride)	Diatrin(e)	(thienyl)	$-CH_2.CH_2.N(CH_3)_2$	25–50 mg 4 times daily
Thenalididine (tartrate)	Sandosten	(thienyl)	(N-methylpiperidine)	Withdrawn because of side effect (agranulocytosis)

2. DIPHENYLEMETHANE DERIVATIVES

Approved name(s)	Proprietary name(s)	R_1	R_2	R_3	Dose and remarks
Buclizine (hydrochloride)	Bucladin-S	H	$-N$ (piperazine) $N.CH_2$— (with $H_3C-C(CH_3)-CH_3$ substituted phenyl)	Cl	50 mg 2–4 times daily. Sedative. Used in motion sickness
Cyclizine (hydrochloride, lactate)	Marzine; Valoid	H	$-N$ (piperazine) $N.CH_3$	—	25–50 mg 3 times daily. Used in motion sickness, Ménière's disease, etc.
Chlorcyclizine (hydrochloride)	Diparalene; Perazil	H	$-N$ (piperazine) $N.CH_3$	Cl	50–100 mg twice daily
Diphenhydramine (hydrochloride)	Benadryl	H	$-O.CH_2.CH_2.N(CH_3)_2$	—	50–100 mg 3 times daily. Used in motion sickness

[In Bromdiphenydramine (Ambodryl), R_3 is Br. The compound is twice as potent as diphenhydramine and has fewer side effects]

Table 21.3 (continued)

Approved name(s)	Proprietary name(s)	R_1	R_2	R_3	Dose and remarks
Dimenhydrinate	Dramamine; Gravol	H	—O.CH$_2$ CH$_2$.N(CH$_3$)$_2$		50 to 100 mg 3 times daily. Used in motion sickness

[Note that dimenhydrinate is the diphenhydramine salt of 8-chlorotheophylline]

Approved name(s)	Proprietary name(s)	R_1	R_2	R_3	Dose and remarks
Diphenylpyraline (hydrochloride)	Diafen Hispril; Histryl Lergoban	H	—O⟨ ⟩N.CH$_3$	—	2 mg 3 or 4 times daily Sedative
Meclozine Meclizine (hydrochloride)	Bonamine; Bonine	H	N⟨ ⟩N.CH$_2$ (CH$_3$-aryl)	Cl	25-50 mg once daily. Long acting. Used in motion sickness.
Pyrrobutamine (phosphate)	Pyronil	—	—CH$_2$.CH$_2$.N⟨ ⟩	Cl	15-25 mg 3 times daily

Pyrrobutamine is a phenylbenzylmethane derivative

3. PHENOTHIAZINE DERIVATIVES

Approved name(s)	Proprietary name(s)	R	Dose and remarks
Methdilazine (hydrochloride)	Dilosyn; Tacaryl	—H$_2$C⟨ ⟩N—CH$_3$	8 mg twice daily. Sedative. Some anti-serotonin activity
Promethazine (hydrochloride)	Phenergan Histantil	—CH$_2$.CH.CH$_3$ | N(CH$_3$)$_2$	25 mg once daily. Very long acting. Sedative. Used in motion sickness. Local anaesthetic. Some antiserotonin activity
Pyrathiazine (hydrochloride) and theoclate	Pyrrolazote	—CH$_2$.CH$_2$.N⟨ ⟩	25 mg 4 times daily
Trimeprazine	Temaril; Vallergan	—CH$_2$.CH.CH$_2$.N (CH$_2$)$_2$ | CH$_3$	2.5 mg 3 times daily

Table 21.3 (*continued*)

4. PYRIDINE DERIVATIVES

Approved name(s)	Proprietary name(s)	R_1	R_2	Dose and remarks
Mepyramine Pyrilamine (maleate)	Anthisan; Neoantergan		$-CH_2.CH_2.N(CH_3)_2$	25-100 mg 4 times daily
Tripelennamine (citrate, hydrochloride)	Pyribenzamine		$-CH_2.CH_2.N(CH_3)_2$	50 mg 3 times daily. Very strong sedative
Methapyrilene Thenylpyramine (hydrochloride)	Histadyl		$-CH_2.CH_2.N(CH_3)_2$	50-100 mg 3 or 4 times daily
Chloropyrilene Chlormethapyrilene Chlorothen (citrate)	Tagathen		$-CH_2.CH_2.N(CH_3)_2$	25-50 mg 3 or 4 times daily

[In Bromethen, the Cl in R_1 is replaced by Br]

| Thenyldiamine (hydrochloride) | Thenfadil | | $-CH_2.CH_2.N(CH_3)_2$ | 25 mg 3 or 4 times daily |

Approved name	Proprietary name(s)	R_1	R_2	R_3	Dose and remarks
Chlorpheniramine Chlorprophenpyridamine (maleate)	Chlor-trimeton; Haynon Piriton	H	$-CH_2.CH_2.N(CH_3)_2$	Cl	4 mg 4 times daily

[Related compounds include pheniramine (Trimeton; 25 mg. thrice daily) which contains no Cl and brompheniramine (Dimotane) in which Cl is replaced by Br. The dose of brompheniramine is the same as that of chlorpheniramine. Dextrochlorpheniramine (Polaramine) is taken in doses of 2 mg.]

Carbinomaxine (maleate)	Clistin	H	$-O.CH_2.CH_2.N(CH_3)_2$Cl		5 mg 3 times daily
Doxylamine (succinate)	Decapryn	CH_3	$-O.CH_2.CH_2.N(CH_3)_2-$		12.5 mg 2 or 3 times daily. Strongly sedative

Table 21.3 (*continued*)

Approved name(s)	Proprietary name(s)	R_1	R_2	R_3	Dose and remarks
Triprolidine (hydrochloride)	Actidil	—	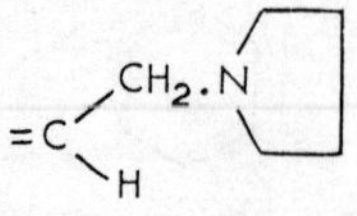	CH_3 (in *meta* position)	2.5-5 mg 3 times daily

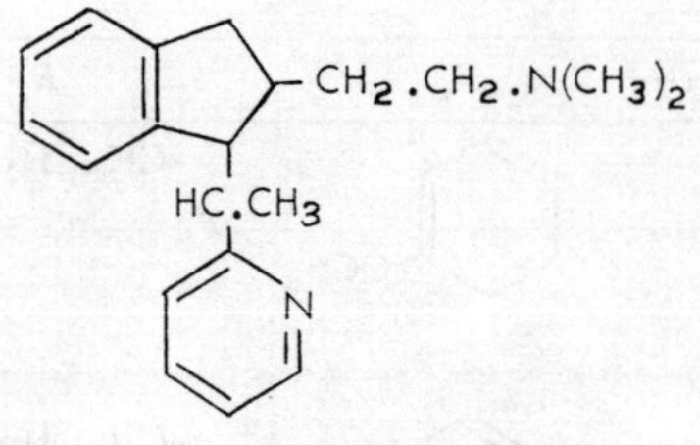

Approved name	Proprietary name(s)	Dose and remarks
Dimethindene (maleate)	Fenostil; Forhistal;	1 mg 3 times daily.

5. PYRIMIDINE DERIVATIVE

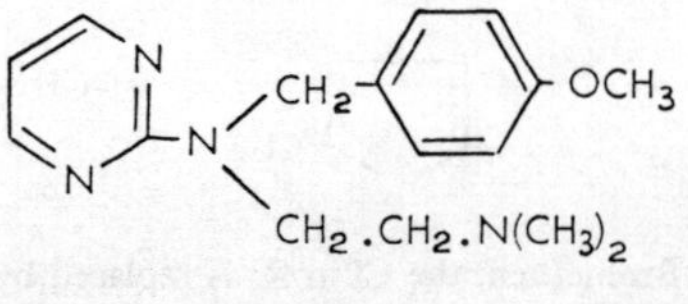

| Thonzylamine (hydrochloride) | Neohetramine; Anahist | 50-100 mg 3 times daily |

6. TETRAHYDROPYRIDINDENE

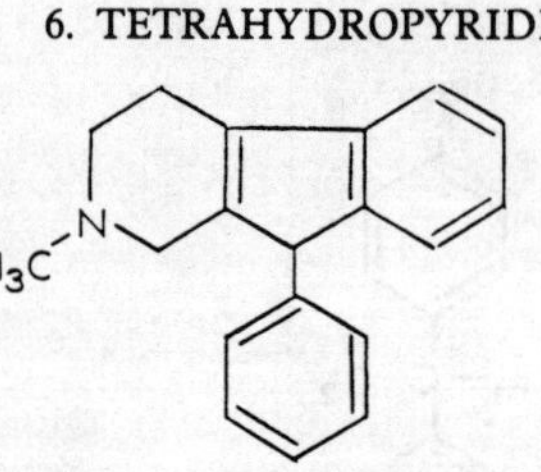

$C_4H_6O_6$

| Phenindamine tartrate | Thephorin | 25-50 mg 3 times daily. Some stimulant activity |

7. OTHER COMPOUNDS

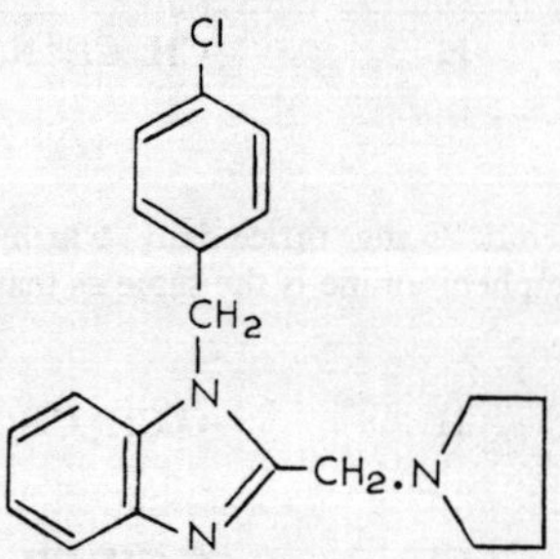

| Clemizole (hydrochloride) | Allercur | 25 mg 3 times daily Sedative |

Cyproheptidine (p. 334) also has some H_1 blocking activity

Trimethobenzamide (p.605) has weak blocking activity

The only major action of histamine that is completely resistant to block by the H_1 antagonists is its ability to stimulate the secretion of gastric acid. In the past, a number of hypotheses were advanced to explain this refractoriness of acid secretion. Among them was that of Ash and Schild (1966) who were the first formally to propose that histamine effects on gastric secretion are mediated by way of a population of receptors different from those that are involved in many other histamine responses. Their hypothesis was completely vindicated by the discovery of drugs that specifically block these 'H_2' receptors. As we have already seen (p. 344) the situation so far as antagonists are concerned is analogous to that which obtains with adrenaline receptors; if the analogy between the two mediators is to be maintained, agonists that act exclusively or preferentially on only one type of receptor should be available and they are, indeed, now beginning to appear. Betazole (Fig. 21.7) has, in comparison with histamine, a more powerful action on gastric secretion and a less powerful stimulant effect on smooth muscle. This preferential action is sufficiently well marked to gain for betazole a recommendation that it should be used instead of histamine in gastric function tests (p. 641). 4-Methylhistamine has, in animal preparations, an even more selective action than betazole on H_2 receptors. Substances with a preference for H_1 receptors include 2-methylhistamine and 2-(2-aminoethyl) pyridine (Durant, Gannelin and Parsons, 1975) (Fig. 21.7, p. 346).

Some H_1 receptor antagonists partly inhibit the secretion of gastric acid but this is almost certainly a consequence of their atropine-like activity.

Although the H_1 antagonists will protect experimental animals against the bronchospasm, arteriolar constriction and capillary dilatation caused by histamine, they do not necessarily antagonize these same responses when they occur in the course of anaphylactic or allergic conditions. The degree of protection is determined, first, by the extent to which histamine participates in the anaphylactic reaction. Thus the guinea pig is almost completely and man partially protected but the rat receives no protection at all. Another factor that may well influence the effectiveness of the H_1 antagonists is the presence of a quota of H_2 receptors in some of the tissues traditionally assumed to be supplied only with H_1 receptors. Their small contribution to the overall response to histamine will be unaffected by the presence of antagonists that can only occlude H_1 receptors. This effect should, of course, be seen in laboratory experiments and careful observation often reveals a residue of histamine activity in preparations in which a superficial inspection indicates that a completely successful blockade has been established. The extent of this contamination by H_2 receptors exhibits species and tissue variation.

It has also to be remembered that the H_1 antagonists act competitively. Some of them probably fit fairly snugly on

the H_1 receptor but others can do more than occupy a minimal area of the receptor surface and so prevent, through steric hindrance, the access of histamine. In both situations the drugs obstruct the passage of histamine more effectively than they can displace it once it has arrived. In therapeutic terms this implies that the antagonists are not very effective if they are given after an anaphylactic attack has begun. Substances such as adrenaline, whose actions are the opposite of histamine's, are much more useful in these conditions.

Dryness of the mouth and throat and disturbances of accommodation are fairly commonly complained of by patients receiving H_1 antagonists. These are manifestations of the atropine-like activity exhibited by most of these drugs. Another feature which is not attributable to histamine antagonism is the ability to cause local anaesthesia. In some circumstances this property adds to the therapeutic value of the drugs. Thus, the primary mechanism by which they prevent itching is by antagonizing the action of histamine on the pain fibres which is the cause of the itch. At the same time, however, their local anaesthetic action will prevent the transmission of nerve impulses generated in these fibres by any histamine that overcomes the antihistamine block. Some agents that block H_1 receptors are so active as local anaesthetics that they have been used as such in individuals who show allergic responses to the more common anaesthetics. There is, in general, no correlation between local anaesthetic and antihistamine activity among the H_1 antagonists.

A common side effect of therapy with the H_1 antagonists is drowsiness. In our present state of knowledge, it is not possible to say whether this is the result of an interference with a central action of histamine. It is true that the sedative effect of the antagonists is not correlated with their ability to antagonize histamine on such preparations as the guinea pig ileum but this is not very good evidence, since so many other factors than simple antihistamine potency could determine the relative effects of different antagonists on central histamine receptors. The balance of opinion certainly favours the view that sedation is not a true antihistamine action but the question must still be regarded as an open one. A similar uncertainty arises in connection with the antiemetic properties of the histamine H_1 antagonists (p. 352).

Uses of the H_1 receptor antagonists
The clinical and laboratory uses of these antihistamine drugs can be understood in the light of the pharmacological properties that have just been discussed.

(i) Drugs that block histamine H_1 receptors are of value in the treatment of those allergic disorders in which the symptoms are attributable largely to histamine release. Thus while they are little use in the treatment of asthma (in which histamine is only one of several substances responsible for the bronchiolar constriction), they bring relief to about 80 per cent of hay fever sufferers. They are rather less effective in perennial vasomotor rhinitis, urticaria and angioneurotic oedema but in all these conditions it is worth trying H_1 antagonists since they are likely to bring some relief in up to 70 per cent of patients. In severe angioneurotic oedema, the laryngeal oedema may be so severe as to constitute an immediate threat to life. In these cases, as we have already noted (p. 351), it would be dangerously foolish to administer antihistamines in the hope that they might be effective. Adrenaline injections are often life saving in these emergencies. Taken by mouth, H_1 receptor antagonists are frequently effective in the treatment of allergic drug rashes. The itching responds more immediately and completely than does the skin rash in these conditions.

(ii) Chlorpheniramine (20 mg) is sometimes injected with penicillin in the hope of preventing anaphylactic reactions in patients known to be sensitive to the antibiotic. Attempts to prevent transfusion reactions by the same method have met with little success.

(iii) Itching is usually the result of histamine injection or release, even when it has not arisen as an allergic response, and it can usually be prevented by blockade of the H_1 receptors. Although they provide relief from itching when they are administered locally in such conditions as pruritis ani or vulvae, dermatitis due to poison ivy or after plant and animal stings, H_1 antagonists should never be applied to the skin: there is the danger, paradoxically enough, that they bring about an allergic sensitization of the skin.

(iv) H_1 receptor antagonists are of proved value for the treatment of motion sickness and for the relief of the nausea and vertigo of Ménière's disease (p. 603). They sometimes very effectively prevent or relieve vomiting after X-irradiation and they provide a rational treatment for this condition inasmuch as there is some evidence that it is caused by histamine liberation from the damaged cells. The drugs can be tried in postoperative and drug-induced vomiting and for the relief of pregnancy sickness. They are of uncertain value in these conditions, although their sedative side effects may contribute to the patient's comfort. When they are used as antiemetics, those that relieve motion sickness should be chosen.

(v) Some H_1 blocking agents have been employed in the treatment of Parkinson's disease. However, the useful members of the group have other attributes—notably an atropine-like activity—to which they probably owe their therapeutic usefulness (p. 593).

(vi) The use of histamine H_1 antagonists as local anaesthetics has already been mentioned (p. 351).

(vii) In the laboratory, H_1 antagonists are used to confirm the identity of histamine in tissue extracts. Doses of extract and equipotent amounts of authentic histamine are added alternately to the test preparation. The responses produced will, of course, be all approximately the same. An antagonist in a dose estimated to be sufficient to reduce, but not to abolish, the contractions caused by the chosen dose of extract is then added to the organ bath and is allowed to remain there for about two minutes. It is then washed out and the alternating additions of extract and histamine are resumed. The response to the extract and the authentic histamine will return to their initial value at the same rate if histamine provides all the activity in the extract and in such circumstances a series of regularly increasing contractions will be traced. If the response to the extract returns at a different rate from that to histamine, it is not justifiable to assume that the activity of the extract is solely derived from histamine even if larger doses of the antihistamine completely abolish its effect on the test organ. Mepyramine is the drug most often used for this confirmatory test. A dose of 2 μg per ml of bath fluid is a suitable one to use.

Mepyramine and similar antagonists can also be used to detect the presence of H_2 receptors. If histamine evokes a response in tissues that are exposed to fully blocking doses of an H_1 receptor antagonist we must conclude that H_2 receptors have been activated.

The choice of a suitable antagonist for the treatment of human subjects is governed by several factors. The patient's own response to the drug and particularly his sensitivity to side effects, is an important consideration. An individual antagonist may send one person to sleep and have no sedative action at all on another. Side effects apart, some members of the group may relieve symptoms in some subjects and be useless in others. Placebo effects exert a powerful influence and the patient may himself strongly favour a particular drug because of benefits, real or fancied, he has derived from it in the past. Notwithstanding these facts, a few general statements can be made:

(i) In the treatment of motion sickness, buclizine, cyclizine, promethazine and meclozine are particularly useful. Meclozine and chlorcyclizine are used when long lasting protection is required.

(ii) Drowsiness is most often experienced with clemizole, diphenhydramine and tripelennamine and least often with antazoline and phenindamine.

(iii) Diphenhydramine, tripelennamine and methapyrilene are useful for topical application on the rare occasions when it is permissible to employ this form of treatment. Dimenhydrinate and promethazine have been used, in suppositories, for the local treatment of pruritus. Antazoline can be used in eye drops since it is much less irritant than the other antihistamines.

(iv) Chlorpheniramine and mepyramine are valuable in hay fever. They rapidly abort acute attacks. Chlorcyclizine is long acting and it gives good protection against attacks of hay fever. It is especially useful when taken before exposure to the offending allergen and the patient can often secure day-long protection by taking the drug before venturing out of doors in the morning.

(v) Some H_1 blockers have been used in cough mixtures. Any value they have lies in their atropine-like action on secretions and in their sedative action. The idea that the drugs are useful in the treatment of the common cold is a piece of latter day folk lore.

Side effects of antihistamine treatment

Most of these have already been mentioned in earlier sections and they need only be enumerated here. They are listed in order of their frequency of occurrence.

(i) Sedation is the most common side effect. In some instances (in the treatment of motion sickness, for example) the sedation actually contributes to the usefulness of the drug. At other times it may be inconvenient or positively dangerous, as in the ambulant patient in charge of a car or dangerous machinery. The other side effects are:

(ii) dryness of the mouth and disturbances of ocular accommodation;

(iii) skin rashes and drug sensitization;

(iv) dizziness, nervousness, tremor and other signs of central nervous stimulation;

(v) nausea, vomiting and other forms of gastrointestinal upset.

(vi) hypersensitivity reactions

(vii) blood dyscrasias including leucopenia and agranulocytosis.

The central nervous actions of the H_1 antagonists are accentuated by alcohol. Drivers and those who work with potentially dangerous machinery should be told of this and be warned not to drink alcohol when they have taken an H_1 antagonist.

When the H_1 receptor antagonists were first introduced, they were freely available without prescription and they became popular occupants of many a family medicine box. Since they were often compounded into attractively-coloured tablets, they provided a constant temptation to young children and several cases of antihistamine poisoning were reported. It has already been mentioned that although the antagonists generally have a sedative action, they sometimes stimulate the central nervous system. After very large doses, central excitation is the usual response, particularly in young children. The acutely poisoned child shows motor incoordination and excitement accompanied by hallucinations. Violent convulsions occur in severe poisoning. Dilated pupils, a flushed face and a high fever are other features: combined with the signs of central excitation, they produce a syndrome similar to that seen in atropine poisoning partly, no doubt, because at high dose levels the atropine-like side effects of the drugs begin to exert a dominant influence. In adults, the effects of toxic doses of the blocking agents are less dramatic: depression is more usual than excitation of the central nervous system and the atropine-like effects are not so prominent. The treatment of acute antihistamine poisoning is restricted to gastric lavage and the control of any

convulsions that occur. Respiratory depression is unlikely and the maintenance of respiration does not therefore constitute a problem.

SUBSTANCES THAT CAUSE BLOCKADE OF HISTAMINE H_2 RECEPTORS

We have already mentioned some of the principal events that led to the emergence of this new group of histamine antagonists. The formulae of the three agents that have so far been developed—burimamide, metiamide and cimetidine—are displayed, alongside those of representative H_1 antagonists in Fig. 21.7 (p. 346). Both groups of compounds have structural analogies with histamine but whereas the H_1 antagonists generally feature an ethylamine residue, the H_2 antagonists are characterized by retention of the imidazole ring.

Early attempts to modify the histamine molecule so as to effect a transformation from an agonist to an H_2 antagonist involved the introduction of structural modifications—the addition of a benzene to the imidazole ring for instance (cf. Table 18.1, p. 303)—similar to those that changed isoprenaline into an adrenaline β antagonist. These attempts proved fruitless and attention had then to be directed to the possibility of effecting the required change by manipulating the side chain. This approach was ultimately rewarded with success and Black and his colleagues, who had initiated the search for H_2 antagonists, were able to announce, in 1972, the birth of burimamide (Black et al, 1972). The fact that they had to synthesize and test some 700 compounds before finding one that met their requirements says as much for their complete faith in the concept of specific H_2 receptors as it does for their industry and patience.

Burimamide differs from histamine in two ways: it possesses a longer side chain and the terminal nitrogen, instead of being strongly basic, is uncharged by virtue of the presence of the thiocarbonyl ($>C = S$) group.

Burimamide is not well absorbed from the alimentary tract and most of the pioneer studies in the field of H_2 receptor antagonism utilized metiamide, burimamide's immediate successor. It enjoyed a brief period of clinical application until a few patients who had received the drug developed an agranulocytosis. The blood picture returned rapidly to its normal state when treatment with metiamide was interrupted but the drug was withdrawn and replaced by cimetidine, a drug that differs from its two predecessors in not possessing the thiourea group, the presumed cause of the agranulocytosis precipitated by metiamide.

Cimetidine (Tagamet)

Cimetidine inhibits the secretion of hydrochloric acid by the stomach in response to histamine, pentagastrin, test meals and other chemical stimulants such as 2-deoxyglucose. This is clearly the consequence of histamine receptor blockade.

Cimetidine is already fulfilling an early promise that it would become a most useful drug for the treatment of peptic ulcer. By suppressing the secretion of gastric acid it creates a local environment that favours the spontaneous healing of the ulcer. It also makes life more comfortable for the duodenal ulcer patient by relieving him of the nocturnal and sleep-disturbing pains that otherwise occur when hydrochloric acid, secreted in response to a lack of food in the stomach, passes into the ulcerated duodenum. It is certainly a more effective curative agent than carbenoxolone (p. 642), an earlier claimant for the title of the most useful antiulcer drug.

Cimetidine produces symptomatic relief in victims of the Zollinger-Ellison syndrome, a rare condition in which tumours of non-specialized cells in the pancreatic islets elaborate polypeptides that cause a profuse secretion of gastric acid and a serious ulceration. It has also proved its worth in cases of pancreatic insufficiency. By reducing the acidity of the gastric contents, cimetidine prevents the too rapid destruction of the oral preparations of pancreatic enzymes that have to be taken by victims of this condition.

The usual oral dose of cimetidine is 200 mg taken immediately after the three principal meals of the day and 400 mg at bedtime. After the ulcer has healed, it is advisable to continue cimetidine treatment for some time to guard against the possibility of recurrence. A suitable maintenance dose for this purpose is 400 mg given once daily at bedtime. It can also be given intravenously to control severe gastrointestinal haemorrhage in patients with ulcers or erosions in the stomach or duodenum. The drug is given by intravenous infusion at an hourly rate of 50 to 150 mg, until bleeding stops so that treatment can be continued with orally administered cimetidine or until appropriate surgery can be undertaken.

At this stage of its history cimetidine seems to be a safe drug: in one multicentre double-blind trial involving almost one hundred patients, adverse side effects occurred more frequently with the placebo than with cimetidine itself! Conclusions concerning the safety of cimetidine are, of course, necessarily tentative and must remain so until a more substantial body of clinical experience has been accumulated. It is worth mentioning in this connection that a few recent reports have indicated the possibility that cimetidine treatment may lead to an increased secretion of prolactin and a consequent galactorrhoea (p. 776) (Delle Fave et al, 1977; Bateson, Browning and Maconnachie, 1977). In view of the fact that cimetidine is reputed not to pass the blood brain barrier, it comes as something of a surprise to discover recent reports of serious mental confusion, dizziness and ataxia among those who have taken, by accident or intent, too high a dose of the drug. Potentially more sinister is the suspicion that cimetidine can cause agranulocytosis and that the absence from its molecule of the thiourea group does not prevent its being able to exert a toxic effect on the bone marrow. Byrom

(1977) has suggested that the activity of the stem cells of the bone marrow might be dependent on stimulation of their histamine H_2 receptors so that blockade of these receptors would compromise the production of leucocytes. If this hypothesis were to be substantiated it would imply that no H_2 receptor antagonist of the present type would be free of potentially toxic effects on the bone marrow.

Cimetidine is well absorbed from the alimentary tract, particularly the duodenum and ileum. Its plasma half life amounts to some two hours. It is excreted in the urine, up to 80 per cent as unchanged cimetidine, free or conjugated. The remainder appears as metabolites, chiefly the sulphoxide (produced by oxidation of the side chain sulphur) and, to a much smaller extent, a derivative in which a hydroxymethyl group occupies position 4 of imidazole ring.

Distribution and significance of histamine H_2 receptors

The possibility that cimetidine and its successors will have other therapeutic uses depends on the outcome of exploratory work designed to establish the localization and physiological importance of the H_2 receptors. So far, it has been established that the stimulant action of histamine on the atrium and its inhibitory action on the uterus are mediated through H_2 receptors. Capillary dilatation seems to involve both H_1 and H_2 receptors suggesting that allergic and other skin reactions might respond particularly well to a combined therapy that causes blocade of both types of receptor. Some other cells and tissues (particularly the basophils and lymphocytes) that participate in anaphylactic reactions also carry H_2 receptors. Some areas of the brain appear to be supplied with both types of receptor.

We have already seen (p. 338) that histidine decarboxylase is subject to feed back inhibition by histamine. This regulatory mechanism is mediated through histamine H_2 receptors and H_2 antagonists increase the activity of the enzyme. They may also inhibit imidazole-N-methyltransferase.

The responses to stimulation of histamine H_2 receptors are mediated through activation of adenyl cyclase, providing yet another analogy between histamine H_2 and adrenaline $ß$ receptors.

Two recent symposia (1973, 1977) provide detailed information concerning histamine H_2 antagonists.

The screening and evaluation of antihistamine drugs

In blind screening procedures, the ability to block H_1 receptors ·is routinely looked for: it manifests itself by preferential inhibition of histamine-induced contractions of the isolated guinea pig ileum or of histamine-induced depression of blood pressure in the anaesthetized cat. For the evaluation of known or suspected antihistamines of this type the guinea pig is the animal of choice. In one type of test, it is placed in a transparent box and an aerosol produced from a two per cent solution of histamine is passed into the chamber. This dose of histamine is normally fatal to the guinea pig but death is preceded by dyspnoea and convulsions and, by careful observation of the animal's breathing the experienced worker can tell with reasonable accuracy, when convulsions are imminent. If he removes the guinea pig from the box at this stage, convulsions and death are prevented and the animal can be used for the next part of the test. The time from the introduction of the aerosol into the box to the onset of the preconvulsive state is noted. Two days later the same animal receives the substance under test by intraperitoneal injection. Twenty minutes after the injection, it is exposed to the histamine aerosol and the preconvulsive time is again determined. Finally, after another two days, the experimental animal is once more exposed to the histamine alone. The prolongation of the preconvulsive time produced by the drug is compared with that caused by a standard antihistamine. The method just described was originally proposed by Armitage, Boswood and Large (1961). A number of essentially similar methods have been elaborated by others. It is sometimes desirable to assess the activity of the test drug against histamine released during anaphylaxis. For this purpose the microshock method of Herxheimer and Stresemann (1960) is used. Guinea pigs are sensitized to egg albumin. Three weeks later they will respond by anaphylaxis to an albumin aerosol and the activity of the drug under test can be assessed by measuring its effect on the preconvulsion time by the same technique as that used for measuring its effectiveness against histamine. It should be added that the term microshock is something of a misnomer since the animals are completely sensitized to the albumin and they would die if they were not removed from the aerosol chamber before convulsions set in. Since antihistamines may be used to treat skin reactions, those which might be introduced into clinical practice should also be tested for their ability to reduce the size of a cutaneous weal produced by the intradermal injection of histamine.

Tests to detect activity against histamine H_2 receptors do not yet constitute a routine item in blind screening programmes, nor is it necessary that they should, since the whole history of the development of the antihistamines makes it clear that while H_1 receptor antagonism is exhibited by a wide range of compounds, the ability to occupy H_2 receptors is a much rarer phenomenon except among substances that are deliberately synthesized for this purpose. Investigations with this type of compound involve examination of antihistamine effects on preparations whose responses to histamine are mediated exclusively through H_2 receptors. These include (the effect of histamine is noted in parentheses) the stomach in *vitro* and *in vivo* (acid secretion), isolated atria (acceleration) and the isolated uterus (inhibition). Suitable preparations for this purpose are supplied by the rat.

BIBLIOGRAPHY

Books, monographs and reviews

Buffoni, F. (1966). Histaminase and related amine oxidases. *Pharmac. Rev.*, **18**, 1163-1199.

Dale, H. H. (1953). *Adventures in Physiology*. London: Pergamon.

Kahlson, G. and Rosengren, Elsa (1971) *Biogenesis and Physiology of Histamine*. London: Edward Arnold

Lewis, T. (1927). *The Blood Vessels of the Human Skin and their Responses*. London: Shaw.

Paton, W. D. M. (1957). Histamine release by compounds of simple chemical structure. *Pharmac. Rev.*, **9**, 269-328.

Pearlman, D. S. (1976) Antihistamines: pharmacology and clinical use. *Drugs*, **12**, 258-273.

Schayer, R. W. (1959). Catabolism of physiological quantities of histamine *in vivo*. *Physiol, Rev.*, **39**, 116-126.

Schayer, R. W. (1966) Catabolism of histamine *in vivo*. In: *Handbook of Experimental Pharmacology*. ed. Eichler, O and Farah, A. vol 18/1 pp. 688-726. Berlin: Springer.

Shepherd, D. M. and Mackay, D. (1967). The histidine decarboxylases. In, Ellis, G. P. and West, G. B. (Eds.) *Progress in Medicinal Chemistry*, Vol. 5, 199-250. London: Butterworths.

Symposium (1973) International Symposium on Histamine H_2 Receptor Antagonists (eds. Wood, C. J. and Simkins, M. Alison). London: Smith, Kline and French.

Symposium (1977) Cimetidine—Second International Symposium on Histamine H-Receptor Antagonists (eds. Burland, W. L. and Simkins, M. Alison). Amsterdam and Oxford: Excerpta Medica.

Original papers

Abdel-Aziz, A. M. and Boullin, D. J. (1964). Effect of pyridoxine deficiency on intestinal histaminase in the rat. *Biochem. Pharmac.*, **13**, 803-805.

Armitage, A. K., Boswood, J. and Large, B. J. (1961). Thioxanthines with potent bronchodilator and coronary dilator properties, *Br. J. Pharmac. Chemother.*, **16**, 59-76.

Ash, A. S. F. and Schild. H. O. (1966). Receptors mediating some actions of histamine. *Br. J. Pharmac. Chemother.*, **27**, 427-439.

Barsoum, G. C. and Gaddum, J. H. (1935). Pharmacological estimation of adenosine and histamine in blood. *J. Physiol.*, **85**, 1-14.

Bateson, M. C., Browning, M. C. D. and Maconnachie. A. (1977). Galactorrhoea with cimetidine. *Lancet* (**ii**) 247-248.

Black, J. W., Duncan, W. A. M., Durant, G. J., Ganellin, C. R. and Parsons, M. E. (1972). Definition and antagonism of histamine H_2-receptors. *Nature, Lond.* **236**, 385-390.

Burn, J. H. and Dale, H. H. (1926). The vasodilator action of histamine and its physiological significance. *J. Physiol.*, **61**, 185-214.

Byrom, J. W. (1977). Cimetidine and the bone marrow. *Lancet*, (**ii**), 555-556.

Carlsten, A. (1950). On the sources of the histaminase present in thoracic duct lymph and other papers. *Acta physiol. scand.*, **20**, suppl. 70, 5-46.

Crossland, J. (1961). Biologic estimation of histamine. In, Quastel, J. H. (ed.) *Methods in Medical Research*, Vol. 9, 186-191. New York: Year Book Medical Publishers, Inc.

Crossland, J., Woodruff, G. N. and Woodruff, Judith M. (1966). The histamine content of brain during bulbocapnine induced catalepsy. *Life Sci.*, **5**, 193-197.

Delle Fave, G. F., Tamburrano, G., de Magistris, Laura, Natoli, Clara, Santoro, M. Luisa, Carratu, R. and Torsoli, A. (1977). *Lancet* (i) 1319.

Douglas, W.W., Feldberg, W., Paton, W.D.M. and Schachter, M. (1951). Distribution of histamine and substance P in the wall of the dog's digestive tract. *J. Physiol.*, **115**, 163-176.

Durant, G. J., Ganellin. C. R. and Parsons, M. E. (1975). Chemical differentiation of histamine H_1- and H_2- receptor agonists. *J. med. Chem.*, **18**, 905-909.

Herxheimer, H. and Stresemann, E. (1960). Protection against anaphylactic shock by ephedrine-theophylline combinations. *Archs int. Pharmacodyn. Ther.*, **125**, 383-403.

Jonson, B. and White, T. (1964). Histamine metabolism in the brain of conscious cats. *Proc. Soc. exp. Biol. Med.*, **115**, 874-876.

Kremzner, L. T. and Pfeiffer, C. C. (1966). Identification of substances interfering with the fluorimetric determination of brain histamine. *Biochem. Pharmac.*, **15**, 197-200.

Snyder, S. H., Glowinski, J. and Axelrod, J. (1966). The physiologic disposition of H^3 histamine in the rat brain. *J. Pharmac. exp. Ther.*, **153**, 8-14.

Shaw, G. G. (1972) Observations on the fluorimetric assay of histamine, spermidine and spermine in brain. *Eur. J. Pharmac.*, **20**, 389-392.

Shore, P. A., Burkhalter, A. and Cohn, V. H. (1959). A method for the fluorimetric assay of histamine in tissues. *J. Pharmac. exp. Ther.*, **127**, 182-186.

Trendelenburg, U. (1954). The action of histamine and pilocarpine on the superior cervical ganglion and the adrenal glands of the cat. *Br. J. Pharmac. Chemother.*, **9**, 481-487.

Waton, N. G. (1956). Studies on mammalian histidine decarboxylase. *Br. J. Pharmac. Chemother.*, **11**, 119-127.

White, T. (1959). The formation and catabolism of histamine in brain tissue *in vitro*. *J. Physiol.*, **149**, 34-42.

White, T. (1960). Formation and catabolism of histamine in cat brain tissue *in vivo*. *J. Physiol.*, **152**, 299-308.

Zeller, E. A. (1963). Identity of histaminase and diamine oxidase. *Fed. Proc.*, **24**, 766-768.

22. Some polypeptides of pharmacological interest

The polypeptides discussed in this chapter are those whose properties would seem to justify their classification as humoral substances in the broadest sense of that term. Other well known polypeptides such as oxytocin and vasopressin are true hormones and as such they are more properly discussed elsewhere (p. 771). The endorphins and related compounds find a place in Chapter 26 (p. 437).

Substance P

In 1931, von Euler and Gaddum reported that extracts of brain and intestine contained material which caused contraction of the isolated rabbit intestine. The material was clearly not acetylcholine, since its action was not abolished by atropine. Since the rabbit intestine is insensitive to histamine and to choline, it was concluded that the active extracts contained a hitherto undetected substance. Von Euler and Gaddum named their unidentified material substance P. This name was given quite arbitrarily (the vessel containing the extract had been labelled P) but it proved to be surprisingly appropriate when it was found that the activity of the extracts disappeared on incubation with trypsin, indicating that substance P was polypeptide in nature.

Substance P stimulates the smooth muscle of the gut but causes relaxation of the arterioles: it is in fact the most powerful hypotensive agent known. When injected into the cerebral ventricles, substance P has a depressant action on the brain. Of the many smooth muscle preparations that have been used for the assay of substance P in tissue extracts, the most useful are the hen's rectal caecum and the isolated intestine of the goldfish.

The physiological function of substance P is not yet known. It occurs only in the central nervous system, in sensory nerves and in the gastrointestinal tract. It has been found in a wide range of mammalian species and in fish. Its distribution in the brain is patchy. Uneven distribution is usually regarded as presumptive evidence that the substance concerned has an important functional role in the central nervous system but the part played by substance P in the regulation of nervous activity is still obscure. Its possible transmitter role is discussed in more detail elsewhere (p. 194).

The amounts of substance P in the gastrointestinal tract are much greater than those in brain. There is as yet, however, no evidence that it is involved in the regulation of intestinal activity, though it is known that its stimulant action on the intestine is exerted directly on the muscle cells and is not inhibited by ganglion blocking agents or by antagonists of acetylcholine, histamine or serotonin.

Angiotensin

For at least 200 years, physicians have suspected that a relationship exists between the development of hypertension and events in the kidney and as long ago as 1898 Tiegerstedt and Bergman showed that saline extracts of the kidney increased blood pressure in experimental animals. The material responsible for this effect was called *renin* and in 1934 Goldblatt demonstrated that the application of a clamp to the kidney caused hypertension as was then thought, by the release of renin. The 'Goldblatt clamp' technique became an accepted method for the production of experimental hypertension. It is now known that renin does not produce hypertension directly but that it is an enzyme (not to be confused with the gastric enzyme, rennin) which liberates a hypertensive agent from a precursor in the α-2-globulin fraction of plasma. The hypertensive principle is now generally known as angiotensin—a happy blend of the two earlier names, hypertensin and angiotonin. Its precursor in plasma is called *angiotensinogen*. The first result of the angiotensinogen-renin interaction is angiotensin I, which has no hypertensive action. Angiotensin II, the active agent, is produced from angiotensin I by a converting enzyme. A plasma peptidase is responsible for the eventual inactivation of angiotensin II. Angiotensin I is a decapeptide; angiotensin II is an octapeptide (Fig. 22.1). In the following paragraphs, the pharmacologically active material will be referred to simply as angiotensin.

Renin is synthesized and secreted by the specialized cells of the afferent arterioles in the 'juxtaglomerular apparatus' of the kidney (p. 617). Secretion is most readily evoked by a reduced pressure in the arterioles but other stimuli such as circulating catecholamines, potassium depletion and an increased activity of the sympathetic nervous system are also effective. Renin release involves activation of the cyclic AMP system in response to stimulation of adrenaline β receptors (p. 322).

Renin like activity has been detected in extracts of the brain, adrenal glands and uterus but the physiological significance of these observations is obscure.

Angiotensin II is the most powerful vasoconstrictor agent known; it acts directly on the smooth muscle of the

```
                             ┌─────────── I ───────────┐
        Leu — his — phe — pro — his — isoleuc — tyr — val — arg — asp
              └──────────── II ────────────┘
```

The angiotensins

```
        ┌──────────────── Kallidin 10 ────────────────┐
        Lys — arg — pro — pro — gly — phe — ser — pro — phe — arg
              └─────────── kallidin 9 (bradykinin) ───────────┘
```

The kallidins

arg — arginine; asp — aspartic acid; gly — glycine; his — histidine;
isoleuc — isoleucine; leu — leucine; lys — lysine; phe — phenylalanine;
pro — proline; ser — serine; tyr — tyramine; val — valine

Fig. 22.1 The angiotensins and the kallidins

vessel walls. The renal arterioles are particularly sensitive to this vasoconstrictor action. In man, an obvious increase in blood pressure occurs in response to a dose of angiotensin as low as 0.1μ g per kilogram of body weight. The dose of noradrenaline required to produce the same effect is about 4μ g per kilogram. For purposes of comparison it may be added that the minimum hypotensive dose of substance P is 0.5μ g per kilogram.

The action of angiotensin on smooth muscle is not confined to blood vessels, although smooth muscle elsewhere is less sensitive than that in the vessels. On the isolated guinea pig ileum, the spasmogenic action of angiotensin is due partly to a direct action on the smooth muscle cells and partly to its stimulating parasympathetic elements in the wall. Other smooth muscle preparations only exhibit a direct response: some of them are so sensitive that they can be used for bioassay purposes. The isolated stomach and strips of rabbit aorta are particularly useful in this respect.

Angiotensin stimulates the release of aldosterone from the adrenal cortex, promoting thereby the absorption of sodium and the retention of water. This represents one of the most important *physiological* actions of angiotensin.

Angiotensin seems to be able to potentiate the action of the sympathetic nervous system by virtue of its action at a number of sites. Thus it stimulates the medullary centres, sympathetic ganglia and the adrenal medulla and it increases the output of transmitter from the stimulated sympathetic nerves.

So far as its physiological function is concerned, angiotensin can be regarded as the mediator of a homeostatic mechanism directed towards the maintenance of sodium balance and blood pressure. The mechanism probably operates as follows. If there is a loss of sodium from the body, the blood volume and the blood pressure fall. In this event (or if the blood pressure falls independently of a primary sodium loss) the secretion of renin from the kidney increases and the concentration of angiotensin in the plasma rises. This causes vasoconstriction and stimulates the release of aldosterone. The vasoconstriction, though generalized, will particularly affect the kidney and the loss of sodium and water will be reduced. The increased aldosterone secretion will also favour sodium retention. Thus three responses—generalized vasoconstriction, renal vasoconstriction and aldosterone release—all contribute to the return to normal of the plasma sodium and the blood pressure. As the blood pressure rises, the stimulus to renin release is reduced and the pressure is stabilized again at its normal level.

Another possibility is that renin is released from the kidney if that organ is damaged and that the increased amounts of angiotensin so produced ensure that the arterial pressure in the glomeruli remains sufficiently high to enable filtration to continue at its normal rate.

The extent to which angiotensin participates in the development of hypertension is a matter of controversy which is discussed elsewhere (p. 314). Angiotensin and the renal prostaglandins have opposite effects on blood flow in the kidney. Since angiotensin promotes prostaglandin synthesis and release in that organ it seems likely that the two agents operate together in the balanced way that is characteristic of so many other pairs of mutually antagonistic influences that exert fine regulatory controls on local physiological activities.

Angiotensin has been used clinically for its hypertensive effect but its value in this field is limited.

Plasma kinins
Some fifty years ago, Frey reported that urine contained a substance capable of causing contraction of the isolated

intestine and generalized vasodilatation. Soon afterwards, it was found that much of this urinary material was derived from the pancreas and it was therefore called *kallikrein* from kallikreas, the Greek for pancreas. (There is some etymological confusion here, for the English word pancreas is itself of Greek origin: it means 'all flesh' and it indicates that the pancreas secretes enzymes which digest all types of food. The Greeks themselves, unaware of the digestive actions of the pancreatic secretion, called the organ kallikreas or 'beautiful flesh', cf. the English sweetbread).

Kallikrein was also found in the plasma and saliva as well as in urine. It was soon recognized that kallikrein itself was an enzyme and that the pharmacological effects seen when it was injected into experimental animals were those of a substance formed by the action of the enzyme on a plasma component. The active substance was called *kallidin* and the plasma component from which it was formed was called *kallidinogen*. Kallidinogen, like angiotensinogen, is a member of the α-2-globulin fraction of the plasma proteins but the two substances are not identical.

Since kallidin activity is not normally present in plasma *in vivo*, it is clear that kallikrein, the enzyme which produces it, must also be normally inactive. It is present in the form of an inactivate precursor *(kallikreinogen)* which is activated when the plasma comes into contact with a foreign surface. It can also be activated in laboratory conditions if plasma is incubated with trypsin. Blood contains enzyme systems capable of destroying both kallikrein and kallidin. The interrelationships of the various factors involved in the production and destruction of kallidin are shown in Fig. 22.2.

Kallidin attracted relatively little attention until 1949, when Rocha e Silva and his colleagues reported that when plasma was incubated with trypsin or with certain snake venom, it developed vasodilator properties and also became capable of causing a slowly developing contraction of the isolated intestine. Because of this last-named property, the material responsible was called *bradykinin* ('slow moving'). It will be clear that the mechanism of production of bradykinin is very similar to that of kallidin and it was soon realized that the two substances were very closely related. Kallidinogen and bradykininogen appear to be the same substance. Bradykinin (sometimes called kallidin 9) is a nine-membered peptide chain while the kallidin produced in the body by kallikrein is a mixture of a decapeptide (kallidin 10) and bradykinin itself. In the following discussion 'kallidin' refers to the pure decapeptide, kallidin 10. A plasma carboxypeptidase is capable of converting kallidin 10 into kallidin 9. These two kallidins are together known as the *plasma kinins:* their structures are indicated in Fig. 22.1.

The production of the plasma kinins is rather more complex than is indicated by the simple scheme in Fig. 22.2. In particular, the activation of kallikreinogen by contact with a foreign surface involves a separate sequence of reactions. The reader will inevitably be reminded of the complex events leading to coagulation which are set in motion when blood comes into contact with a foreign surface. It is now known that the factor which is activated by contact (the Hageman factor) is responsible not only for the activation of kallikreinogen but also for the initiation of the reactions which lead to the production of thromboplastin (p. 662). A number of individuals (of whom Hageman was the first to be identified) lack this contact factor and their blood shows both coagulation defects and an impaired ability to produce the plasma kinins.

Bradykinin is a powerful vasodilator substance and at doses of from 0.05 to 0.5 μg per kilogram it causes a fall of blood pressure in anaesthetized animals. The rabbit is the most sensitive species. Bradykinin causes vasodilatation of the skin blood vessels in man and it is a potent pain

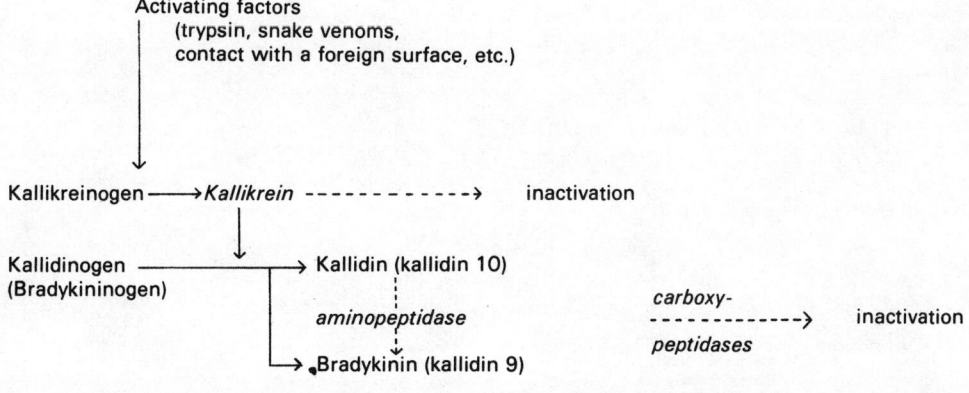

Enzymes are in *italics*.

Fig. 22.2 Factors involved in the production and destruction of the plasma kinins.

producing agent (p. 417). The characteristically slow contraction produced in isolated intestinal preparations is not inhibited by atropine, by antihistamines or by ganglion blocking agents. Bradykinin is much less effective in stimulating intestinal or uterine smooth muscle in the intact animal than it is in isolated preparations.

Bradykinin causes powerful bronchoconstriction in the guinea pig and it produces the characteristic signs of an inflammatory reaction (increased capillary permeability and the migration and accumulation of leucocytes) in a variety of species. It is released during anaphylactic and peptone shock and in inflammatory reactions. A number of antipyretic, analgesic and antirheumatic drugs antagonize the bronchoconstrictor action of bradykinin but they have a less regular effect on inflammatory reactions produced by bradykinin.

The actions of kallidin are qualitatively the same as those of bradykinin but some quantitative differences are apparent. Thus, in the rat, kallidin is a more powerful hypotensive agent than bradykinin but it is much less active in causing contraction of the isolated ileum of the guinea pig.

The physiological functions of the plasma kinins are not yet established. The possibility that they are involved in functional vasodilatation, the production of pain, the mediation of inflammatory reactions or the initiation of anaphylactic and allergic responses is fully discussed elsewhere in this book as are their relationships with the prostaglandins.

The plasma kinins are of little therapeutic use. A preparation of kallikrein known as Padutin has been used in efforts to relieve arterial spasm but it is of doubtful utility.

BIBLIOGRAPHY

Books, monographs and reviews

Conference (1962). Bradykinin and vasodilating polypeptides. *Biochem. Pharmac.,* **10**, 1-94.

Conference (1963). Structure and function of biologically active peptides: bradykinin, kallidin and congeners. *Ann. N. Y. Acad. Sci.,* **104**, 1-464.

Erdos, E. G. (1966). Hypotensive peptides: bradykinin, kallidin and Eledoisin. *Advances in Pharmacology,* **4**, 1-90.

Gross, F. (1971). Angiotension. *In: Pharmacology of Naturally Occurring Polypeptides and Lipid Soluble Acids (International Encyclopedia of Pharmacology and Therapeutics.)* 73-286. Oxford: Pergamon Press.

Khairallah, P. A. (1971). Pharmacology of angiotensin. *In:* Fisher, J. W. (ed.) *Kidney Hormones,* 129-171. London: Academic Press.

Law, H. D. (1965). Polypeptides of medicinal interest. In: Ellis, G. P. and West, G. B. (eds.), *Progress in Medicinal Chemistry,* Vol. 4, 86-170. London: Butterworths.

Lewis, G. P. (1968). Pharmacologically active polypeptides. In: Robson, J. M. and Stacey, R. S. (eds.), *Recent Advances in Pharmacology.* 4th ed. London: Churchill.

Regoli, D., Park, W. K. and Rioux, F. (1974). Pharmacology of angiotensin. *Pharmac. Rev.,* **26**, 69-124.

Vander, A. J. (1967). Control of renin release. *Physiol. Rev.,* **47**, 359-382.

23. The prostaglandins

Although it had been coined thirty years earlier, the word 'prostaglandin' appeared nowhere in the 1965 edition of this book, nor, indeed in any of its contemporaries. By then pluralized, the prostaglandins were able to gain a foothold in the 1970 edition and those few pages have now been able to demand expansion into the present chapter which, though substantial, does but scant justice to recent developments in this field.

Textbooks react, if sometimes sluggishly, to events in the world they describe. Before 1957, papers concerned with prostaglandin activity appeared only sporadically. From then until about 1962, they were published more regularly but at a rate of never more than six each year. In 1963, more than thirty prostaglandin papers saw the light of day and thereafter interest grew at a spectacular rate until in 1974 an estimated 7500 publications appeared.

The event that triggered recent interest in the prostaglandins was their chemical identification. We have noticed before how small is the impact made by the discovery of pharmacological activity in tissue extracts when that activity cannot be assigned to an identifiable chemical substance and how radically the picture changes as soon as the active material is identified, particularly if its concentration in tissue extracts and body fluids can be easily measured. Workers attracted into the prostaglandin field by these circumstances were very soon convinced that these novel compounds had fundamentally important physiological functions. Their results attracted the attention of countless other investigators—not all of them, let it be said, as distinguished or as cautious as the original workers—and this led to the explosive expansion of publications and ideas to which, for once, the word escalation can be justifiably applied. The diligent reader can hardly fail to recognize the parallels between the history of the prostaglandins and that of 5-hydroxytryptamine (p. 327).

This chapter attempts to provide from the mass of recent literature a concise, coherent and cohesive account of the pharmacological actions of the prostaglandins, to assess their place in normal physiology and in disease processes and to speculate on their possible future (and that of their analogues and antagonists) as therapeutic agents. Confusion and contradictions abound in the literature and this account will inevitably be oversimplified, not to say biassed. The wise reader will wish to counter these defects by reading some of the abundant literature for himself. He can reach this through the reviews and mono-graphs listed on p. 390. He should not be daunted by the sheer number of recent books devoted to the prostaglandins for many of them differ only marginally from one another. And he will, of course, choose to read particularly the writers who have made the most significant contributions to the subject. Their names will emerge in the course of this chapter. Finally, though the point is surely self evident, it should be added that the rate at which information is accumulating and opinions are changing inevitably means that not a little of what is written here (and, *a fortiori*, in the review articles listed in the bibliography) will need modification by the time it is read.

HISTORY OF THE PROSTAGLANDINS

von Euler, the Swedish physiologist and Nobel laureate, is usually (and justly) credited with the discovery of the prostaglandins though an assiduous search through the literature will uncover reports of a number of earlier observations similar to those made by von Euler. He himself has drawn attention to these precedent publications (von Euler, 1967) and we shall have occasion to refer to some of them. Nevertheless, only he and his colleagues had the enthusiasm and vision to exploit their original observations and until 1963 virtually all the work on prostaglandins emanated from Swedish laboratories. Particular reference must be made to Bergström who, stimulated by von Euler, embarked on the arduous task of identifying the prostaglandins. The successful completion of this project initiated, as we have seen, a world-wide enthusiasm for prostaglandin research. The extent of earlier indifference is perhaps best illustrated by reference to a well known and otherwise impeccable history which summarizes, with the aid of extracts from their published work, the achievements of the world's leading pharmacologists. In the section devoted to von Euler the prostaglandins find no mention though the book appeared as late as 1963 and was compiled by two Swedes! (Holmstedt and Liljestrand, 1963).

In 1934, von Euler found that extracts of human seminal fluid caused vasodilatation and contraction of the isolated intestine and uterus. The material responsible for these actions differed in its properties from all the pharmacologically active substances then known and von Euler called it prostaglandin because he believed that it was a single substance and that it was produced by the prostate gland. In fact, the word is a misnomer because the active material, as we now know, comes from the seminal vesicles. By the time this fact was established it was too late for semantic corrections, 'prostaglandin' having become firmly entrenched in the world's scientific vocabulary.

In view of the importance that now attaches to the seminal prostaglandins, it is a surprising fact—and one that needs to be remembered—that von Euler was only able to detect prostaglandin material in the semen of man, sheep and goat. The seminal fluid and vesicular glands of monkeys yielded a vasodilator substance that was devoid of any action on the smooth muscle of other organs. It was called vesiglandin (von Euler, 1936).

Nearly thirty years were to elapse before the chemical nature of prostaglandin was established but in 1962, Bergström and his collaborators (Bergström et al., 1962) were able to report that the prostaglandin of seminal fluid was in fact a mixture of five related substances. They were designated prostaglandins E_1, E_2, E_3, $F_{1\alpha}$ and $F_{2\alpha}$. A year later, a sixth prostaglandin ($F_{3\alpha}$) was identified by the Bergström team. Prostaglandin $F_{3\alpha}$ is not present in semen but it occurs in some other tissues such as the lung. By 1966 two new series of compounds (prostaglandins A and B) had been found in tissue extracts. Prostaglandins A_1, A_2, B_1 and B_2 are constituents of human seminal fluid which also carries the 19-hydroxy derivatives of these four compounds as well as those of prostaglandins E_1 and E_2. A comparison of their properties indicates that vesiglandin consists largely of prostaglandins A.

Prostaglandins C, D, G and H next appeared. The two last named compounds (only G_2 and H_2 have yet been identified) had been known for some years before but they were not classified as prostaglandins until 1974 when they were isolated in the pure state (Nelson, 1974).

The newest prostaglandin is labelled I_2. It is also known as prostacyclin. At first dubbed prostaglandin X, prostacyclin was first identified, in 1976, by Vane and his colleagues (Moncada et al., 1976) who reported their discovery in a communication the very title of which (p. 392) succinctly describes—a rare event indeed in scientific papers—the substance of their message. Thromboxanes A_2 and B_2, which we shall have to consider in relation to the prostaglandins proper, emerged at about the same time (Hamberg, Svensson and Samuelsson, 1975).

Those who are new to the prostaglandins may well wonder why the first prostaglandins to be identified were assigned the letters E and F while all their successors (A to D; G, H and I) have been labelled sequentially in the order of their discovery. The reason is simply that, in the course of their original work into the nature of the active material in sheep vesical glands, Bergström and his collaborators partitioned a concentrated tissue extract between ether and a phosphate buffer. Activity appeared in both of the fractions so formed and it had clearly to be attributed to two substances. The one soluble in ether was labelled E from the initial letter of the solvent. Similarly the one soluble in the phosphate buffer was called F. The Swedish word for phosphate is 'fosfat'. So were born prostaglandins E and F and when other members of the family appeared (rather unexpectedly at first, as is the way with children) it seemed reasonable to continue the process of identifying them by letters and first to fill in the early blanks in the alphabetical list. Readers who have kept the tally will be aware that human seminal fluid contains no fewer than 15 different prostaglandins—three of the E series, two each of prostaglandins F, A and B and the six 19-hydroxy derivatives of the A, B and E compounds. They are present in relatively large amounts, the concentration of the three prostaglandins E together averaging about 50 μg per ml and that of the F group reaching about 8 μg per ml. Concentrations as high (and mixtures as complex) as this are not found in organized tissues because prostaglandins are associated with cell membranes. Consequently, tissues cannot acquire 'stores' of prostaglandins in the way, for instance, that nerve terminals accumulate stores of transmitter. Stimuli that call forth the release of prostaglandins from tissues also stimulate synthesis at a level that enables the release rate to be maintained in the absence of any reserve store. This is a unique and important feature of prostaglandin behaviour which should be kept in mind. There is of course no structural constraint on the accumulation of prostaglandins in semen and other body fluids. In this connection it should be noted that quite high values for the prostaglandin content of individual organs are sometimes quoted in the literature and these may appear to falsify the assertion that the organized tissues of the body cannot store more than trivial quantities of the several prostaglandins. Many of these values are, however, spuriously high and they reflect the fact that synthesis occurs during the maceration and homogenization of the tissue that is an essential step in the extraction process. Synthesis can continue because the newly formed prostaglandins escape into the extraction medium.

Before the chemical nature of the prostaglandins had been established, a number of workers had been studying the behaviour of materials in tissue extracts which, though unidentified, seemed likely to be of physiological importance. Thus, W. Vogt (1957) found that, when a piece of intestine was left in an organ bath without change of fluid, it liberated material capable of initiating contraction in a freshly set up intestinal preparation. The material was called Darmstoff ('intestine substance'). Again, Ambache who was interested in the mechanisms whereby local trauma provoked inflammatory changes in the eye, found material in extracts of rabbit iris that caused inflammation and pupillary constriction when it was injected into the eyes of other rabbits. The active substance was called irin (Ambache, 1957). Pickles had the idea that a substance capable of inducing the contraction of uterine muscle might be liberated in that organ during menstruation and that its appearance in abnormally large amounts might cause painful spasms of the uterine muscle (*dysmenorrhoea*). Testing his hypothesis, Pickles found that human menstrual fluid was indeed capable of causing uterine contractions (Pickles, 1957). Finally, it has been known for some time that extracts of the renal medulla contain an antihypertensive principle (*medullin*). All these substances—Darmstoff, irin, medullin and the menstrual stimulant—are now known to be different prostaglandin mixtures, a finding that emphasizes both the widespread distribution of the prostaglandins and the varied nature of the effects they produce. More recent work has established the virtual ubiquity of prostaglandins in the tissues of the body.

CHEMISTRY AND METABOLISM

It is beyond the competence of this writer to provide information about the chemistry of the prostaglandins beyond that likely to be demanded by his average reader. Any chemist who has unwittingly strayed into these pages in search of enlightenment should refer to more specialized reviews such as those by Schneider (1972, 1976), Weinshenker and Andersen (1973) and Samuelsson (1978).

From a structural point of view, prostaglandins can be regarded as derivatives of prostanoic acid, a compound that has been synthesized but which does not occur naturally. As can be seen by reference to Fig. 23.1 *a*, it is a long chain fatty acid that includes within its structure a cyclopentane (five-membered) ring. The conventional way of representing prostanoic acid (and hence the prostaglandins) indicates that the chain of carbon atoms 1 to 7, which is shown attached to the ring by an interrupted line, is below the plane of the ring while chain C_{13} to C_{20} is above it. Similarly, the hydrogen atom on C8 is above the ring and that on C12 is below it.

So long as trivial names are adhered to, the nomenclature of the prostaglandins and their derivatives is simple. With the exception of those labelled G and I, prostaglandins differ from one another only in the nature of their cyclopentane rings and in the number of double bonds in the open chain part of their molecules. The letter (E, F, A, B, C, D or H) identifies the ring structure and the suffixes ($_1$, $_2$ or $_3$) indicates the number and implies the position of the double bonds. The individual ring structures are displayed in Fig. 23.1 *b* and Fig. 23.2.

Prostaglandins G_2 and I_2 (and, presumably, any other members of these series that eventually emerge) provide exceptions to the general labelling principle that has just been enunciated, both compounds having unique structural features. Prostaglandin G_2 carries an -OOH group at position C15 instead of the hydroxyl group found in that position in all other prostaglandins including

prostaglandin I_2. Its cyclopentane ring is identical with that characteristic of prostaglandin H_2.

The cyclopentane ring in prostacyclin I_2 is similar to that in prostaglandins of the E series but the structure of the molecule is changed by reason of the fact that the oxygen of the ring is additionally bonded to carbon atom 6 (Fig. 23.3 *a*).

During laboratory syntheses of the prostaglandins, two F series appear. In one the hydroxyl group in position 9 is below the plane of the ring and F prostaglandins with this configuration are designated α. In the β series the hydroxyl group is above the plane of the ring. Naturally occurring F prostaglandins belong to the α series and it is conventional to indicate this in the trivial name although this is not strictly necessary.

The positions of the double bonds in the prostaglandin molecule are completely uniform irrespective of the series. All prostaglandins have a double bond in the C13—C14 position. Those with no other double bond in the chains carry the suffix 1. Those with the suffix 2 have, in addition, a double bond at position C5—C6 and those labelled 3 have a further double bond linking carbon atoms 17 and 18. Double bonds restrict the free rotation of the groups they connect and this introduces the possibility of the compound's occurring in *cis* and *trans* stereoisomeric forms (Fig. 23.1 *c*). In the prostaglandins, the configuration at the double bond 1 (that linking C13 and C14) is *trans* and at the other two it is *cis*. The conventional way of representing these configurations should be evident from a comparison of the formulae of prostaglandins E_1 and E_3 (Fig. 23.1 *d*).

The hydroxyl group, already referred to, that is carried on the open chain of all prostaglandins except prostaglandins G (which bear the -OOH group instead) appears at position 15.

Reference to Fig. 23.1 *b* will make it clear why prostaglandins of the G and H series are known as the prostaglandin endoperoxides.

The formulae of prostacyclin and the thromboxanes appear in Fig. 23.3.

With the information presented here and the illustrative examples in Fig. 23.1, no reader should experience difficulty in deriving the formulae of individual prostaglandins for himself.

Trivial names for prostaglandin metabolites and synthetic analogues have also been coined. Some of the more common conventions are illustrated in Fig. 23.2. If the open chain is reduced in length by one, two, three or more methylene groups the appropriate prefix nor, dinor, trinor etc. is attached to the name of the corresponding prostaglandin. A further prefix, α or ω, is attached to indicate whether the shortening has been applied to the carboxyl-containing (α) or to the hydroxyl carrying (ω) chain. Lengthening of the chain is denoted by the prefix homo, appropriately qualified as α or ω.

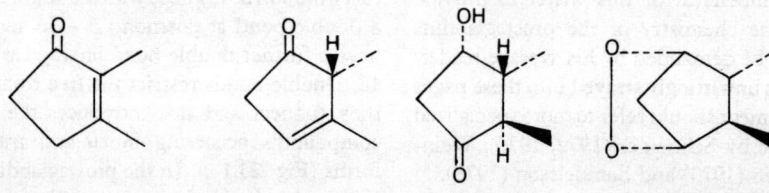

Fig. 23.1 Aspects of prostaglandin structure

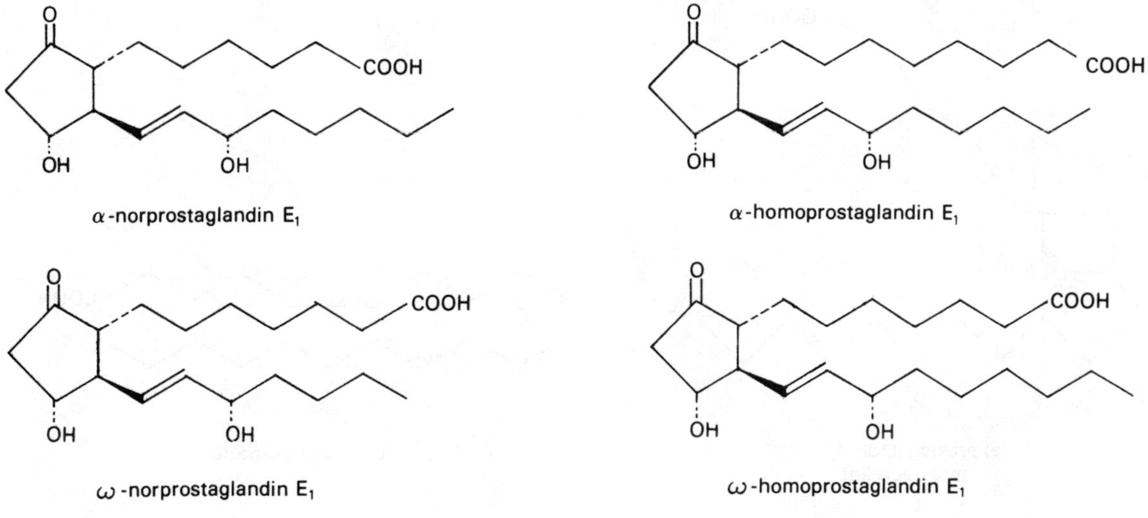

α-norprostaglandin E₁

α-homoprostaglandin E₁

ω-norprostaglandin E₁

ω-homoprostaglandin E₁

Fig. 23.2

The full chemical names of the prostaglandins are logical, unambiguous, informative and clumsy. Thus prostaglandins E_1 and E_2 are properly called $11\alpha, 15\alpha$-dihydroxy-9-oxo-13-*trans*-prostenoic acid and $11\alpha,15\alpha$-dihydroxy-9-oxo-5-*cis*-13-*trans*-prostadienoic acid but these names are rarely needed by the pharmacologist. In 1969, Andersen introduced a new system of abbreviations intended to emphasize the stereochemical specificities of the prostaglandin molecules. According to this scheme, prostaglandins E_2 and $F_{1\beta}$, to take two examples, became $PG(E\alpha\alpha)_2$ and $PG(\beta\alpha\alpha)_1$ respectively. The scheme has its value, particularly in the chemistry laboratory, but it has not been extensively adopted and most of us can thankfully retain the old and comfortable nomenclature.

Individual prostaglandins occur naturally in only one structural form, but many stereoisomers can be created in the laboratory. There are, for instance, 128 possible stereoisomers of prostaglandin $F_{2\alpha}$. Quite apart from his being able to produce isomers of known compounds, the chemist has almost unlimited prospects of creating entirely new prostaglandins and prostaglandin analogues. The veriest tyro has only to look at the formulae displayed in Fig. 23.1 and 23.2 to appreciate the vast number of compounds that could be produced, for instance, by altering chain lengths, the number and position of double bonds, the nature of the ring and the number and nature of the substituents on the ring and open chains. As we shall see, there are many indications that compounds with more selective actions than the native prostaglandins would have a considerable therapeutic promise and we can be certain that natural curiosity, commercial pressures and the desire to produce something useful for his fellow men will together ensure that the synthesizing chemist will exploit to the full the opportunities offered to him by the prostaglandins.

The thromboxanes (whose chemical formulae are displayed in Fig. 23.3) owe their name to the facts that they are formed (though by no means exclusively) in the platelets (thrombocytes) and that they incorporate oxane rings in their molecules. Lacking the prostanoic acid skeleton they cannot be called prostaglandins but they are derived from the same endoperoxide precursors that give rise to the prostaglandins proper. Moreover their physiological role is so interwoven with that of at least some of the prostaglandins that it is necessary as well as appropriate that the two groups of compounds should be considered together in our discussions.

The formulae of a number of other substances that have to be considered in the context of prostaglandin synthesis are also included in Fig. 23.3. These substances are 12-L-hydroxy-5,8,10,14-eicosatetraenoic acid (HETE), its 12-hydroperoxide analogue (HPETE), 12-L-hydroxy-5,8,11-heptadecatrienoic acid (HHT), malondialdehyde (MDA) and 6-oxoprostaglandin $F_2\alpha$.

Biosynthesis of prostaglandins and thromboxanes
Prostaglandin synthesis can be achieved in vitro by incubating extracts of sheep seminal vesicles with open chain unsaturated fatty acids with chain lengths of 20 carbon atoms. Three such acids—8,11,14-eicosatrienoic acid (dihomo-γ-linolenic acid), 5,8,11,14-eicosatetraenoic acid (arachidonic acid) and 5,8,11,14,17-eicosapentaenoic acid —give rise to prostaglandins with, respectively, 1, 2 and 3 double bonds in their side chains (Fig. 23.4). They are the precursors of the prostaglandins synthesized in vivo. The first two of these acids are derived from linoleic acid and the last from linolenic acid. Dihomo-γ-linolenic acid can be changed into arachidonic acid and it may be that some hormones can effect this change (insulin and thyroid

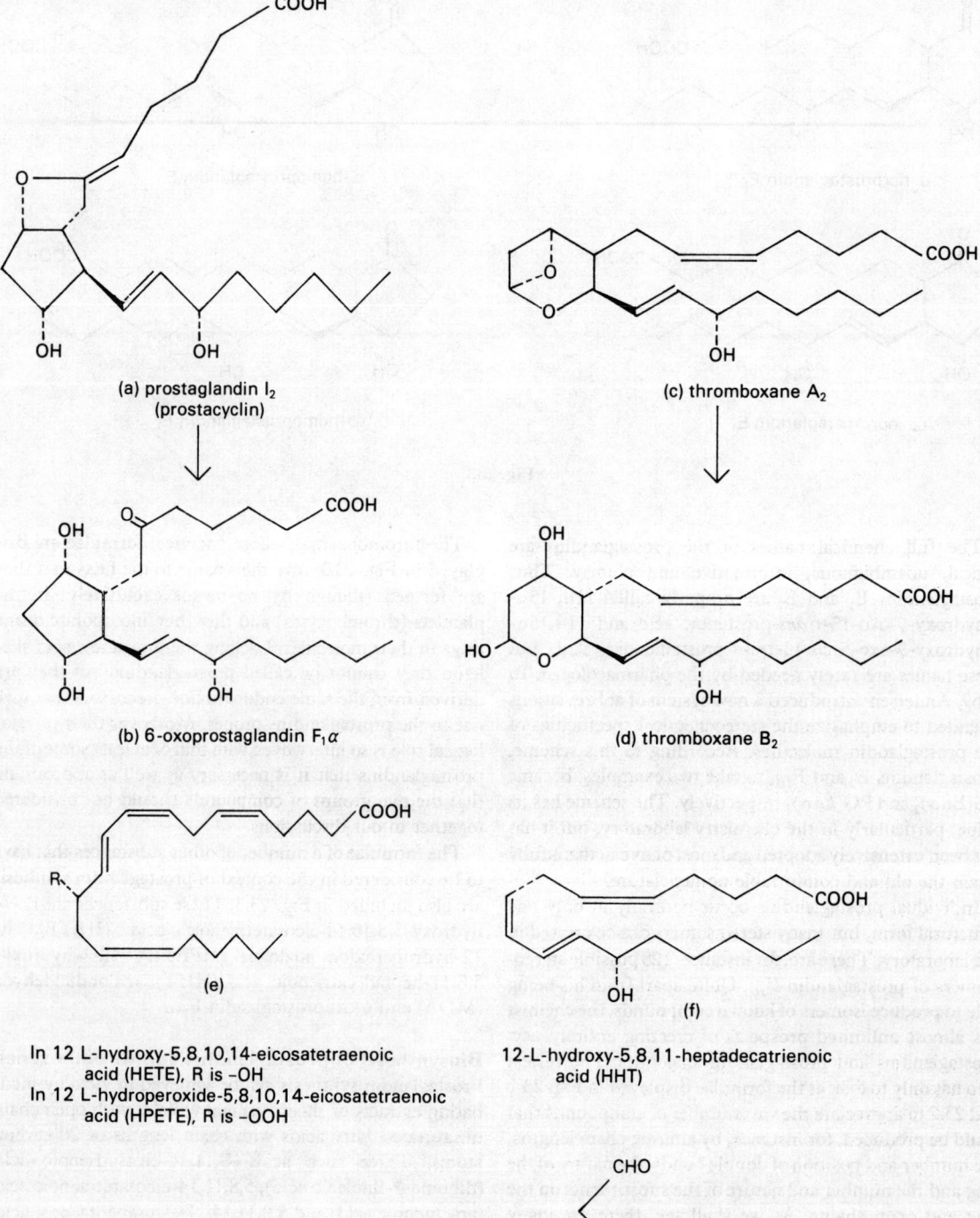

Fig. 23.3 Some substances produced from arachidonic acid.

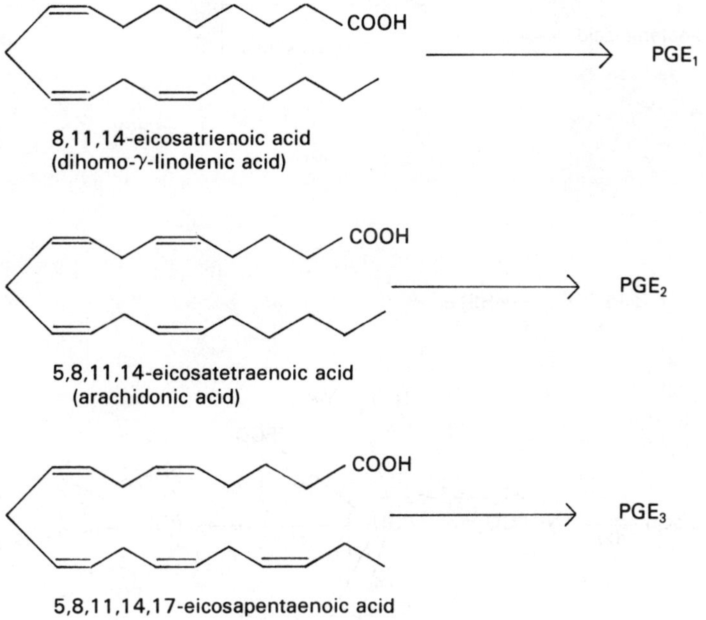

8,11,14-eicosatrienoic acid
(dihomo-γ-linolenic acid)

→ PGE₁

5,8,11,14-eicosatetraenoic acid
(arachidonic acid)

→ PGE₂

5,8,11,14,17-eicosapentaenoic acid

→ PGE₃

Fig. 23.4 Prostaglandin precursors

hormone have been mentioned in this connection) and so alter the balance of the '1' and '2' prostaglandins and their respective derivatives.

Long before anyone had become aware of the existence of the prostaglandins it became clear that linoleic and linolenic acids were essential components of the diet. We can now see, if prostaglandins are the vital physiological regulators we believe them to be, why an intake of the essential fatty acids (which cannot be synthesized in the body) is indispensible to an animal's well being. Conditions referable to a deficiency of one or other of the essential fatty acids are not seen as often as those consequent on a vitamin deficiency (largely because mammals normally carry large stores of the acids) but they can be induced in laboratory animals and even in human beings linoleic acid deficiency is a recognized, if rare, clinical entity. As would be expected of a condition arising from a depressed synthesis of substances with such wide ranging actions as the prostaglandins, linoleic acid deficiency gives rise to a multisymptom complex characterized by disordered function of the gastrointestinal, reproductive, endocrine and urinary systems, by loss of hair and lesions of the skin. On the other hand, as far as this author is aware, no pathological condition readily attributable to a deficiency of linolenic acid has ever been reported, and this would suggest, perhaps, that prostaglandins with three double bonds in the open chain are of smaller biological significance than those of the 1 and 2 series. Although PGE_3 and $PGF_{3\alpha}$ do occur naturally in some species (in seminal fluid and lung tissue respectively) their pharmacological actions are not impressive and the reader will find very little mention of the 3 series prostaglandins in the following pages or in any of the other reviews to which he has been directed. This is not to say, of course, that naturally occurring members of the group other than PGE_3 and $PGF_{3\alpha}$ might not eventually come to light nor that synthetic compounds of this type are not worthy of study. Indeed as this volume went to press the discovery of prostaglandin I_3 was reported.

The fatty acid precursors of the prostaglandins occur in an esterified form, particularly as phospholipids, in the cell membrane and when prostaglandin synthesis occurs the precursors are freed by the action of phospholipase A_2. The subsequent series of events are summarized, as far as they have been elucidated, in Fig. 23.5, which relates to the synthesis of prostaglandin E_2 and related compounds from arachidonic acid.

Arachidonic acid released from the cell membrane is offered two fates. One of them, catalysed by lipoxygenase, involves its conversion into HETE by way of HPETE. The possible significance of these two compounds will be mentioned in an appropriate context later (p. 377). The other path that arachidonic acid can follow is controlled by a group of enzymes known as prostaglandin synthetase (or synthase). Cyclooxygenase converts arachidonic acid into the cyclic endoperoxides (PGG_2 and PGH_2) which stand at the origin of no fewer than six branches of the prostaglandin synthesis pathway. The components of the prostaglandin synthetase system that serve these branches are named in Fig. 23.5. Which of the available paths is

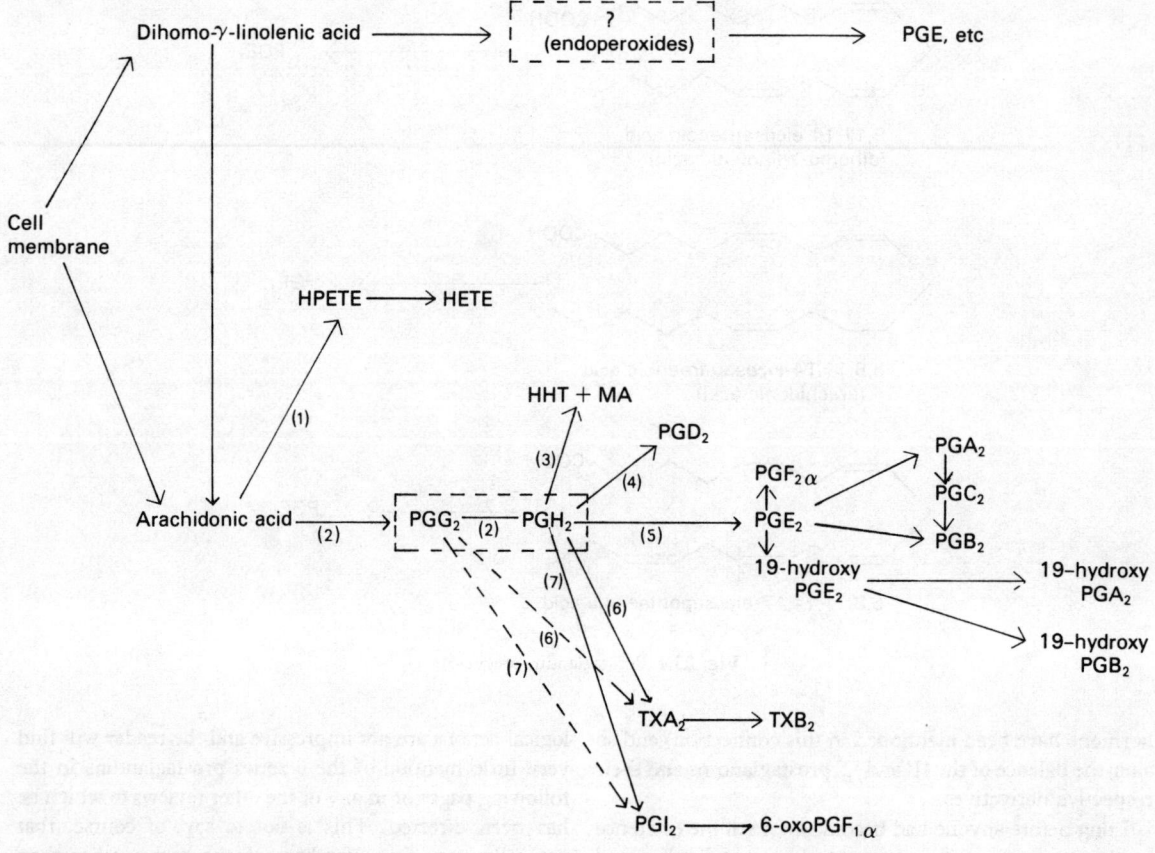

Enzymes involved
(1) lipo-oxygenase
(2) cycloxygenase (prostaglandin endoperoxide synthetase)
(3) serum albumin glutathione-S-transferase
(4) prostaglandin endoperoxide reductase
(5) prostaglandin endoperoxide E isomerase
(6) prostaglandin endoperoxide-thromboxane A isomerase (thromboxane A_2 synthetase)
(7) prostaglandin endoperoxide I isomerase

Names and formulae of the substances represented by initials are given in Figs 23.1 and 23.2

Fig. 23.5 The formation of prostaglandins and their derivatives

followed in a particular tissue is determined by the nature of the enzymes and co-factors that can be offered by the tissue as well, probably, as by other local conditions.

The endoperoxides are relatively unstable compounds with half lives of about five minutes. Although they are key intermediates in prostaglandin synthesis the endoperoxides probably have important physiological actions in their own right. Prostacyclin and thromboxane A_2 are unstable with half lives of approximately two minutes and 30 sec. respectively. Prostacyclin changes into 6-oxo $PG1_\alpha$ while thromboxane A_2 changes into thromboxane B_2. Both these breakdown products are devoid of pronounced pharmacological activity.

The conversion of prostaglandin E_2 into prostaglandins A_2, B_2 and (possibly) C_2, as indicated in Fig. 23.4, is of doubtful physiological significance, although enzymes that facilitate these conversions are certainly present in some tissues. However, the changes can also occur spontaneously and it is possible that when prostaglandins A, B or C are found in tissue extracts they represent nothing more than extraction artefacts and that they do not exist in the living animal. The resolution of doubts concerning the importance of these prostaglandins awaits the outcome of further work.

Prostaglandins E_1 and $F_{1\alpha}$ are formed, as we have already noted from dihomo-γ-linolenic acid and we must suppose that in vivo synthesis proceeds by way of prosta-glandin endoperoxide intermediates and that perhaps branch pathways to thromboxanes, a prostacyclin and so on are also available. It must be added, though, that the existence of such substances as prostaglandins G_1, H_1 and I_1 and of thromboxanes A_1 and B_1 has not yet been established.

Inhibitors of cyclo-oxygenase activity

Pharmacologists are always (and properly) anxious to study the effects in the living animal of substances that prevent the synthesis of endogenous compounds, believ-ing that any deficiency syndrome produced in this way will throw light on the physiological role of the missing sub-stance. The alternative way of elucidating physiological function, by recording the effects of administration of the compound, can never entirely escape the criticism that the responses are merely pharmacological in nature and do not portray the physiological situation. Eagerness to discern the likely physiological functions of the prostaglandins provoked an early interest in the development of inhibitors of prostaglandin synthesis. A number of such compounds became available and were used in experimental work but the situation was dramatically changed in 1971 when Vane discovered that a group of drugs that had been known and used for many years actually owe their therapeutic and most of their toxic actions to an ability to prevent prosta-glandin synthesis (Vane, 1971). These compounds are the nonsteroidal antiinflammatory drugs of which aspirin, one of our oldest and most valuable therapeutic agents, can be taken as the archetype.

The known inhibitors of prostaglandin synthesis can be grouped as indicated in the following paragraphs. It should however be noted that, among different tissues, the synthetase is not uniformly sensitive to inhibition by a particular agent. It should also be noted that it is the cyclo-oxygenase moiety of the prostaglandin synthetase complex that is most susceptible to the action of the inhibitors which thus prevent the production of the prostaglandin endoperoxides and all the compounds that are formed from them. The lipoxygenase is, however, unaffected so that, in those tissues where it is proceeding, the production of HETE is not interrupted by the inhibitors. Substances that selectively inhibit stages in the synthesis of prosta-glandins and thromboxane beyond the point at which the enderoperoxides are formed are now being recognized. They are mentioned separately in the next column.

a. Substrate analogues compete competitively for the synthetase but are not themselves changed in any way. A number of analogues display activity of this type but the most powerful are 8,12,14-eicosatrienoic acid and 5,8,12,14-eicosatetraneoic acid (Fig. 23.6). The close simi-larity of these compounds to the prostaglandin precursors dihomo-γ-linolenic acid (8,11,14-eicosatrienoic acid) and arachidonic acid (5,8,11,14-eicosatetraenoic acid)

respectively is evident from both the names and the chemical formulae of the precursors (Fig. 23.6).

Some prostaglandins also inhibit the synthetase but others increase its activity.

b. Oleic, linoleic and linolenic acids and some highly unsaturated fatty acids inhibit cyclooxygenase by a bipha-sic process that results in the actual destruction of the catalytic centres in the enzyme.

c. The nonsteroidal antiinflammatory acids have already been mentioned. Their actions are discussed in detail in later pages of this chapter as well as in the sections of the book that are concerned particularly with the drugs' therapeutic uses.

d. Zinc, cadmium and cupric ions inhibit the synthesis of prostaglandins E *in vitro* but, with copper at least, the falling off of E production is accompanied by an increased synthesis of prostaglandins F.

e. Other substances that inhibit prostaglandin synthetase include sulphasalazine, gold, silver and nutmeg. The last named substance has been successfully applied to the treatment of diarrhoea (Bennett, Gradidge and Stamford, 1974).

Inhibitors of other components of prostaglandin synthetase

As we hinted earlier, compounds that inhibit the various enzymes that service the synthetic pathways beyond the prostaglandin endoperoxides are now making their appearance. Imidazole inhibits thromboxane synthetase and as we shall see it has been used successfully to help establish the physiological role of thromboxane A_2. Other well known drugs that in small doses inhibit thromboxane synthetase include dipyridamole (a substance employed to prevent platelet aggregation), furosemide and bumetanide. The formation of prostaglandin I_2 can be inhibited by 15-hydroperoxy-arachidonic acid while copper and zinc ions can hinder the formation of prostaglandin E_2 by inhibiting prostaglandin endoperoxide E isomerase.

Many substances can promote synthesis of prostaglan-dins. They are reviewed by Horrobin (1978).

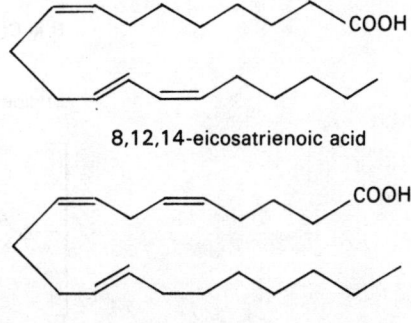

8,12,14-eicosatrienoic acid

5,8,12,14-eicosatetranoic acid

Fig. 23.6 Substrate analogue inhibitors of prostaglandin synthetase

Prostaglandin antagonists

In addition to those that prevent prostaglandin synthesis, some substances oppose the action of the prostaglandins by behaving as antagonists. They may be competitive or non-competitive antagonists in the strictly pharmacological sense (p. 100) or they may simply exert a physiological antagonism by virtue of their being able to bring about changes opposite to those induced by the prostaglandins themselves.

Until some ten years ago only three types of prostaglandin antagonist were known: 7-oxa prostaglandin analogues, dibenzoxazepine hydrazide derivatives and a high molecular weight polyester of phloretin and phosphoric acid (polyphloretin phosphate). The 7-oxa analogues display a confusing mixture of pharmacological activities that include both competitive and non-competitive antagonism, inhibition of prostaglandin synthesis, prostaglandin-like agonist activity and a degree of competitive antagonism against both acetylcholine and histamine. The dibenzoxazepine hydroxide derivatives are almost purely competitive antagonists with only a slight antagonism towards 5-hydroxytryptamine to prevent their being described as specific antagonists. Polyphloretin phosphate is a competitive inhibitor with, it seems, a specifically antiprostaglandin action. It is to be noted that the antagonists are not equally active against all the prostaglandins nor

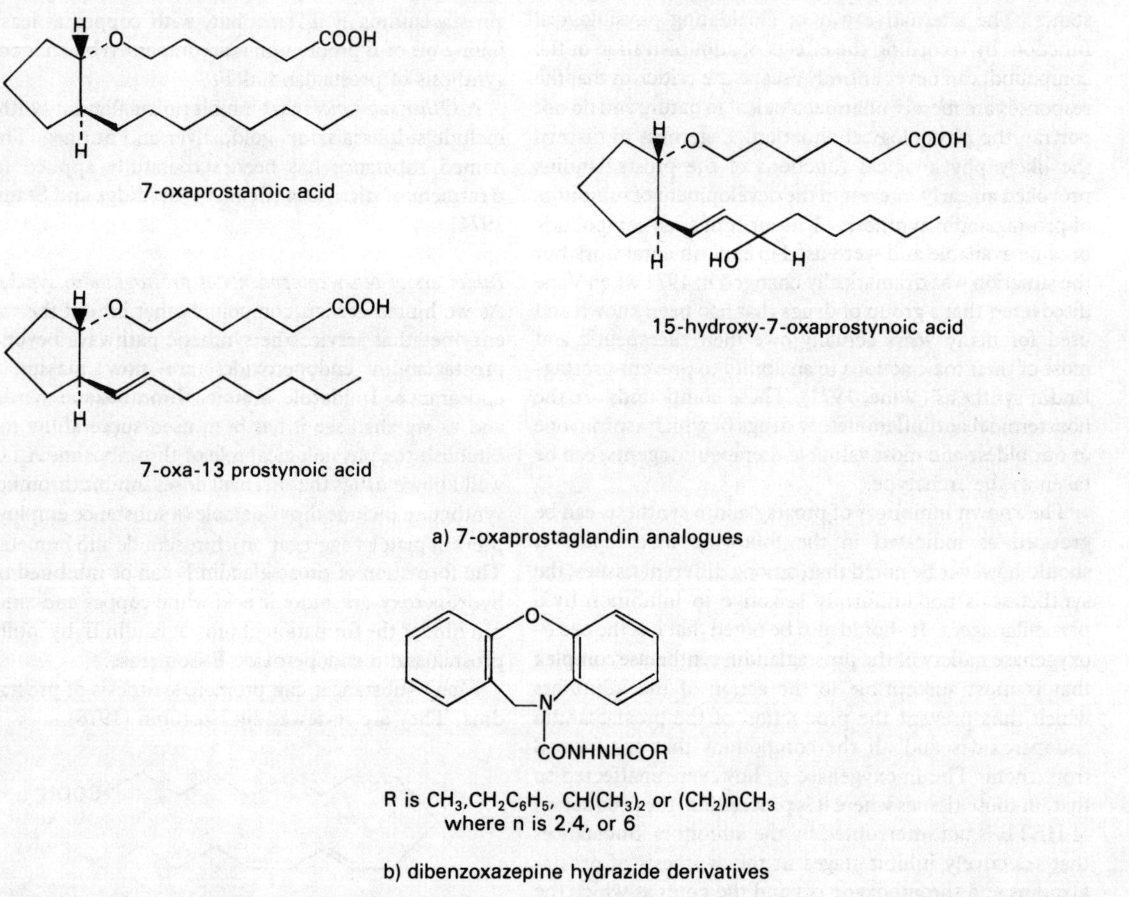

7-oxaprostanoic acid

15-hydroxy-7-oxaprostynoic acid

7-oxa-13 prostynoic acid

a) 7-oxaprostaglandin analogues

R is CH$_3$,CH$_2$C$_6$H$_5$, CH(CH$_3$)$_2$ or (CH$_2$)$_n$CH$_3$
where n is 2,4, or 6

b) dibenzoxazepine hydrazide derivatives

c) polyphloretin phosphate

Fig. 23.7 Prostaglandin antagonists

against all the actions on different tissues of a single prostaglandin.

New prostaglandin antagonists are now appearing at an accelerated rate. They include morphine, substances like p-hydroxymercuribenzoate that bind to sulphydryl groups and some membrane stabilizing substances such as quinidine, chloroquine and procaine. It must be noted, too, that some species of prostaglandin can act as competitive or as physiological antagonists of certain of their fellows.

We have seen already that some drugs inhibit thromboxane synthetase rather specifically. Some other drugs act as rather specific antagonists of thromboxane activity: they include both the benzodiazepine anti-anxiety drugs and the tricyclic antidepressant agents, as well as striated and smooth muscle relaxants, adenosine and creatine. Much of this more recent work has to be credited to Horrobin and his colleagues whose most recent prostaglandin review (Horrobin, 1978) should be consulted for further details concerning this topic. Reviews relating to earlier work are provided by Weeks (1972), Bennett (1974) and Sanner (1974).

Catabolism of prostaglandins

A number of enzymes operate in a concerted sequence to bring about degradation of the prostaglandins. So far as prostaglandins E are concerned, the first change to occur is oxidation of the hydroxyl group on C15. It is catalysed by the activity of 15-OH dehydrogenase, a widely distributed enzyme that reaches a particularly high concentration in the lungs. This reaction is the rate limiting step in the breakdown of the prostaglandins. The resulting compound is a 15-keto prostaglandin. The next step is saturation of the double bond at C13, to give a 15-keto-13,14, dihydroprostaglandin, the result of action by a Δ^{13} reductase. This reaction too takes place predominantly in the lungs. The two ends of the carbon chain are next attacked: β oxidation occurs twice (in β oxidation, the second carbon atom from the carboxyl group is oxidized),

each of the compounds so formed being a dinor. This action occurs primarily in the liver as does ω-oxidation, the final catabolic change. Prostaglandin $F_{2\alpha}$ is known to be metabolized along similar pathways.

The catabolic changes mentioned in the foregoing paragraph are summarized in Fig. 23.8

PHARMACOLOGICAL, PHYSIOLOGICAL AND THERAPEUTIC ASPECTS OF PROSTAGLANDIN ACTION

The rest of this chapter provides a summary, system by system, of the pharmacological actions of the prostaglandins and it considers the implications for physiology and for therapeutics. Before the details are presented some general points are listed. They bear on all the material in the remaining sections of the chapter and the reader who keeps them constantly in mind should be the better equipped to make a critical appraisal of the evidence that is placed before him, here and elsewhere.

1. Until quite recently, the only prostaglandins that were available in the quantities demanded by the laboratory worker were those of the E series. This inevitably means that these compounds have been more intensively studied and more frequently written about than others that may be of equal pharmacological significance.

2. Much of the early work (in this context, 'early' can be taken to mean 'before 1977') was carried out in ignorance of the existence of such recently discovered substances as prostacyclin and the thromboxanes. This circumstance led, in several instances, to an attribution to prostaglandins E and F of actions and roles that should properly have been credited to others.

3. The pharmacological actions of the prostaglandins are influenced by a variety of factors: the preparation used and the species that provides it, the nature and depth of the anaesthetic and the presence of other drugs in whole-animal preparations, the type, dose and route of administration of the prostaglandin used and so on. The reader

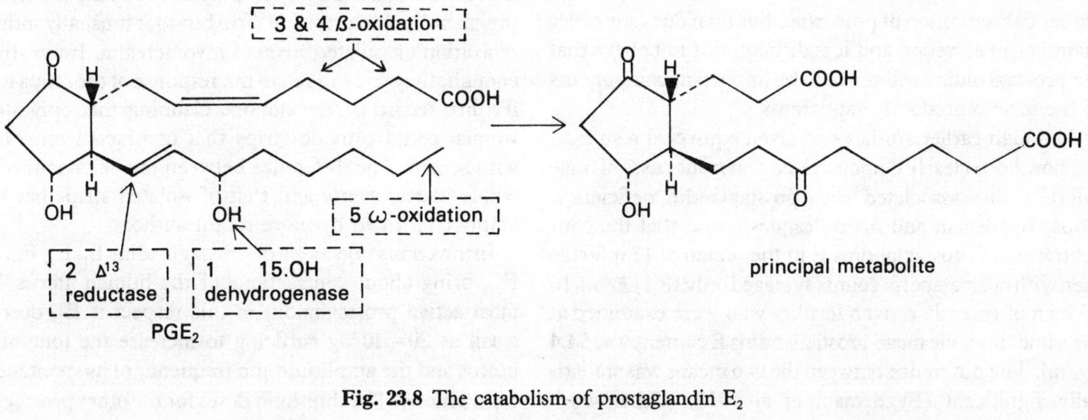

Fig. 23.8 The catabolism of prostaglandin E₂

who is not alive to these sources of variation may find the literature more contradictory and confusing than it need be. These confusions are especially likely to arise in descriptions of experiments on intact animals in which the observed response to prostaglandin adminstration is often the resultant of several mutually independent effects which are themselves susceptible to the sources of variation we have mentioned.

4. Some prostaglandins disappear from the blood very rapidly but their pharmacological effects may be more prolonged. This may be the result of their having liberated other active substances from the tissues or it may be that they have been converted into more stable, but still active, metabolites.

5. We often have no precise knowledge of the relative amounts of the different prostaglandins and their metabolites that are liberated into the tissues during normal physiological activity so that, in view of the qualitative and quantitative differences between the actions of different prostaglandins, few conclusions concerning their physiological role can be regarded as other than tentative or highly speculative.

6. Finally we must reiterate the general principle that pharmacological activity does not necessarily reflect or predict physiological function: the fact that a naturally occurring substance modifies physiological activity when it is applied in an experimental situation cannot, in the absence of collateral evidence, be taken as incontrovertible evidence that the substance has a similar—or any—action if it is liberated endogenously in the normal animal.

The reproductive system

So far as the prostaglandins are concerned, the secretions of the male genital tract proved to be seminal in the widest sense of that word because it was the detection and eventual isolation of the prostaglandins of seminal fluid that seeded the spectacular growth that is the subject of this chapter. It is only appropriate, therefore, that our enquiry into the possible significance of the prostaglandins should begin with the material that started it all.

Human seminal plasma carries a wider variety and a higher concentration of prostaglandins than does any other mammalian secretion and it is difficult not to believe that the prostaglandins will prove to be important components of the male reproductive apparatus.

Although earlier studies had given equivocal results, it has now been clearly demonstrated that some cases of male infertility are associated with prostaglandin deficiency. Thus, Bygdeman and his colleagues found that the concentration of prostaglandins E in the semen of 17 infertile men with normal sperm counts averaged only $18.1 \mu g/ml$. In 29 men of recently proven fertility who were examined at the same time, the mean prostaglandins E content was 54.4 $\mu g/ml$. The difference between the two means was statistically significant (Bygdeman, et al 1970). Other work

indicates that prostaglandins F may also be deficient in infertile males but prostaglandins A and B are not, apparently, affected.

It is not easy to discern the role of the prostaglandins in the male reproductive process. We have seen that they are synthesized in the seminal vesicles. Accordingly, they appear in highest concentration in the last portion of the seminal ejaculate and it would not be unreasonable to assume that they might thus be able to encourage fertilization by ensuring the complete emptying of the seminal vesicles during coitus. Unfortunately for this hypothesis, the only species of animal whose seminal vesicles have been shown to contract on exposure to prostaglandins— the guinea pig— is one whose semen contains very little of any prostaglandin. Moreover, prostaglandin E_2 actually causes relaxation of vesicular muscle in the rabbit, an animal species that is not notoriously infertile. Nor do prostaglandins influence the motility or metabolism of spermatozoa and we are forced into the position of having to consider the intriguing possibility that they may support male fertility by an action on the female reproductive system. The ways in which this might be brought about are discussed later.

The testis can synthesize prostaglandins E_1, $F_{1\alpha}$ and $F_{2\alpha}$ and there is evidence that the prostaglandins can stimulate the production and secretion of testosterone (Eik-Nes, 1969). Prostaglandin E_1 inhibits the tone and spontaneous contractions of the smooth muscle that constitutes the testicular capsule. Prostaglandin $F_{1\alpha}$ has the opposite effect. The significance of these observations is not clear.

THE FEMALE REPRODUCTIVE SYSTEM

It is both convenient and prudent to discuss separately the pharmacological actions, the physiological significance and the therapeutic uses of prostaglandins in the female.

Pharmacological actions

As long ago as 1930, Kurzrok and Lieb reported that human seminal fluid caused contraction of the intact, nonpregnant human uterus *in vitro* but that it usually induced relaxation of isolated *strips* of myometrium. Interestingly enough, they tried to relate the response of the strips to the fertility record of the donors, claiming that only sterile women could provide strips that contracted on contact with semen. The difference between the behaviour of the whole uterus *in situ* and that of isolated strips has been amply confirmed by more recent authors.

Intravenous injections of prostaglandins E_1, E_2, $F_{1\alpha}$ and $F_{2\alpha}$ bring about contractions of the human uterus. The most active prostaglandin in this respect is E_2, doses as small as 20 – 40 μg sufficing to increase the tone of the uterus and the amplitude and frequency of its spontaneous contractions. The threshold doses for the other prostaglandins are two to ten times higher than this. Infusion of the prostaglandins is accompanied by increases of uterine activity that persist throughout the period of the infusion and for an hour or longer thereafter. The sensitivity of the uterus to prostaglandins increases towards the end of pregnancy.

Strips of uterine myometrium *in vitro* relax when they are exposed to prostaglandins E (particularly E_1) but contract in response to F prostaglandins. The response to seminal fluid is, as we have seen, usually inhibitory and this is clearly a reflection of the relative concentration and activity of the E components of the seminal mixture. It is not clear why the intact uterus should behave so differently from strips of the same organ but it provides an illustration of the complications that abound in the prostaglandin field and which can so easily confuse the unwary reader.

In 1969 Pharriss and Wyngarden found that prostaglandin $F_{2\alpha}$ caused luteolysis (breakdown of the corpus lutem) in the rat and since then a number of other workers have demonstrated a similar effect in other mammalian species. Although there is no direct evidence that the prostaglandin can induce luteolysis in the human female there is every reason to believe that it does do so: it certainly does in other primates.

It is known that mechanical irritation of the uterus such as that produced by the insertion of a foreign body can result in luteolysis and this effect was hitherto attributed to the liberation of a hormone with the predictable name of luteolysin. It is now clear that luteolysin is prostaglandin $F_{2\alpha}$. It has been suggested that intrauterine contraceptive devices owe their effectiveness to luteolysin liberation (Chaudhuri, 1971).

A number of explanations have been offered for the luteolytic behaviour of prostaglandin $F_{2\alpha}$. It constricts the ovarian veins—this effect seems to be rather specific for these vessels—and could in this way cause a partial failure of the ovarian circulation and a consequent destruction of the corpus luteum. However, prostaglandin $F_{2\alpha}$ depresses progesterone synthesis in cultures of corpora lutea and there is also evidence that it can antagonize the action of the luteinising hormone which normally ensures the integrity of the corpus luteum (p. 738). More than one of these postulated mechanisms might be involved in luteolysis.

Before leaving this topic the inevitable contradiction must be pointed out. More than one group of workers have shown that prostaglandins (of both the E and F varieties) stimulate the production of progesterone in ovarian tissue *in vitro* and it has even been suggested that prostaglandins might provide a link between luteinising hormone release and progesterone synthesis. It is not easy to explain these discrepant findings: perhaps one is a pharmacological response and the other a physiological one. There is also evidence that the secretion of luteinizing hormone is dependent on the synthesis of prostaglandin $F_{2\alpha}$ in the brain.

Physiological significance

a. *The induction of labour*. During labour, prostaglandins E_1, E_2, $F_{1\alpha}$ and $F_{2\alpha}$ appear in quantity in amniotic fluid and the maternal blood. The most abundant are the F prostaglandins, total concentrations of more than 150 ng/ml having been noted (Karim, 1966). Before labour sets in, only small amounts of only one prostaglandin (E_1) can be detected. The prostaglandins in amniotic fluid and the maternal bloodstream presumably represent an overflow from a site, probably the uterine endometrium, that is synthesizing them at a more than usually rapid rate. Since the four prostaglandins that appear are all capable of causing uterine contraction and since the sensitivity of the uterus to prostaglandins increases in late pregnancy it seems possible that prostaglandin release may be a factor— if only one of many—contributing to the initiation of labour. It is very interesting in this connection that Karim has found prostaglandins in the amniotic fluid of foetuses that have been spontaneously aborted as early as the fourteenth week of pregnancy, although they are normally virtually absent from the amniotic fluid, as we have seen, until full term is reached and labour begins. Thus an aberrant outburst of activity on the part of the uterine prostaglandin synthesis system might be a factor in the precipitation of spontaneous abortion although we have as yet no clue as to what might cause the disturbance of uterine biochemistry.

Aspirin, as we have already noted, inhibits prostaglandin synthesis and it was found some time ago that both the period of gestation and the duration of labour were significantly prolonged in women who had been taking aspirin during the last six months of pregnancy (Lewis and Schulman, 1973). The intake of aspirin was large (more than 3 g daily) and the average durations of pregnancy and of labour were 286 days and 12 hr respectively. In another group of arthritic subjects who were not taking aspirin, gestation and labour occupied, respectively, 275 days and 7.3 hr. These results not only confirm the importance of prostaglandins in parturition but they also provide evidence that prostaglandin release is the cause and not the consequence of the contractile activity in the uterus. They also hint at the possibility of using antiinflammatory drugs to prevent abortion in susceptible women.

There is a belief in some quarters that sexual intercourse during pregnancy involves the risk of abortion or of premature labour. This belief is not an illogical one since prostaglandins are readily absorbed from the vagina and can thereby influence uterine activity. However, it appears that prostaglandins are less readily absorbed from the vagina (or are more rapidly inactivated) during pregnancy than at other times. Thus, in the interests of the foetus, the uterus rejects the material it would otherwise welcome. Nevertheless, it is clearly possible that intercourse could be hazardous if the uterus were unduly sensitive, the concentrations of seminal prostaglandin were unusually high, if the vaginal defences were weakened or if acts of intercourse followed too rapidly on one another.

b. Menstruation and dysmenorrhoea. We have already seen that Pickles detected a spasmogenic substance in menstrual fluid and that he believed that an excessive production of this material might be responsible for dysmenorrhoea. Following identification of the menstrual stimulant as a prostaglandin, Pickles and his colleagues were able to examine the composition of the mixture in the menstrual discharge. They found that the concentration of prostaglandin $F_{2\alpha}$ in the menstrual fluid of a group of subjects with dysmenorrhoea averaged 9.6 $\mu g/ml$, a value significantly greater than the 3.4 $\mu g/ml$ found in the discharge of those whose menstruation was comfortable. Unfortunately for Pickles' original hypothesis, the subjects with dysmenorrhoea produced smaller amounts of prostaglandins E (which, as we have seen, are powerful uterine stimulants) than normal subjects so that the total prostaglandin content and, probably, the total spasmogenic activity of the fluid from the two groups was similar. But we must recall the luteolytic action of prostaglandin $F_{2\alpha}$. Menstruation is associated with the withdrawal of progesterone and it is by no means unlikely that a too precipitate breaking down of the corpus luteum might lead to a disorganized and painful menstruation. The physiological trigger for menstrual luteolysis might well be prostaglandin $F_{2\alpha}$.

It is often, and rightly, said that the best cure for dysmenorrhoea is marriage. It is not easy to see why this is so if dysmenorrhoea is attributable to the presence of greater than normal amounts of prostaglandin $F_{2\alpha}$, a major component of seminal fluid. Marriage evidently involves more than the transfer of prostaglandins.

c. Male prostaglandins and the female reproductive system. We saw earlier that prostaglandins have relatively little influence on the male genital system, a surprising fact in view of the rich variety of prostaglandins in seminal fluid. There is, however, abundant evidence that prostaglandins can be absorbed from the vagina in sufficient quantity for them to be able to exert an action on the uterus and its appendages. One such action is on the Fallopian tubes: the portion nearer the uterus is constricted and the more distal part is dilated by prostaglandins E_1 and E_2. Other prostaglandins have a less selective action: prostaglandin E_3 dilates the tube along its whole length and prostaglandins $F_{1\alpha}$ and $F_{2\alpha}$ have an overall constrictor action. If sufficient amounts of prostaglandins E_1 and E_2 are absorbed from the vagina after coitus to exert the effect seen in laboratory experiments, the ovum might be held in an advantageous position for fertilization in the Fallopian tube. If it is confirmed that seminal prostaglandins do exert an action on the female reproductive organs, we shall be able to classify the prostaglandins as 'pheromones'— substances produced by one individual but influencing activity in another. This would be the first example of a pheromone in man.

Clinical applications
The powerful actions of the prostaglandins on the female reproductive tract have prompted their use for the induction of labour and as abortifacient and contraceptive agents. Much of the work in this field was initiated by Karim and his colleagues to whose writings the interested reader is referred (see, for instance, Karim, 1975).

For the induction of labour, prostaglandin $F_{2\alpha}$ given by intravenous infusion was used at first and it proved to be as effective as oxytocin (Anderson, 1973). In some respects the prostaglandin was preferable to the hormone: it was more often successful in patients with rigid cervices and its lack of antidiuretic activity constituted a distinct advantage. Prostaglandin E_2 is more potent than the F variety. It is effective at infusion rates of 0.5 to 2 μg per minute and in obstetrics it is now generally employed in preference to prostaglandin $F_{2\alpha}$. The prostaglandins are also effective by the oral route but care has to be taken lest prostaglandin action on the gastointestinal tract cause unacceptable nausea, vomiting and diarrhoea. Because of its higher potency on the uterus, prostaglandin E_2 (in two-hourly oral doses of 0.5 to 2 mg) is less likely than prostaglandin $F_{2\alpha}$ to have undesirable effects on gastrointestinal function.

Prostaglandins E_2 and $F_{2\alpha}$ will, of course, induce abortion when they are given intravenously but in the interest of minimizing side effects, intravaginal administration (or direct injection into the uterine cavity by way of an intravaginal catheter) is to be preferred when the prostaglandins are employed to secure an abortion. After the first three months of pregnancy, the prostaglandins can be injected through the abdominal wall directly into the amniotic cavity. Effective doses of prostaglandins E_2 and $F_{2\alpha}$ by this route are of the order of 5 and 25 mg respectively. As well as being abortifacients in their own right, prostaglandins can also be given to dilate the uterine cervix as a preliminary to evacuation of the uterus by mechanical means.

In recent years, the 15-methyl esters of prostaglandins E_2 and $F_{2\alpha}$ have been made use of in preference to the prostaglandins themselves.

The use of prostaglandins as post-coital contraceptive agents is mentioned on p. 751.

Platelet function
When a small blood vessel is punctured, platelets in the region of the injury adhere to one another and to the damaged vessel wall, forming a temporary plug for the hole. The aggregate of platelets so formed releases factors that initiate coagulation and others that encourage further aggregation. The fibrin of the clot further strengthens the plug which continues to extend until the vessel is blocked

by an impermeable mass (the thrombus) which effectively prevents further bleeding. It will be evident to the reader that the initial aggregation of the platelets is the key event in the whole process.

Although thrombus formation serves an obvious physiological purpose it is also the source of serious disease and disabilities. In arteriosclerosis (atherosclerosis), for instance, the blood flow through the arteries is disturbed by reason of the narrowing of the vessels brought about by the atheromatous plaques. This forms a stimulus to thrombus formation (Goldsmith, 1972). Arterial thrombosis can give rise, depending on the location of the affected vessel, to strokes, gangrene of a limb or the intestine and kidney disease. Myocardial infarction is sometimes the result of thrombosis of a coronary artery though not as commonly as might be supposed from the older name (coronary thrombosis) for this condition. In addition to that arising in the organ supplied by a thrombosed artery, damage can also be caused by fragments of the thrombus that break off from the main mass and, being swept into the blood stream, then become impacted in smaller vessels elsewhere causing a sudden arrest of function in the area they supply. A myocardial infarction can arise in this way and other organs with a rich blood supply derived from a number of small arteries (kidney, lung and brain) are particularly vulnerable to the effects of this kind of embolism.

The extent to which platelet aggregation is an important factor in the development of venous thrombosis is a matter of some controversy.

Aggregation begins when the platelets come into contact with collagen exposed in damaged tissues (or with atheromatous plaques or other foreign surfaces) and it causes the release of a number of substances in addition to the specific coagulation factors. These substances include 5-hydroxytryptamine (serotonin), noradrenaline, adenosine diphosphate (ADP), the prostaglandin endoperoxides, prostaglandins (E_2 and $F_{2\alpha}$) and thromboxane A_2. The first wave of aggregation is followed by a second that is initiated by ADP and sustained and augmented by serotonin, noradrenaline and thrombin. More important than any of these substances, however, are the prostaglandins and compounds related to them.

It has been known for some time that prostaglandin E_2 (but not prostaglandin E_1) will promote the aggregation of platelets under *in vitro* pharmacological conditions as can its precursors such as phospholipase A_2 and arachidonic acid. That a similar aggregation mechanism operates *in vivo* is strongly suggested by the fact that ADP, serotonin, noradrenaline and thrombin all promote prostaglandin synthesis. Even more convincing, perhaps, is the discovery of a human subject with a cyclooxygenase deficiency and the observation that his platelets did not suffer aggregation when they were exposed to arachidonic acid but did so in response to the prostaglandin endoperoxides (Malmsten *et al.*, 1975). None of these observations, however, is inconsistent with the idea that the physiological aggregating factor might be some prostaglandin compound other than E_2. An obvious claimant for the role is thromboxane A_2 in view of the fact that the platelets are the richest source of this material. Careful comparisons between the kinetics of the natural thrombotic process and that induced by thromboxane A_2 or prostaglandin E_2 support thromboxane's claim (Samuelsson, 1977) as does the observation that imidazole, which selectively inhibits thromboxane synthetase (p. 369) inhibits platelet aggregation (Puig-Parellada and Planas, 1977). The last mentioned finding has not, however, been confirmed by all those who have attempted the exercise and it seems likely that other substances (prostaglandins D_2 and E_2 and the prostaglandin endoperoxides themselves) may supplement the action of thromboxane A_2.

Although prostaglandin E_2 promotes platelet aggregation in *in vitro* experiments, prostaglandin E_1 has the opposite effect, concentrations as low as 10 ng per ml being sufficient to prevent aggregation in a platelet suspension exposed to ADP. However, of the substances that are involved in the control of thrombotic processes in the living animal, the most potent inhibitor of aggregation is prostacyclin which is produced in quantity by the arterial walls. Thus the ability of our platelets to synthesize proaggregation factors in response to tissue damage and of our vessels to produce prostacyclin and so to maintain the fluidity of the blood when there is no damage maintains a finely balanced system that should maintain our vascular health. But when we succumb to atherosclerosis or to any of the conditions already mentioned as being associated with the production of thrombotic diseases this balance is upset. Thus in atherosclerosis the production of prostacyclin is inhibited by components of the plaques. It is in these conditions that therapeutic benefit might accrue from an inhibition of cyclooxygenase that would prevent the synthesis of the proaggregation components of the prostaglandin system and so go at least some way to restoring the balance between the factors that promote and those that prevent aggregation and thrombosis. Considerable interest has been aroused in recent years by the suggestion that men at least might be able, by taking daily doses of aspirin, to prevent, or delay the onset of, the thrombotic catastrophes that lie in wait for so many of us. The early results of trials designed to test this proposition have been promising (Dale *et al.*, 1977; Yatsu, 1977). Sulphinpyrazone, a drug employed in the treatment of gout (p. 458) also inhibits prostaglandin synthesis and a recent report indicates that its regular use by individuals who have suffered a myocardial infarct reduces the likelihood of reinfarction.

An alternative way of preventing thrombotic accidents might be to encourage the production of prostaglandin E_1 by increasing the dietary intake of linoleic or of dihomo-γ-linolenic acid. Recent work by Sim and McCraw (1977), among others, indicates that this approach might indeed prove therapeutically fruitful.

A large number of drugs influence platelet activity, many of them by affecting prostaglandin synthesis (Mustard and Packham, 1975) and this action must be included among their side effects.

Inflammatory and allergic reactions

Inflammation is the most basic of pathological changes representing, as it does, the body's primary defensive response to physical or microbial attack. As such it is discussed in more detail in those sections of this book that discuss the drugs that counter its more damaging effects. For the purposes of the present discussion it need only be said that the cardinal signs of an acute inflammatory change are pain, redness (erythema), local heat and oedema and that these signs imply that damaged tissues release vasoactive substances with algogenic (pain producing) activity. However, inflamed tissue also carries large numbers of leucocytes and we might postulate that the ability to attract polymorphonuclear leucocytes into an area of tissue damage is another quality invested in the mediators of inflammation.

A vast range of substances have been developed over the years as antiinflammatory drugs but they can be conveniently segregated into two categories, the steroidal and the nonsteroidal antiinflammatory agents respectively. The discovery by Vane and his colleagues that aspirin (and many other members of the last named group of drugs) inhibited the synthesis of prostaglandins led to the inescapable conclusion that inflammatory changes are dependent to at least a major extent on prostaglandin release. There is now overwhelming evidence that this is indeed so, although uncertainty still exists concerning the precise part played by the individual prostaglandins (and other substances) that occur in inflamed tissues.

The release of prostaglandins into the inflamed or damaged skin of human subjects, into the synovial fluid of patients with rheumatoid arthritis and at other sites of inflammation has been repeatedly demonstrated. Other substances, particularly histamine and bradykinin, are liberated too and we must attempt now to determine the extent to which each of the prostaglandins and other substances contribute to the overall inflammatory reaction.

Pain

It has been known for some time that bradykinin is a pain producing substance in both man and animals and the observation that aspirin and similar analgesic agents prevented this algogenic effect seemed to establish the kinin's role as the body's major endogenous pain producer. However, this simple view had to be modified in the light of the later discovery that the aspirin-like analgesics inhibit the synthesis of prostaglandins without preventing the appearance of bradykinin. Prostaglandins themselves can cause pain and although they are not particularly effective in this respect they do, it is now known, enjoy an important synergistic relationship with bradykinin. Bradykinin stimulates the synthesis and release of prostaglandins which, in their turn, sensitize the pain nerve endings to the kinin. Inhibition of prostaglandin synthesis severs this regulatory loop so that pain is attenuated or abolished.

Histamine (which is a mediator of itch as well as of pain) is also more effective in the presence of prostaglandins (Ferreira, 1972) and prostaglandins can stimulate histamine release.

The prostaglandins most likely to be involved in pain production in inflamed tissues are prostaglandin E_2, prostacyclin and perhaps thromboxane A_2.

Erythema

Erythema and the local heat associated with it are caused by dilatation of the smaller arterioles and venules, brought about by relaxation of the smooth muscle in their walls. Even in nanogram quantities, the E prostaglandins produce a long lasting vasodilatation. Prostaglandin $F_{2\alpha}$ has a similar effect though microgram quantities are needed. The evidence indicates that of all the substances liberated in the inflammatory response, prostaglandins E and F contribute most to the erythema.

Oedema

Inflammatory oedema is the result of an increased permeability of the small vessels. It is sometimes stated or implied that this is purely a sequel to vasodilatation but this is not so. The production of oedema seems to depend primarily on an active contraction of the endothelial cells in the smallest venules so that the intercellular spaces are opened up. Erythema on the other hand is dependent on relaxation of vascular smooth muscle. Moreover, while oedema formation occurs largely as a sequel to events in the immediately postcapillary venules, both arteriolar and venular dilatation contribute to the erythema. Thus it is not to be expected that the two conditions will be provoked by identical combinations of mediators.

Like pain, oedema is probably caused by a number of mediators, the most important of which include histamine, the plasma kinins and, possibly, serotonin. The effect of these primary mediators is certainly potentiated by prostaglandins particularly prostacyclin and prostaglandins E but this synergism is evidently not as important as that which takes place at nociceptive nerve terminals for inhibition of prostaglandin synthesis obtunds the pain of inflammation more effectively than it clears the oedema.

That the prostaglandins play a more prominent role in the initiation of vasodilatation than they do in the production of oedema is indicated by the observation that indomethacin prevents inflammatory vasodilatation but not the formation of oedema in the rabbit skin preparation (Williams and Peck, 1977). This experiment also underlines the independence of oedema formation from vasodilatation.

Other changes in inflammation

The migration of leucocytes into the injured area is a prominent feature of the inflammatory response. It is the result of a chemotactic influence exerted by some of the substances that appear at the inflammatory site. Prominent among these is prostaglandin E_1 but thromboxane B_2 (a substance that is usually assumed to be little more than a breakdown product of the more illustrious thromboxane A_2) has some chemotactic activity. Much more powerful in this respect is HETE. It is interesting to see that a biological role may have been found for the one product of arachidonic acid metabolism whose formation is not obstructed by the nonsteroidal antiinflammatory agents.

As well as being attracted there by prostaglandins, the white cells at sites of inflammation can themselves, like platelets, synthesize prostaglandins and thromboxanes.

A number of observations introduce a complication into the possibly oversimplified view that prostaglandins and related compounds operate exclusively as mediators of inflammation. Polymorphonuclear leucocytes assembled at inflammatory sites liberate lysosomal enzymes that play their part in initiating inflammatory responses. The release of these enzymes is inhibited by cyclic AMP and hence by substances, including prostaglandin E_1, that promote the formation of the nucleotide (Weissmann, Goldstein and Hoffstein, 1976). This antiinflammatory action of prostaglandin E_1 can be demonstrated in experimental animals. Prostaglandin $F_{2\alpha}$ stimulates the accumulation of cyclic GMP and this *promotes* the release of lysosomal contents.

The division of antiinflammatory agents into steroidal and nonsteroidal groups suggested (as indeed was once thought to be so) that the two categories of drugs exert their therapeutic action by way of two essentially different mechanisms but it is now known that the corticosteroids prevent the release, if not the synthesis, of prostaglandins in inflamed tissues (Lewis and Piper, 1975).

The special case of inflammation in the eye is the concern of the next section of this chapter.

ALLERGIC PHENOMENA

Allergic phenomena are discussed in detail in Chapter 24 (p. 393) where it is pointed out that there are close analogies between acute inflammation and some forms of atopic disease. These parallels extend to the mediators of these conditions and the position of the prostaglandins in this respect is discussed in Chapter 24. The special case of asthma is additionally considered later in this chapter (p. 381).

Another aspect of the immune response is the participation of lymphocytes and there is some evidence (which at this date can only be categorized as 'suggestive') that prostaglandins (particularly the E_1 species) are involved in the maturation and perhaps the functioning of T lymphocytes. The topic is reviewed by Pelus and Strausser (1977) and by Horrobin (1978).

The eye

We have already noted that Ambache's original interest in the material he called irin arose from a desire to explain the origin of the inflammatory changes produced in the eye by mechanical trauma.

Irin is a mixture of prostaglandins E_2 and $F_{2\alpha}$ (Ambache and Brummer, 1968; Cole and Unger, 1973) and the mammalian iris can synthesize prostaglandins *in vitro*. Other ocular structures, the conjunctivae apart, are largely devoid of this ability. The small amounts of irin liberated from the irides of normal eyes are probably removed by active transport mechanisms across the ciliary processes (the anatomical structures mentioned in this section are displayed in the diagram on p. 225) but mechanical trauma leads to the liberation of larger amounts of irin and its accumulation in the aqueous humour (Ambache, Kavanagh and Whiting, 1965). The increased liberation of prostaglandins reflects increased synthesis.

The observable responses of the eye to trauma vary a little from one animal species to another but pupillary constriction, vasodilatation and an increased permeability of the blood-aqueous humour barrier are among the more important and constant responses. They underlie ocular inflammatory changes but they may also have dangerous sequelae such as a seriously elevated intraocular pressure and retinal detachment. Prostaglandins, injected into the anterior chamber of the eye can reproduce all these effects in at least some species of experimental animal.

Mechanical or chemical injury to one eye sometimes induces inflammatory changes in the other eye (the consensual reaction) as well as in the one that was directly injured. A consensual response to injury or to the intraocular injection of prostaglandins has been produced in experimental animals (Ambache, Kavanagh and Whiting, 1965; Beitch and Eakins, 1969). The response, which may be of reflex origin is itself mediated by irin release. There is thus a considerable body of evidence that links irin release with inflammatory changes in the eye and the possibility of using suitable inhibitors of prostaglandin synthesis to treat these often intractable ophthalmic conditions is now being actively explored. On the other face of the coin there is the theoretical danger that inflammatory conditions in the eye might arise iatrogenically in patients receiving intravenous infusions of a prostaglandin for the induction of abortion or labour. This danger may, however, be more apparent than real in view of the rapidity with which the prostaglandins are inactivated in the body.

Like some other organs, the eye is generally more sensitive to the E than to the F prostaglandins. The activity of prostaglandin $F_{2\alpha}$ approaches that of the E series but prostaglandin $F_{1\alpha}$ is without effect.

It should be noted that, although prostaglandins certainly seem to mediate the inflammatory responses to mechanical trauma in the eye they are not involved in the reaction to at least some forms of chemical insult. The reader should also remember that, while the increased intraocular pressure in the traumatized eye is the result of an accelerated secretion of aqueous humour, nontraumatic glaucoma (p. 225) is the consequence of a restricted drainage of the fluid. Prostaglandins do not influence this process.

In addition to their role as mediators of ocular inflammation, iridal prostaglandins possibly have a physiological function. There is experimental evidence for the view that they maintain the tone of the *sphincter pupillae*.

The cardiovascular system
The ability to bring about a fall in blood pressure was one of the identifying actions of the 'prostaglandin' originally described by von Euler and it is now evident that the prostaglandins as a group have a variety of actions on the cardiovascular system. These actions have attracted the attention of a large number of investigators and it is perhaps inevitable at this early stage in the history of the prostaglandins that the multiplicity of studies has sometimes led to more obfuscation than illumination. The following paragraphs attempt to fit together the more well authenticated reports into an intelligible whole. The reader who needs more detailed information is referred to recent reviews such as that by Malik and McGiff (1976).

Prostaglandins E and I_2
Prostaglandins E are uniformly depressor in man and laboratory animals, the E_1 variety being effective in doses as low as 0.1 μg per kilogram in some species (cf. bradykinin, p. 359). They dilate the arterioles in a number of vascular beds, particularly those that contribute most to the peripheral resistance. In some situations they also bring about constriction of the portal vein so that the return of blood to the heart is reduced. The consequent fall in cardiac output contributes to the overall hypotensive effect. When the portal vein is not constricted the venous return is sometimes accelerated by reason of the reduced arteriolar resistance. In these circumstances, the cardiac output increases but this change is not sufficient to offset more than minimally the hypotension initiated by the arteriolar dilatation. A similar remark applies to the increased cardiac output that sometimes occurs as a result of the prostaglandins' ability to increase myocardial contractility (see below).

The vasodilatation produced by the E prostaglandins is attributable to a direct effect on the blood vessels. It is unaffected by agents that block autonomic ganglia and by those that modify the actions of acetylcholine, noradrenaline, histamine or 5-hydroxytryptamine. The possibility of employing prostaglandins E in the treatment of peripheral vascular disease is being explored but investigations are restricted by the lack of adequate supplies of the prostaglandins.

Prostaglandins E have a direct action on cardiac muscle, increasing thereby both its rate and its power of contraction. These effects may be mediated by activation of adenyl cyclase.

In addition to their direct actions on the heart and blood vessels, prostaglandins E interact with activity in noradrenergic neurones and indirectly influence vascular responses in a way which suggests that they may be important modulators of sympathetic nervous activity. This point is taken up later.

Although they are generally vasodilator in their actions, prostaglandins E bring about vasoconstriction in certain restricted regions. A very good example of this is provided by the mucous membrane of the nose.

So far as their direct actions on the cardiovascular system are concerned, prostaglandins E_1 and E_2 are approximately equipotent and much more active than E_3.

The heart synthesizes prostaglandins, chiefly prostacyclin. Like the E type prostaglandins, prostacyclin is a vasodilator substance. It is particularly effective in the coronary circulation and it seems likely that the heart's endogenous prostacyclin serves to maintain coronary flow in the face of factors (including other prostaglandins and thromboxane A_2) that tend to cause constriction of the coronary vessels.

Prostaglandins F
The cardiovascular actions of prostaglandins F are, to some degree, species dependent. They lower the blood pressure of cats and rabbits but they are pressor in the rat, dog, monkey and man. The depressor action, like that of prostaglandins E, is attributable primarily to a direct dilatation of the resistance vessels. Supplementary contributions to the overall hypotensive effect may be provided by pulmonary vasoconstriction and an increased vagal tone but the importance of these mechanisms is species dependent.

Two mechanisms subscribe to the pressor response to prostaglandins F: stimulation of the myocardium and constriction of peripheral veins. Venous constriction accelerates the return of blood to the heart and induces thereby an increase in cardiac output. Central activation of the sympathetic nervous system is a possible minor factor in the hypertensive response. The careful reader will, no doubt, have noted the niceties of physiological argument—prostaglandins E bring about constriction of the portal vein and this adds to their hypotensive action while prostaglandins F cause constriction of veins elsewhere and this contributes to their hypertensive action.

The venoconstrictor action of prostaglandin $F_{2\alpha}$ has more than cardiovascular implications. As we have already noted (p. 373) it might be the cause of prostaglandin luteolysis.

Prostaglandins E and F are rapidly metabolized in the lungs, liver and elsewhere. Nevertheless, when it is infused in quite low doses, prostaglandin E_1 produces a clear fall in blood pressure with tachycardia and associated symptoms such as a throbbing headache. These changes persist for 15 min or longer after the infusion has been stopped and it may be that other and more stable vasodilator substances are liberated in the course of the infusion (5-hydroxytryptamine could be one such additional substance) and that they add their own effect to that of the prostaglandin itself.

Prostaglandins A

Like the members of the E series, from which they are derived, prostaglandins A_1 and A_2 produce sharp falls of blood pressure in man and experimental animals. These two prostaglandins (which are approximately equipotent) are more active than those of the E series. The threshold hypotensive doses of prostaglandin A_2 by intravenous injection in cat and man are of the order of 10 ng and $50 \mu g$ respectively (Horton and Jones, 1969; Lee, et al 1965). The hypotensive response is accompanied by tachycardia and an increased cardiac stroke volume. This would seem to be a reflex response to the hypotension when it is evoked by prostaglandin A_2 (it is, for instance, completely blocked if sympathetic activity is prevented by propranolol from exerting its cardiac actions) but the A_1 compound has, in addition, a direct stimulant action on the myocardium.

The hypotensive response to injections or infusions of prostaglandins A stems largely from a direct vasodilatatory action but there is a delay of some seconds before the fall of blood pressure is complete and it may be that these prostaglandins operate at least partly by liberating vasodilator substances. Alternatively, they may be converted into prostaglandins C (which are vasoactive) by prostaglandin A isomerase.

Infusions of prostaglandins A induce diuresis and increased sodium excretion and this may have implications for renal physiology as is discussed later (p. 382).

Although prostaglandins A have more potent cardiovascular actions than their parent prostaglandins E, the converse statement applies to their activity on most other systems.

Prostaglandins and hypertension

The hypotensive effect of the prostaglandins prompts the question as to whether they or their analogues may have a future as antihypertensive drugs and whether deficient prostaglandin production may be a factor in the development of hypertension in man. The second of these two questions is particularly challenging in view of both the direct hypotensive effects of the prostaglandins and their apparently close relationships with the renin-angiotensin system (p. 358). Recent work in laboratory animals has shown that the continued ingestion of indomethacin and other antiinflammatory agents that inhibit prostaglandin synthesis is accompanied by a progressive increase in the animals' blood pressure.

Prostaglandins and migraine

Migraine attacks (p. 418) are associated with dilatation of the extracranial blood vessels. The importance of this vasodilatation as an immediate causal factor, at least for the intense headache of migraine, is testified to by the fact that ergotamine, a powerful vasoconstrictor agent, often alleviates the headache. Ergotamine has enjoyed many years of popularity on this account but it is by no means a perfect drug. Its incautious use can lead to gangrene in the limbs (itself a consequence of the vasoconstrictor action that underlies its therapeutic effect), epileptiform seizures occasionally attend its use, tolerance to its therapeutic effects may develop after some years and the occurrence of unpleasant side effects (particularly nausea) may make it less than completely acceptable to the patient. A number of other drugs are available for those who do not respond favourably to ergotamine but recent studies indicate that attention should be redirected to the aspirin like analgesic drugs. There is evidence that the characteristic extracranial vasodilatation is caused by prostaglandins E and it seems likely that the other stigmata of migraine—including even the prodromal cerebral vasoconstriction—may also be attributable to prostaglandin release (Sandler, 1972; Horrobin, 1978). Although aspirin is effective in some patients it has not hitherto been highly regarded as an antimigraine drug. The fenamic acids (p. 446), on the other hand, are gaining a favourable reputation and a very recent report indicates that tolfenamic acid, the newest of them all, is as effective as ergotamine (Hakkarainen et al., 1979). The fenamic acids antagonize the actions as well as the synthesis of prostaglandins and this may account for their apparent superiority over aspirin at modest dose levels.

Some of the other drugs favoured by migraine patients may owe their effectiveness to an interference with prostaglandin activity. Thus methysergide (p. 334), a serotonin antagonist, may prevent the synthesis of prostaglandins in response to serotonin.

Prostaglandins and the ductus arteriosus

In the foetus the lungs are not in use and much of the blood that enters the pulmonary artery from the right ventricle passes by way of the ductus arteriosus to the aorta. At birth, when the lungs take on their oxygenating function, the ductus normally closes but sometimes it remains partially or fully open. After birth the blood pressure in the systemic circuit is higher than that in the pulmonary system so that in cases of persistent ductus arteriosus some of the blood entering the aorta is passed back into the pulmonary artery and thus has to make a quite unnecessary repeat trip through the lungs in the company, of course, of blood that is making its first circuit round the pulmonary system. Thus the volume of blood returning for ejection

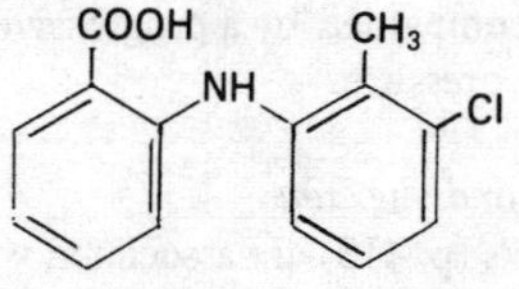

Fig. 23.9 Tolfenamic acid

by the left ventricle is increased. Although a persistent ductus arteriosus is not incompatible with life it is a potent cause of later heart failure by reason of the extra demands made on the resources of a heart that has, at every beat, to eject a larger volume of blood than it would have been called upon to do had the ductus closed. Hitherto the treatment of persistent ductus arteriosus has consisted of ligation of the vessel but some success has attended recent attempts to avoid surgery by giving a prostaglandin antagonist or a synthetase inhibitor. Chloroquine and indomethacin, respectively, have been the drugs favoured for this purpose (Heymann, Rudolph and Silverman, 1976; Collins et al., 1976). The rationale of the method is that the ductus arteriosus synthesizes prostacyclin and it is likely that it is this substance that maintains the patency of the vessel before birth and after birth in those neonates in whom closure does not occur. Neither indomethacin nor chloroquine is entirely above suspicion from the point of view of producing seriously toxic side effects but these early attempts to right a congenital defect by a method that does not involve surgical intervention are clearly encouraging. From a more theoretical standpoint, the fact that indomethacin brings about closure in one day provides convincing support for the view that the patency of the ductus arteriosus really does depend on the continued production of a prostaglandin.

There are occasions on which benefit could accrue from the retention of a patent ductus after birth. Congenital defects expressed as a narrowing or deformation of the pulmonary artery or of the adjacent region of the right ventricle may seriously impede blood flow through the lungs and in these circumstances a patent ductus arteriosus, by providing the blood with an alternative entry to the pulmonary circulation might relieve the circulatory embarrassment. There are several recent reports that infusions of prostaglandin E_2 in newborn children with serious oxygenation defects have resulted in re-opening of the almost closed ductus arteriosus with such an improvement in oxygenation that remedial surgery could be carried out. The doses used by Coceani and his colleagues (Coceani, Olley and Bodach, 1976) were of the order of 0.12 μg per kilogram and minute and infusions were continued for up to fifteen hours.

The respiratory system

The relationships between prostaglandins and the respiratory system are important and interesting from several points of view: the lungs synthesize and liberate a variety of prostaglandins (particularly in pulmonary anaphylactic states) and related substances, the prostaglandins influence both pulmonary blood flow and the tone of bronchial muscle and the lungs constitute a major site of prostaglandin catabolism.

Until recently it was known only that pulmonary tissue could synthesize prostaglandins E_2, $F_{2\alpha}$ and, perhaps, E_3. Lung parenchyma produces much more prostaglandin $F_{2\alpha}$ than the E_2 variety but in the bronchi the opposite state of affairs prevails. It is now known that pulmonary tissue can also synthesize prostacyclin, prostaglandin D_2 and thromboxane A_2. Indeed it seems possible that the three last named substances, particularly thromboxane A, may play a major regulatory role in the respiratory system.

Prostaglandins of the E series relax bronchial muscle in vitro and they also reverse the contraction provoked by acetylcholine, histamine, serotonin, bradykinin, barium and prostaglandins F. This effect has been demonstrated in bronchial tissue from every animal species so far studied, including man (Main, 1964; Sweatman and Collier, 1968). In intact animals, prostaglandins E induce bronchodilatation: in guinea pigs they exert a much more powerful effect than isoprenaline when both drugs are given by aerosol. In man, prostaglandin E_1 is as effective as isoprenaline or salbutamol (Cuthbert, 1969; Herxheimer and Roetscher, 1971).

Prostaglandin A also relaxes bronchial muscle. It is much less potent than the E prostaglandins but its action is more prolonged by reason of the fact that it is much more slowly metabolized.

What might prove to be an important aspect of the E prostaglandin's action on the lungs is the fact that when inhaled it produces irritation as well as bronchodilatation. Human subjects receiving prostaglandin E_1 in this way often cough and they may also complain of irritation of the throat and of pain and soreness in the chest.

In contrast to prostaglandins of the E series, prostaglandin $F_{2\alpha}$ induces contraction of bronchial muscle in vitro and bronchospasm in vivo. Evidence for this action in the human being comes from observations made in women receiving infusions of this prostaglandin for the induction of abortion. In one such study, impaired respiratory exchange attributable to bronchoconstriction was seen in five of a group of eight patients. Surprisingly, a similar response frequently occurs when prostaglandins of the E series are infused. A probable explanation of this apparently anomalous effect may be that a constrictor metabolite is produced from the prostaglandin during the infusion.

The other prostaglandins (particularly the endoperoxides) also cause bronchoconstriction, as does thromboxane A_2, perhaps the most powerful of them all.

Prostaglandin E_1 (and, presumably, E_2 too) promotes dilatation of capillaries in the lungs. Cardiac output is also stimulated, at least in some species, so that the pulmonary blood flow is augmented. F prostaglandins cause pulmonary vascular constriction with a consequent rise in pulmonary arterial pressure. Infusions of prostaglandins E are accompanied by a considerable degree of respiratory stimulation. Several factors probably underlie this response. They include a direct action on the respiratory centre, reflex responses and cortical stimulation resulting from the unpleasant sensations engendered by the infusion.

Up to 95 per cent of a dose of a prostaglandin E given by intravenous injection in animals is inactivated during its first passage through the lungs though the proportion in the human being is probably little more than 70 per cent. Prostaglandin $F_{2\alpha}$ is less readily metabolized in the pulmonary circuit and prostaglandins A are attacked to an even smaller extent. This rapid inactivation of prostaglandins should serve to re-emphasize two points—that the lungs are important metabolism sites (though this point is often forgotten) and that the prostaglandins in general operate as local regulators of activity in the tissues in which they are found rather than as blood-borne hormones.

The fact that so many of the naturally occurring prostaglandins have a bronchoconstrictor action suggests immediately that prostaglandin release might underlie the constrictor spasms of asthma, a possibility that is rendered the more likely by the finding that a range of prostaglandins is liberated in asthmatic attacks (p. 407). It is known too that many asthmatic subjects are extraordinarily sensitive to the bronchoconstrictor action of inhaled prostaglandin $F_{2\alpha}$ (Mathe et al., 1973).

The reader may well ask why aspirin and the other inhibitors of cyclooxygenase are not employed as antiasthma drugs if the prostaglandins, as we have asserted, are such important precipitants of asthmatic bronchospasm. He may find himself even more confused if he knows that, in a small minority of individuals, the taking of aspirin is itself followed by a severe bronchospasm.

There are several possible answers to this conundrum. In the first place it must be remembered that bronchospasm is only one of the elements in the asthma syndrome and even this one element is not entirely attributable to prostaglandin release. The force of the latter point is, it must be admitted, somewhat reduced by the fact that the action of some of the other mediators (histamine and the plasma kinins, for example) is dependent on the presence of prostaglandins just as it is in inflammatory responses (p. 376). Another answer to our problem, however, is that aspirin *is* occasionally effective in asthma patients, some of whom have by chance discovered this fact for themselves. Others have taken one of the European proprietary preparations that contain aspirin and have been sold over many years as asthma cures. It is also known that aspirin antagonizes the bronchoconstrictor response to inhaled prostaglandin $F_{2\alpha}$ in some asthmatic patients (Orchek et al., 1977). Having said all this we are still left, of course, with the subjects who suffer asthmatic attacks when they take aspirin and it is tempting to resolve our difficulties by resorting to the speculation that the calibre of our bronchi is normally regulated by both bronchodilator and bronchoconstrictor prostaglandins the relative amounts of which presumably fluctuate in response to varying physiological demands. We can imagine that in individuals in whom, for one reason or another, the bronchodilator prostaglandins (those of the E group) exert a dominant influence, inhibition of prostaglandin synthesis will result in brochospasm whereas in those in whom the bronchoconstrictor prostaglandins exert the major control, bronchodilatation will be produced by inhibition of synthesis. In the majority of us on the majority of occasions the effects of the constrictor and the dilator prostaglandins are presumably properly balanced so that removal of their influence will have no obviously adverse effect.

It should be noted that we could proffer other equally valid explanations of the finding that asthmatic attacks sometimes follow the ingestion of aspirin: the drug might, for instance, be capable of acting, in concert with a plasma protein, as an antigen and so of bringing about an allergic reaction. It should also be added that we have not taken into account possible differences in the doses of aspirin required to effect the two opposite reactions. To ignore quantitative factors of this kind is always a dangerous procedure. It is doubly so where prostaglandins are involved.

Whether or not the speculation we have indulged in will be shown to have a basis in fact, it will probably still be necessary to conclude that the physiological significance of the pulmonary prostaglandins is as local regulators of bronchial diameter or of lung blood flow or both.

From the therapeutic point of view we have to consider the possibility that therapeutically effective bronchodilator drugs might be developed from analogues of prostaglandin E_2 free of the irritant effects displayed by the prostaglandin itself.

The gastrointestinal tract

Given intravenously, prostaglandins E_1 and E_2 and, more particularly, the methyl analogues of prostaglandin E_2 all inhibit the gastric secretion evoked by food, histamine, pentagastrin and 2-deoxyglucose. This effect has been demonstrated in dogs, rats and man. Prostaglandin A_1 behaves in a similar fashion but F prostaglandins are ineffective.

The incidence of gastric ulceration in rats subjected to pyloric ligation is reduced if the animals are also given subcutaneous injections of prostaglandin E_1 (Robert, Nezamis and Phillips, 1968).

There has been some difference of opinion concerning the mechanism by which prostaglandins inhibit gastric secretory activity. Some authorities have maintained that the prostaglandins simply reduce the blood flow through the stomach but it seems more likely that we must invoke (as so often) inhibition of adenylate cyclase activity as the responsible mechanism. It is certainly true that histamine exerts its secretory effect by activation of the enzyme.

There is no evidence that prostaglandins act as physiological regulators of gastric secretory activity (although there is no *a priori* reason why they should not be able to exert a negative feedback control as they do in some other systems) but the possibility of their having therapeutic uses has to be considered. The prostaglandins do not inhibit secretory activity when they are taken by mouth but methylated derivatives (methyl- and dimethyl prostaglandins E_2) are active by the oral route and they are much more potent than the parent compound. Cimetidine and the other histamine H_2 antagonists (p. 353) also prevent the secretion of gastric acid but their action does not duplicate that of the prostaglandins. Thus only the histamine antagonists prevent the secretion of pepsin as well as acid and only the prostaglandins prevent damage to the gastric mucosa independently of their action on acid secretion. It is possible therefore that peptic ulcers might yield more completely or more rapidly to combined treatment with a prostaglandin analogue and cimetidine than they do to the latter drug alone.

Prostaglandins E cause contraction of the longitudinal muscles of the gastrointestinal tract (as von Euler demonstrated so long ago) and relaxation of the circular muscle. Prostaglandins F have a more uniformly stimulant action on the intestine (as they have in several other parts of the body) bringing about contraction of both the longitudinal and the circular muscle fibres. The contractions of the longitudinal muscle are partly blocked by atropine indicating that the prostaglandins stimulate cholinergic terminals in the muscle. For the most part, however, the responses depend on the stimulation of specific receptors in the muscle itself.

Since they are released into the lumen of the gut when the latter is distended it is possible that the prostaglandins are involved in the physiological regulation of peristalsis. A similar role has been postulated, and for similar reasons, for 5-hydroxytryptamine (p. 330). Whether or not prostaglandins do initiate peristalsis there can be no doubt concerning their ability to produce diarrhoea. We have already seen that diarrhoea, severe enough to necessitate withdrawal of the drug, not infrequently complicates attempts to induce abortion or labour with the prostaglandins. Volunteers who took prostaglandins by mouth passed bulky and extremely watery faeces some two to four hours later (Misiewicz *et al.*, 1969). The faeces were so reminiscent of those produced in cholera that it has been suggested that the cholera enterotoxin might stimulate prostaglandin synthesis and that inhibitors of synthesis might be employed to control some forms of diarrhoea (Bennett, 1971, 1978). So yet another use for aspirin-like drugs—and nutmeg (p. 93)—might have been found! It should be added that the diarrhoea induced by the prostaglandins is not simply the consequence of hastened peristalsis. There is also a mass movement of water into the intestinal lumen.

The actions of the prostaglandins on the gastrointestinal tract that have been mentioned in the foregoing paragraphs may well be of a purely pharmacological nature and it is not yet possible to say whether the prostaglandins have any physiological function in the digestive system. The gut can certainly synthesize prostaglandins—prostaglandins D_2, E_2 and $F_{2\alpha}$, thromboxane B_2 and, particularly, 6-oxoprostaglandin $F_{1\alpha}$—have all been detected in homogenates of the gastointestinal tract. In the stomach, the ability to synthesize prostaglandins is, apparently, restricted to the mucosal tissue but in the rest of the intestine both the muscle and the mucous membrane sythesize prostaglandins. It is not unreasonable to assume that such activity presupposes a physiological function for at least some of the material that is synthesized.

We note elsewhere (p. 823) that sulphasalazine is employed in the treatment of ulcerative colitis and that its success has been attributed to the 5-aminosalicylic acid that it liberates on hydrolysis. 5-Aminosalicylic acid, like all salicylates, inhibits prostaglandin synthesis and the idea that this provides the key to the therapeutic action of sulphasalazine in ulcerative colitis has been considerably strengthened by the recent observation that in this condition prostaglandin synthesis by the intestinal mucosa proceeds at an unusually high rate (Harris and Swan, 1977).

The urinary system

The kidney is an active synthesizer of prostaglandins, particularly the E_2 and $F_{2\alpha}$ varieties. Until recently it was generally believed that the most abundant renal prostaglandin was prostaglandin A_2 and this substance was thought to be identical with *medullin*, the postulated natriuretic hormone (p. 625). This was an attractive hypothesis because prostaglandin A_2, unlike those of the E and F series, is not extensively broken down in the lungs. Released into the blood stream it would be able to survive there, as befits a hormone, even after passing through the lungs. Present doubts concerning the reality of prostaglandin A_2's existence other than as an extraction artefact demand a re-examination of the hormonal status of the renal prostaglandins and it may well transpire that they will prove to be essentially local hormones, operating only in the immediate vicinity of the area in which they are produced.

In the kidney, the medulla synthesizes prostaglandins much more vigorously than does the cortex while the papillary regions are more active still. The enzymes that promote the breakdown of the prostaglandins are, on the other hand, much more active in the cortex. Whether this represents a device to protect the cortex against the possibly unwelcome effects of prostaglandins generated elsewhere in the kidney is a question that must remain open until further evidence is forthcoming.

The most reasonable interpretation of the mass of often conflicting evidence that has accumulated since attention first fell upon the renal prostaglandins is, in this author's opinion at least, that these substances operate primarily as regulators of local blood flow in the kidney or as modulators of the action of other flow regulators. Prostaglandins E bring about dilatation of the renal vasculature as a result of their inhibiting the release of noradrenaline from the renal nerves. Inhibitors of prostaglandin synthesis prevent the increase in blood flow that otherwise would occur after the relief of renal compression or following the administration of a powerful diuretic agent such as furosemide. Moreover, substances such as angiotensin II, noradrenaline and vasopressin (all of which cause constriction of renal vessels) stimulate prostaglandin synthesis.

Although all the findings recorded in the foregoing paragraph imply that the overall effect of the kidney's prostaglandins is one of vasodilatation it remains a fact that prostaglandin $F_{2\alpha}$ causes vasoconstriction even though, like the E prostaglandins, it inhibits the release of the sympathetic transmitter. Its vasoconstrictor effect, we must conclude, is entirely attributable to an action on the vessel walls. The significance of the fact that the kidney synthesizes both an E and an F prostaglandin is not immediately obvious but it may be that, in certain regions of the kidney, conditions sometimes arise that demand and can effect local vasoconstriction while blood flow through the rest of the organ is augmented.

Prostaglandins stimulate the formation of renin and one or more of the prostaglandins elaborated by the kidney serves to mediate the renin response to other stimuli.

Among the renal actions of prostaglandins that are not related to modifications of blood flow are to be noted their ability to antagonize the increased permeability of the collecting tubules induced by vasopressin and to increase the activity of the bladder.

Obstruction of the ureter is a powerful stimulus to the production of prostaglandin G and thromboxane A_2 by the kidney (Morrison, Nishikawa and Needleman, 1977).

The nervous system

In the laboratory, prostaglandins can be shown to influence nervous activity in several ways and there seems to be little doubt that these actions for the most part reflect physiological functions.

The following paragraphs provide a brief review of prostaglandin actions on the nervous system in a way that focuses on those that seem, at the time of writing, to be the most indicative of their likely physiological functions.

THE AUTONOMIC NERVOUS SYSTEM

Holmes, Horton and Main (1963) found that the vasoconstrictor action of noradrenaline and of sympathetic nerve stimulation was reduced during intravenous injections or infusions of prostaglandin E_1. This effect, which has been repeatedly confirmed, is not simply a reflection of the prostaglandin's known ability to cause vasodilatation by a direct action on blood vessels because it can be easily demonstrated in preparations in which the prostaglandin is exerting its maximum vascular action. This first indication of an interaction between prostaglandins and noradrenaline was taken up by others, notably Hedqvist and his colleagues who have produced very persuasive experimental support for the notion that prostaglandins serve to regulate activity in at least the sympathetic division of the autonomic nervous system (Hedqvist, 1973, 1977).

That prostaglandins E do modify the vasconstrictor response to sympathetic stimulation partly by a direct action on the vessels themselves is evident from the fact that, as we have noticed, they antagonise the action of noradrenaline as well as that of sympathetic nerve stimulation. However, amounts of prostaglandin E_1 too small to have a direct effect on the vessels will still produce an obvious reduction in the vasoconstrictor response to nerve stimulation and this suggests that part of the inhibition recorded by Horton and his colleagues was the result of an interference with the liberation of noradrenaline. Recent studies have provided ample evidence that this is indeed so.

Prostaglandins E_1 and E_2 have been found to modify the result of sympathetic stimulation in almost every one of the large number of preparations that have so far been studied. Their actions on the effector organs themselves are variable: whether they antagonize, potentiate or leave unaffected the response to noradrenaline depends on the organ that is examined and on the species and the dose of the prostaglandin that is used. On the other hand, and with but a few exceptions, they depress the liberation of noradrenaline from stimulated nerve. This inhibition of transmitter release—which is easily demonstrated if tritium labelled noradrenaline has been previously incorporated into the nerve—occurs with very small amounts of prostaglandin. Thus, bath concentrations of prostaglandin E_2 as low as 0.01 μg per ml markedly reduce the response to transmural nerve stimulation in the isolated vas deferens of the guinea pig.

Stimulation of sympathetic nerves evokes the release of prostaglandins from the innervated tissues. This was first shown for the spleen (Davies, Horton and Withrington, 1968), it is known to occur in adipose tissue, the kidney, the heart, the vas deferens and the seminal vesicles and there is no reason to believe that it will prove to be other than an invariable accompaniment of sympathetic activity. Moreover, the amounts of prostaglandin that are liberated by a quite short burst of sympathetic stimulation are demonstrably sufficient to produce a sharp reduction in transmitter release. The physiological significance of this observation is further underlined by the fact that inhibitors of prostaglandin synthesis bring about substantial increases in the output of noradrenaline from sympathetic nerves. Phenoxybenzamine blocks the release of prostaglandins by its presynaptic action and it too promotes thereby the release of noradrenaline.

The experimental facts assembled in the foregoing paragraphs are best interpreted on the hypothesis that prostaglandins provide a feedback control on the release of the sympathetic transmitter. As Hedqvist visualizes it, the noradrenaline released by sympathetic nerve stimulation induces the synthesis and release of prostaglandin E_2 in a dose dependent manner. The liberated prostaglandin in its turn partially inhibits noradrenaline release by a mechanism that has not yet been established with certainty but which probably involves a reduction in the influx of calcium ions into the nerve terminal, an event that is an essential preliminary to noradrenaline release. Thus, the more active the sympathetic nerves the more their effect is inhibited by their own activity.

Other prostaglandins likely to be released by sympathetic nerves (prostaglandins G_2, H_2 and D_2) are also capable of inhibiting noradrenaline release but they are so much less effective in this respect than prostaglandin E_2 that it seems likely that their limited action is entirely attributable to their conversion to the more powerful prostaglandin (Hedqvist, 1976). It should be added that some authorities believe that the noradrenaline released by stimulated sympathetic nerves directly affects noradrenaline release. On this view, small amounts of transmitter act on presynaptic β receptors and increase transmitter release while larger amounts, operating on α receptors, inhibit release (Langer, 1977).

For many years past, pharmacologists have referred to modulators of transmission, usually in the context of processes within the central nervous system (p. 180). A modulator is a substance that modifies but does not itself initiate the transsynaptic transmission of nerve impulses. The influence of prostaglandins on peripheral noradrenergic transmission clearly falls into the category of modulation and we cannot exclude the possibility that noradrenergic neurones in the central nervous system are also subject to the modulating influence of the prostaglandins. It is interesting to note in this connection that noradrenaline stimulates prostaglandin synthesis in the brain.

Recent evidence suggests that prostaglandins can exert a negative feed back control over acetylcholine release by at least some parasympathetic nerves (Hedqvist, 1977; Wennmalm and Hedqvist, 1971). The heart and its nerves has been the most intensively studied system in this connection.

Prostaglandins and fever

The maintenance of body temperature in homoiothermic animals depends to a considerable extent on the activity of the two components of the autonomic nervous system regulated by the temperature controlling centres in the hypothalamus. The fact that prostaglandins can upset the balance between heat production and heat loss to the extent of inducing fever is perhaps most strongly hinted at by the actions of the nonsteroidal antiinflammatory agents. These drugs, whose actions are so strongly dependent on their ability to inhibit cyclooxygenase, are valuable antipyretic agents but they are incapable of depressing body temperature below its normal level. Strong corroborative evidence for the view that prostaglandins are involved in the genesis of fever is provided by the observation that both arachidonic acid and prostaglandins E induce fever when they are injected into the anterior hypothalamus but whereas the response to arachidonic acid is delayed and can be prevented by aspirin that caused by the prostaglandins is immediate and is not prevented by aspirin. Prostaglandin E_1 is the most powerful pyrexia producing substance yet to be discovered. The release of prostaglandins into the cerebrospinal fluid is increased, sometimes as much as tenfold, during pyrexia occurring in the course of a bacterial infection or following the intravenous administration of a pyrogen. Fevers have also been noted in women undergoing abortions induced by prostaglandins E_2 or $F_{2\alpha}$. In general, the E prostaglandins contribute much more to the development of pyrexia than do those of the F series.

Normal body temperature is apparently maintained by the balanced activity of opposing groups of neurones controlled by serotonin and noradrenaline respectively (p. 188) although other neurotransmitters might also be involved to variable degrees. It is not clear how prostaglandins can intervene in this system but there is some evidence that they act directly on the regions that respond to the monoamines and other evidence that cholinergic links might also form an integral component of the mechanism.

It may also be that some forms of pyrexia stem directly from disturbances of the temperature regulating centres that do not involve prostaglandin production.

THE CENTRAL NERVOUS SYSTEM

The brain synthesizes prostaglandins (particularly prostaglandins E_2 and $F_{2\alpha}$) which are released from the organ during normal cerebral activity. The neuropharmacological actions of the prostaglandins are thus of considerable interest.

The actions of prostaglandins on the central nervous system vary (as they do in other systems, of course) with the prostaglandin and the animal used, with the dose of prostaglandin and its route of administration and with the nature of the experimental preparation. Generally, however, prostaglandins of the E series depress central nervous activity. Among the array of responses that have been reported are profound sedation with loss of righting reflexes at higher dose levels, reduced exploratory activity, prolongation of barbiturate sleeping time and even, sur- prisingly enough, a degree of analgesia. Given in small doses into the cerebral ventricles of the cat, prostaglandins E cause catatonia—the animal remains in any posture in which it is placed but it does not lose consciousness and its righting reflex is preserved. These prostaglandins have a dual action on spinal reflexes: they potentiate some reflexes by an action at the level of the cord but they also act on the higher centres of the brain to inhibit the reflexes. Usually the latter effect annuls or overwhelms the former one. The prostaglandins bring about an increase in blood pressure if they are applied directly to the cardiovascular centres in the brain stem.

The direct action of prostaglandins E on individual neurones is usually excitatory although the neurones that are stimulated are often inhibitory in nature.

Prostaglandin $F_{2\alpha}$ is less active than the E prostaglan- dins. On intracerebroventricular injection in the cat it produces sedation without catatonia and the sedation following intravenous injection is usually less profound than that caused by prostaglandins E_1 and E_2. Prostaglan- din $F_{2\alpha}$ usually facilitates spinal reflexes.

The prostaglandin receptors in the central nervous system are specific in the sense that each prostaglandin seems to have its own population of receptors: tachyphyl- axis develops readily but cross tolerance among different prostaglandins is not seen.

Some of the central nervous sequelae of prostaglandin administration may be the result of the prostaglandin's triggering self-perpetuating changes because the effects evoked by very small doses may persist long after the prostaglandin itself must have disappeared from the brain.

The functional significance of the cerebral prostaglan- dins is still a matter of conjecture. The inevitable sugges- tion that they may act as mediators of synaptic transmission has been duly put forward but the evidence supporting this idea is slender in the extreme. The sugges- tion that they act as modulators of transmission has, as we have seen, much more to recommend it. An alternative suggestion is that they act as modifiers of the chemical environment in the nervous system and so modify the effects of other chemical or physical agents. Their effect on the response of pain receptors to the plasma kinins (p. 376) provides an example of this type of activity. But a complete delineation of their mode of interaction with fundamental processes in the nervous system must await the outcome of much more experimental work. In the meantime the reader is counselled to preserve an open mind on the subject.

The role of prostaglandins in the nervous system has been reviewed by Coceani and Pace-Asciak (1976), among others.

PROSTAGLANDINS AND NERVOUS DISEASE
The refractoriness of many nervous and mental diseases to

treatment of any kind has prompted many workers to devote their efforts to a search for aetiological factors, which seem so reluctant to declare themselves, in the hope that they might thereby be shown the way to the develop- ment of rational forms of therapy. The prostaglandins have not escaped investigation from this point of view and it has been seriously suggested that disturbances of their metab- olism may be a contributory, if not the sole, aetiological factor in the genesis of a wide range of apparently disparate conditions including, among others, the muscular dystro- phies, multiple sclerosis, myasthenia gravis, Parkinson's disease, Huntington's chorea, epilepsy, migraine and virtually the full spectrum of mental disorders including, especially, anxiety neurosis, depression and, of course, schizophrenia! The topic is reviewed by Horrobin (1978), a staunch advocate of the view that 'abnormalities in prostaglandin metabolism may underlie the majority of human diseases including infections, degenerative diseases and cancer' (loc.cit.). One is reminded of the enthusiasm that once attached to the hypothesis that a wide variety of diseases were referable to a breakdown of adrenocortically mediated adaptation processes.

The evidence so far adduced to support the prostaglan- din hypothesis of disease is almost entirely circumstantial and much of it can be interpreted on other grounds than the ones favoured by those who espouse the prostaglandin cause. Nevertheless it may well be that, in some conditions at least, the prostaglandin hypothesis might provide the best interpretation of the facts. The reader is recom- mended, once again, to keep an open mind.

The relationship between prostaglandins and schi- zophrenia is mentioned again later (p. 544).

Metabolic systems
Prostaglandins can influence a variety of metabolic sys- tems in ways that hint at the likelihood of their being physiological regulators of metabolic processes.

PROSTAGLANDINS AND LIPID METABOLISM
That the prostaglandins can intervene in lipid metabolism is a fact that was established very soon after they had been chemically identified.

Sympathetic stimulation, a number of hormones (corti- cotrophin, glucagon and thyrotrophin) and drugs like theophylline all accelerate the breakdown of neutral fat (lipolysis) and the consequent liberation of free fatty acids and glycerol from adipose tissue. Lipolysis is effected by lipase after the latter has been activated by cyclic AMP. Theophylline promotes lipolysis because it inhibits phosphodiesterase, the enzyme that breaks down cyclic AMP. The other substances mentioned induce the forma- tion of cyclic AMP from adenosine triphosphate (ATP) by activating adenylyl (adenylate) cyclase (p. 321).

Lipolysis can be conveniently studied in vitro and Bergström and his colleagues (Steinberg et al., 1963) using the rat epididymal pad preparation demonstrated that very low concentrations of prostaglandin E_1 (20–100 ngs per ml) inhibited the fat mobilizing action of theophylline and the lipolytic hormones without modifying that of cyclic AMP. It would appear that the prostaglandin had prevented the activation of adenylyl cyclase by the lipolytic hormones and had thus halted the production of cyclic AMP. The antagonism between prostaglandin E_1 and theophylline is explained simply by the fact that a substance that operates by inhibiting the destruction of another can have little effect if there is nothing to preserve. Other workers, measuring the amount of cyclic AMP in adipose tissue, showed that its concentration increased when noradrenaline was present and that this stimulant effect was prevented by prostaglandin E_1 (Butcher, Pike and Sutherland, 1967).

The position in the intact animal is a little more complicated. Prostaglandin E_1, given in small intravenous doses to anaesthetized dogs, actually *promoted* lipolysis but this effect was probably an indirect one attributable to a central stimulation of sympathetic centres by the prostaglandin or by one of its metabolites. Slightly larger doses of the prostaglandin had the expected antilipolytic acid. The lipolytic effect of small doses of prostaglandin E_1 has also been demonstrated in human beings but it is likely that larger doses, if they could be given, would have an antilipolytic action because the prostaglandin certainly inhibits lipolysis in preparations of human subcutaneous fat *in vitro* (Bergström and Carlson, 1965).

Prostaglandin E_2 is an even more potent antilipolytic agent than the E_1 variety. Members of the F and A series, on the other hand, exert virtually no influence on the breakdown of fats.

The likelihood that the results of the essentially pharmacological experiments discussed in the foregoing paragraphs reflect physiological events is increased by a number of observations. Adipose tissue can synthesize prostaglandins (largely the E_2 variety) and the synthesis can be promoted by stimulation of sympathetic nerves and by the lipolytic hormones. Thus the greater the lipolytic stimulus the greater the output of inhibitory material. It has been shown, in dogs, that the output of prostaglandins from adipose tissue during sympathetic stimulation is more than adequate to induce a significant inhibition of lipolysis. Moreover lipolysis is enhanced in animals placed on diets that lack linoleic acid.

It would seem that we are once again presented with an example of the prostaglandins' acting as mediators of a system of negative feed back control. A word of caution against too uncritical an acceptance of this view would not, however, be out of place since in the majority of tissues prostaglandins $\dot{E}$ promote rather than prevent the activation of adenylate cyclase.

Another aspect of prostaglandin action is that prostaglandins E apparently limit cholesterol synthesis.

Prostaglandins and obesity

Destruction of the satiety centre in the hypothalamus of rats is followed by incessant eating and an inevitable obesity. The fatty tissue in these obese animals contains prostaglandin-like material (Haessler and Crawford, 1966) in a higher concentration than in the fat from normal animals. Moreover, it is known that fatty tissue in some forms of experimental obesity is not very responsive to lipolytic agents. Taken together, these observations raise the interesting possibility that human obesity might sometimes be associated with the production of abnormally large amounts of prostaglandins and that prostaglandin antagonists might help in the management of those afflicted with this disfiguring and dangerous consequence of the affluent life. Perhaps the aspirin we are sometimes bidden to take to ward off our thrombosis would contribute even further to our cardiovascular health by helping us to keep down our weight!

PROSTAGLANDINS AND THE METABOLISM OF CARBOHYDRATE AND PROTEIN

We have seen that prostaglandin E_1 inhibits lipolysis. Insulin has a similar action and this similarity between the actions of the two substances extends to their both being able to stimulate the uptake of glucose. On the other hand, glucose inhibits the biosynthesis of the prostaglandins and this action is potentiated by insulin while, in their turn, prostaglandins inhibit the secretion of insulin. These actions (and several others not mentioned here) indicate that prostaglandins might be involved in the regulation of blood sugar concentration. The precise nature and significance of their intervention has not yet, however, been elucidated.

The synthesis of collagen (the principal component of fibrous connective tissue) is inhibited by prostaglandins, particularly prostaglandins E_2 and $F_{2\alpha}$, and it proceeds at an enhanced rate in animals that have received inhibitors of cyclooxygenase (Parnham *et al.*, 1977). It is well known that diphenylhydantoin (the antiepileptic drug, p. 523) stimulates the formation of collagen fibres and it is interesting that the drug has been found to be a prostaglandin antagonist. Collagen can stimulate the production of prostaglandins and this may prove to be a feed back link in a system that operates to restrain collagen synthesis.

The incorporation of sulphur into mucopolysaccharides appears to be stimulated by prostaglandins. Mucopolysaccharides are important components of joint structures (particularly the synovial fluid) and it has even been suggested that osteoarthritis, which is essentially a degenerative disease, may be associated with a prostaglandin deficiency unlike some other forms of arthritis such as the rheumatoid variety which, being essentially inflammatory in nature, are the result, partly at least, of prostaglandin action.

PROSTAGLANDINS, HORMONES AND THE CYCLIC NUCLEOTIDES

There can be no doubt that the prostaglandins can intervene, certainly at the pharmacological level and, as most of us believe, at the physiological level too, in a large number of the regulatory mechanisms that guarantee homeostasis in the healthy animal. These regulatory mechanisms are largely dependent, of course, on the activity of the endocrine and the autonomic nervous systems and the foregoing pages should have made abundantly clear the points in these systems that are susceptible to prostaglandin action.

Many hormonal regulatory mechanisms appear to operate by influencing the synthesis of cyclic AMP or cyclic GMP (chapter 19, p. 321). The requirement for homeostasis demands control by opposing but balanced factors and while we might be reluctant to accept the idea that the two major cyclic nucleotides invariably mediate mutually antagonistic actions in a 'Yin-Yang' system (p. 325) it is undeniable that they do sometimes appear in this capacity: for instance, many of the actions of the sympathetic nervous system are ultimately mediated by cyclic AMP while the opposite actions displayed by the parasympathetic nervous system often depend on the synthesis of cyclic GMP. But we have seen that the ubiquitous prostaglandins also have diametrically opposite effects in different systems and the nature of the relationship between the prostaglandins and the cyclic nucleotides raises fascinating questions.

Generally speaking, prostaglandins of the E series promote the synthesis of cyclic AMP by activating adenylyl (adenylate) cyclase though we encountered a major exception to this generalization only a page ago (p. 386) when we noted that prostaglandin E_1 inhibited the formation of cyclic AMP in adipose tissue. Rather less substantial evidence than that which relates to prostaglandin E_1 indicates that prostaglandin $F_{2\alpha}$ promotes the formation of cyclic GMP. It is also clear that the newer prostaglandins also have their effect on the formation of the nucleotides. It seems that the prostaglandin endoperoxides and thromboxane A_2 inhibit, while prostacyclin stimulates, the synthesis of cyclic AMP. The endoperoxides also stimulate the synthesis of cyclic GMP. It may be, indeed, that these last named substances, rather than prostaglandins E and F, may be the physiological regulators of nucleotide synthesis. It will be noted that a shift in synthesis from the lipoxygenase to the cyclooxygenase pathway could bring about a change in the relative amounts of the two cyclic nucleotides and hence in the direction of the regulatory actions they promote.

In view of the insight he should now have gained into prostaglandin mediated mechanisms, the reader should not be surprised to learn that, in their turn, the cyclic nucleotides influence the synthesis of prostaglandins.

Cancer

One of the most interesting developments in the prostaglandin field in recent years has related to the growth and spread of tumours. Tumour homogenates generate prostaglandins much more actively than homogenates of the corresponding tissue. This has been shown for many different types of tumour in several animal species, including man. Particular attention has been directed towards neoplasms of the human breast. Not only do tumours synthesize prostaglandin-like material at a higher rate than normal mammary tissue but malignant growths are more effective than benign tumours (Bennett *et al.*, 1975, 1977). Malignant tumours of the breast often spread to bone and it seems that the extensive resorption of bone caused by these metastases is also attributable, to some extent at least, to the action of prostaglandins. Prostaglandin E_2, the prostaglandin endoperoxides G_2 and H_2 and 13,14-dihydroprostaglandin E_2 (a metabolite of prostaglandin E_2, p. 371) all stimulate osteoclastic activity (Raisz, Dietrich and Simmons, 1977). Another substance released by tumour cells was described by Dowsett and his colleagues (Dowsett *et al.*, 1976). It too may operate through activation of osteoclasts. It is not a prostaglandin but its activity may well be potentiated by prostaglandins. If this should prove to be so, an interesting parallel will have been established with prostaglandin's activity in the processes that cause inflammation (p. 376). The osteoclast activating factor (and perhaps parathyroid hormone too) may stimulate the synthesis of prostaglandins in the body metastases.

Other tumours that metastasize in bone also synthesize prostaglandins. These tumours occur particularly in the lungs, the kidney and the prostate gland. The reader may be relieved to learn that prostate tissue can synthesize prostaglandins so that the word is not so much of a misnomer after all.

Those tumours of the breast that synthesize prostaglandins most vigorously are the ones that are most likely to spread to bone.

The observations recorded in the foregoing paragraphs inevitably prompt the question whether inhibition of prostaglandin synthesis could prevent the growth and spread of primary tumours or minimise the damage done by secondary growths in bone or elsewhere. This question cannot yet be answered with any degree of confidence. There are some, indeed, who believe, not without some justification, that the increased ability of tumour tissue to synthesize prostaglandins represents an augmented defence reaction and that to prevent this synthesis would be to encourage tumour growth. Animal experiments designed to clarify the nature and extent of prostaglandin intervention in the several processes associated with the growth and spread of tumours have as yet yielded only equivocal results. Thus, while we emphasize nowadays the immune system's anticancer role (p. 395) there is no agreement concerning the influence of prostaglandins on this function, for while some investigators (Plescia, Grinwich and Plescia, 1976, for instance) have obtained what appears to be convincing evidence that prostaglandins suppress immune responses, others (Loose and Di Luzio, 1973, for instance) are equally clear that prostaglandins promote them. Again some of those who have studied the effect of prostaglandins and their antagonists on the growth of soft tissue tumours have concluded that prostaglandins inhibit tumour growth (Jacobson, 1974; Santoro, Pillpot and Jaffé, 1976, *inter al*) while others (Strausser and Humes, 1976, for instance) reach the opposite conclusion. Nevertheless, there is no evidence that human subjects who have received large doses of antiinflammatory drugs over long periods of time are more likely to develop tumours, or if they do develop them, to succumb more rapidly than those who have not been deprived of their prostaglandins. The balance of evidence certainly seems to justify the clinical trials that have recently been initiated to assess the possible value of aspirin as a therapeutic agent in breast cancer patients with bony metastases. Perhaps yet another step has been taken to establish the once humble aspirin as a panacea for (nearly) all our ills—a rare distinction for a drug that has never even received the accolade of popular respectability that comes from being a 'prescription only' drug!

Recent developments in our knowledge of prostaglandin participation in tumour growth has been succinctly reviewed by Bennett (1978), himself an original contributor to the subject.

Horrobin has recently put forward the suggestion that the primary event in tumour aetiology is an impaired synthesis of thromboxane A_2. This admittedly speculative hypothesis is supported by some highly circumstantial evidence. It is set out in detail in Horrobin's book (Horrobin, 1978) which can be recommended as a valuable source of reference for the student who is seriously interested in the prostaglandins but who also approaches his reading in a constructively critical frame of mind.

PROSTAGLANDIN ASSAY

The accurate identification and quantitative determination of prostaglandins in tissue fluids is fraught with difficulties and the quite remarkable advances in our knowledge of the nature, metabolism and function of the prostaglandins and thoromboxanes that have been achieved in the face of these difficulties is a tribute to the ingenuity, skill and resourcefulness of those who have contributed to these advances.

It need hardly be said that it is no part of this chapter's intention to provide practical instructions for the extraction and assay of prostaglandins nor even to direct the reader to sources (if, indeed, any exist) that supply these instructions in a sufficiently detailed form to enable him to perform these procedures for himself in a laboratory in which they have not hitherto been practised. The aim is, rather, to direct his attention to possible defects in the methodology—and hence in the quantitative results—of some of those whose publications he will consult. Reviews that discuss these methods in more detail than is possible here are provided *inter al.* by Horton (1976) and Salmon and Karim (1976) and in volume 1 of the work edited by Samuelsson and Paoletti (1976).

We have mentioned on more than one occasion that prostaglandins are not found in solid tissues in a preformed state but that tissue damage is a potent stimulus to the initiation of synthesis by the breached cell membrane. To speak of the prostaglandin content of a tissue is, consequently, meaningless and any prostaglandin-like material that exerts a physiological action presumably does so either from the interstitial fluid in which the cells are bathed or by way of the blood, cerebrospinal fluid or, of course, the seminal fluid, that major repository of prostaglandins. But even so simple a technique as taking a blood sample has to be carried out with the utmost care if the intention is to assay prostaglandins in the sample. This is necessary because platelet damage will set into motion synthetic processes that will produce a mixture and a concentration of substances in the blood quite different from those present when the needle was first inserted. In order to circumvent this difficulty it is usual nowadays only to use needles and syringes that have been rinsed with a solution containing indomethacin or another inhibitor of prostaglandin synthetase.

Another problem is related to the instability of many of the products of prostaglandin synthesis. Thromboxane A_2 and prostacyclin are particularly unstable (p. 368) and it is usual to assay them in terms of their more stable breakdown products, thromboxane B_2 and 6-ketoprostaglandin $F_{2\alpha}$ respectively. The products of the catabolism of prostaglandins E_2 and $F_{2\alpha}$ are sometimes also measured for the same reason. Of course, to assay individual prostaglandins and thromboxanes is not to answer the question as to whether they are active compounds in their own right or simply precursors or breakdown products of the compounds that really do the work. The A prostaglandins provide the best known examples of active compounds that are possibly nothing more than postmortem breakdown products of other substances (prostaglandins E in this instance) with no existence in the intact organism. There are some, indeed, who believe that even the E prostaglandins are less functionally important than their endoperoxide precursors.

The actual assay of the material that is eventually won also presents difficulties. In our present state of knowledge we cannot be sure that we know the precise nature of the prostaglandin-like substances present in a particular biological fluid or extract. Hitherto undetected prostaglandins or prostaglandin-like material might well be present in the extracts and if they influence the assay preparation in any way it will result in the return of spurious estimates of the prostaglandin content of the fluids under test. Finally, it is necessary to point to the relatively low sensitivity of many of the available methods of assay. It is clear that, under physiological conditions, prostaglandins will be present in body fluids in extremely small amounts. Concentrations of the order of 10^{-12}M have been quoted so that some attempt to concentrate the material under test has often to be made. This will inevitably involve physical or chemical manipulations and the attendant dangers of losing active material or of changing one prostaglandin into another.

Assays can be performed by biological or by chemical methods. Vane and his colleagues have made productive use of the technique of differential bioassay (p. 210) using a battery of three preparations, usually the rat stomach, the rat colon and the chicken rectum. The sensitivity of these preparations is enhanced by the use of the superfusion procedure (p. 148), the material to be assayed being allowed to drip, cascade-like, over each tissue in turn (Gilmore, Vane and Wyllie, 1968). The tissues respond to several of the other active substances likely to be present in biological fluids and an embarrassingly large number of antagonists (atropine, methysergide, phenoxybenzamine, propranolol and mepyramine) has often to be added to the fluid under test to annul the effects of these other substances. The antagonists may adversely influence the sensitivity of the chain of assay preparations. Moreover, it is by no means certain that none of them antagonizes or otherwise modifies the tissues' response to one or more of the prostaglandins. A further potential complication is presented by the fact that the test tissues can themselves synthesize and release prostaglandins in response to active substances in the superfusate to which they are exposed. These prostaglandins would, of course, be added to the fluid and be carried to the next tissue in the chain. To thwart the efforts of the enzyme in the test tissue, indomethacin has to be added to the other antagonists in the pharmacological cocktail that the superfusate has become. In spite of the problems presented by this bioassay method it has, in the hands of its originators, contributed substantially to our knowledge of the prostaglandins.

Many investigators would, understandably, prefer always to use chemical methods to assay biologically active substances and one of the most versatile of contemporary techniques for this purpose is radioimmunoassay. It has already been applied to the measurement of prostaglandins but is has not yet been developed to the stage of being suitable for the accurate assay of the components of a prostaglandin mixture of the kind found in biological fluids, in spite of assertions to the contrary by some workers in the field. The success or otherwise of the method depends on the production of specific antibodies for each of the likely components of the mixture to be assayed. There seems to be no doubt that this essential task will soon be achieved and that radioimmunoassay will then become an assay method of choice. Until then, quantitative results obtained by radioimmunoassay of prostaglandins in biological material must be regarded as suspect.

The present state of the art as applied to prostaglandin assay has been critically reviewed by Granstrom (1978), himself an exponent of the method.

Other methods of prostaglandin determination include gas chromatography with mass spectrometry or mass fragmentography. They have proved useful in investigations designed to study metabolic pathways affecting known prostaglandins and precursors in vitro and they have the potential to be developed into assay methods for prostaglandins in biological fluids. But even in laboratories where the necessary equipment is available, the technique has not yet been perfected to a stage that will permit it to be employed for routine use.

CONCLUSION

This chapter has recorded, and discussed the results of, a small number of the investigations conducted during the past twenty or so years that have led to the recognition of the prostaglandins and the thromboxanes and to some appreciation of their pharmacological actions and possible physiological significance. Brief though the selection is, it is hoped that it is a representative one and that the general themes and conclusions that emerge from a study of the foregoing pages would not have been substantially different if space had permitted a more exhaustive survey of the relevant experimental material.

Aside from their ubiquity in tissue extracts (if not in intact organs) the most striking property of the prostaglandins is surely their ability to modify, but not usually to initiate, regulatory reactions in a wide range of physiological systems. The prostaglandins are, indeed, modulators (p. 180) par excellence. This modulation is often achieved as a result of their forming an essential link in negative feedback systems. The fact that a number of different prostaglandins (and related substances) with differing biological actions can be produced in varying proportions by physiological and pathological stimuli, provides the conditions that will ensure the precise modulation effect demanded by the needs of the moment.

Inhibition of prostaglandin synthesis by the nonsteroid antiinflammatory agents has a number of actual or potential therapeutic consequences and an earlier reference (p. 388) to aspirin's being a panacea for all our ills was not made entirely with facetious intent. The fact that it has such a wide spectrum of therapeutic activity has important implications, the most important of which is that many apparently diverse diseases arise, at least partially, because of the malfunctioning of a single chemical control system and that their clinical diversity is simply a manifestation of the fact that disease processes exert, for reasons not necessarily connected with their final mode of action, a degree of selectivity in the tissues and hence in the physiological systems they attack. If we also recall that the virtual ubiquity of the prostaglandins is matched only by that of the cyclic nucleotides (with which, as we have seen, the prostaglandins are to some extent associated) we can begin to appreciate that the healthy functioning of the organism probably depends on the operation of only a small number of fundamental mechanisms such as those that maintain the functional integrity of the cell membrane or ensure the accurate replication of tissue proteins. The wonder is that, in spite of this biological conservatism, we have been able to develop a huge range of diverse and relatively selective drugs for the treatment of a multitude of clinical conditions. It is clear that much of this apparent selectivity is attributable to variations in the physiochemical properties of drugs (such as their stability, ease of penetration of membranes and of attachment to receptors and other proteins) and not to differences in their fundamental modes of action.

The prostaglandin system is only one of a number of fundamental biological mechanisms and it would be stupid in the extreme to suggest that our science will soon have to be called prostaglandinology. Nevertheless it is clear that in the next years much time will be devoted to the search for selective inhibitors of the several pathways involved in the synthesis of the different prostaglandins and thromboxanes and for new analogues and antagonists of these substances. In this author's opinion, it will be time well spent.

BIBLIOGRAPHY

Books, monographs and reviews

Bennett, A. (1974) Prostaglandin antagonists. *Adv. Drug Res.*, **8**, 83-118.

Bennett, A. (1978) Prostaglandins. In *Recent Advances in Clinical Pharmacology*, pp. 17-30. Turner, P.J., Shand, D.G. (eds) Edinburgh, London and New York: Churchill Livingstone.

Bindra, J.S. and Bindra, Ranjna (1977) *Prostaglandin Synthesis.* New York, San Francisco and London: Academic Press.

Coceani, F. and Pace-Asciak, C.R. (1976) Prostaglandins and the central nervous system. In *Prostaglandins: Physiological, Pharmacological and Pathological Aspects*, pp. 1-36. Karim, S.M.M. (ed) Lancaster: UTP.

Crabbé, P. (ed) (1977) *Prostaglandin Research.* New York, San Francisco and London: Academic Press.

Curtis-Prior, P.G. (1976) *Prostaglandins.* Amsterdam: North Holland

Cuthbert, M.F. (ed) (1973) *The Prostaglandins. Pharmacological and Therapeutic Advances.* London: Heinemann.

Granstrom, E (1978) Radioimmunoassay of prostaglandins. *Prostaglandins*, **15**, 3-17.

Hedqvišt, P. (1977) Basic mechanisms of prostaglandin action on autonomic neurotransmission. *Ann. Rev. Pharmac. Toxicol.*, **17**, 259-279.

Holmstedt, B. and Liljestrand, G, (1963) *Readings in Pharmacology.* Oxford and London: Pergamon Press.

Horrobin, D.F. (1978) *Prostaglandins: Physiology, Pharmacology and Clinical Significance*, Edinburgh: Churchill Livingstone.

Horton, E.W. (1972) *Prostaglandins.* London: Heinemann, and Berlin: Springer-Verlag.

Horton, E.W. (1976) The measurement of prostaglandins. In *The Role of Prostaglandins in Inflammation.* Lewis, G.P. (ed). Berne: Huber.

Kahn, R.H. and Lands, W.E.M. (eds) (1973) *Prostaglandins and Cyclic AMP.* New York and London: Academic Press.

Karim, S.M.M. (ed) (1975) *Prostaglandins and Reproduction.* Oxford and Lancaster: MTP.

Karim, S.M.M. (ed) (1976) *Prostaglandins: Chemical and Biochemical Aspects.* Lancaster: MTP.

Karim, S.M.M. (ed) (1976) *Prostaglandins: Physiological, Pharmacological and Pathological Aspects.* Lancaster: MTP.

Kharasch, N. and Fried, J. (eds) (1977) *Biochemical Aspects of Prostaglandins and Thromboxanes.* New York, San Francisco and London: Academic Press.

Langer, S.Z. (1977) Presynaptic receptors and their role in the regulation of transmitter release. *Br. J. Pharmac.*, **60**, 481-497.

Moncada, S. and Vane, J.R. (1979) Mode of action of aspirin-like drugs. In *Advances in Internal Medicine*, pp. 1-22. Stollerman, G.H. (ed). Chicago and London: Year Book Medical Publishers.

Nickander, R., McMahon, F.G. and Ridolfo, A.S. (1979) Nonsteroidal anti-inflammatory agents. *Ann. Rev. Pharmac. Toxicol.*, **19**, 469-490.

Salmon, J.A. and Karim, S.M.M. (1976) Methods for analysis of prostaglandins. In *Prostaglandins: Physiological, Pharmacological and Pathological Aspects.* pp. 25-86. Karim, S.M.M. (ed) Lancaster: MTP.

Samuelsson, B. (1978) Prostaglandins and thromboxanes. *Recent Prog. Horm. Res.*, **34**, 239-253.

Samuelsson, B. and Paoletti, R. (1976) *Advances in Prostaglandin and Thromboxane Research* Vols 1 and 2. New York: Raven Press.

Sanner, J.H. (1974) Substances that inhibit the actions of prostaglandins. *Archs. intern. Med.*, **133**, 133-146.

Schneider, W.P. (1972) The chemistry of the prostaglandins. In *The Prostaglandins* pp. 293-392. Karim, S.M.M. (ed) Lancaster: MTP.

Schneider, W.P. (1976) The chemistry of prostaglandins. In *Prostaglandins: Chemical and Biochemical Aspects.* pp. 1-23 Karim, S.M.M. (ed) Lancaster: MTP.

Weeks, J.R. (1972) Prostaglandins. *Ann. Rev. Pharmac.*, **12**, 317-336.

Weinshenker, N.M. and Andersen, N.H. (1973) Chemistry. In *The Prostaglandins*, vol. 1, pp. 5-82. Ramwell, P.W. (ed) New York: Plenum Press.

Original Papers

Ambache, N. (1957) Properties of irin, a physiological constituent of the rabbit iris. *J. Physiol.*, **135**, 114-132.

Ambache, N. and Brummer, Hilary C. (1968) A simple chemical procedure for distinguishing E from F prostaglandins with application to tissue extracts. *Br. J. Pharmac.*, **33**, 162-170.

Ambache, N., Kavanagh, L. and Whiting, Judith (1965) Effect of mechanical stimulation on rabbit's eyes: release of active substances in anterior chamber perfusates. *J. Physiol.*, **176**, 378-408.

Andersen, N.H. (1969). Preparative thin-layer and column chromatography of prostaglandins. *J. Lipid. Res.*, **10**, 316-319.

Andersen, G.G. (1973) Induction of labour with intravenous PGF$_{2\alpha}$: a review. *Prostaglandins*, **4**, 765-774.

Beitch, B.R. and Eakins, K.E. (1969) The effects of prostaglandins on the intraocular pressure of the rabbit. *Br. J. Pharmac.*, **37**, 158-167.

Bennett, A. (1971) Cholera and prostaglandins. *Nature, Lond.*, **231**, 536.

Bennett, A., Charlier, E.M., McDonald, A.M., Simpson, J.S., Stamford, E.F. and Zebro, T. (1977) Prostaglandins and breast cancer. *Lancet*, **(ii)**, 624-626.

Bennett, A., Gradidge, C.F. and Stamford, E.F. (1974) Prostaglandins, nutmeg and diarrhoea. *New Engl. J. Med.*, **290**, 110-111.

Bennett, A., McDonald, A.M., Simpson, J.S. and Stamford, I.F. (1975) Breast cancer, prostaglandins and metastases. *Lancet*, **(i)** 1218-1220.

Bergström, S. and Carlson, L.A. (1965) Inhibitory action of prostaglandin E$_1$ on the mobilization of free fatty acids and glycerol from human adipose tissue in vitro *Acta physiol. Scand.*, **63**, 195-196.

Bergström, S., Ryhage, R., Samuelsson, B. and Sjovall, J. (1962) The structure of prostaglandins E, F$_1$ and F$_2$. *Acta chem. Scand.*, **16**, 501-502.

Butcher, R.W., Pike, J.E. and Sutherland, E.W. (1967) The effect of prostaglandin E$_1$ on adenosine 3',5'-monophosphate levels in adipose tissue. In *Prostaglandins*, pp. 133-138 Bergström, S. and Samuelsson, B. (eds) Stockholm: Almqvist and Wilksell.

Bygdeman, M., Fredricsson, H., Svanberg, K. and Samuelsson, B. (1970) The relation between fertility and prostaglandin content of seminal fluid in man. *Fertility and Sterility*, **21**, 622-630.

Chaudhuri, G. (1971) Intrauterine device: possible role of prostaglandins. *Lancet*, **(i)**, 480.

Coceani, F., Olley, P.M. and Bodach, E. (1976) Prostaglandins: a possible regulator of muscle tone in the ductus arteriosus. In *Advances in Prostaglandin and Thromboxane Research*, **Vol. 1**, pp. 417-420. Samuelsson, B. and Paoletti, R. (eds) New York: Raven Press.

Cole, D.F. and Unger, W.G. (1973) Prostaglandins as mediators of the responses of the eye to trauma. *Exp. Eye Res.*, **17**, 357-368.

Collins, G., Outerbridge, E., Manku, M.S. and Horrobin, D.F. (1976) Chloroquine as prostaglandin antagonist in treatment of patent ductus arteriosus. *Lancet* **(ii)**, 810.

Cuthbert, M.F. (1969) Effect on airway resistance of prostaglandin E$_1$ given by aerosol to healthy and asthmatic volunteers. *Br. med. J.* **(iv)**, 723-726.

Dale, J., Myhre, E., Storstein, O., Stormorken, H. and Efskind, L. (1977) Prevention of arterial thrombo-embolism with acetylsalicylic acid. *Am. Heart J.*, **94**, 101-111.

Davies, B.N., Horton, E.W. and Withrington, P.G. (1968) The occurrence of prostaglandin E$_2$ in splenic venous blood of the dog following nerve stimulation. *Br. J. Pharmac.*, **32**, 127-135.

Dowsett, M., Easty G.C., Powles, T.J., Easty, D.M. and Neville, A.M. (1976) Human breast tumour-induced osteolysis and prostaglandins. *Prostaglandins*, **11**, 447-460.

Eik-Nes, K.B. (1969) Patterns of steroidogenesis in vertebrate gonads. *Gen. comp. Endocrin.* Supp. **2**, 87.

von Euler, U.S. (1963) On the specific vasodilating and plain muscle stimulating substances from accessory genital glands in man and certain animals (prostaglandin and vesiglandin) *J. Physiol.*, **88**, 213-234.

von Euler, U.S. (1967) Welcoming address. In *Prostaglandins. Proceedings of the Second Nobel Symposium.* pp. 17-20 Bergström, S. and Samuelsson, B. (eds) Stockholm: Almqvist and Wiksell.

Ferreira, S.H. (1972) Prostaglandins, aspirin-like drugs and analgesia. *Nature New Biol.*, **240**, 200-203.

Gilmore, N., Vane, J.R. and Wyllie, J.H. (1968) Prostaglandins released by the spleen. *Nature, Lond.*, **218**, 1135-1140.

Goldsmith, H.L. (1972) The flow of model particles and blood cells and its relation to thrombogenesis. In *Progress in Haemostasis and Thrombosis*, **1**, pp. 97-139 Spaet (ed) New York: Grune and Stratton.

Haessler, H.A. and Crawford, J.D. (1966) Lipolysis in homogenates of adipose tissue: an inhibitor found in fat from obese rats. *Science*, **154**, 909-910.

Hakkarainen, H., Vapaatalo, H., Gothoni, G. and Parantainen, J. (1979) Tolfenamic acid is as effective as ergotamine during migraine attacks. *Lancet* **(ii)**, 326-328.

Hamberg, M., Stevensson, J. and Samuelsson, B. (1975) Thromboxanes. A new group of biologically active compounds derived from prostaglandin endoperoxides. *Proc. natn. Acad. Sci. USA.* **72**, 2994-2998.

Harris, D.W. and Swan, C.H.J. (1977) Increased synthesis of prostaglandins in ulcerative colitis. *Lancet* **(ii)**, 196.

Hedqvist, P. (1973) Prostaglandin mediated control of sympathetic neuroeffector transmission. *Adv. Biosci.*, **9**, 461-473.

Hedqvist, P. (1976) Prostaglandin action on transmitter release at adrenergic neuroeffector junctions. In *Advances in Prostaglandin and Thromboxane Research*, **vol. 1**, pp. 357-363. Samuelsson, B. and Paoletti, R. (eds). New York: Raven Press.

Herxheimer, H. and Roetscher, I. (1971) Effects of prostaglandin E$_1$ on lung function in bronchial asthma. *Eur. J. clin. Pharmac.*, **3**. 123-125.

Heymann, M.A., Rudolph, A.M. and Silverman, N.H. (1976) Closure of the ductus arteriosus in premature infants by inhibition of prostaglandin synthesis. *New Eng. J. Med.*, **295**, 530-533.

Holmes, S.W., Horton, E.W. and Main, I.M.H. (1963) The effect of prostaglandin E$_1$ on responses of smooth muscle to catecholamines, angiotensin and vasopressin. *Br. J. Pharmac.*, **21**, 538-543.

Horton, E.W. and Jones, R.L. (1969) Prostaglandins A$_1$, A$_2$ and 19 hydroxy A$_1$, their actions on smooth muscle and their inactivation on passage through the pulmonary and hepatic portal vascular beds. *Br. J. Pharmac.*, **37**, 705-722.

Jacobson, H.I. (1974) Oncolytic action of prostaglandins. *Cancer Chemother. Rep.*, **58**, 503-511.

Karim, S.M.M. (1966) Identification of prostaglandins in human amniotic fluid. *J. Obstet Gynaecol. Brit. Cwlth.*, **73**, 903-908.

Katler, E. and Weissmann, G. (1977) Steroids, aspirin and inflammation. *Inflammation*, **2**, 295-307.

Kurzrok, R. and Lieb, C.C. (1930) Biochemical studies of human semen - II. Action of semen on human uterus. *Proc Soc. exp. Biol. Med.*, **28**, 268-272.

Lee, J.B., Covino, B.G., Takman, B.H. and Smith, E.R. (1965) Renomedullary vasodepressor substance medullin: chemical characterization and physiological properties. *Circulation Res.*, **17**, 57-77.

Lewis, G.P. and Piper, Priscilla J. (1975) Inhibition of release of prostaglandins as an explanation of some of the actions of anti-inflammatory corticosteroids. *Nature, Lond.*, **254**, 308-311.

Lewis, R.B. and Shulman, J.D. (1973) Influence of acetylsalicylic acid, an inhibitor of prostaglandin synthesis on the duration of human gestation and labour. *Lancet*, (ii), 1159-1160.

Loose, L.D. and Di Luzio, N.R. (1973) Effect of prostaglandin E_1 on cellular and humoral immune responses. *J. reticuloendothelial Soc.*, **13**, 70-77.

Main, I.H.M. (1964) The inhibitory actions of prostaglandins on respiratory smooth muscle. *Br. J. Pharmac.*, **22**, 511-519.

Malik, K.U. and McGiff, J.C. (1976) Cardiovascular actions of prostaglandins In *Prostaglandins: Physiological, Pharmacological and Pathological Aspects* pp. 103-200 Karim, S.M.M. (ed) Lancaster: MTP.

Malmsten, C., Hamberg, M., Svensson, J. and Samuelsson, B. (1975) Physiological role of an endoperoxide in human platelets. Haemostatic defect due to platelet cyclo-oxygenase deficiency. *Proc. natn. Acad. Sci. USA*, **72**, 1446-1450.

Mathe, A.A., Hedqvist, P., Holmgren, A. and Svanborg, M. (1973) Bronchial hyperreactivity to prostaglandin $F_{2\alpha}$ and histamine in patients with asthma. *Br. med. J.*, (i), 193-196.

Misiewicz, J.J., Walker, S.L., Kiley, N. and Horton, E.W. (1969) Effect of oral prostaglandin E_1 on intestinal transit in man. *Lancet* (i), 648-651.

Moncada, S., Gryglewski, R., Bunting, S. and Vane, J.R. (1976) An enzyme isolated from arteries transforms prostaglandin endoperoxides to an unstable substance that inhibits platelet aggregation. *Nature, Lond.*, **263**, 663-664.

Morrison, A.R., Nishikawa, K. and Needleman, P. (1977) Unmasking of thromboxane A_2 synthesis by ureteral obstruction in the rabbit kidney. *Nature, Lond.*, **267**, 259-260.

Nelson, N.A. (1974) Prostaglandin nomenclature. *J. med. Chem.*, **17**, 911-918.

Orchek, J., Gayrard, P., Grimaud, C. and Charpin, J. (1977) Bronchial response to inhaled prostaglandin $F_{2\alpha}$ in patients with common or aspirin-sensitive asthma. *J. Allergy clin. Immunol.*, **59**, 414-419.

Parnham, M.J., Shoshan, S., Bonta, I.L. and Neiman-Wollner, S. (1977) Increased collagen metabolism in granulomata induced in rats deficient in endogenous prostaglandin precursors. *Prostaglandins*, **14**, 709-714.

Pelus, L.M. and Strausser, H.R. (1977) Prostaglandins and the immune response. *Life Sci.*, **20**, 903-913.

Pharris, B.B. and Wyngarden, L. (1969) The effect of prostaglandin $F_{2\alpha}$ on the progestogen content of ovaries from pseudopregnant rats. *Proc. Soc. exp. Biol. Med.*, **130**, 92-94.

Pickles, V.R. (1957) A plain muscle stimulant in the menstrual fluid. *Nature, Lond.*, **180**, 1198-1199.

Plescia, O.J., Grinwich, K. and Plescia, A.M. (1976) Subversive activity of syngeneic tumour cells as an escape mechanism from immune surveillance and the role of prostaglandins. *Ann. N.Y. Acad. Sci.*, **276**, 455-465.

Puig-Parellada, P. and Planas, J.M. (1977) Action of selective inhibitor of thromboxane synthetase on experimental thrombois induced by arachidonic acid in rabbits. *Lancet*, (ii), 40.

Raisz, L.G., Dietrich, J.W. and Simmons, H.A. (1977) Effect of prostaglandin endoperoxides and metabolites on bone resorption in vitro. *Nature, Lond.*, **267**, 532-534.

Robert, A., Nezamis, J.E. and Phillips, J.P. (1968) Effect of prostaglandin E_1 on gastric secretion and ulcer formation in the rat. *Gastroenterology*, **55**, 481-487.

Samuelsson, B. (1977) The role of prostaglandin endoperoxides and thromboxanes in human platelets. In *Prostaglandins in Hematology*, pp. 1-10 Silver, M.J., Smith, J.B. and Kocsis, J.J. (eds) New York: Spectrum.

Sandler, M. (1972) Migraine: a pulmonary disease. *Lancet* (i), 618-619.

Santoro, M.G., Pilpott, G.W. and Jaffé, B.M. (1976) Inhibition of tumour growth in vivo and in vitro by prostaglandin E. *Nature, Lond.*, **263**. 777-779.

Sim, A.K. and McCraw, A.P. (1977) The activity of γ-linolenate and dihomo-γ linolenate methyl esters in vitro and in vivo on blood platelet function in non-human primates and man. *Thrombosis Res.*, **10**, 385-387.

Steinberg, D., Vaughan, M., Nestle, P.J. and Bergström, S. (1963) Effects of prostaglandin E opposing those of catecholamines on blood pressure and on triglyceride breakdown in adipose tissue. *Biochem. Pharmac.*, **12**, 764-766.

Strausser, H.R. and Humes, J.L. (1975) Prostaglandin synthesis inhibition: effect on bone changes and sarcoma tumour induction in BALB/c mice. *Int. J. Cancer*, **15**, 724-730.

Sweatman, W.J.F. and Collier, H.O.J. (1968) Effect of prostaglandins on human bronchial muscle. *Nature, Lond.*, **217**, 69.

Vane, J.R. (1971) Inhibition of prostaglandin synthesis as a mechanism of action for aspirin-like drugs. *Nature (New Biol.)*, **235**, 232-235.

Vogt, W. (1957) Pharmacologically active lipid soluble acids of natural occurrence. *Nature, Lond.*, **179**, 300-304.

Weissmann, G., Goldstein, Ira and Hoffstein, Sylvia (1976) Prostaglandins and the modulation by cyclic nucleotides of lysosomal enzyme release. In *Advances in Prostaglandin and Thromboxane Research*, **vol. 2**, pp. 803-814. Samuelsson, B. and Paoletti, R. (eds) New York: Raven Press.

Wennmalm, A. and Hedqvist, P. (1971) Inhibition by prostaglandin E_1 of parasympathetic neurotransmission in the rabbit heart. *Life Sci.*, **10**, 465-470.

Williams, T.J. and Peck, M.J. (1977) Role of prostaglandin-mediated vasodilatation in inflammation. *Nature, Lond.*, **270**, 530-532.

Yatsu, F.M. (1977) Stroke therapy: status of anti-platelet aggregation drugs. *Neurology*, **27**, 503-504.

24. Pharmacological aspects of allergy

Most of us had measles when we were children and we know that it is most unlikely that we shall succumb to the disease again. We have become *immune*. An attack of many other infectious diseases confers a similar kind of immunity which lasts, depending on the individual and on the illness, for anything between a few weeks and a lifetime. The immunity arises because the infecting organism acts as an *antigen* which stimulates the production of a specific antagonist. The antagonist is most often an *antibody* (the nature of which we shall discuss later) that circulates with the blood. When the illness has passed, the concentration of circulating antibody falls to a very low level but the mechanisms that produced it retain an *immunological memory* of the antigen so that they immediately 'recognize' it if they encounter it again. On these subsequent occasions, antibody is produced much more quickly and in much larger quantities than it was on the occasion of the original infection (Fig. 24.1) so that the new invaders are overwhelmed before they can do any harm.

On the occasions when immune reactions are not effected by antibodies they are the result of an interaction of the antigen with specific cells. These *cell mediated* responses are as specific as those mediated by antibody.

Immunity against some infectious diseases can develop as a result of an initial exposure to a dose of pathogenic organisms so trivial that it does not lead to recognizable symptoms of the disease. This finding is exploited in artificial immunization which involves the administration of small amounts of antigen (*active immunization*) or of the corresponding antibody (*passive immunization*) and spares the patient the inconvenience, discomfort or danger of the illness itself. Prophylactic measures (*prophylaxis* means

'favouring protection') of this kind have been extensively employed ever since 1796 when Jenner successfully, and with considerable personal courage, instituted the practice of vaccination against smallpox. Vaccination is active immunization with vaccinia (cowpox) virus. Its introduction as a prophylactic technique arose from the long standing observation that milkmaids, who by the very nature of their calling must have suffered at least subclinical attacks of cowpox, did not succumb to smallpox and so retained that unsullied milkmaid complexion, so lauded by poets, that placed them at such an advantage with the young men of their time.

We receive further protection from immune reactions by virtue of the antibodies we develop against the microorganisms that are the normal inhabitants of our gastrointestinal tract (*commensal* organisms) and the protection so provided extends to other, potentially harmful, organisms that produce similar antigens. The importance of this protection is illustrated by the fact that animals that are bred into, and brought up in, completely germ free surroundings rapidly succumb to infection if they are transferred to a more normal environment. They might even die as a result of being attacked by bacteria that are completely innocuous to their fellows that have been brought up in less sheltered conditions.

There can be no doubt then that immune reactions have a vital part to play in the maintenance of health but they are sometimes the reverse of protective as Richet and Portier recognized in 1902 when they coined the word *anaphylaxis* (which means 'removal of protection') to describe the untoward result of what we now recognize as an antigen-antibody reaction. Richet and Portier were investigating the toxin secreted by the Portuguese man of war, a jelly fish that produces an urticarial rash (p. 403) in those with whom it comes into contact. They found that a single injection of the toxin had no adverse effect in dogs but that a second injection given some days later provoked violent systemic reactions that proved fatal. Although 'anaphylaxis' did not enter the medical vocabulary until 1902 the phenomenon had been noticed and accurately described many years earlier. In 1839, the great Magendie (who also formulated the 'law' that sensory and motor impulses travel in the posterior and anterior spinal nerve roots respectively) showed that rabbits, which were not troubled by a single injection of egg albumin died following a second injection of that substance.

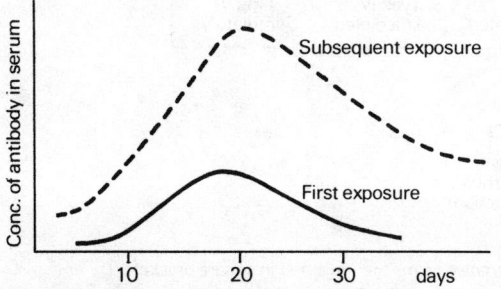

Fig. 24.1 Antibody response to the first (continuous line) and subsequent (broken line) exposures to antigen

At the time when Richet and Portier first drew attention to the phenomenon of anaphylaxis in animals, von Pirquet was studying the responses of patients given prophylactic injections of horse serum. Some of those who received a second injection of serum some days after a first (which had caused no adverse reaction) suffered severe attacks of urticaria or asthma. Von Pirquet realized that he had encountered a similar situation to that described by Magendie and by Richet and Portier but he took exception to its being called anaphylaxis, pointing out that those who survived the attack were as well protected as those who suffered no ill effect from the inoculation. He proposed, instead, that the immediate reactions should be described as *allergic*, the word signifying an unexpected or altered reaction. Von Pirquet's word has been adopted by his successors, most of whom, however, have forgotten its true meaning. To be strictly accurate, *all* immune reactions have to be described as allergic since the failure of an immunized person to respond by pathological changes to an attack by invading organisms is, in its way, as unexpected a reaction as is a violent urticarial response to a second injection of horse serum. Following Ward (1970), an attempt is made to effect a return to this semantically correct nomenclature throughout this chapter. According to the scheme set out in Fig. 24.2, allergy is manifested as either immunity or as hypersensitivity, while anaphylaxis is just one type (albeit an important one) of hypersensitivity reaction. Although von Pirquet, were he with us, would certainly applaud the use of 'allergic' in the sense in which it is used here he might be driven to protest over the retention of 'anaphylaxis' to describe a condition that is not necessarily fatal.

The reader should be aware that the terminology favoured in this chapter is not the most widely popular. In particular, many writers use 'allergy' as an alternative to our 'hypersensitivity' but there exists a degree of confusion, 'allergy' and 'anaphylaxis' often being used interchangeably.

To return now to the mainstream of our discussion, we have to note that, like horse serum, some other therapeutic agents provoke anaphylactic reactions of varying degrees of severity in sensitive individuals. The number of fatalities from this cause has increased with the recent growth in the variety of available drugs and in the enthusiasm with which they are prescribed. A big offender in this respect is penicillin, otherwise the most valuable and benign of drugs.

The anaphylactic states we have mentioned as sometimes occurring in response to the injection of serum or the ingestion of some drugs are most often seen—as are some related conditions such as hay fever and contact dermatitis—as a result of exposure to antigens in pollens, hair, house dust, chemicals and foodstuffs. The word *allergen* (from 'allergic antigen') is sometimes applied to substances that detonate hypersensitivity responses of this type. The disorders so caused are categorized as allergies or *atopic* diseases. The last mentioned adjective is also used to describe individuals sensitive to the allergens.

Although anaphylactic reactions are truly immune responses in the sense that they result in the destruction or

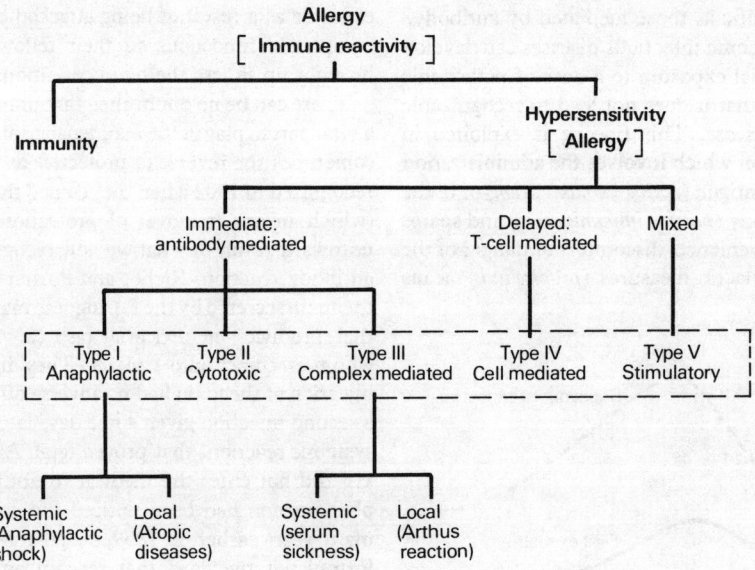

Acceptable alternative terms are indicated in square brackets

Fig. 24.2 Allergic phenomena

immobilization of antigen it is surely remarkable that in securing the defeat of the antigen they may seriously inconvenience or even kill the individual in whose tissues the battle has taken place. What makes the situation even more perplexing, at least at first sight, is that there is no evidence to indicate that the common allergens would do any real harm if they were permitted to gain access to the tissues. In this way they contrast sharply,of course, with many microbial antigens. Anaphylactic reactions to apparently innocuous materials provide a classical example of throwing out the baby with the bathwater: the body abhors foreign cells and substances to such an extent that it will, if necessary, kill itself rather than admit them into its tissues.

It has become clear in recent years that immune reactions have now to be considered in a much wider context than that encompassed by a consideration of allergic diseases, anaphylactic shock and resistance to infection. Mention must also be made of transplant rejection, autoimmune disease and the aetiology and treatment of cancer.

An *allograft*—tissue transplanted from one individual to another of the same species—experiences a very cold reception in its new situation unless donor and recipient are closely related. The recipient treats the graft as it would an invading pathogen: immune reactions are set in train that lead to the death and rejection of the transplanted tissue. It is clear that successful transplantation is contingent on the suppression of these immune reactions. This can sometimes be achieved by the deployment of *immunosuppressive* agents and some organs can now be transplanted under the umbrella of these drugs with some assurance that they will not be rejected.

Immune reactions, then, are a manifestation of the body's anathema to foreign material, particularly proteins. A corollary of this is that these defence mechanisms, like a well trained watch dog, shall recognize and not react against the body's own cells and products. Ehrlich, the progenitor of chemotherapy and of the 'receptor' concept, recognized this selectivity of immune reactions in 1900 when he spoke of an organism's *horror autoxicus*, a phrase that needs no translation. It has, however, become evident that our watch dog (or self recognition system) is not always as vigilant or as perceptive as we would wish, *horror autoxicus* notwithstanding, and it may turn against the very organism it should be defending. Conditions attributable to the breakdown of the self recognition system are called *autoimmune* diseases and it may surprise the previously uninformed reader to discover how many cases of human illness have an autoimmune basis. Some autoimmune diseases are mentioned in the appropriate chapters of this book—the chapters that discuss the individual organs and systems that may be affected—and they are collected together in the Index, but to indicate their range it should be said here that autoimmunity is responsible for at least some cases (the majority in many instances) of rheumatic fever, systemic lupus erythematosis, myasthenia gravis, ulcerative colitis, thyrotoxicosis, Addison's disease, nephritis, Hodgkin's disease, multiple sclerosis, viral encephalitis and some skin conditions, to select but a few from a list whose length emphasizes the extent of the hazards we face from our own defence system.

Inflammation is a usual reaction in tissues that have been damaged by physical agencies or pathogenic organisms. The events that consitute the inflammatory response are described elsewhere (p. 440) and it is there pointed out that some of the substances that are liberated from damaged cells and are responsible thereby for the inflammatory response are also set free by, and are responsible for some of the effects of, immune reactions. Moreover, the body reacts against its own dead cells in much the same way that it responds to the presence of foreign cells. It is evident that there is a considerable degree of congruence between inflammatory and immune reactions. An appreciation of this relationship should resolve the confusion that is sometimes created in the mind of the nonspecialist who reads, for instance, that the ability to prevent or attenuate an anaphylactic reaction is one of the properties that is looked for by laboratory workers engaged in evaluating compounds for possible antiinflammatory activity.

Although neoplastic (cancerous, p. 912) growths are derived from the victim's own tissues, they do acquire an antigenic individuality that should qualify them for rejection by the body just as a foreign tissue graft is rejected. The question as to why they are apparently not rejected has found a variety of possible answers. At one extreme, there is the view that cancer cells, their specific antigens notwithstanding, cannot initiate effective immune reactions. At the other, the *immunosurveillance* hypothesis, championed by Burnet, maintains that the whole *raison d'être* of the immune system is to defend us against cancer (Burnet, 1970). According to the immunosurveillance concept, neoplastic cells are repeatedly formed in the tissues but are promptly eradicated by the operation of immunological mechanisms. If these mechanisms fail, the new growth establishes and extends itself. It is unlikely that the immunosurveillance hypothesis will survive in its original form but there seems to be no doubt that cancers do provoke weak immunogenic rejection mechanisms and that attempts to develop agents that will improve the effectiveness of these reactions constitute a promising development in the field of cancer chemotherapy.

Those who have read this chapter to this point can be forgiven if they have reached the conclusion that immune reactions are on the whole more burdensome than beneficial. It would, however, be a false conclusion. The risk of allergic and autoimmune diseases, widespread and crippling though these are, is a small price to pay for the protection our immune systems provide against pathogenic organisms and perhaps against cancer too. The value of this protection is testified to by the rapidity with which animals bred into a germ free environment succumb if they are transferred into more 'normal' surroundings.

IMMUNITY MECHANISMS

Immunology is a subject that, in recent years, has developed apace and it can now be regarded as a science in its own right. With this development it has acquired its own vocabulary (not to say jargon), its own hypotheses and a variety of specialized experimental techniques all of which combine to leave many novices bewildered and confused. Attempts to remedy this situation have been signalled by the appearance of a plethora of elementary textbooks all of them purporting to and some of them actually succeeding in making the subject intelligible to the beginner. A few of the better ones (one or two of which contrive to be both informative and entertaining) are listed in the bibliography to this chapter. The serious student is referred to them but he should be forewarned that those aspects of immunology that particularly attract the pharmacologist constitute a very minor part of the subject as a whole. It is a part, moreover, that does not seem noticeably to capture the interest of the majority of immunologists and it receives scant attention in even the best textbooks.

In the pages that follow, an attempt is made to provide the reader with a superficial survey of the elements of immunology that should enable him to understand the background of the scene against which our pharmacological studies play their parts.

Immune reactions are invariably initiated by antigens and we can therefore define an antigen as a substance that provokes a specific immune response. The response most often involves the production of circulating antibodies (*humoral immunity*) but it is sometimes brought about by the production of specifically modified cells (*cell mediated immunity*) whose mode of action is mentioned later (p. 401). Whole cells (bacteria, viruses, erythrocytes etc.), proteins and large polysaccharide molecules can initiate immune responses but substances with molecular weights below the 5000 to 8000 range are uniformly devoid of antigenic activity. This last statement is in no way vitiated by the well known observation that some drugs and chemicals of simple structure and low molecular weight

are capable of eliciting undoubtedly allergic reactions. They do this by becoming linked in the body with a carrier protein such as serum albumin. The resulting complex acts as the antigen proper, the low molecular weight component being the *antigenic determinant* which confers specificity on the complete antigen molecule. It is also known as a *hapten*, a word of Greek origin introduced into immunology by Landsteiner (of blood group fame), signifying an attachment.

ANTIBODIES

Antibodies can only be defined in a somewhat circular fashion as proteins generated by and capable of reacting with antigens. Antibody molecules are of a highly specific nature every antigenic substance inducing the appearance of antibodies that react only with molecules of that (or sometimes a closely related) antigen. Antibodies are sometimes named (as agglutinins, precipitins, etc.) in accordance with the type of response that follows their combination with antigen. A *reagin* is an antibody involved in anaphylactic responses.

Antibody proteins are associated with the gammaglobulin fraction of the plasma and for that reason they are known as *immunoglobulins* (Ig). Five types of immunoglobulin (labelled G, M, A, D and E) have so far been recognized and the existence of a sixth (IgT) has been postulated. The principal features of the known immunoglobulins are summarized in Table 24.1 and discussed briefly in the following paragraphs.

Some 80 per cent of the immunoglobulin fraction of serum is in the form of IgG and most of the body's antibodies are proteins of the IgG type. They pass the blood-placental barrier and they are responsible for the immunity the newborn display against almost all infectious diseases.

Immunoglobulin M is the first antibody type to be elaborated in response to antigenic stimulation and it was also the first to appear in the course of evolution. Many IgM antibodies are short lived, being replaced after some days by IgG molecules of similar specificity. Not all IgM antibodies have to accept so short a life, however. Among the long lived members of the species are the anti-A and the anti-B blood group agglutinins α and β.

The IgM antibodies are large molecules that do not

Table 24.1: The human immunoglobulins

	IgG	IgM	IgA	IgD	IgE
Light chain (L)	All Ig molecules carry κ or λ light chains				
Heavy chain (H)	γ	μ	α	δ	ϵ
Make up of molecule	$\gamma_2 L_2$	$(\mu_2 L_2)_5$	$(\alpha_2 L_2)_{1,2}$ or $_3$	$\delta_2 L_2$	$\epsilon_2 L_2$
Molecular weight	c. 150000	900000	160000	185000	200000
Concentration in normal serum (mg/ml)	8–16	0.5–2	1.4–4	0.1–0.4	v. low

cross the bloodplacental barrier. They combine readily with foreign particles and because they appear early and do not leave the blood stream they serve the valuable function of preventing the rapid dissemination of infecting organisms throughout the body. Individuals who lack IgA antibodies are exposed to the threat of a serious septicaemia if pathogenic microorganisms enter their blood.

Immunoglobulins A occur in the blood in only small quantites but much higher concentrations appear in tears, saliva, bronchial and gastrointestinal secretions and other serous fluids. These antibodies seem to be particularly concerned with resisting infection of the eyes and the gastrointestinal and upper respiratory tracts.

The function of IgD antibodies is still obscure but they seem to be particularly associated with the function of lymphocytes of the B type (p. 398). The postulated immunoglobulin T, if it exists, is thought to be associated with T type lymphocytes.

Immunoglobulins E (the reaginic antibodies or reagins) are of particular interest to the pharmacologist because their union with antigens' (allergens) initiates the events that lead to anaphylactic shock and atropic diseases. Because they are attached to tissue cells, immunoglobulins E are normally present in negligibly trivial amounts in the blood but larger quantities are found in atopic ('allergic') individuals.

Immunoglobulin structure

The structure of a molecule of immunoglobulin G is depicted in Fig. 24.3. It consists of two identical 'heavy' (H) chains each with a molecular weight of about 50000 daltons and two identical 'light' (L) chains with molecular weights of about 25000 daltons. The molecule has a Y-shaped form, the constituent chains being held together by disulphide bridges. The whole molecule can be split by papain (a proteolytic enzyme) into two 'antigen binding' fragments (Fab) and a 'crystallizable' fragment (Fc). Pepsin cleaves the molecule at a different point leading to the production of a conjoined bivalent antigen binding fragment that can be conveniently represented as F (ab')$_2$.

The other classes of immunoglobulin have essentially the same form as IgG except that IgM and IgA molecules are made up of aggregates of the basic four-chain units assembled in forms that will be mentioned later. The fine structure of the 'heavy' and 'light' chains does, however, vary among and within the different immunological classes. There are five types of 'heavy' chain designated γ, μ, α, δ; and ϵ, these labels indicating that the chains are found in immunoglobulins G, M, A, D and E respectively. Throughout the range of immunoglobulins only two types of 'light' chain (κ and λ) are known. Both chains are represented in all the immunoglobulin types but an individual antibody molecule carries 'light' chains of only one species. In the human being, immunoglobulin molecules bearing κ chains outnumber those carrying the λ

chain by about two to one but the $\kappa : \lambda$ ratio exhibits a large interspecies variation.

Since antigens provoke the production of specific antibodies, a huge variety of minor modifications in immunoglobulin structure must be possible within the otherwise very similar molecules. These minor variations in structure all occur within the 'variable' part of both the 'heavy' and the 'light' chains (Fig. 24.3) the rest of the molecule conforming to that characteristic of the two species of chains (γ, μ, α, δ or ϵ associated with κ or λ) from which it is made. The variable part of all chains, 'light' or 'heavy' is about 110 aminoacid residues long (this is approximately half the length of the L chain and one quarter or one fifth the length of the H chain) and the opportunities for minor structural variations provided by this arrangement are obviously enormous. It is self evident that antigen binding must be to the variable part of the Fab portion of the immunoglobulin molecule. The Fc fragment determines the type of response that is to be initiated by the antigen-antibody complex.

The basic four chain units are aggregated into groups of five to make up IgM molecules. The individual units are united by disulphide bridges provided by a linking polypeptide and known as the J (for joining) chain (Fig. 24.3B). The J-chain, rich in cysteine, has a molecular weight of about 15000 daltons. Many IgA molecules occur as simple

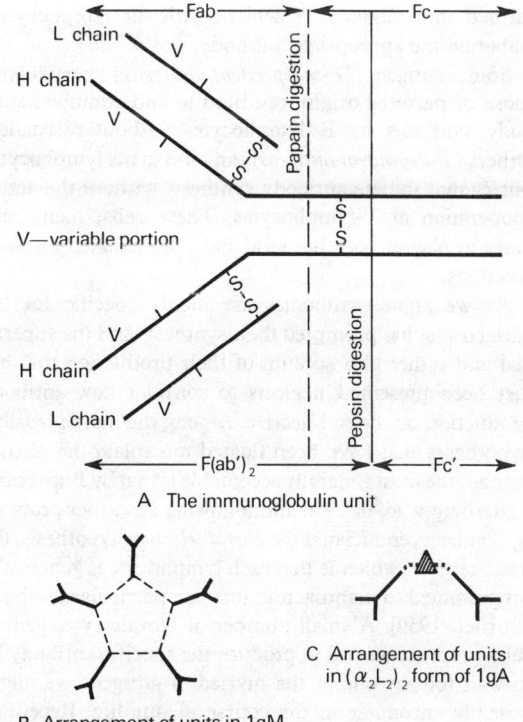

A   The immunoglobulin unit

B   Arrangement of units in 1gM

C   Arrangement of units in ($\alpha_2 L_2$)$_2$ form of 1gA

Fig. 24.3 Immunoglobulin structure (schematic)

monomers (like all the other immunoglobulins save IgM) but others appear as aggregates of two or three units that also incorporate both a J-chain and a somewhat larger polypeptide with a molecular weight of some 60 000 daltons (the secretory component) that probably protects the molecule from proteolysis during its secretion into the body fluids.

Antibody synthesis

Lymphocytes play a key role in the production of antibodies. In the adult animal all blood cells are produced in the bone marrow. Presumed precursors of the mature lymphocytes migrate to the thymus where they differentiate into the so-called T lymphocytes. Other precursor cells are converted into B lymphocytes. In birds this change takes place in the bursa of Fabricius, a collection of lymphoid tissue in the region of the cloaca, but in mammals the B lymphocytes are probably elaborated in the bone marrow itself.

The major sites of antibody production are the spleen and the lymph nodes: the anatomy of the situation is such that intravenous antigen is taken up primarily by the spleen (but also by the bone marrow) while if it is given by the subcutaneous or intradermal routes it finds itself in the antigen trapping meshes of the lymph nodes. In the lymphoid tissue the antigen is held by *macrophages* (these are fixed, mononuclear phagocytic cells) and exposed to circulating B lymphocytes. Some of the latter are transformed into *plasma cells* which, with the lymphocytes, elaborate the appropriate antibody.

Some antigens (*T-independent antigens*), particularly those of bacterial origin, can bind to and stimulate antibody synthesis by B lymphocytes without assistance. Others (*T-dependent antigens*) can bind to the lymphocytes but cannot initiate antibody synthesis without the active cooperation of T-lymphocytes. These cells, then, have parts to play in both humoral and cell mediated immune reactions.

As we know, antibodies are highly specific for the antigen that has prompted their synthesis and the superficial and rather glib account of their production that has just been presented neglects to consider how antibody production can be so selective. Among the more plausible hypotheses that have been floated to explain the phenomenon, the most generally acceptable is that by Burnet and Lederberg who, in 1958 and following an earlier proposal by Talmage, enunciated the *clonal selection* hypothesis, the basic tenet of which is that each lymphocyte is genetically programmed to manufacture just one particular antibody (Burnet, 1959). A small number of lymphocytes genetically preprogrammed to produce the specific antibody lie in wait for any one of the myriad of antigens we might possibly encounter in the course of our life. Receptors incorporated in the cells' surface membranes—the most effective and consequently the most likely receptor would

be the antibody molecule itself—permit union with the antigen. Following union, the lymphocytes divide, some are transformed into plasma cells and the resulting small *clone* of cells (lymphocytes and plasma cells) sets about the manufacture of antibody molecules. Some of the new cells retain antibody when the immune reaction ceases and return to their original lymphocyte status. Thus more cells will be immediately available to resume antibody production should the antigen return to the scene of its previous defeat. This is the basis of the body's *immunological memory* and it explains why the production of antibody molecules is so much more brisk when an antigen enters the body on a second (and any subsequent) occasion than when it first activates the immune mechanisms.

The clonal selection hypothesis has been extended to explain why the body's immune mechanisms do not operate against its own cells. It is suggested—and this view is supported by a substantial body of experimental evidence—that the ability of a lymphocyte to direct the manufacture of antibody is suppressed if the cell encounters antigen before or immediately after birth. The only antigens likely to be met at this time are, of course, the body's own. The idea that in *immune tolerance* the ability to manufacture antibody is only suppressed and not abolished is an attractive one inasmuch as it sees autoimmune disease as the simple consequence of a breakdown of the suppression metabolism.

By suitable experimental manipulation, immune tolerance can be induced in adult animals.

THE COMPLEMENT SYSTEM

An understanding of the pharmacological aspects of allergy does not (fortunately) demand more than the superficial acquaintance with the complement system that is provided by the following paragraphs.

If red blood cells are suspended in fresh serum containing the appropriate red cell antibody they will suffer haemolysis. It has been known since the very early days of immunology that haemolysis fails to occur if the serum has been preheated or allowed to stand for some time before the red cells and their antibody are added to it. Haemolysis, therefore, is effected by the conjoint activity of antibody and a heat labile factor in the serum known as *complement*. Originally believed to be a single substance, complement is now known to consist of a mixture of eleven mutually interacting protein components. Under normal circumstances the complement factors are inactive but when a cellular antigen combines with an immunoglobulin molecule of the IgM or IgG series, conformational changes take place in the Fc moiety of the antibody which thereby develops the ability to combine with a complement component. This component is designated C1 although it is actually a complex of three closely related proteins. When it is bound to antibody, C1 can interact with two other components (C2 and C4) to form an enzyme complex (C3 convertase) that splits component C3 into a small unit (C3a) which is released into the body fluids and a larger unit (C3b) which remains in association with C3 convertase to form another converting enzyme (C5 convertase) which cleaves the complement component C5 into small and large fragments, C5a and C5b respectively. The C3 and C5 convertases thus have analogous actions. The larger C5 fragment, like the similar C3 unit, remains in association with its progenitors (C1, 2, 4 and 3) and the resulting complex (which is conventionally designated C12435, the horizontal line indicating a complexing together of the named components) incorporates the remaining complement fractions (C6 to C9) into a complex with phospholipase activity that erodes tiny holes in the cell membrane and so causes haemolysis of red cells or the death of bacterial cells.

The sequence of events just outlined (and further summarized in Fig. 24.4) constitutes the so-called *classical pathway* of complement activation but a miscellaneous group of substances—bacterial endotoxins, insulin, agar, F (ab')$_2$ fractions, immunoglobulins A and G etc.—can bring about the formation of a C3 activator (which has the same function as C3 convertase) without the intervention of C1, C2 or C4. Because the initiation of this change does not require the activation of C1, substances that operate through the *alternative pathway* do not have to be first bound to antibody.

Activation of complement, like the coagulation of blood involves a cascade of reactions, a single molecule formed at one stage of the process activating several molecules each of which, in its turn, also deals with a number of substrate molecules. Inhibitory factors, activated by reaction products, are the instruments of a feedback system that prevents the cascade from developing into an uncontrolled torrent.

Some of the components of the complement system exert actions independently of the concerted effort that leads to haemolysis and cell death. The fragments C3a and C5a attract leucocytes by chemotaxis and they also promote the formation of the *anaphylatoxins* (p. 405). Combinations of the C1423 complex with components C5, C6 and C7 also have leucocyte chemotactic activity; C1, C2 and C3 are *opsonins* (p. 400); component C3b seems to be involved in the activation of macrophages and B-lymphocytes while components C1, C4 and C2 may take part in the production of the plasma kinins and increased vascular permeability.

Complement fixation tests, the best known of which is the Wassermann reaction for syphilis, are employed to diagnose the presence and nature of pathogenic antigens. The basis of the technique is that a suspension of red cells in serum will not undergo haemolysis in the presence of erythrocyte antibody if complement is missing. This situation will arise if the serum used in the test contains antibody which, in a preliminary incubation with the corresponding antigen has formed an antigen-antibody complex which has reacted with complement. In the test the antigen is selected, of course, on the basis of the provisional clinical diagnosis.

IMMUNE REACTIONS

We can now refer back to Fig. 24.2 and review briefly the several immune reactions enumerated there.

IMMUNITY

The primary value of the immune system is that it provides mechanisms that enable us to resist infection by pathogenic organisms.

The natural defence against infection by microorganisms is vested in the phagocytes—erudite readers, recalling Shaw's bitter play *The Doctor's Dilemma* will remember that these cells came into their own, following the work of Metchnikoff, at the turn of the century—but many virulent organisms have contrived means of circumventing

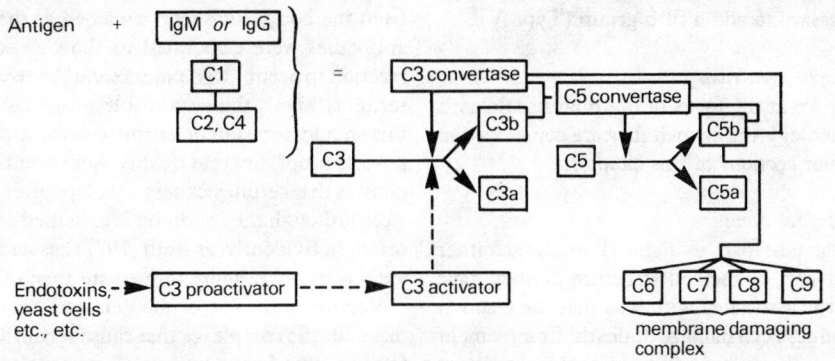

The alternative pathway is indicated by broken lines.

Fig. 24.4 Principal reactions involved in complement activation: for details see text.

these defences. Some species refuse to adhere to the phagocytes while others manufacture antiphagocyte substances. However, when virulent species are coated with their specific antibodies (whether these have been acquired actively or passively) they become much more adherent to phagocytes and their defences are often further weakened by the intervention of components of the complement system (p. 398). Complement intervention results in *opsonization* (the relevant components are known as opsonins) a delightful word whose inspired etymology implies that the bacteria have been rendered so palatable that the phagocytes engulf them with relish.

Even after phagocytosis some organisms (tubercle and leprosy bacilli for instance) continue to thrive but they are still exposed to attack by cell mediated immune reactions mounted by T-lymphocytes.

The mechanisms just outlined do not by any means constitute the full repertoire of our immune defence reactions. Some Gram negative bacteria are bounded by an outer wall with a structure reminiscent of that of the mammalian erythrocyte. They are similarly susceptible to the lethal action of antibody acting in concert with complement activated through the classical pathway. Moreover, and as we have already seen, bacterial endotoxin can activate complement in the absence of antibody by way of the alternative pathway. Bacterial exotoxins can be neutralized by antibodies (antitoxins) independently of the operation of immune reactions that might at the same time be attacking the microorganism itself while IgA antibodies (p. 397), in addition to acting as antitoxins, may also discourage the adhesion of bacteria to the intestinal wall. Mention must also be made of *interferon* (p. 859), a natural antivirus agent, although its generation is not contingent on the activity of immune reactions.

HYPERSENSITIVITY REACTIONS

In 1968, Coombs and Gell segregated hypersensitivity reactions into four groups (Types I to IV) a classification that has been generally adopted although most immunologists find it necessary to add a fifth group (Type V).

Type I (anaphylactic) reactions

Type I reactions lie at the focus of the pharmacologist's interest in immunology and as such they are considered in some detail in later sections of this chapter.

Type II (cytotoxic) reactions

The antigens that take part in Type II reactions either form an integral part of the cell structure or they have become secondarily associated with it so that the reaction with antibody induces cell damage or death. Complement is usually involved: the reader will recall, indeed, that our discussion of complement centred on just such a cytotoxic reaction that culminated in haemolysis. Type II reactions can, of course, be truly protective when the antigens are of

bacterial origin but they also underlie some idiosyncratic drug responses and they are, therefore, justifiably included with the other hypersensitivity reactions. The classical example of a drug hypersensitivity mediated by a Type II reaction is provided by apronal (Sedormid), a once popular hypnotic drug that had to be abandoned because it occasionally caused thrombocytopenic purpura, a condition characterized by the occurrence of subcutaneous and intraarticular haemorrhages and attributable to platelet deficiency. Apronal was absorbed on to platelets, acted there as a hapten and thereby induced the production of specific antibody and a Type II reaction that caused platelet destruction. Haemolytic disease of the newborn, the reactions that accompany incompatible blood transfusions and an autoimmune variety of haemolytic anaemia, are also dependent on Type II reactions. It seems likely, moreover, that the haemolytic phenomena that complicate several other diseases and the treatment of yet others have a similar origin.

Type III (toxic complex) reactions

Type III reactions result from the binding of antigen to circulating antibody in and around blood vessels and to the events set in motion by the toxic complex so formed. Two varieties of Type III reaction are recognized: one, associated with antigen excess and the production of soluble complexes that cause a systemic response, is serum sickness and the other, associated with antibody excess and a local response, is the Arthus reaction.

Serum sickness, as we have already noted, was the first condition to be described as 'allergic'. Von Pirquet, after the fashion of the time, had been treating diphtheria with large doses of horse serum containing antitoxin. Some of his patients developed urticaria, joint pains and oedema of the face about a week after they had received their injection. It is clear what had happened: following the injection of the serum, antibodies slowly appeared in the patients' plasma. Because of the high dose of antitoxin that had been given and the relatively slow rate at which it was eliminated from the body, sufficient remained at the time when the antibodies were elaborated to allow an antigen-antibody reaction to occur. Two points should perhaps be added. In serum sickness, the responsible antigen is an antibody but this should occasion no surprise since antibody molecules possess properties that qualify them as antigens. The other point is that serum sickness develops after a lag of at least a week although the condition is classified as an 'immediate' reaction. Evidently, as Roitt (1977) has said, some immediate reactions are more immediate than others!

Varying numbers of antigen and antibody molecules make up the complexes that cause serum sickness and this fact accounts for the varied symptomatology of the disease. The larger complexes can bring about the direct release of histamine and the other vasoactive substances (though not so readily as do the IgE antibodies of anaphylaxis) and so cause oedema, urticaria and rashes while others can become lodged in the capillaries of various tissues particularly in the kidney and the joints where they induce complement activation and provoke inflammatory changes: glomerulonephritis and painful joints (or a frank arthritis) are commonly seen in serum sickness. The myocardium is also vulnerable to inflammatory changes.

Large doses of serum are no longer given for therapeutic purposes but serum sickness is still seen. The glomerulonephritis that accompanies some cases of malaria and some virus infections have their origin in the action of toxic complexes, as have many of the symptoms of systemic lupus erythematosus. Penicillin and the sulphonamides have also sometimes provoked Type III reactions.

The Arthus reaction occurs at the site of injection when antigen is given intradermally into subjects with a high concentration of the corresponding IgG antibody. The complex that is formed at the site of injection binds complement and causes thereby anaphylatoxin release, platelet aggregation and an influx of polymorphonuclear leucocytes. The overt manifestations of these changes are oedema and erythema which appear immediately, reach their peak some eight hours after exposure to the antigen and pass off over the next sixteen hours or so.

The conditions for the appearance of an Arthus reaction are sometimes created in themselves by diabetic patients who, using the less purified insulin preparations (p. 727) inadvisably make repeated use of the same injection site.

Arthus type reactions also occur in the bronchi and the pulmonary alveoli. They are probably the cause of 'farmer's lung', a condition characterized by the onset of respiratory difficulty six to eight hours after exposure to mouldy hay and of 'pigeon fancier's disease', a somewhat similar condition provoked by exposure to dust from the birds' desiccated faeces.

Type IV (delayed hypersensitivity) reactions

The appearance of Type IV reactions is delayed for some 12 to 24 hours following the introduction of antigen into the body. They are mediated, not by humoral antibodies, but by specific T-lymphocytes.

It has been known for many years that animals previously infected with tuberculosis are much more sensitive than noninfected animals to the local action of the tubercle bacillus or to protein extracted from it. If a very small dose of the protein is injected intradermally into previously infected animals a local delayed reaction occurs. It takes the form of a raised nodule on the skin which may even undergo necrosis. It can be evoked in any part of the body but it is always restricted to the immediate area of injection. The fact that the tuberculin reaction—an *allergy of infection*—can only be produced in previously infected animals forms the basis of the *Mantoux test* applied to human beings: a positive response to tuberculin indicates a previous infection with the tubercle bacillus (most likely a subclinical infection) so that a prophylactic inoculation is not necessary. Reactions of a similar type—*reactions of immunity*—sometimes make their appearance at the injection site in individuals who have recently been inoculated against certain diseases. Transplant rejection also depends on Type IV mechanisms.

Another form of delayed hypersensitivity is *contact dermatitis*. It occurs in those who come into frequent contact with particular chemical agents that eventually cause sensitization. Thereafter, contact with the sensitizing chemical provokes an eczema like condition in the skin. Agents that can cause contact dermatitis include (among others) some metals (especially nickel and chromium), dyestuffs, certain plants (poison ivy is a particularly notorious offender in this respect), hair colouring agents and penicillin.

Type IV reactions are not uniformly deleterious. The influx of cells (lymphocytes and macrophages) into an inoculation site is essentially a protective response and Type IV reactions are also involved, as we have already noted (p. 400), in the elimination of some phagocytes that have ingested organisms but have not killed them. T-lymphocytes can also generate cells that attack virus particles. Efforts are being made to apply delayed hypersensitivity reactions to the treatment of skin cancers.

In delayed hypersensitivity, the antigen first reacts with T-lymphocytes. These cells are as specific for individual antigens as are humoral antibodies and it must be assumed that this specificity is bestowed on the lymphocyte by some subtlety of the membrane structure that enables the cell to recognize and seek out its mate. Once united with their antigen the lymphocytes multiply and their offspring enlarge to form lymphoblasts. Some of the latter become modified into the rather dramatically named *killer cells* which can attack virus particles and are also responsible for tissue graft rejection. Other blast cells, when united with antigen, liberate *lymphokines*. These are small proteins, with molecular weights in the region of 25000–50000 daltons, and they serve a variety of functions. Thus they attract previously 'uncommitted' (unspecific) lymphocytes to inflammatory sites and there stimulate them into metabolic and reproductive activity. Two other lymphokines (the *macrophage migration inhibition factor* or *MIF* and the *macrophage arming factor* or *MAF*) ensure that macrophages are retained at the site of the hypersensitivity reaction and that their phagocytic activity is properly aroused. Other lymphokines may promote the production of interferon (p. 859), influence the activity of the B-lymphocytes, increase the permeability of capillaries and exert cytotoxic actions. This by no means exhaustive list should be sufficient to indicate the preeminent importance of lymphokines in Type IV reactions.

Type V (antibody dependent cell mediated) reactions

In this type of reaction, antibodies combine with antigen

on a cell surface and this leads to stimulation of the cell's activities rather than to the cytotoxic effects that usually follow the combination of antigen and antibody. A good example of a Type V reaction is provided by thyrotoxicosis. In this autoimmune disease, antibodies have been developed against antigens on the surface of the thyroid gland. Activation of these receptors by combination with antibody has the same effect as has stimulation by thyroid stimulating hormone, the 'natural' agonist. Type V reactions are 'mixed' in nature, both antibodies and cellular activity contributing to the final response.

ANAPHYLACTIC REACTIONS

Anaphylactic shock and the atopic diseases together comprise the Type I hypersensitivity reactions. The distinguishing and common feature of these reactions is that they depend predominantly on the union of antigen with IgE antibodies.

Anaphylactic shock is a state of systemic anaphylaxis while atopic diseases are the result of anaphylactic responses in more restricted areas (local anaphylaxis).

Anaphylactic shock is best described in terms of specific examples and it is only proper that the first of these examples should be provided by the guinea pig, the animal species that, by reason of its sensitivity to the mediators of anaphylaxis, has contributed most to our understanding of the phenomenon.

If a guinea pig is given a small amount of a foreign protein by intraperitoneal injection, no obvious change occurs but we know (Fig. 24.1) that the animal's immune system will have generated small quantities of the appropriate antibodies and, more important, that it will have acquired a 'memory' of the antigen (the guinea pig has become *sensitized*) so that if it encounters the antigen again it will respond by the immediate production of a new and large batch of antibody molecules. A period of about three weeks must elapse before our guinea pig becomes properly sensitized but thereafter a second injection of the foreign protein will precipitate anaphylactic shock. The nature of the anaphylactic reaction depends on the route by which this second injection is administered. If it is given intravenously, the effects are dramatic, the animal dying in acute respiratory distress within a few seconds of receiving the protein. Post mortem examination reveals that the cause of death is invariably an intense bronchospasm. This persists after death so that on removing the lungs from the thorax they remain inflated. If the shocking dose of protein is given by the subcutaneous or intraperitoneal route, the anaphylactic reaction is less dramatic but more protracted: dyspnoea resulting from bronchoconstriction is certainly seen but, in addition, there is a gradually increasing degree of circulatory collapse with gastrointestinal haemorrhages

and hypothermia. The animal also itches as is evidenced by its violent scratching.

The major manifestations of anaphylactic shock differ in other species. In the dog, a precipitous fall of blood pressure occurs. This is caused by constriction of the hepatic vein, which thus has the effect of excluding a large proportion of the animal's blood volume from the circulation. The overriding importance of this mechanism in the dog is shown by the fact that anaphylactic shock does not occur in animals whose liver is excluded from the circulation. In the rabbit there is generalized arterial constriction which particularly affects the pulmonary system. Hypotension is a secondary effect, consequent on myocardial failure produced by the intense arterial vasoconstriction. These differing major manifestations of anaphylactic shock are closely similar to those produced by toxic doses of histamine in the corresponding species (p. 336).

Anaphylaxis is more difficult to produce in other laboratory species. When it does occur, it is characterized in the rat by respiratory embarrassment, hypotension, gastrointestinal haemorrhages and hypothermia. Mice become cyanosed and partly paralysed but the paralysis gives way to convulsions which usher in death.

Like most immune reactions, anaphylactic shock is both a specific and a sensitive response. If an animal is sensitized to, say, egg albumin, anaphylaxis can only be evoked by a shocking dose of egg albumin. All other proteins including, for example, serum albumin will be ineffective. The sensitivity of the response is attested to by the fact that some workers have found it possible to sensitize a guinea pig with as little as 10^{-6} ml of horse serum although larger amounts than this are needed to produce anaphylactic shock in the sensitized animal.

Anaphylactic shock is not entirely a laboratory phenomenon. In human beings it can complicate the administration of antisera and of drugs (penicillin is a particular offender in this respect) and some unfortunate individuals suffer severe or even fatal anaphylactic shock if they are bitten or stung by an insect to whose venom they are sensitive.

Atopic diseases include such distinct clinical entities as asthma, hay fever and urticarial dermatitis but some drugs and items of the diet can cause gastrointestinal upsets of anaphylactic origin. A number of drugs also provoke truly immune reactions in the skin (the drug molecule serving as a hapten) but it is to be noted that not all drug rashes are attributable to the operation of this kind of mechanism.

In atopy, the specific antibodies are often present in the serum from birth, though the allergy may not make its appearance until relatively late in life. There is a strong hereditary predisposition to atopic conditions and psychological factors often play an important part in the precipitation of individual attacks. It is well known, for instance, that a patient who is allergic to a particular item of food may suffer an attack if he sees a realistic picture of that foodstuff, and many attacks of asthma are precipitated by emotional factors. Another feature of some forms of atopy is that an allergic response does not invariably follow exposure to the allergen. This is particularly noticeable in urticarial responses to foods: sometimes, indeed, the sensitive individual may only respond once in his lifetime to the offending foodstuff. More than one atopic condition may coexist in the same person or as he grows older he may exchange one allergy for another. A typical occurrence is the development of hay fever in the adolescent who had asthma as a child. Later still he may also lose his hay fever, as there is a natural tendency for atopic conditions to disappear with age. A point which may cause some confusion is that allergic responses are produced by dietary protein which would be expected to be completely broken down by the normal digestive processes before absorption into the circulation. However, only minute quantities of protein are needed to provoke an allergic response and small amounts of protein can escape digestion and enter the blood stream unchanged. This occurs particularly easily in childhood and children suffer food allergies more than adults.

Hay fever and asthma sufferers are usually sensitive to more than one antigen—a whole range of pollens, for instance—and it seems possible that this type of hypersensitivity is often inborn, no post-natal contact with the allergen being necessary to provoke the formation of the antibodies. Responses to drugs, on the other hand, are usually confined to one particular compound and in these cases allergic reactions do not occur until sensitization has been produced by previous contact with the drug. This contact need not involve the actual taking of the drug: the mere handling of a penicillin preparation, for instance, is sufficient to produce sensitization in some subjects. Allergic responses then occur either when the drug is handled again or when it is taken for therapeutic purposes.

In atopy, as we shall see, the blood eosinophil count is increased (*eosinophilia*). This constitutes a useful diagnostic feature in cases in which there is doubt whether the condition is atopic or not.

One consequence of the occurrence of circulating antibodies in atopy is that the offending allergen can be detected by skin testing even when the atopic condition does not itself cause skin lesions. Thus, if extracts of different pollens are injected intradermally into a hay fever patient, a weal and flare reaction will occur in response to those pollens which on inhalation cause hay fever. The facts that hypersensitivity can be passively transferred and that skin reactions occur in hypersensitive subjects form the basis of the Prausnitz-Küstner reaction, so named after the individuals in whom it was first demonstrated. Prausnitz was allergic to cooked fish. A small amount of his serum was injected intradermally into Küstner, who thereafter himself responded with a weal and flare reaction to an intradermal injection of fish extract. This type of

passively induced hypersensitivity is relatively short lived and desensitization (p. 408) is caused by one positive Prausnitz-Küstner reaction but it can be usefully employed to determine the reagin content of the serum of a sensitive individual.

The clinical features of the main forms of atopy need to be briefly described. *Asthma* is characterized by the occurrence of paroxysmal attacks of difficult respiration caused by constriction of the bronchi. The condition is further aggravated by oedema of the bronchial mucosa. There is a short inspiration followed by a prolonged and distressing expiratory effort accompanied by wheezing as air is forced past the narrowed bronchial tubes. After a number of these abortive respiratory efforts, cyanosis may be evident.

Two categories of asthma are commonly recognized. *Extrinsic asthma*, which usually makes its first appearance no later than early adult life, is precipitated by recognizable allergens. In *intrinsic asthma*, allergens cannot be identified. This is not to say that external allergens are never involved in this form of the disease: indeed it seems to be established beyond reasonable doubt that some cases of intrinsic asthma arise from the operation of allergens that have escaped identification. In some other cases, the condition is of autoimmune origin and involves Type II reactions. There remains a residue of patients with hyperresponsive bronchial systems that are goaded into generating asthmatic responses by stimuli such as climatic changes, emotional stress, exercise and irritant vapours that operate independently of immune mechanisms.

Allergens commonly responsible for asthmatic attacks include feathers, the fur and hair of animals, mites (of the family *Dermatophagoides*) that inhabit house dusts and some foodstuffs.

Hay fever occurs in people sensitive to a variety of pollens: it is therefore a summer disease. Sneezing, running nose, itching and irritation of the nose and eyes, profuse lachrymation and photophobia all occur, the relative intensity of these symptoms varying with the individual. Some patients who are sensitive to material of nonseasonal incidence, such as dust and feathers, may show hay fever like symptoms at any time: they are said to suffer from perennial paroxysmal rhinorrhoea (which only means that they have irregular attacks of running nose throughout the year). On this nomenclature, hay fever is *seasonal paroxysmal rhinorrhoea. Urticaria* is popularly called nettle rash. The popular name is a literal translation of the medical term (urticara = nettle) and both are appropriate, since the skin lesions of urticaria have very similar causes to those of the nettle sting (p. 420). In urticaria there is a widespread eruption of firm, pink or white weals accompanied by intense itching. A characteristic feature of urticaria is its evanescent nature, the lesions appearing very suddenly and disappearing within a few hours. It is a common manifestation of an allergic sensitivity to foods and drugs, though it sometimes also occurs in people who are not apparently hypersensitive to any article of diet but who are under some form of emotional stress— that engendered, for example, by the prospect of having to speak or perform in public. Among the dietary constituents that provoke urticarial reactions, the most common offenders are the proteins of shell fish, eggs, milk and some fruits such as strawberries and bananas. Allergic reactions to drugs are not uncommon but it is important to remember that not all drug rashes are of an allergic type.

Anaphylactic mechanisms

In anaphylaxis, the primary victim is the mast cell. Apart from those that inhabit the blood stream (the basophil leucocytes) mast cells are fixed in connective tissues and

the antibodies that attach to them are often described as being *homocytotrophic*. As we noted earlier they are also known as reagins (or reaginic antibodies) while the antigens that inspire their production can be described as allergens. Throughout this chapter these several synonyms are used interchangeably and indiscriminately.

Reaginic antibodies belong predominantly to the IgE class of immunoglobulins although IgG antibodies can exert a degree of reaginic activity. It is not completely clear why allergens provoke the production of predominantly IgE antibodies but it is presumably related to the fact that sensitization to these antigens results from contact with mucous surfaces.

Fig. 24.5 summarily depicts the mechanisms that sub-

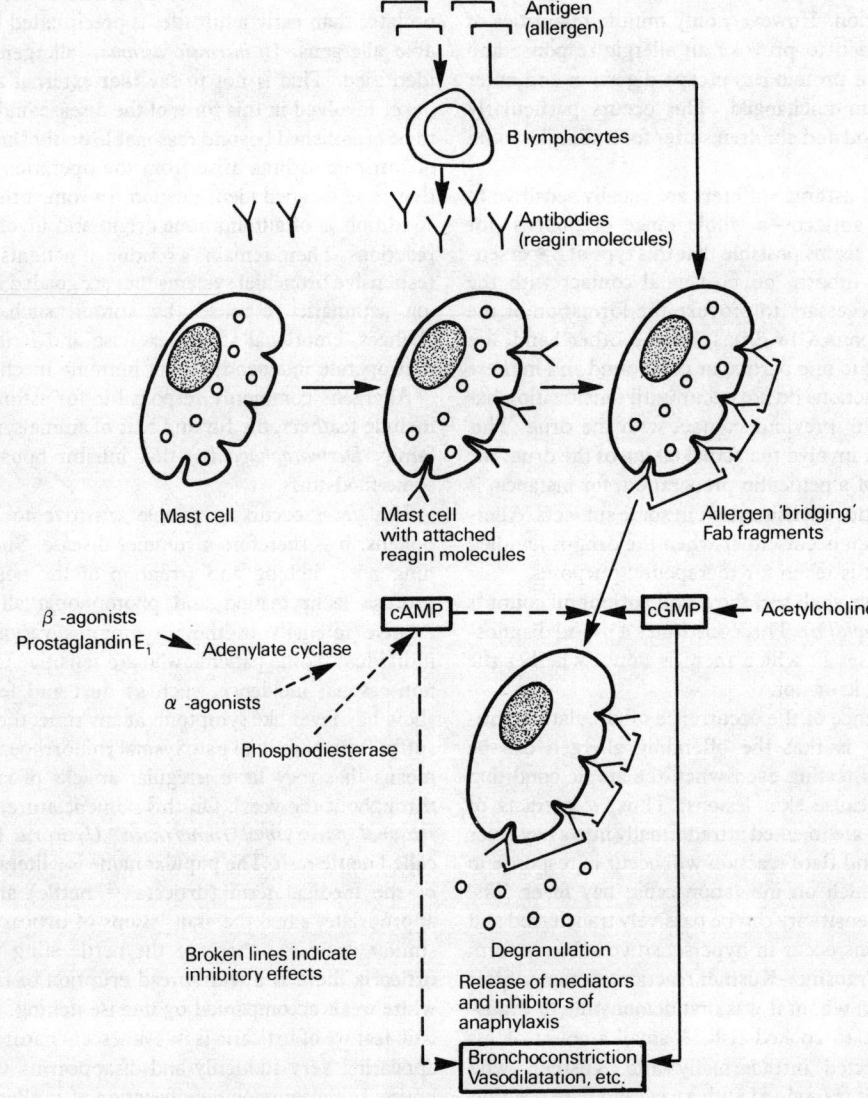

Fig. 24.5 Processes involved in the production of Type 1 (anaphylactic) reactions.

serve and influence anaphylactic reactions. In sensitized individuals, some of the mast cells will already carry the appropriate antibodies that will be able to react with allergen molecules immediately the latter gain access to the body. Further supplies of antibody will, of course, be produced by B lymphocytes in the usual way and they too will become attached to mast cells. Because the cells are fixed in the tissues the ones chiefly affected in a particular case will be determined by the route by which antigen enters the body. Thus a pollen which will normally come into contact with the conjunctivae and the nasal mucous membrane will induce the reactions in these tissues that typify hay fever. On the other hand, an antigen given by the intravenous route will be distributed more widely and the humoral mediators of anaphylaxis will appear in the systemic circulation to produce the more generalized explosive reactions of anaphylactic shock. Even in anaphylactic shock, of course, some tissues respond more violently than others by reason of their particular sensitivity to the mediators.

Reaginic antibodies attach themselves by their Fc constituents to the mast cells and the allergic antigens unite with the resulting complex in such a fashion that adjacent antibody molecules are *bridged* (Fig. 24.5). This leads to distortion of the surface membrane of the cell and the influx of calcium ions that trigger the release of material from the intracellular granules into the extracellular fluid. The mast cells thereby become degranulated. Changes in the local concentration of cyclic AMP probably take place at the same time. It is to be noted that molecules that can combine with the Fab components of the IgE antibody but cannot effect a bridge with the Fab of an adjacent molecule ('univalent' anti-IgE antibodies fall into this category) can protect sensitized mast cells against specific allergen but do not cause degranulation.

The material released on degranulation include heparin, humoral mediators of the anaphylactic response, platelet activating factor and chemotactic substances that encourage the migration of polymorphs and eosinophils to the site of the reaction. Eosinophils release substances, detailed below, that antagonize some of the mediators of anaphylaxis. Thus, in the way of so many physiological systems, substances that promote particular changes appear in the company of others that limit these changes. The fact that eosinophilia is a feature of the atopic condition testifies to the importance of the 'eosinophil brake'.

The extent of mast cell degranulation depends on more factors than the mere combination of allergen and IgE antibody. The most important of these other factors is cyclic AMP which stabilizes the membrane and so tends to oppose degranulation and the consequent anaphylactic changes. Circumstances that increase the amount of available cyclic AMP will prevent or attenuate the response and it may, conversely, be that some inbuilt instability of the mast cell membrane, occasioned by a relative deficiency of cyclic AMP, may determine why some of us are highly sensitive to a variety of extrinsic allergens while others are totally unmoved by their presence.

Substances liberated in anaphylactic reactions

Although it is clear to the modern reader that many of the changes that characterize anaphylactic reactions are very similar to those which follow the administration of histamine, this fact was not so obvious when the anaphylactic state first became a subject for study. It will be recalled that Richet introduced 'anaphylaxis' into our vocabulary in 1902 but that Barger and Dale's classical paper on the properties of histamine did not appear until 1910 and the occurrence of histamine in mammalian tissues was not established until 1927. Until that date, therefore, it was not possible to suggest that histamine was responsible for anaphylactic reactions, which were thought by many to be caused by anaphylatoxin (see below). After 1927, the importance of histamine was universally recognized but during the past twenty five years or so it has become clear that other substances also participate in anaphylactic reactions.

ANAPHYLATOXIN

In 1909 Friedemann suggested that the antigen-antibody combination was subjected to proteolysis in the blood to release a substance—anaphylatoxin—which was finally responsible for anaphylactic responses. Although this view was to be eclipsed as a result of the later demonstration that histamine is released in anaphylaxis, anaphylatoxin is still discussed, though in a rather different context, in contemporary textbooks of immunology. Three anaphylatoxins, with molecular weights that range from 7500 to 10000 daltons, are recognized. They are found in complement fractions C3a and C5a and are responsible for causing the release of histamine from mast cells in the course of Type III hypersensitivity reactions (p. 400).

HISTAMINE

An essential feature of the anaphylatoxin hypothesis in its original form was that the antigen-antibody complex was subjected to attack by a serum enzyme. As early as 1913, Dale showed that anaphylactic reactions could occur in isolated tissues suspended in a saline medium in which, of course, serum-mediated reactions cannot occur. Dale took the isolated uterus of a sensitized guinea pig in the traditional organ bath and showed that it contracted strongly when a small dose of the protein to which the animal had been sensitized was added to the bath. It was quite insensitive to other proteins. Because Schultz independently demonstrated it, the response of isolated tissues to the allergen is sometimes known as the 'Schultz-Dale reaction'. A tracing from Dale's paper is reproduced in Fig. 24.6. The experiment not only illustrated the specificity of anaphylactic reactions but it also formed the basis of Dale's view that anaphylaxis occurred primarily as a result

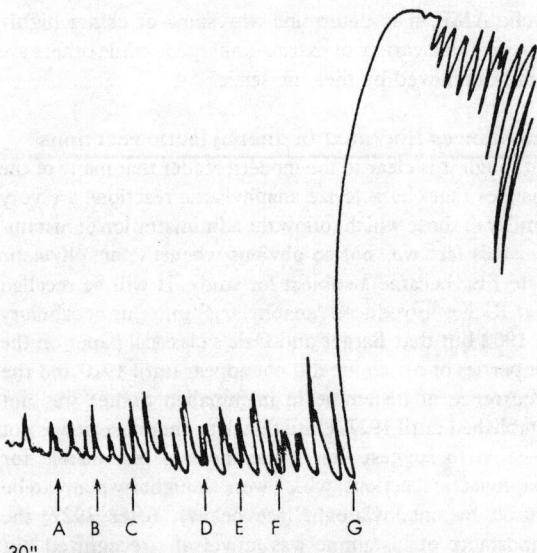

Fig. 24.6 Response of the isolated guinea-pig uterus (sensitized to horse serum) to 0.1 ml doses of A: sheep serum, B: cat serum, C: rabbit serum, D: dog serum, E: human serum, F: egg white, G: horse serum. Reproduced by kind permission from H.H. Dale 'The anaphylactic reaction of plain muscle in the guinea pig', *J. Pharmae exp. Ther.* **4**, 167-223 copyright 1913, The Williams and Wilkins Co., Baltimore, Md. 21202, USA.

of intracellular events. For several years, vigorous argument centred on the relative merits of the anaphylatoxin and the intracellular theories of anaphylaxis. Dale was aware that the reactions of sensitized tissues to the specific proteins were similar to those produced by histamine but, since this substance was not then known to occur in mammalian tissues, he was reluctant to suggest that it was responsible for anaphylactic reactions. In his own later words he seemed to take 'great pains to avoid a possibility which was almost clamouring to be recognized'.

After 1927, evidence that histamine was indeed liberated during anaphylaxis came not only from Dale but also from others such as Feldberg and Schild. It was shown, for instance, that a material pharmacologically identifiable as histamine is liberated when the appropriate antigen is added to a saline solution perfusing the isolated lungs of a sensitized guinea pig. It was also demonstrated that the liberated histamine exists in a pre-formed state in the lung and is not formed in response to the presence of the antigen. These demonstrations, indeed, are so simple that every modern student of pharmacology performs them for himself. Other equally convincing evidence of histamine release was obtained for other tissues.

For some years the histamine theory of anaphylaxis went almost completely unchallenged and when the antihistamine group of drugs was developed it was widely believed that they would provide the means of treating all atopic diseases. These optimistic expectations went unful-

filled, for although the antihistamines were extremely successful in relieving the symptoms of hay fever and allergic drug rashes, they provided very little relief in asthma. Dale was inclined to explain this on the proposition that histamine liberated in the tissues in which it actually evokes a response—*intrinsic histamine*—is less accessible to the action of antagonists than is *extrinsic histamine* which is liberated at a site remote from its points of action. This hypothesis never received strong support from the available experimental evidence and it soon succumbed to the alternative view that more substances than histamine contributed to hypersensitivity reactions, particularly asthma.

SLOW REACTING SUBSTANCE OF ANAPHYLAXIS (SRS-A)

Kellaway and Trethewie (1940) perfused the isolated lungs of sensitized guinea pigs and showed that when antigen was added to the perfusate the material leaving the lungs contained not only histamine but also a substance which caused a delayed and much slower contraction of the isolated ileum. They also showed that this second substance appeared later than histamine but that its liberation continued for some time after that of histamine had ceased. Kellaway and Trethewie realized that this second substance was similar to a 'slow reacting substance' that Feldberg and Kellaway had detected some years before in isolated lungs perfused with a solution to which cobra venom had been added. The material liberated in anaphylaxis is now known as the 'slow reacting substance of anaphylaxis'. The name is an adequate description of the unidentified material liberated from sensitized lung provided it is remembered that other tissue constituents—such as bradykinin whose very etymology attests to the fact—also cause slow contractions of isolated preparations.

In the years that have elapsed since Kellaway and Trethewie's original observation it has become clear that the slow reacting substance of anaphylaxis is liberated from the sensitized lungs of many animal species on antigen challenge. Not all species are equally responsive to its actions but the most sensitive—among which we must number the human being (Brocklehurst, 1962)—react to much less than a nanogram of the material. It is powerfully bronchoconstrictor in its action but that from at least some species also induces contraction of smooth muscle in the veins (particularly the pulmonary vein) and in the gastrointestinal tract.

Forty years on, the chemical identity of SRS-A remains obscure. It has a molecular weight of some 500 daltons and the properties of an unsaturated acid. It is inactivated by arylsulphatase, an observation that indicates the possibility that it is a sulphate ester, but the most fascinating aspect of its synthesis and structure concerns its relationships with the prostaglandins, prostacyclins and thromboxanes. Like these latter compounds (and unlike histamine) SRS-A does not exist in lung tissue in a preformed state: it is synthesized in response to the stimulus provided by the interaction of antigen and antibody. There is a reciprocal relationship between the synthesis (and hence the release) of the slow reacting substance of anaphylaxis and that of the prostaglandins and their relatives. Thus, antiinflammatory drugs, which inhibit prostaglandin synthetase (cyclooxygenase) promote the release of the slow reacting substance (and also, incidentally, that of histamine) while diethylcarbamazine, a drug that inhibits the release of SRS-A, similarly promotes the output of the prostaglandins (Engineer, et al., 1978; Piper, 1978). It may be that the key to these interactions lies in the possibility that SRS-A stimulates arachidonic acid metabolism by activating phospholipase (p. 367). There is recent evidence to suggest that arachidonic acid is incorporated in the molecule of SRS-A.

The slow reacting substance described by Feldberg and Kellaway can be released from lung tissue *in vitro* by physical insults such as repeated freezing and thawing and the evidence indicates that, unlike SRS-A, it exists in the lungs (and other tissues) in a preformed state. Nevertheless there is reason to believe that this substance (SRS) is closely related to that liberated in anaphylaxis (SRS-A).

PLASMA KININS

The plasma kinins are referred to in more detail elsewhere (p. 358). Some of their actions are similar to those which might be expected of mediators of anaphylaxis (they cause bronchoconstriction and increased capillary permeability, for instance) and there is certainly evidence that they are involved in the mediation of inflammatory responses. As was mentioned earlier, the properties of bradykinin (one of the plasma kinins) recall those of the slow reacting substance of anaphylaxis and one report (Beraldo, 1950) suggests that bradykinin is liberated during anaphylaxis. There is, however, no substantial evidence that the kinins are in any way concerned in the initiation of anaphylactic responses.

SEROTONIN

It was pointed out earlier (p. 332) that some of the properties of 5-hydroxytryptamine (serotonin) are intriguingly similar to those of histamine and it is even possible to produce an anaphylactic like shock in guinea pigs by exposing them to an aerosol containing serotonin. However, the serotonin content of guinea pig lung is low, its bronchial muscle is less sensitive to serotonin than it is to histamine and doses of serotonin antagonists that protect guinea pigs against serotonin shock do little to alleviate the anaphylactic state.

Mice and rats differ from the other common laboratory animals in that their mast cells contain serotonin as well as histamine. Since much of the histamine liberated during anaphylaxis is derived from mast cells, the possibility has to be considered that serotonin may also be liberated and that, in mice and rats, it may have a part to play in the initiation of anaphylactic reactions. There is no evidence that this is so: neither the depletion of serotonin stores nor the administration of serotonin antagonists modifies anaphylaxis in these species. It is, however, possible that serotonin rather than histamine is involved in the production of *anaphylactoid* responses. Anaphylactoid reactions occur in response to injections of protein in *unsensitized* animals. Dextran and glycogen can also precipitate anaphylactoid reactions. The reactions are evoked easily in rats but not at all in rabbits or guinea pigs. Anaphylactoid reactions take the form of oedema of the extremities. They are not seen in rats that happen to suffer anaphylactic shock in response to the injection because the fall in blood pressure that epitomizes the shock precludes the formation of oedema fluid.

Mouse and rat capillaries are much more sensitive to serotonin than to histamine and prior depletion of serotonin from the skin diminishes the intensity of anaphylactoid reactions. Depletion of histamine is without effect. Moreover, substances with antiserotonin action inhibit the anaphylactoid reaction, while antihistamines do not. Other substances may well be liberated in the course of anaphylactoid reactions (Spencer and West, 1965).

Serotonin is liberated from platelets in anaphylaxis and the urinary excretion of 5-hydroxyindoleacetic acid rises. Nevertheless, there is little evidence to suggest that serotonin plays any but a minor role in anaphylaxis.

HEPARIN

Heparin (p. 663) is a normal constituent of mast cells and it is liberated when these cells undergo degranulation in the course of allergen-reagin reactions. It does not contribute to the symptomatology of atopic diseases but the blood of animals that have died in anaphylactic shock is often incoagulable.

THE PROSTAGLANDINS

As we discuss in detail elsewhere (p. 380), prostaglandins and some related substances take part in the humoral regulation of bronchial tone. There is also no doubt, as we saw above, that they are released, reciprocally with the slow reacting substance, in anaphylactic reactions. The question that really concerns us here, however, is whether anaphylaxis brings about any change in the relative amounts, or in the relative activities, of the bronchoconstrictor and bronchodilator prostaglandins that appear in the lung. Some asthmatic patients, but by no means all, are more than usually sensitive to prostaglandin $F_{2\alpha}$ (a bronchoconstrictor agent) and there is evidence that there may be a shift in the emphasis of prostaglandin synthesis from E_2 to $F_{2\alpha}$ in asthmatic subjects. On the other hand, drugs that inhibit prostaglandin synthesis do not usually influence the course of atopic diseases. Aspirin, for instance, precipitates asthmatic attacks in some individuals and relieves them in others but for the most part it leaves the condition unaffected.

PLATELET ACTIVATING FACTOR

The platelet activating factor which emanates from the mast cells along with the other mediators and inhibitors of anaphylaxis promotes the release of histamine and 5-hydroxytryptamine from the platelets.

EOSINOPHIL CHEMOTACTIC FACTOR

The eosinophil chemotactic factor of anaphylaxis (ECF-A) is a tetrapeptide of mast cell origin. As its name implies, it attracts eosinophils to the site of an anaphylactic reaction and in so doing it serves to attenuate the reaction by reason of the enzymes secreted by the eosinophils. These include a histamine degrading enzyme (probably histaminase), aryl sulphatase (which disposes of the slow reacting substance of anaphylaxis) and a phospholipase D that destroys the platelet activating factor.

The treatment of anaphylactic shock and atopic diseases

From the foregoing discussions it will have become clear that a number of substances and processes are involved in the initiation of anaphylactic reactions. Their importance relative to one another varies with the disorder and with the patient. This complexity of the anaphylactic response finds an echo in the large number of drugs and therapeutic manoeuvres that can be recruited for the treatment of the anaphylactic state. These various agents are enumerated and discussed below but it should be made clear at the outset that the therapist's choice of weapons is to a greater or lesser extent determined by the needs of the moment. Anaphylactic shock and status asthmaticus are medical emergencies that demand the immediate institution of life saving measures but in the less desperate situations presented by chronic or recurring atopic disease there is time to try a variety of drugs and expedients until the most suitable combination is found. Again, some atopic conditions such as hay fever are relatively easy to treat while others (particularly asthma) often pose considerable therapeutic problems. Finally we must remember that some clinical states (and asthma again provides us with the best example) can be of either allergic or nonallergic origin. Some drugs are equally efficacious in both forms of the disease but others attack only the allergic variety.

Many of the agents that receive a mention in the paragraphs that follow are discussed in more detail in other parts of this book.

AVOIDING THE ALLERGEN

If the atopic patient never again meets the antigen to which he has become sensitized he will never suffer an anaphylactic response. Individuals who have discovered that they are hypersensitive to a particular drug, a cosmetic agent or an item of diet or that their atopy is precipitated by contact with the fur of their pets or the feathers that stuff their pillows can avoid untoward reactions by shunning the offending antigen. Those sensitive to pollens can some-

times attenuate their annually recurring attacks of hay fever (or asthma) by taking such simple and pleasurable avoiding actions as going on a seaside holiday or refusing to mow their lawns during the period when the pollens to which they are sensitive would otherwise foul their conjunctivae and nasal mucosae. In many instances, however, a policy of avoiding the allergen is hardly practicable although the successful management of childhood asthma still occasionally demands (as it did more frequently in the past) the extreme remedy of their removal to countries able to provide clinics in a totally unpolluted environment.

DESENSITIZATION

The next best thing to avoiding the antigen altogether is to render it incapable of initiating an immune response. Desensitization (nowadays more often called *hyposensitization*) attempts to achieve this end by depriving the allergen of its opportunity of combining with its reagin. The desensitization procedure, which has been applied to the management of asthma and hay fever since the beginning of the century, involves the subcutaneous injection, usually at monthly intervals, of the pollen or pollens to which the patient is sensitive. The culprit pollens are identified by skin testing. The injections are timed to end just before the pollens are scheduled to appear in the atmosphere and a single course often provides protection for several years.

The rationale of the hyposensitization procedure is that the hyposensitizing injections stimulate the production of IgG antibodies (*blocking antibodies*) that will immediately mop up the allergen should it gain access to the body. In this way they prevent its coming into contact with the mast cells. An alternative, and probably a more likely, explanation is that the repeated injections of allergen induce the formation of 'tolerant' T lymphocytes which have lost their ability to support the synthesis of IgE antibodies. Recent developments in this field include the administration of antigens to which the patient is not sensitive with the idea that the antibodies they generate will occupy the mast cell receptors to the exclusion of the specific IgE antibodies. An even more recent advance has utilized a synthetic pentapeptide (Asp-Ser-Asp-Pro-Arg) whose structure corresponds to that of a fragment of the Fc moiety of IgE and which, consequently, is capable of occupying the mast cell receptors so that they are no longer accessible to the reagins.

SYMPATHOMIMETIC AMINES

Long before its mode of action was properly understood, adrenaline was introduced for the treatment of anaphylactic shock and asthma. We now know that, by its action on β receptors, adrenaline stimulates the formation of cyclic AMP and so inhibits the degranulation of mast cells (Fig. 24.5). It also has a direct bronchodilatatory action, again as a result of its stimulating β receptors.

Adrenaline is still employed on the rare occasions when

a patient suffers an anaphylactic shock but it has been superseded as an antiasthma agent by sympathomimetic drugs with a more selective action on the bronchi. The story of the progression from adrenaline through isoprenaline to salbutamol and similar compounds is retailed elsewhere (p. 272).

In anaphylactic shock, adrenaline in a 1 in 1000 solution is administered by the intramuscular route. Up to 1 ml can be given followed by up to 100 mg of hydrocortisone (or the equivalent amount of another glucocorticoid) intravenously. General measures to counter shock have also to be instituted. In some asthmatic subjects, attacks of bronchoconstriction are sometimes so severe and prolonged that they constitute an emergency—*status asthmaticus*—almost as grave as that presented by anaphylactic shock. This condition too can be treated with adrenaline which is usually given subcutaneously, sometimes as often as every fifteen minutes. If it becomes clear that adrenaline is having an insufficient effect, treatment is supplemented with aminophylline (see below), which can be given intravenously. An alternative treatment is to give hydrocortisone by intravenous injection in doses of 100 mg every three hours or so. A glucocorticoid active by mouth can with benefit be given for up to a week after the initial emergency has been surmounted.

Ephedrine, a compound that has a mixed action, stimulating adrenaline receptors (both α and β) directly as well as evoking the release of noradrenaline from sympathetic nerve endings, also enjoyed a vogue as a therapeutic agent in both asthma and hay fever. It is active by mouth and is only slowly inactivated. Like adrenaline, ephedrine has been largely supplanted as an antiasthma drug by sympathomimetic amines that have a more selective action on β_2 receptors. In hay fever, the agonist action of ephedrine on α receptors causes a vasoconstriction that brings much relief to the sufferer's tortured nose and conjunctivae and much more than compensates for the tendency of α stimulation to inhibit the formation of cyclic AMP (Fig. 24.5). Moreover, the central nervous stimulation induced by ephedrine often provides (except at bed time) a welcome contrast to the sedation that mars the otherwise beneficial effects of so many histamine H_1 antagonists. It is a pity that this same effect on the central nervous system can lead to an amphetamine like dependence (p. 91) among those tempted to abuse ephedrine so that its pharmacological advantages have to count for little against the wisdom of severely curtailing the distribution of the drug.

GLUCOCORTICOIDS

There can be no doubting the fact that the glucocorticoids can provide relief in anaphylactic states even when other therapies have failed. This is partly because of their antiinflammatory properties and partly because of their ability to potentiate the effects of β receptor stimulation.

Their value in anaphylactic shock and *status asthmaticus* has already been alluded to. They are certainly as effective in the management of more chronic atopic disease states. Unfortunately the side effects of the glucocorticoids are serious and far reaching if they are taken systemically over a period of time. This arises by reason of the drugs' interference with adrenocortical function (p. 767) so that it has become usual to regard the glucocorticoids, as far as their long continued use is contemplated, as drugs to be called upon when other treatment fails. While this is wise counsel so far as systemic corticosteroids are concerned, it is less so if they are applied locally. Recent surveys have demonstrated that beclomethasone, taken in this way, is therapeutically effective in amounts that have no systemic effect. Aerosol inhalers and nasal drops provide suitable vehicles for beclomethasone in individuals with asthma and hay fever respectively (Brogden *et al*, 1975 *a* and *b;* Wilson and McPhillips, 1978). Dexamethasone (p. 762) can be used in the same fashion as beclomethasone.

HISTAMINE H_1 ANTAGONISTS ('ANTIHISTAMINES')

The reader should by now be aware that histamine liberation is involved to varying degrees in the different forms of anaphylaxis (and probably among different patients too) so that histamine antagonists are quite effective in some atopic diseases such as hay fever and virtually useless in others, particularly asthma. The clinical uses of the histamine antagonists are discussed in detail elsewhere in this volume (p. 351).

XANTHINE DERIVATIVES

Theophylline and aminophylline (p. 321) inhibit phosphodiesterase and thereby permit the accumulation of cyclic AMP. Consequently their actions resemble those of the β agonists in respect both of the inhibition of mediator release from stimulated mast cells and the induction of bronchodilatation. Aminophylline can be given intravenously to supplement the actions of parenteral injections of adrenaline in stubborn cases of status asthmaticus. Adult patients can receive up to 300 mg and older children up to 100 mg of aminophylline on a single occasion. Theophylline, in oral doses of about 250 mg thrice daily, can bring relief from coughing and bronchospasm in asthma of all types and in chronic bronchitis.

DIETHYLCARBAMAZINE

This drug is an antifilarial agent and as such it is described on p. 893. In addition to its anthelmintic properties, diethylcarbamazine inhibits the release of SRS-A from mast cells and it might therefore be expected to have potential value as an antiasthma drug. Some investigators have indeed claimed that in doses of about 10 mg per kilogram of body mass the drug can benefit asthmatic patients who have proved refractory to other drugs but most authorities remain unconvinced of its value.

Oddly enough, anaphylactic side effects not infrequently occur in those who have received diethylcarbamazine for their filariasis. This response is simply a reaction to the mass of dead worms which overwhelms any protection that might be provided by the drug's effect on the mast cells.

SODIUM CROMOGLYCATE

Sodium cromoglycate (cromolyn sodium, Aarane, Inostral, Intal, Lomudal, Lomusol, Nasmil), one of our newer drugs—it was first synthesized in 1968—has proved to be a boon to many atopic patients as a consequence of its ability to prevent, rather than merely to relieve, their attacks.

Khellin (p. 706) is the active principle in an Egyptian folk medicine long employed to relieve the smooth muscle spasm of renal colic, ureteral spasm and asthma. In the course of a modern investigation designed to discover khellin like substances that might be more active but less toxic than their parent, there emerged a compound (chromone-2-carboxylic acid) with unique properties. The new substance partially relaxed the bronchospasm of asthma but it was otherwise devoid of muscle relaxing

the mode of action of a range of drugs—those with anaesthetic, antiepileptic and arrhythmic activity for instance—but it is not a very illuminating one unless some idea of the nature of the particular stabilization process can be provided. So far as sodium cromoglycate is concerned we cannot say more at this stage of our knowledge than that it probably operates through enzyme inhibition.

It is possible that a minor part of sodium cromoglycate's activity is not a consequence of its ability to inhibit mediator release. In particular it inhibits, in some circumstances, the bronchoconstriction induced by stimulation of adrenaline α receptors. While it is always possible that, in atopic asthma, the effects of α receptor stimulation are mediated entirely by way of the mast cell mechanism there is some evidence that cromoglycate can counter the bronchoconstriction of exercise asthma, a condition that is not dependent on the participation of mast cells.

Only trivial amounts of sodium cromoglycate are absorbed from the gastrointestinal tract but the drug in the form of a fine powder is readily absorbed from the lungs.

sodium cromoglycate

activity. Sodium cromoglycate was the most successful of a group of compounds whose synthesis was inspired by the desire to produce a more powerful but still selective antiasthma agent.

Sodium cromoglycate is not a bronchodilator or an antiinflammatory agent and it does not antagonize or destroy any of the known mediators of anaphylaxis. What it does do is to prevent the release of mediators after allergen has united with reagin. Consequently it is only effective when it is given before exposure to the antigen: it may prevent but it cannot relieve acute attacks of atopy.

Early studies indicated that sodium cromoglycate was absolutely specific in its action, preventing the release of mediators only from mast cells and then only if the thwarted stimulus to release was a type I reaction. More recent work has, however, made it clear that sodium cromoglycate is also capable of preventing type III reactions and the release of histamine from mast cells exposed to such nonantigenic stimuli as phospholipase, compound 48/80 and dextran. Finally, in some species at least, it can inhibit the anaphylactic release of histamine from basophils. It seems that cromoglycate stabilizes the cell membrane. This is a pharmacologically respectable view that can also be invoked (and not unreasonably so) to explain

For this reason, asthma patients often take their sodium cromoglycate by inhalation of the powder, using for this purpose a device (Spinhaler) that permits the contents of a capsule to be dusted into the lungs in response to an inspiratory effort. An aerosol preparation (Lomusol) is also available. This can be taken, in a metered dose, from the more conventional type of inhaler.

Sodium cromoglycate is not metabolized in the body and the side effects most frequently reported (cough, slight bronchospasm, dryness of the mouth and throat) are those that might be expected to follow the inhalation of any dry powder. If it is troublesome the bronchospasm can be relieved by adding a small amount of isoprenaline to the cromoglycate powder. Minor gastrointestinal side effects, an occasional skin eruption and, infrequently, severe bronchoconstriction and nasal congestion have also been noticed in those taking the drug.

A capsule of sodium cromoglycate contains 20 mg of the drug, sometimes admixed with 100 μg of isoprenaline. The usual dose is one capsule taken at four- or six-hourly intervals although it is occasionally necessary to take the drug every three hours. The usual care must be exercised (p. 272) by patients who use preparations that contain isoprenaline.

When sodium cromoglycate treatment is instituted in patients who have previously been maintained on glucocorticoids it is often possible gradually to reduce the intake of the corticosteroid. It must however be remembered that a too complete or too sudden removal of this protection might place the patient in a dangerously vulnerable position should circumstances arise (an attack of bronchitis, for instance) that prevent the proper inhalation of the cromoglycate.

Preparations for the prophylaxis of allergic rhinitis include solutions (Rynacrom and Opticrom respectively) for application to the nose and eyes. Sodium cromoglycate has also been employed with success in some cases of urticaria and of infantile gastrointestinal allergy to milk.

DRUGS THAT BLOCK ADRENALINE α-RECEPTORS

We have already noted (p. 405) that a deficiency of adenyl cyclase might lie at the root of some forms of asthma. This failure of the adrenaline β system leaves the bronchi under the now dominant control of constrictor responses mediated through α receptors. Stimulation of α receptors also promotes mediator release by decreasing the amount of available cyclic AMP. Drugs that effect a blockade of α receptors might therefore be useful in asthma. Preliminary work has indicated that thymoxamine (Opilon) has some bronchodilator activity in asthmatic subjects but that it is not as active in this respect as the adrenaline β agonists. Thymoxamine is most effective (in doses of 200 μg per kilogram of body mass) by the intravenous route and the possibility of its developing into a useful and popular antiasthma drug is not very promising.

DRUGS THAT BLOCK MUSCARINE RECEPTORS

Stimulation of muscarine receptors has much the same effect as α receptor stimulation on both bronchiolar diameter and mediator release from mast cells. There is, moreover, evidence for parasympathetic involvement in the bronchoconstrictor responses in some cases of asthma in children (Cropp, 1975). Antimuscarine agents would therefore be expected to have useful therapeutic possibilities in these cases and atropine has indeed figured in many of the proprietary preparations once offered to asthma sufferers. Taken by mouth, however, effectively bronchodilator doses of atropine produce a number of unwelcome effects (p. 226) that led to its being excluded from antiasthma preparations. It is, however, now staging something of a come back since it was found to be effective, yet innocent of side effects, when taken by inhalation. A related drug is N-isopropylnortropine (ipratropium, Atrovane). It is taken by inhalation in doses of up to 40 μg four times daily and it is used in the treatment of both chronic bronchitis and asthma.

BIBLIOGRAPHY

Books, monographs and reviews

Amos, H. E. (1976). *Allergic Drug Reactions*. London: Edward Arnold.

Brocklehurst, W. E. (1962) Slow reacting substance and related compounds. *Prog. Allergy*, **6**, 539-558.

Brogden, R. N., Speight, T. M. and Avery, G. S. (1974). Sodium cromoglycate (cromolyn sodium): a review of its mode of action, pharmacology, therapeutic efficacy and use. *Drugs*, **7**, 164-282.

Burnet, F. M. (1959). *The Clonal Selection Theory of Acquired Immunity*. Cambridge: University Press.

Burnet, F. M. (1970). *Immunological Surveillance*. Oxford: Pergamon Press.

Cunningham, A. J. (1978). *Understanding Immunology*. New York, San Francisco and London: Academic Press.

Davies, G. E. (1962). Anaphylactic reactions. In *Progress in Medicinal Chemistry*, Vol. 2, pp. 176-198. Ed. Ellis, G. P. and West, G. B. London: Butterworths.

Humphrey, J. H. and White, R. G. (1970). *Immunology for Students of Medicine*. 3rd edn. Oxford and Edinburgh: Blackwell Scientific Publications.

Roitt, I. (1977). *Essential Immunology*, 3rd edn. Oxford, London, Edinburgh and Melbourne: Blackwell Scientific Publications.

Spencer, P. S. J. and West, G. B. (1965). Experimental hypersensitivity reactions. In *Progress in Medicinal Chemistry*, vol. 4, pp. 1-17. Ed. Ellis, G. P. and West, G. B. London: Butterworths.

Various Authors (1967). Delayed hypersensitivity: specific cell-mediated immunity. *Br. med. Bull.*, **23**, 1-97.

Ward, F. A. (1970). *A Primer of Immunology*. London: Butterworths.

Weir, D. M. (1977). *Immunology. An Outline for Students of Medicine and Biology*, 4th edn. Edinburgh, London and New York: Churchill Livingstone.

Wilson, A. F. and McPhillips, J. J. (1978). Pharmacological control of asthma. *A. rev. Pharmac.*, **18**, 541-561.

Original papers

Brogden, R. N., Pinder, R. M., Sawyer, Phyllis R., Speight, T. M. and Avery, G. S. (1975*a*). Beclomethasone dipropionate inhaler: a review of its pharmacology, therapeutic value and adverse effects. I: Asthma. *Drugs.* **10**, 166-210.

Brogden, R. N., Pinder, R. M., Sawyer, Phyllis R., Speight, T. M. and Avery, G. S. (1975*b*). Beclomethasone dipropionate: II: Allergic rhinitis and other conditions. *Drugs.* **10**, 211-217.

Cropp, G. (1975). The role of the parasympathetic nervous system in the maintenance of chronic airway obstruction in asthmatic children. *Am. Rev. resp. Dis.*, **112**, 599-605.

Dale, H. H. (1913). The anaphylactic reaction of plain muscles in the guinea pig. *J. Pharmac. exp. Ther.*, **4**, 167-223.

Engineer, Dinaz M., Niederhauser, U., Piper, Priscilla J., and Sirois, P. (1978). Release of mediators of anaphylaxis: inhibition of prostaglandin synthesis and the modification of release of slow reacting substances of anaphylaxis and histamine. *Br. J. Pharmac.*, **62**, 61-66.

Kellaway, C. H. and Trethewie, E. R. (1940). The liberation of a slow-reacting smooth muscle-stimulating substance in anaphylaxis. *Q. Jl. exp. Physiol.*, **30**, 121-145.

Piper, Priscilla P. (1978). SRS of anaphylaxis. *Ann. R. Coll. Surg.*, **60**, 201-204.

PART III

SYSTEMATIC PHARMACOLOGY

25. Pain and itch

The pharmacologist has a twofold interest in pain. He is concerned on the one hand with the mode of action of drugs which prevent or relieve pain and on the other with the nature of substances which are involved in the production of pain. The physiology of pain and the pharmacology of pain-producing substances are discussed in this chapter. Itch, a condition closely related to pain, is also discussed here. Drugs used in the prevention or treatment of pain form the substance of the three succeeding chapters.

The nature of pain

It is important to remember that pain is a subjective

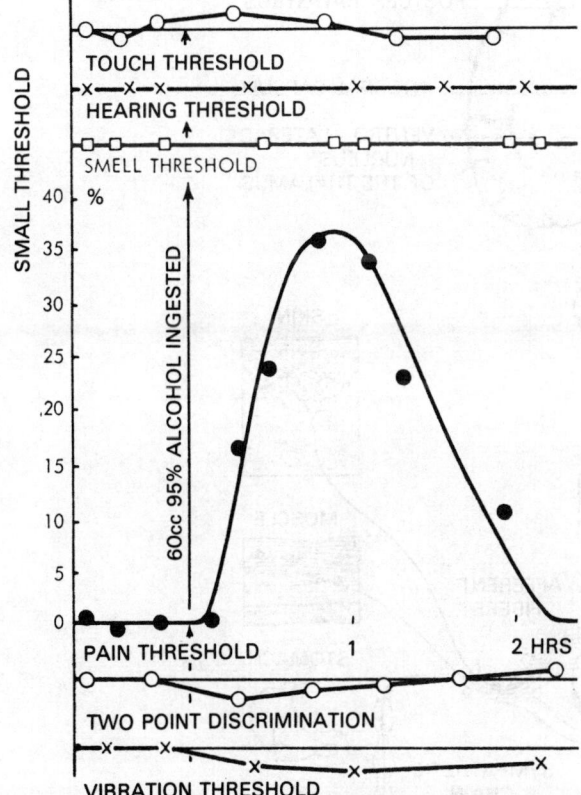

Fig. 25.1 Independence of the sense of pain. Alcohol increased the threshold to pain but not to the other modalities of sensation. Reproduced from *H.G. Wolff and Stewart Wolf, Pain, 1958.* By courtesy of Dr Stewart Wolf and of Charles C. Thomas, (publisher) Springfield, Illinois.

sensation. Like all subjective experiences, it cannot be quantitatively measured with any accuracy. We have, indeed, no real evidence that pain 'feels' the same in others as it does in ourselves. On the other hand, we do know that pain is experienced as a result of the stimulation of identifiable nerve fibres that travel to the brain along well-defined paths. Impulses in these fibres are generated by stimuli that damage the tissues (noxious stimuli) and pain can be regarded as having a *nocifensive* function—that is, it helps the organism to defend itself against harmful stimuli. Noxious stimuli may activate other nocifensive mechanisms. Thus, in the decapitate animal (which cannot experience pain), pinching the foot causes a prompt reflex withdrawal of the limb—a nocifensive reflex. Pain, then, can be defined as the effect produced in consciousness by the arrival in the brain of nerve impulses generated by noxious stimuli. This definition is not entirely satisfactory, since it does not include pain which is experienced in the absence of noxious stimuli. It would be wrong to dismiss this 'central' pain as 'imaginary' since the physical events in the brain that underlie this type of pain are probably the same as those produced by the arrival of nocifensive impulses and pain arising in the absence of damaging stimuli is as real as (and often more agonizing than) pain arising from tissue damage.

Although the actual sensation of pain in response to a given stimulus may vary considerably from one individual to another, the *pain threshold*—the intensity of the stimulus required to cause a just perceptible sensation of pain—is relatively constant among normal people. It is extremely important to recognize that the pain threshold and the intensity of the subjective pain response can alter independently of one another. In some neurological states, for instance, a patient may experience very severe pain even though physiological experiments indicate that his pain threshold is actually increased. In other conditions, pain sensations may be much less intense than usual though pain thresholds are depressed.

If a moderately hot object is placed in contact with the skin the sensation of heat is experienced. If the temperature of the object is progressively increased, the sensation of heat becomes more intense until pain is felt. Experiences such as these might suggest that pain simply arises as a result of excessive stimulation of receptors for the other modalities of sensation. This is not so. The independence of pain sensation is shown by the simple pharmacological experiment illustrated in Fig. 25.1. The ingestion of ethyl alcohol caused a marked increase in pain threshold while the threshold to other sensory stimuli remained unaffected.

Low intensity stimulation of pain receptors produces a sensation rather different from frank pain, since it lacks the latter's quality of unpleasantness. If, for instance, one sits in a bath containing very hot water, the sensation of heat is pleasurable though it certainly has some of the quality of pain. This condition of pleasurable pain has been called 'painless pain' but a better term is *metaesthesia*, proposed by Keele (see Keele and Armstrong 1964). Metaesthesia (*meta*—passing through, *aesthesia*—feeling) properly suggests a transitional state between 'no pain' and unpleasant pain.

The anatomical receptors for pain are bare nerve endings. It now seems likely that bare nerve endings (as well as more specialized receptors) are also involved in the reception of touch, pressure, heat and cold stimuli though these presumably differ from one another, and from those subserving pain, in submicroscopic detail.

The traditional description of the pain sense and of the nerve pathways that subserve it are presented in the following paragraphs but it is now clear that modifications need to be introduced into this simple scheme if all the facts concerning pain and its relief are to be adequately explained. Attempts to provide acceptable modifications are detailed later (p. 423).

Anatomical pathways for pain

Impulses generated by noxious stimuli travel, *via* the posterior spinal roots to the posterior horn of the grey matter in the spinal cord. These fibres form synapses with neurones whose axons cross to the other side of the cord into the lateral white matter, in which they ascend, as the lateral spinothalamic tract, through the cord and brain stem to the thalamus. A smaller number of fibres travel in the anterior white matter as the anterior spinothalamic tract. Sensory fibres in the cranial nerves also pass to the thalamus. From the thalamus a third set of neurones carries the impulses to the postcentral gyrus (Area 3) in the

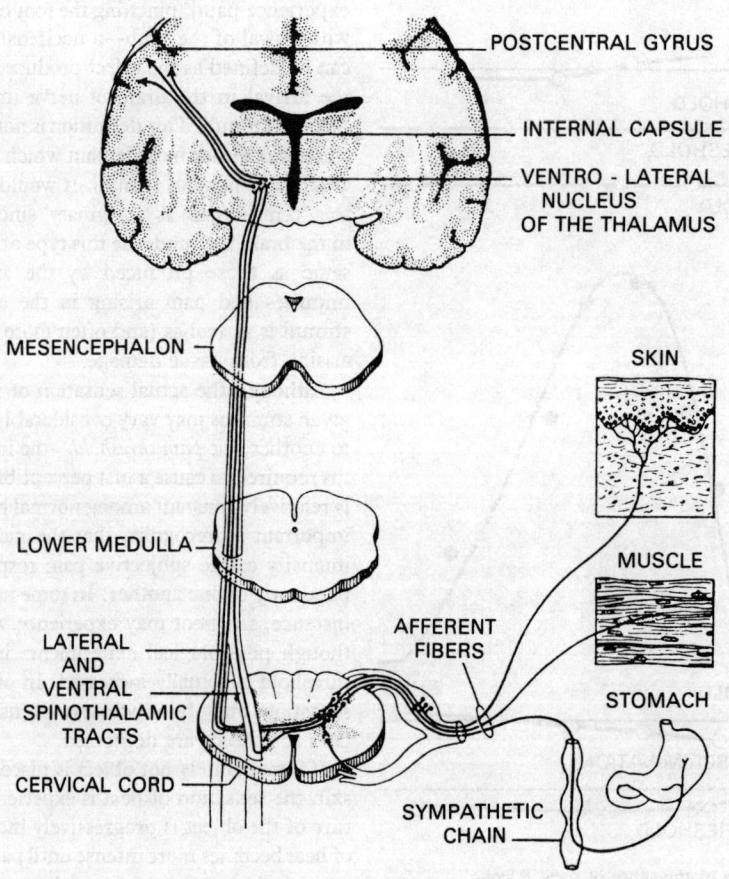

Fig. 25.2 Diagrammatic representation of pathways for pain. (E.H. Broedel after F. Netter). *Reproduced from H.G. Wolff and Stewart Wolf, 1958, Pain by* courtesy of Dr Stewart Wolf and of Charles Thomas, (publisher) Springfield; Illinois.

parietal lobe of the cerebral hemispheres. These pathways are shown in Fig. 25.2

It seems that the cerebral cortex exerts its own influence on the thalamus, limiting the inflow of impulses into the cortex and reducing the intensity of the pain sensation.

Nerve fibres subserving the sensation of pain are of two sizes. Some are large diameter, myelinated, rapidly-conducting fibres (type A in Erlanger and Gasser's classification, see p. 157); others are small, nonmyelinated and slowly-conducting (type C). Thus, when a noxious stimulus excites a group of nerve endings, impulses will arrive at the sensory cortex in two waves, the first along A fibres and the later one (which may be up to 1 sec. later) along C fibres. A consequence of this is that two pains are often experienced in response to a noxious stimulus of short duration. These two pains are of different character: the first, reflecting the sudden arrival of a synchronous burst of impulses, is sharp, intense and 'bright'. The second pain, a reflection of the more dispersed arrival of nerve impulses, is less intense, more prolonged and 'dull' in character. With stimuli of longer duration the two types of pain will be intermingled but one or the other will predominate depending on the distribution of nerve fibre types in the area stimulated and on the nature of the noxious stimuli. Small nerve fibres are more susceptible than large ones to the action of local anaesthetics, so that the 'dull' pain is more easily prevented by these agents than is the 'bright' pain.

Substances causing pain and itch

Many, if not all, pains appear to be caused by the production or liberation of chemical substances by the noxious stimulus. These substances may produce pain in several ways: they may themselves stimulate the nocifensive nerve terminals, they may cause other compounds to do so, they may have a local vascular action or they may cause spasm of visceral muscle.

In the course of his pioneer work into the nature of the local vascular responses to cutaneous irritation, Sir Thomas Lewis observed that itching occurred when histamine was pricked into the skin (Lewis, 1942). In more recent years, it has been found that a large number of other substances cause sensations of pain or itch when they are allowed to come into contact with bare nerve endings. Much of this knowledge results from the work of Keele and his colleagues; more complete details of their work are available in the monograph by Keele and Armstrong (1964).

In the type of experiment designed by Keele a cantharidin plaster is applied to the skin of the forearm and is left in place for about five hours. After a few more hours, a painless blister develops. The blister fluid is removed by a fine syringe, the raised part of the blister is cut away and the exposed blister base is then used for assessing the ability of different substances to produce pain or itch. Substances are applied in a warm isotonic solution at the

physiological pH. The subject grades the intensity of any pain produced on a scale of 0 (no pain) to 4 (very severe pain). As the pain flucturates in intensity, he moves a pointer to the appropriate number of the scale. The pointer is connected to a lever writing on a conventional kymograph which thus produces a record of the time course and intensity fluctuations of the subjective sensation. The type of record obtained is illustrated in Fig. 25.3, which contrasts the sharp pain produced by acetylcholine with the more intense, prolonged and fluctuating pain evoked by a saline extract of rat skin. Keele's method also permits itch to be recorded. For this sensation a scale of 0–2 and another pointer is used. A record of itch is also shown in Fig. 25.3. It can be seen that the rat skin extract produced itch as the intensity of the pain fell. Substances producing pain on application to a blister base can be grouped as follows. The approximate threshold doses of some of the substances are also indicated:

(i) acids (pH less than about 3), bases (pH greater than 11), potassium ions (10 mEq. per litre)

(ii) hyptonic and hypertonic solutions

(iii) *neurohumours:* acetylcholine (10 μg. per ml.), histamine (10 μg. per ml.), 5-hydroxytryptamine (0.1 μg. per ml.), histamine liberators.

(iv) some naturally-occurring polypeptides particularly substance P and the plasma kinins (0.1 μg per ml.).

(v) Although the prostaglandins are not very potent pain producers some of them do potentiate the *algogenic* (pain-producing) action of other substances, particularly the plasma kinins (p. 358), to such an extent that inhibition of prostaglandin

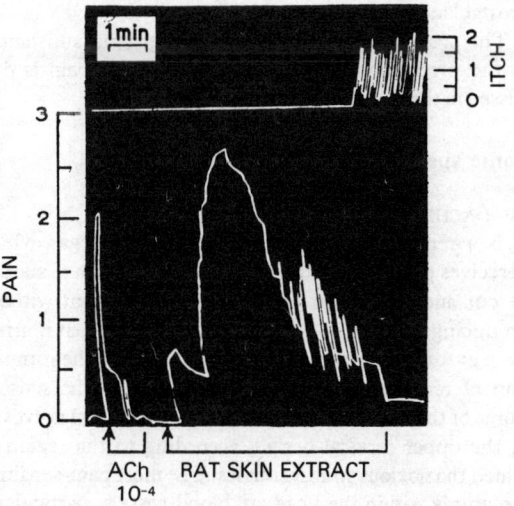

Fig. 25.3 Response of the exposed blister base to acetylcholine and to an extract of rat skin. Reproduced from Desirée Armstrong, R.M.L. Dry, C.A. Keele and J.W. Markham, *J. Physiol.* 1953 **120**, 326-351 by kind permission of the authors and of the Cambridge University Press.

synthesis ensures analgesia even when the kinins are being produced in quantity. This point is discussed in detail in a later chapter (p. 376).

The receptors stimulated by acetylcholine are nicotinic in type: the algogenic action of acetylcholine is not reproduced by acetyl-β-methylcholine or by pilocarpine and it is blocked by tubocurarine and by decamethonium iodide. Nicotine itself first produces pain and then blocks both its own algogenic action and that of acetylcholine. An apparent anomaly is provided by atropine, which prevents the pain-producing action of acetylcholine when both are applied to a blister base. However, the concentration of atropine required (100 μg per ml) is such as to suggest that in this situation it is acting as a local anaesthetic, blocking the conduction, but not the initiation, of impulses.

Histamine produces itching. This has been demonstrated by a large number of workers who have administered it by a variety of routes. Substances that liberate histamine in the skin also produce itching and the itch of urticaria, anaphylaxis and other conditions in which histamine is liberated is undoubtedly caused, at least in part, by this substance. However other substances produce itch and in some experimental situations—for instance, when it is injected intradermally in a concentration of about 1 mg per ml—histamine produces pain. Histamine also produces intense headache by its vascular action (see below).

Since the skin is the site of many injuries, it is important to consider the nature of any pain-producing substances it contains, since they may be liberated by injurious stimuli. Histamine is certainly present in the skin but the substance responsible for producing the pain response illustrated in Fig. 25.3 seems to be a lipid soluble acid, perhaps a prostaglandin-like substance.

The possible role of the individual algogenic substances in the production of some specific types of pain is discussed in the following sections

Some specific types of pain

HEADACHE

It is a remarkable fact that the brain, the organ which perceives pain, is itself insensitive to pain. Brain tissue can be cut and stimulated in the conscious patient without producing any discomfort. Headache, even when it arises from events within the cranial cavity, involves the stimulation of receptors that generate impulses in the sensory fibres of the fifth, seventh, ninth or tenth cranial nerves or in the upper cervical nerves, according to the region in which the noxious stimulus arises. The most pain-sensitive structures within the head are blood vessels, particularly the large venous sinuses and the main branches of the larger arteries. Headache occurs when the vessel walls are stretched either by traction from without or by distension from within. Thus, headache frequently follows the removal of a sample of cerebrospinal fluid for diagnostic

examination. The slight reduction in the volume of fluid allows the brain to slip downwards. In so doing, it pulls on the vessels, which are more securely attached to the skull. That the resulting traction is the cause of the headache is shown by the fact that the headache is alleviated if the patient's bed is tilted head downwards. It is also relieved if the cerebrospinal fluid volume is restored by the introduction of an amount of saline solution equal to that of the withdrawn fluid. Brain tumours produce headache if they are large enough to displace and distort normal tissue and thus to produce tension on the vessel walls.

Many headaches are caused by an active dilatation of blood vessels. The sensitivity of the intracranial blood vessels is illustrated by the action of histamine, which on intravenous injection causes dilatation of cerebral arteries and an intense headache. The headache can be relieved if the dilatation is counteted by increasing the intracranial pressure. A common and disabling form of headache is *migraine*. Its name, which is a corrupted contraction of 'hemicrania' ('half-head') indicates one of the characteristic features of migraine: its restriction to one side of the head or face. Attacks of migraine are commonly preceded by a visual aura, the victim seeing vivid and oscillating zig zag lines separated by black areas. These so-called fortification figures or scintillating scotomas result from *constriction* of blood vessels in the visual areas of the brain and they disappear if small doses of a vasodilator substance such as amyl nitrite are given. The headache of migraine, on the other hand, is attributable to arterial dilatation. Since the aura and the headache of migraine have different underlying causes, they can occur independently of one another. Some people suffer the headache without prodromal symptoms, a few experience the aura but have no headache.

The blood vessels involved in the production of migraine headache are different from those affected by histamine. Migraine cannot be relieved by increasing the intracranial pressure, an indication that the affected vessels are situated outside the skull. They are probably branches of the external carotid artery, for if the carotid artery on the affected side is occluded by pressure on the neck, the intensity of the headache is reduced.

There is good evidence that the vascular dilatation underlying migraine is brought about by the release of a humoral factor. During an attack of migraine there is often localized tenderness as well as headache and it is possible to remove subcutaneous tissue fluid from the area of tenderness. Wolff and his colleagues (Chapman *et al*., 1960) have shown that this fluid contains an active substance ('neurokinin') which is absent in samples collected during a period of freedom from headache. When neurokinin is injected into normal skin it causes vasodilatation and oedema (localized oedema occurs in migraine) and it reduces the pain threshold. It may also have pain producing properties. Its liberation in the tissues of the head would be expected to produce similar effects and pain would result from pressure exerted by the dilated blood vessels on the hypersensitive pain receptors. Any pain producing activity possessed by the neurokinin itself would clearly contribute to the headache but the relief produced by vasoconstrictor agents testifies to the predominant importance of the vascular response. The fluid collected during a migraine headache also contains a proteolytic enzyme capable of producing neurokinin from plasma substrates and it is possible that the circumstances that precipitate an attack of migraine operate by activating the enzyme, perhaps by a nervous mechanism.

Neurokinin itself is a polypeptide. Its identity has not been completely established but its actions are very similar to those of the plasma kinins which are thought to participate in inflammatory reactions (see below). It may well prove to be a mixture of some of these substances.

The possibility has also to be considered that the liberation of 5-hydroxytryptamine is also involved in the aetiology of migraine. Some drugs that antagonize this neurohumour provide relief for migraine sufferers.

Headaches are more severe in hypertensive subjects, since the elevated blood pressure increases the tension exerted by the distended arterial walls.

Continued tension in the muscles of the head and neck such as occurs during prolonged study and which will be exaggerated by any accompanying emotional stress, gives rise to headache as a result of stimulation of pain receptors in the muscles. Tension in eye muscles has similar consequences. In these conditions, the substance stimulating the pain receptors arises as a result of impaired blood flow (*ischaemia*) in the muscles (see below).

The view that constipation can produce headache is unfounded.

MUSCLE PAINS

In some forms of arterial disease, spasm of the arteries in the legs may occur when the patient walks a short distance. This causes pain, which is relieved by a short rest, only to appear again a short time after the walk is resumed. This condition is *intermittent claudication* (from *claudere*—to close), and the pain is again caused by ischaemia. Many other muscle aches are probably the consequence of ischaemia; it is common knowledge that they respond to local warming which will encourage vasodilatation as well as having a counter irritant action. Counter irritation is discussed below. It is an old hypothesis, originally propounded by Sir Thomas Lewis, that muscle pain is attributable to a humoral agent. Lewis himself called it 'factor P' (not to be confused with substance P).

Ischaemia will permit the accumulation of metabolites and possibly the release of cellular constituents. Among the substances possibly responsible for ischaemic muscle pain are lactic acid, adenosine triphosphate and potassium. Potassium will certainly be liberated in pain-producing quantities in more serious conditions when muscle tissue is actually destroyed (*myonecrosis*). One of the most agonizing pains experienced by man is that accompanying coronary thrombosis. The myocardial infarction so produced causes destruction of muscle and liberation of potassium. Other substances derived from cardiac muscle may contribute to the pain. In addition, 5-hydroxytryptamine, a potent pain-producer, is released from platelets, which disintegrate in large numbers.

INFLAMMATION AND INJURY

Tissue damage results in inflammation, oedema and pain. Sometimes the oedema is sufficient in quantity to form blisters. Injury results in the liberation of many algogenic substances such as potassium from the erythrocytes, 5-hydroxytryptamine from the platelets and histamine from the tissues, but a very important source of pain, vasodilatation and oedema are the kinins liberated from plasma, and operating in concert with prostaglandins. The kinins are produced as the culmination of a sequence of events that is initiated by contact of plasma with damaged tissue and which is described in detail elsewhere (p. 359).

It may be that other mechanisms contribute to kinin production. There is considerable evidence for the view that the vascular responses to irritation of the skin are mediated partly by axon reflexes (p. 337). It is, therefore, possible that bradykinin and kallidin are formed by axon reflexes. If the kinins are formed in this way, the chemical mediator of antidromic vasodilatation might give rise to pain directly, as well as indirectly through the kinins. Although the nature of the antidromic mediator is still unknown it is interesting to note that all the compounds that have been considered as possible mediators (substance P, ATP and histamine, p.180) have pain producing properties. It should be added that, whereas vascular dilatation is the most important cause of headache, pain from other parts of the body seems to depend on direct stimulation of the bare nerve endings by algogenic substances, although vasodilatation certainly adds to their effect by reducing pain threshold. Since the evidence suggests that bradykinin and neurokinin are closely related, if not identical, compounds, it must be concluded that the same substance can produce pain by different mechanisms, depending on its site of action.

STINGS AND BITES

A number of animals and plants inject pain-producing substances into their human victims. The nature of these substances (so far as they have been identified) are indicated, for a few offensive species, in Table 25.1 To those whose only previous knowledge of this subject was that ants produce formic acid, the variety of substances mentioned must be surprising. Interest in the active components of stings was stimulated by the demonstration by Emmelin and Feldberg (1947) that acetylcholine and histamine occur in the sting of the common nettle. They suspected that a third substance was present and their suspicion was confirmed when Collier and Cheshire (1956) identified 5-hydroxytryptamine in nettle sting. A report that dock leaves contain a 5-hydroxytryptamine antagonist has never been confirmed. The three substances in the sting, acting in concert, produce the initial sharp pain, histamine produces the blister and itching. It is possible that a fourth substance is present and that this is responsible for the prolonged pain of a nettle sting. The concentrations of acetylcholine, histamine and 5-hydroxytryptamine in mgs per ml of nettle hair fluid, are of the order of 10, 1 and 0.5 respectively. These concentrations thought high (contrast them with the amounts in brain tissue) are low in comparison with those found in the venom of the hornet, another species which makes use of these neurohumoral substances. In hornet venom, acetylcholine and histamine reach concentrations of up to 40 mg per gram; 5-hydroxytryptamine is present in about one half of this amount.

It can be seen by reference to Table 25.1 that some stings and venoms, including some which cause agonizing pain (those of the weever fish and the black widow spider, for instance) do not contain acetylcholine, histamine or 5-hydroxytryptamine. Moreover, those which do contain these compounds usually have other components which evoke a longer lasting pain than do the neurohumoral substances, whose action is relatively evanescent. Many of these other pain-producing substances arise as a consequence of the tissue destruction which is the end to which the venomous activities of the more offensive organisms are directed.

These other pain-producing substances can be grouped as follows:

(i) kinins or kinin-liberating substances
(ii) phospholipase which splits lysolecithin from phospholipids. Lysolecithin causes histamine release from the tissues and it disrupts mast cells which will liberate their contained 5-hydroxytryptamine.
(iii) proteolytic enzymes and non-enzymatic protein toxins which break down tissue, liberating potassium from muscle, bradykinin from plasma, etc. Haemolysins affect only blood cells, causing haemolysis and the liberation of potassium.

In addition to the pain-producing substances proper, stings and venoms may contain hyaluronidase which facilitates the dispersal of the injected material

Counter irritants

In order to make intense pain more tolerable, the sufferer

Table 25.1 Algogenic and pruritogenic substances in some stings and venoms (Based on information in Keele & Armstrong, 1964)

	Formic acid	Acetyl-choline	5-hydroxy-tryptamine	Histamine	Histamine liberators (phopholipase)	Kinins or kinin producers	Unidentified toxic proteins or peptides	Others
Common nettle		+	+	+			+?	proteolytic enzyme (?)
Itching powder		+						proteolytic enzyme 'mucunain'
Stinging ant						Kinin former(?)		
Red ant	+							
Scorpion			+				+	haemolysin proteolytic enzyme hyaluronidase
Spider							+	proteolytic enzymes trypsin activator
Snake					+			hyaluronidase proteolytic enzymes etc.
Bee			+	+	+		+	hyaluronidase
Wasp		+	+	+		+		
Hornet	+	+	+	+		+		
Jelly fish					+			slow reacting substance
Octopus		+	+	+			+	
Weever fish							+	

will bite his lips or clench his fists, digging his nails into the palm of his hand. The elevation of the pain threshold achieved by this means is most satisfactorily explained on the basis of the 'gate theory' that is expounded below (p. 423). For our present purpose all that needs to be said is that the phenomemon is a particular example of the general one of *extinction*: the elevation of the threshold to one type of sensory stimulus if another is applied at the same time.

Counter irritants, which are applied to skin to relieve deep-seated pain, operate on the same principle. They can all cause pain, though they are most effective when they are applied in a form which does not provoke frank pain. A prominent feature of counter-irritant action is vasodilatation: this produces a comfortable feeling of warmth and it may also affect the more deep-seated tissues and so permit the dispersal of pain producing substances. Both these effects add their contribution to the general sensation of increased comfort evoked by the extinction effect.

The use of counter irritants dates from antiquity and a large number of physical agents have been employed for this purpose. Radiant heat, hot water bottles, short wave diathermy and galvanic electrical currents are the modern representatives of these ancient remedies. Similarly a large number of chemical irritants have been used: a few survivors are described below.

Substances which irritate the skin are conventionally divided into *rubefacients* (which cause redness), *vesicants* (which cause blistering) and *pustulants* (which cause more severe irritation with pus formation). The vesicants and pustulants cause too much pain and damage to be of therapeutic value, though they were extensively used in the past. They have also been employed as offensive weapons: mustard-gas (p. 913) achieved notoriety in this respect in the 1914-18 war. The difference between rubefacients, vesicants and pustulants is one of degree: a rubefacient applied to the skin in a sufficiently high concentration for a sufficiently long period of time will cause blistering, a dilute solution of a pustulant applied briefly will cause simple reddening of the skin and so on.

Cantharidin, a vesicant, is a lactone obtained from cantharides which consists of a dried beetle (*Cantharides vesicatoria*) also known as the Spanish fly. Cantharidin is severely irritant when taken internally; it causes vomiting, purging and severe pain. Any absorbed from the gastrointestinal tract is excreted unchanged in the urine, causing irritation of the kidney and urinary tract. Urethral irritation accounts for the reputation cantharidin once had as an aphrodisiac.

Capsaicin

Capsaicin is a crystalline compound obtained from various species of *Capsicum* many of which are well-known for their use as spices. Chillies (red peppers) are the fruit of the species *Capsicum minimum*. The hot taste of chillies arises from the ability of their contained capsaicin to stimulate taste, pain and heat receptors in the mouth. When applied to the skin, capsaicin produces a sensation of 'burning' pain. In experimental animals it has also been shown to stimulate other sensory endings—vagal stretch receptors in the lungs, chemoceptors in the heart and lungs, the carotid sinus receptors and so on. Since acetylcholine also has this ability to stimulate a wide variety of receptors, it is natural to enquire whether capsaicin produces pain by stimulating acetylcholine receptors in the bare nerve endings. Jancsó and his colleagues (quoted by Keele and Armstrong, 1964) have investigated this problem. They found that if nerve endings were desensitized to acetylcholine by nicotine or by hexamethonium, they still responded to capsaicin. On the other hand, if the endings were selectively desensitized to capsaicin by repeated local applications of the drug, the nerve endings no longer responded to acetylcholine. The easiest interpretation of these results is that stimulation of capsaicin receptors is a necessary intermediate event between stimulation of acetylcholine receptors and the generation of sensory nerve impulses. If this is so, the nature of the capsaicin receptors and of their normal physiological stimulus becomes of considerable theoretical importance. This is underlined by the observation, also by Jancsó, that the parenteral administration of capsaicin will desensitize the pain receptors of rats and guinea pigs to all algogenic compounds throughout the body. This desensitization is very long lasting, persisting for months or years. The animals remain sensitive to other sensory stimuli and also to pain produced by physical stimuli.

The pain-producing effect of capsaicin is intensified if the area to which it has been applied is heated. This suggests that it may cause the formation or release of other pain-producing substances. The vasodilatation produced

Nonylic acid
vanillylamide

Cantharidin

by capsaicin will also sensitize the nerve endings to its own irritant action.

Nonylic acid vanillilamide is similar in its properties to capsaicin.

Methyl salicylate also known as oil of wintergreen is an ingredient of many proprietary rubefacient ointments and liniments. Methyl salicylate is too irritant and too toxic for internal use as a salicylate: absorption also takes place through the skin and the drug should be used with some caution. A number of other salicylates have been used as rubefacients.

Methyl salicylate

Esters of nicotinic acid include among others, tetrahydrofurfuryl nicotinate, ß-butoxyethyl nicotinate and benzyl nicotinate.

Tetrahydrofurfuryl nicotinate

ß-Butoxyethyl nicotinate

Benzyl nicotinate

Camphor is a rubefacient and is used in the form of liniment of camphor B.P. (camphorated oil), and other preparations to relieve painful conditions of the joints and muscles.

Mustard. Black mustard seeds contain a glycoside, sinigrin, and when the seeds are crushed and moistened, the glycoside undergoes enzymatic hydrolysis with the formation of allyl isothiocyanate. It is this substance (also called volatile oil of mustard) which is responsible for the irritant properties of mustard plasters. The enzyme present in the seeds is called myrosin. Mustard is irritant to mucous membranes and if taken internally in large quantities it causes vomiting. A suspension of mustard in tepid water is sometimes employed in emergencies as an emetic.

White mustard seeds contain myrosin and a glycoside (sinalbin) which is chemically related to sinigrin; its properties and actions are similar to those of black mustard.

Other counter irritants include oil of turpentine, iodine and various expensive proprietary preparations. Some of the latter contain ephedrine, adrenaline or histamine (as well as a rubefacient) on the superficially sound principle that they will increase skin or muscle blood flow. The likelihood that they do so when applied topically in this way is remote.

Referred pain

Disease processes in certain viscera produce pain which appears to originate in the body wall some distance away from the diseased organ itself. Thus in the early states of appendicitis, pain is felt in the region of the umbilicus; in attacks of angina pectoris pain may be felt, not in the chest overlying the heart but in the arm; in gall bladder disease pain may be felt in the tip of the right shoulder. The pain originating in the organ is, in fact, 'referred' to another area of the body. The anatomical basis of referred pain is simple: afferent nerves from the stimulated organ enter the spinal cord at the same point as those from the region of the body to which the pain is referred. Since the healthy individual often experiences pain as a result of minor injuries to the body surface, the brain interprets all pain impulses entering a particular segment of the spinal cord as originating from the appropriate part of the body surface. The reason why nerves from a viscus and from a relatively distant area of the body may enter the cord at the same point is a consequence of the differential growth of the viscera and the body wall during embryonic development. Not all visceral pain is referred, since not all organs move relatively to the part of the body wall in whose area they originally developed.

It appears that in attacks of referred pain, non-painful stimuli from the area of the body to which pain is referred actually contribute to the pain. If a local anaesthetic is infiltrated into the skin of the shoulder, pain from a diseased gall bladder is alleviated. It may be that the impulses from the diseased viscus sensitize the central nervous system to impulses arriving by that route so that impulses such as those initiated, for instance, by the pressure of clothes become painful. The situation is the opposite of that in counter irritation, when pain, or near pain, is deliberately produced in the body wall to *relieve* pain in deep-seated structures. In the latter instance the inflow of impulses into the cord is intense enough to 'swamp' those from the viscera.

The treatment of pain

Intractable pain is sometimes treated surgically. The appropriate posterior spinal roots can be cut near their entrance to the cord (the operation of *rhizotomy*); the spinothalamic tracts can be sectioned (*cordotomy*) or localized regions of the thalamus can be destroyed by electro-

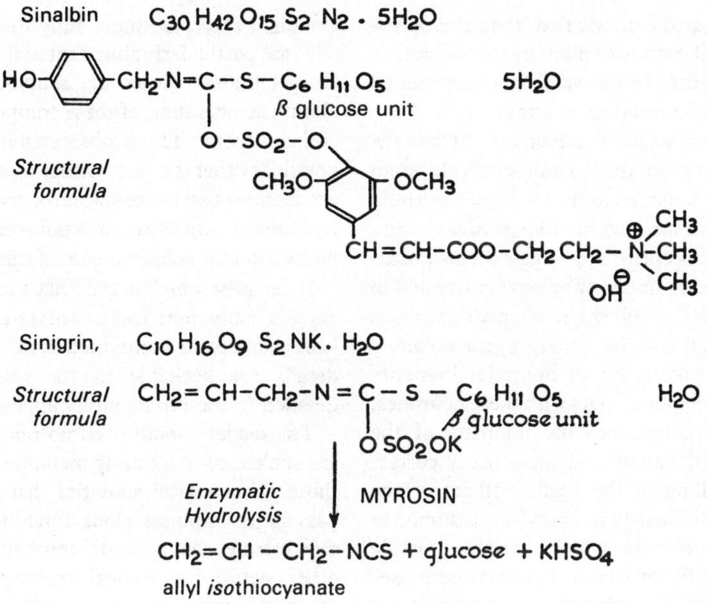

Sinalbin $C_{30}H_{42}O_{15}S_2N_2 \cdot 5H_2O$

$$HO-\langle\ \rangle-CH_2\text{-}N=C-S-C_6H_{11}O_5 \qquad\qquad 5H_2O$$
$$\overset{|}{O-SO_2-O}\qquad\beta\ glucose\ unit$$

Structural formula

$$CH_3O-\overset{OCH_3}{\underset{}{\langle\ \rangle}}$$

$$CH=CH\text{-}COO\text{-}CH_2\ CH_2-\overset{\oplus}{\underset{\underset{OH}{\ominus}}{N}}\overset{CH_3}{\underset{CH_3}{\diagup}}CH_3$$

Sinigrin, $C_{10}H_{16}O_9S_2NK \cdot H_2O$

Structural formula

$$CH_2=CH\text{-}CH_2\text{-}N=C-S-C_6H_{11}O_5 \qquad\qquad H_2O$$
$$\overset{|}{O\ SO_2OK}\qquad\beta\ glucose\ unit$$

Enzymatic Hydrolysis   MYROSIN

$$CH_2=CH-CH_2\text{-}NCS\ +\ glucose\ +\ KHSO_4$$

allyl *iso*thiocyanate

Fig. 25.4

coagulation. Rhizotomy is rarely performed, since section of the posterior roots leads to the loss of all sensation from an area of skin and muscles. Since the proper performance of skilled movements depends on a continued flow of impulses from the proprioceptors of the muscles and joints, rhizotomy has a more extensive disabling effect than might be thought. Rhizotomy can, however, be used for treating trigeminal neuralgia, a condition in which even slight stimulation of the face may bring on an almost unbearable pain. Cordotomy is more satisfactory than rhizotomy, since apart from pain, only the sensations of heat and cold (which travel by the same pathway as pain) are lost. Thalamotomy is technically difficult. Leucotomy (p. 166) was a relatively common method of relieving intractable pain when that operation was in vogue. It is usually said that the operation did not reduce the pain felt by the patient, only the reaction he made to the pain—'he no longer worried about the pain'. It is difficult to see what is meant by statements such as these, since the 'reaction to the pain' is in fact an integral part of the subjective sensation we call pain. It is true that leucotomy does not reduce pain threshold but, as we have pointed out earlier, the sensation of pain is not necessarily determined by the pain threshold. Moreover, it is just possible that some impulses from the viscera (but not from the body wall) pass to the frontal lobes and were cut when leucotomy was performed. It is certainly true that leucotomy was more successful in relieving pain from internal organs than that from the body wall. This, of course, may be partly attributable to the fact that we can see lesions of our body wall and are well aware whether or not they are improving. If leucotomy does interrupt some sensory impulses from the

viscera, this would not be reflected in the pain threshold, which is measured by applying stimuli to the skin. (p. 460)

Resort is made to surgery for the symptomatic relief of pain only when the underlying clincial condition is one that will not itself yield to surgery and when it is deemed inadvisable to condemn an active and otherwise healthy patient to a lifetime of taking high doses of analgesic drugs.

In most instances, pain is prevented or relieved by drugs. *Anaesthetics*, as their name implies, block all forms of sensory stimulation. They find their principal use in preventing the pain of surgical operation. General anaesthetics operate centrally and cause unconsciousness; local anaesthetics block nerve fibres in the area in which they are applied. *Analgesics* selectively impair the appreciation of pain. Anxiolytic drugs (p. 561) are also useful in calming the patient and reducing the stress and worry associated with pain.

The 'gate' theory of pain

Up to this point, pain has been discussed entirely in terms of the classical theory of sensory perception according to which specific stimuli evoke nerve impulses that travel by specific routes and give rise to specific sensations, the intensity of which is determined by the impulse frequency in the afferent pathways. Although an application of the classical theory yields explanations of pain phenomena that are superficially satisfactory, a closer study reveals deficiencies in the classical description that have led to the emergence of more sophisticated ideas concerning pain sensation. The best known and most cogently argued of these newer hypotheses is that due to Melzack and Wall (1965) and known generally as the gate theory. It is necessary to point out at the outset that, though impressive, the gate theory still convinces more by the theoretical arguments in its favour than by the weight of experimental evidence that has been adduced in its support.

Briefly, the gate theory asserts that pain arises when the inflow of nervous activity into the thalamo-cortical system that subserves this sensation exceeds a critical threshold value. This inflow is regulated, within the nervous system, by processes that are conceptualized as gates. It is postulated that some of the more important gates are situated in the substantia gelatinosa, a collection of small neurones that caps the posterior horn of the spinal grey matter along its whole length. The posterior root fibres (or branches from the roots) make synaptic contact with these neurones, the activity of which determines the intensity of the impulse traffic to the thalamus and the sensory cortex. Nerve impulses travelling in the smaller fibres of the posterior roots (the traditional 'pain fibres') are assumed to facilitate this onward traffic (they 'open the gates') while impulses in the larger fibres (those that carry impulses generated by stimulation of touch and pressure receptors) tend, it is supposed, to 'close the gates'. Thus the gate theory provides a ready explanation of the fact, already alluded to, that we can blunt our pain sensation by deliberately stimulating our touch and pressure receptors as we do, for instance, if we grip the arms of the dentist's chair. It also at least partly explains the relief from pain that can undoubtedly be provided by acupuncture. The beneficial effect of stimulating nerves subserving the sensations of touch and pressure has, in recent years, been profitably exploited to provide some relief to sufferers from intractable pain whose misery has not been alleviated by cordotomy or for whom that operation was deemed to be inadvisable. They have been provided with equipment that permits them to stimulate at will by way of indwelling electrodes the nerve tracts in the posterior white matter of the spinal cord. These fibres carry impulses subserving the sensations of touch and pressure but when they are electrically stimulated the intensity of pre-existing pain is often reduced to a welcome extent. Stimulation of the periaqueductal grey matter has the same effect.

Other influences also operate the neural gates. In particular, nerve impulses descending from higher centres of the brain can 'open' or 'close' gates in the spinal cord and, presumably, in other locations such as the thalamus. It has, for instance, long been known that certain lesions of the thalamus give rise to the *thalamic syndrome* in which trivial stimuli, not usually regarded as pain producing, give rise to feelings of intense pain. It seems that the nerve lesion has interrupted descending impulses that operate to prevent too wide an opening of the gates.

Considerable interest has been evoked in recent years by the finding that analgesic substances, pharmacologically similar to morphine, occur naturally in the central nervous system. There is evidence that these endogenous compounds (which are more fully discussed in Chap. 26, p. 437) are particularly abundant in the region of the substantia gelatinosa. Moreover, acupuncture seems to bring about the liberation of these compounds from nerves that contain them. These observations raise the intriguing possibility that the endogenous morphine-like compounds act as transmitter substances (or modify the action of other transmitter substances) at a point or points along the nerve pathways that subserve gate closing activity.

It is to be emphasized that the gate theory serves to explain many more features of the activity of pain mechanisms than can be mentioned in this brief account. Further details are available in the appropriate monographs detailed in the bibliography appended to this chapter.

The reader should need no reminder that neural gates are spoken of in a purely metaphorical sense to represent those physiological activities that promote or inhibit the passage of impulses along functional pathways and that they feature, though in different guises, in explanations of other neurophysiological phenomena. Thus, ion flow across the membrane of nerve fibres can be quantitatively expressed in terms of the activity of a group of four gates located in channels through which the ions flow (p. 157).

The measurement of pain in man and animals
This topic is discussed in Chapter 27 (p. 460).

ITCH

Itch (or *pruritus*) arises only in skin. The itch receptors are the most superficial of the slow pain fibres and they produce the sensation of itching when they are lightly stimulated. Tickling is allied to itch and it occurs when the itch producing stimulus moves rapidly from spot to spot.

Since itch arises from stimulation of pain fibres, it is not surprising that many of the substances that produce pain in experimental situations are also capable of provoking itch. Under normal conditions, however, some substances are more likely to cause itching than others, presumably because they are liberated in, or are injected into, the most superficial layers of the skin.

Histamine is the best-known itch-producing substance and itching caused by histamine release can be a distressing side effect of several otherwise very useful drugs. (p. 342).

Potent though histamine is as a pruritogenic agent, other compounds also provoke itch. Itching powder, the schoolboys' favourite, (which consists of the trichomes of cowhage, *Mucuna prurians*) contains neither histamine nor a histamine liberator. It does contain 5-hydroxytryptamine but its principal pruritogenic component is a proteolytic enzyme called, because of its origin, mucunain. It presumably liberates an itch-producing substance (not necessarily histamine) as a result of its proteolytic action.

Other proteolytic enzymes produce itch if they are administered intradermally or applied to an exposed blister base. Many stings and venoms contain proteases (Table 25.1) which must contribute to the irritation they produce. Bradykinin may also cause itching.

Itching occurs in certain diseases such as diabetes mellitus and obstructive jaundice. The responsible agents have not yet been clearly identified.

BIBLIOGRAPHY

Books and monographs

Haddington, Edda (1974). *Migraine.* London: Priory Press
Keele, C. A. and Armstrong, D. (1964). *Substances Producing Pain and Itch.* London: Arnold.
Keele, K. D. (1957). *Anatomies of Pain.* Oxford: Blackwell.
Lance, J. W. (1969). *The Management and Mechanism of Headache.* London: Butterworths
Lewis, T. (1942). *Pain.* New York: Macmillan.
Melzack, R. (1973). *The Puzzle of Pain.* Harmondsworth: Penguin.

Prescott, F. (1964). *The Control of Pain.* London: English Universities Press.
Wolff, H. G. (1948). *Headache and other Head Pain.* London: Oxford University Press.
Wolff, H. G. and Wolf, S. (1958). *Pain,* Springfield, Ill.: Thomas.

Original papers

Chapman, L. F., Ramos, A. O., Goodell, H., Silverman, G. and Wolff, H. G. (1960). A humoral agent implicated in vascular headache of the migraine type. *Archs Neurol., Chicago,* **3**, 233.
Collier, H. O. J. and Chesher, G. B. (1956) Identification of 5-hydroxytryptamine in the sting of the nettle. *Br. J. Pharmac.,* **15**, 290-297.
Emmelin, N. and Feldberg, W. (1947). The mechanism of the sting of the common nettle. *J. Physiol.,* **106**, 440.
Macarthur, J. G. and Alstead, S. (1953). Counter-irritants. A method of assessing their effect. *Lancet* **2**, 1060.
Melzack, R. and Wall. P. D. (1965). Pain mechanisms: a new theory. *Science.* **150**, 971-979.
Mendell, L. M. and Wall, P. D. (1965). Presynaptic hyperpolarization: a role for fine afferent fibres. *J. Physiol.,* **172** 274-294.

26. Morphine and related analgesics

The analgesic properties of opium have been recognized since the dawn of history and it is not surprising that man, whose life until quite recently has been dominated by misery and pain, seized upon opium as a God-given gift sent to relieve the sufferings of his mind and body. The most important constituent of opium is morphine, a drug which has been responsible for easing the pain of millions who would otherwise have suffered in agony. Unfortunately the qualities of morphine that brought not only analgesia but also a leavening of happiness into the lives of our forefathers are those that are likely to induce drug dependence (p. 86), a state that is less acceptable in today's complex and highly conforming society than it was in the past. It is of no importance in those dying from an incurable disease and it is unlikely to arise in those who have received single injections of morphine to relieve the acute and distressing pain of, say, severe trauma or a cardiac infarct. It does, however, preclude the extended use of morphine in less serious conditions. For this reason, a large number of compounds related to morphine has been synthesized in efforts to produce drugs which, while possessing the analgesic strength of morphine, do not cause dependence. As we shall see, this aim has been partly realized.

Morphine and its congeners are often known collectively as the 'narcotic' or the 'strong' analgesics, but neither of these terms is entirely satisfactory. It is difficult to state precisely what is intended by 'narcotic'. Literally, it means 'sleep-producing' but not all hypnotic substances are classified as narcotics. Because the word was first applied, in its literal sense, to morphine, it was later used to describe other analgesics with similar properties. One of the most characteristic properties of these substances, as we have already hinted, is their ability to produce drug dependence and 'narcotic' was extended to include some other (but by no means all) of the drugs that cause dependence. Until recently, it could have been said, indeed, that narcotic had become virtually synonymous with 'addictive' or 'drug of addiction' (cf. the Narcotics Bureau in the United States). However, as is explained elsewhere (p. 86) the word addiction itself falling into disuse, since it can no longer be adequately defined. The position is further complicated by the fact that morphine derivatives with little tendency to produce dependence are now known. A word whose meaning was never very clear has evidently outlived its usefulness and 'narcotic' should, in the writer's opinion, be abandoned.

Although morphine and some related drugs are capable of relieving extremely severe pain, others are less active in this respect. Thus, not all of the drugs related to morphine can justifiably be called strong analgesics. In this book, therefore, the designation *morphine-like* is used instead of 'narcotic' or 'strong'.

Another and entirely different class of drugs combine analgesic with antiinflammatory activity. They are, in general, weaker than morphine and, because their action is predominantly peripheral and not central, they do not produce sedation, euphoria or dependence. They are suitable for relieving pain in a wide variety of conditions including some for which the morphine-like analgesics have been traditionally used. These analgesics as a class are often referred to as non-narcotic analgesics. However, if 'narcotic' is an unsuitable term, so equally is 'non-narcotic'. Nor is it accurate to describe them as 'weak' analgesics since some members of the group are more effective than some of the less potent morphine derivatives. The archetypal member of the group is aspirin and we shall adhere in this book to the term 'aspirin-like' to describe these analgesics.

Aspirin-like analgesics and antiinflammatory agents form the subject of the next chapter (p. 440).

Morphine

If the unripe seed capsules of the poppy (*Papaver somniferum*) are opened, a milky juice exudes which solidifies in the air to give opium. The word opium is itself derived from the Greek for juice. Opium was certainly known and used in the third century B.C., but there is some evidence that it was employed as early as 4000 B.C. Throughout its long history, opium has been used for both its analgesic and its psychotropic effects but opium smoking is not, apparently, as ancient a practice as is sometimes believed,

Morphine

since there is little evidence that it was indulged in before the eighteenth century.

A tincture of opium is known as laudanum: it was first prepared in the sixteenth century. It was very popular as an analgesic until quite recently, as readers of Victorian novels will know. It also provided a ready source of opium for the addict—the so-called opium eaters were usually laudanum drinkers.

The identification of the active constituents of opium began in the early years of the nineteenth century. The first to be isolated was morphine (Morpheus is the God of sleep) but its structure was not elucidated until 1925. Morphine is present in opium to the extent of about 10 per cent. The other alkaloids of opium are noscapine (6 per cent.) and papaverine (1 per cent.) with smaller amounts of codeine, thebaine and narceine.

The principal results of morphine administration in man—and those for which it and opium have been most widely used in the past—are analgesia, euphoria and constipation.

Therapeutic doses of morphine cause drowsiness or sleep. If the patient remains awake, he usually finds concentration difficult and he may be mentally confused. The relief of pain and the subjective effects of morphine (which cause a sensation of detachment from the physical world) combine to produce euphoria in the previously distressed patient. The desire to recall this euphoric state was the immediate cause of many cases of morphine dependence when the drug was more widely used than it is today. When morphine is given (in preanaesthetic medication, for instance) for the first time to patients who are not in pain, the sense of detachment is often less pleasant and a distinct *dysphoria*—a sense of anxiety and uneasiness—may be produced.

Morphine causes depression of respiration (particularly in man) and it also depresses many spinal reflexes. It is clear, therefore, that it is essentially a central nervous system depressant but its actions are not uniformly inhibitory in type. It stimulates the chemoceptive trigger zone (though it depresses the vomiting centre proper) and therapeutic doses of morphine sometimes produce nausea or vomiting. The related compound, apomorphine (p. 600) is a powerful emetic agent. The 'Straub tail' produced in mice (p. 138) is also a manifestation of morphine's central stimulant action. Morphine causes release of the antidiuretic hormone and it sometimes produces hyperglycaemia. These two effects are manifestations of hypothalamic stimulation. The effect on body temperature, however, is variable, depending on the species and dose. Morphine usually produces hyperthermia in cats and hypothermia in dogs. It slows the heart, probably by a direct stimulant action on the vagus centre.

In many mammalian species, morphine causes constriction of the pupil. This is particularly marked in man in whom morphine produces characteristically 'pin point' pupils. This tightly constricted pupil is seen even in those who have otherwise become tolerant to the effects of morphine. It is central in origin but it is not known whether it results from a direct excitation of the parasympathetic component of the oculomotor nucleus (the Edinger-Westphal nucleus) or from a depression of a centre that normally restrains activity in that nucleus. In the cat and monkey morphine causes pupillary dilatation.

All the stimulant effects we have so far mentioned are seen with therapeutic doses of morphine: higher doses produce signs of more generalized excitation, including restlessness and perhaps convulsions. In cats, this generalized excitation is seen after quite small doses and every experimental pharmacologist is taught that attempts to sedate a cat with morphine will lead to the production of a frightened and wildly excited animal. On rare occasions, therapeutic doses of morphine produce excitement in the human subject.

Constipation is a regular consequence of morphine administration and preparations of opium have been used for the treatment of diarrhoea for at least as long as they have been employed as analgesics. Morphine reduces the motility but increases the tone of gastrointestinal smooth muscle with closing of the sphincters. The dose required to cause these effects is smaller than that which produces analgesia. Morphine also reduces the glandular secretions of the digestive tract. These actions extend to associated structures such as the pancreas (whose secretions are diminished), the gall bladder and the bile duct (the sphincter of Oddi is contracted). As a result of the operation of all these factors, gastric emptying is delayed, the rate of passage of the intestinal contents is reduced and more time is available for the absorption of water. Solidification of the intestinal contents is further promoted by the reduced volume of secretions. One potentially hazardous consequence of the gastrointestinal actions of morphine should be noted. If the victim of an accident who is given morphine to relieve his immediate pain has recently eaten a meal, his stomach emptying will be delayed. If he then needs emergency surgery, he may have to be anaesthetized while his stomach is still full. The anaesthetist must be aware of, and should guard against, the risk that his patient will regurgitate gastric contents, some of which may be aspirated into the lungs.

In addition to its actions on the nervous system and gut, morphine stimulates the uterus, dilates the capillaries and tends to cause constriction of the bronchi.

When morphine is used as an analgesic over a period of time, the constipation produced can be regarded as a side effect. Another common side effect is itching, particularly of the nose and cheeks. It is usually assumed that this is attributable to the release of histamine but not all workers accept this explanation, even though morphine is known to be a powerful histamine liberator (p. 342). The itching caused by morphine is prolonged, while histamine release is usually completed in a very short time. Alternative explanations for the origin of the itch are not very satisfactory. It seems unlikely that morphine, as some have suggested, lowers the threshold for itching as a result of its central action, since itch and pain are subserved by similar mechanisms and morphine certainly raises the pain threshold. A reduction of the threshold for itch by a peripheral action cannot be entirely excluded, since morphine causes cutaneous vasodilatation with sweating. The areas affected—the face and neck—are similar to those in which itching occurs.

Therapeutic uses of morphine

Morphine is the prototype of the 'strong' analgesics. The therapeutic uses to which it has been put will be considered in this section. The particular advantages of the newer derivatives and analogues are detailed later.

First and foremost, morphine has been valued for its unsurpassed ability to relieve pain. The fact that physical dependence on the drug is a very likely consequence of its continued administration demands that extreme caution should be exercised before morphine is prescribed. Many cases of morphine dependence in the past were the direct result of injudicious administration of the drug to patients whose emotional condition was such that dependence was even more easily produced than in the normal subject. To use recent terminology, these cases of dependence were of *iatrogenic* origin (literally 'produced by the physician'). Another disadvantage of morphine is that if it is given to a subject who has suddenly collapsed with acute pain, it may, by removing the pain, erase a vital diagnostic sign. It is an axiom of medical treatment that morphine should not be given in acute conditions until the diagnosis has been established, although in some instances the administration of small doses of morphine may actually assist diagnosis by relieving the patient's distress and enabling him to give a more coherent history of his condition. Neither of the disadvantages mentioned provides sufficient grounds for withholding morphine in all circumstances. In the dying patient whose pain has not responded to other analgesics, there is clearly no justification in denying him the solace provided by morphine. Moreover, drug dependence is less likely to occur when morphine is given by mouth rather than parenterally and small doses are less prone to produce dependence than larger ones. Mixtures of small doses of morphine with other analgesics, 'tranquillizers', sedatives or antispasmodics are valuable in a variety of conditions. Acute pain, postoperative discomfort and labour are all states in which the use of morphine (or one of the newer morphine-like drugs) may be justified. In patients with biliary colic, the analgesic effect of morphine must be weighed against its constricting action on the sphincter of Oddi which may cause an increase in intravesicular pressure and an aggravation of the pain. The concurrent administration of an antispasmodic agent is an obvious way of avoiding this complication. Morphine itself should not be given to women in labour. It causes respiratory depression and the foetus is even more susceptible than the mother. Some of the newer morphine-like drugs such as pethidine (p. 430) are less liable to cause respiratory embarrassment.

For the relief of extreme pain in victims of myocardial infarction (coronary thrombosis) and serious accidents of all types, morphine is a boon.

By the subcutaneous route, 10 mg of morphine (usually as the sulphate) is often sufficient to relieve severe pain in the adult patient. In emergencies of extreme gravity, up to 20 mg may be required and the dose may have to be repeated within an hour. When taken by mouth, the action of morphine is more prolonged than it is by the parenteral route but much higher doses have to be taken to produce the same analgesic effect.

In the treatment of diarrhoea, opium rather than morphine itself is used. Powdered opium or tincture of opium is given in oral doses containing the equivalent of about 10 mg of morphine.

A facet of morphine's depressant action on the respiratory centre is that it suppresses cough. This is sometimes a useful and sometimes a troublesome effect in patients whose condition otherwise demands morphine. There is no justification in using morphine primarily as an antitussive agent but codeine has been used for many years for the treatment of cough.

Side effects and toxic reactions to morphine

Itching and constipation have already been mentioned as common side effects of morphine administration. Because it releases histamine, the subcutaneous injection of morphine sometimes causes the production of weals. In some instances, skin reactions are more extensive, suggesting that an allergic response has occurred. Morphine should not be. given to patients suffering an attack of asthma. Nausea and vomiting caused by stimulation of medullary centres and dizziness due, perhaps, to a transient hypotension have also been reported. Morphine dependence is described in detail elsewhere (p. 86).

The lethal oral dose of morphine is at least 120 mg and accidental overdosage is not very common. In acute morphine poisoning, there is coma; respiratory depression may be extreme. The co-existence of severe respiratory depression and pin point pupils is almost pathognomonic of morphine poisoning but when the respiratory depression is so severe that tissue oxygenation is being seriously interfered with, the pupils may become dilated because energy is no longer available for maintaining contraction of the circular muscle of the iris. The most important measures to be adopted in the treatment of acute morphine poisoning are the establishment of effective artificial respiration and the administration of one of the morphine antagonists, (p. 434). They are given intravenously and

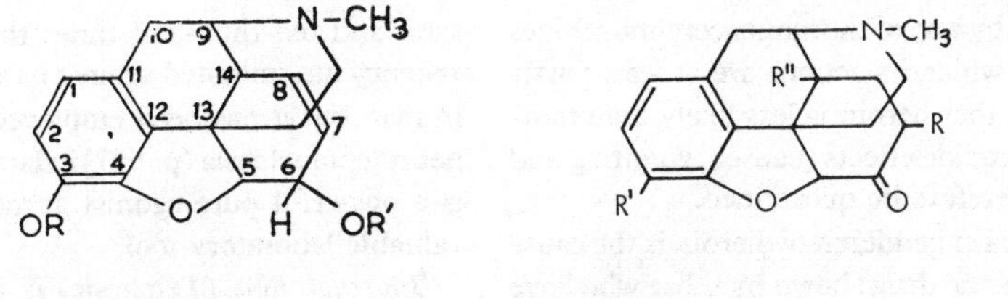

R = R' = H, morphine
R = CH₃, R' = H, codeine
R = CH₃, R' = H, single bond at 7-8: dihydrocodeine
R = R' = CH₃, double bond at 5-6: thebaine
R = C₂H₅, R = H, ethylmorphine
R = R' = COCH₃, diacetylmorphine

R = H, R' = OCH₃, R″ = H dihydro-codeinone
R = H, R' = OH, R″ = H dihydro-morphinone
R = CH₃ R' = OH, R″ = H metopon
R = H, R' = OH, R″ = OH oxymor-phone
R = H, R' = OCH₃, R″ = OH oxy-codeine

Fig. 26.1 Morphine and some naturally occurring and semisynthetic congeners.

their effectiveness is such that it has been asserted that if a dose of 15 to 20 mg of nalorphine does not cause a significant improvement in the patient's condition, the diagnosis of morphine poisoning should be questioned.

MORPHINE-LIKE COMPOUNDS

Constituents of opium

CODEINE
The structure and properties of codeine (methylmorphine, Fig. 26.1) are very similar to those of morphine into which codeine is converted in the body by demethylation. Its analgesic, euphoriant and respiratory depressant activities are low but its ability to suppress cough is relatively less inferior to that of morphine. Codeine is a useful antitussive agent and it is also used to relieve diarrhoea. The usual dose for these purposes is 10 to 60 mgs repeated as necessary at intervals of 4 to 6 hours. Large doses of codeine can produce physical dependence but it is not very popular among addicts. Nevertheless, even if it is marginal, the drug's ability to produce dependence should be recognized.

Although it is not a very powerful analgesic, codeine, particularly in association with aspirin or paracetamol (or both) finds its way into a number of popular analgesic preparations. Compound Codeine Tablets (which contain codeine phosphate, phenacetin and aspirin) were once widely used but are no longer recommended in view of their content of phenacetin, a drug whose toxicity is now well established, particularly when it is given with aspirin.

THEBAINE
The small differences in chemical structure between morphine and thebaine (Fig. 26.1) are associated with marked differences in pharmacological activity. Thebaine is virtually devoid of analgesic and other central depressant actions but it has excitatory properties and can produce

convulsions reminiscent of those caused by strychnine. Some thebaine derivatives, however, are powerful analgesics (p. 430). It has already been seen that morphine has both excitatory and inhibitory actions and it is clear that their relative intensities can be altered by small structural changes in the molecule.

PAPAVERINE, NOSCAPINE AND NARCEINE
Morphine, codeine and thebaine are all phenanthrene derivatives. In addition to possessing central actions, they all produce some degree of muscle spasm. The other three alkaloids of opium are benzylisoquinoline derivatives. They have depressant actions on the central nervous system but they cause relaxation of smooth muscle. Papaverine, indeed, is used as a vasodilator drug and noscapine (narcotine) is a cough suppressant.

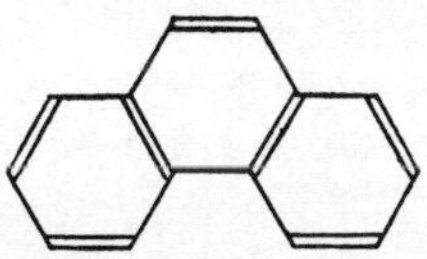

Phenanthrene

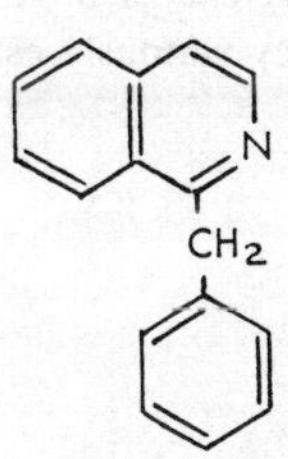

Benzylisoquinoline

Semisynthetic compounds
These substances are obtained by producing small changes in the structure of the naturally-occurring alkaloids.

DIACETYLMORPHINE
Diacetylmorphine (diamorphine, heroin) is a stronger analgesic than morphine. It is also a more powerful depressant of the respiratory and cough centres and it produces a more intense euphoria. Its duration of action is rather shorter. These purely quantitative differences between morphine and heroin are attributable to the ease with which the latter drug crosses the blood brain barrier.

Heroin is metabolized by way of the monoacetylmorphines to morphine through which its actions are at least partly mediated. Statements that heroin is less likely than morphine to cause systemic side effects (nausea, vomiting and constipation) must therefore be questioned.

The intense euphoria engendered by heroin is the cause of both the craving for the drug shown by those who have become dependent on it and the readiness with which dependence develops. The import and manufacture of heroin is now forbidden in many countries (including the United States) but many clinicians believe that heroin still has a valuable, if limited, place for relieving pain in the terminal stages of fatal diseases if morphine is contraindicated for any reason. When given by subcutaneous injection, the therapeutic dose of heroin is 5 to 10 mg repeated, if necessary, at three-hourly intervals. Liquid preparations (elixirs) of heroin with cocaine or with cocaine and chlorpromazine are available for oral administration.

OTHER MORPHINE DERIVATIVES
Dihydrocodeine, dihydromorphinone (hydromorphone, Dilaudid), dihydrocodeinone (hydrocodone, Codone, Dicodid, Hycodan), oxymorphone (Numorphan) and methyldihydromophinone (metopon) all have generally similar properties to morphine itself. Their chemical formulae are indicated in Figure 26.1.

THEBAINE DERIVATIVES
The oripavines (Fig. 26.2) are thebaine derivatives and are therefore to be regarded, formally at least, as semisynthetic compounds. They are numbered among the most recently developed morphine-like compounds.

Etorphine is a very powerful analgesic drug with a potency variously estimated as being between one thousand and ten thousand times that of morphine. Its very potency has militated against its acceptance as an analgesic in man but it has been employed to secure analgesia and neuroleptanalgesia (p. 507) in large animals and, because it is a powerful pure agonist at morphine receptors, it is a valuable laboratory tool.

Buprenorphine (Temgesic) is at least fifty times more potent than morphine in animal tests and it has a longer duration of action. It is used in parenteral (intramuscular or intravenous) doses of 0.2 to 0.6 mg to relieve postoperative or postinfarction pain. Median doses give analgesia that persists for about six hours.

The cyclopropylmethyl group in buprenorphine confers morphine antagonist properties on the molecule (see below, p. 434) that become evident at doses greater than about 1 mg. For this reason, patients are unlikely to become dependent on the drug. Buprenorphine does not exhibit the psychotomimetic activity that mars some other compounds that would otherwise be therapeutically useful by virtue of their possessing both agonist and antagonist properties. Side effects of buprenorphine treatment include drowsiness (this has been reported in 70 per cent of treated patients) and, much less frequently, nausea and vomiting.

Buprenorphine is metabolized by N-dealkylation and glucuronidation, the metabolites being excreted primarily in the bile.

Diprenorphine is a powerful and specific morphine antagonist. It has not yet been employed clinically.

Synthetic compounds
PETHIDINE AND RELATED COMPOUNDS
Pethidine (meperidine) is one of the most widely used of the 'strong' analgesics. Its popularity is reflected in the

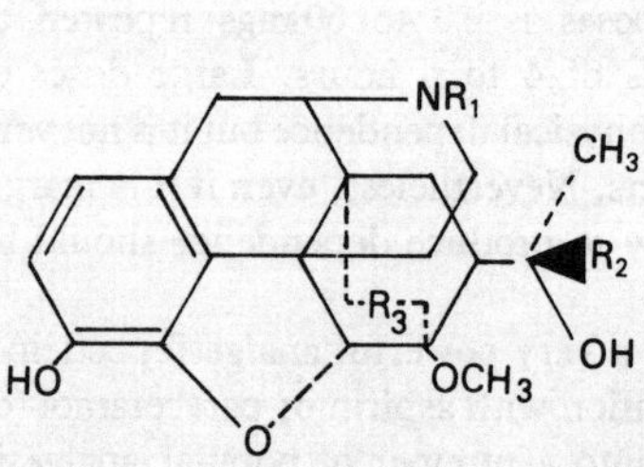

	R₁	R₂	R₃
Etorphine (Agonist)	CH_3	$(CH_2)_2CH_3$	$CH=CH$
Buprenorphine (Partial agonist)	$CH_2CH\langle{}^{CH_2}_{CH_2}$	$C(CH_3)_3$	CH_2CH_2
Diprenorphine (Agonist)	$CH_2CH\langle{}^{CH_2}_{CH_2}$	CH_3	CH_2CH_2

Fig. 26.2 The oripavines

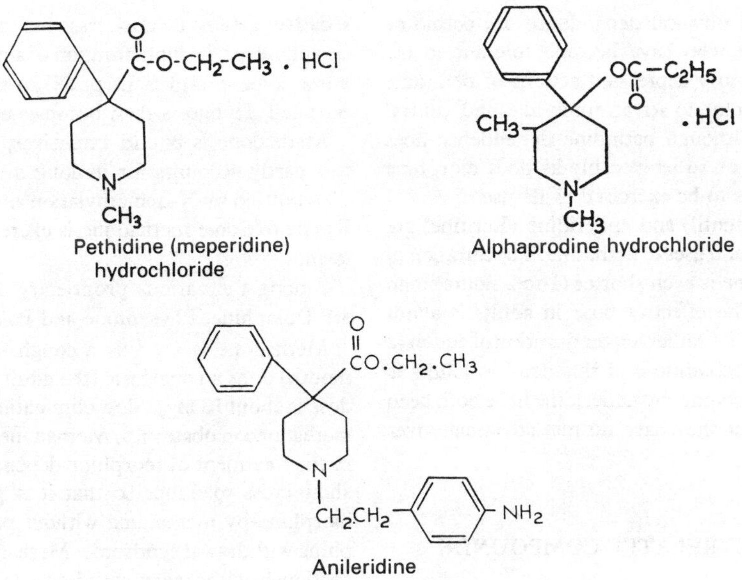

Fig. 26.3 Pethidine and some related compounds.

multiplicity of proprietary names under which it is supplied. These include Dolantin, Dolosal, Demerol and Isonipecaine.

Pethidine was originally developed (in 1939) as an antispasmodic and it has some atropine-like properties. It soon became evident, however, that it was more valuable as an analgesic. Like many other atropine-like substances, pethidine has some local anaesthetic activity but this property has not been exploited since pethidine can cause irritation when it is applied locally.

Pethidine has very similar properties to morphine: it even has a contractile action on smooth muscle which overrides the spasmolytic action conferred by its atropine-like properties. It causes pupillary constriction rather less readily than does morphine, presumably because of its antimuscarine action. In general, pethidine is rather more likely than morphine to produce excitatory side effects. Nervousness, hallucinations, muscle twitches and frank convulsions have all been reported. Other side effects include feelings of weakness, dizziness and fainting. These are the result of a transient vasodilatation which may be caused either by histamine release or a short-lived ganglion blockade. Thirst and dryness of the mouth are manifestations of pethidine's atropine-like actions.

Although excitatory side effects are not uncommon after toxic doses of pethidine, profound depression of the nervous system with respiratory depression and coma is also seen. These variable responses arise partly at least from the fact that the excitatory effects of pethidine are caused by the demethylated metabolite (norpethidine). The actions of pethidine itself are more purely depressant so that the final state of excitation of the nervous system is

determined by the relative amounts of norpethidine and pethidine present.

Even low doses of pethidine sometimes produce alarming side effects in patients who are also receiving monoamine oxidase inhibitors. These compounds inhibit both the N-demethylation of pethidine and the hydrolysis of norpethidine. Consequently their administration concurrently with pethidine can cause either violent excitation or a deep coma. These exaggerated side effects provide evidence of yet another incompatibility between monoamine oxidase inhibitors and common drugs. Respiratory depression tends to be very marked if pethidine and a phenothiazine are given together.

Pethidine has a much shorter duration of action (2 to 4 hours) than morphine. This is an advantage when the drug is used as an analgesic in labour, since respiratory depression in the foetus or new born infant is not so prolonged as it would be if morphine were used. A further advantage of pethidine as an obstetric analgesic is its relative lack of inhibitory action on the uterine musculature. Pethidine is also used to remove apprehension in those about to undergo surgery and it is useful in the relief of postoperative pain. In the latter instance its brief duration of action constitutes a disadvantage since repeated injections of the drug may be necessary. The therapeutic dose of pethidine is 100 mg by the subcutaneous or (preferably) the intramuscular route. Pethidine is usually rather less effective by mouth.

Pethidine has no antitussive action, it does not induce sleep and, by reason of its spasmogenic action on the sphincter of Oddi, its use is contraindicated in patients with biliary colic.

Tolerance to, and physical dependence on, pethidine does occur. Patients who have become tolerant to the analgesic and respiratory depressant actions of pethidine are usually not tolerant to its atropine-like and central excitatory effects. Although pethidine dependence does not arise so readily or so irrevocably as does morphine dependence, care has to be exercised in its use.

Alphaprodine (Nisentil) and anileridine (Leritine) are similar in properties and uses to pethidine. The duration of action of alphaprodine is even shorter (1 to 2 hours) than that of pethidine. The effective dose in adults is about 50 mg. Anileridine has a rather longer duration of action (2 to 3 hours). The effective dose of this drug in adults is about 50 mg. Alphaprodine and anileridine have both been used in obstetrics but they have no real advantage over pethidine.

METHADONE AND RELATED COMPOUNDS

Methadone (amidone Fig. 26.4) and morphine have very different structures but very similar properties. In comparison with morphine, methadone is a slightly more potent analgesic and a considerably more powerful depressant of the respiratory and cough centres. Methadone, like

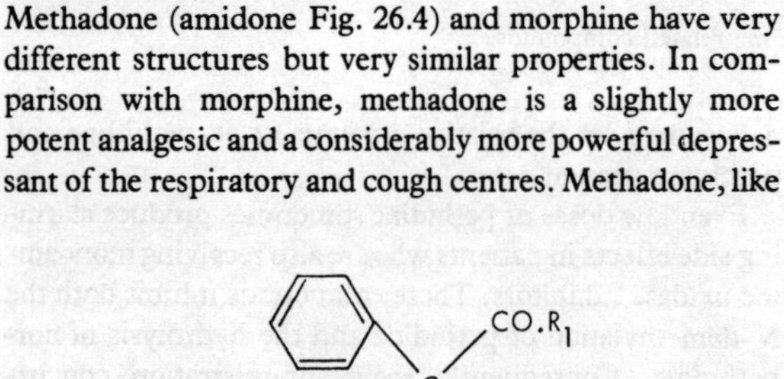

R	R_1	R_2
Methadone	C_2H_5	$-CH_2.CH.N(CH_3)_2$ / CH_3
Isomethadone	C_2H_5	$-CH(CH_3)CH_2N(CH_3)_2$
Dipipanone	C_2H_5	$-CH_2.CH(CH_3)N$
Phenadoxone	C_2H_5	$CH_2.CH(CH_3)N$ O
Dextromoramide	$-N$	$CH(CH_3)CH_2N$ O

Fig. 26.4 Methadone and some related compounds.

pethidine, relaxes smooth muscle in isolated preparations but in the intact animal it increases intestinal tone and delays intestinal emptying. It may thus cause constipation but in this respect it is less powerful than morphine. Its

sedative action is also less well marked than that of morphine but its long duration of action (3 to 4 hours) may allow some cumulation (p. 68) to take place if doses are repeated. Hypnosis then becomes evident.

Methadone is bound extensively to tissue protein and this partly accounts for its long duration of action. It is metabolized by N-demethylation and by cyclization of the R_2 chain. Some methadone is excreted in the unchanged form.

Among the various proprietary names for methadone are Dolophine, Physeptone and Polamidon.

Methadone is used as a cough suppressant (2 mg by mouth) or as an analgesic (the adult oral or intramuscular dose is about 10 mg). Slow elimination precludes the use of methadone in obstetrics. Methadone finds a valuable place in the treatment of morphine dependence. The two drugs show cross tolerance so that it is possible to substitute morphine by methadone without precipitating the morphine withdrawal syndrome. Methadone can then itself be cautiously withdrawn: withdrawal symptoms are mild and easily dealt with (p. 87).

Unlike the other analgesics so far discussed, methadone is as active by mouth as it is by parenteral injection.

Dipipanone (Pipadone), dextromoramide (Palfium) and phenadoxone (Heptalgin) have properties and uses similar to those of methadone itself. A preparation containing dipipanone and cyclizine (p. 347) goes under the name of Diconal.

The side effects of methadone and its congeners are similar to those listed for pethidine. A few cases of a paranoid psychosis with hallucinations have been reported among those taking the drugs, the most recent involving dipipanone (Bound and Greer, 1978).

DEXTROPROPOXYPHENE

Dextropropoxyphene (propoxyphene) is structurally similar to the methadone derivatives just described. It is rather more active by parenteral injection than it is by the oral route but it is available in a combined form with other analgesics for oral administration.

Combined preparations of dextropropoxyphene hydrochloride with paracetamol or with amylobarbitone are marketed as Distalgesic and Doloxytal respectively. Depronal is a sustained release preparation of the hydrochloride. Doloxene is the proprietary name for dextropropoxyphene napsylate and this compound, together with aspirin, also appears in Dolasan and Napsalgesic.

Dextropropoxyphene is given in single doses of 50 to 100 mg whether it is used alone or as one member of a combined preparation. The dose is customarily given three or four times daily but Depronal needs to be taken (in amounts of 150 mg) no more frequently than once every twelve hours or so. Propoxyphene is employed for the relief of moderate pain which does not respond to aspirin or for patients who cannot tolerate the salicylate. The incidence of toxic side effects is low and drug dependence is only occasionally produced. Nevertheless, it must be remembered that dextropropoxyphene does have essentially the same actions as morphine. Tolerance of and physical dependence on the drug are easily produced in experimental animals: that dependence is not more often seen in human subjects is a reflection of the fact that dextropropoxyphene does not normally induce a significant degree of euphoria.

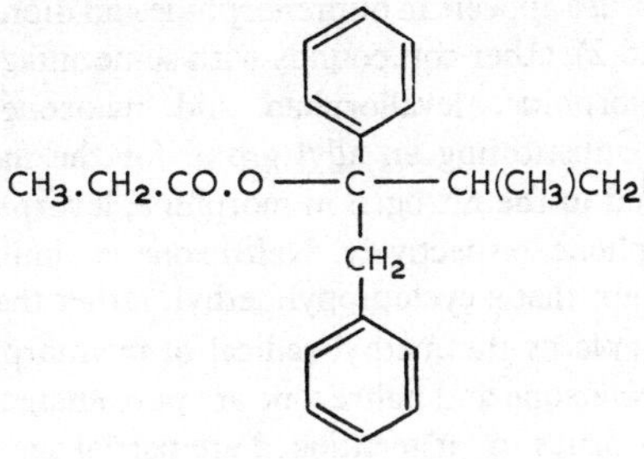

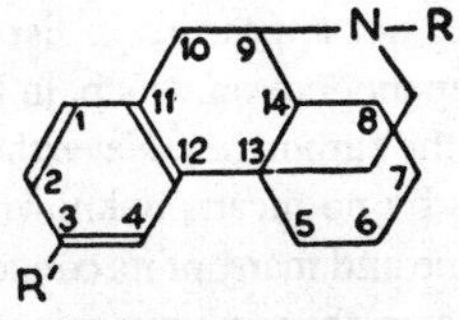

R = R′ = H,   morphinan
R = CH_3, R′ = OH, . levorphanol

Fig. 26.5

Dextropropoxyphene

Dextropropoxyphene is sometimes taken with suicidal intent and cases of poisoning have been reported with increasing frequency in recent years. Morphine antagonists provide the best antidote.

MORPHINAN DERIVATIVES

Morphinan (Fig. 26.5) has little or no analgesic activity but some of its derivatives are very potent.

Levorphanol (levorphan, methorphinan, Dromoran) has similar properties to morphine but it is about twice as potent. The dextrorotatory form has no activity and the racemic form (racemorphan) is consequently equipotent with morphine.

Levorphanol, unusually among compounds related to morphine, is as active by mouth as it is by parenteral routes. A single oral dose (1 to 5 mg) is effective for up to eight hours. A useful analgesic agent (with all the advantages and disadvantages of morphine) levorphanol has also been used as an adjunct to nitrous oxide anaesthesia.

BENZOMORPHAN DERIVATIVES

Benzomorphan itself is devoid of analgesic properties but many of its derivatives, the most important of which are shown in Figure 26.6, have morphine like properties. In addition, pentazocine displays some and cyclazocine a considerable degree of antagonist activity. Cyclazocine, indeed, is properly classified as a morphine antagonist. Pentazocine and cyclazocine are, in receptor terminology, partial agonists.

Phenazocine (Narphen) is a more powerful analgesic than morphine but dependence develops relatively slowly. Oral (5 to 20 mg) and parenteral (1 to 3 mg) doses have analgesic effects that persist for up to six hours. A useful feature of phenazocine's actions is its minimal tendency to cause spasm of the sphincter of Oddi so that it can be recommended for the treatment of biliary pain.

Pentazocine (Fortagesic, Fortral, Talwin) is rather less powerful an analgesic than phenazocine but it is considerably more active than pethidine and, because it has antagonist as well as agonist activity, its tendency to induce dependence is very small: indeed, pentazocine (unlike

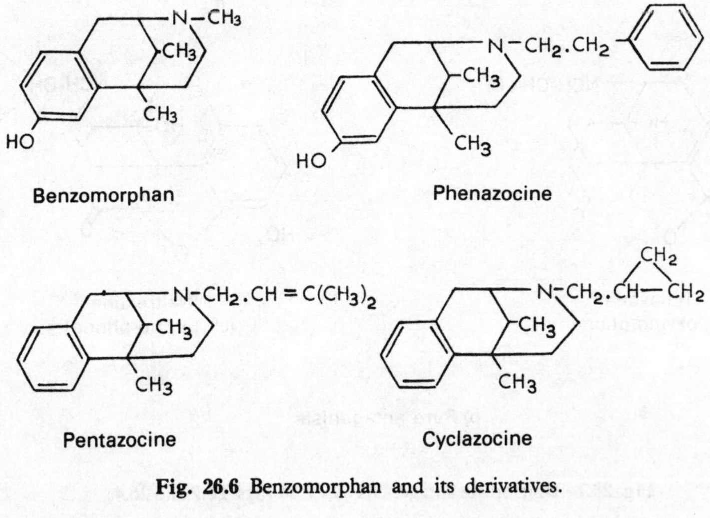

Benzomorphan

Phenazocine

Pentazocine

Cyclazocine

Fig. 26.6 Benzomorphan and its derivatives.

phenazocine) does not appear in the list of morphine like drugs detected dependence on which, in Britain, demands registration with the authorities. Nevertheless dependence on pentazocine is by no means unknown.

Unlike morphine and many of its congeners which have depressant actions on the cardiovascular system, pentazocine causes, through peripheral catecholamine release, increases in the heart rate and blood pressure. Although these changes are small in extent, some authorities believe that they may constitute a hazard if pentazocine is given injudiciously to victims of recent myocardial infarctions.

Visual hallucinations, sometimes with paranoid delusions, are sometimes experienced by those who have taken pentazocine. Some other partial agonists at the morphine receptor have psychotomimetic activity that prevents their being the valuable analgesic agents they would otherwise certainly be. Side effects are otherwise similar to those recorded for pethidine.

Like phenazocine, pentazocine does not cause spasm of the biliary ducts so that it can be usefully given to patients with biliary colic. Otherwise its therapeutic uses are similar to those of pethidine.

Adult doses by mouth and parenterally are the order of 50–100 mg and 30–60 mg respectively. Doses may have to be repeated at three to four hourly intervals.

MORPHINE ANTAGONISTS

Apparently trivial changes in the structure of a morphine like compound can bring about marked changes in its properties. In particular the agonist molecule can be converted into a partial agonist or a pure antagonist. We have already seen that this transformation can be effected in the case of the phenazocine molecule by replacing the phenylethyl group attached to the nitrogen by allyl or cyclopropylmethyl substituents (Fig. 26.6). The last named group also appears in buprenorphine and diprenorphine (Fig. 26.2), other compounds with some antagonist activity. Nalorphine, levallorphan and naloxone are obtained by substituting an allyl group for the methyl group attached to the nitrogen in morphine, levorphanol and oxymorphone respectively. Naltrexone is similar to naloxone except that a cyclopropylmethyl, rather than an allyl group replaces the methyl radical of oxymorphone (Fig. 26.7). Naloxone and naltrexone are pure anatgonists but the other drugs so far mentioned are partial agonists.

NALORPHINE
In 1915 and 1916 respectively, Pohl and von Braun showed that N-allylnorcodeine was a morphine antagonist. These observations aroused little or no interest until 1941 when

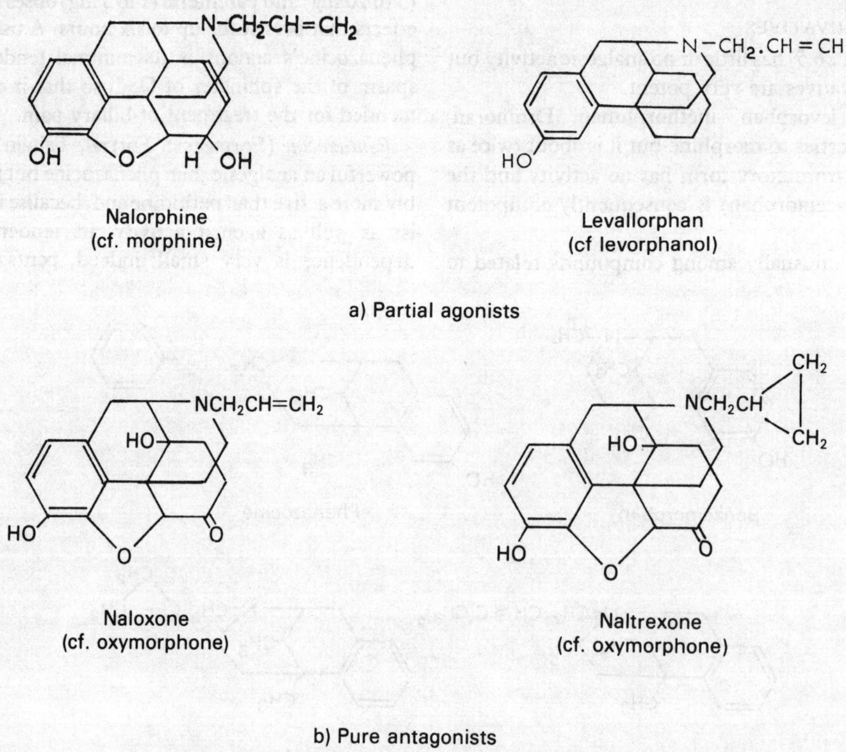

Nalorphine
(cf. morphine)

Levallorphan
(cf levorphanol)

a) Partial agonists

Naloxone
(cf. oxymorphone)

Naltrexone
(cf. oxymorphone)

b) Pure antagonists

Fig. 26.7 Some opiate antagonists (*See also* Figs. 26.2 and 26.4).

N-allylnormophine (nalorphine; Lethidrone; Nalline) was synthesized and shown to be a powerful morphine antagonist.

Used alone, nalorphine has morphine-like properties. Thus it is an analgesic, a respiratory depressant and a cough suppressant and it causes constriction of the pupils. On the other hand, it causes relaxation rather than tonic contraction of intestinal muscle and it produces dysphoria more regularly than does morphine. The dysphoria may be associated with dreams or hallucinations, often of an unpleasant nature. Physical or psychological dependence on nalorphine is unknown but it is not possible to use the drug as an analgesic because of the dysphoria it induces.

Morphine-like when given alone, nalorphine is a morphine antagonist in animal or human subjects who have already received morphine. It antagonizes almost all the actions of morphine, although in some species one or more actions may be resistant. In man, for instance, it has been reported that nalorphine does not antagonize the antidiuretic, cough suppressant and hypothermic effects of morphine and its congeners. When nalorphine is given to subjects who have developed morphine dependence, a typical morphine withdrawal syndrome is precipitated.

LEVALLORPHAN

Levallorphan (Lorfan) has similar properties to nalorphine except that it has only trivial morphine-like activity. It is some three times as powerful a morphine antagonist as nalorphine.

NALOXONE AND NALTREXONE

Because it is not an agonist, naloxone (Narcan) has virtually no action in individuals who are not dependent on an opiate. Since it does not depress the respiratory centre, no harm is done if naloxone is given in fruitless attempts to revive respiratory activity in patients whose depressed respiration is erroneously believed to be the result of an opiate overdose. Under these circumstances, partial agonists such as nalorphine might further (and perhaps fatally) depress the respiration. Naltrexone resembles naloxone in its properties and uses.

Therapeutic uses of the opiate antagonists

The opiate antagonists are valuable restorative agents in cases of poisoning with any of the morphine like agents. It must, however, be noted that while nalorphine and levallorphan will reverse the action of morphine and the other agonists they (being partial agonists themselves) are useless when the poisoning is the result of an overdose of one of the partial agonists such as pentazocine. The effects of this latter class of drug are countered only by a 'pure' antagonist such as naloxone. The antagonists are given by slow intravenous injection: initial doses of 0.5 (naloxone), 1.0 (levallorphan) or 5.0 mg (nalorphine) may be repeated at four-minute intervals, as required, but if respiratory movements do not show early signs of revival, the suspi-

cion must be aroused that the toxic signs arise from causes other than an opiate overdose. As we have already noted, the repeated administration of a partial agonist is likely to aggravate the respiratory embarrassment caused by any agent other than a 'pure' agonist.

Opiate antagonists are particularly useful in obstetrics if the mother has received a morphine-like analgesic during labour. If they are given just before delivery, the baby's respiratory centre will not be depressed at the vital time when independent respiration is needed. The antagonists can also be given to the baby immediately after delivery by injection into the umbilical vein. The method has the obvious advantage that it does not impair the analgesia in the mother for which the morphine-like drug was originally given.

The subcutaneous injection of nalorphine (3 mg) or levallorphan (1 mg) is also used in the diagnosis of morphine dependence. Within half an hour of the injection, addicted patients will usually exhibit the morphine abstinence syndrome. The method has the obvious disadvantage that it produces an extremely distressing condition in the patient. A description of the likely consequences of nalorphine injection is, if graphic enough, often sufficient to induce the patient to confess to his addiction and thus to render the injection unnecessary. A less horrific version of this manoeuvre is the nalorphine pupil test. A subcutaneous injection of 3 mg of nalorphine causes a measurable dilatation of the pupil in those under the influence of an opiate analgesic. This dilatation appears within an hour or so of the injection.

MODE OF ACTION OF THE MORPHINE LIKE ANALGESICS

There can be no doubt that, in contradistinction to the aspirin-like compounds, morphine and its congeners produce analgesia by an action on the central nervous system. The euphoria and other signs of excitation and depression induced by the opiates bear adequate witness to this central action and more formal experiments provide unequivocal evidence that these drugs relieve pain by modifying the response to, rather than the initiation of, nociceptive nerve impulses.

Part of morphine's action is referable to its ability to reduce the anxiety and distress associated with pain. It achieves this by a direct action on the limbic system (p. 167) and on structures (particularly the frontal lobes of the brain) associated with it. In this latter respect, it has the same kind of action as alcohol or prefrontal leucotomy (p. 166), an operation that was, in the quite recent past, not infrequently performed for the relief of chronic and otherwise intractable pain.

However important the actions of morphine on the highest centres may be, it seems to be established that it also depresses activity in the pain pathway. It has a clear analgesic effect in human volunteers when the pain-producing stimulus is a simple pin prick which is hardly likely to cause anxiety or worry. Similarly, it inhibits the overt responses of animals to many of the simple physical stimuli used in the laboratory (p. 461). The elevation of pain threshold is quite specific, since morphine does not alter the perceptive threshold for two-point tactile discrimination, hearing, smell, touch or vibration. Some increase in visual threshold has been reported after prolonged administration of morphine.

Considerations of structure-action relationships among the large number of available morphine like compounds and the close structural similarities between the morphine antagonists and the corresponding agonists strongly suggest that the opiates exert their effects by interacting with specific receptors. An early hypothesis concerning the gross features of the postulated morphine receptor was that by Beckett and his associates (Beckett and Casy, 1954). In general terms this representation of the receptors is still valid and the structure of many of the newer analgesic agents would enable them to be accommodated on this kind of receptor surface (see, for example, Bentley and Lewis, 1972). Beckett and Casy proposed that the aromatic part of the molecule is held to the flattened part of the receptor by Van der Waal's forces (Fig. 26.8). Alongside this is a hollow which accommodates the two carbon link between the tertiary nitrogen and the quaternary carbon. Finally, an anionic site holds the basic part of the analgesic molecule which is assumed to be ionized at physiological pH values. The orientation of the three components of the receptor explains the stereospecificity of the morphine like analgesics.

It is far easier to postulate than it is to demonstrate the existence of a specific receptor but advances made in recent years have revealed that the opiate receptor is much more than a useful concept.

As we have seen, among the opiates and their antagonists, only the *laevo* enantiomers are pharmacologically active. Goldstein suggested that parts of the brain carrying opiate receptors could be identified by incubating a suitably labelled opiate with a homogenate of nervous tissue in the presence of an excess of either levorphanol or its inactive *dextro* isomer (dextrorphanol). Binding to the opiate receptors would be prevented by levorphanol but not by dextrorphanol. In this way it would be possible to distinguish stereospecific binding to the physiological receptors from nonspecific binding to other sites. Exploitation of this principle by several independent groups of workers revealed that the opiates do indeed bind to stereospecific and irregularly distributed sites in the central nervous system. These sites do not bind other substances and they are saturated by very low concentrations of opiates. Moreover the affinity of the several analgesic agents for the binding sites parallels, in a very striking fashion, both their activity on isolated pharmacological preparations (the electrically stimulated guinea pig ileum and the rat vas deferens) and their clinical effectiveness (Snyder and Pert, 1975; Akil, 1977; Simon and Hiller, 1978). The reader will readily appreciate that the interactions of the opiates with their binding sites fully meet the criteria for agonist-receptor combinations (p. 98).

The irregular distribution of the opiate receptors in the central nervous system is interesting and significant. Among the regions that contain the greatest numbers of the receptors, some (the amygdaloid and septal nuclei, the temporal and frontal lobes of the cortex) are involved in the activity of the limbic system, others (the substantia gelatinosa, some thalamic nuclei and the grey matter surrounding the third ventricle and the neighbouring aqueduct) are associated with the 'pain pathways' while yet others (the *locus coeruleus* and the area postrema of the fourth ventricle) play important roles in the processes of sleep and vomiting, respectively. This distribution of the opiate receptors is entirely consistent with the fact that their agonists induce euphoria, relieve pain, encourage sleep and sometimes cause vomiting.

Opiate antagonists, as well as the agonists, bind to the stereospecific receptors. It is a fact of some interest that in the presence of sodium the conformation of the receptor alters into a form that binds the antagonists more strongly than the agonists.

If we agree that the opiate analgesics bind to specific receptors we have to ask what substance acts as the physiological agonist at these receptors. It is hardly conceivable that the pressures of the evolutionary process have

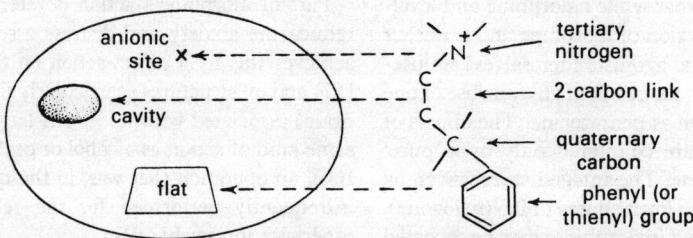

Fig. 26.8 The analgesic receptor and its relationship to the analgesic molecule.

equipped mammals (opiate receptors are not found in non-mammalian species) with receptors specifically adapted to respond to the product of a not very common flowering plant. Until the nature and distribution of the receptors was more precisely delineated it was fashionable to assume that the natural agonist at the then only hypothetical receptor was one (or perhaps more) of the established neurotransmitter substances. Chemists, armed with their usual ingenuity and molecular models, demonstrated structural affinities between morphine and acetylcholine and there is compelling evidence that acetylcholine and other transmitter substances are involved in opiate action. This point will be taken up again later. In the meantime it can be asserted with some confidence that the opiate receptors are not physiologically activated by any of the traditional transmitter substances. Their distribution does not correspond to that of the terminals of any individual neurohumoral system nor are they affected by procedures that selectively destroy cholinergic, noradrenergic, dopaminergic or serotoninergic neurones. Moreover none of the likely transmitter substances so far studied (acetylcholine, noradrenaline, dopamine, serotonin, histamine and substance P) is capable of displacing opiates from their combination with the receptors (Terenius, 1973). The failure to identify a specific agonist among the known humoral substances prompted the bold hypothesis that the physiological agonist is a substance with morphine-like properties occurring naturally in brain tissue. This hypothesis, once formulated, soon received a great deal of experimental support that culminated in the identification of a number of endogenous morphine like substances.

In 1975, Hughes became the first of a number of independent investigators to report the presence in brain extracts of material that behaves like morphine on pharmacological preparations. Hughes made use of the rat vas deferens preparation and he showed that the morphine like actions of his extracts (inhibition of the contractions induced by electrical stimulation) were readily reversed by naloxone. Shortly afterwards, Hughes and Kosterlitz and their coworkers found that the active material in brain extracts consisted of a mixture of two pentapeptides differing from another solely in the nature of the terminal aminoacid residue (Hughes, 1975; Hughes et al, 1975). The compounds were called *enkephalins* (Fig. 26.9) although this is perhaps not an entirely happy choice in view of the use of the term 'encephalins' to describe lipid substances in nervous tissue. For obvious reasons, the two active peptides are called leucine (or leu-) and methionine (or met-) enkephalin. The enkephalins have been found in the brains of all the mammalian species so far examined and their distribution broadly corresponds to that of the opiate receptors. The free pentapeptides are broken down very rapidly *in vivo*—this occurs through rupture of the tyrosine-glycine link and degradation of the terminal carboxyl group—but it is, nevertheless, possible to show

that the enkephalins suitably administered (intracerebroventricular or rapid intravenous injection) do exert analgesic actions demonstrable by such classical means as the hot plate test (p. 461).

ß-Lipotropin is a polypeptide made up of 91 aminoacid residues. It is present in (and probably fabricated by) the partes intermedia and distalis of the pituitary body. ß-Lipotropin may well be the prohormone of the melanocyte stimulating principle but it is interesting in the present context because the sequence of aminoacid residues that occupy positions 61 to 65 of the molecule is identical with that found in met-enkephalin. Moreover a number of polypeptide fractions of the ß-lipotropin molecule, all beginning with residue 61, have enkephalin like activity. These fractions are known as *endorphins* ('endogenous morphines') although this term has recently been extended to include all endogenous opiates including the enkephalins. The lipotropin endorphin chains are labelled α (residues 61 to 76), ß (61 to 91) and γ (61 to 77 and 61 to 86). The most potent of these polypeptides is endorphin ß, also known as c-fragment. It is analgesic when given by intravenous injection but it differs from the enkephalins in having a prolonged action. Because of their relative stability the endorphins appear in the blood and cerebrospinal fluid. There is recent evidence that the endorphins can be elaborated by the brain as well as by pituitary tissue (Jeffcoate et al, 1978).

The facts that the enkephalins are found in association with the opiate receptors, that they have analgesic properties, that they are rapidly destroyed and that, on microiontophoretic application to single neurones, they have generally depressant actions qualifies them for consideration as transmitter substances in neuronal systems devoted to the suppression of pain. We know that such a system exists, that it corresponds to the large fibre 'gate closing'

H–Tyr Gly Gly Phe Lev –OH

Leucine enkephalin

H–Tyr Gly Gly Phe Met –OH

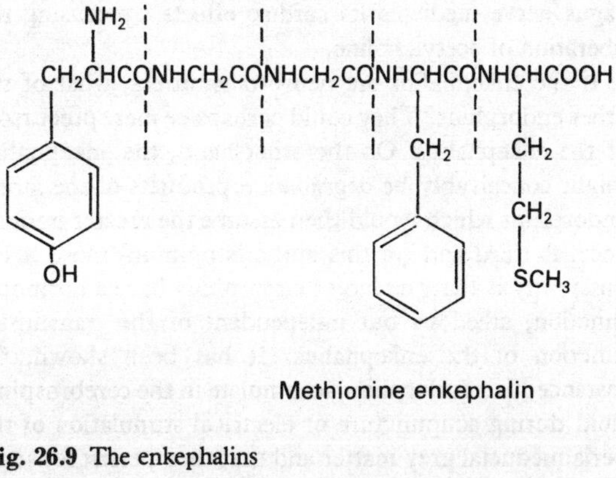

Methionine enkephalin

Fig. 26.9 The enkephalins

tracts demanded by the Melzack and Wall hypothesis (p. 423) and that it can be activated by stimulation of the dorsal columns of the cord and the central grey matter and probably also by such manoeuvres as acupuncture and the application of counter irritants. We have already seen that the opiate receptors are distributed in a fashion that is consistent with their being stationed along this pain suppression pathway, among other sites. It seems that we shall not be doing any great violence to the experimental facts if we tentatively conclude that the enkephalins are transmitter substances liberated in response to stimulation of fibres that suppress pain. In this connection, it is interesting to note that the analgesic consequence of electrical stimulation of the periventricular and periaqueductal grey matter is antagonized by naloxone.

Our knowledge of other transmitter substances persuades us that individual transmitters are rarely, if ever, confined to a single functional system and we can therefore expect to find that the enkephalins are involved in the mediation of other neurophysiological activities. We must, of course, immediately include functions subserved by the limbic system (in view of the euphoria induced by many opiates, the enkephalins may perhaps have to be thought of as endogenous pleasure substances) and there is some evidence that disorders of enkephalin function might be associated with some forms of mental illness. We must not exclude the possibility that the enkephalins may also be involved as transmitter substances at more restricted or prosaic sites in the nervous system.

If the 'enkephalinergic' system—if this term is not being introduced prematurely—were tonically active, antagonists such as naloxone should have more obvious effects than they are usually reported to have in subjects who are not dependent on opiate drugs. In fact, naloxone is not entirely devoid of pharmacological activity in these circumstances (Frederickson, 1977) but even if it were, the apparent lack of tonic activity in the proposed enkephalinergic system need not engender the concern it sometimes does. Atropine, for instance, has very little effect on the heart rate of the untrained individual or the sedentary type of animal but we do not, on that account, doubt that the vagus nerve mediates its cardiac effects by causing the liberation of acetylcholine.

If the enkephalins are neurotransmitters, what of the other endorphins? They could perhaps be mere precursors of the enkephalins. On the other hand, the enkephalins might conceivably be degradation products of the larger endorphins which would then assume the greater importance. A third and (in this author's opinion) more likely possibility is that the larger endorphins have a hormonal function, allied to but independent of the transmitter function of the enkephalins. It has been shown, for instance, that endorphins accumulate in the cerebrospinal fluid during acupuncture or electrical stimulation of the periaqueductal grey matter and that they persist for some

time after stimulation has ceased. There is a corresponding persistence of the analgesic effect and it would seem a reasonable possibility that the larger endorphins might potentiate and prolong some of the effects of stimulation of the 'enkephalinergic' nerves just as adrenaline potentiates and prolongs some of the effects of stimulation of sympathetic nerves. The reader will not need to be warned that these suggestions can be no more than tentative and that new experimental facts that are emerging daily may well demand their early revision or rejection.

Finally, we must turn to the evidence that supports the view that acetylcholine, serotonin and other mediators of synaptic transmission are involved in the action of opiates.

It is known that the morphine like analgesics inhibit the release of acetylcholine from the intestine whether this occurs spontaneously or is induced by electrical stimulation of the nervous elements (Paton, 1957). This type of action could well explain the inhibitory action of the analgesics on intestinal motility and secretions. Moreover, there is evidence that morphine and related agents similarly inhibit the release of acetylcholine from neurones in the brain and to an extent that is commensurate with their analgesic potencies. Finally, as we discuss more fully on p. 94 it is possible to demonstrate consistent changes, at least in the rat, in the release of acetylcholine during the development of tolerance to and after withdrawal from morphine (Crossland & Slater, 1968; Crossland, 1972). Serotonin also seems to be rather similarly involved in morphine's action—in the mouse, indeed, serotonin seems to be more important than acetylcholine in this respect (Way, 1972)—and a role for noradrenaline cannot be excluded. Finally we must recall that when morphine causes vomiting it probably does so by activating dopaminergic neurones in the medullary centres. We have to enquire how we can accommodate these observations into a concept that sees the endorphins playing a crucial role. It must be remembered that, just as no one transmitter substance is restricted to serving a single physiological function, few if any functions depend on the activities of a single transmitter substance. If activity in the enkephalinergic neurones directly or indirectly inhibits cholinergic or serotoninergic neurones we can readily explain why morphine inhibits the release of acetylcholine and serotonin respectively and why substances that interact with these transmitter substances might have similar effects to substances that similarly interact with enkephalins or their receptors. More complicated possibilities, such as an interaction between enkephalins and acetylcholine (or other transmitter substances) at presynaptic loci, though they have been postulated and supported by some experimental evidence (Knoll, 1977) are, perhaps, rather less likely in view of the evidence that the enkephalins are contained in neurones quite distinct from those that carry acetylcholine or the monoamines.

The possibility that the endorphins might be involved in

the development of opiate dependence is discussed elsewhere (p. 94).

THE TESTING OF MORPHINE LIKE ANALGESICS

Methods available for the screening of compounds of potential value as analgesics are discussed in the next chapter (p. 461). Tests directed to an assessment of a drug's liability to cause dependence in man are considered in Chapter 7 (p. 95).

BIBLIOGRAPHY

Books, monographs and reviews

Barchas, J. D., Berger, P. A., Ciaranello, R. D. and Elliott, G. R. (eds) (1977). *Psychopharmacology from Theory to Practice.* New York: Oxford University Press.

Beckett, A. H. and Casy, A. F. (1954). Synthetic analgesics: sterochemical considerations. *J. Pharm. Pharmac.*, **6**, 986-1001.

Beckett, A. H. and Casy, A. F. (1962). The testing and development of analgesic drugs. In *Progress in Medicinal Chemistry*, Vol. 2, 43-87. ed. Ellis, G. P. and West, G. B. London: Butterworths.

Beckett, A. H. and Casy, A. F. (1965). Analgesics and their antagonists: biochemical aspects and structure-activity relationships. In *Progress in Medicinal Chemistry*, Vol. 4, 171-218. ed. Ellis, G. P. and West, G. B. London: Butterworths.

Frederickson, R. C. A. (1977). Enkephalin pentapeptides—a review of current evidence for a physiological role in vertebrate neurotransmission. *Life Sci.*, **21**, 23-42.

Hughes, J. (ed) (1978) *Centrally Acting Peptides.* London and Basingstoke: Macmillan.

Kosterlitz, H. W., Collier, H. O. J. and Villaveal, J. E. (1972) *Agonist and Antagonist of Narcotic Analgesic Drugs.* London and Basingstoke: Macmillan.

Kosterlitz, H. W. (ed) (1976) *Opiates and Endogenous Opioid Peptides.* Amsterdam, New York, Oxford: North Holland Publishing Co.

Martin, W. R. (1963) Strong analgesics. In *Physiological Pharmacology*, Vol 1, pp. 275-313. ed. Root, W. S. and Hofmann, F. G. New York and London: Academic Press.

Simon, E. J. and Hiller, J. M. (1978) The opiate receptors. *Ann. rev. Pharmac. Toxicol.*, **18**, 371-394.

Snyder, S. H. and Matthysse, S. (eds) (1975) *Opiate Receptor Mechanisms.* Cambridge, Mass. and London: The MIT Press.

Terenius, L. (1978) Endogenous peptides and analgesia. *Ann. rev. Pharmac. Toxicol.*, **18**, 189-204.

Original papers

Akil, H. (1977) Opiates: biological mechanisms. In: Barchas, J. D. *et al* (q.v.) pp. 292-303.

Bentley, K. W. and Lewis, J. W. (1972) The relationship between structure and activity in the 6, 14-*endo*ethenotetrahydrothebaine series of analgesics. In: Kosterlitz, H. W., Collier, H. O. J. and Villareal, J. E. (q.v.) pp. 7-16.

Bound, Denise and Greer, S. (1978) Psychotic symptoms after dipipanone. *Lancet ii*, 480.

Braendon, O. J., Eddy, N. B. and Halbach, H. (1955). Synthetic substances with morphine-like effect. Relationship between chemical structure and analgesic action. *Bull. Wld Hlth Org.*, **13**, 937-998.

Crossland, J. (1972) Acetylcholine and morphine dependence. *In* Kosterlitz, H. W., Collier, H. O. J. and Villareal, J. E. (q.v.) pp. 232-234.

Crossland, J. and Slater, P. (1968). The effect of some drugs on the 'free' and 'bound' acetylcholine content of rat brain. *Br. J. Pharmac. Chemother.*, **33**, 42-47.

Hughes, J. (1975). Isolation of an endogenous compound from the brain with pharmacological properties similar to those of morphine. *Brain Res.* **88**, 295-308.

Hughes, J., Smith, T. W., Kosterlitz, H. W., Fothergill, L. A., Morgan, B. A. and Morris, H. R. (1975). Identification of two related pentapeptides from the brain with potent opiate agonist activity. *Nature*, **258**, 577-579.

Jeffcoate, W. J., Rees, Lesley, McLoughlin, Lorraine, Ratter, Sally, Hope, J., Lowry, P. J. and Besser, G. M. (1978). ß-Endorphin in human cerebrospinal fluid. *Lancet* (ii), 119-121.

Knoll, J. (1977). Two kinds of opiate receptors. *Pol. J. Pharmac. Pharm.*, **29**, 165-175.

Paton, W. D. M. (1957). The action of morphine and related substances on contraction and on acetylcholine output of coaxially stimulated guinea pig ileum. *Br. J. Pharmac. Chemother.*, **12**, 119-127.

Snyder, S. H. and Pert, C. B. (1975) Regional distribution of the opiate receptor. *In* Snyder, S. H. and Matthysse, S. (q.v.) pp. 35-38

Terenius, L. (1973). Stereospecific uptake of narcotic analgesics by a subcellular fraction of the guinea pig ileum. *Upsala J. Med. Sci.*, **78**, 150-152.

Trendelenburg, U. (1957) The action of morphine on the superior cervical ganglion and on the nictitating membrane of the cat. *Br. J. Pharmac. Chemother.*, **12**, 79-85.

Way, E. L. (1972) Reassessment of brain 5-hydroxytryptamine in morphine tolerance and physical dependence. *In* Kosterlitz, H. W., Collier, H. O. J. and Villareal, J. E. (q.v.) pp. 153-163.

27. Antiinflammatory drugs

The drugs to be discussed in this chapter are gathered together under four heads:

a. aspirin like drugs
b. corticosteroids
c. miscellaneous antiinflammatory agents
d. drugs used for the treatment of gout.

ASPIRIN LIKE DRUGS

All the drugs decribed here as 'aspirin like' have antipyretic and analgesic as well as antiinflammatory activities and they all owe their effectiveness primarily to an ability to inhibit the synthesis of prostaglandins. Aspirin (acetylsalicylic acid) is taken as the prototypical member of the group not only because it was the first to be widely used but also because it has been more thoroughly investigated than any of its fellows.

Unlike morphine and its congeners, which featured in the previous chapter, the aspirin like drugs owe their effectiveness as analgesic agents to an action in the area of origin of the pain and not to an intervention at sites in the central nervous system. Consequently they induce no change in mood and they have no tendency to cause dependence.

Before discussing the antiinflammatory drugs themselves we must pause to consider the nature of the conditions for whose relief they are employed.

Pain has already been discussed in detail (p. 415) and *pyrexia* is a synonym for fever. An antipyretic substance is one that lowers the body temperature during fever; unlike a hypothermic substance it does not depress normal body temperatures.

Although it is not easy to provide a completely satisfactory definition of inflammation, it is possible to describe it in general terms as a local tissue response to injury by chemical or physical agents. In an acute inflammatory change, there is dilatation of the capillaries and of the smaller arterioles and venules at the site of injury. The permeability of the capillary and venular walls increases and this, together with the increased local pressure caused by the arteriolar dilatation, leads to an increased transudation of fluid into the tissue spaces. In some circumstances it seems that the transudate is derived exclusively from the venules, in others it comes only from capillaries while in yet others both types of vessel release fluid. The increased permeability of the vessels is attributable to the opening up of gaps between adjacent endothelial cells.

The vascular changes cause redness (erythema), heat and swelling while tissue components liberated by the original insult cause pain. Thus we arrive at the four cardinal signs of inflammation which must be familiar to all readers of this book. They have been quoted for two millenia in their Latin form—rubor, calor, turgor and dolor respectively—as the pathognomonic features of the inflammatory condition.

The passage of leucocytes and of plasma proteins from the capillaries into the tissue spaces is another feature of the acute inflammatory process. In the early stages, polymorphonuclear leucocytes constitute the predominant cell type in the cellular exudate but mononuclear cells (particularly monocytes) leave the capillaries later. They are joined by fibroblasts and other cells which migrate to the affected area from neighbouring regions in response to chemotactic influences from the damaged cells. Once in the tissue spaces, the monocytes are converted into macrophages, histiocytes, epithelioid and giant cells. The polymorphs are phagocytic: they engulf and remove foreign particles and organisms and often die in the process. In their turn, they and dead tissue cells are removed by the macrophages. After a localized acute inflammatory response, the affected region often returns completely to its previous healthy state, new connective tissue and capillaries being laid down by the fibroblasts and epithelioid cells to replace those destroyed by the original tissue damage. A small amount of fibrous tissue may also be formed.

Some inflammatory agents produce a chronic inflammation in which the observed changes are less intense but more long lasting than those seen in acute inflammation. The predominant feature of a chronic inflammatory process is proliferation of fibrous tissue though the exudative changes characteristic of acute inflammation are also often in evidence and a condition of chronic inflammation may be ushered in by a phase of acute changes.

The most common of the disorders characterized by chronic inflammatory changes are those classified as connective tissue diseases. These include rheumatic fever, rheumatoid arthritis, ankylosing spondylitis, osteoarthritis, systemic lupus erythematosus, polyarteritis nodosa and some less common diseases. In these diseases, the inflammatory changes take place in the connective tissue of the joints and (in rheumatic fever) in the heart. In rheumatic fever particularly, the exudative changes characteristic of an acute inflammatory process coexist with the proliferative changes characteristic of the chronic condition. The proliferative changes result in the formation of nodules of fibrous tissue in each of which are enclosed a few giant cells and other connective tissue elements. In the heart these nodules are known as Aschoff bodies. They occur beneath the endocardium of both the heart wall and the valves, particularly the mitral and aortic valves. The distortion of the valves produced by the Aschoff bodies and the fibrosis they provoke may lead to valvular defects of which the most common are mitral stenosis (narrowing) and aortic incompetence, which causes aortic regurgitation.

A large number of factors is released or activated in response to tissue damage. They provoke, directly or indirectly, the appearance of the mediators of pain and inflammation. The factors include lysosomal enzymes from a number of cell types (mast cells, macrophages, polymorphonuclear leucocytes and platelets), leukokines and lymphokines from the polymorphs and lymphocytes respectively and the Hageman factor (p 359) from plasma. The cyclic nucleotides also play a part. These same factors are also involved in the initiation of immune responses and a more detailed discussion of their nature and significance can be found in Chapter 24 (p. 393).

The mediators of the acute inflammatory reaction include histamine (with, in some species, a small contribution from 5-hydroxytryptamine), the plasma kinins and the prostaglandins. Histamine and 5-hydroxytryptamine appear early in the inflammatory response and exert relatively evanescent effects. The plasma kinins come next and they overlap with the release of prostaglandins whose contribution to the inflammatory process is dominant. The overwhelming importance of the prostaglandins is testified to by the fact that all the clinically useful antiinflammatory drugs share the property of being able to prevent the synthesis or release of these substances.

As we have indicated, immune and inflammatory reactions have much in common but antiinflammatory agents, the corticosteroids apart, are not recruited for the treatment of anaphylactic (allergic) conditions. This is partly because the prostaglandins are not of such primary importance in the mediation of anaphylactic as they are in inflammatory responses, partly because the events that lead to the liberation of the mediators of anaphylaxis are themselves susceptible to attack by drugs which can consequently prevent the actual release of mediators and partly because a range of substances are capable of reversing the reactions in the affected tissues and so relieving the symptoms of anaphylaxis in a way that is not possible with inflammatory changes.

That the corticosteroids are effective in both inflammatory and allergic conditions is a testimony to the multiplicity of their actions.

Salicylates and related compounds

Among ancient folk remedies for pain and fever, extracts of the barks, leaves or fruits of a number of trees had a high reputation. It is now known that many of these herbal remedies owed their effectiveness to their contained salicylates. The word salicylate is itself derived from *Salicaceae*, the botanical name for the willow family. The bark of the white willow *(Salix alba)* contains a glycoside with antipyretic and analgesic properties. The glycoside is known as salicin: it yields salicylic acid (Fig. 27.1) and glucose on hydrolysis. Extracts of willow became part of the physician's therapeutic armentarium more than two hundred years ago. The nature and composition of salicylic acid, the bark's active principle, were established in the middle of the 19th century and Kolbe, who had made major contributions to the earlier studies on the chemistry of the bark,

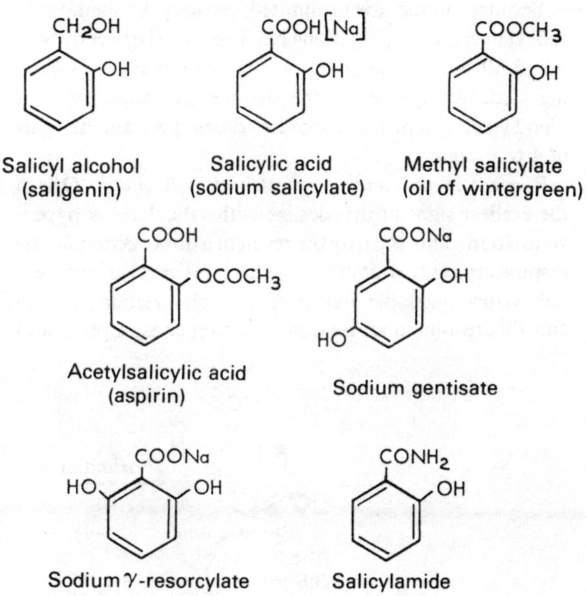

Salicyl alcohol (saligenin)

Salicylic acid (sodium salicylate)

Methyl salicylate (oil of wintergreen)

Acetylsalicylic acid (aspirin)

Sodium gentisate

Sodium γ-resorcylate

Salicylamide

Fig. 27.1 Some salicylates and related compounds.

published methods for the synthesis of salicylic acid in the laboratory and on the industrial scale in 1860 and 1873 respectively. Aspirin made its appearance in 1899. The salicylates, particularly aspirin, remain one of the most widely used group of drugs but in spite of their long history it is only very recently that their mode of action has become established. The salicylates intervene in a number of biochemical systems but their most important action, from the therapeutic point of view at least, is to prevent the synthesis of prostaglandins and thromboxames (p. 369). So high do the prostaglandins rank among the mediators of pain and inflammation that, had our forefathers not stumbled upon the salicylates for us, we would now be busily engaged in looking for them.

General pharmacology of the salicylates

Absorption, metabolism and excretion. The salicylates are active when taken by mouth and they are readily absorbed from the gastrointestinal tract. Although absorption is favoured by the low pH (p. 41), salicylates are more readily absorbed from the small intestine than from the stomach and anything that accelerates gastric emptying promotes their absorption. This is a simple consequence of the fact that the surface available for absorption is so much greater in the small intestine than in the stomach that it outweighs the disadvantage of the unfavourable pH. The fate of salicylates after absorption is shown in Fig. 27.2. It will be seen that much of the salicylate is conjugated with glycine or with glucuronic acid but in alkaline urine the proportion excreted as free salicylate is much higher than that indicated. It can reach 85 per cent of the administered dose.

Because of the liver's limited capacity to metabolize salicylates, the drug's plasma half lives vary between about 3 and 30 hours depending on the amount that has been ingested. With doses in the therapeutic range constant blood levels can be maintained by doses spaced at intervals of 4 to 6 hours.

Respiratory and metabolic effects of the salicylates. One of the earliest signs of overdosage with salicylates is hyperventilation. This is partly the result of a direct action on the respiratory centre but other mechanisms are also involved. Salicylates uncouple oxidative phosphorylation (p. 31) and this results in an increased oxygen consumption and carbon dioxide production which will also contribute to the hyperventilatory stimulus. The salicylates also inhibit a range of dehydrogenase and aminotransferase systems. Although this effect reduces the demands for oxygen and thus partly offsets the increased demands arising from the uncoupling effect, it also causes the accumulation of acid metabolites which themselves tend to cause hyperventilation, though this stimulus will be ineffective unless it is more powerful than that provided by the direct action of the salicylate on the respiratory centre. It will be evident that the pH change produced by large doses of salicylate is variable, depending upon whether the total respiratory stimulation exceeds or falls short of that necessary to compensate for the metabolic acidosis. Generally speaking, salicylate poisoning causes acidosis in very young children while older children and adults suffer an alkalosis (Winters, 1963).

The salicylates affect many other metabolic systems. Quite small doses cause hypoglycaemia in the diabetic patient but larger doses produce hyperglycaemia in the normal subject. The hyperglycaemic response is partly a consequence of increased glycogenolysis in the liver. The response is much reduced by adrenal demedullation, indicating that it arises, in part at least, from adrenaline release. The latter event probably represents the result of a stimulation of hypothalamic sympathetic centres. Stimulation of the adrenal cortex may also be involved. At least one other mechanism contributes to the hyperglycaemic response, for salicylates can be shown to inhibit the prod-

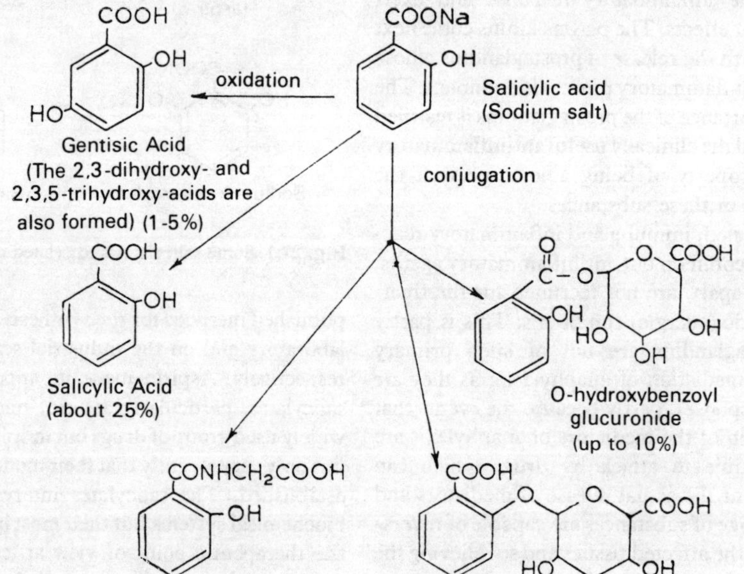

Fig. 27.2 The metabolism and elimination of salicylic acid.

uction of glycogen by the liver *in vitro*. This effect might be a consequence of the uncoupling of oxidative phosphorylation, since other uncouplers have a similar effect and glycogen synthesis is dependent on the presence of ATP.

The hypoglycaemic action of salicylates in diabetic patients has been the subject of intensive investigation because it was at one time believed that the effect might have a therapeutic application. Although the mechanism of the hypoglycaemic action has not been certainly determined, a number of the more obvious possibilities (such as stimulation of insulin release or of glucose excretion or inhibition of its intestinal absorption) have been excluded. It may be that salicylates stimulate the utilization of glucose or inhibit its production from non-carbohydrate sources.

High doses of the salicylates increase nitrogen excretion. This appears to be yet another consequence of the metabolic stimulation resulting from uncoupling and which leads to increased protein breakdown. In addition, enzyme inhibition may impair protein synthesis. An ATP dependent renal mechanism may also be involved, since there is evidence that salicylates interfere with the tubular reabsorption of amino acids.

An interesting facet of the action of salicylates on nitrogen metabolism concerns the response of the glutamine-glutamic acid system. Glutamic acid occupies an important position in several metabolic systems in the body as a result of which it is converted into glutamine, proline, α-oxoglutaric acid and γ-aminobutyric acid. The enzymes responsible for these several reactions are all inhibited (though to different extents) by the salicylates. Salicylates thus cause the accumulation of glutamate and a possible increase in cerebral excitability (p. 193) that could be responsible for the convulsions sometimes seen in salicylate poisoning.

Actions on the central nervous system. Although salicylates in therapeutic doses have an antipyretic action, hyperthermia is a feature of salicylate poisoning, particularly in young children in whom temperatures of up to 108 °F (42 °C) have been recorded. These contrasting effects of salicylate ingestion provide a rather neat demonstration of the operation of what seem to be the two most important aspects of salicylate pharmacology. The antipyretic action arises from inhibition of prostaglandin synthesis and the hyperthermia results from the uncoupling of oxidative phosphorylation.

In bacterial infections, fever arises as a result of prostaglandin action on the hypothalamic heat regulating centres. The salicylates prevent prostaglandin synthesis and so lead to a resolution of the fever. On the other hand, when the dose taken is high enough to uncouple oxidative phosphorylation, oxidative metabolism may be stimulated to such an extent, particularly in children, that heat is produced at a faster rate than it is dispelled. In these conditions, the profuse sweating which normally keeps down the body temperature becomes a distinct liability because it causes the blood volume to be reduced and this interferes with heat loss. This effect will be the more serious in the presence of vomiting (a common occurrence in salicylate poisoning especially in children), which adds further to the water loss and prevents its replacement by mouth.

Another aspect of salicylate action which is probably mediated by the hypothalamus concerns the drug's ability to stimulate the pituitary-adrenal axis. The salicylates produce a number of changes reminiscent of those produced by the adrenocorticotrophic hormone (ACTH). Thus they partially deplete the adrenal glands of their ascorbic acid and cholesterol, they cause a reduction in the number of circulating eosinophils and they increase the plasma concentration of 17-hydroxycorticosteroids. None of these effects is seen in the hypophysectomized animal and it must therefore be concluded that salicylates stimulate the release of ACTH. There has been a good deal of argument concerning the significance of these observations but the balance of evidence (for a summary, see Paulus and Whitehouse, 1973) suggests that pituitary stimulation can only be produced by high, and possibly toxic, doses of the salicylates. For instance, in one series of observations, no elevation of plasma 17-hydroxycorticosteroid concentration was detected in patients who had been receiving up to 1.7 grams of sodium salicylate at four-hourly intervals for up to 16 days (Bayliss and Steinbeck, 1954). On the other hand, raised plasma 17-hydroxycorticosteroid concentrations are regularly found in people who have attempted suicide by taking massive amounts of salicylates.

The convulsant action of large doses of salicylates has already been mentioned.

Individual salicylates and related compounds

SODIUM SALICYLATE

Sodium salicylate finds its chief use in the treatment of rheumatic fever, for which purpose total daily doses of up to 8 grams have to be given, usually in instalments taken at three-hourly intervals. This approaches the toxic dose and symptoms of mild intoxication (nausea, vomiting and *tinnitus*—ringing in the ears) collectively known as *salicylism* may appear in the early stages of treatment. The intelligent patient can be encouraged to adjust his intake of salicylate until it is just below the threshold for salicylism as manifested by the occurrence of tinnitus. In that way he will secure the optimal therapeutic effect and it will be possible the quicker to reduce the dose, as the initial symptoms subside, to a more modest level.

Sodium salicylate is not now used, as it once was, for the treatment of gout.

ACETYLSALICYLIC ACID (ASPIRIN)

Like sodium salicylate, aspirin is used for the relief of pain and inflammation associated with the rheumatic diseases and gout but in addition it is widely employed by the layman for the treatment of minor family ills; ordinary headaches, muscle pains and mild fevers respond very well to the drug and little harm attends its use in the moderation observed by most people. Aspirin is not without value in relieving the pain of more serious conditions and the physician should always consider the possibility of using it in preference to the stronger analgesics.

In the treatment of rheumatic diseases, aspirin is used in the same dose range as sodium salicylate. Although the two drugs are equally effective antiinflammatory agents, idiosyncratic reactions are more common with aspirin. On the other hand, some patients do not tolerate sodium salicylate well but suffer no ill effects from aspirin.

There seems to be no doubt that aspirin is a more powerful analgesic than sodium salicylate, notwithstanding the fact that it is hydrolysed in the body to give salicylic acid. Aspirin appears to be an analgesic in its own right since its effectiveness sharply declines when acetylsalicylate disappears from the plasma, even though salicylate levels remain high (Lester, Lolli and Greenberg, 1946). This point is taken up again later.

In addition to the acid itself, several other preparations of aspirin have been used. They include the sodium, calcium and aluminium salts, the choline ester and buffered aspirin. They are of limited utility.

Side effects of aspirin administration are discussed below.

NEWER SALICYLATE DERIVATIVES

During the past thirty years, strenuous attempts have been made to find salicylate derivatives that will be more effective, longer acting and less toxic than aspirin. It says much for the effectiveness of aspirin that many have thought it worthwhile to concentrate their efforts on the development of aspirin related substances rather than on the exploration of the antiinflammatory potentiality of novel compounds. It says even more for the good fortune (or serendipity) of our forefathers that more than 500 salicylate derivatives had to be synthesized before diflunisal (see below) appeared in 1971.

The difficulty of finding a salicylate derivative that might represent an improvement on aspirin provided the stimulus to investigate compounds formed by the molecular union of aspirin with another antiinflammatory agent. One outcome of this quest was the discovery of benorylate (Fig. 27.3).

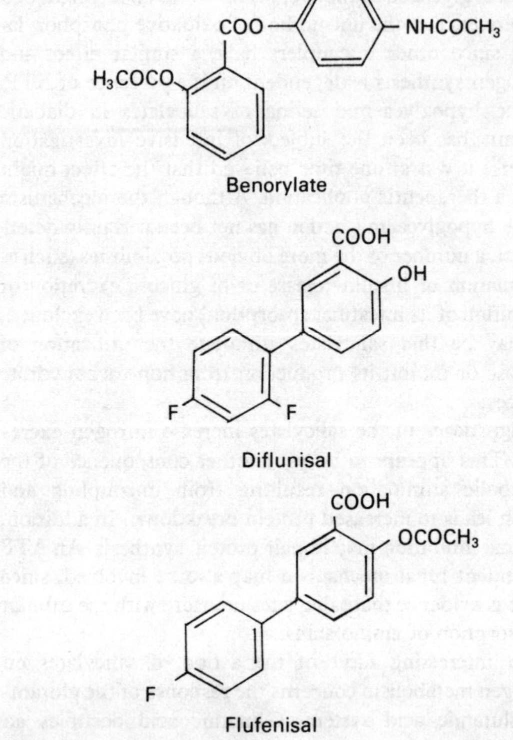

Benorylate (Benoral) is a compound of aspirin and paracetamol. It is said to be less likely than aspirin itself to cause gastrointestinal haemorrhage but an overdose will produce the toxic effects of both component drugs. It has analgesic and antipyretic actions like aspirin itself but it has been employed principally for the treatment of rheumatoid arthritis. For this purpose it is given four times

Fig. 27.3 Some newer salicylate derivatives

daily in oral doses of 2 grams with appropriate reductions for children.

Diflunisal (Dolobid) is the successor to flufenisal (Fig. 27.3), a compound that, despite early promise, proved to be no less toxic than aspirin. The omens for diflunisal (which has only recently become generally available) are more favourable: it is a more potent analgesic and antiinflammatory agent than aspirin but it is much less likely to induce gastric haemorrhage or to inhibit platelet aggregation because it has relatively little action on the prostaglandin synthetase of the platelets. Nevertheless caution should attend its use in patients with a history of peptic ulceration or gastroduodenal bleeding.

Although diflunisal has antiinflammatory activity it is being currently promoted as an analgesic drug. After oral administration, peak plasma levels are reached in some two hours. The plasma half life is about eight hours and this enables round the clock analgesia to be maintained by twice daily dosing—hence the proprietary name! Early trials indicated that diflunisal might prove to be particularly suitable for securing relief from postoperative pain or of pain associated with arthritis, especially in patients with bleeding diseases.

The recommended dose of diflunisal is 250 to 500 mg twice daily.

Diflunisal has been the subject of a recent review (Willoughby, Wright and Turner, 1977)

OTHER COMPOUNDS

Gentisic acid, salicylamide and sodium γ-resorcylate have been employed as antiinflammatory drugs but they can now be regarded as obsolete. Methyl salicylate (oil of wintergreen) is applied locally as a counter irritant (p. 422).

Toxic reactions to the salicylates

Hypersensitivity. About 1 in 500 of the population display hypersensitivity to aspirin. The hypersensitivity reactions take the form of skin rashes, urticaria, angioneurotic oedema and asthma. The angioneurotic oedema sometimes affects the laryngeal mucosa which may become so oedematous as to cause a life-threatening asphyxia. Attacks of asthma provoked by aspirin also occasionally have a fatal outcome. The reactions may follow quite small doses of aspirin and, until recently, most investigators believed that they provided an example of an antigen-antibody reaction provoked by a simple non-protein substance which, acting as a hapten (p. 396), combined with a component of the plasma protein to produce the allergen. In this instance it was thought that the allergen would prove to be an acetylated protein. It now seems unlikely that aspirin hypersensitivity reactions are truly anaphylactic in origin: antibodies have never been detected in the serum of sensitive subjects and intolerance to aspirin lacks the specificity that would be expected if it had an immunological basis. It seems instead that aspirin hypersensitivity is the direct result, like so many of its actions, of an inhibition of prostaglandin synthesis (Vane, 1976). The topic is discussed more fully on p. 381. Sensitivity to salicylates other than aspirin is less common but it does occasionally occur.

Gastrointestinal bleeding and ulceration. Salicylates are prone to cause bleeding from the gastrointestinal mucosa, particularly that of the stomach. The incidence of bleeding has been estimated as 70 per cent. It is the result of a local effect but the daily blood loss in patients receiving four therapeutic doses of salicylate a day is usually no more than 2 to 6 ml (Holt, 1960). Sometimes, though, the blood loss is more severe and the local damage that induces bleeding can also precipitate or exacerbate peptic ulceration. These local influences include denaturation of mucosal cells, inhibition of mucous synthesis, changes in the permeability of the gastric mucosa and an initial stimulation of gastric acid secretion. Hypoprothrombinaemia and inhibition of platelet aggregation may further aggravate the blood loss and convert what would otherwise have been an innocuously trivial ooze into a serious gastrointestinal haemorrhage. Undissolved particles of aspirin irritate the gastric mucosa and may add their own quota of damage. This constitutes something of an argument for using aspirin in a soluble or an enteric coated form. Although overt gastroduodenal haemorrhages are not very common, the repeated loss of small quantities of blood incident on the continued intake of salicylates sometimes leads to an iron deficiency anaemia. It is clear, however, that little danger from blood loss exists for the normal subject who takes occasional doses of aspirin.

Nephrotoxicity. Kidney damage—specifically renal papillary necrosis—is commonly seen in laboratory animals that have received substantial doses of salicylates (or of many other antiinflammatory drugs) over a prolonged period. It is, of course, a much less common occurrence in human patients who will be taking more modest doses of the drugs but the appearance of evidence of impaired kidney function in these patients should properly be regarded as a signal to withdraw the offending drug.

Other side effects. For clinical effectiveness in rheumatic conditions, the intake of salicylates must be maintained at near-toxic levels and signs of salicylate overdosage may appear in patients receiving what were intended to be only therapeutic doses of the drugs. These signs (most of which have been discussed earlier in this chapter) include dyspepsia, nausea, vomiting, tinnitus, hyperventilation and hypoprothrombinaemia.

Drug interactions involving salicylates. This topic is discussed elsewhere (p. 78).

Salicylate poisoning

Because aspirin is so readily available, it is a favourite instrument of suicide and a major cause of accidental poisoning in young children. In Great Britain, salicylate poisoning accounts for the deaths of about 200 people a year. The fatal dose varies considerably with the individual. While some adults have succumbed to as little as 10 grams of aspirin, others have survived doses of as much as 120 grams.

In severe poisoning, there is usually a metabolic acidosis or alkalosis (p. 442) with symptoms of stimulation of the central nervous system. These may progress until delirium and convulsions occur, followed later by signs of depression of the central nervous system with coma and death. There is severe pyrexia.

In the emergency treatment of salicylate poisoning, unabsorbed salicylate is removed from the stomach by gastric lavage. The intravenous infusion of an alkaline glucose solution (5 per cent glucose with 2 per cent sodium bicarbonate in normal saline) is often life-saving. The glucose produces an osmotic diuresis (p. 623) and the bicarbonate facilitates the excretion of free salicylate. If there is a metabolic acidoses the bicarbonate will help to correct it, but many authorities believe that bicarbonate should not be withheld even when alkalosis is present. They argue that the beneficial effect of bicarbonate on salicylate excretion more than offsets its deleterious effect on blood pH. Those who do not favour the administration of bicarbonate to patients in alkalosis recommend the use of an infusion of mannitol and sodium lactate for the production of diuresis. In extreme cases, where kidney

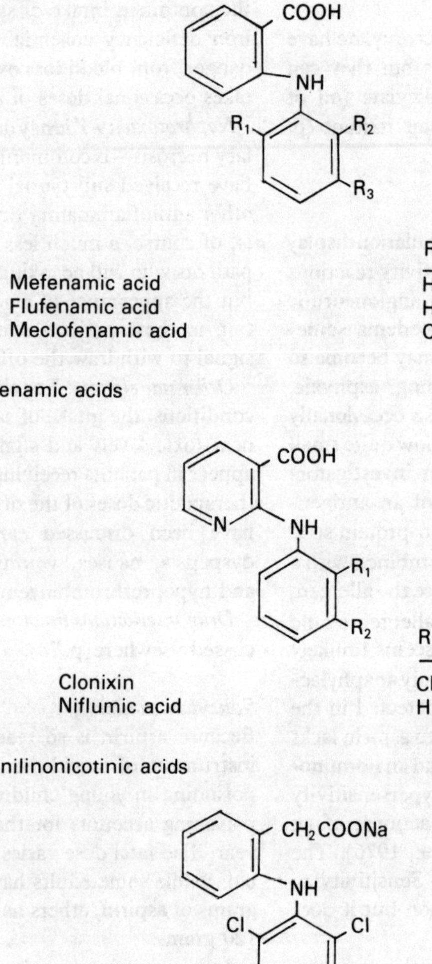

Mefenamic acid
Flufenamic acid
Meclofenamic acid

	R_1	R_2	R_3
Mefenamic acid	H	CH_3	CH_3
Flufenamic acid	H	H	CF_3
Meclofenamic acid	Cl	Cl	CH_3

a) The fenamic acids

	R_1	R_2
Clonixin	CH_3	Cl
Niflumic acid	H	CF_3

b) The anilinonicotinic acids

c) Diclofenac sodium

Fig. 27.4 The N-arylanthranilic acids

function is severely depressed by reason of circulatory failure, attempts to produce a forced diuresis may fail and it is then necessary to resort to haemodialysis using the artificial kidney. In very young children, technical difficulties sometimes prevent the use of the artificial kidney. In these circumstances, exchange transfusion is used.

Efforts to rid the body of salicylates must be accompanied by appropriate treatment to counter excitation or depression of the nervous system. Care must also be taken to ensure that the volume of infusate administered in attempts to force diuresis is such as to prevent depletion of body water which would only aggravate what might already be a dangerously high pyrexia.

The N-arylanthranilic acids

These compounds can be conveniently divided into the fenamic (Fig. 24.7a) and the anilinonicotinic (Fig. 27.4b) acids. The former group is represented by mefenamic, flufenamic and meclofenamic acids and the latter by niflumic acid and clonixin. Diclofenac sodium (Fig. 27.4c) is also included with these drugs although it is actually the salt of a homologue of an N-arylanthranilic acid.

Mefenamic and flufenamic acids have been in clinical use for more than a decade but diclofenac sodium and niflumic acid have only become available very recently. The other members of the group are still undergoing trials.

THE FENAMIC ACIDS

Mefenamic acid (Ponstan, Ponstel) has properties and uses generally similar to those of aspirin but it is markedly more toxic than the salicylates, particularly to the gastointestinal tract. It is rather more likely than aspirin to cause bleeding and ulceration but, in addition, it is prone to produce a severe diarrhoea if it is taken over a longer period than about one week at a time. An autoimmune type of haemolytic anaemia is another possible complication of mefenamic acid treatment, as are various blood dyscrasias.

The analgesic dose of mefenamic acid is 500 mg taken three times daily. Most of the drug is rapidly excreted in the urine (as conjugates of unchanged mefenamic acid and of a dicarboxylic acid metabolite), some is taken into the enterohepatic circulation and so is retained in the body for some time.

Although mefenamic acid would appear to offer no particular advantage over aspirin, some very recent reports indicate that it may prove to be a valuable drug for the relief of the discomfort and pain of dysmenorrhoea (Anderson *et al.*, 1978). There is evidence that this condition is brought about by prostaglandin release (p. 374) and to treat it by inhibiting prostaglandin synthetase is therefore both reasonable and rational. It is, however, not easy to see why the fenamic acids are superior to most other synthetase inhibitors in this respect unless it is because of their reported ability to antagonize some of the actions of prostaglandins. Such a property would add to the drugs' effectiveness by providing a net to catch any prostaglandin synthesized by enzyme molecules that had escaped inactivation.

Flufenamic acid (Arlef) is similar to mefenamic acid. The thrice daily dose is 200 mg and the drug is extensively metabolized into the 6-hydroxy derivative before excretion. Like mefenamic acid, flufenamic acid effectively relieves dysmenorrhoea (Anderson *et al.*, 1978; Kapadia and Elder, 1978).

Meclofenamic acid is still undergoing trials with a view to

its possible application to the treatment of rheumatoid arthritis. It is the most powerful of the fenamic acids, being active at a daily dose level of 100 mg.

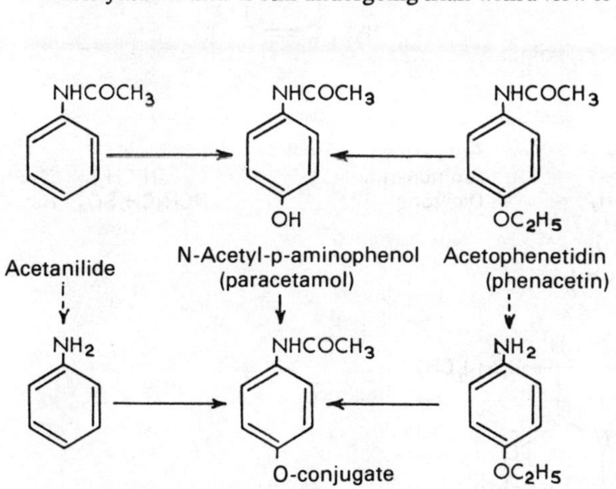

THE ANILINONICOTINIC ACIDS

Clonixin shows promise as an analgesic drug. Preliminary trials have indicated that a dose of 600 mg is as effective as 10 mg of morphine for the relief of postoperative and postpartum pain.

Niflumic acid (Actol, Flaminon, Nifluril) has been used, in daily doses of 500 mg to one gram, to treat rheumatic diseases but this new drug has not yet won wide popularity.

DICLOFENAC SODIUM

Diclofenac sodium (Voltaren) is employed as an antiinflammatory drug. It is usually given by mouth in thrice daily doses of 25 mg. It has a potency similar to that of indomethacin (q.v.). It is contraindicated in the first three months of pregnancy.

Derivatives of *p*-aminophenol

In 1886, an absent-minded pharmacist added acetanilide to a mixture which had been prescribed for a fevered patient. Before the mistake was discovered, the patient had taken some of the mixture, which caused a rapid resolution of his fever. As a result of this accident, acetanilide was introduced into medicine as an antipyretic under the name antifebrin. It proved to be much more toxic than sodium salicylate and less dangerous compounds were therefore sought. Because it was thought (erroneously, as it later transpired) that acetanilide owed its antipyretic action to its conversion in the body to *p*-aminophenol, derivatives of this last named compound were examined. *p*-Aminophenol itself proved to be as toxic as acetanilide but toxicity was reduced if the hydroxyl or amino group received alkyl or acid substituents respectively. The two most successful compounds thus produced were acetophenetidin (phenacetin) and *N*-acetyl-*p*-aminophenol (acetaminophenol, paracetamol). As can be seen by reference to Figure 27.5, phenacetin is metabolized in the body to paracetamol and *p*-phenetidine. Since *p*-phenetidine has toxic properties, paracetamol is obviously to be preferred to phenacetin. Very recently indeed phenacetin has been withdrawn from the British market, an event that was long overdue.

Acetanilide is metabolized into paracetamol and aniline. The toxicity of the latter compound militated against the widespread adoption of acetanilide as a therapeutic agent.

The *p*-aminophenol derivatives are all antipyretics and analgesics. In its time, phenacetin was a popular remedy for headache, lumbago and other muscle pains, neuralgia and dysmenorrhoea, and paracetamol is now filling the breach left by the withdrawal of phenacetin. The single dose of paracetamol is about 300 mg and not more than 2-4 grams should be taken daily.

Fig. 27.5 Interrelations and metabolism of the *p*-aminophenol derivatives

Toxic reactions to the p-aminophenol derivatives

When phenacetin was in vogue, and particularly in the days before paracetamol had begun to replace it, chronic poisoning with the drug was not uncommon. It most often occurred as the result of a reckless consumption of headache powders. It has been said that phenacetin sometimes caused euphoria and some cases of habituation to the drug were certainly reported. A few habituated patients apparently displayed restlessness and hyperexcitability when the drug was withdrawn, a hint that it was even possible to become physically dependent on phenacetin. These facts, if true, constitute something of an exception to the general rule that aspirin like analgesics have no tendency to cause dependence.

Phenacetin and paracetamol have always found less favour than aspirin with potential suicides so that cases of severe acute poisoning with the p-aminophenol derivatives have always been uncommon.

The symptoms of chronic poisoning with phenacetin (or acetanilide) included cyanosis with associated anaemia, weakness and dyspnoea. These effects resulted from the conversion of haemoglobin into methaemoglobin and small amounts of sulphaemoglobin. Since neither compound is a respiratory pigment, they cause a *functional anaemia*. The agents responsible for these toxic changes were, of course, p-phenetidine and aniline (Fig. 27.5).

In addition to the functional anaemia arising from the effective lack of haemoglobin, chronic phenacetin poisoning sometimes caused a true haemolytic anaemia perhaps because the drug is capable of oxidizing vital components of the haemoglobin molecule.

Phenacetin, like the salicylates, sometimes caused renal papillary necrosis but it is not easy to assess the relative toxicities of aspirin and phenacetin in this respect since so many of those who suffered kidney damage after the prolonged ingestion of analgesics had taken preparations containing both drugs.

Pyrazolone derivatives

The compound now known as antipyrine (Fig. 27.6) was first synthesized in 1884. It received its name from an early observation that it had an antipyretic action in human beings. Analgesic and antiinflammatory actions were discovered soon afterwards.

ANTIPYRINE AND AMINOPYRINE

Both antipyrine (phenazone) and aminopyrine (amidopyrine) are effective analgesic and antiinflammatory compounds and until quite recently they were very successfully used for the treatment of rheumatic fever and for the relief of pain of moderate intensity, including lumbago and dysmenorrhoea. An incidental use of anti-

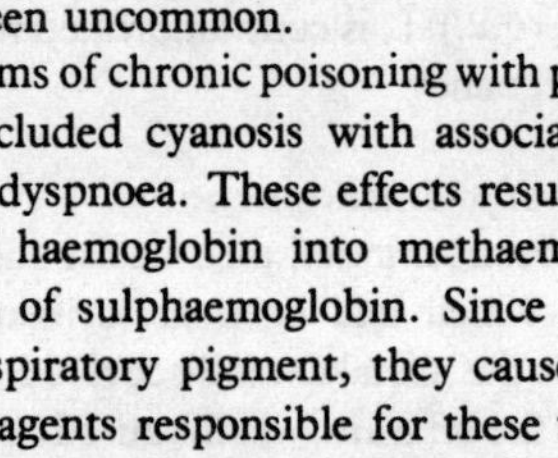

	R_1	R_2		R
Phenylbutazone	H	$(CH_2)_3CH_3$	Antipyrine	H
Oxyphenbutazone	OH	$(CH_2)_3CH_3$	Aminopyrine	$-N(CH_3)_2$
Kebuzone (Kétazone)	H	$(CH_2)_2COCH_3$	Dipyrone	$-NCH_3CH_2SO_3^-$ Na$^+$
G25671	H	$(CH_2)_2SC_6H_5$		
Sulphinpyrazone	H	$(CH_2)_2SOC_6H_5$		
Phenazone	H	$CH_2CH = C(CH_3)_2$		

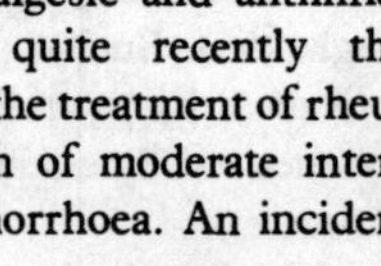

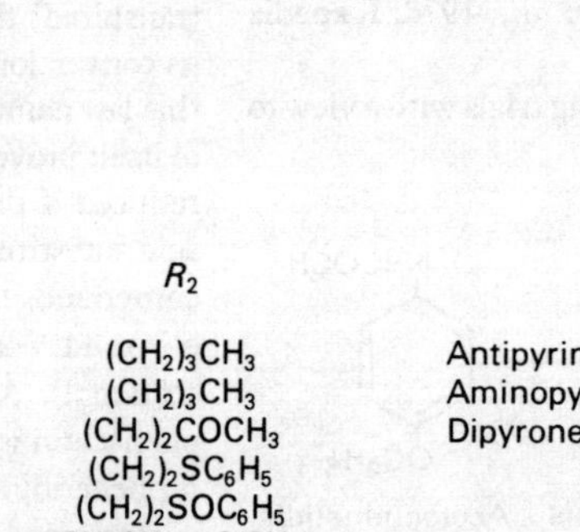

Azapropazone

Fig. 27.6 Pyrazolone derivatives with antiinflammatory activity

pyrine was in the measurement of total body water. The drug is very rapidly and evently distributed throughout the body water, both extracellular and intracellular, and it is relatively slowly excreted. If a known amount of antipyrine is given to a subject, it is possible to determine the total amount of his body water by measuring the concentration of antipyrine in his plasma—which will be the same as that in the other body fluids—after equilibration has taken place.

Aminopyrine is a more effective analgesic than antipyrine. In daily doses of 2 to 3 grams, it was as effective a remedy as aspirin but it is not used nowadays because it can cause a fatal agranulocytosis. Antipyrine is much less prone to cause agranulocytosis but it is also a less powerful analgesic so that it is now used only infrequently. Similar remarks apply to dipyrone.

PHENYLBUTAZONE

Phenylbutazone (Butazolidin, Butacote, Butazone, Ethibute, Flexazone, Oppazone, Tetnor and many others) was first synthesized in 1946 and it has been in clinical use since 1952. It is structurally similar to aminopyrine and because of its toxicity it should only be employed for the short term relief of acute inflammation in patients with rheumatic or allied disorders that do not respond to other agents. Phenylbutazone has had success as a remedy for acute gout (presumably by reason of its uricosuric metabolite mentioned below) but its toxicity precludes the more prolonged use that would be required if it were applied to the treatment of chronic gout.

Phenylbutazone is metabolized very slowly in man. Its half life is about three days, a circumstance which gives rise to the risk of cumulative effects if the drug is administered injudiciously. On the other hand, it also makes it easier to maintain therapeutically effective concentrations of the drug throughout a period of treatment. Phenylbutazone is metabolized much more rapidly by other mammalian species.

The two principal metabolites of phenylbutazone are metabolite I (oxyphenbutazone) and metabolite II (γ-hydroxyphenylbutazone; Fig. 27.7). Metabolite I is as powerful an antirheumatic agent as phenylbutazone and it seems probable that the antiinflammatory properties of phenylbutazone are at least partly attributable to oxyphenbutazone which accumulates in the plasma after phenylbutazone administration and which is cleared only slowly from the body, its half-life being the same as that of phenylbutazone itself. Metabolite II is devoid of antirheumatic activity but it is a powerful uricosuric agent (p. 458). In contrast to metabolite I, it is excreted rapidly with a half-life of eight hours.

Because it seemed that the uricosuric action of metabolite II arose from the increased acidity conferred by the hydroxyl substituent in the side chain, efforts were made to synthesize even more powerful agents by appropriate modification of the side chain of phenylbutazone. The results of these efforts was the discovery of G25671 (Fig. 27.6) and its metabolite, sulphinpyrazone. The latter compound is a very powerful uricosuric agent.

Phenylbutazone, like the salicylates, uncouples oxidative phosphorylation.

The daily dose of phenylbutazone is of the order of 200–400 mg taken with meals. It may be necessary to prescribe an antacid to prevent gastric upsets but if so the preparation used should be free of sodium in view of phenylbutazone's tendency to cause sodium retention. The incidence of gastrointestinal disturbances can be reduced by offering the drug by the rectal route.

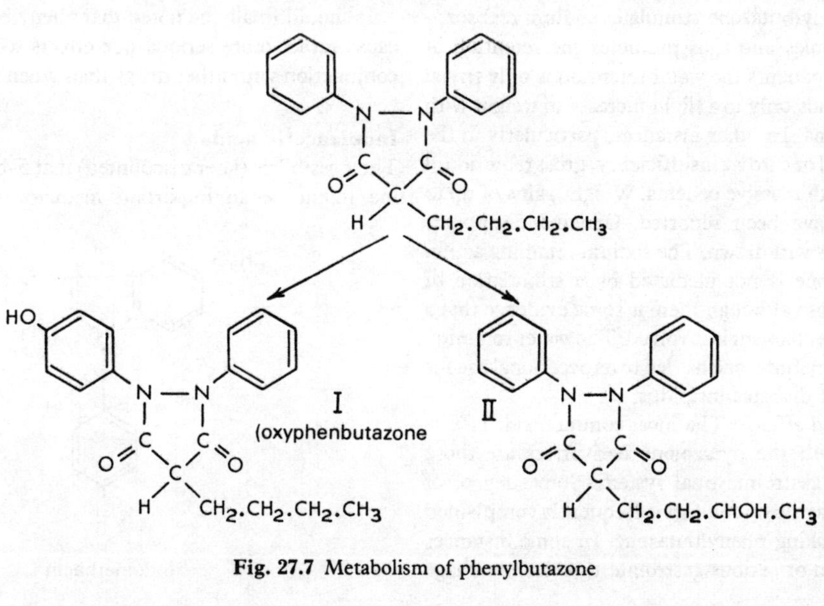

Fig. 27.7 Metabolism of phenylbutazone

OTHER COMPOUNDS

As we have already noted, *oxyphenbutazone* (Tandacote, Tanderil) has properties that duplicate those of phenylbutazone and the two drugs are employed in identical dosage forms and amounts, for similar purposes. *Kebuzone* (Kétazone) is also similar to phenylbutazone. It is popular in some parts of mainland Europe, particularly Czechoslovakia.

Toxic reactions to the pyrazolone derivatives

Blood Dyscrasias. It has already been noticed that the use of amidopyrine is seriously limited by its tendency to cause agranulocytosis and the possibility that structurally related compounds may have the same toxic action has clearly to be eliminated before the drugs can be unreservedly recommended for clinical use. Because of its therapeutic potentiality, phenylbutazone was particularly carefully scrutinized with the conclusion that the danger of agranulocytosis as a result of phenylbutazone treatment was minimal. It was calculated (Rechenberg, 1962) that the number of deaths from all causes attributable to phenylbutazone was no more than one in a million of all patients treated with the drug. This compares very favourably with that caused by other drugs but it does not justify complacency and phenylbutazone should be prescribed only when the patient does not respond well to safer drugs and then it must be given with circumspection. The danger of death from agranulocytosis can be minimized by avoiding high doses or prolonged administration of phenylbutazone and by making sure that the patient immediately reports the occurrence of any unusual symptom, particularly a sore mouth or throat. Regular blood counts, though advisable, are of limited utility, since they may not warn of danger until irreversible changes have occurred in the bone marrow.

Oedema. Phenylbutazone stimulates sodium reabsorption by the tubules and thus promotes the retention of water. In many patients the water retention is only trivial in extent and leads only to a slight increase in weight with no visible oedema. In other instances, particularly in the presence of renal or cardiac insufficiency, gross retention of water occurs with massive oedema. Weight gains of up to 15 kilograms have been reported. Oedema disappears when the drug is withdrawn. The sodium retaining action of phenylbutazone is not mediated by a stimulation of aldosterone release although there is some evidence that a hypothalamic mechanism is involved. The water retaining property of phenylbutazone has led to its occasional use for the treatment of diabetes insipidus.

Gastrointestinal effects. The most common side effects of treatment with the pyrazolone derivatives are those exerted on the gastrointestinal system. Some degree of nausea and epigastric discomfort is frequently complained of by patients taking phenylbutazone. In some instances peptic ulceration or serious gastrointestinal haemorrhage

occurs and pyrazolone derivatives should not be given to patients with a history of peptic ulceration unless no other drug is available.

It will be recalled that gastrointestinal symptoms also occur as side effects of salicylate therapy but whereas salicylates act directly on the gastric and intestinal mucosa, the ulcerogenic action of the pyrazolone derivative is not wholly attributable to a local action: gastrointestinal side effects are seen after parenteral administration of the drug. It seems possible that the gastrointestinal symptoms are the result of the drugs' acting on hypothalamic centres. It has already been mentioned that phenylbutazone acts on this part of the diencephalon and it is known that erosions of the gastric and intestinal mucosa can be produced by other drugs (reserpine is an example) that act on hypothalamic cnetres.

Even though the pyrazolone derivatives appear to produce gastrointestinal symptoms largely through their action on central mechanisms, the incidence of minor degrees of gastrointestinal upset can be considerably reduced when oral preparations are used by taking the drug with, or immediately after, meals. Rectal administration offers similar benefits.

Other side effects. Other reported side effects of treatment with the pyrazolone derivatives include drug rash, vertigo, euphoria, insomnia and tremor. A few cases of convulsions following the intramuscular injection of phenylbutazone have been reported.

Although phenylbutazone uncouples oxidative phosphorylation, pyrexia does not arise as a result of taking toxic doses of the drug. This is rather surprising in view of the fact that the pyrexia of salicylate poisoning is usually said to be a consequence of uncoupling. It may be that doses of phenylbutazone high enough to cause a sufficiently complete uncoupling are not commonly taken.

It should finally be noted that phenylbutazone tends to cause rather more serious side effects when it is taken in conjunction with other drugs than when it is taken alone.

Indoleacetic acids

The possibility (later discounted) that 5-hydroxytryptamine might be an important mediator of inflammation

Indomethacin

inspired an investigation into the antiinflammatory activity of a number of indole derivatives synthesized in the expectation of their having an antiserotonin action. The clues revealed by these studies led to the development of indomethacin, a compound that has been in clinical use since 1963.

Indomethacin (Indocid, Imbrilon) is a powerful analgesic and antiinflammatory agent with antipyretic and uricosuric actions. Because of the frequency with which it evokes untoward side effects, indomethacin is not used as a routine analgesic or antipyretic agent or for the treatment of gout. It is sometimes employed to resolve the pyrexia of Hodgkin's disease that has stubbornly withstood attack from other antipyretic agents but its chief value is for the treatment of cases of rheumatoid arthritis that cannot be given aspirin. Like the fenamic acids it has also been successfully employed for the treatment of dysmenorrhoea.

Indomethacin is readily absorbed from the alimentary tract reaching a peak plasma level about one hour after its ingestion. Its plasma half life is two hours. In man it is largely metabolized by O-demethylation and N-deacylation and some of the transformed molecules are conjugated with glucuronic acid. Excretion is by the kidney and faeces but the conjugates undergo enterohepatic cycling and this is a factor in the production of intestinal side effects.

It has been estimated that up to 50 per cent of those receiving therapeutic doses of indomethacin suffer untoward side effects, severe enough in about 20 per cent of these cases to necessitate the drug's withdrawal. Side effects include blood dyscrasias (including thrombocytopenia and aplastic anaemia), severe frontal headache, peptic ulcer and other gastrointestinal disturbances, dizziness, tinnitus, psychotic disturbances, hallucinations and depression. Some of these reactions are the result of the drug's aspirin-like attributes but the others reflect its antiserotonin action. Like aspirin, indomethacin uncouples oxidative phosphorylation as well as inhibiting the synthesis of prostaglandins.

The initial oral dose of indomethacin is 25 mg. It is given only twice daily in the early stages of treatment but if no untoward reaction occurs within a week, it is permissible to increase the dose to 25-35 mg thrice daily taken with meals in order to reduce the incidence of gastrointestinal complications. Indomethacin is contraindicated in pregnancy and in patients with a history of peptic ulcer.

Derivatives of phenylacetic and phenylpropionic acids

Investigations into the antiinflammatory activity of this group of compounds began some twenty five years ago. What promised to be the first successful outcome of these studies was the appearance of ibufenac (Fig. 27.8) but this compound was found to cause liver damage in experimental animals and it never left the laboratory. Ibufenac's successful successors—which are depicted in Fig. 27.8—are free of hepatoxicity.

A simple modification of the ibufenac molecule gave *ibuprofen* (Brufen, Motrin) which became generally available for clinical use in 1969, since when it has enjoyed considerable success.

Ibuprofen is comparable in its actions and potency to phenylbutazone and indomethacin but it is less likely to cause undesirable side effects. When side effects do occur they are typically aspirin-like and include gastrointestinal upsets (sometimes with bleeding), disturbances of central nervous function (including headache, blurred vision and tinnitus) and blood dyscrasias, particularly thrombocytopenia.

Ibuprofen is readily absorbed after oral administration. Peak plasma levels are reached after some two hours and the drug's plasma half life is also about two hours. About 60 per cent of an administered dose appears in the urine largely in the form of two principal metabolites formed as a result of transformations in the isobutyl moiety of the ibuprofen molecule. These metabolic changes involve hydroxylation of the CH radical and carboxylation of one of the methyl groups respectively. The metabolites appear in both the free and the conjugated forms.

Ibuprofen is used particularly in the treatment of rheumatoid arthritis, ankylosing spondylitis and osteoarthritis while clinical reports indicate its value in juvenile polyarthritis (Still's disease). The daily adult dose is 600-1200 mg in four instalments. Some increase in this dose is permissible to deal with acute arthritic exacerbations. For long term administration, the maintenance dose should be kept as near as possible to the lowest point of the dose range.

The actions, pharmacokinetic characteristics, uses and side effects of *fenoprofen* (Fenopron), *ketoprofen* (Alrheumat, Orudis), *flurbiprofen* (Froben), the other phenylpropionic acid deriviatives, are similar to those of ibuprofen. Fenoprofen is compounded as the calcium salt and is given in daily oral doses equivalent to 300 to 600 mg of the acid. Ketoprofen and flurbiprofen are much more potent than ibuprofen: they are given in three or four doses, each of 50 mg. Flurbiprofen, the newest member of the group, has been used with success to relieve the pain from soft tissue injuries sustained by professional footballers. For this purpose it is, apparently, superior to aspirin.

Some newer derivatives of phenylacetic acid have enjoyed more success than did ibufenac. They include *alclofenac* (Prinalgin, Zumaril), *buflexamac* (Feximac, Parfenac) and, most recently, *fenclofenoc*.

Alclofenac is employed, in thrice daily oral doses of a half to one gram, largely for the relief of muscular and rheumatic pain but the incidence of side effects is high. About one in two of those who receive the drug develop skin rashes. Bufexamac is made up in a 5 per cent cream for the local treatment of pruritis, psoriasis and of the pain resulting from rheumatism or trauma. Bufexamac sometimes causes contact dermatitis. Early experience indicates that fenclofenac will prove to be a useful agent for the management of rheumatoid arthritis and osteoarthrosis. The daily dose, taken in two instalments is 600 to 1800 mg. The incidence of gastrointestinal complications among patients taking fenclofenac is encouragingly low but skin rashes sometimes cause trouble.

Naphthaleneacetic acids

Naproxen (Naprosyn) is the most successful of a series of naphthaleneacetic acids that have analgesic, antipyretic and antiinflammatory actions. It is applied to the treatment of rheumatoid arthritis, osteoarthrosis and ankylosing spondylitis for which purpose it is given in twice daily oral doses of 250 to 400 mg. Its side effects are similar to those of the salicylates and its tendency to cause gastroin-

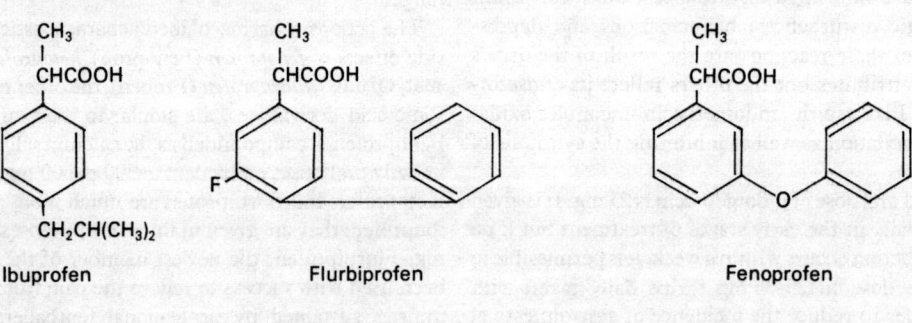

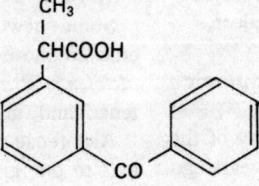

Fig. 27.8 Derivatives of phenylacetic and phenylpropionic acids

Naproxen

testinal bleeding demands that the drug should be given only with the utmost circumspection to those with a history of peptic ulceration.

Naproxen is extensively bound to plasma protein, it has a half life of some twelve hours and it is largely excreted as the glucuronide.

CORTICOSTEROIDS

In 1929 Hench noticed that the condition of his patients with rheumatoid arthritis improved if they became pregnant or jaundiced. He thought that these temporary remissions might be caused by a hormone of the adrenal cortex but he had to wait for twenty years before he was able to test his hypothesis adequately. When cortisone (p. 766) became available in quantity, Hench and his colleagues were able to embark on clinical trials and they soon found that cortisone and the adrenocorticotrophic hormone (corticotrophin, ACTH) both brought about a rapid relief of symptoms in rheumatoid arthritis. The paper in which these results were announced (Hench, Kendall, Slocumb and Polley, 1949) made an immediate and worldwide impact. One consequence was that Hench and two of those who had been most closely associated with the synthesis of cortisone (Kendall and Reichstein) were awarded the Nobel Prize for Medicine in 1950. Another result of Hench's observations was that cortisone and the synthetic corticosteroids which were developed later, were tested as potential therapeutic agents in a large number of diseases. Their success in many of these conditions apparently supported Selye's hypothesis that many human disorders result from a failure of a mechanism which is mediated by the adrenal cortex and controlled by the hypothalamic-pituitary system and whose activity enables the organism to adapt itself to the stresses—physical, chemical or nervous—of everyday life.

The view that corticosteroids boosted this *general adaptation syndrome* won general acceptance and approval when it was first put forward some two decades ago, at a time when the concept of 'stress disease' was in its heyday and corticosteroids were spoken of almost with awe. The observation that large doses of salicylates stimulated the release of corticotrophin, tempted many to conclude at the time that aspirin like drugs too owed their therapeutic efficacy to an effect on the pituitary-adrenal axis which thus became regarded as the primary site of action of all antiinflammatory drugs. More recent events have completely turned the tables for it is now generally believed, as

we shall see, that corticosteroids owe their antiinflammatory action at least predominantly to their possessing properties that permit them to exert aspirin like actions. The corticosteroids are no longer spoken of as being of any more than secondary importance, to be used when other treatments fail or as an adjunct to other forms of treatment. Although it is still usual to divide antiinflammatory agents into steroidal and nonsteroidal groups (with the implication that the former group constitutes a class apart) this division is no longer a useful one and the time is probably not too far distant before the corticosteroids will feature at the bottom of lists of aspirin like agents.

The antiinflammatory effects of the natural corticosteroids is associated exclusively with their glucocorticoid functions and it is, therefore, an advantage when treating inflammatory conditions to use synthetic corticosteroids with glucocorticoid but minimal mineralocorticoid activity. A number of compounds fall into this category: they are listed in Table 44.2 (p. 760).

The most useful steroids for the long term treatment of rheumatoid arthritis are prednisone and prednisolone. The daily dose of these compounds is usually about 10 mg though it may be increased cautiously to 15 mg if required or reduced in those patients who show a marked response to 10 mg of the drug.

Dexamethasone is much the most potent steroid available. A dose of 1.7 mg of dexamethasone is equipotent with 10 mg of prednisone. In general, none of the other compounds mentioned in Table 44.2 is as useful as prednisone or prednisolone, but hydrocortisone can be given by direct intra-articular injection in patients affected in very few joints. Corticotrophin has the same general effects as the corticosteroids but side effects, though similar in type, tend to be more serious.

Toxic reactions to the corticosteroids

Even in therapeutic doses, the corticosteroids may cause toxic side effects. Many of these are simply the inevitable result of the administration of grossly unphysiological quantities of a hormone preparation and in some instances a clinical picture similar to that of Cushing's syndrome is seen. The side effects can be catalogued as follows:

Effects caused by mineralocorticoid activity. The mineralocorticoids cause retention of sodium and chloride. As a result, there is retention of water which may be sufficiently marked to produce frank oedema or a measurable change in body weight. In addition, there may be sufficient loss of potassium to cause muscle weakness, while in elderly patients serious calcium loss may lead to osteoporosis.

Effects caused mainly by glucocorticoid activity. There may be rounding of the face (the 'moon face' effect), abnormal deposition of fat, excessive appetite, marked increase of body weight, increased hair growth, sweating and pigmentation of the skin. The increased glucocorticoid can also precipitate diabetes mellitus.

Other effects. There may be a decreased resistance to infection and latent infections may become active. Dyspepsia and other gastointestinal upsets are not uncommon and peptic ulcer is sometimeś activated or induced. Hypertension may occur.

Effects on withdrawal of the drugs. The administration of corticosteroids will cause the output of corticotrophin from the pituitary to be depressed. Consequently, the activity of the adrenal cortex will be suppressed. If steroid therapy is suddenly stopped, symptoms of acute adrenocortical insufficiency may appear. Withdrawal of steroids must therefore be gradual and corticotrophin may have to be given to stimulate the adrenal cortex into renewed activity.

MISCELLANEOUS ANTIINFLAMMATORY AGENTS

The only justification for gathering together under one heading the drugs to be mentioned in the course of the next few pages is the rather negative one that none of them operates primarily by inhibiting prostaglandin synthesis or release.

GOLD COMPOUNDS

In 1890, Koch reported that low concentrations of gold salts were toxic to the tubercle bacillus and this led to the therapeutic use of gold compounds (*chrysotherapy*). Because it was believed that rheumatoid arthritis was the result of a bacterial infection, chrysotherapy was applied to this condition as well as to tuberculosis. Notwithstanding the erroneous premiss upon which the treatment was based, chrysotherapy achieved a considerable success in the treatment of arthritis until it was superseded by the corticosteroids. However, its eclipse was only temporary for when it became clear that corticosteroids were not suitable agents for the long-term treatment of rheumatoid arthritis, chrysotherapy was partly restored to favour and it now has a place again—albeit a very limited one—in the treatment of carefully selected cases. The use of gold is restricted by the frequency with which it causes seriously toxic side effects and at best it can only be regarded as an adjunct to other forms of therapy. The mode of action of gold compounds is not known; the psychological effect of being treated with a material so traditionally precious and awe inspiring as gold must play some part. Its pharmacological effects are probably related to its ability to inhibit thiol compounds, a fact which explains the effectiveness of dimercaprol in the treatment of gold poisoning. Among the enzymes inhibited by gold compounds are acid phosphatase, cathepsin and β-glucuronidase all of which are present in the lysosomes of polymorphonuclear leucocytes and must be numbered among the likely mediators of inflammation. It is known too that gold is concentrated in the lysosomes.

Gold compounds may also inhibit the synthesis of mucopolysaccharide and so limit the formation of connective tissue.

The gold preparations now in use include sodium aurothiomalate (Myocrisin, Myochrysine), aurothioglucose (Solganal) and aurothioglycanide (Leuron). The formulae of these compounds are presented in Figure 27.9.

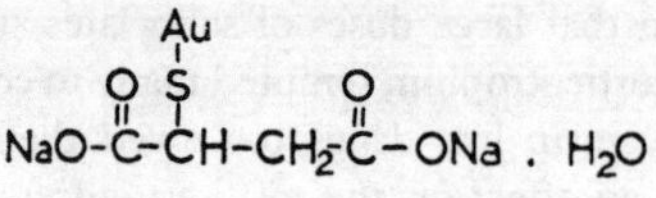

No one gold compound appears to be more satisfactory than another and all are given at the same dose level. Weekly intramuscular injections, each containing 50 mg can be given for three to six months. A careful watch must be kept for toxic side effects, the most dangerous of which are agranulocytosis, exfoliative dermatitis and hepatitis. Patients who suffer from anaemia or from diseases of the skin, liver or kidneys are particularly likely to exhibit toxic reactions to gold.

Skin reactions to metallic gold are very occasionally seen (in ear lobes, fingers etc.) in those who wear gold jewellery.

Gold is of no value in the treatment of rheumatic fever and even in cases in which it is initially successful there may be a relapse when treatment ceases. Repeat courses of treatment can be given, provided that a period of at least three months elapses between courses. Gold is excreted only very slowly and the possibility of producing a dangerous cumulation must always be borne in mind.

IMMUNOSUPPRESSIVE AND IMMUNOREGULATORY DRUGS

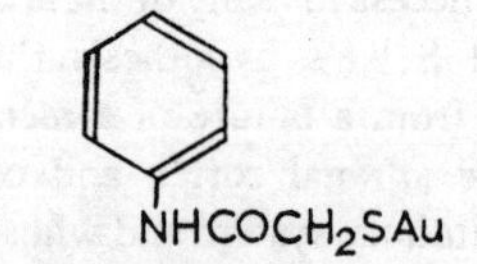

Some drugs that are capable of suppressing immune

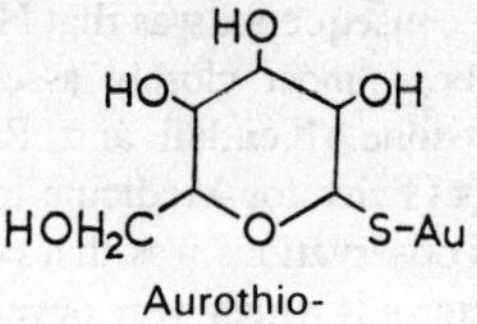

Fig. 27.9 Therapeutically useful gold compounds

reactions also abolish inflammatory responses particularly those of the acute variety. The two activities may be causally related—some inflammatory conditions such as rheumatoid arthritis have, after all, an autoimmune origin (p.395)—or the antiinflammatory effects may arise from an entirely independent property of the immunosuppressive agents. Present opinion leans towards the latter viewpoint. Whatever the true position, immunosuppressive agents certainly have to be found a place in any survey that purports to include all varieties of antiinflammatory drugs.

Immunosuppressive agents in general have been developed as anticancer agents and, as such, they are discussed in detail in Chapter 61 (p. 912). They are quite toxic and the only ones that need to be seriously considered in the present context are azathioprine (p. 919) and cyclophosphamide (p. 915). Neither drug should be used unless other forms of treatment have failed. Both drugs are given in daily doses of 2-3 mg per kilogram of body weight.

An *immunoregulatory* agent, as its name implies, is one that modifies an immune response. Although some drugs of this type inhibit the response (and so behave as immunosuppressive substances) othere actually enhance it. The rationale for exploring the possibility of employing drugs of the latter type for the treatment of rheumatoid arthritis is that further stimulation of the immune response that has actually precipitated the disease should render ineffective the responsible antigen. As yet, levamisole (Ketrax) is the only drug of this type that has actually been used for the routine treatment of rheumatoid arthritis. It is given in daily oral doses of 150 mg.

Levamisole

Levamisole is also employed in the treatment of round worm infection (ascariasis, p. 887).

D-PENICILLAMINE

Penicillamine (a degradation product of penicillin) has become established as the drug of choice for the treatment of Wilson's disease (p. 164). As one of its proprietary names (Cuprimine) indicates, it promotes the excretion of the retained copper which is responsible for the pathological features of that condition. It chelates other heavy metals too and it can be recommended for the treatment of lead and mercury poisoning. This aspect of its therapeutic use is discussed in Chapter 48 (p. 797), where its chemical formula can also be found.

The L-isomer of penicillamine (and consequently the racemic mixture) is more toxic than the D-isomer by reason of its liability to antagonize pyridoxine and to cause optic neuritis. Only the D-isomer should, therefore, be used.

D-Penicillamine has recently attracted the attention of rheumatologists who have shown that it has beneficial actions in rheumatoid arthritis. It seems to have more than a merely palliative effect and rheumatoid arthritis responds rather specifically to penicillamine therapy. The drug can be combined, if necessary, with corticosteroids or aspirin like agents but not with gold compounds whose toxic effects are similar to, and would therefore sum with, those of penicillamine itself. It is unfortunate that penicillamine has a relatively high toxicity particularly since the nature of the condition it may be called upon to treat will inevitably require that it be given over a long period of time. Toxic reactions apart, early clinical reports have been encouraging.

The toxicity of D-penicillamine demands that no arthritic patient should receive a starting dose of more than 250 mg daily. Those who do not exhibit hypersensitivity to this modest dose can be exposed to gradually increasing amounts of penicillamine until the maximal permissible daily dose (1 to 1.5 grams) is reached. Many patients respond satisfactorily to lower maintenance doses. Hypersensitivity reactions—which are sometimes severe enough to warrant treatment with corticosteroids or histamine H_1 antagonists—include vomiting, pyrexia, dermatitis and neutropenia. Hypersensitivity should be expected (though it does not invariably occur) in patients who are known to be sensitive to penicillin. Toxic effects appearing in the course of treatment with normal doses of D-penicillamine include skin rashes, kidney disease (nephrosis and glomerulonephritis have both been reported), temporary loss of taste, blood dyscrasias, systemic lupus erythematosus and, oddly enough, myasthenia gravis.

Penicillamine has been shown to exert a large number of pharmacological actions, any or all of which might be related to its therapeutic effects, so protean are the aetiological factors in rheumatoid arthritis. It certainly has an immunoregulatory action (of the type that potentiates immune reactions) but there is evidence that it is an immunosuppressive substance too. It is, of course, a chelating agent and it is known that concentrations of copper in the serum are elevated in rheumatoid arthritis and other inflammatory states. It is therefore possible (though, on the balance of evidence, not very likely) that chelation of copper contributes to penicillamine's therapeutic usefulness. Penicillamine also inhibits the formation of the insoluble form of collagen which is laid down in the joints in rheumatoid arthritis. Penicillamine affects other aspects of protein metabolism causing, for instance, a depression in the amount of a collagen like protein in the plasma of arthritic subjects. This protein has antigenic properties that certainly contribute to the total rheumatic process.

These, and several other properties of penicillamine, are discussed by Arrigoni-Martelli (1977).

ANTIMALARIALS

In 1953, Haydn used the antimalarial drug chloroquine phosphate (p. 867) for the treatment of rheumatoid arthritis. He obtained encouraging results and suggested that in rheumatoid arthritis the requirements of the tissues for adenosine triphosphate are increased and that chloroquine, which inhibits adenosine triphosphatase, might be active by virtue of that property. While it is unlikely that this is the correct explanation of chloroquine's action, there is no doubt that the drug does possess some antiinflammatory activity and that its use as an adjunct to more established forms of therapy can be considered in appropriate cases. Chloroquine produces adverse side effects in a high proportion of patients unless the dose is carefully controlled. A daily dose limit of 250 mg has been recommended. Hydroxychloroquine sulphate (daily dose 400 mg) appears to be less toxic. Mepacrine has also been used but it is less satisfactory.

The side effects of chloroquine are discussed elsewhere (p. 867) but an additional hazard may be encountered if the drug is administered for the prolonged periods required for the control of rheumatoid arthritis. Chloroquine is concentrated in the structures of the eye to a greater extent than in other tissues and this may lead to opacities of the cornea or to degenerative changes in the retina. Regular examination of the eyes is therefore essential in patients receiving long term treatment with the antimalarials.

OTHER COMPOUNDS

A large number of other substances has been shown to have an antiinflammatory effect in laboratory preparations but few of them have been employed for therapeutic purposes. They are catalogued and their actions are discussed by Adams and Cobb (1967) and they need no mention here. We should, however, refer to *glycyrrhetinic acid*, a compound obtained by the hydrolysis of glycyrrhiz-

Glycyrrhetinic Acid

inic acid, a glycoside obtained from liquorice. It has antiinflammatory activity, as has carbenoxolone, a water soluble derivative of glycyrrhetinic acid. Carbenoxolone is used in the treatment of gastric ulcer and as such it is discussed on page 642.

Mode of action of the antiinflammatory drugs

We have mentioned on several occasions in the course of this chapter that the primary action of the aspirin like drugs is to inhibit the synthesis of thromboxanes and prostaglandins. This topic is discussed in detail in Chapter 23 (p. 361) and it is not necessary to say more at this point beyond the fact that the experimental evidence indicates quite clearly that the antipyretic, analgesic and antiinflammatory actions of the drugs are all dependent, at least to a considerable degree, on this one property. Moreover there is now a substantial body of evidence to indicate that the corticosteroids—whose mode of action has hitherto been believed to be fundamentally different from that of the nonsteroidal agents—also interfere with the release, if not the synthesis, of prostaglandins (see Vane, 1976). Nevertheless, it would be very surprising indeed if it happened that not one from the large range of available antiinflammatory drugs exerted any other action that might usefully contribute to its therapeutic usefulness. Indeed we have already drawn attention (p. 454) to a small group of antiinflammatory agents that do not, apparently suppress the synthesis or release of prostaglandins and we have also concluded (p. 442) that the pyrexia caused by high doses of aspirin depends on its being able to uncouple oxidative phosphorylation.

We can admit that the analgesic and antipyretic actions of the major antiinflammatory agents are entirely attributable to their being able to inhibit prostaglandin synthetase but we need to enquire more closely into the contribution, if any, made by other biochemical actions to the drugs' antiinflammatory efficacy. Since we know that the uncoupling of oxidative phosphorylation is responsible for at least one aspect of aspirin's toxicity it is appropriate to ask whether this action contributes also to the therapeutic action of aspirin and other antiinflammatory agents.

Rheumatism is essentially a disease of connective tissue and a number of attempts have been made to explore the possibility that antiinflammatory agents prevent the continued synthesis of connective tissue components. Several antiinflammatory agents uncouple oxidative phosphorylation and it has been argued that the consequent impairment of adenosine triphosphate synthesis will deprive the cells of the energy supplies needed for the production of mucopolysaccharides, which with collagen fibres constitute the most important component of connective tissue. Impairment of mucopolysaccharide synthesis would not only reduce the formation of scars and other overgrowths of connective tissue but it would also reduce oedema by virtue of the fact that mucopolysaccharides (which are polyanions) tend to cause retention of sodium and hence of water. It has been pointed out (Whitehouse, 1963) that the ability of antiinflammatory drugs to uncouple oxidative phosphorylation parallels their ability to reduce inflammatory changes.

The list of antiinflammatory agents which uncouple

oxidative phosphorylation is impressive. In addition to the salicylates and phenylbutazone it includes indomethacin, some compounds of gold, glycyrrhetinic acid, indomethacin, cinchophen, mefenamic acid and flufenamic acid. It is a matter of some interest that high doses of some drugs that are not usually regarded as antiinflammatory compounds (the antipsychotic agents provide one example) uncouple oxidative phosphorylation and also exhibit rudimentary antiinflammatory activity. It is true that the association between antiinflammatory and uncoupling activity is not an indissoluble one: the classical uncoupling agent is 2,4-dinitrophenol but it exhibits no antiinflammatory activity whatever. Nevertheless it does not seem totally unreasonable to suppose that the uncoupling ability seen in so many antiinflammatory agents does contribute to their overall therapeutic effect particularly when they are applied to the treatment of the more chronic types of inflammatory disorder.

Since the antiinflammatory agents inhibit prostaglandin synthetase it would not be surprising if they proved to have a similar action on other enzymes. One of the early stages in the synthesis of mucopolysaccharide is the production of glucosame 6-phosphate and it has been shown that aurothiomalate, flufenamic acid, phenylbutazone and salicylates all inhibit the formation of this component of connective tissue quite independently of any uncoupling action (Gryglewski and Vane, 1972). Antiinflammatory drugs may also be able to intervene at other loci in the synthetic sequence. The corticosteroids are also known to inhibit collagen synthesis probably by interfering with nucleic acid function.

Some of the antiinflammatory agents may accelerate the breakdown of mucopolysaccharide instead of (or in addition to) inhibiting its synthesis.

The inhibitory effect of the salicylates on proline formation has already been alluded to (p. 443). Since this aminoacid is a constituent of the plasma kinins its failure to appear in adequate amounts may play a subsidiary antiinflammatory role by preventing the formation of these minor mediators of the inflammatory process.

Other mechanisms that probably make a minor contribution to the effectiveness of some antiinflammatory drugs include stabilization of lysosomes and antagonism of some of the less important mediators of inflammation.

Guerra's belief (Guerra, 1946) that hyaluronidase activity is one of the biochemical determinants of the connective tissue disorders has not received much recent support and the ability of the salicylates to inhibit this enzyme is probably quite irrelevant to their therapeutic actions especially since the usual doses of these drugs exert only minor effects.

ACTION IN GOUT
The mode of action of drugs used for the treatment of gout is discussed below.

GOUT

Gout is an arthritic condition resulting from the deposition of urates (chiefly monosodium urate) in the joint cavities and on the articular cartilages. Small joints are affected before larger ones (gout usually appears first in the metatarsal-pharyngeal joint of the big toe) and the urates may also be deposited at an early stage on the cartilage of the external ear to give the telltale *tophaceous* ('stony') irregularities on the external edge of the auricular appendage.

The inflammatory changes that give rise to pain and immobility of the joints in gout are not the direct result of irritation by the crystalline urates. The crystals suffer phagocytosis by polymorphonuclear leucocytes and are thereby brought into contact with lysosomes, the membranes of which are ruptured with the release of destructive enzymes. The phagocytes after ingestion of urate also release chemotactic substances and, probably, lactic acid. The last mentioned substance provokes the further crystallization of urates from the plasma.

The central importance of polymorphs in the production of the inflammatory changes of gout is testified to by the fact that the intra-articular injection of monosodium urate in experimental animals is without effect unless polymorphonuclear leucocytes are also present.

The deposition of urates is the consequence of an increased concentration of uric acid in the blood. This end product of nucleoprotein metabolism has a notoriously low solubility (it is a pity that man could not evolve a system that would have produced a nucleoprotein metabolite more suited to urinary excretion) and only moderate increases in the concentration of urates in the plasma can precipitate an attack of gout. Although gout is probably the result of a metabolic defect it can certainly be precipitated by any factor that increases the production or hampers the excretion of uric acid. It was indeed once regarded as a prerogative of wealth: port and caviare are rich in purines. Gout sometimes complicates conditions such as myeloproliferative disease, leukaemia and polycythaemia rubra vera in which there is an accelerated breakdown (and production) of nucleic acid. The elimination of uric acid can be impaired to an extent that will precipitate gout in those susceptible to it by lead poisoning, the taking of pyrazinamide or of diuretic drugs, particularly the thiazides.

Drugs employed in the treatment of gout can be divided into three groups:

    a. those needed to control acute attacks,
    b. uricosuric agents, which promote the excretion of urates and
    c. allopurinol, which inhibits the formation of uric acid.

Drugs for acute gout
Attacks of acute gout are intensely painful and demand urgent attention. Colchicine is the traditional drug for this purpose but phenylbutazone is also of value.

COLCHICINE

Colchicine is an alkaloid obtained from the autumn crocus, *Colchicum autumnale*. It gives rapid relief from pain in acute attacks of gout although it is not properly an analgesic, except in this special case.

Colchicine is an antimitotic agent (for this reason it has been applied, not very successfully, to the treatment of leukaemia) because it binds to the microtubule elements (p. 17) of the mitotic spindle. This same property underlies its effectiveness in acute gout because microtubules are also involved in many other cellular processes including, in the polymorphonuclear leucocyte, the phagocytosis of urate crystals and the transport of lysosomes to and their subsequent fusion with the phagocytic vacuoles containing ingested urate. These processes culminate in lysosomal disruption which, as we have seen, provides the necessary preface to the inflammatory changes of gout. Thus the use of colchicine rests, after all, on a sound theoretical basis even though its effectiveness was discovered quite empirically.

Colchicine

The difference between the mechanism involved in gout and that operating in other inflammatory conditions is underlined by the fact that colchicine apparently *stimulates* the synthesis of prostaglandins.

In the treatment of acute gout, colchicine is given in an initial dose of 1 mg followed by 0.5 mg every two hours until the symptoms subside. It is usual to prescribe an upper limit of 8 mg to the total dose of colchicine to be taken in the course of any one attack. Side effects include vomiting, diarrhoea, abdominal pain, depression of the bone marrow, alopecia and peripheral neuritis. All these reactions are typical of those provoked by antimitotic drugs (p. 922) and their incidence can be reduced by paying careful attention to dosage.

It may be necessary to supplement colchicine with a regular analgesic to blunt the pain of an acute attack of gout.

PHENYLBUTAZONE

Phenylbutazone is a uricosuric agent, and, as such, it is discussed again below but it clears urate from the blood so rapidly that it can be used to treat acute gout. Because phenylbutazone is less toxic than colchicine it is, in many quarters, now the preferred drug notwithstanding colchi-cine's ability to suppress the very reactions that are responsible for the clinical manifestations of acute gout.

CORTICOSTEROIDS

Corticosteroids and corticotrophin also have a place among the drugs recommended for the control of acute gout. Their particular value is in individuals who do not respond to phenylbutazone. When corticotrophin is used, it is the practice to give colchicine too, lest a recrudescence of symptoms should occur when the corticotrophin is withdrawn.

Uricosuric agents

Uric acid is filtered by the renal glomeruli and it is then almost completely reabsorbed in the proximal tubules. Some is then secreted back into the urine by the distal tubules. Uricosuric drugs impair the process of tubular reabsorption, increase the excretion of uric acid and effect a reduction in its plasma concentration.

Many of the nonsteroidal antiinflammatory agents already discussed in this chapter together with a miscellany of other drugs exhibit a degree of uricosuric activity. Those made use of in the treatment of chronic gout are listed here.

PHENYLBUTAZONE

This drug is discussed in detail elsewhere (p. 449). For acute gout it is given in divided doses totalling 600 to 800 mg daily. Relief can usually be expected within 48 hours. Phenylbutazone elicits a brisk excretion of urate and care must be taken to maintain a high urine volume when it is used so as to guard against a painful crystallization of uric acid in the renal tubules. Phenylbutazone's toxicity is a contraindication to its use in chronic gout.

Indomethacin is as powerfully uricosuric as phenylbutazone but, being even more toxic, it is not recommended even for the therapy of acute gout.

SULPHINPYRAZONE

The development of sulphinpyrazone (Anturan) from the uricosuric metabolite of phenylbutazone has already been mentioned (p. 449). Sulphinpyrazone is considerably less toxic than phenylbutazone and it can usually be given with impunity on a long term basis between attacks of acute gout. It should, however, be withheld from patients who have reacted adversely to phenylbutazone and it is a wise precaution to make occasional checks on the blood counts of those who do receive the drug.

In the therapy of chronic gout, sulphinpyrazone is given by mouth in total daily amounts of 200–600 mg in three or four divided doses with meals. The injunction to ensure high daily urine volumes applies to sulphinpyrazone as strongly as it does to phenylbutazone. An alkaline urine enhances urate solubility.

Sulphinpyrazone is a poor analgesic and, particularly in the early stages of treatment, it may be necessary to supplement it with an analgesic drug. Salicylates are contraindicated for this purpose because they antagonize the uricosuric action of sulphinpyrazone, although if given alone they themselves reduce the concentration of urate in the plasma (see below).

Like probenecid (q.v.) sulphinpyrazone may interact with other drugs. Particular care should be exercised if it is given to patients receiving coumarin anticoagulant agents or orally active hypoglycaemic agents.

Sulphinpyrazone and myocardial infarction. Sulphinpyrazone is known to prolong the life of blood platelets and to inhibit their adhesion and aggregation. These facts prompted an investigation into the possibility that sulphinpyrazone might be used to prevent a second attack in patients who have survived their first myocardial infarction. The first results of this study have recently become available and they indicate that sulphinpyrazone does indeed significantly reduce the likelihood of an early and fatal reinfarction. Nearly 1500 patients were studied in this investigation.

Perhaps sulphinpyrazone (like aspirin, p. 375) should be taken by all those at risk in the hope of warding off even the first infarction!

PROBENECID

Probenecid (Benemid) was first synthesized in 1951 in the course of a project directed towards the production of non-toxic compounds that would inhibit the secretion of penicillin by the kidney tubules and thus permit the maintenance of high concentrations of the antibiotic in the tissues. Probenecid was used for a time in this way and it is still sometimes called upon to perform a similar service for cephalexin or cephalothin but since it is a potent uricosuric agent its main use is in the treatment of chronic gout. It is given orally in doses of 500 mg three or four times daily but lower doses (250 mg twice daily) are often employed in the early stages of treatment to prevent the complications such as an attack of acute gout that might follow the sudden mobilization of large amounts of urate. At the same time it should be remembered that very low doses of probenecid actually cause retention of urate, as they do of penicillin, by inhibiting tubular secretion processes. This occurs at dose levels that do not influence tubular reabsorption.

When probenecid is given the same precautions must be taken as were detailed for sulphinpyrazone and phenylbutazone to ensure the excretion of high volumes of alkaline urine. Salicylates exhibit the same kind of incompatability towards probenecid as they do towards sulphinpyrazone and they should not be given to patients who are also receiving probenecid. Combined therapy with probenecid and sulphinpyrazone is permissible for the probenecid impairs the excretion of sulphinpyrazone and the two drugs thus have an additive effect. Side reactions to probenecid therapy are relatively rare and usually mild. They include gastrointestinal upsets and drug rash

although more severe urticarial reactions sometimes appear. Renal calculi may be formed if the urine is acid and of low volume. Large doses taken with suicidal intent have caused epileptiform convulsions. Probenecid hinders the urinary excretion of some other drugs (including dapsone and indomethacin) and it is extensively bound to plasma protein. Both these circumstances give rise to the possibility of interactions with other substances and some thought should be given to the possible adverse consequences of giving another drug to patients already receiving probenecid.

Probenecid

Probenecid and sulphinpyrazone probably obstruct urate reabsorption by simple competition in the tubules.

A mixture of probenecid and colchicine, marketed as Colbenemid, is also available for the treatment of chronic gout.

SALICYLATES

Salicylates have a complex action on uric acid metabolism and excretion. Small doses inhibit the secretory mechanisms of the tubules and thus cause retention of uric acid. As the dose is increased, tubular reabsorption begins to be impaired and a dose level is eventually reached at which the increased retention of uric acid caused by inhibition of secretory mechanisms just balances the increased loss caused by inhibition of absorption. At this stage salicylates have no effect at all on uric acid secretion. At higher dose levels, there is a progressively increasing uricosuric action as reabsorption is further hindered. Salicylates can therefore be properly classed as uricosuric agents. Moreover they also have allopurinol like actions (see below), inhibiting xanthine oxidase and thereby reducing the production of uric acid. Nevertheless they are of limited utility as antigout agents in any but toxic doses and sodium salicylate is no longer recommended as a treatment of chronic gout.

It was mentioned earlier that the uricosuric action of probenecid and sulphinpyrazole is antagonized by the salicylates. The causes of this antagonism are not entirely clear. It may be that the action of the salicylates on the secretory mechanism causes a retention of urate sufficient to offset the effect of the other drugs on the process of reabsorption. Another explanation is that the salicylates promote binding of the other drug to plasma proteins. This would reduce the drug's effective concentration in the plasma.

The extensive effects of salicylates on urate metabolism and excretion are presumably reflections of their widespread metabolic actions to which attention was drawn earlier.

Allopurinol

Allopurinol (Zyloric, Zyloprim) was originally developed in the hope that it might possess useful antineoplastic activity, like the related mercaptopurine (p. 918). In the event, it proved to be an inhibitor of xanthine oxidase, a rather unspecific enzyme that is responsible for the conversion of hypoxanthine to xanthine and the further transformation of the latter compound into uric acid. Mercaptopurine, azathioprine and similar antineoplastic drugs—the purine antimetabolites—also form substrates for xanthine oxidase and allopurinol at least partly lived up to its creators' expectations because it was used for a time in cancer chemotherapy to potentiate and prolong the action of the purine antimetabolites. It was soon realized, however, that allopurinol's ability to impede the production of uric acid offered greater therapeutic promise and the drug has now enjoyed more than ten years of popularity as a remedy for chronic gout. It seems to be especially useful in cases of gout that, like those associated with leukaemia and myeloproliferative disease, have their origin in an increased turnover of nucleic acids. It is also indicated in patients who do not respond, or show adverse reactions, to probenecid or sulphinpyrazone. It is permissible to combine allopurinol with a uricosuric drug.

Allopurinol is itself a substrate for xanthine oxidase (at low dose levels it is a competitive inhibitor of the enzyme) but the substance into which it is enzymatically transformed (alloxanthine; Fig. 27.10) retains inhibitory activity.

Allopurinol is given in daily amounts of 200–600 mg (in single or divided doses) but in some circumstances—when, for instance, leukaemic patients are about to receive radio- or chemotherapy—higher doses may well be needed. It is a relatively safe drug, mild hypersensitivity reactions constituting the majority of the reported side effects. It inhibits hepatic microsomal enzyme activity and so can potentiate the action of some of the drugs (oral anticoagulant agents provide an example) that might be being taken at the same time. It is hardly necessary to add that if a patient is receiving mercaptopurine or a similar drug, the dose of the antimetabolite has to be sharply reduced if allopurinol is given too.

THE SCREENING OF ANALGESIC DRUGS AND ANTIINFLAMMATORY SUBSTANCES

A very large number of methods has been introduced for the laboratory assessment of analgesic activity. This is partly a reflection of the difficulties inherent in using animal preparations in the search for drugs capable of alleviating pain in man. These difficulties can be summarized as follows:

a. It is impossible to know whether the sensation experienced by animals in response to noxious stimuli is qualitatively similar to the pain felt by human beings in similar circumstances. This point is often stressed but too much should not be made of it. It is not unreasonable to suppose that an animal that cries or struggles in response to a noxious stimulus is undergoing a subjective experience whose underlying mechanism is similar to that operating

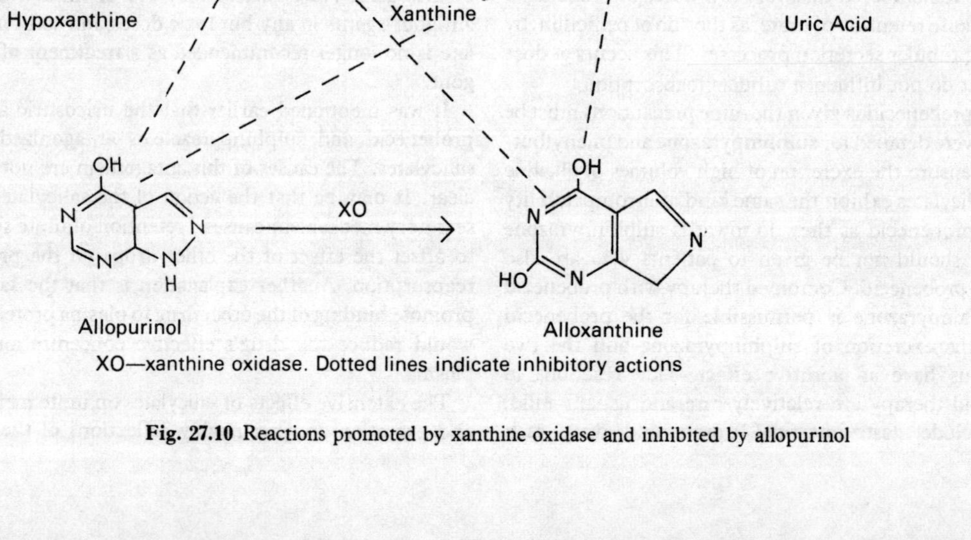

XO—xanthine oxidase. Dotted lines indicate inhibitory actions

Fig. 27.10 Reactions promoted by xanthine oxidase and inhibited by allopurinol

in man in similar circumstances and that a drug which prevents the overt signs of distress in the animal will be analgesic in man.

b. The relief of pain in human beings may involve more than an interference with pain producing mechanisms or an inhibition of activity in the nervous pathways for pain. What may loosely be termed psychological factors play a prominent part, as is evident from the ease with which it is possible to demonstrate a raising of pain threshold, or a relief of existing pain, by pharmacologically inactive placebos. Some part of the beneficial action produced by an analgesic drug may be due to side actions that cause subjective effects sufficient to persuade the patient that he has taken a potent drug. It is not possible to assess by animal experiments the extent to which factors such as these will contribute to the overall analgesic effect.

c. However, much the most serious deficiency concerns the nature of the stimulus used to provoke pain. A pin prick or similar form of mechanical trauma may stimulate pain fibres directly but pain whose relief demands the use of analgesics is more likely to be caused by the action of pain producing substances. Since some analgesics owe their effectiveness to an ability to antagonize pain producing substances, it is not surprising that their action is not revealed if the pain is produced by simple trauma. On the other hand, a drug that inhibits activity in the central pain pathway should be capable of preventing pain whatever the nature of the stimulus. These considerations explain the common finding that the activity of morphine like analgesics, unlike that of those with a peripheral action, is easily detected on a wide range of animal preparations. Unfortunately, a number of substances that have no analgesic action in man give positive results in many animal tests. In some instances, this is because the drug under test interferes with the response (licking the paws, crying, etc.) that signals that discomfort is being experienced. It is therefore always necessary to establish that a drug which appears to have analgesic properties does not cause motor incoordination or muscle paralysis.

In some investigations on analgesics, healthy human volunteers have been used. Most of these experiments are open to the criticism that, as in animal experiments, the stimulus employed bears little relationship to those that produce pain in conditions which demand the use of analgesics. The intraperitoneal injection of bradykinin in human subjects is obviously too heroic a procedure for routine purposes. The exposed blister base (p. 417) is very suitable for detecting pain producing substances but it seems to be less useful for the screening of potentially analgesic drugs.

The many procedures which have been used for testing analgesics can be summarized as follows:

Thermal methods

A popular method, applicable to mice, uses an electrically heated plate at 55°C. on which is placed an open cylinder. The mouse is placed in the cylinder and after a latent period which varies with the criterion selected, it begins to show signs of discomfort: it may raise its hind feet alternately from the place, dance, lick its forepaws or jump out of the cylinder. The two last named signs are the ones usually employed as the end point and if other manifestations of discomfort are ignored, relatively constant reaction times, of the order of ten seconds, are found with mice of any one strain. Analgesics with a central action prolong the reaction time to the thermal stimulus. It has been reported that if the temperature of the plate is increased to 65°C., the analgesic action of salicylates can be demonstrated. Presumably the higher temperature causes a more extensive liberation of pain producing substances.

Radiant heat can be used to provide the thermal stimulus in a range of animals, including man. An electric light bulb provides the thermal stimulus: in animals (dogs, guinea pigs, cats and rats have been used), it is focussed on a shaved area of the back and twitching of the skin indicates that pain is being felt. In man, the heat from an electric lamp is focussed on to an area of the forehead blackened with soot (to increase absorption of the radiant heat) and the subject signals when pain is felt. The test is only applicable to centrally acting analgesics: the more powerful the analgesic, the longer the period which elapses before pain is felt. Alternatively, if the current supplied to the lamp can be varied, the response to the thermal stimulus can be assessed by finding the current that has to be supplied to cause pain after a predetermined period of exposure. Three seconds is the period usually chosen.

Mechanical methods

A number of mechanical methods of stimulation have been developed. One of the more satisfactory involves the application of pressure to the tail of a rat. A constant rate motor or the pressure of gas from a cylinder is employed to drive a plunger on to the tail which is fixed in clamps (Fig. 27.11). In other mechanical methods an artery forceps or a bulldog clip is applied to the tail or toe. Untreated animals cry and attempt to remove the clip by biting it. After adminstration of an appropriate dose of a centrally acting analgesic, they disregard the clip. In order to obtain comparative results using this method, the clips used must all exert the same pressure when they are applied to the tail. Simple devices to measure clip tension can easily be constructed (Collier, 1964). Mechanical methods are of no value for the detection of analgesics that antagonize pain producing substances.

Electrical methods

There are a great many of these, some of them very ingenious. The instrument sometimes known rather pretentiously as a pododolorimeter (the etymology is obvious) consists of a cage capable of accommodating a mouse or rat and having a floor made of a series of metallic roads that can be electrified. The voltage that has to be applied across the rods in order to cause the animal to squeak and struggle is recorded before and after administration of the substance under test. In a modification of the pododolorimeter the floor of the cage consists of a single copper plate which is connected to one pole of the current supply. The other pole is connected to a small electrode inserted into the animal's rectum. In other electrical methods, electrodes are applied to the skin, scrotum, tail or ear of the experimental animal. Electrical stimulation of the skin is applicable to man.

One electrical method worthy of note involves electrical stimulation of metal fillings in the teeth of dog. This causes stimulation of nerves in the tooth pulp. The method can be applied to man. Peripherally acting analgesics, as well as those that act centrally, prevent pain in this test.

Prevention of ischaemic pain
Ischaemic pain can be produced experimentally in man by exercising a limb in which the circulation has been obstructed by means of a sphygmomanometer cuff. Morphine like drugs reduce the intensity of this ischaemic pain and the method has been used to evaluate this type of analgesic agent.

Chemical methods
The use of the exposed blister base (p. 417) and experiments involving the injection of bradykinin into the splenic circulation of animals and the peritoneal cavity of man have already been discussed. It has also been empha-

sized that the production of pain by chemical methods is the most suitable procedure to adopt when peripherally acting analgesics are being studied. The simplest chemical method consists of the intraperitoneal injection of phenylquinone in mice. Benzoquinone, bradykinin or acetic acid can be used instead. In all instances, the response to the irritant solution is a characteristic writhing: it is usual to count the total number of writhes in groups of six mice that have been given the irritant and either the drug under test or a suitable control solution. A large number of animals show no writhing response, even if they have received no analgesic and it is necessary to exclude 'nonwrithers' from the trial before the experiment proper begins. Another disadvantage of the method is that it is far from specific: antihistamines, sympathomimetics, adrenaline blocking agents and central nervous stimulants are only some of the compounds that have been said to inhibit the writhing response. Nevertheless, when taken in conjunction with the results of other studies, the writhing test can provide useful information concerning the possible effectiveness of newly discovered compounds.

Antiinflammatory substances
Since the ability to inhibit prostaglandin synthetase is a feature shared by many groups of antiinflammatory agents it is clearly advisable that the existence or otherwise of this property should be established at an early stage in the investigation of new substances that might have useful antiinflammatory activity. Microsome preparations from extracts of sheep seminal vesicles provide a suitable source of the enzyme and a number of techniques is now available

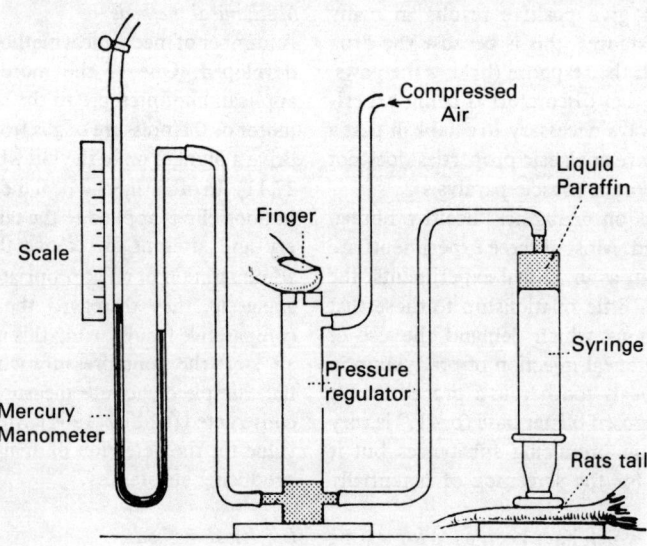

Fig. 27.11 A diagram of apparatus used to estimate analgesic potency by applying pressure to the rat's tail. The plunger of the syringe presses upon the tail as long as the finger is applied to the hole on the top of the pressure regulator. The pressure required to cause a squeak or movement is read on the manometer. (After A. F. Green and P. A. Young (1951). *Brit. J. Pharmac* 6, 572. By kind permission of Dr. Green and the Editors.)

for assaying the rate of formation of prostaglandins by the system.

To investigate the actions of the new compounds on the inflammatory process itself, rather than on the synthesis of its principal mediator, simple tests are available that permit studies to be made of the extent to which a particular compound can attenuate the individual components of acute and chronic inflammatory changes.

ERYTHEMA

Erythema is the earliest visible response to injury of the superficial layers of the skin. In the laboratory it can be induced by exposing the previously depilated skin of the experimental animal (the guinea pig is a favourite species for this purpose) to ultraviolet light for a period of about one minute. The extent of the erythema is read some three hours later in control animals and in those pretreated with the substance under test.

The permeability of the capillaries increases well in advance of the appearance of visible erythema and the change can be detected by the intravenous injection of a dye that is known to bind to plasma protein. Such dyes do not normally penetrate the capillary wall but they do so when the permeability of the vessels is increased in the early stages of the inflammatory process. The extent of the increase in capillary permeability and the degree of protection provided by antiinflammatory drugs can be assessed by excising, and comparing the weights of, the areas of dyed skin in animals that have and have not been treated with the agent under test before exposure to ultraviolet radiation. Rats are commonly employed in this test.

An obvious criticism of the erythema and capillary permeability tests is that they only assess the ability of a drug to prevent or ameliorate the very early phases of the inflammatory state. These are less important in the overall response than are those that develop later. Nevertheless, most of the antiinflammatory agents in common use, with the exception of the corticosteroids, show activity in both the erythema and the capillary permeability tests.

OEDEMA

A suitable irritant material is injected subcutaneously into one hind foot and the difference between the oedema produced in the two feet is measured. The observations are repeated after administration of the drug which is being tested. If the drug is active locally, the test can be modified so that the irritant and the drug are injected into one foot and the irritant and a suitable control solution (vehicle or saline) are injected into the other. Substances that have been used to provoke the inflammatory reaction include formalin (3.5 per cent), dextran (30 mg per kilogram body weight), egg white (0.1 ml), yeast, nystatin (a polymer antibiotic, p. 908) and the likely mediators of inflammation. The most popular agent of all, however, is carrageenin. Carrageenin, which is extracted from a sea moss, consists of a mixture of several salts of two polysaccharides. The injection volume of these solutions should not exceed 0.1 ml. Oedema is measured by plethysmographic methods or (in experiments in which the drug is applied locally) by killing the animal and weighing the amputated hind limbs.

GRANULOMA FORMATION

For the assessment of drugs which might be useful in the treatment of chronic inflammatory conditions, the granuloma pouch method is very useful. Turpentine or croton oil is injected into a cavity produced by the subcutaneous injection of air into the back of the rat. A sterile abscess is formed and the extent of the tissue reaction can be assessed by measuring the thickness of the fibrous wall of the abscess, by measuring the volume of its contained fluid or by excising and weighing the abscess. The size of abscesses in untreated animals is compared with those in rats given the agent under test. Weighed pellets of cotton wool can be used instead of turpentine to produce the inflammatory response. After about one week, the pellets and the granulation tissue attached to them are removed and weighed. Among the drugs currently in use for the treatment of rheumatic diseases, there is a good correlation between their therapeutic activity and their activity in the granuloma pouch tests just described. The tests are particularly suited for assessing antiinflammatory steroids.

ARTHRITIS

At the opposite extreme to assessing the effect of potentially useful drugs on the separate elements of the inflammatory response it is also desirable to be able to glean some idea of their likely usefulness in particular clinical conditions. The most aetiologically and clinically complex of these conditions is arthritis and several animal models of the arthritic state have been developed.

Adjuvant arthritis can be induced in rats by injecting killed *Mycobacteria*, suspended in mineral oil, into a hind paw or the tail. There is an immediate reaction in the injected region but the arthritic response proper does not appear for some ten days. There is swelling of all the paws and, in addition, small hard masses (which are presumably analogous to the arthritic nodules seen in human patients) can be felt in the ears and tail. The extent of these latter changes and the degree of swelling of the paws can be made use of to derive quantitative measures of the severity of the reaction and of the effectiveness of substances under test. Both steroidal and nonsteroidal antiinflammatory drugs demonstrate their therapeutic efficacy in this model as do a range of other agents and manoevres including oestrogens, antilymphocyte globulin (p. 919), thyroidectomy and removal of the lymph nodes in the neighbourhood of the injection site.

Alternative methods of producing the arthritis involve the subcutaneous or oral adminstration of 6-sulphanylamidoindazole in rats and the administration of a suitable antigen (fibrin, albumins and immunoglobulin derivatives have all been used) in rabbits. A theoretical advantage of the last named approach is that the response is an immuno-logical one, an important consideration in view of the fact that rheumatoid arthritis is often of autoimmune origin (p. 395).

GOUT

Animal models of gout have been produced by injecting sodium urate into the paws of rats or mice or into the joints of dogs or birds.

BIBLIOGRAPHY

Books, monographs and reviews

Adams, S. S. and Cobb, R. (1967). Nonsteroidal antiinflammatory drugs. In *Progress in Medicinal Chemistry.* Vol. 5, 59-138. ed. Ellis, G.P. and West, G.B. London: Butterworths.

Arrigoni-Martelli, E. (1977). *Inflammation and Antiinflammatories.* New York: Spectrum Publications, Inc.

Brogden, R. N., Heel, R.C., Speight, T. M. and Avery, G. S. (1977). Alclofenac: a review of its pharmacological properties and therapeutic efficacy in rheumatoid arthritis and allied rheumatic disorders. *Drugs,* 14 241-259.

Collier, H. O. J. (1964). Analgesics, in *Evaluation of Drug Activities,* Vol. 1 ed. Laurence, D. R. and Bacharach, A. L., London and New York: Academic Press.

Davison, C. (1971). Salicylate metabolism in man. *Ann. N.Y. Acad. Sci.,* 179, 249-268.

Domenjoz, R. (1966). Synthetic anti-inflammatory drugs: concepts of their mode of action. *Adv. Pharmac.,* 4 143-217.

Goldberg, A. A. J. and Tudor, R. (1977). A seminar on fenclofenac. *Proc. R. Soc. Med.,* 70 (Supp. 6), 1-52.

Gutman, A. B. (1966). Uricosuric drugs with special reference to probenecid and sulfinpyrazone. *Adv. Pharmac.,* 4 91-142.

Paulus, H. E. and Whitehouse, M. W. (1973). Nonsteroid antiinflammatory agents. *A. Rev. Pharmac.,* 13 107-125.

Randall, L. O. (1963). Non-narcotic analgesics. In *Physiological Pharmacology,* Vol. 1. pp. 314-416. ed. Root, W. S. and Holmann, F. G. New York and London: Academic Press.

Smith, M. J. H. and Smith, P. K. (1966). *The Salicylates.* New York, London and Sydney: Interscience Publishers.

Spector, W. G. and Willoughby, D. A. (1968). *The Pharmacology of Inflammation.* London: English Universities Press.

Vane, J. R. (1976). The mode of action of aspirin and similar compounds. *J. Allergy clin. Immunol.,* 6, 691-712.

Willoughby, D. A., Wright, V. and Turner, P. (eds) (1977). Diflunisal. *Br. J. clin. Pharmac.,* 4 (Supp. 1), 1-52.

Winters, R. W. (1963). Acid-base disturbances and the treatment of salicylate intoxication. In *Salicylates: An International Symposium.* pp. 270-280. ed. Dixon, A. St. J., Martin. B. K., Smith, M. J. H. and Wood, P. H. N. London: Churchill.

Original papers

Brown, D. M. and Robson, R. D. (1964). Effects of anti-inflammatory agents on capillary permeability and oedema formation. *Nature, Lond.,* 202 812-813.

Collier, H. O. J. and Shorley, P. G. (1963). Antagonism by mefenamic and flufenamic acids of the bronchoconstrictor action of kinins in the guinea pig. *Br. J. Pharmac. Chemother.,* 20, 345-351.

Gryglewski, R. and Vane, J. R. (1972). The release of prostaglandins and rabbit aorta contracting substance (RCS) from rabbit spleen and its antagonism by anti-inflammatory drugs. *Br. J. Pharmac.,* 45 37-44.

Guerra, F. (1946). Action of sodium salicylate and sulfadiazine on hyaluronidase. *J. Pharmacol.,* 87 193-197.

Hench, P. S., Kendall, E. C., Slocumb, C. H. and Polley, H. F. (1949). The effect of a hormone of the adrenal cortex (17-hydroxy-11-dehydrocorticosterone; compound E) and of pituitary adrenocorticotropic hormone on rheumatoid arthritis. *Proc. Staff Meet. Mayo Clin.,* 24 181-197.

Holt, P. R. (1960). Measurement of gastrointestinal blood loss in subjects taking aspirin. *J. Lab. clin. Med.,* 56 717-726.

Lester, D., Lolli, G. and Greenberg, L. A. (1946). The fate of acetylsalicylic acid. *J. Pharmac.,* 87 329-342.

Lish, P. M. and McKinney, G. R. (1963). Pharmacology of metholilazine, II - some determinants and limits of action on vascular permeability and inflammation in model systems. *J. Lab. clin. Med.,* 61 1015-1028.

Spector, W. G. and Willoughby, D. A. (1963). Anti-inflammatory effects of salicylate in the rat. In *Salicylates: An International Symposium.* pp. 141-147. ed. Dixon, A. St. J., Martin, B. K., Smith, M. J. H. and Wood, P. H. N. Boston: Little, Brown.

Whitehouse, M. W. (1963). Some effects of salicylates upon connective tissue metabolism. In *Salicylates: An International Symposium,* pp. 55-64. ed. Dixon, A. St. J., Martin, B. K., Smith, M. J. H. and Wood, P. H. N. Boston: Little, Brown.

28. Local anaesthetics

Local anaesthetics (which, for no very convincing reason are sometimes called local analgesics) are used in order to abolish pain sensations from relatively restricted areas of the body. They do this by preventing the generation or propagation of action potentials. This action can be exerted at any point along the nerve so that if a train of normal action potentials enters a region of nerve which is exposed to a local anaesthetic, its further propagation will be prevented. Equally, if the anaesthetic is applied to the fine terminals of a sensory fibre, it will prevent the initiation of impulses.

The mechanism underlying the production and propagation of action potentials is essentially the same in all nerve fibres and local anaesthetics can block impulse conduction in all types of nerve. Thin fibres are, however, more susceptible to the action of local anaesthetics than are those of larger diameter and since pain fibres in general are smaller than many other types of sensory fibre and most motor fibres, they are anaesthetized by concentrations of local anaesthetics which cause neither muscle paralysis nor abolition of the sense of touch and pressure. One group of fibres is more susceptible than pain fibres. These are the postganglionic elements of the autonomic nervous system. Blood vessels are normally subjected to sympathetic vasoconstrictor influences and vasodilatation will be produced when local anaesthetics are applied to sites at which they can gain access to sympathetic fibres. Some local anaesthetics also produce vasodilatation by a direct action on blood vessels.

The fact that the sensitivity of a nerve fibre to a local anaesthetic is inversely related to its diameter is made use of in a diagnostic test. Spastic conditions in muscle can arise as a result of hyperactivity in the nerves of either the α- or the γ-motor system (p. 165). If a two per cent solution of procaine is injected into the neighbourhood of the motor supply to a spastic limb, the spasticity will be reduced if it is the result of overactivity in the γ system. It will not be affected if its origin lies in hyperactivity of the large diameter α fibres (Rushworth, 1960).

SITES OF APPLICATION OF LOCAL ANAESTHETICS

The several locations at which a local anaesthetic may be applied are shown in Fig. 28.1.

TOPICAL ANAESTHESIA

The local anaesthetic is applied in the form of a solution, ointment, cream or powder directly to the site at which anaesthesia is required. The method is restricted to mucous surfaces, damaged skin surfaces, wounds or burns. None of the local anaesthetics has any effect if it is applied directly to the unbroken skin. Skin can be anaesthetized by the application of ethyl chloride which evaporates so rapidly that the skin is frozen and is thereby briefly anaesthetized. Ethyl chloride has been used during very minor surgery—the lancing of an abscess, for example— but it is not a satisfactory anaesthetic since freezing may damage the tissues and render them more susceptible to infection. Moreover the nerves recover their function as soon as the skin warms after the operation and the patient may experience intense post-operative pain. A mixture of volatile fluorochloromethanes has been used for the same purpose as ethyl chloride. Topical anaesthesia proper is used to relieve pain or itching in, for example, haemorrhoids or anal pruritus, or to anaesthetize the cornea.

INFILTRATION ANAESTHESIA

In infiltration anaesthesia a solution of the local anaesthetic is injected at one or more sites in and around the area which is to be incised by the surgeon. The object is to

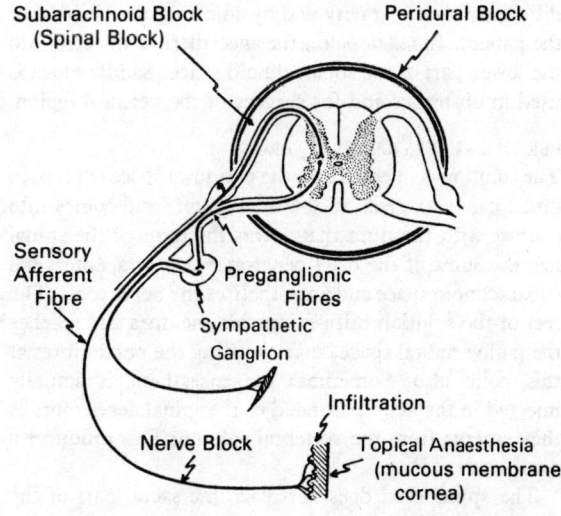

Fig. 28.1 The sites at which local anaesthetics are applied and act.

ensure that the finer nerve endings which supply the region are anaesthetized. This form of local anaesthesia is used for minor operations such as the draining of a carbuncle or the excision of a small superficial cyst. Infiltration anaesthesia is also employed in the treatment of rheumatoid arthritis and muscular rheumatism (fibrositis). The local anaesthetic (procaine is usually used) is infiltrated around the joint or into the fibrositic nodules.

NERVE BLOCK

The anaesthetic is injected as close as possible to the main nerve trunk supplying the area in which anaesthesia is required. Since the fibres in the nerve trunk are considerably thicker than the fine nerve terminals encountered in the skin, somewhat higher concentrations of local anaesthetic than are used in infiltration anaesthesia are required to produce anaesthesia by nerve block. Like epidural block (see below) this technique is being increasingly adopted not only to provide anaesthesia during surgery but also to secure relief from postoperative pain, The intercostal nerves, which are easily accessible to a needle inserted between the ribs and which carry traffic from the thorax and upper abdomen offer a particularly convenient way of preventing pain from some of the regions of the body that most commonly need to suffer assault by the surgeon's knife.

SPINAL ANAESTHESIA

In spinal (or subarachnoid) anaesthesia, the solution is injected into the subarachnoid space so that it reaches the roots of the spinal nerves. The site of injection is chosen so as to block the roots of those nerves supplying the site of the operation. Solutions that possess the same specific gravity as the cerebrospinal fluid act primarily at the site of injection but movement of the anaesthetic up or down the subarachnoid space can be produced by using solutions of different specific gravity and by adjusting the position of the patient. In *saddle block*, the anaesthetic is injected into the lower part of the subarachnoid space. Saddle block is used in obstetrics and for surgery of the perineal region.

PERIDURAL (EXTRADURAL) BLOCK

The solution is injected into the peridural space (the space immediately external to the dura mater) and comes into contact with the dura that covers the roots of the spinal nerves. Some of the drug penetrates the dura, enters the subarachnoid space and anaesthetizes the nerve roots. The rest of the solution diffuses outside the dura and reaches the paravertebral space, anaesthetizing the nerve fibres at this point also. Sometimes the anaesthetic is actually injected in the neighbourhood of the spinal nerve roots as they emerge from the vertebral column. This produces a *paravertebral block*.

The spinal cord does not reach the sacral part of the vertebral canal which contains only the *cauda equina*, the bundle of spinal nerves which supply the pelvic viscera.

Injections of local anaesthesia into the sacral part of the vertebral canal therefore anaesthetize the nerve trunks of the cauda equina. Caudal anaesthesia is used in operations on the pelvic viscera.

In the last few years, the advantages of extradural anaesthesia have become much more widely recognised. It is used in obstetrics and during thoracic and abdominal surgery but it is also employed for the relief of postoperative pain. For this purpose it offers, for many patients, considerable advantages over analgesic drugs: it is more likely to effect a complete relief and because its action is localised it leaves the patient alert, co-operative and mobile to an extent that is rarely achieved by the opiates. Some of the newer local anaesthetics such as etidocaine and bupivacaine have an extended duration of action and they are especially valuable for postoperative use in this way. Shorter acting compounds such as lignocaine, prilocaine and mepivacaine are indicated if an anaesthetic is needed only during surgery.

INDIVIDUAL LOCAL ANAESTHETICS

COCAINE

Cocaine, the prototype of all local anaesthetics, is an alkaloid obtained from the leaves of several species of *Erythroxylon*, the coca plant, which grow in various parts of South America and the Far East. From the earliest days, the natives of these countries have chewed coca leaves, which they use as a stimulant, but the local anaesthetic actions of cocaine were not discovered until 1879, some fifteen years after its isolation in the pure state by Neimann. Its introduction into medicine was delayed until 1884 when Köller proposed its use in ophthalmic surgery.

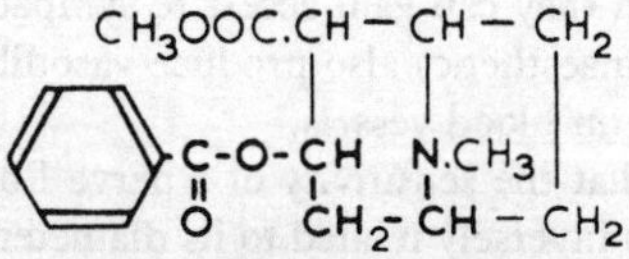

Fig. 28.2 Cocaine. The 'core' of the molecule responsible for its local anaesthetic activity is emphasized.

The experiments which led Köller to make this suggestion were initiated by Sigmund Freud and the story of how Freud had to ask Köller to continue the experiments because he himself wished to spend a holiday with his girl friend is now well known. It would be difficult to imagine a more apt cause for the failure of the father of psychoanalysis to achieve fame in another field.

Cocaine is a very potent local anaesthetic but it is not used nowadays except, very occasionally, to produce surface anaesthesia of the eye or the laryngeal mucous membrane. It is prone to cause toxic side effects if it is given other than topically. Its systemic actions should, however, be noted, because some of them are relevant to the action of local anaesthetics in general and some raise questions of theoretical interest.

Cocaine stimulates the central nervous system though high doses cause depression. As a result of its stimulant action, resistance to fatigue is increased and it was their discovery of this action that originally led native labourers to chew coca leaves. Cocaine also accelerates mental processes, though at the expense of accuracy. Other manifestations of this central stumulant action which are sometimes seen include increased respiration, increased body temperature and vomiting. Toxic doses of cocaine cause hyperexcitability and convulsions unless very high doses have been taken, when depression occurs without previous stimulation. The euphoria and the feelings of increased mental and muscular power produced by cocaine explain its liability to produce dependence. Cocaine dependence is described in more detail in Chapter 7. Here it is only necessary to add that cocaine is unusual among drugs of dependence in that tolerance to its effects does not occur.

Cocaine has some sympathomimetic actions. Under its influence the pupil is dilated, the heart rate and blood pressure increase and the skin is pale. The sympathomimetic effects of cocaine are discussed in more detail elsewhere (p. 269).

Cocaine poisoning is treated by intravenous injection of a muscle relaxant and the use of controlled ventilation. Toxic reactions to cocaine were not uncommon when the drug was widely used as a local anaesthetic: they are now rarely seen.

Synthetic local anaesthetics

A very large number of compounds with local anaesthetic activity has been synthesized. The formulae and names of a small but representative selection are given in Table 28.1. Some of the substances included in the table have clinical uses and a few of these are discussed individually below. For the most part, however, the table is for reference purposes though it also provides the individual items of data on which are based some of the generalizations made in this and succeeding sections.

The general structure of local anaesthetics is discussed in detail later but even a cursory glance at Table 28.1 should make it clear that almost all local anaesthetics contain an aromatic ring linked to an amino residue. The classification of the anaesthetics given in the table is based on the nature of the chain that provides the linkage. Many local anaesthetics, including cocaine, are esters but other linkages which have been incorporated into substances with local anaesthetic activity include the amides (—NHCO— and —CONH—), ureas (—NHCONH—), urethanes (—NHCOO—), ketones (—CO—) and ethers (—O). Another point which is illustrated by Table 28.1 is

that many local anaesthetics are derivatives of p-aminobenzoic acid.

Table 28.1 is based on information provided by Wiedling and Tegner (1963). In the following discussions, Roman numerals relate to the formulae given in Table 28.1.

PROCAINE

Procaine (I) was the first successful synthetic local anaesthetic—hence 'Novocain', its best known proprietary name. Procaine has been in use for more than 70 years. It is poorly absorbed from mucous surfaces and it is therefore of little or no value in topical anaesthesia. It causes vasodilatation by a direct action on the blood vessels so that adrenaline has to be added to procaine solutions intended for use in infiltration and nerve block anaesthesia. The adrenaline serves to localize and prolong the action of procaine. Procaine is a relatively weak local anaesthetic and it is rapidly metabolized in the blood and liver to give p-aminobenzoic acid and diethylaminoethanol. Repeated injections of the drug may therefore have to be given.

p-Aminobenzoic acid antagonizes the action of the sulphonamides (p. 819) and when procaine was given to patients who were also receiving sulphonamides it was necessary to ensure that the dose of the latter was increased sufficiently to counter the antagonistic action of the procaine. Sulphonamides are much less widely used now than formerly so that this particular situation is unlikely to arise today.

Procaine, like cocaine, has some stimulant actions on the central nervous system but it also possesses anticonvulsant properties. Although, again like cocaine, it sensitizes some tissues to adrenaline and to the effects of sympathetic stimulation, it also antagonizes the sympathomimetic amines in some situations. Cyclopropane and some other drugs, for instance, sensitize the myocardium to adrenaline. This sensitization is prevented by procaine. Allied to this is the fact that procaine has a quinidine-like action on the heart (p. 687). Procaine amide (procainamide, XXIII) has similar effects on the heart but it does not have the central excitatory actions of procaine itself and it can be used in the treatment of cardiac arrhythmias. For this purpose, it is given in capsules (each containing 0.25 gram of the drug) or by slow intravenous injection. By the latter route up to one gram can be given, provided that the injection is made slowly and cautiously, in an effort to restore normal rhythm. On isolated preparations such as the frog rectus muscle and the rat phrenic nerve-diaphragm, procaine and procainamide can be shown to have a neuromuscular blocking action. Procainamide is also useful in the symptomatic treatment of the hereditary muscular dystrophies. For this purpose it is given by mouth (one or more capsules four times daily) and it reduces the irritability of the dystrophic muscles. Procaine and procainamide have occasionally been given by intravenous

Table 28.1 Names and chemical formulae of some local anaesthetics

A. *ESTERS*

1. *Aminoalkyl esters of substituted aromatic acids*

	Approved name(s)	Proprietary name(s)	R_1	R_2	R_3
I.	Procaine	Novocain; Planocaine;			
	Ethocaine		NH_2	H	$(CH_2)_2N(C_2H_5)_2$
II.	Hydroxyprocaine	Oxycaine; Oxyprocaine	NH_2	OH	$(CH_2)_2N(C_2H_5)_2$
III.	Butacaine	Butelline; Butyn	NH_2	H	$(CH_2)_3N(C_4H_9)_2$
IV.	Amethocaine	Pantocain; Pontocaine;			
	Tetracaine	Anethaine; Decicain;	C_4H_9NH	H	$(CH_2)_2N(CH_3)_2$
V.	Butethamine	Monocaine	NH_2	H	$(CH_2)_2NH\ CH_2.CH(CH_3)_2$
VI.	Naepaine	Amylsine	NH_2	H	$(CH_2)_2NH(CH_2)_4CH_3$
VII.	Butamin	Tutocaine	NH_2	H	$CH(CH_3).CH(CH_3)CH_2N(CH_3)_2$
VIII.	Dimethocaine	Larocaine	NH_2	H	$CH_2:C(CH_3)_2CH_2N(C_2H_5)_2$
IX.	Parethoxycaine	Intracaine; Maxicaine	C_2H_5O	H	$(CH_2)_2N(C_2H_5)_2$
X.	Propoxycaine	Pravocaine	NH_2	OC_3H_7	$(CH_2)_2N(C_2H_5)_3$

2. *Alkyl esters of amino benzoic acids.*

	Approved name	Proprietary name	R_1	R_2	R_3
XI.	Orthocaine	Orthoform	OH	NH_2	CH_3
XII.	Benzocaine	Anaesthesin	NH_2	H	C_2H_5
XIII.	Butyl amino benzoate	Butesin	NH_2	H	$(CH_2)_3CH_3$

3. *Esters of benzoic acid*

	Approved name	Proprietary name(s)	R_1	R_2
XIV.	Piperocaine	Metycaine	H	
XV.	Cyclomethycaine	Surfathesin; Surfacaine; Topocaine		
XVI.	Hexylcaine	Cyclaine	H	

Table 28.1 *(contd)*

B. AMIDES

1. Aminoacylamides (i.e compounds with an —NHCO—linkage)

Approved name(s)	Proprietary name(s)	R_1	R_2	R_3
XVII. Bupivacaine	Marcain	CH_3	CH_3	
XVIII. Etidocaine	Duranest	CH_3	CH_3	
XIX. Lignocaine Lidocaine	Xylocaine; Xylodase Xylotox;	CH_3	CH_3	$CH_2N(C_2H_5)_2$
XX. Mepivacaine	Carbocaine; Scandicain	CH_3	CH_3	
XXI. Prilocaine Propitocaine	Citanest	CH_3	H	$CH.CH_3.NH(CH_2)_3CH_3$

2 Aminoalkylamides (i.e. compounds with a —CONH— linkage)

XXII *Approved names:* Cinchocaine; Dibucaine
Proprietary names: Nupercaine

XXIII *Approved name:* Procaine amide (Procainamide)
Proprietary name: Pronestyl; Procapan

C. URETHANES *(compounds with a —NHCO₂—linkage)*

XXIV *Approved name(s):* Diperodon, Diperocaine
Proprietary name: Diothane

Table 28.1 *(contd)*

D. *AMINOKETONES*

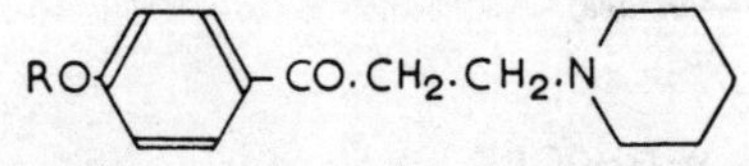

$$RO-\!\!\bigcirc\!\!-CO.CH_2.CH_2.N\!\!\bigcirc$$

Approved name	Proprietary name	R
XXV—	Falicaine	C_3H_7
XXVI Dyclonine	Dyclone	C_4H_9

E. *AMINOETHERS*

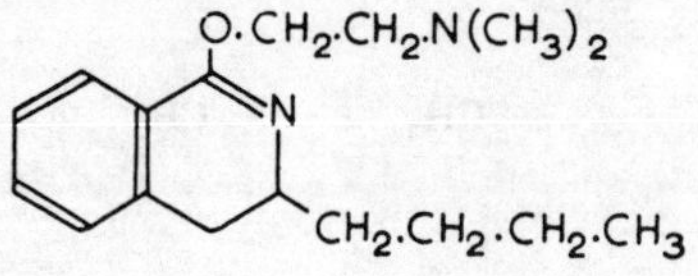

$$\text{O.CH}_2.\text{CH}_2.\text{N(CH}_3)_2$$

$$\text{CH}_2.\text{CH}_2.\text{CH}_2.\text{CH}_3$$

XXVII *Approved name:* Dimethisoquin
       Proprietary name: Quotane

F. *OTHER COMPOUNDS*

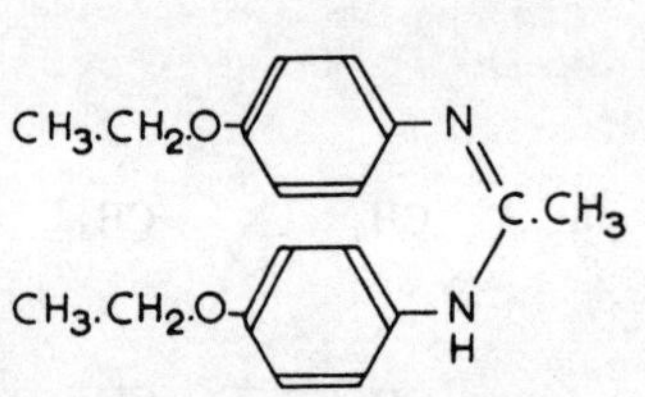

$$CH_3.CH_2O-\!\!\bigcirc\!\!-N$$
$$C.CH_3$$
$$CH_3.CH_2O-\!\!\bigcirc\!\!-N{\atop H}$$

XXVIII *Approved name:* Phenacaine
        Proprietary name: Holocaine

$$C_{12}H_{25}(O.CH_2CH_2.)_n\,OH$$

XXIX *Approved name:* Hydroxypolyethoxydodecane
      Proprietary name: Thesit

---

injection for the purpose of producing generalized analgesia. This analgesic action is of central origin and is independent of the drugs' local anaesthetic activity.

The use of procaine in the treatment of arthritis and fibrositis and in the diagnosis of spastic conditions of muscle has already been mentioned.

The toxicity of procaine is low but accidental overdosage or a too rapid intravenous injection may cause restlessness, headache and even convulsions and loss of consciousness. Toxic side reactions can be controlled to some extent by the injection of sodium thiopentone. Idiosyncratic reactions to procaine are very rare.

LIGNOCAINE (LIDOCAINE, XYLOCAINE, ETC., XIX)
Lignocaine was introduced into clinical practice in 1946 by Löfgren and Lundquist and it is now one of the most widely used local anaesthetics. It is used in an 0.5 to 5.0 per cent solution. Lignocaine is also effective when it is applied topically: it can be applied to the conjunctiva or sprayed on to the glottis and larynx. It is a favourite dental anaesthetic. It causes vasodilatation and it has to be mixed with adrenaline when it is employed for infiltration anaesthesia. It is used as the hydrochloride.

Xylodase is a cream containing lignocaine and hyaluronidase, the 'spreading factor' (p. 420). It can be applied to mucous membranes and skin wounds.

Lignocaine is more potent than procaine and it has a longer lasting effect since, being an amide, it is not susceptible to the hydrolytic action of the blood and tissue esterases.

Like procaine and other local anaesthetics, lignocaine has a number of actions not directly related to its local anaesthetic properties. Some of these are more prominent than in procaine. In particular, lignocaine has well marked depressant actions on the central nervous system causing sedation, analgesia and potentiation of anaesthesia. It is an anticonvulsant and it has been used in the treatment of status epilepticus. For this purpose it is given by intravenous injection. Notwithstanding its anticonvulsant properties, toxic reactions to lignocaine given by other routes sometimes take the form of convulsions. Lignocaine will arrest cardiac arrhythmias in the same way as procaine.

The multiple actions of local anaesthetics is a topic that is taken up again later in this chapter (p. 473).

The other local anaesthetics have general properties which are qualitatively similar to those of procaine and lignocaine, though none of them is used for purposes other than the production of anaesthesia. The particular applications in this field of a few of them are detailed below.

AMETHOCAINE (IV)

Amethocaine (IV) is about ten to fifteen times more active than procaine. It is well absorbed from mucous surfaces and it is particularly useful for local application to the conjunctiva and the mucous membranes of the nose, mouth and throat. It is an ester and is therefore destroyed quite quickly. Like lignocaine it is used as the hydrochloride. Gingicain contains amethocaine in an aerosol spray, for use, as etymologists will appreciate, in dentistry. Weight for weight, it is more toxic than procaine but since it is effective in lower concentrations toxic side effects are relatively rare. It sometimes causes skin reactions.

CINCHOCAINE (DIBUCAINE XXII)

Cinchocaine is an anaesthetic amide with a prolonged and powerful action. It is a potentially dangerous substance: although local anaesthesia can be achieved with small and safe amounts of cinchocaine, accidental overdosage is attended by the risk of toxic sequelae similar in nature to, but more severe than, those seen with cocaine and the anaesthetic has lost much of its earlier popularity, although it is still sometimes used as a topical anaesthetic. A 1 or 2 per cent solution is needed to anaesthetize the mucous membranes of the ear, nose and throat but great care has to be taken to prevent the application of solutions of this concentration to the cornea, urethra, bladder or open wounds which would be severely irritated by the drug. A dilute solution (0.1 per cent) is quite adequate for the production of anaesthesia in these tissues.

Cinchocaine is a stable inhibitor of cholinesterase and the extent to which the hydrolysis of benzoylcholine by the enzyme is inhibited by a standard concentration of the anaesthetic (10^{-5}M) is used as a measure of cholinesterase activity. It is expressed as the 'dibucaine number'.

BUPIVACAINE (XVII)

Bupivacaine (XVII) is one of the newer local anaesthetics. We have commented earlier (p. 466) on the increasing attention that is being paid to extradural nerve blockade as a means of relieving pain in labour and during the postoperative period. The success of the method depends on the availability of safe local anaesthetics with a sufficiently prolonged action. An added requirement in obstetric practice is that the chosen agent shall not expose the foetus

to greater risks than it meets during more conventional procedures. Bupivacaine goes a long way towards satisfying these requirements although if injudiciously used it can cause a foetal bradycardia severe enough to demand the intravenous administration of atropine.

For extradural anaesthesia, bupivacaine is given in an 0.25 to 0.5 per cent solution with adrenaline but the concentration may have to be increased to secure complete muscle relaxation during surgery. It can also be used to secure anaesthesia by nerve trunk block.

ETIDOCAINE (XVIII)

Etidocaine (XVIII) has come into use even more recently than bupivacaine. It has similar properties and uses.

BENZOCAINE (XII)

Benzocaine (XII) is very insoluble in water. It is usually employed as a dusting powder or in the form of ointments or lozenges. It is non-irritant and non-toxic and it can therefore be applied to mucous surfaces to relieve the pain of wounds, burns, ulcers, and inflammation and to alleviate itching. Suppositories containing benzocaine are used for the relief of pain from haemorrhoids. It is too insoluble for use by injection. Like procaine, benzocaine antagonizes the antibacterial activity of the sulphonamides.

BUTACAINE (III)

Butacaine (III) is used almost exclusively as a topical anaesthetic especially for the eye. It has largely replaced cocaine as an anaesthetic in ophthalmic surgery. It is equally effective but is much less likely to cause irritation; it also lacks the mydriatic properties of cocaine. It is too toxic for use by injection.

THE MODE OF ACTION OF LOCAL ANAESTHETICS

Local anaesthetics do not affect the resting potential of nerve but they prevent the development of the action potential—in other words they stabilize the nerve membrane, making it less excitable. In physiological terms, this means that they do not interfere with the activity of the sodium pump but that they do prevent the increase in sodium permeability that is the necessary preliminary to the influx of sodium ions which constitutes the first phase of the action potential (p. 157). So much is incontrovertible. What is in doubt is the nature of the mechanisms, chemical or physical, by which local anaesthetics bring about membrane stabilization.

Contemporary theories of local anaesthesia postulate a direct action (obstruction or distortion) by the anaesthetic molecules on the membrane channels through which sodium enters the nerve. Earlier hypotheses visualized instead an interference with the liberation or action of a chemical that was itself responsible for the changes in membrane permeability that initiate nerve action potentials. These obsolescent views can be disposed of briefly but they need to be mentioned, partly for historical reasons and partly because they still have a few adherents that results in their being occasionally referred to in the literature.

Procaine has a formal resemblance to acetylcholine (Fig. 28.3) and it was for long believed that local anaesthetics might owe their effectiveness to an interaction with acetylcholine receptors in the nerve fibre. It is true that procaine is an acetylcholine antagonist and we know that local anaesthetic activity is displayed by atropine and many related compounds that certainly can occupy acetylcholine receptors. On the other hand, many local anaesthetics in no way resemble acetylcholine and Wiedling (1959) has convincingly demonstrated that, among those that do, there is but a poor correlation between anaesthetic activity and the ability to antagonise acetylcholine. Moreover—and most important of all—no explanation that is based on acetylcholine antagonism can be seriously entertained unless it can be shown that acetylcholine is critically involved in the initiation and transmission of action potentials in nerve fibres. Although Nachmansohn has argued over many years that this is so, his hypothesis has never been generally accepted. A formidable amount of evidence can be arrayed against it and his own experiments, ingenious and voluminous though they are, provide only equivocal support for his views.

Many local anaesthetics antagonize the actions of histamine, some drugs classified as antihistamines behave as local anaesthetics (and have indeed occasionally been used clinically for this purpose) and histamine is present in at least some peripheral nerves. The evidence that histamine plays a part in the initiation of the nerve impulse and that local anaesthetics prevent this action of histamine is no stronger—nor is it weaker—than that relating to acetylcholine. An even more remote possibility is that local anaesthetics act on a thiamine dependent mechanism: many years ago, von Müralt, the Swiss physiologist, provided some evidence that thiamine was in some way involved in the propagation of the nerve impulse and Eckert (1962) showed that a variety of local anaesthetics

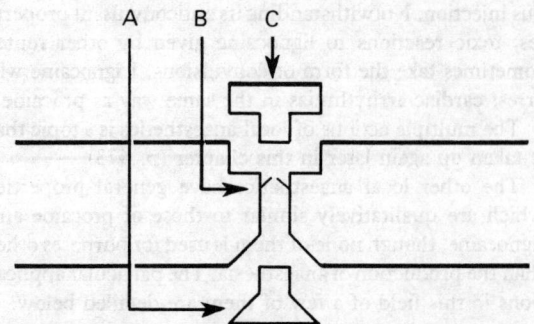

Fig. 28.4 Schematic illustration of the notion that local anaesthetics might operate by obstructing the inner (A) or the outer (C) ends of the sodium channels or by distorting them from within the plasma membrane (B)

can form complexes with thiamine. No further evidence to support this view of local anaesthetic action has been forthcoming and it can probably be safely disregarded particularly since the direct role of thiamine in the generation of the action potential can at most be a minor one. It is, perhaps, worth adding that the mutual actions of local anaesthetics and thiamine on nerve fibres are sometimes complementary and sometimes antagonistic.

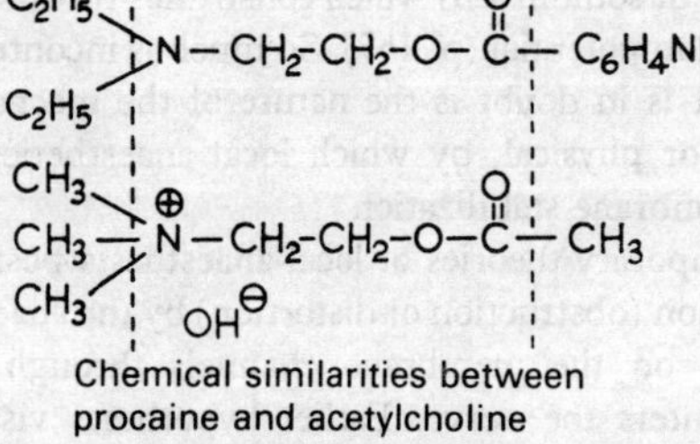

The very multiplicity of the compounds that produce local anaesthesia makes it unlikely that all local anaesthetics interact with a single chemical agent and the alternative hypothesis of a direct action on the sodium channels is intrinsically more attractive. Theoretically at least the channels might be blocked from either the inside or the outside of the nerve or they might be closed or constricted from within the substance of the plasma membrane itself. These three possibilities are somewhat fancifully illustrated in Figure 28.4, the features of which should be clarified by the discussion that follows.

Many local anaesthetics are amines (Table 28.1) and so can exist in either a charged or an uncharged form (Fig. 28.5). They are more effective in an alkaline than in an acid solution because increasing the pH increases the proportion of uncharged molecules and these penetrate the tissues more readily than the protonated molecules (Chapter 4). This is not to say that the pharmacological activity of these anaesthetics resides in the uncharged molecules and we now know indeed that, once they have arrived at their site of action, some of them are only active in the protonated form. This was elegantly demonstrated by Ritchie and Greengard (1961) who exposed unmyelinated nerve fibres

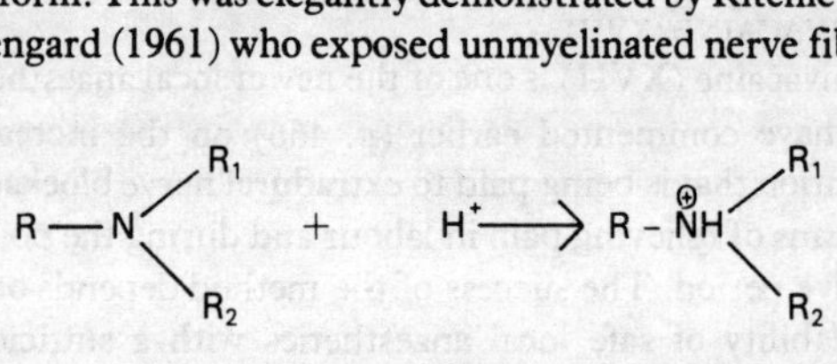

$$C_2H_5$$
$$C_2H_5 \Big\rangle N - CH_2 - CH_2 - O - \overset{\overset{O}{\|}}{C} - C_6H_4NH_2$$

$$CH_3$$
$$CH_3 \Big\rangle \overset{\oplus}{N} - CH_2 - CH_2 - O - \overset{\overset{O}{\|}}{C} - CH_3$$
$$CH_3 \quad OH^{\ominus}$$

Chemical similarities between procaine and acetylcholine

Fig. 28.3 Chemical similarities between procaine and acetylcholine

$$R - N \Big\langle \overset{R_1}{\underset{R_2}{}} \quad + \quad H^+ \quad \rightleftharpoons \quad R - \overset{\oplus}{N}H \Big\langle \overset{R_1}{\underset{R_2}{}}$$

Fig. 28.5 The uncharged and charged (protonated or cationic) forms of an amine.

to cinchocaine until a conduction block was established. The bathing solution was then replaced by one that contained no cinchocaine but enough of the long acting anaesthetic remained adsorbed on to the nerve to ensure maintenance of the block. However, when the pH of the solution was increased to 9.6 (so that the number of charged molecules was reduced) the nerve fibres regained their ability to conduct impulses only to lose it again immediately the solution was made neutral. This process of blocking and unblocking the nerve could be repeated at will, simply by making the appropriate shift from a neutral to an alkaline pH.

Anaesthetics that are only effective in the cationic form probably act from within the nerve fibre. This view has received much support from Hille and his colleagues (among others) who have made use of quaternary analogues of local anaesthetic agents. By their very chemical nature, these substances can only exist in solution as cations. One such compound, which is clearly related to lignocaine, is shown in Fig. 28.6. It behaves like lignocaine provided that it is introduced directly into the nerve: if it is applied to the external surface of nerve fibres it is entirely without effect. All the available evidence indicates that lignocaine occupies the same sites on the inner surface of the nerve membrane as those to which the quaternary analogue can become attached: uncharged molecules of lignocaine are able to penetrate the nerve membrane but the slightly more acid conditions within the fibre (themselves a consequence of the metabolic activity of the nerve) will encourage the production of charged molecules.

The existence of well marked structure-action relationships among anaesthetics that are believed to operate from within the fibre, together with the fact that only protonated molecules are effective at this site, argues for the presence of specific receptors on the internal surface of the plasma membrane.

Present day knowledge of the nature of the nerve impulse owes much to the work of Hodgkin and his associates (p. 157). Among the refinements of the Hodgkin view of the nerve impulse is the concept of 'gates' (which have to be thought of as unspecified molecular events rather than discrete physical structures) which close the internal entrances to the sodium channels. Excitation of the nerve is associated with opening of the gates which thereby permits the ingress of sodium ions notwithstanding the continued activity of the sodium pump. Recent experiments have made it clear that anaesthetic molecules only become attached to the nerve membrane when the gates are open, a clear indication that the postulated receptors are themselves located in the vicinity of the gates, perhaps in the sodium channels themselves (Fig. 28.5).

Benzocaine is an effective local anaesthetic but, as a glance at its formula (XII, Table 28.1) will make plain, it can exist in only the uncharged form. Consequently it can penetrate into and through nerve membranes with ease but it cannot occupy the sodium channel receptors which, as we have seen, are available only to charged molecules. Instead it may be able to constrict or otherwise distort the sodium channel by an action from within the membrane. A number of hypotheses have been proposed to explain how this might occur: in general they postulate that the anaesthetic molecules cause an expansion of the membrane (and thus narrow the channels) by increasing the movements of the lipid molecules or by altering the conformation of the protein moiety. They can certainly exert an expansion effect on organised lipid layers in vitro but direct experiments on nerves have yet to be performed.

Some local anaesthetics evidently have a dual mode of action. Thus, procaine in its charged form can certainly occupy the membrane receptors but the conduction of impulses in nerve fibres exposed to a procaine solution is more readily blocked if the solution is alkaline than if it is neutral. This is the opposite effect to that we described above for cinchocaine and it indicates that the uncharged molecules of procaine, which must act from within the substance of the membrane, are more effective than the protonated molecules which occupy the membrane receptors. Among substances that have this dual action, there are likely to be considerable variations in the relative contributions to the total anaesthetic effect made by the charged and the uncharged molecules.

We can summarise the foregoing paragraphs by saying that some local anaesthetics (like cinchocaine and lignocaine) bring about conduction block primarily by occupying specific receptors on the inner surface of the membrane, others (such as benzocaine) do so because they expand the membrane from within its substance while another group (typified by procaine) has a mixed action.

In addition to their primary actions, local anaesthetics may have others which may contribute to their effectiveness. They have, for instance, variable effects on membrane bound calcium, an ion that is an important regulator of membrane function in nerve and muscle fibres while some of them also influence the activity of sodium-potassium ATPase (p. 44).

We opened this discussion by declaring that local anaesthetics operate by stabilizing the nerve membrane but all cell membranes are essentially similar and it should

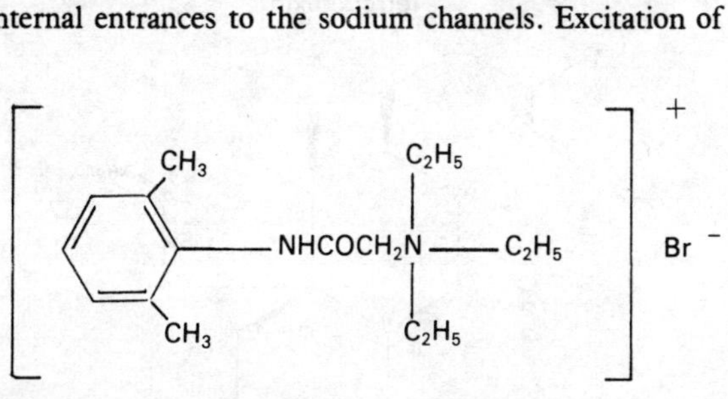

Fig. 28.6 Compound QX314, a quaternary analogue of lignocaine

occasion no surprise that local anaesthetics have effects on structures other than peripheral nerve fibres, particularly nerve cell bodies and muscle fibres. Conversely, a large number of drugs whose characteristic action can be attributed to a stabilization of cell membranes in the brain or elsewhere would be expected to exhibit local anaesthetic activity. Alcohols, inhalation anaesthetics, barbiturates, antiepileptic drugs, antihistamines, tranquillizers such as chlorpromazine and reserpine and antidepressants such as imipramine, to name but a few, can all be shown to block conduction in isolated nerves. In experimental conditions, chlorpromazine indeed is a much more potent local anaesthetic than procaine. This inevitably raises the question as to why all groups of membrane stabilizers do not have an identical range of actions in the intact animal and why each has its own distinctive and well defined clinical use. This is not an easy question to answer but we can identify a number of possible factors that might be responsible for conferring a degree of specificity on each of these potentially pluripotent drugs (Seeman, 1972). These include, among others, differences in lipid and water solubility, the occurrence of specific receptors, selective uptake into different organs or into different regions of the brain, and the possession of additional properties that counteract the drug's action on some membranes and potentiate it on others. It is unfortunate that limitations of space preclude further discussion of this important topic which warrants more attention than it customarily receives from authors and teachers. It illustrates a principle that is often overlooked because of our preoccupation with the minutiae of drug action—the principle that there are relatively few basic mechanisms with which drugs can interfere.

The fact that membrane stabilization underlies the action of several different classes of drug at least partly explains why none of them has a truly specific action and why they all may display a variety of side effects. It also explains why, in a few patients, particular drugs sometimes provide a surprisingly effective treatment for conditions other than those for which they are intended. The whole topic of membrane stabilization has been comprehensively reviewed by Seeman (1966, 1972).

Obstruction of sodium channels from outside the membrane

All the local anaesthetics in current clinical use have their loci of action within, or on the internal surface of, the plasma membrane but there is a group of substances that prevent excitation by an action on the external surface of the nerve membrane. The best known representatives of the group are tetrodotoxin and saxitoxin.

Tetrodotoxin is present in the ovaries and liver of the Japanese puffer fish. Puffer fish poisoning (tetrodon poisoning or *fugu*) awaits those who eat the fish without first making sure that its evisceration has been performed with the necessary care. Among uninformed travellers who

have suffered tetrodon poisoning and have survived to tell the tale the most famous is probably Captain Cook.

Although the existence of puffer fish toxin was apparently first reported in an ancient Chinese pharmacopoeia published more than 4500 years ago, its chemical composition was not finally established until 1964.

Saxitoxin is produced by several species of algae (one of them, *Saxidomus giganteus*, gives its name to the toxin) that may be consumed by shell fish. It is the cause of paralytic shellfish poisoning, outbreaks of which occur from time to time all over the world. Although the total number of reported cases is not large, there was a celebrated outbreak in San Francisco in 1927 that claimed 102 victims, all of whom had eaten mussels. Among explorers, some of Captain Vancouver's men died from saxitoxin poisoning just as Captain Cook's had succumbed to tetrodotoxin. The chemical composition of saxitoxin was firmly determined in 1971.

A fascinating account of the early history of the two toxins is provided by Kao (1966) who also reviews their pharmacological actions.

Both toxins are extremely potent: in nanogram quantities they induce total paralysis by rendering nerves and muscles completely inexcitable. There seems to be no doubt that the two toxins have identical modes of action. They cannot penetrate into or through the plasma membrane but even if they could they would be incapable, it seems, of obstructing the sodium channels from the inside of the membrane. Tetrodotoxin has been introduced by microinjection directly into the interior of the squid's giant axon but it did not influence the nerve action potential even when it was given in a concentration 10 000 times greater than that which, applied externally, would produce

tetrodotoxin

saxitoxin dihydrochloride

a complete conduction block (Moore, 1965). The only known action of the toxins is to block the sodium channels from outside. This is a highly specific effect—so specific, in fact, that it has enabled tetrodotoxin to be used as a tool for counting the sodium channels. One outcome of this work has been the revelation that the channels are quite sparsely distributed throughout the nerve membrane: Figures of 30 channels per μm^2 have been quoted for the vagus nerve of the rabbit and much smaller ones for fish nerves (Ritchie, 1975) and this explains why tiny doses of the toxins produce complete inexcitability of the nerves. Tetrodotoxin is, for instance, 160 000 times more potent than cocaine.

Because the biotoxins do not penetrate lipid membranes (and therefore do not cross the blood-brain barrier) they do not exhibit any effect other than that which can be achieved by blocking the sodium channels and it ought to be possible to exploit these properties to develop a long acting and completely non toxic local anaesthetic. Indeed, an attempt to use tetrodotoxin itself for this purpose was reported as long ago as 1913. It was not very successful because that very lack of lipid solubility that prevents entry into brain and penetration of the nerve membranes also hinders the toxin's penetration to its site of action. This need not be a serious disadvantage in an anaesthetic that is to be employed for spinal anaesthesia and a chemically stable analogue of tetrodotoxin or saxitoxin might well provide a valuable addition to the range of local anaesthetic agents.

The external orifice of the sodium channel in nerve is said to have dimensions of 0.3×0.5 nm and to be lined with a ring of six oxygen atoms. The guanidine groups of tetrodotoxin and saxitoxin may slip into the channels (where it is possible that they become attached to a specific binding site) leaving the rest of the molecule to be fixed by hydrogen bonding to the oxygen atoms (Kao and Nishiyama, 1963).

STRUCTURE-ACTIVITY RELATIONSHIPS IN THE LOCAL ANAESTHETICS

Notwithstanding the multiplicity and apparent variety of local anaesthetics, it is possible to make a few generalizations concerning the relationship between structure and activity in this group of compounds. As Löfgren first pointed out, almost all local anaesthetic agents are composed of lipophilic and hydrophilic components separated by an intermediate chain. The lipophilic centre is usually a carbocyclic or heterocyclic ring and the hydrophilic centre is almost invariably a secondary or a tertiary amino group. This general structure is shown by some other compounds (see, for instance, the formulae of the atropine-like and antihistamine drugs in Chapters 15 and 21 respectively) but as has already been pointed out this is not surprising

since many types of pharmacological activity are exerted via the cell membrane.

Hydroxypolyethoxydodecane (XXIX) provides an obvious exception to the statements just made concerning the general structure of local anaesthetics. In this compound the lipophilic component is a higher alkyl group and the hydrophilic centre is a hydroxyl group.

The original concept of Löfgren has been extended by others. It is now recognized, for instance, that the lipophilic and hydrophilic centres must be in balance: if the hydrophilic portion is dominant, the local anaesthetic action is weak, probably because the molecule cannot penetrate to the plasma membrane. On the other hand, dominance of the lipophilic portion makes for low solubility. In a properly balanced molecule, however, the two centres do more than determine lipid and water solubility, for both are involved in attaching the molecule to the nerve membrane. Büchi and Perlia (1960) have particularly emphasized this in their electron theory analysis of the structure of local anaesthetics. They suggest that local anaesthetics are bound to the nerve membrane by three types of force—van der Waals forces, dipole interactions and electrostatic binding—which are illustrated in Figure 28.7. Büchi and Perlia also point out that if the substituent R is an electron donating group (NH_2, NHR, OR etc.), there will be an increase in the density of electrons at the carbonyl oxygen with a consequent increase in the attachment of the anaesthetic to the receptor. Conversely, a group (such as $-NO_2$) that withdrew electrons would reduce the attachment. The presence of methyl groups in the intermediate chain also tends to cause an increase in the activity of the local anaesthetic by increasing the electron density at the carbonyl oxygen. In practice these expectations are borne out as can be seen by inspecting the formulae of useful local anaesthetics shown in Table 28.1. The same general considerations apply when the intermediate chain is an amide or some other group.

The triple importance of the lipophilic aromatic portion of the local anaesthetic molecule should be evident: it permits lipid solubility, it facilitates binding to the receptor and it allows the production of a strong anionic reaction site in the chain.

It should also be noted, as is pointed out by Ritchie and Greengard (1966), that there may be additional features in the structure of the local anaesthetic molecule which

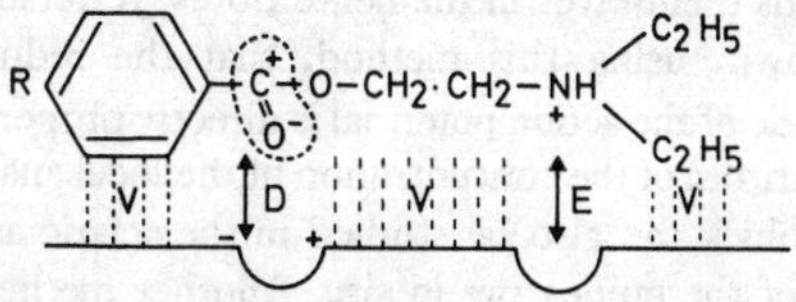

Fig 28.7 Binding of local anaesthetic. V = van der Waals forces, D = dipole attraction, E = electrostatic forces. After Büchi and Perlia, 1960.

determine its activity other than by simple binding to the receptor site. For instance, the methyl groups of lignocaine and mepivacaine (XIX and XX) may hinder their attachment to hydrolytic enzymes.

THE SCREENING AND EVALUATION OF LOCAL ANAESTHETICS

The mere detection of local anaesthetic activity in a compound being newly screened is easy and a large number of simple preparations is available for this purpose. It is desirable in the preliminary screening to subject the anaesthetic to a battery of tests, since a compound which is ineffective when it is applied to mucous membranes by reason of its inability to penetrate to the sensory nerve endings, may be quite active in producing nerve block. The evaluation of a new anaesthetic in relation to established compounds is rather more difficult than the preliminary screening, since the apparent relative potency of two anaesthetics varies according to the method used. There is now, however, general agreement that, for quantitative work, methods employing nerve block and spinal anaesthesia give the most reliable estimates of anaesthetic potency. Attention must also be paid, of course, to the results of testing procedures in which the anaesthetic is administered by the route which is most likely to be used if the drug proves clinically useful.

Surface anaesthesia
Solutions of the drug to be tested are applied to the cornea of the rabbit or guinea pig and after a short interval of time the cornea is touched lightly with a hair. If it is anaesthetized, the animal no longer responds by blinking. When this method is used it is also possible at the same time to see whether the drug causes irritation of the cornea.

Nerve block
Nerve block can be demonstrated on the simple frog sciatic nerve-gastrocnemius preparation. Since local anaesthetics block all types of nerve, it is possible to detect local anaesthetic action by stimulating the nerve, exposing it, between the electrodes and the muscle, to a solution of the drug under test and noting whether and when muscle contraction is abolished. A more up to date and satisfactory version of the same technique is to record the action potentials themselves in the nerve fibres. Jefferson (1963) has shown, using this method, that the reduction in amplitude of the action potential is directly proportional to the logarithm of the concentration of the local anaesthetic. Nerve block can also be studied in the sciatic and other nerves of the guinea pig in situ. Another method which uses frogs is that introduced by Sollmann and modified by Bübring and Wajda. Frogs are decapitated and pithed and the abdominal viscera removed. The animal is pinned on to

a board in a vertical position with its legs dangling. When the legs are allowed to dip into small beakers containing dilute (N/5) hydrochloric acid, they are rapidly and reflexly withdrawn. The solution of the local anaesthetic is then poured into the abdominal cavity and so comes into contact with the lumbar plexus. After a short time the legs are again dipped into the beakers. The time taken for the drug to abolish the reflex response to the noxious stimulus is measured at different concentrations of the drug. By plotting the logarithm of the dose against the time taken to cause plexus anaesthesia, it is possible to compare the potencies of drugs against a standard.

Infiltration anaesthesia
A very widely used method for the assessment of infiltration anaesthesia is the guinea pig intradermal weal technique. In this test, six animals are used and weals are produced by the intradermal injection of local anaesthetics into two sites on the shaved back of each animal. At intervals of five minutes, the weals are each pricked six times and a note is made of the number of occasions on which the guinea pig does not respond by twitching or by some other movement which indicates that the pain of the prick has been felt. The test continues for half an hour. For quantitative comparisons of different anaesthetics, the total number of negative responses is plotted against the logarithm of the dose. This method is not very useful if the anaesthetic under test has a vasoconstrictor action. It has the advantage that it can be used in man, injection being made into the flexor surface of the forearm which will accommodate four to six weals. The subject reports whether or not he experiences pain in response to the pin prick.

Spinal anaesthesia
This can be produced in rabbits and dogs. When rabbits are used, the anaesthetic is dissolved in a very small volume (0.02 ml/cm length of the spine) and it is injected into the subarachnoid space near the union of the sacrum with the rest of the vertebral column. In the method as originally developed, anaesthesia was judged to have been produced when electrical stimulation of the skin produced no increase in respiratory movements (Bieter, Cunningham, Lenz and McNearney, 1936).

It should be remembered that although adrenaline can usefully be added to many local anaesthetics, it increases the toxicity of some of them. This possibility must always be considered when new local anaesthetics are being studied with a view to offering them for clinical use.

BIBLIOGRAPHY

Books, monographs and reviews

Fink, B. R. (ed) (1975). *Molecular mechanisms of anaesthesia.* New York: Raven Press.

Grasshof, H. (1962)ʻ. Zusammenhänge zwischen Konstitution und Wirksamkeit bei Lokalanaesthetica. *Prog. Drug. Res.* **4**, 353-405.

Kao, C. Y. (1966).Tetrodotoxin, saxitoxin and their significance in the study of excitation phenomena. *Pharmac. Rev.*, **18**, 997-1049.

Ritchie, J. M. (1975). Mechanism of action of local anaesthetic agents and biotoxins. *Br. J. Anaesth.* **47**, 191-198.

Seeman, P. M. (1966). Membrane stabilization by drugs, tranquilizers, steroids and anaesthetics. *Int. Rev. Neurobiol.* **9**, 145-221.

Seeman, P. M. (1972). The membrane action of anaesthetics and tranquilizers. *Pharmac. Rev.*, **24**, 583-655.

Watson, P. J. (1960). The mode of action of local anaesthetics. *J. Pharm. Pharmac.*, **12**, 257-292.

Wiedling, S. (1959). *Xylocaine. The Pharmacological Basis of its Clinical Use.* Uppsala: Almqvist and Wiksell.

Wiedling, S. and Tegnér, C. (1963). Local anaesthetics. In: *Progress in Medicinal Chemistry*, Vol. 3. 332-398, ed. Ellis, G. P. and West, G. B. London: Butterworth.

Original papers

Bieter, R. N., Cunningham, R. W., Lenz, O. and McNearney,

J. J. (1936). Threshold anaesthetic and lethal concentrations of certain spinal anaesthetics in the rabbit. *J. Pharmac. exp. Ther.*, **5**, 221-224.

Büchi, J. and Perlia, X. (1962). Benziehungen zwischen den physikalischchemischen Eigenschaften und der Wirkunk von Lokalanästhetica. *Arzneimittel-Forsch*, **10**, 1-8, 117-124, 174-177, 297-301, 456-467, 554-559.

Eckert, T. (1962). On the pi-electron-donor-acceptor complex of local anaesthetics with aneurin (thiamine). A contribution to the problem of the mechanism of action of local anaesthetics. *Arzneimittel-Forsch.* **12**, 8-12.

Jefferson, G. C. (1963). The assessment of conduction anaesthesia. *J. Pharm. Pharmac.*, **15**, 92-99.

Kao, C. Y. and Nishiyama, A. (1963). Actions of saxitoxin on peripheral neuromuscular systems. *J. Physiol.*, **180**, 50-66.

Kuperman, A. S., Okamoto, M., Beyer, A. M. and Volpert, W. A. (1964). Procaine action: antagonism by adenosine triphosphate and other nucleotides. *Science*, **144**, 1222 1223.

Moore, J. W. (1965). Voltage clamp studies on internally perfused axons. *J. gen. Physiol.*, **48**, part 2, 11-17.

Ritchie, J. M. and Greengard, P. (1961). On the active structure of local anaesthetics. *J. Pharmac. exp. Ther.*, **133**, 241-245.

Rushworth, G. (1960). Spasticity and rigidity: an experimental study and review. *J. Neurol. Neurosurg. Psychiat.* **23**, 99-118.

29. Sleep and the drugs that influence it

Sleep is so common an experience that we need not define it. It is one of the more favoured topics in dictionaries of quotations and neither poet nor common man ever questions the desirability of sleep. Only the physiologist remains uneasy and wonders *why* we sleep and what good comes of it. Theories abound: Freemon (1972) suggests that there are as many as there are workers in the field since, for every investigator who proffers no theory there is another who proposes two. The enquiring reader finds a literature so replete with metaphor and analogy (he is asked to think, among many other things, of computers, storage tapes, water cisterns and patrolling sentries) that he is in danger of forgetting that the skull contains a brain and that it is in terms of neuronal activity that sleep must ultimately be explained. But, whatever the reason for sleeping, all of us seem to yearn for the blessed but reversible oblivion of sleep, that nightly rehearsal for death, and this is where the subject becomes of intense interest for the pharmacologist. In the quest for sleep (or perhaps for too much sleep) the consumption of hypnotic drugs has reached alarmingly high proportions and we must enquire into the nature and mode of action of these drugs and into the dangers associated with their use. These discussions can only take place against the background of the information we possess concerning the nature of sleep and of the nervous mechanisms that subserve it.

THE PHYSIOLOGY AND PHARMACOLOGY OF SLEEP

The electroencephalogram (EEG) exhibits a characteristic slowing when the activity of the brain decreases from whatever cause. This change is seen in sleep: as consciousness is lost, slow (1–3Hz) high amplitude waves (the delta rhythm) begin to dominate the record, replacing the faster (8–13Hz) alpha rhythm which is the sign of relaxed wakefulness. This shift from alpha to delta activity is associated with partial muscle relaxation and the almost total abolition of eye movements. Those who make intensive use of the electroencephalograph in their investigations into sleep recognise four stages in the transition from an alpha to a delta record. It is not necessary to discuss the stages in detail here beyond stating that an early one (stage 2) is identified by the appearance of K complexes, that 'sleep spindles' are seen in stages 2, 3 and (to a lesser

extent) 4 and that delta activity begins to intrude prominently into the record in stage 3. K complexes are single, sharp, high amplitude negative waves each one followed by a positive one. They appear in response to external stimuli (noises etc.) and to signals from the bladder, gastrointestinal tract or other viscera. Sleep spindles are bursts of high frequency (12–15Hz) waves with spindle shaped envelopes that are interspersed among gradually lengthening periods of delta activity.

It seems that tissue regeneration processes are particularly active during sleep stages 3 and 4 which are always accompanied by a considerable increase in the secretion of growth hormone.

That delta activity occurs during sleep is a discovery almost as old as that of the electroencephalograph itself but it was not until all-night records were taken that it became clear that there are two kinds of sleep, only one of which is associated with delta activity, and that we shift from one kind to the other and back again several times during the course of a night's sleep. For the first one or two hours, sleep takes the form we have already described, with delta waves, muscle relaxation and immobile eyes but then a quite sudden change occurs, signalled by the disappearance of the slow waves and their replacement by the fast, low voltage activity that indicates desynchronization and hence an 'alerting' response (p. 162). The inference that sleep is becoming lighter is, at first sight, confirmed by the fact that recording electrodes, placed near the orbit, will reveal that the previously quiescent eyes are now moving rapidly beneath their closed lids. Moreover, a sleeper woken during this period is much more likely to declare that he is in the middle of a dream than if he is disturbed when his electroencephalogram is in a phase of delta activity. However, the evidence provided by these signs of arousal loses much of its impact when it is set against electromyographic recordings that make it clear that the muscles have become even more relaxed than they were previously and the observation that it is more difficult to rouse the sleeper at this time. For these reasons, this kind of sleep is frequently and fittingly described as *paradoxical sleep*. An alternative acceptable name is *r.e.m. sleep* (r.e.m. signifying 'rapid eye movement') but both this kind of sleep and that associated with delta activity have attracted a large number of descriptive epithets—25 each on this author's last count! It is not surprising, perhaps, that the nomenclature has become confused: to some workers, for instance, paradoxical sleep is synonymous with light sleep (so that the other form becomes deep sleep) while others use the opposite terminology. The author's preference is for 'delta', 'slow wave' or 'synchronized' sleep on the one hand and 'paradoxical', 'r.e.m.' or 'desynchronized' sleep on the other. He recommends them to his readers while pleading with them to reject the temptation, fashionable in some quarters, to manufacture an acronym from the inoffensive initials r.e.m.

After a period spent in paradoxical sleep, the sleeper drifts back into delta sleep where he remains for about one and a half hours until his eyes begin to move again as they announce another burst of paradoxical sleep. This alternation of delta and paradoxical sleeps continues throughout the night. The duration of the successive bursts of paradoxical sleep increases progressively from a few minutes to an hour or more as the night wears on but each interval of delta sleep lasts for between one and one and a half hours. Thus, the longer our sleep the greater the proportion of it that is of the paradoxical variety. In a 'normal' eight hours period of uninterrupted sleep, there will be four or five instalments of delta sleep occupying a total of some five and a half hours and the same number of episodes of paradoxical sleep taking up the remaining two and a half hours. During the periods of delta activity the depth of sleep oscillates among the four stages mentioned earlier.

During paradoxical sleep, bursts of high amplitude waves appear in the electroencephalographic record immediately before each of the eye movements that characterize this phase of sleep. Their name—*PGO waves*—derives from the fact that they are most prominent in the pons (in the reticular formation in that area), the lateral geniculate body and the occipital cortex.

It is a simple matter to deprive volunteer subjects of their r.e.m. sleep: we monitor their eye movements, muscle tone and electroencephalographic activity throughout the night and rouse them every time the polygraphic records proclaim the onset of r.e.m. sleep. When our subjects return to sleep they will, as we have noted earlier, enter delta wave sleep so that it is possible completely to deny them their ration of r.e.m. sleep for several nights in succession. Because the technique is so simple and the topic so interesting (particularly for psychologists who have always been in the vanguard of those who wish to read into sleep a deeper significance than that of mere refreshment) many groups of workers have been able to report the effects of this deprivation and on one point, at least, they have reached unanimity. This is that individuals who have been denied paradoxical sleep will compensate for their loss by spending a longer period in this state when they are allowed to sleep undisturbed. Evidently there is a physiological need for paradoxical sleep but in our present state of knowledge and, despite much speculation, it is quite impossible to discern clearly the nature of this need. There is not even unanimity of opinion concerning the effect next

day of a partial or complete loss of a night's paradoxical sleep. There are those who aver that this deprivation is a partial cause of the 'hangover' (p. 486) engendered by so many hypnotic drugs, others who assert that it has subtle psychological sequelae not easy to measure and still others who deny that it has any effect at all. The reader will recall that dreams occur during paradoxical sleep and there are those who would claim that our need is not for paradoxical sleep but for the dreams it brings. These topics cannot be pursued further here but it is worth noting that a great many drugs (including most of those commonly used as hypnotic agents) partially or totally suppress paradoxical sleep.

Sleep secured with the aid of a hypnotic drug will be deficient in the paradoxical component but the extent of this deficiency will become progressively smaller if the drug is taken every night. This is, of course, a simple manifestation of tolerance (p. 83) and the parallel with a dependence phenomenon is completed by the considerable 'rebound' of paradoxical sleep that occurs when the drug is withdrawn. The rebound activity reaches its peak when the final traces of the drug have been eliminated from the brain. At this stage, paradoxical sleep may occupy 50 per cent or more of the total sleeping time. The proportion of the night spent in paradoxical sleep gradually falls but several weeks may need to elapse before it finally sinks to its predrug level. The dreams experienced during the early nights of the rebound state are likely to be much more vivid and disturbing than usual and they frequently take on a nightmare quality. These unpleasant withdrawal symptoms doubtless explain why patients readily become dependent on agents such as the barbiturates, withdrawal of which precipitates particularly prominent rebound effects.

Nightmares in individuals who have not been recently withdrawn from a hypnotic drug usually occur during stage 4 of slow wave sleep.

Sleep mechanisms

A considerable literature related to sleep mechanisms and to the effects of drugs on these mechanisms has accumulated in recent years but there is a dearth of accounts that attempt to explain these findings in terms of easily understood hypotheses capable of comprehending both the physiological and the pharmacological data. The brief account that follows attempts to remedy this deficiency.

We can begin by reminding ourselves of the work of the pioneers in this field and particularly of the finding (p. 162) that collateral fibres from the sensory tracts that ascend to the thalamus relay to a postulated waking centre (or to reciprocally paired waking and sleep centres) in the hypothalamus and thence to all areas of the cerebral cortex. These collateral fibres constitute the most important components of the ascending reticular system and, as we saw, cutting them induces sleep. Conversely, activating the system by sensory stimulation promotes wakefulness. This simple picture can still provide us with the core of an understanding of sleep though it needs elaboration in two respects. First, the idea of discrete waking and sleep centres in the hypothalamus has been replaced by the view that a number of areas scattered throughout the neuraxis, but functionally interconnected, together fulfil the role of controlling centres. The most important of these components (each of which probably plays a distinctive role) are located in the hypothalamus, the thalamus, the basal forebrain areas and the reticular core in the pons and midbrain. Secondly, it has to be appreciated that nerve impulses directed *from* the cerebral cortex to the reticular system can help, by a positive feedback mechanism, to maintain activity in the system once it has been initiated. Similarly, tonic activation of the peripheral musculature by way of the descending fibres of the reticular system also ensures continuing activation of the system by impulses from the muscles.

It is a matter of common experience that a reduction in the activity of the ascending reticular system helps to induce sleep. That, of course, is why, when we wish to sleep we switch off the lights, try to exclude sound and swathe ourselves in warm bedclothes to reduce sensory stimulation. Conversely we can be roused from sleep by bright lights, the noise of an alarm bell and so on. Sleep can be encouraged by drugs that are known to inhibit the transmission of impulses in the reticular system.

It is clear, however, that we cannot attribute sleep solely to a reduction in the activity of the activating systems brought about by the deliberate withdrawal of sensory stimulation. If this were the only factor involved we would be able to stay awake indefinitely by the simple expedient of exposing ourselves to continuous sensory stimulation. That we are unable to do this implies that the mere act of being awake creates the conditions that induce sleep by inhibiting activity in the reticular system (or in areas of the brain to which its fibres project) even in the face of external stimuli that would normally excite it. Some authorities incline to the view that sleep is essentially a passive state and that, after a period of wakefulness, neuronal mechanisms become fatigued. An alternative (or additional) hypothesis—to which this author subscribes—holds that, during waking hours, 'hypnogenic' material is generated in the brain. This substance (or group of substances) accumulates until it inhibits neuronal activity either by a direct action on the transmission systems responsible for maintaining consciousness or by stimulation of the sleep centres and perhaps also by reciprocal inhibition of waking centres. The hypnogenic material, it must be assumed, is dispersed or metabolized during sleep so that consciousness can return. This hypothesis sees sleep as an active state.

Whichever hypothesis is correct, it is easy to understand how exogenous and endogenous factors can facilitate or antagonize one another so that, within limits, we can postpone and shorten or bring forward and prolong the loss of consciousness that is the inevitable consequence of the waking state.

Under normal circumstances, sleep is always ushered in by a period of slow wave activity that only later gives way to paradoxical sleep. It appears, then, that delta sleep serves as a delayed trigger for paradoxical sleep. The mechanism by which the change is brought about is unknown but an appealingly simple view is that paradoxical sleep represents nothing more than a cyclical resurgence of activity in the activating systems. In this connection it is worth noting that regular fluctuations in the activity of the reticular system have been recorded even in the fully awake individual. These fluctuations have a cycle length of some ninety minutes just as they have in sleep. The characteristic association of increased brain activity with diminished muscle activity in paradoxical sleep can be explained if we assume that, concurrently with activation of the ascending reticular fibres, there is activation of the descending inhibitory system.

As we have already observed, the significance of paradoxical sleep is obscure. A physiological speculation (as opposed to the many psychological ones on current offer) is that the cyclical bursts of enhanced activity serve the purpose of testing the intrinsic excitability of the activating systems. If the test indicates that the excitability is too low, another period of delta sleep is indulged in but when the test signals a restored excitability, waking occurs (Guyton, 1976). Another speculation to which reference is made below (p. 481) is that paradoxical sleep is an occasion for 'refreshing' the noradrenergic system.

Transmission of information among the neurones constituting the systems that subserve sleep and wakefulness is obviously dependent on the release of neurohumoral substances. Drugs that influence the activity of any of these transmitters would be expected to affect sleep processes. The identification of these transmitters is therefore of both academic and therapeutic importance. This process is far from complete notwithstanding the many investigations that have been undertaken in recent years.

The following paragraphs summarize some of the more significant conclusions concerning neurohumoral mechanisms in sleep but it must be emphasized that many of them have been hotly contested by those whose experimental results have led them to champion other points of view. The findings reported here may appear to dovetail together into a firm conceptual structure but this is partly because they have been deliberately selected to this end from the mass of available literature. The wise reader will consult additional sources of information if he wishes to acquire a panoramic view of contemporary studies in this field.

5-Hydroxytryptamine

One of the largest concentrations of 'serotoninergic' neurones in the central nervous system is to be found in the raphé nuclei which are located in the midline areas of the pons and midbrain and which are closely associated with the ascending reticular formation. Many workers—but by no means all those who have studied the problem—have reported that destruction of the raphé nuclei causes insomnia in experimental animals as do manoeuvres such as the administration of p-chlorophenylalanine (p. 327) that prevent serotonin synthesis. Slow wave sleep has also been induced in some mammalian species (including man) by tryptophan, a precursor of 5-hydroxytryptamine. Electrical stimulation of the raphé nuclei does not, however, usually induce sleep. Indeed it sometimes evokes an alerting response.

Although raphé lesions are sometimes followed by an insomnia that persists for a week or more their effects are never permanent. Similarly, animals whose serotonin synthesis is chronically suppressed by p-chlorophenylalanine eventually escape from insomnia into sleep. Presumably the withdrawal of the sleep inducing influences previously exerted by the raphé system is eventually followed by compensatory changes in the activity of the other controlling centres so that normal sleep rhythms are re-established. Evidence in partial support of this supposition comes from the observation that the insomnia induced by raphé lesions can be readily reversed by the administration of drugs that prevent the synthesis or the action of catecholamines.

In animals deficient in serotonin, PGO spikes appear in the waking state and in slow wave sleep as well as during paradoxical sleep, implying that serotoninergic neurone activity serves to suppress at least this aspect of paradoxical sleep. This observation is consistent with the further finding that loss of slow wave sleep is the first effect of raphé lesions and the conclusion that slow wave sleep is dependent, at least partly, on neurones that release serotonin.

Dopamine and noradrenaline

It is a well known fact that drugs such as amphetamine and its congeners that bring about the liberation of dopamine and noradrenaline cause sleeplessness—indeed a slang word for amphetamine is 'wakeamine'. The results of experimental work using compounds such as piribedil and clonidine (which rather specifically stimulate dopamine and noradrenaline receptors respectively) indicate, though not absolutely unequivocally, that while dopaminergic activity inhibits slow wave sleep, noradrenaline is particularly involved in the operation of systems that suppress paradoxical sleep.

The most prominent aggregation of dopaminergic fibres in the central nervous system is the nigrostriatal system (p. 186) the best known function of which is to control muscle tone. However, there is also evidence that activity in the system maintains behavioural arousal. Moreover it is known that it receives inhibitory connections from, and may itself send inhibitory projections to, the raphé neurones. Thus when the raphé neurones are stimulated into activity (perhaps by hypnogenic substances, if such there be) the dopaminergic neurones will be inhibited while reduction in the activity of the raphé neurones can be expected to free the activating dopaminergic system.

The inhibitory effect of noradrenaline on paradoxical sleep is striking. Sleep following the administration of substances that result in catecholamine deficiency uniformly includes a more than average quota of paradoxical sleep. Substances in this category include α-methyl-p-tyrosine (which inhibits catecholamine synthesis), 6-hydroxydopamine (which selectively destroys neurones that contain catecholamines) and reserpine. The last named drug depletes the brain of serotonin as well as the catecholamines. A number of experiments attest to the view that the emergence of paradoxical sleep is attributable to the withdrawal of noradrenaline and not to the loss of dopamine. Thus, after fusaric acid—a compound that inhibits dopamine-β-hydroxylase (p. 258) and so causes noradrenaline deficiency without affecting dopamine stores—experimental animals experience sleep with an increased proportion of the paradoxical variety while dopamine antagonists such as pimozide and the antipsychotic drugs induce sleep that includes a virtually normal complement of the paradoxical variety. It has also been shown that the amount of (3-methoxy-4-hydroxyphenyl) ethanediol (p. 260) in the urine is inversely proportional to the duration of paradoxical sleep during the period over which the urine is formed. This metabolite is derived predominantly from noradrenaline.

The fact that paradoxical sleep appears to be a consequence of the removal of tonic restraint imposed by noradrenergic neurones has prompted Hartmann (1978) to propose yet another hypothesis relating to the significance of paradoxical sleep. He suggests that this form of sleep occurs when noradrenaline supplies become exhausted and that it allows replenishment of these supplies.

Two small nuclear areas in the dorsal part of the middle pons constitute the locus coeruleus. If the locus is completely destroyed, paradoxical sleep can no longer occur. The effects of partial destruction suggest that the rostral and caudal segments of the locus coeruleus control cortical activation and muscle relaxation respectively.

The neurones of the locus coeruleus are noradrenergic in type, a fact that seems to conflict with our previous conclusion that noradrenaline inhibits paradoxical sleep. However the neurones in the locus appear to be of two kinds: the so-called 'D-on' cells initiate and the 'D-off' cells inhibit paradoxical sleep. We can suppose that, in the presence of adequate amounts of transmitter, the activity of the 'D-off' cells keeps paradoxical sleep at bay but that if their effect is reduced (by depletion of noradrenaline or the use of antagonists) the 'D-on' cells might gain dominance.

We have to assume, of course, that the 'D-on' cells are more resistant than the 'D-off' cells to lack of noradrenaline.

The periodic appearances of episodes of paradoxical sleep in the course of a normal night's rest are presumably the result of cyclical fluctuations in the relative activities of 'D-off' and 'D-on' cells. The origin of these fluctuations is unknown but the proposal, mentioned earlier, that they might be attributable to successive depletions and replenishments of noradrenaline cannot yet be rejected, speculative though it is.

Interconnections between the locus coeruleus and the raphé system provides an anatomical basis for the mutual inhibition between slow wave and paradoxical sleep.

There is evidence of a reciprocal functional connection between the 'D-off' cells and cholinergic neurones in the tegmental area of the midbrain. Stimulation of the tegmental neurones reproduces all the features of paradoxical sleep—atonia, PGO spikes and cortical arousal—but these neurones cannot, apparently, fire if the 'D-off' cells are active. Thus paradoxical sleep, though initiated by events in the locus coeruleus may actually depend on tegmental activity.

Acetylcholine

The effects of cholinomimetic substances (pilocarpine, anticholinesterases, tremorine etc.) and of acetylcholine antagonists (atropine, scopolamine etc.) are generally consistent with the notion, already discussed, that paradoxical sleep is regulated, partly at least, by cholinergic neurones which are themselves activated by impulses from the locus coeruleus. The cholinergic neurones are muscarinic in type.

Hypnogenic factors

The active theory of sleep requires that the neurones that initiate slow wave sleep be stimulated by some sleep inducing (hypnogenic) factor that accumulates during waking hours. As long ago as 1913, Pieron found that cerebrospinal fluid, taken from dogs that had been kept awake for more than a week, caused sleep when it was injected into the cerebral ventricles of fully alert recipient dogs. The sleep so induced persisted for several hours; fluid taken from dogs that had not been denied sleep had no hypnogenic effect. These observations did not, apparently, excite much interest at the time (indeed they were not unequivocally confirmed until some ten years ago) although the idea that sleep might be caused by chemical substances produced during nervous activity was quite an old one. Now that Pieron's observations have been repeatedly confirmed on a variety of animal species there is an eagerness to identify the hypnogenic factor. That isolated from the brains of goats and sheep deprived of sleep seems to be a peptide with a molecular weight in the region of 500. There is some evidence that this substance (Factor S)

is also elaborated by the human brain. Monnier and his colleagues have recently isolated another hypnogenic substance. They found it in cerebral venous blood. This 'sleep factor delta' is a nonapeptide; unlike Factor S, which only induces sleep some two hours after the start of an intraventricular infusion, the new factor produces a prompt but shorter lasting response (Monnier *et al*, 1977). 'Alerting' factors have also been described, the work of Pappenheimer and his colleagues indicating that sheep, goats and man each produce two polypeptides of this type. They have higher molecular weights than Factor S and sleep factor delta.

The hypnogenic and alerting peptides cannot yet be firmly accepted as substances of physiological importance but none of the evidence so far amassed conflicts with the notion that they do have a role to play in the control of sleep-waking cycles, and that they will soon take their place alongside the other low molecular weight polypeptides that have recently assumed such importance in physiology, particularly in relation to their regulatory roles in the central nervous system.

HYPNOTIC AGENTS

Insomnia is complained of more frequently than almost any other bodily symptom. In many instances, sleeplessness is the simple consequence of the insomniac's seeking more sleep than he needs: a belief that a nightly ration of eight hours of sleep is a normal requirement ignores the meaninglessness of the word 'normal' (p. 115) and is the cause of many sleepless and unproductive hours in bed. At the same time, it must be accepted that anxieties about such important matters as work, health and family are a potent cause of sleeplessness and of a daytime tiredness and inefficiency that impairs the insomniac's ability to deal with the problems that led to the sleeplessness in the first place. And it has to be remembered, too, that sleep disturbances are commonplace in several psychiatric conditions (particularly the depressive syndromes), in incipient cardiac failure and in the elderly.

The wise physician will try to secure sound sleep for his patient by enlightened psychotherapy and by recommending simple bedtime measures—hot milk drinks have a not unjustified reputation as inducers of sound sleep—before resorting to the prescription of drugs. Unfortunately, such is the average patient's fear of losing sleep and his belief in, and demand for, drugs that this last resort situation will often arise and if a placebo is not effective a hypnotic drug will have to be given.

The beginning of the present century saw the discovery of the barbiturates and, until very recently, they were the favourite hypnotic drugs of patient and practitioner alike. Energetic attempts are now being made to replace them by less dangerous hypnotic agents but old habits die hard and barbiturate preparations are still being far too widely prescribed. Among the better informed, the benzodiazepines (particularly nitrazepam and flurazepam) constitute the hypnotic drugs of first choice. However, many other agents (most of which are less dangerous than the barbiturates) are also available.

However undesirable they may be as sedatives and hypnotics, the barbiturates still constitute an important group of drugs: thiopentone remains the best available intravenous anaesthetic (p. 504), phenobarbitone still has its advocates as an antiepileptic agent (p. 522) and the group as a whole has properties and actions that are of interest and importance to the pharmacologist. In the account that follows the barbiturates are considered as a group and they have, consequently, to occupy what might appear to be a disproportionate amount of space in a chapter that is nominally devoted solely to a consideration of modern hypnotic agents. On the other hand, the benzodiazepines are dismissed almost abruptly, important though they are, because they enjoy a variety of therapeutic uses and are more conveniently discussed in detail elsewhere (Chap. 32). The other drugs mentioned, with the notable exception of chlorpromazine, find employment only as hypnotics.

The barbiturates

All the barbiturates possess the barbituric acid nucleus but barbituric acid is not itself a hypnotic. Barbituric acid can be obtained by the condensation of urea and malonic acid (Fig. 29.1) and the barbiturates themselves are prepared by substitution of the hydrogen atoms on C(5). These substituents may both be alkyl or one may be aryl. In some compounds, the hydrogen on one of the nitrogen atoms is also replaced by an alkyl group and the oxygen at C(2) is sometimes replaced by sulphur.

The word barbiturate is derived from 'Barbara' and 'urea' but whether the Barbara refers to St Barbara or to a Munich barmaid seems to be a matter of dispute (Sharpless, 1965).

The first barbiturate to be used clinically was barbitone. It was called Veronal and it was introduced in 1903 by Fischer and von Mering. The next to appear (in 1912) was phenobarbitone (Luminal, Gardenal, Parabal) which is still widely used as an antiepileptic drug. Following the

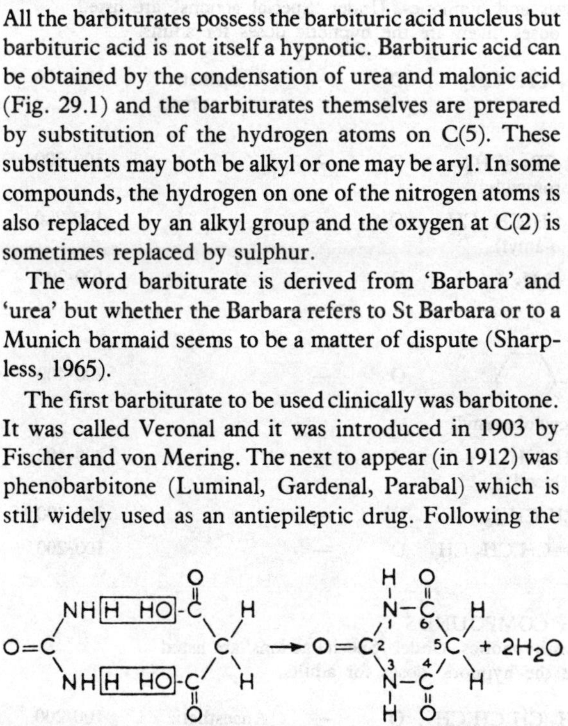

Fig. 29.1

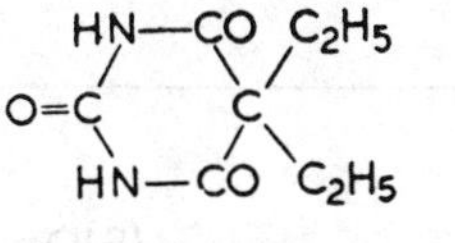

Barbitone 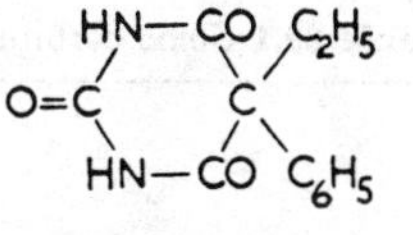   Phenobarbitone

success of Veronal and Luminal, a very large number of other barbiturates were synthesized and tested and about fifty survivors have been used clinically. The names and formulae of the better known of these are set out in Table 29.1; the relationship of chemical structure to pharmacological action is discussed in a later section.

The carbonyl group at position 2 of the barbiturate molecule exhibits lactam-lactim tautomerism. The lactim (acidic) form predominates in alkaline solution and permits the formation of salts. The sodium salt is usually preferred. The sodium is associated with the oxygen atom, as indicated in Fig. 29.2. The salts are more soluble than the parent barbiturates and they yield alkaline solutions. When barbiturates are required for injection or for any other purpose for which water solubility is desirable, they are used in the form of the salts. The less soluble forms are suitable for oral administration.

In the British Isles, the official names of the barbiturates end in -one (as in phenobarbitone). In the United States, the terminal syllable is -al (as in phenobarbital). In Table 29.1 only the British form is given except when the drug is used only in the United States when the '-al' form is preferred.

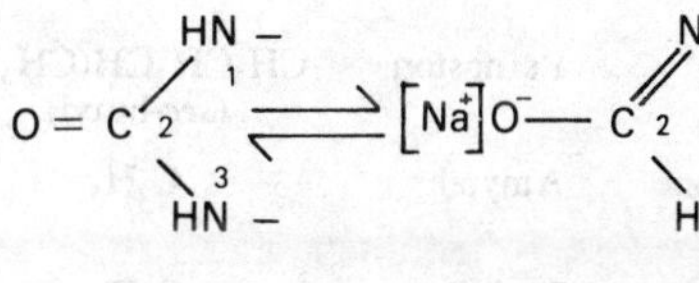

Fig. 29.2 Tautomerism in the barbiturate molecule.

Like the other hypnotics and anaesthetics, the barbiturates produce a descending depression of the central nervous system but the respiratory centre is particularly vulnerable to their action and respiratory depression is a feature of barbiturate anaesthesia. In anaesthetic doses, barbiturates cause a marked hypotension because they depress the vasomotor centre. A direct action on the blood vessels and some degree of ganglion blockade may contribute to the hypotensive action.

A small number of the barbiturates have an anticonvulsant action and a few can cause convulsions. These exceptions apart, it is true to say that all the barbiturates are capable of producing the same effects (sedation, hypnosis or anaesthesia) depending on the dose that is given and the choice of a drug for a particular purpose is determined largely by its duration of action.

Barbiturates have no analgesic action and in hypnotic doses will not cause sleep when insomnia is associated with

Table 29.1 Some barbiturates

$$(S)O=\overset{\displaystyle HN-\overset{6}{C}=O}{\underset{\displaystyle HN-\overset{4}{C}=O}{\overset{|}{\underset{|}{C}2}}}\overset{5}{C}\overset{\displaystyle H^a}{\underset{\displaystyle H^b}{}}$$

Approved name(s)	Proprietary name(s)	Nature of substituent on				Special actions	Dose (mg)
		Ha	Hb	C(2)	N(1) or N(3)		

LONG ACTING COMPOUNDS
All the compounds in this group were used as sedatives and hypnotics. Under 'Special actions'
are listed additional uses. Except where otherwise stated, doses given are the hypnotic doses for adults.

Approved name(s)	Proprietary name(s)	Ha	Hb	C(2)	N(1) or N(3)	Special actions	Dose (mg)
Aprobarbitone	Alurate	$-CH_2.CH=CH_2$ (allyl)	$(CH_3)_2CH-$ (isopropyl)	O	—		40–160
Barbitone	Veronal	C_2H_5	C_2H_5	O	—		300–600
Methylpheno-barbitone Mephobarbital	Mebaral Prominal Phemitone	C_6H_5	C_2H_5	O	CH_3	Antiepileptic	500 daily (for epilepsy)
Phenobarbitone	Luminal	C_6H_5	C_2H_5	O	—	Antiepileptic	30–120 (for epilepsy 100 twice daily)

INTERMEDIATE ACTING COMPOUNDS
All the compounds in this group were used as sedatives and hypnotics. Under 'Special actions' are listed
additional uses. Except where otherwise stated, doses given are the hypnotic doses for adults.

Approved name(s)	Proprietary name(s)	Ha	Hb	C(2)	N(1) or N(3)	Special actions	Dose (mg)
Allobarbitone Diallylbarbituric acid	Dial	$-CH_2-CH=CH_2$	$-CH_2-CH=CH_2$	O	—	Anaesthetic in animals	100–300
Butallylonal	Pernoston	$CH_3CH_2CH(CH_3)-$ (sec-butyl)	$-CH_2CBr=CH_2$ (β-bromoallyl)	O	—		100–200
Amylobarbitone	Amytal	C_2H_5	$-(CH_2)_2CH(CH_3)CH_3$ (iso-amyl)	O	—		100–200
Butobarbitone Butethal	Butisol Neonal Soneryl	C_4H_9 (sec-butyl)	C_2H_5	O	—		100–200
Cyclobarbitone	Cyclodorm Phanodorm	C_2H_5	(5.Δ¹.cyclohexenyl)	O	—		200–400
Hexethal	Ortal	C_2H_5	$CH_3(CH_2)_5$ (hexyl)	O	—		200–400
Probarbital	Ipral	C_2H_5	$-CH(CH_3)_2$	O	—		200–400
Vinbarbitone	Diminal	C_2H_5	$-C(CH_3)=CH.CH_2.CH_3$	O	—		100–200

SHORT ACTING COMPOUNDS
The compounds in this group were used only as hypnotics. Under 'Special actions' are listed
additional uses. Doses given are the hypnotic doses for adults.

Approved name(s)	Proprietary name(s)	Ha	Hb	C(2)	N(1) or N(3)	Special actions	Dose (mg)
Pentobarbitone	Nembutal	C_2H_5	$-CH.(CH_3)CH_2CH_2CH_3$ (1-methylbutyl)	O	—	Anaesthetic in animals	100–200
Quinalbarbitone Secobarbital	Seconal	$-CH_2CH=CH_2$ (allyl)	$-CH.(CH_3)CH_2CH_2CH_3$ (1-methylbutyl)	O	—		100–200

Table 29.1 (contd)

| Approved name(s) | Proprietary names | Nature of substituent on | | | | Special actions | Dose (mg) |
		Ha	Hb	C(2)	N(1) or N(3)		
		COMPOUNDS WITH A VERY BRIEF PERIOD OF ACTIVITY					

The compounds in this group are used as anaesthetics. Under 'Special actions' are listed additional uses. The dose administered depends upon the circumstances of each case; about 200 mg is used for anaesthetic induction.

Approved name(s)	Proprietary names	Ha	Hb	C(2)	N(1) or N(3)	Special actions	Dose (mg)
Buthalitone	Transithal	$-CH_2CH=CH_2$ (allyl)	$(CH_3)_2CH.CH_2$ (isobutyl)	S	—		
Hexobarbitone	Cyclonal Evipal Evipan	CH_3	(5.Δ^1.cyclohexenyl)	O	CH_3	Also used as hypnotic	250-500 (for hypnosis)
Methohexitone	Brevital	$-CH_2.CH=CH_2$ (allyl)	$-CH.C(CH_3)\equiv C.C_2H_5$ (1-methylbutyl)	O	CH_3		
Thialbarbitone	Kemithal	$-CH_2CH=CH_2$ (allyl)	(5. Δ^1.cyclohexenyl)	S	—		
Thiamylal	Surital	$-CH_2CH=CH_2$ (allyl)	$-CH.(CH_3)CH_2CH_2CH_3$ (1-methylbutyl)	S	—		
Thiopentone	Pentothal Intraval	C_2H_5	$-CH.(CH_3)CH_2CH_2CH_3$ (1-methylbutyl)	S	—		

pain. In these circumstances, they sometimes cause restlessness and confusion.

Barbiturates do not cause damage to the kidneys but during barbiturate anaesthesia the urine flow is often very low. This is caused partly by a reduction in the glomerular filtration rate consequent on the fall in blood pressure and partly perhaps by a barbitone-induced release of antidiuretic hormone.

The barbiturates inhibit the transmission of impulses in the reticular activating system, an action that explains their hypnotic and anaesthetic properties. In the sense discussed elsewhere (p. 493), barbiturates operate nonspecifically and do not, apparently, directly influence the formation or function of any of the neurohumoral substances that participate in the mechanisms that maintain consciousness.

It has been common practice to divide the barbiturates into four groups on the basis of their supposed duration of action. For information purposes, this grouping is preserved in Table 29.1, but it is now widely recognized that it implies fine differences in the duration of action of individual barbiturates that are not realized in practice. Many of the pharmacokinetic data on which the groupings were originally based were derived from animal experiments and they obviously cannot be transferrred directly to the human situation. They certainly cannot be used as a basis for establishing such tenuous distinctions as that, say,

between the so-called 'intermediate acting' and the 'short acting' compounds.

Since the barbiturates have begun their journey into history the old classification is retained in Table 29.1 to explain, for instance, why it was customary to prescribe a 'short acting' barbiturate (such as hexobarbitone or quinalbarbitone) for patients who had difficulty in falling asleep and then slept soundly. Those who complained of waking up frequently, or for long periods, during the night were given a barbiturate such as amylobarbitone or butobarbitone from the 'intermediate acting' group.

It remains true, of course, that the compounds appearing at the extremities of Table 29.1 exhibit at least the qualitative differences in their duration of action that is implicit in their position. Even here, however, a caution has to be entered. The 'ultra short acting' drugs are employed only as basal anaesthetics (p. 504) and the adjective refers to their sojourn in the brain and not to that in the tissues generally. Because of its high solubility and the richness of the brain's blood supply, a large part of a single intravenous dose of one of these agents is taken up immediately by the brain. In the succeeding few minutes much of it is redistributed to the other fatty tissues which, by reason of their paltry blood supply, were unable to take up much of the drug when it first appeared in the blood stream. Thus consciousness is regained while substantial amounts of the barbiturate remain in the tissues. The 'ultra short acting' barbiturates are not metabolized particularly quickly: while the half life of thiopentone in the brain is no more than 20 to 30 minutes, it reaches 8 hours or so in the body generally. This is still considerably lower than that found for barbiturates not classified as 'ultra short acting'.

An early critic of the system of classifying barbiturates on the basis of their supposed duration of action was Mark (1969) to whose paper the interested reader is referred.

The use of barbiturates as basal anaesthetics, psychotropic drugs and antiepileptic agents is discussed on pages 504, 563 and 522 respectively.

METABOLISM OF BARBITURATES
The metabolic fate of the barbiturates varies from compound to compound. The more chemically stable the compound, the less extensively is it broken down. Barbitone is not metabolized at all and almost 100 per cent appears unchanged in the urine. About 50 per cent of a dose of phenobarbitone also appears unchanged but only traces of the more unstable compounds such as thiopentone can be demonstrated in the unchanged condition. The changes that do occur include (i) oxidation of the radicals on C(5) to form carboxy, hydroxy or keto derivatives, (ii) opening of the barbiturate ring, (iii) loss of N-alkyl radicals and (iv) desulphuration of thiobarbiturates. Some further details are given on page 53.

SIDE EFFECTS AND TOXICITY OF BARBITURATES
Some patients exhibit an inborn idiosyncrasy or acquire an allergic hypersensitivity to the barbiturates. The idiosyncratic response takes the form of gastrointestinal disturbances, dizziness, a feeling of weakness and emotional upsets. Excitement, restlessness or delirium instead of sedation may be produced, particularly in patients who are in pain, and there are reports of barbiturates having actually caused pain of an arthritic type. Allergic responses to the barbiturates may take several forms but an oedema of the eyelids and face is commonly seen. As would be expected, these responses tend to occur most frequently among those who have a history of allergic disorders. Phenobarbitone has sometimes caused exfoliative dermatitis.

Even single doses of a hypnotic barbiturate can be followed by a 'hangover' effect on the following day since some of the drug persists in the brain. The overnight suppression of paradoxical sleep may contribute to the hangover, which takes the form of a feeling of depression followed by nausea, dizziness and disorientation later in the day. Hangovers are especially likely to occur in neurotic patients.

Individuals (particularly if they are elderly) who wake in the night after taking a barbiturate often feel confused. In their confusion they may take another dose of the drug believing that their disturbed sleep has resulted from their having forgotten to take their drug before retiring. Fatal overdoses have resulted from this confusion.

As we have seen, barbiturates suppress paradoxical sleep. Although tolerance to this effect develops rapidly there is a sharp and prolonged rebound when the drug is withdrawn (p. 479). In the early days of withdrawal, nightmares occur rather often and in the desire to avoid or to arrest these unpleasant sequelae the barbiturate taker is likely to resist drug withdrawal or to return to the drug once it has been withdrawn. Because tolerance develops rapidly, dose levels are soon increased and dependence is readily induced. The incidence of barbiturate dependence, in the days when the drugs were widely prescribed, was much higher than many physicians appreciated and overgenerous prescribing allowed many a patient to acquire the large stocks of drugs he needed to indulge his dependence.

Barbiturates are bound to plasma proteins—individual members of the group to different extents—and they stimulate microsomal enzymes. For these reasons, the possibility that interactions will occur with other drugs being taken at the same time has always to be borne in mind when barbiturates are prescribed (p. 80).

Barbiturate poisoning is almost invariably the result of an attempt at suicide. Symptoms include coma with cyanosis and a severely depressed respiration. Respiratory failure may be followed by cardiovascular collapse and death. The most important necessity in treatment is the institution of artificial respiration. If the drug has been taken soon before the patient is found, gastric lavage or the induction of vomiting may be usefully employed to remove the barbiturate but if much has been absorbed it may be necessary to institute forced diuresis or peritoneal dialysis. The weight of current opinion does not favour the use of respiratory stimulants in barbiturate poisoning.

The barbiturate antagonists, bemegride (Megimide) and amiphenazole (Daptazole) may be used to treat less severe degrees of barbiturate overdosage and to speed recovery from barbiturate anaesthesia. Bemegride is the more useful. As can be seen, it has a structure which is somewhat reminiscent of that of the barbiturates themselves. Amiphenazole is a less powerful barbiturate antagonist than bemegride but it does directly stimulate the respiratory centre.

Bemegride   Amiphenazole

STRUCTURE-ACTION RELATIONSHIPS IN THE BARBITURATES
1. For hypnotic or sedative activity both of the hydrogens on C(5) must be replaced by alkyl groups (as for

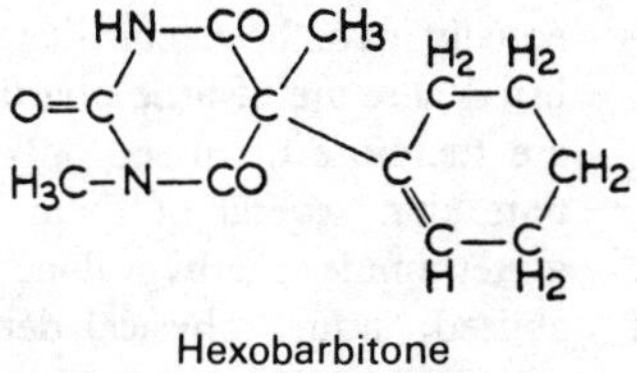

Hexobarbitone

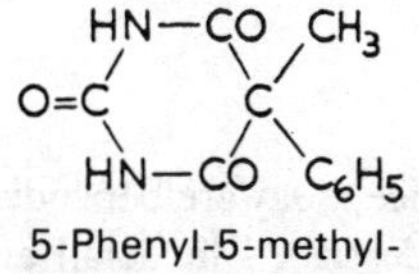

5-Phenyl-5-methyl-barbituric acid

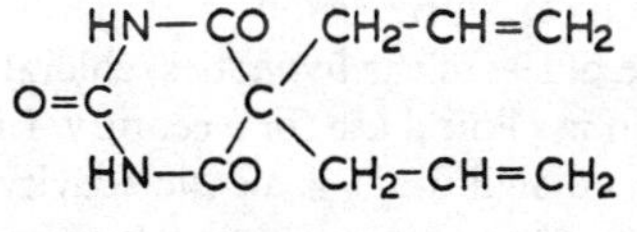

Allobarbitone

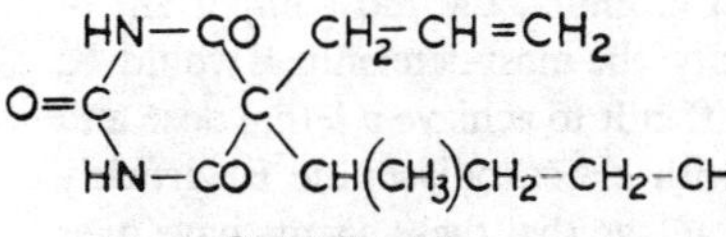

Quinalbarbitone

example in barbitone) or by one alkyl and one aryl group (as in hexobarbitone).

2. The presence of a phenyl group of C(5) confers anticonvulsant properties upon the compound (e.g. phenobarbitone and phenylmethylbarbituric acid).

3. Increase in length of one or both of the alkyl side chains on C(5) increases hypnotic potency (cf. allobarbitone and quinalbarbitone) but if the chain length is greater than five or six carbons, hypnotic activity is reduced and may be replaced by convulsant activity.

4. When the alkyl side chains on C(5) are branched, depressant activity is of shorter duration than when they are straight (e.g. amylobarbitone and quinalbarbitone).

5. Unsaturated side chains on C(5), especially short unsaturated side chains, increase potency (e.g. allobarbitone and quinalbarbitone).

6. Substitution with alkyl groups on both of the nitrogen atoms at positions 1 and 3 produces compounds with convulsant activity. When there is only one substitu-ent on N(1) or N(3), duration of hypnotic activity is shortened (e.g. hexobarbitone, methylphenobarbitone).

7. Substitution of one of the hydrogen atoms on C(5) by cyclohexenyl or cyclopentenyl rings produces compounds with a short but intense action which may make them suitable for use as anaesthetics, e.g. hexobarbitone.

8. When the oxygen atom on C(2) is replaced by sulphur, forming thiobarbituric acid, stability is reduced and the compounds have a shorter duration of action (e.g. thiopentone, thialbarbitone, buthalitone).

9. When the substituents on C(5) are derived from secondary alcohols (e.g. pentobarbitone) they may be more potent than those derived from primary alcohols (e.g. amylobarbitone).

10. Duration of activity is related to chemical stability within the body. The most stable, and therefore longest acting compounds, have straight, saturated, unbranched side chains or a phenyl ring on C(5) (e.g. barbitone, phenobarbitone). The least stable barbiturates are either derivatives of the less stable thiobarbituric acid or have an

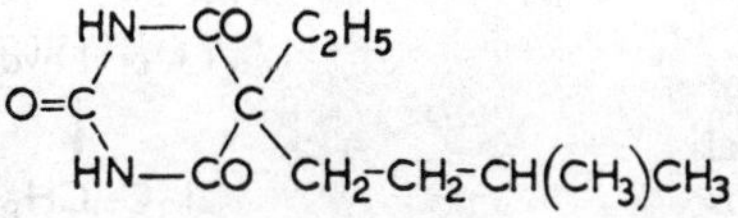

Amylobarbitone

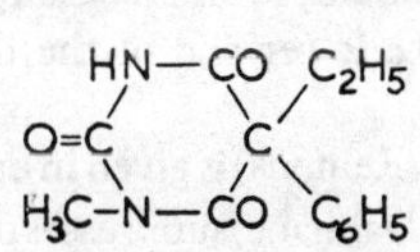

Methylphenobarbitone (phemitone)

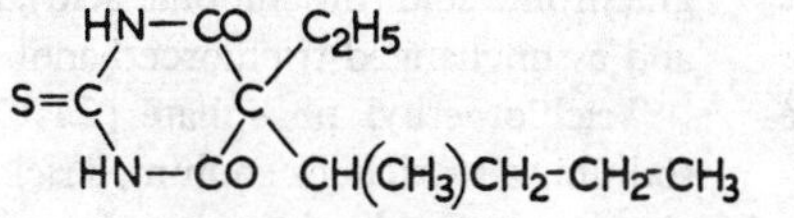

Thiopentone

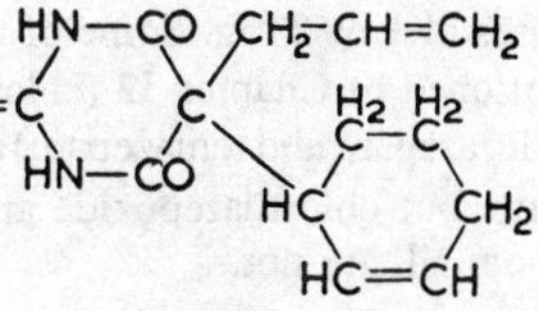

Thialbarbitone

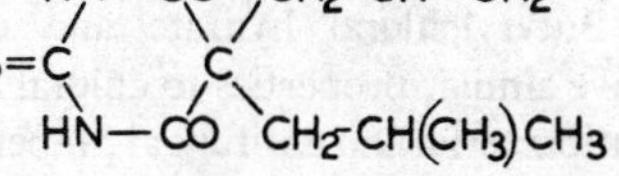

Buthalitone

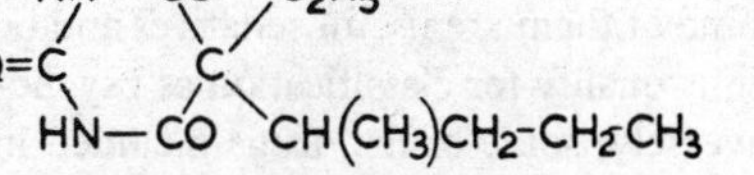

Pentobarbitone

alicyclic substituent on C(5) (e.g. thialbarbitone, thiopentone, hexobarbitone).

The benzodiazepines

The hypnotic drugs of choice today are benzodiazepines. The benzodiazepines are described in detail elsewhere; only their use as hypnotic agents is mentioned here.

The benzodiazepine hypnotics are to be preferred to the barbiturates on several grounds, the most important of which is their low toxicity: the most determined would-be suicide would find it difficult to achieve a lethal dose and accidental poisoning with a benzodiazepine is virtually unknown. Another advantage that these agents have over the barbiturates derives from the fact that they do not induce hepatic microsomal enzymes. This greatly reduces the possibility of adverse interactions between benzodiazepines and other drugs being taken at the same time. Finally, although cases of a barbiturate-like dependence have been reported, the benzodiazepines are much less liable than the barbiturates to be abused.

Like the barbiturates, the benzodiazepines tend to suppress paradoxical sleep to some extent with a rebound effect following their withdrawal after chronic use. Unusually among hypnotic drugs, they also inhibit stages 3 and 4 of slow wave sleep. Although restorative processes are active during these stages of sleep, they may be attended by less welcome activities such as bed wetting, sleep walking and nightmares. Those who suffer these embarrassments might well benefit from a nightly dose of a benzodiazepine.

The benzodiazepines secure sound sleep for some 7 to 8 hr after an induction period of about half an hour. Their persistence in the brain for some time after wakening causes a hangover effect against which patients (particularly those who are skilled workers) should be warned. They are also prone to produce a degree of mental confusion in the elderly who should, for this reason, always be prescribed doses from the lower end of the therapeutic range.

Nitrazepam (Mogadon, Remnos) is given in oral doses of 2.5 to 10 mg. *Flurazepam* (Dalmane) suppresses paradoxical sleep to a smaller extent than does nitrazepam and is probably to be preferred as a hypnotic agent. The recommended dose is 10 to 30 mg. *Flunitrazepam* (Rohypnol) has similar actions in doses of 1 or 2 mg. Some of the other benzodiazepines mentioned in Chapter 32 (chlorazepate, desmethyldiazepam, lorazepam and temazepam) are effective as hypnotic agents but chlordiazepoxide and diazepam, the oldest of them all, are not.

Other hypnotics

All the compounds listed in this section are hypnotics but in smaller doses some of them are useful sedatives and on this score they might qualify for classification as psychotropic drugs. Conversely, some of the drugs included in the discussion on psychotropic drugs (p. 536) might equally have been considered here. Most of the drugs listed here are of little pharmacological interest and they are therefore discussed only briefly. The reader should note that several of them (ethchlorvynol, ethinamate, glutethimide, methyprylone and methaqualone) can, if abused, induce physical dependence of the barbiturate type.

CHLORAL HYDRATE

The oldest of the hypnotics, chloral hydrate (Noctec) has been in clinical use for a century. Like the barbiturates, it has no significant analgesic activity and it will not overcome sleeplessness caused by severe pain. In hypnotic doses (1.5 to 2 grams) it is almost non-toxic: it gives sleep lasting for about 8 hours but the patient can be readily awakened and he suffers no 'hangover' effect next day. It is a particularly useful hypnotic agent for the very young and the very old. Unusually among hypnotic drugs it does not suppress paradoxical sleep. Tolerance to chloral hydrate develops rapidly and cases of dependence on the drug were not uncommon in the days when it was used more widely than it is today. The most famous chloral hydrate addict was Rossetti. Chloral hydrate is useful in insomnia associated with worry and excitement and it has been employed as a sedative in convulsions, delirium, mania, whooping cough and alcoholism. It has an unpleasant taste which has to be disguised by an acceptable diluent such as orange juice. Dilution of chloral hydrate is, in any event, necessary because it has an irritant action on the skin and mucous membranes. Large doses, even when diluted, may so irritate the gastrointestinal tract that they cause vomiting but this eventuality can be avoided by giving the drug by the rectal route.

After administration, chloral hydrate is converted into trichloroethanol which is the immediate cause of the hypnotic effect. Trichloroethanol is metabolized in the

$$Cl_3C.CH(OH)_2$$
Chloral hydrate

$$\downarrow$$

$$Cl_3C.CH_2OH$$
Trichloroethanol

liver and it is eliminated in the urine as a conjugate with glucuronic acid (urochloralic acid), as trichloroacetic acid and as unchanged trichloroethanol.

Trichloroethyl phosphate ($Cl_3C.CH_2$) H_2PO_4, or its sodium salt (triclofos sodium, Tricloryl) can be used as an alternative to chloral hydrate. It is tasteless and it does not cause gastrointestinal irritation. The hypnotic dose of triclofos sodium is 2.5 to 3.5 grams.

Butyrylchloral hydrate and chlorbutol (chloretone) have similar properties to chloral hydrate. Chlorbutol has antibacterial and antifungal properties and it is more often employed as a disinfectant than as a hypnotic agent.

$$CH_3CHClCCl_2CH(OH)_2 \qquad CCl_3C(CH_3)_2OH$$

Butyl chloral hydrate   Chlorbutol
                            (trichlortertiary
                            butanol)

Dichloralphenazone is a complex of chloral hydrate and phenazone (p. 448) which dissociates into its constituents after absorption. It has essentially the same actions and uses as chloral hydrate: the hypnotic dose is 500 mg to 2 grams. Proprietary names include Bonadorm, Dormwell and Welldorm.

CHLORPROMAZINE

Although chlorpromazine is primarily an antipsychotic drug, it is also in some circumstances a useful hypnotic agent. Both its hypnotic and its antipsychotic actions are attributable to its ability to antagonize dopamine. It does not markedly depress paradoxical sleep: some reports indeed claim that it induces sleep with an enhanced proportion of this component. Chlorpromazine is discussed in more detail on p. 548.

ETHCHLORVYNOL

Ethchlorvynol (Placidyl, Serensil) is a mildly hypnotic drug which in effective oral doses (500 mg to one gram) has a hypnotic effect that extends over some five hours. It has also been given preoperatively to reduce apprehension.

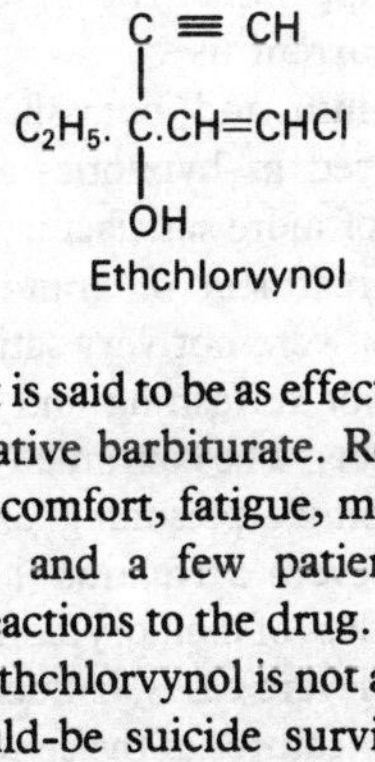

C ≡ CH
|
C_2H_5. C.CH=CHCl
|
OH
Ethchlorvynol

For this purpose it is said to be as effective as diazepam but less so than a sedative barbiturate. Reported side effects include gastric discomfort, fatigue, mental confusion and thrombocytopenia and a few patients have displayed hypersensitivity reactions to the drug. In its favour it must be admitted that ethchlorvynol is not a very useful suicide weapon: one would-be suicide survived a dose of 125 grams!

ETHINAMATE

Ethinamate (Valamin, Valmid) has similar actions and uses to ethchlorvynol. Even the recommended hypnotic dose (0.5 to 1 gram) is the same.

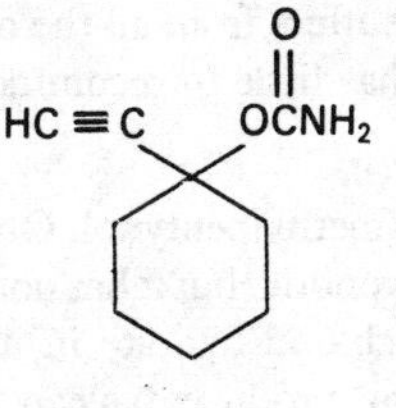

Ethinamate

GLUTETHIMIDE

When glutethimide (Doriden, Gludorm) was first introduced (in 1954), it was hailed as a drug which would replace the hypnotic barbiturates since it was reputed to be free of toxic side effects and unlikely to cause dependence. Neither of these hopes was realized. Glutethimide can cause epileptiform convulsions and neurological and haematological disorders particularly in older patients and it produces psychic and physical dependence at least as readily as do the barbiturates. Those who take glutethimide are likely to experience a 'hangover' effect. A state of intoxication similar to that produced by alcohol has been described and the only indication for its use is as a hypnotic in those who are intolerant of the better hypnotics. Glutethimide is related to thalidomide (Fig. 29.3) but its metabolic fate is different and no case of foetal deformity following its use has been reported. The oral hypnotic dose of glutethimide is 500 mg.

Methyprylone (Noludar) is similar to glutethimide in its properties, uses and side effects. The recommended dose is 400 mg for hypnosis.

METHAQUALONE

Methaqualone (Methalone, Quaalude, Revonal) is taken alone or in association with diphenhydramine, the mixture (250 mg of methaqualone and 25 mg of the histamine H_1 antagonist) being known as Mandrax. The antihistamine drug potentiates methaqualone's hypnotic action.

Methaqualone and (especially) Mandrax have attracted a certain notoriety as drugs that are sought after for nontherapeutic purposes and numerous cases of dependence on the drug have been reported.

The hypnotic dose of methaqualone is 150 to 400 mg. Once sleep supervenes it usually persists for six to eight hours. When taken as Mandrax, a single tablet (which contains 250 mg of methaqualone) is usually sufficient to secure sleep.

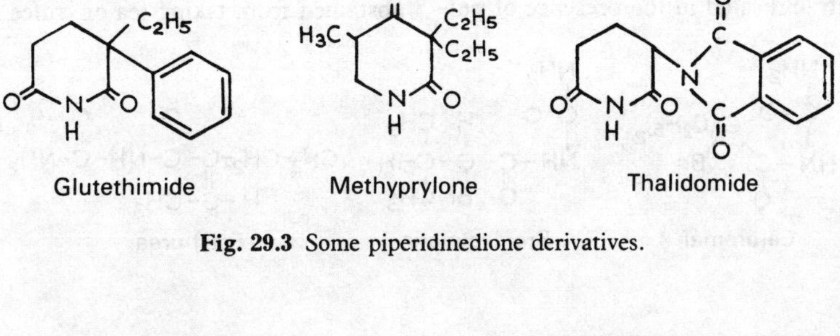

Glutethimide   Methyprylone   Thalidomide

Fig. 29.3 Some piperidinedione derivatives.

Methaqualone suffers from all the disadvantages of the barbiturates and has little to recommend it.

METHYLPARAFYNOL

Methylparafynol (methylpentynol, Oblivon, Dormisol) is a relatively new hypnotic, but it has not won wide popularity. It resembles chloral hydrate in its actions. The oral dose (0.5 to 1 gram) produces a sleep that endures for six hours or so with no subsequent 'hangover'.

Paraldehyde

Methylparafynol

PARALDEHYDE

Paraldehyde (Paral) is a powerful hypnotic agent with marked anticonvulsant properties. It is no longer widely used, due largely to its unpleasant and persistent odour and taste and to the fact that better hypnotic and anticonvulsive drugs are avilable. Some 20 to 30 per cent of a dose of paraldehyde is excreted, in an unchanged form, by the lungs so that its offensive smell is as evident to the immediate neighbours of the person who has been given paraldehyde as it is to the patient himself. The breath remains tainted for up to 24 hours after a single dose of paraldehyde. That which is not excreted in the expired air is metabolized in the liver. As with ethanol, acetaldehyde is first formed and paraldehyde should not be given to patients who are also receiving disulphiram (p. 90).

When it is used for securing sleep, paraldehyde is given by mouth or intramuscular injection in doses of 5 to 10 ml. A period of six to eight hours of undisturbed sleep can be expected. The dose required to induce basal anaesthesia is 15 to 30 ml (0.5 ml per kilogram of body mass in children, for whom paraldehyde is a suitable drug), suitably diluted and given by the rectal route. A similar dose, given by intramuscular injection is required to control patients in the throes of delirium tremens, status epilepticus or tetanus but no more than 5 ml of paraldehyde is to be injected at any one intramuscular site. Intravenous injection carries the risk of cardiovascular collapse and can only be permitted when it is justified by the gravity of the emergency.

Paraldehyde is contraindicated in the presence of pulmonary or hepatic disease but it is otherwise a safe drug. Notwithstanding its foul taste it is sometimes drunk by drug abusers (particularly alcoholics), a sad if telling commentary on the lengths to which man is sometimes driven to achieve the solace which comes, strangely enough, from inhibition of the highest centres of his brain.

UREA DERIVATIVES

Two monoureides which were extensively used in the past but are now obsolescent, are carbromal (bromadal) and bromvaletone (bromisovalum, Bromural). It will be recalled that the barbiturates are cyclic diureides: they are correspondingly more powerful hypnotic agents than the monoureides. Carbromal and bromvaletone may cause signs of bromism (see below) in sensitive individuals. When it is felt necessary to use either of these compounds they are given in doses of about 500 mg. They are quick acting, producing a light hypnosis which lasts for about four hours and which is attended by no after effects. Carbrital contains carbromal and pentobarbitone sodium.

Ectyl urea (Levanil, Nostyn) does not contain bromine. Large doses are required to produce hypnosis but sedation can be obtained with doses of the order of 250 mg.

BROMIDES

Bromides are no longer used clinically but they retain some attraction for the pharmacologist and these comments are added by way of an appendix to our discussion concerning hypnotic drugs in current use.

Ammonium, sodium and potassium bromides were once widely employed as hypnotics and sedatives and, until the discovery of more satisfactory agents, they were also used for the treatment of grand mal epilepsy. As hypnotics, bromides were not very satisfactory: the sleep they induced was not refreshing and they often caused unpleasant after effects. The continued ingestion of bromides often led to bromide poisoning (*bromism*) which was characterized by a severe dermatitis (bromide rash), gastrointestinal upsets, loss of memory, confusion, inability to concentrate and, in severe cases, hallucinations, delusions and delirium. Other features of the condition were dilated pupils, tremors, muscle weakness, an unsteady gait and depression of reflexes. These features are reminiscent of the drunken state and misdiagnoses of alcoholism or other forms of mental disturbance in patients who were, in fact, victims of bromism were not uncommon.

Bromides have the unearned reputation of being powerful inhibitors of sexual drive and many a soldier has abstained from taking tea or coffee in his barracks in the

Carbromal

Bromvaletone

Ectyl urea

belief that his beverages had had bromides added. This widespread misconception concerning the effect of bromides on the libido had one interesting and beneficial consequence. In less enlightened times, boys were often told that masturbation led to epilepsy, a view which was accepted by some medical authorities. Among these, Locock argued that, if this were so, the administration of bromides should prevent or relieve epilepsy. In 1857 he exposed his theoretical argument to the test of experiment and thus discovered, by accident, a method for the treatment of epilepsy which provided untold relief and comfort to epileptics until more powerful antiepileptic drugs were discovered in 1912.

SLEEP DISORDERS

Some recognized sleep disorders other than simple insomnia deserve a brief mention.

Snoring. Many of us snore occasionally as our bedmates are only too ready to tell us but in some unfortunate individuals the condition reaches pathological proportions and may lead to daytime sleepiness. It is attributable to obstruction of the upper reaches of the respiratory tract occasioned by loss of tone in muscles that normally maintain its patency. In the most serious cases it may be necessary to resort to tracheostomy to bring relief to the victim. Snoring normally occurs only in periods of slow wave sleep.

Nocturnal myoclonus. Although this condition was not formally described and labelled until 1953 many people before that date must have been aware of it. In nocturnal myoclonus, repeated series of involuntary jerks occur in the muscles, usually in the lower limbs, when on the threshold of sleep. Myoclonus must be distinguished from the isolated lower limb jerks most of us occasionally experience as we are drifting into sleep. Nocturnal myoclonus proper may recur at intervals throughout the night and it is a potent cause of insomnia. It usually responds to treatment with a hypnotic benzodiazepine. Many patients who suffer from nocturnal myoclonus also complain of uncomfortable and sometimes painful sensations in the lower limbs that provoke restless movements and thereby delay the onset of sleep. Among the drugs recommended for treatment of the *restless legs syndrome*, the best is probably carbamazepine (Tegretol, p. 526).

Drug dependency insomnia. The continued ingestion of hypnotic drugs can itself lead to insomnia as tolerance to the drug develops. Treatment is by education and reassurance.

Other states. Nocturnal enuresis, somnambulism, night terrors and nightmares were mentioned earlier in this chapter; narcolepsy and cataplexy are discussed in Chapter 17 (p. 275).

BIBLIOGRAPHY

Books, monographs and reviews

Freemon, F. R. (1972) *Sleep Research. A critical Review.* Springfield, Ill: Charles C. Thomas.

Gillin, J. C., Mendelson, W. B., Sitaram, N. and Wyatt, R. J. (1978). The neuropharmacology of sleep and wakefulness. *A. rev. Pharmac. Toxicol.,* **18**, 563-579.

Guyton, A. C. (1976) *Organ Physiology Structure and Function of the Nervous System* 2nd ed. Philadelphia, London, Toronto: W. B. Saunders.

Hartman, E. (1978). Effects of psychotropic drugs on sleep: the catecholamines and sleep. In: Lipton, M. A., DiMascio, A. and Killam, K. F., eds., *Psychopharmacology: A Generation of Progress* pp. 711-728. New York: Raven Press.

Johns, M. W. (1975) Sleep and hypnotic drugs. *Drugs,* **9**, 448-478.

Kagan, F., Harwood, Theresa, Rickels, K., Rudzik, A. D. and Sorer, H. (eds) (1975) *Hypnotics: Methods of Development and Evaluation.* New York: Spectrum Publications.

Kleitman, N. (1963). *Sleep and Wakefulness* 2nd ed. Chicago: University of Chicago Press.

Margolin, S. (1963) Non-barbiturates. *Physiol. Pharmac.,* **1**, 239-273.

Petre-Quadens, Olga and Schlag, J. (eds) (1974) *Basic Sleep Mechanisms.* New York and London: Academic Press.

Sharpless, S. K. (1965) The barbiturates. In: Goodman, L. S. and Gilman, A. (eds) *The Pharmacological Basis of Therapeutics.* 3rd ed., pp. 105-128. New York: Macmillan.

Original papers

Mark, L. C. (1969) Archaic classification of barbiturates. *Clin. pharmac. ther.* **10**, 287-291.

Monnier, M., Dudler, L., Gaechter, R., Maier, P. F., Tobler, H. J. and Schoenenberger, G. A. (1977) The delta sleep inducing peptide (DSIP). Comparative properties of the original and synthetic polypeptide. *Experientia,* **33**, 548-552.

Pappenheimer, J. R., Koski, G., Fencl, V., Karnovsky, M. L. and Krueger, J. (1975). Extraction of sleep-promoting Factor S from cerebrospinal fluid and from brains of sleep-deprived animals. *J. Neurophysiol.,* **38**, 1299-1311.

30. General anaesthetics

Of all the benefits which medical science has provided for mankind, none has surpassed the general anaesthetic. It is difficult for modern man to imagine the torture that surgery meant little more than a century ago or the bravery of those who voluntarily submitted to it. Then, surgical skill was synonymous with speed and the only type of operation which could be contemplated was that which, involving only the crudest amputations or excisions, could be completed within minutes. General anaesthetics brought the patient relief from the agonies of surgery but they did much more. In order to perform more intricate surgical manoeuvres, the surgeon needed time and he needed a patient whose muscles were relaxed. General anaesthetics provided him with both and the era of modern surgery arrived.

Paracelsus, the bombastic alchemist of the 16th century, demonstrated that ether, which even then had been known for 300 years, was capable of producing insensibility in animals and he suggested that it might be used to relieve pain in man. His suggestion was ignored and forgotten and another two centuries were to pass before ether was used as an anaesthetic. Sir Humphry Davy and Sir Michael Faraday almost discovered the anaesthetic powers of nitrous oxide and ether respectively but most of those to whom they expressed their ideas were much more interested in the exciting subjective effects produced by inhalation of these substances. When Humphry Davy first inhaled nitrous oxide he became so euphoric that he burst out laughing and from that day the substance has been called 'laughing gas'. Hundreds of the fashionable set of his day flocked to his demonstrations, eager to savour the hallucinatory experiences and the erotic imagery conjured up by small doses of nitrous oxide. Ether enjoyed the same doubtful reputation and 'ether frolics' were a feature of the social scene in the United States and Europe in the early years of the 19th century. Observations made at one of these frolics led to the first authenticated use of general anaesthesia in surgery. In 1841 Long, a young American physician, noticed that participants in an ether frolic who had inhaled ether vapour to the point of becoming stuporous, seemed to suffer less pain than would have been expected when they received injuries in the course of their uninhibited horse play. Many other people must have noticed a similar insensitivity in those intoxicated with alcohol (indeed alcohol was sometimes given in efforts to obtund the horrors of surgery) but Long was the first to carry what must have been an ancient observation to its logical conclusion. Shortly after making his observations at the ether frolic, Long excised two cysts from the neck of a friend previously rendered unconscious with ether. Long performed other simple surgical operations under ether anaesthesia but news of his discovery was slow to spread. Others made their own independent observations and carried out operations under anaesthesia but difficulties of communication, failure to follow up the original findings, personal animosities and professional prejudices conspired to prevent the rapid dissemination of the news which was to prove so important. William Morton, an American dentist, is rightly given the credit for demonstrating, with a conviction that could not be ignored, that surgery could be painlessly performed on the anaesthetized patient. After preliminary experiments on a number of animal species including himself and the family dog, Morton extracted a tooth from a patient anaesthetized with ether. That was in September of 1846 and in November of that year a London dentist, hearing of Morton's success, also successfully removed a tooth from a patient under ether anaesthesia. Chloroform was first used in 1847 by Dr. James Simpson of Edinburgh who gave it to a woman to relieve the pains of labour. He was attacked and denigrated by the ministers of the Scottish church (all men, of course) and by not a few of his fellow doctors who believed that it was woman's God-given privilege to suffer in childbirth but he persisted in his use of chloroform and all opposition to his activities mysteriously disappeared when Queen Victoria herself received chloroform during the birth of her seventh child in 1853. The early days of anaesthesia are vividly described by Prescott (1964).

At first, to be anaesthetized was a hazardous experience. The induction of anaesthesia was often unpleasant to the patient, toxic reactions to the anaesthetic agent were frequent and death under the anaesthetic or shortly after regaining consciousness was not a rare occurrence. As anaesthetics became more pure and the importance of suitable pre-anaesthetic preparation of the patient became appreciated, anaesthesia became a safer undertaking. Another advance was the development of agents to promote relaxation of the skeletal musculature (p. 236). These drugs cause the muscle relaxation which could previously only be provided by large doses of anaesthetic so that it is now possible to undertake surgery on the patient who, though he has received only a relatively small amount of anaesthetic, has a completely relaxed musculature. As a result of these advances, the dangers and unpleasantness of anaesthesia have largely disappeared and the modern patient faces the prospect of undergoing surgery with equanimity.

Anaesthesia enables the surgeon to perform operations that were previously unthinkable. As his experience widened, he demanded new anaesthetic agents and methods which allowed him to develop even more elaborate procedures but the two oldest anaesthetic agents—nitrous oxide and ether—have not been abandoned.

Gaseous and volatile anaesthetics are still widely used. Some other agents can be given by intravenous injection and they induce anaesthesia very rapidly. They are used either as *basal anaesthetics* (substances used to cause loss of consciousness before a volatile or gaseous anaesthetic is given) or as an anaesthetic agent proper for surgical operations of short duration.

$$\underset{\substack{H_2C \\[-2pt] H_2C \text{———} CH_2}}{}\quad \text{cyclopropane}$$

Hydrocarbon

$$CH_2 = CH - O - CH = CH_2 \quad \text{vinyl ether}$$
$$C_2H_5 - O - C_2H_5 \quad \text{ethyl ether}$$

Ethers

$CHCl_3$	chloroform
CH_3CH_2Cl	ethyl chloride
$CHCl = CCl_2$	trichloroethylene
$CF_3CHCl\,Br$	halothane
Br_3C-CH_2OH	tribromoethanol
$Cl_3C-CH(OH)_2$	chloral hydrate
$CF_3CH_2O-CH = CH_2$	fluoroxene
$CHCl_2.CF_2.OCH_3$	methoxyflurane

Halogenated compounds

Fig 30.1

THEORIES OF ANAESTHESIA

It has already been mentioned that pharmacologically active compounds can be divided into two major groups—the *structurally specific* and the *structurally non-specific*. The evidence indicates that drugs in the first group bring about their action by combining with a specific receptor and that there must be a relationship between the chemical properties of the drug molecule and those of the receptor which can only be varied within relatively narrow limits if activity is not to be lost or very considerably reduced. The structurally non-specific drugs do not act on specific receptors. Instead, they penetrate into the cell or accumulate in cellular membranes where they interfere, by chemical or physical means, with enzyme systems, with ion transport or with some other fundamental cellular process. A prerequisite for this type of activity is the possession of physiochemical properties which permit the drug to reach its site of action. Consequently all members of the group of structurally non-specific drugs have similar physiochemical properties whatever their ultimate action on the chemical systems of the cell.

The group of structurally non-specific drugs is exemplified by general anaesthetics of the type illustrated in Figure 30.1. They are lipid soluble compounds of simple but unrelated structure. The overriding importance of physicochemical properties among the structurally non-specific drugs is illustrated by the action of xenon. Under physiological conditions the only form of activity shown by this inert gas is the formation of Van der Waal's bonds. Yet it is capable of inducing surgical anaesthesia.

It is possible to specify some structural features which preclude the possession of general anaesthetic activity. Thus, compounds which ionize at physiological pH values, compounds which are very soluble in water and compounds which are changed after administration into ionized or very water-soluble derivatives cannot cause anaesthesia. Neither the properties which are a prerequisite for anaesthetic activity nor those which preclude it are associated with rigidly defined chemical structures so that compounds with the same sort of pharmacological action may be very different chemically. This is strikingly illustrated by the fact that, with one exception, all gases and volatile liquids so far investigated, whatever their structure and chemical reactivity, display anaesthetic activity if they are supplied in a sufficiently high concentration. The exception is provided by *n*-decane whose lack of anaesthetic activity may be attributable to its being metabolized at a rate that prevents its achieving a sufficiently high concentration at the site of anaesthetic action. It must not, however, be assumed that the nonspecific nature of their pharmacological action makes it impossible to derive structure-action relationships among the members of any group of general anaesthetics. Small changes in the structure of both the barbiturates and the steroid anaesthetics may produce marked changes in anaesthetic activity. These changes may influence both the ease with which the anaesthetic gains access to its site of action and its effectiveness when it gets there. Even if anaesthetic action involves no more than a simple physical effect on the plasma membrane (such as an occlusion of transmembrane channels) it is evident that, by their very shape, some molecules will be more capable than others of bringing about this effect..

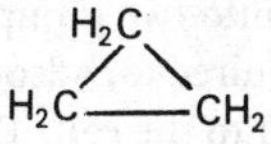

Many hypotheses have been advanced to explain the mode of action of anaesthetics. None is entirely satisfactory and it may well be that not all anaesthetics operate by the same mechanism. The hypotheses are discussed below.

It will be appreciated that they fall into two groups. Some simply formulate the conditions required for adsorption to cell membranes or for penetration into the cell. The other hypotheses are more directly concerned with the nature of the drugs' interaction with fundamental neuronal processes.

THE OVERTON-MEYER RULE
In 1901, Overton and Meyer independently pointed out that anaesthetics were soluble in lipids and that anaesthetic potency was directly related to the partition coefficient of the drug in an oil-water system. The nervous system has a high lipid content and the Overton-Meyer theory (or rule) does no more than indicate that anaesthetic action is exerted in a lipid phase of the neurone. It does not, of course, explain the origin of the anaesthetic activity.

FERGUSON'S PRINCIPLE
Ferguson suggested, in 1939, that the potency of structurally non-specific drugs was determined by their thermodynamic activity. This quantity is a measure of the proportion of the molecules which are free to react with enzyme systems, nerve membranes and similar biologically important sites. The molecules which are not free to act in this way are reacting with one another, with the molecules of solvent or with molecules of other solutes which may be present. The thermodynamic activity of a drug in solution is therefore not determined entirely by its concentration. In the case of volatile anaesthetics administered with air or oxygen, the thermodynamic activity is proportional to the partial pressure of the drug in the gas mixture divided by the saturated vapour pressure of the pure drug at the same temperature. Analogous calculations can be used to determine the activity of drugs in solution. Ferguson's theory predicts that a particular group of structurally non-specific drugs will show the same degree of biological activity if their concentrations are adjusted so that their thermodynamic activites are equal. The prediction is in general borne out by the experimental evidence. An important implication of Ferguson's theory is that the potency of a structurally non-specific drug is inversely proportional to its solubility in water. This extends the scope of the Overton-Meyer generalization, since high lipid solubility is not the only property which is associated with low solubility in water.

The main value of the Ferguson principle lies in the fact that it has provided a method of deciding whether a particular drug belongs to the structurally specific or the non-specific group. It is, of course, applicable to substances other than anaesthetics and it was indeed originally applied to insecticides and antibacterial substances. Its relevance to theories of anaesthetic action lies simply in the support it provides for the idea that anaesthetic molecules have purely physical actions (distortion of cell membranes, occlusion of channels etc.) on the cell.

MULLINS' HYPOTHESIS
Mullins formulated his hypothesis in 1954. It is essentially an extension of the Ferguson principle but it is capable of accommodating some of the experimental data that had previously provided something of an obstacle to a complete acceptance of Ferguson's views. One such awkward fact is that the thermodynamic activity of the members of a homologous group of substances associated with the production of a particular degree of anaesthesia increases as the series is ascended.

Mullins suggested that the phase in the central nervous system in which an anaesthetic acts is a nonaqueous polar lattice. For theoretical purposes the lattice can be looked upon as being composed of solid cylindrical rods packed together to form a three dimensional structure. Such a structure will have channels running through it. These form what is called the 'free space' and may serve to permit the inward and outward flux of the ions associated with neuronal activity. The molecules of the anaesthetic, providing that they are not greater than a certain maximum size, will fit into these channels and partially or wholly block them. The smaller the molecules the more easily will they fit into the spaces but unless they can form aggregations, the less effectively will they occlude them. Mullins also suggested that because cell membranes are not static structures but are constantly showing thermal motion, larger molecules will sometimes be accommodated in enlarged spaces formed by distortion of the membrane molecules. When the occlusion of the free space in the membrane reaches a certain fraction of the whole, membrane permeability is depressed to a level at which neuronal activity is also reduced and anaesthesia results.

This theory suggests that the size of the molecules is as important as the number which reach the site of action and it is interesting that it has been shown that the product of the thermodynamic activity of an anaesthetic multiplied by its molar volume is a constant.

THE ICE COVER AND MICROCRYSTALLINE HYDRATE THEORIES.
In 1961, Miller and Pauling put forward independent but related hypotheses which sought to explain how anaesthetic agents could interfere with nervous activity by physical means. Both hypotheses are based on the idea that anaesthetic activity is the result of clathrate formation.

In experiments carried out between 1945 and 1950, Palin and Powell showed that hydroquinone could combine with certain gases and vapours. In these complexes, three molecules of hydroquinone form, by hydrogen bonds, a cage-like structure which encloses a cavity in which are trapped the molecules of the other substance. This is an example of a *clathrate*—a complex formed by the complete enclosure of the molecules of one chemical species within a cage-like structure formed from the molecules of the second. When such a complex is formed from water and a gas or a vapour it is often described as a *gas hydrate*.

Miller pointed out that many gaseous and volatile anaesthetics were capable of forming gas hydrates and he showed that the partial pressure of an anaesthetic agent required to maintain anaesthesia was proportional to the dissociation pressure of its hydrate at 0°C However, under normal conditions, gas hydrates are unstable in body tissues and both Miller and Pauling proposed modifications of hydrate structure that would render them more stable. Miller investigated gas hydrates by X-ray crystallography and was able to show that the molecules of water which immediately surround a gas molecule are arranged in a more orderly fashion than those in the bulk of the solution. This water has a crystal configuration similar to that of ice and Miller suggested that a proportion of the dissolved molecules of an anaesthetic gas were surrounded with these regularly arranged water molecules. The molecules of the complex have been picturesquely described as 'gas-filled icebergs'. Miller suggested that the 'icebergs' could be formed near an enzyme or other surface and he calculated the fraction of such a surface that would be covered with structured water in different conditions. This is the so-called *ice cover*. At a given temperature, the extent of the ice cover is proportional to the partial pressure of the anaesthetic. Even in the absence of any anaesthetic, some ice cover is present, and its extent increases as the temperature falls. Miller's hypothesis thus provides an explanation of the anaesthesia resulting from simple hypothermia. In its general form the hypothesis can be summarized in the statement that the presence of an anaesthetic increases the extent of the ice cover normally present at a given temperature. Cherkin and Cathpool (1964) have provided experimental support for Miller's hypothesis They showed in goldfish adapted to different environmental temperatures, that the partial pressure of an anaesthetic required to produce a given depth of anaesthesia increased with the temperature. This relationship was observed with a number of different anaesthetics, including ether, chloroform and halothane.

Pauling pointed out that the stability of a clathrate increased with the size of the entrapped molecule and he suggested that the stability of gas hydrates might be increased if the complexes included not only the anaesthetic molecule but also molecules of salts and the charged side chains of proteins present in the brain tissue. Pauling called this type of clathrate a *micro-crystalline hydrate*.

Micro-crystalline hydrates or ice cover could presumably effect anaesthesia by directly interfering with ionic mobility, enzyme activity or some other fundamental process.

A number of objections can be raised against both the Pauling and Miller hypotheses. Now that a wider range of anaesthetic agents has been investigated it emerges that the relationship between anaesthetic potency and hydrate stability at 0°C is not nearly as close as Miller had believed. Another serious objection concerns the fact that the stability of clathrates and the extent of the ice cover decrease with increasing temperature. The increased stability of micro-crystalline hydrates over that of the simple hydrates is hardly likely to be capable of preventing their breakdown at the high body temperature maintained by homeothermic animals. Similarly, the maintenance of a sufficiently extensive ice cover at 37°C. would require the delivery of the anaesthetic at several atmospheres pressure and even then, anaesthesia might not be produced because high pressure reverses anaesthetic action. Thus although Miller's and Pauling's hypotheses may provide an explanation of the effects of hypothermia on the activity of anaesthetic agents, they are less capable of explaining how anaesthesia is produced at normal body temperatures. Other criticisms of these hypotheses include the facts that it has never been possible to persuade some substances, including ether and halothane, actually to form hydrates and that the complexes described by Miller and Pauling are not formed by barbiturates. This last mentioned fact need not, however, constitute an insuperable objection to the hypotheses since there is no real necessity to postulate that all anaesthetics have a common mode of action. Finally, it should be noted that both hypotheses visualize anaesthetic action as something that occurs in an aqueous phase of the cell although so much other evidence locates it firmly in the lipid phase.

BIOCHEMICAL THEORIES OF ANAESTHESIA

All the hypotheses concerning anaesthetic action we have so far considered are essentially 'physical' in nature in the sense that they attribute anaesthesia to a nonspecific action on cell membranes. It is easy to visualize, in general terms at least, how this might arise. Thus, the anaesthetic molecules might occlude ion transport channels, distort the fine structure of the membrane, modify enzyme activity or directly influence ion movements and such changes might clearly lead to a physiological stabilization of the membrane and hence to a blockade of nerve impulse transmission. It has been demonstrated, indeed, that a range of drugs—tranquillizers and sedatives as well as local and general anaesthetics—do exert membrane actions of this type (Seeman, 1972). Moreover it is a well established fact that high pressure, certainly a 'physical' event, inhibits anaesthetic action. However, none of the foregoing implies that the only membrane susceptible to anaesthetic agents is the plasma membrane of the nerve fibre even though this is certainly the locus of action of local anaesthetic agents (p. 471). General anaesthetics, however, are given by inhalation or injection and even when total insensibility has been produced the drug concentration in the immediate neighbourhood of nerve fibres is insufficient to cause conduction block. There can be little doubt that general anaesthetics operate at the synaptic level, a region that is very sensitive to drug action and is also, of course, particularly well endowed with membrane bound structures. Physical effects on, say, the mitochondria might influence enzyme action and so induce biochemical changes. To advocate biochemical theories of general anaesthesia is, therefore, in no way to deny the validity of the conclusion that all anaesthetics, local and general alike, operate through structurally non-specific mechanisms. Nor does it militate against the hypothesis that local and general anaesthetics operate at different sites and by different mechanisms.

An early biochemical theory of anaesthesia was based on the fact that many anaesthetics can uncouple oxidative phosphorylation (p. 31) and so depress the synthesis of adenosine triphosphate (ATP). Since the continued synthesis of acetylcholine (and possibly of other transmitter agents) demands the presence of ATP, uncoupling agents might be expected to interfere with the synthesis of acetylcholine and thus to impair synaptic transmission in the brain. Superficially this provides a plausible explanation of anaesthetic action and, once very popular, this hypothesis still finds favour in some quarters. It is not entirely without experimental support. It is, for instance, an old observation that ether inhibits the synthesis of acetylcholine by brain slices unless ATP is added to the incubation medium. Moreover, acetylcholine is an important transmitter substance in the reticular activating system, a part of the brain that is particularly involved in the maintenance of consciousness. However, the concentration of ether required to depress acetylcholine synthesis is very much in excess of that which would be reached in the brain of the living anaesthetized animal and there is other evidence against the view that anaesthetics act by virtue of their being able to uncouple oxidative phosphorylation. The amount of acetylcholine in the brain actually increases during anaesthesia. This is almost certainly a secondary effect consequent on the reduced release of transmitter (Crossland and Merrick, 1954) but it is clear that there can be no question of any acetylcholine deficiency occurring in the anaesthetic state. Nor has it been possible to demonstrate any lack of ATP in the brains of anaesthetized animals—indeed, some anaesthetics cause small increases in the brain's content of high energy phosphates (ATP and creatine phosphate) in both *in vitro* and *in vivo* conditions. Finally, many other drugs that uncouple oxidative phosphorylation are devoid of any anaesthetic effectiveness.

Another hypothesis which has been much canvassed in the past is that anaesthetics act by inhibiting oxidative processes. The concentration of anaesthetic required to demonstrate this effect *in vitro* is very high but McIlwain has shown that if brain slices are stimulated electrically their oxygen uptake increases. Under these circumstances, oxygen uptake is depressed by concentrations of barbiturate anaesthetics which much more closely approach those found in the brain of the living anaesthetized animal.

There is no doubt that anaesthetics inhibit the uptake of oxygen by the brains of animals and man *in vivo* but this is more likely to be the result, rather than the cause, of anaesthesia.

A more recent biochemical hypothesis, not unrelated to the foregoing, is due to Krnjević and his colleagues (Krnjević, 1972, 1974) who suppose that general anaesthetics interfere with the uptake of calcium by mitochondria so that free calcium ions will accumulate in the axoplasm. This will occur in both the presynaptic and the postsynaptic elements. At the former site an increased availability of calcium ions would be prejudicial to transmitter release while postsynaptically it would lead to an increased potassium conductance and hence to a diminished neuronal excitability (p. 179). It is known that the excitatory action of acetylcholine on cortical neurones is antagonized by deep anaesthesia and that the effects of other putative excitatory mediators such as glutamic acid are less vulnerable to anaesthetics. It may well be, therefore, that general anaesthetics depress central nervous activity by mechanisms that inhibit both transmitter release and transmitter action. It is not unreasonable to assume that inhibition of transmitter release would lead to an accumulation of transmitter in the neurones (if their storage capacity permits this) so that both the earlier and the more recent work is fully consistent with the view that inhibition of acetylcholine release might be a key event in the induction of anaesthesia. It cannot be regarded as the only factor in anaesthetic action because a variety of other neurochemical changes can be expected if calcium movement into the mitochondria is hindered.

PHYSIOLOGICAL ASPECTS OF ANAESTHESIA

So far as their site of action is concerned, it seems to be established that anaesthetics interfere primarily with activity in the ascending reticular system (p. 162) thus depressing the overall level of excitability of the cortex.

Anaesthesia is associated with characteristic changes in the electroencephalogram. At first (during the period described below as Stage I of the anaesthesia) the normal α-rhythm disappears and is replaced by a faster low voltage rhythm. As Stage II is entered, the electroencephalographic picture changes, becoming dominated by slow, high-voltage waves. As anaesthesia deepens, the waves undergo an even more marked reduction in frequency associated with a further increase in amplitude. This slowing of the electroencephalographic rhythm is seen in other conditions (such as natural sleep) in which cerebral excitability is reduced.

Further deepening of the anaesthesia causes the appearance of brief periods of electrical silence which alternate with the slow, previously continuous, slow wave activity. The periods of electrical silence occupy a progressively increasing fraction of the record until, when the activity of the brain is depressed to the point of death, complete electrical silence prevails and the pen of the electroencephalograph traces an unwavering line.

The electroencephalographic changes which occur in the earlier stages of anaesthesia are sufficiently closely correlated with the concentration of the anaesthetic agent in the brain to enable them to be used to maintain anaesthesia automatically in experimental animals. As anaesthesia lightens, the changed electrical output from the brain actuates a syringe which injects more anaesthetic until the previous level of electroencephalographic activity is restored. It is possible to arrange this apparatus to maintain any predetermined level of anaesthesia.

STAGES OF ANAESTHESIA

General anaesthetics cause a descending depression of the central nervous system, the higher cortical centres being affected first. The vital medullary centres are, fortunately, the last to be depressed. By adjusting the amount of anaesthetic delivered to the patient, the degree of central depression can be held at any desired level but for this purpose it is necessary to be able easily to assess the depth of anaesthesia which has been reached. In 1937, Guedel

pointed out that this could be done by simple observation principally of the eyes and the movements of respiration. He divided anaesthesia into four *stages*, the most important one of which (Stage III) he further subdivided into four *planes*. Guedel arrived at his description of the features of the several stages and planes of anaesthesia by observing the behaviour and responses of patients undergoing anaesthesia with ether. In such circumstances, the passage of the patient through each stage of anaesthesia is easily observed. Nowadays, however, anaesthesia is often induced by an an intravenous anaesthetic (p. 504) whatever substance is to be used to continue the anaesthesia and the transition from complete consciousness to surgical anaesthesia is so rapid that none of the earlier stages of anaesthesia can be seen. Moreover, preanaesthetic medication blurs the classical Guedel picture by preventing, or altering the intensity of, some of the identifying signs of the several stages of anaesthesia. Thus atropine dilates the pupil and pethidine constricts it independently of any effect of the anaesthetic itself. Nevertheless a knowledge of Guedel's description of the progress of anaesthesia is still useful, more particularly, perhaps, for the laboratory worker.

The most important features of each stage of anaesthesia are described below and they are also summarized in Table 30.1. It should be noted that not all anaesthetics produce

Table 30.1 Effects of volatile anaesthetics on the eye and respiration in the unpremedicated patient

| | Pupil Size | Eyeball Movement | Eye Reflexes | | Respiration |
			Corneal	Conjunctival	
Stage I	Normal	Normal (voluntary)	Present	Present	Regular
Stage II	Dilatation	Increased	Present	Present	Irregular
Stage III					
Plane 1	Constriction: abolition of inhibitory impulses	Further increased	Present	Absent	Regular but faster
Plane 2	Constriction ↓ Normal	None	Present ↓ Disappears	Absent	Slow and regular
Plane 3	Dilatation	None	Absent	Absent	Thoracic respiration depressed; abdominal respiration regular
Plane 4	Maximal dilatation	None	Absent	Absent	Thoracic respiration ceases; abdominal respiration depressed
Stage IV	Maximal dilatation	None	Absent	Absent	Ceases

precisely the same overall pharmacological effects at a particular stage of anaesthesia. Thus, cyclopropane and the barbiturates cause arrest of respiration more readily than does ether and different anaesthetics vary in the degree of analgesia they produce in Stage I and in the extent of the delirium they provoke in Stage II.

Stage I—the stage of analgesia
Consciousness is maintained but there is analgesia and the sense of smell disappears. Respiration is unaffected and reflexes are preserved. Because of the depression of the higher centres, the patient may experience visual or auditory hallucinations or vivid dreams. Small noises (such as those made in the setting out of surgical instruments) are often magnified.

Stage II—the stage of delirium
Stage II is entered when consciousness is lost. The further removal of cortical inhibition leads to a great increase in motor and autonomic activity and the patient may shout and struggle violently. Attempts to restrain him at this stage often make the struggling more violent, since it is largely the result of uninhibited reflex activity which will be increased if sensory stimulation is increased. For the same reason, any noise at this stage is likely to increase the patient's struggles. During the last war, it was often noticed that a sudden unexpected noise occurring at this stage of anaesthesia would evoke reactions of terror in patients on the edge of consciousness. The noise was dimly perceived and it caused an unrestrained and almost automatic pattern of response of the type which had been established by the sound of bombs or gunfire. The violence of the delirium in Stage II depends to some extent on the degree of self control exerted by the patient when in a fully conscious state. Thus the brave man who steeled himself not to show his fear when under fire was more likely than the obviously timid person to show violent responses when cortical restraint was removed. The extent of the delirium in the unmedicated patient given ether is also influenced by the skill of the anaesthetist.

In Stage II of anaesthesia, breathing is irregular and the eyes move rapidly.

Stage II is not seen during the induction of anaesthesia with a suitable basal anaesthetic but all patients will pass through this stage on their return to consciousness. Although it is not nearly so evident on the return to consciousness as it is during induction with some anaesthetics, the possibility that a brief period of restlessness may occur in the immediately post-operative period must be recognized and the patient must not, therefore, be left unattended at this time.

Stage III—the stage of surgical anaesthesia
Entry into Stage III is signalled by the return of regular breathing. Eye reflexes (blinking if the lashes or conjunc-

tiva are gently touched) disappear but, in the first place of Stage III anaesthesia, irregular movements of the eyeballs are even more in evidence than they are in Stage II. They disappear as the second plane is reached. Passage from the second to the third plane is shown by the depression of thoracic respiration. This disappears altogether as plane 4 is entered and respiration is now dependent entirely on the movements of the abdominal muscles. As anaesthesia is deepened still further, even the abdominal respiration becomes depressed and breathing ceases altogether as Stage IV is entered.

Complete relaxation and the abolition of reflex activity in voluntary muscles is not seen until plane 3 is reached and in the past major surgery could only be successfully carried out if anaesthesia had reached planes 3 or 4. For this reason, these planes were sometimes known as the 'planes of surgical anaesthesia'. The advent of neuromuscular blocking agents however, has made it possible to obtain a sufficient degree of muscle relaxation without the necessity of reaching the lowest planes of surgical anaesthesia.

Stage IV—the stage of medullary paralysis
A patient who reaches this stage of anaesthesia is in the hands of an incompetent anaesthetist. The medullary centres are paralysed so that respiration ceases. There is cardiovascular collapse and the tissues rapidly become anoxic. With some anaesthetics, respiration ceases well in advance of any severe depression of the cardiac and vasomotor centres and artificial respiration will usually keep the patient alive until sufficient anaesthetic has been expired or metabolized to permit the return of spontaneous respiration. The situation is considerably more dangerous if the cardiovascular centres or the heart itself are seriously depressed by amounts of anaesthetic which cause cessation of respiratory movements.

Reference to Table 30.1 will make it clear that pupillary size is a useful index of the stage to which anaesthesia has progressed in the patient or animal who has not received atropine. The dilatation seen in Stage II is caused by adrenaline release and the constriction of the pupil which occurs in the earlier planes of Stage III is a manifestation of parasympathetic dominance at this time. As the activity of the brain becomes more deeply depressed, all nervous control is removed and the pupil dilates under the stretch exerted by the elastic tissue component of the iris.

GASEOUS AND VOLATILE ANAESTHETICS

Although anaesthesia is often induced with a basal anaesthetic, it is frequently maintained with a gaseous or volatile anaesthetic. An obvious advantage of these agents is that they permit the depth of anaesthesia to be easily varied during the course of a surgical operation. Moreover, recovery from the anaesthetic begins immediately the anaesthetic supply is cut off and it continues rapidly since the anaesthetic is excreted in the expired air.

There are several methods of administration. In the *open drop method* a gauze mask supported on a wire frame is used. The volatile anaesthetic is dropped on to the mask which is applied to the patient's nose and mouth. The anaesthetic vaporizes and the vapour, mixed with air, is inhaled. The open drop method is only used for short operations, or when no other equipment is available. In the *semi-closed method*, a breathing bag connected to an anaesthetic mask is used. Oxygen and the anaesthetic gas or vapourized liquid pass into the bag and the patient breathes into the mask. He takes the anaesthetic from the bag but valves on the bag and mask direct his expired air into the atmosphere. In the completely *closed method*, the patient takes anaesthetic in the same way as in the semi-closed method, but his expired air passes into a container of soda lime which absorbs the carbon dioxide. The rest of the expired air (oxygen and unused anaesthetic) rejoins the stream of oxygen and anaesthetic vapour passing to the breathing bag. Modern anaesthetic apparatus (of which Boyle's is the best known type) has provision for passing oxygen mixed with any of a number of other gases into the breathing bag. The relative proportions of the different gases in the mixture is controlled by adjustable valves and measured by flowmeters. If a volatile anaesthetic is to be added to the gas mixture, the latter can be directed through one or more bottles of the anaesthetic. A plunger in the bottle directs the gases close to or into the volatile anaesthetic. The lower the plunger is placed, the greater the quantity of anaesthetic vapour which is added to the gas mixture. The anaesthetic bottle can be surrounded with warm water, if necessary, to aid evaporation.

It is usual to give premedication to patients who are to receive a general anaesthetic. They are given a hypnotic on the night before so that they can be assured of a good night's sleep. One or two hours before surgery, atropine (or hyoscine) is usually administered in order to prevent excess secretion of saliva or mucus which might impede the work of the anaesthetist and be hazardous to the patient. Atropine also helps to prevent cardiac arrest due to stimulation of the vagal centre but not all anaesthetists approve of its being given when non-irritative anaesthetics are used. Hyoscine is sometimes preferred to atropine because of its additional sedative and amnesic properties. Morphine (or pethidine) is also given to allay fear and apprehension. Its analgesic properties are also valuable for reducing the intensity of post-operative pain.

Other preanaesthetic medication may be required because of special circumstances connected with the physical condition of the patient or with the nature of the particular anaesthetic being used. Some of these circumstances are mentioned in the following discussions.

Volatile liquids

The boiling point of a volatile anaesthetic and its solubility in plasma are, among other properties, important determinants of its acceptability to the anaesthetist and his patient. The higher its boiling point, the more difficult it is to achieve a high concentration of vapour in the air that is supplied to the patient while if the anaesthetic is very soluble in plasma its partial pressure in the pulmonary alveoli will rise only slowly. Consequently it will at first be delivered to the tissues in a low concentration (the solubility of a gas in a liquid is directly proportional to the partial pressure to which it is exposed) so that its passage into the brain will proceed only sluggishly notwithstanding its initially rapid influx into the blood. Thus the induction of anaesthesia with a highly soluble vapour is slow and, if the vapour is irritant or otherwise unpleasant, can be very harassing for patients who have not been given a basal anaesthetic (p. 504). Recovery of consciousness after the anaesthetic has been withdrawn is also slow. At the same time, anaesthetics of this type can be more safely given, in emergencies, by the novice.

So far as they refer to the consequences of solubility in plasma, the foregoing considerations apply equally, of course, to volatile anaesthetics and to those that exist as gases at ordinary temperatures.

The speed with which it induces unconsciousness is no indication of an anaesthetic's potency. The most potent anaesthetics are those which, by virtue of high lipid solubility, are most avidly taken up by the brain.

ETHER

Diethyl ether (boiling point 35°) is a colourless, volatile liquid which yields a pungent irritant vapour which some people seem to find peculiarly attractive. Ether vapour forms an explosive mixture with air or oxygen and care must be taken to avoid fire or explosion when it is employed as an anaesthetic. Electrocautery, for instance, cannot be used and in very dry climates explosions have occurred in operating theatres as a result of a spark discharge of static electricity from the surgeon or his assistants igniting an ether-oxygen mixture. Ether oxidizes readily on exposure to air, light or moisture to form peroxides and acetaldehyde. The peroxides are unstable and may cause a spontaneous fire or explosion. They also increase the toxicity of the ether vapour. The oxidation of ether is inhibited by copper: for this reason, ether is sometimes stored in copper cans and the plunger mechanism in the ether bottle of the Boyle's apparatus is made of copper.

Induction of anaesthesia with ether alone is unpleasant and frightening and Stage II of the anaesthesia is often very prolonged. Respiration may cease in the early stages of anaesthesia proper. This is a reflex effect resulting from stimulation of nerve endings in the upper respiratory passages. The irritant nature of the ether vapour also causes profuse bronchial secretion. This can cause obstruction of the air passages, preventing the easy passage of the anaesthetic vapour to the alveoli. It also predisposes the patient to postoperative pulmonary collapse. For this reason, it is essential to premedicate the patient with atropine. Ether has been known to cause convulsions in children anaesthetized to Stage III. In most of the reported cases the child has been in a toxic, dehydrated and pyretic condition and in these unfavourable circumstances other inhalation anaesthetics precipitate convulsions almost as readily as does ether.

Recovery from ether anaesthesia is slow and it is frequently followed by nausea and vomiting. Since ether causes vasodilatation, oozing of blood from the cut edges of the skin may be troublesome during and after surgery. Almost 90 per cent of any ether in the body is excreted unchanged by the lungs. The rest is degraded in the liver, the principal metabolites being ethyl alcohol and acetic acid.

Ether is usually administered in a nitrous oxide—oxygen mixture: the addition of carbon dioxide to the mixture during the early stages of induction promotes deep breathing. This causes rapid induction of anaesthesia (nitrous oxide is one of most insoluble of anaesthetics) with a welcome shortening of Stages I and II. A high concentration of ether (12-14 per cent.) is required for induction but surgical anaesthesia, once attained, can be maintained with much lower concentrations of anaesthetic. Ether is not a very potent anaesthetic.

CHLOROFORM

Chloroform (boiling point 61°) is a heavy, colourless liquid the vapour of which has a characteristic sweet and sickly odour and taste. It is not highly inflammable nor does it form an explosive mixture with air. Chloroform is chemically more stable than ether. The most dangerous potential impurity is phosgene, to which chloroform is readily oxidized on heating. To prevent the accumulation of phosgene, a small quantity (0.5 to 1.0 per cent.) of ethanol is added to anaesthetic chloroform. Induction with chloroform is rapid and not unpleasant, it is much less irritant to the respiratory passages than is ether and, since it is a much more potent anaesthetic, it need be supplied at only a low concentration to maintain anaesthesia. Chloroform produces good muscle relaxation. On all these counts, chloroform has advantages over ether and it was a popular anaesthetic for many years. Experience has made it clear, however, that chloroform is a highly toxic substance and a very dangerous anaesthetic and it is now rarely used by anaesthetists who can call upon the resources of modern drugs and equipment. On the other hand, it must be remembered that anaesthetics have sometimes to be given under adverse conditions and away from a properly equipped operating theatre. Under these circumstances, there may still be a place for chloroform. Alstead and Macarthur (1967) have pointed out that for the single handed practitioner working in a tropical station, chloroform is not without its advantages. Because of its potency, it need be carried only in small amounts, there is no danger of its exploding or igniting in the hot conditions, it can be given by open mask and it is not rapidly lost, as ether would be, by evaporation from the mask. There is a suspicion that the toxic actions of chloroform have been somewhat exaggerated but there is no cause to advocate its use except in special circumstances of the type which have been mentioned.

The parts of the body most susceptible to the toxic actions of chloroform are the cardiovascular system and the liver. Chloroform sensitizes the heart to the actions of adrenaline and to the effects of sympathetic nerve activity. This may cause dangerous disorders of cardiac rhythm and sudden fatal cardiac arrest ('chloroform syncope') has occurred during the induction of chloroform anaesthesia. Chloroform had been largely abandoned before the discovery of drugs that could have prevented these fatalities by blocking adrenaline β receptors (p. 302). In addition to its direct action on the heart, chloroform depresses the vasomotor centre and may cause serious falls of blood pressure. Depression of the vasomotor and respiratory centres proceed together so that if breathing stops in the patient under chloroform anaesthesia it is of much more serious import than is cessation of breathing due to anaesthetics which spare the vasomotor centre.

Chloroform causes depletion of liver glycogen and it inhibits bile secretion. It may also interfere with the utilization of glucose. These changes are usually of a temporary nature but chloroform anaesthesia, especially if prolonged, may cause hepatitis with fatty infiltration of the liver and a permanent impairment of liver function. This may manifest itself as delayed chloroform poisoning in which a catastrophic failure of liver function suddenly makes its appearance during the first week after recovery from the operation. Delayed chloroform posioning (which produces a clinical picture reminiscent of diabetes) is usually seen in children: its incidence is much reduced if the patient is fed well in the days immediately preceding operation.

TRICHLOROETHYLENE

Trichloroethylene (Trilene, boiling point 87°) is a colourless liquid with an odour reminiscent of chloroform. It is usually stabilized by the addition of thymol (0.01 per cent.) and it is coloured blue for identification purposes. Trichloroethylene cannot be used in a closed circuit apparatus because soda lime reacts with it to form the highly toxic phosgene and dichloroacetylene. Trichloroethylene is decomposed by light and it is therefore marketed in amber glass bottles or metal cans. In the body, some trichloroethylene is metabolized in the liver to give trichloroacetic acid and trichloroethanol. The last named substance is conjugated with glucuronic acid before it appears in the urine.

Trichloroethylene cannot be administered by the open mask method because of its relatively low volatility. It is usually given with nitrous oxide and oxygen.

The solubility of trichloroethylene vapour in plasma approaches that of ether so that it induces anaesthesia quite slowly. However, like ether, it is usually given in a nitrous oxide-air mixture and this will accelerate induction in a patient who has not received a basal anaesthetic.

Trichloroethylene is the most lipid soluble and hence the most potent of all anaesthetic agents and anaesthesia can be maintained with concentrations as low as one or two per cent in the nitrous oxide-air mixture. At lower concentrations (about 0.5 per cent in air) trichloroethylene is a useful analgesic.

Induction of anaesthesia with trichloroethylene is not unpleasant despite its slowness and post-anaesthetic nausea and vomiting is unusual. The anaesthetic does not produce good muscular relaxation and it is not suitable for prolonged operations. It is, however, of value in dental surgery, in operations on the ear, nose and throat, for the dressing of painful wounds and in obstetrics. For the latter purpose, trichloroethylene can be used in an inhalation apparatus which permits the patient to administer her own anaesthetic when the intensity of her labour pains demands relief. Trichloroethylene has also been used to provide relief from the pain of trigeminal neuralgia. It will be appreciated that in the last two instances trichloroethylene is used for its analgesic action.

The toxic effects of trichloroethylene are qualitatively similar but less intense than those of chloroform. Cardiac arrhythmias occur not infrequently during trichloroethylene anaesthesia but they are rarely serious and they respond well to propranolol (p. 302)

HALOTHANE,

Halothane (Fluothane, boiling point 43°) is the newest volatile anaesthetic. It was discovered as the result of a deliberate effort to produce a non-explosive volatile anaesthetic. Although the research was undertaken by a team, halothane itself was actually discovered by Suckling and its pharmacological properties were first described in 1956 by Raventos. Halothane has an odour not unlike that of chloroform. It is relatively stable but prolonged exposure of halothane to sunlight may lead to discolouration and for this reason it is kept in amber glass bottles with thymol.

Induction of anaesthesia with halothane is pleasant and it is not attended by irritation of the bronchial mucous membrane. Halothane is as powerful an anaesthetic as chloroform. It is usually added to a nitrous oxide-air mixture in which it need attain a concentration of no more than two per cent to maintain surgical anaesthesia. It is the least soluble of the volatile anaesthetics and so would induce anaesthesia quite rapidly if it had to be given alone.

Halothane causes muscle relaxation and in operations in which muscle relaxants are indicated, it permits the use of minimal doses of the chosen relaxant. On the other hand, halothane causes bradycardia (which is prevented by atropine) and hypotension and it therefore potentiates the action of anticholinesterases so that care has to be taken when neostigmine is used to reverse the action of a muscle relaxant in patients under halothane anaesthesia. The cardiovascular actions of halothane are the result of actions on the vasomotor centre, the autonomic ganglia and perhaps the blood vessels. Cardiac arrhythmias have been observed during halothane anaesthesia. Their incidence is increased by adrenaline and decreased by propranolol.

Halothane has enjoyed considerable popularity since it was first introduced and it is now the most widely used of all volatile anaesthetics. Because of its high activity, halothane has to be delivered from special equipment which permits a fine regulation of the dose given. For the same reason, it is an anaesthetic which can only safely be administered by the most experienced anaesthetists. Halothane is expensive and it is therefore administered by a closed circuit method.

About 85 per cent of the halothane taken into the body is excreted unchanged by the lungs. The rest is transformed in the liver and the metabolites (which include trifluoroacetic acid, bromide and fluoride) appear in the urine over a period of up to two weeks.

Halothane is given in only small amounts and in many ways it is one of the least toxic of anaesthetics. Nevertheless it has some of the toxic actions of chloroform, particularly on the liver and the question of its safety has aroused considerable interest and not a little controversy. Jaundice or other signs of liver damage are more likely to appear in those who have undergone prolonged or repeated exposures to halothane than it is in patients who have been given the anaesthetic in the course of an isolated and uncomplicated surgical operation. Liver necrosis has occurred in a few pregnant women who have received repeated doses of halothane. Pregnancy (and labour) should, therefore, be regarded as contraindications to the use of halothane even on a single occasion. Another group of patients who seem to be peculiarly vulnerable to halothane are those with cancers requiring treatment by radiation (Wright et al., 1975; Trowell, Peto and Crampton-Smith, 1973). It may be that the irradiation process provokes the production of toxic breakdown products of halothane. Particular care is needed when halothane is used in patients on insulin therapy and in those with a low volume of circulating blood. Because of its hypotensive action it should not be given in combination with barbiturates. It should hardly be necessary to add that any suspicion of an impaired liver function in a patient needing surgery constitutes grounds for avoiding halothane.

We have seen that the metabolic degradation of halothane results in the production of a number of substances, including bromides, and that these metabolites are retained in the body for days or weeks. It is not impossible that anaesthetists and others exposed to low concentrations of halothane for prolonged periods may accumulate bromides in their tissues perhaps even to the extent that it causes ill effects such as a deterioration in mental activity (Cass, 1976).

The whole question of halothane's toxicity is still, in quantitative terms, unanswered and it will remain so until more solid information has been collected. It would appear reasonable, nevertheless, to classify it as a safe anaesthetic provided that it is withheld from those in whom it is clearly contraindicated on the grounds we have already discussed. It is worth recalling that as long ago as 1966 the overall incidence of hepatitis in those who had received halothane was no more than one in 700 000 (Bunker 1966).

FLUOROXENE

Fluoroxene (Fluoromar) is inflammable and explosive and it must be delivered from a closed circuit system. It is only suitable for the production of light anaesthesia. Not surprisingly it has not attracted much attention.

METHOXYFLURANE

Methoxyflurane (Penthrane) is a non-explosive anaesthetic. It is less irritating than ether and apart from possessing a tendency to produce cardiac arrhythmias, it is relatively safe though some cases of kidney damage following its use have been reported. A curious feature of its action is that the pupils are constricted throughout all the stages of anaesthesia. Methoxyflurane has analgesic as well as anaesthetic properties and it has been employed, like trichloroethylene, to provide analgesia during labour.

VINYL ETHER.

Vinyl ether (Vinesthene, boiling point 28°) is a colourless liquid with a slight purplish fluorescence. As would be expected from its chemical structure, vinyl ether resembles diethyl ether in its odour, its properties and its actions. It is, however, very much more volatile and inflammable than diethyl ether: its volatility is such that its rapid evaporation may cause freezing of water vapour if it is given by the open drop method. It is more unstable than diethyl ether, being decomposed by air, heat or light to form peroxides and polymerization products. It is stored in amber glass bottles under nitrogen and decomposition is further prevented by the addition of ethanol (4 per cent) and a small quantity of phenyl-α-naphthylamine. The ethanol also reduces the rate of evaporation of the anaesthetic if it is given by open mask but if this method of administration is chosen it is advisable to mix vinyl ether with three times its volume of diethyl ether. The inflammability and high volatility of vinyl ether (even when mixed with ether) precludes its use in hot climates and it is always preferable to administer the anaesthetic with oxygen from an anaesthetic inhaler.

Vinyl ether is a very potent anaesthetic. Deep anaesthesia is rapidly attained with a smooth passage through Stage II and with minimal irritation of the respiratory passages. Muscle relaxation is not very satisfactory. The fact that anaesthesia is attained rapidly carries the implication that the depth of anaesthesia may quickly vary if vinyl ether is not administered with great care. This is so and patients anaesthetized with vinyl ether by any but the most expert anaesthetist may show alarming and rapid fluctuations from the brink of Stage IV to almost complete consciousness and back again as the anaesthetist strives to achieve the correct maintenance dose.

Vinyl ether should only be used for operations of short duration; it is usual to restrict its use to cases where anaesthesia will not be needed for a longer period than half an hour. If anaesthesia is prolonged beyond about that time, there is a real danger of causing irreversible liver damage. It is obvious that vinyl ether should not be given to those with impaired liver function. Apart from the possibility of producing liver damage by injudiciously protracted administration of the anaesthetic, vinyl ether is relatively non toxic. Cardiac arrhythmias attributable to the anaesthetic do not cause worry during the operation and postanaesthetic nausea and vomiting is uncommon.

Vinyl ether is also used in obstetrics and dentistry and it has sometimes been given together with nitrous oxide to induce anaesthesia in patients who are to undergo surgery under ether, but it is clearly of very limited utility.

ETHYL CHLORIDE

Ethyl chloride is unique in that it can be used either as a local or as a general anaesthetic. It is a colourless, highly volatile liquid with an ethereal odour. It is supplied in glass vessels, usually of 60 ml capacity, the narrow necks of which are closed by means of a spring-loaded cap. When the cap is released, the pressure of ethyl chloride vapour within the container is sufficient to expel a fine jet of the liquid. If the liquid is directed on to the skin, it evaporates so rapidly that freezing and local anaesthesia of the skin occurs. The local anaesthesia so produced is sufficient for such minor operations as the incision of carbuncles or the removal of splinters from beneath the finger nails. Attempts to produce local anaesthesia of longer duration by repeated applications of ethyl chloride are to be discouraged because the rapid thawing and re-freezing is likely to damage the skin and subcutaneous tissues.

When ethyl chloride is used as a general anaesthetic it can be administered either by the open drop method or by means of an inhaler. In the latter method a predetermined amount of ethyl chloride from the usual type of container is sprayed through a valvular opening in a breathing bag to which is attached an anaesthetic mask.

Ethyl chloride is only used for short operations, particularly in dentistry and for the induction of anaesthesia which is to be continued with ether. Induction is pleasant and very rapid but ethyl chloride has chloroform-like actions on the cardiovascular system and liver and the patient should therefore only be exposed to it for the minimal period of time.

Ethyl chloride is very useful for inducing anaesthesia in experimental animals. It is sprayed on to a gauze mask in a small frame held close to the animal's nose and mouth. Provided that the mask does not actually come into contact with the animal (which would find the intense cold distressing) anaesthesia is produced rapidly and smoothly.

Gases

The two commonly used gaseous anaesthetics are nitrous oxide and cyclopropane. They are supplied as compressed liquids in metal cylinders coloured (in Britain) blue and orange respectively. The liquid gasifies when the pressure is released.

NITROUS OXIDE

Nitrous oxide, one of the oldest of the anaesthetics, remains one of the safest. It is a colourless gas with a sweet smell and taste. It is not itself inflammable but it supports combusion better than does air.

Until quite recently nitrous oxide was used alone for minor dental operations. The patient breathed the pure gas until he was completely unconscious, giving the dentist about 30 seconds to perform his operation before the patient struggled back to consciousness. The person who has inhaled pure nitrous oxide to the point of unconsciousness is anoxic and cyanosed and there is no doubt that his anaesthetic state is partly attributable to oxygen lack. Because even a brief period of anoxia exposes the patient to the risk of brain damage, nitrous oxide is now never given without an admixture of oxygen, which should constitute at least 20 per cent of the mixture. At this concentration, nitrous oxide produces light anaesthesia which is certainly not attributable to oxygen lack. If it were, a mixture of an inert gas such as nitrogen with 20 per cent of oxygen (*i.e.* atmospheric air!) should have anaesthetic properties.

Thus nitrous oxide is a true anaesthetic. It is also a useful analgesic: a mixture of equal parts of nitrous oxide and oxygen, delivered by an apparatus that permits self medication is employed in obstetrics to relieve the pains of labour. The same analgesic mixture can be used to dull the pains of cardiac ischaemia and physical injuries and to make more tolerable such painful procedures as the dressing of burns.

Even though it is incapable, by itself, of providing the deep anaesthesia required in major surgery, nitrous oxide is a valuable anaesthetic agent. The analgesia and light anaesthesia it does produce can easily be converted into full surgical anaesthesia by adding another more potent anaesthetic (such as ether or halothane) to the gas-oxygen mixture. The amount of supplemental anaesthetic that will be needed under these circumstances is much smaller (and

therefore much safer) than if the drug were given in the absence of nitrous oxide. The use, in addition, of a muscle relaxant would probably reduce the anaesthetic requirement still further. A mixture of nitrous oxide, oxygen and ether (or halothane) still provides one of the most valuable means of maintaining anaesthesia during prolonged or complicated surgical procedures.

Induction of anaesthesia with nitrous oxide is both rapid and pleasant. In the early stages of induction, hallucinations, feelings of exhilaration or realistically erotic dreams may occur. However, apart from the obvious dangers if prolonged anoxia is produced, nitrous oxide is remarkably free of toxic actions

CYCLOPROPANE

Cyclopropane is a dense, colourless gas with a sweetish odour and taste which is unpleasant for some people but attractive to others. It is the most plasma-insoluble of anaesthetics and in an admixture with oxygen, it produces a rapid and smooth induction of anaesthesia. The plane of deep surgical anaesthesia can be reached within one minute of beginning cyclopropane administration. The anaesthetic is non-irritant and it does not produce excessive stimulation of the salivary or bronchial secretions but it does depress respiration. Deep anaesthesia can be maintained with a concentration of cyclopropane in oxygen of no more than 20 per cent, so that the drug is particularly valuable for anaesthetizing patients with cardiac or pulmonary disease. It is also very useful for anaesthetizing the aged. Cyclopropane does not always produce the hoped-for degree of muscle relaxation but its action may be supplemented by the administration of a suitable muscle relaxant.

If anoxia is guarded against, cyclopropane is a safe anaesthetic. It tends to cause reflex bradycardia (which can be prevented by atropine) and cardiac arrhythmias. Like those caused by chloroform and trichloroethylene, the latter effects are due to sensitization of the myocardium to sympathomimetic amines, the liberation of which is greater with cyclopropane than with most other anaesthetics by reason of the accumulation of carbon dioxide consequent on the depressed respiration. The incidence and impact of cardiac arrhythmias can be reduced by premedication or treatment with drugs that block adrenaline β receptors.

Cyclopropane is a valuable anaesthetic agent when major surgical procedures are to be undertaken. Its disadvantages include the fact that it forms an explosive mixture with air, that it causes capillary oozing (although it constricts other vessels) and that it sometimes produces a sudden postoperative shock with a precipitous fall of blood pressure. This is the so-called 'cyclopropane shock'. Cyclopropane is transferred from blood to brain in the form of an association with erythrocytes with virtually none dissolved in the plasma. It is rapidly excreted in an uncharged form by the lungs.

ETHYLENE

The actions of ethylene are very similar to those of nitrous oxide and it has been used for the same purposes. As an anaesthetic it has no particular advantage over nitrous oxide and it is highly inflammable, forming a dangerously explosive mixture with air or oxygen. It is said to have caused more deaths through explosions than it has as a result of its actual administration and in view of the large number of other anaesthetics now available there seems to be no good reason why ethylene should ever be used as an anaesthetic agent.

INTRAVENOUS ANAESTHETICS

Some anaesthetic substances can be given by the intravenous route. They induce a brief period of anaesthesia within seconds of being injected. The main purposes for which they are used are:

a. As the only anaesthetics for operations or procedures of very short duration. These include minor surgery, simple dental extractions, orthopaedic manipulations, electroconvulsive therapy and the insertion of endoscopes, bronchoscopes and other instruments.

b. To induce anaesthesia that will then be continued by an inhalation anaesthetic. The speed with which the intravenous anaesthetics produced unconsciousness was a real boon in the days when the alternative was to endure the experience of being thrust slowly and uncomfortably from full consciousness to oblivion by gas and ether or some other such mixture. The modern anaesthetist is so skilled, and has such a range of drugs and devices at his disposal that he should be able to ensure comfortable inductions even with an inhalation anaesthetic and, but for patient demand, intravenous inductions should be needed less often today than they were in the past.

c. To increase the effectiveness of a weak inhalation anaesthetic. In these circumstances the intravenous anaesthetic is given repeatedly in small doses throughout the period during which effective anaesthesia is required.

d. As a basal anaesthetic during the establishment of a nerve block in patients whose protection from pain will be secured primarily by the local anaesthetic.

e. To arrest convulsions arising from the action or withdrawal of other drugs, provided that the violence of the muscle activity does not prevent access to a vein.

f. As an adjunct to psychiatric diagnosis and treatment, intravenous barbiturates are given at dose levels just insufficient to produce unconsciousness, so that the patient can be subjected to *narcoanalysis*. In his semi-anaesthetized state he becomes much more accessible to his psychiatrist, losing his inhibitions and his grasp on the elaborate mental mechanisms he has invented to conceal even from himself his real thoughts and motives. Narcoanalysis has also been instrumental in bringing back the memory in many cases of neurotic amnesia. Unfortunately, not all the applications of narcoanalysis are equally admirable: in the hands of unscrupulous interrogators the intravenous anaesthetics can be employed as 'truth drugs'. The drugs that find favour as narcoanalytical agents are amylobarbitone and pentobarbitone but thiopentone is also used.

The advantages of intravenous anaesthetics are so obvious that it is easy to forget their attendant disadvantages. It is not always easy to know what dose of anaesthetic to use but, once given, the drug cannot be recalled. An accidental overdose may cause profound respiratory and cardiovascular collapse. By contrast, the depth of anaesthesia produced by an inhalation anaesthetic can be regulated rapidly and at will so that overdosing is avoided by simply adjusting the amount of anaesthetic in the gas mixture. Other hazards of intravenous anaesthesia are those asso-

Table 30.2 Properties of intravenous anaesthetics

Property	Thiopentone	Methohexitone	Propanidid	Althesin	Ketamine
Therapeutic index (rats)	6.9	7.4	8.1	30.6	8.5
Typical adult dose (mg/kg)	4-8	1-2	5-10	40-80 μl	1-2
Approx. duration of anaesthesia after single dose (min)	20	10	5	15	15
Approx. duration of clouded consciousness after recovery (min)	60	20	20	35	15-60
Effect on cardiovascular system	Slight D	Slight S	D	Slight D	S
Effect on respiratory system	D	D	S	None	D
Effect on succinylcholine paralysis	None	None	Potentiated	None	Potentiated
Tendency to cause involuntary movements	V.low	High	Moderate	Low	Moderate
Approx. per cent of patients who suffer postanaesthetic vomiting	20	25	40	10	35

D = depression   S = stimulation

ciated with the intravenous technique itself. Needles can break, infection may be introduced into the blood stream, incompetence can lead to the deposition of irritant substances (such as thiopentone) into the subcutaneous tissues or into the arterial blood stream with possible dire consequences such as tissue necrosis or gangrene respectively while clumsy manipulations of the limb, made in efforts to locate a suitable vein, can cause damage to the nerves of the upper arm.

The intravenous anaesthetics proper can be grouped into the barbiturates, the eugenols and the steroids but some other agents which produce states bordering on anaesthesia will also have to be considered.

Barbiturates

These compounds feature as a group in Chapter 29 (pp. 483 to 488) where their chemical formulae and a discussion of their chemical properties will be found. Here we need to consider only the relevant properties of those that are used as intravenous anaesthetics.

HEXOBARBITONE

Hexobarbitone (Evipan) can lay claim to being the first drug properly to be used as an intravenous anaesthetic. First employed in 1932, it enjoyed tremendous popularity until thiopentone appeared on the scene in 1935. Thereafter it was used progressively less frequently and was withdrawn from the British market some ten years ago.

THIOPENTONE

Thiopentone (Intraval, Pentothal) has been in use for more than forty years but it is still deservedly popular notwithstanding the advent of new intravenous anaesthetics and the falling into disfavour of the hypnotic barbiturates.

The anaesthetic (the sodium salt is used, of course) is usually presented as a 2.5 per cent solution; more concentrated solutions are available but should be avoided. The anaesthetic dose is 250-500 mg. Given over a period of 15 seconds, it induces surgical anaesthesia within 15 to 30 seconds of the beginning of the injection. Smaller doses (no more than 300 mg or so) suffice when the only purpose of the injection is to secure unconsciousness preparatory to the administration of an inhalation anaesthetic. The anaesthetized subject wakes up again some 20 minutes after a single dose of thiopentone but his consciousness remains clouded for up to another 45 minutes or more and he should not be left unattended during at least the first hour after waking up.

When thiopentone is used, involuntary muscle movements, tremors and twitches are less likely to disturb the induction process than they are when other intravenous anaesthetics are given. Recovery from thiopentone anaesthesia is usually uneventful with nausea and vomiting occurring in no more than 20 per cent of those who have had the drug. In this respect, thiopentone is inferior only to Althesin. On the other hand, thiopentone does depress respiration, reduce cardiac output and cause peripheral vasodilatation. These potentially dangerous effects are accentuated in shocked patients, the elderly and those with cardiovascular disease. In these groups the administration of thiopentone (or indeed of any other intravenous anaesthetic) should be undertaken only with the utmost circumspection if at all. It was once remarked that, for the shocked patient, intravenous anaesthesia constitutes the ideal form of euthanasia (Halford, 1943).

As is emphasized elsewhere (p. 485), a single dose of thiopentone produces only a brief period of unconsciousness because it is rapidly redistributed from the brain to other tissues. If a second and later doses of the anaesthetic are given each time an anaesthetized subject begins to recover consciousness, the period of anaesthesia can be extended but after a time the peripheral tissues will become saturated with thiopentone and the rapid redistribution from brain to tissues will no longer be possible. In these circumstances, clearance of the anaesthetic from the brain will depend on metabolic processes. These are not very brisk and recovery of consciousness after the last of a succession of thiopentone injections will be delayed by up to one hour. This effect is partly offset by the rapid development of tolerance towards thiopentone. After a few successive doses have been given, the patient wakes up when the amount of anaesthetic remaining in the brain is quite incompatible with consciousness during recovery from a single dose of the barbiturate.

Unlike some anaesthetics, thiopentone is not an analgesic. In subanaesthetic doses, indeed, it actually increases sensitivity to deep pain (*hyperalgesia* or *antanalgesia*) and this increased awareness of painful stimuli is sometimes seen immediately after an anaesthetized patient recovers consciousness.

A very few cases of hypersensitivity to thiopentone have been recorded and occasional reports of a delayed reaction appear. This delayed reaction includes general malaise, joint pains and fever. It may make its appearance as late as 24 hours after the anaesthetic has been given. Large doses of thiopentone cause histamine release.

Thiopentone is absolutely contraindicated in cases of porphyria.

METHOHEXITONE

The actions of methohexitone (Brietal, Brevital) are very similar to those of thiopentone except that single doses produce an even shorter period of anaesthesia. Involuntary muscle movements occur more often with methohexitone than with thiopentone and postanaesthetic pain is sometimes experienced along the course of the injected vein by those who have received methohexitone.

For several years methohexitone has been popular in some quarters as a dental anaesthetic. For this purpose it is given in repeated doses, sufficient to maintain very light ('ultralight') anaesthesia.

OTHER BARBITURATES

Some other sulphur-containing barbiturates—thiamylal, thialbarbitone and thiobutobarbitone—are similar to thiopentone in their properties but, for no very good or obvious reason, they have never enjoyed the popularity that has been the lot of thiopentone and methohexitone. Two other thiobarbiturates, buthaliton and methitural, were always recognized as being less useful than thiopentone and they are no longer available.

We have already noted that amylobarbitone and pentobarbitone (Nembutal) are employed in narcoanalysis. Pentobarbitone is also a useful intravenous anaesthetic in the animal laboratory.

Eugenols

Eugenol is a principal constituent of oil of cloves. Some twenty years ago, a number of derivatives of eugenol were prepared and some of them were found to possess anaesthetic activity. One or two of them survived toxicity and other tests and worked their way through into the clinic but only one of them (propanidid) has stood the test of time.

PROPANIDID

Propanidid (Epontol, Fabontal) enjoys some popularity as an intravenous anaesthetic. Unusually among anaesthetics it stimulates respiration, perhaps as a reflex response to stimulation of peripheral chemoceptors.

The duration of the anaesthesia induced by single doses of propanidid does not exceed six minutes and the patient regains his preoperative state of mental alertness within half an hour. The evanescent nature of propanidid's anaesthetic action (which is attributable to its hydrolysis by serum cholinesterase) may constitute something of a disadvantage since it sometimes predisposes to undue haste on the part of the surgeon. On the other hand, the rapid clearing of consciousness following propanidid renders it an ideal anaesthetic for patients who need or wish to return home, perhaps at the wheel of a car, immediately after undergoing a minor surgical procedure under outpatient conditions. It is unfortunate that postoperative vomiting occurs more frequently with propanidid than with any other intravenous anaesthetic: an unclouded consciousness is no boon to a nauseated patient. One survey revealed that nausea and vomiting occurred in more than 40 per cent of those who had received propanidid.

Involuntary muscle movements, hiccoughs and tremor during the induction of anaesthesia are seen more frequently with propanidid than with thiopentone but less so than with methohexitone. Propanidid has a depressant action on the myocardium and the resulting hypotension is sometimes added to by histamine release. In some individuals, who have an inborn or acquired hypersensitivity to propanidid, injection of the anaesthetic provokes a cardiovascular collapse that demands emergency treatment.

Anaesthetists and others who handle propanidid frequently, sometimes develop oedema of the face, itching rashes and other stigmata of hypersensitivity.

The insertion of bronchoscopes, endoscopes and similar instruments is made easier for the examiner and less harassing for the examinee if recourse is made to an intravenous anaesthetic and a short acting neuromuscular blocking agent. Succinylcholine (p. 243) is ideal for producing muscle relaxation in these circumstances but its action is likely to be unexpectedly prolonged if it is used in combination with propanidid. This is because propanidid (which as we have already noted, is also a substrate for the enzyme) can temporarily inhibit cholinesterase activity and so interfere with the mechanism on which depends the brevity of the paralysis produced by succinylcholine. The action of propanidid itself may be prolonged in individuals with abnormal cholinesterases (p. 74). Against these disadvantages must be set the fact that propanidid reduces the incidence of the postoperative muscle pains that are otherwise likely to occur as a sequel to succinylcholine use.

Under the influence of serum cholinesterase in plasma and liver the ester linkage in propanidid is ruptured. A very small proportion of the resulting acid is further degraded by loss of the diethylamino group.

Unlike thiopentone and the other barbiturates, propanidid can be given to patients with porphyria.

Steroids

As long ago as 1942, Hans Selye, the best known, not to say the most controversial, contemporary advocate of steroid therapy, found that a number of steroid hormones and their congeners had anaesthetic actions in experimental animals. Following this observation attempts were made to find steroids that could be used as anaesthetics in man. A few compounds that seemed to combine anaesthetic potency with low toxicity in animals were investigated in detail but the claims of all the early contenders for a place in the anaesthetist's armoury crumbled in the face of rigorous trials and it was not until 1971 that an acceptable steroid anaesthetic emerged from the laboratories.

ALTHESIN

Althesin is a mixture of alphaxalone and alphadolone acetate (Fig. 30.2) dissolved in a polyoxyethylated castor oil (Cremophor EL). The alphadolone acetate increases the solubility of alphaxalone. Each 100 ml of Althesin contains 900 mg of alphaxalone and 300 mg of alphadolone acetate. The anaesthetic dose is 40–80 μl per kilogram of body mass given by an intravenous injection occupying 15 to 30 seconds. Under these conditions, unconsciousness supervenes within 40 seconds of the beginning of the anaesthetic and lasts for a rather shorter time than does that induced by thiopentone.

Like propanidid, Althesin is rapidly metabolized although a measure of redistribution may be partly respon-

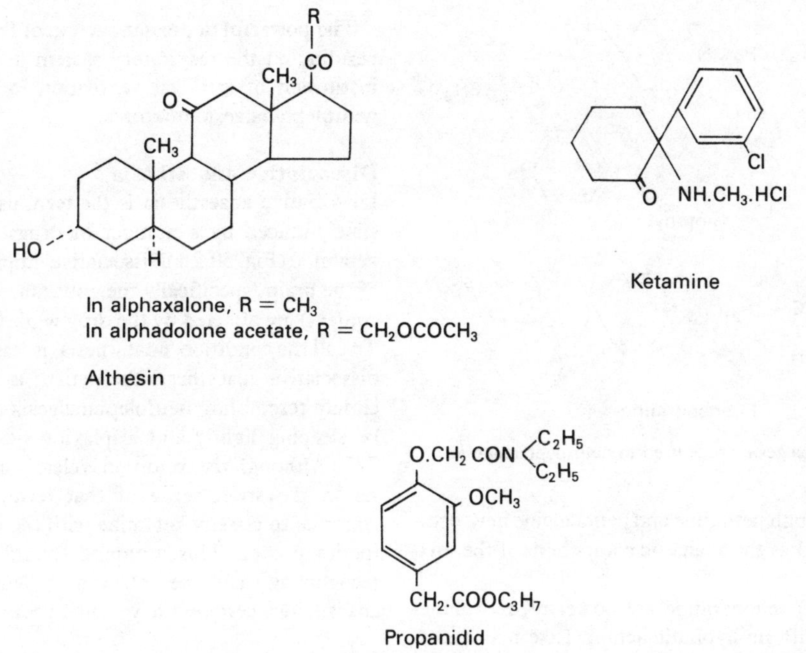

In alphaxalone, R = CH₃
In alphadolone acetate, R = CH₂OCOCH₃

Althesin

Ketamine

Propanidid

Fig. 30.2 Some intravenous anaesthetics

sible for the brevity of its anaesthetic action. It is metabolized in the liver, both steroid components of the Althesin mixture undergoing hydroxylation in a number of positions. For the most part, the metabolites are rapidly excreted, to a large extent in the bile. A proportion of the metabolites are probably retained for a time in the enterohepatic circulation. About 20 per cent of the metabolites appear in the urine as conjugates.

Althesin seems to be a very safe anaesthetic. In animals its therapeutic index, according to Child *et al.* (1971) is 30.6 which compares very favourably with those of thiopentone (6.9) and propanidid (8.1). There is no reason to believe that it is any less safe in human beings. The work of Clarke *et al.* (1971), to which oblique reference has already been made in other contexts, indicates that postoperative nausea and vomiting occur in no more than about 12 per cent of those who have been anaesthetized with Althesin. This is a lower incidence than that recorded for any other intravenous anaesthetic.

Althesin has some tendency to cause tremor or muscle twitches, especially at the higher dose levels but the frequency with which this occurs is lower than it is with all other intravenous anaesthetics save thiopentone. Some cases of hypersensitivity towards Althesin have been reported.

Althesin can be given by continuous infusion to supplement other anaesthetics during surgery. Its depressant action on cerebral metabolism, brain blood flow and cerebrospinal fluid pressure may make it particularly suitable for use during neurosurgery.

The anaesthetic is contraindicated in those with liver disease.

The reader should remember that Althesin is still a relatively untried drug and that many of the statements concerning its actions and potentialities are still necessarily tentative and might need revision in the light of continuing experience.

Table 30.2 brings together some of the more important features of the major intravenous anaesthetics. Like the paragraphs on which it is based, it owes much to Dundee and Wyant (1974), a monograph that should be consulted by those who wish to obtain more information on this topic.

STATES RELATED TO ANAESTHESIA

The last few years have witnessed the exploitation of some systemic drugs and drug combinations so as to provide alternatives or adjuncts to general anaesthesia. In essence, these newer procedures secure analgesia linked with complete tranquillity and, sometimes, an element of amnesia. Two separate, but closely related states are described. They are *neuroleptanalgesia* and *dissociative anaesthesia*.

Neuroleptanalgesia
In neuroleptanalgesia, a neuroleptic drug (p. 547) and an analgesic agent are given together. A usual combination is droperidol (a butyrophenone tranquillizer, p. 561) and either fentanyl (Sublimaze) or phenoperidine (Lealgin,

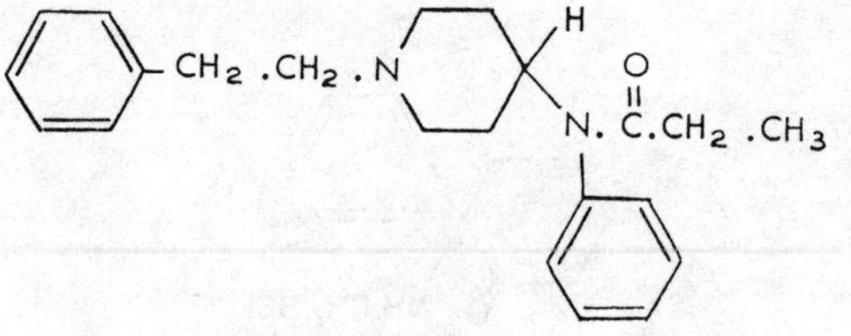

Fentanyl

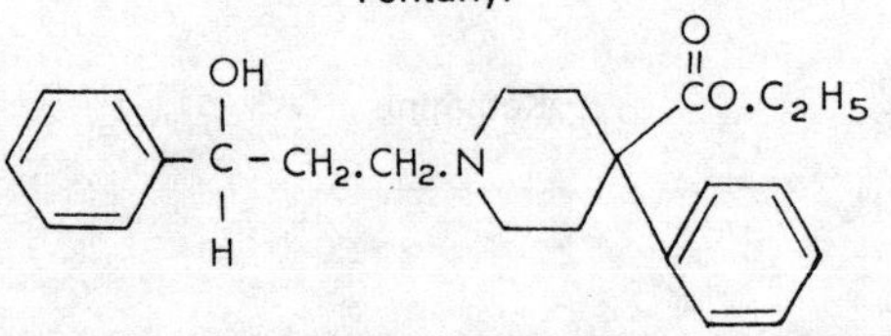

Phenoperidine

Fig. 30.3 Some analgesic drugs used in neuroleptanalgesia.

Operidine) although pethidine and pentazocine have occasionally appeared as the analgesic component of the mixture.

Fentanyl and phenoperidine are powerful, morphine-like analgesics with no hypnotic action. Like many compounds of their class they are prone to cause vomiting but in neuroleptanalgesia this tendency is offset by the antiemetic action of the tranquillizing component of the medication.

Neuroleptanalgesia gives total insensitivity to pain and is so completely tranquillizing that, under its influence, the patient stays motionless and apparently quite indifferent to his surroundings and to the surgical manipulations he is experiencing. Nevertheless he retains consciousness and will respond, albeit sluggishly, to orders. In some quarters, neuroleptanalgesia is used as an alternative to a general anaesthetic even during major surgery. It is said to be particularly suitable for very old or seriously debilitated patients. More usually its application is restricted to obstetric and minor surgical procedures, particularly those that demand cooperation from the patient. The neuroleptanalgesic misture is also given in association with conventional anaesthetics as an induction agent, as part of a regime to secure 'balanced anaesthesia' (p. 509) or as a supplement to low potency anaesthetics. In these latter instances, the effect of the mixture is more properly called neuroleptanaesthesia.

Suitable intravenous doses of the 'neurolept' drugs for induction of anaesthesia are of the order of 0.3 mg of fentanyl and 15 mg of droperidol. If phenoperidone is used instead of fentanyl, the dose is 3 mg. When the effect of the drugs is to be maintained over a period of time, further doses of the analgesic will be needed, the duration of useful action of fentanyl and phenoperidine extending to 20 and 45 minutes respectively. Droperidol is longer acting. Thalamonal and Innovar are proprietary names for a commercial mixture of droperidol (2.5 mg) and fentanyl (0.05 mg).

The powerful depressant action of fentanyl and phenoperidine on the respiratory system usually demands the institution of artificial ventilation in patients receiving neuroleptanalgesic mixtures.

Dissociative anaesthesia

Dissociative anaesthesia is the term used to describe the state induced by a number of drugs, most particularly ketamine (Fig. 30.2). 'Dissociative' implies that some parts of the brain (specifically the midbrain areas in the present context) are affected by the drug while the rest are spared. To call the condition 'anaesthesia' is less easily justified: in dissociative anaesthesia the patient is in a physical state closely resembling neuroleptanalgesia except that he will be sleeping lightly and displaying signs of catalepsy (p. 275). Although the condition is clearly not one of anaesthesia in the strict sense of that term, some authorities continue to classify ketamine with the intravenous anaesthetics proper. This grouping should be avoided while recognizing that the intravenous and the dissociative anaesthetics certainly have some properties in common.

KETAMINE.

Ketamine (Ketalar, Ketaject) is structurally related to phencyclidine (p. 588) and has similar properties. Phencyclidine, indeed, was the first drug to be used as a dissociative anaesthetic but it had to be abandoned because of the frequency with which hallucinations and maniacal outbursts occurred during the anaesthetized patient's return to consciousness.

Ketamine can be administered by either the intravenous or the intramuscular route. A single intravenous dose (1.5 mg per kilogram of body mass) induces sleep in about half a minute (this is a longer delay than that experienced with the intravenous anaesthetics proper) and consciousness returns after another 5 to 10 minutes. The intramuscular dose is larger (5 to 10 mg per kilogram) and consciousness is not lost for some three to six minutes after injection.

Ketamine has a stimulant action on the cardiovascular system, increasing both heart rate and blood pressure. These effects are attributable partly to a cocaine like effect (p. 269) on the sympathetic terminals and partly to a desensitization of the baroreceptors in the carotid sinus and elsewhere. By their activity, which increases if the blood pressure rises, these receptors normally exert a 'buffering' restraint on the heart rate and vascular tone. Cardiac arrhythmias do not occur.

Ketamine does not noticeably depress respiration but it sometimes causes small increases in intraocular pressure. Involuntary muscle movements occur more frequently during the administration of ketamine than they do when anaesthesia is induced with intravenous barbiturates.

Although they do not constitute as serious a problem as did those that led to the abandoning of phencyclidine, psychic disturbances not infrequently occur during recovery from the effects of ketamine. The overall incidence of these so-called 'emergence reactions' has not been accurately assessed but they probably affect, to some degree, about one third of those who receive ketamine without special pre- or postanaesthetic medication while up to 10 per cent suffer so badly that they need special postoperative treatment. The possibility that sequelae of this kind will appear after ketamine must inevitably raise doubts concerning the advisability of encouraging a more widespread use of what is still essentially an untried drug.

Emergence reactions include affective changes, confusion, disorientation, delirium, hallucinations, vivid dreams (unpleasant dreams outnumber pleasant ones by two to one) and disturbances of perception. Premedication with morphine, pethidine, chlorpromazine or diazepam reduces the incidence of emergence reactions which can also often be prevented or attenuated by intravenous injections of diazepam or droperidol as consciousness returns or signs of untoward reactions develop. It is, unfortunately, not always possible to prevent or to blunt emergence reactions—particularly the terrifying dreams—however elaborate the pre- and postanaesthetic medication.

Postanaesthetic disturbances of all kinds seem to be quite uncommon in women who are given ketamine during labour. Perhaps her newborn baby provides the mother with a powerful contact with reality. Very young children constitute another group who only rarely suffer untoward psychic changes after ketamine. We might speculate that this is the result of their subconscious minds being less crowded with suppressed memories of their past behaviour than is that of their wicked elders.

Theoretically at least, ketamine can be given in any of the situations that call for or permit the use of an intravenous anaesthetic (p. 504) but at this early stage in the drug's history, prudence suggests that it should only be used when it can offer distinct advantages over other available anaesthetics. Procedures that may benefit from dissociative anaesthesia include minor surgery and diagnostic investigations in very young children, particularly those with inaccessible veins (ketamine can be given intramuscularly), for painful treatments, such as the application and removal of surgical dressings from burned or extensively damaged tissue, that need to be repeated frequently (repeated doses of ketamine have no deleterious effect on the liver or kidney), in obstetrics (ketamine does not exert adverse effects on the foetus) and in old people.

Ketamine is contraindicated in patients with hypertension, increased intraocular pressure or a history of mental illness.

DIAZEPAM

Diazepam is a benzodiazepine and, as such, it is described in detail alongside other members of this group of drugs in Chapter 32 (p. 536). We are concerned here only with its

place on the anaesthetics scene and it is not inappropriate to discuss it at this point although it is not a dissociative anaesthetic.

Like all the benzodiazepines, diazepam is a tranquillizer but it also has antiepileptic, hypnotic and muscle relaxant properties, all of which are put to good use in the drug's several therapeutic roles (p. 573). We have already seen that it can be used, as a pre- or postoperative medicament, to prevent or relieve some of the more unpleasant aftermaths of ketamine administration and it sometimes finds a place as a preanaesthetic sedative when more conventional anaesthetics are to be given. In intravenous doses of about 10 to 20 mg it forms a satisfactory substitute for thiopentone in patients in whom this drug is contraindicated by reason of its cardiovascular actions. Diazepam also finds employment as a sedative in patients who have to submit to minor surgical procedures under local anaesthesia. In this connection, it has been particularly welcomed by dentists and their more apprehensive patients, many of whom remain nervous and uncooperative even when an effective local anaesthetic has been given. In dentistry, diazepam is given by slow intravenous injection until the patient seems to be drowsy. About 15 mg of the drug will be needed and more can be given during the operation if necessary. Diazepam causes amnesia as well as sedation so that, having no recollection of the local anaesthetic's being given, the patient willingly returns for further treatment.

Although recovery from diazepam is usually uneventful, those who have received the drug intravenously may remain sedated or confused for some time. They must not be left on their own until they are safely home and they should not drive, operate dangerous machinery or consume alcohol during the rest of the day.

BALANCED ANAESTHESIA

In the early days of the specialty, anaesthesia involved the inhalation of a single vapour from an open mask. As more sophisticated means of delivering anaesthetics were developed, the surgical patient could be given mixtures of inhalation anaesthetics with added oxygen. The value of premedication as a means of making anaesthesia more comfortable and of preventing postoperative complications was also recognized, atropine and morphine being almost universally employed for this purpose for many years. Then the intravenous anaesthetics arrived to provide the patient with an even more comfortable induction and to initiate the modern age of anaesthesia in which the individual receives a variety of drugs, selected from an impressively long menu, in accordance with his particular needs as revealed by careful studies of his physical state and the nature of the surgical intervention that is contemplated. The modern anaesthetist, unlike his more humble predecessors, has to be a pharmacologist of no mean order.

One wit has remarked that, whereas in the past the surgeon dictated the anaesthetic to be used, the anaesthetist now tells the surgeon which operation is best suited to the anaesthetic medication he has chosen!

The several agents used in the individual patient should be selected so as to give 'balanced anaesthesia', each drug being selected for one specific purpose and the whole combination providing the most effective and comfortable but the least hazardous anaesthetic experience for the patient and the best operating conditions for the surgeon. As an example of a combination of drugs chosen to achieve balanced anaesthesia we may quote that given by Cutting (1972), as follows:

'Premedication with a basal anaesthetic (barbiturate), a narcotic analgesic (meperidine), and a vagal inhibitor (atropine); induction by a short-acting barbiturate (thiopental); maintenance of unconsciousness, analgesia and reflex inhibition by an anaesthetic gas (75 to 80 per cent nitrous oxide) and an intravenous narcotic analgesic (meperidine); maintenance of muscle relaxation by a curare-type agent (gallamine)'

Certainly the modern anaesthetist must be a pharmacologist if he is properly to appreciate the possible actions and interactions of the members of any group of drugs he might select, with the aim of providing balanced anaesthesia, from the large numbers available to him.

MISCELLANEOUS COMPOUNDS

The substances collected together in the following paragraphs have in common only the feature that they cannot properly be discussed elsewhere in this chapter.

FLUROTHYL
Flurothyl (hexafluorodiethyl ether, Indoklan) was synthesized in the expectation that it would have anaesthetic activity like the halogenated anaesthetics its structure recalls (Fig. 30.1, p. 493). It proved instead to be a powerful convulsant agent and it has been employed as an alternative to electroshock to induce therapeutic convulsions. For this purpose it is given by intravenous injection

$$NH_2$$
$$|$$
$$C = O$$
$$|$$
$$O - C_2H_5 \qquad\qquad F_3C.CH_2OCH_2.CF_3$$

Urethane (ethyl ester of   Flurothyl
   carbamic acid)

or, better, by inhalation. A recommended regime for convulsive therapy suggests that 0.5 to 0.75 ml of flurothyl, vaporized in oxygen, should be given to patients anaesthetized with sodium methohexitone and paralyzed with succinylcholine (Small and Small, 1972).

CHLORALOSE
Chloralose is prepared by heating together anhydrous chloral (p. 488) and anhydrous glucose. It is never used in man but it is a traditional anaesthetic for experimental animals (particularly the cat) and it still has a place in the laboratory. It is sometimes administered by intraperitoneal injection in a warm and very dilute solution (the solubility of chloralose in water is low) but it is better to dissolve it in a hot 10 per cent solution of polyethylene glycol in water. It remains in solution on cooling and the anaesthetic is then given by intravenous injection to animals that have already been anaesthetized with ether. The ether is withdrawn as soon as the chloralose has been given. The inconvenience of this method of anaesthesia does not detract from the value of chloralose as an anaesthetic, for the animal's blood pressure and reflex activity are well maintained. Chloralose has some of the attributes of a convulsant drug. Animals under chloralose anaesthesia sometimes exhibit muscular twitchings and spike activity diagnostic of central nervous stimulation appears on the electroencephalographic record, even though the animal remains anaesthetized. The dose of chloralose is 60 to 80 mg per kilogram of body weight.

URETHANE
Urethane is another substance whose hypnotic actions are made use of only in the laboratory. It is a useful anaesthetic for rabbits to which it is administered in intravenous doses of 0.5 to 1 gram per kg.

Although urethane is not used in man as a hypnotic, it is employed in the treatment of some forms of leukaemia because it depresses the activity of the bone marrow and lymphoid tissue.

BIBLIOGRAPHY

Books, monographs and reviews

Alstead, S. and Macarthur, J. G. (1967). *Clinical Pharmacology* (Dilling), 21st edn., pp. 251-253. London: Bailliere Tindall and Cassell.

Artusio, J. F., Jr. (1963). *Halogenated Anaesthetics*. Oxford: Blackwell Scientific Publications.

Cutting, W. C. (1972). *Handbook of Pharmacology*, 5th edn. p. 492. New York: Appleton-Century-Crofts.

Dundee, J. W. and Wyant, G. M. (1974). *Intravenous Anaesthesia*. Edinburgh & London: Churchill Livingstone.

Faulconer, A., Jr. and Bickford, R G. (1960). *Electroencephalography in Anesthesiology*, Springfield: Thomas.

Greene, N. M. (ed) (1968). *Halothane*. Philadelphia: F. A. Davis.

Guedel, A. E. (1937). *Inhalation Anaesthesia*. New York: Macmillan.

Halsey, M. J., Millar, R. A. and Sutton, J. A. (eds) (1974). *Molecular Mechanisms in General Anaesthesia*. Edinburgh, London and New York: Churchill Livingstone.

Hewer, C. L. (ed.) (1972). *Recent Advances in Anaesthesia and Analgesia*, 11th edn. Edinburgh and London: Churchill Livingstone.

Johnstone, M. (1961). Halothane: the first five years. *Anesthesiology*, **22**, 591-614.

Krnjević, K. (1972). Excitable membranes and anaesthetics. In: *Cellular Biology and Toxicity of Anesthetics*, Fink, B. R. (ed.) pp. 3-9. Baltimore: Williams and Wilkins.

Krnjević. K. (1974). Central actions of general anaesthetics. In: Halsey, M. J., Millar, R. A. and Sutton, J. A. (eds) pp 65-90. *op. cit.*

Mullins, L. J. (1954). Some physical mechanisms in narcosis. *Chem. Rev.*, **54**, 289-323.

Prescott, F. (1964). *The Control of Pain*. London: English Universities Press.

Quastel, J. H. (1952). Biochemical aspects of narcosis. *Curr. Res. Anesth.*, **31**, 151-163.

Seeman, P. (1972). The membrane actions of anesthetics and tranquillizers. *Pharmac. Rev.*, **24**, 583-655.

Vandam, L. D. (1966). Anaesthesia. *Ann. Rev. Pharmac.*, **6**, 379-404.

Van Der Waals, J. H. and Platteeuw, J. C. (1960). Clathrate solutions. *Advanc. Chem. Phys.*, **11**, 1-57.

Wood-Smith, F. G., Vickers, M. D. and Stewart, H. C.(1973). *Drugs in Anaesthetic Practice*. 4th edn. London: Butterworth.

Wylie, W. D. and Churchill-Davidson, H. C. (eds) (1972). *A Practice of Anaesthesia*, 3rd edn., London: Lloyd-Luke (Medical Books).

Original papers

Bunker, J. P. (1966). Summary of the National Halothane Study. *J. Am med. Ass.*, **197**, 775-788.

Cass, N. (1976). Comment on paper by Tinker, Gandolfi and Van Dyke (1976) (*op. cit.*), *Drugs*, **12**, 455.

Cherkin, A. and Catchpool, J. F. (1964). Temperature dependence of anaesthesia in goldfish. *Science*, **144**, 1460-1462.

Child, K. J., Currie, J. P., Davis, B., Dodds, M. G., Pearce, D. R. and Swissell, D. J. (1971). The pharmacological properties in animals of CT 1341—a new steroid anaesthetic agent. *Br. J. Anaesth.*, **43**, 2-13.

Clarke, R. S. J., Montgomery, S. J., Dundee, J. W. and Bovill, J. G. (1971). Clinical studies of induction agents. XXXIX:CT 1341, a new steroid anaesthetic. *Br. J. Anaesth.*, **43**, 947-952.

Crossland, J. and Merrick, A. J. (1954). The effect of anaesthesia on the acetylcholine content of brain. *J. Physiol., Lond.*, **125**, 56-66.

Ferguson, J. (1939). The use of chemical potentials as indices of toxicity. *Proc. Roy. Soc. B*, **127**, 387-404.

Halford, F. J. (1943), A critique of intravenous anaesthesia in war surgery. *Anesthesiology*, **4**, 67-69.

Miller, K. W. (1969). How do anesthetics work? *Anesthesiology*, **30**, 127-128.

Miller, S. L. (1961). A theory of gaseous anaesthetics. *Proc. Nat. Acad. Sci. USA*, **47**, 1515-1524.

Pauling, L. (1961). A molecular theory of general anesthesia. *Science*, **134**, 15-21.

Small. J. G. and Small, I. F. (1972). Clinical results: Indoklon versus ECT. *Seminars in Psychiatry*, **4**, 13-26.

Tinker, J. H., Gandolfi, A. J. and van Dyke, R. A. (1976). Elevation of plasma bromide levels in patients following halothane anaesthesia. *Anesthesiology*, **44**, 194-196.

Trowell, J., Peto, R. and Crampton-Smith, A. (1975). Controlled trials of repeated halothane anaesthetics in patients with carcinoma of the uterine cervix treated with radium. *Lancet*, (i), 821-823.

Wright, R., Chisholm M., Lloyd, B., Edwards, J C., Eade, O. E., Hawksley, M., Moles, T. M. and Gardner, M. J. (1973). Controlled prospective study of the effect on liver function of multiple exposures to halothane. *Lancet*, (i), 817-820.

31. Epilepsy and the pharmacology of convulsions and of anticonvulsant drugs

A convulsion is a violent involuntary spasmodic contraction of the skeletal musculature. In their most severe forms, convulsions are the result of the most powerful degree of stimulation to which motor neurones in the central nervous system can be subjected.

The course of a complete major convulsion can best be described by reference to the sequence of events which follows electrical stimulation of the brain delivered by an electroshock machine of the type which is used to produce experimental convulsions in laboratory animals or therapeutic convulsions in psychiatric patients. A very suitable apparatus for laboratory use is that described by Woodbury and Davenport (1952). It enables currents of variable strength and duration to be applied to the heads of animals through corneal electrodes (small metallic discs moistened with saline solution and applied one to each cornea) or through simple clips attached to the ears. A current of 50 milliamps passed for one fifth of a second is sufficient to cause maximal seizures in the rat. Under these circumstances, the first observable effect is a powerful flexion of the fore limbs. This is the so-called *tonic flexor spasm* and it commences almost immediately after passage of the current. It very soon gives way to the *tonic extensor spasm*. First the forelimbs and then the hind limbs are thrust slowly backwards in a powerful, sustained contraction. There is tonic contraction of the thoracic and abdominal muscles (so that breathing ceases) and the tail is rigidly extended (Fig. 31.1). Consciousness is lost during the tonic extensor spasm. Examination of the limbs at this stage will reveal that the flexor muscles as well as the extensor muscles are rigidly contracted: the whole animal, indeed, is rigid and board-like. This tonic phase is the result of a powerful stimulation of all the motor neurones in the brain. The fact that the spasm is extensor in type is a reflection of the inherently greater power of the extensor muscles. These are the antigravity muscles whose normal activity enables the animal to maintain its posture in the face of gravitational attraction which, if unopposed, would make the animal collapse. The sloth uses its flexor muscles to enable it to counter the effects of gravity and electrical stimulation of the brain of the sloth causes a powerful and prolonged tonic flexor spasm.

The extensor tonic spasm is held for some seconds and the animal then gradually relaxes and becomes completely flaccid. Breathing returns and after a variable period of quiescence there ensues a phase of *clonic convulsions* which may persist for up to one minute. In clonic convulsions, flexor and extensor movements occur alternately and contraction of one set of muscles is accompanied by relaxation of the antagonists as it is in normal muscle activity. The clonic convulsions seen after a full tonic extensor spasm are frequently feeble and of short duration. This is because of the exhaustion produced by the violent tonic spasm and the accompanying apnoea. Towards the end of the period of clonic convulsions the animal may partially regain consciousness but it remains profoundly depressed *(post-ictal depression)* for many minutes after the convulsions proper have ceased.

If the intensity of electrical stimulation is rather less than that required to produce a maximal seizure of the type just described, the extensor spasm will be less intense and it may affect only the fore limbs. On the other hand, the clonic phase will be more intense because of the smaller degree of exhaustion occasioned by the less severe tonic spasms. Weaker stimuli produce still milder seizures with no tonic phase at all. Anticonvulsant drugs will also attenuate the effects of a shock which would cause maximal convulsions in the unmedicated animal.

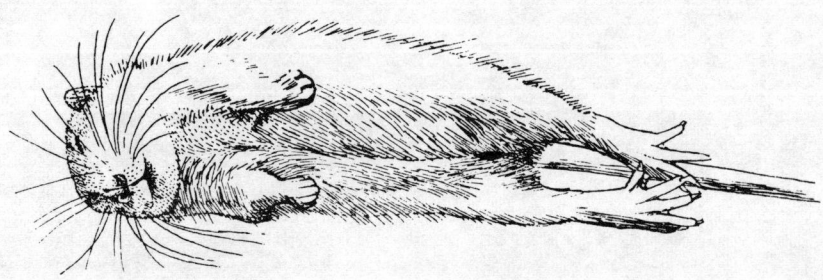

Fig. 31.1 Tonic extensor spasm in the rat.

Because of the relatively clear cut nature of the different responses to stimuli of increasing intensity, it is possible to grade the effects of electroshock on a numerical scale which is particularly useful for the assessment of anticonvulsant agents, since it enables quantitative comparisons to be made between the effects of different drugs. Individual workers like to devise their own scales in the light of the responses they see in the particular circumstances of their own laboratory and experimental techniques but the grading is usually of the following type:

0 no response
1 excited running behaviour
2 stunning, with catatonia (p. 594) and maintenance of an upright posture
3 clonic convulsions
4 front leg tonic extensor spasm followed by clonic convulsions
5 complete extensor tonic spasm followed by clonic convulsions.

The convulsions which are produced by those convulsant drugs which act on the motor cortex (p. 514) take a similar form to the seizures which follow the application of an electric shock but they are modified by reason of the fact that the stimulation of the brain increases steadily over a period of time as the drug is absorbed. As a result, the convulsions progressively increase in severity until they reach the level determined by the dose of the drug. Thus, after a maximal convulsant dose of a chemical convulsant, only tremors and hyperexcitability are seen at first. There may be catatonia. Clonic convulsions then set in and they increase in severity (though they may be interrupted by periods of quiescence) until they give way to a full tonic extensor spasm. The animal then becomes completely flaccid before clonic convulsions reappear. The convulsions that occur in this second phase of clonic activity are weaker than those which ushered in the extensor tonic phase and they are followed by a phase of post-ictal depression.

ANALEPTIC AND CONVULSANT DRUGS

The word *analeptic* (= take up), if its etymological origin is to be respected, means 'reviver' and it is used of those drugs which by stimulating the vital centres in the medulla can overcome the depression of the nervous system produced by an overdosage of drugs such as morphine or the barbiturates. Although the medullary centres are particularly sensitive, the stimulant action of the analeptics is not confined to the medulla and in appropriate doses they will stimulate all parts of the brain and give rise to frank convulsions. Thus the terms analeptic and convulsant are virtually synonymous except that convulsant substances which have never been used to revive the deeply unconscious patient are not ordinarily called analeptics. Substances such as caffeine, amphetamine and many other drugs which stimulate the central nervous system but which do not cause convulsions (or do so only when they are given in very large doses) are simply designated as central nervous stimulants and are more appropriately dealt with elsewhere in this book.

Gross interference with the metabolic state of the brain (as might be produced, for instance, by poisons, by large doses of insulin, or the antidiuretic hormone) may also lead to convulsions as may the sudden withdrawal of some depressant drugs from patients who have become habituated to them (p. 90). In grand mal epilepsy (p. 517), convulsions arise spontaneously.

The traditional analeptics no longer occupy an important place in medicine: reliance is placed on artificial respiration, oxygen administration, peritoneal dialysis and forced diuresis for the treatment of patients poisoned by depressant drugs. Nevertheless, convulsant drugs are of considerable pharmacological interest and utility.

STRYCHNINE

Strychnine is an alkaloid obtained from the seeds of the Indian plant *Strychnos nux vomica*. It has an intensely bitter taste and a traditional but quite unjustified reputation as a 'tonic', whatever that might be (p. 640). Though useless as a therapeutic agent, strychnine is used for poisoning rats, moles and other animal pests and it is a useful laboratory tool. If strychnine is applied to a localized area of the brain, it stimulates the neurones in that area and the excitation so produced is transmitted to parts of the nervous system in functional connection with the stimulated area. This technique of *strychnine neuronography* enables neuronal connections to be delineated in areas where the complexity of the nervous network prevents their detection by direct examination. The area secondarily excited from the strychnine-stimulated area can be localized by exploring electrodes.

Strychnine convulsions differ in three important respects from those induced by most other agents: they are not accompanied by loss of consciousness, they are essentially reflex in nature and they involve simultaneous contraction of agonist and antagonist muscles. All these features are a consequence of the fact that strychnine antagonizes the action of glycine. This substance is a mediator of postsynaptic inhibition in the spinal cord but not, to any appreciable extent, in the higher reaches of the

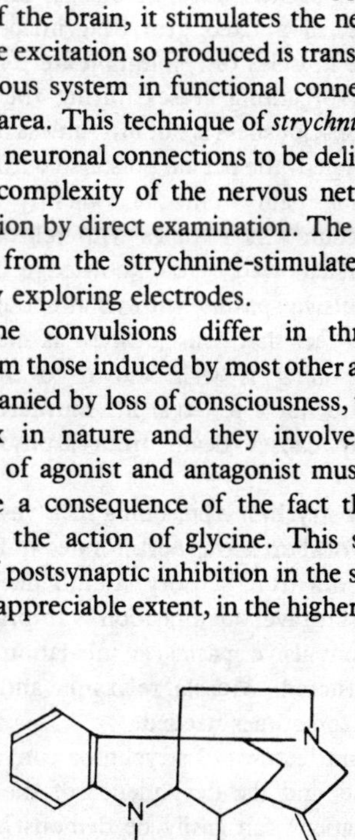

Strychnine

central nervous system (p. 192). In convulsions produced by agents that activate the motor cortex, contraction of agonist muscles is accompanied (except during the tonic extensor spasm) by inhibition of antagonistic muscles. Convulsive movements of the limbs, therefore, though violent, are co-ordinated. In strychnine poisoning, relaxation of the antagonists (which depends on inhibitory processes in the cord) is prevented and convulsive movements of the limbs take the form of powerful *extensor thrusts*—both hind limbs, for instance, are forcibly extended simultaneously and the flexor muscles (the normal antagonists) will also contract strongly though the more powerful extensor muscles determine the extended position of the limbs. With these facts established, the course of strychnine poisoning can be described. The symptoms may be sudden in onset or they may develop more gradually. In the latter case, there is stiffness of the jaw, face and neck, increased reflex activity and muscular twitching. The convulsive spasms which follow are of reflex origin but they can be induced by the slightest sensory stimulus. This is a clear consequence of the fact that strychnine acts primarily to reduce inhibition in the spinal cord. Convulsions produced by other agents proceed independently of sensory stimulation, although strong sensory stimulation will often precipitate convulsions when a slightly subthreshold dose of the convulsant has been given. During a strychnine convulsion, the body is arched rigidly backwards (*opisthotonus*) and the facial muscles are set in a fixed grin or grimace—the *risus sardonicus*. The muscles of respiration are tonically contracted so that breathing ceases during the convulsive spasm. Since consciousness is not lost (unless the period of apnoea is prolonged) the person poisoned with strychnine suffers agonizing pain from the violently contracting muscles. The calm which comes with relaxation of the muscles is overshadowed by the knowledge that another period of convulsive spasms, with its attendant agony, is inevitable. The fact that consciousness is maintained in strychnine poisoning is well known to the torturers of fiction and to not a few real life murderers. Strychnine eventually causes death from asphyxiation and exhaustion.

Treatment of strychnine poisoning involves the intravenous injection of short acting barbiturates and the protection of the victim from sensory stimuli likely to cause convulsions. If intravenous injection is impracticable by reason of the convulsive spasms, an inhalation anaesthetic can be administered. Muscle relaxants and controlled ventilation are sometimes needed.

The important features of strychnine convulsions (the extensor thrusts and the dependence of the spasms on sensory stimulation) can easily be demonstrated on the decapitate frog. A dose of 0.25 mg of strychnine injected subcutaneously is sufficient to produce convulsions in the frog.

PICROTOXIN

Picrotoxin is obtained from the seeds (Levant berries) of an East Indian shrub (*Anamirta cocculus*). The seeds are also known as fish berries, since if they are thrown into water they will poison any fish in the vicinity, a method of catching fish which has been used in the East. Picrotoxin is a molecular compound of picrotoxinin and picrotin. The convulsant properties of picrotoxin are attributable to its picrotoxinin moiety, picrotin being inert.

Picrotoxinin   Picrotin

Picrotoxin antagonizes the action of γ-aminobutyric acid, a major mediator of postsynaptic inhibition in the higher levels of the central nervous system. Although it has some action on the spinal cord (p. 179) this is not intense enough seriously to attenuate the inhibitory processes that permit antagonist muscles to relax in concert with contraction of the agonists so that picrotoxin convulsions are similar in nature to those provoked by the generality of convulsive agents that stimulate (or remove the inhibition from) the brain. The form of these convulsions has already been described (p. 513).

Small doses of picrotoxin stimulate the medullary and midbrain centres. When larger amounts are given, excitation spreads upwards into the cortex and downwards into the cord. Clonic convulsions with loss of consciousness occur and tonic spasms are seen if the convulsions are severe.

Picrotoxin is a respiratory stimulant and it was once the analeptic of choice in the treatment of severe barbiturate poisoning. It was given intravenously in a solution containing 2 mg per ml until corneal and pupillary reflexes were restored. Total doses of up to 3 g had sometimes to be given and the possibility of overdosage converting the comatose condition into a convulsive state had always to be reckoned with. Picrotoxin is now out of favour.

LEPTAZOL

Leptazol (pentamethylenetetrazole, pentylenetetrazol, Cardiazol, Metrazol) is an analeptic and a convulsant drug. It has a widespread stimulant action on central neurones but it causes convulsions by stimulating the cortex. As the name Cardiazol indicates, leptazol was once used as a cardiac stimulant but it has little action either on the heart or on the cardiovascular centres and it is no longer employed in the treatment of heart failure. Leptazol is still

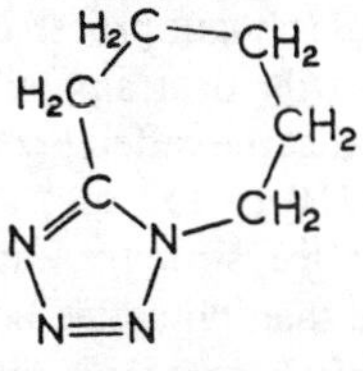

Leptazol

sometimes employed as a respiratory stimulant and as an aid to diagnostic electroencephalography (p. 520). As a generator of therapeutic convulsions it has been superseded by the electric current.

Although convulsant doses of leptazol produce violent convulsions with tonic as well as clonic phases, the convulsions can be more easily prevented by drugs which are effective against petit mal epilepsy than by those which are used in the prevention of grand mal seizures. For this reason leptazol is of considerable value in the screening of new compounds for antiepileptic activity. The convulsant dose of leptazol is of the order of 500 mg in the adult human subject.

Leptazol, it seems, does not interact with any known inhibitory transmitter substance although the convulsions it precipitates are similar in form to those released by picrotoxin. Evidently not all convulsant agents operate by inhibiting inhibitory systems.

NIKETHAMIDE

Nikethamide (Coramine), the diethylamide of nicotinic acid, is closely related to nicotinic acid and nicotinamide and it shares to some extent the nutritional activity of those B-complex vitamins. It can relieve the symptoms of pellagra (p. 791).

Nikethamide is a moderately powerful analeptic. It acts initially on the medulla and midbrain: its effects then spread to the spinal cord and cortex. The respiratory stimulant action arises from a direct action on the respiratory centre, sensitization of the centre to afferent nerve impulses and reflex stimulation from an action on sensory receptors in the carotid sinus. Large doses cause convulsions.

Nikethamide is not as powerful an analeptic as picrotoxin or leptazol but it is of some value in the treatment of moderately severe respiratory failure arising in the course of such pulmonary conditions as chronic bronchitis. It is administered intravenously and aminophylline can be given at the same time. Nikethamide is employed in a 25 per cent solution: two millilitres is usually sufficient to rouse the patient and his medullary centres to productive coughing.

ETHAMIVAN

Ethamivan (Clairvan) has a brief duration of action but otherwise its properties and uses are similar to those of nikethamide to which it bears a strong structural resemblance.

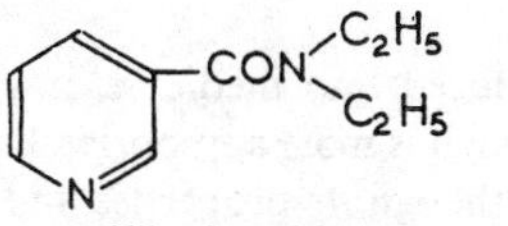

Nikethamide

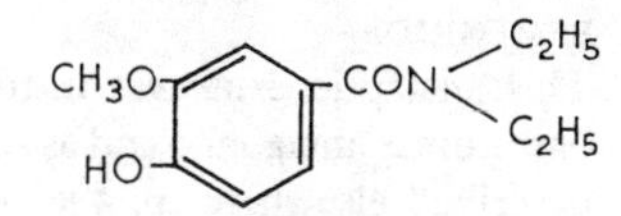

Ethamivan

Ethamivan is given in intravenous doses of 200 to 350 mg or as a continuous infusion. The analeptic effect of a single dose persists for no more than ten minutes.

DOXAPRAM

Doxapram (Dopram), the latest addition to the list of useful analeptic agents, has an even shorter duration of action than ethamivan so that it is usually given as an intravenous infusion. Its particular value is in the treatment of respiratory depression following anaesthesia, for which purpose the initial infusion rate is 5 mg per minute. This is reduced to 2 mg per minute as the respiratory centre begins to reassert itself. Hypertension, cardiac arrhythmias, vomiting and convulsions have been reported as side effects and the drug is contraindicated in patients with hyperthyroidism, hypertension or epilepsy.

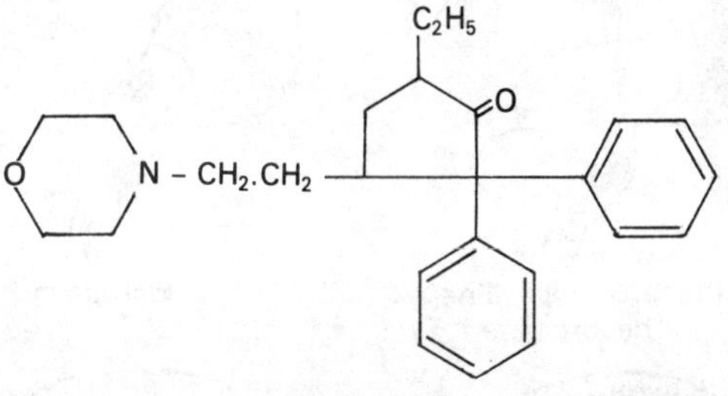

Doxapram

AMIPHENAZOLE

Amiphenazole (Daptazole) can be given by intramuscular or intravenous injection and can also be taken by mouth. The last named route is suitable in cases of mild respiratory insufficiency. The oral dose, taken three or four times daily, is 100 to 150 mg. In more urgent situations parenteral administration will be called for.

Amiphenazole can counter the respiratory depression caused by morphine and this property can be turned to advantage when severe and intractable pain demands the administration of larger than usual doses of morphine. For the purpose of utilizing this beneficial interaction, amiphenazole is given in doses of 30 mg by intramuscular injection each time morphine is needed.

Side effects of amiphenazole treatment include muscle twitchings and idiosyncratic skin rashes. Continued administration may cause depression of the bone marrow.

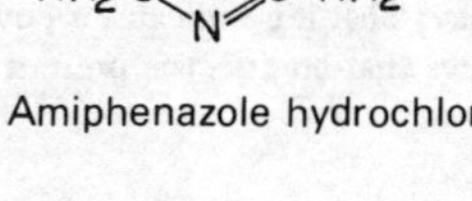

Amiphenazole hydrochloride

BEMEGRIDE

This analeptic drug was introduced into medicine as a barbiturate antagonist and as such it is more appropriately described elsewhere (p. 486) although its properties and uses are not very different from those of nikethamide.

CAFFEINE, THEOPHYLLINE AND THEOBROMINE

These related substances have a variety of actions and uses, most of which are mentioned in more detail elsewhere (p. 624, 706). Only their central stimulant actions are discussed here.

Throughout the world man has, for centuries past, made drinks from plants (tea, coffee, cocoa, coca, etc.) that contain one or more of the xanthine derivatives and a large part of the human race has developed a psychological dependence on these drugs. The dependence is of a benign form which causes neither physical nor psychological harm. Caffeine, in particular, stimulates the cerebral cortex and the reduction in mental and physical fatigue

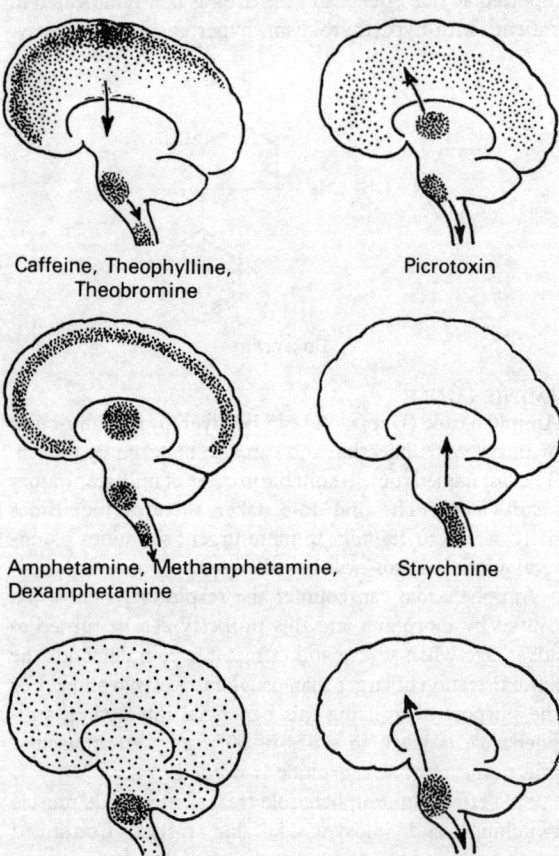

Caffeine, Theophylline, Theobromine

Picrotoxin

Amphetamine, Methamphetamine, Dexamphetamine

Strychnine

Leptazol

Nikethamide

Fig. 31.2 The sites of action of some drugs that act on the central nervous system. The arrows point in the direction of spread of effect. Heavy shading indicates a powerful effect. Lighter shading shows that an effect is present in these areas but is less marked.

and the stimulation of thought processes which this brings is the clear reason for the drug's popularity. It should be remarked in passing that the caffeine content of a cup of tea is about the same (100 to 150 mg) as that of a cup of moderately strong coffee, since tea leaves contain considerably more caffeine than do coffee beans.

The caffeine taken in beverages is sufficient to stimulate the cortex. If higher doses (200 to 250 mg) are administered by intravenous injection the respiratory and vasomotor centres of the medulla are also stimulated. Part of the action of caffeine in the respiratory system may be the result of sensitization of the medulla to carbon dioxide. Caffeine is included in some analgesic preparations and it potentiates the action of ergotamine in relieving migraine (p. 297).

Theophylline has essentially similar properties to caffeine, except that it is a less powerful diuretic and it produces a smaller degree of cortical stimulation than does caffeine in doses that affect the medullary centres. For these reasons theophylline (in the form of aminophylline, p. 706) is preferred as a respiratory stimulant. Aminophylline is also used in congestive cardiac failure, in chronic renal failure and as an antispasmodic.

The central stimulant and the diuretic actions of theobromine (the xanthine derivative found in cocoa) are weak.

EPILEPSY

Epilepsy is derived from the Greek epilambanein (to seize) and it is a fitting name for the convulsions (seizures) which occur in the *grand mal* form of the disorder. Epilepsy takes several other overtly less spectacular forms, however, and it is impossible to provide a complete definition of the condition. Among the more extreme and unhelpful (but nonetheless serious) definitions which have been put forward we have 'Epilepsy is the tendency to recurring epileptic seizures' and 'Epilepsy is the manifestation of an unconscious desire for unconsciousness'. Attempts to provide a neurologically-based definition have been scarcely more helpful and have produced nothing more precise than 'Epilepsy is a symptom complex characterized by recurrent paroxysmal aberrations of brain function, usually brief and self limited'. Epilepsy is probably best understood from a description of the principal features of its more common forms but these must first be catalogued.

The classification that follows is based on, but is by no means identical with, that proposed in 1969 by the International League against Epilepsy. The 'official' classification, though valuable to those with a predominantly clinical or neurological interest in the nature of epilepsy, is unnecessarily cumbersome for the pharmacologist since it is not yet possible to provide a specific drug for each one of the clinically recognizable subvarieties of epilepsy. The

International League's classification also involves changes in nomenclature which abolish some terms (such as petit mal, grand mal and focal epilepsies) that have become hallowed by age and are so firmly entrenched in the medical vocabulary that many non specialists still use them. Indeed many specialists frequently slip back into the old terminology in the very articles that advocate its replacement. In the following account the new and the old nomenclatures are employed interchangeably and indiscriminately.

We can distinguish between *generalized* and *focal* (or partial) epilepsy. In generalized attacks, the neuronal discharge originates in the thalamus and midbrain (hence the alternative name *centrencephalic* epilepsy) and then spreads widely by way of the reticular activating system (p. 162) into the cortex of both cerebral hemispheres. The overt manifestations of this spreading discharge assume a variety of forms that include the epilepsies designated as *grand mal (tonic-clonic seizures), petit mal (absences), infantile spasms, myoclonic seizures* and *akinetic seizures.*

In focal epilepsy, the discharge originates from a localized area of the cerebral cortex or subcortex and its spread may be limited. The brains of individuals with focal epilepsy often display, at operation or on post mortem examination, evidence of brain damage or of tumour growth in a position corresponding to the point of origin of the epileptic discharge. The abnormal tissue presumably produces the seizures by reason of its irritant action on the surrounding neurones. Cases of focal epilepsy in which the abnormal brain tissue is sharply localized may be amenable to surgical treatment, excision of the abnormal zone effecting a complete cure. Although epileptic foci can occur anywhere in the cortex they are most often located in one or both temporal lobes or, less frequently, in the motor or sensory areas that border the central cortical sulcus. The most usual manifestation of a temporal lobe seizure is psychomotor epilepsy while attacks originating in the sensorimotor cortex classically induce either sensory epilepsy or Jacksonian fits depending on whether the focus lies in the sensory or the motor cortex.

The dichotomy between focal and generalized epilepsies is not as sharp as might be assumed from the foregoing descriptions. Temporal lobe attacks sometimes occur secondarily as a result of a spread of activity from the frontal or occipital lobes of the brain and in about 50 per cent of cases generalized grand mal attacks have developed from an initially focal discharge.

We have noted that focal epilepsy is usually the consequence of recognizable pathological changes in the brain. It is sometimes possible to identify aetiological factors (tumour, trauma, gross metabolic disturbances, drug withdrawal, etc.) in other forms of epilepsy but this frequently cannot be done and the seizures have to be labelled 'idiopathic'. As in the parallel situation presented by many patients with mental illnesses, it has to be assumed that so called idiopathic disturbances are the result of subtle anomalies of biochemical or neuronal function. The nature of these abnormalities is the subject of much speculation but little firm knowledge (p. 532).

We can now describe the more important varieties of epilepsy in some detail.

GENERALIZED EPILEPSY
Grand mal (major or tonic-clonic) seizures
This is the most common and the most dramatic form. It has been known since the earliest times and the superstitious dread with which the ancients regarded this condition (which they imagined was due to the victim's being possessed with devils) has even now not been completely eradicated.

Epilepsy attacks some 0.5 per cent of the population in Western countries so that it claims no fewer than 250 000 victims in Great Britain alone. Of these, about 100 000 experience grand mal attacks: they share their disability with a considerable number of famous figures of the past including St Paul, Julius Caesar, Caligula and Dostoievsky. In several of the latter's novels there are some striking character sketches of epileptic subjects and vivid descriptions of the sensations they experience before and after fits.

Grand mal seizures begin in about 50 per cent of cases with a warning sign or *aura* which may take the form of a sensation in the epigastrium, hallucinatory voices or other sounds, a taste, a smell or a psychic sensation that may range, in different subjects, from a feeling of spiritual exaltation to one of uncontrollable aggressiveness. An aura is evidence that the generalized attack has begun focally and its nature provides a clue to the location of this focus. It never ushers in a primarily centrencephalic attack.

An aura is a short lived phenomenon but some grand mal fits follow prodromal changes of mood (or even physical changes such as the development of a rash) that may have persisted for hours or even days. Unlike the aura proper, this experience is not restricted to grand mal attacks that have developed from initially focal discharges.

During the fit a pattern of activity similar to that seen in animals subjected to electroshock can be recognized: consciousness is lost, the victim falls to the ground with the muscles in tonic spasm and, after a short period of quiescence, clonic convulsive movements of the limbs and jaws begin. Urine and faeces may be voided and the clonic movements of the jaws may cause the tongue to be bitten. In those who happen to be supported by a chair or bed when a seizure begins, the slow development of the tonic phase can often be seen.

Exhaustion and sleep frequently follow grand mal attacks but there may also be postictal behavioural changes such as *fugues* (aimless wanderings) and the outbursts of violent rage and destructiveness described as *furor.*

The frequency of attacks varies with the individual.

Even in the unmedicated subject, seizures may occur only rarely. In severe cases, on the other hand, they may occur at the rate of several daily.

Although most grand mal seizures are of the tonic-clonic type, it sometimes happens that only one kind of response is in evidence and the attacks are then designated as 'tonic' or 'clonic', whichever adjective is appropriate.

The full blown grand mal seizure is the most easily understood variety of epileptic attack. It is closely similar in form to the response provoked by mass stimulation of cortical neurones such as that induced by electroshock. Moreover if the excitability of central neurones is deliberately or unintentionally increased (by exposure, for instance, to any of the manoeuvres mentioned on p. 520) a grand mal attack may ensue in the absence of any artificially applied external stimulus and this can occur even in individuals who have not been diagnosed as epileptic. A latent tendency to epilepsy probably resides in every one of us so that, as Gibberd (1976) has recently reminded us, there is really no such thing as an epileptic patient. There are only epileptic attacks.

Although grand mal epilepsy represents the ultimate in cerebral excitation, the spread of the epileptic discharge is favoured by quiescent conditions in the brain. Some people only experience epileptic attacks when they are asleep while others, having been warned by an aura that a generalized attack is impending, are able to prevent its further spread by indulging in some form of intense mental activity. All varieties of epilepsy involve synchronized neuronal activity but the keynote of mental alertness is desynchronized cortical activity (p. 478).

Petit mal (or minor) epilepsy
This form of epilepsy is seen particularly in children and adolescents who may suffer up to a hundred fits (or absences) a day. These take the form of a momentary loss of consciousness which is usually so brief that the child does not fall to the ground: an onlooker may notice nothing more than a brief lapse of attention. Since even normal children exhibit lapses of attention, the child with petit mal epilepsy may go undiagnosed for a time. Frequently, however, the interruptions of consciousness are accompanied by some rigidity or by staring of the eyes.

Myoclonic epilepsy
This form of epilepsy takes the form of episodes of jerky muscular movements of the head, limbs or body. Each episode lasts for about one second and it recurs at about five-second intervals for a period of half a minute or so. Patients who experience attacks of myoclonus not infrequently suffer grand mal attacks too. Myoclonic epilepsy is often associated with brain damage.

Akinetic seizures
Muscle movements do not feature in these seizures as is indeed indicated by their very name. In an akinetic attack, there is a sudden but only transitory loss of tone in the postural (antigravity) muscles so that the victim collapses to the ground. Normal muscle tone returns rapidly and consciousness is not lost. Some individuals suffer both myoclonic and akinetic seizures.

Infantile spasms
This type of attack typically begins in the early months of life and takes the form of brief periods of head nodding, body flexion or the picturesquely named salaam attacks in which the child raises its arms and then bends forward from the trunk. The attacks, during which consciousness is momentarily lost, sometimes begin with a cry.

Infantile spasms are usually associated with gross abnormalities of brain structure and function, mental retardation and grand mal attacks but a few cases result from a relative deficiency of pyridoxine and can be cured if this deficiency is remedied.

FOCAL (PARTIAL) EPILEPSY

Psychomotor epilepsy
We have already noted that psychomotor attacks are usually generated by temporal lobe activity but that they are sometimes attributable to focal activity elsewhere in the brain.

The incidence of psychomotor epilepsy is second only to that of the grand mal condition. A person suffering a psychomotor attack exhibits compulsive and sometimes bizarre behaviour (automatism) associated with marked emotional changes such as fear, hate or pleasure. There may also be hallucinations, changes in sensory perception and clouding of consciousness. In an individual patient the type of behaviour tends to be stereotyped. When psychomotor epilepsy has its origin in the temporal lobe of the brain the compulsive activity may take the form of an unprovoked violence towards other people or other forms of antisocial behaviour. Occasionally, clouding of consciousness and behavioural disturbances persist for days or weeks after a psychomotor attack.

Motor (Jacksonian) epilepsy
In a Jacksonian attack involuntary movements start unilaterally in the thumb, the angle of the mouth or the big toe and progress systematically to neighbouring muscles, until the whole of the one side of the body is caught up in the epileptic activity. There may be an aura but consciousness is usually not lost. It sometimes happens that the neuronal discharge remains sharply localized to the small area of cortex in which it arises but when this happens the circumscribed discharge and the corresponding motor activity (the movement of a thumb, for instance) may persist for many days. This state is clumsily if accurately described as *epilepsia partialis continuans*. At the other extreme of activity the focal attack may develop into a

grand mal seizure. After the grand mal seizure a paralysis (*Todd's paralysis*) sometimes affects the side of the body that was involved in the focal attack. Like the petit mal variant, Jacksonian epilepsy is essentially a disorder of childhood.

Sensory epilepsy

In this condition, focal activity arises in the sensory cortex and develops in a fashion entirely analogous to that seen in motor epilepsy. The overt manifestations of the epileptic discharge are *paraesthesiae* ('pins and needles') or a sensation of burning or pressure. The sensory changes may remain localized or may spread unilaterally to involve the whole of one side of the body. In the latter event, the attack often blossoms into a grand mal seizure with residual

paraesthesiae that constitute the sensory equivalent of Todd's paralysis.

The reader will not be surprised to learn that mixed motor and sensory attacks are sometimes experienced.

Other forms of focal epilepsy

Epileptic activity in the temporal lobe does not necessarily produce a psychomotor attack. Depending on the location and extent of the cortex that is activated, temporal lobe epilepsy may cause no more than a feeling of constriction or heaviness in the epigastrium, a smell or a sound, a sensation of *déjà vu*, autonomic effects (sweating, a feeling of coldness, gastrointestinal movements, etc.) or stereotyped motor activity such as smacking the lips. Changes such as these are likely to occur, of course, in psychomotor

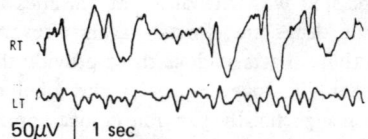

(iii) Slow wave activity in records from right and left temporal region of a child with temporal lobe epilepsy. The record was obtained after 1 minute's overbreathing.

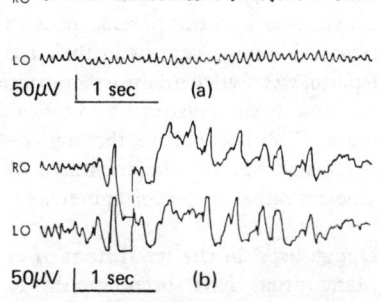

(i) Records from right and left occipital regions of a patient with grand mal epilepsy. (a) essentially normal interseizure record. (b) record after chemical activation. During the 'spiking' generalized twitchings were seen.

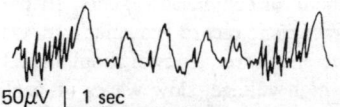

(iv) Mixture of 'spiking' and slow wave activity recorded between seizures from the temporal region of a patient with grand mal epilepsy. Similar tracings were obtained from other electrodes in the temporal and parietal regions. Shakings of the head were seen during the 'spiking'.

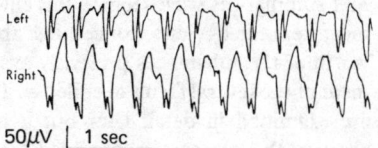

(ii) Spike and waves (3 per sec.) recorded from parieto-temporal region of patient with petit mal epilepsy. The record was obtained after 3 minutes' overbreathing.

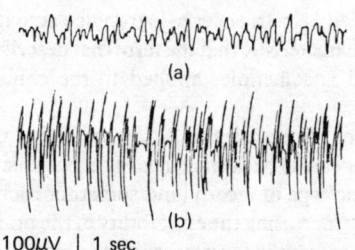

(v) EEG record from an anaesthetized rabbit before (a) and after (b) the administration of a convulsive dose of leptazol.

Fig. 31.3 Some typical electroencephalographic records. The tracings from the human subject are abstracted from multichannel recordings supplied through the kindness of Dr. W. Fabisch. The rabbit record is from an experiment by Dr. G. G. Shaw.

epilepsy but one or more of them occurring in isolation may provide the only evidence of a temporal lobe discharge that does not escape from its area of origin. They will, however, constitute the aura of a grand mal attack if, as is usually the case, the initial focus of activity secondarily detonates a generalized discharge.

Focal activity in the occipital lobes can produce transient blindness or sensations of brightly coloured flashes of light. Like the effects produced by temporal lobe activity, these visual hallucinations can occur in isolation but they usually provide the aura of a grand mal attack that supervenes when the underlying focal activity generates a spreading discharge.

It is not unusual for more than one kind of epilepsy to coexist in the same individual. Moreover, there are similarities (as well as differences) in the electroencephalographic changes associated with the different varieties of epilepsies and some drugs are effective against several types of seizure activity. Facts such as these provide the justification for grouping together under the label of epilepsy a number of superficially disparate clinical conditions.

ELECTROENCEPHALOGRAPHIC CHANGES IN EPILEPSY
Epileptic attacks are accompanied by characteristic changes in the electroencephalogram (Fig. 31.3). In grand mal attacks, high frequency spikes are seen; a similar electroencephalographic record accompanies major convulsions caused by chemical convulsant agents. In petit mal seizures, the characteristic record is a spike and wave ('spike and dome') pattern at a frequency of about 3 Hz. In psychomotor attacks high voltage, slow waves (4–6 Hz) dominate the record. They may be located over the temporal lobe. In the epileptic subject between attacks the electroencephalographic record may be normal, though there is often evidence (whatever the form of epilepsy) of slow wave or spike and wave activity in the record. Patients who are prone to attacks of myoclonic and akinetic epilepsy may display spike and wave activity at a lower frequency (about 2 Hz) than that seen in those who have petit mal seizures. Infants who suffer from infantile spasms have a grossly disorganized electroencephalographic activity. This change is so characteristic that the term that describes it (hypsarrhythmia) is sometimes applied to the clinical condition itself.

In cases where the clinical diagnosis is in doubt and the electrical record appears to be normal, it is often possible to uncover an epileptic type of record (and sometimes actually to cause fits) by increasing the excitability of the brain. To this end the patient is asked to overbreathe or he may be given antidiuretic hormone (p. 637) or a subconvulsive dose of leptazol (p. 515). Alternatively, a record may be made during sleep induced by a barbiturate. Another routine manoeuvre is to flash a light into his eyes through his closed lids. If a stroboscope is used for this purpose its flash frequency can be continuously varied until a rate is found which affects the electroencephalographic record. The ability of a flickering light to precipitate epileptic attacks is high. Patients sometimes suffer attacks at the cinema or when watching television and there are well-authenticated instances of drivers losing consciousness when driving at a steady speed along a straight tree-lined road. Under such circumstances the alternation of sunlight and shadow can have, if the frequency of change is appropriate, the same effect as a stroboscope. Some cases of self induced grand mal attacks have been reported among children who reproduce the stroboscope effect by looking into the sun and moving their spread fingers rapidly to and fro before their eyes. They presumably do this because of the attention and sympathy that the ensuing fit brings them.

THERAPEUTIC CONVULSIONS
In 1934 a Hungarian psychiatrist (von Meduna) pointed out that epileptics were rarely schizophrenic. On the basis of this observation (which, most authorities believe, was almost certainly a mistaken one) he induced epileptiform convulsions in schizophrenic patients and he claimed a remarkable improvement in their recovery rate. At first leptazol was used to produce therapeutic convulsions but it has now been replaced by electrical stimulation of the brain. Electroconvulsive therapy is still widely used in psychiatry but for the treatment of severe depressive illnesses rather than schizophrenia.

Drugs used in the treatment of epilepsy
Many drugs have been applied to the treatment of epilepsy. Although some of them are of undoubted efficacy there are differences of opinion concerning the others, in some instances because the drugs have not yet been fully evaluated and in the rest because many prescribers are not yet aware that long standing reputations, based on the subjective impressions of patients and their physicians, have crumbled in the cold light of controlled clinical trials. Table 31.1 summarizes what seem to this author at least to be the most reputable views concerning the use and relative worth of the substances presently available for the treatment of the several forms of epilepsy. The individual drugs are examined in detail later but it is first necessary to sharpen the perspective provided by the information in Table 31.1 by drawing attention to a number of general points concerning antiepileptic therapy.

a. It is clear that, from the point of view of treatment, two forms of epilepsy—petit mal and hypsarrhythmia—stand apart in that they respond best to drugs that have little place in the treatment of other types of seizure. It is also clear that several of the other drugs have quite a wide spectrum of antiepileptic activity and may be equally effective against several different kinds of attack.

b. Antiepileptic drugs can prevent, or reduce the fre-

Table 31.1 Drugs that control epilepsy

Type of epilepsy	Drugs of choice	Less useful, obsolete or obsolescent drugs
Generalized epilepsy		
Grand mal	Phenobarbitone	Bromides
	Phenytoin	Primidone
	Carbamazepine	Methoin
		Sulthiame
		Aminoglutethimide[1]
Petit mal absences	Ethosuximide	Trimethadione
	Phensuximide	Acetazolamide
	Nitrazepam	
	Clonazepam	
	Sodium valproate[2]	
Myoclonic and akinetic seizures	Phenobarbitone	Primidone
	Nitrazepam	
	Clonazepam	
	Sodium valproate[2]	
Infantile spasms (hypsarrhythmia)	ACTH	
	Nitrazepam	
	Clonazepam	
	Pyridoxine[3]	
Partial epilepsy		
Sensorimotor, temporal and other focal attacks	Phenobarbitone	Primidone
	Phenytoin	Methoin
	Carbamazepine	Sulthiame
Psychomotor[4]	Phenytoin	Methoin
	Methsuximide	Primidone
	Carbamazepine	Phenacemide
		Pheneturide

[1] This drug is not described in the text
[2] This drug is still under investigation (see text)
[3] This drug is only effective in special cases (see text)
[4] Psychomotor epilepsy is often refractory to drug treatment

quency of, seizures in those susceptible to them but in many cases they should offer more than palliation. A totally successful treatment is curative in the sense that fits no longer occur even when anticonvulsive medication has been withdrawn. Success of this order waits on early diagnosis and prompt and prolonged treatment. There are those who even urge the institution of antiepileptic therapy during any feverish illness in the young children of families with a history of febrile convulsions and to accident victims whose brain may have been injured. Many others, who would hesitate to adopt such extreme measures against what they would regard as very flimsy threats to their patients' wellbeing, would nevertheless agree with the injunction that 'as a general rule, anticonvulsant therapy should begin at the time of the first recognised epileptic manifestation, unless there is adequate reason for believing that further .epileptic attacks are unlikely' (Eadie and Tyrer, 1974). This seems to be a more realistic approach than the one (which still has its adherents) that advocates a 'wait and see' policy on the grounds that a single seizure might prove to be an isolated event in the patient's life and

that what will inevitably be a prolonged treatment with potentially toxic drugs should not be inaugurated until he has experienced at least two attacks.

In the present context hypsarrhythmia is a case apart. It is usually associated with such serious abnormalities of brain function that all would agree the only hope of alleviating the condition at all is to initiate treatment as soon as the diagnosis is made.

c. Adequate treatment is as important as early diagnosis. It has only recently become clear that antiepileptic medication has often failed because the drugs used have not attained a therapeutically effective concentration in the brain. Recommended doses have been adhered to but we now appreciate that for many antiepileptic (and other) drugs that are taken by mouth, there is a very poor correlation between the dose of drug and the amount that reaches the tissues. The accounts that follow quote, for each important drug, the plasma concentrations associated with therapeutic effectiveness. The appropriate dose of any of these drugs should be determined for the individual patient in the light of the plasma concentrations produced by test doses. Only in this way is it possible to ensure that antiepileptic drug therapy will be as effective as possible and that toxic responses will be avoided.

As long ago as 1968, Rodin estimated that grand mal seizures had been suppressed in 50 to 60 per cent of those who had received the appropriate medication. There is little doubt that this figure will have been bettered in recent years and that it will improve still further as an appreciation of the importance of maintaining an adequate concentration of drug in the tissues becomes more widely disseminated.

d. It is usual to embark on the treatment of epilepsy by giving one of the drugs of choice. If adequate control cannot be achieved by the one drug or if side effects prove troublesome a second drug can be used to supplement or replace the first. Although it is sometimes preferable, in any condition, to give modest doses of two drugs rather than a large dose of a single agent (p. 76), combined therapy in epilepsy may give rise to drug interaction problems. These are detailed in the sections devoted to the individual drugs.

e. Some forms of epilepsy (particularly hypsarrhythmia and psychomotor epilepsy) are much less amenable than the others to drug therapy and even the drugs of choice listed in Table 31.1 will often fail to provide much relief for these conditions.

BROMIDES

In the interests of historical accuracy, mention should be made of the bromides which, during more than half a century between their introduction into medicine and the discovery of the barbiturates, provided the only hope of relief from attacks of grand mal epilepsy. The pharmacology of the bromides and their use as antiepileptic agents is discussed elsewhere (p. 491).

BARBITURATES

Phenobarbitone

Like the other barbiturates, phenobarbitone (Luminal, Gardenal) was introduced into medicine as a sedative and hypnotic but it was soon found that the drug had useful anticonvulsant activity at dose levels which did not heavily

Barbiturates

R=H, R'=C₂H₅, R''=C₆H₅,
Phenobarbitone
R=CH₃, R'=C₂H₅, R''=C₆H₅,
Mephobarbitone
R=CH₃, R'=C₂H₅, R''=C₂H₅
Methabarbitone

sedate the patient. It was first employed in the treatment of grand mal epilepsy in 1913 and it is still widely used for this purpose, often in conjunction with phenytoin or another antiepileptic agent.

It is also of value in the treatment of some of the focal epilepsies, particularly those that lead to generalized convulsions, but it has enjoyed no more than minimal success in psychomotor epilepsy.

Adequate control of grand mal attacks demands the maintenance of a phenobarbitone concentration in the plasma of about 20 μg per ml and this requires, in adults, a once-daily dose of about 2 mg per kilogram of body mass. Children metabolize the drug more rapidly than do adults and so need to take proportionally higher amounts of phenobarbitone and in twice-daily doses.

Though not powerfully sedative in its actions, phenobarbitone may produce unwelcome sedation and drowsiness. This effect often passes off with prolonged treatment and it is, of course, less evident when the dose of phenobarbitone can be reduced by using an additional anticonvulsant drug. Children, paradoxically enough, may become irritable and hyperactive and sometimes their intelligence becomes blunted. Confusion and disorientation have been reported among old people.

Phenobarbitone may cause a number of other and potentially more serious toxic reactions (folate deficiency, hypocalcaemia, foetal abnormalities and coagulation defects in the newborn) but these same adverse effects can also arise during treatment with phenytoin and they are further considered in the paragraphs that discuss the last named drug (p. 524). Similarly, both phenobarbitone and phenytoin induce hepatic microsomal enzymes. This point too is taken up later (p. 525).

Other barbiturates

Methylphenobarbitone (mephobarbitone, phemitone; Mebaral, Prominal) and metharbitone (Gemonil) have some slight anticonvulsive action on their own account but they are demethylated in the liver to give phenobarbitone and barbitone respectively and there seems to be no good reason why either drug should ever be preferred to phenobarbitone.

Primidone

Although primidone (Primaclone, Mysoline) is not itself a barbiturate (it is a pyrimidinedione), its principal metabolite is phenobarbitone. Neither primidone itself nor phenylethylmalonamide, its other metabolite (Fig. 31.4) has more than minimal anticonvulsive effectiveness and there is now little doubt that primidone is active only by virtue of the phenobarbitone it produces. Appreciable quantities of phenobarbitone do not appear in the plasma until primidone has been given for some two to three days and the onset of the drug's therapeutic action is similarly delayed.

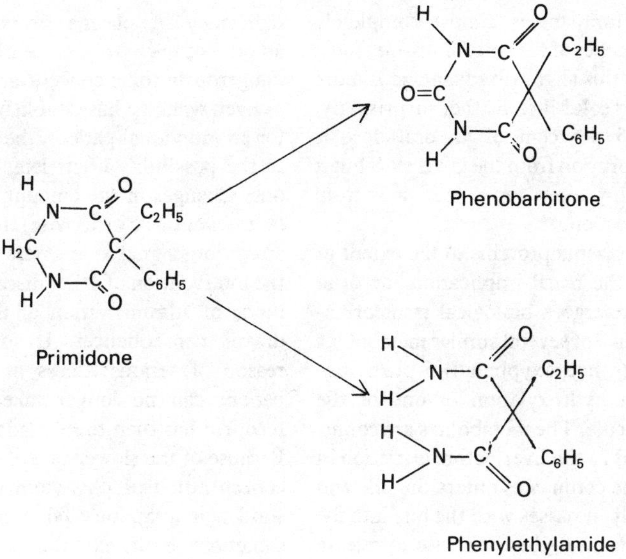

Fig. 31.4 Primidone and its principal metabolites

Not surprisingly, the toxic actions of primidone are generally similar to those of phenobarbitone but, in addition, a heavy drowsiness is sometimes experienced by those beginning treatment with primidone. Since this is an immediate response, blame for it can hardly be laid at the door of phenobarbitone. Indeed it is said to be antagonized by the barbiturate and this may at least partly explain why the drowsiness only persists for a day or two: after this time there may be enough phenobarbitone in the plasma to counter the soporific effect of the primidone.

Primidone gained a secure foothold in the list of favoured antiepileptic drugs before it became clear that it simply acts as a source of phenobarbitone. With our present knowledge there would seem to be no reason for prescribing primidone instead of phenobarbitone itself. Nevertheless, some highly reputable authorities still recommend the use of primidone (but not phenobarbitone) for the treatment of psychomotor epilepsy. This recommendation would seem to be based on the results of a few uncontrolled trials that were performed in the days when primidone was thought to be different from phenobarbitone. It is difficult to believe that primidone would emerge with credit from any rigorously controlled trial of its effectiveness in psychomotor epilepsy.

Primidone is therapeutically active when it provides a phenobarbitone concentration in the plasma of 10 to 25 μg per ml and to achieve this the daily oral dose has to be of the order of 10 to 15 mg per kilogram body mass.

THE HYDANTOINS
Phenytoin
Phenytoin (diphenylhydantoin; Dilantin, Epanutin) is one of the few drugs used in medicine whose discovery was the outcome of laboratory research rather than the result of incidental observation of the effects of a substance being used clinically for some other purpose. In the work which led, in 1938, to the discovery of phenytoin, Merritt & Putnam examined a large number of compounds for their ability to raise the threshold of electrically induced seizures. Phenytoin was found to be particularly effective in preventing the tonic extensor spasm, an observation which suggested that the drug would be able to control the fits of grand mal epilepsy. This proved to be so and for the past thirty years phenytoin has been the most extensively used of all antiepileptic drugs. It does not suppress or prevent convulsions precipitated by chemical agents such as strychnine, leptazol or tetanus toxin.

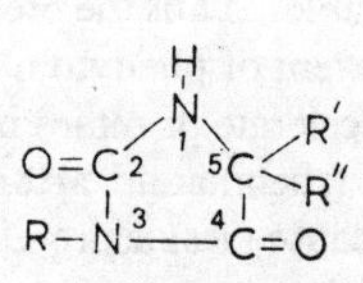

Hydantoins

R = H, R'=C_6H_5, R''=C_6H_5
Phenytoin (diphenylhydantoin)
R = CH_3, R' = C_6H_5, R'' = C_2H_5
Methoin (mesantoin)
R = H, R' = C_6H_5, R'' C_2H_5,
5,5-phenylethylhydantoin

Phenytoin is used as the sodium salt which produces a very alkaline solution and the drug is therefore presented in capsules that are taken with meals.

Although phenytoin is a weak acid with a pK_a of 9.2 it is not, contrary to expectation (p. 41), well absorbed from the stomach because the unionized compound that is formed in an acid environment is almost completely insoluble. In the upper reaches of the small intestine, some of the drug is ionized but this slight disadvantage is more than offset by an improved solubility. Rather surprisingly, perhaps, all but about 5 per cent of an oral dose is eventually absorbed. Absorption from the gut is slow but it is nevertheless considerably more rapid than it is from intramuscular sites of injection.

Phenytoin is bound to plasma proteins to the extent of about 90 per cent with the usual implication for drug interactions (p. 78). It undergoes biological transformation in the liver, the principal of several similar metabolites being the compound 5-(p-hydroxyphenyl)-5-phenylhydantoin formed by *para* hydroxylation of one of the benzene rings in the molecule. The metabolites are conjugated with glucuronic acid in the liver before excretion in the urine. A fraction of the conjugates enters the bile and circulates enterohepatically: it passes with the bile into the small intestine and is split by β-glucuronidase to release the free metabolites which are then reabsorbed.

Many patients suffer only occasional seizures, so that clinical response cannot usually be used to assess the adequacy of their antiepileptic medication. With many antiepileptic (and other) substances there is only a fragile relationship between oral dose and plasma concentration and there is no doubt that, in the past, a blind reliance on recommended doses led to many patients being given either too little drug so that their condition remained uncontrolled or too much so they had to suffer unnecessarily severe toxic effects. The situation has been particularly serious with phenytoin, partly because its therapeutic ratio is low (a therapeutic effect is achieved at plasma concentrations of 10 to 20 μg per ml but toxic effects begin to make their appearance at concentrations of 20 to 40 μg per ml), partly because of the drug's many toxic actions and partly because the amount of phenytoin in the plasma is influenced by many variables. Thus the presence of other drugs might reduce the extent of phenytoin's binding to plasma protein or might accelerate or retard its metabolism while concurrent disease (rheumatoid arthritis, uraemia, liver disease, etc) might cause plasma protein deficiency. Moreover, the metabolizing system for phenytoin becomes saturated at plasma drug concentrations within the therapeutic range. Once the system is saturated, a small increment in phenytoin intake will produce a large increase in plasma concentration that may be sufficient to effect a transition from an innocuous to a dangerously toxic dose. There is no real choice in the new patient but to monitor plasma concentrations in order to decide what his initial level of drug intake should be. It must, however, be pointed out that most of the methods available for the determination of phenytoin in the plasma do not differentiate between free and protein-bound drug. The free form (which is no more than 10 per cent of the total) is the pharmacologically active moiety so that in patients with a deficiency of plasma proteins, an apparently modest amount of phenytoin in the plasma may in fact represent a dangerously toxic concentration of the drug.

Even when he has established a satisfactory dose regime for an individual patient, the physician must remain alive to the possibility of its later becoming an unsatisfactory one. Changes in the amount or nature of the other drugs (antiepileptic or otherwise) that are being taken constitute an obvious signal to re-assess the phenytoin dosage as does the intervention of other disease processes. Changes in the mode of administration of the phenytoin can also have drastic consequences. It sometimes happens that, by reason of serious illness or an impending operation a patient can no longer take phenytoin by mouth and recourse has then to be made to the intramuscular route. Because of the slower rate of absorption from this site the concentration of phenytoin in the plasma may suffer a sudden if temporary fall when the changeover is made, sometimes to the extent of precipitating status epilepticus (p. 530). This eventuality can be guarded against by making the first intramuscular doses some 50 per cent higher than the oral doses on which the patient has been stabilized. Finally, it is salutary to remember a recent *cause célèbre:* in Australia in 1968, a drug manufacturer changed the excipient used in the production of a phenytoin mixture from calcium sulphate to lactose. The supposedly inert calcium sulphate that was at first used had in fact interfered with the absorption of phenytoin so that when the change to lactose was made and the unsuspecting patients continued to take their usual dose of drug they suffered phenytoin intoxication.

Daily doses of phenytoin needed to produce effective plasma concentrations are of the order of 300 to 500 mgs.

Side effects of phenytoin administration. Many thousands of people all over the world have been treated with phenytoin and since many of these patients have received the drug over long periods of time it is not surprising that a large number of toxic effects has been reported and that new ones keep emerging. Some of these side effects are peculiar to phenytoin but others are seen with other antiepileptic drugs particularly phenobarbitone and, of course, primidone.

Of those confined to phenytoin, a quite common side effect is a horizontal nystagmus which occasionally appears when the amount of phenytoin in the plasma is as low as 20 μg per ml. It tends to be associated with ataxia, dizziness, difficulty in articulation and other stigmata of cerebellar malfunction. These signs disappear if the drug is withdrawn or its dose reduced. Permanent damage to the cerebellum (degeneration of the Purkinje cells) has been detected post mortem in patients who have taken high doses of phenytoin over long periods of time but the consensus of informed contemporary opinion is that this change, unlike the reversible ones just referred to, is the result of the seizures rather than their treatment. It is known that the Purkinje cells are very susceptible to anoxia.

Other central nervous sequelae of phenytoin medication (though these are also seen during treatment with other antiepileptic drugs) include drowsiness, depression and frank psychoses. Some of these changes are sometimes accompanied by a slowing of the electroencephalographic rhythms and this may foreshadow an escape from the restraining influence of the antiepileptic drugs. Peripheral neuropathy and myasthenia gravis have also been reported as complications of phenytoin treatment.

One of the best known and certainly the most character-istic side effect of phenytoin treatment is hyperplasia (overgrowth) of the gums—sometimes to the point of almost burying the teeth—with associated soreness and bleeding. This condition is less often seen now that phenytoin is given in capsules so that the drug does not come into immediate contact with the mouth. However, it is partly excreted in the saliva so that the use of capsules does not entirely prevent the drug's acting on the gums. Attention to oral hygiene will minimize the effects of this contact.

The hypertrophy of the gums may be the result of phenytoin's having inhibited collagenase (the enzyme that breaks down the collagen of connective tissue) and this action might also explain the coarseness of the features that sometimes develops, usually in association with the gin-gival changes. Hirsutism may also appear to the embar-rassment particularly of women patients.

Like so many other drugs, phenytoin sometimes causes allergic skin rashes. A more rare idiosyncratic response is characterized by a generalized but painless enlargement of the lymph nodes accompanied by a skin rash and malaise. This condition (pseudolymphoma) though harmless in itself may progress to malignant lymphoma. Its appearance (and when it occurs it does so after only a few weeks of treatment) is an obvious indication to replace phenytoin by another drug. Pseudolymphoma has also been seen in patients receiving phensuximides or troxidone.

Of the side effects that are common to phenytoin and the barbiturates (some of them occur in the course of treat-ment with other drugs) the most important and certainly the most interesting from a theoretical point of view is folic acid deficiency with sometimes a consequential megalo-blastic anaemia. The origin of this complication is in doubt: it is possible that drugs that cause it impair the absorption of the vitamin from the gut. Alternatively they may increase the body's demands for folate by inducing the formation of microsomal enzymes in the liver which use folate as a co-factor. The possible relationship between folic acid deficiency and the mode of action of antiepileptic drugs is discussed later (p. 534).

An appreciable number of patients (probably about 20 to 30 per cent) taking phenytoin or phenobarbitone develop a degree of hypocalcaemia sometimes to the point of developing rickets or osteomalacia (p. 783). It may be that the anticonvulsant drugs induce the liver enzymes that break down vitamin D. An analogous mechanism may explain the blood coagulation defects that are sometimes seen in the newborn infants of epileptic mothers.

Between 5 and 15 per cent of women who receive treatment with phenytoin, phenobarbitone or some other antiepileptic drugs during pregnancy give birth to infants with congenital defects particularly hare lip and cleft palate (South, 1972; Fedrick, 1973 and others). The incidence of malformations in the offspring of mothers without epilepsy is no more than about 3 per cent. These statistics do not justify a recommendation that antiepileptic medica-tion should be withheld during pregnancy since the increased number of seizures that would follow drug withdrawal would pose a much more serious threat to the foetus than would the teratogenicity of a carefully regu-lated treatment programme.

Drug interactions involving phenytoin and phenobarbitone. We have seen that both phenytoin and phenobarbitone induce liver microsomal enzymes and that this may pro-vide the mechanism that underlies some of the toxic effects the two drugs have in common. It might be thought (and it is indeed sometimes asserted) that each will also stimulate the metabolism of the other so that, for instance, the amount of phenytoin in the plasma of a patient who has been receiving only this drug will fall if he begins to take phenobarbitone as well. This is not necessarily so. In 15 groups of patients on phenytoin studied in 7 different investigations, the average concentration of phenytoin in the plasma fell in five, rose in five and was unchanged in five when phenobarbitone was also given. The explanation for this variable behaviour probably lies in the fact that, as well as inducing microsomal enzymes that will lead to the more rapid metabolism of phenytoin, phenobarbitone will also compete with phenytoin for the available enzyme so that some of the latter drug will escape destruction. Some other antiepileptic and other drugs do exert more regularly predictable effects on the amount of phenytoin in the plasma by one or more of the drug interaction mechanisms that are discussed elsewhere (p. 76). Those that lower the concentration include ethanol, carbamazepine and the benzodiazepines (through stimulation of phenytoin catab-olism) while among the many that are reported to increase it are pheneturide, sulthiame, isoniazid (only in slow acetylators, p. 73) and dicoumarol. In all these instances phenytoin metabolism is hindered. The drugs named will, of course, similarly influence the amount of phenobarbi-tone in the plasma.

In their turn, antiepileptic compounds will influence the effectiveness of other drugs. These interactions are best dealt with when the pharmacology of these other sub-stances are discussed but one of them should be mentioned here since it bears directly on the whole problem of the management of epilepsy. A number of pregnancies have been reported among women taking phenytoin and oral contraceptives. This is an uncommon occurrence but the knowledge that her pregnancy is an unlikely one is poor consolation for the victim of contraceptive failure, particularly, when the culprit is a drug used to treat the very condition that constitutes grounds for avoiding pregnancy in the first place. The antiepileptic drugs only promote the metabolism of oestrogenic substances so that progestogens offer better protection to epileptic patients taking phenytoin or phenobarbitone than do the mixed contraceptives.

Methoin (mephenytoin, Mesantoin)

Methoin resembles phenytoin in its pharmacological properties and clinical uses. Weight for weight, methoin is twice as active as phenytoin. It is demethylated in vivo to form 5,5-phenylethylhydantoin and this compound may be responsible for the antiepileptic activity. 5,5-Phenylethylhydantoin has itself been employed as an anticonvulsant drug but toxic side effects are serious and the drug is now no longer used. Oddly enough, methoin is still spoken of with favour in several authoritative textbooks even though it is partly converted into a compound that has fallen into disrepute. The most menacing side effect of both drugs is aplastic anaemia but skin rashes and hepatitis are also seen. They are less likely than phenytoin to cause disturbances of cerebellar function, gum overgrowth and hirsutism.

Other hydantoins

Other antiepileptic hydantoins that have been developed have made little impact on the clinical scene. They include 1-methylmethoin (deltoin; methetoin), 3-ethyl-5-phenylhydantoin (ethotoin) and 3–allyl–5–isobutyl–2 thiohydantoin (albutoin).

CARBAMAZEPINE

First synthesized in 1953, carbamazepine (Tegretol) has only recently attracted the notice it deserves. The results of controlled clinical trials are unanimous in their agreement that, in many cases of major epilepsy, carbamazepine is at least as effective an anticonvulsant agent as phenobarbitone, phenytoin and primidone. The fact that the drug still tends to be given only to patients whose epilepsy is not adequately controlled by the older agents merely reflects a natural and laudable inclination among sober physicians to prefer the familiar to the unfamiliar drug.

In major epilepsy, carbamazepine can be used either alone or as a supplement to other drugs. It is also as effective as phenytoin and primidone in psychomotor epilepsy but this hardly constitutes a powerful recommendation because this condition is notoriously unresponsive to drugs of any kind.

Carbamazepine has also become established as the drug of choice for the treatment of trigeminal neuralgia (p. 423) and there has even been a suggestion that, because of a

presumed action on the hypothalamus, it might be useful in diabetes insipidus (p. 637).

Carbamazepine is a tricyclic compound, not dissimilar in structure to the tricyclic antidepressant agents such as imipramime (p. 580). Whether carbamazepine itself has psychotropic actions is disputed but there are those who maintain that it is capable of elevating mood and that this confers on it a particular advantage if it is employed to control epilepsy in children who are also emotionally retarded.

Presently available evidence indicates that, in order to control epilepsy without provoking undesirable side effects, carbamazepine must attain a plasma concentration of 5 to 7 μg per ml. This necessitates daily oral doses of the order of 500 to 1000 mg in adults and 50 to 500 mg (depending on age) in children up to the age of seven years. The higher daily doses are usually taken in two to four instalments.

Carbamazepine

Like the other antiepileptic drugs, carbamazepine is not entirely benign. Apart from the possibility of its inducing allergic skin rashes, it can cause gastrointestinal upsets, drowsiness, dizziness and double vision. Nystagmus sometimes occurs: it has been seen with plasma concentrations as low as 1.5 μg per ml. Aplastic anaemia has also been reported. This last condition apart, the side effects are more likely to make their appearance during the early stages of carbamazepine therapy and to disappear or diminish as treatment progresses.

It is not yet known whether carbamazepine affects folic acid metabolism in any way.

Carbamazepine induces hepatic microsomal enzyme activity but therapeutic doses do not saturate or inhibit the enzymes. Consequently (and unlike the barbiturates) it will always bring about a reduction in the phenytoin concentration in the plasma of patients who, having been previously given only the hydantoin, begin to take carbamazepine as well.

In experimental animals, carbamazepine has a teratogenic action. It seems likely that the human foetus is less susceptible to the drug, but until more is known about it, prudence would perhaps dictate that carbamazepine should not be given during the first twelve weeks of pregnancy and that it should be withheld altogether from those exposed to the risk of unplanned pregnancies. It has, however, to be remembered that other antiepileptic drugs can cause foetal malformations (p. 525) and that carbamazepine may prove to be no more dangerous than phenytoin or phenobarbitone in this respect.

THE BENZODIAZEPINES

The first benzodiazepine to be introduced into medicine was chlordiazepoxide. This occurred in 1960 and the drug rapidly achieved a reputation as a safe but effective minor tranquillizer. Success bred new members of the family and further success and it soon became evident that the benzodiazepines were almost as versatile as (but much safer than) the barbiturates. The group continues to grow and it has to be mentioned in many therapeutic contexts. The paragraphs that follow are concerned only with the place of the benzodiazepines in the management of epilepsy. Details of their structure and general properties appear elsewhere (pp. 571-577).

Diazepam

Diazepam (Valium, Tensium, Atensine), the first benzodiazepine to be added to the antiepileptic armamentarium, is of particular value in the management of status epilepticus and it is discussed in this context later (p. 530). It also has a place in the treatment of the febrile convulsions of infancy. It is now known that the temporal lobe can suffer damage during these attacks and so leave the child with a legacy of temporal lobe epilepsy. It is therefore vital to abort febrile convulsions at the earliest possible moment. Antipyretic measures must be instituted but until they take effect the prompt administration of diazepam (if circumstances permit intravenous injections) will often arrest the convulsive activity. Doses of up to 1 mg per kilogram of body mass may have to be given.

As a supplement to other forms of antiepileptic medication, diazepam is sometimes useful in patients who show behavioural disturbances. Used as the sole medication for other forms of epilepsy, diazepam is much less effective than nitrazepam and, probably, than the newer clonazepam.

Nitrazepam

Nitrazepam (Mogadon) now provides the first choice medication for myoclonic and akinetic seizures and it has even had some success in controlling the salaam spasms of hypsarrhythmia. Nitrazepam is not conventionally included in the drugs of first choice for controlling petit mal seizures but there is reliable evidence that it can be at least as effective as ethosuximide.

The daily dose of nitrazepam is 5 to 10 mg. Side effects are few but nitrazepam is a sedative drug (it is indeed one of the most widely used of all hypnotics) and therapeutic doses may induce an unacceptable degree of ataxia and drowsiness. The only other well authenticated side effects are allergic rashes and hypersecretion of the salivary and bronchial glands.

Clonazepam

Clonazepam (Rivotril) is the newest antiepileptic benzodiazepine. Presently available evidence indicates that it can replace, and is superior to, both diazepam and nitrazepam whether it is given intravenously in status epilepticus or febrile convulsions or orally in petit mal epilepsy, myoclonic spasms or salaam attacks. If these hopes are fulfilled, clonazepam will have to be recognized as the most versatile of antiepileptic drugs. The adult dose is of the order of 2 mg thrice daily. Side effects are similar to, but even milder than, those produced by nitrazepam.

Other benzodiazepines

Chlordiazepoxide (Librium) and oxazepam (Serax, Serenid) have demonstrable anticonvulsive activity but neither drug is now used for the treatment of epilepsy.

THE SUCCINIMIDES

Suppression of petit mal seizures is more difficult than the prevention of the overtly more dramatic fits of grand mal epilepsy but succinimides have enjoyed more success than other antiepileptic drugs. The three in current use are discussed in the chronological order of their discovery.

Phensuximide

Phensuximide (N-methyl-α-phenylsuccinimide; Milontin) is the most effective member of a series of α-phenylsuccinimides whose action were reported by Chen and his colleagues in 1951. Phensuximide was found to be capable of protecting experimental animals against convulsions induced by leptazol but to be relatively ineffective against electroshock convulsions. In accordance with expectations, the drug proved to be useful in the treatment of petit mal epilepsy. Nausea, vomiting, skin rashes and leucopenia have been reported as side effects. Phensuximide is less likely than ethosuximide to precipitate grand mal attacks in those susceptible to them and for this reason it is sometimes to be preferred to ethosuximide, otherwise the drug of first choice for the treatment of petit mal epilepsy.

Methsuximide

Methsuximide (Celontin) is chemically similar to phensuximide but it has been used for the treatment of psycho-

R = H, R' = C$_6$H$_5$, R'' = CH$_3$
Phensuximide
R = CH$_3$, R^1 = C$_6$H$_5$, R'' = CH$_3$
Methsuximide

The Succinimides

motor as well as petit mal epilepsy. However, methsuximide is much more toxic than phensuximide. Anorexia is a prominent side effect: more serious toxic actions include damage to the liver, the kidney and the bone marrow. Methsuximide is of limited value.

Ethosuximide

Ethosuximide (Zarontin, Capitus; Emeside), the latest member of the group, is more selective against petit mal than are the other two succinimides. It may increase the severity of grand mal seizures and it should therefore only be given to petit mal patients who are also subject to grand mal attacks if the latter can be controlled by normal doses of phenobarbitone or phenytoin. Ethosuximide is not as toxic as methsuximide but gastrointestinal upsets, anorexia, headache and skin rashes do occur and a few instances of blood dyscrasias have been reported. Plasma concentrations of 40 to 80 μg per ml are necessary properly to control petit mal attacks: daily oral doses of 20 mg per kilogram can be expected to produce plasma concentrations of the order of 60 μg per ml. The long half life of ethosuximide (60 hr in children, 30 hr in adults) permits once-daily administration.

THE OXAZOLIDINEDIONES

Like so many other antiepileptic drugs, these compounds were originally developed as hypnotics or analgesics but it was soon found that their outstanding property was to reduce the frequency of petit mal seizures. Those that have been used clinically are trimethadione, paramethadione and allylmethyloxazolidinedione. They all reduce the susceptibility of experimental animals to leptazol seizures.

Trimethadione came into clinical use in 1947 and was the drug of first choice for the treatment of petit mal epilepsy until it had to yield pride of place to the succinimides which are both more effective and less toxic though they are less successful in raising the threshold for the induction of convulsions by electric shock.

Oxazolidinediones
R=CH₃, R'=CH₃, R''=CH₃,
Trimethadione (troxidone)
R = CH₃, R' = CH₃, R'' = C₂H₅,
Paramethadione
R=CH₂CH=CH₂,R'=CH₃,R''=H,
Allylmethyloxazolidinedione

Trimethadione

Trimethadione (troxidone; Tridione) does not begin to exert its full clinical effect until it had been taken for two or three days. It is given by mouth and is apparently completely metabolized. N-demethylation takes place in the liver with the formation of 5,5-dimethyloxazolidine-2,4-dione. This compound is only slowly excreted and accumulates in the blood. It has been suggested that the delay in onset of the antiepileptic activity of trimethadione is accounted for by the slow accumulation of the metabolite and that the metabolite or the combination of drug and metabolite, or perhaps a further breakdown product, is responsible for the activity.

Troxidone is taken in doses of 300 to 600 mg four times daily to give a steady plasma concentration of 700 μg per ml. Side effects include drowsiness, increased sensitivity to light (photophobia) with blurring of vision in bright light, gastric upsets and skin rashes. The most serious side effect, which is rare, is aplastic anaemia and regular examination of the blood is advisable in patients who are treated for long periods with trimethadione. Skin rashes may be troublesome. Large toxic doses cause ataxia, hypnosis, loss of consciousness and respiratory depression. Like ethosuximide, troxidone may precipitate grand mal activity.

The only indication for the use of troxidone is the occurrence of petit mal attacks that cannot be controlled by a succinimide.

Paramethadione

Trimethadione is a white crystalline powder but paramethadione (Paradione) is an oily liquid. Its pharmacological properties, therapeutic uses and side effects are essentially similar to those of trimethadione but it is rather less likely to cause the uncomfortable glare responses to bright light. Patients who suffer badly in this respect when they take trimethadione may nevertheless tolerate paramethadione very well.

Allylmethyloxazolidinedione

This compound, also known as aloxidone, is not now used.

SODIUM VALPROATE

Sodium valproate (sodium dipropylacetate, Epilim, Depakine) has been used for some years on the European mainland but it has only recently attracted serious attention in Britain. It is a simple compound with none of the structural features that have hitherto been thought to be determinants of antiepileptic activity.

Sodium valproate

In vitro experiments reveal that sodium valproate inhibits glutamic acid decarboxylase and γ-aminobutyric acid-glutamate transferase, the enzymes responsible, respectively, for the formation and breakdown of γ-aminobutyric acid. The transaminase is more powerfully inhibited than the decarboxylase. The results of in vivo experiments are consistent with the findings in vitro: the amount of γ-aminobutyric acid in the brains of rats given sodium valproate is greater than that in untreated animals. In one investigation, the increase amounted to almost 50 per cent (Godin, Heiner, Mark and Mandel, 1969). It must however not be too readily assumed that the drug's antiepileptic activity is necessarily the result of its permitting the accumulation of γ-aminobutyric acid in brain, tempting though that hypothesis may be (p. 191).

Clinical experience has demonstrated the effectiveness of sodium valproate in many epileptic patients who have proved refractory to the more established antiepileptic agents: petit mal absences, myoclonic attacks and tonic-clonic (grand mal) fits have all been controlled by the drug but it has been less successful in cases of temporal lobe, psychomotor and focal motor epilepsy (Jeavons and Clark, 1974; Richens and Ahmad, 1975). It has been usual to give sodium valproate in association with other antiepileptic medicaments and part of its beneficial action, like that of sulthiame (p. 530) may derive from an ability to maintain effectively high serum concentrations of the other drugs. Thus Richens and Ahmad (1975) demonstrated a 27 per cent increase in the concentration of serum barbiturate when sodium valproate was given to patients maintained on phenobarbitone. Nevertheless the drug has antiepileptic activity in its own right: it attenuates experimental convulsions in animals and it can bring benefit to patients with myoclonic epilepsy even when all other drugs are withdrawn. Moreover, in the trial already referred to, Richens and Ahmad found that even when it was effective, sodium valproate did not increase the amount of phenytoin in the serum of patients receiving that drug.

The daily dose of sodium valproate is of the order of 1200 mg but it has to be carefully determined for the individual patient in the light of the other drugs he is receiving and of his response to the combined medication. Side effects are unusual and those that do occur (nausea, ataxia, drowsiness) are more likely to be the result of the increased effectiveness of another drug. Consequently, side effects that emerge when sodium valproate is given are often best dealt with by reducing the intake of its partner, particularly if this happens to be phenobarbitone or primidone.

ACETYLUREAS

This group of compounds was originally tested for hypnotic activity but they were found in laboratory tests to be more effective as anticonvulsants. They show a structural resemblance to the clinically useful barbiturates and hydantoins, as can be seen by reference to Figure 31.5

For some years the acetylureas were regarded as valuable agents for the treatment of psychomotor epilepsy but this reputation was lost when the drugs were subjected to

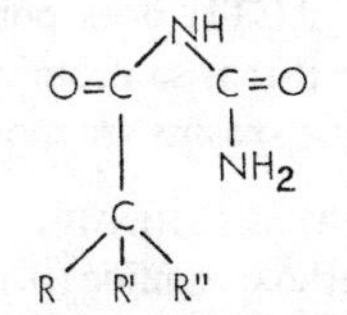

R = C_6H_5, R' = H, R'' = H
Phenacemide (phenacetylurea; Phenurone)
R = C_6H_5, R' = C_2H_5, R'' = H
Pheneturidine (Benuride)

Fig. 31.5 The acetylureas

properly controlled trials. Moreover they are highly toxic, the liver, the bone marrow and the psyche being particularly vulnerable. The high toxicity of phenacemide came as something of a surprise because in the tests to which phenacemide was subjected before it was released for clinical use, it appeared that it was of remarkably low toxicity: dogs, for instance, received up to 600 mg per kg daily and after eighteen months they showed no abnormality of the liver or bone marrow. However carefully laboratory tests on animals are performed, they do not reduce the necessity for extreme vigilance in clinical trials.

The acetylureas inhibit the metabolism of other antiepileptic drugs and this might partly explain why they appear to be effective medicaments when they are given in combination with other drugs. Such a combination is Trinuride, a mixture of pheneturide, phenobarbitone and phenytoin: the acetylurea helps to maintain the concentration of the other drugs in the tissues.

The acetylureas are still available but they clearly qualify only as 'last resort' drugs.

PYRIDOXINE (VITAMIN B_6)

We have already seen (p. 518) that a small proportion of those with hypsarrhythmia suffer from pyridoxine deficiency and benefit from the addition of the vitamin to their diet. In order to determine whether a particular patient falls into this category, it is only necessary to assess the immediate clinical and electroencephalographic responses to an intravenous injection of pyridoxine. If these are favourable, pyridoxine should be added to the diet on a long term basis. The usual diagnostic intravenous dose of pyridoxine is 1 mg per kg; the daily dietary supplement is 14 mg per kg.

It is pointless to give pyridoxine to patients with other kinds of epilepsy or to hypsarrhythmic infants who do not respond to the test dose of the vitamin.

ADRENOCORTICOTROPHIC HORMONE (ACTH)

This hormone and its multifarious uses are fully discussed elsewhere (p. 775). It is an empirical observation that it brings about clinical improvement in some (but by no means all) cases of hypsarrhythmia. The reason for this is not known. Unless treatment is initiated early in the history of the case, ACTH does not usually arrest the mental deterioration that is so prominent a feature of the disease but the muscle spasms are more easily controlled.

ACETAZOLAMIDE AND SULTHIAME

Acetazolamide and ethoxzolamide (p. 631) have both been used in the treatment of grand mal and petit mal epilepsy, usually as an adjunct to more powerful antiepileptic medication. There is considerable experimental support for the view that carbonic anhydrase in some way regulates the excitability of central neurones and that inhibition of carbonic anhydrase reduces the susceptibility to seizures. When carbonic anhydrase is inhibited so is the union of carbon dioxide and water. It may be that carbon dioxide retention will produce an acidosis sufficient to retard the passage of sodium ions into the neurones and so to stabilize the membrane. Evidence that this explanation is not an unreasonable one is provided by the well known fact that alkalosis (induced, for example, by expelling carbon dioxide from the body in a spell of overbreathing) is associated with an increased excitability of nerve cells. In spite of the apparently rational reason for using the drugs, carbonic anhydrase inhibitors are not notably successful as antiepileptic agents and tolerance arises quite rapidly. Sulthiame (Ospolot), like acetazolamide, is another sulphonamide derivative with some ability to inhibit carbonic anhydrase. It has been used particularly in the treatment of psychomotor epilepsy, usually in association with other drugs.

Sulthiamine.

As well as inhibiting carbonic anhydrase, sulthiame inhibits oxygen consumption by the brain. Both properties have been invoked to provide an explanation of its therapeutic activity. However, it now seems likely that in the doses used in man, sulthiame has no antiepileptic activity at all in its own right (Green *et al*, 1974) and that, like the acetylureas, it simply delays the metabolism of other anticonvulsive agents. This explains why it always seemed to be at its best when it formed one of a mixture of antiepileptic drugs. There seems to be no good reason for retaining sulthiame in the list of recommended medicaments, particularly since many of those who take it suffer distressing side effects. The most prominent of these (hyperventilation, paraesthesiae and drowsiness) are clearly referable to carbon dioxide retention but they are not so commonly seen in patients taking acetazolamide.

KETOGENIC DIETS

It has been known for many years that the severity of petit mal epilepsy is reduced in children fed a high fat diet which leads to increased blood levels of acid metabolites such as acetoacetic acid. This type of diet sometimes forms a useful adjunct to anticonvulsant medication.

Status epilepticus

Single major fits, though distressing to onlookers and embarrassing to the victim, are not dangerous (surprisingly enough, serious accidents rarely befall the epileptic during an actual fit) but *status epilepticus*, in which one grand mal seizure follows another without the patient's regaining consciousness, constitutes a medical emergency, with a mortality of more than 20 per cent. Status epilepticus is also seen in patients with petit mal and focal epilepsies. Petit mal status epilepticus is not necessarily accompanied by any immediately overt sign of an alteration in the patient's condition other than ataxia, muscle twitches or a lack of coordination in voluntary movements but if not promptly treated it may lead to disturbances of behaviour and intellectual deterioration. The encephalographic record (continuous spike and wave or slow wave activity) is diagnostic. Focal status epilepticus is synonymous with epilepsia partialis continuans, a condition that has already been described (p. 518).

Status epilepticus may occur because the victim has failed to adhere to the therapeutic regimen prescribed for him. When it is known that this has occurred, a logical way of dealing with the situation is to re-establish an adequately anticonvulsant concentration of drug in the plasma. This must be done quickly and the drug has therefore to be given by intravenous injection. In grand mal status, the continuing major convulsions sometimes make intravenous injections impossible particularly if the circumstances are such that the physician has to work single handed. Other means of quieting the convulsive activity must then be sought. A time honoured method of achieving this is to give paraldehyde (p. 490) by intramuscular injection. Some authorities believe that, alone among antiepileptic drugs, sodium phenobarbitone can be absorbed rapidly enough from intramuscular injection sites to justify its use as an alternative to paraldehyde.

Because of the danger of giving a toxic overdose, antiepileptic drugs like phenytoin and phenobarbitone should not be given in cases where it is not clear that status epilepticus has been precipitated by failure to take an adequate dose of one or other of these substances. Diazepam should be given instead: the drug, indeed, is now accepted as the drug of choice for the management of all forms of status epilepticus although it seems likely that it will shortly have to yield pride of place to clonazepam, its younger sibling. Sodium thiopentone has also been popular but it has the disadvantage that it depresses respiration. Moreover, sodium thiopentone may also cause laryngeal spasm, a dangerous condition since the victim will already be suffering some degree of anoxia.

Lignocaine (p. 470) has also been given, by the intravenous route, to interrupt the convulsions of status epilepticus. When status epilepticus has been relieved, it is desirable to keep the patient heavily sedated for some time and to allow him to recover consciousness only slowly. Rapid withdrawal of medication may cause the reappearance of the status epilepticus.

The screening and investigation of antiepileptic drugs

Several methods, enumerated later, are available for producing chonic epilepsy in experimental animals but they do not lend themselves to the provision of the large numbers of small-animal preparations required for the routine screening of potentially antiepileptic drugs. For this purpose, it is usual to study the actions of the compounds under test on convulsions caused by electroshock or leptazol. The mouse is the animal of choice for preliminary screening procedures.

From what has already been said, it should be clear that many antiepileptic drugs have actions (depressant or excitatory) on the nervous system which may give rise to troublesome side effects and in the preliminary screening of a new drug it is advisable to record the dose required to produce the first signs of toxicity (ataxia, excitement or depression) as well as that which protects the animal from the effect of the convulsive stimulus. Other toxic effects will, of course, be looked for during routine toxicity tests.

Different classes of drug affect the several phases of electrically induced convulsions in different ways. Their relative effectiveness against electroshock and leptazol seizures also differs. These different patterns of activity permit some predictions to be made concerning the possible clinical usefulness of individual substances. For this reason, each new drug should be subjected to a variety of tests. In all of them it is usual to perform the test one and two hours after the oral adminstration of the substance being investigated. For quantitative work, the ED_{50} and the TD_{50} of the compound under test (TD = toxic dose) are compared with those of established drugs.

The sequence of events which follows the application of a brief electric shock to the heads of mice has already been described. The effect of anticonvulsant drugs on this response can be assessed by reference to several parameters as follows:

(i) *the maximal electroshock response.* A stimulus at least five times greater than the threshold shock is applied. Substances which abolish the tonic phase of the resulting convulsion may be effective against grand mal seizures though not all drugs of proved utility in this condition abolish the tonic spasms. Instead of determining the dose of drug necessary to prevent the tonic spasm, the effect of a particular dose can be scored by reference to the severity of the convulsions produced (p. 513).

During the performance of this test, it is useful also to measure the *extensor seizure latency* (the time interval between the application of the stimulus and the appearance of the extensor spasm) which can be done very accurately if a stop watch is triggered by the switch on the electroshock machine (Toman and Everett, 1958). Drugs which abolish the tonic phase of the seizure will, in smaller doses, lengthen the extensor seizure latency and to this extent measurement of the latency adds nothing to the information supplied by the rest of the test if the compound being studied has a strong anticonvulsive action. On the other hand, if other classes of centrally acting compounds (tranquillizers, analgesics, hypnotics, etc.) are under test, prolongation or curtailment of the extensor seizure latency, signals the likelihood that these compounds have, as incidental actions, some anticonvulsant or convulsant properties respectively.

(ii) *the minimal electroshock threshold.* The effect of the substance being tested on the voltage necessary to produce minimal seizures is measured. Minimal seizures consist of brief clonic convulsions with the animal maintaining an upright posture, followed by a period of catatonia. In a variant of this method, mice are stimulated by low frequency (6 Hz) high amplitude (50-100 volts) shocks for six seconds. The dose of drug required to curtail the resulting minimal seizures is determined. In the method as originally developed, an effective dose of the drug was defined as that which brought the period of immobility to an end within ten seconds of the delivery of the shock.

Because the animal remains upright but stunned and because of the nature of the accompanying electroencephalographic discharge, the minimal seizure in the mouse has been regarded as analogous to a psychomotor attack in human beings. Although some of the drugs that may exert some beneficial effect on the course of psychomotor epilepsy certainly protect mice against minimal seizures, the test is not specific enough to do more than provide a hint that a new drug has been found. The drug treatment of psychomotor epilepsy is so unsatisfactory that it is not yet possible to develop a reliable screening test for substances that might control it because no existing drug is sufficiently efficacious to serve as a suitable reference compound.

It is important to remember that electroshock thresholds depend on the emotional state of the animal and if consistent results are to be obtained in this type of test the mice must be handled very gently. Further, the application of an electric shock to the head causes long lasting alterations in the excitability of its cerebral neurones and, on this account, no mouse should be used more than once a day.

As we have already pointed out, drugs which are active against petit mal are usually more successful in protecting mice against seizures induced by leptazol than they are in reducing the intensity of maximal electroshock convulsions. Those that prevent grand mal attacks usually exhibit the opposite pattern of activity. There are, however, exceptions to these generalizations. Carbonic anhydrase inhibitors, for instance, though effective in petit mal, do not reduce the severity of convulsions induced by leptazol.

For the production of convulsions in mice, leptazol is administered by the subcutaneous route in doses of 100 mg per kilogram of body mass. Other chemical convulsants give less satisfactory results. Screening tests have also been developed which depend on the initiation of convulsions by hyperthermia produced by a diathermy machine or by depletion of sodium from the brain, produced by the intraperitoneal injection of a hypertonic glucose solution. Although they are of little value as routine screening procedures, these methods are sometimes useful when the modes of action of convulsant and anticonvulsant drugs are being investigated. Another test which is useful in the same type of investigation is that due to Toman (1952). If isolated nerves are subjected to repeated stimulation for about two seconds with a shock of ten times threshold strength, they become transiently more excitable so that, for a brief period following the rapid stimulation, their threshold is lowered. Anticonvulsant compounds which are active against grand mal epilepsy, provided that they contain an aromatic group, prevent this post-stimulation facilitation without altering the stimulus threshold of the resting nerve. This test can be performed quite easily using frog nerves in a conventional moist chamber. The substance under test is applied directly to the nerve.

In sophisticated studies it is useful to be able to use animals which exhibit spontaneous epileptiform convulsions. Some strains of mice have major fits when they are subjected to auditory stimuli and these are useful for some purposes. In larger animals, lesions that give rise to convulsions can be produced by a variety of agents of which the best known is alumina cream: it is injected in a small volume (usually 0.1 ml) through a trephine hole and the dura mater on to the motor area of the cortex. Alternatively, it is applied in a small gauze disc. Monkeys are particularly suitable animals for this purpose. Convulsions begin to occur about six weeks after application of the cream and they may persist for several years. This method of producing chronic 'artificial' epilepsy is due to Kopeloff and his colleagues (1954). Localized freezing with ethyl chloride has a similar effect but, although the convulsions occur within a few hours of freezing, the hyperexcitable state of the cortex is maintained for only a few weeks. Freezing and the application of alumina cream can be combined. Other substances, such as crystalline penicillin, tetanus toxin and powdered heavy metals, also produce convulsions when they are applied to the motor cortex but their action continues only for as long as they remain in actual contact with the cortex. It is interesting that convulsions will also occur in an animal sensitized to a specific protein, if that protein is applied to the motor cortex.

Another method of investigating the mode of action of anticonvulsant drugs is to measure their ability to raise the threshold stimulus required for the production of evoked cortical potentials in the conscious rabbit. The animal carries needle electrodes implanted in the skull: one pair of electrodes serves to receive the electrical stimulus from an appropriate stimulator and the evoked potential is recorded from another pair of electrodes.

Further details of the methods described in this section can be found in the reviews by Toman and Everett (1964) and Millichap (1965).

Clinical trials of antiepileptic drugs. Readers of the detailed descriptions of the antiepileptic drugs featured in this chapter cannot have failed to notice the recurrent hints that claims concerning the effectiveness of several of the drugs are based on anecdote rather than on the results of properly controlled clinical trials. It is essential to make sure that new drugs are both effective and safe before they are launched on to a trusting public and this is particularly so with antiepileptic drugs which, by their very nature, are likely to be more potentially dangerous than most and will have to be taken over protracted periods of time. Those who wish to assess the reliability of published trial reports (or, more important, to organize trials themselves) should carefully examine the extent to which the procedures meet the criteria for drug trials in general, as set out on pp. 143-146 of this volume, or for antiepileptic drugs in particular as detailed by Richens (1976).

The origins of epilepsy and the mode of action of antiepileptic drugs

The overt signs and the electroencephalographic features of grand mal seizures are so similar to those elicited by many convulsant agents that it is natural to assume that common mechanisms underlie idiopathic and chemically evoked convulsions.

In a major convulsion, excitation spreads over a wide area of the brain. Central synapses make use of a number of different transmitter substances but it should be clear that the spread of an excitatory process is likely to be encouraged by circumstances that increase the availability of only one of the excitatory transmitters (or decrease that of an inhibitory one) even if that transmitter does not operate at all the synapses that lie in the path of the spreading discharge: if one neurone is exposed to an increased amount of transmitter derived from the nerve endings that converge on it, it will itself be able to pass on the increased excitation to the neurones with which it is in synaptic contact, irrespective of the nature of the transmitter substance that mediates this excitation.

It is not difficult to accept the idea that different convulsant agents are likely to act on different transmitter systems. Picrotoxin, as we have seen, antagonizes the action of γ-aminobutyric acid in the brain while drugs that induce a central deficiency of this presumed mediator of inhibitory transmission are likely to precipitate convulsions (p. 191). On the other hand, physostigmine, atropine and nicotine, all of which are convulsant agents when given in appropriate doses, intervene in the acetylcholine transmitter system while many other substances (leptazol and nikethamide for instance) seem to evoke convulsions independently of any direct influence on either the γ-aminobutyric acid or the acetylcholine system.

These observations give no hint as to which transmitter substance is likely to be primarily involved in the initiation of idiopathic major seizures. It might indeed be misleading to assume that defects in a transmitter system are necessarily responsible for epileptic activity. One approach to the solution of the problem is to investigate the actions of antiepileptic drugs of proven efficacy. Any common pharmacological actions they exert should provide pointers to the aetiological culprits in epilepsy. In the paragraphs that follow, the transmitter and other systems that have so far been investigated in any detail in the epilepsy context are considered separately. It should be added that most of the studies relate to grand mal seizures. The other types of epilepsy pose even more difficult problems for the laboratory investigator.

ACETYLCHOLINE

Although interference with the acetylcholine system can lead to major convulsions, there can be little support for the view that acetylcholine is critically involved in the aetiology of epilepsy and in the action of more than a few convulsant agents. It is true that acute changes in the acetylcholine content of brain have been demonstrated during convulsions produced by a variety of agents (Richter and Crossland, 1949; Crossland, 1953) but these changes are almost certainly the consequence, rather than the cause, of convulsions. Considerable interest was aroused some years ago by the report that when human cerebral cortex containing an epileptic focus was incubated *in vitro*, its ability to produce 'bound' acetylcholine was much less than that of normal cortex although the synthesis of 'free' acetylcholine was unimpaired (Tower and Elliott, 1952). Unfortunately, a later study (Pappius and Elliott, 1958) completely failed to confirm the original observation, notwithstanding the fact that one of the investigators participated in both studies. Since then, all the experiments which have sought to establish what role is played by acetylcholine in the initiation of convulsions have led to the conclusion that although it may be necessary for the maintenance of convulsive activity, acetylcholine has no part to play in the initiation of seizures and disturbances in its metabolism cannot be the cause of convulsions.

The chronic administration of phenytoin and trimethadione has been reported to cause a decrease in the acetylcholine content of brain (Bose *et al.*, 1958), but the significance of this observation is difficult to assess. Other antiepileptic agents have little or no effect on the brain's acetylcholine.

γ-AMINOBUTYRIC ACID

There is nothing to suggest that γ-aminobutyric acid, any more than acetylcholine, is involved in the initiation of all forms of seizure activity. There is, certainly, a report in the literature that the concentration of γ-aminobutyric acid in focal epileptic tissue in human subjects is lower than that in the surrounding normal tissue (van Gelder, Sherwin and Rasmussen, 1972) but the change affected other amino acids too and the finding still awaits confirmation. In the meantime, it has to be said that none of the therapeutically useful anticonvulsant agents, sodium valproate apart, has any biochemical action that might be expected to make more γ-aminobutyric acid available in the brain (Tapia, 1976).

The reader will recall that some cases of hypsarrhythmia are associated with, and are apparently caused by, a relative deficiency of pyridoxine, a situation that would be expected to hinder the production of γ-aminobutyric acid. However the salaam attacks that are so characteristic a feature of hypsarrhythmia bear no resemblance to the convulsive attacks that occur in other pyridoxine deficiency states or that are produced by drugs that prevent the formation of γ-aminobutyric acid. Pyridoxine is involved in more than the production of the inhibitory transmitter (p. 793): in particular it acts as a cofactor in tryptophan metabolism and it is this activity that seems to be disrupted in pyridoxine dependent hypsarrhythmia.

The question as to whether sodium valproate is an antiepileptic agent by virtue of its permitting the accumulation of γ-aminobutyric acid in the brain is discussed elsewhere (p. 528).

There is some evidence that the amount of glutamic acid in the brains of human epileptic subjects is less than that in normal brain tissue. A similar finding has been reported in cats with experimental epilepsy. Glutamic acid is essentially an excitatory substance (p. 193) and it is not easy to see how a deficiency of glutamic acid can be associated with an increase in excitability. One explanation which has been put forward (Tower, 1960) is that the depletion of glutamic acid mirrors a reaction directed to the maintenance of normal amounts of γ-aminobutyric acid in the brain in the face of processes tending to deplete the supplies. However, this is not a very satisfactory explanation since, whatever the reason for the glutamic acid loss, it should still be associated with a depression of cerebral excitability if supplies of γ-aminobutyric acid are maintained.

Among the anti-epileptic drugs, phenytoin has been reported to decrease and acetazolamide to increase the glutamic acid content of brain.

The relationship of γ-aminobutyric and glutamic acids to convulsive activity in general is discussed in more detail elsewhere (p. 191).

5-HYDROXYTRYPTAMINE

It has been reported that several anticonvulsant drugs (bromides, phenytoin, phenurone, primidone and trimethadione) increase the 5-hydroxytryptamine content of brain (Bonnycastle *et al.*, 1957). Not all later workers have been able to confirm these findings but they are of interest in view of the fact that 5-hydroxytryptamine has predominantly inhibitory actions in the brain (p. 187). It may also be significant that a number of different anticonvulsant drugs share a common pharmacological action. These facts and the disturbance of tryptophan metabolism in infantile spasms indicate that a considerable profit might accrue from a more detailed investigation into the relationship between 5-hydroxytryptamine and epileptic activity.

INORGANIC IONS
If the activity of the sodium pump is reduced, the concentration of sodium ions outside the nerve falls. A similar result follows an increase in the sodium permeability of the neuronal membrane. In either case the excitability of the neurones increases. A variety of biochemical mechanisms controls the energy-providing reactions on which the continued activity of the sodium pump depends and interference with any of these might lead to a hyperexcitability of a sufficient degree to initiate convulsive activity. Anoxia, hypoglycaemia and poisoning with substances, such as fluorocitrate, which block the Krebs cycle, are all conditions in which convulsions occur and in which energy supplies for the proper operation of the sodium pump are interfered with.

Phenytoin increases sodium efflux from nerve and acetazolamide inhibits its influx into nerve. Ketogenic diets also lead to a reduced influx of sodium. Thus the anticonvulsant actions of these drugs are easily explained on the ionic hypothesis of convulsions. There is as yet, however, little evidence that epilepsy has its roots in a biochemical lesion of this type and none of the actions of chemical convulsants is such as to suggest that these substances are interfering with the processes which support the operation of the sodium pump.

FOLIC ACID
As we have seen, folic acid deficiency is likely to occur in the course of treatment with a number of antiepileptic drugs including phenobarbitone, primidone, phenytoin and phenuride. The origin of this deficiency is uncertain. It may be that antiepileptic drugs interfere with the absorption of folic acid from the gut but it is perhaps more likely that they accelerate its breakdown by inducing hepatic microsomal enzymes. Whatever the origin of the deficiency state, it is so regular an accompaniment of antiepileptic medication that Reynolds (1973) believes that a drug's ability to suppress grand mal seizures is inseparable from its antifolate effect. There is some experimental evidence in support of this view which implies that epileptic attacks are linked in some way with an excess, or an increased activity, of folate in the brain. Thus, folic acid causes convulsions when it is applied topically to the cerebral cortex and a mutual antagonism between folic

acid and anticonvulsant drugs of the phenobarbitone-phenytoin type has been demonstrated in a number of biochemical and pharmacological preparations (Spector, 1972; Jenkins and Spector, 1973).

We have noted already that psychotic disturbances are not infrequent occurrences among patients who have received treatment for grand mal epilepsy and there arises the intriguing possibility (for which there is a substantial body of experimental support as well as an equal amount of contradictory evidence) that the psychotic changes are a consequence of folic acid deficiency. If this were so, grand mal epilepsy and some forms of psychiatric upset might prove to be mutually antagonistic conditions, the occurrence of one precluding the intrusion of the other. In other words, von Meduna (p. 520) might have been right all the time!

Folic acid is the precursor of tetrahydrofolic acid (p. 678) which is itself, through such adducts as methyltetrahydrofolic acid, involved in a number of reactions in the brain and elsewhere. Inhibition of these reactions might lead, *inter alia*, to an accumulation of dopamine in the brain (Leading Article, 1975). The role, if any, of folic acid in the aetiology of epilepsy might be an indirect one and a study of its relationship with transmitter and other regulatory substances in the brain might pay handsome dividends.

BIBLIOGRAPHY

Books, monographs and reviews
Eadie, M. J. and Tyrer, J. H. (1974). *Anticonvulsant Therapy.* Edinburgh and London: Churchill Livingstone
Eadie, K. J. (1976). Plasma level monitoring of anticonvulsants. *Clin. pharmacokin*, **1**, 52-66.
Millichap, J. G. (1965). Anticonvulsant drugs. In *Physiological Pharmacology*, vol. 2, pp. 97-173, ed. Root, W. S. and Hofmann, F. G. New York: Academic Press.
Richens, A. (1976). *Drug Treatment of Epilepsy.* London: Henry Kimpton.
Rodin, E. A. (1968). *The Prognosis of Patients with Epilepsy.* Springfield: Thomas
Spinks, A. and Waring, W. S. (1963). Anticonvulsant drugs. In *Progress in Medicinal Chemistry*, vol. 3, pp. 261-331, ed Ellis, G. P. and West, G. B. London: Butterworth
Sutherland, J. M., Tait, H. and Eadie, M. J. (1974). *The Epilepsies.* Edinburgh and London: Churchill Livingstone
Tapia, R. (1975). Biochemical pharmacology of GABA in CNS. In Inversen, L. L., Iversen, Susan D. and Synder, S. H. (eds). *Handbook of Psychopharmacology*, New York and London: Plenum Press, Vol. 4, pp. 1-58.
Toman J. E. P. (1952). Neuropharmacology of peripheral nerve. *Pharmac. Rev.*, **4**, 168-218.
Toman, J. E. P. and Everett, G. M. (1964). Anticonvulsants. In *Evaluation of Drug Activities: Pharmacometrics.* Vol. 1, pp. 287-300, ed Laurence, D. R. and Bacharach, A. L. New York: Academic Press.
Tower, D. B. (1960). *The Neurochemistry of Epilepsy.* Springfield, Ill.: Thomas.
Woodbury, D. M., Penry, J. K. and Schmidt, R. P. (eds) (1972). *Antiepileptic Drugs*, New York: Raven Press.

Original papers

Bonnycastle, D. D., Giarman, N. J. and Paasonen, M. K. (1975). *Br. J. Pharmac.*, **12**, 228-231.

Bose, B. C., Gupta, S. S. and Sharma, S. (1958). Effect of anticonvulsant drugs on the acetylcholine content in rat tissues. *Archs. int. Pharmacodyn.*, **117**, 248-253.

Crossland, J. (1953). The significance of brain acetylcholine. *J. ment. Sci.*, **99**, 247-251.

Fedrick, J. (1973). Epilepsy and pregnancy: a report from the Oxford Record Linkage Survey, *Br. med. J.*, **2**, 442-448.

Van Gelder, N. M., Sherwin, A. L. and Rasmussen, T. (1972). Amino acid content of epileptogenic human brain: focal versus surrounding regions. *Brain Res.*, **40**, 385-393.

Gibberd, F. B. (1976). Who is epileptic? *Practitioner*, **216**, 426-430.

Godin, Y., Heiner, L., Mark, J. and Mandel, P. (1969). Effect of DL-n-propylacetate, an anticonvulsive compound, on GABA metabolism. *J. Neurochem*, **16**, 869-873.

Jeavons, P. M. and Clark, Jean E. (1974). Sodium valproate in the treatment of epilepsy. *Br. med. J.*, **2**, 584.

Jenkins, D. and Spector, R. G. (1973). The actions of folate and phenytoin on the rat heart *in vivo* and *in vitro*. *Biochem. Pharmac.*, **22**, 1813-1816.

Kopeloff, L. M., Chusiv, J. G. and Kopeloff, N. (1954). Chronic experimental epilepsy in *Macaca mulatta*. *Neurology*, **4**, 218-227.

Leading Article (1975). Folate-responsive schizophrenia. *Lancet*, **1**, 1283-1284.

Merrit, H. H. and Putnam, T. J. (1938). A new series of anticonvulsant drugs tested by experiments on animals. *Archs. Neurol. Psychiat.*, *Chicago*, **39**, 1003-1015.

Pappius, H. M. and Elliott, K. A. C. (1958). Acetylcholine metabolism in normal and epileptogenic brain tissue; failure to repeat previous findings. *J. appl. Physiol.*, **12**, 319-323.

Reynolds, E. H. (1973). Anticonvulsants, folic acid and epilepsy. *Lancet*, **1**, 1376-1378.

Richens, A. and Ahmad, S. (1975). Controlled trial of sodium valproate in severe epilepsy. *Br. med. J.*, **4**, 255-256.

Richter, D. and Crossland, J. (1949). Variation in acetylcholine content of brain with physiological state. *Am. J. Physiol.*, **159**, 247-255.

South, J. (1972). Teratogenic effect of anticonvulsants. *Lancet*, **2**, 1154.

Spector, R. G. (1973). The influence of anticonvulsant drugs on formyl tetrahydrofolic acid stimulation of rat brain respiration *in vitro*. *Biochem. Pharmac.*, **21**, 3198-3201.

Toman, J. E. P. and Everett, G. M. (1958). Comparison of laboratory methods in the search for new drugs of potential value to psychiatry. In *Psychopharmacology*, pp. 247-266, ed. Pennes, H. H. London: Cassell.

Tower, D. B. and Elliott, K. A. C. (1952). Activity of acetylcholine system in human epileptogenic focus. *J. appl. Physiol.*, **4**, 669-676.

Woodbury, L. A. and Davenport, V. D. (1952). Design and use of a new electroshock seizure apparatus and analysis of factors altering seizure threshold pattern. *Archs. int. Pharmacodyn.*, **92**, 97-107.

32. Psychotropic drugs

A *psychotropic, psychoactive* or *phenotropic* drug is one that inhibits, sharpens or alters emotional and behavioural responses. Whole new ranges of these drugs have been developed during the past thirty years or so and many of them have been employed for the symptomatic treatment of neurotic and psychotic conditions. Before this therapeutic explosion took place, virtually the only drugs available, in the present century, for the control of mental illness were the barbiturates. Much earlier in history, however, man had made use of some of the drugs that are today often regarded as being of recent origin. Reserpine was first employed by contemporary psychiatrists in 1950 but extracts of the root of *Rauwolfia serpentina* (from which reserpine is derived) had been used to calm maniacal persons in the eighteenth century in Europe and centuries before that in Asia. Ancient man knew many of the psychoactive substances that raise such acute social problems today. Centuries ago, and in many parts of the world, he discovered natural sources of drugs such as opium, cocaine and alcohol which enabled him to meet the tribulations of this world while his visions of the next were provided by priests and holy men whose sensitivity, percipience and insight appeared to be intensified by the mescaline and other compounds present in the cacti, seeds and fungi whose ritual ingestion formed the focal point of many primitive ceremonies.

The present chapter surveys the main groups of psychotropic drugs and discusses the properties and mode of action of some of those that are currently in use for therapeutic or experimental purposes.

TYPES OF MENTAL ILLNESS

It is not possible to present more than a superficial account of the principal features of the common forms of mental illness within the space that is available for this introduction to the psychotropic drugs. The reader is introduced to little more than a vocabulary of the subject treated in a fashion so simple that the expert might be inclined to dismiss it as misleading. Those without expert knowledge who wish to be more properly informed about mental illness should consult a manageable textbook (such as that by Anderson and Trethowan, 1973) that discusses psychiatric conditions in an up-to-date way.

Mental defect and psychopathic states result from failure of intellectual and emotional development respectively. Mental deficiency is inevitably accompanied by some failure of emotional development but the psychopath—who betrays his emotional immaturity by his grossly antisocial conduct—may be intellectually normal. The majority of psychiatric disorders, however, occur in those whose maturation processes have progressed in a normal fashion and they represent a disturbance of function in a previously healthy organ.

Psychiatric illnesses can be divided into the *neuroses* and the *psychoses*. There is some overlap between these two categories but it is broadly true to say that the reactions and emotions of a patient suffering from a neurotic illness are simply an exaggeration of those exhibited by normal individuals whereas the psychotic patient lives in a world of his own, the victim of his delusions and hallucinations, and with only a tenuous hold on the world of reality. To put this in another way, the neurotic usually retains sufficient insight to realise that he is ill; the psychotic usually believes that only his own actions are completely rational. This simple dichotomy, it need hardly be said, grossly underestimates the complexities of psychiatric disorders. It is not to be expected that irregularities in the functioning of the mechanisms of the mind will invariably produce conditions that can be cleanly allocated to one or other of these major classes of mental disorder. It is equally difficult to draw clear boundaries between individual neuroses and psychoses.

THE NEUROSES

Although the neuroses are described here as separate symptom complexes, it must be appreciated that the individual patient may exhibit elements of more than one of these complexes.

Anxiety states. Anxiety or fear is a normal response to a situation in which the health or safety of the individual is threatened. An anxiety state can only be regarded as a neurosis if the degree or duration of the anxiety is out of proportion to the stress that evokes it. The patient with an anxiety neurosis is tense, tremorous, restless and excitable. The activity of his nervous system is increased so that there may be sweating, a dry mouth, palpitations and loss of appetite. Headache and fatigue may be complained of. In some patients the anxiety state may arise from, or be associated with, abnormal fears (*phobias*) of specific objects or conditions. The wise pedestrian has a fear of motor traffic but the patient with a phobic anxiety neurosis may be quite incapable of leaving his home for fear of being involved in a road accident if he does. Anxiety neuroses constitute a high proportion of the neurotic conditions encountered in general and hospital out-patient practice.

Hysteria. The hysterical patient produces his own illness in order to escape from an unwelcome situation. Quite dramatic symptoms, such as total muscle paralysis or complete blindness may be produced in this way but the hysterical illness is always related to the stress situation in which the victim finds himself. The worker in a chemical factory, for instance, may develop an incapacitating dermatitis and so escape from the factory floor into duties that are more congenial to him. It is important to realize that the hysterical patient is quite unconscious of the fact that he has manufactured his own illness. He is not a conscious malingerer and his symptoms, though they are of psychogenic origin, are every bit as 'real' as if they had arisen from identifiable physical causes.

Individuals who draw attention to themselves by histrionic outbursts, overdramatization of trivial events and bouts of violent emotion are said to have a hysterical personality and it is in this sense that the layman understands the word hysterical. He also usually associates 'hysterical' behaviour with the female sex and in this he is semantically—if not medically—correct, for 'hysteria' comes from the Greek *hystera* (the uterus: hence hysterectomy) because of an ancient belief that the condition arose in that organ. However, individuals who develop hysterical illnesses do not necessarily have a hysterical personality and those with a hysterical personality do not necessarily succumb to hysterical illnesses.

Obsessional neuroses. The life of the obsessional neurotic is dominated, and his activities are restricted, by irrational obsessions. In the belief that they are dirty, some obsessional neurotics wash their hands countless times a day, others are driven to count, touch or avoid trivial and common objects, others elevate simple everyday acts into elaborate rituals, and so on.

Depression. Depression may occur in both neurotic and psychotic conditions. Neurotic depression is usually 'reactive' in nature—that is, it is an abnormally severe or prolonged response to a stress (such as a bereavement) that would be expected to cause some degree of misery even in a normal individual.

The depressed neurotic is miserably unhappy and his depression is not infrequently accompanied by feelings of guilt and by a variety of bodily symptoms such as headache, constipation and weariness.

THE PSYCHOSES
The psychoses are usually dichotomized into the functional and the organic psychoses. Those in the former category (schizophrenia and the affective psychoses) arise from no presently identifiable physical cause; the organic psychoses are the consequence of recognizable disease of the brain or other organs. It is to be hoped that the day is not too distant when increasing knowledge will permit the transfer of the 'functional' psychoses to the 'organic' category.

Schizophrenia. Schizophrenia (the most common of all psychoses) is the name given to a group of psychoses characterized by disturbances of thought processes, a blunting of normal emotional responses, hallucinatory disturbances of perception, changes in motor activity and withdrawal from reality. These different features of schizophrenia occur to varying degrees in the several forms of the illness. 'Schizophrenia' means 'split mind' and it should be taken to indicate that the victim displays dissociations between his thoughts and his behaviour, inappropriate associations of ideas and actions that seem to belie his apparent emotional state. He himself believes that his actions are perfectly rational, often because he is reacting to voices and visions that he regards as real while we describe them as hallucinatory.

It is usual, following Bleuler, to recognize four types of schizophrenia:

a. paranoid schizophrenia (*paraphrenia*);
b. catatonic schizophrenia;
c. hebephrenic schizophrenia;
d. simple schizophrenia.

In *paraphrenia*, the patient believes that he is being subjected to a relentless persecution. In extreme cases he may believe that every situation in which he finds himself presents an organized threat to his safety. If he enters a strange room, he may believe, for instance, that the furnishings have been arranged in a way to facilitate his murder or to provide a coded message for an assailant. Hallucinations are common in this condition and some paranoid schizophrenics believe that they are historical figures, saints or saviours, and that the world is plotting to hinder them from achieving their objectives. In *catatonic* schizophrenia, motor activity is distorted or inhibited. Sometimes the catatonic schizophrenic may behave 'like a madman', indulging in extraordinary posturings or violent hyperactivity; at other times he is stuporous, motionless and withdrawn. In *hebephrenic* schizophrenia, blunting of emotional responses is the characteristic feature. Hallucinations may occur but they do not loom so large in the clinical picture as they do in paranoid and catatonic schizophrenia. *Simple* schizophrenia is probably best thought of as a milder form of hebephrenic schizophrenia.

The more serious varieties of schizophrenia occur in acute and chronic forms. Acute attacks of schizophrenia constitute a medical emergency demanding immediate treatment by large doses of an antipsychotic drug (p. 548). In the past, of course, physical methods of restraint had to be used. Chronic schizophrenia runs a more benign course but treatment is less easy.

The affective psychoses. A number of clinically recognizable conditions comprise this group of psychoses. They include endogenous depression, involutional melancholia, acute mania and manic-depressive states. In *endogenous depression* (unlike the reactive variety) there is no obvious precipitating cause and the condition may persist, if untreated, for several years. The depressed patient is not miserable all the time and the clinical picture is sometimes complicated by the concurrent occurrence of symptoms of anxiety so that the patient may appear restless or agitated. Other features of endogenous depression include feelings of unworthiness, insomnia and hypochondria. As in schizophrenia, paranoid symptoms with hallucinations and delusions may occur. The victim's delusions may make him believe that he has committed sins of unpardonable wickedness. This adds to his depressed state and may lead to suicide attempts, an outcome of endogenous depression that has always to be guarded against. The depressed patient may fear that he is going to murder his children or other close relatives and his delusions may lead to his actually committing the act he fears. Labels that indicate the dominant feature of the illness may be attached to individual cases of depression. Thus, agitated, depersonalized, hypochondriacal, obsessional, paranoid and phobic depressions are recognized. *Involutional melancholia* arises in middle age. All the usual features of depression may be encountered in this condition. A bizarre but not entirely uncommon feature is that the patient may believe himself to be a dead man among dead people. *Mania* is the opposite to depression. In a mild form it is usually described as *hypomania.* The hypomanic subject is euphoric, elated and full of energy. He talks fast and continuously and he is perpetually busy, ignoring his bodily needs in order to undertake a succession of sometimes pointless and almost always uncompleted tasks. This condition is not easy to diagnose because it merges with what is the usual behaviour pattern of many worthy and psychiatrically normal people. Hypomania can be regarded as a psychotic condition when it progresses to the state when the patient's uninhibited excesses of energy make him lose all sense of reality and of the needs of the moment. In *mania* proper the symptoms of hypomania are present in a more extreme form. The talk becomes gibberish and the energy may be spent in homicidal assaults on those who attempt to restrain the manic's unbounded exuberance. Delusions and hallucinations may occur and physical collapse may be brought on by lack of sleep and inadequate nourishment. In *manic-depressive disease,* periods of mania alternate with periods of depression; in the *mixed affective state* symptoms of mania and depression coexist. When depression appears as an element in a mixed affective state it is said to be of a *bipolar* type. In *unipolar* depression, the depressive episodes are not temporally separated by phases of mania.

Bipolar states are sometimes further subdivided into bipolar I and bipolar II types. In type I, mania constitutes the major psychiatric problem; in type II, depression predominates.

Some patients display the symptoms of both schizophrenia and the affective psychoses. Sometimes the two groups of symptoms coexist and sometimes they alternate with one another. In either event the condition is fittingly described as a 'schizoaffective' psychosis.

Psychiatric organic states. A number of symptoms occur with some regularity in the organic psychoses whatever the nature of the underlying pathology. These include clouding of consciousness, delirium, loss of recent memory, hallucinations, failure of attention, a tendency to move with great rapidity and with little obvious reason from one emotional extreme to another, disorientation in space and time and intellectual confusion. Superimposed on these symptoms may be others more specifically related to the precipitating disease.

Organic psychotic states run an acute or a chronic course and the list of organic diseases that may have psychotic concomitants or sequelae is a long one. It includes, among others, brain disease (meningitis, encephalitis, etc.), metabolic disturbances, endocrine dysfunction, pregnancy toxaemias and arterial disease. The chronic organic psychotic state is usually known as *dementia.* Arteriosclerosis affecting the cerebral arteries is responsible for many of the cases of dementia that arise in the later years of life. Dementia is also a feature of Huntington's chorea (p. 164).

HUMORAL THEORIES OF MENTAL ILLNESS

The ancients believed that temperament and mood were determined by humours. Four such controlling humours—blood, black bile, choler and phlegm—were postulated and 'good humoured' individuals were those whose humours were thought to be in balance with one another. A preponderance of any one humour was, it was supposed, reflected in what we would now call the affective state producing, respectively, sanguine, melancholic, choleric and phlegmatic individuals. These primitive beliefs were among the first to be swept away by the avalanche of scepticism and experiment initiated by the birth of scientific medicine. But the ancient doctrines were not to be buried for ever. After centuries of submersion, humoral theories have reappeared and this time, it seems, they are here to stay. All that has really altered is the identity of the humours although the word itself is rightly preserved so that we can still speak of the humoral substances that control mental processes. We have even had to resort, as the ancients did, to 'imbalance' concepts of mental illness.

The new humoral theory is no more than thirty years old and it has not yet been wholeheartedly embraced by all psychiatrists largely because, as is inevitable in one so young, it lacks the precision and sophistication of scientific theories of longer standing. Those inclined to scoff at these still ill formed 'chemical theories' should ask themselves whether the idea that a serious mental illness arises from the breakdown of a chemical controlling system is any less likely than the traditional psychiatric view that the gross abnormalities of thought and behaviour exhibited by psychotic individuals can be attributed to relatively trivial deficiencies in their early environment.

The appearance of the contemporary humoral theories coincided with, and indeed was demanded by, the emergence of the modern range of psychotropic drugs. These agents are capable of effecting a considerable amelioration in the condition of psychiatric patients, a fact that implies an interaction with chemical processes in the brain and requires a complete identification of these processes if even more successful psychoactive agents are to be created.

For convenience of discussion the humoral theories of schizophrenia will be discussed separately from those relating to the affective disorders but this is not to suggest that the biochemical mechanisms operating in the one condition are necessarily totally different from those that underlie the others.

Before considering the details of the biochemical hypotheses, however, attention must be directed to some general points that were often disregarded by the early investigators and are not always fully appreciated even today. Many of the studies have necessarily involved a comparative examination of blood or urine from psychotic and normal individuals and the following should be noted.

a. None of the psychoses can be regarded as a single disease entity and because varying criteria for selection may be adopted, the nature of the clinical and biochemical abnormality in one group of subjects may well differ from those chosen for participation in another investigation.

b. Some of the substances that appear in the urine are derived directly from food or drugs. It is rarely possible to ensure that the subjects in a particular investigation have been fed a diet identical with that taken by the normal subjects that constitute the 'control' group or that they have been withdrawn from drugs for a sufficiently long period to ensure that all drug metabolites have completely disappeared from the urine.

c. Only a small proportion of an individual urinary metabolite is elaborated in the nervous system and quite marked changes in cerebral metabolism may produce changes of urinary composition too subtle for detection by presently available methods. A novel metabolite produced only by the brain and only by one type of patient would, of course, be more readily detectable and this is the type of substance that most investigators have sought.

Schizophrenia

The ideas concerning the biochemical aetiology of schizophrenia that have emerged in recent years can be divided into two main groups. One group sees the disease as the result of the production of an abnormal metabolite (a *schizogen* or *schizotoxin*) while the other maintains only that there is an abnormality in the production or liberation of one or more of the neurotransmitter agents.

Hallucinations are neither confined to, nor are they invariably experienced, in schizophrenia. Nevertheless, they often constitute so striking a feature of the disease that many workers have been convinced that an understanding of the mode of action of drugs that induce hallucinogenic activity is the key to an understanding of the biochemical aetiology of schizophrenia. This conviction was at the root of both main biochemical hypotheses—this in spite of the fact that the hallucinogenic (*psychotomimetic*) drugs usually generate visual hallucinations while the hallucinations occurring in psychotic patients are predominantly auditory in nature.

Before discussing the transmethylation hypothesis some other ideas that relate schizophrenia to the production of an endogenous schizogen should be briefly noted.

The first suggestion was that disturbances of catecholamine metabolism might lead to the production of adrenochrome or adrenolutin (Fig. 32.1). Interesting facets of this hypothesis were the observations, in *in vitro* experiments, that lysergide and mescaline promoted the enzymatic conversion of adrenaline to adrenolutin and that both adrenochrome and adrenolutin inhibited the enzymatic decarboxylation of glutamic acid. Thus the action of two very different hallucinogens was linked with deficient production of a known inhibitory substance (γ-aminobutyric acid) and this made it appear the more likely that schizophrenia itself might have the same origin. Unfortunately for this attractive hypothesis, it never proved possible to establish the presence of adrenochrome or adrenolutin in the blood or urine of either normal or schizophrenic subjects.

Caeruloplasmin is a copper-containing enzyme found in plasma. It participates in some oxidative reactions and some years ago it was found that the plasma of schizophrenic patients contained a generally higher concentration of caeruloplasmin than did that of normal subjects. This finding hinted at the nature of a mechanism that might be responsible for the production of abnormal—or abnormal amounts of—oxidative metabolites. However, elevated concentrations of caeruloplasmin were subsequently found in a number of other pathological (but nonpsychotic) conditions. These observations do not entirely exclude the possibility of there being a qualitative difference between the caeruloplasmin from normal and schizophrenic subjects. Heath and his colleagues, for instance, have obtained evidence for the presence in the plasma of schizophrenic subjects of a substance ('taraxein') that induces behavioural and electroencephalographic changes in monkeys and human beings. Taraxein may be an abnormal caeruloplasmin or a compound derived from it

Compounds related to the catecholamines

Phenylethylamine: formula on p. 279

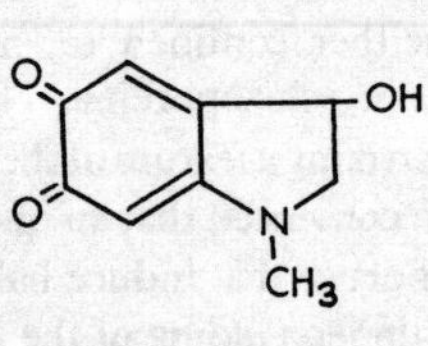

Adrenochrome

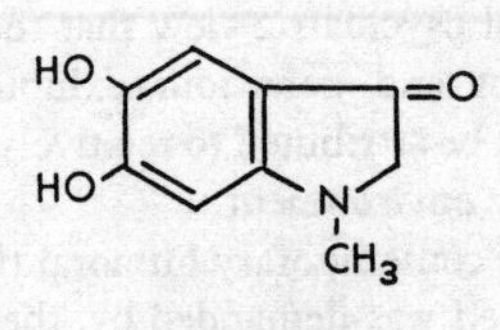

Adrenolutin

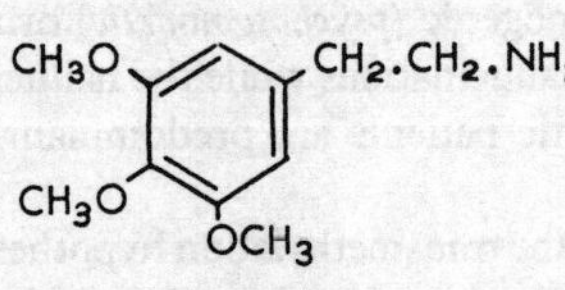

Mescaline

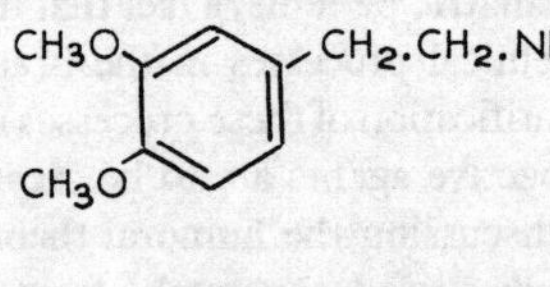

3,4 Dimethoxyphenylethylamine
(DMPEA)

Compounds related to serotonin

Lysergic acid diethylamide (LSD 25) : formula on p. 290

Harmine and harmaline : see Table 32.7 (p. 577)

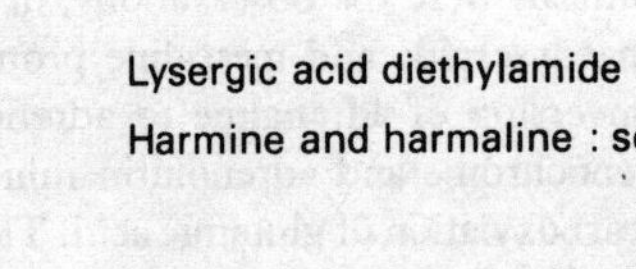

N,N-Dimethyltryptamine

5-methoxydimethyltryptamine

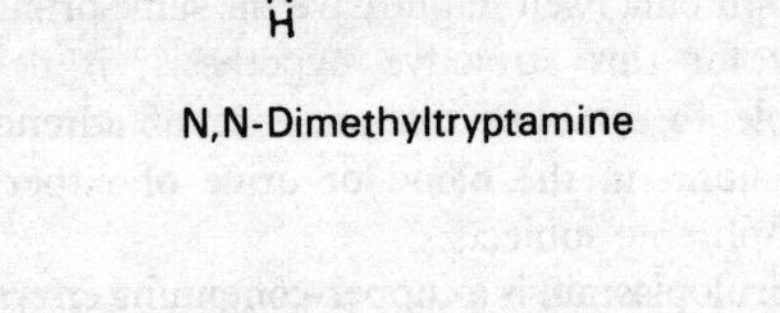

Bufotenin

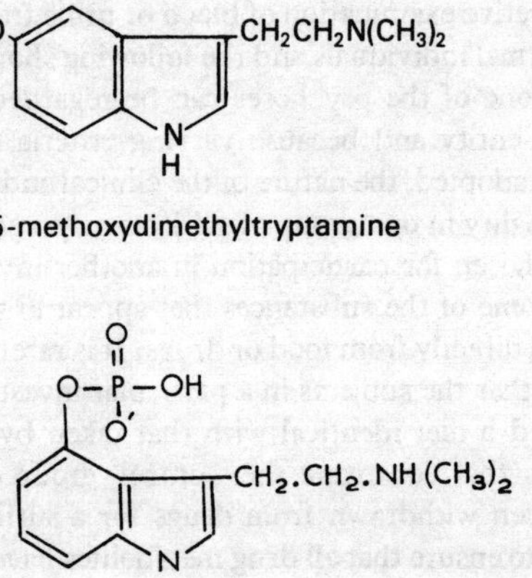

Psilocybin

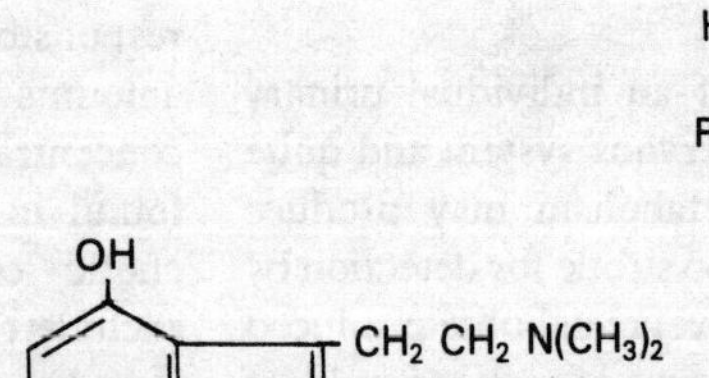

Psilocin

Fig. 32.1 Substances that might act as, or be related to, endogenous schizogens.

but its nature is not clear and not all investigators have been able to confirm the observations on which the taraxein hypothesis was founded.

A recent hypothesis attributes schizophrenia to the production of phenylethylamine (Sandler and Reynolds, 1976). This substance, which has amphetamine-like activity, is a product of normal metabolic activity but it is rapidly oxidized by monoamine oxidase so that it normally exerts no pharmacological activity. In schizophrenia, it is suggested, its destruction is retarded so that its amphetamine-like properties can now manifest themselves. The fact that some authorities have detected depressed monoamine oxidase activity in schizophrenic subjects may be relevant to this hypothesis.

The transmethylation hypothesis

In 1952, Osmond and Smythies pointed out, in what must now be regarded as a classical paper, that mescaline (Fig. 32.1), a powerfully hallucinogenic substance, has structural affinities with the catecholamines. The distinguishing feature of mescaline is the presence of methoxy groups in the ring and Osmond and Smythies pointed out that since an N-methylating enzyme is in any event required for the physiological conversion of noradrenaline to adrenaline, it would be in no way surprising if some individuals were found to carry an aberrant form of the enzyme that could effect ring O-methylation as well as N-methylation in the side chain and so bring about the production of mescaline or an analogous substance such as 3,4 dimethoxyphenylethylamine (DMPEA) from, say, dopamine or phenylalanine. And we must also bear in mind the possibility that catechol-O-methyltransferase (p. 260) might sometimes be capable of effecting a double O-methylation of the catechol nucleus instead of the single change it normally catalyses. Other investigators suggested that an N-methylating enzyme might be able to bring about the methylation of serotonin to bufotenin or of tryptamine to dimethyltryptamine. This latter belief was bolstered by the knowledge that many potent hallucinogens (lysergic acid diethylamide, psilocybin and psilocin, for example) are methylated indolealkylamine derivatives. And so the transmethylation hypothesis was born.

The seeds implanted by the transmethylation concept germinated first in 1962 with the arrival of the 'pink spot' hypothesis and the generation of a good deal of excitement and argument. Friedhoff and van Winkle subjected urine samples from schizophrenic patients to paper chromatography. When the paper was sprayed with ninhydrin and a modified Ehrlich reagent a pink spot appeared: it could not be detected in the chromatograms of urine collected from non-schizophrenic subjects. The pink spot was later shown, to the delight of those who sponsored the transmethylation hypothesis, to be caused by DMPEA. Unfortunately the pink spot soon fell on hard times. It was not possible to detect psychotomimetic activity in DMPEA

but, worse still, it became evident that the pink chromatographic spot could be produced by a number of drugs and their metabolites (including the very phenothiazines that had previously been given to the schizophrenic subjects in the original investigation!) and by some articles of diet. Later studies that took account of these and other complicating factors completely failed to substantiate the belief that DMPEA is uniquely restricted to the urine of schizophrenic subjects. Some very recent work by Friedhoff and his colleagues has indicated that this condemnation of the pink spot experiments was perhaps a little hasty (Friedhoff *et al*, 1977) but even the complete demise of the pink spot would not signal the end of the transmethylation hypothesis. Dimethyltryptamine and 5-methoxydimethyltryptamine, for instance, are powerful hallucinogens in man (unlike DMPEA) and both substances have been detected in human urine. Although it is true that schizophrenic subjects seem to excrete no more of these hallucinogens than do normal individuals (indeed, some reports indicate that they excrete less) this is not to say that all areas of the brains of schizophrenic individuals necessarily elaborate the same amount of the schizotoxins as do those of non-schizophrenic subjects or that they respond to them in the same way. Moreover, transmethylation reactions could theoretically generate a large number of putative schizotoxins which have not yet been identified.

We have already referred to difficulties of using urine analysis to detect the production of brain constituents and a number of other approaches have been made in efforts to test the transmethylation hypothesis. One such approach was initiated by Pollin, Cardon and Kety (1961) who argued that if schizophrenia were associated with the production of a methylated metabolite it should be possible to being about an exacerbation of the disease by manoeuvres that encourage methylation. Their expectations seemed to be realized by experiments in which methionine (a methyl donor) together with a monoamine oxidase inhibitor was given to schizophrenic subjects whose condition invariably became worse as a result. This study is almost unique in the annals of psychochemical research in that many other workers have confirmed the effect of methionine and none has been able to contradict it. Unfortunately the observation does not provide unequivocal evidence that the aggravation of the schizophrenic condition is the result of accelerated methylation reactions. Moreover, hopes that methionine-free diets or the administration of large doses of nicotinamide (which might be expected to inhibit methylation reactions by itself taking up the methyl groups) would exert a beneficial effect in schizophrenic patients, have not been fulfilled.

Since serotonin derivatives appear to be rather better candidates for the role of endogenous schizotoxin than do those related to the catecholamines, considerable efforts have been made to identify enzymes that might specifically effect the N-methylation of indolealkylamines. Axelrod

(1961) did identify an enzyme capable of transferring methyl groups from S-adenosylmethionine (p. 67) to tryptamine and 5-methoxytryptamine *in vitro*. The significance of the enzyme in the intact animal is still obscure but there is certainly no evidence that it is more (or less) active in schizophrenic subjects.

Reference has already been made to the possibility that catechol-O-methyltransferase might be involved in methylation reactions leading to the production of schizotoxins and it is interesting that the activity of this enzyme in the ghosts of red cells taken from schizophrenic patients is higher than it is in those from normal subjects. Such a difference has not, however, been detected in the activity of the enzyme in the brain.

Thus, the transmethylation hypothesis, attractive though it is, is not strongly supported by the available experimental evidence but a final judgment must await the outcome of more extensive investigations into the subject.

Transmitter hypotheses

The view that schizophrenia is the result of disturbances in transmitter function was first mooted at about the time when the transmethylation hypothesis first saw the light of day. In 1954, Gaddum and Woolley independently pointed out that lysergic acid diethylamide (lysergide; LSD) antagonized the action of serotonin on isolated tissues. They argued that a similar antagonistic action exerted at serotonin receptors in the brain might account for the powerfully psychotomimetic state induced by lysergide and that, therefore, schizophrenia itself might arise as a result of a breakdown in transmission processes mediated by serotonin. The argument received some reinforcement (as, of course, did the transmethylation hypothesis) from the structural similarities between serotonin and a number of other hallucinogenic substances. The later discovery that 2-bromolysergic acid diethylamide (BOL)—a serotonin antagonist as judged by its action on isolated tissues—had no psychotomimetic activity did not seriously weaken the serotonin hypothesis because it was shown that regions of the brain sensitive to lysergide were not so readily accessible to the halogenated compound. On the other hand (and in spite of brave attempts to prove that it was possible) the properties of the then newly discovered anti-schizophrenia drugs could not be convincingly accommodated in theories that attributed schizophrenia to serotonin deficiency: reserpine depletes the brain of its serotonin while chlorpromazine has some antiserotonin activity. Moreover the administration of tryptophan (which might be expected to increase supplies of serotonin at the synapse) does not improve the condition of schizophrenic patients though it is sometimes effective in depressive states. The totality of present evidence indicates that defects in the serotonin system play no more than, at most, a minor role in the genesis of schizophrenia.

As interest in serotonin's role waned that in dopamine's role waxed and evidence that has been amassed during the past few years provides persuasive—if not yet fully convincing—support for the view that schizophrenia is associated with the presence of greater than normal amounts of dopamine at central synapses that utilize this transmitter substance.

Observations relating to the dopamine hypothesis can be conveniently grouped into a number of separate categories as follows:

a. Large, or frequently repeated doses, of amphetamine induce a toxic psychosis that strongly resembles paranoid schizophrenia. Amphetamine, an indirectly acting sympathomimetic amine, owes the major part of its activity to an ability to increase the amount of transmitter at noradrenergic and dopaminergic synapses. There is a general belief that, so far as the generation of schizophrenia like signs is concerned, the accumulation of dopamine is more important than that of noradrenaline although not all the experimental evidence that is customarily invoked to support this belief is as totally convincing as is sometimes supposed. For instance, in an experiment frequently referred to, Snyder (1973) demonstrated that the two stereoisomers of amphetamine were apparently equally well taken up by dopamine synaptosomes from the corpus striatum whereas only the dextrorotatory compound displayed a high affinity for noradrenaline synaptosomes. Since the two isomers appear to induce a toxic psychosis with equal ease, Snyder's results provided powerful support for the dopamine hypothesis. Unfortunately, though, recent attempts to confirm his findings have so far been unsuccessful. But other support for dopamine's role in the production of the amphetamine psychosis has been forthcoming.

In experimental animals, amphetamine stimulates locomotor activity and also causes stereotypy (p. 277). The latter response—which recalls similar behaviour in schizophrenic patients and can therefore be regarded as having the same origin as human schizophrenia—is attributable solely to dopamine: head turning, compulsive chewing and other characteristic stereotyped movements can be evoked by injecting dopamine directly into the basal ganglia. Apomorphine, an agonist at dopamine receptors, has a similar action but noradrenaline is without effect (Barnett, 1975). Drugs effective in the treatment of schizophrenia (antipsychotic or neuroleptic agents, p. 548) abolish stereotypy in animals given amphetamine.

b. There is evidence that L-DOPA can precipitate schizophrenic attacks or aggravate a pre-existing psychosis and that α-methyl-p-tyrosine (which inhibits catecholamine synthesis, p. 290) potentiates the action of antipsychotic drugs. The supposition that these responses are the results of effects on dopamine synthesis (rather than on that of noradrenaline) is based largely on other evidence that seems to implicate dopamine and not noradrenaline in the aetiology of schizophrenia. It must, in any event, be remembered that studies of this type are inevitably of an indirect nature: because a drug is known to have a particular action (an influence on catecholamine synthesis in this instance) it is rather gratuitously assumed that all the responses it evokes are necessarily a consequence of its known action. This need not be so and the dopamine hypothesis would receive a much more powerful boost from a successful direct demonstration of enhanced dopamine activity in the schizophrenic patient. Unfortunately, all attempts to provide this direct demonstration have so far failed. The concentration of homovanillic acid (the principal metabolite of dopamine) in the cerebrospinal fluid of schizophrenic subjects appears to be no different from that in normal individuals and examination of post mortem material has yielded no evidence of any difference in the activity of the enzymes involved in the synthesis and catabolism of the catecholamines apart from one provocative, but so far unconfirmed suggestion that dopamine-ß-hydroxylase (the enzyme that promotes the conversion of dopamine to noradrenaline) is significantly deficient in schizophrenic subjects (Wise, Baden and Stein, 1974).

c. We have already seen that the neurotransmitter hypothesis of schizophrenia was born from the observation that lysergic acid diethylamide is a serotonin antagonist. Although the particular speculation to which this observation gave rise was found to be untenable, lysergide has now been brought back into the fold by the finding that it too is a dopamine agonist (Pieri, Pieri and Haefely, 1974).

d. Much the most compelling evidence in favour of the dopamine hypothesis comes from a consideration of the properties of the antipsychotic drugs. It seems that they all cause blockade of dopamine receptors (or in the case of reserpine and its congeners deplete dopaminergic neurones of their transmitter) and while it is true that many of them also antagonize the actions of other neurotransmitter agents some very effective drugs such as haloperidol and pimozide are rather specific dopamine antagonists. The antipsychotic drugs also abolish the stereotypy caused by amphetamine or apomorphine and attributable, as we have seen, to an action on dopamine receptors. Moreover, except to the extent that anticholinergic activity counters the effect (p. 551), the drugs also give rise to Parkinsonian side effects, a condition that is caused by dopamine deficiency. Dopamine exerts its central actions by way of a specific adenylate cyclase (p. 186) and the antipsychotic drugs can be shown to bind to this enzyme many of them to an extent that parallels their therapeutic efficacy. Further evidence that the drugs influence dopamine receptors comes from the observation that they sometimes induce galactorrhoea in response to prolactin release. Prolactin release is normally inhibited by dopamine.

All the antipsychotic drugs increase the turnover of dopamine in the brain, an effect that probably represents a compensatory increase in synthesis in response to an effective deficiency of dopamine at the receptors. There is a very high degree of correlation between the ability of an antipsychotic drug to antagonise apomorphine activity and its stimulant effect on dopamine synthesis. This stimulation of dopamine synthesis is partly responsible for the tardive dyskinesia (p. 552) that may arise as a late complication of antipsychotic drug therapy.

In view of the near overwhelming evidence that antipsychotic agents owe their effectiveness to an antidopamine action it is difficult to escape the conclusion that schizophrenia is the result, at least partly, of overactivity on dopaminergic synapses. The origin of this activity is still a matter for speculation. Some possibilities are discussed below but we must remember also that it might, after all, be generated by a methylated metabolite!

Other agents. It would be unwise to conclude that dopamine is the only mediator of processes whose disturbance provokes schizophrenia. All forms of complex nervous activity require the participation of a multiplicity of synapses and it must be rare indeed for all the synapses that subserve a particular function to be of only one chemical type. It is by no means impossible that a disturbance of transmission processes mediated by agents other than dopamine could have equally catastrophic effects. Moreover disturbances in dopaminergic activity might themselves be secondary to dysfunction in another transmitter system. The fact that all our present day antipsychotic agents are dopamine antagonists might be no more than coincidental and later generations of antipsychotic drugs might antagonize other synaptic transmitter substances. After all, drugs that block adrenaline ß-receptors did not appear until many years after a whole range of α blocking agents had made their appearance.

Some authorities believe, as did the ancient philosophers, that the harmonious functioning of the brain depends on the maintenance of a proper balance between opposing neurohumoral systems. This condition certainly seems to obtain in the extrapyramidal system where opposing cholinergic and dopaminergic mechanisms work together to maintain normal muscle tone. Dopamine deficiency upsets the balance so that the cholinergic mechanisms become dominant. The consequence of this is the appearance of Parkinsonism (p. 588). The proper balance can be restored, and the Parkinsonism relieved, either by promoting dopamine synthesis or by giving atropine-like drugs to counter the actions of the unopposed cholinergic system. A similar cholinergic-dopaminergic balance elsewhere in the brain may well be upset in schizophrenia: it is known for instance that physostigmine (p. 213) which permits the accumulation of acetylcholine at cholinergic synapses, potentiates the therapeutic effect of antipsychotic drugs.

We must now glance, however briefly, at some of the other humoral hypotheses that have sought to explain the origin of schizophrenia.

Attempts have been made to conscript almost all the newly discovered endogenous substances—and some older ones—into the ranks of the substances that might play an aetiological role in schizophrenia. Among these candidates are melatonin, the prostaglandins, folic acid and the endorphins.

Melatonin is elaborated in the pineal body (p. 332) and it has been pointed out that disturbances of serotonin metabolism there might lead to the production not of melatonin but of hallucinogenic substances structurally similar to harmaline (Fig. 32.1). Melatonin is the 'lightening factor' which prevents excessive melanin deposition in the skin and some slight corroboration of the melatonin hypothesis comes from the observation that schizophrenic patients tend to show deeper pigmentation of the skin than do non-schizophrenic individuals. Unfortunately for the melatonin hypothesis, melanin deposition is a not uncommon consequence of antipsychotic drug therapy so that in some instances at least the skin pigmentation of the schizophrenic is a consequence of the treatment he has received and is not a witness to the cause of his trouble.

The prostaglandins are involved in so many regulatory functions in the body and such a number of conditions with highly diverse antecedents are designated as 'schizophrenia' that it is hardly surprising that it has been possible to demonstrate several abnormal responses to the prostaglandins in schizophrenic subjects. Thus, schizophrenic patients are said to be less likely than psychiatrically normal individuals to develop inflammatory conditions, such as arthritis, that are known to be mediated by the prostaglandins while their platelets form cyclic AMP less readily on exposure to prostaglandin E_1. It has also been pointed out that prolactin secretion, which is usually regarded as a side effect of antipsychotic drug therapy, stimulates the formation of prostaglandins and might therefore play a part in the therapeutic action of these drugs.

The hypothesis that schizophrenia arises from, or is aggravated by, folic acid deficiency is derived from the old observations that schizophrenia is rather less likely to develop in victims of grand mal epilepsy than it is in the rest of the population, that the action of antiepileptic drugs hints at a common mechanism directed towards preventing the accumulation of excessive amounts of folic acid in the brain and that schizophrenia-like symptoms have appeared in some individuals who have received prolonged treatment with anticonvulsant drugs. This hypothesis is mentioned elsewhere in this book (p. 534): in its present rather naive form it links folic acid excess and deficiency with epilepsy and schizophrenia respectively.

There is some evidence that the endorphins (p. 437) reach higher than average concentrations in the cerebrospinal fluid of schizophrenic patients and that average values are regained when clinical recovery occurs. The supposition that schizophrenia is related to an excessive production or release of endorphins receives some indirect support from an unexpected quarter: for many years some victims of schizophrenia have avoided wheat products in the firm belief, which has received but scant support from their scientific and medical advisers, that this dietary abstention leads to an amelioration of their psychosis. It now transpires that opioid like substances are produced by the intestinal breakdown of gluten. If they escape final digestion they will, presumably, be absorbed into the blood and brain.

Finally, mention has to be made of views still held by a few authorities that link schizophrenia with zinc deficiency or with disordered histamine metabolism in the brain.

Very recently, Horrobin has made a commendable but probably premature attempt to link the much favoured dopamine hypothesis and a number of the fringe hypotheses to provide a comprehensive thesis (Horrobin, 1979). He suggests (and he has some experimental evidence to support all his proposals) that zinc deficiency, melatonin lack and the opioids derived from wheat all suppress the synthesis of prostaglandin E_1 and that the resulting prostaglandin deficiency releases dopaminergic activity. Another consequence of the prostaglandin deficit might be hyperactivity of B-lymphocytes (p. 398) with the production of the hypersensitivity to a variety of allergens which has long been recognized as a feature of the schizophrenic condition.

It is a pity that so many of the observations that Horrobin invokes to support his challenging hypothesis have not been generally confirmed and that, in any event, they can be interpreted in several different ways.

The affective psychoses

Since about 1960, transmitter hypotheses of the affective psychoses have attracted increasing attention. Like those relating to schizophrenia, they have received their most solid support from studies on the mode of action of drugs that have been discovered to exert a useful influence on the course of these disorders.

Over the years, the most widely used antidepressant drugs have been the monoamine oxidase inhibitors, the tricyclic antidepressant agents and (until relatively recently) amphetamine. All these compounds in their various ways bring about the accumulation of noradrenaline, serotonin and (less often) dopamine at central synapses. Conversely, drugs such as reserpine which are known to deplete neurones of monoamine transmitters can produce a profound depression in individuals with no previous history of psychiatric disorder. It is but a short (if not absolutely logical) step from these observations to a conviction that the types of depression that respond to antidepressant drug therapy are themselves the result of a deficiency of one or other of the monoamine transmitters at strategic sites in the brain.

The hypothesis that noradrenaline is a key transmitter in the systems responsible for generating the affective state was first formally proposed by Schildkraut in 1965. He is still a major champion of the hypothesis but he has always conceded—and indeed has emphasized—that other mediators are likely to be involved too. From what has already been written it will be evident that the most likely alternative (or additional) mediator is serotonin.

The most direct evidence supporting the view that at least some forms of depression are associated with and may well be caused by a noradrenaline deficit has been provided by measuring the amount of 3-methoxy-4-hydroxyphenylglycol (3-methoxy-4-hydroxyphenylethanediol, MHPG, p. 260) in urine and cerebrospinal fluid. This compound, it is generally agreed, is the principal metabolite of neuronal noradrenaline and it has been estimated that—usually among transmitter metabolites—half of the MHPG in the urine comes from the brain. In a number of investigations, Schildkraut and his colleagues have demonstrated that in bipolar depression (p. 538), MHPG excretion falls during depressed phases, rises during manic phases and resumes a normal value during periods of spontaneous remission (Greenspan and Schildkraut, 1970). Several independent groups of investigators (but not all those who have studied the problem) have confirmed these findings and some have been able to show, in addition, that the successful drug therapy restores normal patterns of metabolite excretion. It is particularly interesting that these changes in excretion precede obvious clinical improvement. Thus it cannot be claimed that the increased MHPG excretion is the result of increased noradrenergic activity consequent on the patient's more lively behaviour.

Depression is not a single or a simple condition and attempts have been made to relate depressed MHPG excretion to particular clinical types of depression. It seems that in addition to patients in the depression phase of a bipolar illness, those with depression arising in the course of schizophrenia also excrete lower than normal amounts of the noradrenaline metabolite. On the other hand, other patients, among whom are included those suffering from reactive depression, are more likely to exhibit no sign of abnormal noradrenaline activity. Whether or not it is finally confirmed that MPHG excretion is related to the clinical diagnosis, measurement of the metabolite may well prove to be a guide to the type of drug therapy most likely to be successful in individual patients. Some of the antidepressant drugs have a preferential action on one or other of the monoamine transmitters and there is some evidence that compounds that inhibit noradrenaline re-uptake more readily than that of serotonin might be more effective in patients whose MHPG excretion is low than it is in those who eliminate normal amounts of the metabolite in the urine. By the same token, drugs that preferentially inhibit serotonin reuptake are, according to some authorities, better for patients with lower than normal concentrations of 5-hydroxyindoleacetic acid (see below) in their cerebrospinal fluid (Maas, 1975).

On the apparently reasonable grounds that the cerebrospinal fluid is nearer to the brain and is less likely to be contaminated with material from other sources, some workers have examined monoamine metabolites in the lumbar spinal fluid instead of in the urine. Many of their studies have involved patients who have been given probenecid (p. 459). This drug prevents the egress of substances from the cerebrospinal fluid so that the rate of accumulation of metabolites after probenecid reflects the 'turnover' of the parent amine. This approach to the study of cerebral metabolites is not without its drawbacks, the most serious of which is that the spinal cord contributes very significantly to the total metabolite content of the lumbar fluid. In addition, probenecid stimulates the synthesis of the monoamines and both practical and ethical considerations preclude the collection of fluid as frequently as would be desirable in a well ordered study. Considerations such as these might explain why studies of the MHPG content of cerebrospinal fluid in depressed patients have yielded less consistent results than have the urine studies (Schildkraut, 1978).

If depression and mania are the respective results of noradrenaline deficiency and excess at critical central synapses, it should be possible to influence the course of these maladies by means of substances that promote or prevent the production of the catecholamine. L-DOPA, the precursor of dopamine and noradrenaline (p. 258), α-methyl-p-tryosine, which inhibits catecholamine synthesis (p. 290) and fusaric acid, which inhibits dopamine-ß-hydroxylase and thus the conversion of dopamine to noradrenaline, have all been studied from this point of view. Such effects as have been observed have been in general accordance with expectations based on the catecholamine hypothesis but none of the compounds has a sufficiently regular or powerful action to warrant its use as a therapeutic agent.

In recent years, the concentration of monoamines and of some of the enzymes responsible for their synthesis and catabolism have been measured in various parts of the brain of recently deceased depressed patients. As far as noradrenaline and its enzymes are concerned, the results can be described, at best, as suggestive but it must be remembered that investigations of this kind are bedevilled by a number of uncontrollable complicating factors (age at and cause of death, previous drug treatment, time since death, etc.) that militate against the emergence of unequivocal conclusions from the results of a relatively few experiments. Similar remarks apply to the few studies that have hinted at reductions in the activity of catechol O-methyltransferase in the erythrocytes and an increase in the activity of monoamine oxidase in the platelets of depressed patients.

The observations that led to to the original formulation of the catecholamine hypothesis could be equally readily explained on the supposition that depressive illnesses might reflect a deficiency of serotonin and we must now enquire into this possibility. Measuring the amount of 5-hydroxyindoleacetic acid (the ultimate serotonin metabolite, p. 528) in the urine of depressed patients has proved to be less profitable than the corresponding exercise with MHPG. However, no more than 10 per cent of the urinary metabolite is derived from cerebral sources and the disappointing outcome of urinary studies probably reflects inadequacies in the experimental method rather than in the serotonin hypothesis itself. A little more success has attended investigations into the 5-hydroxyindoleacetic acid content of lumbar spinal fluid notwithstanding the disadvantages of this type of study to which attention has already been drawn. A compilation of the results of 14 recent inquiries (Murphy, Campbell and Costa, 1978) reveals that all but two of them reported lower concentrations of the metabolite in depressed patients than in normal subjects, the deficit averaging some 33 per cent. The impact of these figures is somewhat blunted by the facts that only four of the reported differences between the two groups of subjects reached statistical significance and that the largest study of them all revealed virtually identical concentrations of 5-hydroxyindoleacetic acid in the cerebrospinal fluid of normal and depressed individuals. It may well be, of course, that the figures are rendered less impressive by virtue of the possibility that only particular groups of depressed patients owe their condition to serotonin deficiency. It is interesting to note, in this connection, recent evidence that low levels of 5-hydroxyindoleacetic acid occur more frequently in male than in female subjects and are especially likely to be found among depressed patients who have attempted suicide (Asberg, Traskman and Thoren, 1976). It also seems that patients afflicted with bipolar depressive illnesses are the most likely to show evidence of reduced serotonin activity.

Like urinary MHPG, 5-hydroxyindoleacetic acid concentrations in spinal fluid may have some value as predictors of therapeutic responses: von Praag (1975) showed that depressed patients whose lumbar fluid accumulated the metabolite only slowly after probenecid were more likely to show a favourable response to chlorimipramine (which operates predominantly on the serotoninergic system) than were those with an apparently normal serotonin metabolism.

The effects of substances that promote or prevent the synthesis of serotonin are rather more striking than are those of substances that similarly influence the production of noradrenaline. Some investigators have found tryptophan, the natural precursor of serotonin to be so active that they have used it, alone or in association with chlorimipramine, as a therapeutic agent. It is said (by those who believe that it is pharmacologically active) to be more effective in bipolar patients: it would be interesting to know whether it is also more effective in those with depressed levels of 5-hydroxyindoleacetic acid in their cerebrospinal fluid. Strangely enough, 5-hydroxytryptophan, the immediate precursor of serotonin (p. 328) seems to have very little effect on the course of depressive illnesses of any type perhaps because it is taken up and decarboxylated rather indiscriminately by central neurones whether or not they are serotoninergic in function. *p*-Chlorophenylalanine (p. 327) inhibits tryptophan hydroxylase and so interferes with the synthesis of serotonin. A number of reports indicate that it can reverse the therapeutic effect of antidepressant drugs and suppress the mania that sometimes develops in the course of antidepressant drug therapy. α-Methyl-*p*-tyrosine, which inhibits the synthesis of noradrenaline, is apparently inactive in these respects. It must not, however, be too readily assumed that the effects of *p*-chlorophenylalanine are the exclusive result of an interference with serotonin synthesis because the drug has actions that are independent of its ability to inhibit tryptophan hydroxylase. It must also be added that neither *p*-chlorophenylalanine nor methysergide (a serotonin antagonist, p. 334) appear to be able to influence the manic phases in patients suffering from manic depression.

Post mortem analyses of the brains of successful suicides have provided some evidence that serotonin and 5-hydroxyindoleacetic acid appear in subnormal quantities in some or all parts of the brain of depressed subjects. Some workers assert, while others deny, that the platelets of depressed patients accumulate smaller quantities of serotonin than do those of healthy subjects.

There is some disputed evidence that the concentrations of homovanillic acid, the final product of dopamine metabolism (p. 262), in lumbar fluid taken from depressed and manic patients are respectively lower and higher than those in psychiatrically normal subjects. If it transpires that dopamine really is involved in the generation of affective disorders this will not be incompatible with its presumed aetiological role in schizophrenia. The two groups of disorder may well have different loci of origin and it is interesting that the antipsychotic drugs that owe their therapeutic action to dopamine antagonism can be applied to the control of severely manic patients. Moreover, depressive episodes not uncommonly occur in schizophrenic subjects, suggesting perhaps that a disturbed dopamine metabolism might sometimes result in the production of interludes of dopamine deficiency in a brain that at other times is suffering the consequences of dopamine excess. Another parallel between schizophrenia and the affective disorders is provided by the observation that the cerebrospinal fluid of manic subjects, like that of schizophrenic patients, contains enhanced concentrations of the endorphins. On the other hand it is true to say that inhibition of dopamine uptake is not a property of the most successful antidepressant drugs.

It is not too difficult to understand how a sudden and unforeseeable breakdown of a metabolic mechanism could cause the appearance, apparently completely out of the blue, of a psychotic state as is the way with endogenous depressions. Reactive depression, however, a condition in which there is an apparently obvious precipitating cause, presents us with a more complex problem when we ask how an external event such as the unexpected death of a near relative can produce a prolonged state of profound depression. It might be that humoral mechanisms are not involved at all (much of the evidence that supports the monoaminergic hypothesis comes from an examination of patients with endogenous disorders) or, alternatively, that the nervous activity generated by the stimulus and which reveals itself even in normal individuals as a feeling of intense misery is prolonged and potentiated as a result of an inherent deficiency in inhibitory systems, presumably humorally mediated, whose function is to keep the evoked activity within bounds.

The hypothalamus is a focal point of the limbic system (p. 167). It is here that external and internal stimuli can interact and here that, by way of the hypothalamo-hypophyseal link, activity in the nervous and endocrine systems is coordinated. It is well known that changes in endocrine activity can be brought about by external events that induce stress of any kind and it could be postulated that these endocrine changes might secondarily influence activity in neurohumoral systems. However, the disturbances in endocrine activity seen in depressed patients seem to be the result rather than the cause of a failure of monoamine (particularly catecholamine) function (Sachar, 1975).

To summarize the present status of the monoamine hypothesis of the affective disorders, it seems fair to say that the noradrenaline and the serotonin hypotheses have attracted equally persuasive experimental support—or equally unimpressive support if doubting readers prefer to express it so. It would seem that at least some forms of depressive illness are associated with a deficiency of either noradrenaline or of serotonin and that it might soon be possible to plan rational therapeutic regimes for individual patients on the basis of a knowledge of their particular biochemical deficiencies. Whether each of the several types of depression will be found to be associated with a unique biochemical lesion must remain an open question for the time being. Just what is implied by a transmitter deficiency excess in terms of the performance of the brain as a whole, what is the origin of the biochemical lesion and how the external factors that precipitate reactive depression can interact with the monoamine systems are questions that will probably have to wait even longer for satisfactory answers.

CLASSIFICATION OF THE PSYCHOTROPIC DRUGS

Before 1950, the few drugs available for the treatment of psychiatric disorders could be simply dichotomized into sedatives (or hypnosedatives) such as the barbiturates and the stimulants such as amphetamine. With the arrival of reserpine this simple situation became more complex because the new drug was able to calm the agitated patient without markedly depressing his level of consciousness. Reserpine was followed by many other depressant drugs reported to have minimal or only mild hypnotic activity in therapeutic doses and it became usual to describe drugs of this kind as *tranquillizers*. Many authorities further distinguished between 'major' and 'minor' tranquillizers. The former term embraced drugs of value in the treatment of severely agitated psychotic patients while the latter referred to tranquillizers of therapeutic use only in the neuroses. This separation of tranquillizers from other types of depressant drug was never entirely satisfactory: chlorpromazine, for long the favourite major tranquillizer, certainly has hypnotic activity while the properties of some of the barbiturate hypnotics are virtually indistinguishable from those of some of the drugs that were generally classified as minor tranquillizers. Consequently the word 'tranquillizer' is now falling into disuse except when it is employed in a very general sense. Some of its more bizarre synonyms—*ataractic, pacific calmative* and *peace pill*, for instance—are also moribund but *neuroleptic* and *psycholeptic* (both of which relate to drugs that would previously have been categorized as major tranquillizers) still enjoy some currency.

Almost simultaneously with the early tranquillizers, new agents for the treatment of depression arrived on the scene. Unlike amphetamine, these substances had no stimulant action in the normal individual. They were named *antidepressant* drugs. This quite rational terminology has been retained and, because drugs specific for particular psychiatric conditions are now being developed, it is becoming usual to extend it and to classify all psychotropic drugs as far as possible in terms of the disorders for which they are indicated. It is not yet possible to assign every psychotropic drug to a unique therapeutic category in this way but the classification is more satisfactory than any of its predecessors and it is sufficiently flexible to accommodate, with minor modifications, all the new drugs likely to appear in the near future.

The classification is as follows:

1. *Antipsychotic drugs.* The substances included in this group are, broadly speaking, those that were previously referred to as the major tranquillizers. They are used primarily for the treatment of schizophrenia and mania though many of them have anxiolytic actions too. The term is not entirely satisfactory on either semantic or medical grounds: 'antipsychosis' would be preferable to 'antipsychotic' and schizophrenia and mania are not the only types of psychosis. As we have already noted 'psycholeptic' and 'neuroleptic' are synonyms of 'antipsychotic' that are still commonly used.

2. *Antimania drugs.* Membership of this group should properly be restricted to those drugs that are used specifically for the treatment of mania and hypomania but, as we have noted, some of the antipsychotic drugs have a broad spectrum of activity that enables them to be employed as antimania agents.

3. *Anxiolytic drugs.* As the rather unhappy adjective implies, these drugs are prescribed for the relief of anxiety. Anxiety is the most common of the neuroses and the drugs categorized as anxiolytic are those previously described as the minor tranquillizers. This category of drugs is again not completely exclusive: propranolol and chlorpromazine, for instance, can claim to be considered as both antipsychotic and anxiolytic agents. 'Antianxiety' is now gaining a foothold as a synonym for 'anxiolytic'. This change is to be welcomed and its extension encouraged.

4. *Antidepressant drugs.*

5. *Psychotomimetic drugs.* Psychotomimetic drugs (also described as *psycholytic, psychodelic* or *hallucinogenic* agents and as *schizogens*) are now of restricted therapeutic value but they are included here among the psychotherapeutic agents because they still find favour as diagnostic tools by some psychiatrists.

ANTIPSYCHOTIC DRUGS

The antipsychotic agents are best classified in terms of their chemical structures. In the following list, and for the benefit of those to whom chemical names are anathema, the prototypical member of each class is named in brackets.

1. The phenothiazines (*chlorpromazine*)
2. The *Rauwolfia* alkaloids (*reserpine*)
3. The butyrophenones (*haloperidol*)
4. The thioxanthenes (*chlorprothixene*)
5. Propranolol
6. Newer drugs

The phenothiazines

More than 3000 phenothiazine derivatives have been synthesized and at least one hundred of them are in clinical use though not all as psychotropic drugs. In this chapter, chlorpromazine, the most extensively used and intensively studied member of the group, is discussed in detail and some of the others are accorded a superficial treatment.

CHLORPROMAZINE

During the development of the antihistamine drugs (p. 345) it was found that promethazine exerted both sedative and antihistamine actions. Promethazine is a phenothiazine derivative and a systematic study of other compounds

of this class by Charpentier and his colleagues revealed that chlorpromazine (Table 32.1) had even more pronounced sedative properties with relatively little antihistamine activity. Chlorpromazine was introduced into clinical medicine by Laborit in 1950. At first it was added to mixtures of pethidine and atropine or promethazine to produce the so-called *lytic cocktail* which was popular in France as a preoperative medication and for producing hypothermia for major surgery. Observations on patients given this mixture, or chlorpromazine alone, made it clear that the new drug differed from the sedatives that had been used previously in that it did not noticeably depress the level of consciousness. Nevertheless, the patient became calm and apparently unperturbed by his surroundings, or by the ordeal that faced him. His air of indifference was reminiscent of that seen in patients who had been leucotomized. Considerations such as these led to the introduction of the term 'tranquillizer' to describe chlorpromazine and some other psychotropic drugs. As we have already seen (p. 547), the term was always suspect and it has now virtually disappeared from the psychopharmacologist's vocabulary.

The therapeutic potentiality of chlorpromazine was first fully appreciated by Delay in 1952. He used the drug to quieten maniacal patients and later to treat other forms of psychosis. The success of this early work led to the widespread use of chlorpromazine; it has been estimated that during the ten years following its debut as a psychotropic drug, it was mentioned in 10000 publications and was administed to no fewer than 50 million patients throughout the world. It is impossible to exaggerate the impact that chlorpromazine has made on the treatment of psychiatric conditions, if only because of the way in which it has enabled hospital staffs to control disturbed and violent patients without having to have recourse to more distasteful methods of restraint.

An exhaustive but interesting account of the discovery of chlorpromazine and its antipsychotic and other properties is provided in a recent monograph (Swazey, 1975).

Pharmacological properties of chlorpromazine

Although the therapeutic actions and some of the side effects of all the antipsychotic drugs are undoubtedly attributable to their ability to interact with dopamine receptors in the brain (p.543), they also have other actions. This is particularly so in the case of chlorpromazine. Indeed, in respect of its pharmacological properties, chlorpromazine is the most protean of drugs. This fact is even commemorated in its best known proprietary name: Largactil is ingeniously derived from 'large (number of) actions'.

Except where the text indicates otherwise, it can be assumed that all the phenothiazine drugs mentioned in this chapter have properties that are at least qualitatively the same as those of chlorpromazine itself. Nevertheless, not all of them are employed as antipsychotic agents. As is indicated in Table 32.2, some of them are used as hypnotics, others for the relief of anxiety and yet others as antiemetic agents.

Antihumoral activity. Chlorpromazine is structurally similar to promethazine (see pp. 348 and 554) and it has some antihistamine activity. It is a weak antagonist of acetylcholine and 5-hydroxytryptamine. On the other hand, it is a moderately active antagonist of adrenaline and noradrenaline at α receptors, its potency in this respect equalling that of ergotamine. The metabolic actions of adrenaline are unaffected by chlorpromazine.

Blockade of α receptors by chlorpromazine can be demonstrated in isolated preparations and its effects can also be seen in the intact animal. In therapeutic doses, the drug sometimes causes postural hypotension as a result of its suppressing the carotid sinus pressor reflex. The resting blood pressure may also be depressed. These effects arise entirely from blockade of the peripheral α receptors and not to an interference with ganglionic transmission.

A particularly interesting example of chlorpromazine's antiadrenaline action is provided by the observation that it antagonizes the excitatory actions of the catecholamines—but not those of acetylcholine, histamine and 5-hydroxytryptamine—on single neurones in the central nervous system.

Actions on the nervous system. Chlorpromazine influences activity at a number of sites in the nervous system. It is a more potent local anaesthetic than procaine and it has some neuromuscular blocking activity. It inhibits monosynaptic reflexes in the intact animal but this probably arises from an action on the higher reaches of the nervous system.

In the *medulla,* by virtue of its antidopamine action, chlorpromazine depresses the chemosensitive trigger zone of the vomiting centre but other medullary centres are spared.

A number of the effects of chlorpromazine administration are referable to a depression of function in the *hypothalamus.* These include hypothermia, suppression of sham rage reactions, galactorrhoea, inhibition of growth hormone and gonadotrophin release from the pituitary gland and an increased appetite. The last mentioned effect is probably caused, at least in part, by a depression of the satiety centre which is located in the hypothalamus while the galactorrhoea results from the removal of the restraint that dopamine normally exerts on prolactin secretion (p. 777). Large doses of chlorpromazine inhibit the release of corticotrophin from the pituitary gland but this is of no functional significance. More moderate doses may stimulate the release of corticotrophin and a number of investigations have led to the conclusion that chlorpromazine increases the ability of animals to resist stress.

In the control of emotional responses, the hypothalamus is closely associated with the *reticular* and the *limbic*

systems. Chlorpromazine inhibits dopamine action in the limbic system but it depresses the activity of the reticular activating system. This last mentioned effect presumably accounts for the hypnotic effect of large therapeutic doses of the drug. Chlorpromazine also influences activity in descending reticular fibres as is evidenced by the fact that symptoms similar to those that occur in Parkinson's disease are not infrequently seen in patients receiving chlorpromazine. The effects of the phenothiazines on muscle tone are considered in more detail later (p. 551).

As might be predicted from its actions on the reticular activating system, chlorpromazine augments the hypnotic effect of barbiturates. Thus it prolongs the sleeping time of animals that have been given hexobarbitone. This action occurs independently of the hypothermia that is also produced. Chlorpromazine also prolongs the anaesthetic state induced by some general anaesthetics and the hypnosis caused by alcohol. It potentiates and prolongs the analgesic effect of morphine and aspirin and of compounds derived from them. Although it protects animals against audiogenic convulsions, chlorpromazine does not regularly behave as an anticonvulsant drug. Indeed, it sometimes accentuates the electroencephalographic abnormalities of epilepsy.

Chlorpromazine causes the appearance of slow wave activity in the electroencephalographic record similar to that which occurs during sleep. It does not modify the electrical activity of isolated slabs of the cerebral cortex, indicating that the electroencephalographic response in the whole animal originates in subcortical structures.

Behavioural effects. In doses equivalent to those used therapeutically in man chlorpromazine reduces the spontaneous motor activity of experimental animals. Animals otherwise fierce and difficult to handle become placid and tractable when they are given chlorpromazine. 'Startle' responses, defaecation and other responses to stress are inhibited. Human beings, as has already been indicated, become less apprehensive of impending surgical manipulations and other threats to their comfort and they show some indifference to their surroundings.

In contrast to the barbiturates (but like morphine), chlorpromazine abolishes conditioned avoidance responses without affecting the reactions to the unconditioned stimulus. Thus, rats can be trained to avoid an electric shock applied to their feet from the floor of their cage by jumping on to a rope at the sound of a bell signalling that the shock is about to be given. After chlorpromazine the animals no longer respond to the bell but they still climb on to the rope when they experience the shock. Chlorpromazine is particularly effective in blocking avoidance responses when the conditioned stimuli are auditory or visual in type.

Chlorpromazine relieves experimental neurosis and depresses operant behaviour. These actions are discussed below in connection with the procedures that are used to detect psychotropic activity in drug screening programmes.

Metabolic effects. Chlorpromazine exerts a number of actions on the metabolism of brain (and other tissues) *in vitro.* Several of these effects can only be demonstrated if the concentration of chlorpromazine in the medium is increased beyond that which is produced by therapeutic doses of the drug and they may, therefore, have little relevance to its pharmacological actions.

Unphysiologically high concentrations of chlorpromazine (and other depressant drugs) inhibit the uptake of oxygen by brain slices. However, concentrations as low as those that are present in the brain after therapeutic doses, partially or completely prevent the increase in metabolism induced by electrical stimulation of the brain slices, according to the techniques originally devised by McIlwain (see McIlwain, 1963). These results on isolated preparations suggest that chlorpromazine depresses the utilization of energy by the brain but does not affect energy production. This action is shared by other depressant drugs but chlorpromazine is active in concentrations as small as 10-20 μM.

Larger doses of chlorpromazine inhibit the activity of mitochondrial cytochrome oxidase, adenosine triphosphatase and succinic oxidase. They also uncouple oxidative phosphorylation—that is, they inhibit the formation of high energy phosphates without affecting the oxidative processes. These observations might suggest, contrary to the conclusions reached from the experiments with stimulated brain slices, that chlorpromazine is capable of interfering with energy production. There is little evidence that this is so in the intact animal: phosphocreatine stores are not depleted in animals treated with chlorpromazine and any changes that occur in the adenosine triphosphate concentration are trivial.

Chlorpromazine has some anticholinesterase activity and it has been suggested that this might explain why a few patients are, paradoxically, excited by the drug.

Chlorpromazine stabilizes cell membranes so that, to take just a few examples, nerve fibres become less easily excited, mitochondrial swelling in isotonic sucrose solution is less easily elicited and erythrocyte fragility is reduced.

More complete accounts of the metabolic effects of chlorpromazine and other depressant drugs are provided, *inter alia,* by Decsi (1964), Seeman (1966), Gordon (1967) and by Shepherd, Lader and Rodnight (1968).

Metabolism of chlorpromazine

Chlorpromazine is rapidly absorbed from the gastrointestinal tract. When it is taken by this route some of the administered dose is conjugated in the liver. It also passes rapidly into the brain. Not all parts of the brain accumulate chlorpromazine with equal avidity. Although the literature is not entirely unanimous on this point, there is evidence that the hypothalamus and brain stem take up more of the drug than does the rest of the brain.

About 90 per cent of the chlorpromazine in blood is bound to plasma protein.

The chlorpromazine that is conjugated in the liver is re-excreted in the bile into the small intestine from which it is again taken up by the liver. This portion of the administered dose (which amounts to about 30 per cent of the whole) is gradually excreted in the faeces. The remainder appears in the urine as conjugates and metabolites. Chlorpromazine can be broken down in several ways and the number of metabolites that could in theory be produced is very large indeed: at the latest count it amounted to 168. The major metabolic pathways in man involve hydroxylation in positions 3 or 7 of the phenothiazine ring (Table 32.1) and removal of one or both methyl groups from the side chain. Oxidation of the sulphur atom (which can be combined with one or more of the other changes mentioned) takes place to a limited extent. Extensive conjugation of the metabolites occurs. Urine and faeces are equally important vehicles for the excretion of chlorpromazine metabolites.

Although the plasma half-life of chlorpromazine itself is quite short (5 to 6 hours), traces of some of its metabolites can be detected in the urine for up to six months after the drug has been withdrawn.

Clinical uses of chlorpromazine

Chlorpromazine and the other psychotropic drugs became available at a time when new and more enlightened attitudes towards the treatment of mental illness were becoming widespread. Consequently some of the credit for the improved outlook for the mentally ill that has been given to pharmacotherapy may properly belong elsewhere. Nevertheless, there need be no doubt concerning the value of the psychotropic drugs. The paragraphs that follow enumerate the therapeutic uses of chlorpromazine but, as we have already indicated, most of them apply equally to the other phenothiazines.

1. The symptomatic treatment of acute schizophrenia. For this purpose, daily doses of up to 1000 mg of chlorpromazine may be required. Occasionally daily doses as high as 3000 mg are called for to control severely agitated patients. It need hardly be said that amounts as large as this should be reduced as soon as this becomes practicable and maintenance doses of chlorpromazine often need be no higher than 300-400 mg daily. At the beginning of treatment it is usual to divide the daily dose into instalments given at four-hourly intervals but later the ration for the day can be taken in one dose at bed time. While the normal route of administration is the oral one, more satisfactory results are sometimes obtained in the acutely disturbed patient if chlorpromazine is given by intramuscular injection. It should be noted that the drug causes pain when it is given by this route. Moreover, the possibil-

ity that a large intramuscular dose may cause a profound hypotension must be kept in mind and noradrenaline should always be available to deal with this emergency should it arise. In this connection it should be remembered that chlorpromazine causes α receptor blockade. Consequently, noradrenaline must be given in amounts adequate to overcome the blockade by displacing chlorpromazine from the α-sites. It should also be clear that adrenaline should never be given in attempts to correct a phenothiazine-induced hypotension lest its action on β receptors in the blood vessels fatally intensifies the hypotension.

In recent years, the intramuscular route has also been utilized for the administration of long acting phenothiazine preparations intended for the treatment of chronic schizophrenia. The best known of these drugs are fluphenazine, oenanthate and decanoate: they need to be given no more frequently than once every two to four weeks.

Chlorpromazine is less effective in chronic schizophrenia than it is in the acute condition but it certainly appears that the chronic schizophrenic given chlorpromazine becomes more tractable and accessible to other forms of therapy.

2. The manic and hypomanic symptoms associated with some other psychotic conditions usually respond well to chlorpromazine. For this purpose the drug is often given in association with lithium, the chlorpromazine being withdrawn as the initial emergency abates and as lithium begins to exert its full effect.

3. Chlorpromazine obtunds the unpleasant symptoms that attend the withdrawal of alcohol and barbiturates from those dependent on the drugs (p. 87).

4. We have noted earlier (p. 542) that amphetamine intoxication produces a state almost indistinguishable from acute schizophrenia and that many aspects of this state are attributable to dopamine action. The use of chlorpromazine, an antidopamine drug, to treat amphetamine poisoning is therefore a rational one. Symptoms respond to intramuscular doses of 50 mg of chlorpromazine.

5. Chlorpromazine prevents or relieves vomiting caused by drugs that act on the chemosensitive trigger zone of the vomiting centre. The vomiting associated with radiation sickness, labyrinthine disease, pregnancy and uraemia also respond to chlorpromazine. It is relatively ineffective against motion sickness in man but it does protect dogs against swing sickness.

For the control or prevention of vomiting, chlorpromazine is given in oral doses of 25 mg four times daily.

6. Although some forms of extrapyramidal disease are associated with dopamine deficiency, in Huntington's chorea there appears to be increased dopamine activity in the basal ganglia and some cases of the disease respond well to chlorpromazine. Dose regimes have, of course, to be carefully regulated lest relief from one extrapyramidal condition is bought at the expense of precipitating another.

7. Chlorpromazine is sometimes employed to induce sleep when the more usual hypnotic agents are contraindicated for any reason. It is unique among recognized hypnotics in that it increases the duration of paradoxical sleep (p. 478).

8. To confound our brave but oversimplistic theories concerning the biochemical origin of mental illness and the mode of action of psychotropic drugs, it should be noted that some authorities aver that chlorpromazine is as effective as the recognized antidepressant drugs for the treatment of depression (Hollister, 1973). This is, of course, as much a commentary on the difficulty of treating depression as it is on the pluripotency of chlorpromzine.

9. The use of chlorpromazine as a preoperative sedative and for the production of hypothermia for surgical purposes has been mentioned earlier. For the last named use, it is supplemented with promethazine, autonomic blocking agents and physical methods of body cooling.

10. Miscellaneous uses for chlorpromazine include the treatment of tetanus, the relief of itching and the control of behavioural disturbances associated with some forms of epilepsy. The possibility that chlorpromazine may accentuate the dysrhythmia underlying the last mentioned condition must always be borne in mind. Chlorpromazine, in small doses, is also useful for the treatment of disturbed or agitated geriatric patients.

The extrapyramidal side effects of chlorpromazine therapy.
As we have already noted, the antipsychotic drugs owe at least the major part of their therapeutic effectiveness to inhibition of central dopamine activity. This action is by no means selective and the dopaminergic neurones that subserve activity in the extrapyramidal system (p. 163) are as responsive to antipsychotic drugs as are similar neurones in the limbic system and hypothalamus. Some degree of extrapyramidal dysfunction is, consequently, an almost inevitable accompaniment of successful therapy with antipsychotic drugs. It may take several forms including motor restlessness (*akathisia*), incoordinated movements or abnormal postures (*dystonia*) or a syndrome of increased muscle tone, tremor and immobility of facial expression similar to that seen in Parkinson's disease (p. 588).

It may at first sight seem surprising that equieffective doses of different antipsychotic drugs do not induce equal degrees of extrapyramidal disturbance. This apparent anomaly finds a ready explanation when we consider the other properties of the drugs. Chlorpromazine has antiacetylcholine activity and by partially blocking central muscarine receptors it offsets to some extent the extrapyramidal changes resulting from interference with dopaminergic function. That this explanation is valid for other antipsychotic drugs has been demonstrated by Snyder and his colleagues (Snyder, Greenberg and Yamamura, 1974) who showed that the ability of drugs of this class for muscarine receptors *in vitro* is inversely related to the frequency with which they induce extrapyramidal side effects. Clozapine and thioridazine have the greatest affinity for the receptor and the smallest tendency to cause extrapyramidal disturbances. Haloperidol occupies the opposite extremity of the scale; among the phenothiazines acetophenazone, perphenazine and trifluoperazine are most likely to disturb extrapyramidal activity. They are, however, less culpable in this respect than halperidol.

A different abnormality of extrapyramidal function may appear, particularly in the elderly, if treatment with chlorpromazine (or the other antipsychotic drugs) is protracted. This condition is *tardive dyskinesia*, and it is characterized by the persistent repetition of purposeless and stereotyped movements such as chewing, smacking the lips, writhing movements of the arms, legs or pelvis and so on. Like Huntington's chorea, tardive dyskineasia is the result of *increased* activity in the dopaminergic fibres of the extrapyramidal motor system. It seems that continued blockade of the dopamine receptors eventually leads to a compensatory increase in dopamine synthesis and release, to an increased sensitivity of the dopamine receptors and perhaps to the formation or uncovering of new receptors. The whole situation provides an example of denervation hypersensitivity.

Tardive dyskinesia is a serious condition and the possibility of its occurrence should constitute a warning against unnecessary or unnecessarily prolonged deployment of the antipsychotic drugs. Withdrawal of the offending drug does not always relieve tardive dyskinesia once the condition has become established and treatment is not easy. Increasing the dose of the drug will temporarily ameliorate the condition but this course of action is obviously not a wise one. Attempts to inhibit dopamine synthesis by giving α-methyl-p-tryosine (p. 290) or to reduce neuronal stores of the catecholamine by giving reserpine (p. 287) have met with little success. More recently, deanol (p. 205), a drug that from time to time appears on the therapeutic scene begging for a role, has been applied to the treatment of both tardive dyskinesia and Huntington's chorea (Miller, 1974) but it is not yet clear that it is of real value: any benefit that it does confer is presumably attributable to its being able to promote the synthesis of acetylcholine (p. 204). The recent evidence that γ-aminobutyric acid inhibits activity in dopaminergic systems (p. 589) and that the benzodiazepines facilitate the transmitter action of γ-aminobutyric acid has led to the use of diazepam for the treatment of tardive dyskinesia. It is sometimes helpful. L-Tryptophan, tetrabenazine and lithium carbonate also have their advocates.

Other side effects of chlorpromazine therapy. A multiplicity of other side effects have been reported in patients receiving chlorpromazine. This is a reflection of the vast number of patients that have received the drug as well as of the drug's ability to influence a wide variety of pharmacological systems. A complete list of the recorded side effects would be less than helpful since it would have to include leucopenia as well as leucocytosis, agitation as well as depression and pyrexia as well as hypothermia. Only those most frequently seen or those of particular pharmacological interest will, therefore, be discussed here.

Chlorpromazine causes lethargy and somnolence when it is first used although these effects do not usually persist. Patients who have received large amounts of the drug may become confused and disorientated and this may necessitate a reduction in the dosage.

The antiacetylcholine activity of chlorpromazine may give rise to dry mouth, blurred vision, paralytic ileus, megacolon, urinary retention and glaucoma; its antiadrenaline properties may cause a troublesome postural hypotension and its antidopamine activity may induce galactorrhoea and gynaecomastia.

Obesity is a not uncommon side effect of continued chlorpromazine therapy. It is probably of hypothalamic origin (p. 162). Other less common side effects referable to depression of hypothalamic function include cessation of menstruation in women and impotence in men.

The side effects so far catalogued can occur in any patient. In addition, some individuals show idiosyncratic hypersensitivity reactions, the three most common being an obstructive jaundice, agranulocytosis (sometimes fatal) and skin rashes. The latter may be associated with photosensitization, a purplish deposit of melanin appearing on parts of the body exposed to sunlight. Melanin is sometimes deposited on the conjunctiva, cornea and lens of the eye of patients who have received chlorpromazine in large doses over a long period of time. These deposits do not usually interfere with vision but thioridazine (apparently uniquely among the phenothiazine drugs) sometimes causes the deposition of pigment on the retina and this can have serious consequences including blindness.

A few instances of sudden and unexpected death have been reported among patients receiving chlorpromazine. This appears to have been caused by ventricular fibrillation. A number of non-fatal cardiac abnormalities and irregularities has also been recorded.

Chlorpromazine sometimes causes a contact dermatitis and those who handle the drug regularly should take care that it does not come into contact with unprotected skin.

OTHER PHENOTHIAZINES

The names, chemical formulae and doses of a number of phenothiazines, including all those in common clinical use, are displayed in Table 32.1. It will be seen that they can be conveniently divided into three groups, according to the nature of the side chain attached to the nitrogen atom.

The reader will appreciate that, when they are being employed to treat attacks of acute schizophrenia, the phenothiazines sometimes need to be given in much larger doses than those indicated in Table 32.1.

All the phenothiazines have qualitatively similar pro-

Table 32.1 Some clinically-useful phenothiazines (After Crossland, 1967, by kind permission of Messrs. Butterworths)

COMPOUNDS WITH A DIALKYLAMINO GROUP IN THE SIDE CHAIN

Approved name(s)	Proprietary name(s)	R	R'	Dose	Remarks
Antipsychotic drugs Chlorpromazine	Largactil, Thorazine, Chloractil Megaphen, Promazil, Sanoprol, Onazine and many others	$-(CH_2)_3.N(CH_3)_2$	$-Cl$	50–200 mg thrice daily by mouth or by intramuscular injection	Fully discussed in text
Triflupromazine, Fluopromazine	Psyquil, Vesprin, Vespral and others	$-(CH_2)_3.N(CH_3)_2$	$-CF_3$	5–50 mg thrice daily	Liable to produce extrapyramidal effects
Methoxypromazine, Mepromazine	Mopazine, Tentone, Vetomazine and others	$-(CH_2)_3.N(CH_3)_2$	$-OCH_3$	10–150 mg thrice daily	Not now used
Acepromazine, Acetylpromazine	Antran, Notensil, Plegicil, Soprontin and others	$-(CH_2)_3.N(CH_3)_2$	$-COCH_3$	10–30 mg thrice daily	Rarely used
Methotrimeprazine, Levomepromazine	Hirnamin, Neurocil, Nozinan, Veractil, Levoprome and others	$-CH_2.CH.CH_2.N(CH_3)_2$ $\quad\mid$ $\quad CH_3$	$-OCH_3$	2–7 mg thrice daily	Also has anal-gesic properties
Hypnotic Propiomazine	Dorevane, Indorm, Largon, Phenoctyl and others	$-CH_2.CH.N(CH_3)_2$ $\quad\mid$ $\quad CH_3$	$-COC_2H_5$	20 mg by intramuscular injection for preoperative sedation	
Antiemetic drug Promazine	Atarzine, Prazine Propazine, Sparine, Sterazin	$-(CH_2)_3.N(CH_3)_2$	H	25–50 mg thrice daily	More useful for elderly than for young patients

Table 32.1 (*contd*)

Approved name(s)	Proprietary name(s)	R	R'	Dose	Remarks
Anti-Parkinsonism Drugs Diethazine	Antipar, Diparcol	$-(CH_2)_2.N(C_2H_5)_2$	H	50–500 mg thrice daily	Both drugs have strong antiacetyl-choline and weak antihistamine activity. Now rarely used
Ethopropazine, Isothazine, Profenamine	Lysivane, Pardidol, Parsidol, Phenopropazine,	$-CH_2.CH.N(C_2H_5)_2$ CH_3	H	15–150 mg thrice daily	
Promethazine	Avomine, Histantin Phenergan, and many others	$-CH_2CH.N(CH_3)_2$ CH_3	H	10–100 mg thrice daily	

(See also Table 21.3, p. 348)

COMPOUNDS WITH A PIPERIDINE RING IN THE SIDE CHAIN

Approved name(s)	Proprietary name(s)	R	R'	Dose	Remarks
Antipsychotic drugs Mepazine, Pecazine	Pacatal, Paxital and others	[piperidine ring structure, $-CH_2$–, $N-CH_3$]	H	10–35 mg thrice daily	Not now used
Mesoridazine	Inofal, Lidanil, Serentil	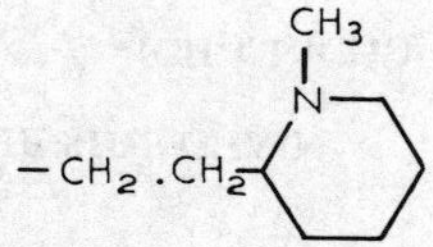 [structure, $-CH_2.CH_2$–, $N-CH_3$]	$\overset{O}{\underset{\parallel}{}}-S.CH_3$	100–400 mg daily for schizophrenia 30–200 mg daily for other purposes	Mesoridazine is a metabolite of thioridazine supplied as the benzene sulphonate
Piperacetazine	Quide	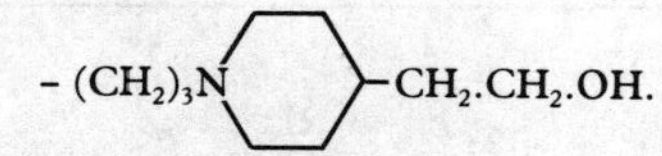 [structure, $-(CH_2)_3N$, $CH_2.CH_2.OH.$]	$\overset{O}{\underset{\parallel}{}}-C.CH_3$	20–150 mg (oral administration. Up to 60 mg (intramuscular injection) daily in divided doses.	Prone to produce extrapyramidal disturbances.
Thioridazine	Mallorol, Melleril Mellaril	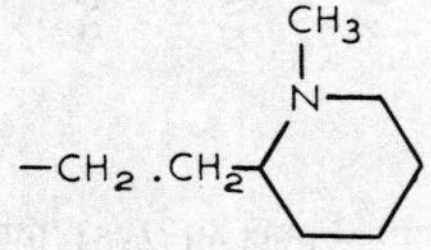 [structure, $-CH_2.CH_2$–, $N-CH_3$]	$-S.CH_3$	30–175 mg thrice daily	

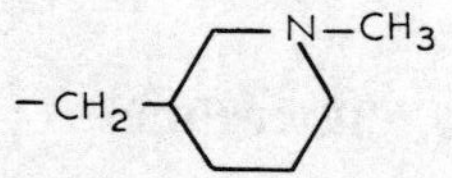

Table 32.1 (contd)

Approved name(s)	Proprietary name(s)	R	R'	Dose	Remarks
Antiemetic Pipamazine	Mornidine Nausidol	$-(CH_2)_3-$ ...CCNH$_2$	Cl	5 mg thrice daily	Useful in pregnancy sickness

COMPOUNDS WITH A PIPERAZINE RING IN THE SIDE CHAIN

Approved name(s)	Proprietary name(s)	R	R'	Dose	Remarks
Antipsychotic drugs Prochlorperazine	Chlormeprazine, Compazine, Nipodal, Stem(m)etil, Vertigon	$-(CH_2)_3-$ N⌷N·CH$_3$	Cl	5-35 mg thrice daily	Also useful as an antiemetic
Acetophenazine	Tindal	$-(CH_2)_3-$ N⌷N·CH$_2$·CH$_2$·OH	$\overset{O}{\overset{\|}{-C}}$·CH$_3$	40-120 mg daily in divided oral doses	
Butaperazine	Randolectil Repoise	$-(CH_2)_3-$ N⌷N·CH$_3$	$\overset{O}{\overset{\|}{-C}}(CH_2)_2CH_3$	50-100 mg daily by mouth in 3 divided doses; 10 mg thrice daily by intramuscular injection	Also used as an antiemetic drug
Carphenazine	Proketazine	$-(CH_2)_3-$ N⌷N·CH$_2$·CH$_2$ OH	$\overset{O}{\overset{\|}{-C}}CH_2CH_3$	40-400 mg daily in divided doses	
Trifluoperazine	Calmazine, Jatroneural, Stelazine and others	$-(CH_2)_3-$ N⌷N·CH$_3$	$-CF_3$	2-10 mg thrice daily	

Table 32.1 (contd)

Approved name(s)	Proprietary name(s)	R	R'	Dose	Remarks
Thioproperazine, Thioperazine	Majeptil	$-(CH_2)_3 \cdot N \underset{N \cdot CH_3}{\bigcirc}$	$-SO_2.N(CH_3)_2$	10-20 mg thrice daily	
Perphenazine	Chlorpiperazin, Etaperazin, Fentazin, Trilafon	$-(CH_2)_3 \cdot N \underset{N \cdot CH_2 \cdot CH_2 \cdot OH}{\bigcirc}$	Cl	2-10 mg thrice daily	Also useful as an antiemetic
Fluphenazine	Anatensol, Flumezine, Modecate, Moditen, Permitil, Prolixin, Tensofin and others	$-(CH_2)_3 \cdot N \underset{N \cdot CH_2 \cdot CH_2 \, OH}{\bigcirc}$	$-CF_3$	1-5 mg thrice daily	The oenanthate and decanoate are available for use as long-acting (2-4 weeks) i.m. preparations
Thiopropazate	Dartal, Dartalan	$-(CH_2)_3 \cdot N \underset{N \cdot CH_2 \cdot CH_2 \, O \cdot COCH_3}{\bigcirc}$	Cl	5-10 mg thrice daily	
Thiethylperazine	Torecan	$-(CH_2)_3 \cdot N \underset{N \cdot CH_3}{\bigcirc}$	$-S.C_2H_5$	5-10 mg thrice daily	

Prothiopendyl, (Dominal, Tolnate) is an isothiazine derivative

Its pharmacological properties are similar to those of chlorpromazine perties but the relative intensity of these properties (and hence the therapeutic uses of the drugs) varies among the different members of the group. Some of these differences are indicated in the following generalizations concerning structure-activity relationships among the phenothiazines.

1. Substitution in position 2 of the phenothiazine ring produces more active compounds than does substitution elsewhere. All the compounds in clinical use that carry substituents in the rings do so in position 2. Among these substituents, the —CF₃ radical produces the most active compounds and chlorine the next most active. Thus while chlorpromazine is an antipsychotic drug, promazine is only an antiemetic. The other substituents commonly employed do not increase pharmacological activity beyond that of the corresponding non-substituted compound.

2. So far as the side chain attached to the nitrogen in position 10 is concerned, antihistamine activity is most marked in compounds in which a dimethylamino group is separated from the ring nitrogen by a chain of two carbon atoms as in promethazine. In diethazine and ethopropazine a diethylamino group is separated by this same

distance from the ring nitrogen. These compounds are weak histamine H₁ antagonists but they also have pronounced antiacetylcholine activity and, so far from causing extrapyramidal symptoms, they are actually used in the treatment of Parkinsonism. If a three-carbon chain separates a dialkylamino group from the ring nitrogen, antihistamine and antiacetylcholine activity fall but antinoradrenaline and antidopamine potencies rise.

3. Phenothiazines with a piperazine ring in the side chain produce a more intense catatonia and are more powerfully antiemetic than the other members of the group. Pipamazine and thiethylperazine are employed as antiemetics, pipamazine being a useful drug for treating morning sickness.

4. Propiomazine is a true hypnotic, prothipendyl has both tranquillizing and sedative properties and methotrimeprazine is an analgesic.

The rauwolfia alkaloids

RESERPINE

Reserpine is no longer used as a psychotropic drug. It

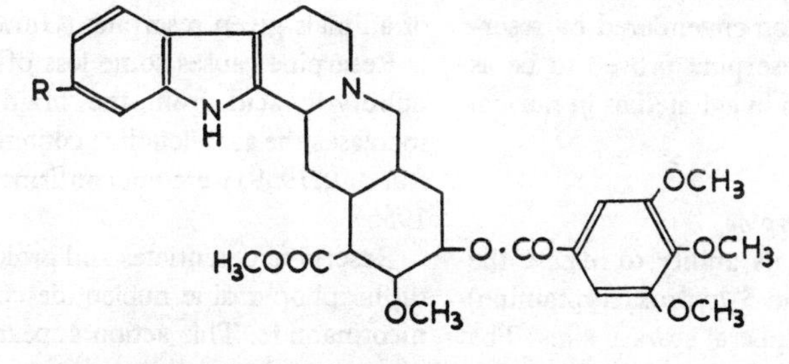

R = H, Deserpidine (Harmonyl)
R = CH₃O, Reserpine (Serpasil)

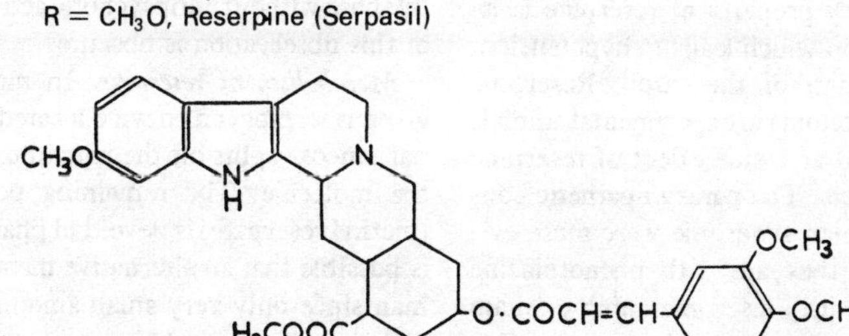

Rescinnamine (Anaprel, Moderil)

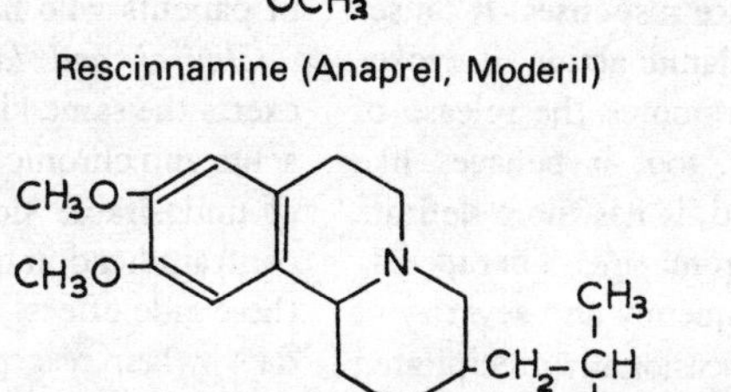

Tetrabenazine (Nitoman)

Fig. 32.2 Reserpine and related compounds.

retains its place here partly for historical reasons—its introduction into psychiatry signalled the start of the modern therapeutic revolution in this field—partly because a study of its mode of action has contributed substantially to our understanding of the biochemical aetiology of the psychosis and partly because it is still a valuable pharmacological tool.

Some thirty years ago, extracts of *Rauwolfia serpentina* began to be used for treating hypertension. The original extract contained a number of alkaloids, but in 1950 the most active principle—to which the name reserpine was given—was isolated and identified (Fig. 32.2).

Hypertensive patients receiving reserpine not infrequently became depressed, sometimes to the point of attempting suicide. It was argued that if psychiatrically normal patients became depressed, agitated ones might be calmed. This prediction was borne out and reserpine thereby found employment as an antipsychotic drug. In this way a very ancient form of therapy was rediscovered.

The use of reserpine in psychiatry slightly antedated that of chlorpromazine and its popularity waned rapidly once the phenothiazines became established. These drugs are as clinically effective as reserpine and are not as prone to cause the feelings of depression engendered by reserpine: contrary to expectation, reserpine proved to be as likely to cause serious depression in agitated as in normal individuals.

Pharmacological properties of reserpine
Reserpine's unique property is its ability to release the monoamines (catecholamines and 5-hydroxytryptamine) from both their central and peripheral storage sites. The mechanism of this action is fully discussed elsewhere (p. 287). The other noteworthy property of reserpine is its parasympathomimetic action which leads to hypotension, bradycardia and constriction of the pupil. Reserpine produces some degree of catatonia in experimental animals and Parkinsonism occurred as a side effect of reserpine treatment in human subjects. The parasympathetic concomitants of the Parkinsonian syndrome were more evident with reserpine than they are with phenothiazine therapy. Like chlorpromazine, reserpine inhibits sham rage reactions, it makes aggressive animals more tractable and it inhibits conditioned avoidance responses. It causes hypothermia because of a hypothalamic action, it evokes the release of prolactin and it promotes the release of corticotrophin. In these respects, too, it behaves like chlorpromazine. On the other hand, it has more definite excitatory actions than has chlorpromazine. Therapeutic doses sometimes increased the frequency and severity of seizures in epileptic subjects and occasionally precipitated convulsions in patients with no previous history of epilepsy. In experimental animals, reserpine increases the potency of convulsant drugs that act on the brain, it lowers the threshold for maximum electroshock seizures and it reduces the protective effect exerted by anticonvulsant drugs.

Patients who were given reserpine complained of sedation or somnolence less frequently than those who received chlorpromazine.

Metabolic effects of reserpine. It has already been mentioned that reserpine depletes monoamine stores in the brain and peripheral structures. A single dose of reserpine (5 mg per kilogram of body weight) is sufficient to bring about a 90 per cent reduction in the amounts of noradrenaline and 5-hydroxytryptamine in the brain. The maximum response is not seen for some six hours following administration of the drug and complete replenishment of the stores is not seen for at least ten days.

Monoamine depletion is entirely attributable to storage failure, synthesis not being interrupted. Indeed, after repeated administration of reserpine, catecholamine synthesis increases as a result of a feedback stimulation of tyrosine hydroxylase. After reserpine treatment the newly synthesized monoamines cannot be sequestered in their normal storage sites and so they are exposed to enzymatic destruction. The amounts of 5-hydroxyindoleacetic acid and of noradrenaline metabolites rise sharply in the brains of animals given reserpine (Glowinski *et al.*, 1966).

Reserpine causes some loss of histamine and of γ-aminobutyric acid from the brain. Early reports that it increases the acetylcholine content of brain (Malhorta and Pundlik, 1959) were not confirmed in a later study (Slater, 1966).

Reserpine potentiates and prolongs the elevation of liver diphosphopyridine nucleotide content brought about by nicotinamide. This action appears to be shared by reserpine derivatives that have antipsychotic properties but not by those without antipsychotic activity but the significance of this observation is obscure.

Metabolism of reserpine. In most mammalian species given reserpine, an enzyme located in the liver and intestinal mucosa splits off the trimethoxybenzoate fragment of the molecule. The remaining portion of the molecule (methyl reserpate) is devoid of pharmacological activity. It is possible that an alternative metabolic pathway exists in man since only very small amounts of methyl reserpate, and virtually no unchanged reserpine, appear in the urine of patients who have received the drug.

Clinical and laboratory uses of reserpine. Reserpine exerts the same kind of effects as do the phenothiazines in acute and chronic schizophrenic patients but the incidence of undesirable side effects is so high as to constitute a contraindication to the use of the drug. The most serious of these side effects, as we have noted, is depression. In the days when reserpine was in clinical use this iatrogenic depression was sometimes so severe that it had to be countered by electroconvulsive therapy. It is a poor form of treatment that necessitates the application of so drastic a corrective, particularly since electroconvulsive therapy appears to be attended by special risks in patients who are also receiving reserpine. Other side effects of reserpine therapy included insomnia, vivid dreams and a number of signs (bradycardia, hypotension, salivation, diarrhoea and the production of peptic ulcers) referable to stimulation of the parasympathetic nervous system. As we have already noted, some of these parasympathomimetic effects made Parkinsonism a more distressing complication of reserpine therapy than it is in those taking phenothiazines.

In low doses, reserpine is still occasionally employed in the treatment of hypertension (p. 316), although there have been reports that its use may be associated with the development of carcinoma of the breast.

The use of reserpine in the laboratory has led to considerable advances in our knowledge of the processes of monoamine storage, of the mode of action of sympathomimetic drugs and of some of the fundamental processes involved in the activity of the autonomic nervous sytem. Reserpine has also been employed to induce experimental peptic ulcers in laboratory animals.

COMPOUNDS RELATED TO RESERPINE

Deserpidine and *rescinnamine* have similar actions to reserpine but neither drug achieved popularity. *Tetrabenazine* (Nitoman) enjoyed rather more success largely because it was reputed to have little action on the gastrointestinal tract. As an antipsychotic drug it has now suffered the same fate as reserpine and it has never been used as an antihypertensive drug. It is occasionally employed in the treatment of Huntington's chorea and tardive dyskinesia.

Mode of action of reserpine and chlorpromazine

As we have already noted, reserpine brings about the depletion of a number of neurotransmitter substances from neurones that contain them and until quite recently a considerable controversy surrounded the question as to which of these depletions underlay reserpine's therapeutic actions. The controversy has been largely resolved by the evidence that now implicates dopamine in the genesis of psychotic states. Reserpine leads to the loss of dopamine from neurones while chlorpromazine antagonizes dopamine action so that the mode of action of both compounds can now be firmly attributed to antidopamine activity. This same property also accounts for most, if not all, of the side effects the two drugs have in common. This is not to say that other pharmacological actions do not contribute at all to the drugs' therapeutic effects or to the production of adverse side reactions. We have already seen, in this connection, that the antimuscarine activity of chlorpromazine partly prevents the discomforting extrapyramidal disorders that otherwise result from dopamine antagonism and there seems to be little doubt that reserpine's ability to deplete serotoninergic neurones of their transmitter accounts partly if not wholly for the readiness with which the drug induces depression. The antiserotonin activity of

chlorpromazine is much smaller than that of reserpine and the drug is correspondingly less likely to induce depression.

Readers who wish to inform themselves of the earlier debate concerning the relative importance of serotonin and the catecholamines as mediators of reserpine action are referred to the previous edition (pages 760-763) of this book.

The butyrophenones

One of the most productive and successful industrial research teams in the immediately postwar years was headed by Janssen. In the course of investigations directed towards the production of analgesic drugs of the pethidine type, the team produced the drug that was to become known as haloperidol. Much to its creators' surprise, it proved to have antipsychotic but no analgesic activity. Haloperidol became available in 1958 and since than a number of other butyrophenones have found clinical application. The names and formulae of the four that have proved most popular are displayed in Table 32.2. A complete list with an exhaustive discussion of the drugs' properties is provided by Janssen himself (1967) but haloperidol is the butyrophenone antipsychotic drug of choice. The butyrophenones have been used quite extensively in veterinary medicine as well as in psychiatry.

HALOPERIDOL

The pharmacological properties, therapeutic uses and side effects of haloperidol are surprisingly similar to those of the phenothiazines except that the antinoradrenaline and antimuscarine activities are less pronounced. The relative lack of blocking activity at muscarine receptors explains why haloperidol is particularly prone to provoke extrapyramidal side effects while the sparing of noradrenaline receptors accounts for the fact that, unlike chlorpromazine, haloperidol only infrequently evokes troublesome autonomic side effects such as postural hypotension. This latter circumstance confers a distinct advantage on the drug particularly when acute schizophrenia demands the parenteral administration of a large dose of an antipsychotic agent. The extrapyramidal complications can be countered, when necessary, by giving atropine or a similar antimuscarine drug (p. 590).

Another point of difference between chlorpromazine and haloperidol is that the butyrophenone has a tendency to cause insomnia (another consequence perhaps of its lack of action on central α receptors) so that the two daily doses recommended in Table 32.2 should be given in the morning and afternoon so as to minimise the risk of disturbing the patients' nocturnal sleep.

For the most part, the therapeutic uses of haloperidol duplicate those of chlorpromazine and its congeners but it has also been applied with some success to the treatment of the rare *Gilles de la Tourette* syndrome, a condition charac-

Table 32.2 Some butyrophenones

$$F-\underset{}{\bigcirc}-\overset{\overset{O}{\parallel}}{C}.CH_2 . CH_2 .CH_2 R$$

Approved name(s)	Proprietary name(s)	R	Daily dose (oral or parenteral)
Haloperidol	Haldol, Aloperidin. Serenace and variations		3-10 mg (in two doses) Larger doses may be needed to control acute schizophrenia
Trifluperidol	Triperidol		1-5 mg
Fluanisone Haloanisone	Sedalande		40-200 mg
Droperidol Dehydrobenzperidol	Droleptan, Inapsin(e)		5-20 mg (Single dose for neuroleptanalgesia)

terized by sudden movements or twitches of the face, head or an arm accompanied by the uttering of meaningless sounds (grunts, cries, hisses, etc.) or a string of obscenities. The last sign is dignified in psychiatric circles by being called *coprolalia*. Haloperidol was also included in the first neuroleptanalgesic mixtures but it has now been superseded by droperidol (Table 32.2).

The effects of haloperidol are delayed for some time after the drug's administration but they are more prolonged than are those of the phenothiazines. The parenteral route is therefore to be preferred if immediate control of an agitated patient is required. The oral route is used for maintenance therapy in chronically schizophrenic patients.

Haloperidol is excreted partly in the bile and partly in the urine. It is denied the multiplicity of metabolic pathways that are offered to chlorpromazine.

TRIFLUPERIDOL
Trifluperidol is a more powerful psycholeptic agent than haloperidol but it is more likely to induce extrapyramidal side effects. It is said to be more effective for treating the

withdrawn schizophrenic while haloperidol is preferable for controlling the agitated schizophrenic subject.

FLUANISONE

Fluanisone has a more rapid onset and a shorter duration of action than have haloperidol and trifluperidol. It has some sedative action and it may cause postural hypotension. It is rarely used.

DROPERIDOL

Droperidol (Droleptan, Inapsine) and fluanisone have similar properties but droperidol has found its major use as a neuroleptanalgesic agent. Fentanyl (Sublimaze) or phenoperidine (Lealgin, Operidine) forms the other component of the neuroleptanalgesic mixture. A mixture of fentanyl (0.05 mg) and droperidol (2.5 mg) is available commercially under the name Thalamonal.

Our discussion of antipsychosis and antimania drugs is resumed, with the thioxanthenes on p. 564.

ANTIANXIETY DRUGS

Over the years many substances have been employed as anxiolytic agents. The oldest of them all is undoubtedly ethanol, a drug that still holds millions of us in its grip and whose influence is so pervasive that it demands to be considered as a special class of psychotropic drug. Ethanol apart, the anxiolytic agents in vogue before 1960 have been overshadowed recently by newer drugs to whom they have now finally abdicated their claim to be considered as drugs of choice.

The anxiolytic drugs, old and new, can be grouped as follows. A typical member of each group is added, by way of illustration, in parentheses.

Older drugs
1. Ethanol
2. Barbiturates (*amylobarbitone*)
3. Propanediols (*meprobamate*)
4. Diphenylmethane derivatives (*hydroxyzine*)

Newer drugs
1. Antipsychotic agents (see p. 547)
2. Antidepressant drugs (*doxepin*)
3. Drugs that block adrenaline ß receptors (*propranolol*)
4. The benzodiazepines (*flurazepam*)

Ethanol
Ethanol is one of a trio of psychoactive drugs (the other two are nicotine and opium) that have been known since the earliest times. To the extent that it is still resorted to in times of anxiety and stress it is appropriate to discuss it here although no physician would ever actually prescribe it (it is devoutly to be hoped) for his patients.

Ethanol (commonly just 'alcohol'), is a depressant of the central nervous system. It has few therapeutic uses but ever since man first enjoyed the taste and the after effects of fermented fruit he has sought it. Some find in it a means of temporarily lightening the load of daily worries, others use it to lubricate the mechanism of social intercourse and yet others become so enslaved to the drug that their lives are ruined by it.

Alcohol causes an irregular descending depression of the central nervous system and in this respect it resembles the general anaesthetics. Large doses of alcohol do produce anaesthesia (hence the phrase 'dead drunk') followed by medullary paralysis. In the days before the anaesthetics proper had been discovered surgeons sometimes gave their patients alcohol in an attempt to reduce the agonies they were to be called upon to endure. It has been pointed out earlier that a period of excitation may occur during the induction of anaesthesia. This is caused by the removal of the inhibition normally imposed by the higher centres. Alcohol has the same effect and under its influence restraints and inhibitions disappear. The person who has had to train himself to exert a tight control over his labile emotions is the one who is likely to show the most obvious changes in personality when under the influence of even small amounts of alcohol. He may weep, laugh outrageously or become frighteningly aggressive. It has been truly said that 'sobriety disguises a man' and perhaps we should respect most those whose personality deteriorates the most when they take alcohol (or those who show fear during the induction of anaesthesia) for it is clearly these who exercise the greatest degree of self control when sober. When alcohol is taken in small doses its depressant action has an obvious social value: the shy introvert who becomes talkative, the pompous man who forgets his self importance, the puritan who sheds his prejudices for a while and the saint who temporarily forgets the miseries of mankind make better company than they do when they are occupied with the more serious aspects of life.

Social acceptability is one thing; responsibility, delicacy of judgment and accuracy in calculations are others and it is as necessary to condemn the use of alcohol when the latter qualities are needed as it is to laud it as an aid to the former. Very small amounts of alcohol cause a detectable deterioration of skilled performance. It is often said—usually in self justification—that the skills at which a man is most proficient are those which suffer least when he takes alcohol. This is true, but the fact remains that these skills *do* suffer. This was strikingly shown in an investigation in which skilled professional truck drivers (all of whom were accustomed to alcohol) were set a series of tasks which involved the precise judgment of distances and the negotiation of a number of hazards. After taking enough alcohol to raise their blood levels to no more than 50 mg per 100 ml of blood the drivers performed the same tasks more rapidly but they made many more errors of judgment and their reaction time was increased (Burn,

1956). These results epitomize the effect of alcohol on skilled performance and it is clearly referable to the removal of control by the higher centres. In their light, the permitted level of blood alcohol in English drivers (80 mg per cent) seems to be excessively generous, while that allowed in Eire (120 mg per cent) is unbelievable. In Norway the permitted level is 50 mg per cent (a reasonable limit, in this writer's opinion) while in some Eastern European countries none is allowed. It is perhaps worth adding that in some inexperienced drivers, impaired ability and judgment can be demonstrated when the blood alcohol level reaches 15 mg per cent, a concentration that is produced by drinking half a pint of beer!

What is true for cars is equally obviously true for other pieces of complex machinery and no one in charge of potentially dangerous equipment should take alcohol before operating it. The effects of alcohol are potentiated by certain anxiolytic drugs and antihistamines. In such circumstances, a very small quantity of alcohol may lead to a marked depression of the central nervous system.

Table 32.3 summarizes the behavioural effects corresponding to different concentrations of blood alcohol. The amounts of whisky or beer required to produce these blood alcohol levels are also indicated though the figures for beer are unreliable by reason of the fact that the alcohol content of different beers ranges from about 6 to 19 grams per half pint (322 ml). Maximum concentrations of blood alcohol are attained about one hour after drinking. The effect of repeated drinks will clearly be influenced to some extent by their spacing but alcohol is metabolized relatively slowly (see below). As a result, a number of drinks spread over, say, two hours will have almost the same effect as if they were taken in rapid succession. The quantitative details given in Table 32.3 are only approximate (quite apart from the varying quantities of alcohol in beer) since

the rate of absorption varies with the individual, with the nature of the drink taken and with the amount of food in the stomach. The response to alcohol after absorption also varies, the degree of tolerance being the most important determinant of the behavioural response.

Alcohol causes a well marked diuresis because it suppresses the secretion of antidiuretic hormone.

In alcoholic intoxication associated with excitement, the pulse rate and blood pressure are often increased but the most prominent effect of alcohol on the cardiovascular system is the production of vasodilatation. This occurs with quite small doses of alcohol and it is the result of a depressant action on the vasomotor centre. It accounts for the pleasant feeling of warmth produced by alcohol. Unfortunately, in a cold atmosphere the vasodilatation which produces the sensation of warmth also causes a loss of body heat and a fall of body temperature. The traditional 'one for the road' is therefore not a wise drink to take, even by a pedestrian. On the other hand, if alcohol is taken in a warm room by someone who had just come in from the cold, the vasodilatation will enable him to absorb heat more rapidly and will thus promote his bodily comfort.

Absorption and metabolism of alcohol

Alcohol is readily and rapidly absorbed from the gastrointestinal tract and a considerable amount (up to 20 per cent) is absorbed from the stomach where it causes a reflex secretion of the acid gastric juices. The rest of the alcohol ingested is absorbed through the wall of the small intestine and the secretion of the pancreatic juice is stimulated. Large quantities of alcohol depress the secretion of both the gastric and pancreatic juices. Alcohol also causes a reflex secretion of saliva. The presence of food, especially fats in the gastrointestinal tract slows the absorption of alcohol. After absorption, alcohol enters the

Table 32.3 Behavioural state and blood alcohol level

Blood alcohol concentration	Amount of alcohol needed		State
mg %	Double whiskies	Pints of beer	
Up to 50			In control: feelings of comfort and self satisfaction
50	1	1½	Beginning to be reckless; takes liberties
100	2	3	Incoordinated; speech begins to be slurred
200	4	6	Drunk but mobile
300	6	9	Drunk and stuporous
400	8	12	Dead drunk, anaesthetized and comatose

1 double whisky (1 English double = 48 ml) contains approx 16 grams of alcohol
1 pint of beer(643 ml) contains 12–34 grams of alcohol

blood and is then absorbed by the brain and other organs. About 95 per cent of the alcohol absorbed is oxidised, largely in the liver, while the remainder appears unchanged in the urine and in the expired air. Oxidation takes place by way of acetaldehyde formation. The acetaldehyde is itself oxidized by a liver aldehyde oxidase and probably by other enzymes. Peak blood levels are reached in about one hour but traces of alcohol can be demonstrated for up to 24 hours. Small amounts appear in the sweat and milk. Alcohol can be used by the body as a source of energy. One gram of alcohol produces 7 Calories, so that as a source of energy it lies midway between the carbohydrates and proteins (4 Calories per gram) and fat (9 Calories per gram). The oxidation of alcohol is a zero order reaction (p. 68) so that its rate of metabolism remains relatively constant at some 10 to 15 ml an hour irrespective of its concentration in the tissues. This figure indicates the rapidity with which alcohol will accumulate in the blood if repeated drinks are taken.

Uses of alcohol

Alcohol is an excellent solvent and it is used as such in the preparation of tinctures, solutions and liquid extracts. Other uses include its injection into the region of nerve tissues or ganglia to relieve severe pain in carcinoma and trigeminal neuralgia and its external application as a skin antiseptic, rubefacient, astringent or cooling lotion. Ethanol is used to prevent bed sores and to remove phenol which has been accidentally spilled on the skin. It is still occasionally prescribed to improve digestion and appetite in invalids and old people.

Alcohol dependence

This topic is discussed elsewhere (p. 87).

METHANOL

Methanol is not used as a drug but it is an important industrial chemical and it is employed (in the form of industrial methylated spirits) as a solvent in liniments, embrocations, perfumes etc. Pharmacological interest in methanol lies largely in its poisonous properties which are seen when impoverished addicts turn to it as a cheap substitute for ethanol. Methanol is oxidized more slowly and less completely than ethanol and in consequence its cumulative effects are much greater and its actions are more prolonged. The presence of ethanol retards the oxidation of methanol and when the two alcohols are taken together (as in industrial methylated spirits), oxidation of methanol is very slow. Symptoms of poisoning are therefore less severe. The oxidation products of methanol include formate and formaldehyde which are believed to be responsible for the selective toxic actions of methanol on the optic nerve. The presence of high levels of formic acid in the blood gives rise to an acidosis which is responsible for many of the severe symptoms seen in methanol

intoxication. The acidosis can be corrected by the use of intravenous infusion of sodium bicarbonate solution. Methanol also causes symptoms of depression of the central nervous system but these are less prominent than those seen in ethanol intoxication.

Barbiturates

Restlessness by day and sleeplessness by night are prominent symptoms of acute anxiety and of neurotic syndromes that feature an anxiety component. These symptoms can be controlled by sedatives and hypnotics and until the advent of the more specifically psychotropic drugs the barbiturates provided almost the only form of drug therapy for mental illness. They were by no means ineffective and from the point of view of therapeutic results in neurotic patients they held their ground for a time against such prominent early members of the new generation as chlorpromazine, reserpine, meprobamate and chlordiazepoxide (Raymond *et al.*, 1957; Stotsky and Borozne, 1972). Their employment as psychotropic drugs has, however, virtually ceased with the wider appreciation of the perils that attend their use (p. 486).

Propanediols

Tense muscles often betray a tense mind. If the muscles relax, feelings of anxiety and stress may become less intense even though the underlying mental state is unaffected. This consideration led to the use of mephenesin (p. 248), a muscle relaxant, as a psychotherapeutic agent. Mephenesin came into vogue for this purpose several years before reserpine or chlorpromazine. A number of compounds have been derived from mephenesin: their names and formulae are displayed in Figure 16.6 (p. 250).

The psychotropic action of mephenesin is not entirely a consequence of its ability to induce muscle relaxation. Some mephenesin derivatives have more psychotropic and less muscle relaxing activity. Foremost amongst these is meprobamate.

MEPROBAMATE

Until recently meprobamate was widely used, particularly in the United States, as a minor tranquillizer. It was given in doses of one to two grams daily but, notwithstanding its popularity in some quarters, meprobamate was not a very effective drug.

This lack of a potent psychotropic action is disappointing in view of the fact that meprobamate exerts a combination of actions on the central nervous system which might be expected (p. 168) to confer powerful tranquillizing potentiality. Thus it weakly stimulates the ascending reticular fibres and it does not depress cortical activity (thus the level of consciousness is unimpaired) but it selectively depresses the thalamus and inhibits evoked seizure discharges in the limbic system (thus reducing emotional tension).

Proprietary names include Aneural, Equanil, Har-monin, Miltown, Perequil and Restenil.

Although meprobamate weakly stimulates ascending reticular fibres, drowsiness was not infrequently com-plained of by patients receiving the drug. It may have been a consequence of the somatic and mental relaxation induced by meprobamate and these same effects presuma-bly explain why the drug was sometimes useful for the treatment of insomnia.

Meprobamate is rapidly falling into complete disuse. It is less effective than the benzodiazepines, the lethal and therapeutic doses of the drug are dangerously close to one another, some patients show hypersensitivity reactions to it while others succumb to its by no means negligible tendency to induce a barbiturate-like physical depen-dence.

TYBAMATE

Tybamate (Nospan) is closely related to meprobamate and had similar therapeutic uses. It is said to be less likely than meprobamate to induce sleepiness or physical dependence

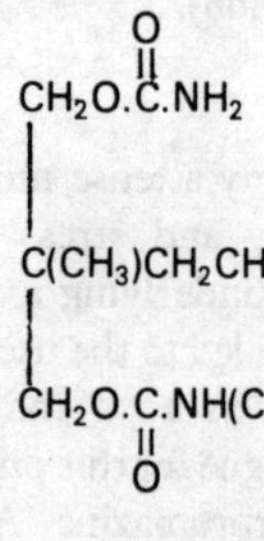

$$CH_2O.\overset{\overset{\displaystyle O}{\|}}{C}.NH_2$$

$$C(CH_3)CH_2CH_2CH_3$$

$$CH_2O.\underset{\underset{\displaystyle O}{\|}}{C}.NH(CH_2)_3CH_3$$

tybamate

but it never achieved the earlier drug's popularity. There may be an argument in favour of retaining tybamate for the few elderly patients who experience an incommoding

ataxia when they take a benzodiazepine. The dose of tybamate is similar to that of meprobamate.

The thioxanthenes

These drugs (Fig. 32.3) are structurally analogous to the phenothiazines with which they share similar properties, uses and side effects although the different ring structure is associated with a somewhat reduced antipsychotic pot-ency. The only real point of difference between the two groups of drugs is that the thioxanthenes are less likely than the phenothiazines to cause photosensitivity reactions and skin pigmentation and this constitutes a recommenda-tion for their use in sensitive patients.

Thiothixene is the most potent and the most commonly used thioxanthene. It is usually given thrice daily in total oral doses of 6 to 60 mg but (as with the phenothiazines) higher doses are sometimes resorted to for the control of very disturbed hospitalized patients. Thiothixene can also be given, if necessary, by the intramuscular route: the normal daily intramuscular dose is 15 to 30 mg.

The principal modes of metabolism of the thioxanthenes is by oxidation of their sulphur and their terminal nitrogen atoms. Unlike the phenothiazines they do not, apparently, suffer ring hydroxylation.

Propranolol

The use of this ß-blocking agent as an antipsychotic drug is discussed later (p. 571).

Newer drugs

The names and formulae of a number of recently intro-duced and relatively untried antipsychotic drugs, some of them with structures very different from those represented in the older drugs are displayed in Fig. 32.4. The diphenyl-butylpiperidine derivatives—which bear an obvious rela-tionship to the butyrophenones—are remarkable by

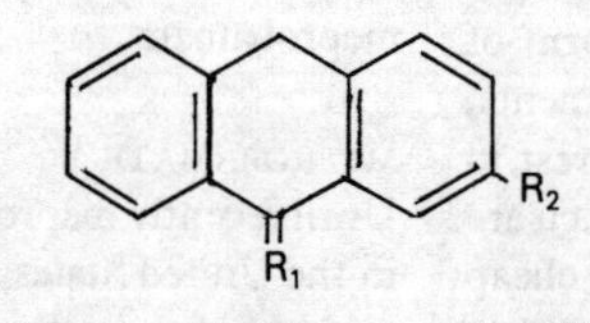

	R₁	R₂
chlorprothixene (Taractan, Truxal)	CH(CH₂)₂N(CH₃)₂	Cl
clopenthixol (Ciatyl, Sordinol)	-CH(CH₂)₂N⟩⟨N(CH₂)₂OH	Cl
thiothixene (Navane, Orbinamon)	-CH(CH₂)₂N⟩⟨NCH₃	-SO₂N(CH₃)₂

Fig. 32.3 The thioxanthenes.

INDOLES

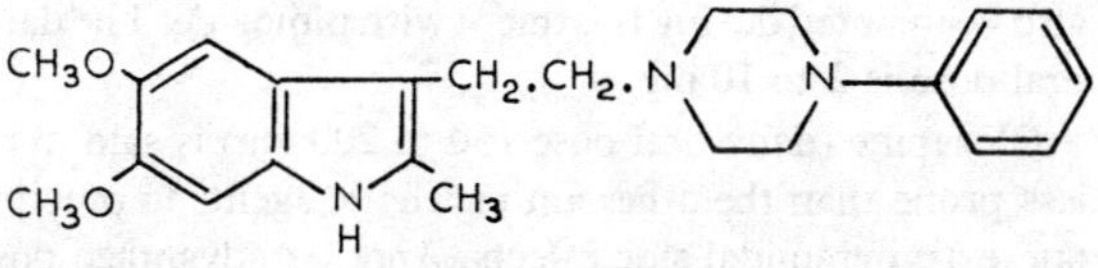

oxypertine (Integrin)

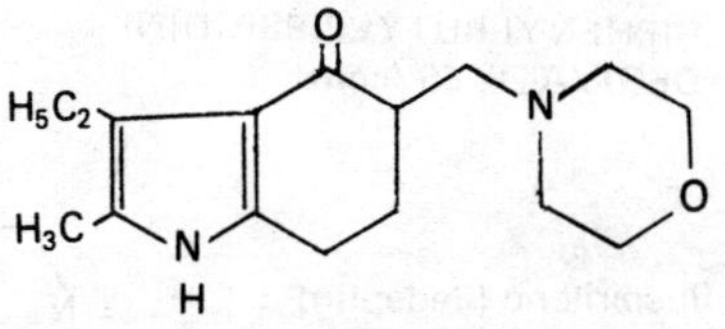

molindole (Moban)

DIBENZOXAZEPINE DERIVATIVES

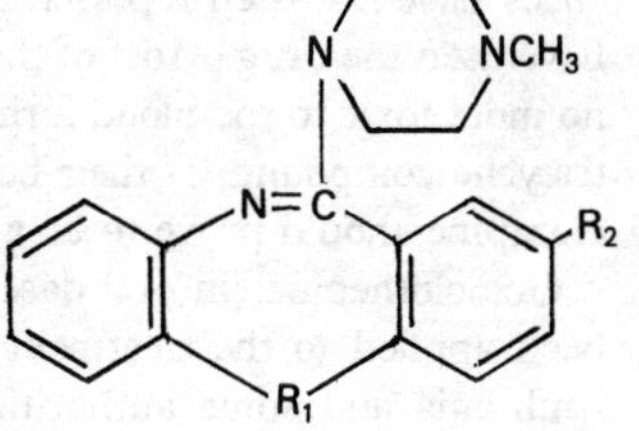

	R_1	R_2
clothiapine (Etopine)	S	Cl
clozapine (Leponex)	N H	Cl
loxapine (Loxitane)	O	Cl
metiapine	S	CH_3

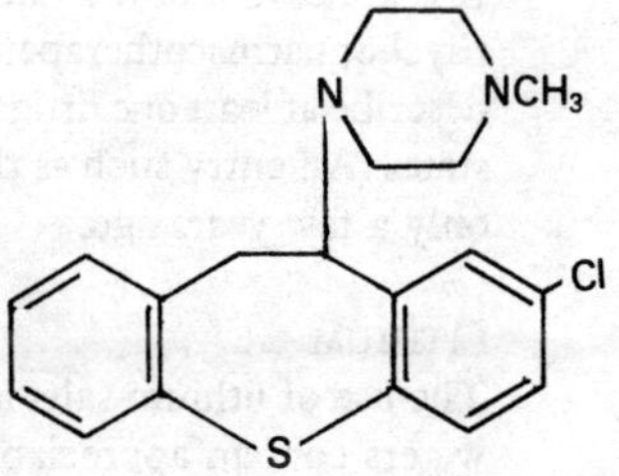

octoclothepine

DIPHENYLBUTYLPIPERIDINE DERIVATIVES

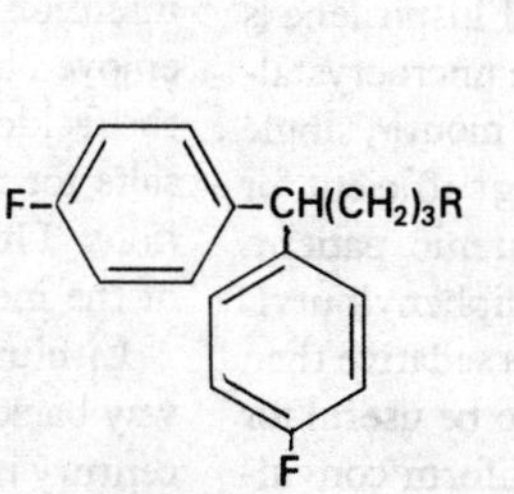

F—⟨ ⟩—CH(CH$_2$)$_3$R

Fig. 32.4 Some newer antipsychotic drugs

DIPHENYLBUTYLPIPERIDINE DERIVATIVES (cont)

fluspirilene (Redeptin)

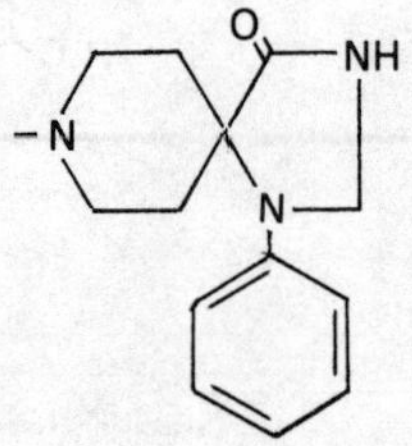

penfluridol (Semap)

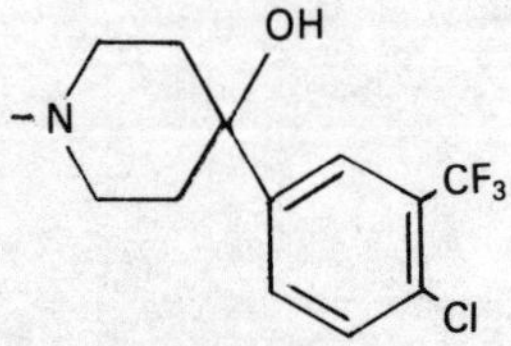

pimozide (Orap)

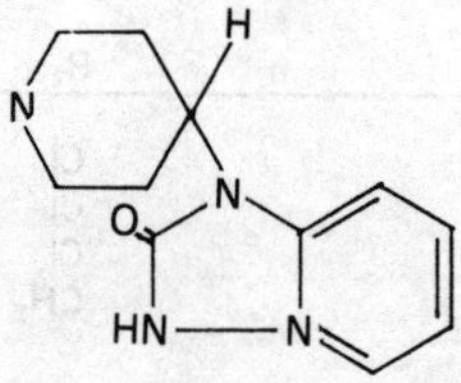

ORTHOPRAMIDES

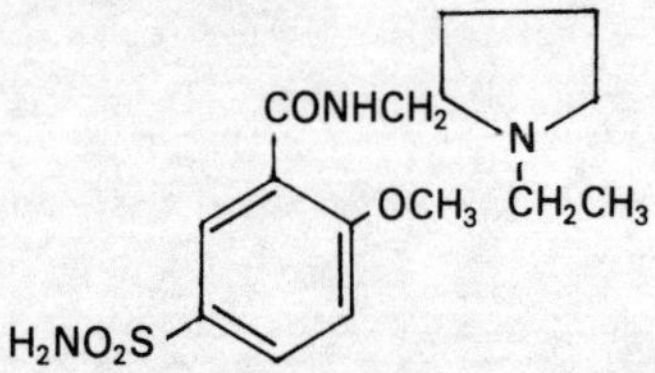

sulpiride (Dogmatil, Eglonyl)

Fig. 32.4 *(contd)*

reason of the long duration of their action. Fluspirilene is given in intramuscular doses (1 to 3 mg) in a microcrystalline suspension but penfluridol is active by mouth, single weekly doses of 30 to 60 mg (or higher) being sufficient for the maintenance of the chronic schizophrenic patient. Pimozide is shorter acting than the other diphenylbutylpiperidine derivatives but it is said to be less sedative than many other antipsychotic drugs. It may also be useful for the control of acute schizophrenia. Epileptiform convulsions have been known to occur in patients withdrawn from pimozide and in our present state of knowledge epilepsy should probably be regarded as a contraindication

to the use of the drug. Disturbances of liver function have also been noted during treatment with pimozide. The daily oral dose is 2 to 10 mg.

Clozapine (daily oral dose 150 to 200 mg) is said to be less prone than the other antipsychotic agents to precipitate extrapyramidal side effects. Another advantage possessed by the drug is its ability to relieve the symptoms of tardive dyskinesia. In the early stages of treatment it sometimes causes heavy sedation but the effect soon passes off. A more disturbing feature of clozapine therapy is the high incidence of agranulocytosis and leukaemia reported in one group of Finnish patients but such dismal consequences have not been reported by workers elsewhere who have used the drug. Most of them would declare that it is no more toxic to the blood forming tissues than any other tricyclic compound. If their belief proves to be justified, clozapine should prove to be a very useful drug.

Octoclothepine (in oral doses of from 5 to 50 mg) has been applied to the treatment of mania as well as schizophrenia and some authorities even claim that it has useful antidepressant activity.

The other drugs featured in Fig. 32.4 require no special mention: none of them has actions, uses or side effects any different from those of the older antipsychotic agents.

ANTIMANIA DRUGS

It is a measure of the rate of recent advance in the field of psychopharmacotherapeutics that it is now possible to describe at least one drug that has a specific effect on manic states. An entry such as this would have been unthinkable only a few years ago.

LITHIUM

The use of lithium salts in medicine is not new. Some spa waters contain appreciable quantities of lithium and they acquired a certain therapeutic reputation among the elderly wealthy who flocked to English and Continental watering places a century and more ago. The waters seemed to be particularly beneficial in gout—that bane of elderly wealthy Victorians—apparently because they promoted the excretion of urates. With the laudable intention of bringing to the not so wealthy the boons enjoyed by those who could afford to indulge themselves in the fashionable spas, physicians began to prescribe lithium salts for the relief of gout and other inflammatory conditions. This form of treatment was soon abandoned because of the incidence of seriously toxic side effects.

Lithium made two unsuccessful attempts to force its way back on to the medical stage. In the early years of the century it was employed for a short time as an antiepileptic agent and some forty years ago it reappeared yet again to enjoy an equally brief vogue when it came to be used as a replacement for sodium in the salt-free diets prescribed for hypertensive patients. On both occasions the toxic effects of lithium (which were responsible for a number of deaths among hypertensive patients) led to its being hastily hustled off the scene.

The potential value of lithium as a psychotropic drug first emerged in 1949 as a result of a series of studies launched by Cade after he had noticed sleepiness in guinea pigs that had received lithium urate (Cade, 1949). Oddly enough, Cade was originally interested in the possibility that uric acid might be involved in the genesis of mania. He employed lithium urate in his early experiments simply because the salt's high solubility allowed him to deliver large amounts of urate to his animals.

Following Cade's first clinical studies, more rigorous trials soon established the therapeutic value of lithium for the treatment and prevention of manic episodes though, not surprisingly in view of its earlier unfortunate history, acceptance of the drug's new role came only slowly. As recently as 1970, for instance, the previous edition of this textbook was noticeably cool about lithium's prospects as a psychotherapeutic agent. It is now clear, however, that it can justifiably claim an honourable place in the roll of useful psychotropic drugs. The incidence of the serious side effects that led to its earlier eclipses has been drastically reduced by an insistence that the concentration of lithium in the plasma shall be carefully monitored while dose levels are being established.

Diligent searches among ancient writings have disclosed (need it be said?) that the value of lithium has been known all the time. It is said that, in the opening years of the Christian era, Sorenus of Ephesus used a natural water, now known to contain lithium, to treat maniacal patients (Fieve, 1978).

Lithium is the only antimania drug whose action can be said to be specific in the sense that it is effective against mania but not against the more generalized agitation that characterizes some other psychiatric conditions and which responds to neuroleptic drugs such as chlorpromazine. The neuroleptic drugs are equally effective against mania and the other agitated states but they control mania at the cost of making the patient lethargic and somnolent. Lithium escapes this criticism.

The specificity of lithium is by no means absolute. In addition to its being able to control mania proper it can, it seems, reduce the frequency of major outbursts of destructive aggression in psychopathic individuals (Sheard et al, 1976). More surprising, perhaps, is the fact that lithium is something of an antidepressant agent having scored successes in the treatment of unipolar endogenous depression as well as of the depressive phases of manic depressive states. Equivocal results have been recorded in studies designed to assess the value of lithium treatment in schizophrenia, alcoholism, character disorder and premenstrual tension.

Lithium is usually given in the form of its carbonate (Camcolit, Litho-Carb, Lithonate) simply because this compound contains, weight for weight, more lithium than the other simple salts. It is taken by mouth in doses that may amount, in the early stages of treatment of severe mania, to two grams daily. Its effects are not immediate, a period of 5 to 10 days commonly elapsing before the patient is adequately controlled. During this latent period, chlorpromazine or another neuroleptic drug can be given to curb the mania should the urgency of the situation demand it.

As soon as possible after the initiation of treatment, the daily dose of lithium should be reduced to a level (usually of the order of one gram of the carbonate) that will maintain its plasma concentration between 1.0 and 1.5 milliequivalents per litre. The required daily dose is usually taken in three instalments unless a slow release preparation (Camcolit Slow, Phasal, Priadel) is used. Until the maintenance dose is firmly established, frequent determinations of the amount of lithium in the plasma are mandatory. Flame photometry or atomic absorption spectrometry is used for this purpose. Since lithium will prevent attacks of mania as well as quelling a present attack it can be given—with continuing checks on its plasma concentration—over long periods of time. On the other hand, it is not necessarily wise to attempt to prevent hypomanic attacks in the mildly afflicted patient. Phases of hypomania often represent periods of high creativity in gifted individuals. Those who prescribe psychotropic drugs of any kind should be alive to the dangers of imposing a uniform, drab and nonproductive 'normality' on all and sundry.

Side effects of lithium therapy
In the initial stages of treatment, the lithium treated patient almost invariably experiences incommoding but innocuous side effects. These include thirst, polyuria, gastrointestinal upsets, tremor and a feeling of weakness. Lithium is concentrated particularly in the thyroid gland and thyroid function is not uncommonly depressed in the early stages of treatment. Physiological compensatory mechanisms (primarily an increased secretion of thyroid stimulating hormone) usually ensure that the disturbance is only a transient one but it is sometimes more troublesome, particularly in those with pre-existing thyroid dysfunction and it may then be necessary to give thyroid hormone to counter the effects of the lithium.

Toxic effects proper, which occur when plasma concentrations exceed two milliequivalents per litre, are exerted primarily on the central nervous system. Among the many signs of central nervous involvement are muscle twitches, ataxia, blurred vision and epileptiform convulsions. In more serious poisoning cerebral anoxia can lead to coma and death.

The replacement of sodium in the tissues by lithium can of itself have toxic repercussions by reason of the upsetting of ionic balances. Arrhythmias, sometimes fatal, fall into this category as do increases in the secretion of glucagon and insulin which can lead to appreciable gains in weight accompanied by either hypo- or hyperglycaemia.

Acute (but reversible) renal failure, temporary skin rashes and an apparently harmless leucocytosis also feature in the list of the side effects of lithium treatment.

The renal excretion of lithium is impaired in the absence of sodium. Sodium lack also accentuates those toxic effects of lithium that are attributable to disturbances of ionic balance. For both these reasons, lithium should only be given with the utmost circumspection, if at all, to patients taking diuretic drugs or salt free diets. We have already seen how disastrous can be the consequences of ignoring this admonition. Extra care should also be exercised in patients who have renal, cardiac or central nervous disease.

Lithium is contraindicated in early pregnancy since it can induce developmental defects in the cardiovascular system.

Mode of action of lithium

Pharmacological experiments have uncovered a number of actions which may be relevant to the mode of action of lithium and also, perhaps, to the aetiology of mania. In view of the interest that attaches to the notion that disturbances of monoamine function underlie affective disorders, we must first direct our attention to the evidence that lithium can intervene in the processes that control monoamine action at the synapses.

Lithium increases the ratio of deaminated to O-methylated noradrenaline metabolites in the brain. This suggests that more of the transmitter is being destroyed within the neurone and that less is released into the synaptic gap. There is, indeed, direct evidence that lithium depresses the evoked release of noradrenaline from brain slices and the splenic nerve. Lithium also promotes the reuptake of noradrenaline into synaptosomes. It has a postsynaptic action too. Applied iontophoretically to a number of central neurones, lithium blocks the action of noradrenaline similarly applied. This action may be related to lithium's ability to inhibit the activity of adenylate cyclase. All the evidence cited in the foregoing paragraph is consistent with the idea that lithium, by various means, hinders the operation of both noradrenergic and noradrenoceptive neurones.

Lithium also promotes the synthesis, and perhaps the release, of 5-hydroxytryptamine but these changes do not persist for longer than a few days. Its actions on the dopamine system are not yet very well established. The available evidence tends to indicate that lithium reduces both the release of dopamine from neurones that contain it and the action of that which is released.

In the flush of enthusiasm for monoamine hypotheses it is easy to forget that behavioural and psychological activities certainly involve a number of other transmitter systems, interference with which can have profound effects even if the primary drive comes from a monoaminergic system and we must not ignore the fact that lithium inhibits acetylcholine synthesis, hinders the release of acetylcholine from stimulated nerves and reduces the sensitivity to acetylcholine of postsynaptic receptors. There is also evidence that lithium affects the production, release and disposition of both γ-aminobutyric and glutamic acids. Some part of this action may be attributable to the fact that lithium has successfully competed with sodium and has thereby inhibited the sodium dependent high affinity uptake system for the aminoacid transmitters.

It is possible that lithium intervenes in neuronal processes at a more intimate level than is implied by suggestions that it modifies transmitter synthesis, release or action. It may partially but imperfectly substitute for sodium and so bring about subtle changes in the structure of cell membranes and their receptors or interfere with ion transport in both nervous and nonnervous tissue. The 'membrane transport hypothesis' of mental illness provides an alternative to hypotheses that lay primary stress on disturbances of transmitter function.

More detailed discussions concerning the mode of action of lithium are provided *inter al* by Gershon and Shopsin (1973), Fieve (1978) and Gerbino, Oleshansky and Gershon (1978).

OTHER COMPOUNDS

A severely manic patient needs urgently to be controlled if he is not to damage himself or others. The strait jackets and padded cells of old were introduced for this purpose but even when these devices were in vogue they often had to be supplemented by drugs: a really determined patient could bite through the straps of his strait jacket though at no small cost to his teeth. Virtually all the older hypnotics and sedatives, but particularly the bromides and the barbiturates, have been employed to bring about this additional restraint as also have hyoscine and hyoscyamine (p. 229), but since 1950 the immediate control of the acutely manic patient has been entrusted to the psycholeptic drugs. Chlorpromazine, indeed, has been described, perhaps a little unkindly, as a chemical straitjacket. Very recently, methysergide (p. 334) and dipropylacetamide (the amide of valproic acid, p. 528) have attracted a few advocates as antimania drugs. Their clinical success has been, at best, only moderate but their relationship to serotonin and γ-aminobutyric acid respectively may hold a lesson for the pharmacologist.

Although the psycholeptic drugs can be used to control acute maniacal outbursts, lithium has no antipsychotic activity. This observation may imply that the psycholeptic drugs, presumably by virtue of their antidopamine properties, control manic behaviour by a nonspecific effect much as the hypnotics did in the past while lithium operates more specifically on regulatory systems that are disturbed in mania but not in schizophrenia. This tentative and facile hypothesis has, however, to meet such challenges as the fact that, in at least some manic-depressive patients, dopamine receptor agonists such as piribedil can precipitate manic episodes. To complicate this issue still further, mention must be made of the fact, testified to by several reports, that piribedil can actually be employed to control manic outbursts! This paradox, however, is probably more apparent than real because in the doses recommended for this purpose (60–100 mg daily by mouth) piribedil is likely to be operating presynaptically to reduce the liberation of dopamine. Only at higher doses does it exhibit appreciable postsynaptic agonist activity (Post, 1978).

We can now return to the antianxiety drugs.

Diphenylmethane derivatives
Several classes of centrally acting drugs, ranging from depressants to stimulants, feature the diphenylmethane structure. For convenience of reference, Table 32.4 includes all the diphenylmethane derivatives that need to be considered in the context of the present chapter. Only a few of them have useful anxiolytic activity and of these the most effective is hydroxyzine.

HYDROXYZINE
Hydroxyzine is a histamine H_1 antagonist, a fact that is at least partly responsible for its anxiolytic (and its antiemetic) effects. Like many of the traditional antihistamines hydroxyzine also displays some antiacetylcholine activity. Hydroxyzine is anticonvulsive but it may also precipitate epileptiform attacks. It prolongs and potentiates the action of hypnotic drugs, it produces hypothermia and hypotension and it depresses activity in the reticular activating system. Extrapyramidal side effects are not seen, presumably because of the drug's antiacetylcholine action which also explains such side effects as dryness of the mouth and the occasional occurrence of central excitation.

Hydroxyzine is used to treat anxiety states particularly those that follow the withdrawal of alcohol and other depressant drugs from those dependent on them. It is also useful for the management of patients with urticarial and other skin conditions that have been provoked or aggravated by emotional factors. Some reports even indicate that it is an effective antidepressant agent.

The single dose of hydroxyzine is 25 to 100 mg but higher doses can safely be given if circumstances demand it; in emergencies it is permissible to administer the drug by the intramuscular route. The reported antidepressant activity of hydroxyzine appears at lower dose levels than those needed to control anxiety states.

OTHER COMPOUNDS
The other anxiolytic agents named in Table 32.4 are now rarely used. Diphenhydramine is described as an antihistamine largely on the grounds of its usual clinical uses but it has some anxiolytic action which in some quarters is as highly regarded as that of hydroxyzine.

Antidepressant drugs
Doxepin is a tricycle antidepressant drug similar in its structure and actions to imipramine. As we note elsewhere (p. 582) it also possesses (as do the other tricycle antidepressant agents) a degree of tranquillizing activity that renders it especially suitable for the treatment of anxious depressed patients. For this purpose it is given in doses of 75 to 150 mg daily in divided doses. Some of the monoamine oxidase inhibitors particularly phenelzine (p. 576) have also been applied to the treatment of anxious depression.

Drugs that block adrenaline ß receptors
Since their introduction into medicine some fifteen years ago, the ß-blocking agents have been applied to the treatment of an ever increasing number of conditions, a full list of which is to be found on p. 306. Their employment as psychotherapeutic agents is a relatively recent development but they are rapidly finding niches for themselves both as antianxiety and, most recently, as antipsychotic drugs. These two aspects of their activity do not necessarily rest on identical pharmacological mechanisms but it is convenient to discuss them together.

Anxiety states are accompanied by somatic manifestations (increased heart action, muscle tremor and tenseness, dizziness and so on) awareness of which contributes to and sharpens the sensation of anxiety and thereby further accentuates the somatic changes. Psychologists will remember the once popular James-Lange theory according to which the subjective emotions consisted of no more than the conscious perception of the bodily changes. Be that as it may, it was certainly reasonable to propose the use as anxiolytic drugs of substances that would attenuate the peripheral accompaniments of the anxiety state—particularly those affecting the heart, a notable target and progenitor of emotional states—just as it earlier seemed reasonable to use muscle relaxants in a similar way (p. 563). Although many would still maintain that the sole mode of anxiolytic action of the ß blocking drugs is the suppression of some of the more important concomitants of the anxiety state there is satisfactory evidence that central actions are certainly involved. That the drugs (or their metabolites) do act centrally is evident from the fact that they themselves can induce psychotic changes (most often a depressive state, sometimes severe enough to provoke suicide attempts) that cannot possibly be ascribed to an inhibition of peripheral ß receptors.

Table 32.4 Some diphenylmethane derivatives (after Crossland, 1967, by kind permission of Messrs. Butterworths)

Approved name	Proprietary name(s)	R_1	R_2	R_3	R_4
Anxiolytic agents					
Hydroxyzine	Atarax, Vistaril	Cl	H	$-N$ piperazine $N.(CH_2)_2.O.CH_2.CH_2OH$	H
Azacyclonol	Frenquel	H	H	piperidyl NH	OH
Benactyzine	Suavitil	H	H	$-CO.O.(CH_2)_2N(C_2H_5)_2$	OH
Captodiamine	Covatine	C_4H_9S	H	$-S(CH_2)_2N(CH_3)_2$	H
Histamine H_1 antagonists					
Diphenhydramine	Benadryl	H	H	$-O(CH_2)_2.N(CH_3)_2$	H
See also Table 21.3 (p. 347)					
Anti-Parkinsonian agents					
Benztropine	Cogentin	H	H	$-O.CH$ tropane $N.CH_3$	H
Chlorphenoxamine	Phenoxene, Clorevan	Cl	H	$-O(CH_2)_2.N(CH_3)_2$	CH_3
Orphenadrine	Disipal, Norflex	H	CH_3	$-O(CH_2)_2.N(CH_3)_2$	H
Central stimulant					
Pipradrol	Meratran	H	OH	piperidyl $N\!H$	H
Psychotomimetic					
N-methyl-3-piperidyl benzilate	—	H	OH	$-CO.O$ piperidyl $N-CH_3$	H

There is no very strong evidence that activation of central ß receptors plays any part in the genesis of anxiety and it may well be that the blocking agents operate through a mechanism that is independent of their principal pharmacological action. It is known, for instance, that a metabolite of propranolol (propranolol glycol) has a marked sedative action in experimental animals (Saelens, Walle and Privitera, 1976). Compounds of this type might contribute to anxiolytic effectiveness. There is evidence, too, that propranolol, and presumably its congeners, can behave as serotonin antagonists (Weinstock, Weiss and Gitter, 1977) but this finding is probably more relevant to the drug's antipsychotic action.

$$OCH_2CH(OH)CH_2OH$$

propranolol glycol

The adrenaline ß-receptor antagonists have been used with some success to reduce the anxiety associated with imminent examinations (in some institutions they are now more frequently offered than chlordiazepoxide to students under stress), an appearance before an audience or participation in a hazardous sport such as motor racing. Some publicity was given to a recent experiment in which a ß-blocking drug was made available to participants in an important violin competition. In all these situations these drugs are preferred to the benzodiazepines because they are unlikely to impair intellectual or psychomotor performance. In more severe anxiety states the ß-blocking agents seem to be rather less effective than the benzodiazepines except in patients in whom tremor and cardiac symptoms such as palpitations are prominent.

Other reported therapeutic successes of the ß-receptor antagonists include the amelioration of the symptoms precipitated by the withdrawal of alcohol or opiate analgesics from those dependent on these drugs—the latter notwithstanding the fact that some have claimed that propranolol is a narcotic antagonist which would be expected to exacerbate the abstinence syndrome—and the prevention of tremor in patients receiving lithium carbonate.

The blocking agents most frequently employed for their anxiolytic action are propranolol (in doses of 20–40 mg), alprenolol (50–100 mg), oxprenolol (40–50 mg) and sotalol (20–80 mg).

Propranolol in schizophrenia
Very recently, several groups of investigators have come to believe that propranolol used either alone or in association with other psychotropic drugs has useful antipsychotic activity. This conclusion has not been unanimously accepted and there have been many critics of the design and interpretation of the studies on which it is based. Nevertheless a sober appraisal of the arguments and counter arguments leaves this author at least with the impression that propranolol's case is a strong one.

The doses of propranolol employed in the therapy of schizophrenia are quite high: in one recent trial in chronically schizophrenic subjects who had not responded satisfactorily to more conventional antipsychotic agents they approached 500 mg daily even though the drugs with which the patients had previously been treated were not withdrawn (Yorkston *et al*, 1977).

The mode of antipsychotic action of propranolol is unknown but the relatively high doses that have to be used might permit the emergence of nonspecific actions that are not usually evident.

All the antipsychotic drugs encountered earlier are characterized by an ability to antagonize dopamine, a property with which propranolol has not been formally credited although there is at least one report in the literature that the stereotyped behaviour induced in rats by amphetamine (and usually attributed to dopamine liberation) can be prevented by propranolol (Herman, 1967). We must also recall the serotonin antagonism displayed by propranolol under some circumstances (see above)—anomalies of serotonin function may play an aetiological role in schizophrenia (p. 542)—and the fact that it also exerts a nonspecific membrane stabilizing action (p. 303) that may have far reaching neurophysiological and behavioural consequences in schizophrenic subjects.

The benzodiazepines
The benzodiazepine structure had been known to chemists for almost a century when Sternbach and his associates decided to synthesize a whole series of benzodiazepines on the chance that some members of the group might prove to have interesting pharmacological properties. The result of this study was the discovery, in 1960, that chlordiazepoxide (Table 32.5) possessed psychotropic activity. The drug rapidly became extremely popular with physicians and patients alike. Its success heralded the development of a whole range of other benzodiazepines which is still being extended twenty years after the arrival of chlordiazepoxide. The Western world's apparently insatiable thirst for drugs to relieve the anxiety and stresses that seem to become more acute and widespread with every increase in the material wealth and creature comforts that should abolish them, has led to a cascading demand for psychotropic drugs to the extent that anxiolytic agents, particularly the benzodiazepines, now feature in almost a half of all the prescriptions written in the developed countries. Unfortuantely, it seems that our indulgence in the benzodiazepines does nothing to damp our desire for more dangerous drugs, particularly alcohol. We can perhaps

Table 32.5 The benzodiazepines

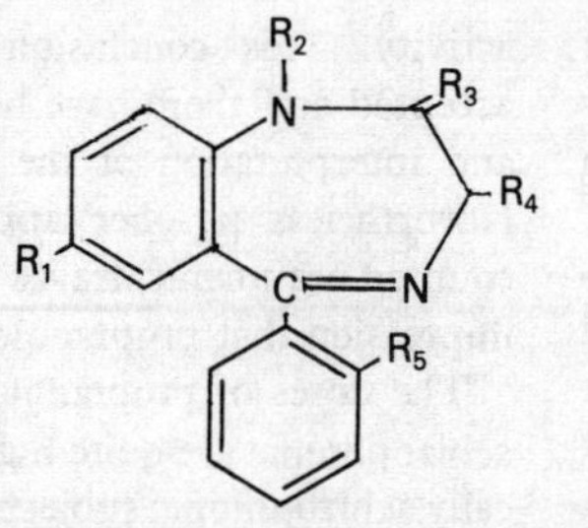

Approved name	Proprietary name(s)	R_1	R_2	R_3	R_4	R_5	Average adult daily dose mg
chlordiazepoxide	Librium Calmoden Tropium			see below			15–100
diazepam	Valium Atensine	Cl	CH_3	O	H_2	—	5–35
nitrazepam	Mogadon	O_2N	H	O	H_2	—	2.5–10*
oxazepam	Serenid	Cl	H	O	OH	—	25–50
medazepam	Nobrium	Cl	CH_3	H_2	H_2	—	25–50
clorazepate	Tranxene Tranxilium			see below			15–30
flurazepam	Dalmane	Cl	$(CH_2)_2N(C_2H_5)_2$	O	H_2	F	15–30*
prazepam	Demetrin	Cl	cyclopropylmethyl		H_2	—	10–30
temazepam		Cl	CH_3	O	OH	—	20–100
lorazepam	Ativan Tavor Temesta	Cl	H	O	OH	Cl	2–3
clonazepam	Rivotril Clonopin	O_2N	H	O	H_2	Cl	5–10
bromazepam				see below			20–25
flunitrazepam	Rohypnol	O_2N	H	O	H_2	F	1–2*

*Hypnotic dose

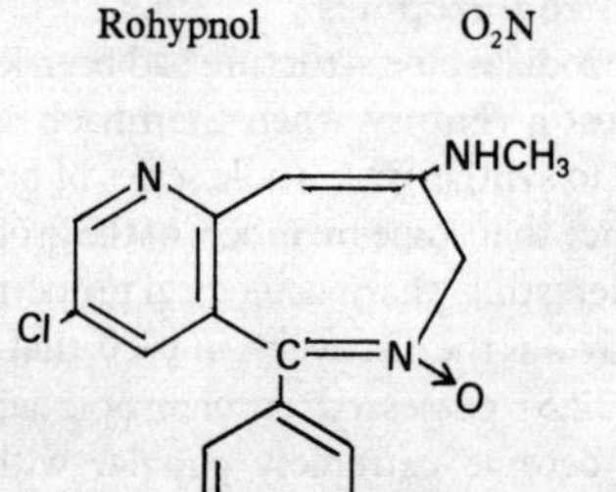

chlordiazepoxide

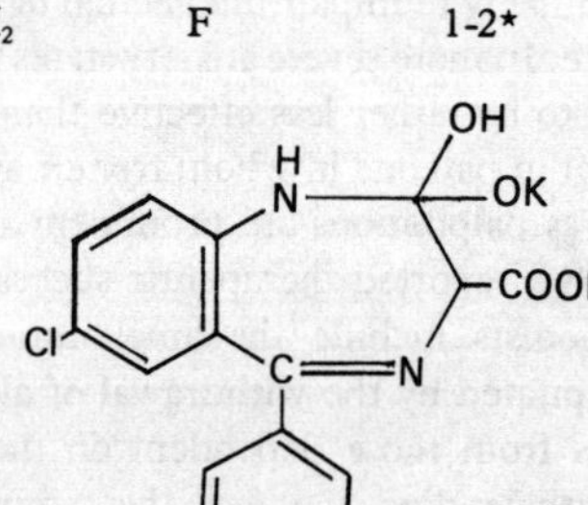

clorazepate

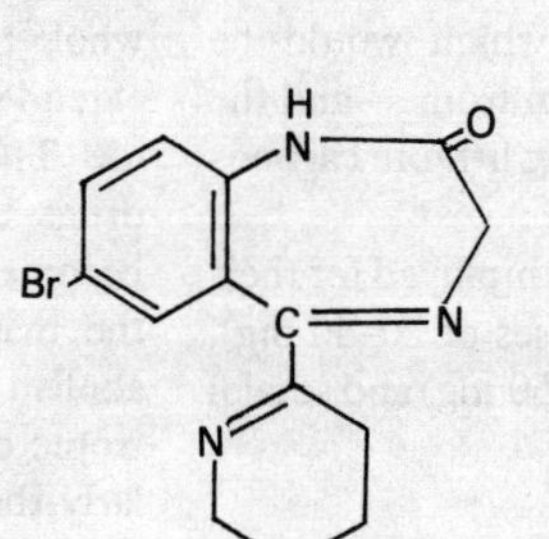

bromazepam

take a crumb of sorry comfort from the reflection that the benzodiazepines are considerably less dangerous than the barbiturates and the amphetamines whose place as the most popular psychotropic agents they have now occupied.

The names and chemical formulae of some of the benzodiazepines now available are set out in Table 32.5.

An account of the early development of the pharmacologically active benzodiazepines and some related compounds is provided by Sternbach, Randall and Gustafson (1967).

Although the benzodiazepines are still thought of primarily as anxiolytic drugs they are employed for a variety of therapeutic purposes. Some of them are recommended for particular purposes but in general the different members of the group differ from one another only quantitatively and no useful purpose would be served by attempting to divine and define the peculiar advantages of each of the compounds that features in Table 32.5. Instead the properties and uses of a few key benzodiazepines will be described. These descriptions should together provide a fairly complete summary of benzodiazepine pharmacology.

Chlordiazepoxide

Like meprobamate (p. 563) chlordiazepoxide (Librium) is a muscle relaxant by virtue of its ability to inhibit polysynaptic reflexes. It is a useful anticonvulsive agent: in its presence the thresholds for leptazol and electroshock seizures are considerably increased. In practice, however, other benzodiazepines such as diazepam and clonazepam are now preferred for the treatment of epileptic conditions. It blocks conditioned avoidance responses but its most characteristic property lies in its ability to calm excited animals and to blunt rage responses, whether these arise naturally or are experimentally induced. It does this without reducing locomotor activity. This effect has been demonstrated in a wide range of mammalian species ranging from mouse to tiger and the drug has been extensively used by veterinary surgeons and animal trainers. Man is less sensitive than most other species but chlordiazepoxide is used as a preoperative sedative in patients who are about to undergo minor surgery as well as for the treatment of anxiety neuroses and the anxiety states associated with impending examinations and similar testing events. It is also of value in the management of alcoholics: it prevents or ameliorates the unpleasant symptoms experienced by the patient who has just been withdrawn from his alcohol and it may serve to curb the anxiety and restlessness which is experienced during the early months of total abstinence. It has to be noted, however, that it is possible to become psychologically and perhaps even physically dependent on chlordiazepoxide itself and the drug must be given to alcoholics with some circumspection lest they exchange one form of dependence for another.

Because of its muscle relaxant properties, chlordiazepoxide has also found employment for the treatment of tetanus and spastic disorders, particularly those in which athetoid movements (p. 164) are a feature. Chlordiazepoxide is sometimes given to depressed patients who are also receiving monoamine oxidase inhibitors or other antidepressant drugs. It helps to allay the symptoms of anxiety often displayed by depressed patients and it is particularly useful in the early weeks of treatment before the antidepressant agents have begun to exert their full therapeutic action.

Chlordiazepoxide is normally taken by mouth but it can also be given by intramuscular or intravenous injection. The last named route is utilized in emergencies such as delirium tremens (p. 89). It is less rapidly and completely absorbed after intramuscular than after oral administration as a result of its binding to tissue proteins at the site of injection. Other members of the benzodiazepine group behave in a similar fashion.

Chlordiazepoxide is metabolized by demethylation to give desmethylchlordiazepoxide, a compound that retains the pharmacological activity of the parent compound. Some of the demethylated metabolite undergoes oxidative deamination to demoxepam, another active substance.

Chlordiazepoxide may induce substantial increases in the appetite and obesity must be guarded against. Confusion, disorientation and drowsiness are fairly common side effects. Interference with extrapyramidal function is not very usual. Chlordiazepoxide increases the aggressiveness of mice housed together in a group (but not that of animals caged singly) and similar paradoxical responses are occasionally seen in human patients or normal volunteers who may respond to therapeutic doses of the drug by becoming agitated or overtly aggressive.

The mode of action of the benzodiazepines is discussed later (p. 574).

Diazepam

Diazepam (Valium) resembles chlordiazepoxide but it is more potent and it is probably the most widely used of all anxiolytic drugs. The gibe that we live in a Valium-dominated society contains at least a gram of truth.

The other uses of diazepam are similar to those found for chlordiazepoxide but in addition its quite pronounced anticonvulsant properties render it a valuable drug for the control of status epilepticus (p. 530). For this purpose the drug is given intravenously. Moreover, while chlordiazepoxide can be used for preanaesthetic sedation, intravenous diazepam has found favour as an anaesthetic in its own right. In doses smaller than those needed to induce complete anaesthesia, intravenous diazepam produces tranquillity, an indifference to what might otherwise be daunting surroundings and a degree of amnesia that make it as useful as an anaesthetic proper for many patients undergoing relatively trivial operative procedures. It is also a valuable adjunct to local anaesthetics for those who might otherwise be distressed by minor operations even though they can be assured that they will feel no pain. Minor dental and other operations, obstetric manipulations, cardioversion and the insertion of endoscopes and other diagnostic instruments are all indications for the use, in suitable cases, of full or subanaesthetic doses of diazepam.

Like chlordiazepoxide, diazepam is metabolized by demethylation. The principal metabolite is desmethyldiazepam (nordiazepam) a little of which is hydroxylated to give oxazepam. Both metabolites are pharmacologically active, oxazepam indeed being included in the list of useful benzodiazepines (Table 32.5).

Diazepam sometimes causes paradoxical aggressiveness as do the other benzodiazepines. Patients taking diazepam should be warned that it potentiates the actions of alcohol and other drugs that depress the activity of the central nervous system.

Nitrazepam

Nitrazepam (Mogadon) has more pronounced hypnotic actions than the other benzodiazepines and it has proved to be a useful replacement for the barbiturate hypnotics. Its use is not infrequently followed by drowsiness and a degree of mental confusion and this feature of the drug's action combined with the potentiating interaction of residual drug with other centrally depressant drugs that might be being taken, should serve as a caution against its indiscriminate use as a hypnotic agent by those who will have to drive vehicles or operate potentially dangerous machinery on the morrow.

After a lapse of a half to one hour, effectively hypnotic doses of nitrazepam secure a sleep that persists for up to eight hours. Currently available evidence suggests that death is an unlikely sequel to overdosage but the possibility that the prolonged use of nitrazepam may lead to physical dependence of the barbiturate type must be constantly borne in mind.

Flurazepam and flunitrazepam

These newer benzodiazepine hypnotics seem, as far as can presently be judged, to offer some advantages over nitrazepam. They are, apparently, less prone to leave 'hangover' effects and their dependence liability has so far proved to be minimal. Flunitrazepam has also been employed as an anaesthetic induction agent.

Clonazepam

Clonazepam has achieved considerable success as an antiepileptic drug. Its use in this capacity is described elsewhere (p. 527). Clonazepam has also been applied to the treatment of tardive dyskinesia (p. 552).

CHLORMETHIAZOLE

As a postscript to our discussion of the benzodiazepine

chlormethiazole

group of drugs, mention should be made of chlormethiazole (Heminevrin, Hemineurin). It is not a benzodiazepine but it has a spectrum of activity—sedative, hypnotic, anxiolytic and anticonvulsive—that almost duplicates that of diazepam and a number of physicians have, for no very good reason, taken up the drug as a preferable alternative to diazepam. Its formal relationship with thiamine, a substance that plays an important part in neurophysiological actions, perhaps confers a certain glamour on chlormethiazole not enjoyed by the benzodiazepines but there is no evidence that it intervenes in the activity of the central nervous system at any more fundamental level than do chlordiazepoxide and its congeners.

Chlormethiazole has been principally employed for the treatment of status epilepticus, acute mania, eclampsia (toxic convulsions) of pregnancy, delirium tremens, sleeplessness and the abstinence states precipitated by abrupt withdrawal of opiates or alcohol from dependent subjects. When used as a hypnotic, chlormethiazole is taken in single doses of 0.5 to 1 gram but daily amounts of 1 to 4 grams, in divided doses, may be needed for the other conditions. The drug can also be given by intravenous infusion.

It has been known for some years that chlormethiazole can induce physical dependence if it is taken for more than one or two weeks. In spite of this, many patients have been permitted to take it for continuous periods of a year or more. Recent reports indicate that organic psychosis and suicidal depression characterize the abstinence syndromes that follow withdrawal of chlormethiazole from those who have become physically dependent on the drug (Hession, Verma and Bhakta, 1979).

There seems little reason to use chlormethiazole in preference to a benzodiazepine except, perhaps, for the emergency treatment of convulsive disorders that have not responded to diazepam.

MODE OF ACTION OF THE BENZODIAZEPINES AND OTHER ANXIOLYTIC DRUGS

In an earlier chapter we concluded (p. 168) that emotional states are determined partly by the nature of the activity generated in the limbic system and partly by the intensity of the arousal response evoked in the cerebral cortex by the flow of impulses along the ascending reticular system. These states ought, then, to be capable of modification by drugs that act at points within the limbic system and equally but rather less specifically by those that depress the arousal response. Some of the older anxiolytic drugs such as meprobamate and the barbiturates act in this latter capacity but the benzodiazepines have loci of action within the limbic system as is evidenced by the fact, among others, that the behaviour of experimental animals that have been given a benzodiazepine is strikingly reminiscent of that exhibited by animals that have been subjected to amygdaloidectomy (p. 168). Moreover, the spontaneous activity of limbic neurones is inhibited by benzodiazepines. In this respect, the limbic neurones are distinctly more sensitive than those elsewhere in the brain.

The limbic system incorporates a balanced complex of excitatory and inhibitory components and it is perhaps not surprising that on occasion the benzodiazepines stimulate the mechanisms that evoke anxiety and aggression instead of inhibiting them as they usually do.

The benzodiazepines presumably exert their pharmacological and therapeutic effects by intervening in transmission processes but in the absence of precise knowledge concerning the nature of the mediators involved in the operation of the several elements of the limbic system and of firm biochemical hypotheses relating to the aetiology of anxiety it is not possible at this time to do more than summarize the known facts concerning the effects of the benzodiazepines on transmitter systems and to add a few tentative speculations concerning the significance of these facts.

Acetylcholine

The benzodiazepines attenuate the toxic effects of anticholinesterase agents as a result, it is usually assumed, of their depressing the turnover of acetylcholine. A few investigators have found confirmation of this hypothesis in observations that the benzodiazepines increase the acetylcholine content of some areas of rat and mouse brain and that this increased content is associated with a reduced liberation of labelled acetylcholine previously incorporated into the brain. However, the time course of those changes that have been detected bears little relationship to that along which the drugs' pharmacological activity develops. Moreover the effects of the benzodiazepines on the acetylcholine system can be duplicated by muscimol (p. 577). Since this drug stimulates γ-aminobutyric acid receptors, it is difficult to escape the conclusion that any change in cholinergic activity induced by the benzodiazepines represents just another consequence of the stimulation of a system that is activated primarily by γ-aminobutyric acid.

The monoamines

When the synthesis of the brain's noradrenaline and dopamine is arrested by the administration of substances such as α-methyl-p-tyrosine that inhibit tyrosine hydroxylase (p. 290) the rate at which the catecholamines then disappear from the brain provides a measure of the rate at which they are each being utilized. p-Chlorophenylalanine, an inhibitor of tryptophan-5-hydroxylase can be similarly employed to measure the turnover rate of 5-

hydroxytryptamine in the brain. Using these techniques it can be shown that the benzodiazepines depress noradrenaline and serotonin release in the brains of experimental animals and prevent or minimize the increased release of these monoamines brought about by procedures that induce model anxiety states (p. 595). Repeated administration of the benzodiazepines discloses a qualitative difference in the response of the two transmitters, for while serotonin release remains depressed throughout the period of drug administration, the noradrenaline response is only transitory. It generally occupies the period during which the benzodiazepines are causing sedative side effects (in addition to their anxiolytic actions proper) to which the experimental animal soon develops tolerance.

The implication that the depressed release of noradrenaline is associated with the sedative action of the benzodiazepines is supported by the observation that the barbiturates and meprobamate (which, as we have seen, owe their anxiolytic effectiveness essentially to their hypnosedative activity) also inhibit noradrenaline release but not that of serotonin.

The association between anxiolytic action and reduced serotonin turnover is further underlined by the fact that substances that block serotonin receptors (bromlysergic acid, cinanerin and methysergide), inhibit serotonin synthesis (p-chlorophenylalanine) or destroy serotoninergic nerve terminals (dihydroxytryptamine) all potentiate the anxiolytic and anticonvulsant actions of small doses of the benzodiazepines.

The response of dopamine to the benzodiazepine group of anxiolytic drugs is similar to, but less well marked than that of noradrenaline.

Glycine

Snyder and his colleagues have championed the claim of glycine to be considered as a mediator of anxiolytic responses but the weight of evidence in its favour is not yet very impressive.

Strychnine binds to sites in the central nevous system which are presumed to correspond to glycine receptors. Benzodiazepines displace strychnine from these binding sites and there is a correlation (but by no means a perfect one) between their anxiolytic effects and their affinity for the receptors (Young, Zukin and Snyder, 1974). It has not, however, proved possible to demonstrate any effect of the benzodiazepines on the convulsant action of strychnine nor does strychnine antagonize the anxiolytic effect of the benzodiazepines or selectively influence the behaviour of experimental animals in model anxiety states.

γ-Aminobutyric acid

In the past few years, a considerable degree of enthusiasm for the idea that benzodiazepines exert their therapeutic action as a result of an intervention in activities mediated by γ-aminobutyric acid has generated a mass of experimental support for the concept. A summary of this evidence is provided by Guidotti (1978).

The benzodiazepines are effective antagonists of convulsions, such as those produced by bicuculline, picrotoxin and thiosemicarbazide, that are supposedly caused by a deficiency of γ-aminobutyric acid. They are much less effective against convulsions induced by agents such as strychnine and leptazol that operate independently of the γ-aminobutyric acid system.

Benzodiazepines, as we have noted, cause relaxation of skeletal muscle and the available evidence indicates that they do this because they increase presynaptic inhibition in the spinal cord, the cuneate nucleus and elsewhere. It is believed by many that γ-aminobutyric acid mediates presynaptic inhibition and the fact that the muscle relaxing effects of the benzodiazepines are antagonized by picrotoxin and bicuculline lends added strength to the supposition that they behave like γ-aminobutyric acid. A further

Table 32.6 Monoamine oxidase inhibitors: hydrazine derivatives.

$R_1NH.NHR_2$

Approved name	Proprietary name(s)	R_1	R_2	Daily dose mg
Iproniazid	Marsilid	pyridin-4-yl-CO	$-CH(CH_3)_2$	100-150 (initial); 25-50 (maintenance) not recommended
Nialamide	Niamid	pyridin-4-yl-CO-	$-CH_2.CH_2CONH.CH_2-$(phenyl)	150-200 then 75-100
Pivazide	Tersavid	phenyl-CH_2-	$-CO.C(CH_3)_3$	Withdrawn
Isocarboxazid	Marplan	phenyl-CH_2-	(5-methylisoxazol-3-yl-carbonyl) $-C(=O)-$(isoxazole with CH_3)	10-30 then 10-20
Mebanazine	Actomol	phenyl-$CH(CH_3)-$	H	Withdrawn
Phenelzine	Nardil	phenyl-$CH_2.CH_2-$	H	15-60 then 10-30
Pheniprazine	Catron Cavodil	phenyl-$CH_2.CH(CH_3)-$	H	Withdrawn
Phenoxypropazine	Drazine	phenyl-$O.CH_2.CH(CH_3)-$	H	Withdrawn

resemblance between the anxiolytic drug and the inhibitory transmitter has been disclosed by the finding that γ-aminobutyric acid, diazepam and muscimol (an agonist at γ-aminobutyric acid receptors) all reduce the concentration of cyclic GMP (p. 324) in the cerebellum. A range of other drugs seem to be without effect.

The precise nature of the interaction between the benzodiazepines and the γ-aminobutyric acid system has not yet been fully elucidated but it may be that the γ-aminobutyric acid receptors are rendered more sensitive or that the inactivation of the transmitter at the synapse is hindered by the benzodiazepines.

We have repeatedly reminded ourselves that few, if any, neurological functions are likely to be effected by neurones all of which utilize the same transmitter substance. Even if it should eventually transpire, therefore, that the benzodiazepines really do operate primarily to enhance activity in a γ-aminobutyric acid system this need not necessarily invalidate the conclusion that serotonin is a mediator of the drugs' pharmacological actions: stimulation of a neurone by γ-aminobutyric acid or a benzodiazepine could well influence activity in serotoninergic neurones.

It should be noted that the experimental evidence that supports the γ-aminobutyric acid hypothesis of benzodiazepine action is not quite as convincing on close examination as it appears at first sight. Its most obvious weakness lies in the fact that so few of the experimental observations relate to the anxiolytic actions of the drugs and those that do produce rather discouraging results. Attempts to demonstrate a synergistic anxiolytic action between diazepam and aminooxyacetic acid (a substance that promotes the synthesis of γ-aminobutyric acid) have failed as have—contrary to earlier reports—attempts to detect an antagonism between picrotoxin and the benzodiazepine (Sepinwall and Cook, 1978). Moreover, the benzodiazepines have useful anticonvulsive activity in idiopathic epilepsy but there is no substantial evidence that deficiency of γ-aminobutyric acid is in any way involved in the aetiology of that condition (p. 533). Finally, much is made of the similarity between the effects of the benzodiazepines and aminooxyacetic acid. While it is true that the latter substance does stimulate the synthesis of γ-aminobutyric acid, it is by no means certain that all its actions are attributable to this property (p. 192).

ANTIDEPRESSANT DRUGS

Authorities on the subject agree that depressive illnesses pose very difficult therapeutic problems. The large num-

Table 32.7 Monoamine oxidase inhibitors: non-hydrazines (Tables 32.6 and 32.7 are taken, with modifications, from Crossland (1967) by kind permission of Messrs. Butterworths).

Approved name(s)	Proprietary name	Formula	Daily dose mg
Tranylcypromine	Parnate Tylciprine	phenyl—CH—CH.NH$_2$ (with CH$_2$ bridge)	20-30
Pargyline	Eutonyl	phenyl—CH$_2$.N.CH$_2$.C$\equiv$CH, with N—CH$_3$	25-100 once daily
Etryptamine α-Ethyltryptamine	Monase	indole—CH$_2$.CH.NH$_2$ with C$_2$H$_5$	withdrawn
Harmine		CH$_3$O-substituted β-carboline with CH$_3$	hallucinogen
Harmaline		CH$_3$O-substituted dihydro-β-carboline with CH$_3$	hallucinogen

ber of antidepressant drugs on the market bears impressive witness both to the size of the population in need of treatment and to the continuing demand for more effective agents. It has to be admitted that the newer drugs offer few, if any, advantages over those that appeared more than thirty years ago and it is a sad commentary on our ignorance of the true nature of depressive illness (the monoamine hypotheses notwithstanding) and of the way in which it should be controlled that many psychiatrists have found it necessary to return to the use of electroconvulsive therapy for the management of serious depression.

It is no easier to classify the antidepressant drugs by reference to a number of mutually exclusive pharmacological categories than it is to perform the same operation for other groups of psychoactive drugs. The classification that follows should be taken as providing an aide memoire rather than a formal segregation into uniquely defined groups. It is also to be noted that the drugs are not arranged in any order of therapeutic merit: their positions were dictated largely by historical and textual considerations.

The classification is as follows:

1. Monoamine oxidase inhibitors
   a. hydrazine derivatives
   b. others
2. Drugs that inhibit the reuptake of monoamines at the synapse
   a. imipramine-like tricyclic compounds
   b. other reuptake inhibitors
3. Drugs with novel actions on monoamine systems
4. Drugs directly related to the monoamines
   a. amphetamine and other sympathomimetic agents
   b. tryptophan and 5-hydroxytryptophan
   c. L- 3,4-dihydroxyphenylalanine (DOPA)
5. Other drugs

Monoamine oxidase inhibitors

Isoniazid (isonicotinic acid hydrazide) was introduced into medicine in 1952 for the treatment of tuberculosis. It proved to be a most valuable drug in that field (p. 846). Iproniazid, its isopropyl derivative (Table 32.6) was also employed for a time in the same capacity but it had to be discarded by reason of the hyperactivity it produced in patients who took it. Since it also induced a noticeable degree of euphoria, it seemed possible that it might have a future as an antidepressant drug. This hope was realized, if not as completely as at first seemed likely. Zeller and his associates had found, at the time when the drug first entered medicine, that iproniazid inhibited the activity of monoamine oxidase in the brain (Zeller et al, 1952) and this led to the development of other monoamine oxidase inhibitors in the expectation that they too might have useful thymoleptic activity. Some of the inhibitors that were eventually used as psychotropic drugs were hydra-

zine derivatives (Table 32.6) like iproniazid itself. Others (Table 32.7), of which tranylcypromine can be taken as the prototype, have different structures.

PHARMACOLOGY OF THE MONOAMINE OXIDASE INHIBITORS

The most characteristic pharmacological action of the monoamine oxidase inhibitors is their ability to prevent or reverse reserpine depression and hypothermia and to potentiate the excitatory effects of sympathomimetic amines and the aminoacid precursors of the biogenic monoamines. The monoamines themselves do not, of course, pass the blood brain barrier and do not exert excitatory effects after parenteral administration.

When they are given alone, in single doses, the monoamine oxidase inhibitors produce no obvious hyperactivity in experimental animals and they may even depress locomotor activity. After prolonged administration, sympathetic and locomotor hyperactivity is seen in rabbits but not in dogs or cats. Even in rabbits, however, the excitatory responses are not so marked as when the inhibitors are given with 5-hydroxytryptophan. The slow onset of any behavioural response to a monoamine oxidase inhibitor reflects the fact that complete inhibition of the enzyme is a sluggish process. The therapeutic effects of the drug make their appearance at a similarly slow rate. The enzyme is inhibited irreversibly and after withdrawal of a monoamine oxidase inhibitor some ten to fourteen days must elapse before adequate supplies of newly synthesized enzyme become available to reestablish the physiological status quo. The monoamine oxidase inhibitors have a hypotensive action that is sufficiently pronounced to have led to one of them (pargyline) being used clinically as antihypertensive agents. The monoamine oxidase inhibitors have also been employed for the treatment of angina pectoris. The origin of the drugs' antihypertensive and antianginal actions is a matter of controversy which is more appropriately discussed in the sections of this book that consider the treatment of hypertension and angina pectoris. For the present it suffices to say that monoamine oxidase inhibitors are of only limited utility in cardiovascular conditions.

The hydrazine derivatives interact with pyridoxal phosphate and thereby inhibit the formation of γ-aminobutyric acid. This may explain why convulsions sometimes occur in patients and animals given monoamine oxidase inhibitors of this type (p. 191).

The enzyme inhibitory effect of the hydrazides apparently resides in their breakdown products. Continuing metabolism inactivates these active moieties. Acetylation plays an important part in this process and inactivation of the hydrazide drugs is retarded in slow acetylators (p. 73). This may account for the fact that some individuals display unexpectedly marked responses to modest doses of the hydrazide inhibitors. It must also be remembered, however, that the simple term, monoamine oxidase, refers to a whole family of closely related isoenzymes. Differences in the response of individual isoenzymes to the inhibitors and variations in the nature of the isoenzymes among patients will also lead to unpredictable irregularities in the responses to the drugs.

The hydrazides do not enjoy a prolonged sojourn in the body although their effects, as we have noted, are persistent by reason of their irreversible action on the enzyme.

The hydrazide inhibitors have some excitatory actions in human subjects, if not in all species of experimental animal (p. 578). Nialamide is said to be less active than its hydrazide fellows in this respect but the difference is not sufficiently well marked to enable a specification to be presented of patients who should be given nialamide in preference to one of the other hydrazides.

Iproniazid and its congeners are toxic substances and a number of hydrazides have had to be withdrawn from the market. Tranylcypromine was the outcome of efforts to find useful monoamine oxidase inhibitors that would spare the liver. Tranylcypromine is structurally related to amphetamine and at the upper end of the recommended dose range its actions (which are otherwise similar to those of iproniazid) are complicated by the emergence of amphetamine-like responses. There is increased activity of the sympathetic nervous system and a desynchronization ('alerting') of the encephalographic record.

Although tranylcypromine is less likely than the hydrazides to cause liver damage it is by no means a safe drug (see below) and in 1964 it was actually withdrawn from the market in the USA only to be allowed back some years later.

Etryptamine had stimulant actions similar to those of tranylcypromine but pargyline is devoid of amphetamine-like activity. Harmine and harmaline have psychotomimetic properties.

CLINICAL USES OF THE MONOAMINE OXIDASE INHIBITORS

Among authorities in this field, opinion concerning the value of the monoamine oxidase inhibitors in the treatment of depression range from the unenthusiastic to the frankly condemnatory. Nevertheless psychiatrists still find it necessary, on occasion, to recommend the drugs, if only when all other treatments (including, some would say, electroconvulsive therapy) have been tried and have failed. Those who feel that the risk of a severe toxic reaction is too high a price to pay for treatment with drugs of limited clinical value should remember that the patient whose depressive illness remains uncontrolled may well commit suicide. Circumstances such as these justify the use of any agent that might be able to prevent so tragic an outcome of our therapeutic shortcomings.

As we have noted earlier, some days must elapse after withdrawal of a monoamine oxidase inhibitor before new supplies of the enzyme can be synthesized in amounts adequate to ensure the restoration of monoaminergic neurone activity. During this period it is unwise to initiate treatment with other antidepressant drugs so that the patient has to be denied the solace of any drug at all. On the other hand, treatment with monoamine oxidase inhibitors can start as soon as other drugs are withdrawn. This provides another reason why monoamine oxidase inhibitors should be prescribed only when other treatments have been tried and found wanting.

It has been mentioned that tranylcypromine has excitatory actions. Some psychiatrists recommend a mixture of tranylcypromine and a phenothiazine for the treatment of patients who are both anxious and depressed but the combination of drugs seems to produce no better a clinical response than does phenothiazine alone.

The monoamine oxidase inhibitors of clinical choice in depression are phenelzine and tranylcyptomine. Pargyline is the preferred inhibitor for antihypertensive use. Parstelin is a proprietary mixture of tranylcypromine and trifluoperazine.

Side effects of monoamine oxidase inhibitors

The hydrazine derivatives can cause severe liver damage, perhaps as a result of lowering the organ's resistance to viral infection. It was because of their hepatoxicity that pheniprazine and phenoxypropazine were withdrawn from the market. Pheniprazine also caused red-green colour blindness, which was sometimes irreversible. Iproniazid itself is severely hepatotoxic in some patients and the drug is no longer available in the United States, although it can still be obtained in Great Britain. The non-hydrazine inhibitors are less likely to cause liver damage but they are toxic in other ways: etryptamine has been withdrawn because of the agranulocytosis that occurred in some of the patients who took the drug, while tranylcypromine is more likely than the hydrazides to cause hypertensive crises as a result of interactions with foods and drugs.

Autonomic disturbances (postural hypotension, dry mouth, sweating, constipation or diarrhoea, etc.) are not unusual among patients taking monoamine oxidase inhibitors of either type. The hypotension is likely to be particularly troublesome in elderly patients. Other signs of toxic involvement of the nervous system include headache, dizziness, muscle weakness and restlessness and the patient may become seriously agitated. Oedema of the ankles is a not unusual side effect.

Patients treated with monoamine oxidase inhibitors have suffered severe (and occasionally fatal) hypertensive attacks after taking certain items of food, notably cheese, beans, Chianti wine and yeast extracts. These hypertensive crises arise because pressor amines in the offending foods (such as tyramine in cheese) escape destruction and are absorbed into the blood stream if the monoamine oxidase of the intestine and liver is inhibited. The response is most severe with tranylcypromine, which increases the blood pressure directly, through its sympathomimetic action, as well as indirectly by inhibition of monoamine oxidase.

The monoamine oxidase inhibitors also interact with a large number of common drugs. When given to patients who are receiving monoamine oxidase inhibitors, reserpine may cause violent excitation, and some indirectly acting sympathomimetic amines including the drugs employed in the treatment of obesity (p. 283) may cause hypertensive crises similar to those produced by dietary amines. The monoamine oxidase inhibitors are not very specific and can interact with other drugs as a result of their inhibiting other enzymes. Thus the hypoglycaemic action of insulin and the sulphonylureas is potentiated and the depressant actions of alcohol, barbiturates and pethidine are intensified. It is to be noted that the risk of reactions between adrenaline (as might for instance be contained in a local anaesthetic) and monoamine oxidase inhibitors is minimal. Adrenaline is not taken up by neurones and so does not come into contact with monoamine oxidase. It is, of course, metabolized by catechol-O-methyltransferase.

It is customary at this point to issue a warning against the combination of a monoamine oxidase inhibitor with a tricycle antidepressant drug. The aim of this treatment is to secure a full antidepressant effect with subtoxic doses of each drug. Instead, agitation, convulsions and death may occur. Nevertheless, many highly experienced, well informed and compassionate psychiatrists have employed the two drugs together with safety and apparent therapeutic success. They would maintain that this combination is sometimes the only means of alleviating what might otherwise be a completely intractable condition. Careful supervision, preferably in hospital, of patients receiving this combined medication is necessary but it is clear that this approach to antidepressive therapy need not be so rigidly proscribed as it so often is by armchair commentators.

The hypertensive response to foodstuffs containing tyramine among patients receiving monoamine oxidase inhibitors was the first adverse drug interaction to become widely known. It led to the recognition of a whole range of other drug interactions, the importance and extent of which are discussed elsewhere (p. 76). In view of the now widespread knowledge of the cheese-monoamine oxidase inhibitor interaction (it almost qualifies for inclusion in a list of 'what every schoolboy knows') it is not without interest that the first report of the phenomenon came from an observant pharmacist who noted the coincidence of cheese eating and hypertensive episodes in his own wife. His suggestion that there was a causal link between the two events was at first greeted with something approaching derision even by those who were well aware that hypertensive crises sometimes complicated therapy with monoamine oxidase inhibitors (Ayd and Blackwell, 1970).

Drugs that inhibit the uptake of monoamines

Until recently all the substances that increased the availability of the monoamines at the synapse by inhibiting their reuptake into presynaptic neurones rather than by preventing their intraneuronal destruction were tricyclic compounds related to imipramine. It was thus possible to make a simple division of the major antidepressant drugs into the monoamine oxidase inhibitors and the tricyclic antidepressant agents. The latter soon became known as the 'tricyclic antidepressants' and then, alas, as the 'tricyclics'. However, some of the new uptake inhibitors do not show the tricyclic structure and it is no longer possible to use 'tricyclic' as a synonym for a drug that prevents the reuptake of a monoaminergic transmitter. This is a real blessing for those of us who not only care for the English language (the use of 'tricyclic' as a noun is a semantic abomination) but who try also to ensure that the words we use are as accurately descriptive as possible. Only very few tricyclic compounds display pharmacological activity and to use 'tricyclic' to describe a category of psychoactive drugs is as scientifically slipshod as it is grammatically offensive.

Some of the drugs to be described preferentially inhibit noradrenaline uptake while others show a partial selectivity towards serotonin. Because this difference might have therapeutic implications (p. 545) indications are given in table and text of the preferences of individual drugs insofar as they have yet been determined. It should be noted that total agreement concerning these preferences has not yet been reached and the reader may well encounter statements that conflict with those given here. Except when a statement to the contrary is entered it can be assumed that the drugs are without effect on transmitter reuptake at dopaminergic synapses.

IMIPRAMINE-LIKE TRICYCLIC COMPOUNDS

Imipramine, the original member of this group of drugs, was first synthesized in 1948. Interestingly enough in view of recent developments (p. 586) it was first intended as an antihistamine drug and its psychotropic activity did not emerge until 1957 in the course of an investigation into the pharmacological properties of compounds structurally analogous to chlorpromazine. Psycholeptic activity was being looked for (imipramine's structure is strikingly reminiscent of that of chlorpromazine) but when it was found that it had the properties of an antidepressant agent, attention was directed towards the development of related compounds with the same therapeutic potentiality. The members of the group that have come into clinical use are listed in Table 32.8.

On isolated preparations, imipramine antagonizes acetylcholine, dopamine, histamine, 5-hydroxytryptamine and noradrenaline. In the intact animal, small doses of imipramine will potentiate the action of those neurohumours whose reuptake is impeded but slightly larger doses (which are still within the therapeutic range) may still

Table 32.8 The tricyclic antidepressant drugs

Approved name(s)	Propriatary name(s)	R	Daily oral dose (in 3-4 divided doses)	Uptake preferentially inhibited NA - noradrenaline HT - serotonin

Approved name(s)	Propriatary name(s)	R	Daily oral dose	Uptake
Imipramine	Tofranil	$-CH_2(CH_2)_2N(CH_3)_2$	75-200 mg	Neither but $HT > NA$
Desipramine	Norpramin Pertofran	$-CH_2(CH_2)_2NHCH_3$	50-200 mg	NA
Trimipramine Trimepropimine	Surmontil	$-CH_2.CH.CH_2.N(CH_3)_2$	75-200	
Clomipramine (Chlorimipramine)	Anafril	As in imipramine but with Cl in position indicated by asterisk	30-150 mg	HT

Approved name(s)	Propriatary name(s)	R	Daily oral dose	Uptake
Amitriptyline	Amizol, Elavil, Domical, Larozyl, Lentizol, Tryptanol, Trypitizol	$=CH.(CH_2)_2.N(CH_3)_2$	75-200 mg	HT
Nortriptyline	Allegron, Aventyl	$=CH.(CH_2)_2.NHCH_3$	20-100 mg	Neither but NA > HT

Approved name(s)	Propriatary name(s)	R	Daily oral dose	Uptake
Opipramil	Insidon Ensidon	(full formula)	100-150 mg	

Approved name(s)	Propriatary name(s)	R	Daily oral dose	Uptake
Protriptyline	Concordin Vivactyl	(full formula)	10-40 mg	NA

Table 32.8 (contd)

Approved name(s)	Proprietary name(s)	R	Daily oral dose (in 3-4 divided doses)	Uptake preferentially inhibited NA - noradrenaline HT - serotonin

$$H_2C-O$$

$$CH(CH_2)_2N(CH_3)_2$$

| Doxepin | Sinequan | (full formula) | 75-150 mg | HT |

$$(CH_2)_2N(CH_3)_2$$

$$N-C=O$$

$$N$$
$$CH_3$$

| Dibenzepin | Noveril | (full formula) | 150-600 mg | |

display some at least of the antagonistic actions seen on isolated preparations. The two effects often coexist. Thus imipramine usually potentiates the responses to amphetamine and other indirectly acting sympathomimetic amines (p. 274) but doses that do this may also cause hypotension and dryness of the mouth as a result of their antagonizing noradrenaline and acetylcholine respectively. Again, imipramine can inhibit the catatonia induced by phenothiazines but it can itself cause tremors and other extrapyramidal side effects.

Imipramine reverses the depressant action of reserpine without restoring monoamines to the brain. It prolongs barbiturate sleeping time and has a marked anticonvulsive potency.

In the otherwise unmedicated animal, imipramine has even fewer behavioural effects than the monoamine oxidase inhibitors: the responses that have been recorded are reminiscent of those produced by chlorpromazine. Although the drug blocks the arousal response detected by electroencephalographic recording, it also sometimes increases the electrical activity of the cortex itself.

Desipramine and nortriptyline are the monodemethylated derivatives of imipramine and amitriptyline respectively. Although the demethylated substances are formed in the course of the normal metabolism of the parent compounds, the pharmacological and therapeutic actions of the latter are not totally attributable to those of their metabolites and the tri- and dimethyl compounds produce sufficiently different effects in the human subject to justify their listing as separate drugs. It should be particularly noted (Table 32.7) that whereas imipramine preferentially

inhibits serotonin reuptake, its metabolites are more effective against noradrenaline.

Apart from demethylation, the tricyclic antidepressant drugs are catabolized by oxidation and by hydroxylation in position 2 of the ring. The plasma half life of the drugs is of the order of 24 hours. The parent drugs and the pharmacologically active demethylated compounds are extensively bound to plasma proteins.

Clinical uses of the tricyclic antidepressants
The tricyclic antidepressant drugs generally achieve more satisfactory clinical results than the monoamine oxidase inhibitors. Imipramine and amitriptyline are the most widely used members of this group of compounds. Both drugs are more effective in endogenous than in reactive depression.

We have noted that the tricyclic agents exhibit differing degrees of preference for the noradrenaline and serotonin uptake mechanisms. Clomipramine is the most selective inhibitor of serotonin uptake; the most selective against noradrenaline seems to be maprotiline, a tetracyclic agent (see below).

Some of the tricyclic antidepressant agents such as clomipramine and amitriptyline (all of which show a stronger preference for serotonin uptake mechanisms) are tertiary amines and cause sedation in contrast to some of the secondary amines such as desipramine and nortriptyline which inhibit noradrenaline uptake mechanisms more strongly and tend to cause a degree of central stimulation.

There is, as yet, no clinical evidence to suggest that any of the newer tricyclic agents are to be preferred to imi-

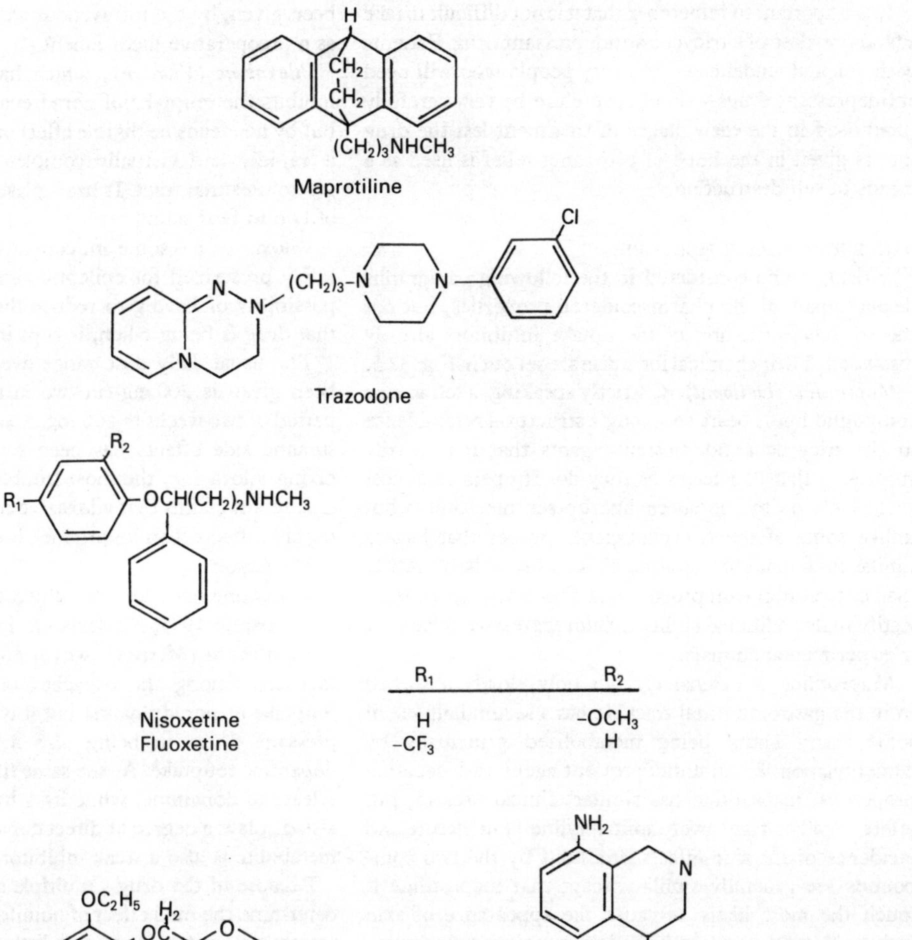

H

CH₂

CH₂

(CH₂)₃NHCH₃

Maprotiline

(CH₂)₃-N   N   Cl

Trazodone

R₂

R₁   OCH(CH₂)₂NHCH₃

| R₁   R₂
| --- | --- | --- |
| Nisoxetine | H | –OCH₃ |
| Fluoxetine | –CF₃ | H |

NH₂

N

OC₂H₅
OC   O
H₂
N
H

Viloxazine

Nomifensine

Fig. 32.5 Some monoamine re-uptake inhibitors not of a tricyclic structure.

pramine and amitriptyline which remain the most favoured antidepressant drugs. Of the two, amitriptyline because of its sedative properties is to be preferred in elderly or anxious patients.

Since quite high doses of the tricyclic drugs may have to be given, autonomic side effects resulting from their antagonizing noradrenaline and acetylcholine are quite common. These include hypotension, dryness of the mouth, retention of urine and constipation. Particular care has to be taken to guard against the development of glaucoma (p. 225) in old patients. Tremors or more definite signs of Parkinsonism may appear and injudicious administration of the drugs may lead to an agitated excite-

ment. Notwithstanding their anticonvulsant action in laboratory tests, imipramine and amitriptyline can precipitate epileptic attacks in susceptible patients. This point—which applies also to many other members of this group of drugs—should always be borne in mind when epileptic patients need antidepressant therapy.

Amitriptyline may cause excessive drowsiness and in a few instances imipramine treatment has been associated with the development of agranulocytosis. Imipramine has been reported to have teratogenic activity in rabbits.

The danger of combined treatment with monoamine oxidase inhibitors and the tricyclic antidepressants has already been alluded to.

It is important to remember that it is not difficult to take a fatal overdose of a tricyclic antidepressant drug. Patients with suicidal tendencies—the very people who will need antidepressant drugs—should therefore be very carefully supervised in the early stages of treatment lest the drug that is given in the hope of providing relief is used as a means of self destruction.

OTHER REUPTAKE INHIBITORS

The drugs to be considered in the following paragraphs display many of the pharmacological properties, but not the tricyclic structure, of the uptake inhibitors already discussed. Their chemical formulae are set out in Fig. 32.5.

Maprotiline (Ludiomil) is, strictly speaking, a tetracyclic compound but it bears so strong a structural resemblance to the tricyclic antidepressant agents that it is hardly surprising that it behaves as they do. It operates almost exclusively on the noradrenaline uptake mechanism but unlike some of the tricyclic agents proper that have a similar preference for noradrenaline, it has sedative rather than central stimulant properties. Laboratory experiments testify to its additional ability to calm aggressive behaviour in experimental animals.

Maprotiline is extensively but only slowly absorbed from the gastrointestinal tract. It has a serum half-life of some thirty hours being metabolized principally by demethylation. As an antidepressant agent with sedating properties, maprotiline has similar clinical uses to, but offers no advantages over, amitriptyline. The nature and incidence of the side effects produced by the two compounds are generally similar except that maprotiline is much the more likely to cause the appearance of skin rashes. Notwithstanding its sedating action, maprotiline very occasionally causes epileptiform convulsions even in patients who have shown no previous evidence of epilepsy.

The average daily dose of maprotiline is 25 to 150 mg but this can be cautiously increased, if necessary, to a maximum daily maintenance dose of 300 mg. Because of the drug's sedative action it is often useful to suggest that the major part of the day's dose should be taken at bed time. A recent review of maprotiline is provided by Pinder et al. (1977).

Trazodone (Trittico), in contrast to maprotiline, operates exclusively on serotonin mechanisms, preventing the monoamine's reuptake into brain without noticeably affecting the concentrations of either serotonin or 5-hydroxyindoleacetic acid. It also prevents the uptake of serotonin into platelets. Trazodone has anxiolytic as well as antidepressant properties but it is devoid of antipsychotic activity.

For the treatment of depression the doses of trazodone so far employed have ranged from 50 to 600 mg daily. The side effects most commonly reported have been related to the drug's anticholinergic actions. Trazodone has also

been given, by the intravenous and intramuscular routes, as a preoperative medicament.

Viloxazine (Vivalan), which has a bicyclic structure, inhibits the reuptake of noradrenaline and has a smaller, but by no means negligible effect on serotonin reuptake. It is rapidly and virtually completely absorbed from the gastrointestinal tract. It has a plasma half life of the order of two to four hours.

Viloxazine has some anticonvulsant action and it may be safely prescribed for epileptic patients provided that the possibility of having to reduce the dose of phenytoin, if that drug is being taken, is kept in mind.

The usual daily dose range over which viloxazine has been given is 200 mg (in two instalments) rising over a period of two weeks to 400 mg. A variety of autonomic and somatic side effects has been reported among patients taking viloxazine, the most troublesome being vomiting. One report claims that viloxazine causes fewer incommoding side effects than imipramine but this conclusion awaits confirmation.

Viloxazine has been the subject of recent major reviews (Symposium 1975; Pinder et al, 1977).

Nomifensine (Merital), which might perhaps have been included among the tricyclic compounds, inhibits the reuptake of noradrenaline but it is unique among antidepressant drugs in being also a powerful inhibitor of dopamine reuptake. At the same time it also promotes the release of dopamine, while its 4-hydroxylated metabolite also displays a degree of direct dopaminergic activity. This metabolite is also a weak inhibitor of serotonin uptake.

Because of the drug's multiple actions it is difficult to determine the final effect of nomifensine on the dopamine system. Nomifensine is of little value in Parkinson's disease which might be taken to imply that its dopaminergic activity is negligible. On the other hand it induces stereotypy of the amphetamine type in rats and it can reverse the depletion of dopamine from the brain induced by 6-hydroxydopamine, indicating that nomifensine increases the availability of synaptic dopamine. Whatever the true state of affairs, there is as yet no evidence that nomifensine's unique pharmacological profile confers unique therapeutic qualities on the drug.

The daily dose of nomifensine is 50–200 mg. A recent review concerning the drug's pharmacology and therapeutics is available (Nicholson and Turner, 1977).

Nisoxetine and *fluoxetine* are an interesting pair of structurally related compounds that challenge our understanding of structure-activity relationships among the antidepressant drugs for while nisoxetine selectively inhibits the reuptake of noradrenaline, fluoxetine does the same for serotonin. Neither drug has yet undergone extensive clinical investigation.

Drugs with novel actions on monoamine systems
The drugs to be considered in the following paragraphs are

not potent inhibitors of monoamine oxidase or of monoamine reuptake and yet they probably owe their undoubted antidepressant actions to an intervention somewhere in the system that determines the amount of transmitter that shall be available at monoaminergic synapses in the brain. Their names and formulae are brought together in Fig. 32.6.

Mianserin (Bolvidon, Norval), a tetracyclic compound, was originally developed as an antiserotonin drug in the hope that it might find employment in the treatment of migraine. Its mood elevating effect emerged during early clinical trials and it was soon established that it had antidepressant activity comparable to that residing in the tricyclic antidepressant agents. At the same time, however, it became equally evident that mianserin has no effect on monoamine reuptake processes in the brain.

The mode of action of mianserin proved to be a matter of considerable pharmacological interest. It transpired that it occupies adrenoceptors located on presynaptic terminals. These so called α_2 receptors (which are pharmacologically distinct from the α- or α_1-receptors located on postsynaptic membranes and elsewhere) normally respond to noradrenaline appearing at the synapse in the course of neuronal activity by restraining the further release of transmitter. They are thus essential components in a negative feed back system that regulates transmitter output. Blocade of α_2 receptors by mianserin interrupts the feed back cycle and leads to an increased noradrenaline liberation. This interpretation of mianserin's action is consistent with the observation that, unlike other antidepressant drugs, mianserin increases the turnover and decreases the content of noradrenaline in the brain.

Mianserin has a slight blocking action at α_1 receptors and some of the tricyclic antidepressant drugs have a minimal action at α_2 receptors. Among the conventional α

blocking agents (p. 293), phenoxybenzamine occupies both α_1 and α_2 receptors but the others have an affinity for only the α_1 variety.

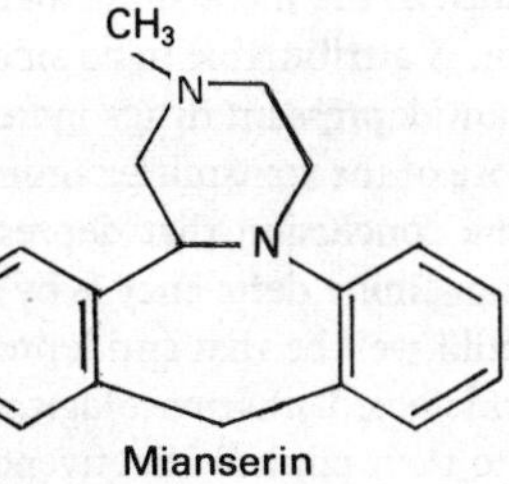

In clinical use, mianserin displays therapeutic activity comparable with that of the established tricyclic antidepressant drugs. It has some sedating action and its side effects are similar to those encountered with the imipramine-like drugs apart from the fact that antimuscarinic activity is usually less evident. When taken by mouth, mianserin is readily absorbed: maximum blood levels are reached some three hours after ingestion and the drug is disposed of by aromatic hydroxylation and demethylation.

Mianserin is a relatively potent drug and is effective in daily doses of the order of 15 to 60 mg.

Mianserin is the subject of a recent symposium (Peet and Turner, 1978).

Iprinodole (Prondol) is clearly a tricyclic compound. It is also an antidepressant drug but it cannot properly be designated as a tricyclic antidepressant agent because it does not significantly impede the reuptake of monoamine transmitters. Nor does it, unlike mianserin, occupy presynaptic α_2 receptors. Just how the drug does relieve depression still constitutes something of a mystery and a challenge. Some have denied that iprindole has any true antidepressant activity (an assertion that is difficult to sustain in the light of the results of recent well designed clinical trials) while others maintain that all antidepressant drugs owe their therapeutic activity to a mechanism that is radically different from any that has so far been postulated. A glimpse of a possible alternative mechanism has been provided by the observation that the brains of rats that have been treated with antidepressant drugs produce cyclic AMP in response to noradrenaline less readily than do the brains of untreated animals. All the antidepressant drugs so far tested (including iprindole) show this effect as, indeed, do electrically induced convulsions similar to those employed in electroconvulsive therapy (Vetulani *et al.* 1976). An interesting feature of this action is that, like the therapeutic response to the antidepressant drugs, the inhibitory effect on cyclic AMP formation does not appear until the drugs have been given for some three or four weeks. This is the first pharmacological property shown by antidepressant drugs that develops with approximately the same time course as the therapeutic response. It should be noted, however, that a logical consequence of embracing the idea that iprindole acts by virtue of its effect on cyclic AMP formation is the conclusion that depressive illnesses are associated with an excess of synaptic noradrenaline or with an increased sensitivity to the transmitter.

Iprindole is used in daily oral doses of 30 to 180 mg, indicating a potency of the order of that shown by mianserin. Although it is said to possess little atropine-like activity, dry mouth, blurred vision and hypotension not infrequently appear in the list of side effects of treatment. However, iprindole treatment is associated with fewer side

CH$_3$

Mianserin

(CH$_2$)$_3$N(CH$_3$)$_2$

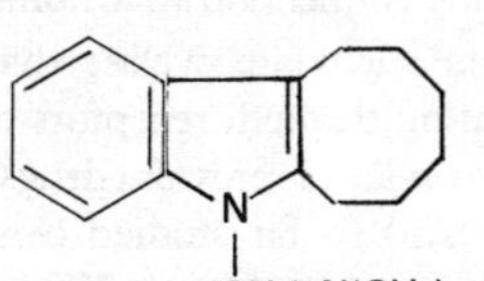

Iprindole

Fig. 32.6 Antidepressant drugs with novel actions on monoamine systems.

effects than is treatment with almost any other antidepressant agent.

Drugs directly related to the monoamines

If depressive disorders arise as a result of a deficiency of one or more of the monoamine transmitters, it should be possible to secure some remission for their victims by supplying them with additional supplies of transmitter. Since the monoamines cannot surmount the blood-brain barrier, only the administration of precursors that can do so has any prospect of remedying the transmitter deficiency. In recent years, much effort has been expended in attempts to demonstrate that restoration of transmitters in this way influences the course of affective disorders. These exertions have been inspired as much by an urge to obtain support for an aetiological role for one or more of the monoamine transmitters as by a desire to improve the therapy of these conditions.

Precursor loading, as the technique is usually called, has most often involved the administration of L-DOPA, tryptophan or 5-hydroxytryptophan but it is important to note that the consequences of giving relatively large amounts of these substances are not nearly so simple as the originators of the method originally assumed. The conversion of the precursors into the transmitters depends on an enzyme (L-aromatic acid decarboxylase, p. 258) that is common to all monoaminergic neurones. Thus the administration of, say, tryptophan, is likely to be followed by the formation of serotonin in noradrenergic as well as in serotoninergic neurones. Moreover the precursors are likely to undergo metabolic changes inside or outside the brain other than a simple transformation into transmitter substances. These other metabolites may well contribute to or interfere with any therapeutic effect exerted by the precursors. Finally it is not clear that simply increasing the production of transmitter necessarily remedies the synaptic deficiency caused by the biochemical lesion that led to the deficiency in the first place.

The results of attempting to treat depression by precursor loading are equivocal but a number of psychiatrists claim that tryptophan, in daily doses of 3 to 6 grams, taken in association with a monoamine oxidase inhibitor is sometimes effective when other treatments have failed. This approach is certainly a logical one inasmuch as it is reasonable to expect that the effects of an enzyme inhibitor will be potentiated if it is provided with adequate amounts of its substrate.

A proprietary name for tryptophan is Pacitron.

AMPHETAMINE

In the past, amphetamine was a very popular prescription for the treatment of bouts of depression (usually of the reactive variety) too trivial to warrant attention by a psychiatrist. Amphetamine is an indirectly acting sympathomimetic amine (p. 274) and, unlike the antidepressant drugs proper, it is a stimulant drug. To the extent that it was sometimes effective its action provides some support for the catecholamine hypothesis of depressive conditions.

Other drugs

A number of drugs that do not formally belong to the category of antidepressant drugs, nevertheless find occasional use for the treatment of depression, a circumstance that illustrates once again the impossibility of fitting the protean variety of mental illnesses and the drugs that alleviate them into a rigid classification system.

Flupenthixol is an antipsychotic drug (p. 564) but in much smaller doses than those employed in the treatment of schizophrenia it seems to have useful antidepressant activity particularly in patients in whom anxiety accompanies the depression. Antidepressant doses of flupenthixol range from 1 to 4 mg daily and the therapeutic response, if any is going to appear, is usually apparent after no more than two or three days. The origin of flupenthixol's antidepressant action is unknown.

Chlorpromazine and some other phenothiazine compounds are also endowed with some antidepressant properties (p. 551) and they are sometimes particularly effective when they are given together with a tricyclic antidepressant drug.

Although *lithium* exerts its principal therapeutic effect on the manic phases of manic-depressive illnesses it is sometimes, and rather surprisingly, able to offer relief to individuals suffering from pure unipolar depressive states.

Concluding remarks

Before completing our discussion of the antidepressant drugs some final remarks are called for though these may be less relevant to the action of our current drugs than they are to the development of the next generation of antidepressant agents.

The dominance of the monoamine deficiency hypothesis of depression is attributable in no small measure to the fact that most antidepressant drugs increase the availability of one or more of the transmitter amines at the synapse. The logic of the conclusion that depression is therefore caused by a monoamine deficiency is by no means impeccable and it could well be that antidepressant drugs have some so far undetected pharmacological actions that are more relevant to their clinical effectiveness. It is interesting to note in this connection that homogenates of brain tissue contain an adenylate cyclase that is activated by histamine operating through receptors of the H_2 type (p. 344). All the known antidepressant drugs (including iprindole and mianserin) so far studied behave as histamine antagonists at these receptor sites (Kanof and Greengard, 1978). It is, perhaps, rather unfortunate for an otherwise promising finding that a few drugs with no pretensions to antidepressant activity also antagonize histamine H_2 receptors.

One well-known (but not unanswerable) objection to the monoamine hypothesis of depression is that whereas the antidepressant drugs do not exert their therapeutic action until treatment has been under way for some three weeks, the pharmacological changes upon which this action supposedly depends occurs immediately. The indication that antidepressant drugs reduce the sensitivity of noradrenaline responses and that this change occurs no more rapidly than the therapeutic response (p. 578) gives a hint that future refinements of the monoamine hypothesis might place more stress on receptor responsiveness. The idea that depression might be a consequence of an increased traffic at noradrenergic synapses (with the diminished synthesis of noradrenaline representing a partially compensatory response) would turn the present catecholamine hypothesis on its head. But such a volte face would not be a unique event in the annals of psychopharmacology. We must remember that the pharmacological actions of reserpine were variously attributed in the past (by authorities having identical knowledge of the experimental facts) to an excess and to a deficiency of monoamines at the synapse.

PSYCHOTOMIMETIC DRUGS

Psychotomimetic substances are those which induce changes in mood, perception or behaviour that mimic some of those seen and experienced in the schizophrenias. In particular, they induce disturbances of perception of an hallucinogenic nature. 'Psychotomimetic' has a number of synonyms including schizogen, psychotogen, phantastica, psychosomimetic and psycholytic, to name but a few.

Many drugs (amphetamine, atropine and cocaine are examples) have psychotomimetic side effects if they are taken in high doses or over a prolonged period of time but because this is not their primary action in low doses they are not usually grouped with the psychotomimetic drugs proper.

The reader should recognize that the resemblance between the symptoms induced in healthy subjects by the psychotomimetic drugs and those occurring naturally in psychotic patients is far from complete. Although the psychotomimetic drugs are said to be hallucinogenic, they do not regularly produce hallucinations in the true sense of the term—sensory experiences that arise in the absence of any physiological stimulation of the corresponding sense organs. The visual sensations that may be experienced by subjects under the influence of the psychotomimetic drugs may be vivid, brightly coloured and quite bizarre but they often represent distorted or accentuated images of some actual object in the visual field. Similar remarks apply to the distortions of auditory and tactile sensations that are induced by the psychotomimetic drugs. When true hallucinations do occur, the subject's surroundings—a quasi-

religious ceremony, for instance—are often such as to induce heightened emotional tension and suggestibility. The relative rarity of true hallucinations in subjects given psychotomimetic substances is probably not merely the reflection of an inherent difference between the responsiveness of the normal and the psychotic individual, for true hallucinations frequently occur in normal subjects in experimental situations in which perceptual stimulation has been reduced to a minimum.

Because the criteria of psychotomimetic action are rather imprecise, there are some differences of opinion concerning the classification of some of the less active substances but the names and formulae of a number of compounds generally recognized as psychotomimetic are set out in Figures 32.1 & 32.7.

Clinical and laboratory uses of the psychotomimetic drugs
Psychotomimetic drugs are not employed as therapeutic agents but lysergic acid diethylamide is sometimes given to revive repressed memories whose psychogenic influence can thus be recognized and dealt with by the patient and his psychiatrist. In general, however, psychiatrists have been more impressed with the possibility of increasing their knowledge of psychiatric conditions by using the drugs to produce 'model psychoses' in normal subjects who can report on their subjective experiences. The interest of the neurochemist and the pharmacologist, as we have seen, is directed towards establishing the nature of the drugs' interaction with humoral mechanisms and thus to obtain some insight into the biochemical aetiology of schizophrenia.

Pharmacological properties and possible modes of action of the psychotomimetic drugs
In the course of discussions concerning the biochemical aetiology of schizophrenia we have already come across a number of psychotomimetic compounds that are related to the monoamine transmitters (p. 324). Those that contain

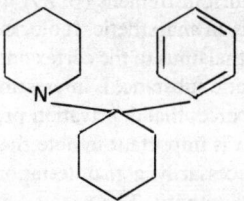

Phencyclidine
(Sernylan, Sernyl)

N-methyl-3-piperidyl benzilate: see Table 32.4
Tetrahydrocannabinol: formula on p. 92

Fig. 32.7 Some psychotomimetic substances (see also Fig. 32.1 p. 540).

an indole nucleus—including adrenochrome and adrenolutin which are derived from adrenaline—have structural affinities with serotonin and they can all be shown to behave as serotonin antagonists on suitably chosen preparations. On the other hand, it can also be congently argued that the actions of lysergide, almost the prototypical serotonin antagonist, arise from an interaction with processes dependent on noradrenaline rather than 5-hydroxytryptamine. Signs of sympathetic stimulation occur after administration of lysergide and there is a suggestion that it may accelerate or induce the production of hallucinogenic metabolites from adrenaline and noradrenaline. In addition to its very marked sympathomimetic actions, lysergide also exerts some effects that more specifically recall those of amphetamine. Thus it impairs the appetite and produces an amphetamine-like desynchronization of the electrical activity of the brain. While it is possible, therefore, that some hallucinogenic agents intervene in mechanisms subserved by noradrenaline or serotonin it is not yet possible to come to any conclusion concerning the ways in which disturbed monoaminergic function might manifest itself as a hallucinatory experience. Moreover some psychotomimetic substances bear no resemblance at all to the monoamine transmitters.

N-Methyl-3-piperidyl benzilate (Table 32.6) has antiacetylcholine activity. That this is the origin of its psychotomimetic properties is suggested by the fact that hallucinations may occur in atropine poisoning or, in sensitive individuals, after therapeutic doses of the drug. Thus in this instance at least, the psychotomimetic response may well be a consequence of interference with transmission processes in cholinergic synapses. It does not, of course, exclude the possibility that the same sort of response may follow interference with other types of transmission system.

True hallucinatory activity (which particualrly affects the visual and auditory systems) occurs much more often with piperidyl benzilate than it does with the other psychotomimetic drugs. In many subjects it produces a condition reminiscent of delirium tremens (p. 89).

Phencyclidine is an anaesthetic. It blocks impulse transmission from the thalamus to the cortex and the fact that it is a psychotomimetic substance is interesting in view of the observation that perceptual deprivation produces hallucinations in man. It is important to note that hallucinatory activity is not necessarily a manifestation of a directly increased cerebral activity. The exclusion of meaningful sensory information from the brain may release restraints and precipitate distorted thought processes as effectively as if the drug acted directly on the cortex. Indeed it may well be that this psychophysiological concept will lead to the most satisfactory explanation for the origin of hallucinatory activity since it does not demand the participation (or exclusion) of a particular transmission system. It is clear that a deficit of incoming patterns of sensory information

might follow interference with any one of several types of chemical mediator.

Reviews of psychotomimetic drug action have been provided by Eduison and his associates (1964), Hoffer and Osmond (1967), Brawley and Duffield (1972) and by Brimblecombe (1973).

THE NEUROPHARMACOLOGY OF EXTRAPYRAMIDAL DISEASE

Parkinson's disease is a condition that attracts a perhaps disproportionate amount of attention from most pharmacology teachers (and the authors of their textbooks) by reason of the fact that it is one of the very few disease states that are associated with a recognizable pharmacological lesion the discovery of which led to the introduction of a rational and successful form of drug therapy. Lest this success goes to our collective head it must be mentioned that other forms of treatment were discovered long ago by purely empirical methods.

Parkinson's disease was first described in the early years of the 19th century by James Parkinson. It is a disorder of extrapyramidal function characterized, as we saw earlier (p. 164), by tremor, impassivity of facial expression, a festinant gait, an increased muscle tone giving rise to rigidity and speech difficulties and signs (such as profuse salivation) of excessive parasympathetic activity.

Parkinson's disease proper (paralysis agitans) is an idiopathic condition that most often makes its appearance in late middle life although it is not unknown in much younger indivduals. It is essentially a degenerative disease and its onset may be accelerated by trauma, tumour, cerebral arteriosclerosis and other conditions that jeopardize the proper nourishment of the brain. Paralysis agitans may appear as a sequel to encephalitis lethargica, a virus disease that occurs only sporadically: in Britain the last epidemic occurred in 1916. Some of the features of Parkinson's disease are not infrequently seen in patients receiving treatment with some of the psychotropic drugs, particularly the phenothiazines and the butyrophenones. This symptom complex is often described as Parkinsonism to distinguish it from true paralysis agitans but the two conditions share the same biochemical aetiology.

It has long been known that an invariable pathological lesion in Parkinson's disease is degeneration of the substantia nigra and in 1966 Hornykiewicz reported that extracts of the caudate nucleus (a major portion of the corpus striatum) taken, post mortem, from the brains of individuals who had had Parkinson's disease were seriously deficient in dopamine often containing no more than 5 or 10 per cent of that found in subjects who were free of the disease (Hornykiewicz, 1966). The obvious conclusion to be drawn from these observations (and it has been amply confirmed by other lines of evidence) is that a tract of dopaminergic fibres courses from the substantia nigra to the caudate nucleus. Moreover, since the degeneration of these fibres gives rise to a condition characterized by an increased muscle tone it has to be further concluded that the dopaminergic fibres activate neurones that have an inhibitory effect on muscle tone and that a reassertion of this nigrostriatal influence could be brought about by supplying exogenous dopamine at the caudate nucleus to replace that no longer being supplied by the activity of its normal source. As even the veriest tyro pharmacology student knows, this conclusion has been triumphantly vindicated by the success of L-DOPA treatment.

It is often forgotten that Hornykiewicz also detected a gross deficiency of serotonin as well as of dopamine in the caudate nuclei of victims of Parkinson's disease but this finding has not been exploited.

Long before we had any knowledge of dopaminergic fibres (or indeed of the existence of any kind of chemical transmitter system) Parkinson's disease was treated with drugs that are now known to block the muscarinic actions of acetylcholine. Belladonna itself was originally used (it was first introduced by the great Charcot in 1890) but it was, of course, later replaced by atropine and hyoscine (p. 229) and later still by the synthetic antimuscarine drugs. Although these drugs were originally introduced on empirical grounds it is now possible to understand the basis of their therapeutic action if we assume that cholinergic fibres activate neurones that augment resting muscle tone. It can be seen by referring to the schematic diagram presented in Figure 32.8 that degeneration of the dopaminergic fibres will lead to a state in which the impulses that augment muscle tone are no longer balanced by those that diminish it (the ancient Hippocratic 'balance' hypothesis raises its head again!) and that partial rectification of the condition can be achieved by antagonizing the now unopposed cholinergic activity as readily as by reintroducing dopamine into the system. It must not, however, be assumed that the two systems have equally important roles in all the muscle control mechanisms that may be affected in Parkinson's disease. Poverty of movement (akinesia or hypokinesia) is, for instance, more readily remedied by L-DOPA than it is by the antimuscarine drugs. Furthermore, some of the therapeutic benefits that accrue from the use of the antimuscarine agents may, as we shall see, be the consequence of their action on the dopamine system. Nevertheless, the freedom from the tendency to cause Parkinsonian side effects that is enjoyed by some of the antipsychotic drugs is attributable to their being able to exert atropine-like actions (p. 551).

To complete our simple picture of the state of affairs in the nigrostriatal system, we should refer to fibres that utilize γ-aminobutyric acid as their transmitter agent and which course from the caudate nucleus to the substantia nigra (Fig. 32.8). When they are stimulated they inhibit activity in the dopaminergic fibres. This provides another

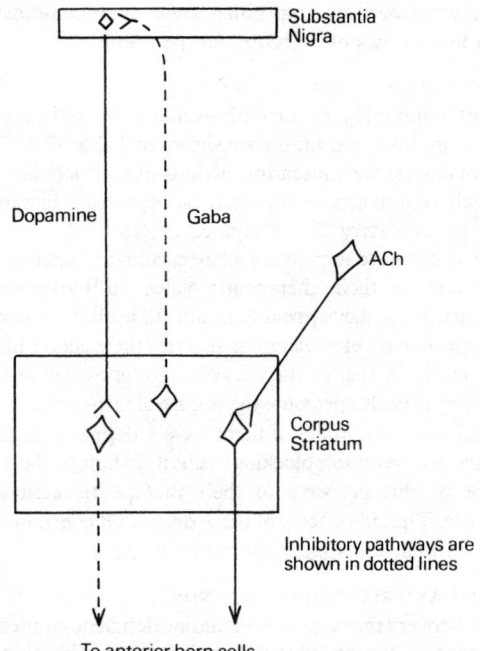

Fig. 32.8 Some neuronal interconnections within the basal ganglia.

example of the interaction between γ-aminobutyric acid and the monoamines that we previously encountered in the course of discussing the mode of action of the benzodiazepines.

The striatonigral fibres are not relevant to our discussion of Parkinson's disease but their degeneration is the key lesion in at least some cases of Huntington's chorea (p. 164). Loss of these fibres will presumably increase the activity of the nigrostriatal dopaminergic fibres. Another lesion seen in Huntington's chorea is a deficiency of choline acetyltransferase with a consequent reduction in the activity of the cholinergic fibres that converge on the caudate nucleus. Thus both lesions lead effectively to an overactivity in dopaminergic neurones and Huntington's chorea is rationally (if not very successfully) treated with phenothiazines which are dopamine antagonists and benzodiazepines which mimic the actions of γ-aminobutyric acid. Treatment with an anticholinesterase agent, though theoretically in order, is impracticable by reason of the incommoding side effects caused by the accumulating acetylcholine.

The treatment of paralysis agitans and Parkinsonism

Notwithstanding the success of the L-DOPA treatment of paralysis agitans, some patients do not respond to treatment as well as they might be expected to while others find the side effects of treatment to be incommoding or embarrassing. For these patients, the older forms of treatment using atropine-like drugs either alone or in combination with lower doses of L-DOPA can be prescribed.

ATROPINE-LIKE DRUGS

Drugs in this category currently available for the treatment of Parkinsonian conditions are shown in Table 32.9. They all antagonize the muscarinic actions of acetylcholine but in their central actions they may be depressant like hyoscine or excitatory like atropine. Interestingly enough, these drugs have some other pharmacological actions that may add to their therapeutic value in Parkinsonian patients. Thus they appear to be able to inhibit the uptake of dopamine by presynaptic neurones (their action in this respect recalls that of the tricyclic antidepressant agents) and they may also promote the release of transmitter in the corpus striatum. Some of them have a degree of antihistamine (H_1-receptor blocking) activity, though the relevance of this property to their therapeutic actions is obscure. The side effects of these drugs and contraindications to their use appear elsewhere (p. 229).

L-DOPA AND RELATED COMPOUNDS

The discovery that a state of dopamine deficiency underlies Parkinson's disease led to the obvious suggestion that the condition might respond to replacement therapy. Because dopamine does not cross the blood-brain barrier, it was necessary to use a precursor that does so in order to effect the replacement. L-DOPA, the immediate precursor of dopamine, meets this requirement but the first trials with the new drug gave discouraging results. It was not until Cotzias and his colleagues took the bold step of using much higher doses of L-DOPA that the earlier hopes were fulfilled. As it became more widely used, L-DOPA came to be known as levodopa, a more euphonious and less clumsy name.

Levodopa does more than merely fill the remnants of the nigrostriatal dopaminergic system with dopamine. The conversion of L-DOPA to dopamine is a step in the biosynthesis of noradrenaline and the enzyme that promotes this conversion (aromatic-L-aminoacid decarboxylase) is also present in serotoninergic fibres. Consequently levodopa in the high doses in which it is customarily given might give rise to increased amounts of transmitter in noradrenergic fibres, both central and peripheral, as well as causing the production of dopamine in sites such as serotoninergic neurones where it is not normally found. Such increased loads of catecholamine transmitters could hardly fail to contribute both psychological and physiological side effects in patients receiving levodopa. Considerations such as these led to the practice of giving levodopa in association with an inhibitor of aromatic-L-aminoacid decarboxylase that does not pass the blood brain barrier. In this way, the production of dopamine in peripheral tissues is prevented without affecting that in the brain, an effect that is doubly useful, for it minimizes side effects of peripheral origin and permits the use of lower doses of levodopa. Suitable enzyme inhibitors are carbidopa and benserazide (Fig. 32.9). Proprietary mixtures of levodopa and one of the inhibitors are Sinemet and Madopar respectively. Sinemet tablets contain 250 mg of levodopa and 25 mg of carbidopa while the proportions in Madopar are 100 mg of levodopa to 25 mg of benserazide.

Treatment with levodopa is begun at an oral dose level of 250 mg and is progressively increased at a rate determined by the patient's response to a maximum daily dose of 2 to 8 grams. Taken in combination with a decarboxylase inhibitor, however, the maximum effective dose need be no more than 1 to 2 grams. The dose can also be lower if amantadine (see below) or an atropine like drug is being taken concurrently.

A large number of side effects have been reported in patients receiving therapeutically useful doses of levodopa. Nausea and vomiting can be troublesome, particularly in patients who are not receiving a decarboxylase inhibitor (it should be remembered that dopamine is the physiological

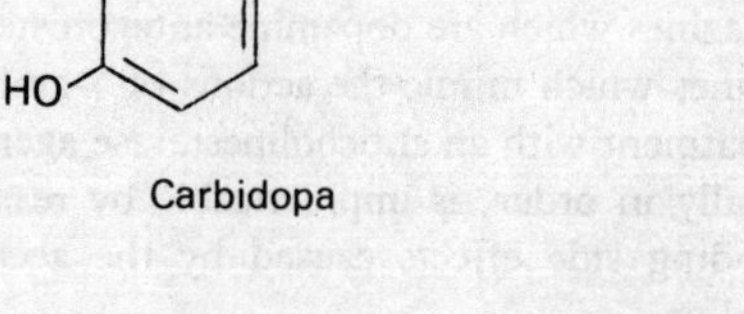

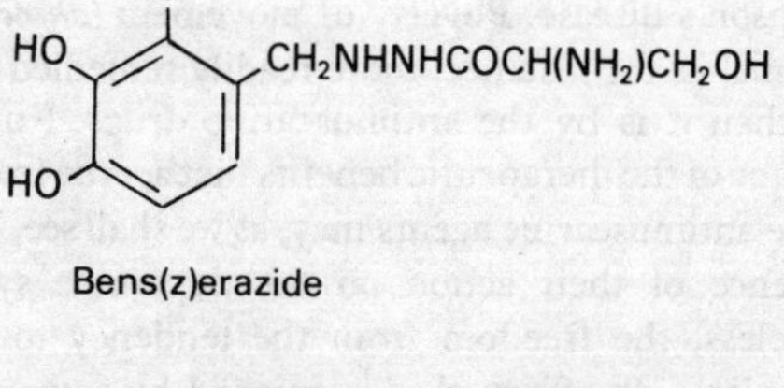

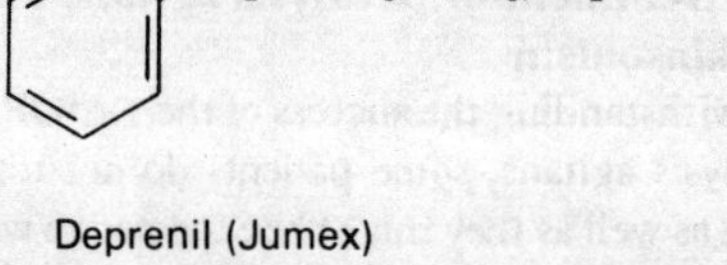

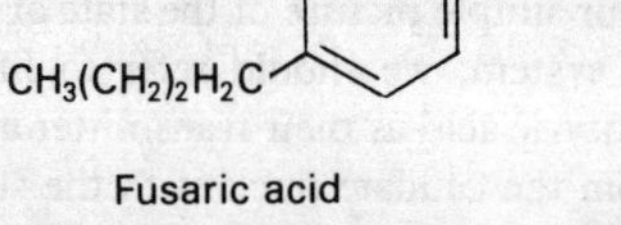

Fig. 32.9 Enzyme inhibitors used as adjuncts in the treatment of Parkinson's disease.

Table 32.9 Some drugs used in the treatment of Parkinson's disease (Modified from Crossland, 1967, by kind permission of Messrs. Butterworths)

Approved name(s)	Proprietary name(s)	Formula	Major Properties	Dose
Benzhexol, Trihexyphenidyl	Artane,	(structure) C–OH, CH$_2$.CH$_2$.N piperidine, HCl	Atropine-like	5-6 mg thrice daily
Benapryzine	Brizin	(structure) OH, CCOOCH$_2$CH$_2$N with CH$_2$CH$_3$ and CH$_2$CH$_2$CH$_3$	Similar to benzhexol	50 mg three times daily
Cycrimine	Pagitane	(structure) C–OH, CH$_2$.CH$_2$.N piperidine	Similar to benzhexol	2-5 mg four times daily
Biperiden	Akineton	(structure) C–OH, CH$_2$.CH$_2$.N piperidine, CH$_2$	Similar to benzhexol	1-4 mg four times daily

agonist at the vomiting centre) as can other disturbances of gastrointestinal function. Cardiovascular side effects include postural hypotension, cardiac arrhythmias and, occasionally, hypertension. The systems that regulate muscle tone are multiple, interrelated and delicately balanced and relief of Parkinsonism can often only be bought at the expense of precipitating other extrapyramidal disturbances such as involuntary movements of the facial muscles, myoclonic jerks (p. 491) and choreoathetosis (p. 164). As might have been expected, psychiatric disturbances including agitation, manic elation, euphoria, paranoid delusions, hallucinations and severe depression have all appeared (or have been revealed) in the course of treatment with levodopa. Minor degrees of euphoria and elation may, of course, be not entirely unwelcome in victims of a disease that sometimes brings depression in its train. The occurrence of these beneficial side effects has, indeed, attracted considerable publicity which has tended to obscure the unfortunate fact that depression occurs more frequently than elation (Mindham, Marsden and Parkes, 1976) and the drug should be withheld from severely psychotic patients.

It should not be necessary to stress that care must be exercised if levodopa is given to patients who are also receiving other drugs that influence dopamine systems. It is not to be given in association with monoamine oxidase inhibitors. Other conditions that constitute an absolute or relative contraindication to the use of levodopa are glaucoma (which is also a contraindication to the use of treatment with antimuscarine drugs), severe systemic disease (particularly if it affects the liver, kidneys, the cardiovascular or the endocrine systems) and pregnancy.

Pyridoxine antagonizes the action of levodopa.

Amantadine

Amantadine (Symmetrel) began life as an antiviral agent and it was when it was being used in this capacity that its ability to ameliorate hypokinesia and rigidity in Parkinsonian patients came to light. Its mode of action is not entirely clear but it can certainly release dopamine from

Table 32.9 (contd)

Approved name(s)	Proprietary name(s)	Formula	Major Properties	Dose
Ethopropazine, Profenamine	Parsidol, Lysivane	See Table 32.1 (p. 553)	Similar to hyoscine	See Table 32.1
Procyclidine	Kemadrin		Similar to ethopropazine	2-10 mg three times daily
Benztropine	Cogentin	See Table 32.4 (p. 570)	Similar to ethopropazine but also has antihistamine activity	1-5 mg once daily
Orphenadrine	Disipal, Norflex	See Table 32.4		50-150 mg thrice daily
Chlorphenoxamine	Phenoxene, Clorevan,	See Table 32.4	Antihistamine and atropine like	50-100 mg thrice daily
Methixene	Tremonil, Tremaril Trest		Similar to orphenadrine	2.5 mg three to six times daily

central neurones (albeit in large doses) and it may also have an agonist action at dopamine receptors. Amantadine can be used alone but it is more often given together with one of the antimuscarine drugs or with levodopa. When it is employed to augment the effects of levodopa the dose of levodopa and therefore the incidence and severity of its side effects can be reduced but amantadine's own side effects may be added to the picture. These may include oedema, hallucinations, anxiety and a mottling of the skin, fittingly called livedo reticularis. Epileptiform convulsions have been reported and a history of epilepsy should be taken as an absolute contraindication to treatment with amantadine. Other indications for circumspection in the use of the drug are similar to those mentioned for levodopa.

The daily oral dose of amantadine is 200 to 400 mg after an introductory week in which the dose should not exceed 100 mg.

The use of amantadine as an antiviral agent is discussed on p. 858.

Apomorphine and similar substances

The therapeutic action of levodopa is, we all believe, dependent on its conversion into dopamine, the chemical mediator of activity in the nigrostriatal tract. If this is so it should be possible to achieve a broadly similar therapeutic effect by giving drugs that directly stimulate dopamine receptors in the corpus striatum and it was on this basis that apomorphine, a specific agonist at dopamine receptors, was added to the list of agents that might be used to treat Parkinson's disease. It proved to be effective, either alone or in association with levodopa, but its use has hitherto been limited by its short duration of action and, more seriously, by its causing hypotension, hormonal changes and (not surprisingly since apomorphine is a powerful emetic agent) vomiting. Corsini and his colleagues have recently reported that these side effects are abolished or attenuated when apomorphine is given together with domperidone, a dopamine receptor antagonist that does not cross the blood brain barrier. In these circumstances, apomorphine only stimulates dopamine receptors within the barrier (the vomiting centre fortunately lies outside it) and the only troublesome side effect that still appears is yawning (Corsini, del Zompo, Gessa and Mangoni, 1979). Bromocriptine and piribedil, two more dopamine agonists have also been thought of as

Domperidone

possible anti Parkinsonism drugs but their use too has been restricted by the incidence of side effects. It is possible that their value might also be boosted by combining them with domperidone (Agid et al., 1979).

Other substances
Attempts have been made to find acceptable drugs that might be able to improve the effectiveness and increase the selectivity of levodopa by retarding the destruction of the dopamine it produces or by preventing dopamine's further conversion into noradrenaline. Substances in this category include deprenil and fusaric acid (Fig. 32.9). Deprenil inhibits monoamine oxidase B (the version of the enzyme that operates preferentially on dopamine) while fusaric acid inhibits dopamine ß -hydroxylase which promotes the conversion of dopamine to noradrenaline. Another interesting approach has utilized L-propyl-L-leucineglycine, a hypothalamic tripeptide that inhibits the release of melanocyte stimulating hormone and potentiates the action of dopamine. It is too early to hazard a prediction concerning the likely future of these new agents.

Other compounds that have attracted some recent attention include histamine H_1 receptor antagonists and the ubiquitous propranolol but the value of these drugs in the treatment of Parkinsonism is limited.

THE SCREENING OF DRUGS FOR PSYCHOTROPIC ACTIVITY

The difficulties inherent in attempts to forecast the therapeutic potential of a new drug on the basis of simple experiments on healthy animals are encountered in their most acute form when psychotropic activity is being sought.

Screening for possible psychotropic activity is usually performed by giving experimental animals the new drug and subjecting them to a battery of tests designed to reveal effects known to be exerted by the psychotropic drugs already in use. In this way the pattern (or 'profile') of activity of the new drug can be compared with those of established drugs. Unfortunately there is often no means of knowing which, if any, of the actions revealed by these tests on normal animals is related to the drug's psychotherapeutic activity and potentially useful compounds whose properties happen not to coincide with those of drugs already in use may escape detection. Additional information can sometimes be gleaned by using animals in which a model psychosis or neurosis has been established but it should not be necessary to stress that animal models of human psychiatric conditions are so far removed from the real thing that their value is severely limited.

Brief details of the experimental techniques employed in psychotropic screening tests are given in the succeeding paragraphs. They are followed by a summary of the actions of each of the principal groups of psychotropic drugs as exhibited in these tests. More detailed examinations of the tests, of the ways in which they are conducted and of their predictive significance can be found in texts devoted to drug screening procedures, some of which are listed in the bibliography to Chapter 10 (p. 137).

Preliminary screening test. Simple observation of the overt effects of administration of the drug to an intact animal should never be omitted. If this preliminary test is conducted according to the scheme devised by Irwin (p. 138), useful information concerning the drug's properties can be obtained before embarking on more elaborate tests.

Spontaneous motor activity. Several techniques are available for measuring spontaneous locomotor activity in rats and mice. In one of the more widely used the animal (or a group of animals) is placed in a cage across which a thin beam of light passes. The light falls on to a photoelectric cell in the cage wall and a counter connected to the cell records the number of times the beam is interrupted as the animal crosses and recrosses it in the course of its ambulations. An advantage of this method is that animals can live permanently in the activity cages so that they suffer only the minimum of disturbance when drug effects are being measured. Spontaneous activity is still sometimes measured by placing animals in a *jiggle* cage. This device (which is oddly called a jingle cage by some workers) consists of a cage suspended or mounted on springs. When the animals move the cage oscillates. Traditionalists record the oscillatory movements with a lever system but electronic recording is preferable and easily arranged. More sophisticated devices are also available. With the aid of some of them it is possible to monitor the movements of single animals from among a group housed together.

Ambulatory and exploratory activity. A simple maze (the so-called Y maze) can be used to assess this kind of activity. Three runways of equal size are connected together in the form of an equilateral Y. A rat, placed in the centre of the maze for the first time, will indulge in very little exploratory activity. This immobility is engendered by the stress attendant on the animal's being in a novel situation. Stress is further indicated by preening movements and by defaecation. After the animal has been placed in the maze on a number of occasions, it becomes accustomed to the previously strange surroundings. Exploratory activity (expressed for the purpose of experiment in terms of the number of times the animal enters any of the arms of the maze) is increased and the other signs of stress diminish in intensity. Exploratory activity can also be measured in an 'open field', a large board marked off into smaller areas being available for exploration.

Motor coordination and muscle tone. Ataxia will usually reveal itself in the preliminary screening test but its extent can be quantitatively assessed to some extent by the rotating rod test. Mice are placed on a horizontally mounted rod some 2 to 3 cm. in diameter. The rod rotates ten times a minute. Normal animals should be able to maintain a position on the rod for at least five minutes. Ataxic animals fall off earlier.

In catatonia, muscle tone is increased and there may be increased parasympathetic activity. The most characteristic feature, however, is that the animal will maintain any position in which it is placed however 'unnatural' that might be. It is easily detected: in one method the animal's front paws are allowed to rest on a horizontal wooden rod placed at such a distance from the bench top that the rat has to 'stretch' to reach it. To maintain this uncomfortable position, the muscles must be quite strongly contracted. Untreated animals refuse to do so but catatonic animals remain up to 30 or more minutes in the position in which they are first placed. (Rogers, 1966).

Conditioning experiments. One method of assessing the action of drugs on conditioned avoidance responses was described earlier (p. 549). The same type of information, and much more besides, can be obtained by making use of *operant conditioning*. The originator of operant conditioning was Skinner: his boxes (first used in 1955) feature prominently among the furnishings of modern psychopharmacology laboratories. An animal in a Skinner box receives food, drink or other rewards in response to his pressing a lever or performing some other task. The reward does not appear every time the lever is pressed. It may be delivered at fixed or variable time intervals irrespective of the total number of times the lever is operated during this interval, provided of course that it is pressed when the reward is due. These constitute the *fixed and variable interval schedules.* Alternatively, it can be arranged that the reward appears after the lever has been pressed for a predetermined number of times (*fixed and variable ratio schedules*) or at a predetermined rate. Shocks can be applied to the feet of the animal from the grid that forms the floor of the box and the animal can be trained to avoid the shock by depressing another lever. Other sophistications include the provision of sound or light signals to indicate to the animal that the experimental schedule is about to be changed—from fixed interval to fixed ratio, for example. In some laboratories, electrodes are implanted in the appropriate area of the hypothalamus and are connected to a stimulator that is linked into the control mechanism of the box. The reward or deterrent thus consists of hypothalamic self stimulation which, depending on the position of the electrodes, is either pleasurable or unwelcome (p. 165).

The behaviour of unmedicated animals in Skinner boxes is predictable for each of the reinforcement schedules that are commonly used. If an animal is rewarded on a fixed interval schedule, it will learn to press the lever more frequently as the end of the interval approaches. With a variable interval schedule, it will operate the lever at a moderately high rate all the time since it cannot know when the reward will come. On the other hand, if the animal is trained to a ratio schedule it will press the lever repeatedly and rapidly in order to obtain a reward as often as possible.

Aggressive and neurotic behaviour. Aggressive behaviour can be induced in mice and rats by applying repeated small electric shocks to the floor of their cages or by making lesions in parts of the limbic system, particularly the septal nucleus. Some rats display violent aggression towards mice placed in their cage. Animals made aggressive in any of these ways can be utilized for screening tests. Aggressiveness is, however, a very complex response and the ability to suppress this state is not the unique prerogative of any particular group of psychoactive drugs.*Experimental neuroses* can be induced in animals in several ways. A simple method, suitable for routine laboratory use, involves training the animal to perform a simple task for a food reward. When the conditioned response has become established, it is arranged that the animal shall be 'punished' by means of an electric shock to its feet whenever it goes for food. Although the animal's attempts to acquire food are inhibited by the prospect of punishment (in the jargon of the psychologist its 'conflict behaviour consists of responding that has been suppressed by the response-contingent delivery of aversive stimulation') the drive for food remains and a state, superficially similar to an anxiety neurosis in man is thereby induced.

Amphetamine toxicity. Mice are much more sensitive to the toxic effects of amphetamine when they are kept together in small groups than when they are housed in individual cages. Some psychotropic drugs potentiate while others annul this aggregation effect.

Other tests. Other screening tests mentioned in the following summary are either described elsewhere in this book or their nature is self evident.

DEPRESSANT DRUGS

Depressant drugs in general reduce spontaneous locomotor activity and prolong barbiturate sleeping time. All, particularly the hypnotics and sedatives, are likely to produce a degree of ataxia. The most characteristic action of the antipsychotic drugs is their ability to inhibit conditioned avoidance reponses. They reduce exploratory activity in the Y-maze and open field but they also inhibit rearing and defaecation. In higher doses, they are likely to produce catatonia. However, not all compounds in this class produce catatonia and some that do produce this condition are patently not antipsychotic agents. It can be said, though, that a drug that produces catalepsy in animals will probably have Parkinsonian side effects in man.

The depressant drugs (particularly the antipsychotic drugs) antagonize the excitatory actions of amphetamine and inhibit the aggregation effect on amphetamine toxicity.

ANTIANXIETY DRUGS

The antianxiety drugs have a taming action in animals rendered aggressive by septal lesions but an action that is more closely related to their therapeutic potentiality is their ability to restore normal behaviour in animals suffering from the effects of the conflict produced when their drive for food rewards is thwarted by stimuli that 'punish' their efforts. Cook and Sepinwall (1975) have demonstrated a very close correlation between the clinically effective dose of an antianxiety drug and its ability to suppress conflict behaviour. They used phenobarbitone, amylobarbitone, meprobamate, chlordiazepoxide, diazepam and oxazepam to establish this relationship.

There are reports that antianxiety drugs increase the exploratory activity of animals placed in a Y-maze for the first time but that the activity of experienced animals is not affected (Marriott and Spencer, 1965).

ANTIDEPRESSANT DRUGS

A characteristic property of the antidepressant drugs is their ability to reverse the hypothermic and behaviourally depressant actions of reserpine. They potentiate the actions of amphetamine, an effect which is best demonstrated in operant behaviour studies. Other effects vary with the nature of the drug. Thus, monoamine oxidase inhibitors bring about an accumulation of noradrenaline and 5-hydroxytryptamine in the brain, and frank stimulants (such as amphetamine) increase spontaneous motor activity and operant behaviour.

It is almost as difficult to predict, from simple tests on animals, that a new drug will have a useful therapeutic effect in depressed patients as it is to treat the condition with existing drugs and many attempts have been made to induce in animals a more satisfactory picture of depression than that provided by the traditional reserpine model. These newer and more or less complex models are reviewed by Everitt and Keverne (1979) but none of them can yet be exploited for the routine testing of potentially antidepressant agents.

DRUGS FOR THE TREATMENT OF PARKINSONISM

In experimental animals, tremorine produces the Parkinsonian triad of asynergia, tremor and akinesia together with intense parasympathetic stimulation and hypo-

Tremorine

Oxotremorine

thermia. Oxotremorine is a more potent substance with similar actions: the pharmacological activity of tremorine is the result of its conversion to oxotremorine in the body. Both drugs are employed in screening tests for anti-Parkinsonian activity but in view of the complexities of extrapyramidal disease, care has to be taken not to imply too close a parallel between the acute condition induced by the drugs and the chronically progressive state produced by the degenerative lesions of Parkinson's disease.

Tremorine does not markedly affect the dopamine or the 5-hydroxytryptamine content of brain; in some species it brings about a small increase in the noradrenaline content. It does have a noticeable action on the acetylcholine system and among anti-Parkinsonian drugs (levodopa apart) there is a good correlation between antitremorine and antiacetylcholine activity. In doses just sufficient to produce tremor and rigidity, tremorine causes an increase of up to 50 per cent in the acetylcholine content of brain but it also stimulates muscarine receptors directly.

The use of tremorine will only reliably detect drugs that relieve Parkinsonism by virtue of their antimuscarine activity but, as we have seen, future advances in the treatment of Parkinsonism will probably be brought about by the exploitation of agents that affect dopaminergic transmission processes. To detect and assess these substances new models of extrapyramidal disease will be needed. The most promising to date involves the use of 6-hydroxydopamine (p. 292) to destroy dopaminergic neurones in selected parts of the extrapyramidal system.

BIBLIOGRAPHY

Books, monographs and reviews

Anderson, E. W. and Trethowan, W. H. (1973). *Psychiatry*, 3rd ed. London: Balliere Tindall.

Ayd, F. J. and Blackwell, B. (eds) (1970) *Discoveries in Biological Psychiatry*. Philadelphia: Lippincott.

Barchas, J. D., Berger, P. A., Claranello, R. D. and Elliott, G. R. (1977). *Psychopharmacology from Theory to Practice*. New York: Oxford University Press.

Barnett, A. (1975). Dopamine receptors and their role in brain functions. In: Essman, W. B. and Valzelli, L. (eds). *Current Developments in Psychopharmacology*, vol. 1 pp. 1-35 New York: Spectrum Publications.

Brawley, P. and Duffield, J. C. (1972) The pharmacology of hallucinogens. *Pharmac. Rev.* **24**, 31-66.

Brimblecombe, R. W. (1973). Psychotomimetic drugs: biochemistry and pharmacology. *Adv. Drug Res.*, **7**, 165-206.

Costa, E. and Greengard, P. (eds) (1975) *Mechanism of Action of Benzodiazepines*. New York: Raven Press.

Cook, L. and Sepinwall, J. (1975) Behavioural analysis of the effects and mechanisms of actions of benzodiazepines. In: Costa, E. and Greengard, P., *Mechanisms of Action of Benzodiazepines*, pp. 1-28.

Crossland, J. (1967) Psychotropic drugs and neurohumoral substances in the central nervous system. In: Ellis, G. P. and West, G. B. (eds). *Progress in Medicinal Chemistry*, vol. 5, 251-319. London: Butterworths.

Decsi, L. (1964). Biochemical effects of drugs acting on the central nervous system. In: Jucker, E. (ed) *Progress in Drug Research*, vol. 8, 54-194. Basle: Birkhaüser.

Eduison, S., Geller, E., Yuwiler,˙A. and Eduison, B. T. (1964). *Biochemistry and Behaviour*. Princeton: Van Nostrand.

Ehrenpreis, S. and Kopin, I. J. (eds) (1978). *Reviews of Neuroscience*, vol. 3. New York: Raven Press.

Everitt, B. J. and Keverne, E. B. (1979). Models of depression based on behavioural observations of experimental animals. In: Paykell, E. S. and Coppen, A. pp. 41-59.

Fieve, R. R. (1978) Lithium and affective disorders. In: Ehrenpreis, S. and Kopin, I. J. (1978). pp. 131-156.

Garattini, S., Mussini, E. and Randall, L. O. (eds) (1973). *The Benzodiazepines*. New York: Raven Press.

Gerbino, L., Oleshansky, M. and Gershon, S. (1978). Clinical use and mode of action of lithium. In: Lipton, M. A., DiMascio, A. and Killam, K. F., pp. 1261-1275.

Gershon, S. and Shopsin, B. (eds) (1973) *Lithium: Its Role in Psychiatric Research and Treatment*. New York: Plenum Press.

Glick, S. D. and Goldfarb, J. (eds) (1976) *Behavioural Pharmacology*. Saint Louis: C. V. Mosby Ço.

Gordon, M. (ed) (1964 and 1967) *Psychopharmacological Agents*, vols I and II. New York and London: Academic Press.

Guidotti, A. (1978) Synaptic mechanisms in the action of benzodiazepines. In: Lipson, M. A., DiMascio, A. and Killam, K. F. pp. 1349-1357.

Hoffer, A. and Osmond, H. F. (1967) *The Hallucinogens*. New York and London: Academic Press.

Hollister, L. (1973) *Clinical Use of Psychotherapeutic Drugs*. Springfield, Ill.: Charles C. Thomas.

Hornykiewicz, O. (1966). Dopamine (3-hydroxytyramine) and brain function. *Pharmac. Rev.*, **18**, 925-964.

Janssen, P. A. J. (1967). Haloperidol and related butyrophenones. In: Gordon, M. (ed) *Psychopharmacological Agents*, vol. II, 119-248. New York and London: Academic Press.

Jarvik, M. E. (ed) (1977) *Psychopharmacology in the Practice of Medicine*. New York: Appleton-Century-Crofts.

Lipton, M. A., DiMascio, A. and Killam, K. F. (eds) (1978). *Psychopharmacology: A Generation of Progress*. New York: Raven Press.

Maxwell, D. R. (1968) Principles˙of animal experimentation of psychopharmacology. In: Joyce, C. R. B. (ed) *Psychopharmacology: Dimensions and Perspectives*, 57-93. London: Tavistock Publications.

McIlwain, H. (1963) Chemical Exploration of the Brain; a Study of Cerebral Excitability and Movement. Amsterdam: Elsevier.

Mendels, J. (ed) (1975) The Psychobiology of Depression. New York: Spectrum Publications, Inc.

Murphy, D. L., Campbell, I and Costa, J. L. (1978) Current

status of the indoleamine hypothesis of the affective disorders. In: Lipton, M. A., Dimascio, A and Killam, K. F., pp. 1235-1247.

Nicholson, P. A. and Turner, P. (eds) (1977) Nomifensine. *Br. J. clin. Pharmac.*, **4**, 53S-248S.

Paykel, E. S. and Coppen, A. (eds) (1979) *Psychopharmacology of Affective Disorders*. Oxford, New York and Toronto: Oxford University Press.

Peet, M. and Turner, P. (eds) (1978) Mianserin. *Br. J. clin. Pharmac.*, **5**, 1S-99S.

Pinder, R. M., Brogden, R. N., Speight, T. M. and Avery, G. S. (1977). Maprotiline: a review of its pharmacological properties and therapeutic efficacy in mental depressive states. *Drugs*, **13**, 321-352.

Pinder, R. M., Brogden, R. N., Speight, T. M. and Avery, G. S. (1977) Viloxazine: a review of its pharmacological properties and therapeutic efficacy in depressive illness. *Drugs*, **13**, 401-421.

Pinder, R. M., Brogden, R. N., Sawyer, Phyllis R., Speight, T. M., Spencer, Rosalind and Avery, G. S. (1976) Pimozide: a review of its pharmacological properties and therapeutic uses in psychiatry. *Drugs*, **12**, 1-40.

Post, R. M. (1978) Frontiers in affective disorder research: new pharmacological agents and new methodologies. In: Lipton, M. A., DiMascio, A. and Killam, K. F., pp. 1323-1335.

Sachar, E. J. (1975). A neuroendocrine strategy in the psychobiological study of depressive illness. In: Mendels, J. (ed) *The Psychobiology of Depression*, pp. 123-132. New York: Spectrum Publications.

Schildkraut, J. J. (1970) *Neuropharmacology and the Affective Disorders*. Boston: Little Brown.

Schildkraut, J. J. (1978) Current status of the catecholamine hypothesis of affective disorders. In: Lipton, M. A., DiMascio, A. and Killam, K. F., pp. 1223-1234.

Seeman, P. M. (1966) Membrane stabilization by drugs: tranquillizers, steroids and anaesthetics. In: Pfeiffer, C. C. and Smythies, R. J. (eds). *International Review of Neurobiology*, vol. 9, 145-221. New York and London: Academic Press.

Seiden, L. S. and Dykstra, L. A. (1977). *Psychopharmacology: A Biochemical and Behavioural Approach*. New York: Van Nostrand Reinhold Company.

Sepinwall, J. and Cook, L. (1978) Behavioural pharmacology of antianxiety drugs. In: Iversen, L. L., Iversen, Susan D. and Snyder, S. H. (eds) *Handbook of Psychopharmacology*, vol. 13, pp. 345-393. New York & London: Plenum Press.

Shepherd, M., Lader, M. and Rodnight, R. (1968) *Clinical Psychopharmacology*. London: The English Universities Press.

Sternbach, L. H. (1978) The benzodiazepine story. *Prog. Drug. Res.*, **22**, 229-266.

Sternbach, L. H., Randall, L. O. and Gustafson, S. R. (1967). 1,4-Benzodiazepines (chlordiazepoxide and related compounds). In: Gordon, M. (ed). *Psychopharmacological Agents*, vol. II, 138-224. New York and London: Academic Press.

Swazey, Judith P. (1975) *Chlorpromazine in Psychiatry—a Study of Therapeutic Innovation*. Chicago: The University Press.

Symposium (1975). International Vivilan Symposium. *J. int. med. Res. 3* (Supp. 3), 1-125.

Symposium (1976) *Advances in the Drug Therapy of Mental Illness*. Geneva: World Health Organization.

Whitlock, F. A. and Price, J. (1974) Use of ß adrenergic receptor drugs in psychiatry. *Drugs*, **8**, 109-124.

Original papers

Agid, Y., Pollak, P., Bonnet, A. M., Signoret, J. L. and Lhermitte, F. (1979). Bromocriptine associated with a peripheral dopamine blocking agent in treatment of Parkinson's disease. *Lancet*, (i), 570-572.

Åsberg, M., Träskman, L. and Thorén, P. (1976) 5-HIAA in the cerebrospinal fluid. A biochemical suicide predictor? *Arch. gen. Psychiat.* 33, 1193-1197.

Axelrod, J. (1961) Enzymatic formation of psychomimetic metabolites from normally occurring metabolites. *Science*, 124, 343-344.

Cade, J. F. J. (1949) Lithium salts in the treatment of psychotic excitement. *Med. J. Aust.*, 36, 349-352.

Corsini, G. U., del Zompo, M., Gessa, G. L. and Mangoni (1979). Therapeutic efficacy of apomorphine combined with an extracerebral inhibitor of dopamine receptors in Parkinson's disease. *Lancet* i), 954-956.

Friedhoff, A. J. and Van Winkle, E. (1962). The characteristics of an amine found in the urine of schizophrenic patients. *J. nerv. ment. Dis.*, 136, 550-555.

Glowinski, J., Axelrod, J. and Iversen, L. I. (1966). Regional studies of catecholamines in the rat brain. IV Effect of drugs on the disposition and metabolism of H^3-noradrenaline and H^3-dopamine. *J. Pharmac. exp. Ther.*, 153, 30-41.

Greenspan, K., Schildkraut, J. J., Gordon, Edna K., Baer, L., Arouoff, M. S. and Durell, J. (1970) Catecholamine metabolism in affective disorders—III. MHPG and other catecholamine metabolites in patients treated with lithium carbonate. *J. psychiat. Res.*, 7, 171-183.

Herman, Z. S. (1967) Influence of some psychotropic and adrenergic-blocking agents upon amphetamine stereotyped behaviour in white rats. *Psychopharmacologia*, II, 136-142.

Hession, M. A., Verma, Sarla and Bhakta, K. G. M. (1979) Dependence on chlormethazole and effects of its withdrawal. *Lancet* (i), 953-954.

Horrobin, D. F. (1979) Schizophrenia: reconciliation of the dopamine, prostaglandin and opioid concepts and the role of the pineal. *Lancet* (i), 529-531.

Kanof, P. D. and Greengard, P. (1978) Brain histamine receptors as targets for antidepressant drugs. *Nature, Lond.* 272, 329-333.

Lapin, I. P. and Oxenkrug, G. F. (1969) Intensification of the central serotoninergic processes as a possible determinant of the thymoleptic effect. *Lancet*, I, 132-136.

Maas, J. W. (1975) Biogenic amines and depression: biochemical and pharmacological separation of two types of depression. *Arch. gen. Psychiat.*, 32, 1357-1361.

Marriott, A. S. and Spencer, P. S. J. (1965) Effects of centrally acting drugs on exploratory behaviour in rats. *Br. J. Pharmac.*, 25, 432-441.

Malhorta, C. L. and Punklik, P. G. (1959) The effect of reserpine on the acetylcholine content of different areas of the central nervous system of the dog. *Br. J. Pharmac. Chemother.*, 14, 46-47.

Miller, E. M. (1974) Deanol: a solution for tardive dyskinesia? *N. Eng. J. Med.*, 291, 796-797.

Mindham, R. H. S., Marsden, C. D. and Parkes, J. D. (1976). Psychiatric symptoms during L -DOPA therapy for Parkinson's disease and their relationship to physical disability. *Psychol. Med.*, 6, 23-33.

Osmond, H. and Smythies, J. (1952) Schizophrenia: a new approach. *J. Ment. Sci.*, 98, 309-315.

Pieri, L., Pieri, M. and Haefely, W. (1974). LSD as an agonist of dopamine receptors in the striatum. *Nature*, 252, 586-588.

Pollin, W., Cardon, P. V. and Kety, S. S. (1961) Effects of amino acid feeding in schizophrenic patients treated with iproniazid. *Science*, 133, 104-105.

van Praag, H. M. (1977) Significance of biochemical parameters in the diagnosis, treatment and prevention of depressive disorders. *Biol. Psychiat.*, 12, 101-131.

Prien, R. F., Caffey, A. M. and Klett, C. J. (1972) Comparison of lithium and chlorpromazine in the treatment of mania. *Arch. gen. Psychiat.*, 26, 146-153.

Raymond, M. J., Lucas, C. J., Beesley, M. L., O'Connell, B. A. and Fraser-Roberts, J. A. (1957) A trial of five tranquillizing drugs in psychoneuroses. *Br. med. J.*, 2, 63-66.

Rogers, K. J. (1966) Neurochemical Aspects of Experimental Catatonia. PhD. Thesis, University of Nottingham.

Saelens, D. A., Walle, T., Gaffney, T. E. and Privitera, J. (1977) Studies on the contribution of active metabolites to the anticonvulsant effects of propranolol. *Eur. J. Pharmac.*, 42, 39-46.

Saelens, D. A., Walle, T. and Privitera, P. (1976) Quantitative determination of propranolol, propranolol glycol and N-desisopropylpropranolol in brain tissue by electron-capture gas chromatography. *J. Chromatography.* 123, 185-192.

Sandler, M. and Reynolds, G. P. (1976) Does phenylethylamine cause schizophrenia? *Lancet*, (i), 70-71.

Sheard, M. H., Marini, J. L., Bridges, Carolyn I. and Wagner, E. (1976). The effect of lithium on impulsive aggressive behaviour in man. *Am. J. Psychiat.*, 133, 1409-1412.

Slater, P. (1966). Studies on Acetylcholine. PhD. Thesis, University of Nottingham.

Snyder, S. H. (1973) Amphetamine Psychosis: a 'model' schizophrenia mediated by catecholamines. *Am. J. Psychiat.*, 130, 61-67.

Snyder, S., Greenberg, D. and Yamamura, H. (1974) Antischizophrenic drugs and brain cholinergic receptors. *Arch. gen. Psychiat.*, 31, 58-67.

Spector, S., Shore, P. A. and Brodie, B. B. (1960) Biochemical and pharmacological effects of the monoamine oxidase inhibitors, iproniazid, 1-phenyl-2-hydrazinopropane (JB 516) and 1-phenyl-3-hydrazinobutane (JB 835). *J. Pharmac. exp. Ther.*, 128, 15-21.

Stotsky, B. A. and Borzone, J. (1972) Butizol sodium vs. Librium among geriatric and younger outpatients and nursing home patients. *Dis. Nerv. Syst.*, 33, 254-267.

Vetulani, J., Stawarz, R. J., Dingell, J. V. and Sulser, F. (1976). A possible common mechanism of action of antidepressant treatments. *Naunyn-Schmiedebergs Arch. exp. Path. Pharmak.*, 293, 109-114.

Watt, J. A. G., Ashcroft, G. W., Daly, R. G. and Smythies, J. R. (1969) Urine volume and pink spots in schizophrenia and health. *Nature, Lond.*, 221, 971-972.

Weinstock, M., Weiss, C. and Gitter, S. (1977). Blockade of 5-hydroxytryptamine receptors in the central nervous system by ß-adrenoceptor antagonists. *Neuropharmacology*, 16, 273-276.

Wise, C. D., Baden, M. M. and Stein, L. (1974) Post-mortem measurement of enzymes in human brain: evidence of a central noradrenergic deficit in schizophrenia. *J. psychiat. Res.*, II, 185-198.

Young. A. B., Zukin, D. R. and Snyder, S. H. (1974) Interaction of benzodiazepines with central nervous glycine receptors: possible mechanism of action. *Proc. natn. Acad. Sci. USA*, 71, 2246-2250.

Yorkston, N. J., Gruzelier, J. H., Zaki, S. A., Hollander, Doris, Pitcher, D. R. and Sergeant, H. G. S. (1977) Propranolol as an adjunct to the treatment of schizophrenia. *Lancet*, (ii), 575-578.

Zeller, E. A., Barsky, J., Fonts, J. R., Kirchheimer, W. F. and van Orden, L. S. (1957). Influence of isonicotinic acid hydrazide (INH) and I-isonicotinyl-2-isopropyl hydrazide (IIH) on bacterial and mammalian enzymes. *Experientia*, 8, 349-350.

33. Vomiting: emetics and antiemetics

Vomiting (less commonly called *emesis*) has been defined as the forceful expulsion of the gastrointestinal contents through the mouth (Wang, 1965). It is usually preceded by signs of autonomic stimulation, particularly salivation, pallor and 'cold sweating', by an unpleasant sensation ('feeling sick') called *nausea* and sometimes by yawning. 'Nausea' has the same etymological origin as 'nautical'; the connection is obvious. The degree of nausea does not necessarily parallel the intensity of the vomiting; severe nausea can occur in the absence of vomiting and severe vomiting can occur without nausea. Nevertheless, it is generally true to say that nausea and vomiting have similar origins and drugs used in the treatment of vomiting (*antiemetics*) are also effective against nausea. The movements of vomiting can take place without the expulsion of gastric contents. From a neurophysiological point of view this event is still vomiting, though it is commonly described as *retching*, a term which should properly be restricted to the irregular and spasmodic respiratory movements that normally precede vomiting but which may occur in its absence.

Vomiting can arise in a variety of circumstances. It may follow the ingestion of toxic or irritant substances; it may occur as a symptom of gastrointestinal or general disease; it may appear as a side-effect of drug action, after exposure to ionizing radiation or during recovery from general anaesthesia; it may be a complication of pregnancy. Vomiting is a common and distressing component of the motion sickness syndrome. It should perhaps, be noted that in Britain, 'sickness' and 'vomiting' are used by laymen as synonyms. In other English speaking countries 'sickness' is used to mean 'illness'. In this chapter, the term sickness is applied to syndromes such as motion sickness. Nausea or vomiting is a usual, but not the exclusive, feature of all the syndromes mentioned.

Vomiting due to the ingestion of toxic material clearly has a protective, even a life-saving, function and it is self-limiting, ceasing when the offending material has been removed. When vomiting is a symptom of disease, it is treated with the underlying disorder, and when it is due to drugs it is sometimes possible to replace the offending substance by one to which the patient is less sensitive. When no alternative drug is available and when vomiting is not due to ingestion of toxic material or to readily cured disease, removal of the underlying cause is usually impossible, impracticable or inadvisable. In these conditions vomiting, far from having a protective action, becomes at best an uncomfortable embarrassment and at worst a real obstacle to treatment and a danger to life. It is then that the antiemetics are useful.

Although many otherwise valuable drugs cause vomiting as a side-effect, few can be called *emetics* in the sense that their primary action, and the reason for their employment, is the production of vomiting. On the rare occasions when the stomach must be emptied of its contents and a stomach tube is not available or cannot be used, recourse usually has to be made to simple domestic emetics such as vinegar, mustard in water or a concentrated solution of common salt. The only drug commonly used for its emetic effect in man is apomorphine which is employed in some addiction centres in the treatment of alcoholism. Apomorphine is administered at the same time that alcohol is offered. Violent vomiting follows and, after a time, a conditioned response is set up so that alcohol taken alone produces nausea and vomiting. The hope is that this 'aversion therapy' will prevent the patient's return to alcohol when he leaves the clinic; it is sometimes successful. Emetics (chiefly apomorphine and copper sulphate) are also used to provoke vomiting in animals when the mode of action of emetics and antiemetics is being studied.

THE MECHANISM OF VOMITING

Although the final result of vomiting is the emptying of the stomach and part of the small intestine, active 'antiperistaltic' movements of these organs play little or no part in the vomiting mechanism. It is an old observation that vomiting still occurs in dogs whose stomach and intestines have been replaced by a balloon. The only occasion when antiperistalsis occurs in the human being is in over-fed infants. The effortless expulsion of food which is then seen is more properly called regurgitation; it cannot be regarded as vomiting.

In vomiting, a deep breath is taken, the glottis closes and the cardiac orifice of the stomach dilates, the musculature of the stomach and oesophagus relax and that of the diaphragm and abdomen contract strongly, compressing the stomach and forcing out its contents. It can be seen that the muscles primarily involved in vomiting are the respiratory muscles and vomiting, like respiration itself, is to a limited extent under voluntary control—it can, for

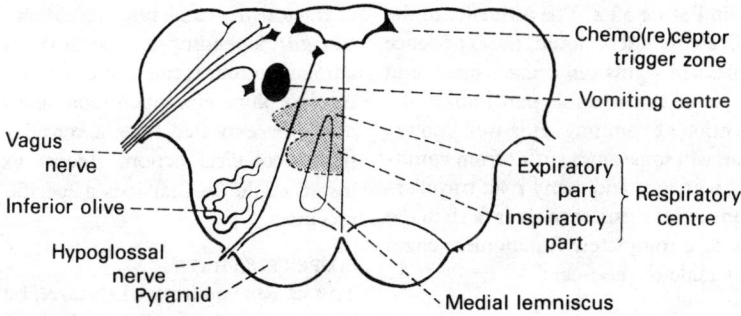

Fig. 33.1 Section of the medulla
To show the position of the vomiting centres in relation to other important structures. The cells and fibres of the reticular system are dispersed between the floor of the fourth ventricle and the pyramids. Note the relationship of the vomiting and respiratory centres.

instance, be suppressed for a short time while the victim seeks seclusion.

The various influences which may promote vomiting are integrated in a small area, the *vomiting centre*, which is located in the lateral reticular formation of the medulla (Fig. 33.1).

In experimental animals, vomiting is provoked by electrical stimulation of the vomiting centre while localized destruction of the centre prevents vomiting. The vomiting centre is located close to the medullary areas which control other functions such as salivation, respiration and vascular responses. These activities are all involved in the act of vomiting but, in other circumstances, they can be influenced independently of one another.

Closely associated with the vomiting centre is the *chemoceptor chemoreceptor,* or *chemosensitive trigger zone.* The trigger zone is located in the area postrema of the fourth ventricle (Fig. 33.1). Many substances which cause vomiting after absorption or injection into the blood

stream stimulate the trigger zone which then sends impulses to the vomiting centre itself. The description 'chemoreceptive' is perhaps not entirely appropriate, for the integrity of the trigger zone is essential for the production of motion sickness, a condition in which no obvious chemical substance is involved. Moreover, a few chemical substances cause vomiting by stimulating areas of the brain other than the trigger zone. Nevertheless, the trigger zone plays a very important part in the initiation of vomiting by many emetic drugs and by conditions which liberate emetic substances into the blood stream.

Although most of the experimental work leading to the discovery of the trigger zone was carried out on animals, particularly the dog, there seems to be no doubt that it is present in human beings. Selective destruction of the area postrema has, indeed, been successfully used for the relief of severe and otherwise intractable vomiting (Lindstrom & Brizzee, 1962).

The various ways in which the vomiting centre can be

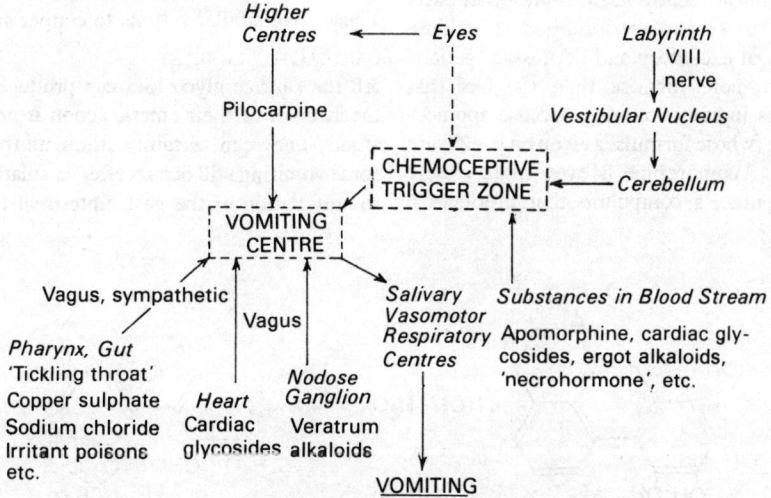

Fig.33.2 Sites of action of emetic substances

stimulated are shown in Figure 33.2. The influence of the higher centres of the brain should be noted: the experience or recollection of unpleasant sights can cause nausea, and psychological factors play a considerable part both in the production and prevention of vomiting. It is well known, for instance, that a man will sometimes suffer from vomiting during his wife's pregnancy and many road travellers owe their freedom from travel sickness to their faith in the prophylactic qualities of a completely functionless chain hanging from the underside of their cars.

Vomiting due to drugs

APOMORPHINE

There is no doubt that apomorphine acts exclusively on the chemoceptive trigger zone. The existence of the zone was, in fact, established by the use of apomorphine: removal of a localized area of the medulla completely protected dogs against the drug's emetic action, though the animals remained susceptible to the action of substances such as copper sulphate which cause reflex stimulation of the vomiting centre by irritating the gastric mucosa.

When apomorphine is injected into the fourth ventricle, thus bringing it into direct contact with the area of the trigger zone, it induces vomiting, in the dog, in doses as small as $0.005 \mu g$ per kg. The trigger zone of the cat is nearly a thousand times less sensitive than that of the dog. In man, a subcutaneous injection of 1 mg of apomorphine will usually induce vomiting within 15 to 20 minutes, but the dose requirement is rather critical. If the amount given is below the individual's emetic threshold it may produce only nausea and a feeling of lethargy but a dose that is substantially supraliminal may also fail to induce emesis. This effect of high doses of apomorphine is presumably a reflection of the drug's ability to depress as well as to excite the trigger zone. Alternatively it may be the result of depression of the vomiting centre itself. Some other parts of the central nervous system are inhibited at all dose levels. This mixture of excitatory and depressant actions should occasion no more surprise than the fact that morphine sometimes induces vomiting because apomorphine and morphine (whose formula is given on p. 429) are structurally similar. Apomorphine is even more closely similar to bulbocapnine, a compound that produces a characteristic cataleptic condition in animals (p. 594) though, depending on the dose given and the route of administration, it can also cause convulsions or vomiting. Apomorphine is a much more interesting substance than might be expected from a consideration of its principal pharmacological action. Recent experiments have, for instance, shown that it is a specific agonist at dopamine receptors.

COPPER SULPHATE

This causes vomiting when taken by mouth and it does so by irritating the gastrointestinal tract. Afferent impulses travel by way of both the vagus and the sympathetic nerves to the medulla. Ablation of the chemoceptive trigger zone does not abolish the emetic action of intragastric copper sulphate, indicating that the nerve impulses travel from the intestine directly to the vomiting centre and are not relayed *via* the trigger zone. Copper sulphate itself can, however, stimulate the trigger zone directly so that it will still cause vomiting if it is administered intravenously. If the gastrointestinal tract of an experimental animal is denervated, vomiting does not immediately follow the introduction of irritant substances into the stomach so they are absorbed into the blood stream. In these circumstances, copper sulphate reaches the trigger zone and causes vomiting after a long latency (of the order of two hours) due to the low rate of absorption. In the intact animal, vomiting occurs within 15 minutes following the ingestion of copper sulphate. In this time, insufficient absorption takes place to permit any direct stimulation of the trigger zone. The emetic action of copper sulphate in the normal animal is thus effectively only due to its action on the gastrointestinal tract. With substances absorbed more rapidly, both peripheral and central actions may contribute to their emetic properties.

ZINC SULPHATE AND MERCURIC CHLORIDE

These have similar actions to copper sulphate.

CARDIAC GLYCOSIDES

All the cardiac glycosides can produce vomiting but the mechanism of their emetic action is not yet fully understood. They can certainly stimulate the trigger zone but some vomiting still occurs after its ablation. This is not due to stimulation of the gastrointestinal tract since it is not

Apomorphine hydrochloride

Bulbocapnine

prevented by complete denervation of the gut. There is evidence that reflex stimulation of the vomiting centre from the heart itself may be responsible; the duration of action of these drugs on the heart and on vomiting is similar and their emetic effect is reduced by denervation of the heart.

THE VERATRUM ALKALOIDS

Doses of the veratrum alkaloids sufficient to reduce blood pressure frequently cause vomiting. This is due to their stimulating the nodose ganglion of the vagus and hence the vomiting centre. No other emetic drug is known to act on vagal ganglia. In addition, the veratrum alkaloids may have a direct stimulant action on the trigger zone.

PILOCARPINE

Pilocarpine is unique among drugs which provoke vomiting by a direct action on the brain in that it exerts its effect by stimulating the frontal lobes of the cerebral hemispheres. The impulses generated there pass directly to the vomiting centre and the emetic action of pilocarpine is, consequently, unaltered by excision of the trigger zone.

OTHER DRUGS

A large number of other drugs and agents can produce vomiting. The mechanisms of action of a few of them can be summarized as follows:

Acting on the trigger zone: ergot alkaloids, aconitine, guanidine, nicotine, lobeline, *Staphylococcus* enterotoxin. In some species the last three named also stimulate receptors in the gut.

Acting on both the gut and the trigger zone: sodium salicylate, tartar emetic, ipecacuanha.

Acting on the gut: quinine, quinidine, organisms causing peritonitis.

In addition, several neurohumoral substances produce vomiting when they are injected in small doses into the cerebral ventricles. They include histamine, adrenaline, dopamine and acetylcholine.

Motion sickness

Motion sickness can develop during any form of travel but the most effective stimulus—a repetitive and rhythmic change in the speed or direction of travel—is provided on board ship. Seasickness is, consequently, the most common form of motion sickness and many travellers who are completely unaffected by other forms of transport succumb to the 'beat and quiver of the sea'. As is well-known, individuals vary very much both in their susceptibility to travel sickness and in the ease with which they adapt, after initial sickness, to continuing motion. Almost everyone will develop seasickness if the sea's motion is severe enough.

Motion sickness frequently begins with a brief period of exhilaration or euphoria but this is quickly followed by uneasiness, drowsiness and yawning. The face becomes pale and a cold sweat breaks out; nausea, salivation and vomiting then occur, possibly with headache and a desire to defaecate. Severe fatigue follows a prolonged bout of travel sickness.

Stimulation of the labyrinth is the most important factor causing motion sickness. This organ consists of the three semicircular canals and the otolith organs which, together with the cochlea (which contains the sensory apparatus of hearing) constitute the inner ear (Fig. 33.3). Each semicircular canal opens, at both its ends, into a common *vestibule*. One end of each canal is enlarged into the *ampulla* near its entrance into the vestibule. The semicircular canals are orientated in three planes, of which two are vertical and one is horizontal. They, and the vestibule, are filled with fluid, the *endolymph*. The sensory receptors of the semicircular canals are located in the ampullae; they consist of a

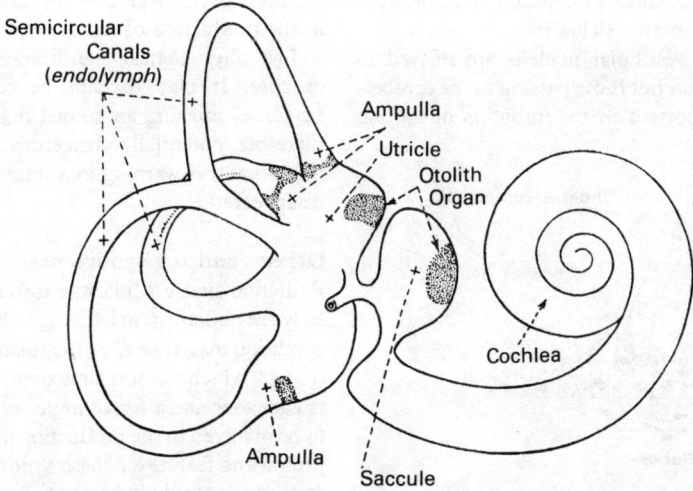

Fig. 33.3 The inner ear to show the position of the otolith organs and sensory membranes. (After Garven.)

patch of sensory epithelium (the *crista*) bearing hair-like projections which are covered by a gelatinous membrane, the *cupula*. The cupula stretches across the ampulla like a swing door. When the head is subjected to angular acceleration (that is, to rotational movements) the inertia of the endolymph causes its movement to lag momentarily behind that of the canals with each change of direction. This relative movement between the canals and their contents causes movement of the cupula and stimulates the sensory receptors. Whereas the semicircular canals signal changes in angular velocity, the position of the head, together with vertical and linear accelerations, is recorded by the otolith organs (otolith=ear stone) which are also located in the vestibule. The otoliths (or *otoconia*) are embedded in a membranous cupula which is similar to those seen in the ampullae; like them, it is in contact with sensory 'hairs' (Fig. 33.4). The two otolith organs are known respectively as the *utricle* and the *saccule;* their sensory epithelium is known as the *macula*.

The impulses generated in the sensory organs of the non-auditory labyrinth travel, *via* the vestibular division of the VIIIth cranial nerve, to the vestibular nucleus (*Dieter's nucleus*) in the pontine part of the floor of the fourth ventricle. The non-auditory labyrinth is an important proprioceptive organ, providing the central nervous system with information concerning the position and velocity of the head in space. This information, added to that provided from other proprioceptors, provides the stimulus for various postural reflexes and changes of muscle tone whose nature and significance are not relevant to the present discussion. That the otolith organs rather than the semicircular canals are of major importance in the production of seasickness is indicated by the fact that this condition occurs less readily when the traveller is supine, a position in which stimulation of the maculae, particularly those of the utricles, is reduced to a minimum. The otolith organs are not necessarily equally important in the production of other forms of motion sickness.

Impulses from the vestibular nucleus are relayed to several parts of the brain but those passing to the cerebellum are the most important in the initiation of motion

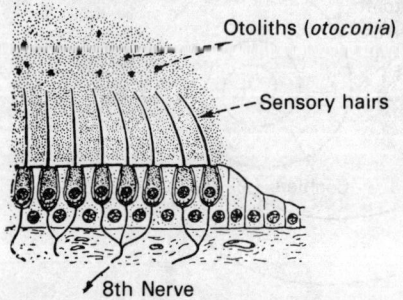

Fig. 33.4 The sensory membrane to show sensory hairs and the position of the otoliths (otoconia). (After Garven.)

Otoliths (*otoconia*)

Sensory hairs

8th Nerve

sickness. That this is so is shown by the fact that removal of two small regions (the *nodule* and the *uvule*) in the anterior lobe of the cerebellum completely protects dogs against the effects of motion. Removal of the chemoceptive trigger zone also prevents motion sickness in dogs and it must therefore be concluded that the vestibular impulses responsible for causing motion sickness are relayed to the vomiting centre by way of both the cerebellum and the trigger zone. The participation of the trigger zone constitutes, as has already been indicated, a curiosity; in vomiting due to causes other than motion the zone is stimulated only by blood-borne emetic substances. Presumably the chemosensitive cells are stimulated by a substance liberated by incoming nerve impulses, though it is difficult to see why this substance should differ from neurohumoral transmitter substances liberated by other nerves which do not require specialized chemoceptive cells to transmit their effects.

Notwithstanding the importance of the vestibular machinery, stimulation of other receptors which help to orientate the body in space play a part in the production of motion sickness in man. If the succession of railway sleepers close to a carriage is observed from a fast moving train, nausea very quickly ensues. Moreover, motion sickness can be produced in the absence of labyrinthine stimulation in subjects seated on a swing which remains quite stationary in a closed chamber which is itself swung about a horizontal axis so as to give the visual impression that the swing is moving in a stationary chamber. Under these conditions, motion sickness must be due entirely to retinal stimulation. Devotees of the ballet will have observed that, during a rapid pirouette, the ballerina keeps her head stationary for as long as possible and then swings it round quickly to a new position. In this way a continuously changing retinal image is avoided and nausea is prevented.

Purely psychological factors are also of great importance in the production of motion sickness in man.

The physiological significance of motion sickness is obscure. It may perhaps be regarded as a primitive response, warning an animal that is on an unstable, and therefore potentially dangerous, support. Any survival value that this warning may once have had has long since disappeared.

Other vomiting syndromes

Radiation sickness follows exposure of the body, particularly the abdomen, to ionizing radiations. A closely similar condition may arise after treatment with nitrogen mustard (p. 913) which has similar actions to X-radiation. Both the trigger zone and afferent impulses from the viscera appear to be involved in the production of the vomiting which is a prominent feature of these syndromes. Since the trigger zone is involved, it has been suggested that irradiation leads to the production of a chemical substance with emetic properties. The idea was put forward by Caspari as long ago as 1923. He called the hypothetical emetic substance a 'necrohormone'. Ellinger (1951) has suggested that histamine may be a necrohormone. He bases this view on the facts of histamine's ubiquitous occurrence and the similarity of some of its actions to the secondary effects of radiant energy. To this we can now add the further point that histamine can certainly induce vomiting if it is injected into the cerebral ventricles (p. 196). Vomiting occurs in uraemia. This condition can be reproduced in experimental animals by the administration of toxic doses of guanidine and since this substance stimulates the chemoceptive trigger zone, it seems possible that uraemic vomiting also arises in this way. In addition, gastrointestinal irritation probably plays a part in uraemic vomiting. Vomiting ('morning sickness') often occurs in otherwise healthy women during the early months of pregnancy. It seems reasonable to believe that this is due partly to a circulating emetic substance and partly to pelvic stimulation. Impulses from the higher centres also participate, apprehension, pleasure and the effects of old wives' tales combining to increase the responsiveness of the vomiting centre. Detailed knowledge concerning the aetiology of pregnancy vomiting is lacking, since the condition cannot be reproduced in animals. When it is severe or prolonged, morning sickness receives the accolade of a Latin name—*hyperemesis gravidarum*, the translation of which should be obvious.

Ménière's syndrome is a condition in which apparently spontaneous outbursts of activity occur in the semicircular canals or in the sensory nerves leading from them. The result is dizziness *(vertigo)*, loss of balance (which may be sufficiently severe to cause the victim to fall to the ground), nausea and sometimes vomiting. A condition indistinguishable from Ménière's syndrome may also occur in association with vascular disease affecting the brain stem.

We have already noted that vomiting may occur as a side effect of drug treatment. It is a rather frequent (and, when it happens a particularly unwelcome) consequence of general anaesthesia.

Finally it is to be noted that intense stimulation of the sensory nerves that supply the thoracic and abdominal viscera can also induce vomiting which may, consequently, be seen as a complication of myocardial infarction, peptic ulcer and peritonitis.

ANTIEMETICS

As we have already emphasized, placebo effects are responsible for much of the benefit conferred by many drugs and devices used in the treatment of vomiting, particularly that associated with pregnancy and with motion sickness. Only those drugs which have been shown by controlled clinical trials to be more effective than placebos are discussed in this section. The effectiveness of an individual preparation, however, is likely to vary from patient to patient.

BARBITURATES AND OTHER DEPRESSANTS OF THE CENTRAL NERVOUS SYSTEM.

Barbiturates have been used to prevent vomiting, particularly that of motion sickness. Their activity is probably due partly to a direct depression of the cortex and the vomiting centre (which is located in an area of the central nervous system particularly susceptible to depression by barbiturates) and partly to their sedative action which induces the traveller to lie down. Other central depressants (chloral hydrate, bromides, etc.) have, in the past, been used as antiemetic drugs. Even apomorphine in some situations has antimetic properties because its depressant action on the vomiting centre more than counters its stimulant action on the trigger zone: a very dilute solution of apomorphine, sipped at frequent intervals during a voyage, was once a favourite remedy for seasickness.

ATROPINE AND HYOSCINE

The use of belladonna alkaloids for the treatment of seasickness was proposed as long ago as 1869 and their effectiveness as antiemetic agents is now soundly established. Hyoscine (scopolamine) which has central depressant properties (Chap. 15) is more effective than atropine; only the L -isomer is effective. Extensive use of hyoscine was made by sea- and airborne invasion troops in the 1939-45 war and it remains the most potent remedy for motion sickness in voyages of short duration. Although the belladonna alkaloids inhibit movements of the gastrointestinal tract, this action is not the major cause of their effectiveness as antiemetic drugs since, as has already been pointed out, active stomach contractions play little or no part in the production of vomiting. Relaxation of the gastrointestinal tract may be of some benefit, since it will reduce the intensity of the afferent discharge from the mucosa but the antiemetic effort of atropine and hyoscine is largely a consequence of their central action. This suggests that a cholinergic mechanism is involved in the vomiting process. In view of the widespread distribution of cholinergic synapses, this conclusion is not, perhaps, surprising. It will be recalled that acetylcholine and pilocarpine can cause vomiting. It should be remembered that many central synapses are non-cholinergic in type so that both cholinergic and non-cholinergic links may well be involved in the initiation of vomiting. If this is so, compounds blocking transmission in the non-cholinergic links might prove to be effective antiemetics.

Atropine and hyoscine are relatively ineffective in the treatment or prevention of vomiting due to causes other than motion. The relevance of these facts to the problem of their site of action is discussed below (p. 606).

In the prevention of motion sickness, hyoscine is effective at a dose level of 0.65 to 0.75 mg atropine and (—)

hyoscyamine are effective in doses of 1 mg. Side actions, at these levels, include dry mouth, blurred vision and giddiness. At higher dose levels, or when repeated doses have been taken they may also cause more severe effects, including hallucinations and disorientation. Hyoscine is less likely than atropine to produce side effects. It is useful if it is taken about one hour before travelling and it offers protection for about six or seven hours without serious side effects. Because side effects become more serious after repeated doses, antihistamines are to be preferred if protection is required for longer periods.

THE ANTIHISTAMINES (HISTAMINE H_1 ANTAGONISTS)

In 1947, the then recently discovered antihistamine drugs were appearing in large numbers and the newest of them all—dimenhydrinate (Dramamine)—was used to treat an allergic condition in a patient who, by chance, also suffered from car sickness (Gay and Carliner, 1949). The patient noticed that, whenever she took the drug, her susceptibility to car sickness disappeared and Dramamine was therefore applied to the treatment of motion sickness in general. It was an immediate success and some other antihistamines have since proved equally successful. The most effective are buclizine, cylizine (Marzine, Marezine, Valoid), chlorcyclizine (Diparalene, Perazil), dimenhydrinate (Dramamine, Gravol), meclozine (Bonamine, Navicalm, Postafen) and promethazine (Avomine, Lergigan, Phenergan). Cyclizine is the shortest-acting of these compounds: it is taken in doses of 50 mg three times daily. Meclozine has the longest duration of action, a single dose of 50 mg providing protection for 24 hours or longer. The formulae of these compounds are given in Chapter 21 where the general properties of the antihistamines are discussed. Antihistamines have a place in the therapy of Ménière's syndrome. They do not relieve the nausea and vomiting if they are taken after an attack has started but appropriate daily doses (Table 21.3, p., 347) may prevent attacks or reduce their frequency. Antihistamine treatment is a rational one in view of the similarities between Ménière's syndrome and travel sickness in respect both of their symptoms and their origin. Antihistamines like promethazine that have a pronounced sedative effect often provide the best relief but some recent successes have been claimed for cinnarazine (Midronal, Stugeron). However, Ménière's syndrome can be most intractable and it is often impossible to predict which drug, if any, will be best for the individual patient. Some patients show a better response to a phenothiazine antiemetic such as prochlorperazine than they do to a regular antihistamine. Moreover (for such is the lack of respect for pharmacological theories that is displayed by disease processes) some victims of Ménière's syndrome find relief only in betahistine (Serc), a drug that potentiates the action of histamine.

The antihistamines are more useful than the belladonna alkaloids but less useful than the phenothiazines in the treatment of radiation sickness, pregnancy vomiting and in the vomiting which occurs during recovery from general anaesthesia and in the course of drug treatment. In other respects, however, their actions seem to parallel those of the belladonna alkaloids. Although the antihistamines are of only limited value for the treatment of drug induced emesis, dimenhydrinate has been recommended in cases of vomiting caused by oral contraceptive agents. Antihistamines are also sometimes still prescribed for the relief of pregnancy sickness but this is a potentially dangerous practice since some members of the group (cyclizine and meclozine) are known to be teratogenic and others may be. Promethazine, however, which is a phenothiazine derivative (p. 554) escapes this suspicion.

It has been suggested that the antihistamines owe their antiemetic activity to the sedative action commonly seem with this group of compounds. However, their antiemetic effect is out of proportion to their sedative action and some of the antihistamines which commonly cause sedation are of no value as antiemetics.

It is possible that antihistamines and the belladonna alkaloids share a common mechanism of antiemetic action since some, at least, of the effective antihistamines antagonize acetylcholine *in vitro*. Even more relevant is the observation that those antihistamines which prevent motion sickness also prevent the circling movements which are produced in rabbits by the intracarotid administration of the anticholinesterase compound, DFP (Freedman and Himwich, 1949). Meclozine and cyclizine, which show no antiacetylcholine activity *in vitro*, are as effective in this respect as are those antiemetic antihistamines that do have atropine like actions on isolated preparations. Atropine and hyoscine, as would be expected, also prevent the circling movements induced by DFP but antihistamines that do not prevent motion sickness (chlorpheniramine and tripellenamine are examples) do not inhibit circling. Whether or not their antiacetylcholine action provides a complete explanation of the antiemetic property of the antihistamines, it is clear that it will materially contribute to their effectiveness.

Another possibility is that the antihistamines do, after all, oppose the central actions of histamine. While very little is yet known about the function of histamine in the central nervous system, it is known that it stimulates the cerebellum—an important station on the motion sickness pathway—and it may be that some histamine is liberated in the region of the cerebellum as a result of the powerful stimulation of the eighth nerve that occurs during irregular motion. The fact that some antihistamines are ineffective

$CH_2.CH_2.NHCH_3$

Betahistine

as motion sickness remedies does not invalidate this hypothesis, for it could well be that some compounds that antagonize the action of histamine at peripheral sites might be without effect on its central actions. Nevertheless, this view of the mode of action of the antihistamines (which is accepted by few other than the author) remains highly speculative.

PHENOTHIAZINE DERIVATIVES

This group of compounds is discussed in detail in Chapter 32. Only the antiemetic properties are concerned here.

In their famous paper detailing the protean actions of chlorpromazine, Courvoisier and his colleagues (1953) reported that the drug prevented apomorphine induced vomiting in the dog. Chlorpromazine is thus unlike the antiemetics previously discussed in that it depresses the trigger zone. Clinical experience suggested that it was as potent a trigger zone depressant in man as in the dog, since it was much more effective than either hyoscine or the antihistamines in the treatment of vomiting due to drugs, pregnancy, uraemia and systemic infection. It was, however, found to be quite ineffective against motion sickness in man or dog. This was surprising, in view of the evidence that the trigger zone is concerned in the production of motion sickness. Moreover, chlorpromazine has both anti-acetylcholine and antihistamine actions and these might have been expected to add to its value as a motion sickness remedy. A final complication is that chlorpromazine is a quite effective remedy for the vomiting caused by inflammation of the labyrinth, in which condition the nervous pathways involved must be similar to those activated in motion sickness. The possible reasons why a drug which depresses the trigger zone does not necessarily prevent motion sickness are discussed below (p. 606). In the absence of any other action on the motion sickness mechanism, the antiacetylcholine and antihistamine properties of chlorpromazine are, of themselves, insufficient to endow the drug with any protective quality.

The means by which chlorpromazine brings about depression of the trigger zone is not yet known.

Some of the newer phenothiazine derivatives, particularly those carrying a piperazine ring on the side chain, are more powerful anitemetics than chlorpromazine itself. They include triflupromazine (Vesprin), perphenazine (Fentazin, Trilafon), pipamazine (Nausidol), prochlorperazine (Compazine, Stemetil) and triethylperazine (Torecan). Their tranquillizing properties probably contribute to their antiemetic action though triethylperazine is devoid of significant tranquillizing activity. All the phenothiazines are likely to produce side effects, especially on the extrapyramidal system. They may also cause hypotension and agranulocytosis. They have, therefore, to be used with caution and avoided in children. When vomiting occurs in pregnancy it does so in the early months when the foetus is most vulnerable to teratogenic influences. Drugs of any kind should, ideally, be avoided at this time and simple sedatives, re-assurance and an explanation that the vomiting will spontaneously disappear constitute the only really safe therapy for this admittedly distressing condition. It is often successful but in severe cases of hyperemesis gravidarum this counsel of perfection has perforce to be ignored. In such circumstances the safest effective drugs are the phenothiazines including promethazine. The reader will already have noticed that Mornidine appears among the proprietary names attached to this group of compounds.

Promethazine is chemically a phenothiazine derivative, but functionally it is an antihistamine. Like the other antihistamines, and unlike the phenothiazine derivatives mentioned previously, it does not depress the trigger zone and it is effective against motion sickness.

TRIMETHOBENZAMIDE

This drug depresses the trigger zone, though it is less active than chlorpromazine in this respect. It is not a sedative and extrapyramidal side effects have not been reported. Trimethobenzamide (Tigan) is said to be useful in the prevention and treatment of all forms of vomiting and, though not as well tried as hyoscine or the antihistamines, it was the antiemetic carried by American astronauts. Its lack of side effects that might reduce the efficiency of space pilots is clearly an advantage.

METOCLOPRAMIDE

This relatively new antiemetic drug (p. 645) depresses the chemosensitive trigger zone but it also has an action like that of acetylcholine on the gastrointestinal tract so that it promotes emptying of the stomach. This action is antagonized by atropine. The clinical uses of the drug are similar to those of the phenothiazine derivatives. Like the latter, metoclopramide may bring about changes in muscle tone as a result of an action on the extrapyramidal motor system.

PYRIDOXINE

In recent years it has become rather fashionable to prescribe preparations containing pyridoxine (p. 792) to control vomiting, particularly morning sickness. Benadon contains only pyridoxine but Ancoloxin is a mixture of

Trimethobenzamide

meclozine and pyridoxine while Debendox contains pyridoxine, an antihistamine (doxylamine) and an antispasmodic agent (dicyclomine). A somewhat esoteric mixture of pyridoxine, benzocaine, nicotinamide and pentobarbitone appears as Nidoxital. Lipoflavonoid is a mixture of B vitamins. It is true that pyridoxine deficiency can cause vomiting but there is no evidence that this condition is a normal accompaniment of pregnancy or that drugs and toxins that cause vomiting do so by inducing a deficiency of pyridoxine. Any beneficial response to these proprietary preparations must be attributed either to a placebo effect or (with some of them) to the other components of the mixture. Pyridoxine itself probably does no harm but some of the mixtures of which it is a component (particularly Debendox) have recently come under the (probably unjustified) suspicion of being teratogenic agents.

To summarize briefly the discussion in the preceding section, it can be said that hyoscine is probably the best drug for the treatment of motion sickness which is likely to be short-lasting, that the antihistamines (particularly meclozine) are most suitable for treating Menière's disease and motion sickness which is likely to be prolonged and that acute attacks of vomiting, such as occur during recovery from anaesthesia or in general disease, are best treated by the phenothiazine drugs. The nature of the likely side-effects of antiemetic therapy should, however, be carefully considered in the light of the circumstances in which it is to be instituted. Blurring of vision due to hyoscine, for instance, though it might be tolerated by those on a pleasure trip, would be unacceptable to assault troops.

THE SITE OF ACTION OF ANTIEMETIC DRUGS

The phenothiazine derivatives depress the trigger zone and it is not, therefore, surprising that they are much more effective than the belladonna alkaloids or the antihistamines in the treatment of vomiting in conditions (such as drug treatment, radiation sickness and pregnancy) in which the trigger zone is stimulated by circulating emetic substances. The trigger zone, however, is also involved in the production of motion sickness, though the phenothiazines are useless in the treatment of this condition. Indeed, it is true to generalize that drugs which ameliorate motion sickness have no effect on the trigger zone (so far as this can be assessed on the basis of their not being able to prevent the emetic action of apomorphine) and that drugs, with the possible exception of Tigan, that do depress the trigger zone are incapable of suppressing motion sickness.

It is not yet possible to say with certainty why the phenothiazines have no action against motion sickness. Although the evidence implicating the trigger zone in this condition came from experiments on dogs, there is no reason to doubt that it is also involved in man. Moreover,

chlorpromazine is as ineffective a prophylactic in dogs as it is in human beings.

It is possible that, although the phenothiazines are capable of antagonizing the effect of circulating emetic substances, they cannot compete against substances liberated from stimulated nerves. Such material might be expected to be liberated in very close proximity to the cells of the trigger zone. This explanation is not very likely, particularly since chlorpromazine is active against the vomiting of labyrinthitis. It might be argued that the phenothiazine derivatives compete with emetic substances for the trigger zone receptors and that in motion sickness, but not in labyrinthitis, the amount of emetic material liberated is sufficient to displace the antiemetic drug. There is, however, no real evidence to support this hypothesis. Another, and more likely, explanation is that the trigger zone contains cells of differing chemical sensitivity. On this view, it has to be assumed that those cells which are stimulated by circulating emetic substances are inhibited by drugs like chlorpromazine but that those which are involved in the production of motion sickness are neither stimulated by apomorphine nor inhibited by chlorpromazine. There is nothing inherently unlikely in the idea that cells stimulated by blood-borne emetic substances should be different from those responding to stimulation by incoming nerves. A somewhat analogous situation exists in the respiratory centre, where it is known that the cells which are stimulated by carbon dioxide in the blood are different from those stimulated by nervous impulses coming from the carotid body. Moreover, there is some evidence that cells of the trigger zone show some specialization even in their sensitivity to circulating emetic substances. In the dog, for instance, chlorpromazine prevents vomiting due to apomorphine but is ineffective against the digitalis gylcoside, lanatoside C, though the emetic action of both drugs is mediated through the trigger zone (Glaviano and Wang, 1955).

It is not necessary to postulate that the trigger zone cells involved in the production of motion sickness are necessarily depressed by drugs such as hyoscine and the antihistamines, for these drugs may operate at other points in the nervous system—on the vestibulocerebellar pathway or on the cerebellum itself, for instance.

All the influences which lead to vomiting are funnelled through the vomiting centre (Fig. 33.2). Any drug which specifically depressed this centre would, therefore, be effective against all forms of vomiting. No really potent drug of this nature has yet been found and it may indeed, be doubted whether it would be possible to suppress the activity of the vomiting centre without also producing an unacceptable depression of respiration. The antiemetic drugs currently in use have their major sites of action at points outside the vomiting centre and since different types of vomiting arise from activity in different nervous pathways it is not surprising that individual groups of antiemetics are effective against particular forms of vomiting.

THE SCREENING AND CLINICAL TESTING OF ANTIEMETIC DRUGS.

Animals differ in their susceptibility to emetic agents. Some species do not vomit, though they may respond in a predictable manner to compounds that cause vomiting in other species. In response to apomorphine injection, for instance, rats develop snuffling, licking and chewing movements, while some species of bird show repetitive pecking movements. The inhibition of these stereotyped movements can be used as an index of antiemesis but it is preferable, when screening antiemetic drugs, to use animals in which frank vomiting occurs. Among such animals the dog is the species of choice. It responds to the same emetic agents as does man and its vomiting centre and trigger zone are very sensitive. Cats and monkeys are much less useful; some individuals of these species are completely refractory to apomorphine and other emetic agents.

It is usual, in animal tests, to assess the effectiveness of antiemetic drugs against the vomiting produced by orally administered copper sulphate and by subcutaneous apomorphine in order to determine whether the antiemetic action is exerted on the vomiting centre or on the chemoceptive trigger zone respectively. As was emphasized in the preceding section, however, the fact that a drug does not provide protection against apomorphine does not necessarily signify that it depresses no cell in the trigger zone.

When potential remedies for motion sickness are being studied in the dog, the appropriate type of vomiting can be produced by rotation or by swinging. Swing sickness is less useful, for this purpose, than rotation sickness.

The design of clinical trials presents difficulties. The subjects used in a trial should be suffering from vomiting of the type against which it is proposed to use the antiemetic drug. Vomiting frequently runs a very acute course and it may prove difficult to collect together, at the appropriate time, a sufficiently large number of cases to provide clear cut evidence concerning the activity of the drug. Because of the well marked placebo effect, 'double blind' methods (p. 144) are essential. The acute course of vomiting usually precludes any possibility of employing cross-over techniques. The organization of a clinical trial of antiemetic drugs is illustrated in a paper by Sparks, Browne and Ferrans (1962).

Clinical trials of motion sickness remedies have usually made use of members of the armed forces undergoing air- or sea-borne assault training or undertaking long sea voyages. The physical and psychological state of these subjects is likely to be different from that of the tourist and only experience will tell whether a remedy which has been found to be effective in clinical trials of this sort will be of equal value in general use.

Various laboratory devices, of varying usefulness, are available for producing motion sickness in man; they include lifts, swings, rotors and artificial rafts rocked in a way which simulates the motion caused by the sea. The methods available for testing motion sickness remedies are critically reviewed by Brand and Perry (1966).

BIBLIOGRAPHY

Reviews

Brand, J. J. and Perry W. L. M. (1966). Drugs in motion sickness. *Pharmac Rev.* **18**, 895-924.
Chinn, H. I. and Smith, P. K. (1955). Motion sickness. *Pharmac. Rev.* **7**, 33-82.
Wang, S. C. (1965). Emertic and anti-emetic drugs. In: *Physiological Pharmacology*, vol. 11, pp. 256-328, ed. Root, W. S. and Hofmann, F. G. New York and London: Academic Press.

Original papers

Courvoiser, S., Fournel, J., Ducrot, R., Kolsky, M. and Koetschet, P. (1953). Proprietes pharmacodynamiques du chlorhydrate de chloro-3 (dimethylamino-3' propyl)-10 phenothiazine (4560 R.P.) *Archs int. pharmacodyn. Ther.*, **92**, 305-361.
Ellinger, F. (1951). Die Histaminhypothese der biologischen Strahlenwirkungen. *Schweiz. med. Wschr.*, **81**, 61-65.
Freedman, A. M. and Himwich, H. E. (1949). DFP: Site of injection and variation in response, *Am. J. Physiol.* **156**, 125-128.
Gay, L. N. and Carliner, P. E. (1949). The prevention and treatment of motion sickness I. Seasickness. *Bull. Johns Hopkins Hosp.*, **84**, 470-487.
Glaviano, V. V. and Wang., S. C. (1955). Dual mechanism of antiemetic action of 10-(γ dimethyl aminopropyl) 2-chlorophenothiazine hydrochloride (chlorpromazine) in dogs. *J. Pharmac. exp. Ther.*, **114**, 358-366.
Lindstrom. P. A. and Brizzee, K. R. (1962). Relief of intractable vomiting from surgical lesions in the area postrema. *J. Neurosurg.*, **19**, 228-236.
Sparks, R. D., Browne, D. C. and Ferrans, V. F. (1962). Triethylperazine: effect on postoperative vomiting and localization in central nervous system of fluorescence techniques. *Am. J. Gastroent. N. Y.*, **37**, 404-414.

34. Cough: expectorants and antitussives

Cough is an activity directed towards the removal of an obstruction or irritant from the respiratory tract. The potentially beneficial value of such a mechanism is obvious and there are circumstances when it is undesirable to suppress cough lest it results in the retention of infected material in the lung. On the other hand, cough, notwithstanding its basically protective function, can have dangerous sequelae. Long-continued coughing, particularly in older people, imposes a severe load on the circulatory system and it may also lead to the breaking down of elastic tissue in the lung (*emphysema*). In young children, too, prolonged coughing can be very exhausting. In these circumstances it may be necessary to take steps to suppress the cough before the disease causing it is itself cured. The difficult decision whether to treat a cough associated with disease of the respiratory system has to be determined by the circumstances of the individual case. The majority of coughs, however, occur in the absence of real disease or serious infection and suppression of the cough provides comfort for the patient and protection for his associates, without postponing his recovery. The popularity of proprietary cough mixtures testifies to the trivial nature of most coughs.

The essential feature of a cough is that air is expelled from the lungs at a high velocity. The glottis is closed and a forcible expiratory movement causes a sharp rise of pressure in the lungs. The glottis then relaxes suddenly, allowing the air to escape. Some degree of bronchospasm accompanies coughing and this has the effect of further increasing the velocity of the air flow.

The characteristic 'coughing' sound is caused by the explosive release of air which follows the abrupt relaxation of the glottis. It sometimes happens that the glottis narrows without actually closing. This is the natural state of affairs in some animals and it occurs in human beings when the glottal muscles or the nerve supplying them (the recurrent laryngeal branch of the vagus) are paralysed. Incomplete closure of the glottis does not prevent the expulsion of air from the lungs at a sufficiently rapid rate to remove irritant material but the characteristic sound is absent.

When expiratory efforts are made with the glottis closed, the pressure inside both the abdomen and the thorax increases. This hinders the return of blood to the heart and may cause circulatory embarrassment. It also causes the redness of the face seen during prolonged bouts of coughing.

The particular pattern of respiratory muscle activity that constitutes coughing is initiated in the medulla and coughing can be produced in animals by medullary stimulation (Borison, 1948). It is, therefore, generally assumed that a cough 'centre' exists in the medulla though it has never been precisely delineated. Expiratory muscle activity is also involved in vomiting and the vomiting centre and the cough 'centre' are associated. When the latter is violently stimulated, excitation sometimes spreads to the vomiting centre. Some cough stimulants are also emetics. Coughing and vomiting also occur together in whooping cough; in this condition the cough terminates, unlike other coughs, in a deep inspiration which is responsible for its 'whooping' nature.

Like vomiting, coughing is to some extent under voluntary control: anyone can cough at will and it is often possible temporarily to suppress a cough. Coughing sometimes represents a nervous tic or an affectation and the outbreak of coughing heard in a concert hall between movements of a symphony is as much a manifestation of the embarrassment created by the intrusion of an interval in which neither applause nor conversation is deemed proper as it is a release of previously suppressed coughs. Nevertheless, coughing is usually initiated by reflexes from the respiratory tract which responds to irritation by discharging impulses to the cough 'centre'. Sensory impulses from the respiratory tract are carried by the vagus, glossopharyngeal and trigeminal nerves. Stimulation of other sensory nerves, particularly those of the ear and abdomen, may also induce coughing. The larynx and trachea are particularly susceptible to mechanical irritants but chemical irritants are effective over a larger part of the respiratory tree as far as the smaller bronchioles.

ANTITUSSIVE DRUGS

Antitussive drugs suppress or alleviate coughing. Coughing can, in theory, be inhibited by depressing the activity of any component of the cough reflex. The site of action of most antitussive drugs has not been adequately investigated but it seems that, with the notable exception of benzonatate (see below), most of them depress the cough

Table 34.1 The pharmacodynamic actions of some antitussive drugs. (Adapted and abridged from Bucher, 1965.)

Drug	Usual single dose mg	Effect on respiration (stimulation +) (inhibition –)	Effect on bronchi (constriction +) (dilatation –)	Local anaesthesia
Dimethoxanate	25	–	+	
Pipazethate	30		–	+
Narcotine	30		+	
Oxeladin	10			
Oxolamine	100		–	+
(cf. Codeine)	30			

'centre' although this is not necessarily their only locus of action. Since the cough and respiratory centres are closely associated, antitussive activity sometimes involves depression of respiration. This is an undesirable effect in many respiratory conditions.

In addition to depressing cough, some antitussives have potentially useful side-effects such as bronchodilatation, sedation, local anaesthesia or respiratory stimulation (Table 34.1). The desirability or otherwise of these side-effects should dictate the use of particular antitussive drugs in the individual case.

THE OPIATES

The opiates (which are fully discussed in Chapter 26) have long been employed in the treatment of cough. Among their other actions, they depress the activity of the medullary centres and this is clearly the basis of their antitussive action. The famous Dover's powder (a mixture of opium and ipecacuanha) first became available in the early years of the eighteenth century while codeine has probably been the most widely-used of all antitussive drugs. Morphine itself, ethylmorphine and methadone (amidone, phenadone, Physeptone) have also been employed as cough suppressants but the temptation to use them for other than strictly medicinal purposes has led to their being abandoned (except in terminal illnesses when their liability to induce dependence is of no consequence) in favour of less addictive opiates. Among these more innocuous drugs, pholcodine has been widely used as an antitussive drug. It is not likely to cause dependence at the dose level at which it is usually prescribed (5-15 mg.). Like all the other opiates it may cause constipation. Dextromethorphan is another effective cough depressant which is not likely to be abused and which has little tendency to

produce undesirable side-effects. It is effective in oral doses of 10-20 mg. Its laevorotatory isomer, however, is highly addictive. Other members of this group of drugs include dihydrocodeinone (hydrocodone, Dicodid) and laevopropoxyphene napsylate.

The antitussive agents mentioned in the foregoing paragraph appear in countless proprietary mixtures, neither the names nor the composition of which need concern the reader.

BENZONATATE (TESSALON)

This drug is unique in that it was developed from the outset as a cough depressant. The antitussive action of the other commonly-used drugs was detected incidentally during the routine screening of compounds not specifically developed for this purpose. The investigations which led to the development of benzonatate were directed towards the discovery of a compound which would selectively

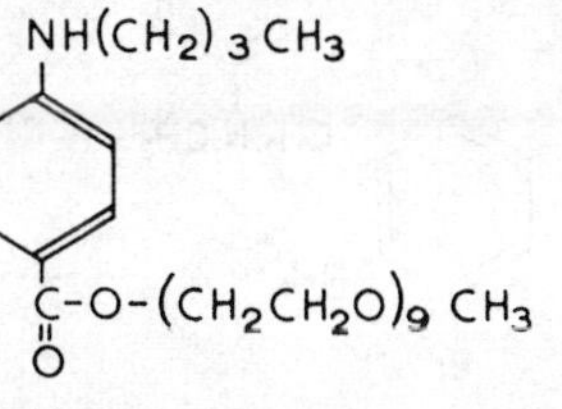

Benzonatate

anaesthetize the stretch and touch receptors in the lungs and thus depress coughing by a peripheral action. This was achieved: the para-n-butylaminobenzoate residue in benzonatate possesses local anaesthetic activity and this is combined with the nonaethylene glycol monomethyl ether

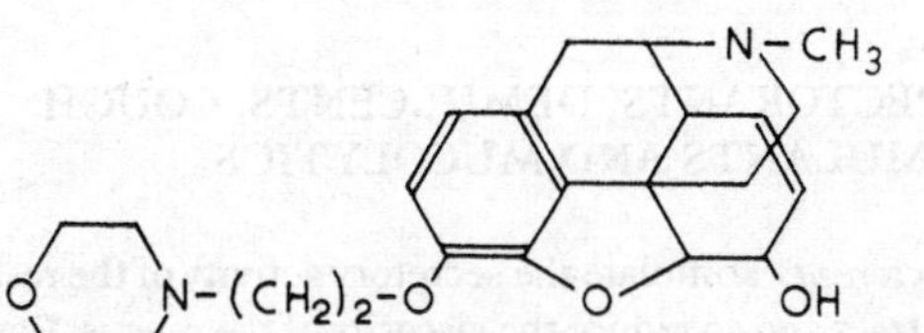

Pholcodine

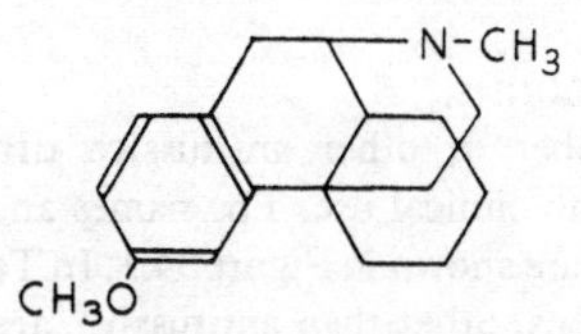

Dextromethorphan

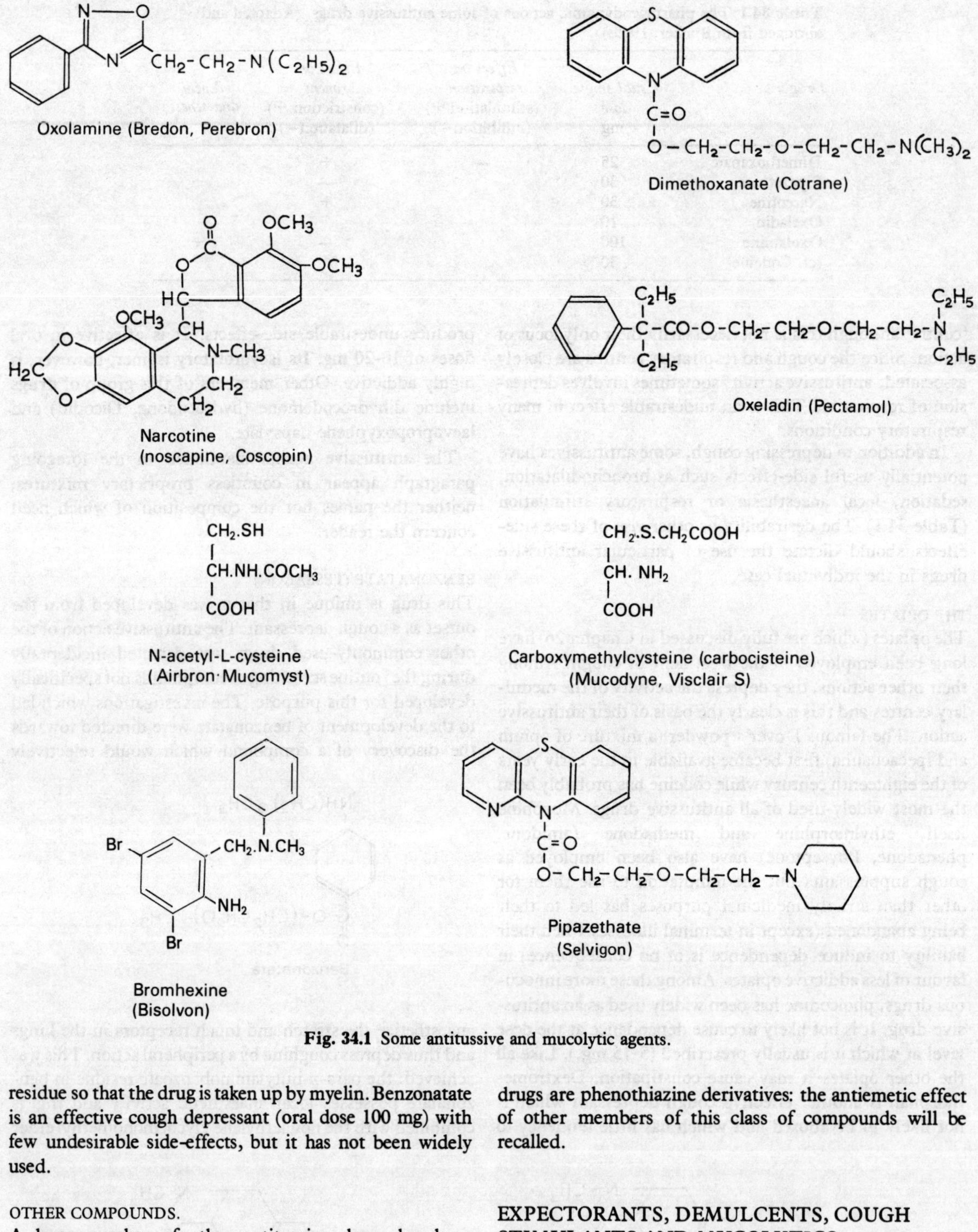

Oxolamine (Bredon, Perebron)

$CH_2-CH_2-N(C_2H_5)_2$

Dimethoxanate (Cotrane)

$O-CH_2-CH_2-O-CH_2-CH_2-N(CH_3)_2$

Narcotine
(noscapine, Coscopin)

OCH_3
OCH_3
OCH_3

Oxeladin (Pectamol)

C_2H_5

$C-CO-O-CH_2-CH_2-O-CH_2-CH_2-N$
C_2H_5
C_2H_5
C_2H_5

$CH_2.SH$
$CH.NH.COCH_3$
$COOH$

N-acetyl-L-cysteine
(Airbron·Mucomyst)

$CH_2.S.CH_2COOH$
$CH. NH_2$
$COOH$

Carboxymethylcysteine (carbocisteine)
(Mucodyne, Visclair S)

Br
$CH_2.N.CH_3$
NH_2
Br

Bromhexine
(Bisolvon)

Pipazethate
(Selvigon)

$C=O$
$O-CH_2-CH_2-O-CH_2-CH_2-N$

Fig. 34.1 Some antitussive and mucolytic agents.

residue so that the drug is taken up by myelin. Benzonatate is an effective cough depressant (oral dose 100 mg) with few undesirable side-effects, but it has not been widely used.

OTHER COMPOUNDS.

A large number of other antitussive drugs has been introduced into clinical use. The names and formulae of some of them are shown in Figure 34.1. In Table 34.1 their principal actions, other than antitussive, are summarized for reference. It will be seen that some of the antitussive

drugs are phenothiazine derivatives: the antiemetic effect of other members of this class of compounds will be recalled.

EXPECTORANTS, DEMULCENTS, COUGH STIMULANTS AND MUCOLYTICS

Expectorants stimulate the secretory activity of the respiratory tract and so reduce the viscosity of the mucus. For this reason they benefit (according to the textbooks at least) hard, 'dry', irritating coughs, converting them into 'productive' coughs that are less exhausting and less painful to the patient. In addition, the increased amounts of mucus act as a demulcent and provide some protection for the inflamed and irritated surfaces. *Demulcents* proper, which protect the mucous membrane without increasing the bronchial secretions, can be used to relieve 'tickling' coughs. *Mucolytics* are used in patients whose mucous secretions though profuse are very viscous. By reducing the viscosity of the secretions the mucolytics make coughing easier and reduce the attendant physical strain.

Among the many simple substances that have been used as expectorants are iodides, citric acid and citrates, sodium bicarbonate, sodium chloride and ammonium salts, but it must be doubted whether they have any value. Iodides are excreted partly by the mucous glands of the respiratory tract. The excretion of the iodide necessitates the excretion of increased amounts of water so the volume of the glandular secretions is increased. Ammonium salts probably owe their expectorant action to a reflex stimulation of the bronchial secretion following irritation of the gastrointestinal tract. This irritative action sometimes causes vomiting and some emetic drugs, such as ipecacuanha and squill, have also been used as expectorants.

Demulcents are frequently included in cough mixtures. Syrups, mucilages, glycerol and extract of liquorice all have demulcent properties. Liquorice is a favourite, as in liquorice lozenges B.P.C. (Brompton Cough Lozenges).

Expectorants, as we have seen, make coughs more 'productive' by increasing the volume of bronchial secretions. Some substances which have a direct irritant action on the upper respiratory tract are also used in mixtures or as inhalations with the intention of promoting easier coughing when the volume of respiratory tract secretions is low. When taken in the form of inhalations the steam itself gives symptomatic relief. Cough stimulants are many in number, reflecting the variety of nominally different proprietary cough mixtures. They include tolu, methol, eucalyptus guaiacol, terpin hydrate, benzoin and oil of turpentine. These substances deserve a mention only because their use has been hallowed by time: it is doubtful whether they have anything but a placebo action.

It has already been mentioned that demulcents and cough stimulants are frequently included in cough mixtures. Expectorants, bronchodilators and antitussives may also be present. The components of any particular mixture have not necessarily been selected on any rational pharmacological grounds and it is not unusual, for instance, to find an antitussive and a cough stimulant in the same preparation.

Among substances that have been used as mucolytics are proteolytic enzymes (pancreatic deoxyribonuclease, trypsin, streptokinase), detergents (2-ethylhexylsulphate) and reducing agents which depolymerize mucopolysaccharides (ascorbic acid, sodium percarbonate). Recently, however, compounds such as bromhexine, S-carboxymethylcysteine and N-acetyl-L-cysteine have become popular. Bromhexine seems to break down the mucopolysaccharide fibres that are found in quantity in the sputum of patients with asthma or chronic bronchitis. The recommended dose is 12 mg three times daily.

The cysteine derivatives probably operate by breaking the disulphide bridges that link together adjacent strands of mucus. They are not entirely free of toxicity, gastrointestinal upsets being the side effect most often experienced.

THE SCREENING AND CLINICAL TESTING OF DRUGS AFFECTING COUGH

Antitussive activity can be looked for in the course of routine screening procedures and a variety of simple methods is available for provoking cough in experimental animals. They can be exposed to ammonia vapour or aerosolized sulphuric acid; coughs can be recorded by a throat microphone or, in anaesthetized animals, by recording the expiratory activity by a conventional pneumograph. Small unanaesthetized animals can be placed in a bottle sealed with a diaphragm containing an air-leak. The sudden changes in pressure caused by coughing cause the diaphragm to move; because of the leak, the gentler pressure changes accompanying normal respiration do not affect the diaphragm.

Newer and ingenious methods are now available for producing cough in unanaesthetized animals. In one, a small piece of iron is suspended in the trachea in a preliminary operation. Thereafter coughing can be induced by causing the metal to vibrate against the trachea in response to an electromagnet placed outside the throat (Tedeschi, 1959). In a similar method, electrodes are placed in the trachea and their leads are brought to the surface of the animal, permitting electrical stimulation when required (Stefko and Benson, 1953).

These methods do not determine either the point of action of the antitussive agents or their effects on the several components of the cough mechanism. In a more sophisticated analysis this information is required. In anaesthetized animals the superior laryngeal branch of the glossopharyngeal nerve can be stimulated directly to produce cough. If a drug which is known to possess antitussive activity does not affect cough induced by this method it is a reasonable conclusion that its depressant action is exerted on the peripheral receptors. This can be tested directly by recording the action potentials in the appropriate sensory nerve following direct stimulation of the respiratory tract. A peripherally-acting antitussive agent should prevent, or reduce, the discharge of afferent impulses. If a drug *does* depress coughing produced by electrical stimulation of the superior laryngeal nerve it either has a central action or it inhibits cough by depressing the activity of the expiratory musculature. The latter possibility is unlikely but the central site of action can be confirmed by studying the effect of the drug on coughing produced by electrical stimulation of the medulla (Chakravarty *et al.* 1956).

Butcher (1965) has proposed the use of anaesthetized pigeons to determine the effect of antitussive drugs on respiratory processes. The bird's trachea is obstructed and this soon causes increased respiratory activity. Measurements are made of the maximum expiratory and inspiratory pressures and the time which elapses between tracheal obstruction and the appearance of increased expiratory activity. Antitussive drugs differ in their relative effects on these quantities and it should be possible to utilize this method to develop drugs with a more selective action on respiratory mechanics than has been possible hitherto.

Before antitussive drugs are released for clinical trial it is usual to test them on healthy volunteers in whom cough has been induced. The substances most widely used for this purpose are citric acid, acetylcholine (both given as aerosols) and lobeline (5 mg. by intravenous injection).

As with the antiemetics, placebo effects play a large part in determining the efficiency of antitussive drugs and 'double blind' techniques are essential when their clinical usefulness is being tested. Since coughs tend to be persistent, time is usually available, when clinical trials proper are begun, for a cross-over test to be undertaken. The effect of drug and placebo treatment can be assessed either by observation or by continuously recording the patient's coughing from a throat microphone.

BIBLIOGRAPHY

Reviews

Bickerman, H. A. (1962). Clinical pharmacology of antitussive agents. *Clin. Pharmac Ther.*, **3**, 353-368.

Bucher, K. (1958). Pathophysiology and pharmacology of cough. *Pharmac. Rev.*, **10**, 43-58.

Bucher, K. (1965). Antitussive drugs. In *Physiological Pharmacology*, vol. 2, pp. 175-200. Ed. Root, W. S. and Hofmann, F. G. New York and London: Academic Press.

Chappel, C. I. and von Seeman, C. (1963). Antitussive drugs. In *Progress in Medicinal Chemistry*, vol. 3, pp. 89-145. Ed. Ellis, G. P. and West, G. B. London: Butterworth.

Doyle, F.P. and Metha, M.D. (1964). Antitussives. *Adv. Drug Res.* **1**, 107-160.

Original papers

Borison, H. L. (1948). Electrical stimulation of the neural mechanism regulating spasmodic respiratory acts in the cat. *Am. J. Physiol.*, **154**, 55-62.

Chakravarty, N. K., Matallana, A., Jensen, R. and Borison, H. L. (1956). Central effects of antitussive drugs on cough and respiration, *J. Pharmac. ext. Ther.*, **117**, 127-135.

Nicholls, F. B. and Pasquariello, G. (1962). Controlled clinical trials of antitussive agents: an experimental evaluation of different methods. *J. Pharmac, exp. Ther.*, **136**, 183-189.

Stefko. P. L. and Benson, W. M. (1953). A method for evaluation of antitussive agents in the unanaesthetised dog. *J. Pharmac. exp. Ther.*, **108**, 217-223.

Tedeschi, R. E. (1959). A new antitussive method involving mechanical stimulation in unanaesthetised dogs. J. *Pharmac, exp. Ther.*, **126**, 338-344.

Widdicombe, J. G. (1954). Receptors from trachea and bronchi of the cat, *J. Physiol.*, *Lond.*, **123**, 71-104.

35. The respiratory system

Most of the drugs that affect the respiratory system (bronchodilators, respiratory stimulants, antitussives, expectorants, etc.) have been dealt with in earlier chapters, as have the allergic conditions which may disturb respiratory function. It remains only to discuss the respiratory gases and to consider the methods available for studying the action of drugs on the respiratory system.

THE RESPIRATORY GASES

The therapeutic uses of oxygen and carbon dioxide can only be adequately discussed if the pathophysiological changes underlying conditions of oxygen want are properly understood.

ANOXIA (HYPOXIA)

Lack of oxygen in the tissues and in blood is described as *anoxia* and *anoxaemia* respectively. If anoxaemia occurs, anoxia must follow but anoxia can occur independently of anoxaemia. Cyanides and other substances that poison the respiratory enzymes prevent the utilization of oxygen even when the blood is fully saturated with oxygen.

Anoxia is sometimes called hypoxia on the reasonable grounds that the condition described is one of deficiency, rather than a complete lack, of oxygen. However, no one appears to have yet suggested that the condition characterized by a diminution in the number of red cells should be called hypaemia instead of anaemia. Even those who speak of hypoxia recognise a condition of anaemic hypoxia. 'Anoxia' is therefore retained in this chapter.

Anoxia is traditionally divided into four types:

Anoxic anoxia. In this condition, the blood passing through the lungs does not become completely oxygenated. Anoxic anoxia occurs in the normal person who has recently arrived at a high altitude. As a result of the overall reduction in atmospheric pressure, the partial pressure of oxygen in his alveoli and the degree of oxygenation of his blood are reduced. After a brief sojourn at the higher altitude, compensatory mechanisms re-establish adequate oxygenation of the tissues.

In patients with some forms of pulmonary or congenital cardiac disease, anoxic anoxia arises even at ordinary altitudes. Entry of air to some of the pulmonary alveoli may be obstructed by exudate, bronchiolar constriction or pulmonary collapse and the haemoglobin in the blood leaving the lungs is therefore incompletely saturated with oxygen. A similar state of affairs arises when some of the blood destined for the lungs is shunted directly into the arterial circulation as a result of the persistence of foetal communications between the right and left sides of the heart or between the pulmonary and subclavian arteries. Anoxic anoxia will also occur if the activity of the muscles of respiration is seriously depressed.

Anaemic anoxia. Anaemic anoxia arises when insufficient haemoglobin is available for the transport of oxygen to the tissues. The deficiency may take the form of an actual lack of haemoglobin due to anaemia. In other instances, the haemoglobin content of the blood is within normal limits but some has been rendered unavailable by virtue of its being converted to carboxyhaemoglobin (in carbon monoxide poisoning) or to sulphaemoglobin or methaemoglobin (in drug poisoning).

Stagnant anoxia. In stagnant anoxia, the blood and hence the tissues become depleted of oxygen because the circulation rate is too sluggish to maintain an adequate rate of oxygen transport from the lungs to the tissues. Stagnant anoxia may be a purely local phenomenon as when the venous return from the whole or part of a limb is obstructed or it may affect the whole body as a result of gross impairment of cardiovascular function.

Histotoxic anoxia. This is the condition already referred to in which anoxia occurs with anoxaemia. Histotoxic means 'tissue poisoning'.

It is often stated or implied that the four types of anoxia produce essentially identical symptomatologies. This is incorrect in several respects. About 95 per cent of the oxygen in the blood is transported in the form of oxyhaemoglobin but the immediate source of oxygen for the tissues is that dissolved in the plasma and the rate at which oxidative reactions take place is determined by the concentration of this dissolved oxygen. The amount of gas which dissolves in a liquid is dependent on the partial pressure of the gas (Henry's Law) and in anoxic anoxia the concentration of oxygen in the plasma of the blood leaving the lungs is low because of the reduced oxygen pressure in the alveoli. In other forms of anoxia, alveolar oxygen pressure is not depressed and the oxygen concentration in the arterial plasma is as high as it is in the normal subject. The concentration in the venous plasma will be depressed because the blood has to give up more than its normal proportion of oxygen but the mean pressure at which the gas is delivered to the tissues will be higher than it is in equivalent degrees of anoxic anoxia. Quite mild degrees of anoxic anoxia may produce obvious signs of respiratory distress.

Differences in the intensity of the symptoms produced are observed even in different forms of the same general type of anoxia. A true anaemia produces less severe symptoms of anoxia than does a haemoglobin deficit resulting from poisoning with carbon monoxide or other substances that render haemoglobin incapable of carrying oxygen. In true anaemia, the reduced number of erythrocytes renders the blood less viscous. This permits the maintenance of a more rapid circulation so that each corpuscle makes more circuits of the cardiovascular system in unit time than do those of nonanaemic blood. Consequently the total amount of oxygen delivered to the tissues is not seriously affected unless quite marked degrees of anaemia have developed. This form of compensatory response is not possible in circumstances not attended by a reduction in the total erythrocyte count. An interesting situation arises when the total number of red cells is pathologically increased (polycythaemia rubra). Notwithstanding the greatly enhanced oxygen carrying capacity of his blood, the polycythaemic patient is likely to suffer from stagnant anoxia because his blood circulates so slowly.

The cardinal symptom of anoxia is breathlessness (dyspnoea). In mild degrees of anoxia it occurs only on exertion but in more severe forms of the condition it is present at rest. Cyanosis is produced if large amounts of reduced haemoglobin are present in the venous blood. It is important to remember that the intensity of the cyanosis is determined by the absolute amount of reduced haemoglobin present and not by the relative quantities of reduced and oxygenated haemoglobin. Cyanosis will not, therefore, be seen in anaemic patients. Conversely, in anoxic anoxia of long standing, cyanosis is likely to be very marked. This arises because the number of red cells, and hence the amount of available haemoglobin, increases in partial compensation of the anoxic state. In polycythaemia it is extreme.

THERAPEUTIC USES OF OXYGEN

Oxygen may have to be used in individual cases of anoxia of all types but it is most generally useful in acute anoxic anoxia arising from inadequate oxygenation of blood in the lung, in anaemic anoxia caused by carbon monoxide poisoning and in the state of cardiovascular shock that follows myocardial infarction.

When respiratory movements are seriously depressed, the concentration of oxygen in the alveoli falls because replenishment of the air in the lungs is interfered with. Under these circumstances, the administration of oxygen leads to an improvement in the degree of oxygenation of the blood, even if ventilation is not mechanically assisted. However, oxygen is often beneficial when respiratory movements are not depressed. Because of the shape of the oxyhaemoglobin dissociation curve, atmospheric air at normal pressures should be sufficient to saturate the haemoglobin in the blood leaving the lungs and it is not immediately apparent why the administration of oxygen is beneficial in conditions of anoxic anoxia not associated with a reduction of alveolar oxygen tension. There is in fact a two-fold explanation. If the alveoli contain exudate, the transfer of oxygen into the blood will be restricted. The replacement of atmospheric air by pure oxygen will serve to increase the oxygen pressure gradient between alveolar air and pulmonary blood and thus will improve the rate of oxygen diffusion into the blood. In some conditions (such as arise when blood is shunted directly from the venous to the arterial side of the circulation or when a proportion of the alveoli are non-functional) the blood which leaves the left ventricle will be deficient in oxygen by virtue of the fact that it contains an admixture of blood which has not been oxygenated in the lungs. If pure oxygen is administered, the haemoglobin of the blood which does pass through functional lung tissue will not carry any more oxygen than it does when only air is breathed. More than the usual amount of oxygen will, however, dissolve in the plasma and some of it will be transferred to the haemoglobin of the non-oxygenated blood when the oxygenated and non-oxygenated streams meet.

The affinity of carbon monoxide for haemoglobin is many times greater than that of oxygen so that small amounts of carbon monoxide are capable of immobilizing large quantities of haemoglobin. Because carbon monoxide and oxygen compete for haemoglobin, the dissociation of carboxyhaemoglobin is favoured by increasing the concentration of oxygen in the inspired air. Carbon dioxide reduces the affinity of carbon monoxide for haemoglobin and it is useful to add 5 per cent of carbon dioxide to the oxygen used for the resuscitation of victims of carbon monoxide poisoning.

Oxygen administration is not without its dangers and it is important to recognize that the effect of oxygen inhalation depends on the carbon dioxide content of the blood. Anoxic anoxia may be caused by a depression of the respiratory movements. This occurs, for instance, in poliomyelitis or when an overdose of a drug that depresses the respiratory centre or the muscles of respiration has been taken or given. The excretion of carbon dioxide is inadequate and as its concentration in the blood increases the respiratory centre becomes progressively less sensitive to it. Control of respiration then becomes vested in the carotid body mechanism which is stimulated by oxygen lack. If a high percentage of oxygen is added to the inspired air, the stimulus delivered to the respiratory centre from the carotid body is diminished, respiration becomes even more depressed and the accumulation of carbon dioxide in the blood (hypercapnia) becomes greater. In these circumstances, over enthusiastic administration of oxygen will exacerbate the patient's condition instead of relieving it. This unfortunate sequel can be avoided only by carefully adjusting the oxygen concentration so that respiration is not further depressed or by assisting the respiration mechanically. When the anoxia is caused by conditions such as pneumonia, pulmonary oedema or lung collapse which do not depress the activity of the respiratory musculature, the respiration is stimulated (because of the oxygen deficit) and there is no accumulation of carbon dioxide. The respiratory centre thus retains its sensitivity and continues to maintain its overriding control so that high concentrations of oxygen can (and indeed should) be administered.

Long continued administration of oxygen under pressure may result in oxygen poisoning, although the likelihood of this occurrence is much smaller than was at one time supposed. Two factors contribute to oxygen toxicity. If the amount of oxygen dissolved in the plasma is increased to the extent that it can supply all the tissues' demands, little or no oxyhaemoglobin will dissociate in the peripheral circulation and the blood's capacity for carbon dioxide carriage will consequently be reduced. Hypercapnia may result. In addition, the high concentration of dissolved oxygen in the blood, and hence in the tissues, inhibits the activity of oxidative enzymes.

In addition to the administration of oxygen, specific forms of treatment may be required in anoxia and the respiratory movements may need mechanical assistance. The use of nitrites for the treatment of cyanide poisoning is discussed in Chapter 40 (p. 701).

A variety of methods is available for the administration of oxygen. These include nasal tubes, oxygen masks and oxygen tents. The type of equipment used is determined by the demands of the individual case. Close fitting masks permit the maintenance of the high oxygen concentrations required in treating carbon monoxide poisoning and myocardial infarction. Devices which enable the concentration of the gas to be regulated with some degree of accuracy are required when there is a danger that the administration of oxygen will lead to respiratory depression and hypercapnia. A concentration of about 30 per cent of oxygen can be maintained in oxygen tents, which have the advantage of sparing the patients the encumbrance of a face mask. Tents are unsuitable in conditions which require the continuous administration of high concentrations of oxygen because the tent has to be opened in order to attend to the needs of the patient. Apparatus for administering oxygen is described and illustrated by Grant (1974).

THERAPEUTIC USES OF CARBON DIOXIDE

Because carbon dioxide is a respiratory stimulant, it was at one time usual to add 5 per cent of the gas to the oxygen used for the treatment of anoxia. From what has already been said it will be obvious that this practice is at best illogical and at worst dangerous. It is permissible to administer carbon dioxide for a short time to patients recovering from an inhalation anaesthetic. Respiration is stimulated and excretion of the anaesthetic is hastened. Carbon dioxide is sometimes useful in terminating attacks of hiccough. The stimulus it provides to the respiration leads to large excursions of the diaphragm which swamp the spasmodic contractions of that muscle. Apart from these minor uses, the only real therapeutic value of carbon dioxide is in the treatment of carbon monoxide poisoning.

THE LABORATORY ASSESSMENT OF DRUGS THAT AFFECT THE RESPIRATORY SYSTEM

In the physiology laboratory, the investigation of respiratory function now involves the use of apparatus of considerable complexity. The requirements of the pharmacologist are usually satisfied by less elaborate equipment.

In routine examinations of the general pharmacological activity of drugs and tissue extracts, it is usual to record respiratory and cardiovascular effects concurrently. Only in this way is it possible to decide whether an effect on one of the systems is the result of an action on the other (a fall of blood pressure, for instance, stimulates respiration) or whether it arises independently. Respiratory activity is measured either by recording the volume of air which enters and leaves the lungs with each breath or (and preferably) by assessing the movements of the chest wall. It has to be remembered that the volume of gas exchanged at each breath (the *tidal air*) is only a fraction of the total lung capacity and a drug may alter the degree of distension of the lungs without affecting the tidal volume. This kind of response can only be reliably detected and followed by means of equipment which indicates changes in size of the thorax. Notwithstanding the clear advantage of making records in this way and the variety of simple ways of doing it, many workers still rely on measurements of tidal volume. In anaesthetized animals a tracheal cannula fitted with inspiratory and expiratory valves is connected to an empty bottle which has a small air inlet. The animal takes air from the bottle and expires into the atmosphere. Because of the restricted inlet, the pressure in the bottle falls during inspiration and rises again during expiration since the air leak allows refilling of the bottle. Pressure changes in the bottle are recorded by connecting the bottle to a diaphragm (tambour) type of recorder. For stethographic recordings (*stethograph*=chest writer) in animals, a piece of thread may be used to connect the xiphisternum or a slip of the diaphragm directly to a writing lever. The stethograph used in simple experiments in the human physiology laboratory consists of a piece of corrugated rubber tubing, the two ends of which are closed and joined by a cord or chain whose length is adjusted so that the apparatus fits snugly around the chest. The movements of respiration cause the tube to lengthen and shorten concertina-wise and the accompanying changes in volume can be measured by attaching a tambour recorder to a tube which passes through the stopper closing one end of the corrugated tubing. This device is easily scaled down for use in the animal laboratory but the most convenient way of recording respiratory movements in animals is undoubtedly the body plethysmograph. The whole of the animal, save its head, is enclosed in a box, an outlet from which passes to a volume recorder. A comfortable but airtight seal surrounds the neck of the animal as it emerges from the box. Changes in the volume of air in the box, which are reciprocally related to changes in thoracic volume occasioned by the respiratory movements, are recorded. Each of the two methods just described can be used for studying respiratory changes in the fully conscious animal and each can be easily adapted for transducer recording.

If a volume of air is delivered to an animal in which spontaneous respiration has ceased, the pressure change within the lungs will depend on the extent to which the component parts of the respiratory apparatus 'give' in the face of the incoming air. This 'give', or *compliance*, of the lung can be measured either by recording the pressure change which occurs in response to the admission of a fixed volume of air or the volume change which follows a fixed change of pressure. Sometimes the *elastance* (or 'stiffness' of the lungs), the reciprocal of the compliance, is measured. In pharmacology laboratories a popular method for detecting changes in lung compliance is that developed by Konsett and Rössler (1940). An animal is anaesthetized or given a neuromuscular blocking agent so that spontaneous ventilatory movements cease. Artificial respiration is then instituted, using the type of pump which delivers the same volume of air with each stroke. The air passes to the lungs through a pressure relief arrangement so that when the pressure in the pump-lung system exceeds a predetermined value, the rest of the air delivered by that stroke is diverted to a volume recorder. The lever of the recorder returns to baseline between the strokes of the pump. It can be seen that the excursions of the lever will decrease if the lung compliance falls so that more air enters the lungs.

A number of factors regulate compliance and when changes are detected by the Konsett-Rössler apparatus, collateral evidence must be considered before coming to any conclusion concerning the origin of the change. Nevertheless, the apparatus has a useful place in the laboratory: it records events occurring in the intact animal and it may be used for the screening and comparative assay of bronchodilator drugs (which increase lung compliance), for the detection of pathological changes such as lung collapse and for studying the action of drugs that affect the respiratory system by mechanisms which are not revealed by experiments on isolated preparations.

A suitable preparation for studying the action of drugs which affect the bronchiolar musculature is provided by rings of trachea or bronchi tied together to form a chain which is set up in the conventional type of isolated organ bath. In one of several variants of this procedure, the volume changes within an intact piece of trachea mounted in an organ bath are measured.

Preparations for investigating the action of drugs which act on other parts of the respiratory system are described in Chapters 21 and 34 (pp. 354 and 611).

BIBLIOGRAPHY

Books, monographs and reviews

Bass, B. H. (1974). *Lung Function Tests*, 4th ed. London: Lewis.
Campbell, E. J. M. (1968). Respiration. In *Clinical Physiology*, 3rd ed. Ed. Campbell, E. J. M., Dickinson, C. J. and Slater, J. D. H. Oxford: Blackwell.
Widdicombe, J. G. (1963). Regulation of tracheobronchial smooth muscle. *Physiol. Rev.*, **43**, 1-37.

Original papers

Grant, I. W. B. (1974). Oxygen therapy and artificial pulmonary ventilation. In *Textbook of Medical Treatment*, 13th ed. Ed. Alstead, S. and Girwood, R. H. Edinburgh: Livingstone.
Konsett, H. and Rössler, R. (1940). Versuchsanordung zu Untersuchungen an der Bronchialmuskulatur. *Arch. exp. Path. Pharmak.*, **195**, 71-74.

36. The kidney: diuretic and antidiuretic agents

The kidney has a variety of functions, all directed towards the preservation of homeostasis. Thus it does much to maintain the osmotic pressure of the body fluids by regulating the loss of water, it is important in the regulation of ionic balance and the acid-base equilibrium and it is the principal channel of excretion of the non-utilizable products of metabolism and foreign substances including drugs. These functions are not mutually independent: if, for instance, the kidney is excreting a heavy load of metabolites, water elimination will inevitably be increased as well. Many other examples of this interdependence of kidney functions will be found in the following pages.

A diuretic drug causes diuresis—an increased flow of urine. Diuretics form an important group of substances that are employed to remove excessive accumulations of fluid (oedema) from the tissue spaces. They are also used in the treatment of hypertension and diabetes insipidus as well as a number of miscellaneous conditions that will be mentioned when the individual drugs are discussed.

Before the pharmacology of the diuretic drugs can be discussed, it is necessary to remind the reader of the basic facts of renal physiology.

Each kidney is an assemblage of about one million nephrons, all of which have essentially the same structure. Each nephron is a tube terminating blindly at one end and opening at the other end into a collecting tubule which after uniting with other collecting tubules, opens into the pelvis of the kidney, which itself leads into the ureter. The enlarged closed end of the nephron is invaginated by a tuft of capillaries. The dilated end of the tubule with its attendant capillaries is the *glomerulus* or Bowman's capsule. The rest of the tubule includes, successively, the first convoluted tubule, the descending and ascending limbs of the loop of Henle and the distal convoluted tubule. These are represented schematically in Figure 36.1

It has already been said that all nephrons have essentially the same structure but they differ in detail and two main types can be recognized. Those (the *cortical nephrons*) which occupy approximately the outer two thirds of the cortex have a relatively short loop of Henle so that the tubule lies entirely within the cortex. The accompanying blood vessels surround the limbs of the loop in a tortuous manner. The glomeruli of the remaining nephrons are deep in the cortex and the loops of Henle occupy the medulla. For this reason the units are called *juxtamedullary nephrons*. The limbs of the loop are long and straight and

the accompanying blood vessels (the *vasa recta*) also form simple loops. As can be seen in Figure 36.1, part of the ascending limb of the loop of Henle is much narrower than the rest. In many nephrons this thin segment (which is of considerable functional importance) extends to include much of the descending limb too.

Arterioles derived from the renal artery (the *afferent arterioles*) divide into the glomerular capillaries. On leaving the glomerulus, the capillaries re-unite to form the *efferent arterioles*. These latter vessels continue to the tubules, where they break up into capillaries again, eventually emptying into the renal veins. The afferent arterioles of the glomerulus are relatively short and wide. The efferent arterioles of the cortical nephrons are long and narrow. This arrangement ensures that a high pressure is maintained within the glomerular capillaries. Both types of arteriole are quite sensitive to the action of chemical agents so that many drugs whose actions are not exerted primarily on the kidney nevertheless affect glomerular blood flow.

One further morphological point needs to be made. It will be clear to the reader that the junctions between the distal convoluted tubules and the collecting ducts occur in a part of the kidney (the cortex) that is replete with glomeruli. In many instances, the tubule comes into actual contact, close to the glomerulus, with the afferent glomerular arteriole. It is at such points of contact that the *juxtaglomerular apparatus* is located. Closely packed cells (the *macula densa*) occupy the small space between the tubule and the glomerular capsule while changes also occur in the histological structure of the afferent arteriole over the area of contact. Large cells with a densely granular cytoplasm appear in the vessel wall. They have the appearance of secretory cells and they are now recognized as the cells that give rise to *renin* (p. 357).

The mechanism by which the kidney produces urine can be quite simply stated as filtration by the glomeruli followed by differential reabsorption and secretion by the tubules. It is possible to collect samples of glomerular filtrate by means of a micropipette. When this is done it is found that the fluid in the glomerulus is a simple protein-free ultrafiltrate of plasma. The differences in composition between the plasma ultrafiltrate and urine are brought about by changes which occur in the tubules. Thus, substances such as glucose which, though present in plasma are normally absent from the urine, are completely reabsorbed in the tubules while non-utilizable metabolic

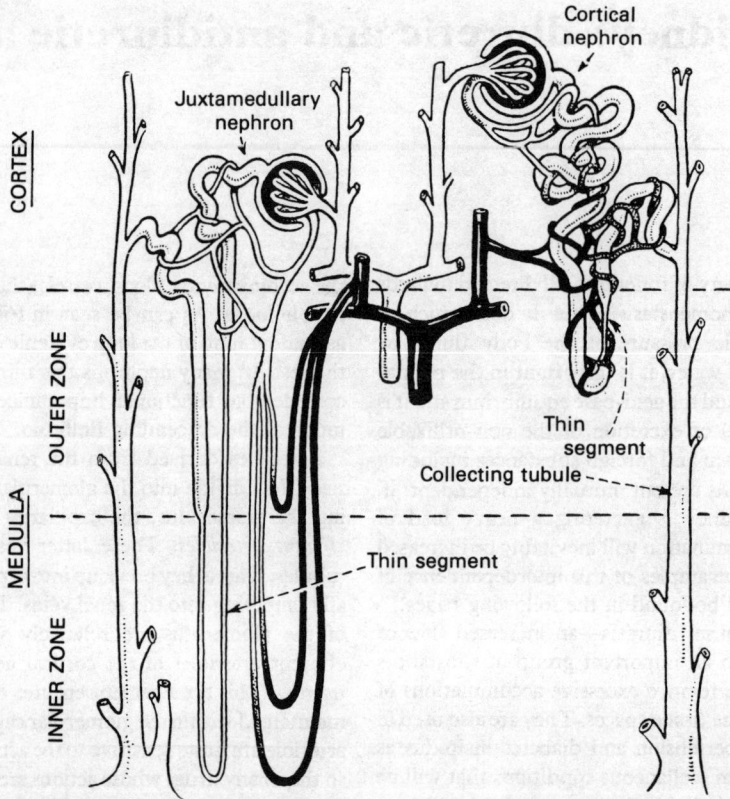

Fig. 36.1 To illustrate the differences between cortical and juxtamedullary nephrons. (Reproduced, by kind permission of the authors and publisher from Koch, A. in Ruch, T. C. and Patton, H. D.: Physiology and Biophysics, 19th Edition (1965), Philadelphia: W. B. Saunders Co.)

products such as urea are only minimally absorbed. The only constituent of normal human urine which is transferred from the blood to the urine by the secretory activity of the tubule cells is creatinine. A number of drugs (*p*-aminohippuric acid, penicillin and many diuretics are examples) are also excreted by this route. They do not pass through the glomerular capillaries but are abstracted from the blood as it circulates past the tubules.

Healthy human kidneys produce about 150 litres of glomerular filtrate daily. At least 85 per cent. of the water in this filtrate is reabsorbed in the tubules with the other plasma constituents. This reabsorption of water is an osmotic effect and it is an inevitable consequence of the reabsorption of the solutes. It can therefore be termed the *obligatory reabsorption*. Removal of 85 per cent. of the glomerular filtrate leaves a potential urine volume of about 23 litres. In fact, the healthy adult normally excretes about 1.5 litres of urine daily and in conditions of water deprivation this can be reduced to as little as 500 ml. The urine volume cannot be reduced below this latter figure (the *obligatory excretion*) because of the necessity of excreting metabolic products which must be dissolved in water and which cannot exceed a maximum concentration imposed

by the limits of the kidney's ability to maintain a concentration gradient between urine and blood. It is clear that a considerable volume of water is absorbed in the tubules by processes independent of those which cause the reabsorption of other components of the glomerular filtrate. The extent of this water reabsorption (which is called the *facultative reabsorption*) is determined by vasopressin (the antidiuretic hormone) which is secreted by the posterior pituitary gland. If the water content of the body falls, as a result of reduced intake or excessive loss, the osmotic pressure of the blood will rise. This causes an increased stimulation of *osmoreceptors* in the hypothalamus. A tract of nerve fibres (the supraoptico-hypophyseal tract) communicates the result of this stimulation to the posterior pituitary which liberates increased amounts of vasopressin. It will be evident, in view of the relatively low daily urine volume, that even under normal circumstances there is a considerable secretion of vasopressin. If the pituitary gland is incapable of secreting the hormone, daily urine volumes do reach very high values. Normal individuals who have drunk large quantities of water achieve urinary volumes over short periods of time which, if they could be maintained for 24 hours, would reach the theoretical daily maximum of approximately 23 litres. Thus the rate of urine excretion can range in the same individual from 20 ml to 1 litre an hour, a fact which indicates the extent to which the kidney is capable of compensating for variations in fluid intake and loss.

It is now realized that the facultative reabsorption of water is not an active process directly controlled by vasopressin. Absorption of water is passive in nature, the primary event being the active absorption of sodium. The extent to which water accompanies the sodium depends on the permeability of the cells of the distal convoluted tubules and the collecting ducts. The permeability of the tubule cells is controlled by the pituitary hormone. Sodium absorption is itself controlled by aldosterone (p. 754). As will be seen, the dependence of water reabsorption on the absorption of sodium is of considerable pharmacological importance.

The limbs of the loop of Henle and the corresponding blood vessels of the juxtamedullary nephrons form a counter current multiplier system, the effects of whose operation is to allow the production of a concentrated urine without necessitating the establishment of high osmotic gradients across any section of the tubule wall. The details of this system can be found in any up to date text book of physiology but the material in this chapter can be understood without reference to these details.

Thresholds, clearances and the assessment of renal function

It has already been pointed out that glucose in the plasma passes into the glomerular filtrate but that it is completely reabsorbed into the blood during its passage along the tubules. However, if the concentration of glucose exceeds about 180 mg per 100 ml of plasma, the excess cannot be absorbed and glucose appears in the urine. This *threshold* value is exceeded in the normal subject only on rare occasions: glucose is an example of a high threshold substance. Urea, which appears in the urine even when its plasma concentration is low, is an example of a substance with a low renal threshold. Substances with a high renal threshold are those whose retention in the body is physiologically advantageous. It should be clear that differences in threshold reflect differences in the rate and extent of tubular reabsorption.

Some foreign substances are not reabsorbed in the tubules at all—they have a renal threshold of zero—and they can be used to measure the rate of formation of glomerular filtrate and thus the effectiveness of the glomerular apparatus. One such substance is the polysaccharide, inulin. Let it be supposed that, after receiving a quantity of inulin, a subject's rate of urine formation (assessed by measuring the urine excreted in one hour) is V ml per minute, Let it be further supposed that the concentrations of inulin in the plasma and urine over the period of observation average P grams per ml and U grams per ml

respectively. Since the glomerular fluid is essentially an ultrafiltrate of plasma, it can be assumed that the concentration of inulin in the filtrate will closely approach that in the plasma. It will therefore be clear that the inulin in each millilitre of the voided urine must have been contained in $\frac{U}{P}$ ml of plasma or glomerular filtrate and that the rate of formation of the filtrate must be $\frac{UV}{P}$ ml per minute.

The quantity $\frac{UV}{P}$ can, of course, be calculated for any substance in plasma, irrespective of the extent to which it is absorbed in the tubules. It is known as the *clearance* value: it can be defined for any particular substance as the volume of plasma that would have contained the amount of the substance excreted in one minute. Only in the special case of inulin and other zero threshold substances is the clearance a measure of glomerular filtration. In other instances it provides an index of the rate at which the substance is excreted. It is to be noted that no substance which is excreted solely via the glomeruli can have a higher clearance than inulin. If clearances higher than this are found, it indicates that the substance in question is eliminated partly or wholly by tubular secretion.

Tubular function can be assessed by measuring the ability of the tubules to absorb glucose or to secrete *p*-aminohippuric acid. The maximum load of glucose which can be absorbed by the tubules (the 'tubular maximum for glucose') is measured by giving an intravenous infusion of a glucose solution whose concentration is gradually increased until glucose appears in the urine. At this stage, the tubular maximum (Tm) has been reached and

$$Tm\ (glucose) = plasma\ glucose\ concentration \times glomerular\ filtration\ rate.$$

The glomerular filtration rate is measured with inulin. Normal values for Tm (glucose) are of the order of 300 mg of glucose per minute.

In order to measure secretory activity, *p*-aminohippuric acid (PAH) is given in increasing amounts until the rate of excretion can no longer keep pace with the rate of administration. At this stage the amount of *p*-aminohippuric acid being handled each minute by the tubules is given by the product of the plasma concentration and the per minute blood flow through the tubules. The last named quantity is equal to the total plasma flow through the kidneys less that which is filtered off in the glomeruli before reaching the tubules. Thus

$$Tm(PAH) = plasma\ PAH\ concentration\ (renal\ plasma\ flow—glomerular\ filtration\ rate).$$

Renal plasma flow itself can be calculated from the amounts of *p*-aminohippuric acid in the plasma and urine because it is known that the compound is removed from the blood in one passage through the kidney. If therefore, *p*-aminohippuric acid is excreted at the rate of X mg per minute when its concentration in the plasma is Y mg per ml renal plasma flow is clearly $\frac{X}{Y}$ ml per minute. The usual value for Tm(PAH) is about 80 mg per minute.

Base conservation by the kidney

Metabolic processes in the body result in the production of acid substances but these do not appreciably alter the pH of the plasma which is kept constant by a number of buffer systems. The most important of these buffers is the sodium bicarbonate-carbonic acid system whose action can be understood by reference to the following equations:

$$H_2CO_3 \rightleftharpoons H^+ + HCO_3^-$$

$$NaHCO_3 \rightleftharpoons Na^+ + HCO_3^-$$

$$HA \rightleftharpoons H^+ + A^-$$

Carbonic acid is a weak acid and is consequently only weakly ionized in solution. Sodium bicarbonate is, like all salts, almost completely dissociated in solution. It can also be assumed that the metabolite, symbolized as HA, is also a relatively strong acid.

If the acid HA is added to the bicarbonate buffer system the added hydrogen ions will favour the reaction

$$H^+ + HCO_3^- \rightarrow H_2CO_3$$

The carbonic acid is excreted in the expired air and the final result of the buffering operation is therefore the loss of bicarbonate and the formation of the sodium salt of the added acid. In the kidney, bicarbonate is re-formed, base (sodium) is returned to the blood and an acid urine is produced. The renal mechanisms which bring about these changes are as follows:

a. *Production of carbonic acid.* The cells of the renal tubule contain the enzyme carbonic anhydrase which promotes the combination of carbon dioxide and water to carbonic acid. The hydrogen ions thus made available exchange with the sodium ions and the latter, together with the bicarbonate formed in the tubule pass back into the blood (Fig. 36.2).

b. *Ammonia production.* The sodium-hydrogen exchange just described leads to a progressive fall in the pH of the urine. When it falls below 6, another base conservation mechanism comes into play. Ammonia is formed in the tubule cells from glutamine under the influence of glutaminase. A little ammonia is also formed as a result of deamination of amino acids. The ammonia exchanges with sodium ions.

Another important buffering system is that provided by the sodium phosphates. Disodium hydrogen phosphate (Na_2HPO_4) can be regarded as the sodium salt of sodium dihydrogen phosphate (NaH_2PO_4) and the two phosphates together form a system analogous to the carbonic acid-

bicarbonate buffer. Buffering involves the formation of the dihydrogen phosphate and the sodium salt of the buffered acid.

$$Na_2HPO_4 \rightleftharpoons Na^+ + NaHPO_4^-$$

$$HA \rightleftharpoons H^+ + A^-$$

In the plasma, the disodium phosphate is present in larger quantities than the dihydrogen salt but because of the buffering the reverse situation obtains in the tubules, the contents of which are acid. Base conservation by the kidneys involves the exchange of sodium for hydrogen by means of the carbonic anhydrase and ammonia mechanisms already discussed. The sodium conserved is that associated with the anion of the buffered acid. In addition, disodium hydrogen phosphate present in the tubular fluid is converted by the same mechanism into the dihydrogen salt so that loss of sodium is even further reduced.

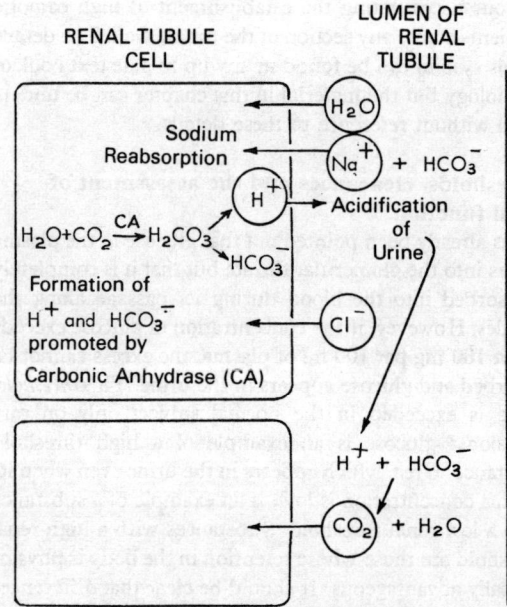

Fig. 36.2 Acidification of the urine by the actions of carbonic anhydrase. Inhibition of carbonic anhydrase prevents acidification of the urine, reabsorption of bicarbonate as carbon dioxide and of sodium ions in exchange for hydrogen ions.

A measure of the total amount of base conservation by the kidney (and also therefore of the total amount of acid buffered) is provided by the sum of the titratable acidity and ammonia content of the urine. The titratable acidity is simply the amount of acid present, as assessed by titration to pH 7 against sodium hydroxide.

OEDEMA

A hypothesis concerning the mechanism by which tissue fluid is formed was first put forward by Starling in 1909. Starling's hypothesis is accepted today substantially in the form in which it was originally set out. It can be summarized by reference to Figure 36.3, which represents a number of cells, a blood capillary and a lymph vessel. Extracellular fluid occupies the whole of the interstitial space between and around the cells and vessels.

At the arteriolar end of the blood capillary, a hydrostatic pressure of some 32 mm of mercury tends to force a protein-free filtrate of plasma from the capillary into the tissue spaces. This outward force is partially offset by the osmotic pressure of the plasma proteins. This reaches a value of about 25 mmHg. The hydrostatic and osmotic pressures of the tissue fluid itself contribute a little (in opposite directions) to the forces tending to move fluid into or out of the capillary but these may be neglected so that there remains a net outward pressure of about 7 mmHg at the arteriolar end of the vessel and fluid passes into the tissue spaces. At the venous end of the capillary the hydrostatic pressure has fallen and (because of the loss of water) the osmotic pressure has very slightly risen. There is now a net inward pressure of 10 mmHg which causes tissue fluid to move back into the capillary. There is thus a continuous movement of fluid out of, and back into, the capillaries. For various reasons, the capillaries cannot take in all the extracellular fluid which needs to be returned to the circulation. However, the lymphatic system provides an additional channel of return. The lymphatic system also conveys back to the bloodstream any protein (fibrinogen and albumin) which may have escaped from the capillaries. Tissue fluid in the lymphatic vessels becomes *lymph* after lymphocytes have been added during its passage through lymph nodes.

NUTRITIONAL OEDEMA
In conditions of severely restricted protein intake the concentration of the plasma proteins may fall. This causes a reduction in the osmotic pressure of the plasma and the loss of fluid from the blood capillaries is increased. At the same time its return to the capillaries is hindered and fluid collects in increased amounts in the tissue spaces, producing oedema. It seems likely that the loss of plasma protein is not the only cause of nutritional oedema, for there is some evidence that aldosterone secretion is increased in conditions of starvation. This will increase the reabsorption of sodium and hence the retention of water. There may also be an increased secretion of vasopressin. Finally, as the victim's own tissues begin to break down, protein and other large molecules will serve to increase the osmotic pressure of the extracellular fluid and to cause even more fluid retention. In severe starvation the victim (particularly if a child) may become so oedematous that he takes on a bloated appearance which may, to the untutored eye, mask the severity of the underlying wasting.

Oedema also occurs in beri beri (p. 790).

The treatment for nutritional oedema is obvious. Diuretic agents have little place unless it is felt desirable to eliminate the oedema fluid rapidly before an adequate nutritional status has been established. It is perhaps worth pointing out that nutritional oedema may be considerably reduced before any change in the plasma protein content has been effected. This is probably because the mere act of placing the patient in a situation in which he knows he is to be cared for reduces the stress to which he is exposed and tends to reverse the hormonal factors which have contributed to the oedema.

PREMENSTRUAL OEDEMA
Slight oedema at the time of menstruation is not uncommon. In some cases it is sufficiently severe to necessitate treatment by diuretic drugs. This form of oedema is caused primarily by sodium retention. Although this may be predominantly the result of sex hormone activity, there may also be an increased secretion of aldosterone. Retention of fluid also occurs in pregnancy. This probably arises from the action of progesterone which is known to inhibit sodium excretion. In addition, localized oedema (particu-

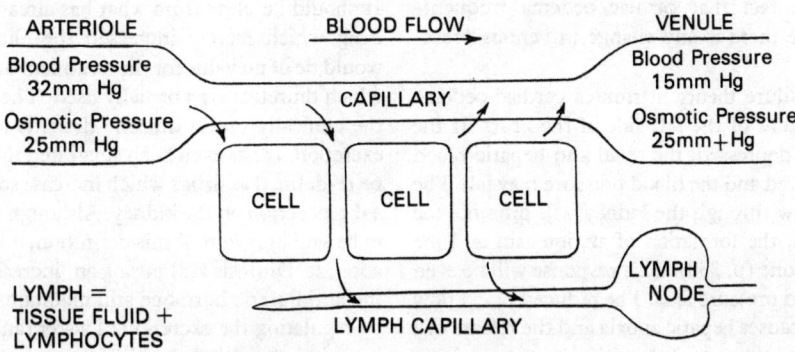

Fig. 36.3 The formation of tissue fluid and lymph.

larly in the ankles) occurs in pregnancy. This is because pressure of the enlarged uterus on the veins in the pelvis increases venous pressure. The filtration pressure in the capillaries is therefore increased and this hinders the return of blood from the tissue spaces. In pregnancy toxaemias the oedema is more extreme.

OEDEMA AND CIRRHOSIS OF THE LIVER.

A number of circumstances may lead to oedema and *ascites* (the accumulation of free fluid in the abdominal cavity) in hepatic disease. The cirrhotic process impairs blood flow though the portal vein and thus increases venous pressure. The liver's ability to manufacture plasma proteins is also likely to be reduced. The plasma may contain abnormally large amounts of aldosterone due to the liver's inability to metabolize it at the normal rate. Diuretics are of little use in this condition.

NEPHROTIC OEDEMA

Nephrotic oedema occurs as a consequence of membranous glomerulonephritis, a condition in which the permeability of the glomerular capillaries is increased and there is a serious loss of protein in the urine. The loss of plasma protein causes oedema. Nephrotic oedema responds to diuretics but it is necessary also to ensure that an adequate concentration of proteins is maintained in the plasma.

CARDIAC OEDEMA

The most common form of oedema is that occurring in cardiac disease and it is the condition for which diuretic therapy is most extensively used. The origin of cardiac oedema has been the subject of dispute for many years, some authorities supporting the *backward failure* theory while others favoured the *forward failure* theory. After some swings of opinion, most workers now favour the forward failure theory.

According to the backward failure theory, cardiac oedema is a simple consequence of the fact that the right side of the heart becomes incapable of expelling all the blood which is returned to it along the veins. As a result, the venous pressure—and hence the filtration pressure in the capillaries—rises and oedema occurs. Against this hypothesis is the fact ·that cardiac oedema frequently develops before there is any change in venous pressure.

The forward failure theory attributes cardiac oedema primarily to a failure of the left side of the heart. If the cardiac output is depressed, the renal and hepatic blood flows will be reduced and the blood pressure may fall. The reduced blood flow through the kidney will promote the secretion of renin, the formation of angiotensin and the release of aldosterone (p. 358). This response will be even greater if the blood pressure falls. The reduced blood flow through the liver causes hepatic anoxia and the release of a substance which stimulates the pituitary to release increased amounts of vasopressin. The destruction of aldosterone by the liver may be inhibited as a result of the impaired blood flow through the organ.

It will be apparent that, according to the forward failure theory the principal cause of cardiac oedema is sodium retention. While there can be little doubt that this is so, it is by no means certain that the only, or even the major, cause of sodium retention is the increased secretion of aldosterone. In many instances of cardiac oedema there is no detectable increase in the amount of aldosterone in the general circulation and aldosterone antagonists have not been conspicuously successful diuretic agents. It can be understood why the rational treatment of cardiac oedema will involve:

   a. Restoration, as far as is possible, of normal cardiac output (Chap. 31).

   b. Restriction of sodium intake.

   c. Promotion of sodium loss by the appropriate diuretic agents.

   d. Aspiration of fluid from the thorax and abdomen (*thoracocentesis and paracentesis* respectively) when necessary.

In failure of the left side of the heart, blood flow in the pulmonary circuit is hindered, pulmonary venous pressure rises and *pulmonary oedema* occurs. This condition may also occur as a result of pathological changes in the lungs occurring in the absence of cardiovascular disease.

OTHER FORMS OF OEDEMA

Stings, bites and burns produce weals which are areas of localized oedema caused by increased capillary permeability which is itself the result of the liberation in, or the injection into, the skin of histamine and other substances.

IDIOPATHIC OEDEMA

This condition arises spontaneously, usually in women. Its pathology is obscure but it resolves spontaneously in a short time. It is sometimes treated with diuretic agents but the treatment may aggravate the condition (p. 630).

DIURETIC AGENTS

It should be clear from what has already been said that a drug which merely increased the elimination of water would be of no value for the treatment of the conditions for which diuretics are normally used. The primary action of the clinically useful diuretic drugs is to increase sodium excretion. It has even been suggested that diuretics should be re-defined as drugs which increase sodium excretion by a direct action on the kidney. Although there is something to be said in favour of this definition, it would be unwise to adopt it. Diuresis still means an 'increased flow of urine', the antidiuretic hormone still maintains osmotic pressure by regulating the excretion of water (and not sodium) and it is still justifiable to speak of water as a diuretic substance even though the diuresis produced does not result in increased sodium excretion. Nevertheless it is convenient to distinguish between diuretic agents that act primarily by inhibiting the tubular reabsorption of sodium and chloride (*saluretics*) and those that influence other mechanisms. The latter group is smaller and less important than the saluretic group and it will be dealt with first..

WATER

If large volumes of fluid are drunk, large volumes of urine are excreted as a result of the operation of the mechanisms which regulate osmotic pressure. In the strict sense of the definition, water is a diuretic agent—indeed, it is the only physiological diuretic substance—but the increased output of water is never greater than the volume drunk, so that water is of no value in the treatment of oedema. On the other hand, it does no harm in this condition since it does not add to the oedema fluid.

There are circumstances in which a high urine output is needed for its own sake. Some of the sulphonamide drugs, for instance, are of low solubility and unless a high urine volume is maintained there is a danger that the drugs or their metabolites will come out of solution in the kidney tubules (p. 820). The diuresis required to keep the drugs in solution can be adequately provided by water. Similarly, part of the treatment of gout is directed towards increasing the urinary elimination of uric acid. This substance is not very soluble and large quantities of water must be given to prevent precipitation of uric acid in the urine.

It must be remembered that diuresis cannot occur unless water is available to provide the urine volume. Although most cases needing diuretic therapy are embarrassed by an excess of fluid, there are occasions when diuretics must be used in patients with a reduced blood volume. In these cases water must be provided to maintain the diuresis.

OSMOTIC DIURETICS

Substances which are not absorbed by the renal tubules—or substances which are absorbed but whose concentration has exceeded the 'tubular maximum' for reabsorption—prevent by their osmotic effect the reabsorption of water. The diuresis thus produced is proportional to the concentration of non-absorbable material in the tubules. Osmotic diuresis occurs naturally in diabetes mellitus (p. 719). In this condition the blood glucose reaches high concentrations, the tubular maximum is exceeded and the resulting excretion of glucose necessitates the excretion of an osmotically equivalent volume of water. Thus the more severe the diabetes, the greater the diuresis and the more intense the attendant thirst.

An osmotic diuresis can be produced artificially by the administration of a foreign substance (which is not therefore absorbed by the tubules) or of a normal constituent of the plasma such as urea whose tubular reabsorption is of limited extent. A very large number of substances has been used for this purpose but no point would be served in

listing them since they have little or no place in modern medicine. The one survivor is mannitol but a newcomer is isosorbide.

Mannitol is not utilized by the body and all of an administered dose is filtered into the tubules from which none is reabsorbed. It is given intravenously in a 25 per cent solution. The total daily dose may have to reach 100 grams. Since mannitol has to be given by intravenous infusion, it is only really suitable for the treatment of hospitalized patients. It finds some use in cases of depressed kidney function associated with low plasma volumes, such as may occur after severe trauma or extensive surgery. In these patients the accumulation of toxic metabolites in the kidney threatens tubular function. The use of an osmotic diuretic dilutes the contents of the proximal tubules and promotes diuresis so that the danger to the kidney is reduced. An incidental advantage of mannitol treatment is that the infusion helps to provide the fluid needed to keep up the diuresis.

Although its effect on osmotic pressure is the principal source of the diuresis induced by mannitol, a number of other actions are probably involved. Thus, mannitol dilates the afferent glomerular arterioles and so increases filtration pressure and it may also reduce the sensitivity of the mechanisms that evoke renin release and hence the retention of sodium (p. 358).

Isosorbide is readily absorbed from the intestine but not from the renal tubules so that it can, when appropriate, be taken by mouth. By this route it has recently been employed for the reduction of intraocular and cerebrospinal pressures. In other circumstances, the advantages of the alternative route or the condition of the patient may dictate intravenous administration. The formula of isosorbide is provided on p. 700 where the drug is discussed in another context.

In the past, urea had a period of popularity as an orally effective osmotic diuretic but its foul taste militated against its continued use.

DIGITALIS ALKALOIDS

It is well known that the discovery of the cardiotonic action of this substance came from the old observation that foxglove cured the 'dropsy' (p. 691). In cardiac oedema an improvement in the cardiac output will increase circulation through the kidney so that glomerular filtration will increase. Thus in this condition digoxin (the most widely used cardiac glycoside) does behave as a diuretic agent, since it causes an augmentation of urine output. It has little diuretic action in patients whose cardiac performance is adequate.

Digoxin is not, of course, given primarily to relieve cardiac oedema but some diuresis is an inevitable consequence of successful digitalization in patients with cardiac failure. Because cardiac oedema is not entirely the result of a reduced cardiac output, the administration of diuretics proper is necessary for the complete relief of oedema even when digoxin is also given.

Recent work has indicated that the digitalis glycosides may also promote the tubular secretion of sodium and potassium. Although this action would obviously contribute to the drugs' overall diuretic effect it cannot be regarded as being of more than trivial importance and it certainly does not imply that the glycosides can have any place in the treatment of any form of oedema that is not of cardiac origin or that they could reasonably be classified as saluretic substances.

XANTHINES AND RELATED COMPOUNDS

It has been common knowledge for centuries that tea, coffee and cocoa cause diuresis. At the turn of the present century it was found that all these popular beverages contain caffeine and that tea and cocoa also have a complement of theophylline and theobromine respectively. All three substances inhibit phosphodiesterase so that (for reasons that are set out on p. 321) they potentiate the action of adrenaline on its β receptors and consequently have central nervous stimulant, bronchodilator and cardiotonic effects. Caffeine has the most powerful central actions but in other respects theophylline is the most potent of the three xanthine derivatives. It is used principally in the form of aminophylline (theophylline ethylene diamine) a drug that still has a place in the treatment of asthma and congestive heart failure.

It is an old observation that caffeine increases the number of active glomeruli in frogs but it is known that this diuretic mechanism cannot operate in mammals and the diuretic action of the xanthine derivatives finds its most ready explanation in the drugs' cardiotonic action. Nevertheless they have some ability to reduce the tubular reabsorption of sodium and chloride so that (as most of us know to our inconvenience) they exert some diuretic action even in those whose cardiac function is unimpaired.

So far as its employment as a diuretic agent per se is concerned theophylline has been used largely, as we shall see, in combination with the organomercurial agents but it

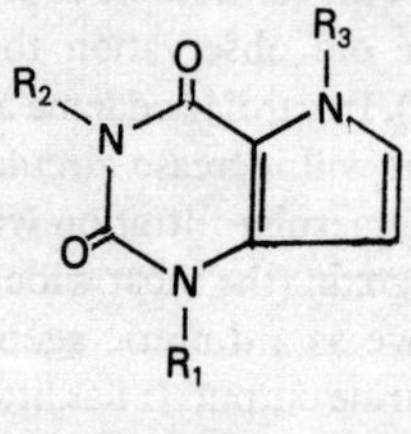

	R_1	R_2	R_3
Xanthine	H	H	H
Caffeine	CH_3	CH_3	CH_3
Theophylline	CH_3	CH_3	H
Theobromine	CH_3	H	CH_3

Fig. 36.4 Xanthine and some derivatives.

has also been employed as an adjunct to other forms of diuretic therapy, particularly in patients with cardiac oedema who are not responding well to the single diuretic. For this latter purpose, it is usual to give the theophylline intravenously at the time when the other diuretic should have been exerting its maximal effect. It is thereby possible to synchronize the actions of the two drugs. In this situation the cardiac action of theophylline undoubtedly contributes to the establishment of the diuresis.

Many hundreds of xanthine derivatives have been synthesized during the past fifty years in the hope of finding one more active than theophylline. None has been found, but one compound, Xanturil, found temporary favour in France.

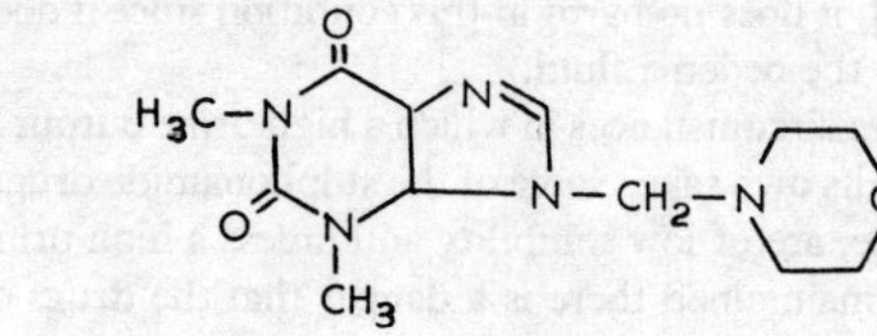

Xanturil

Pyrimidines are essential intermediates in the synthesis of the xanthines and it was natural to enquire whether the pyrimidines themselves had diuretic properties. Some had; from them were developed aminometradine (Mictine) and amisometradine (Rolicton). These compounds are effective when taken orally and they are more active than theophylline but they have never achieved more than a fleeting popularity.

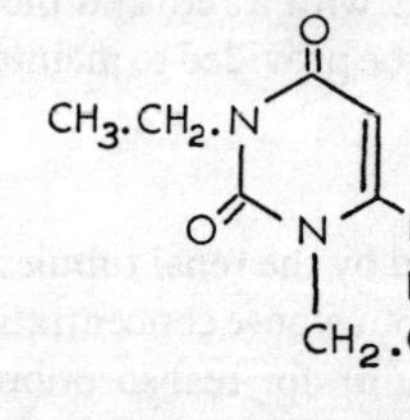

Aminometradine 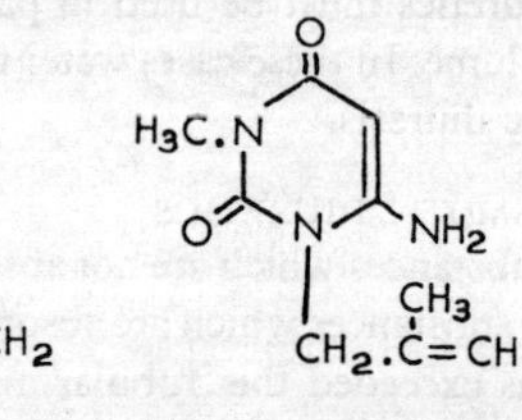   Amisometradine

In 1944, Lipschitz and Hadidian pointed out that a feature common to the xanthine derivatives and to some other substances with diuretic activity was the possession of the $=N.C.N.=$ grouping. They tested a large number of other compounds containing this group and they found that several behaved as diuretics. One such compound was formoguanamine and this observation led eventually to the synthesis by others of the triazines, amanozine and chlorazanil. Chlorazanil (Orpidan) has been used clinically, alone or in combination with other drugs, in the treatment of hypertension but inconvenient side effects have prevented its general acceptance into a therapeutic field that already carries a superfluity of useful agents.

Chlorazanil

Formoguanamine

Amanozine

Diuretic agents and sodium excretion

We can now turn to a consideration of those drugs that bring about diuresis as a result of their being able to promote the excretion of sodium and other ions. These, the saluretic agents, include (for reasons that have already been made plain) most of the diuretic drugs used in clinical practice.

Sodium is absorbed from several regions of the kidney tubule and recent advances in experimental techniques and analysis have made it clear that saluretics differ among themselves in the extent to which they influence the absorption processes at these several sites. A knowledge of the loci of action of diuretics is as important to the clinician as it is essential to the pharmacologist because it enables us to allocate each agent to one of a small number of categories. The members of a particular group resemble one another in respect of the extent of the diuresis and the pattern of electrolyte excretion they produce, their clinical usefulness and many of their side effects.

Sites of action of diuretic substances

Figure 36.5 is a schematic diagram of a single nephron that indicates the sites of sodium reabsorption. One consequence of the operation of the counter current exchange and multiplyer systems (p. 619) is the fact that the osmotic pressure of the extracellular fluid that surrounds the kidney tubules (and blood vessels) increases progressively from cortex to medulla. This is indicated on the diagram by the changing separation of the horizontal lines.

Site 1: Glomerular filtrate is delivered to the proximal convoluted tubule where about two thirds of the 'filtered load' of sodium is absorbed. This absorption is an active process but it necessarily involves the passive transfer of an equal number of anions (chiefly chloride and bicarbonate) and it induces, by osmosis, the passive absorption of an osmotically equivalent volume of water. Thus both the fluid left in the tubules and that transferred into the interstitial fluid and thence into the blood remain isotonic with plasma. About three quarters of the sodium that is reabsorbed is accompanied by chloride while the rest is exchanged for hydrogen ions by a process that involves the reabsorption of bicarbonate that has been previously secreted into the tubule. This sodium-hydrogen exchange, which is sustained by carbonic anhydrase, forms part of the organism's base conservation mechanism and as such it is described elsewhere (p. 620). In the discussions that follow we shall designate as site 1*a* and 1*b* processes the

absorption mechanisms that are, respectively, dependent on and independent of carbonic anhydrase.

Sodium and water absorption from the proximal tubule is reduced if the plasma and extracellular fluid volumes are increased. Although this is largely attributable to the operation of purely physical factors such as changes in osmotic pressure, there is some evidence for the existence of a *natriuretic hormone* which is released, perhaps from the brain, in response to the stimulus of volume expansion. It seems likely that the postulated hormone operates at more distal sites in addition to its presumed locus in the proximal convoluted tubule.

The glomerular filtrate that is not absorbed in the proximal convoluted tubule is delivered to the descending limb of the loop of Henle. Sodium is not absorbed along this length of the nephron. Some, indeed, passes passively *into* the tubular fluid and there is also a passive outflow of water. As a result, the osmotic pressure of the tubule's contents by the time they reach the loop is as high as that of the interstitial fluid in this region (Fig. 36.5). The novice reader who might be puzzled by what might appear to be the return to the tubular fluid of material that has just been absorbed from it should remember that, because of the narrowness of the tube, the total *amount* of sodium (and water) that is transferred is quite small.

Sites II and III: About 25 per cent of the total filtered load of sodium is absorbed as it moves along the thick portion of the ascending limb of Henle's loop. This stretch of the tubule is quite impermeable to water so that the tubule fluid becomes diluted again as it ascends the limb. Nevertheless, the events in this segment of the nephron constitute the mechanism by which urine is concentrated. This is because the loss of sodium to the interstitial fluid causes an increase in osmotic pressure and hence a transfer of water from the urine in the collecting ducts. This final concentrating process can only occur if the walls of the collecting ducts are freely permeable to water, a condition that will be met if antidiuretic hormone is available.

As the tubular fluid approaches the renal cortex it reaches a point where it again becomes isotonic with plasma. Further absorption of sodium in the remainder of the ascending limb and the early reaches of the distal convoluted tubule leads to hypotonicity of the urine. Because the surrounding extracellular fluid remains isotonic with plasma, this movement of sodium ions (unlike that from the more proximal portion of the tubule) plays no part in the urine concentrating process: it is indeed the

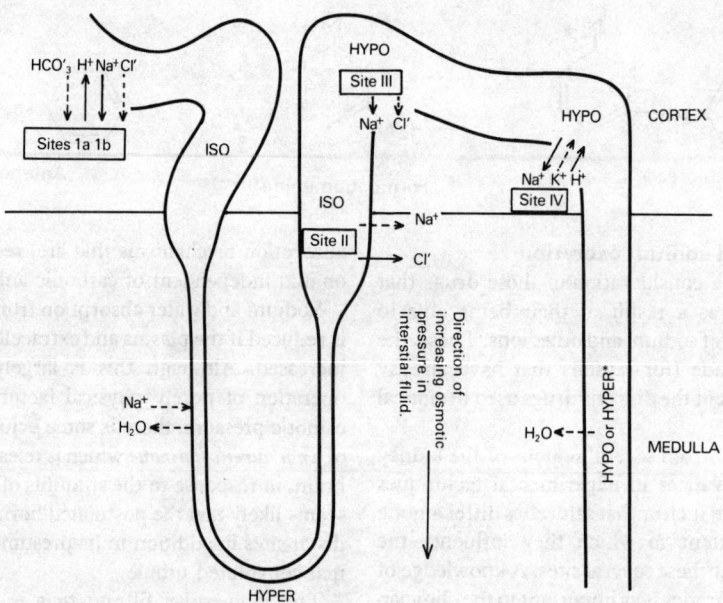

*Depending on the level of antidiuretic hormone activity
The extracellular and tubular fluids may be isotonic (ISO), hypertonic (HYPER) or hypotonic (HYPO)

Fig. 36.5 Schematic diagram to indicate the sites of sodium absorption in the nephron (*for details see text*).

urine diluting site. The reader should remember that the normal kidney is called upon to produce both highly concentrated and very dilute urines according to the circumstances so that concentrating and diluting mechanisms are equally important.

As we shall see, sodium absorption in the medullary portion of the ascending limb seems to be a passive response to an active absorption of chloride (Rocha and Kokko, 1973) but in the distal convoluted tubule, sodium itself is actively reabsorbed, chloride following passively.

The concentrating and diluting segments are designated sites II and III respectively. Agents that have their locus of action at either site will promote the excretion of both sodium and chloride.

Site IV: We have now reached the most distal part of the tubule and the cortical portion of the collecting tubule where the last phase of sodium reabsorption (which accounts for about 5 per cent of the original filtered load) takes place. Most of the sodium is taken up by an active mechanism that depends on aldosterone (an adrenocortical hormone, p. 753) and it is linked with the secretion into the tubule of potassium and hydrogen ions. Thus if sodium absorption at this site is prevented the secretion of potassium will cease and there will be conservation of the body's supplies of this ion. It is convenient to divide site IV activity into that dependent on aldosterone (IVa) and that which does not demand the presence of the hormone (IVb).

Diuretic agents that inhibit tubular activity at sites, I, II or III will increase the concentration of sodium in the fluid

that bathes site IV. The rate of sodium absorption here will, consequently, be somewhat increased so that the sodium-potassium exchange will be more brisk and the amount of potassium in the urine will increase. This explains why all saluretics except those that operate at site IV lead to the increased excretion of both sodium and potassium.

Site IV diuretic activity will also, of course, be associated with a reduced rate of hydrogen ion secretion into the distal tubule. There will, consequently, be a smaller demand for bicarbonate ions (Fig. 36.2), the excretion of which will therefore show a slight rise. This is a much smaller effect than that produced by drugs such as acetazolamide and the benzothiadiazines that interfere with the activity of carbonic anhydrase.

Determination of the sites of action of diuretic agents
If site I mechanisms are inhibited, there will be a considerable increase in the volume of glomerular filtrate that is delivered to the rest of the tubule. In the absence of antidiuretic hormone, this will result in a corresponding increase in urine production. Site I diuretics will, therefore, promote an additional urine flow in a water loaded subject. Phosphate is absorbed at site I and the appearance of phosphate in the urine may signify the operation of a site I diuretic.

Diuretic drugs whose locus of action is site II will obviously impair renal concentrating activity but they will also reduce the effectiveness of the diluting mechanism too because of the unmanageable load of sodium that is delivered to the diluting segments. Site III diuretics, on the other hand, interfere only with the kidney's diluting mechanisms.

Drugs that cause diuresis by an action at site IV will lead to the production of urine whose potassium concentration is low in relation to that of sodium.

Many diuretic agents exert an action at more than one of the absorption sites. To determine which, requires a rather more complicated experimental analysis than that presented here.

Individual saluretic agents

It is convenient to group these drugs into those that bring about, respectively, a marked, a moderate or a mild diuresis. This classification is adopted in Table 36.1. which lists the more important diuretics, indicates their likely sites of action and summarizes their effects on electrolyte excretion patterns.

DRUGS THAT PRODUCE A MARKED DIURESIS
Single doses of the agents in this category induce an excretion of 20 to 25 per cent of the filtered load of sodium. Apart from the organomercurial compounds (which have a more extensive locus of action), these drugs act principally at site II in the ascending limb of the loop of Henle and for this reason they are often designated as *loop diuretics*. An alternative description is *high ceiling diuretics*.

Organomercurial compounds

Until quite recently the most powerful of the available diuretics were the organomercurial compounds and textbooks of pharmacology provided long lists of those in common use: the previous edition of this book logged eleven of them. They are now obsolescent but it would be unwise to disregard them completely, partly because some of them are still occasionally used, partly because they were in a real sense the antecedents of the present generation of high ceiling diuretics and partly because a knowledge of their mode of action can contribute to a better appreciation of the pharmacology of diuresis in general.

The diuretic action of mercurous chloride was discovered in the sixteenth century but the modern use of organic compounds of mercury arose from clinical observations in the early days of chemotherapy. Ehrlich achieved great success in the treatment of sleeping sickness and syphilis with organic compounds of arsenic and this stimulated research into the chemotherapeutic potential of other types of organometallic compounds. Mercury compounds were found to be particularly active and as soon as relatively non-toxic ones were synthesized they were applied to the treatment of syphilis. It was not known that the drugs also had diuretic activity (the earlier use of mercurous chloride had been forgotten) until 1919, when an observant medical student noticed an association between diuresis and mercury treatment in syphilitic

Table 36.1 Sites of action of saluretic agents

| Agent | Effect on sodium absorption sites | | | | | | Effect on electrolyte excretion | | | |
	Ia	Ib	II	III	IVa	IVb	Na⁺	K⁺	Cl⁻	HCO₃⁻
Drugs that produce a marked diuresis										
Organomercurial compounds	S	P	S	S			↑	↓	↑	→
'Loop diuretics'										
Ethacrynic acid		P	S				↑	↑	↑	→
Frusemide	S	P	S				↑	↑	↑	→
Bumetanide	S	P	S				↑	↑	↑	→
Drugs that produce a moderate diuresis										
Carbonic anhydrase inhibitors	P						↑	↑	→	↑
Benzothiadiazines	S			P			↑	↑	↑	↑
Drugs that produce a mild diuresis										
Potassium-sparing diuretics										
Aldosterone antagonists						P	↑	↓	→	→
Triamterene						P	↑	↓	→	→
Amiloride	S			S		P	↑	↓	↑	↑
Acidifying salts	Increase chloride load at absorption sites						↑	↑	↑	→

Notes: a. P and S refer to the principal and subsidiary sites of action respectively. They explain the patterns of electrolyte excretion. Many diuretic agents have some slight degree of activity at sites other than those indicated.

b. ↑., ↓ and → indicate, respectively, an increase, a decrease or no change in urinary electrolyte excretion. They have qualitative significance only.

Table 36.2 Some organomercurial diuretic agents

$$R - CH_2 - CH - CH_2.Hg^+ R_2$$
$$| \atop OR_1$$

Official name	Proprietary name	R	R_1	R_2
Mersalyl	Salyrgan	[benzene ring with O.CH$_2$.COONa and CONH—]	CH_3	Theophylline
Mercurophyllin	Novurit	[ring structure with CH_3 CH_3, H_3C, NaOOC, CONH—]	CH_3	Theophylline
Mercaptomerin	Thiomerin	— As for mercurophyllin —		$- S.CH_2.COOH$

patients. Thereafter a very large number of organomercurial compounds was examined for diuretic activity and several of them dominated the diuretic field for a quarter of a century and more. Mersalyl, the oldest of them all, is also the principal survivor in the clinic; in the laboratory it is joined by some other survivors, particularly mercaptomerin and chloromerodrin for studies of drug effects on transport processes across cell membranes.

When used clinically, the mercurial diuretics (apart from chloromerodrin which is active by mouth) are given by deep intramuscular injection in doses that will provide 20 to 80 mg of mercury daily. The substituent R_2 (Table 36.2) increases the rate of absorption of the drug and reduces the local irritation produced by the injection.

These mercurial compounds undergo a high degree of binding to plasma proteins and so cannot pass to any appreciable extent into the glomerular filtrate. They are actively secreted by the tubules and the most powerful diuretic agents are those that are eliminated most rapidly by this route. There is now general agreement that the organomercurial drugs combine with the sulphydryl (-SH) groups, and so impair the activity, of enzymes concerned in the regulation of tubular absorption processes. Dimercaprol, which contains sulphydryl groups, might be expected to restore enzyme activity and it certainly prevents mercurial diuresis or arrests it if it is already under way. Controversy still surrounds the question as to which enzyme system succumbs to the mercury diuretics. Candidates include sodium-potassium activated ATPase (p. 44) and the enzyme systems that promote glycolysis or the formation of cyclic AMP (p. 321).

The principal site of action of the organomercury compounds is the thick portion of the ascending limb of the loop of Henle (site II). The drugs bring about the excretion of large quantities of chloride and rather less sodium and it was this observation that provided the original basis for the view that loop diuretics operate by inhibiting the reabsorption of chloride. Recent experiments with isolated perfused nephrons have provided solid support for this view by demonstrating that chloride is indeed actively transported across the tubule wall at site II and that this transport system is impeded by the organomercury diuretic agents (Burg and Green, 1973).

Since the organomercurial compounds combine with a chemical grouping that is common to many enzymes it is not surprising that they influence activity at several loci in the nephron in addition to that at their presumed primary site of action. They partially inhibit the reabsorption of glucose but have no effect on the excretion of bicarbonate. This argues for an action at site Ia. In addition, they exert a distinct potassium sparing action, a fact that indicates inhibition of sodium-potassium exchange in the distal tubules (site IVa).

The mercurial diuretics are more active during acidosis, and if a patient ceases to respond to a mercury compound, or if he is unresponsive from the beginning of treatment, diuresis can often be restored or established by the administration of an acidifying diuretic such as ammonium chloride. The diuresis thus produced is much greater than that which would be produced by the ammonium chloride acting alone. The basis of this synergistic action of ammonium chloride is not clear: it is not due to its acidifying effect *per se* since the diuretic action of the mercurials is not affected if acidosis is produced by carbon dioxide inhalation. It may be that ammonium chloride replenishes the supply of chloride ions so that more are available to be excreted. Against this is the fact that ammonium nitrate is as effective as ammonium chloride (although it may be that nitrate can substitute for chloride) and that the action of mercurial diuretics is not inhibited by all conditions that cause a reduction in plasma chloride.

Another problem concerns the form in which the mercurials exert their action in the kidney. Some authorities believe that all the active organomercurial compounds liberate mercuric ions (Mudge and Weiner, 1958). Others point to the fact that the diuretic activity of the mercurial diuretics depends on their possessing a distinct type of structure (Kessler, Lozano and Pitts, 1957). It is certainly true that only very small amounts of the mercury compound are excreted in the inorganic form but it is not unreasonable to assume that a minute quantity of an ion as toxic as mercury is all that will be required to inhibit enzyme activity. The fact that diuretic activity is linked to a distinctive organic structure may simply imply that the structure is required to ensure the transport of the mercury to its particular site of action (Heller and Ginsburg, 1961).

Ethacrynic acid

When it became clear that the action of the mercury-containing diuretics was probably attributable to their being able to combine with the sulphydryl groups of tubule enzymes, attention became focussed on the possibility of finding powerful but nontoxic diuretic agents among compounds deliberately synthesized as sulphydryl group binders. Ethacrynic acid, which was first used in 1963, was found in this way: unsaturated ketones combine with sulphydryl groups and the aryloxyacetic acid structure ensure that the compound will be concentrated in the kidney.

Ethacrynic acid

There can be little doubt that ethacrynic acid and the organomercury compounds share the same major site of action in the nephron. Indeed, they occupy the same receptors, as is demonstrated in experiments that disclose their mutual competition and by the fact that ethacrynic acid interferes with the tubular excretion of mercury compounds (Nigrovic, Koechel & Cafruny, 1973). Ethacrynic acid does not, however, influence activity at other absorption sites to the extent that is exercised by the organomercury agents. Thus the diuresis it brings about is associated with an increased loss of potassium in the urine and we can conclude that ethacrynic acid does not interfere with sodium-potassium exchange in the distal tubule. Its more localized action justifies its classification as a loop diuretic.

Ethacrynic acid has some effects that are not related to its interacting with sodium absorption mechanisms. It influences blood flow through the kidney, diverting blood to the outer part of the cortex and it is possible that it also antagonizes the antidiuretic action of vasopressin. These actions will clearly augment the drug's diuretic activity. It is important to be aware of the possibility that some diuretic agents may possess these (or other) additional properties that go some way to explaining why substances that have apparently identical actions on the sodium absorption mechanisms nevertheless have different effects on the composition and volume of the urine that is finally voided.

Ethacrynic acid is bound to plasma protein to a considerable extent so that only a little appears in the glomerular filtrate. The rest is secreted into the proximal convoluted tubule.

Ethacrynic acid is an extremely powerful diuretic and clinical reports have mentioned the excretion of up to eight or nine litres of urine in the twenty-four hours following a single dose of the drug. The loss of sodium is correspondingly dramatic and, if given injudiciously, ethacrynic acid may cause a serious dehydration. On the other hand, in emergencies it can produce a very rapid decrease in the volume of oedema fluid in patients who do not respond to the thiazides or the organomercurial diuretics.

Ethacrynic acid is not without toxic side effects including hypotension, gastrointestinal upsets and hyperuricaemia (p. 457). It should, perhaps, still be regarded as a diuretic to be tried when other drugs have failed.

Ethacrynic acid is active by mouth: the daily dose range is 20 to 200 mg.

Frusemide (furosemide)

Although it has only been available for a few years, frusemide (Lasix, Dryptal, Frusid) is now one of the most widely used members of the group of potent diuretics. Like the thiazide diuretics (which are discussed below, p. 631), frusemide carries an unsubstituted sulphonamido group but this common structural feature does not confer common properties.

Frusemide (furosemide, Lasix)

Frusemide shares with the other potent diuretic agents the power of inhibiting chloride transport (and hence that of sodium) across the wall of the thick part of the ascending limb of the loop of Henle: it is, in other words, primarily a loop diuretic. Unlike ethacrynic acid, however, it also induces a loss of bicarbonate because of its not unexpected ability partially to inhibit carbonic anhydrase activity

(Puschett and Goldberg, 1968). Frusemide shares with ethacrynic acid the ability to shunt blood into the glomerular regions of the kidney.

Frusemide is bound to plasma protein but it is readily excreted into the kidney tubules. Its action is rapid and urine losses of up to six litres have been recorded in the two hours following an oral dose of the drug. It is almost completely cleared from the body (most of it in an unchanged form) within a further two hours.

The diuresis following the administration of frusemide is so profuse that, as with ethacrynic acid, some care has to be observed in its use if cardiovascular collapse is to be avoided. The oral and intravenous doses are 100 to 200 mg (or more) and 25 to 50 mg respectively.

The use of frusemide in modest doses is rarely attended by serious side effects. Most of those that are seen—hypokalaemia, hypotension, hyperuricaemia and disturbances of carbohydrate metabolism—are just as likely to arise in the course of treatment with the benzothiadiazines (p. 635) which are much less powerful diuretics. An untoward response that is rather more characteristic of frusemide (although it has also been reported among patients taking ethacrynic acid) is deafness caused by damage to the acoustic division of the auditory nerve (*ototoxicity*). It occurs occasionally in patients with renal insufficiency who have been given high doses of frusemide by intravenous infusion.

An interesting reaction to the *withdrawal* of frusemide has recently been reported in women treated with the drug for idopathic oedema (p. 622). As soon as treatment ceased a 'rebound' oedema developed. More severe than that for which the drug was originally prescribed, this secondary oedema cleared spontaneously within a few days. It appears that the vigorous diuresis induced by frusemide prompted the activation of compensatory sodium retention mechanisms (presumably those operated by the renin-angiotensin system) which ran on for a few days after the diuretic agent was withdrawn. During this period they could exert their action unopposed (MacGregor, Tasker and de Wardener, 1975). The patient who wished not to suffer the withdrawal oedema would have no choice but to continue taking frusemide indefinitely: she would indeed be as dependent on her drug as the alcohol or opiate addict who fears the consequences of abstinence. Not only is the situation similar, but the postulated mechanism—a delay in the reversal of compensatory changes—is strongly reminiscent of at least some of those that have been put forward to explain withdrawal phenomena in those dependent on the more familiar drugs of 'addiction' (p. 94).

The number of cases of withdrawal oedema so far reported is small. There seems to be no reason why it should not develop in response to other powerful diuretic agents administered to patients whose oedema is not associated with excessive sodium retention.

Since idiopathic oedema usually disappears spontaneously there would seem to be no good reason for treating it with diuretic drugs.

Bumetanide

Bumetanide (Burinex) is one of the latest arrivals on the diuretic scene. It resembles frusemide in structure, actions and uses.

Like ethacrynic acid and frusemide, bumetanide is bound to plasma proteins (though to a rather smaller extent than are the other two compounds) and in most animal species it is rapidly excreted into the tubules in an unchanged form. In the rat, however, the drug undergoes a metabolic transformation that prevents its being an effective diuretic agent.

Up to 30 per cent of an oral dose of bumetanide is lost in the faeces and through other extrarenal channels.

Bumetanide

Bumetanide is primarily a loop diuretic but it also hinders absorption processes in the proximal convoluted tubule (site Ib). It has no influence on site Ia processes so that its effect on the pattern of electrolyte excretion resembles that of ethacrynic acid rather than frusemide.

An oral dose of 1 mg of bumetanide is equivalent to about 60 mg of frusemide but the maximum diuresis it can produce (13 to 25 per cent of the filtered load) is no greater than that achieved by frusemide. The effect of a single dose, which reaches its peak 60 to 90 min after oral and 15 to 45 min after intravenous administration, is spent within six hours. The response to an oral dose is so rapid that no useful purpose is served by giving the drug intravenously unless there are obvious contraindications—unconsciousness, local conditions in the gastrointestinal tract, etc.—to the oral route.

The continued administration of bumetanide sometimes adversely influences carbohydrate metabolism in diabetic subjects. This complication is rather less likely to occur with frusemide. On the other hand, early reports suggest that even large doses of bumetanide produce only small degrees of hyperuricaemia.

The usual oral dose of bumetanide is 1 to 4 mg.

DRUGS THAT PRODUCE A MODERATE DIURESIS

Single doses of the diuretic agents in this category induce an excretion of 5 to 10 per cent of the filtered load of sodium. The oldest members of the group are the carbonic anhydrase inhibitors. Their success led directly to the development of the now very popular benzothiadiazines ('the thiazide diuretics') and to their own almost total eclipse.

Carbonic anhydrase inhibitors

We saw earlier in this chapter that the exchanges of sodium for hydrogen ions in the renal tubules provides an important base conservation mechanism. The sodium is derived from sodium bicarbonate and the hydrogen ions come from carbonic acid formed in the cells of the tubule under the influence of carbonic anhydrase. If this enzyme is inhibited the sodium-hydrogen exchange is no longer possible and large amounts of sodium and bicarbonate ions and an osmotically equivalent quantity of water are excreted. Thus inhibitors of carbonic anhydrase are diuretics. They also cause an increased excretion of potassium as well as of sodium: in the normal kidney, potassium and hydrogen ions compete with one another in the sodium exchange and when the availability of hydrogen ions is reduced, there is a correspondingly greater transfer of potassium from the tubule cell into the lumen.

Although it is easy to explain the action of carbonic anhydrase inhibitors, their use as diuretic agents was not prompted by these considerations but by the accidental observation in the early days of chemotherapy that patients undergoing treatment with the sulphonamides developed a metabolic acidosis with diuresis. As soon as it was appreciated that this was due to inhibition of carbonic anhydrase, a search was instituted for more powerful inhibitors. Some were found and were used as diuretic agents: the best known are acetazolamide (Diamox), dichlorphenamide (Daranide, Oratrol) and ethoxzolamide (Cardrase). It will be seen that all the compounds contain an unsubstituted sulphonamido ($-SO_2NH_2$) group, a feature which seems to be essential for enzyme inhibitory activity and which we have already met in diuretic agents whose mode of action is quite different from that of the carbonic anhydrase inhibitors.

The metabolic acidosis that occurs as a result of administration of carbonic anhydrase inhibitors is caused by the loss of bicarbonate. As the supply of bicarbonate in the tubules (which itself depends on the activity of carbonic anhydrase) becomes depleted, the diuretic action of carbonic anhydrase inhibitors ceases. This occurs after about twenty-four hours of diuresis and it seriously limits the usefulness of these diuretics for the treatment of oedema or hypertension, particularly as the diuresis, even at its height, is never voluminous. They do, however, still have a limited use in conditions in which a large diuresis is not required, especially if they can be given intermittently so that the bicarbonate supplies can be restored between doses. Such conditions include premenstrual oedema, glaucoma and petit mal epilepsy. Acetazolamide is given by mouth in doses of 250 to 500 mg: the daily dose may reach two grams. Dichlorphenamide is more potent, effective doses being of the order of 25 to 100 mg. This last named drug causes the excretion of more chloride and less bicarbonate than does acetazolamide. Consequently, a longer period elapses before its diuretic effectiveness wanes.

Because of the self-limiting action of the carbonic anhydrase inhibitors, attempts were made to develop compounds of similar structure with a more prolonged action. This led to the discovery of the thiazide diuretics that form the subject of the next section.

The benzothiadiazines and related compounds

We have seen that this most valuable group of compounds was developed during the search for more useful carbonic anhydrase inhibitors and they (or their metabolites) all contain the free sulphonamido group which characterizes the enzyme inhibitors. Nevertheless, the diuretic action of the thiazides is not due primarily to their ability to inhibit carbonic anhydrase. In general, they are relatively weak inhibitors of the enzyme.

The first thiazide diuretic was chlorothiazide. It was discovered by Sprague in 1958. Shortly afterwards, de Stevens and his colleagues (1958) synthesized hydrochlorothiazide, a more powerful diuretic but a less effective inhibitor of carbonic anhydrase. The two drugs soon proved their value and a very large number of related compounds has become available in recent years. This proliferation is a response to commercial rather than therapeutic pressures and all the benzothiadiazines exhibit

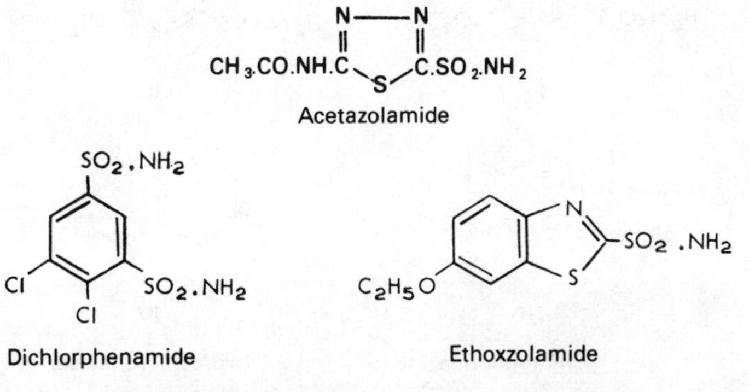

Acetazolamide

Dichlorphenamide

Ethoxzolamide

Fig. 36.6 Some carbonic anhydrase inhibitors.

essentially the same spectrum of properties and enjoy the same range of clinical applications. They all carry a 3-sulphamoyl-4-halogenated benzene ring (see Table 36.3) and all have an identical mode and site of action. Analysis of their effects on water and electrolyte excretion indicates that their principal locus of action is in the diluting segment of the loop of Henle (our site III). This identity of action is underlined by the fact that a patient who is found to be resistant to one benzothiadiazine will almost certainly prove to be equally resistant to them all. The one way in which the several benzothiadiazines differ from one another is that some of the newer compounds have a more prolonged duration of action than have the older members of the group. These differences in duration of action are probably attributable to differences in their lipid and water solubilities. Those with a brief duration of action are not very soluble in lipids so that they are distributed largely in the extracellular fluid whence they can be rapidly cleared. The longer acting members of the group have a high lipid solubility and are taken up into both the extracellular and intracellular fluids. In addition they may be absorbed by the tubule cells. This recycling effect will help to prolong their action still further.

The benzothiadiazines are classified chemically in Table 36.3 which also displays formulae and effective doses and indicates the drugs' duration of action. It should not be necessary to add that Table 36.3 is intended only for reference purposes. The toiling student should encourage himself with the thought that to know one benzothiadiazine is to know them all. Specific mention should, however, be made of one particular compound. As is indicated by both its name and its chemical structure, mefruside is related to frusemide but it is properly included among the benzothiadiazines. Frusemide itself, of course, carries the 3-sulphamoyl-4-halogenated benzene ring but its other structural features confer properties that lift it from the class of moderately potent to that of the very powerful diuretic agents.

The derivation of the thiazides and chlorothiazides from the sulphonamides via active carbonic anhydrase inhibitors can be understood by reference to Figure 36.7. Compound I (5-chloro-2,4-disulphamylaniline) is a benzene disulphonamide clearly similar to dichlorphenamide. It is itself, as would be expected, a carbonic anhydrase inhibitor though some of its properties foreshadow those of the thiazides. When this compound is treated with formaldehyde compound III (chlorothiazide) is produced, presumably by way of compound II which, we must assume, enjoys only a transitory existence. Thus the thiazide has been formed from the sulphonamide by simple ring closure. Hydrochlorothiazide is chlorothiazide in which the diazine ring is saturated and a similar relationship exists between other thiazides and the corresponding hydrothiazides. It will be appreciated, by reference to Table 36.3 that the hydrothiazides are all more active than the thiazides.

That the thiazide diuretics do not operate through the medium of carbonic anhydrase inhibition is indicated by the effect they have on excretion patterns (Table 36.1). At low dose levels they cause increased excretion of sodium and chloride and only when the dose is increased is the urinary output of bicarbonate augmented. This stands in marked contrast to the effects produced by the carbonic anhydrase inhibitors.

An unexpected property of the thiazide and hydrothiazide diuretics is that, like some of their successors, they produce an *antidiuresis* in patients with diabetes insipidus. The reason for this is not completely known. The thiazides do slightly depress glomerular filtration rate as a result of their vasodilator action on the renal vessels. This does not normally do more than slightly offset their diuretic action but its effect would clearly be more evident in diabetes insipidus when the reabsorption of water is completely inhibited and urine output is determined entirely by the glomerular filtration rate. Another possible reason is that sodium depletion renders the thirst of diabetes insipidus

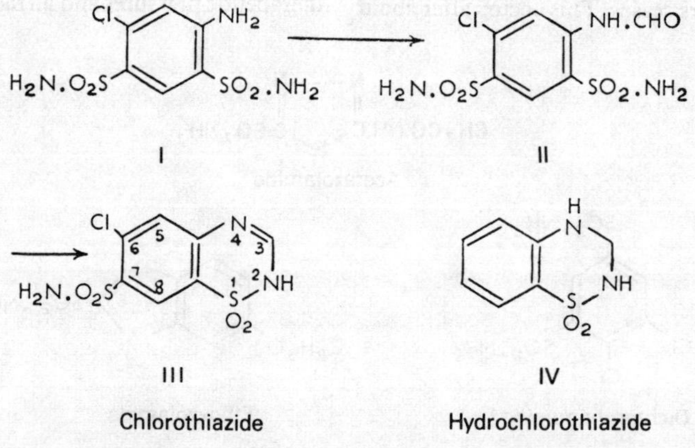

Fig. 36.7 Origin of chlorothiazide from a carbonic anhydrase inhibitor.

Table 36.3 Benzothiadiazine diuretic agents

THIAZIDES

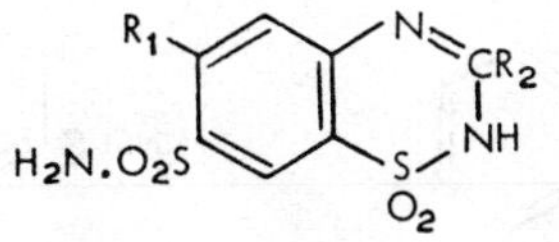

Approved name	Proprietary name(s)	R_1	R_2	Approx daily dose mg	Duration of action hr
Chlorothiazide	Saluric; Diuril; Chlotride;	Cl	H	1000	10-12 (major action 4-6)
Flumethiazide	Ademol	CF_3	H	1000	10-12 (major action 4-6)
Benzthiazide	Fovane;	Cl	$CH_2.S.CH_2-$	100	10-12 (major action 4-6)

HYDROTHIAZIDES

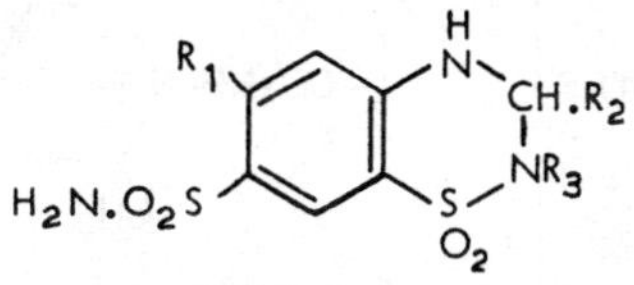

Approved name(s)	Proprietary name(s)	R_1	R_2	R_3	Approx daily dose mg	Duration of action hr
Hydrochlorothiazide	Esidrex; Esidrix; HydroSaluric; HydroDiuril	Cl	H	H	50-100	10-12 (major action 4-6)
Hydroflumethiazide	NaClex; Hydrenox; Saluron	CF_3	H	H	50-100	10-12 (major action 4-6)
Hydrobentizide		Cl	$CH_2.S.CH_2-$	H	10-100.	10-12 (major action 4-6)
Benzhydroflumethiazide / Bendrofluazide	Aprinox; Berkozide; Centyl; Neo-NaClex; Naturetin	CF_3	CH_2-	H	2.5-5.0	at least 24
Cyclopenthiazide	Navidrex	Cl	CH_2-	H	1-3	at least 24
Trichlormethiazide	Naqua; Metahydrin	Cl	$-CHCl_2$	H	5-12	at least 24
Polythiazide	Nephril Renese	Cl	$-CH_2.S.CH_2.CF_3$	CH_2	1-5	at least 24
Methyclothiazide	Enduron	Cl	CH_2Cl	CH_2	5-10	at least 24

QUINAZOLINONES

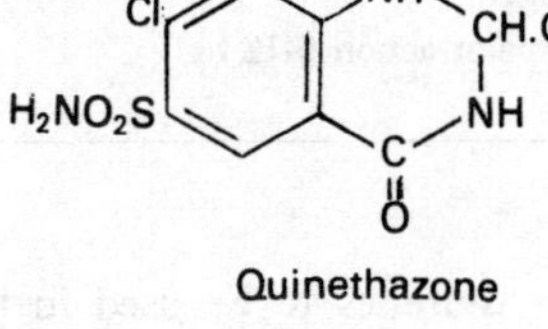

Quinethazone

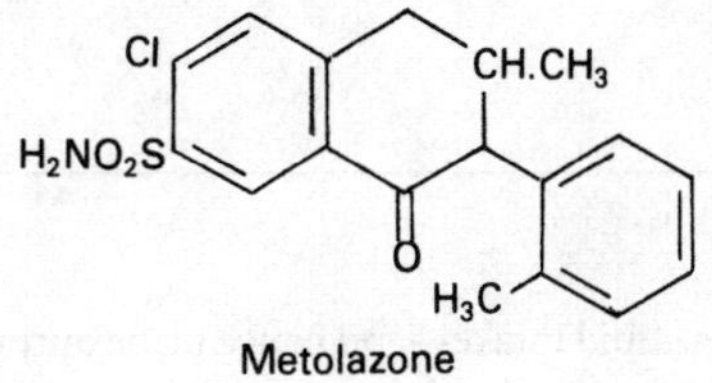

Metolazone

Approved name	quinethazone	metolazone
Proprietary name	Aquamox	Zaroxolyn
Approx daily dose	50-100 mg	10-12 mg
Duration of action	18-24 hr	18-24 hr

Table 36.3 (contd.)

PHTHALIMIDES

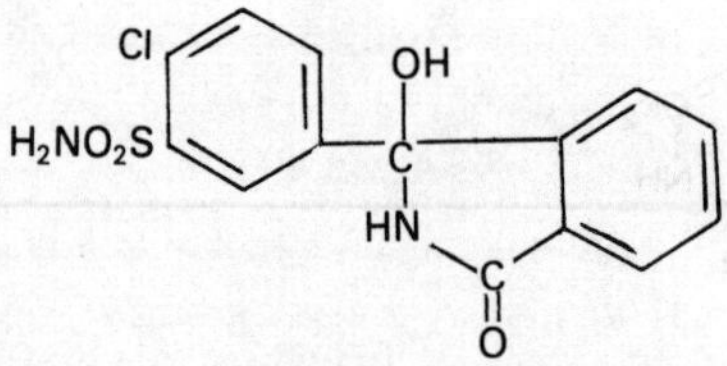

Chlorthalidone

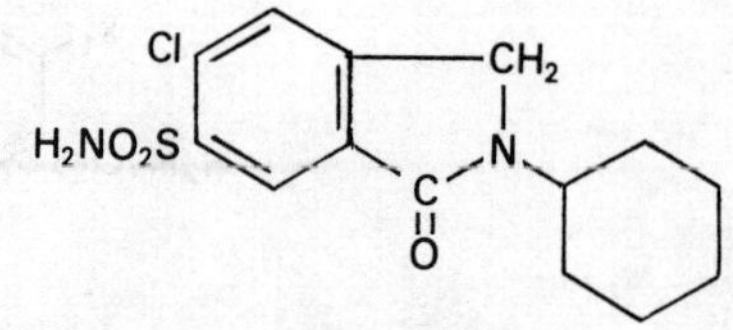

Clorexolone

Approved name	chlorthalidone	clorexolone
Proprietary name	Hygroton	Nefrolan
Approx daily dose	50-100 mg	20 mg
Duration of action	72 hr	72 hr

CHLOROBENZAMIDES

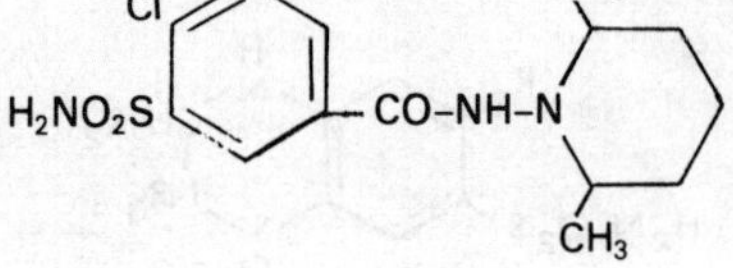

Clopamide

Approved name	clopamide
Proprietary names	Aquex, Brinaldix
Approx daily dose	20-40 mg
Duration of action	24 hr (major action 8-10 hr)

BENZENE DISULPHONAMIDES

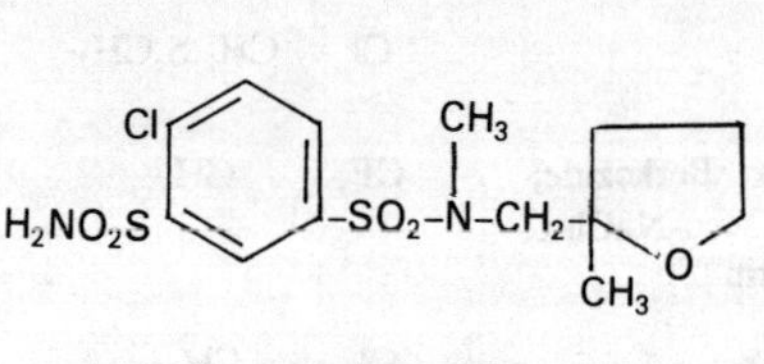

Mefruside

Approved name	mefruside
Proprietary name	Baycaron
Approx daily dose	25-50 mg
Duration of action	24 hr (major action 6-12 hr)

less intense so that fluid intake—and hence urine output—is reduced. A final, and perhaps the most likely, possibility is that in addition to their diuretic action, the thiazides are capable of increasing the permeability of the tubules to water. It is clear that this property might only be able to show itself when tubular permeability is at its lowest, because of the absence of vasopressin or of the failure of the kidney to respond to it. Whatever the mechanism, it

enables diuretics to be used in the treatment of some patients with diabetes insipidus.

Although the diuretic action of the thiazides is not self limiting in the same sense as that of the carbonic anhydrase inhibitors or the organomercurial compounds, prolonged administration does result in a gradual reduction of diuretic effect. The origin of this 'escape' is not yet clear: it may arise from an increase in the depressant effect on glomerular filtration rate, to a compensatory increase of aldosterone secretion or to mechanisms that have not yet been detected.

The thiazides and hydrothiazides have proved to be very useful in the treatment of oedema, particularly that of cardiac origin. They are also valuable in the treatment of hypertension. It was thought at first that they simply potentiated the effect of other types of hypotensive agent but it is now clear that they have a hypotensive effect independently of any interaction with other drugs. Many cases of mild hypertension are treated by diuretics alone. The origin of this hypotensive action is discussed elsewhere (p. 317).

It has already been mentioned that hypokalaemia is a likely accompaniment of thiazide therapy, and it is usually necessary to give potassium supplements to patients receiving thiazides. A useful regime, when a relatively prolonged treatment is envisaged, is to give the thiazide three times weekly and to supply potassium chloride (500 mg twice daily) on the intervening days. Enteric coated tablets containing both thiazide and potassium chloride are available but their use is to be deprecated. Not only does the use of combined tablets prevent the independent adjustment of the doses of the constituents but the tablets have been known to cause gastrointestinal ulceration and haemorrhages which do not occur when potassium chloride is taken alone in a dilute solution.

Hypokalaemia is a potentially dangerous hazard in two conditions which demand treatment by diuretics. In the digitalized cardiac patient, hypokalaemia increases the sensitivity of the heart to digitalis and may cause digitalis intoxication. In cirrhosis of the liver, hypokalaemia may precipitate coma. In addition to these dangers, hypokalaemia causes muscle weakness in all subjects.

Apart from the effects of hypokalaemia, side effects from thiazide therapy are relatively uncommon. Like ethacrynic acid, the thiazides impair the excretion of uric acid and they are therefore contraindicated in the gouty patient. Gastrointestinal disturbances sometimes occur, while agranulocytosis and skin haemorrhages have been reported on a few occasions. Pancreatitis has been seen and diabetes may be precipitated in potentially diabetic subjects. The hypotensive effect of the thiazides may cause circulatory embarrassment in normotensive patients. This fairly long list of side effects is less of an indication of an inherently high toxicity than a reflection of the number of

intensive observations that have been made in patients treated with the now popular drugs.

Finally, a word may be said concerning structure activity relations in the thiazide diuretics. The extensive work which has been carried out in this field has been directed towards the development of thiazides that will cause a smaller degree of hypokalaemia. However, as one of the foremost workers in the field has himself said 'this work has evolved a structure activity relationship which in some aspects has provided useful generalizations but in other respects is replete with inconsistencies' (de Stevens, 1963). To summarize the 'useful generalizations': For diuretic activity there must be a free sulphonamido group in position 7 (see Fig. 36.7). This can be substituted, but the substituent must be capable of removal *in vivo* to yield a compound containing a free sulphonamido group. Substitution in position 6 with -Cl or $-CF_3$ does not alter the type of activity but it increases potency. Saturation of the 3-4 double bond of the heterocyclic ring also sharply increases potency and reduces carbonic anhydrase inhibiting activity. Substitution in position 3 of the heterocyclic ring increases potency still further. For a more extensive discussion of this topic, the reader is referred to the review by de Stevens (1963).

DRUGS THAT PRODUCE A MILD DIURESIS

The diuretic agents in this category provoke the excretion of no more than 2 to 4 per cent of the filtered load of sodium. Apart from the acidifying salts, which ought properly to be classified as mild diuretics (but which are considered separately below) all these drugs operate distally, at site IVa where, as we have seen, sodium is absorbed under the influence of aldosterone and is 'exchanged' for potassium. If sodium is not absorbed here, potassium is not excreted and drugs that operate at site IV can be described as potassium sparing diuretic agents. Two types of compound can be recognized—those that inhibit the production, release or physiological action of aldosterone and those that interfere with potassium transport.

Aldosterone antagonists

Since some forms of oedema result largely, as has already been mentioned (pp. 621-2) from an increased section of the hormone, aldosterone antagonists should provide a rational form of therapy. For this reason, a considerable

Amphenone B

SU 4885 (metyrapone)

effort has been devoted to the discovery of substances which can oppose the action of aldosterone but none of those so far developed is as useful as had been hoped.

Amphenone B inhibits the synthesis of aldosterone but it also interferes with the production of glucocorticoids and it is too toxic for clinical use. SU 4885 or metyrapone (Metopirone) does not affect the synthesis of glucocorticoids but it does inhibit the production of hydrocortisone as well as aldosterone. As a result, the output of adrenocorticotrophic hormone (ACTH) from the pituitary is increased. Under normal conditions, ACTH calls forth an increased secretion of aldosterone but when aldosterone synthesis is blocked another corticoid (11-deoxycorticosterone) appears in the adrenal secretions. This compound, which is normally secreted only in minute amounts, has a much more powerful sodium retaining action than aldosterone itself. Thus the administration of metyrapone causes antidiuresis instead of the expected diuresis. If the output of ACTH is prevented by giving prednisolone, metyrapone does have a diuretic action but so far it has found little use as a diuretic agent in clinical practice.

Rather more success has attended the use of spironolactone (Aldactone). This compound bears a structural resemblance to aldosterone (p. 753) and this bestows the property of competitively inhibiting the action of aldosterone on the renal tubules. Because of its potassium sparing action, spironolactone is potentially useful in patients for whom hypokalaemia would be a hazard. They include those with hepatic cirrhosis and those receiving digitalis.

Spironolactone

Spironolactone is given by mouth in thrice daily doses of 100 to 200 mg. In smaller doses (25 to 50 mg) it can be used to supplement other diuretics. Reported side effects are trivial. They include drowsiness and skin rashes.

Triamterene and amiloride

Triamterene (Dyrenium, Dytac) was developed as an aldosterone antagonist and it was at first thought to behave in this way. It increases the excretion of sodium and chloride, depresses potassium excretion and is most active in conditions of heightened aldosterone secretion. Nevertheless, it also causes diuresis in the totally adrenalectomized animal and we have to conclude that triamterene does not owe its activity to aldosterone antagonism.

This conclusion is reinforced by the observation that the diuresis induced by maximally effective doses of spironolactone is augmented if triamterene is also given.

The indications for triamterene are the same as for spironolactone. It is given in thrice daily doses of 500 mg. Some reduction in the granulocyte count has been reported in patients receiving triamterene but this does not appear to be of serious import. Combinations of triamterene with benzthiazide or hydrochlorothiazide are available under the proprietary names of Dytide and Dyazide respectively.

The actions and uses of amiloride (Midamor, Modamide) are similar to those of triamterene, a not surprising fact in view of its chemical structure. However, it seems that amiloride has some action at sites Ib and III as well as the site IV activity it shares with triamterene (see Jacobson and Kokko, 1976). The oral dose is 10 mg daily but in smaller doses it can be used as an adjunct to other forms of diuretic therapy. Moduretic is a proprietary mixture of amiloride and hydrochlorothiazide.

Triamterene

Amiloride

Recorded side effects of amiloride therapy include nausea and mental confusion.

Although the potassium sparing action of the mild diuretic agents is often an advantage, the drugs can cause a serious degree of hyperkalaemia in patients whose condition is associated with potassium retention or who are taking potassium supplements for any reason.

ACIDIFYING SALTS

Ammonium chloride, ammonium nitrate and calcium chloride all cause a transient diuresis. They are not now used as diuretic agents themselves but they may be given in conjunction with the organomercury compounds (p. 627). All the acidifying salts have essentially the same mode of action. The ammonium ion is converted into urea in the liver while calcium is partly excreted as the phosphate or carbonate and is partly taken up by bone. Although some of the chloride (or nitrate) ion thus left is reabsorbed by the kidney tubules, much of it is excreted, taking with it an equivalent amount of sodium and the appropriate amount of water. Thus both sodium and water are excreted. The excretion of sodium means that the alkali reserve is depleted and this is ultimately reflected in an increasing urinary acidity since the amount of disodium hydrogen phosphate falls and the amount of the acid salt increases. As the acidity of the urine increases, the kidneys' additional base conserving mechanisms come into operation. Ammonia is formed and this exchanges with sodium in the tubules. The net result is that ammonium chloride (or nitrate) is excreted and when compensation is complete the amount of ammonium chloride or nitrate which is excreted is exactly the same as (or, in the case of calcium chloride, exactly equivalent to) that ingested. Sodium loss no longer occurs and the diuretic action ceases. This state of affairs is reached after only one or two days of treatment; it explains the very limited usefulness of the acidifying salts.

Ammonium chloride and nitrate are given by mouth in the form of capsules or enteric coated tablets to prevent the nausea and vomiting they otherwise cause.

ANTIDIURETIC AGENTS

The only clinical condition requiring treatment by antidiuretics is diabetes insipidus. Two forms of this disease are recognized. The first is caused by a primary lack of vasopressin and it is treated by supplying the missing hormone. In the second type—*nephrogenic diabetes insipidus*—vasopressin is secreted normally but the kidney is incapable of responding to it. This type of diabetes insipidus is treated by giving a diuretic drug, usually one of the longer acting members of the benzothiadiazide group.

VASOPRESSIN
The pharmacology of vasopressin is discussed in more detail elsewhere (pp. 618 and 773). In this section, only the therapeutic uses of vasopressin are considered.

In diabetes insipidus, vasopressin is administered as a daily intramuscular injection of a suspension in oil. Alternatively, posterior pituitary powder can be taken as a nasal snuff. By this latter route the dose has to be repeated at intervals of twelve hours or less. The dose of vasopressin or pituitary powder has to be adjusted for the individual patient: it is of the order of one unit of vasopressin daily.

Vasopressin causes vasoconstriction and a resulting facial pallor. Increased intestinal movements and painful uterine cramps may also occur. None of these effects is of serious consequence in the majority of patients, but in those with coronary arterial disease vasopressin may produce serious anginal attacks. When diabetes insipidus coexists with arterial disease, diuretics should be used instead of vasopressin.

In the non-diabetic subject, vasopressin can be used to test the ability of the kidney to concentrate urine. Another use for vasopressin is in the radiographic examination of the kidney. A suitable contrast medium is injected intravenously. If vasopressin is also given, a concentrated urine is assured, the contrast medium in the ureter and the pelvis of the kidney shows up more clearly and the examination (*intravenous pyelography*) is facilitated. Vasopressin is sometimes used to determine whether epilepsy is present in cases where diagnosis is otherwise difficult. Hydration of the brain increases its excitability and if water retention is artificially produced by the injection of vasopressin, the previously normal electroencephalographic record may show signs of hyperactivity in those with a tendency to epileptic attacks.

DIURETIC DRUGS
The possible mechanisms by which the benzothiadiazide diuretics reduce urine flow in patients with diabetes insipidus have already been discussed (p. 632). It is only necessary to add here that these drugs provide the only means of treating nephrogenic diabetes insipidus and that they are strongly indicated when arterial disease develops in patients with the pituitary form of diabetes insipidus. The drugs are given in the same doses as when they are used to induce diuresis. Too great a loss of potassium ions can be guarded against by giving amiloride as well as the benzothiadiazide.

CHLORPROPAMIDE
Chlorpropamide is best known as an oral hypoglycaemic agent that achieves its therapeutic action by stimulating the synthesis and release of insulin by the failing pancreas. It is similarly capable of boosting vasopressin secretion in those individuals with the pituitary form of diabetes insipidus who nevertheless retain a minimal degree of posterior lobe function. Given alone or in association with vasopressin, chlorpropamide is often useful in properly selected cases of diabetes insipidus. The drug is described in more detail elsewhere (p. 728).

BIBLIOGRAPHY

Books, monographs and reviews
Brogden, R. N., Speight, T. M. and Avery, G. S. (1974). Mefruside: a preliminary report of its pharmacological properties and therapeutic efficacy in oedema and hypertension. *Drugs*, **7**, 419-425.

Brogden, R. N., Speight, T. M. and Avery, G. S. (1975). Bumetanide: a preliminary report of its pharmacological properties and therapeutic efficacy in oedema. *Drugs*, **9**, 4-18.

Burg, M. (1974). The mechanism of action of diuretics in renal tubules. In: *Recent Advances in Renal Physiology and Pharmacology*. ed. L. Wesson, G. Fanelli. Baltimore Md: Univ. Park Press.

Cafruny, E. J. (1968). The site and mechanism of action of mercurial diuretics. *Pharmac. Rev.*, **20**, 89-116.

Davies, D.L. and Wilson, G. M. (1975). Diuretics: mechanism of action and clinical application. *Drugs*, **9**, 178-226.

De Stevens, G. (1963). *Diuretics: Chemistry and Pharmacology*. New York: Academic Press.

De Wardener (1973). *The Kidney*. Edinburgh and London: Churchill Livingstone.

Fisher, J. W. (ed.) (1971). *Renal Pharmacology*. London: Butterworths.

Heller, H. and Ginsburg, M. (1961). *Diuretic Drugs*. In, Ellis, G. P. and West, G. B. (eds.) Progress in Medicinal Chemistry, Vol. 1, 132-186. London: Butterworths.

Jacobson, H. R. and Kokko, J. P. (1976). Diuretics: sites and mechanisms of action. *A. rev. pharmac.* **16**, 201-214.

Starling, E. H. (1909). *The Fluids of the Body*. London: Constable.

Original papers

Burg, M. B. and Green, N. (1973). Function of the thick ascending limb of Henle's loop. *Amer. J. Physiol.*, **25**, 119-124.

de Stevens, G., Werner, L. H., Halamandaris, A. and Ricca, S. (Jr.), (1958). Dihydrobenzothiadiazine dioxides with potent diuretic effect. *Experientia*, **14**, 463.

Kessler, R. H., Lozano, R. and Pitts, R. F. (1957). Studies on structure—diuretic activity relationships of organic compounds of mercury. *J. Clin. Invest.* **36**, 656-668.

Lipschitz, W. L. and Hadidian, Z. (1944). Amides, amines and related compounds as diuretics. *J. Pharmac. exp. Therap.*, **81**, 84-94.

Macgregor, G. A., Tasker, P. R. W. and De Wardener, H. E. (1975). Diuretic-induced oedema. *Lancet* (i) 489-492.

Mudge, G. H. and Weiner, I. M. (1958). The mechanism of action of mercurial and xanthine diuretics. *Ann. N. Y. Acad. Sci.*, **71**, 344-354.

Nigrovic, V., Koechel, D. A. and Cafruny, E. J. (1973). Renal interaction between ethacrynic acid and mercurial diuretics. *J. Pharmac. exp. Ther.* **186**, 331-334.

Puschett, J. B. and Goldberg, M. (1968). The acute effects of furosemide on acid and electrolyte excretion in man. Differences from ethacrynic acid and evidence for a proximal action. *J. Lab. Clin. Med.*, **71**, 666-677.

Rocha, A. S. and Kokko, J. P. (1973). Sodium chloride and water transport in the medullary thick ascending limb of Henle. *J. Clin. Invest.* **52**, 612-623.

Sprague, J. M. (1958). The chemistry of diuretics. *Ann. N. Y. Acad. Sci.*, **71**, 328-343.

37. The pharmacology of the gastrointestinal tract

Disturbances of gastrointestinal function are responsible for much human illness and discomfort. Some of the drugs with actions on the gastrointestinal tract are considered in this chapter; vomiting and drugs used in its treatment form the subject of Chapter 33.

THE SALIVARY GLANDS

Saliva contains an amylase (ptyalin) which passes with the food into the stomach where it begins the digestion of starch. Saliva serves a number of other useful functions: by keeping the mouth and lips moist it aids articulation and by moistening and lubricating the food it facilitates swallowing. Cessation of salivary secretion causes the sensation of thirst which signals a fall in the body's water content. The importance of the non-digestive functions of saliva is illustrated by the discomfort and inconvenience experienced as a side effect of atropine medication which causes a prolonged inhibition of salivary secretion (p. 226).

Vasodilatation in the salivary glands

The most interesting pharmacological problem associated with salivary gland function concerns the mechanism of the vasodilatation which accompanies secretion. The discussion which follows applies also to the functional hyperaemia seen in some other glands such as the pancreas and the sweat glands but it is appropriate to discuss the problem here since most of the relevant experimental work has involved a study of salivary secretion, particularly in the cat.

The salivary glands are supplied by parasympathetic nerves which are conveyed by the chorda tympani branch of the facial nerve (which supplies the submaxillary and sublingual glands) and by the glossopharyngeal nerve, which supplies the parotid gland. Stimulation of these nerves causes salivary secretion and dilatation of the blood vessels in the activated gland. The vasodilatation clearly serves a useful purpose during the increased functional activity associated with the secretory process and it would not be surprising if it were found that the parasympathetic fibres supplied both the gland cells and the blood vessels. An alternative view is that the vasodilatation is a secondary response to the increased secretory activity. This hypothesis was originally put forward in 1914 by Sir Joseph

Barcroft: it was stimulated by the observation first made as long ago as 1872 by Heidenhain and repeatedly confirmed since, that atropine prevents the secretory response to stimulation of the chorda tympani but only partly blocks the accompanying vasodilatation. Barcroft suggested that the vasodilatation was caused by metabolites and he showed that, in the atropinized animal, stimulation of the secretory nerves increased the oxygen consumption of the salivary glands, though secretion itself was prevented. Barcroft assumed that the vasodilator metabolites were of a non-specific nature (carbon dioxide, lactic acid, etc.) but in 1936 kallikrein was discovered in the salivary glands. Kallikrein is a proteolytic enzyme which liberates vasodilator polypeptides (the plasma kinins, p. 358) from plasma. Ungar and Parrot suggested that kallikrein was the metabolite responsible for functional hyperaemia in the salivary glands. This important idea was completely ignored for almost twenty years but in 1955 Hilton and Lewis published the first of a series of papers which led to the conclusion that vasodilatation in salivary glands is indeed brought about by the liberation of kallikrein on stimulation of the secretory nerves.

The principal arguments put forward by Hilton and Lewis (for further details see Hilton and Lewis 1955a and b, 1956; Hilton, 1960; Lewis, 1967) can be summarized as follows:

Stimulation of the chorda tympani in cats causes the liberation of a vasodilator substance in the submandibular salivary gland. This substance cannot be acetylcholine, for if the arterial blood supply to the gland is obstructed during chorda stimulation, the vasodilator material collects in the tissue spaces and appears in the blood when the blood flow is re-established. By this technique it can be shown that the vasodilator substance persists for several minutes after nerve stimulation has ceased: acetylcholine, on the other hand, would be destroyed very quickly. The vasodilator material can be collected in the outflow from a perfused gland. On re-injection into the circulation of another gland (where it will come into contact with plasma proteins) it produces vasodilatation. However, the material does not have any action on isolated preparations unless it is first incubated with plasma proteins, when it produces the slow contraction of smooth muscle characteristic of that due to plasma kinins. Thus the material produced by chorda stimulation is of an enzymic nature, liberating a vasodilator polypeptide from the plasma proteins. The enzyme (kallikrein) can also be shown to occur in saliva itself.

Kallikrein occurs in several other glands—it was in fact first detected in the pancreas—and Hilton and Lewis believed that functional vasodilatation in glandular tissues generally (though not in muscle) might be the result of kallikrein liberation. Two general considerations lend some attraction to this view. In the first place, it is well-known that, in the body generally, vasodilator nerves are uncommon: vasodilatation is usually brought about by a relaxation of sympathetic vasomotor tone. If the kallikrein mechanism were shown to operate in all tissues showing functional hyperaemia, it would not be necessary to postulate the existence of vasodilator fibres anywhere in the body except, perhaps, in skeletal muscle. Secondly, it is known that plasma kinins mediate other vasodilator responses: the evidence suggests that they play an important part in inflammatory responses and in the production of some forms of vascular headache (p. 418). Nevertheless, the kallikrein hypothesis has been challenged, particularly by Schachter and his associates (Bhoola et al., 1965; Morley, Schachter and Smaje, 1966; Schachter and Beilenson, 1967) on the following grounds.

Most of the experiments which sought to establish a vasodilator role for kallikrein were carried out on the cat. Some other species behave differently. In the rabbit, both salivary secretion and the accompanying vasodilatation are blocked by atropine. Anticholinesterase drugs restore both activities in the atropinized animal. In sheep, vasodilatation in the parotid gland is inhibited by atropine but that in the submaxillary gland is resistant to atropine. In the guinea pig, chorda stimulation causes the release of kallikrein which is capable of liberating kinins from the plasma of several species but not, unfortunately, from guinea pig plasma. Even in the cat, vasodilatation caused by nerve stimulation is still present after the gland has been almost depleted of its contained kallikrein and it is not affected by the enzyme carboxypeptidase which destroys plasma kinins. These and other observations have led Schachter to propose that the vasodilatation is under the immediate control of cholinergic parasympathetic fibres. The inability of atropine to block the vasodilator response in some species is explained as a manifestation of the well known variation in the sensitivity to atropine of muscarinic receptor sites among different species and in different parts of the body. There is histochemical evidence for the existence of cholinergic fibres (or at any rate of fibres containing cholinesterase) ending in relation to blood vessels in salivary glands. The origin of the functional vasodilatation in active glands must therefore be regarded as unsettled but it certainly appears likely that the kallikrein mechanism will prove to be of less widespread occurrence than was once believed.

Another large polypeptide that appears in saliva after nerve stimulation is sialotonin (Moriwaki, Beilenson and Schachter, 1968; Barton, et al., 1976.) Unlike kallikrein, which appears in response to stimulation of both sympathetic and parasympathetic nerves, sialotonin is found only in saliva collected during stimulation of the chorda tympani. Injections of sialotonin evoke a short lived vasoconstriction but the physiological significance of sialotonin is still a matter of conjecture.

Stimulation of the sympathetic nerves to the salivary glands produces both vasoconstrictor and vasodilator responses. The vasoconstriction is blocked by agents that block adrenaline α-receptors but the vasodilator response is not affected by blockade of either the α- or the β-receptors. Sympathetic vasodilatation may therefore also be a consequence of the secretory response.

Drugs that stimulate salivary secretion

Food in the mouth stimulates the secretion of both saliva and gastric juice. When the appetite is depressed, as after an illness, the reflexes are also depressed. The taking of substances with a bitter taste which stimulate the taste buds increases the secretion of saliva and gastric juice and improves appetite and digestion. Among bitters (stomachics) that have been used to restore appetite are the alkaloids strychnine, quinine and extracts of gentian, quassia and calumba. The tinctures of cinchona and nux vomica also contain alkaloids. The so-called tonics (which have no tonic action in any physiological sense of that term) rely largely on their content of bitters to maintain their reputation among laymen (and family physicians) as useful preparations for restoring health and vigour after an illness. Their other constituents (which may include glycerophosphates, iron, vitamins and liver extracts) are added for no particular reason. The so-called 'neurophosphates' exert no beneficial action on the central nervous system.

Appetite suppression

In the treatment of obesity it is necessary to persuade the patient to reduce his calorie intake. One way of achieving this is to administer drugs that reduce the appetite. These drugs (together with other devices for promoting weight loss) are discussed in detail elsewhere (p. 281).

THE STOMACH AND DUODENUM

The constituents of gastric juice most important in digestion are pepsin (a proteolytic enzyme) and hydrochloric acid which together initiate the digestion of protein. Salivary amylase also operates in the stomach until hydrochloric acid penetrates the food mass and arrests amylase activity. Digestion of protein and starch continues, and that of other substances is started, in the duodenum, which receives the pancreatic secretions, and in the rest of the small intestine, which secretes the succus entericus.

Hydrochloric acid is produced by the oxyntic (or parietal) cells of the stomach. These cells also secrete Castle's intrinsic factor, the substance on which depends the absorption of vitamin B_{12} (p. 675). Hydrogen ions, derived from water, are secreted by the glands against a concentration gradient using energy obtained from a series of oxidative reactions. The hydroxyl ions combine with carbon dioxide under the influence of carbonic anhydrase and the resulting bicarbonate ions pass into the blood, exchanging with chloride ions which accompany the hydrogen ions into the glandular lumen. The final result, therefore, of this separation of the hydrogen and hydroxyl ions of water, is the production of hydrochloric acid in the stomach and of bicarbonate in the blood. It will be readily appreciated that the more vigorous the secretion of acid the more alkaline will be the blood leaving the stomach. This is the cause of the 'alkaline tide' in the blood which accompanies gastric digestion. For more complete details of the reactions involved in the production of gastric acid, the reader is referred to standard textbooks of physiology (see, especially, Davson, 1970) but the pharmacologist should note that a very high degree of carbonic anhydrase inhibition is required before any detectable change in acid secretion occurs. Kidney function is more susceptible to carbonic anhydrase inhibition and inhibitors such as acetazolamide (p. 631) can be used as diuretic agents without seriously interfering with the formation of acid in the stomach.

Carbonic anhydrase is also present in the pancreas, where it promotes the formation of sodium bicarbonate, the principal nonenzymic constituent of pancreatic juice. Its occurrence in the blood, brain and kidney is referred to in the appropriate places in this book.

Pepsinogen is produced by the zymogen (or chief) cells of the stomach while gastrin (see below) comes from the so-called G cells of the pyloric mucosa. Cells in both the cardiac and pyloric regions of the gastric mucosa secrete mucus. Gastrin is also manufactured by specialized cells in the pancreatic islets (p. 719).

The secretion of gastric juice occurs in three phases. In the first or *cephalic phase*, food in the mouth causes a reflex secretion of gastric juice—the so-called 'appetite juice'— the vagus nerves constituting the efferent part of the reflex pathway. In the second or *gastric phase* of secretion, food (particularly protein and its digestion products) in the stomach releases gastrin from the pyloric mucosa. Gastrin passes into the blood stream and is recirculated to the stomach where it stimulates the secretion of an acid-rich juice. The circulating gastrin also supplements the actions of some of the other gastrointestinal hormones. Thus it evokes the secretion of enzymes and bicarbonate by the pancreas and causes contraction of the gall bladder. A possible therapeutic future for gastrin is foreshadowed by the observation that it increases the tone of the sphincter at the oesophago-gastric junction and may thus provide a useful means of preventing regurgitation of the stomach contents into the oesophagus of patients who experience this symptom.

The physiological action of gastrin is eventually arrested by the hydrochloric acid it has itself been instrumental in producing. In the final *intestinal phase* of gastric digestion, food (particularly fat) in the duodenum and jejunum causes the release of another hormone—enterogastrone— which inhibits the secretion of both acid and pepsin. Urogastrone is a similar substance to enterogastrone: it is extracted from urine. Enterogastrone has not yet been isolated or identified and the possibility that it is identical with one of the other gastrointestinal hormones cannot yet be excluded.

Food in the duodenum also calls forth the secretion of hormones involved in intestinal digestive processes (see below).

Although the gastric phase of secretion involves hormonal stimulation of the stomach, the secretory action of gastrin is inhibited by atropine and is enhanced by concurrent stimulation of the vagus. Conversely, it seems that stimulation of the vagus can cause the release of gastrin and that gastrin can only be released by food if vagal excitation is occurring. The experiments which led to these conclusions are summarized by Gregory (1962). They suggest to the present author the possibility that gastrin may influence synaptic transmission in the local autonomic plexuses in the stomach wall and that gastrin (like pepsin) secretion depends ultimately on nervous activity.

HISTAMINE AND GASTRIN

Histamine is a powerful stimulant of acid secretion and it has been used in clinical investigations in order to assess the ability of the stomach to secrete acid. Pentagastrin (see below) is now preferred for this purpose. If no acid is produced in response to pentagastrin the condition of *achlorhydria* or *achylia gastrica* exists. This occurs occasionally in otherwise normal subjects but it more often accompanies pernicious anaemia (p. 676). Some individuals have hypertrophied gastric mucosa and they produce more gastric acid than the normal subject in response to pentagastrin. Insulin injection produces gastric juice which is rich in both pepsin and acid: the hypoglycaemia stimulates the vagal centres in the brain.

Gastrin was first detected by Edkins in 1905 and for many years thereafter it was believed that it would prove to be identical with histamine. A suspicion that this belief was untenable became a certainty when it was finally established (in 1964) that gastrin is a heptadecapeptide. Nevertheless it is difficult to believe that histamine has no place in gastric physiology: it is a powerful stimulant of acid secretion, it is present in the stomach, particularly in the neighbourhood of the oxyntic cells, and the gastric mucosa has no histaminase, suggesting that the preservation of histamine is of functional importance. Histamine, of course, is also present in the rest of the intestine. The stimulant effect of histamine on gastric secretion (unlike that to gastrin and to vagal stimulation) is not affected by atropine. These findings are perhaps best interpreted in the light of a hypothesis, first proposed by Babkin in 1938, to the effect that the immediate stimulus to the secretion of gastric acid is histamine liberation. Vagal stimulation, it is suggested, releases acetylcholine which in its turn releases histamine. Thus atropine will inhibit the action of acetylcholine (and of gastrin if this operates, as has been suggested above, via the autonomous plexuses) but will not affect the response to histamine. We can perhaps say (by borrowing a famous phrase used by Sherrington in an entirely different context) that histamine provides the 'final common path' to the oxyntic cells for the several factors that influence the secretion of acid by the stomach. The effects of histamine on gastric secretion are mediated through H_2 receptors (p. 344).

Although gastrin contains seventeen aminoacid residues, only the four at the acid end of the molecule are responsible for its physiological activity. A number of substances based on the active terminal residues have been synthesized. Pentagastrin (Peptavlon) is one such compound. When it is used to assess acid secretory activity in the stomach it is given in intramuscular doses of 6 μg per kilogram.

There is evidence that gastrin (like so many other substances) promotes the formation of the ubiquitous cyclic AMP.

PANCREATIC SECRETION
Pancreatic secretion is under the control of two hormones which are liberated when the acid contents of the stomach pass into the duodenum. *Secretin* evokes a copious flow of watery juice containing sodium bicarbonate; *cholecysto-kinin-pancreozymin* induces contraction of the gall bladder and calls forth the secretion of the enzyme components of the juice. Until recently it was believed that these activities were separately controlled by two different hormones, the original and respective names of which are retained in the present awkwardly double barrelled neologism. It is to be hoped that a simpler and more euphonious name will soon be available for the single substance. The presence of food in the mouth causes the reflex secretion of pancreatic as well as gastric juice. Secretin was the first substance to be given (in 1902) the name 'hormone'.

Drugs used in the treatment of peptic ulcer
Ulceration can occur in both the stomach and the duodenum. It arises as the result of the digestive action of pepsin and acid against which the normal stomach and duodenum are protected by their mucous secretions. It is not necessary to discuss here the reasons why this protec-

tion has failed in the peptic ulcer patient but it should be pointed out that some drugs (aspirin and adrenocortical hormones, for instance) tend to cause peptic ulcers. The treatment of peptic ulcer is directed towards reducing the amount and acidity of the gastric juice and the intensity of gastro-duodenal movements. This produces symptomatic relief and also provides the conditions which promote healing of the ulcer. Attention is directed towards the diet but drugs have a more important place in treatment. They include sedatives, atropine-like compounds, carbenoxolone, antacids and, most recently of all, antagonists of H_2 histamine receptors. Another new drug is metoclopramide. Sedatives are given because of the strong psychosomatic element in peptic ulceration and because there is little doubt that nervous tension can hinder the healing of an ulcer. The use of atropine-like drugs in the treatment of gastrointestinal conditions is discussed elsewhere (p. 228). Among the more useful compounds in this group are propantheline—which is said to be particularly active in suppressing excessive secretory activity—and tricyclamol, which inhibits motility.

CARBENOXOLONE
Liquid extract of liquorice is frequently used to sweeten and flavour saline mixtures and it was the accidental observation that the ulcers of patients taking liquorice-flavoured mixtures seemed to heal more quickly which led to the introduction of carbenoxolone. Carbenoxolone is a pentacyclic triterpene extracted from liquorice root and well-controlled clinical trials have established that it does indeed accelerate the healing of gastric and duodenal ulcers. (Doll, *et al.*, 1962; Pinder *et al*, 1976). The drug is given in the form of the sodium salt.

Carbenoxolone (Biogastrone) taken by mouth is rapidly absorbed, largely by the stomach. More than 99 per cent of that reaching the blood is bound to plasma proteins (particularly albumin) and in this form it is transported to the liver where it is conjugated with glucuronic acid. The glucuronide passes into the duodenum in the bile and thence into the faeces. A little is reabsorbed and circulates enterohepatically. The drug is not metabolized to any appreciable extent. It has a plasma half life in the young adult of about twelve hours but this increases progressively with age.

Although gastric ulcers can be treated with simple tablets of carbenoxolone, 'positioned release' capsules (Duogastrone) which do not release their contents until they have left the stomach are sometimes preferred when the ulcer is in the duodenum. The introduction of this formulation has been at least partly responsible for the more sanguine attitude that now prevails concerning the value of the drug in duodenal ulcer; until recently it was recommended only for gastric ulcers.

The basis of carbenoxolone's therapeutic action has not yet been precisely delineated but contributions are probably made by a number of its properties. Thus, it promotes the secretion of the mucus that provides a protective coating for the gastric and duodenal mucosa, it prolongs the life of the mucosa's epithelial cells and it reduces the peptic activity of gastric juice. It also has some mineralo-corticoid-like properties which are responsible for the drug's side effects but which might also be relevant to its therapeutic effectiveness: lauroyl glycyrrhetinic (BX 24), which is completely devoid of mineralocorticoid activity but is in other respects very similar to carbenoxolone, is not a very effective antiulcer agent while spironolactone (p. 636), a mineralocorticoid antagonist, impairs the effectiveness of carbenoxolone.

The usual dose of carbenoxolone for patients with peptic ulcers is of the order of 100 to 200 mg three or four times daily. The higher dose regimes are recommended for duodenal ulcers. Side effects are by no means uncommon and may be serious if carbenoxolone treatment is not carefully supervised. The side effects, as we have noted, are manifestations of mineralocorticoid activity and they

Carbenoxolone sodium

include retention of sodium and water and depletion of potassium with oedema and hypertension. If carbenoxolone treatment is to be continued these side effects will need to be countered by giving diuretics and potassium. Spironolactone should be avoided, notwithstanding its potassium sparing diuretic activity because it is a carbenoxolone antagonist.

Although carbenoxolone certainly accelerates the healing of ulcers, the evidence that its continued administration will prevent their occurrence is not very convincing. The reader should remember, when he is attempting to assess the worth of any antiulcer drug that spontaneous healing and repeated recurrences are characteristic of peptic ulcers. He should also not forget that, advances in pharmacology notwithstanding, many ulcer patients only free themselves permanently of their complaint by a visit to the surgeon.

Bioral is a proprietary preparation of carbenozolone suitable for the treatment of ulcers in the mouth.

Other drugs that have been promoted as ulcer healers are Caved-S (a preparation that contains deglycyrrhinized liquorice, among other constituents) and geranyl farnesyl

acetate. They seem to offer no particular advantage over carbenoxolone.

ANTACIDS

Antacids have long been used in the treatment of peptic ulceration. They are also employed, particularly by the layman and with more enthusiasm than discretion, to relieve dyspepsia and 'heartburn'.

Antacids are midly alkaline compounds which react with gastric acid to form neutral salts. It is usually assumed that those which form colloidal adsorbent gels in the stomach also adsorb both pepsin and acid. In fact this mechanism is of little importance.

To be useful in the treatment of peptic ulcer, the antacid used should neutralize free acidity to a degree adequate to prevent the proteolytic activity of pepsin and to prevent the irritant actions of a high concentration of free acid on the ulcerated area. In therapeutic doses a good antacid should not cause systemic alkalosis or other toxic effects. It should not cause the formation of large amounts of gas, it should not cause constipation or diarrhoea and there should be no risk of a compensating increase in acid secretion or 'acid rebound' after its us use.

Sodium bicarbonate

Sodium bicarbonate is a popular and widely used antacid; its actions are rapid but short-lived, and it is used to give rapid relief from heartburn and dyspepsia. The reaction which takes place in the stomach is as follows:

$$NaHCO_3 + HCl \rightarrow NaCl + H_2O + CO_2$$

The carbon dioxide evolved during the reaction distends the stomach and may cause belching *(eructation)*.

The most undesirable feature associated with the use of sodium bicarbonate is the possibility of a systemic alkalosis in patients with impaired renal function. Large amounts of bicarbonate ion are absorbed from the intestine. Although the kidney normally responds to the increased blood alkalinity by secreting an alkaline urine, any impairment of kidney function may lead to a systemic alkalosis. Sodium bicarbonate is an ingredient of a great many proprietary antacid mixtures.

Compounds of magnesium

Magnesium oxide (magnesia, MgO), magnesium hydroxide $(Mg(OH)_2)$ light magnesium carbonate $(3MgCo_3 . Mg(OH)_2 . 3H_2O)$ and heavy magnesium carbonate $(3MgCO_3 . Mg(OH)_2 . 4H_2O)$ are all insoluble compounds which are not absorbed in significant quantities from the stomach or intestine. All the compounds have a more prolonged action than sodium bicarbonate and they have the further considerable advantage of not being absorbed even when present in excess. They are not liable, therefore, to cause a systemic alkalosis. Moreover, the oxide and hydroxide neutralize the stomach contents without liberating carbon dioxide. A disadvantage of the magnesium compounds is that magnesium chloride, formed as a result of their interaction with the hydrochloric acid of the stomach, and the carbonate (produced when the chloride reacts with the bicarbonate of the pancreatic juice) may have a purgative action (p. 649) though this can be offset by mixing the magnesium compound with calcium carbonate. *Cream of magnesia* is a 7.9 per cent suspension of magnesium hydroxide in water: it is used as an antacid-laxative preparation for young children. Fluid magnesia is a solution of magnesium bicarbonate ($Mg(HCO_3)_2$) saturated with carbon dioxide.

Magnesium trisilicate is a hydrated magnesium silicate with the formula $2MgO.3SiO_2.xH_2O$. The reaction that takes place in the stomach is:

$$2MgO.3SiO_2.xH_2O + 4HCl \rightarrow$$
$$2MgCl_2 + 3SiO_2 + (x+2)H_2O$$

The reaction of the trisilicate with hydrochloric acid is slow and prolonged and the silica formed is in the gelatinous colloidal state. The antacid action is accordingly slow in onset but it is prolonged and powerful. The silica gel may also provide a protective coating over the walls of the stomach. Since it possesses antacid, adsorbent and protective properties, magnesium trisilicate has been one of the most useful of drugs for relieving the pain of peptic ulcer. Like the other magnesium compounds it may give rise to diarrhoea. Magnesium trisilicate is also used as an adsorbent to remove toxic substances from the intestine in intestinal toxaemia.

Calcium Compounds

Calcium carbonate and calcium hydroxide are useful antacids. They are used alone or in mixtures with magnesium antacids. Neutralization of the gastric contents involves the formation of calcium chloride which is converted into calcium carbonate in the intestine. The carbonate precipitates in the intestine and causes constipation, an effect which counters the purgative action of the corresponding magnesium salt when calcium and magnesium antacids are given together or alternately. A particularly effective antacid mixture is the compound powder of magnesium trisilicate which contains magnesium trisilicate, heavy magnesium carbonate, calcium carbonate and sodium bicarbonate.

Aluminium compounds

Aluminium hydroxide has neutralizing and adsorbent actions. The alumina gel prescribed under the name 'colloidal aluminium hydroxide' is actually a mixture of the hydroxide, the hydrated oxide and a small amount of the basic carbonate. Aluminium hydroxide does not completely neutralize the stomach contents but the pH achieved (3.5-4.0) is sufficient to inhibit the proteolytic action of pepsin. There is also some evidence that the aluminium ion may inhibit pepsin action independently of its pH effect. Aluminium hydroxide may cause constipation and for this reason it is often used in combination with magnesium antacids. Aluminium salts are not absorbed from the gastrointestinal tract so that systemic toxic effects do not arise during treatment with aluminium hydroxide. There is, however, the danger of producing phosphorus deficiency if its administration is prolonged since the aluminium chloride produced in the stomach reacts with dietary phosphate to produce the insoluble aluminium phosphate. Dietary supplements will prevent phosphate deficiency.

Aluminium glycinate, an aluminium phosphate gel and basic aluminium carbonate have also been used in the treatment of peptic ulcer: their properties are similar to those of the hydroxide.

Milk

Milk is a weak antacid which also possesses some protective action, and a 'milk drip' containing aluminium hydroxide gel facilitates healing in peptic ulcer of the oesophagus or of the stomach. A Ryle's tube is passed through the nose and into the oesophagus and the milk-antacid mixture is allowed to flow continuously over the damaged area. This form of therapy can only be employed in patients who are in bed, but more recently, antacid tablets (Nulacin) have been prepared which contain dried milk together with calcium carbonate and the trisilicate, oxide and carbonate of magnesium. These are allowed to dissolve slowly in the mouth. It is claimed that their action closely resembles that of the 'milk drip' with the advantage that they can be used in the ambulant patient. The possibility of producing an excess of calcium in blood with a resulting hypoparathyroidism and irreversible kidney damage (the milk alkali syndrome) has to be guarded against when milk and calcium compounds are given together. This condition is most likely to occur if preexisting renal insufficiency has permitted the establishment of an alkalosis. In extreme cases, the milk alkali syndrome appears when milk or calcium compounds are taken singly.

Tripotassium dicitrato bidmuthate

In the past, bismuth carbonate and subnitrate enjoyed a reputation as antacids although their ability to neutralize acid is minimal. It is probable that any benefit they conferred arose partly as a placebo effect and partly from their being able to cover the gastrointestinal mucosa with a dry, inert and protective coating. Interest in bismuth has revived recently and there is some enthusiasm for tripotassium dicitrato bismuthate (De-Nol), the most successful member of the new generation of bismuth compounds.

As we have already emphasized, antacids generally have no more than a palliative effect in peptic ulcer but the new bismuth compound actually promotes the healing of ulcers and (if work in experimental animals can be taken as a guide) it may also prevent their recurrence.

Tripotassium dicitrato bismuthate comes as a colloidal solution in an ammoniacal buffered base and it is taken, in quantities of 5 to 10 ml, half an hour before each meal. It is devoid of unpleasant or hazardous side effects. Like the more simple bismuth compounds of yore, tripotassium dicitrato bismuthate provides a protective coating for the gastrointestinal mucosa but it has other useful actions. At an acid pH, it chelates protein and so acts as an antipepsin, it stimulates the secretion of mucus, it inhibits microbial activity in the gut and so minimizes gas production, it inhibits gastrointestinal activity and thereby reduces the incidence of painful spasms and it has some antacid action. The last mentioned property is associated with the production of bismuth oxychloride but this compound is not absorbed from the intestine so there is no danger of a patient's receiving a toxic dose of bismuth.

Carminatives

Carminatives are used to relieve feelings of discomfort and distension after meals and they may do this by causing eructation and by giving a sensation of warmth. Many of the liqueurs customarily taken after dinner exert a carminative action and do so probably by virtue of their content of volatile oil. A large number of different carminatives have been employed in practice but they are of little pharmacological or therapeutic importance.

HISTAMINE H_2-ANTAGONISTS

The background to the recent discovery that histamine activates two classes of receptors is sketched elsewhere (p. 344). One of the most important responses to stimulation of the newly recognized H_2-receptors is the secretion of hydrochloric acid by the stomach and the development of specific H_2-receptor antagonists kindled the immediate hope that a new generation of antiulcer drugs might have been born. These early hopes appear to have been realized. The first two antagonists (metiamide and burimamide) had to be discarded but the third (cymetidine) has survived rigorous pharmacological and clinical scrutiny and it has just been released, bearing the name Tagamet, for clinical use. Early trials established that cymetidine can suppress acid secretion for several hours and among its successes is to be listed the fact that it can bestow the boon of an undisturbed night's sleep on patients with duodenal ulcer who, without the drug's help, would have been woken up every few hours by the pain resulting from acid secretion provoked by an empty stomach. Cymetidine (which is more fully discussed on p. 353) is certainly the antacid *par excellence*.

METOCLOPRAMIDE

This new drug—its proprietary names include Maxeran, Maxolon and Primperan—has a variety of uses in gastrointestinal therapeutics. It is usefully antiemetic, partly

$$CI \quad \quad CONH.CH_2.CH_2.N(C_2H_5)_2$$

$$H_2N \quad \quad OCH_3$$

Metoclopramide

because of a peripheral action but chiefly because it antagonizes dopamine at the chemoceptor trigger zone (p. 599). It also accelerates the passage of material through the stomach and the small intestine. This effect on intestinal motility is blocked by antimuscarine drugs such as atropine and potentiated by carbachol. These observations indicate that metoclopramide has an influence on cholinergic mechanisms in the gut. The possibilities are that acetylcholine release is potentiated and that muscle cells become sensitized to the transmitter (Hay, 1975). There is some evidence that dopaminergic mechanisms are involved too, at least in the oesophagus, since the increase in oesophageal tone brought about by metoclopramide is antagonized by L-dopa as well as by atropine.

Metoclopramide does not affect the secretion of pepsin or gastric acid.

As an antiemetic agent, metoclopramide finds application in the prevention of postoperative vomiting particularly when a morphine-like drug such as pethidine (which sometimes induces vomiting by stimulating the chemoceptor trigger zone) has been incorporated in the premedication programme. It is even more useful when the surgery has to be performed under emergency conditions when food is likely to be present in the stomach. This constitutes a potentially dangerous situation because vomiting, with subsequent inhalation of vomited matter, may occur under anaesthesia. In these circumstances, metoclopramide's ability to accelerate gastric emptying adds another dimension to its antiemetic activity. The drug can also be given in association with the barium meals that are used in diagnostic radiography where it is doubly useful: it hastens the passage of the meal and so shortens the time needed for the examination and it blunts the nausea that a barium meal induces in some patients. Metoclopropamide also facilitates the passage of catheters into the duodenum and beyond. In all these procedures it is often given in single intramuscular doses of 20 mg. When a more prolonged treatment is called for—as in radiation sickness and pregnancy, for instance—it can be taken in oral doses of 20 mg up to three times daily.

Metoclopramide relieves flatulent dyspepsia and heartburn and there is some not yet very substantial evidence that it promotes the healing of peptic ulcers. The symptomatic relief it affords in dyspepsia is the result of its emptying the stomach whereby feeling of fullness and flatulence disappear. Because it also causes contraction of the oesophageal sphincter, regurgitation of acid into the oesophagus (a common cause of dyspeptic pain) is also prevented. Additional explanations will have to be sought if further clinical experience confirms that the drug really does promote the healing of ulcers.

Metoclopramide is readily absorbed from the gastrointestinal tract and has a plasma half life of one to two hours. Although it is metabolized along a number of routes (deethylation, O-demethylation, oxidation, rupture of the amide bond and conjugation reactions all seem to be involved) a substantial portion of an administered dose is excreted in the urine in an unchanged form.

Because it shortens transit time in the stomach, so hastening the passage of material into the absorption sites in the intestine, metoclopramide may affect the absorption of other drugs taken at the same time. Drugs whose absorption is hastened in this way include ethanol, tetracyclines and L-dopa.

Side effects accompany metoclopramide therapy in a minority of patients. The most usual side effect is drowsiness but disturbances of muscle tone including spasm of muscles in the face and neck, are sometimes seen as might be expected in the light of the drug's known ability to occupy dopamine receptors. Because of this property, the drug is contraindicated in patients receiving the phenothiazine derivatives that themselves have an action on the extrapyramidal system. Metoclopramide evokes prolactin release and this constitutes a bar to employing the drug in patients with breast cancer, the growth of which is stimulated by prolactin.

An extensive recent review of the properties and uses of metoclopramide is provided by Pinder and his colleagues (1976).

THE INTESTINES

The small intestine: malabsorption syndromes

Digestive processes are completed in the small intestine which can then exercise its absorptive function. The small intestine also provides the principal channel of absorption for ingested drugs and other non-nutritive material: the factors that control drug absorption are discussed in detail in Chapter 4 (p. 46).

If intestinal function is disturbed the products of digestion may not be completely absorbed and so they pass into the large intestine. The amount of fluid that necessarily accompanies them may be more than can be absorbed by the colon in which event the faeces will be watery as well as bulky. Diarrhoea, therefore, is characteristic (but not pathognomic) of *malabsorption syndromes* of whatever aetiology. If fat is a prominent component of the bulky faeces, the condition is called *steatorrhoea* but it would be incorrect to assume that malabsorption syndromes invariably feature steatorrhoea: it is quite possible for fat absorption to be unaffected in conditions that seriously hinder the uptake of other nutrients (Creamer, 1974).

Absorption processes can be interfered with in diverse ways and no attempt can be made here to provide either an exhaustive or a systematic list of the conditions that bring malabsorption in their train. Instead, a few of the more clinically important and pharmacologically relevant malabsorption syndromes are briefly described. The reader who requires more detailed information is referred to such authoritative but readable sources as Frazer (1968) and Creamer (1974).

Interference with digestive processes. If nutrients are not digested in the first place they clearly cannot be absorbed. Conditions that are associated with malabsorption from this cause include:

a. diseases of the exocrine pancreas
b. absence of enterokinase
c. the Zollinger-Ellison syndrome
d. lack of disaccharidases

Enterokinase is the enzyme released from the duodenum in response to food there. It converts trypsinogen to trypsin and so ensures that proteolysis can occur when it is needed. As a result of a congenital defect a very few individuals cannot elaborate enterokinase. The Zollinger-Ellison syndrome is caused by a pancreatic tumour that secretes gastrin and thereby provokes the secretion of excessive amounts of hydrochloric acid that renders the intestinal contents so acid that the pancreatic and intestinal enzymes are inactivated. Disaccharidases (which convert the disaccharide moieties of carbohydrate digestion into absorbable monosaccharides) occur in the endothelial cells of the intestinal mucosa. Congenital factors and damage to the mucosa, as in gastroenteritis, may result in disaccharidase deficiency. Another important cause of malabsorption because of disaccharide lack is severe malnutrition.

Exclusion of bile from the intestine. If bile salts cannot reach the intestine the absorption of fat and of fat soluble vitamins is impeded. Circumstances in which this occurs, include, among others, obstructive jaundice and cirrhosis of the liver but bile salt deficiency may occur too in diverticulosis and in Crohn's disease (see below). Drugs that bind to, or otherwise inactivate, bile salts can also induce steatorrhoea. Substances in this category include neomycin and cholestyramine.

Crohn's disease (regional enteritis) is a condition of disputed aetiology in which lengths of small intestine (usually the ileum) suffer inflammatory changes that spread across the whole extent of their walls so that they ultimately become thick and rigid with a much narrowed lumen. Pain, diarrhoea, loss of weight and other stigmata of malabsorption are prominent features of the disease.

Bile salts are normally recycled by continuous secretion into and absorption from the intestine (with a degree of 'topping up' by newly synthesized material) in the enterohepatic circuit. A deficiency of bile salts soon develops if their reabsorption is seriously interfered with since they pass into the colon instead of keeping on the enterohepatic merry-go-round. For this reason steatorrhoea occurs when

Crohn's disease affects an appreciable fraction of the small intestine. The critical length is of the order of half a metre. The bile salts that pass into the colon may seriously depress the absorption of water there so further increasing the diarrhoea. Some relief from this *choleretic enteropathy* can be obtained by taking cholestyramine which binds and inactivates bile salts. This form of treatment will not, of course, afford any amelioration of the steatorrhoea.

Coeliac disease. This well known condition is said to be the most common cause of malabsorption in the British Isles. In the past, a number of other names have been attached to the disease and some of them linger on in the textbooks, to the confusion of all but the gastroenterologists. The most common of these persistent synonyms is *idiopathic steatorrhoea.*

Coeliac disease often becomes manifest in childhood and persists for life, but in some cases overt symptoms have appeared for the first time in middle life. It affects principally the duodenum and jejunum but it occasionally spreads into the upper reaches of the ileum. The epithelial cells of the mucous membrane exhibit widespread damage, the intestinal villi become atrophic and an inflammatory exudate appears in the submucous tissue.

In the infant, intestinal absorption is disturbed to such an extent that the growing body is deprived of its essential nutrients—a situation aggravated by a characteristic loss of appetite—so that coeliac disease presents us with a miserable, anaemic, wasted child passing the pale bulky faeces of steatorrhoea. When the disease first appears in adult life, disorders caused by malabsorption of calcium and folic acid dominate the clinical picture but these disorders are likely to be accompanied by others (including nervous and mental disturbances) that cannot be so obviously related to the deficient absorption of essential components of the diet.

Coeliac disease is treated by imposing on the victim the rule that he must avoid gluten for the rest of his life. This treatment is invariably successful in cases that begin in infancy and usually successful in those that arise in adult life.

The characteristic consistency of flour dough is conferred on it by gliadin and glutenin, high molecular weight proteins whose actual composition varies according to the species of grain from which the flour was derived. They undergo enzymatic hydrolysis in the intestine in the usual way but one of the resulting polypeptides (gluten) is toxic to the intestines of the minority of individuals who develop coeliac disease. The importance of gluten in the aetiology of the disease is established not only by the relief that is provided by a diet that yields no gluten (the so-called 'gluten free' diet) but also by the fact that symptoms immediately reappear if the treated patient allows gluten to enter his body. Although not all glutens are equally toxic, the only safe rule for the patient with coeliac disease is to avoid wheat, oats, barley and all foods made with flour derived from these cereals.

Coeliac disease has a hereditary basis and is probably of autoimmune origin.

Tropical sprue. In this disease, widespread in the tropics, the mucosa of small intestine (particularly the jejunum) suffers extensive atrophic changes so that absorption processes are seriously impaired. The resulting diarrhoea must be dealt with as must any nutritional deficiency resulting from the deranged intestinal function. The aetiology of tropical sprue remains a mystery.

Other conditions. Among the other conditions associated with malabsorption states we must list obstruction of intestinal lymph flow, gastric and intestinal surgery, parasitic infestation of the intestinal tract and some systemic diseases such as diabetes mellitus and Addison's disease.

Diverticulosis (or diverticular disease) has already been mentioned as a possible cause of malabsorption and hence of diarrhoea but it will also be referred to as both a cause and a consequence of constipation. It is clearly a disease of some significance. In it, the colonic musculature becomes hypertrophied and its contractions more powerful. The contractions eventually cause the extrusion of multiple small pockets *(diverticula)* of mucous membrane through naturally weak spots in the intestinal wall. The condition may be symptomless, or it may cause no more than pain and either diarrhoea or constipation but if the diverticula suffer inflammation they may precipitate an acute abdominal crisis with fever, collapse and bleeding.

The treatment of diarrhoea, which features in all malabsorption syndromes, is discussed later in this chapter (p. 651).

Laxatives and purgatives

Many people have an almost obsessional interest in their bowel movements. The origin of this preoccupation with the processes of evacuation is a matter for the psychologist but there is no doubt that it is sustained by the ordinary man's ignorance of physiology, nurtured by well meaning but misinformed articles in popular magazines and exploited by advertising which suggests that clear complexion, bright eyes, freedom from headache and a general feeling of wellbeing are all dependent on the maintenance of a daily 'opening of the bowels'. The taking of purgatives (drugs which cause defaecation) is, consequently, widespread.

It is certainly true that modern diets, which lack the 'bulk' provided by the indigestible fibres in less well refined food, tend to reduce the frequency of defaecation and thereby predispose to the development of some disorders of the large intestine, particularly diverticulosis. The wise man will, without becoming obsessional over the matter, make sure that his bowel movements are reasonably regular. To achieve this usually requires either no effort at all on his part or the adoption of very simple measures such as the taking of gentle daily exercise and a diet in which the proportion of high residue items (see below) has been modestly increased. It does not justify the daily ingestion of either purgative drugs or of large amounts of the oddly-named 'health foods'.

Regularity of bowel performance is recommended as a protection against long term ills: there is no evidence that irregularity or infrequency of defaecation over short periods of time can affect the wellbeing of the otherwise healthy person. Although distension of the rectum does produce vague feelings of discomfort, most of the symptoms of constipation are of psychogenic origin. The long-standing view that constipation can cause headache as a result of distension of the intestinal wall takes a long time to die, although the experimental evidence shows that the view is unfounded. An older idea that absorption of toxic substances can take place from faecal material delayed in the large intestine was shown to be false many years ago, though it, too, still persists and would no doubt be offered as the apparently rational reason for his indulgence by the habitual taker of purgatives. It also forms the guiding principle of many so-called 'health' clinics in which restriction of food intake is combined with the administration of enemas for the purpose of evacuating the large intestine. This provides an uncomfortable and expensive way of achieving an unnecessary end.

It should not be necessary to emphasize that any *change* in the bowel habits not associated with a change in environment, dietary regime or drug intake may indicate the development of a pathological condition in the large intestine. Constipation arising in this way calls for a rigorous physical examination and not for the administration of a purgative drug.

The use of purgatives should be restricted to cases where it is necessary to ensure soft faeces because of local conditions (such as haemorrhoids) of the rectum or anus or after surgical operation in this region; to counteract the constipation which arises as a side effect of some drugs (such as atropine and its congeners, morphine and ganglion blocking agents); to prevent faecal impaction in those susceptible to it; to minimize the cardiac effort involved in the act of evacuation after myocardial infarction or in those otherwise debilitated and to empty the intestine for particular diagnostic or therapeutic reasons.

Constipation and the drugs used in its treatment have attracted a large and not entirely well defined vocabulary. The word constipation itself simply implies a delayed passage of faeces through the intestine, the final act of defaecation being quite normal. In *dyschezia* it is the act of evacuation which is deranged: small amounts of faeces may be passed but the rectum is not completely emptied, even after repeated passage of faeces. Although all substances which cause emptying of the intestine are properly called purgatives (or cathartics) the term is often restricted to those which cause a powerful contraction of the bowel. Laxatives and aperients have a 'gentler' action, producing a soft but well formed stool while drastics and purges (these terms are now obsolescent) have a more violent action, emptying the intestine so rapidly that watery stools are produced. To a large extent, however, the difference between an aperient and a purge is purely quantitative and most purgatives can produce gentle or violent defaecation depending on the dose administered.

Defaecation occurs in response to peristaltic waves which pass some of the contents of the large intestine into the rectum. The ensuing distension initiates further reflex contraction with relaxation of the anal sphincters and emptying not only of the rectum itself but also of the distal half of the colon. The defaecation reflex can be temporarily inhibited by an act of will and on the other hand defaecation is usually aided by voluntary effort; after a short inspiration, an expiratory effort is made with the glottis closed. Pressure rises in the abdominal and pelvic cavities as a result of the powerful contraction of the abdominal muscles with the diaphragm held in its inspiratory position. The increased pressure aids contraction of the rectum: it also restricts the return of blood to the heart and reddening of the face and distension of the neck veins accompanies difficult defaecation. From what has been said concerning the mechanism of defaecation, the mode of action of the main types of purgatives should be readily appreciated.

(i) *Bulk-forming purgatives* increase the bulk of the non-absorbable portion of the intestinal contents. This increases the stimulus for peristalsis.

(ii) *Stimulant or irritant purgatives* increase the irritability of the intestinal muscle so that it responds more readily to distension. They do not necessarily affect the large intestine directly since increased motility in the small intestine may initiate increased activity in the colon.

(iii) *Lubricants* soften the faeces and ease defaecation.

BULK-FORMING PURGATIVES
Diet
The non-absorbable residue in the diet supplies much of the bulk which provides the stimulus for normal defaecation and a high residue diet (containing whole meal bread, cereals, dried fruits and other items supplying 'roughage') encourages defaecation. The use of high residue diets has become something of a cult among the bowel-conscious and it is worth pointing out that over enthusiastic indulgence in these diets can cause the very condition it is hoped to prevent. In the laboratory, every student of pharmacology soon learns that an overstretched muscle loses its responsiveness to drugs and to physical stimuli. Similarly overdistension of the intestine by unabsorbable food residues may lead to atony of the intestine which becomes insensitive to the stimulus which normally causes emptying.

Saline purgatives
Some inorganic salts and salts of inorganic cations with

simple organic anions are used as purgatives. The traditional explanation of their mode of action is that one or both of the ions is not absorbed, or is absorbed very slowly, from the gastrointestinal tract and its osmotic action causes the retention of fluid. As a result the intestinal contents are increased in bulk. However, Harvey and Read (1975) have adduced convincing evidence for the view that the saline purgatives stimulate the secretion of cholecystokinin-pancreozymin which evokes the secretion of intestinal and pancreatic juice and also inhibits the intestinal reabsorption of sodium chloride and water. The motor effects of the local hormone ensure that the large volume of fluid so formed is hurried into the large intestine where it initiates peristalsis by the usual mechanism, facilitated in this instance by the stimulant action of cholecystokinin-pancreozymin on the colonic musculature. Saline purgatives act within one or two hours of their administration; they may cause considerable loss of water and electrolytes from the body and this precludes the use of saline purgatives as serious therapeutic agents. Magnesium ions are toxic after absorption and toxic effects may be encountered in patients with impaired kidney function. The saline purgatives are also potentially dangerous in cases of advanced cardiovascular disease. However, they remain popular self-medication agents. Sulphates have been widely used as saline purgatives. Magnesium sulphate (Epsom salts) was very popular but sodium sulphate is cheaper and just as effective. Magnesium oxide and hydroxide are used primarily as antacids (p. 643) but they also have laxative properties.

The sulphates have a bitter taste and citrates and tartrates are more pleasant to take. They are often presented in the form of powders which produce an effervescent drink. Seidlitz powders, for instance, contain sodium potassium tartrate (7.5 grams) mixed with sodium bicarbonate (2.5 grams). This is dissolved in water and tartaric acid (2.5 grams) from a separate package is added. The result is an effervescing drink and an effective saline purgative, though the layman who takes it is usually unaware that its sole action is that of purgation and that the condition (a headache or a hangover) from which he seeks relief is neither the result, as he imagines, of disturbed liver function nor is it amenable to treatment by purgation. The fresh taste provided by the drink probably contributes as much as the purgation to the relief obtained which is due principally, however, to the passage of time. Similar remarks apply to other 'salt' drinks.

Colloidal purgatives

On ingestion these substances, which are hydrophilic colloids, absorb fluid and swell, keeping the intestinal contents moist and bulky and increasing intestinal motility. They are relatively non-irritant. Substances in this class include agar, sodium alginate, mucilaginous polysaccharides (such as Metamucil, Isogel and Normacol)

obtained from vegetable sources, methylcellulose (Celevac) and sodium carboxymethylcellulose. Cellulose forms much of the indigestible material in the high residue diets already referred to. Apart from producing occasional allergic reactions, all these compounds are non-toxic but their use is limited, though they are of some value in the treatment of chronic constipation.

Enemas

If warm soapy water is introduced into the rectum, it causes the evacuation of the large intestine since it stimulates muscular activity in both the rectum and the colon. One pint of a five per cent solution of soft soap is still widely used in hospitals as a means of evacuating the lower colon and rectum before surgery or radiography of that region of the intestine. It is not a procedure that appeals overmuch to the psychiatrically normal patient who will certainly experience discomfort and may well suffer severe pain. 'Few therapeutic procedures prescribed by the doctor and carried out by the nurse can be so infrequently experienced by either...If medical and nursing students were required to receive a soap enema as part of their training its dramatic demise could be confidently predicted' (Godding, 1971).

Soft soap enemas sometimes do more than cause discomfort: soap sometimes induces anaphylactic reactions, it is irritant to the gut and this can result in severe local reactions or in a fatal cardiovascular collapse while the absorption of potassium ions from the rectum may have disastrous consequences in the patient with advanced cardiovascular disease.

When it is deemed necessary to give an enema, a hypertonic saline solution provides a much safer evacuant solution than soap. Alternatively the lower intestine can simply be irrigated by a large volume of warmed normal saline. Attempts to evacuate the rectum by the use of suppositories containing an ordinary purgative drug have not been very successful.

Some otherwise healthy people are given to patronizing private clinics where 'colonic irrigation' is offered. Some of these individuals are misguided cranks who believe that a 'cleansed' intestine provides a sure road to a healthy body and a pure soul. The motives of the others can only be guessed at.

STIMULANT OR IRRITANT PURGATIVES
Anthraquinone purgatives

All these compounds have a direct action on the colon, stimulating activity in the small intestine by a secondary reflex. Their purgative action is therefore slow in onset, appearing about eight hours after the drug is taken. The anthraquinone glycosides in the crude vegetable preparations mentioned below are slowly broken down in the gastrointestinal tract with the liberation of emodins or similar compounds. The emodins are probably absorbed in the small intestine and secreted by the colon, where they probably stimulate the neurones of the intestinal plexuses (Fig. 37.1). Because of the possibility that they may eventually induce irreversible damage to these neurones, the anthraquinone purgatives should not be taken over a prolonged period of time.

Aloes and aloin Aloin is a mixture of the active principles of aloes. Aloes and aloin tend to cause griping (painful spasm of the intestine) and venous congestion in the pelvic viscera.

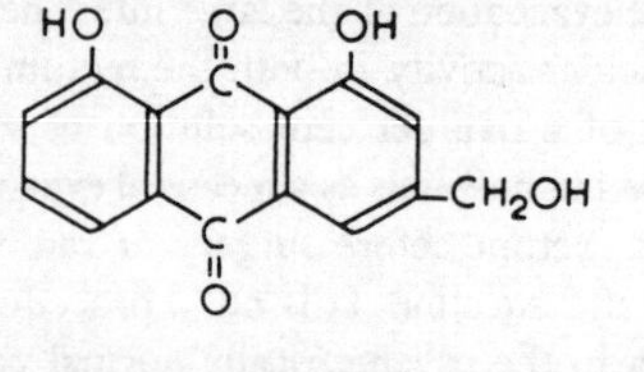

Emodin from aloes

Cascara sagrada is a popular member of many domestic medicine cupboards. It is free of toxic actions but it should not be taken over long periods. It is less prone to cause griping than aloes or senna. Cascara is a mixture of four principal glycosides (the cascarosides) with a small proportion of sennosides and aloin. A standardized preparation of cascara is now available.

Rhubarb preparations contain tannins as well as anthraquinone glycosides. The astringent effects of the tannins may cause constipation following purgation.

Senna. An infusion of senna pods or leaves is another traditional purgative. It may cause griping because of the presence of resins, oils and other impurities in the crude preparations. The chemically pure purgative principles, the sennosides A and B have been isolated. They are glycosides that arise by hydrolysis of the primary glycosides that occur in the unheated plant. Improved methods of making extracts of senna pods preserve the primary glycosides in an intact form and this, combined with accurate assay methods, has permitted the development of a standardized preparation of senna (Senokot). Senna is the principal component of a number of popular preparations the best known of which is compound syrup of figs.

1,8 Dihydroxyanthraquinone (danthron) is a breakdown product and the principal active moiety of the senna glycosides. It is a less potent purgative than senna itself perhaps because some of the small molecules are absorbed

1,8-Dihydroxyanthraquinone
(danthron)

in the upper reaches of the gastrointestinal tract and so can exert no colonic action.

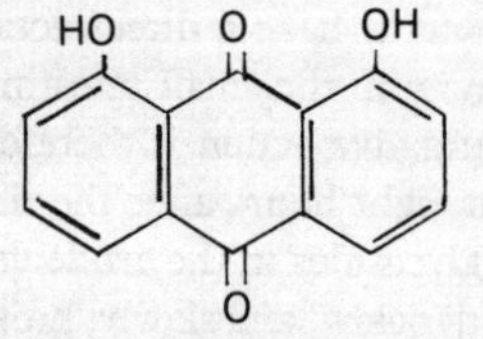

Purgative resins
These substances are powerful irritants which cause an effusion of fluid into the intestine. For this reason they are sometimes referred to as hydragogue purgatives. The purgative resins (which include jalap, ipomoea, elaterin, colocynth and podophyllum) are not now used as purgatives, though podophyllum is employed as a wart remover.

Irritant oils
Croton oil is a highly irritant and very dangerous substance. Acute enteritis and collapse may follow its use as a purgative and death is reported to have occurred after the ingestion of as few as ten drops of the oil. Its use as a purgative is clearly unjustified.

Castor oil is obtained from the seeds of the castor oil plant. For many years it was the schoolroom panacea and because of its unpleasant smell and taste it must claim the doubtful distinction of having caused more unhappiness to no therapeutic avail than any other drug of childhood. Castor oil contains the glycerides of ricinoleic and isoricinoleic acids. The purgative principle is ricinoleic acid which is liberated, as a result of enzymic hydrolysis, in the small intestine; the hydrolysis requires the presence of bile. Ricinoleic acid acts primarily on the small intestine and its purgative action therefore occurs within two hours of its administration. Castor oil is a safe purgative but it may cause griping and its use may be followed by prolonged constipation.

Other compounds
Phenolphthalein is an indicator, turning red in alkaline solution. Its purgative properties have been known since the beginning of the century when the Hungarian government caused it to be added to inferior wines so that they could be readily identified by the addition of a drop of alkali. Phenolphthalein is absorbed by the small intestine whence it is secreted into the bile (and hence the small intestine) and into the colon. The secreted drug is reabsorbed and a prolonged reabsorption-resecretion cycle is set up, maintaining the purgative action for several days. Following this action, constipation occurs and during this

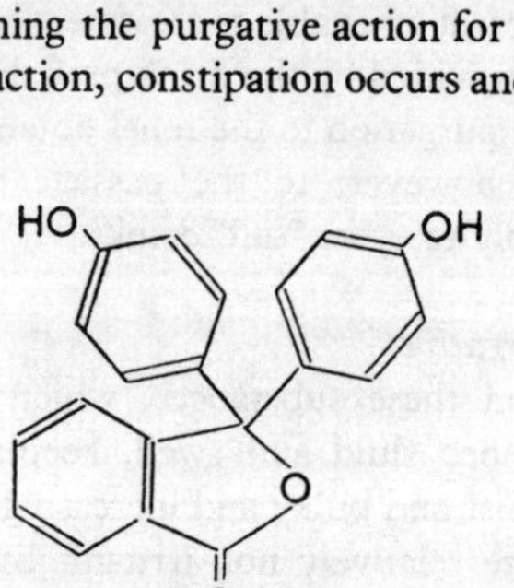

Phenolphthalein

period a further dose of phenolphthalein may be taken thus causing a habit to be formed. The dose of phenolphthalein is 60–300 mg and it is relatively non-toxic, though in susceptible individuals a characteristic purplish skin rash may be produced and isolated fatalities from an allergic encephalitis have been reported. Some people are highly susceptible to the purgative action of phenolphthalein and they may suffer abdominal pain, violent purging and sometimes collapse after quite small doses. Because of its indicator properties, phenolphthalein imparts an alarming pink colour to alkaline urine. It produces copious watery faeces.

Bisacodyl (Dulcolax) is a purgative that was developed in the course of studies into structure-activity relationships in compounds related to phenolphthalein. Bisacodyl, unlike phenolpthalein is not absorbed from the gastrointestinal tract. It is given in the form of enteric coated tablets that prevent its exerting an action in the upper parts of the gastrointestinal tract (p. 33) but alkalis may dissolve the enteric coating. Patients who need to take both bisacodyl and an antacid should take the drugs at different times. The oral dose of bisacodyl is 10 to 15 mg but it is sometimes given in the form of a suppository. It causes no adverse side effect other than occasional griping if the dose is too high.

Bisacodyl

Sulphur Brimstone and treacle is another ancient schoolroom horror, as all Dickens readers know. Sulphur itself has no purgative action but in the intestine it is partly converted into sodium and potassium sulphides which irritate the intestine. Sulphur administration may lead to the production of hydrogen sulphide which is excreted in the faeces; some may also be absorbed, to be excreted in the breath to which it imparts the same unpleasant odour. It is these aesthetically unpleasant consequences of sulphur administration that have led to its being abandoned as a purgative agent.

Obsolete drugs. The toxicity of mercurous chloride (calomel) and oxyphenisatin is too high to justify their continued use as purgatives.

LUBRICANTS (STOOL SOFTENERS)
Liquid paraffin
Liquid paraffin is a mixture of hydrocarbons. Only minute amounts are absorbed and none is digested. In the past, liquid paraffin was a favoured purgative and it is still used in some quarters in spite of the formidable case that has been built up against it in recent years. It may impede the absorption of fat soluble vitamins and cases of vitamin deficiency due to liquid paraffin are still being reported (see, for instance, Sinclair, 1967). It has also been known to cause lipid pneumonia as a result of its accidental passage into the trachea instead of the oesophagus. There is sound evidence that the prolonged use of liquid paraffin might produce carcinoma of the colon or rectum. A minor disadvantage of liquid paraffin is the leakage of oil from the anus. This is not only unpleasant but it may retard the healing of the wounds in that area that were the reason for prescribing the purgative in the first place. There seems to be no good reason why liquid paraffin should ever be used.

Dioctyl sodium sulphosuccinate
Dioctyl sodium sulphosuccinate (Colace; Dio-Medicone) and the corresponding calcium compound (Surfak) have detergent properties and are employed as faecal softeners because they allow water to penetrate into the faeces. They can be taken by mouth (the dose of the sodium compound is about 25 to 55 mg) but there must be considerable doubt concerning the wisdom of introducing surface active agents into the stomach. The stool softeners are sometimes incorporated into retention enemas (small volume enemas that are retained for some six hours before being washed out) intended to soften hard and impacted faeces. Combinations of a stool softener with another purgative such as bisacodyl (as in Dulcodos) are potentially toxic and should be avoided.

Dioctyl sodium sulphosuccinate

The poloxalkols
These nonionic detergents are polymers of polyoxyethylene and polyoxypropylene with similar actions and uses to the sulphosuccinates.

The purgatives of choice today include bulking agents, bisacodyl and the senna glycosides.

The treatment of diarrhoea
If diarrhoea is an identifiable organism, the appropriate chemotherapeutic agent must be used. Many instances of long-continued diarrhoea are functional in origin, no physical cause for the condition being detectable. Treat-

ment must be directed towards the patient's psychological condition. Most cases of diarrhoea, however, are short lived and are the consequence of a very mild infection or the ingestion of something has caused intestinal irritation. In these cases, which occur particularly in children, symptomatic treatment is justified. Care must be taken to prevent depletion of water and salts and a mixture of sodium chloride and sodium bicarbonate in water should be given if water and salt deficiency threatens. Kaolin and chalk form a coating to the intestine which reduces its irritability and may absorb the material causing the diarrhoea. Opium derivatives have a constipating action and therefore allow more time for any adsorbent present in the intestine to exert its action. The B.P.C. mixture is thus useful in the treatment of mild diarrhoea. Other morphine like compounds employed in the treatment of diarrhoea include codeine phosphate (50 mg three times daily) and diphenoxylate hydrochloride, a substance structurally related to pethidine (p. 430). It is given in twice daily doses of 5 mg either alone or as Lomotil, a proprietary mixture of diphenoxylate and atropine. Although constipating in their action, morphine and its congeners actually increase the tone of the circular muscle of the intestine but they inhibit propulsive movements. This has the effect of reducing the rate at which faeces are moved along the intestine so that more time is available for water absorption. The drugs must be given with caution if the diarrhoea is associated with colicky spasms of the intestine or is the result of disorders such as diverticular disease that involve an overall increase in the tone and activity of the colonic musculature. In these circumstances the atropine like antispasmodic drugs (p. 228) are likely to offer more relief than the opiates. Mebeverine (Colofac) may also be beneficial. This drug is a papaverine derivative and as such it brings about intestinal relaxation by a direct action on smooth muscle (p. 705).

Morphine inhibits secretory activity in the gastrointestinal tract and this contributes to its antidiarrhoeal action by helping to bring about the reduction in faecal volume that is the whole aim of treatment. Another way of achieving this end is to give a water absorbing agent such as methylcellulose and this form of treatment is sometimes more effective than those that aim to influence intestinal movements. It is left to the reader to reflect on the versatility of compounds that can be recommended for the treatment of both constipation and diarrhoea!

Many cases of mild diarrhoea respond best to a day's abstinence from food. This provides what is sometimes graphically but inelegantly described as 'gut rest'.

THE PHARMACOLOGY OF THE ISOLATED INTESTINE

The isolated intestine—especially the guinea pig ileum—is still the most widely used preparation in experimental pharmacology. This extraordinarily simple arrangement of an inch of intestine in a saline medium, attached by a cotton thread to the most rudimentary of levers, has provided the experimental foundation for ideas of considerable sophistication, as can be seen by reference, for instance, to contemporary receptor theories.

The activity of the intestine is controlled to a considerable extent by local mechanisms which retain much of their function in the isolated preparation, and substances which have an action on the intestine *in vitro* may act directly on muscle fibres or directly via the surviving autonomous plexuses.

The innervation of the intestine is shown, in a schematic way, in Fig. 37.1. The parasympathetic supply of the intestine as far as the caecum is provided by the vagus nerves while the sacral nerves supply the large intestine. These fibres are, of course, preganglionic in nature. They ramify in two plexuses, one of which is located between the longitudinal and the circular muscle coats (the *myenteric* or *Auerbach's plexus*) while the other (the *submucous* or *Meissner's plexus*) is found immediately deep to the submucosa. Postganglionic fibres arise in the plexuses and are distributed to the intestinal muscles (including that of the villi) and glands. The sympathetic control of the intestine is rather less important. Only the postganglionic fibres of the sympathetic supply survive in the isolated intestine since the preganglionic fibres terminate in the abdomen, in the coeliac and mesenteric ganglia. Finally, some of the sensory fibres arising in the mucous membrane make synaptic connection with the neurones of the autonomous plexuses. This arrangement enables movements of the intestine to be initiated and controlled by reflex mechanisms located entirely within the organ itself. Co-ordination of movements in neighbouring segments of the intestine is effected by the interconnections, along its length, of the neurones in the plexuses.

The actions of drugs on the isolated intestine are discussed in the chapters of this book which deal with the individual compounds but it may be helpful to summarize here the responses to some of the more frequently encountered drugs. They all relate to the unstimulated guinea pig ileum.

Acetylcholine, histamine and 5-hydroxytryptamine all cause contraction of the isolated ileum. The contractions are reduced or prevented by appropriate antagonists, those most usually employed being, respectively, atropine, mepyramine and bromolysergic acid diethylamide (BOL). These antagonists enable the neurohumours to be identified in tissue extracts. Conversely, in a drug screening project, the demonstration that a compound antagonizes the stimulant action of acetylcholine, histamine or 5-hydroxytryptamine gives important information concerning its pharmacological nature. It should be remembered that the antagonists are not entirely specific and when

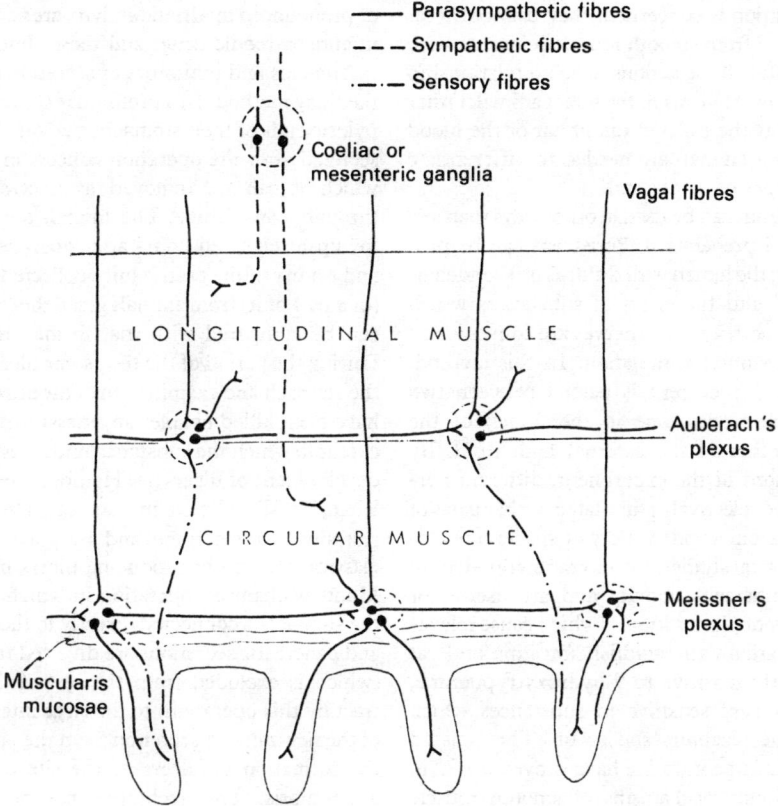

Fig. 37.1 Innervation of the gastrointestinal tract (schematic).

identifying the constituents of a tissue extract, the presence of one of the neurohumours should not be too readily inferred unless, after removal of the appropriate antagonist from the bath, the responses to the neurohumour and to the extract return at the same rate.

Other choline esters also stimulate the ileum. They are generally less active than acetylcholine itself but if they are present in a tissue extract in unknown amounts they can only be differentiated from acetylcholine by the technique of differential bioassay (p. 210).

Nicotine stimulates the ganglion cells in the intestine. Its action can be distinguished from that of acetylcholine by the fact that contractions induced by nicotine are antagonized by ganglion blocking agents such as hexamethonium and by local anaesthetics as well as by atropine. The action of acetylcholine is prevented only by atropine. The antagonism towards nicotine in the isolated intestine forms a useful test for ganglion blocking activity in substances being subjected to pharmacological screening. 5-Hydroxytryptamine also stimulates nerve elements in the intestine so that its action is partly inhibited by atropine, hexamethonium and local anaesthetics.

The pharmacologically active polypeptides and organic acids discussed in Chapter 22 also cause intestinal contrac-

tion. They can be identified in tissue extracts by the facts that some of them cause a characteristically slow contraction, that the activity of the polypeptides is abolished by incubation with trypsin or chymotrypsin and that none of the compounds is susceptible to antagonism by small doses of atropine, mepyramine or bromolysergic acid diethylamide. Further differentiation is made by consideration of the source of the extract and its other pharmacological properties.

Sympathomimetic substances have a predominantly inhibitory action on the intestine but since the isolated ileum shows no spontaneous activity, this inhibitory effect is usually not observed unless the intestine is made to contract by a stimulant substance. As would be expected, the inhibition produced by sympathomimetic substances is characterized by its lack of specificity, a particular dose of the drug inhibiting to an approximately equal extent contractions due to acetylcholine, histamine, 5-hydroxytryptamine or barium chloride. The last named substance, added to the organ bath in a concentration of about 200 μg per ml, is a useful stimulant when the action of inhibitory drugs is being investigated.

Sympathomimetic substances act directly on the smooth muscle of the intestine and, as far as their action on the isolated preparation is concerned, they cannot therefore be distinguished from smooth muscle relaxants such as papaverine (p. 705) whose actions have no relationship to the sympathetic mechanisms in the intact animal. Other preparations (such as the isolated rabbit ear or the blood pressure of the intact animal) are needed to differentiate between the two types of compound.

The guinea pig ileum can be used in other ways than as a simple unstimulated preparation. Peristalsis can be produced by distending the lumen with fluid, as in Trendelenburg's preparation, and the effect of substances which particularly modify activity in the nerves are conveniently studied during transmural stimulation. In this method, due to Paton (1954), a current is passed between two coaxial (parallel) electrodes, one in the lumen of the intestine and the other in the external bath fluid. By altering the conditions of the experiment, different nervous elements can be selectively stimulated. Other parts of the intestine taken from a wide variety of species are also used in pharmacological studies: rat and rabbit duodenum exhibit strong spontaneous activity and are useful for studying the activity of plasma kinins (which cause relaxation in this preparation), the goldfish intestine and rat colon are particularly sensitive to 5-hydroxytryptamine, the rat jejunum is very sensitive to substances which stimulate muscarinic receptors and so on. The isolated taeniae coli from the large intestine have proved useful in the study of the ionic mechanisms of smooth muscle activity.

Presence of humoral substances in the gastrointestinal tract
Acetylcholine, ATP, histamine, 5-hydroxytryptamine, substance P and prostaglandins are all present in the gastrointestinal tract. Their distribution in the different layers and anatomical subdivisions of the gut is considered in the chapters dealing with the individual substances where their possible role as regulators of gastrointestinal function is also discussed. It is evident that the nervous control of intestinal movements is a matter of some complexity. Kosterlitz indeed puts forward the view that in many contexts the isolated intestine can be regarded as a model of the brain. The careful reader of this book will soon appreciate the validity of this claim.

THE SCREENING AND CLINICAL TESTING OF DRUGS THAT ACT ON THE GASTROINTESTINAL TRACT

The most important drugs for the treatment of peptic ulcer are atropine-like drugs, antacids and histamine H_2-antagonists. Antispasmodics can be assessed by their inhibitory action on smooth muscle preparations stimulated to contract by acetylcholine or by acetyl-β-methylcholine. The possession of local anaesthetic action and the absence

of pronounced mydriatic activity are additional advantages in antispasmodic drugs and these should be tested for.

Antacids and inhibitors of secretion can be screened by the Shay method. In a preliminary operation, rats have the pyloric ends of their stomachs tied off. All the gastric juice secreted after the operation collects in the stomach from which it can be removed as necessary by aspiration through a small tube. The animals are allowed to survive for up to eighteen hours after operation and the volume and acidity of the gastric juice collected during this period (or a part of it) from animals given the substance under test can be compared with that formed in control animals. During the period of the test, some ulceration will occur in the stomach and examination of the organ after the animals have been killed enables an assessment to be made of the extent to which the substance under test has prevented the development of ulcers (*see* Hambourger, Calvin and Houlahan, 1952). Ulcers in rats can also be produced by restraint, by reserpine and by cortisol injections. The classical method of producing ulcers in the dog is by the Mann-Williamson operation in which the pyloric end of the stomach is connected directly to the jejunum. The bile and pancreatic secretions are diverted from the duodenum (which is excluded from the rest of the gastrointestinal tract by this operation) to the large intestine. The absence of the neutralizing secretion from the pancreas encourages the formation of ulcers at the site of the gastrojejunal anastomosis. This technique has been extended, with success, to rats (Kuroyanagi and Necheles, 1961). Cats with gastric fistulae (which enable gastric juice to be collected from the stomach via a cannula opening on to the abdominal wall) also make useful chronic preparations for the study of antacids and histamine-H_2 antagonists. Histamine is given to stimulate acid secretion and the inhibitory effect of antacid on this secretion is measured. The same type of study can be carried out on human volunteers whose gastric juice is continuously sampled by way of a stomach tube. In the most recent development of this technique, up to three glass electrodes are placed in the stomach itself. Leads pass from the stomach, through the mouth, to a meter which records the pH of the gastric contents continuously.

Specific methods for assessing antagonism at H_2 receptors are discussed elsewhere (p. 355).

Purgative action in rats is assessed by placing a suitable marker (such as carbon particles), with or without the purgative under test, in the stomach of previously starved rats. The animals are then allowed free access to food for about one hour, after which they are killed and the movement of the marker is determined by direct inspection of the opened intestine. The extent of the movement in those animals given the drug is compared with that in the control animals. In other methods, the number and consistency of the faeces passed by mice is measured. Apart from its use in the screening of purgatives, the rate of passage of faeces is useful for assessing the extent to which emotional stress is occurring in experimental animals.

Purgative action in man is measured by determination of the number of bowel movements and the consistency of the stool. Sometimes the wet and dry weight and the volume of the stool are estimated. From studies of this type it is possible to estimate the average number of stools per day following a purgative and to compare this figure with those obtained with other purgatives and a control series. The consistency of the stools is compared in a similar fashion. Side effects of an undesirable nature such as griping, nausea and distension are also taken into account in assessing the purgative.

BIBLIOGRAPHY

Books, monographs and reviews

Avery Jones, F. and Sullivan, F. M. (Eds) (1972). *Carbenoxolone in Gastroenterology*. London: Butterworths.

Avery Jones, F. and Godding, F. W. (Eds) (1973). *Management of Constipation*. Oxford: Blackwell.

Burgen, A. S. V. and Emmelin, N. G. (1961). *Physiology of the Salivary Glands*. London: Arnold.

Creamer, B. (1974) (Ed.) *The Small Intestine*. London: Heinemann.

Davson, H. (1970) *A Textbook of General Physiology*, 4th ed., pp. 811-836 London: Churchill.

Frazer, A. C. (1968). *Malabsorption Syndromes*. London: Heinemann.

Gregory, R. A. (1962). *Secretory Mechanisms of the Gastrointestinal Tract*. London: Arnold.

Hilton, S. M. (1960). Plasma kinins and blood flow. In *Polypeptides which affect Smooth Muscles and Blood Vessels*, pp. 258-262, ed. Schachter, M. London: Pergamon.

James, A. H. (1957). *The Physiology of Gastric Digestion*. London: Arnold.

Jones, F. A. (1958). *Modern Trends in Gastro-enterology*. London: Butterworth.

Lewis, G. P. (1967). The role of plasma kinins as mediators of functional vasodilatation. *Gastroenterology*, **52**, 406-413.

Pinder, R. M., Brogden, R. N., Sawyer, Phyllis R., Speight, T. M., Spencer, Rosalind and Avery, G. S. (1976). Carbenoxolone: A review of its pharmacological properties and therepeutic efficacy in peptic ulcer disease. *Drugs*, **11**, 241-307.

Pinder, R. M. Brogden, R. N., Sawyer, Phyllis R., Speight, T. M., and Avery, G. S (1976) Metoclopramide: A review of its pharmacological properties and clinical use. *Drugs*, **12**, 81-131.

Schachter, M. and Beilenson, Susanne (1967). Kallikrein and vasodilatation in the submaxillary gland. *Gastroenterology*, **52**, 401-405.

Spencer, R. B. (1960). *The Intestinal Tract*, Springfield: Thomas.

Symposium, (1975). Tri-potassium di-citrato bismuthate. *Postgrad. med. J.*, **51**, (supp. 5), 7-46.

Truelove, S. C. (1966). Movements of the large intestine. *Physiol. Rev.*, **46**. 457-512.

Vaughan Williams, E. M. (1954). The mode of action of drugs upon intestinal motility. *Pharmac. Rev.*, **6**, 159-190.

Original papers

Barton, Susanne, Karpinski, E., Moriwaki, C. and Schachter, M. (1976). Sialotonin: vasopressor substance in saliva and submandibular gland of the cat. *J. Physiol.*, **261**, 523-533.

Bhoola, K. D., Morley, J., Schachter, M. and Smaje, L. H. (1965). Vasodilatation in the submaxillary gland of the cat. *J. Physiol.*, **179**, 172-183.

Campbell-Mackie, M. (1959). The treatment of bowel dysfunction in infants and young children. *Practitioner*, **183**, 732-736.

Doll, R., Hill, I. D., Hutton, C. and Underwood, D. J. (1962). Clinical trial of a triterpenoid liquorice compound in gastric and duodenal ulcer. *Lancet*, **2**, 793-796.

Fairbairn, J. W. (1959). The cathartic action of anthraquinones. *The Pharmacology of Plant Phenolics*, pp. 39-49. London: Academic Press.

Godding, E. W. (1973). In: *Management of Constipation*. ed. Avery Jones, F. and Godding, F. W., p. 69. Oxford: Blackwell.

Hambourger, W. E., Calvin, L. D. Houlahan, D. A. (1952). A quantitative anti-ulcer assay using the Shay rat. *J. Pharmacol. exp. Ther.*, **106**, 392-393.

Harvey, R. F. and Read, A. E. (1973) Saline purgatives act by releasing cholecystokinin. *Lancet*, **ii**, 185-187.

Hay, A. M., (1975). The mechanism of action of metoclopramide. *Gut*, **16**, 403.

Hilton, S. M. and Lewis, G. P. (1955a). The cause of the vasodilatation accompanying activity in the submandibular salivary gland. *J. Physiol.*, **128**, 235-248.

Hilton, S. M. and Lewis, G. P., (1955b). The mechanism of the functional hyperaemia in the submandibular salivary gland. *J. Physiol.*, **129**, 253-271.

Hilton, S. M. and Lewis, G. P. (1956). The relationship between glandular activity, bradykinin formation and functional vasodilatation in the submandibular salivary gland. *J. Physiol.*, **134**, 471-483.

Kuroyanagi, Y. and Necheles, H. (1961). Mann-Williamson rat. *Proc. Soc. exp. Biol.*, **108**, 771-773.

Macgregor, A. G. and Williams, M. J. (1961). Antacid therapy. *Practitioner*, **198**, 447-452.

Moriwaki, C., Beilenson, S. and Schachter, M. (1968). Sialotonin: vasopressor substance in cat submaxillary saliva. *Nature, Lond.*, **217**, 270-271.

Morley, J. Schachter, M. and Smaje, L. H. (1966). Vasodilatation in the submaxillary gland of the rabbit. *J. Physiol.*, **187**, 595-602.

Paton, W. D. M. (1954). The response of the guinea pig ileum to electrical stimulation by coaxial electrodes. *J. Physiol.*, **127**, 40-41P.

Sinclair, L. (1967). Rickets from liquid paraffin. *Lancet*, **2**, 792.

Seed, J. C. and Harris, R. (1954). Some factors in the design of aperient studies. *Ann. N. Y. Acad Sci.*, **58**, 426-435.

38. Drugs that act on the liver

Since many drugs are detoxified by the liver and some are stored there, it is not surprising that liver damage is often a prominent feature of the body's reaction to toxic drugs. Conversely, of course, liver damage from any cause may prevent the metabolic transformation of drugs and of endogenous hormones and other regulatory substances. Thus, profound systemic disturbances may arise from damage to a single organ.

Hepatotoxic reactions sometimes arise acutely, they sometimes occur only during prolonged treatment with a drug or they may have a delayed onset, appearing some time after treatment has ceased.

Acute liver damage may take the form of necrotic or fatty changes or both; the part of the liver lobule which suffers damage varies to some extent according to the nature of the agent responsible for the damage. Chloroform, carbon tetrachloride and a number of other chlorinated aliphatic and aromatic compounds are particularly liable to cause acute liver injury. A single period of chloroform anaesthesia may be followed by delayed fatty and necrotic changes. These delayed reactions were responsible for many post-operative deaths in the early days of anaesthesia when chloroform was the only available anaesthetic agent. Carbon tetrachloride is even more toxic and serious damage to the liver has followed accidental inhalation of carbon tetrachloride in the course of its use for cleaning purposes.

In acute hepatitis, the liver cells undergo necrotic and inflammatory changes: cirrhosis of the liver is a manifestation of a more chronic injury process. It may follow the repeated administration of chloroform and it occurs, as is well known, in the course of chronic alcohol poisoning. In cirrhosis the liver substance undergoes fibrosis and enlargement. This causes narrowing of the intralobular sinusoids of the liver, the blood flow is reduced and the cirrhotic condition is thereby made even worse.

It is known that the nutritional deficiency that is the usual accompaniment of alcoholism plays a contributory part in the development of alcoholic cirrhosis but the importance of this factor must not be overestimated. In spite of frequent statements to the contrary, alcohol itself cannot escape responsibility as the principal immediate cause of alcoholic cirrhosis. Indeed there are those who maintain that malnutrition in the alcoholic actually provides a degree of protection against cirrhosis by reducing the metabolic work imposed on the organ.

Phosphorus and arsenic cause both acute and cirrhotic changes in the liver.

A large number of other substances cause liver damage and many a promising drug has had to be abandoned because of its hepatotoxic effects.

Much effort has been expended in attempts to discover ways in which liver damage can be prevented or reversed. Diets rich in carbohydrate appear to exert some protective action and it has also been suggested that choline and methionine might be of value in the treatment of liver injury caused by drugs or chemicals. There is, however, little experimental evidence to support this latter view.

CHOLERETIC AGENTS

The bile is formed by the liver and flows into the intestine *via* the bile duct, which opens, in common with the pancreatic duct, into the duodenum. Bile is an emulsifying agent and because of this, and because it activates pancreatic lipase, it aids the digestion and absorption of fats and the absorption of fat soluble vitamins. Bile is formed continuously by the liver and—in man and those other animals which possess the organ—it is stored in the gall bladder. Its release from the gall bladder is stimulated by *cholecystokinin-pancreozymin*, a gastrointestinal hormone (p. 642).

The most important constituents of the bile are cholic acid and desoxycholic acid. They are found as the sodium salts and, in combination with glycine and taurine respectively, as glycocholic and taurocholic acids. Salts of the last named acids are known as the bile salts.

Drugs that cause an increase in bile production are known as *choleretics* or *cholagogues*. Choleretics that evoke the secretion of a watery bile are sometimes referred to as *hydrocholeretics*.

Choleretics are employed to improve the supply of bile and so to improve digestion and absorption of fats and to lessen digestive discomfort after meals. They are particularly useful in conditions in which fat absorption is pathologically deranged. Because they increase the flow of bile down the biliary ducts, the choleretics are also sometimes used to treat *cholecystitis* (inflammation of the gall bladder), to wash away small gall stones and to prevent the formation of others. Most cases of gallstones, however, have to be treated by surgical excision of the gall bladder (*cholecystectomy*). Pathological conditions of the gall bladder are often associated with spasm of the sphincter of Oddi, which is situated at the junction of the bile and pancreatic ducts. The spasm can be relieved by atropine and it is advisable to ensure that spasm of the sphincter is not present when choleretics are being given. If there is obstruction or unrelieved spasm of the biliary tract, the use of choleretics may lead to an unwelcome increase of pressure behind the obstruction.

Instead of choleretics, bile itself or sodium tauroglycocholate can be given if fat absorption is impaired. These preparations are particularly useful when there is obstruction of the bile ducts or when the bile ducts are being drained. An extract of bile is available under the name of Desibyl.

Dehydrocholic acid (Decholin) is a potent hydrocholeretic obtained by the oxidation of cholic acid.

1-Phenylpropanol is a synthetic choleretic. It is a colourless oil which is presented in capsules.

Florantyrone (Zanchol) is a synthetic hydrocholeretic.

1-phenylpropan-1-ol

Florantyrone

SUBSTANCES USED IN THE INVESTIGATION OF LIVER FUNCTION

Sulphobromaphthalein sodium (Bromsulphalein, Bromthalein) is a dye which, if injected intravenously, combines with plasma proteins, from which it is then removed by the liver to be excreted in the bile. In the healthy subject, no more than 10 per cent of the administered dose (5 mg per kilogram) should remain in the blood 45 minutes after its injection. The bromsulphthalein test is extensively used to detect liver damage in experimental animals. Although it is

Sulphobromaphthalein sodium

also used in clinical investigations in man, some authorities question the wisdom of employing a diagnostic test which may impose an extra task on an already damaged liver.

Other diagnostic procedures are the galactose tolerance and the hippuric acid excretion tests. The first measures the ability of the liver to convert an orally administered dose of galactose into glucose. In the second test, sodium benzoate is taken by mouth. It is conjugated with glycine in the liver (and to a small extent in the kidney) to form hippuric acid. In the healthy individual about half the dose of sodium benzoate (6 grams) should be excreted in the urine, as hippuric acid, during the four hours after its ingestion. In the damaged liver the production and hence the excretion of hippuric acid is depressed. These tests, like the bromsulphthalein test, are open to the criticism that they may place an unnecessary burden on a malfunctioning liver. Another way of diagnosing liver damage involves the measurement of enzyme activities in the serum. This does not require the administration of material which has to be handled by the liver itself. The enzymes measured are glutamate-oxaloacetate transaminase (SGOT) and glutamate-pyruvate transaminase (SGPT). Additional information can sometimes be obtained by also measuring glutamate dehydrogenase and alkaline phosphatase. The activity of all these enzymes increases if the liver is damaged. By determining the extent and time course of the increased activity in the individual enzyme systems, it is possible to differentiate between the several forms of liver disease. The measurement of serum enzyme activities is also useful in the diagnosis of disease in other organs.

For further details concerning these and other liver function tests, the reader is referred to standard textbooks of clinical biochemistry.

CHOLECYSTOGRAPHIC MEDIA

In order to examine the gall bladder and bile duct radiologically, it is necessary to administer a contrast medium which is eliminated in the bile. The shape of the relaxed gall bladder can only be seen if the patient is on a fat free diet. A method often employed is to give a fatty meal several hours before the contrast medium is taken: this empties the gall bladder of concentrated bile and leaves it free to accommodate the diagnostic medium. Late at night on the same day, the contrast medium is taken but no more fat is allowed until just after cholecystography. This enables the shape of the gall bladder to be seen: after a fatty meal the gall bladder contracts and begins to expel its contents. Further films can then be taken of the contracting gall bladder and the bile ducts can also be seen.

All the contrast media in current use as cholecystographic media contain iodine. Sodium tetraiodophenolphthalein was widely used but because of its tendency to produce undesirable side effects (nausea, vomiting and diarrhoea) it has now been replaced by the compounds mentioned below.

Pheniodol is given by mouth in the form of granules or tablets. After its excretion by the bile it is eliminated in the urine.

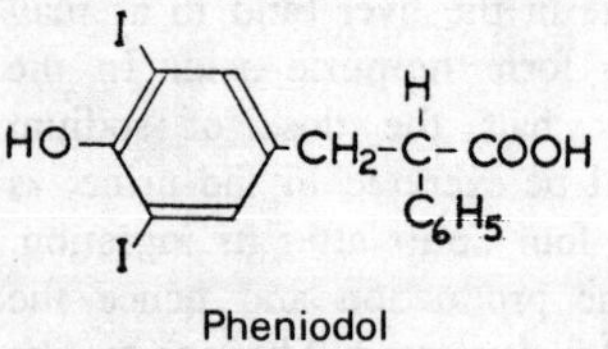

Pheniodol

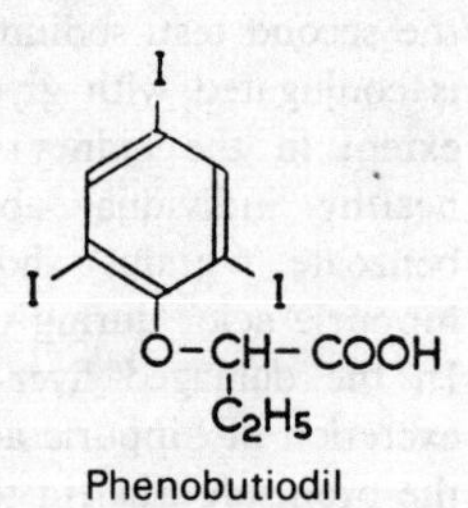

Phenobutiodil

Phenobutiodil is used for cholecystography and for cholangiography (visualization of the gall bladder vessels) and it also enables the bile ducts to be well seen. It is given by mouth. Side effects are mild but they may include polyuria, nausea, and diarrhoea. *Iopanoic acid* and *sodium ipodate* have similar properties and uses. *Sodium iodipamide* is a water soluble compound introduced to allow visualization of the intrahepatic ducts in patients who have undergone cholecystectomy. In addition, since it is given by intravenous injection, sodium iodipamide is employed in investigations in patients who cannot absorb orally administered media. It is useful when the gall bladder can no longer concentrate bile or when a rapid result is needed. This compound is also used in the form of the methyl glucaminate. A modified preparation of the methyl glucaminate (Biligrafin, Cholografin, Endografin) is employed

in the radiological examination of the bladder, urethra and uterus.

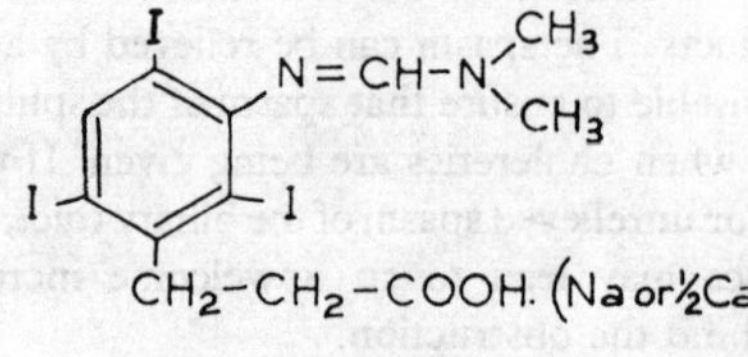

Sodium ipodate

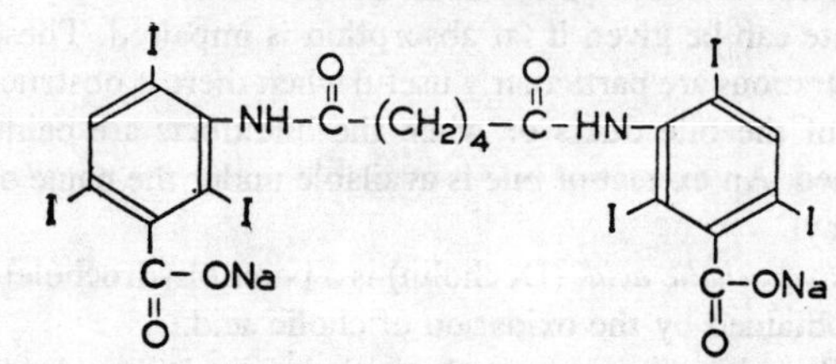

Sodium iodipamide

BIBLIOGRAPHY

Monographs and reviews

Conference (1963). Hepatotoxicity of therapeutic agents. *Ann. N.Y. Acad. Sci.*, **104**, 819-1092.

Drill, V. A. (1952). Hepatotoxic agents: mechanism of action and dietary interrelationship. *Pharmac. Rev.*, **4**, 1-42.

Schaffner, F., Sherlock, Sheila and Leevy, Carrol M., (eds.) (1974) *The Liver and its Diseases*. New York: Intercontinental Medical Book Corporation.

Original paper

Fare, G. (1966). The effect of cupric oxyacetate on rat liver damage associated with five poisons of unrelated chemical structure. *Br. J. Cancer*, **20**, 569-581.

39. Drugs that act on the blood and on blood forming tissues

In a very real sense, iron occupies a position of central importance in haemoglobin, that most essential of molecules. The foetus initially obtains its iron from the mother towards the end of pregnancy and her stores of iron, apart from those with which she herself was born, are obtained from dietary sources. The organism carefully conserves iron and it recycles most of that which it possesses. Despite careful conservation, women lose iron by blood loss during menstruation and parturition. Iron is also lost when it is transferred to the foetus during pregnancy. Women therefore need more iron than men and iron deficiency anaemia is common among underprivileged women in all parts of the world. The recommended daily intake of iron is 12 mg. This should be increased to 15 mg daily in pregnancy and lactation. A good mixed diet will provide this amount of iron; iron preparations that can be taken by mouth should be given to correct iron deficiency in those whose dietary intake of iron is irremediably inadequate.

ABSORPTION AND UTILIZATION OF IRON

Dietary iron is absorbed mainly from the small intestine, particularly the duodenum. Only the ionized forms are absorbed and ferrous iron is much more effectively absorbed than ferric iron. Nonionized compounds are converted into the ionized forms and ferric iron is reduced to ferrous iron. This reaction probably occurs because of the increased availability of thiol (-SH) reducing groups in the stomach following the digestion of protein. In order still further to improve the conversion of ferric to ferrous iron, large doses of ascorbic acid are sometimes given during iron therapy. A diet adequate in protein favours the absorption of iron and iron absorption in those on a protein-poor diet improves if the protein intake is increased. Certain components of the diet, most notably phosphates and phytates, form insoluble salts with iron and so reduce the amount of the element available for absorption. Achlorhydria has a similar effect, probably because acid increases the effectiveness of the reducing agents in the gut.

Not all of the ferrous ions entering or formed in the gut are absorbed into the blood stream. Although the animal body jealously hoards its supples of iron it takes care not to add unnecessarily to them and under normal circumstances it absorbs no more than one tenth of the iron presented to it in the diet. Once within the cells of the intestinal mucosa the ferrous ions are reoxidized and some

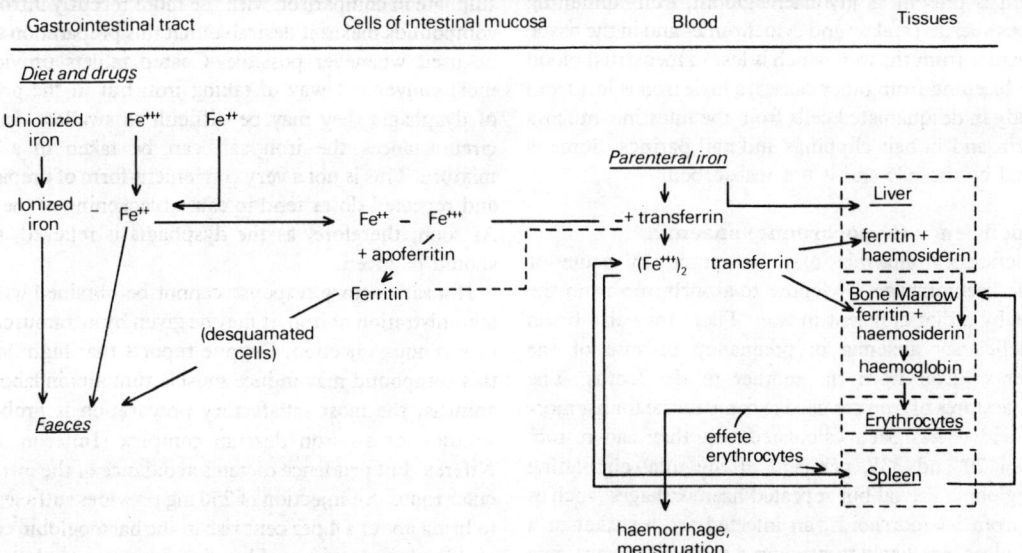

Fig. 39.1 The absorption and metabolism of iron (For details see text).

of the ferric ions so formed combine with apoferritin, a protein. The resulting *ferritin* is sequestered within the mucosal cells. When these die and their remains pass into the gut, the ferritin goes with them and enters the faeces. Ferritin formation clearly constitutes a buffer device that mops up excess ions and so prevents the access to the tissues of toxic quantities of iron. It may also be capable of releasing ferric ions into the bloodstream in times of need.

The iron that escapes the ferritin net passes into the plasma where it forms a complex with a protein of the β-globulin group known as *transferrin* or *siderophilin*. The iron-protein complex is a stable chelate (p. 796) and it is in this form that the metal is transported in the blood: one molecule of transferrin combines with two atoms of ferric ion. The later fate of the bound iron is charted in Figure 39.1, from which it can be seen that iron is finally deposited in the bone marrow (and thence in the erythrocytes), the liver and the spleen. It is held in the tissues as ferritin and haemosiderin. Haemosiderin is an aggregation of ferritin molecules.

Although the intestinal ferritin control system serves an obviously useful purpose, its capacity is, of course, strictly limited and if it is overwhelmed by reason of its having large amounts of iron presented to it an excess of ferric ions will pass into the storage depots to give the condition of *haemosiderosis* (or siderosis). A small minority of individuals absorb iron more completely and avidly than do the rest of us and they too may suffer the effects of an excessive amount of iron in the tissue stores. Although this congenital condition is dignified by a separate name (*haemochromatosis*) it is essentially identical with haemosiderosis.

Of the body's total content of iron, about 60 per cent is present as haemoglobin, 20 per cent is bound as ferritin or haemosiderin in the storage depots and the remaining 20 per cent is present as myohaemoglobin, iron-containing enzymes such as catalase and cytochromes and in the tissue cells. Apart from the iron which is lost in menstrual blood and in bleeding from other causes, a little iron is lost from the body in desquamated cells from the intestinal mucosa and skin and in hair clippings and nail parings. Some is excreted by the bile and is not reabsorbed.

Iron deficiency (hypochromic) anaemia

Iron-deficiency anaemia may be caused by acute or chronic haemorrhage, by failure to absorb iron from the diet or by a diet deficient in iron. There may also be an iron-deficiency anaemia in pregnancy because of the transfer of iron from the mother to the foetus. The available stores of iron are used to compensate for haemorrhage and it has been calculated that they can restore between 20 and $33\frac{1}{3}$ per cent of the total circulating haemoglobin. Trivial but repeated haemorrhages (such as those from haemorrhoids, an infected tooth socket or a peptic ulcer) are likely to produce a more severe anaemia than a single large haemorrhage. It appears that mobilization and increased absorption of iron proceeds more effectively after a large haemorrhage. One factor which is undoubtedly involved in this effect is the establishment of a large concentration gradient between intestine and blood so that absorption is increased.

In iron deficiency anaemia, the ordinary signs of anaemia (pallor, breathlessness on exertion, weakness and loss of appetite) are all present. Other signs, peculiar to iron deficiency anaemia, usually make their appearance. The finger nails become thin and brittle and they break very easily. They may also become hollowed with raised borders so that they will actually hold water like a spoon. This is the condition of *koilonychia*. The tongue becomes smooth, the papillae atrophy and the whole organ may become inflamed (*glossitis*): this is recognized as a precancerous condition. Inflammation at the corners of the mough (*cheilosis*) is common. Difficulty in swallowing (*dysphagia*) may be experienced. The triad of sore mouth, glossitis and dysphagia is known as the Plummer-Vinson syndrome and it is pathognomic of iron-deficiency anaemia.

Iron-deficiency anaemia is treated by iron administration: both ferric and ferrous iron may be employed and the oral route is usually satisfactory. Compounds currently used (with proprietary names and the thrice-daily dose in parentheses) include ferrous sulphate (Ferro-Gradumet, Feospan, Toniron; 200 mg), ferrous fumarate (Fersamal; 200 mg), ferrous succinate (Ferromyn; 250 mg), ferrous gluconate (Cerevon, Fergon, Ferronicum; 300 mg) and ferric ammonium citrate (2 grams). Iron salts are prone to cause gastrointestinal irritation but ferrous salts are less likely to produce side effects than are ferric salts. Ferrous salts of organic acids are more innocuous than salts of inorganic acid. Nevertheless, the cheapness of ferrous sulphate in comparison with the more recently introduced compounds makes it desirable that this preparation should be used whenever possible. Coated tablets provide the most convenient way of taking iron but in the presence of dysphagia they may be difficult to swallow. In these circumstances the iron salt can be taken in a liquid mixture. This is not a very convenient form of preparation and repeated doses tend to cause blackening of the teeth. As soon, therefore, as the dysphagia is relieved, tablets should be given.

If a satisfactory response cannot be obtained with oral administration of iron, it may be given by intramuscular or intravenous injection. Despite reports that high doses of this compound may induce muscle tumours in laboratory animals, the most satisfactory preparation is probably a solution of an iron dextran complex (Imferon, Direx, Niferex) but prudence dictates avoidance of the intramuscular route. An injection of 250 mg provides sufficient iron to bring about a 4 per cent rise in the haemoglobin content of blood and this enables the appropriate dose to be calculated for the individual patient. Imferon contains 50 mg of the complex per ml of solution and it is usual to give the calculated dose in a number of injections of 2 to 4 ml. Iron dextran is broken down in the liver and the liberated iron combines with apoferritin in the usual way. Some of the injected material (up to half if the drug is given by the intramuscular route) is deposited in lymph nodes and although it is permissible to attempt to fill the body's iron stores by slightly exceeding the calculated dose, too much of the drug cannot be given without causing siderosis (p. 660). Saccharated ferric oxide has also been employed and an iron-sorbitol citric acid dextran complex (Jectofer) is available for intramuscular iron therapy. Astrafer is another iron dextran complex suitable for intravenous administration. It is given in doses of 20 to 100 mg. The parenteral route is used if iron absorption is impaired because of achlorhydria, milk diets or antacids, when oral administration causes gastrointestinal upset and in acute or chronic blood loss resulting from haemorrhage, peptic ulcer, colitis, etc. Preparations containing dextran sometimes evoke anaphylactic reactions and deaths from this cause have been reported. The appropriate remedial measures must be available when dextran is administered for the first time and the initial dose should not exceed 50 mg.

It is not always realized that iron in the ionized form is a very toxic substance which has been responsible for many deaths. As we have seen, iron is normally transported and stored in an unionized form but if large quantities of ionizable compounds are taken, the capacity of the carrier molecules may be overwhelmed and ferrous ions then enter the blood stream. They cause severe irritation of the gastrointestinal tract with pain and vomiting, cyanosis, haematuria, depression of the cardiovascular system and liver damage. Until recently, only non-specific forms of treatment were available. These took the form of gastric lavage, blood transfusion and the intravenous injection of fluids. The discovery of the therapeutic potentiality of chelating agents has transformed the treatment of poisoning by heavy metals: desferrioxamine mesylate and diethylene triamine pentaacetic acid are used to effect the rapid removal of ionized iron from the bloodstream (p. 797).

Iron poisoning occurs most often in children who take tablets containing iron in the mistaken belief that they are eating sweets but some of the older preparations of iron, when given parenterally, frequently gave rise to toxic side effects.

THE COAGULATION OF BLOOD

The modern theory of blood coagulation had its origin in the simple scheme proposed by Morawitz in the early years of the present century. It is illustrated in Figure 39.2: when blood is shed, damaged platelets or the injured tissues release an enzyme (thromboplastin) which, in the presence of calcium, produces another enzyme (thrombin) from a precursor (prothrombin) in the plasma. Thrombin converts fibrinogen, another plasma protein, into the insoluble fibrin which forms the essential matrix of the clot.

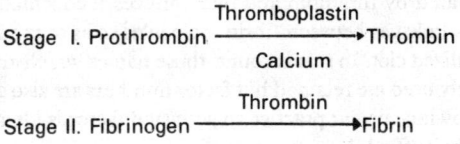

Fig. 39.2 The Morawitz theory of blood clotting.

It is now realized that the thromboplastin produced by tissue extracts is not directly responsible for the formation of thrombin. Tissue thromboplastin forms the starting point of a cascade of reactions that lead to the formation of a substance known as prothrombin activator. It is the last named substance that has the function attributed to thromboplastin in the original Morawitz scheme. However, shed blood clots even when there is no damage to tissues and no liberation of thromboplastin. Contact of the blood with a foreign surface initiates its own series of reactions which culminate in the formation of prothrombin activator. The prothrombin activator produced from plasma constituents activated by contact is called *intrinsic prothrombin activator;* that produced from injured tissues or disintegrated platelets is called *extrinsic prothrombin activator.* It is probable that the two substances are chemically identical but they are produced by different mechanisms and the use of the two names is a convenient way of distinguishing between the two antecedent chains of reactions. Intrinsic prothrombin activator is produced by contact of blood with any surface it does not normally bathe. This includes not only the glass of test tubes but also such ordinary tissue components as connective tissue (collagen) exposed by damage to a blood vessel. Consequently, many types of injury activate both the intrinsic and the extrinsic mechanisms.

Discovery of the additional factors in blood coagulation came from the study of patients with coagulation disorders which could not be attributed to a deficiency of any of the substances then known to be involved in the clotting process. Some of the factors were named after the patients whose conditions first drew attention to the likely existence of a new factor. This is the origin of Christmas factor and Hageman factor: it seems that a new and effortless way of achieving immortality is to have your name attached to something you do not possess! Other factors were given names (antihaemophilic globulin, accelerator globulin, etc.) which suggested their function. Names have now been replaced by numbers which have been allotted by international agreement, to the various factors in a systematic way. Thus fibrinogen, the substance most immediately involved in coagulation, is Factor I, while Hageman factor, which is the first to be activated when blood is shed (and is thus the most distantly removed from the coagulation process) is Factor XII. Factor XIII provides a discordant note in this otherwise harmonious scheme for it triggers the very last act in the coagulation process. It is activated by thrombin and then induces the formation of cross linkages between fibrin molecules so as to produce a stabilized clot. In this account, those names which are still widely used are retained but factor numbers are also given. Following current practice an activated factor is identified by the suffix 'α'.

The initial step in the production of intrinsic prothrombin activator is the activation by contact of the Hageman factor (Factor XII) and its combination with plasma thromboplastin antecedent (Factor XI). It will be recalled that the Hageman factor is also responsible for initiating the reactions which lead to the production of the plasma kinins (p. 359).

It is generally agreed that blood coagulation is the result of a cascade of events, each stage in the cascade initiating the next. It is not surprising that different workers in this complex field proffer coagulation schemes that differ slightly from one another in their details and in the ways in which they are formally presented. That in Figure 39.3 is based on that developed by Macfarlane some ten years ago. Readers who need more details of this or rival schemes or who wish to inspect other and more imaginative methods of representing the coagulation cascade are referred to the specialized monographs. That presented by Biggs (1976) is particularly comprehensive.

The absence of contact with a foreign surface is not the only reason why blood does not coagulate in its vessels. Without this protection the whole of the blood in the cardiovascular system might rapidly solidify once a small intravascular clot had formed. Until quite recently, the mechanisms which maintain the fluidity of the blood have received less attention than those which promote coagulation and it sometimes seems to be forgotten that the prevention of clotting inside the vessels is at least as important as the promotion of clotting outside the vessels. It seems likely that the activity of, every one of the coagulation factors is opposed by a corresponding antifactor activity initiated at the same time but the only antagonists to have been so far identified are six different antithrombin activities, antagonists of activated factors IX, X and XI, and heparin, the oldest established of them all. Of the antithrombin activities, those designated I, II and III have been the most intensively studied. (These Roman numerals bear no relation to the clotting factors that bear these numbers). Fibrin, once formed, absorbs thrombin and this obviously constitutes a potentially valuable means of preventing the further spread of a clot. This is the antithrombin I mechanism. Antithrombin II is the plasma cofactor needed for heparin activation while antithrombin III brings about the actual destruction of thrombin. The anti-XIα factor is sometimes known as antithromboplastin and an excess production of the factor

may be ultimately responsible for the production of some forms of haemophilia.

In the long term, clots are dispersed by the activity of the fibrinolytic system, a topic that is discussed later.

A. *Formation of active Factor X (Factor Xα) from shed blood – the intrinsic pathway*

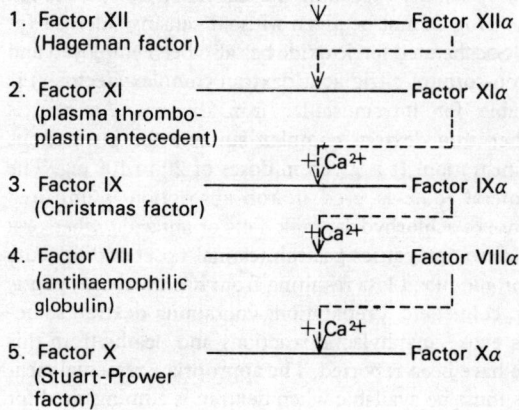

B. *Formation of Factor Xα from damaged tissues or platelets – the extrinsic pathway*

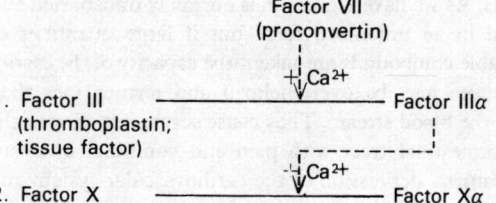

(Process B2 is identical with process A5 except that the activator is Factor III instead of Factor VIII)

C. *The final common pathway*

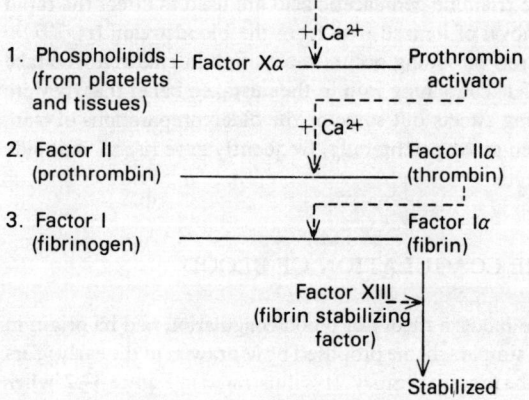

Note: Factor IV is calcium; there is no Factor VI

Fig. 39.3 Reactions involved in blood coagulation.

Even this very brief account should be sufficient to impress upon the reader the complexities and elegance of the finely balanced mechanisms that can both promote and prevent coagulation, according to the demands of the moment, without allowing either process to proceed too far. He should also be impressed by the patience and ingenuity of those who, over a relatively short period of years, have unravelled these complexities to such effect that the underlying patterns of activity can now be so clearly discerned.

Heparin

The best known naturally occurring anticoagulant is heparin. It was discovered as long ago as 1916 and it is widely distributed in the tissues, particularly the lung and the liver. The name heparin commemorates the fact that it was first isolated from the liver though commercial heparin is prepared from mammalian lung. Heparin is localized in the mast cells and little or none is normally present in plasma. Mast cells are, however, found along the course of the blood capillaries and it is possible that tissue damage may liberate heparin from these cells and so limit the spread of any clot formed as a result of the damage. Heparin (together with histamine) is liberated from the mast cells in anaphylactic reactions and it is well known that the blood of some species of animal dying in anaphylaxis is incoagulable .

Heparin inhibits production of intrinsic prothrombin activator and thus antagonizes thrombin production. In addition, it prevents any thrombin which is formed from initiating the conversion of fibrinogen to fibrin—that is, it is an antithrombin as well as an inhibitor of prothrombin activator production. Heparin owes its antithrombin action partly to its ability to increase adsorption of thrombin on to fibrin and partly to a direct combination with thrombin itself. It will be realized that these actions are similar to those shown by the antithrombins and insofar as its antithrombin activity is concerned, heparin may accelerate or potentiate the actions of some of the plasma antithrombins. The precise point in the coagulation sequence at which heparin acts to prevent the formation of the intrinsic prothrombin activator is not yet known.

The chemical composition of heparin was established in 1937 by Jorpes. It is a mucoitin polysulphuric acid in which glucuronic acid and sulphated glucosamine residues alternate. Its molecular weight is at least 8000. It is unique among naturally-occurring mucopolysaccharides in that it contains linkages between sulphate and amino groups. It is only active in the presence of a cofactor (antithrombin II) normally present in the albumin fraction of the plasma. After injection it is rapidly metabolized, largely by the activity of a liver enzyme ('heparinase').

If it is given after a fatty meal, heparin clears the lipaemia rapidly and it thus appears to have a fat solubilizing action. The origin of the clearing action lies in the ability of heparin to release a lipase from the blood vessel walls. Since mast cells are found along the course of blood capillaries, it is possible that they assist in the transfer of fatty acids through the capillary wall.

Heparin

The sodium salt of heparin is stable, and heparin is usually supplied in this form. A calcium salt is also available (p. 666). It has been shown that the molecules of heparin in aqueous solution carry a very strong negative charge. This will enable it to combine with the basic groups of enzyme proteins and this probably forms the basis of its anticoagulant action. The size of the molecule also plays a part, for depolymerization reduces its potency.

The actions of heparin are very specific. It has few pharmacological properties other than that of reducing the coagulability of blood although it is said to have a diuretic action.

Heparin is the only one of the naturally-occurring anticoagulant substances which has so far been used in clinical practice. Its therapeutic potentiality is described in the next section.

Coagulation tests

Over the years a number of laboratory tests has been developed with the aim of measuring the activity of the several coagulation factors in blood. It is not necessary to list them all but some of them are employed to determine the progress of anticoagulant therapy and on these grounds they need to be mentioned here though there is no need to dwell on the experimental details. The *whole blood clotting time* is a simple measure of the time taken for blood to clot in a glass tube: it is determined almost entirely by the time taken to produce intrinsic prothrombin activator, the rest of the coagulation process occurring very rapidly. Prolongation of clotting time occurs if any of the factors involved in the earlier stages of coagulation are absent or abnormal. The so-called *one-stage prothrombin time* (Quick's test) gives an overall assessment of prothrombin and factors VII and X. Plasma is separated from citrated blood and mixed with calcium and a thromboplastin preparation. The time taken to coagulation is noted: it reflects the time required for activation of prothrombin by the extrinsic pathway. The *partial thromboplastin time*, on the other hand, provides a measure of the speed of activation by intrinsic factors. It is essentially a clotting time test in which variations imposed by differences in platelet count are eliminated by adding a platelet substitute such as cephalin.

THROMBOSIS AND ANTITHROMBOTIC DRUGS.

Damage to blood vessels, with leakage of blood into the extravascular space, triggers the cascade of events that culminates in blood coagulation. The clot so formed, though largely extravascular, effectively seals the breach in the vessel wall and prevents further extravasation of blood. This is a normal, physiological and obviously beneficial process. In some circumstances, however, a plug or *thrombus* is formed *inside* the vessel in the absence of damage severe enough to cause blood loss. This process, far from being a beneficial one, is fraught with danger and a major medical problem is posed by the need to prevent thrombosis in those at risk and to minimize its consequences if it should occur.

Thrombi can form in veins, arteries or the chambers of the heart. In venous thrombosis, packets of platelets aggregate together and adhere to the vessel wall, particularly in the neighbourhood of the valves. Localized coagulation follows and the interlacing strands of fibrin so produced form a dense feltwork, the interstices of which contain erythrocytes and more plateletes. The thrombus enlarges and extends, particularly in the direction of blood flow and the vein becomes completely occluded. There is no theoretical upper limit to the length of vein that can be plugged by growth from an initially small focus but most thrombi remain localized to their area of origin. Extensive thrombi cause disturbances of blood flow but the most serious threat presented by thrombi (even small ones) is the possibility of pulmonary or cerebral embolism if small portions of the plug (*emboli*) break off and are swept into the general circulation, later to lodge in the smaller vessels of the lung or brain. A major embolism of this type, which may cause an abrupt arrest of pulmonary or cerebral function, constitutes a medical emergency of the utmost gravity.

Sluggish blood flow is a predisposing factor in the production of venous thrombosis which is, consequently, particularly likely to occur after forms of major surgery that result in the patient's having to suffer a period of postoperative immobilization. Surgery involving the hip joint is a notorious antecedent of venous thromboembolism.

The rate of passage of blood along the veins may be critically reduced even in individuals who have not recently undergone surgery: varicose veins and pressure from a pregnant uterus on the venous trunks that collect blood from the lower limbs are the major culprits in this category.

A retarded blood flow is not sufficient of itself to bring about venous thrombosis. It is merely a precipitating factor which is effective only in those predisposed to thrombosis by reason of advancing age, obesity, damaged veins, cardiovascular insufficiency or (and most important

of all) a hypercoagulability of their blood. Hypercoagulability may result from an increased activity of the coagulation mechanisms themselves or to a deficiency of anticoagulation factors. It is sometimes inborn, sometimes the result of pregnancy and sometimes a consequence of taking drugs, particularly some types of oral contraceptive agents (p. 749). Drugs also influence platelet aggregation.

The blood flows more rapidly in arteries than in veins and platelets are less likely to attach themselves to the arterial wall to form the nucleus of a thrombus unless irregularities in the normally smooth vascular endothelium provide crannies in which they can lodge. Such irregularities are formed by the plaques that develop in atherosclerosis.

Because they are bathed by fast flowing blood, arterial thrombi do not enjoy the same opportunities for growth and extension that are offered to venous thrombi which lie in calmer waters. They are, however, just as dangerous potential sources of emboli which, once they separate from the thrombus will be rapidly swept up and transferred downstream.

The coronary arteries are often the victims of atherosclerotic changes that may lead to a sudden occlusion of one of these major vessels. When this occurs, the heart muscle previously fed by the affected vessel loses its means of nourishment so that cardiac function becomes impaired, perhaps fatally so. A cardiac infarct has occurred and it is signalled by the intense pain, shock and collapse that constitute the heart attack that so many of us are destined to suffer. The arterial occlusion may be caused by a thrombus seeded on an atheromatous plaque, by an embolus broken off from a thrombus elsewhere or by vascular spasm. The fact that 'myocardial infarct' and 'coronary thrombosis' are used synonymously by many people indicates the frequency with which the infarction is the result of thrombosis. Myocardial infarction is one of the scourges of our unnecessarily affluent life style. Overindulgence in food, tobacco, alcohol, the armchair and the motor car predisposes to the development of the atherosclerotic changes that lay foundations for a coronary attack.

Rapidly beating atria make ineffective pumps and some of the blood in fibrillating atria stagnates in the recesses of the chamber instead of being passed into the ventricles. This creates the conditions for thrombus formation and for massive embolism should atrial function improve to the point of effecting a more complete emptying of the chambers.

The rôle of prostaglandins and related substances in the prevention and production of intra-vascular thrombosis is discussed on page 375.

Antithrombotic drugs are employed in attempts to restrict the further growth or a recurrence elsewhere of thrombi that have already appeared and to prevent thrombosis in patients who are to be subjected to these surgical procedures that carry a high risk of postoperative thrombosis.

They can be considered in three groups:

(i) drugs that prevent coagulation (anticoagulant drugs)

(ii) drugs that cause the dissolution of thrombi (*fibrinolytic* or *thrombolytic* agents)

(iii) drugs that prevent platelet aggregation

The rationale for using each of these groups of drugs as antithrombotic agents should be immediately apparent to the reader who should also not need to be reminded that thrombosis can best be avoided by adopting a way of life that discourages the development of hypercoagulability in his blood and atheromatous changes in his vessels.

Anticoagulant drugs

Substances in this category include agents that are added to freshly drawn blood so as to maintain its fluidity until it is needed for transfusion or other processes and drugs that are given to patients for prophylactic purposes. It is convenient to consider the two groups separately.

SUBSTANCES ADDED TO DRAWN BLOOD

The coagulation process is dependent on the presence of calcium ions and blood can be rendered incoagulable by substances which either precipitate calcium from solution or convert it into a non-ionizable form. It is obvious that compounds which act in this way cannot be administered to human beings in sufficient quantity to prevent intravascular clotting without grossly affecting the excitability of nerve and muscle. Sodium citrate (which produces the non-ionizable calcium citrate) is, however, used to prevent coagulation in blood required for transfusion purposes. For experimental or preparative purposes, blood can also be rendered incoagulable by the addition of sodium oxalate (which precipitates calcium as the oxalate) or the disodium salt of ethylene diamine tetraacetic acid (Sequestrene), a chelating agent that binds calcium (p. 796). Ion exchange resins have also been used to remove calcium from blood. Coagulation in drawn blood can also be prevented by substances that destroy or antagonize the actions of other coagulation factors. Among the substances of this type that have been used in laboratory or clinic are dyes (Chicago sky blue and chlorazol pink), trypsin inhibitors and cobra venom.

SUBSTANCES USED TO PREVENT COAGULATION IN VIVO

Drugs in this category include heparin, which has to be given intravenously, and a substantial group of substances that can be taken by mouth. Because of their different mechanisms of action heparin is effective immediately it is given while the oral anticoagulant agents do not exert a therapeutically useful action during the 24–36 hr immediately following their arrival in the bloodstream. When the need for anticoagulant therapy arises there is often a degree of urgency in the situation that demands an immediate and prolonged inhibition of coagulation processes.

In these circumstances, heparin and an orally active drug are employed in tandem, heparin given to relieve the immediate emergency being followed by a course of treatment with an orally active agent with the aim of preventing further thrombotic attacks. In addition to being immediately effective, heparin is a more powerful antithrombotic agent than the oral anticoagulant drugs.

The indications for anticoagulant therapy can be itemized as follows:

(i) To prevent the further growth of venous thrombi and of emboli that might have broken off from them. The immediate mortality from pulmonary embolism can be dramatically reduced by the institution of heparin treatment as soon as the condition is diagnosed while the chances of recurrence are made significantly smaller if a course of treatment with orally active drugs is established once the immediate emergency has been surmounted (Barritt and Jordan, 1960).

(ii) To prevent the development of venous thrombosis after major thoracic, abdominal, pelvic or hip joint surgery. The risk of thromboembolism is very much smaller in those who come to operation with blood of reduced coagulability. This condition is achieved by preoperative treatment with an orally active anticoagulant begun sufficiently in advance of the surgery to ensure maximum effectiveness over the critical operative and postoperative periods. Some authorities now prefer to give small doses of heparin by subcutaneous injection instead of an orally active agent but this alternative form of treatment is not recommended for patients who are to undergo surgery of the hip joint. Clinical evidence indicates that heparin is not a very effective prophylactic agent in these circumstances and that its use carries a significantly greater risk of postoperative bleeding than does oral therapy (Gallus and Hirsh, 1976a). Indeed, the danger of postoperative bleeding, whichever means is adopted to enhance the fluidity of the blood, has militated against the use of prophylactic anticoagulant therapy except in those surgical procedures that carry a high risk of postoperative thrombosis.

(iii) To prevent the development of thrombi and consequent embolism in patients fitted with heart valve replacements and in those with forms of heart disease that are particularly likely to be associated with the appearance of intracardiac thrombi. This latter group of conditions, which demands long term prophylactic treatment, includes among others rheumatic valvular disease and atrial fibrillation.

(iv) To prevent complications in those who have suffered a myocardial infarct. Presently available evidence indicates that immediate anticoagulant therapy reduces the incidence of venous thrombosis during the period of immobilization that necessarily follows such an attack but that long term therapy is of marginal value as a preventative of further infarction. Even a marginal possibility of benefit should not, however, be denied to those who have suffered this most traumatic of medical catastrophes and it is usual to include anticoagulant therapy among the measures taken to minimize the possibility of further attacks.

Heparin

The pharmacology of heparin has already been discussed. Its anticoagulant action appears within ten or fifteen minutes of injection but the effects wear off in about two hours, the plasma half life of the drug averaging about one hour. In the circumstances in which the effect of heparin needs to be maintained for days it is usually convenient to add it to an intravenous drip. The alternative is to give repeated intravenous injections. The needs of ambulant patients requiring anticoagulant therapy are normally met by one of the orally active agents but these drugs may be contraindicated by reason of pregnancy or drug resistance. When this happens, heparin has to be given and the most practicable mode of administration is by subcutaneous injection repeated at least twice daily. The method carries the risk of bleeding at the injection site. Heparin is virtually inactive when taken by mouth.

The dose of heparin is still customarily expressed in units, although it is available in a pure form. One milligram of purified heparin contains about 100 units of heparin. The usual dose of heparin when given in an intravenous drip is of the order of 30 000 units every 24 hours following an initial 'loading' injection of 5000 units. By intravenous injection, the dose is about 5000 units repeated every four hours. Subcutaneous depots, for twice daily replenishment, average 15 000 units in size. In all these instances, the precise requirements should be determined in the light of the changes in coagulability produced in the individual patient. Suitable laboratory criteria for this purpose include the clotting time and the activated partial thromboplastin time.

When it is applied to the prevention of postoperative thrombosis, heparin is given in a subcutaneous dose of 5000 units two hours before surgery. This dose is repeated twelve hours after operation and is thereafter repeated twice or thrice daily until the patient can leave his bed (Gallus and Hirsh, 1976a). Laboratory control is not, apparently, necessary when these modest doses of heparin are given.

In cases of venous thromboembolism and myocardial infarction, heparin therapy is usually continued for one or two weeks.

Heparin has few toxic side effects. The most important is haemorrhage due to overdosage, but in rare instances heparin may cause anaphylactic shock, alopecia or osteoporosis. Heparin is contraindicated in patients who already have bleeding diseases, gastric ulceration or subacute bacterial endocarditis. Those receiving heparin (or other anticoagulant drugs) should not be permitted to take salicylates. These drugs tend to cause gastric bleeding which might assume dangerous proportions if the blood is

$$\left[-(CH_2)_6 \overset{\overset{\displaystyle CH_3}{|}}{\underset{\underset{\displaystyle CH_3}{|}}{\overset{\oplus}{N}}} (CH_2)_3 \overset{\overset{\displaystyle CH_3}{|}}{\underset{\underset{\displaystyle CH_3}{|}}{\overset{\oplus}{N}}} 2Br^{\ominus} \right]_n$$

Hexadimethrine bromide

incoagulable. It should be noted that heparin does not affect the ability of blood vessels to constrict and thus to arrest minor haemorrhages. The patient receiving anticoagulants need not therefore fear that he will suffer a serious haemorrhage as a result of a trivial wound.

It may be necessary to reverse the action of heparin either because of overdosage or because the patient requires urgent surgery. Blood transfusions will bring this about and protamine sulphate or hexadimethrine bromide (Polybrene) have the same effect. Protamine sulphate is a basic compound of high molecular weight. It probably acts by neutralizing the charge on the heparin molecules. It is given by slow intravenous injection in a one per cent solution at a dose level determined by the time which has elapsed since heparin administration ceased. In general 0.5-1 mg of protamine sulphate is sufficient to overcome the action of 1 mg of heparin. Care has to be taken not to give too much protamine sulphate since it is itself an anticoagulant and this action will become evident after all the heparin has been neutralized.

Hexadimethrine is also a strongly basic compound. It is given in the same way and at virtually the same dose level as protamine sulphate. It has little anticoagulant action.

Heparin is usually supplied as the sodium salt. A calcium salt is also available but it offers no particular advantage over the more usual form.

Potential alternatives to heparin

In recent years the possibility of finding alternatives to heparin has been actively explored although there is no compelling reason why heparin should be replaced. The two substances that have attracted most attention in this connection are ancrod (Arvin) and dextran.

Ancrod. The story of ancrod began in 1963 when Reid and his colleagues reported that the Malayan pit viper produced a severe deficiency of fibrinogen in the blood of those it bit without causing severe bleeding. Some years had to elapse before it became clear that the viper's venom contains a substance that *activates* coagulation processes and the paradox was further confounded by the demonstration that administration of the purified coagulation factor rendered the blood incoagulable.

These superficially contradictory observations found a ready explanation when it was found that the coagulation factor (by then called ancrod) converts fibrinogen to fibrin but that, unlike thrombin, it does not activate factor XIII (p. 662). Consequently the fibrin in the clots it forms (though sufficient to prevent immediate bleeding in the victim of a pit viper bite) do not undergo cross linking so that they remain unstable and small enough to be dispersed innocuously throughout the circulation. Given intravenously, ancrod induces clot formation and dispersion (and hence fibrinogen deficiency) for as long as the infusion is maintained. The therapeutic potentialities of ancrod are clearly similar to those of heparin. In the clinical studies so far reported the drug has been given by slow intravenous injection in doses of up to 1 μg per kilogram body mass at twelve hourly intervals.

Ancrod disappears from the blood in a biphasic fashion. The first phase, which results in the clearing of about 90 per cent of the amount of drug initially present has a half-time of about four hours but the later phase is much more sluggish, its half-time reaching ten days. If necessary, the action of ancrod can be reversed by administration of the appropriate antivenom but fibrinogen also has to be given to cover the period during which residual ancrod is being slowly lost from the blood.

Enthusiasts declare that ancrod therapy is attended by even fewer side effects than occur with heparin. Nevertheless, both allergic reactions and subcutaneous haemorrhages have been reported and a sober assessment of the therapeutic future of ancrod must await the outcome of more controlled trials. It has also to be remembered that the laying down of fibrin is an essential element in wound healing and it is possible that ancrod treatment may delay the healing of surgical wounds.

Dextran sulphate. The dextrans are best known as plasma expanders and their use for this purpose (as well as details of their structure and general properties) are discussed later in this chapter (p. 675). They have some antithrombotic action and the possibility of exploiting this property for clinical ends has been the subject of some recent investigations.

Given by intravenous infusion during and for two to three days after surgery, dextran seems to reduce the incidence of postoperative venous thrombosis. The usual daily dose is 1000 ml infused over a period of some four hours: dextran 70 is usually preferred to dextran 40 for this purpose. Possible adverse reactions to the dextrans are discussed elsewhere (p. 675) but an additional complication may arise when they are used to prevent postoperative thrombosis because they increase the plasma volume beyond its normal bounds and this may cause circulatory embarrassment in patients whose cardiovascular performance is not of the best.

The origin of the dextrans' antithrombotic action is obscure. Among the mechanisms that have been proposed are a reduced blood viscosity consequent on the volume expansion, inhibition of platelet aggregation, changes in the fibrin molecule that render clots more susceptible to fibrinolysis and the production of a protective coating on the vascular endothelium and platelets that inhibit the initiating phase of thrombus formation.

No very convincing case can yet be made for preferring dextran to heparin.

Orally active anticoagulant agents
The story of the discovery of the coumarin derivatives is one of the classics of pharmacology. In 1922, Schofield reported that a haemorrhagic disease then afflicting cattle in parts of the United States and Canada was the result of the animals' having been fed improperly cured sweet clover. Further investigations made it clear that the offending clover contained a coumarin derivative. In 1940 this was identified as 3,3-methylene-bis-(4-hydroxycoumarin). It was synthesized in 1943. It is now known as dicoumarol or bishydroxycoumarin and since 1950 it has been used as an anticoagulant agent.

Bishydroxycoumarin (Dicoumarol)

Several other coumarin derivatives were synthesized in the wake of dicoumarol's therapeutic successes. The newer compounds differ from dicoumarol and from one another in the speed of onset and the duration of their anticoagulant action. Their names and formulae together with details of effective dose regimens and durations of action are set out in Table 39.1.

It is difficult to achieve a steady reduction in blood coagulability by the use of ethylbiscoumacetate because of the drug's rapid excretion. At the other extreme, phenprocoumon is cleared so slowly from the body that the effects of even trivial overdosing may be embarrassingly prolonged. The coumarin derivatives to be preferred are those with an intermediate duration of action and there is a unanimity of opinion that declares warfarin sodium to be the oral anticoagulant drug of choice by reason both of its duration of action and its minimal side effects.

The coumarins interfere with the proper synthesis of prothrombin and of Factors VII, IX and X by the liver. This synthesis is normally promoted by vitamin K (p. 673) and coumarin derivatives hinder the utilization of this vitamin. For this reason, patients whose absorption of vitamin K is deficient are particularly sensitive to the action of oral anticoagulants. An important source of vitamin K is provided by the bacterial flora of the intestine and antibiotics may cause a relative deficiency of the vitamin. Disturbances of fat absorption may be associated with defective absorption of vitamin K. Coagulation factors synthesized in the absence of vitamin K lack the carboxyl groups that would enable the molecules to bind to calcium ions.

The effects of the coumarin derivatives on blood coagulation are not fully operative until the body's existing

Table 39.1 Anticoagulant drugs that can be taken by mouth

Approved name	Proprietary name(s)	Chemical formula	Onset of action Hr	Duration of action Days	Daily dose	Remarks
		THE COUMARIN DERIVATIVES				
Ethyl bis-coumacetate	Tromexan	*(structure: two coumarin rings with OH groups, central CH linked to C-OC₂H₅ and C=O)*	24	3	1000 mg initially, then 500-900 mg	Because of its rapid action, it may be useful in emergencies
Cyclocoumarol	Cumopyran	*(structure: H₃C, OCH₃, phenyl, coumarin ring)*	48	6	150 mg followed by 50 mg	Too long-acting for most purposes
Warfarin sodium	Coumadin Marevan Panwarfin Prothomadin	*(structure: ONa, CH linked to phenyl and CH₂COCH₃, coumarin ring)*	48	4	50 mg followed by 20-50 mg	Drug of choice Solubility enables it to be given parenterally as well as orally. Used as pesticide (rats). May cause alopecia
Phenprocoumon	Liquamar	*(structure: coumarin ring with OH, CH linked to phenyl and C₂H₅)*	48	10	30 mg followed by 5-6 mg	
		THE INDANEDIONES				
Phenindione (Phenylindanedione)	Danilone Dindevan Indema Indon Hedulin	*(structure: indane-1,3-dione with phenyl)*	30	2	250 mg followed by 100 mg	May cause fatal hypersensitivity reactions
Diphenadione	Dipaxin	*(structure: indane-1,3-dione with C=O and two phenyl groups, CH)*	36	Up to 20 days	30 mg on first day, 15 mg on second day and 5 mg thereafter	Less toxic than phenindione but note very long duration of action

supplies of prothrombin and of Factors VII, IX and X have been exhausted. Conversely, when the drug is withdrawn its anticoagulant effect will not disappear until the liver has produced and released new supplies of the coagulation factors. These facts have two important consequences. In the first place, dicoumarol and related compounds, given alone, cannot effect the immediate decrease in blood coagulability which is an essential requirement in such emergencies as cardiac infarction. In these conditions, heparin must also be given but it may be withdrawn after a few days when the coumarin-type drug has begun to exert its full effect. The other consequence is that if severe bleeding occurs as a result of overdosage with a drug of this type, normal coagulability will not be immediately restored if the drug is withdrawn. Whole blood will be needed to restore the missing factors.

It will be readily appreciated that the dosage of the coumarin-type anticoagulants must be very carefully controlled. This task is rendered difficult by the fact that the effect of the drugs may fluctuate even in the same patient because of the operation of such factors as variations in the diet and the concurrent administration of other drugs. Disturbances of liver or kidney function and alcoholism are factors which may cause the optimal dose of the drug to vary from patient to patient. The dosage is regulated on the basis of information supplied by estimations of the one-stage prothrombin time which gives an overall assessment of prothrombin and Factors VII and X. The prothrombin time normally averages some 14 seconds. Experience indicates that it must be prolonged to between two and three times this value if intravascular thrombosis is to be prevented. Prothrombin time must be measured at daily intervals while a suitable maintenance dosage is being sought. Thereafter, the measurements need be made less frequently but they must be continued in view of the likelihood of sudden variations in the patient's sensitivity to the drug.

The coumarin-type anticoagulants are taken by mouth: for obvious reasons they have no effect on coagulation processes *in vitro* Their most dangerous side effect is haemorrhage. This usually only occurs when insufficient care has been taken to maintain the prothrombin time within safe limits but it sometimes appears when all precautions to prevent it have been observed. Haemorrhage is treated by withdrawal of the drug and intravenous administration of vitamin K. In cases of emergency it may be necessary to supply the missing coagulation factors by giving a transfusion of whole blood. Less serious side effects, which are not common, include headache, nausea, vomiting, diarrhoea and mild transient purpura (small subcutaneous haemorrhages).

The coumarin-type anticoagulants are contraindicated in patients who have a history of haemorrhage or who are suffering from conditions such as peptic ulcer or ulcerative colitis which may give rise to haemorrhage if blood coagulability is reduced. They are also contraindicated during the first three and the last two months of pregnancy. In early pregnancy they may induce malformation of the foetal nose and, because they cross the blood-plancental barrier they may cause bleeding in the newly delivered infant if they are allowed to enter the foetal circulation during the last two months of foetal life. Care has to be exercised when the drugs are given to patients with kidney or liver disease in whom metabolic and excretory processes are likely to be seriously depressed.

The coumarin derivatives are absorbed from the gastrointestinal tract, they undergo a very high degree of binding to the plasma proteins and they are almost completely metabolized by microsomal enzymes in the liver. In circumstances such as this, there is a high probability that other drugs that can influence one or more of these dispositional processes will cause marked changes in the amount of the active form of the first drug in the blood and patients maintained on orally active coagulation inhibitors constitute one of a small number of groups of individuals in whom adverse drug interactions are particularly likely to occur unless they and their medical advisers are always fully alert to the dangers that may attend the taking of additional drugs, however benign their reputation when taken alone, once a therapeutic programme has been established.

To summarize the most important drug interactions that involve the coumarin derivatives we can adhere to an earlier plan (p., 77) and list these according to the interaction sites as follows:

a. *in the gastrointestinal tract:* some drugs (cholestyramine heptabarbitone) inhibit the absorption of coumarin derivatives, while others (nortriptyline is an example) promote absorption. Drugs that influence the absorption of vitamin K will also interact with the coumarin derivatives. Thus liquid paraffin and cholestyramine hinder the absorption of vitamin K and so potentiate the effects of the oral anticoagulant agents. The reader will note that cholestyramine inhibits the absorption of both vitamin K and the anticoagulant drugs so that its ultimate effect on the coagulation processes in the individual patient has to be measured. It cannot be predicted.

b. *in the blood:* a large number of substances (some antiinflammatory agents, clofibrate, ethacrynic acid, etc.) displace the anticoagulants from plasma proteins and so increase, sometimes to a dangerous level, the anticoagulant effect of the drugs.

c. *in the liver:* some drugs stimulate the biotransformation of the anticoagulant drugs and so reduce their effectiveness while others have the opposite effects. Drugs in the first group include diphenylhydantoin, barbiturates, haloperidol and griseofulvin; representatives of the second group are chloramphenicol and nortriptyline.

d. *in the kidney:* rifampicin is said to promote the excretion of the coumarin derivatives and their metabolites, many of which have some anticoagulant action in their own right.

e. *elsewhere:* drugs that influence platelet function (see below, p. 671) will interact with the coumarins in the sense that they exert an independent antithrombotic effect which will be added to that of the coumarins; some oral contraceptives promote while salicylates inhibit the synthesis of clotting factors. Salicylates are particularly interesting in the present context for they also inhibit platelet aggregation and displace the coumarins from their binding to plasma albumin. Moreover, salicylic acid is a normal metabolite of dicoumarol.

The easiest way of dealing with these interactions is to avoid taking the drugs that provoke them. Benzodiazepines can be used instead of barbiturates, paracetamol instead of aspirin, indomethacin instead of phenylbutazone, etc. If a drug that induces an interaction has to be used, the dose of the interacting drugs must be determined in the light of the information provided by the prothrombin time.

Table 39.1 includes details of two compounds (phenindione and diphenadione) that are not coumarin derivatives. They and some others of related structure (anisindione, bromindione and chlorphenylindanedione) behave in every way like the coumarin derivatives and until quite recently they enjoyed a similar vogue as antithrombotic drugs. It has, however, become clear that a not inconsiderable number of patients (about two per cent of those so far treated with the phenindione derivatives) suffer hypersensitivity reactions. These reactions take a number of forms—skin rashes, diarrhoea, fever, agranulocytosis and liver or kidney damage—some of which may be fatal. The phenindiones are, consequently, rapidly losing favour, though they can, of course, still be prescribed for those who have already begun to take them and have not suffered hypersensitivity reactions. An incidental property of the phenindiones is their tendency to impart a red colour to the urine. Though harmless in itself, this effect can deliver a considerable shock to an unprepared patient who knows that haemorrhage is a potentially dangerous complication of anticoagulant therapy.

Thrombolytic (fibrinolytic) agents

Anticoagulants may prevent the spread of thrombi but they do nothing to disperse those already formed so that an occluded or partially obstructed vessel is not rendered patent again by the use of anticoagulant agents. The development of methods to solubilize thrombi safely would therefore represent a distinct therapeutic advance and attempts to do this have been made recently.

A physiological mechanism causes the gradual lysis of clots formed within the body. Plasma contains *plasminogen,* the precursor of a proteolytic enzyme which is converted into the enzyme proper (*plasmin*) by various activators which are found in many tissues, in plasma and in urine. The activator found in urine (which may or may not be identical with that in the tissues) is called *urokinase*. The amount of activator in the plasma is normally much less than that in the tissues but it is increased by exercise, by the administration of adrenaline and in certain pathological conditions. In particular, plasminogen activators are synthesized by the vascular endothelium and are released from it in the neighbourhood of thrombi. Urine, tears and milk contain relatively large amounts of activator.

Even in the absence of thrombotic activity, small amounts of activator are released into the plasma all the time. Plasmin is by no means specific in its actions and the plasma and tissue proteins would therefore be exposed to the possibility of proteolysis were it not for the presence of enzyme inhibitors in plasma. When blood clots or thrombi form fibrin absorbs plasmin, plasminogen and plasminogen activators but it does not take up the plasmin inhibitors and it thus sets the stage for its own eventual destruction. The high concentration of plasminogen activators in urine, tears and milk presumably serves to prevent blocking of the secretory tubules by fibrin.

Knowledge of the physiological thrombolytic mechanism has prompted attempts to use plasmin or similar compounds for therpeutic purposes. The substances that have been investigated in this connection fall naturally into three groups:

  a. plasmin and other proteolytic enzymes
  b. plasminogen activators
  c. substances that promote synthesis of plasminogen activators

PLASMIN AND OTHER PROTEOLYTIC ENZYMES

Notwithstanding its physiological role, plasmin has not generally been very successful as a therapeutic agent. However, a recent investigation (Storm *et al.* 1974) led to the more favourable conclusion that plasmin is as useful an agent as streptokinase for preventing the spread of deep vein thrombosis in the lower limbs.

Plasma is inactivated in the plasma and it seemed possible that more stable proteolytic enzymes such as trypsin and chymotrypsin might be more useful thrombolytic agents than plasmin itself. This hope was not realized: the tissue proteolysis produced by the enzymes merely resulted in an increased tendency to clotting.

Another proteolytic enzyme that has received some attention is brinase, a protease obtained from *Aspergillus oryzae* but there seems to be little prospect of its replacing the plasminogen activators.

PLASMINOGEN ACTIVATORS

Streptokinase (which is produced by the metabolism of β-haemolytic streptococci) is a powerful plasminogen activator which has recently enjoyed some therapeutic successes.

In the early days of streptokinase therapy, toxic reactions (pyrexia and allergic skin rashes) were not uncommon but these were often produced by contaminants and they occur much less frequently now that pure preparations of the activator are available. Nevertheless, streptokinase is a protein and as such it has antigenic activity. Moreover, because streptococcal infections are so common, most of us have accumulated a quota of streptokinase antibodies by the time we need thrombolytic therapy. Although these antibodies only rarely precipitate anaphylactic reactions when streptokinase is given they will reduce its effectiveness unless they are neutralized by an initial loading dose of the activator.

Strictly speaking, streptokinase itself is not a plasminogen activator. It forms a complex with plasminogen (one molecule of plasminogen combines with one of streptokinase) and it is this complex that activates uncomplexed plasminogen. Consequently, the higher the dose of streptokinase the greater the amount of complex that is formed and the smaller the amount of unchanged plasminogen that is available for activation. In practice, streptokinase therapy is initiated by a large intravenous dose of the activator to ensure neutralization of circulating antibodies and to produce immediate conversion of a large proportion of the plasminogen into activator complex. This initial loading dose is followed by a maintenance infusion that captures any plasminogen that enters the circulation, converting it into activator and so restricting its conversion into plasmin. In this way, the embarrassment of producing a dangerous excess of active plasmin is avoided.

Although the loading dose of streptokinase should ideally be determined for each patient in the light of his antibody titre, a standard loading dose (1.25m units) can be given with impunity. The maintenance dose (usually about 100000 units hourly) is regulated by measuring the clotting and euglobulin lysis times. The last mentioned parameter provides a measure of the amount of plasminogen activator in the blood.

Streptokinase can be used in the treatment of pulmonary embolism and venous thrombosis of the limbs. It will not prevent the spread or recurrence of a coronary thrombosis. It will not promote the lysis of clots unless it is administered within 72 hours of their formation. It is given by intravenous infusion and a careful watch has to be kept for changes in other components of the clotting mechanism. It can be employed in conjunction with heparin. If the dose is not carefully controlled, streptokinase may cause excessive bleeding in response to minor injuries or surgical procedures. The action of streptokinase can be reversed, if necessary, by giving ε-aminocaproic acid or aprotinin (p. 673).

Urokinase has actions and uses similar to those of streptokinase but it is without antigenic activity in man. It does not, therefore, induce allergic reactions nor is its effectiveness threatened by neutralizing antibodies in the blood. A disadvantage of urokinase is the fact that it increases the activity of coagulation factor VIII but this tendency to favour coagulation processes is more than offset by the activator's fibrinolytic activity. Indications for urokinase therapy are the same as those for streptokinase. The therapeutic dose of urokinase, by intravenous infusion per hour and kilogram body mass is 3000–4000 units.

SUBSTANCES THAT PROMOTE THE SYNTHESIS OF PLASMINOGEN ACTIVATORS

Anabolic steroids (p. 736) increase the rate of synthesis of plasminogen activator by the vascular endothelium and attempts have recently been made to use anabolic steroids (often in combination with one of the biguanide group of oral hypoglycaemic agents) as fibrinolytic agents. The usual combination of drugs is ethyloestranol (p. 736) and phenformin (p. 728) and it has been given to reduce the incidence of postoperative venous thromboembolism. As yet, there is no evidence that this form of treatment is superior to that provided by other types of anticoagulant and fibrinolytic drugs.

Drugs that prevent platelet aggregation

'Inhibition of platelet aggregation' has long been listed among the side effects of a number of otherwise disparate drugs but it is only in recent years that the therapeutic possibilities of this side effect have been recognized.

Platelet aggregation, as we have seen, is the first in a sequence of events that culminates in thrombosis and it is not unreasonable to assume that the whole thrombotic process would be effectively thwarted if this triggering event were prevented. Among the drugs whose possible range of usefulness has been extended by exploiting their inhibitory action on platelet aggregation are clofibrate, dipyridamole, hydroxychloroquine, sulphinpyrazole and aspirin. All these substances are better known for their primary pharmacological actions and it is in these contexts that they are fully described elsewhere in this book. Mention should be made here, however, of the fact that the inclusion of aspirin in the list adds yet another facet of interest to this most fascinating of drugs.

The prevention of platelet aggregation as a therapeutic measure is still in its infancy but it is already possible to draw some general conclusions concerning its effectiveness (Gallus and Hirsh, 1976b). Thus, a combination of dipyridamole (400 mg daily) and warfarin or of dipyridamole (200 mg daily), aspirin (300 mg three times daily) and warfarin prevents embolism in patients who have received heart valve replacements. The regimen based on the lower dose of dipyramidole is the less likely to cause side effects such as headache and vomiting. Sulphinpyrazole (200 mg three times daily) often increases the effectiveness of oral anticoagulation agents in patients with venous thrombosis who have not responded well to treatment with the latter drugs alone. It also reduces the incidence of thrombosis in the tubes and vessels at the junction of a patient and his haemodialysis equipment. Aspirin is particularly useful in those whose thrombosis is attributable to their processing an excess of platelets (thrombocytosis) or platelets that exhibit spontaneous aggregation.

HAEMOSTATICS AND COAGULANTS

The arrest of trivial bleeding is brought about by constriction of the damaged vessels. The application of a cold compress arrests bleeding by this mechanism and the homely remedy of putting a large cold door key down the back of the person whose nose is bleeding operates by causing reflex vasoconstriction in response to the shock of feeling the cold object. Bleeding from tooth sockets can be arrested by the firm application of a pledget of cotton wool soaked in a dilute (one per cent) solution of adrenaline hydrochloride. Alum arrests trivial bleeding by virtue of its astringent action (p. 807).

More severe haemorrhage is arrested by promoting coagulation. The method chosen to achieve this is determined by the circumstances under which the haemorrhage occurs as indicated below.

Absorbable gelatin sponge

Absorbable gelatin sponge (Gelfoam, Sterispon) consists of dried sterilized gelatin foam which can be cut or moulded into any desired shape. Tough and porous, gelatin foam can absorb up to fifty times its own weight of blood. It is used in surgery to arrest the loss of blood from oozing surfaces and since it is absorbable it can be left in the wound after closure. It can be moistened with a solution of thrombin. Absorbable gelatin sponge acts so as to form an insoluble protein matrix, somewhat similar to fibrin, which traps the formed elements in its interstices and by damaging the platelets causes liberation of the platelet factors and other components of the coagulation mechanism. Similar effects are brought about when a piece of cotton wool is applied to a cut or a cotton wool plug is inserted into a bleeding dental cavity.

Thrombin

Surgical thrombin is a freeze-dried powder which is used in the form of a freshly prepared solution in normal saline as a coagulant in general surgery and as an adhesive in plastic surgery. It has been used orally to arrest bleeding in gastric haemorrhage and it is employed in obstetrics as an aid to the diagnosis of *afibrinogenaemia* with haemorrhage since it will not cause coagulation in the absence of fibrinogen.

Thrombin is often supplied as a mixture of prothrombin, thromboplastin and a calcium salt. Because it is a powder it can be sprinkled on to pieces of gelatin foam whose haemostatic properties are thereby increased.

Fibrin and fibrinogen

Human fibrin foam is a dried, artificial sponge. Human fibrinogen is also available. Like fibrin, it is used in surgery to arrest haemorrhage but it is also employed to treat afibrinogenaemia when transfusion of whole blood fails to restore fibrinogen supplies.

Oxidized cellulose

Oxidized cellulose (Oxycel, Surgicel) is a special type of surgical cotton or surgical gauze consisting mainly of cellulosic acid. This compound forms an absorbable artificial clot. Oxidized cellulose is used in surgery to control haemorrhage caused by damage to small arteries and veins, especially when suturing is not possible or would not be effective. It can also be applied to surface wounds to arrest bleeding, but since it impairs healing it should not be used as a surface dressing.

Russell's viper venom

Russell's viper venom is a very potent coagulant which coagulates normal and haemophilic blood. The solution in normal saline has been used to control dental bleeding in haemophiliacs and to arrest haemorrhage following tonsillectomy.

Epsilon-aminocaproic acid

A number of synthetic substances that inhibit fibrinolysis have become available in the last twenty years or so. The first of these was ε-aminocaproic acid (EACA, Amicar). It prevents fibrinolysis by competitively inhibiting the naturally occurring plasminogen activators. An obvious and rational use of the drug is to reverse the action of streptokinase and urokinase if they have been given in excess but it has also been given to prevent bleeding in patients who have undergone surgery particularly of the heart or the prostate gland, events that are associated with activation of plasminogen. Some authorities recommend the routine use of aminocaproic acid after prostatectomy so as to prevent activation of urokinase and so minimise bleeding in the urinary tract. The drug has a place too as a preventative of excessive bleeding after minor surgery in haemophilic subjects and it has met with some success in the treatment of menorrhagia (excessive menstrual bleeding).

$$H_2N-(CH_2)_5-COOH$$

ε-Aminocaproic acid

$$H_2N.CH_2-\bigcirc-COOH$$

Tranexamic acid

Aminocaproic acid is often given as an intravenous infusion but it is equally effective if taken by mouth. Daily doses are of the order of 6 to 10 g (in three or four instalments) sometimes preceded by a loading dose. It is important to give adequate amounts because low concentrations of the acid actually potentiate plasminogen activity. Contrary perhaps to expectations, intravascular thrombosis is but rarely seen as a complication of short term therapy with aminocaproic acid. On the other hand, a hazardous situation can arise if bleeding into body cavities such as the thorax or the pericardium occurs in a patient who has undergone cardiac surgery and has been given aminocaproic acid. The clots that subsequently form in the body cavities will not be eroded by fibrinolysis and may fatally impede the action of the lungs and heart.

Dizziness, nausea, vomiting, abdominal pain and orthostatic hypotension have all been occasionally reported in patients given aminocaproic acid.

Tranexamic acid

As can be seen by referring to its formula and alternative name (cyclic aminocaproic acid), tranexamic acid (Transamin) is closely related to ϵ -aminocaproic acid and the two substances have similar actions and uses. Tranexamic acid is ten times more potent than the open chain compound and it seems to be less likely to cause untoward side effects. It may well be destined to replace aminocaproic acid as the favoured antifibrinolytic agent.

Aprotinin

Aprotinin (Trasylol) is another inhibitor of the plasminogen activators: on a molar basis it is almost one hundred times more potent than tranexamic acid. It also has a degree of anticoagulant activity by virtue of its ability partially to inhibit the formation of thromboplastin. Both actions help to conserve the body's supply of fibrin and fibrinogen and would indicate that aprotinin could be applied to the treatment of defibrination syndromes. However when it is necessary to prevent both the formation and lysis of clots it is probably better to use a mixture of heparin and tranexamic acid rather than to rely on the dual action of aprotinin. Considered simply as an antifibrinolytic drug, aprotinin is in no way superior to either aminocaproic or tranexamic acid.

Aprotinin is a polypeptide containing sixteen aminoacid residues. It is obtained from beef lung.

Protamine sulphate

This substance is a heparin antagonist and as such it was discussed earlier (p. 666).

Vitamin K

The initial K is given to this vitamin (K for Koagulationsvitamin) because deficiency leads to clotting defects. Vitamin K promotes the synthesis by the liver of pro-

thrombin, Factors VII and X and the precursor of Factor IX. Deficiency of the vitamin therefore reproduces the action of the dicoumarin-like anticoagulants.

Vitamin K occurs naturally in two forms. Vitamin K_1 is present in dark-green vegetables such as cauliflower, spinach and kale. The ordinary stinging nettle is also a good source of the vitamin. Vitamin K_2 is found in putrefying food and it is also synthesized by bacteria in the intestine. In addition to the natural sources, a number of naphthoquinones also have vitamin K activity: their names and formulae are presented in Figure 39.4.

Vitamin K and the synthetic compounds are fat soluble but certain salt forms (menadiol sodium phosphate and menaphthone sodium bisulphite) are water soluble although the parent compounds are not. The absorption of vitamin K can only occur in the presence of bile salts and a deficiency of the vitamin may occur in obstructive jaundice, a condition in which bile is denied access to the gut. Malabsorption syndromes and an over indulgence in liquid paraffin will also hinder absorption. Vitamin K deficiency is a common occurrence in the immediately neonatal period when the infant has used up all the vitamin bequeathed to him by his mother but has not yet acquired either the bacterial flora or the diet that will provide him with his own supplies. It gives rise to haemolytic disease of the newborn. A condition resembling vitamin K deficiency may also occur even when supplies of the vitamin are adequate if the liver is incapable of synthesizing the coagulation factors. This may occur in acute chloroform poisoning and in the course of viral hepatitis or hepatic cirrhosis.

Vitamin K and related substances are employed to remedy deficiencies of the type we have just discussed and to reverse the actions of the hydroxycoumarin and the indanedione anticoagulants. The water soluble analogues can cause haemolysis in the newborn and in adults whose erythrocytes are congenitally deficient in glucose-6-phosphate dehydrogenase. They also displace bilirubin from its combination with plasma proteins, an event that is liable to have a fatal outcome in premature infants (p. 70). When vitamin K is given to newly born children as a prophylactic measure, small doses (0.5 to 1 mg) and the intramuscular route are chosen.

When it is necessary to reverse the action of a coagulant, vitamin K should always be preferred to the synthetic analogues: in an emergency it can be administered in 10 mg doses in oil by the intramuscular route or in a fine emulsion by the intravenous route. If the situation is less urgent, the same amounts of the vitamin can be taken by mouth. The same plan can be adopted for the treatment of haemorrhagic diseases associated with an impaired absorption of vitamin K but in these instances it is permissible to give a water soluble analogue, such as Synkavit (15 to 30 mg) in non-urgent cases. Patients with obstructive jaundice will need vitamin K, given by a parenteral route, before surgery.

The actions of vitamin K are prolonged and antagonism to the anticoagulants may last for up to 14 days after a single dose of 500 mg of vitamin K. It is, therefore, necessary to monitor the effect of the vitamin as carefully as that of an anticoagulant. Since the latter is used to prevent the occurrence or extension of thromboses, it is obviously undesirable to change a tendency to haemorrhage into a tendency to form clots.

NATURALLY OCCURRING VITAMINS

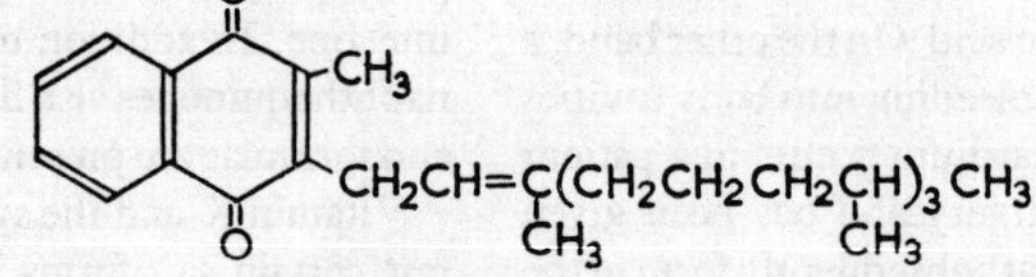

Vitamin K (phytomenadione, Mephyton, Konakion)

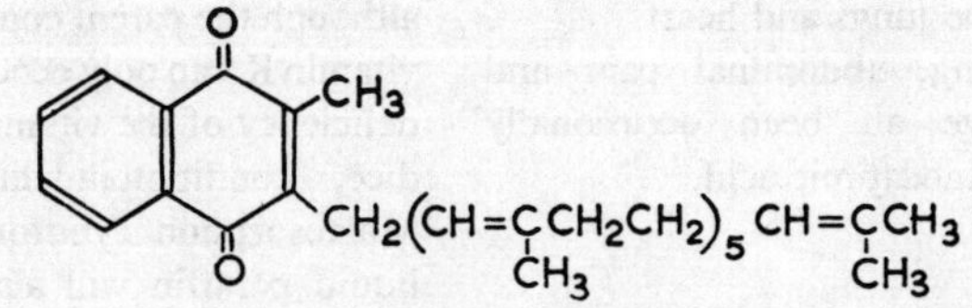

Vitamin K₂

SYNTHETIC ANALOGUES

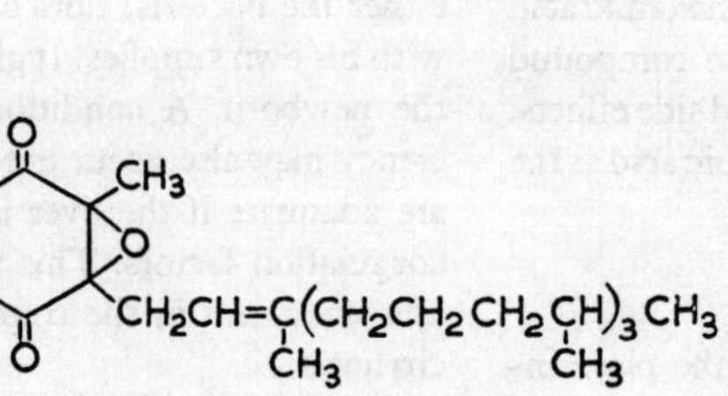

Vitamin K₁ oxide

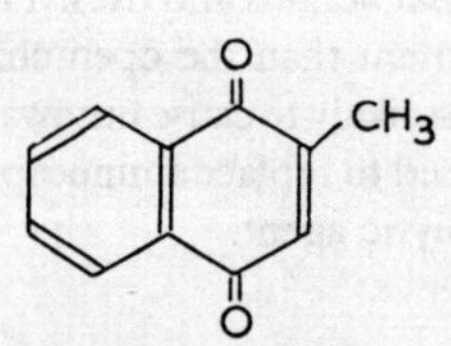

Menaphthone (menadione,)
Hykinone is a proprietary name for menaphthone sodium bisulphite.

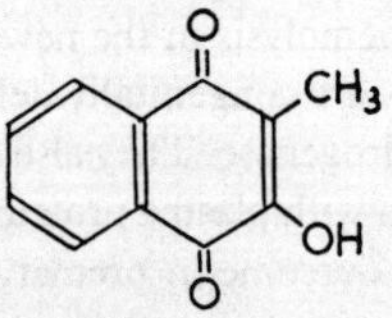

Phthiocol

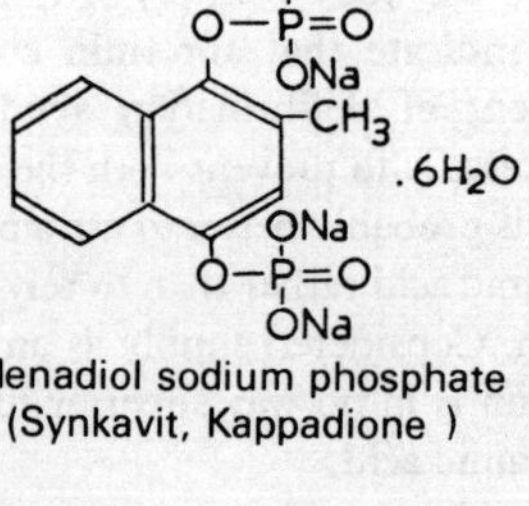

Menadiol sodium phosphate
(Synkavit, Kappadione)

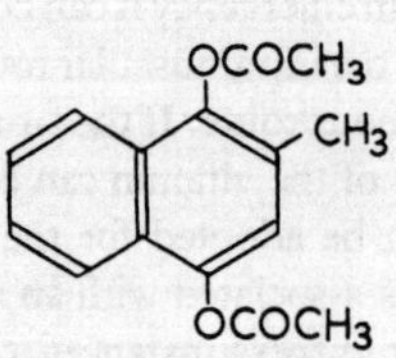

Acetomenaphthone

Fig. 39.4 Vitamin K₁ and some of its natural and synthetic analogues.

PLASMA SUBSTITUTES

Dextran

Dextran is a carbohydrate polymer of high molecular weight. It is synthesized from sucrose by the micro-organism *Leuconostoc mesenteroides,* which possesses an enzyme that polymerizes the glucose residue of the sucrose molecule to form dextran with the liberation of fructose. In the dextran molecule, glucosidic linkages of the α-1.6 type form chains of about 20 000 units. These chains are bound together in loose bundles by a relatively small number of α-1,4 cross linkages (Fig. 39.5). The average molecular weight of the complete dextran molecule is about 40 millions. Dextran in this form is not suitable for clinical use so the large molecules are hydrolyzed and the product is fractionated to give preparations with average molecular weights of 40 000, 70 000, 110 000 and 150 000 daltons. Proprietary preparations include Gentran 40, Gentran 70, Lomodex 40, Lomodex 70, Dextraven 110, Dextraven 150, Perfudex and Rheomacrodex (both dextran 40), Hyskon and Macrodex (both dextran 70). The significance of the numbers attached to some of these names should be obvious.

Solutions of dextran in isotonic sodium chloride are employed to increase blood volume and to maintain the blood pressure in haemorrhagic and traumatic shock. Dextran is employed mainly in emergencies and is not a substitute for whole blood—it contains neither formed elements nor proteins—but it is useful inasmuch as it restores the colloid osmotic pressure and the circulatory volume to normal. Because of its low molecular weight, dextran 40 disappears rather rapidly from the blood so that repeated administrations may be necessary. Moreover it induces an osmotic diuresis and so leads to fluid loss at a time when conservation should be the aim. On the other hand, preparations that contain a substantial proportion of molecules with a weight of the order of 200 000 daltons are undesirable because of the possibility of their inducing antigen-antibody reactions. For this reason, dextran 150 is not to be recommended: its name implies only that the *average* molecular weight of its constituent molecules is 150 000.

Dextran solutions are virtually inert pharmacologically but may in rare instances cause sensitization reactions. Dextran is largely excreted by the kidney at a rate dependent on its molecular size but some is excreted by the gastrointestinal tract and some is metabolized.

The advantages associated with the use of dextran are that in emergencies there is no need to produce matched blood and there is no risk of homologous serum jaundice or infective jaundice.

Solutions of dextran free from sodium chloride are employed in the treatment of hypoproteinaemia, nephrosis and toxaemia of late pregnancy.

Other preparations which have been employed for the restoration of circulating blood volume and plasma colloid osmotic pressure include polyvinylpyrrolidine and gelatin.

HAEMATOPOIETIC DRUGS

Haematopoietic drugs are substances that influence the blood cell forming tissues. They are also known as haematinics and are particularly useful for the treatment of pernicious anaemia.

Pernicious anaemia, known also as Addisonian anaemia, is a deficiency disease. The essential deficiency is that of the *intrinsic factor,* which in normal subjects is secreted by the parietal cells of the gastric mucosa. Patients suffering from pernicious anaemia respond if given gastric juice taken from normal subjects and normal gastric juice has been shown to contain the intrinsic factor. The intrinsic factor is essential for the absorption by the ileum of a heat stable substance present in the diet and described as the *extrinsic factor.*

Early studies showed that dried, defatted hog's stomach contained both the intrinsic and extrinsic factors and was effective in the treatment of pernicious anaemia. Unfortunately a daily dose of about 40 g of this preparation is necessary for maintenance treatment. Raw liver and liver extracts contain the extrinsic factor. When given by mouth these preparations are not effective unless they are given with a source of intrinsic factor such as dried hog's stomach or normal gastric juice. Liver extracts are, how-

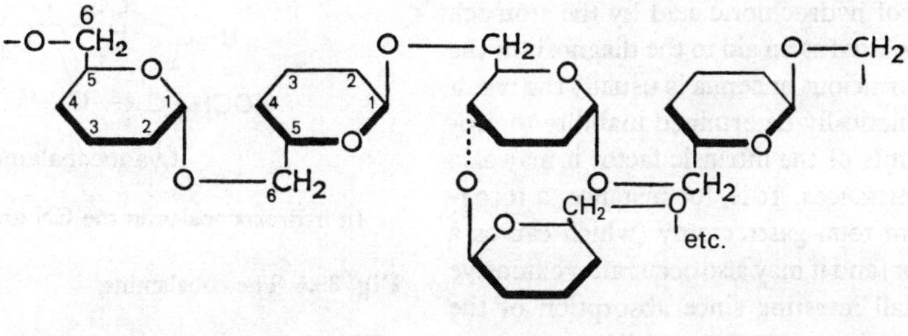

Fig. 39.5 Part of dextran molecule to show α-1:6 and α-1:4 glucosidic linkages. *(For the sake of clarity, hydroxyl groups are not shown).*

ever, effective when given by intramuscular injection. The ultimate precursor of the circulating erythrocyte is the haemocytoblast of the bone marrow. This is converted into the pro-erythroblast and in normal circumstances the latter forms the early normoblast from which the erythrocytes proper are derived. In the foetus all, and in the pernicious anaemia patient some, of the pro-erythroblasts are converted into the early megaloblast and thence into the megalocyte (the macrocytic erythrocyte). In pernicious anaemia, up to 40 per cent. of the circulating erythrocytes are of the macrocytic type: none are detectable in normal blood. Macrocytes, as the name implies, are larger than normal erythrocytes and they contain correspondingly more than the usual amount of haemoglobin. However, the total number of erythrocytes (normal and macrocytic) is considerably depressed and red blood counts as low as 2 000 000 per cu.mm. may be returned by pernicious anaemia patients. In spite of this, the traditional sign of anaemia (breathlessness on exertion) is often not seen, even in those patients whose blood haemoglobin content has reached very low levels. This is so distinctive a feature of the disease that some have suggested that it is diagnostic of pernicious anaemia (Whitby, 1963). Because of their origin, pernicious and similar anaemias are called *megaloblastic anaemias:* they can also be described as *macrocytic anaemias.* Thus the blood contains a small number of large cells instead of a large number of small ones. There is also an overall deficiency of haemoglobin.

Pernicious anaemia is accompanied by a hyperplastic red bone marrow, a histamine-resistant achlorhydria, atrophy of the gastric mucosa causing gastro-intestinal disorders (including soreness and inflammation of the tongue, gastric upset and diarrhoea) and in some cases, by well-marked neurological symptoms including a peripheral neuritis, atrophy of the optic nerve, mental deterioration and subacute combined degeneration of the spinal cord. The intrinsic factor is a glycoprotein with a molecular weight of about 50000. Patients suffering from pernicious anaemia do not manufacture the intrinsic factor and because this defect is attributable to atrophy of the gastric mucosa it is almost always linked with failure to secrete both pepsin and hydrochloric acid. In achlorhydria associated with pernicious anaemia, injection of histamine does not evoke secretion of hydrochloric acid by the stomach and this effect can be used as an aid to the diagnosis of the disease. Although pernicious anaemia is usually the result of an inborn and genetically determined inability to produce adequate amounts of the intrinsic factor it may also arise in other circumstances. It is, for instance, a recognized consequence of total gastrectomy (which causes a loss of intrinsic factor) and it may also occur after extensive excisions of the small intestine since absorption of the complex of intrinsic and extrinsic factor will be prevented. In cases of malabsorption syndrome the absorption of the extrinsic factor may be seriously interfered with, even

though dietary intake is adequate. There is accumulating evidence of an autoimmune element (p. 395) in the pathogenesis of pernicious anaemia.

Cyanocobalamin (cobalamin)

Castle's extrinsic factor has been isolated and identified (Fig. 39.6). Though often called cyanocobalamin, a better name is cobalamin because the cyano group is something of an extraction artefact. Cobalamin is a member of the B group of vitamins and in the nomenclature of the system its appelation is vitamin B_{12}. In the account that follows, 'cobalamin' is used as a synonym of the natural vitamin, 'cyanocobalamin' refers to the pure substance of the composition implied by its name while 'cobalamins' is a group name that identified both of the cobalamins (cyanocobalamin and hydroxocobalamin) in general use. Cobalamin was first isolated by Lester Smith from liver, in which it is present in relatively large amounts. It is synthesized by a number of organisms and the mould *Streptomyces griseus* is now the main commercial source of cyanocobalamin. Intestinal bacteria synthesize cobalamin which is passed to the liver for storage. Thus our own supplies of vitamin B_{12} are ultimately dependent on bacterial activity in our own intestine and in that of the animals whose flesh we eat.

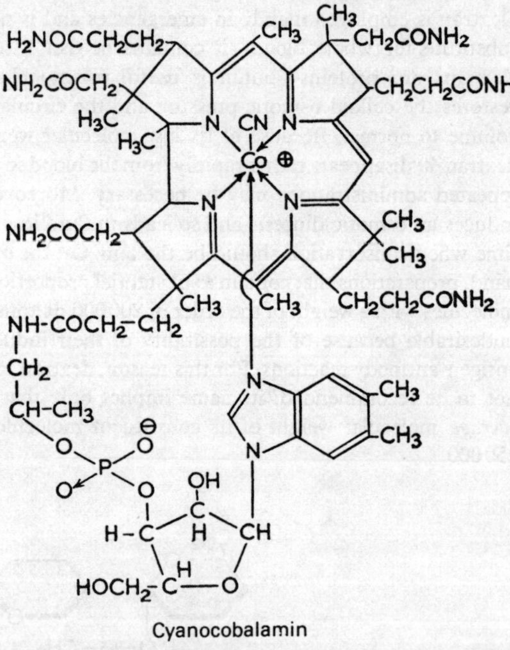

Cyanocobalamin

In hydroxocobalamin the CN group is replaced by OH

Fig. 39.6 The cobalamins.

The richest food sources of vitamin B_{12} are beef, kidney and liver which contain amounts of up to 5, 25 and 50 μg per 100 g of tissue respectively.

Cobalamin in the gastrointestinal tract combines with the intrinsic factor and ileal absorption cannot take place until this combination has occurred. At some, as yet undefined, point in the absorption process free cobalamin is released from the complex and emerges into the blood only to be bound again, this time with one or other of the carrier globulins transcobalamin I and II which convey the vitamin to the liver and other storage sites. It is stored in combination with transcobalamin I.

Cobalamin is needed to correct deficiencies of the vitamin in the tissues. The most common cause of this deficiency is absence (or ineffectiveness) of the intrinsic factor arising idiopathically or as a consequence of gastrectomy but malabsorption syndromes affecting the ileum also hinder cobalamin absorption. Very occasionally the deficiency is of dietary origin: Vegans, who shun all forms of animal food, may develop a grave deficiency if they remain faithful to their beliefs for the two or three years needed to exhaust the stores of cobalamin that existed in their tissues at the time of their conversion to this strange creed. Although pernicious anaemia is the most usual clinical manifestation of vitamin B_{12} deficiency, other conditions with the same aetiology include postgastrectomy and nutritional macrocytic anaemia and idiopathic steatorrhoea. Cobalamins have been applied to the treatment of all these disorders although some of these conditions (particularly steatorrhoea and the nutritional anaemias) are associated with deficiencies of both vitamin B_{12} and folic acid and accordingly demand treatment by both substances.

Cobalamins given by injection at dose levels as low as 50 μg produce a rapid improvement in the anaemia and the blood picture returns to normal. It also prevents the appearance of the neurological symptoms if these have not already become evident and, provided that the damage is not irreversible, it reduces the severity of any neurological complication already present.

Since the function of the intrinsic factor is to promote the absorption of the extrinsic factor in an unchanged state and since pernicious anaemia is caused by absence of the intrinsic factor, it will be clear that the therapeutic effects of cyanocobalamin will be shown only when the drug is injected although massive doses given by mouth are sometimes effective. A mixture of a cobalamin and intrinsic factor is of course, effective if taken by mouth.

Cobalamin is involved in the biosynthesis of the methyl groups of thymidine and methionine and, *via* the latter, of most of the *N*-methyl, *S*-methyl and *O*-methyl groups in compounds of biochemical interest. It is also involved in certain intramolecular shifts of carbon bonds such as occur in the conversion of malonyl coenzyme A to succinyl coenzyme A. In some biochemical systems it may function as a hydrogen carrier. In some of these actions it probably acts as a cofactor to folic acid (p. 678). Whether one of these effects is involved in pernicious anaemia is not known. It is, however, clear that cobalamin has many important metabolic functions, some of which are not well understood. There is no doubt that its presence is essential for normal red cell formation, for the formation of normal epithelial cells in the mouth and gastrointestinal tract, and for the normal functioning of peripheral nerves and the central nervous system.

Hydroxocobalamin and cyanocobalamin do not differ qualitatively in their actions but hydroxocobalamin is the more firmly bound to protein *in vivo*, it has a longer duration of action, it is retained more effectively and utilized more economically. For all these reasons, hydroxocobalamin is now regarded as the drug of choice for the treatment of vitamin B_{12} deficiency. It has an additional use. It is readily converted into cyanocobalamin and so can be given to victims of cyanide poisoning in the hope of mopping up free cyanide in the tissues. Cyanocobalamin would clearly be useless in this situation.

Table 39.2 Proprietary names for the cobalamins

Cyanocobalamin	Anacobin, Cobalin, Cytacon, Cyanovit, Cytamen, Sytobex
Hydroxocobalamin	Alpharedisol, Alpha-Ruvite, Oxobemin, Sytobex-H, Vibeden

In cases of severe deficiency of vitamin B_{12} body stores have first to be replenished and this can be achieved by giving intramuscular injections of hydroxocobalamin in twice weekly doses of 1 mg for three weeks. When the deficiency is caused by lack of intrinsic factor from any cause or by ineffectiveness of absorption processes in the ileum, maintenance doses of the vitamin will be needed for the rest of the patient's life. For this purpose 1 mg can be given every three months. In cases where the deficiency has arisen from adherence to strange dietary habits the physician should be able to play his educational role so as to ensure that, once the initial deficiency has been corrected, further supplies of vitamin B_{12} will be obtained from the supplies that are provided for us in such abundance in a rational diet. The patient may still prefer, of course, to receive four intramuscular injections in each of his remaining years as the price of a clear conscience.

Many manufacturers, aware of the therapeutic value and widespread use of the cobalamins, have entered this particular market. This fact is reflected in the large number of proprietary names borne by both the cobalamins. Some of them are listed in Table 39.2.

Folic Acid
It has been long known that a macrocytic anaemia may develop in malnourished women during pregnancy. This is clearly of dietary origin and it was assumed for many years that it was a true pernicious anaemia but in 1931

Lucy Wills, who had been studying the condition in India, reported that it could not be cured by injections of purified liver extract although this was known to contain adequate amounts of the extrinsic factor. The condition could, however, be cured by the administration of crude liver extracts and by a yeast extract (Marmite) which is not usually effective in pernicious anaemia. It was therefore concluded that the nutritional megaloblastic anaemia was not identical with pernicious anaemia and that it was caused by deficiency of a dietary factor other than vitamin B_{12}. Animal experiments confirmed these conclusions and it was soon shown that the missing factor was folic acid, a substance that had already been known for some time.

Deficiency of folic acid may arise from a number of causes other than a simple absence from the diet. From the physician's point of view, the most important of these causes is the long-continued administration of anticonvulsant drugs such as phenobarbitone, diphenylhydantoin and primidone (Malpas, *et al.*, 1966). In up to 70 per cent of patients receiving anticonvulsant drugs, the amount of folic acid in the blood is abnormally low. Not all of these patients develop a megaloblastic anaemia but a careful watch should be kept on the blood picture of epileptic patients on long term medication. Recently there has appeared the challenging suggestion that some antiepileptic drugs may actually owe their effectiveness to an ability to antagonize the production of folic acid. It is further suggested that folic acid deficiency may induce psychiatric changes. These possibilities have fascinating and important implications concerning the much discussed issue of the relationships between epilepsy and mental illness. This topic is discussed in more detail elsewhere (p. 534); a recent brief summary of the present situation is also available (Leading Article, 1976).

Folate deficiency sometimes occurs in the course of treatment with pyrimethamine (p. 868).

Folic acid antagonists are used for the treatment of leukaemia and the possibility of a megaloblastic anaemia developing in these circumstances must obviously be borne in mind. Vitamin C deficiency may also lead to an effective deficiency of folic acid (see below).

It is a curious fact that, although vitamin B_{12} does not cure anaemia caused by folic acid deficiency, folic acid does relieve some of the symptoms of anaemia caused by vitamin B_{12} deficiency. However, folic acid does not prevent the development of the neurological changes seen in pernicious anaemia nor does it alleviate any that might already have appeared. Indeed, folic acid sometimes precipitates neurological changes. It is for this reason that most textbooks of therapeutics carry injunctions against the use of folic acid or its analogues in pernicious anaemia or in other conditions that will respond equally well to vitamin B_{12}. Moreover, its effect on the blood picture is short-lived, for after some months macrocytes once again appear in the blood. A possible explanation for this action

may be that folic acid is the essential factor required for the proper development of the erythrocyte and that cobalamin is a cofactor. Thus deficiency of either folic acid or cobalamin would cause a macrocytic anaemia. In the absence of folic acid, the development of normal erythrocytes would be prevented however much cobalamin was provided. On the other hand, large amounts of folic acid, even in the absence of the cofactor, might be able, temporarily at least, to restore normal erythropoiesis by a 'mass action'. It may be that vitamin B_{12} is a cofactor in another system not dependent upon folic acid but necessary for maintaining normal nervous function. This would explain why folic acid is without even a temporary effect on the neurological changes seen in pernicious anaemia and why neurological complications are rare in anaemias caused by folic acid deficiency.

Folic acid is thought to act as a coenzyme in a number of reactions involving the transfer of one-carbon units in the synthesis of methionine, thymine and purines. It is also concerned in the catabolism of pyrimidines, purines and histidine. The units involved include the methyl, hydroxymethyl, formimino ($-CH=NH$) and formyl ($-CHO$) groups. Interruption of one or more of these transfers may well underlie the therapeutic action of those antiepileptic drugs that induce folic acid deficiency. The reader will readily appreciate why folic acid antagonists, which interfere with the synthesis of vital components of the cell, have a place in the chemotherapy of cancer (p. 917).

Folic acid was known for many years before it was identified chemically and for this reason it received a number of names which reflect the methods and interests of the many workers who were studying it. Folic acid should properly refer only to pteroylglutamic acid (Fig. 39.7) while the various naturally-occurring derivatives should be grouped together as *folacin*. However, old habits die hard and most authors continue the harmless practice of designating as folic acid both the pure substance and its several derivatives.

Folic acid is found in liver, in fresh dark-green leafy vegetables, particularly spinach (*cf.* vitamin K_1, p. 673) and in some meats. It owes its name to its occurrence in leaves.

The naturally occurring derivatives we have referred to are usually conjugates possessing more than one glutamic acid residue in the molecule. The most common are pteroyltriglutamic acid (which is particularly formed by certain bacteria) and pteroylheptaglutamic acid, which is synthesized by yeasts. In many of these conjugates the folic acid component is in a reduced (dihydro or tetrahydro) form and a proportion of the molecules appear as methyl or formyl derivatives. Dietary folacin contains pteroylglutamic acid in these various forms. During digestion, the extra glutamate residues are removed to leave monoglutamates. During absorption, any of these molecules that are not already in the reduced form are converted, successively, into the dihydro and the tetrahydro derivatives under the influence of *dihydrofolate reductase*. The process of 5-methylation also occurs so that most of the folic acid in the blood is in the form of 5-methyltetrahydrofolate (5-methyltetrahydro pterylglutamate). An analogous molecule containing several glutamate residues provides a storage form.

It has been suggested that before folic acid can bring about its erythropoietic effect it must undergo a chemical change to form a more active but labile form. This was originally thought to be folinic acid (the citrovorum factor) but it now seems likely that the active factor is *N*-5 methyltetrahydrofolic acid. The reduction of folic acid and its derivatives to the tetrahydro forms require vitamin C and this presumably explains why ascorbic acid deficiency may cause a megaloblastic anaemia.

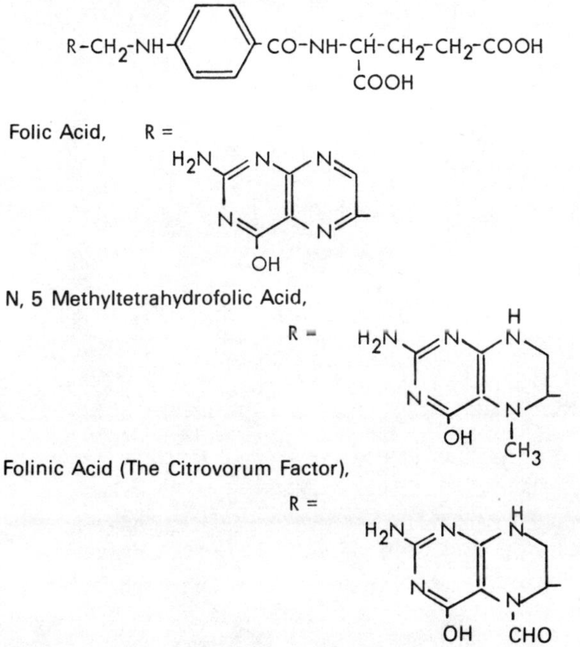

Folic Acid,   R =

N, 5 Methyltetrahydrofolic Acid,

R =

Folinic Acid (The Citrovorum Factor),

R =

Fig. 39.7 Folic (pteroylglutamic acid) and some related substances.

Citrovorum factor was the name used to describe a substance present in liver extracts which was found to be essential for the growth of the micro-organism *Leuconostoc citrovorum* on synthetic media. It was later identified as folinic acid.

Deficiency of folic acid resulting from dietary inadequacies is almost unknown in the more affluent parts of the world but deficiency from the other causes mentioned on page 678 is encountered. Macrocytic anaemia resulting from a simple lack of folacin in the diet can be treated by giving folic acid by mouth (10-30 mg daily) but the vitamin will have to be given by the intramuscular route if

the deficiency is the consequence of malabsorption. Folic acid deficiency caused by drugs needs to be treated with folinic acid (10-20 mg daily). The drugs inhibit dihydrofolate reductase but folinic acid needs no further reduction (Fig. 39.7) before conversion into a physiologically active compound. A proprietary form of folic acid is available under the name of Folvite.

It must be remembered that folic acid may precipitate irreversible damage to the nervous system if it is given to patients suffering from pernicious anaemia. If the diagnosis of a macrocytic anaemia is in doubt, hydroxocobalamin must always be tried first. If the cobalamin effects no improvement in the clinical condition, folic acid can be given. However, the differential diagnosis of pernicious anaemia from an anaemia caused by folic acid deficiency rarely presents difficulty.

BIBLIOGRAPHY

Books, monographs and reviews

Biggs, Rosemary (ed) (1976). *Human Blood Coagulation, Haemostasis and Thrombosis.* 2nd ed. Oxford: Blackwell.

Britton, C. J. C. (1963). *Whitby and Britton's Disorders of the Blood,* 9th ed. London: Churchill.

Conference (1959). Hematopoietic mechanisms. *Ann. N. Y. Acad. Sci.,* **77,** 407-820.

Engleberg, H. (1963). *Heparin: Metabolism, Physiology and Clinical Application.* Springfield: Thomas.

Fletcher, A. P. and Sherry, S. (1966). Thrombolytic agents. *A. Rev. Pharmacol.,* **6,** 89-106.

Friedman, M. (1969). *Pathogenesis of Coronary Artery Disease.* New York: McGraw-Hill.

Gallus, A. S. and Hirsh, J. (1976a). Antithrombotic drugs: Part I. *Drugs,* **12,** 41-68.

Gallus, A. S. and Hirsh, J. (1976b). Antithrombotic drugs: Part II. *Drugs,* **12,** 132-157.

Harris, J. W. (1963). *The Red Cell.* Cambridge, Mass.: Harvard University Press.

Ingram, G. I. C. (1961). Anticoagulant therapy. *Pharmac. Rev.,* **13,** 279-328.

Laurell, C. B. (1952). Plasma iron and the transport of iron in the organism. *Pharmac. Rev.,* **4,** 371-395.

Lester Smith, E. (1960). *Vitamin B_{12}* London: Methuen.

Linman, J. W. and Bethell, F. H. (1960). *Factors Controlling Erythropoiesis.* Springfield: Thomas.

Mustard, J. F. and Packham, Marian A. (1975). Platelets, thrombosis and drugs. *Drugs,* **9,** 19-76.

Nicolaides, A. N. (ed) (1975). *Thromboembolism* Lancaster: Medical and Technical Publishing Company.

Prankerd, T. A. J. (1961). *The Red Cell.* Oxford: Blackwell.

Thompson, R. B. (1975). A Short Textbook of Haematology. 4th ed. Tunbridge Wells: Pitman Medical Publishing Company.

Von Kualla, K. N. (1963). *Chemistry of Thrombolysis: Human Fibrinolytic Enzymes.* Springfield: Thomas.

Wolstenholme, G. E. W. and O'Connor, M. (1960). *Haemopoiesis.* London: Churchill.

Original papers

Barritt, D. W. and Jordan, S. C. (1960). Anticoagulant drugs in the treatment of pulmonary embolism. A controlled trial. *Lancet.* (i), 1309-1312.

Charlton, R. W., Jacobs, P., Torrance, J. D. and Bothwell, T. H. (1963). The role of ferritin in iron absorption. *Lancet*, **2**, 762-764.

Leading Article (1976). Folic acid and the nervous system. Lancet (**ii**), 836.

Malpas, J. S., Spray, G. H. and Witts, L. J. (1966). Serum folic acid and vitamin B_{12} levels in anticonvulsant therapy. *Br. med. J.*, **1**, 955-957.

Reid, H. A., Thean, P. C., Chan, K. E. and Baharom, A. R. (1963). Clinical effects of bites by Malayan viper (Ancistrodon rhodostoma). Lancet (**i**), 617-626.

Storm, O., Ollendorff, P., Drewsen, E. and Tang, P. (1974). Acute deep vein thrombosis treated with porcine plasmin. A double blind trial. *Thrombosis et Diathesis Haemorrhagica*, **32**, 468-482.

Wills, Lucy (1931). Treatment of 'pernicious anaemia of pregnancy' and tropical 'anaemia' with special reference to yeast extract as curative agent. *Br. med. J.*, **1**, 1059-1065.

40. Drugs that act on the cardiovascular system

The drugs that are to be considered in this chapter can be conveniently divided into four groups. The *antiarrhythmic (antidysrhythmic) drugs* are essentially depressant: they depress the excitability of cardiac muscle and that of the specialized conducting tissue and they are used in the treatment of cardiac arrhythmias. The *cardiotonic drugs* are excitatory: they increase the power of contraction of cardiac muscle and they are used in the treatment of cardiac failure. The *antianginal drugs* reduce the oxygen demands of, or increase the blood supply to, the myocardium (or have both of these effects) and they are employed to treat angina pectoris. Finally, the *vasoactive drugs* (vasodilator and vasoconstrictor) have actions located predominantly in the blood vessels. They are used to treat peripheral vascular disorders. These classes are not mutually exclusive. Some arrhythmias are best treated by cardiotonic drugs, the antiarrhythmic drugs indirectly improve the cardiac output when they correct an arrhythmia and some drugs could justifiably be included in more than one category.

ANTIARRHYTHMIC DRUGS

Before the antiarrhythmic drugs themselves are considered it might be helpful to discuss briefly the nature and origin of those disturbances of cardiac rhythm which are most often encountered in clinical practice. It is assumed that the reader is familiar with the elementary facts concerning the origin and propagation of the heart beat in the healthy subject and with the configuration of the normal electrocardiogram.

Disturbances of rhythm are sometimes (and more properly) described as 'dysrhythmias' but the time honoured 'arrhythmias' is retained here. Abnormalities of heart rate are included among the arrhythmias even though the actual rhythm of the beat is not necessarily disturbed in these conditions.

Arrhythmias can arise in the sinoatrial (sinus) node, the atria, the junctional conducting tissue and the ventricles. In the summary account that follows they are classified according to their sites of origin.

Arrhythmias arising in the sinus
The sinus node is the point of origin of the normal heart beat. In certain conditions—fever, hyperthyroidism, anaemia or after taking cardioacceleratory drugs such as sympathomimetic agents—the rate of impulse discharge increases producing a quickening of the beat that is properly described as *sinus tachycardia*. The opposite condition—*sinus bradycardia*—occurs in the trained athlete, in myxoedema, as a consequence of raised intracranial pressure or after taking drugs such as guanethidine or adrenaline β receptor blocking agents. Neither sinus tachycardia nor sinus bradycardia is referable to any pathological change in the heart itself and if treatment is indicated (as it sometimes is in cases of extreme sinus bradycardia) it is to be directed against the factor that provoked the abnormal rate in the first place.

Sinus arrhythmia is common among healthy young people: the heart accelerates on inspiration and decelerates on expiration. It is the result of an 'overflow' of impulses from the respiratory to the adjoining vagal centre. It is of no pathological significance whatever.

Arrhythmias arising in the atria
Atrial flutter will be described first to provide a basis for discussing the other atrial arrhythmias.

ATRIAL FLUTTER
In this condition, the atria beat very rapidly but regularly. The rate of atrial contraction ranges from 250 to 350 but most often it is in the region of 300 beats a minute. Not all of these beats cause ventricular contraction but a regular proportion (usually one half but sometimes one third or even a quarter) are transmitted to the ventricles. Consequently the most usual pulse rate in atrial flutter is close to 150. An attack of atrial flutter may be an isolated event in the patient's cardiac history or attacks may recur at intervals. Atrial flutter is usually the result of organic disease of the heart such as rheumatic fever, myocarditis or thyrotoxicosis.

Atrial flutter is probably often the consequence of a *circus movement*. If an area of the atrial tissue outside the normal pacemaker is stimulated and if some obstacle near the excited focus limits the spread of excitation so that it propagates in only one direction, it may travel round the periphery of the obstacle. Provided that this is large enough to ensure that the original point of excitation has recovered from its refractory period by the time the wave of excitation returns to it, the impulse will continue to travel round the obstacle, circus fashion. The excitation spreading from the normal pacemaker will be suppressed since it will be propagated to muscle which is being driven by the rapid circus movement. Circus movements of this type can be produced in experimental animals by crushing an area of atrial wall (to provide the obstacle) between the superior and inferior venae cavae. If the area of the crushed tissue is too small, the circus movement will not be established because the wave of excitation will return to its point of origin too soon and it will be extinguished as it enters the zone of refractoriness created by its own first passage. When the area of damage becomes just large enough to prevent this, the circus movement which results produces an atrial beat of about 300 a minute, the rate actually observed in the human being. In the human patient the obstacle is provided by an area of the myocardium damaged or disturbed by disease. It will be clear that an established circus movement will be suppressed by anything that causes a sufficiently large increase in the refractory period.

In some cases, atrial flutter may simply be caused by the rapid but regular discharge of impulses from a focus (the *ectopic focus*) outside the pacemaker. It takes over pacemaker function because of its high rate of discharge.

The symptoms of atrial flutter are similar to those of atrial tachycardia (see below) but the condition is of more serious import because it often precipitates failure in an already damaged heart.

SUPRAVENTRICULAR PAROXYSMAL (ATRIAL) TACHYCARDIA
This is often a relatively trivial condition. It is similar to atrial flutter except that the rate of atrial contraction is usually no more than about 200 per minute. Attacks of supraventricular paroxysmal tachycardia may be quite transitory but they often persist for hours. In either event they usually stop spontaneously. Their occurrence may go unnoticed but most patients complain of fear, faintness, dizziness, anginal pain or of a sensation of fluttering in the chest. Vagal stimulation, brought about reflexly by carotid compression or pressure on the eyes, will often terminate an attack of tachycardia, a fact which is often discovered by the patient himself.

Like atrial flutter, atrial tachycardia can provoke cardiac failure when it occurs in a diseased heart. On the other hand, it is quite harmless in otherwise healthy individuals from whom the condition can usually be banished by mere reassurance, a simple sedative or the proscription of tobacco and strong coffee.

The Wolff-Parkinson-White syndrome is the name given to a distinctive electrocardiographic pattern the principal features of which are a short PR interval and a broadened QRS complex with a characteristic notch on its upstroke. The syndrome, which is most often seen in those with a susceptibility to supraventricular paroxysmal tachycardia, reveals the existence of pathways that conduct the cardiac impulse abnormally quickly from atria to ventricles.

ATRIAL FIBRILLATION
In this condition the rate of atrial contraction may reach 500 a minute. At this rate, the wave of contraction cannot spread in an orderly manner through the atria as it is extinguished or delayed by irregular patches of refractoriness. When the next wave arrives, these areas will have recovered their excitability but others which have permitted the passage of the preceding wave will be refractory. This type of response can occur because the refractory period of atrial muscle is not uniform. It results in the atrial beats being irregular and uncoordinated and it is this, rather than the rate of beat, which distinguishes fibrillation from flutter. The term 'beat' is something of a misnomer when it is applied to fibrillating atria. The contractions are so rapid and fragmentary that most of them are mechanically quite ineffectual and few of them survive long enough to reach the atrioventricular node. If fibrillating atria are inspected *in situ*, no more than a few rapid twitchings (*fibrillations*) are seen.

In atrial fibrillation the ventricles beat at no more than one-quarter or one-fifth of the atrial rate but the transmission of the atrial beat is not regular so that the ventricular systoles are irregular and of varying strength. The pulse is similarly affected so that diagnosis becomes a simple matter.

Atrial fibrillation may be chronic or paroxysmal. In the latter event, attacks begin and end very suddenly. The chronic state is likely to have serious consequences. The impaired ventricular performance causes a reduction in cardiac output and so predisposes to cardiac failure. Another likely complication is thrombosis of the virtually stagnant blood in the ineffective atria with the risk of a fatal embolism should a portion of the clot become dislodged and pass into the ventricles and thence into the vascular system.

Atrial fibrillation is usually the consequence of rheumatic heart disease, myocardial infarction, hypertension or thyrotoxicosis. It sometimes arises as a consequence of surgical activity in the heart or lungs and in a small percentage of cases it appears in the absence of any detectable pathological change.

Like flutter, atrial fibrillation may be produced by a circus movement but it is more likely to be due to the rapid discharge of an ectopic focus.

Arrhythmias arising in the junctional tissue
Disturbances in the ability of the cardiac junctional tissue to transmit the cardiac impulse give rise to several varieties of *heart block*.

SINO-ATRIAL BLOCK
In this condition, an occasional impulse from the sino-atrial node fails to reach the atria and a heart beat is missed. Like several other conduction defects, sino-atrial block is often attributable to digitalis poisoning. Minor degrees of block are quite symptomless but fainting will occur if several beats in succession are missed.

Sometimes the sino-atrial node itself fails. Normal cardiac function is restored as soon as another pacemaker takes over.

ATRIOVENTRICULAR BLOCK

In this condition, the conduction of the impulse from atria to ventricles is delayed (first degree block), partially blocked (second degree block) or totally arrested (complete heart block).

First degree block is not attended by any cardiovascular symptoms. It is diagnosed from the electrocardiographic record when the PR interval (which measures the conduction time from the sino-atrial node to the ventricular muscle) exceeds the upper limit of normality (0.2 sec.). It is sometimes seen in rheumatic fever but it most often occurs as a sign of early digitalis intoxication.

In most forms of second degree block, only one in 2, 3, 4 or more of the atrial beats is successfully transmitted to the ventricles. An exception to this generalization is provided by the Wenckebach phenomenon (a type of second degree block) in which the PR interval becomes progressively lengthened with successive beats until an atrial contraction fails to evoke a ventricular response. The process is repeated. The pulse rate, which reflects the ventricular contractions, is irregular. In other forms of heart block the pulse, though slow, is regular. Second degree heart block is a feature of intoxication with cardiac glycosides and of some forms of cardiac disorder particularly myocardial infarction.

In severe cases of second degree heart block the number of ventricular beats may be so small that the cardiac output and the arterial blood pressure fall to such an extent that cardiac failure supervenes. Another hazard associated with this degree of dysfunction is the possibility that it may evolve into a complete block. The transition from second degree to complete heart block may be marked by brief periods of cardiac arrest with dizziness, fainting, cyanosis and, in extreme cases, convulsions (Adams-Stokes attacks). Adams-Stokes attacks are rather less likely to occur once complete block has become established and the responsibility for initating ventricular beats has shifted to an extra-atrial site.

Complete heart block is sometimes a sequel to myocardial infarction, severe rheumatic heart disease or cardiac surgery but it also occurs, particularly in the elderly, as a result of fibrosis in the two branches of the bundle of His. The aetiology of this fibrosis is obscure.

The existence of a state of complete heart block is not necessarily incompatible with a normal life span but the possibility of its precipitating cardiac failure demands that the condition be adequately treated, if necessary by means of an artificial pacemaker.

Heart block sometimes affects only one of the bundle branches. A block restricted to the right branch is symptomless and of little significance but a left bundle branch block is a more serious condition, often associated with coronary arterial disease.

Recently developed methods of recording permit more detailed analyses of the heart's action than has hitherto been possible. In particular, recordings from the bundle of His can discover the sites where conduction of the cardiac impulse is interrupted in individual cases of heart block. The newly coined 'suprahisian', 'intrahisian' and 'infrahisian' are employed to denote the position of conduction blocks in relation to the bundle of His. Readers requiring a more sophisticated exposition than can be given here of the nature and origin of the several forms of heart block (and of the other cardiac arrhythmias) are referred to recent monographs such as that by Krikler and Goodwin (1975).

Arrhythmias arising in the ventricles

Disturbances of rhythm arising in the ventricles include fibrillation, tachycardia and extrasystoles.

VENTRICULAR FIBRILLATION

Although fibrillating atria are incapable of executing effective systoles, this does not impair the transfer of blood from atria to ventricles. Atrial systole in any event only occupies about one eighth of the cardiac cycle and the passage of blood from the veins to the ventricles is a passive event, most of it occurring during the period of atrial diastole. However, when the ventricles go into fibrillation a much more serious situation obtains, for the heart may be quite incapable of expelling blood. Ventricular fibrillation is therefore an extremely dangerous condition which leads to rapid death unless it is immediately corrected. It is the immediate cause of death in many fatal cases of cardiac infarction, electrocution and overdosage with cardiotonic drugs.

VENTRICULAR (PAROXYSMAL) TACHYCARDIA

This is a relatively uncommon condition. It is usually associated with a history of a serious heart disease such as myocardial infarction but it sometimes occurs after exercise in healthy people. The condition results from an increase in the irritability of the ventricles which lead to a rapid series of contractions (*ventricular extrasystoles*) which occur independently of those arriving from the atria. Attacks of ventricular tachycardia are sudden in onset and they usually end suddenly. The rate of ventricular contraction can reach 200 a minute or more and attacks last for varying periods from a few seconds to several days. Diminished cardiac output is often severe enough to give rise to such symptoms of cardiac failure as dyspnoea and chest pains during an episode of ventricular tachycardia. Extrasystoles may also occur singly or at widely spaced intervals. Following a single extrasystole the heart is refractory to the next impulse arriving from the pacemaker so that there is a 'compensatory pause' before the next systole. The patient, unaware of the extrasystole, notices that his heart has apparently missed a beat. This may cause him some alarm but occasional extrasystoles are usually of no significance in young and healthy subjects. They may follow the first indulgence in tobacco smoking, a heavy meal or some similarly trivial event. On the other hand, extrasystoles occurring in older patients with a history of heart disease may herald the onset of a more serious arrhythmia. If they occur in patients receiving a cardiac glycoside, they should be regarded as evidence that toxic dose levels have been reached.

Classification and actions of antiarrhythmic drugs

A potential difference of some 85 mV exists across the plasma membrane of cardiac muscle fibres in diastole, the outside of the fibre being positive with respect to the inside. This demarcation potential is reversed by stimuli that provoke contraction of the muscle. Both the demarcation and the action potentials are qualitatively similar to those recorded from nerve and striated muscle and they have a similar origin (p. 155). Briefly, an active pump mechanism, operating across a membrane of limited permeability, permits the accumulation of sodium ions on the external surface of the membrane until a suitable stimulus brings about such an increase in the permeability of the membrane that sodium enters the tissue, the sodium pump notwithstanding. As in nerve (p. 157) the passage of sodium ions across the membrane can be quantitatively expressed in terms of the activity of hypothetical 'm' and 'h' gates that guard the sodium channels. Nevertheless, ionic movements in cardiac muscle—and the mechanisms that generate them—show some unique features.

The time courses of the action potential in atrial and ventricular fibres on the one hand and in pacemaker tissue on the other are indicated in Fig. 40.1 (a) and (b) respectively.

The plasma membranes of the atrial and ventricular fibres maintain a steady resting potential (phase 4) until the heart is provoked into contraction by the arrival of an impulse from the pacemaker or the application of an external stimulus. When this occurs there is a sudden reversal of the resting potential (phase 0) followed by a more leisurely restoration of the resting condition. Three stages in the restoration process are recognized: a stage of rapid repolarization (phase 1) is followed by a plateau (phase 2) and a final stage of rapid repolarization (phase 3). The whole process occupies some 300 msec and it is thus much more sluggish than the corresponding event in nerve and striated muscle.

Action potentials in nodal tissue and Purkinje fibres differ from those in the generality of cardiac fibres in that phase 4 takes the form of a slow spontaneous depolarization that eventually reaches the threshold point for initiation of the rapid inrush of sodium ions that occurs during phase 0 of the potential changes. The three phases of the repolarization process are less sharply delineated from one

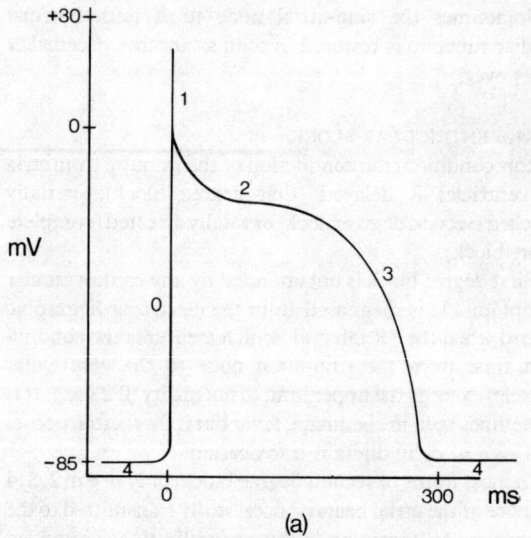

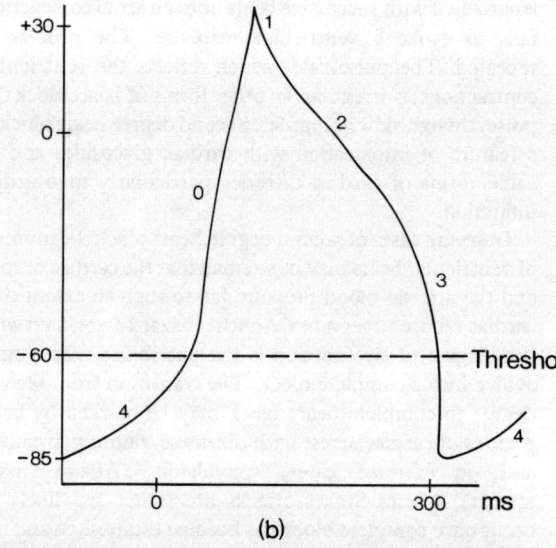

Fig. 40.1 Cardiac action potentials in ventricle muscle (a) and in pacemaker tissue (b)

another in pacemaker tissue than they are in nonautomatic fibres (Fig. 40.1b).

As in other excitable tissues, action currents in cardiac muscle are carried by sodium and potassium ions but an additional and important contribution to the inward flowing current is made by the movement of calcium ions. The calcium current is activated when the demarcation potential falls to some 40 mV. Unlike the sodium current (which only flows for a few milliseconds) the calcium current is extinguished only slowly. It is this continued inward calcium current that is responsible for the delayed repolarization of cardiac muscle and the characteristic form of cardiac action potentials. The ingress of calcium ions evokes the release of further supplies of the free ion from intracellular sites (the sarcoplasmic reticulum) and the resulting increased concentration of free calcium ions is sufficient to activate the contractile mechanisms.

The energy for cardiac contraction is provided by the hydrolysis of adenosine triphosphate (ATP). The instrument responsible for this hydrolysis is an ATPase present in the myosin fibrils and capable of activation by the interdigitating actin fibrils. During diastole this activation is prevented by the troponin-tropomyosin system, a protein complex closely associated with actin. This inhibitory action is annulled by combination with calcium, an ion for which the complex exhibits a considerable affinity. Consequently, the influx of calcium sets in motion a train of processes that culminates in systolic contraction.

The mechanism and route by which calcium crosses the plasma membrane differ from those utilized by sodium. Sodium channels are blocked by tetrodotoxin (p. 474), a substance that has no effect on calcium channels. Verapamil (p. 690), on the other hand, prevents the access of calcium but does not interfere with the movement of sodium ions into the heart. Catecholamines and the methylxanthines activate the calcium current (indicating that the adenylate cyclase system is involved in the activation) but these substances do not influence sodium ingress.

Following the pioneer work of Vaughan Williams and his colleagues (Vaughan Williams, 1975) it has become customary, in pharmacological circles at least, to group antiarrhythmic drugs into four classes according to their principal mode of action. Like all devices of this type the grouping leaves something to be desired since a number of substances defy classification either because they display more than one or because they have none of the properties that characterize the individual classes.

Class I drugs reduce the rate of rise of the action potential. In spontaneously active cells, both phase 4 and phase 0 of the action potential are prolonged. In others, of course, only phase 0 is influenced. The refractory period is also increased and the two effects operate together to slow the heart when the rate is abnormally high particularly when the tachycardia is caused by the activity of ectopic foci. The action of Class I drugs on the rate of depolarization can most readily be explained by the hypothesis that they partially occlude the sodium channels. This same hypothesis can explain the prolongation of the effective refractory period since if sodium movement is hindered it will be necessary for a depolarized membrane to become more completely repolarized than usual (i.e. a bigger sodium gradient must be established) before it can be discharged again. Some Class I drugs (but not all) also slow conduction in the heart, a property that will clearly contribute to their ability to suppress tachycardial arrhythmias.

The prototypical member of this class of drug is quini-

dine. Among the other members are lignocaine, procainamide and diphenylhydantoin. The first two members of this last named trio are also well known as local anaesthetics and the third is in wide use as an antiepileptic agent. These antiarrhythmic, local anaesthetic and antiepileptic properties can all be regarded as manifestations of the drugs' ability to stabilize membranes. Some of the drugs that block adrenaline β receptors (and thus are properly included in the Class II category) are also capable of effecting membrane stabilization but only at dose levels beyond those commonly used for the relief of arrhythmias.

Other Class I drugs include disopyramide, mexiletine, ajmaline and aprindine.

Class II drugs antagonize the action of sympathomimetic agents and they are particularly useful in conditions that are associated with an increased sensitivity of the pacemaker to the endogenous catecholamines. One such condition is the anaesthesia induced by the halogenated hydrocarbons (p. 493). Atrial and ventricular tachycardias and extrasystoles also respond well to Class II drugs.

The most important members of the class are the β blocking agents but other sympathetic antagonists such as bretylium have similar actions.

Class III drugs prolong the cardiac action potential and, consequently, the refractory period. Lack of thyroid hormone has Class III effects. The best known Class III drug is amiodarone.

Class IV drugs exert their pharmacological action as a result of their interfering with the entry of calcium into the sarcofibrils either by obstructing the calcium channels or by depleting calcium stores at the membrane. Verapamil and prenylamine are members of the class.

Class I drugs

The action of drugs of this type on the electrical changes in the heart (see above) result in a decrease in the rate of the accelerated heart and usually reduce the rate of conduction of the cardiac impulse. Oddly enough the drugs occasionally precipitate tachycardias. Quinidine, the longest known member of the group is also the most powerful in respect of both its beneficial and its adverse effects.

QUINIDINE

It was Wenckebach who, in 1914, first proposed the use of quinidine for the treatment of cardiac arrhythmias, although the observation which led to this suggestion came from one of his own patients who suffered from both atrial fibrillation and malaria. The patient had noticed that when an attack of malarial fever necessitated his taking quinine, his atrial fibrillation also improved. Wenckebach investigated the antifibrillatory action of other antimalarial drugs and found that quinidine (the dextroisomer of quinine) was much more effective than quinine itself.

Pharmacological properties of quinidine

Since quinidine prolongs the depolarization-repolarization cycle, it decreases the rate at which cardiac contractions can succeed one another. The effect is the same as if the absolute refractory period had itself been extended and this forms the basis of its effectiveness in the treatment of disorders of cardiac rhythm.

Delay in depolarization reduces the velocity of conduction of the propagated muscle activity as well as the rate at which contractions can be initiated. Another effect of quinidine is to decrease the excitability of cardiac muscle. This is probably brought about by the same mechanism as that which causes the delay in depolarization: the essential event in depolarization is the inward passage of sodium and it seems that quinidine reduces the effectiveness of the sodium carrier mechanism (Szekeres and Vaughan Williams, 1963). This would have the effect of increasing the threshold for the initiation of cardiac activity.

Although quinidine reduces the rate of contraction of fluttering or fibrillating heart chambers, it is likely to increase the rate of beat of the normal heart. This is because it has an atropine like as well as an antiarrhythmic action and it therefore removes the restraint normally imposed by the tonic activity of the vagus nerves. In the arrhythmic heart, the beat is controlled by activity outside the sphere of influence of the vagus nerves and the atropine like effect of quinidine does not usually offset the antiarrhythmic effect. In the normal heart, on the other hand, it often does because the sinus node is much less sensitive to the depressant action of quinidine than is the rest of the atrial tissue. The distinction between the 'normal' and the 'arrhythmic' heart is by no means absolute and the atropine like action of quinidine is responsible for the tachycardias that sometimes complicate its clinical use. Quinidine also causes some fall in blood pressure and this may further increase the heart rate by reflex stimulation of the sympathetic nervous system.

The atropine like actions of quinidine have other implications. Stimulation of the vagus shortens the refractory period of cardiac muscle and abolition of this effect by quinidine will add to the latter's direct antiarrhythmic action. Atropine itself will sometimes restore normal beating in the arrhythmic atrium. On the other hand, vagal stimulation reduces the conductivity of the atrioventricular bundle and thus tends to reduce the ventricular rate in patients with atrial flutter or fibrillation. It has already been pointed out that attacks of paroxysmal supraventricular tachycardia can often be arrested by manoeuvres that increase tonic vagal activity. Quinidine therefore tends to antagonize the beneficial effect of tonic vagal activity on ventricular rate. In short, it may reduce the atrial rate but increase the ventricular rate in the same patient.

In large doses, quinidine has a curare like action as can be easily demonstrated on the frog rectus preparation.

Therapeutic uses of quinidine
Once the most widely used antiarrhythmic weapon, quinidine lost much of its earlier popularity when less dangerous drugs and alternative procedures became available. It is now recommended principally for the treatment of arrhythmias of ventricular origin that have not responded satisfactorily to other drugs or that may need prolonged treatment. Some authorities still favour its use to prevent the recurrence of atrial arrhythmias that have been corrected by electrical treatment (p. 690) and it is still occasionally given to patients who have only recently developed an atrial arrhythmia and in whom there is little or no impairment of ventricular function or evidence of myocardial damage. In this latter circumstance, digitalis (or another cardiac glycoside) is given in conjunction with the quinidine. The glycoside restores normal ventricular contractions while the quinidine looks after the atria.

Quinidine is almost invariably given by mouth. A suitable dose (in patients who have been shown not to be hypersensitive to the drug) is 400 mg three or four times daily. A sustained release of quinidine is provided by Kinidin Durules which need to be taken (in amounts that supply 250 to 500 mg of quinidine) only twice daily.

Quinidine is bound to plasma protein to the extent of approximately 85 per cent. Its half life in blood is some 8 hr and therapeutically effective doses of the drug give plasma concentrations of 2.5 to 6 μg per ml.

Side effects and toxic reactions in quinidine treatment
Quinidine is a dangerous drug. It should be used only when no other drug suffices and then only if the patient can be kept under close clinical surveillance while the dose is being established.

Incommoding, but not usually serious, gastrointestinal upsets (nausea, vomiting and diarrhoea) occur in up to one third of those who take quinidine. Other systemic disturbances are much less common but some hypersensitive individuals experience the alarming array of symptoms that constitute cinchonism (p. 866) if they take even small doses of the drug or they may suffer angioneurotic oedema or other obviously allergic reactions. It should be regarded as mandatory to give a small test dose of quinidine (200 mg) to any patient in whom the use of quinidine is contemplated.

The most potentially dangerous hazard of quinidine therapy is the possibility of cardiovascular complications such as hypotension, cardiac failure, conduction blocks, tachycardias and ventricular fibrillation. Unexpected sudden deaths have been reported among patients receiving small prophylactic doses of quinidine after having had their original arrhythmias corrected by electroversion. It seems that in these unfortunate patients, some circumstance (perhaps a reduction in the acidity of the urine) has led to a reduction in the excretion of quinidine and a consequent increase in its serum concentration to toxic levels.

The neuromuscular blocking action of quinidine sometimes brings complaints of muscle weakness from those receiving the drug. It need hardly be added that muscle relaxing drugs should only be given with circumspection to those who are also taking quinidine.

A potentially serious hazard of quinidine therapy is one which is always quoted but occurs rarely. Fibrillating atria do not themselves expel blood, which simply passes through them from veins to ventricles. Pockets of blood tend therefore to collect in recesses of the atria (particularly the auricular appendages) where they stagnate and may develop into thrombi. An antiarrhythmic drug may, by promoting vigorous atrial contraction, dislodge the thrombi which may then break up, enter the general circulation and cause multiple and perhaps fatal emboli by lodging in the fine vessels of the cerebral and pulmonary circulations.

One advantage can be claimed for quinidine: long term treatment is not associated with the risk of systemic lupus erythematosus as it is with some other antiarrhythmic drugs.

LIGNOCAINE

Lignocaine (lidocaine, Xylocaine) differs from quinidine in one important respect: it does not depress—indeed it sometimes enhances—intracardiac conduction. Nevertheless, because it reduces the rate of rise of phase 4 of the action potential, it is properly regarded as a Class I drug.

Lignocaine is employed principally in the treatment of acute disturbances of the ventricular rhythm (tachycardia and fibrillation) particularly those that may accompany or follow cardiac surgery or myocardial infarction. It is a valuable agent for the treatment of arrhythmias caused by poisoning by the digitalis glycosides. It is extensively and rapidly metabolized in the liver and it is not, therefore, suitable for oral administration, particularly in the emergency conditions in which its use is usually called for. A common practice in these circumstances is to give an intravenous injection of 100 mg of lignocaine and at the same time to set up an infusion that will supply one or two milligrams of the drug a minute. Since its plasma half life is of the order of an hour and a half the drug delivered by the original injection will have been largely eliminated before that coming in from the infusion system reaches its steady state concentration. The latter condition is not attained for some five or six hours and it may be necessary to give a second injection if the arrhythmia threatens to return during the period in which the amount of infused drug in the plasma is still climbing to its plateau level. Should the infusion rate fail to control the heart even when the plateau concentration has been reached it is permissible to increase it so as to provide up to four milligrams of lignocaine a minute provided that signs of toxicity do not develop. Control of the arrhythmia is usually achieved at plasma concentrations of 2 to 5 μg per ml. If the drug proves ineffective or toxic at these levels a change to another agent must be made.

Because lignocaine does not interfere with conduction processes it exerts no adverse effect on the heart. By reason of its high lipid solubility it has a predilection for nervous tissue (hence its value as a local anaesthetic and as a corrective for *status epilepticus*) and signs of lignocaine toxicity are almost all referable to an interference with nervous system function. They include tremors, twitchings, disorientation, paraesthesiae and, oddly enough, epileptiform convulsions.

The use of lignocaine as a local anaesthetic agent is discussed on p. 470.

PROCAINAMIDE

Procainamide (Pronestyl, Procapan) is the amide analogue of procaine. Like lignocaine, procaine is a local anaesthetic but, in its properties and uses, procainamide resembles quinidine rather than lignocaine. Thus it depresses myocardial conduction processes, it does not display a particular avidity for nervous tissue and it is less effective than lignocaine in the treatment of arrhythmias associated with cardiac glycoside poisoning. Procainamide is particularly indicated for the correction of ventricular arrhythmias consequent on myocardial infarction.

$$H_2N \underset{}{\overset{}{\bigcirc}} CONH(CH_2)_2N(C_2H_5)_2$$

Procainamide
(cf procaine, p. 468)

Like procaine itself, procainamide causes vasodilatation and it is prone to induce a serious hypotension if it is given by the intravenous route. Fortunately it is rapidly effective when taken by mouth: it is quickly absorbed from the intestine (peak plasma levels are reached within an hour of its ingestion) and it does not suffer extensive 'first pass' inactivation. The oral route can even be utilized in acute conditions and only in the most dire emergencies should it be necessary to resort to intravenous administration.

The usual (oral) dose of procainamide is one gram initially followed by 500 mg every four hours. The necessity of rousing the patient at such frequent intervals constitutes something of a disadvantage particularly if he is seriously ill and the recent arrival of sustained release preparations (Cardiorytmin Retard etc.) is to be welcomed. With these preparations dosing intervals can be extended to six or eight hours.

Effective doses of procainamide produce plasma concentrations of 4 to 8 μg per ml. The drug is eliminated quite quickly and has a plasma half life of 3.5 h. Most of it (60 per cent) is excreted in an unchanged form in the urine and much of the remainder is converted into *N*-acetylprocainamide, a compound that retains the pharmacological activity of its parent.

Care has to be exercised when procainamide is given to patients in heart failure lest the impaired renal function that is a feature of that condition hinder the elimination of the drug. To guard against the possibility of toxic reactions from this cause it is advisable to monitor the amount of procainamide in treated patients whose renal function is suspect.

Relatively rare complications of procainamide treatment in those who have not been exposed to toxic doses include gastrointestinal upsets, skin rashes and agranulocytosis. A more serious hazard is the possibility that a condition related to systemic lupus erythematosus (p. 767) will develop if treatment with procainamide is continued for more than a few months. For this reason it is prudent to place a limit of four or five weeks on the period over which an individual patient may take procainamide.

PHENYTOIN

Phenytoin (diphenylhydantoin, Epanutin etc.) is a well established antiepileptic drug and as such it is described in detail on p. 523. Its actions on cardiac tissue are identical with those of lignocaine and it is used for the treatment of ventricular tachycardias (including those induced by digitalis) when lignocaine has failed or is contraindicated for any reason.

Phenytoin is given by intravenous infusion or is taken by mouth but by either route large loading doses are followed by more modest maintenance doses. By the intravenous route a suitable loading dose is 250 mg infused over ten minutes followed by a maintenance dose that suffices to keep the arrhythmia in check without causing toxic effects. Oral administration is clearly to be preferred when protracted medication is called for: on the first day, 1 gram can be taken in four instalments but this is reduced to 600 mg on the second day and to 400 mg on the third and subsequent days. This type of dosing regime is recommended because in the circumstances in which phenytoin has to be given it is necessary to establish an effective concentration of the drug in the tissues as soon as possible. Since low concentrations are very readily metabolized, this aim can only be realized by providing a high initial dose. On the other hand, the enzymes that effect this inactivation of phenytoin are easily saturated and when this happens a small increment of dose gives rise to a large increase in the concentration of drug in the plasma and a considerable risk that toxic reactions will be provoked. Thus, after the initial dose of phenytoin has provided a therapeutically effective concentration in the tissues, maintenance doses have merely to replace that which is being lost by the now rather sluggish metabolic processes. Some figures supplied by Richens (1974) vividly illustrate these points: in one of Richens' patients, doses of phenytoin of the order of 200 mg daily produced a serum level of about 25 μM but if the daily dose was increased to 300 mg the serum level climbed to about 120 μM.

Effectively antiarrhythmic plasma concentrations of phenytoin range from 10 to 18 μg per ml; toxic reactions are noted at concentrations over 20 μg per ml.

The many possible side effects of phenytoin therapy are detailed elsewhere (p. 524). It should be noted that phenytoin is one of the drugs that is most likely to precipitate undesirable reactions if it is taken in association with another agent (p. 525).

DISOPYRAMIDE

The action of disopyramide (Rythmodan, Norpace) are very similar to those of quinidine but its use is less often plagued by serious side effects. A relatively new drug, disopyramide has been recommended for the treatment and prevention of atrial and ventricular extrasystoles and tachycardias including that of the Wolf-Parkinson-White syndrome. Like quinidine, disopyramide has atropine like properties and this is responsible for many of the almost invariably mild side effects—retention of urine, dry mouth and paralysis of accommodation—associated with its use. Gastrointestinal upsets are also noted. Because of its muscarinic actions, disopyramide should not be given to patients with glaucoma.

Disopyramide is usually given by mouth in doses of 100 to 200 mg every three or four hours.

MEXILETINE

Mexiletine (Mexitil, Fig. 40.2), a structural analogue of lignocaine, has been applied to the treatment of tachycardial disturbances of ventricular rhythm particularly those that develop after surgery or myocardial infarction.

Mexiletine is given intravenously or (when the condition is not in urgent need of correction) by mouth. The initial intravenous dose is 100 to 250 mg infused over a period of about ten minutes. Thereafter the infusion rate is progressively reduced until it reaches a maintenance level of about 1 mg per minute. The oral dose, initially 500 mg, is reduced to 200 to 250 mg every two hours.

Mexiletine is extensively bound to plasma protein and its half life ranges from 10 to 24 h. The elimination of mexiletine is very much dependent on urinary pH (excretion is delayed in alkaline urine) and care has to be taken lest normally innocuous doses of the drug have toxic effects. The margin between therapeutic and toxic doses is quite narrow.

Untoward side effects of mexiletine include nausea, vomiting, paraesthesiae, dizziness and confusion. Patients with Parkinson's disease may experience an accentuation of their tremor. Cardiovascular effects include bradycardia, hypotension and atrial fibrillation.

OTHER COMPOUNDS

Ajmaline (Fig. 40.2) is a Rauwolfia alkaloid, active parenterally or orally, that has been used for the treatment of tachyarrhythmias including that of the Wolff-Parkinson-White syndrome. *Aprindine* (Fibocil) has local anaesthetic

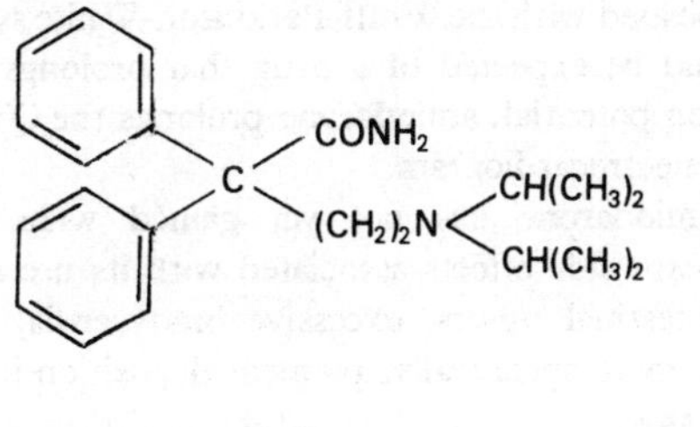

Disopyramide

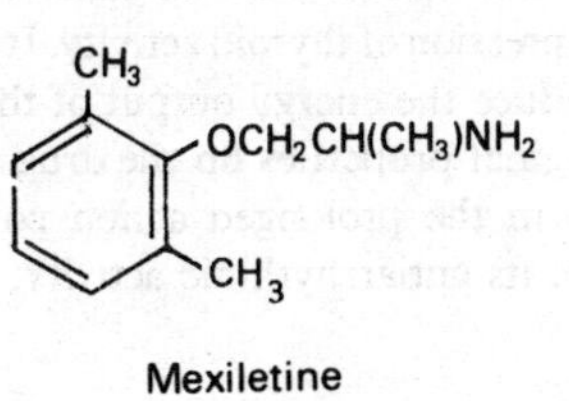

Mexiletine

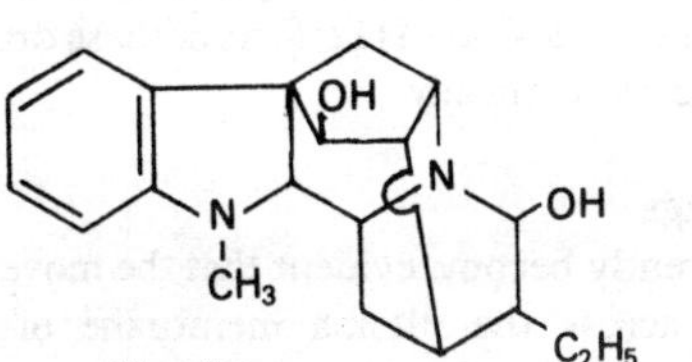

Ajmaline

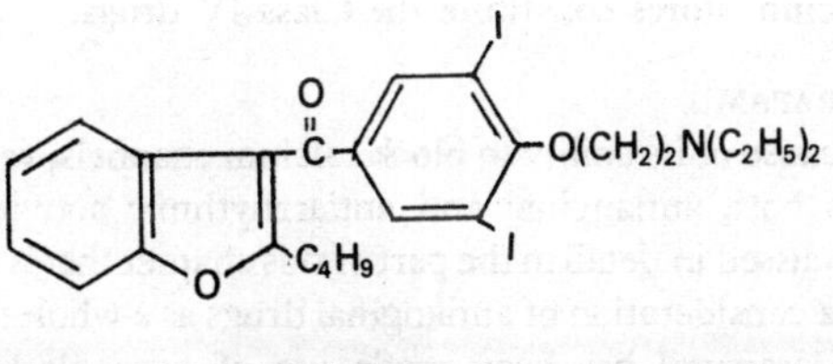

Amiodarone

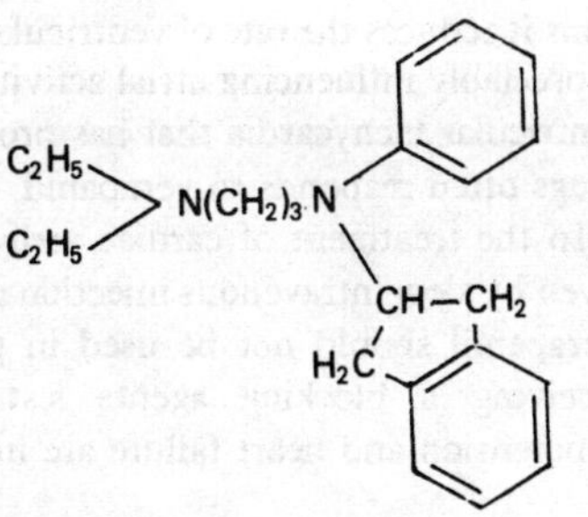

Aprindine

Fig. 40.2 Some newer antiarrhythmic drugs.

properties and other actions reminiscent of those of ligno-caine. Jaundice, agranulocytosis and disturbances of central nervous function have been reported as side effects. Like ajmaline, aprindine is equally active by oral and parenteral routes.

Class II drugs

All the members of this class of drugs oppose the effects of adrenaline and of sympathetic nervous stimulation on the rate and force of contraction of the heart.

ANTAGONISTS OF ADRENALINE β RECEPTORS

We would expect these drugs to be especially valuable for the correction of arrhythmias arising from an increased sensitivity or stimulation of the β receptors. These conditions arise classically during the administration of the halogenated anaesthetics and the giving of 'β blockers' as premedication agents in anaesthesia was the first of what was to prove to become a multiplicity of therapeutic applications.

As far as their influence on cardiac arrhythmias is concerned, the β receptor antagonists have found more applications than was originally envisaged for them. Because of their ability to increase the refractory period of the atrioventricular node and so to slow transmission from atria to ventricles, they have been applied to the prevention or treatment of atrial fibrillation (in which condition they reduce the ventricular rate but do not necessarily influence that of the atria) and of the arrhythmias that may arise during exercise or after cardiac infarction or major cardiac surgery. They are active against disorders of cardiac rhythm brought on by poisoning with cardiac glycosides. Some authorities regard them as drugs of choice for the prevention of the paroxysms of tachycardia that characterize the Wolff-Parkinson-White syndrome (Singh and Jewitt, 1974). Combined therapy with a β blocking agent and another antiarrhythmic drug is often rewarding.

Some of the drugs that block β receptors have membrane stabilizing properties but these do not normally manifest themselves at low dose levels and it is permissible to conclude that Class I activity plays no significant part in the arrhythmic activity of the β blocking agents. Thus there is no valid reason for preferring drugs with membrane stabilizing properties over those that are devoid of this type of activity.

Dose levels for the treatment of cardiac arrhythmias are generally lower than those needed in angina pectoris and hypertension. Thus the recommended oral dose of oxprenolol is 20 to 40 mg three times daily. The drugs should only be given intravenously with the utmost circumspection.

The reader should remember that β receptor blockade deprives the patient of the sympathetic drive on which the continued activity of his heart might well depend. The possibility that cardiac failure may supervene in the course of treatment with these drugs must be constantly borne in mind. The use of atropine, particularly when the β blocking agent is given intravenously, will reduce the likelihood of this unfortunate occurrence.

Details concerning the actions, metabolism and toxic effects of the β receptor antagonists are to be found later in this chapter (p. 702) and elsewhere (p. 302).

BRETYLIUM

Bretylium at first promotes and then prevents the release of noradrenaline from sympathetic nerve endings so that its actions on the heart are analogous to those of the ß blocking agents. Like them it delays the rate of diastolic repolarization. Because of its action on the nerves that control vasomotor tone, bretylium lowers the blood pressure but it no longer finds a place among the antihypertensive drugs partly because of the uncomfortable side effects (particularly nasal congestion and parotid pain) that attend its continued use and partly because patients rapidly become tolerant to its blood pressure lowering action. Recently, however, it has been granted a new lease of life, this time as an antiarrhythmic drug.

The principal present day indication for the use of bretylium is the occurrence of ventricular fibrillation that has proved resistant to electroversion. It can also be employed when the electrical equipment is not available or as a supplement to the electroversion technique.

The recommended dose of bretylium (as the tosylate, the form in which the drug is now usually provided) is 5 mg per kilogram of body mass by intravenous or intramuscular injection. It is given three or four times daily. It is a wise precaution to give a ß receptor blocking drug at the beginning of treatment to annul the effects of the initial noradrenaline release which might otherwise aggravate the condition. The fibrillating patient will obviously not be in a position to suffer the orthostatic hypotension that would otherwise constitute a major disadvantage to the drug's use nor will treatment have to be prolonged enough to permit the development of parotid pain. Nausea and vomiting sometimes complicate bretylium administration. Tolerance to the antiarrhythmic actions of bretylium does not occur.

Bretylium has also been employed to treat other arrhythmias of ventricular origin that have failed to respond to other drugs.

The pharmacology of bretylium is discussed on page 290.

Class III drugs

In thyroid deficiency, the cardiac action potential and, consequently, the absolute refractory period, is prolonged so that the heart rate is lowered. Attempts have been made to find drugs that have a similar action on the heart but do not compromise thyroid function. Drugs of this type might be expected to possess useful antiarrhythmic activity but so far only one has emerged. This is amiodarone.

AMIODARONE

Amiodarone (Cordarone) was originally introduced into therapeutics as an antianginal drug but it has claims to be considered as an antiarrhythmic agent. In daily oral doses of 300 to 600 mg it can ameliorate tachycardial arrhythmias of both atrial and ventricular origin including those associated with the Wolff-Parkinson-White syndrome. As would be expected of a drug that prolongs the cardiac action potential, amiodarone prolongs the QT interval of the electrocardiogram.

Amiodarone has not yet gained wide acceptance. Adverse side effects associated with its use include gastrointestinal upsets, excessive bradycardia, heart block and, more specifically, pigment deposition in the cornea and skin.

Although amiodarone is an iodinated compound (Fig. 40.2) there is no evidence that its mode of action is in any way dependent on depression of thyroid activity. It may be that the ability to reduce the energy output of the heart which confers antianginal properties on the drug may be secondarily reflected in the prolonged action potentials that form the basis of its antiarrhythmic activity.

OTHER COMPOUNDS

High doses of sotalol (p. 304) and bretylium prolong cardiac action potentials as does oxyfedrine after chronic administration but the Class III effects of these drugs have not been exploited clinically.

Class IV drugs

It has only recently become evident that the movement of calcium ions across the plasma membrane of cardiac muscle cells has a vital part to play in cardiac physiology (p. 684). Drugs that occlude the calcium channels or deplete calcium stores constitute the Class IV drugs.

VERAPAMIL

Because of its ability to block calcium channels, verapamil has both antianginal and antiarrhythmic activity. It is discussed in detail in the part of this chapter that is devoted to a consideration of antianginal drugs as a whole (p. 704).

Verapamil has been made use of particularly in the treatment of atrial flutter and fibrillation. In these conditions it reduces the rate of ventricular contraction without appreciably influencing atrial activity. Paroxysmal supraventricular tachycardia that has proved resistant to other drugs often responds to verapamil.

In the treatment of cardiac arrhythmias, verapamil is given by slow intravenous injection in doses of 5 to 10 mg. Verapamil should not be used in patients who are also receiving ß blocking agents lest severe bradycardia, hypotension and heart failure are induced.

PRENYLAMINE

Prenylamine (p. 704), like verapamil, is an antianginal drug with antiarrhythmic properties attributable to its ability to occlude calcium channels. It has been employed in the treatment of angina pectoris but its therapeutic value in arrhythmias remains to be established.

Electrical cardioversion (electroversion)

The passage of short bursts of a direct electrical current

between electrodes applied to the thorax will often bring about a prompt conversion of a tachycardial arrhythmia into a normal rhythm. This form of treatment is indicated when correction of an arrhythmia is a matter of urgency by reason of its causing severe hypotension or cardiac failure. The prompt institution of shock therapy in cases of ventricular fibrillation can be life saving. Electroversion should not, however, be attempted in patients whose arrhythmia is attributable to digitalis or quinidine poisoning. In these conditions electrical stimulation is likely to precipitate ventricular fibrillation.

The timing of electroversion shocks is important. The optimal moment is the beginning of ventricular systole: if the shocks arrive during the repolarization phases of the cardiac cycle, ventricular fibrillation can be produced. One way of ensuring that the shocks are delivered at the appropriate time is to arrange that the shock machine (the defibrillator) is triggered, after a delay of 20 msec, by the R wave of the patient's own electrocardiogram. Proper timing of the shocks is not possible (nor fortunately is it necessary) when the ventricles are fibrillating.

The shocks are allowed to pass for 2 msec but the energy that has to be delivered to restore normal rhythm depends on a number of factors, chief among which is the severity of the cardiac disturbance. It is customary to begin treatment with shocks that supply 25 joules of energy and progressively to increase it, if necessary, to a limit of 250 J.

Patients undergoing electroversion should be given an analgesic drug or be rendered indifferent to pain. Intravenous diazepam is ideal for this purpose (see p. 509) and it can be supplemented if necessary with morphine. Anaesthetics proper should be avoided since they may aggravate the arrhythmia. Electroversion attempts sometimes induce ectopic beats. If this happens, lignocaine should be given.

Anticoagulant drugs should be administered before and for some weeks after electroversion to minimise the embolic effects of any blood clots that might be expelled by the more efficiently contracting heart (p. 687).

CARDIOTONIC DRUGS

The catecholamines, particularly adrenaline and isoprenaline, have a cardiotonic action but they are rapidly destroyed in the body and are therefore of therapuetic value only in emergencies such as sudden cardiac arrest occurring in the course of surgery. Some drugs, however, exert a powerful and sustained effect on the heart. They are all naturally occurring substances and they all exhibit some degree of toxicity if they are given in effectively cardiotonic doses. These toxic effects preclude the use of most of the drugs for therapeutic purposes and the only clinically useful ones are the cardiac glycosides.

The cardiac glycosides

Cardiac glycosides are obtained from a number of plants but some toxic substances obtained from the skin of toads (the bufotoxins) have similar properties. Extracts of plants now known to contain cardiac glycosides were used as arrow poisons in ancient times (this fact underlines their toxicity) but they were also used as medicines and the Romans at least seem to have been aware that they were capable of exerting a beneficial action on the heart. The modern use of the cardiac glycosides dates from the eighteenth century. William Withering heard reports (which he was tempted to dismiss as Old Wives' Tales) that country people were able to cure 'the dropsy' (oedema) with extracts of foxglove. He investigated these reports and found that foxglove had the powers attributed to it. Although Withering erroneously attributed the diuretic effect of foxglove extracts to an action on the kidney, he clearly appreciated both the potentialities and the dangers of treatment with this preparation and his book on the subject, first published in 1785, is rightly regarded as one of the classics of medical writing.

The most important sources of the cardiac glycosides are digitalis (foxglove), strophanthus and squill. Several species of these plants contain one or more of the glycosides.

Precursor glycoside → Cardiac glycoside = aglycone + sugar

DIGITALIS
    Leaves of *Digitalis purpurea* (the common foxglove)
(a) Purpurea glycoside A → Digitoxin = Digitoxigenin + Digitoxose
                                          (3 molecules)
(b) Purpurea glycoside B → Gitoxin = Gitoxigenin + Digitoxose
                                          (3 molecules)
(c)   Gitalin = Gitaligenin + Digitoxose
                                          (2 molecules)
    Leaves of *D. lanata*
(a) Lanatoside A → Digitoxin = as above
(b) Lanatoside B → Gitoxin = as above
(c) Lanatoside C → Digoxin = Digoxigenin + Digitoxose
                                          (3 molecules)

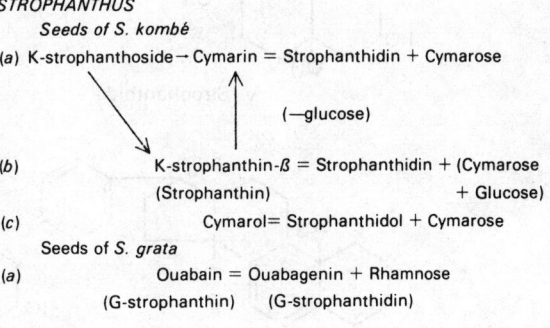

STROPHANTHUS
    Seeds of *S. kombé*
(a) K-strophanthoside → Cymarin = Strophanthidin + Cymarose

                              (—glucose)

(b)   K-strophanthin-ß = Strophanthidin + (Cymarose
              (Strophanthin)   + Glucose)
(c)   Cymarol= Strophanthidol + Cymarose
    Seeds of *S. grata*
(a)   Ouabain = Ouabagenin + Rhamnose
        (G-strophanthin)   (G-strophanthidin)

SQUILL
    Bulb of *Urginea maritima*
(a) Scillaren A → Proscillaridin A = Scillaridin A + Rhamnose

Fig. 40.3 Origin and composition of some cardiac glycosides.

The cardiac glycosides consist of a steroid (the *aglycone*) combined with a sugar residue. Some of the plant sources contain precursors (themselves glycosides) which undergo enzymatic hydrolysis to yield glucose (or glucose and acetic acid) and the cardiac glycoside proper. Some of the precursor glycosides are hydrolysed during drying of the plant preparations but others are more stable and they can be used clinically.

The more important glycosides and their aglycones are displayed in Figure 40.3. The different glycosides have essentially similar properties and in the following account individual compounds are mentioned only when this is necessary by virtue of their having unique properties or clinical uses. This should provide the reader with a guide to those cardiac glycosides whose names he needs to know.

The rest of the information in Figure 40.3 is provided only for reference. The names of the glycosides and their aglycones are confusing and unsystematic and no useful purpose is served by committing them or their interrelationships to memory.

The formulae of the aglycones appear in Figure 40.4: bufotalin is the aglycone obtained from toad poisons. The similarity in structure between the cardiac aglycones and several other compounds of pharmacological interest such as the adrenocortical steroids, cholesterol and the sex hormones will be evident.

The cardiac glycosides all possess hydroxyl groups on C(3) and C(14) and an unsaturated lactone ring on C(17). The sugars are attached to the aglycone at the C(3) hydroxyl group. The numbering of the carbon atoms is

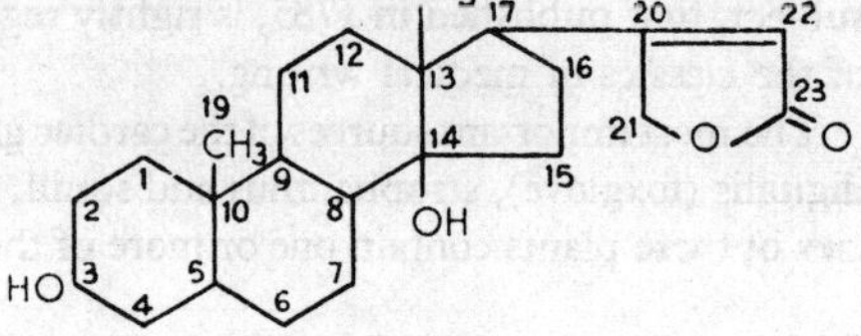

i. Digitoxigenin

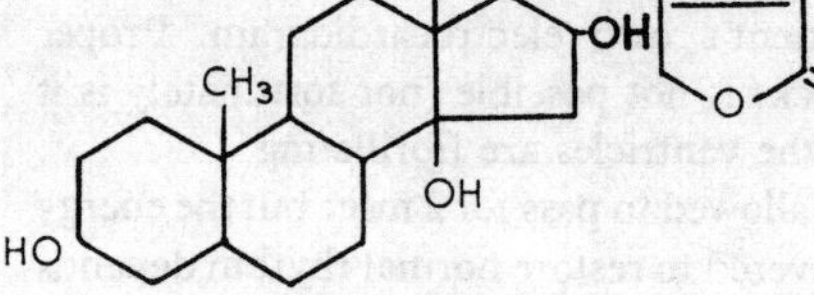

ii. Gitoxigenin
(iia. Gitaligenin = gitoxigenin hydrate)

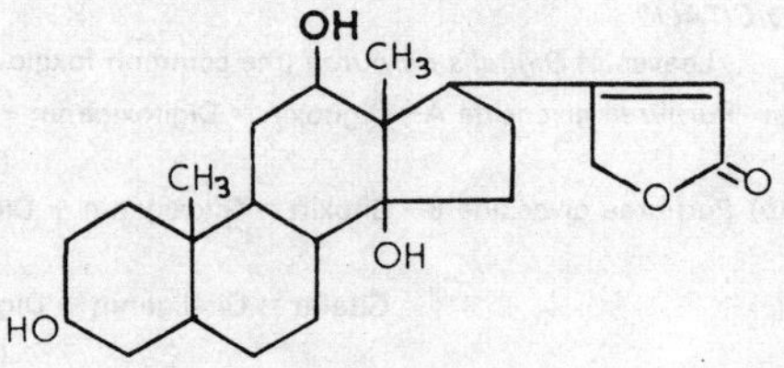

iii. Digoxigenin

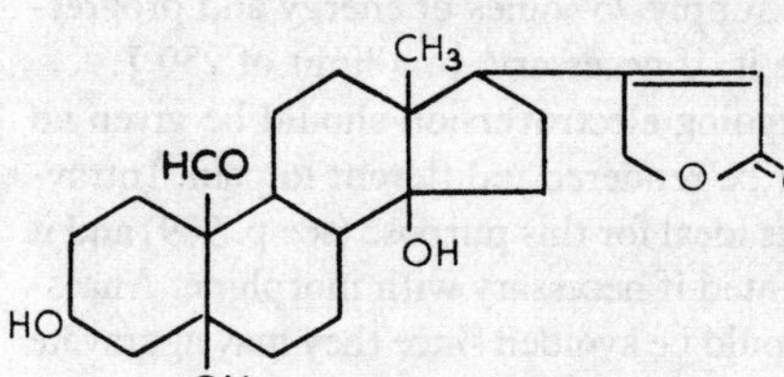

iv. Strophanthidin

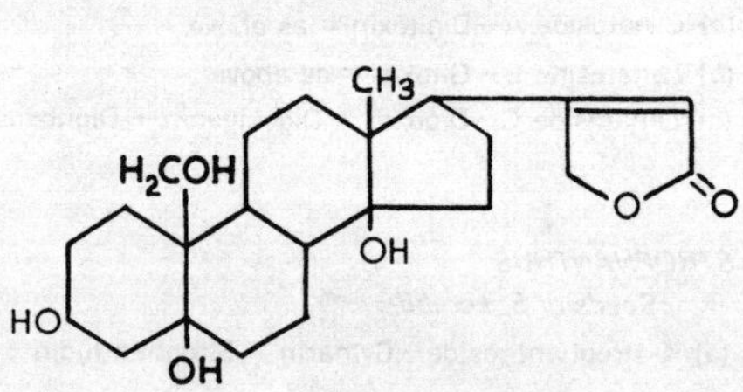

v. Strophanthidol

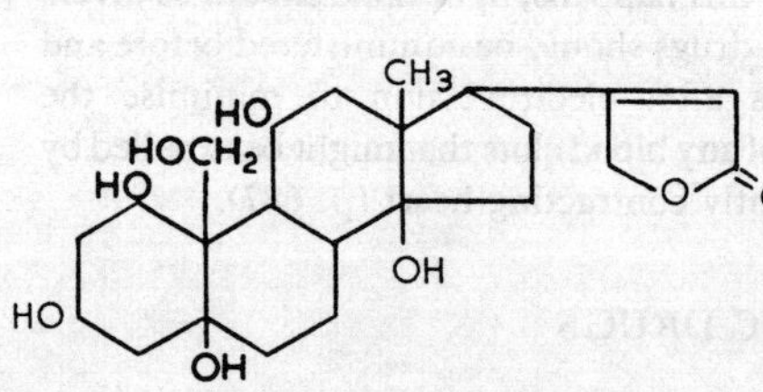

vi. Ouabagenin

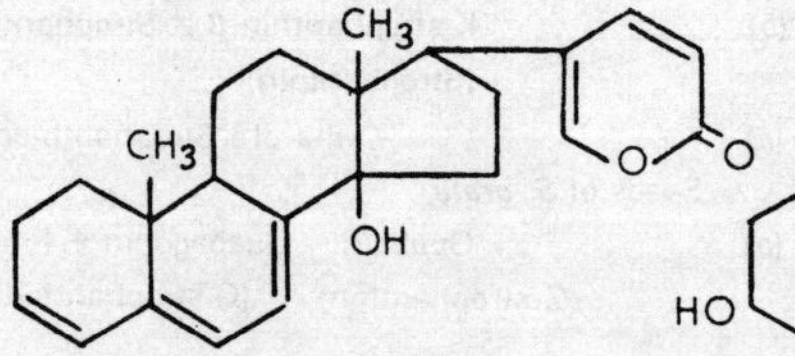

vii. Scillaridin A

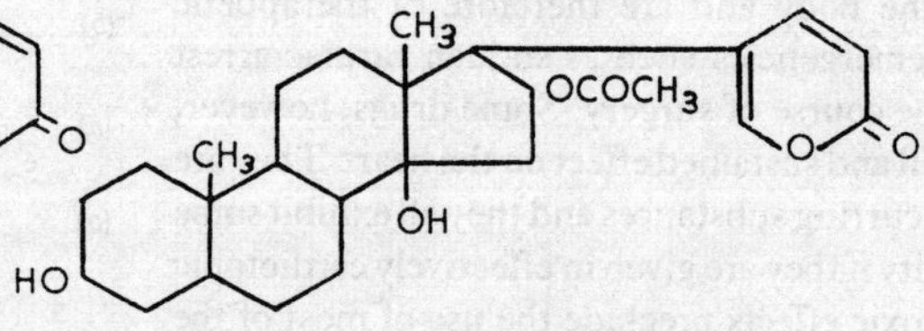

viii. Bufotalin

In formulae ii-vi the radicals shown in heavy type indicate the ways in which the molecular structure differs from that of digitoxigenin.

Fig. 40.4 The cardiac aglycones.

shown in Figure 40.4. It has been suggested (Tanz and Kerby, 1961) that the characteristic actions of the cardiac glycosides depend on two factors—(a) chemical features of the molecules associated with mineralocorticoid activity which are responsible for an immediate but brief action on the force of the beat and (b) the presence of the lactone and hydroxyl groups which are responsible for the prolonged cardiotonic actions. The lactone ring is a very important determinant of pharmacological activity in these compounds: opening of the ring may render the compound completely inert.

The aglycones are less active than the intact glycosides, indicating that the sugar residues are important functional parts of the molecule. They may facilitate absorption and attachment to the heart or they may serve to protect the aglycones against the activity of enzymes that might otherwise inactivate them by changing their steric configuration.

Pharmacological properties of the cardiac glycosides

Differences in therapeutic value among individual glycosides are largely determined by differences in their pharmacokinetic behaviour: their pharmacological properties are essentially identical.

The cardiac glycosides have a direct action on the myocardium causing it to contract more powerfully and thus to expel more blood into the arterial system with each beat. In the jargon of the day, this is described as a positive inotropic action. It is often stated that the cardiac glycosides only affect the failing heart. This should not be taken to mean that they have no action at all on the healthy heart. It is simply that the overall effect of the cardiac stimulation is less obvious in the healthy heart. The reason for this should be clear from the following considerations.

Starling's Law of the Heart expresses the fact that the force of cardiac contractions is governed by the degree to which the cardiac muscle fibres are stretched. With every beat, the normally functioning heart expels as much blood as it has received in the preceding diastole. If the amount of blood returning to the heart is increased, the stroke volume will increase correspondingly because of the increased stetch of the cardiac fibres which will consequently contract more powerfully. Starling's Law does not apply to all degrees of stretch: if the muscle fibres are stretched beyond a critical length, their contractile power falls off and further stretching beyond this point causes a progressive decline in the power of their response. At this stage, therefore, cardiac output is increased if the size of the heart is reduced. In the failing heart the power of contraction is reduced and the heart can no longer eject all the blood which is returned to it. Blood accumulates in the heart which becomes stretched beyond the point of operation of Starling's Law so that failure becomes even more pronounced. Blood also begins to accumulate in the large veins as well as in the heart giving rise to the condition of *congestive cardiac failure*. It is often assumed that many of the concomitants of cardiac failure, such as oedema, are the consequence of this elevation of venous pressure but it seems more likely that they are the result of failure of the left side of the heart to expel an adequate quantity of blood. This problem is discussed in greater detail in another chapter (p. 622); it does not affect the argument presented here.

If a cardiac glycoside is administered to a patient in cardiac failure, the power of cardiac contraction is improved and the failure is partially relieved. Moreover, the increased cardiac output will reduce the size of the heart so that its power of contraction is improved still further. Reduction in heart size has the additional advantage that, by bringing the heart once more within the range of operation of Starling's Law, cardiac output is again subject to the automatic regulatory action of the returning blood. If a cardiac glycoside is given to a normal subject, the force of myocardial contraction is at first increased but the amount of blood which is returned to the heart during the succeeding period of diastole will be insufficient to distend it to its original size. The cardiac output will therefore be reduced by an extent which counteracts the effects of the increased contractility.

The improved cardiac performance produced in the patient with the failing heart improves the blood flow through the kidney. This is the origin of the diuretic effect of digitalis which so impressed Withering. Recent work suggests that the cardiac glycosides also decrease the tubular reabsorption of sodium, perhaps because they compete with the chemically related adenocortical steroids for receptors involved in sodium transport. Increased sodium excretion itself causes diuresis.

The cardiac glycosides slow the heart—the negative chronotropic effect—in two senses: they relieve the tachycardia that is the usual concomitant of cardiac failure and they induce bradycardia in the normally functioning heart. The relief of tachycardia is a reflex response consequent on the enhanced cardiac output (and hence the improved blood pressure) engendered by successful glycoside therapy. In cases of congestive cardiac failure, the relief of pressure in the previously distended right heart will add its contribution to the overall improvement in heart rate. The bradycardia evoked after normal heart rates have been restored is attributable partly to vagal stimulation and an increased sensitivity of the sinus node to the effects of vagal stimulation (so that the discharge rate of the node is reduced) and partly to a direct action on the conducting tissue. A moderate degree of slowing of the glycoside treated heart can be taken as a sign that its condition is improving but a more extreme degree of bradycardia is a warning that the drug is present in near toxic quantities.

The glycosides increase the refractory period of both

atrial and ventricular muscle. They also cause a pronounced vasoconstriction in the healthy cardiovascular system. This response is not seen in patients with cardiac failure because their blood vessels are already maximally constricted.

The mode of action of the cardiac glycosides has been a matter of debate for many years. Recent work, even if it has not yet led to a complete exposure of the responsible mechanisms, has at least provided the evidence that enables us to discard many of the older hypotheses and to focus our attention on the most promising of the newer ones. The hypotheses that can now be discounted include those that suggest that the glycosides increase the efficiency of myocardial contraction, that they promote metabolic processes in the heart or that they stimulate the production of phosphocreatine and adenosine triphosphate. Nor does it any longer seem feasible to suppose that the glycosides owe their pharmacological effect to a direct action on the polymerization of actin or on the contractility of actomyosin. What remains are hypotheses that propose an action on the availability or transport of calcium.

In 1965, Repke showed that therapeutic doses of the cardiac glycosides inhibited the sodium-potassium activated ATPase on which the activity of the sodium pump depends. He further noted that the more cardioactive the glycoside the more potent its ability to inhibit the pump. Later workers (Langer, 1970 and Nayler, 1973 among others) have adduced further evidence to support the view that the most important action of the cardiac glycosides is to inhibit membrane bound ATPase.

Interference with the activity of the sodium pump will allow the ingress of sodium ions into and the loss of potassium ions from the substance of the myocardial fibres. One consequence of this change in the distribution of the ions will be a reduction in the demarcation potential across the plasma membrane and hence an increased tendency to the development of ectopic foci of excitation. Another will be an enhanced ingress of calcium ions which in its turn will promote a greater than normal liberation of the ion from intracellular stores (p. 684). There may well be other factors that increase the availability of calcium. Thus the intracellular sites are known to be able to accumulate sodium as well as calcium and the increased amounts of sodium that arrive in the cell consequent on the partial failure of the pump may displace calcium from its stores and so provide further supplies of the ion. Moreover calcium ions can themselves inhibit the activity of the ATPase and so amplify the effects of the cardiac glycosides that originally promoted their accumulation. The provision of increased quantities of free calcium ions will, of course, promote a more forceful cardiac contraction.

None of the mechanisms discussed in the preceding paragraphs is capable of explaining the antiarrhythmic actions of the cardiac glycosides.

Not all recent experiments have provided unequivocal support for the ATPase inhibition hypothesis of cardiac glycoside action. Some substances (quinidine and the mercurial diuretic agents among others) inhibit the enzyme but exert no inotropic effect while Okita and his colleagues have shown that, in experimental situations, the inotropic action of the glycosides can be reversed while the ATPase remains inhibited (Okita, Richardson and Roth-Schaechter, 1973). It could possibly be that the cardiotonic drugs, which certainly bind to the muscle membrane, have a general effect on membrane proteins one aspect of which is ATPase inhibition while another aspect is the mobilization of calcium stores. On balance, however, it seems that the original hypothesis will eventually prove the more satisfactory. In any event it seems that calcium holds the key to the action of cardiac glycosides.

Clinical aspects of the cardiac glycosides

The cardiac glycosides are used to provide long term support for the failing heart. Different glycosides differ in the speed of onset and in the duration of their cardiotonic action but they can be considered as a group before the characteristics of some individual compounds are mentioned.

Indications for clinical use

The cardiac glycosides find their chief use in the treatment of cardiac failure and some cardiac arrhythmias. For reasons which have already been discussed, they have their most dramatic effect in cases of congestive cardiac failure but they are also useful in any condition in which myocardial contractility is impaired. The rationale of their employment in the treatment of cardiac arrhythmias was also discussed earlier (p. 693). They are contraindicated in cases of ventricular tachycardias which are best treated with quinidine or procainamide. In the treatment of atrial flutter or fibrillation, a cardiac glycoside and quinidine are often given together but one advantage of using only the glycoside should be mentioned. These compounds do not reduce the rate of atrial fibrillation (indeed, they often increase it) and no risk of producing embolism arises when they are used alone.

Dosage

Patients who need treatment with cardiac glycosides often have to have their heart condition improved as a matter of urgency. Once this has been achieved, the improved condition has to be maintained and the drugs have to be given for life. Because many of the glycosides are excreted slowly, the possibility of cumulation arises (p. 68) and the drug dosage has to be very carefully controlled, particularly since the cardiac glycosides only exert their therapeutic effect in doses which verge on the toxic. A heart rate of under 60, or the occurrence of vomiting in patients who have withstood earlier doses of the glycoside, should be taken as danger signals.

Because it is necessary first to establish and then to maintain an effective concentration of the drug in the heart, it is usual to quote two doses (the initial, or digitalizing, dose and the maintenance dose) for the cardiac glycosides. They are given, for the individual drugs mentioned below, in Table 40.1. They are provided for reference purposes and to indicate the relative activities of the different compounds. The actual dose required by the individual patient must be determined by careful observation of his response to treatment.

Bioavailability

It is not easy, as the preceding paragraph has already hinted, to prescribe a dose regime for a cardiac glycoside that is generally applicable to the adult patient and that will ensure that his tissues receive optimally therapeutic but minimally toxic amounts of the drug. A number of factors contribute to this difficulty but the one that has caused the greatest furore in recent years concerns the 'bioavailability' of cardiac glycosides in commercial preparations of the drugs.

The most popular cardiac glycoside is digoxin and in 1971 it was found that nominally identical tablets of digoxin from different commercial sources gave very different concentrations of the drug in the plasma of those who took them. Sometimes even different batches of tablets from the same manufacturer could not be relied on to provide the same amount of drug. These differences in bioavailability were shown to arise from differences in formulation, tablets that disintegrated most readily in the gastrointestinal tract providing high plasma levels of digoxin that showed relatively little variation from patient to patient. Conversely, tablets with a low dissolution rate yielded low and very variable amounts of digoxin to the plasma. In the United Kingdom, digoxin tablets now have to be formulated in such a way that, under *in vitro* test conditions, at least 75 per cent of their contained glycoside is released into solution in one hour. Tablet preparations of other cardiac glycosides will presumably be equally satisfactory from the point of view of bioavailability if they too undergo rapid dissolution.

The incorporation of the cardiac glycosides into formulations that guarantee a high bioavailability has done much to ensure that adherence to a standard dosage regime will produce more uniform concentrations of the drugs in the plasma than was obtainable in the past. However, several other sources of variation remain. These include body size, age, sex and urinary excretion rates, but attempts to incorporate these variables into a formula designed to permit computer calculation of the amount of glycoside needed to maintain its plasma concentration at a predetermined level were not outstandingly successful. In a group of 39 subjects who had been given computer calculated maintenance doses of digoxin the actual concentrations of the drug in the serum ranged from 0.25 to 2.7 ng per ml (Christiansen *et al*, 1973). Evidently there are still other sources of variation. Some of these will appear in subsequent paragraphs.

Absorption and disposal

The cardiac glycosides are readily absorbed from the gut, principally the upper reaches of the small intestine. The amount of drug that is absorbed shows a considerable variation even among subjects with normal gastrointestinal function taking preparations that permit rapid absorption of the glycoside. This clearly constitutes another cause of the variation in plasma concentration among patients who have taken identical doses of the same glycoside. As with many other substances (p. 77) the absorption of glycosides is hindered by the presence of some other drugs in the intestine. These include (as far as the glycosides are concerned) antacids, neomycin and kaolin.

On arrival in the blood stream the cardiac glycosides are bound to very variable degrees to the plasma proteins. Thus digoxin is 20 per cent bound in contrast to digitoxin which is bound to the extent of more than 95 per cent.

Different cardiac glycosides are metabolized to different extents, some of them being almost totally excreted in the urine in an untransformed form. Metabolic processes do, however, have to be considered even when they normally play only a minimal part in the disposition of the drugs. A few individuals, for instance, can convert digoxin (which is not usually metabolized to any significant extent) to the inactive dihydrodigoxin much more readily than can the

Table 40.1 Doses of some cardiac glycosides

		Total initial dose	Daily maintenance dose
Digitalis	oral dose	1–2 g (24–72 hr)	100 – 200 mg
Digitoxin	oral dose	1–2 mg (24–48 hr)	0.1 – 0.2 mg
	intravenous	1–1.5 mg (24 hr)	—
Lanatoside C	intravenous	1–1.5 mg (24 hr)	—
Digoxin	oral dose	1–2 mg (24 hr)	0.25 – 0.5 mg
	intravenous	0.5–1.5 mg (24 hr)	—
Ouabain	intravenous	1 mg (2 hr)	—

The total initial dose is given in divided amounts, usually at 6-hourly intervals (but every 15-30 min for ouabain and every 2 h for lanatoside C) over the period indicated in parentheses.

majority of the population. As a result they can tolerate abnormally high doses of digoxin. Conversion into the dihydro compound occurs more readily with some of the other cardiac glycosides. Digitoxin is transformed, to the extent of about 10 per cent, into digoxin, which, because of its more polar nature, is more rapidly excreted than the parent compound. However the most important pathway for the degradation of the cardiac glycosides involves serial removal of the sugar molecules, the resulting 'genin' being disposed of partly by conjugation and partly by epoxidation.

Toxic reactions
It will be recalled that the cardiac glycosides cause a loss of intracellular potassium and that this contributes to both their toxic and their therapeutic effects. By the very nature of their clinical condition, many patients requiring treatment with a cardiac glycoside are also being given diuretic drugs, many of which cause a loss of potassium from the tissue. Care has therefore to be taken to ensure that potassium intake is maintained.

As has already been indicated, toxic reactions to the cardiac glycosides are exerted particularly on the central nervous system and the heart. In overdosage, the effects on the nervous system are pronounced and a distinct psychosis may be precipitated. On the heart the overdosage can cause a variety of arrhythmias such as heart block, ventricular fibrillation or, more commonly, the appearance of ventricular extrasystoles. Some of these toxic responses such as extrasystoles and fibrillations arise because of an increased excitability of the heart brought about, as we have seen (p. 694), by the mechanism (inhibition of ATPase) that is also responsible for the drugs' inotropic action. Others, such as heart block, represent an exaggeration of the depressant action on conduction processes that confers useful antiarrhythmic properties on the drugs. The mechanism of this latter effect is not well understood.

Drug interactions involving cardiac glycosides
The perceptive reader will have remarked that, at several stages in their journey from mouth to urine, the cardiac glycosides are involved in processes that can be modified by other substances. These processes include absorption from the intestine, binding to plasma proteins and transformation by hepatic enzymes as well as the drugs' primary action on the ionic pump mechanisms. It would be proper to assume, therefore, that the ingestion of a cardiac glycoside would set the stage for the occurrence of a multiplicity of possible interactions with other drugs (p. 77). Although this is undoubtedly so, the incidence of adverse interactions between cardiac glycosides and other drugs is remarkably low always excepting those which arise from the injudicious administration of diuretic agents without adequate potassium supplements. The fact that digoxin, now the most widely used glycoside, is only minimally

bound to plasma proteins and only minimally degraded by liver enzymes contributes to this welcome state of affairs.

Combinations of the glycosides with antiarrhythmic drugs such as lignocaine promote beneficial interactions. The antiarrhythmic drug suppresses the tendency of the glycoside to disturb the cardiac rhythm but leaves it free to exert its inotropic action.

Individual cardiac glycosides

DIGITALIS
The standardized leaf of *D. purpurea* (prepared digitalis) is available as a powder and as tablets. Tincture of digitalis is only rarely used. The onset of the cardiotonic action is slow and a period of 24 to 72 hrs (depending on the dosage and frequency of drug administration) is required for full digitalization. Digitalis is only taken by mouth. There is no longer any justification for using intravenous preparations of digitalis leaf.

DIGITOXIN
Digitoxin (Crystodigin, Digitaline Nativelle, Digitox) is one of the glycosides of *D. purpurea* (Fig. 40.3). It has a prolonged action but a state of full digitalization can be attained quickly. It is normally taken by mouth but in emergencies it can be given by the intravenous route. A single intravenous dose is often sufficient to produce digitalization and maintenance doses can then be taken orally. As can be gathered from the doses given in Table 40.1, digitoxin is very potent. Its prolonged action constitutes something of a hazard since the effect of an overdosage of digitoxin takes a long time to correct. Its plasma half life is of the order of six days. A small amount of the drug, as we have seen, is converted into digoxin but the rest is slowly metabolized to inactive metabolites.

LANATOSIDE C
Lanatoside C (deslanoside, Cedilanid, Lanocide) is a precursor glycoside isolated from *D. lanata*. It acts very quickly but the effect is short lived, the glycoside being completely eliminated from the body within 36 hours of cessation of treatment. Lanatoside C is used in emergencies to produce rapid digitalization. The digitalized state is maintained by other drugs, preferably digoxin. Lanatoside C is poorly absorbed from the intestine and its oral administration is no longer recommended.

DIGOXIN
Digoxin (Diganox, Lanoxin) is the cardiac glycoside produced from Lanatoside C. Like its parent glycoside, it has a short duration of action. It is now the most widely used cardiac glycoside. It is well absorbed from suitably formulated oral preparations (though not as well as digitoxin) and it has a short half life (about 34 hours).

Patients with advanced cardiac failure are much more likely to show signs of intoxication with cardiac glycosides than are those less seriously affected. For this reason, it is advisable to treat them with a short acting compound such as digoxin, so that if signs of a toxic reaction appear the concentration of glycoside in the tissues can be rapidly reduced if the drug is withdrawn or its dosage reduced.

OUABAIN

Ouabain (strophanthin-G, strophanthoside-G) acts exceedingly rapidly, its effect being seen within five to fifteen minutes after intravenous administration. It has a plasma half life of 21 hr. Ouabain is used for producing rapid digitalization, small intravenous doses (250 μg initially and then 100 μg) being given at fifteen minute intervals until a favourable response is secured. Digitalization can thereafter be maintained by digoxin. Ouabain is extensively used in laboratory investigations into the mode of action of the cardiac glycosides.

K-strophanthoside (strophanthin-K) has therapeutic uses similar to those of ouabain.

Biological standardization and laboratory testing of drugs that act on the heart

BIOLOGICAL STANDARDIZATION

Biological standardization of those glycosides which are used in the pure form is not necessary but some impure preparations such as digitalis leaf are still used and they require standardization. None of the available methods is entirely satisfactory, since the response used for standardization purposes is a toxic action of the drug (cardiac arrest or vomiting) and not one which mimics the therapeutic effect. The standard preparation which is used must therefore always be of the same type as that which is being assayed and it should be clear that none of the methods used for biological assay is suitable for the detection of potentially useful cardiotonic activity in newly produced compounds. Screening methods are therefore considered separately.

GUINEA PIG METHOD

Alcohol extracts of the standard and unknown preparations are given, each preparation into several animals, by slow intravenous infusion into the jugular vein of guinea pigs receiving artificial respiration and anaesthetized with urethane. The end point is arrest of the heart, determined preferably by opening the thorax as soon as the beats become very weak. This method forms the basis of the official assay given in the British Pharmacopoeia; it is the successor to the method of Hatcher and Brody which was developed as long ago as 1910 and which used cats anaesthetized with ether or chloralose. Cats are expensive and difficult to come by, so that they are never used when an alternative species is available. In the present instance, the necessity of finding another sensitive animal led to an improvement in the method, for guinea pigs are much less variable than cats in their response.

PIGEON METHOD

The cardiac glycosides cause vomiting by an action on the chemoceptive trigger zone and this effect is made the basis of a standardization technique recognized by the United States Pharmacopoeia. Different doses of the standard and unknown solutions are given intravenously (using a wing vein) into several groups of lightly anaesthetized pigeons. From the log(dose)-response curve, the dose of each preparation required to cause vomiting in 50 per cent of the birds is calculated in the usual way and the potency of the unknown can therefore be expressed in terms of that of the standard.

TREVAN'S METHOD

This is the classical method of digitalis assay. It makes use of frogs, separate groups of which receive the standard or unknown solutions by intraperitoneal injection. The number of frogs which die within the succeeding 12 hours is noted, to give the relative potencies of the test and standard solutions.

EMBRYONIC DUCK (OR CHICK) HEART ASSAY

This method was particularly suitable for the detection of small amounts of cardiac glycosides in biological fluids or tissue extracts before chemical assay methods became available. It is capable of detecting less than 1 μg of many of the glycosides. In its original form, the method used embryonic duck heart but the heart of the embryonic chick can be made as sensitive and this became the favoured preparation. This is historically fitting, for Pickering demonstrated that digitalis affected embryonic chick heart as long ago as 1893. The fertile eggs are incubated until the embryonic heart has reached an appropriate state of development (for details see Thorp and Cobbin, 1967). The heart is then removed from the embryo and placed in a well slide containing a small amount of the tissue extract which is to be assayed. Up to five hearts are placed in each well, which is kept at 35° C. and is observed through a microscope. The time that elapses before atrio-ventricular block appears is recorded and the concentration of glycoside is calculated from a standard curve. Within a range of about four to ten minutes, there is a linear relationship between the logarithm of the glycoside concentration and the time required for the production of conduction block.

CHEMICAL ASSAY OF THE CARDIAC GLYCOSIDES

During the past fifteen years or so a number of methods have become available for the rapid determination of the cardiac glycosides in body fluids and tissues. Their development was the prelude to the investigations that have recently contributed so much to our understanding of the pharmacokinetic behaviour of the cardiac glycosides in human subjects. It is not possible here to do more than name the techniques used (they include double isotope dilution, gas chromatography, radioimmunoassay and measurement of the inhibition of sodium-potassium dependent ATPase) but they are reviewed by Butler (1972).

LABORATORY TESTING OF CARDIOTONIC AND ANTIARRHYTHMIC DRUGS

The best known method of detecting cardiotonic activity is by means of the perfused heart of the kitten, rabbit or guinea pig (the Langendorff preparation, Fig. 40.5). Although this preparation is suitable for the preliminary screening of drugs that may have cardiotonic activity, its responses tend to be irregular, even when more elaborate versions of the original apparatus are used and it is not suitable for quantitative work, such as is needed when the potency of a new drug has to be compared with that of an established agent. The Langendorff preparation sometimes gives 'false positive' results, for a drug without direct cardiotonic activity may improve the power of contraction of the heart if it dilates the coronary vessels and thereby improves the nutrition of the tissues, which is likely to be impaired in the relatively unfavourable conditions which prevail in the saline-perfused heart.

Preparations which are useful both for screening purposes and for comparative assay include the isolated papillary muscle of the cat, isolated guinea pig atria, the excised frog heart and isolated arterial strips. The isolated papillary muscle is particularly useful: it needs only a very small bath and any contractile response obtained must be due to a direct action of the active agent on muscle since the preparation is nerve free and is not dependent on a blood supply. A further advantage is that the preparation has no spontaneous activity, fluctuations of which in preparations of the atria or the whole heart may cause variations in the response to drugs.

For more detailed investigation of the mode of action of cardioactive drugs, a number of more complicated techniques are available. The classical heart lung preparation, originally devised by Starling in 1912, is still useful. In this preparation, defibrinated blood passes into the heart from a reservoir and the systemic circulation is replaced by a system of tubes which enables the peripheral resistance to be accurately controlled and through which blood returns to the reservoir. The blood is oxygenated by the animal's own lungs and the whole arrangement provides an ingenious way of combining a normally functioning heart with an artificial circulatory system not subject to drug induced fluctuations of peripheral resistance which might affect cardiac performance independently of the drug's direct action on the heart. For experiments in intact conscious animals, it is possible in a preliminary operation to sew strain gauges into the ventricular wall and to bring recording leads to the surface of the body.

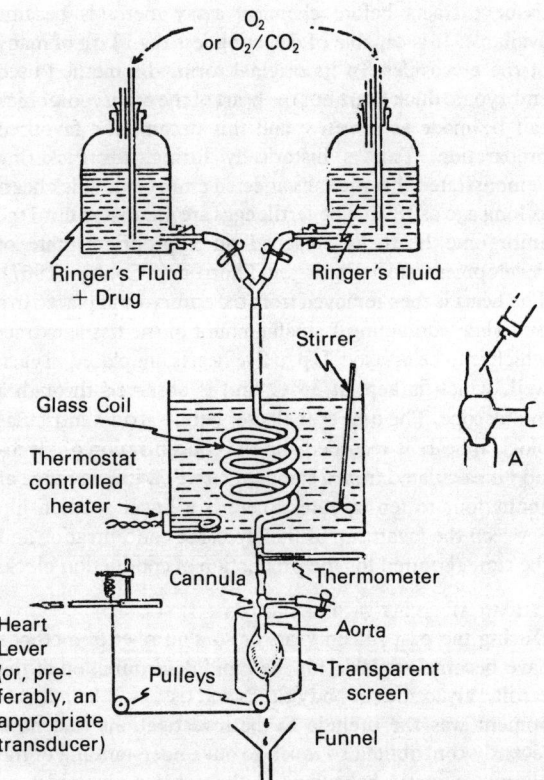

Fig. 40.5 A method for recording the beat of the isolated, perfused mammalian heart. A, shows the injection of a dose of the drug into the rubber tubing above the cannula. Otherwise the drug is added to one of the reservoirs and the heart perfused with a dilute solution.

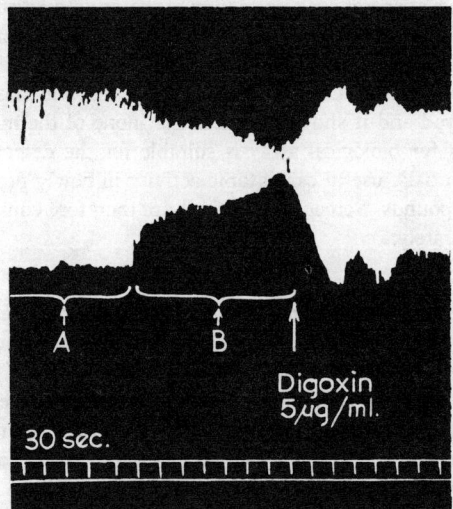

Fig. 40.6 The effect of digoxin on the failing heart. At A the heart was perfused with Tyrode's solution; at B the perfusion fluid was altered in composition so that it contained half the normal amount of calcium chloride. Digoxin was then given by injection into the cannula (see Fig. 40.5) and perfusion with 'half calcium' Tyrode's solution continued.

The essential requirement of a cardiotonic drug is that it should be capable of improving cardiac output in the failing heart. It is possible to reproduce the effects of heart failure in several of the preparations that have just been described. In the Langendorff heart preparation, a reduction in the amount of calcium in the perfusion fluid causes a rapid deterioration in cardiac performance which is restored by cardiac glycosides (Fig. 40.6). There are several ways of inducing cardiac failure in the heart-lung preparation. Delay in establishing cardiac oxygenation by the lungs provides one method and the addition of barbiturate or dinitrophenol to the perfusion fluid is another. Cardiac failure can be induced in intact animals by applying a permanent ligature that partially occludes the pulmonary artery. It should be obvious that studies on failing hearts are likely to give more information concerning the potential value of a new drug than are experiments on normal organs. An additional advantage of these preparations is that they permit the calculation of both the therapeutic and the lethal doses in the same heart.

One method of testing for antiarrhythmic activity is to determine the maximum rate at which isolated atria can be induced to beat in response to electrical stimulation. If a compound with antiarrhythmic properties is added to the bath, the maximum rate of response will be reduced. Electrical stimulation can also be used to produce arrhythmias in the intact animal.

A number of drugs will produce arrhythmias. These include digitalis, aconitine and acetylcholine. Arrhythmias are also evoked by adrenaline, administered to animals anaesthetized with chloroform or cyclopropane. An apparent advantage of this technique is that it reproduces a situation which is a frequent cause of arrhythmia in the human subject. In practice, however, many workers prefer to use benzene to sensitize the heart to adrenaline, since it produces arrhythmias more regularly and predictably than does either chloroform or cyclopropane.

ANTIANGINAL DRUGS AND PROCEDURES

The word 'angina' (from the Greek verb meaning 'to choke') has been with us since 1768 when Heberden introduced it into the medical vocabulary to describe the pain or discomfort (*angina pectoris,* or, nowadays, often plain *angina*) of cardiac origin (Julian, 1977). This meaning is widely understood even by the medical layman but the reader should also be aware of Vincent's angina, a much less well known condition and one that is completely unrelated to angina pectoris. Vincent's angina is a spirochaetal infection of the mouth and throat and the use of angina in this context is clearly wholly appropriate.

Angina pectoris occurs in subjects whose coronary blood flow is impaired by reason of degenerative changes in the arteries and it is symptomatic of an ischaemic condition in the myocardium, the blood flow being inadequate to meet the increased demands of the heart during physical or emotional exertion. The discomfort of angina takes the form of a pain, an ache or a feeling of pressure which is experienced in the region of the sternum and is also often referred (p. 422) to one or both arms or between shoulder blades. Pain in the region of the heart itself is exceptional. Breathlessness sometimes occurs along with the other discomforts and this contributes to the choking sensation that prompted Heberden's apt description of the condition. The description is doubly apt, for angina has the same etymological origin as have words like anxiety and the German *Angst*. The suffocating sensation that typifies so many anginal attacks is often (and not surprisingly) accompanied by anxiety about the outcome and by a feeling of impending death.

Once angina became recognized as a distinct clinical entity a search was begun for agents that might relieve it. At first, and in true 18th century fashion, a bewildering variety of quite useless remedies was offered to those who suffered anginal attacks but as early as 1867 Brunton, through that combination of good luck and serendipity that has given birth to so many advances in medicine, discovered the value of amyl nitrite. Glyceryl trinitrate followed in 1879. Most of the large number of other antianginal drugs that have subsequently made (usually brief) appearances on the therapeutic stage have failed to steal the limelight from glyceryl trinitrate which, a hundred years on, can still claim top listing among the very few drugs of choice for the relief of angina pectoris.

Amyl nitrite, glyceryl trinitrate and some other antianginal drugs are powerful vasodilators but vasodilatatory activity does not, of itself, confer antianginal effectiveness. In the accounts that follow, drugs with pronounced vasodilator activity that are not (or are no longer) used in the treatment of angina pectoris are considered separately (p. 705) from the antianginal drugs proper.

Drug therapy must, of course, be accorded pride of place in a textbook of pharmacology but it is important to note that the proper treatment of anginal patients demands more than the mere administration of drugs. With this in mind we can classify antianginal agents as follows:

1. The nitrites and nitrates
2. Drugs that block adrenaline β-receptors
3. Other drugs
4. Surgical procedures
5. General measures

Nitrates and nitrites
Several organic nitrites and nitrates have been used clinically but the only inorganic nitrite of therapeutic interest is sodium nitrite. Bismuth nitrate has enjoyed some popularity in the treatment of peptic ulcer and it was formerly given to relieve infantile diarrhoea. The administration of nitrates to very young children is, however, fraught with danger that bacterial reduction in the intestinal tract may

Table 40.2 Some nitrites and nitrates

Approved name(s)	Proprietary name(s)	Formula
Sodium nitrite	Erinitrit	$NaNO_2$
Amyl nitrite	Vaporol	$CH_3.CH(CH_3)CH_2.CH_2.NO_2$
Octyl nitrite		$CH_3.(CH_2)_5.CH(C_2H_5)CH_2NO_2$
Glyceryl trinitrate Trinitrin; Glonoin	Anginine; Angised; Nitrong; and many others	$CH_2.O.NO_2$ $\|$ $CH.O.NO_2$ $\|$ $CH_2.O.NO_2$
	Long acting: Nitrocontin, Nitroglyn, Sustac.	
Erythrityl tetra- nitrate Erythritol tetranitrate Erythrol nitrate Tetranitrol	Cardilate; Cardiwell	$CH_2.O.NO_2$ $\|$ $CH.O.NO_2$ $\|$ $CH.O.NO_2$ $\|$ $CH_2.O.NO_2$
Pentaerythritol tetranitrate	Cardiacap; Mycardol; Pentritol; Peritrate; Pentafin; Quintrate and others	$O_2N.O.H_2C \diagdown \quad \diagup CH_2.O.NO_2$ C $O_2N.O.H_2C \diagup \quad \diagdown CH_2.O.NO_2$
Mannitol hexa- nitrate Mannityl hexa- nitrate Nitromannite	Moloid;	$H_2C.O.NO_2$ $O_2N.O.CH$ $O_2N.O.CH$ $HC.O.NO_2$ $HC.O.NO_2$ $H_2C.O.NO_2$
Isosorbide dinitrate Sorbide nitrate	Carvasin; Cedocard; Isordil; Sorbitrate; Sorquad; Vascardin and others	H_2C — — ⌐ $HC.O.NO_2$ O CH HC O $CH.O.NO_2$ CH_2
Triethanolamine trinitrate bi- phosphate Trolnitrate phosphate	Metamine; Nitroduran; Nitretamin	$(CH_2)_2.O.NO_2$ $N{-}(CH_2)_2.O.NO_2 . 2H_3PO_4$ $(CH_2)_2.O.NO_2$

produce nitrite in amounts sufficient to cause methaemoglobinaemia. The peril and origins of this condition are discussed elsewhere (p. 71) in the course of an account of infant deaths caused by nitrate in drinking water.

It is usual to categorize the nitrites and nitrates together as nitrites, with the implication that the nitrites only exert their characteristic action after reduction to nitrites. This custom will be followed here and the term nitrite is taken to include both nitrates and nitrites. The names and formulae of the best known nitrites are set out in Table 40.2. The group will be discussed as a whole before individual members are described.

The nitrites relax the smooth muscle in all types of vessel but the postcapillary vessels (venules and veins) are particularly sensitive. Since capillaries proper have no smooth muscle in their walls, they are not directly affected by the nitrites but the relaxation of the precapillary sphincters (which control the inflow of blood into the capillary beds) will indirectly increase capillary flow in areas where compensatory vasoconstriction does not occur. The vasodilatatory action of the nitrites is very evident after taking amyl nitrite which is the most rapidly acting of this group of compounds and which causes an intense flushing of the face and neck. The nitrites are also prone to cause dilatation of intracranial vessels and an unpleasant headache is often experienced after taking amyl nitrite. Workers in explosives factories also commonly complain of headache which is the result of their continued exposure to glyceryl trinitrate. The nitrites cause dilatation of the retinal and other intraocular vessels (and may therefore cause increased intraocular pressure) but the effects on pulmonary and renal vessels are minimal. The effects of nitrites on the splanchnic vessels (the seat of the peripheral resistance) is normally compensated by a reflex vasoconstriction so that the blood pressure does not fall to the extent that might be expected in the light of the vasodilatation that occurs in other vascular beds. A compensatory reflex cardioacceleration also helps to moderate the fall in blood pressure. Some individuals, however, have an impaired sympathetic response to a fall in blood pressure and they may react violently to nitrites. The blood accumulates in the abdomen and lower limbs, venous return of blood to the heart is grossly reduced and the cardiac output and blood pressure fall precipitously. The reduced supply of blood to the brain may cause fainting preceded by nausea, shivering and cold sweats, the so-called *nitrite syncope.*

The nitrites relax smooth muscle throughout the body and they increase the amplitude and rate of respiration, probably by a direct effect on the carotid body chemoreceptors.

Amyl nitrite, octyl nitrite and glyceryl trinitrate are relatively short acting and they are used primarily to cut short anginal attacks which have already begun or to prevent an attack if precipitating circumstances such as unavoidable exercise are expected. The other nitrites mentioned below and in Table 40.2 were developed in attempts to produce long lasting vasodilatation and so to provide long term protection for the anginal patient. A longer acting form of glyceryl trinitrate is also available. However, none of the nitrites is really suitable for use as a prophylactic agent. Other means (the blockade of β receptors and the general measures detailed below) should be adopted for this purpose, reserving the nitrites for the relief of acute anginal attacks that are prone to occur occasionally even in those receiving prophylactic treatment.

As has already been hinted, the most likely side effects of nitrite therapy are methaemoglobinaemia, serious hypotension and headache. Some of the nitrites also cause gastrointestinal upsets.

Sodium nitrite is of little value in the treatment of angina, as it is likely to cause hypotension. It is, however, a valuable antidote in cyanide poisoning. Until recently, indeed, sodium nitrite provided the only real hope for those with acute cyanide poisoning. The lethal action of cyanide is the result of its inactivating cytochrome oxidase but in the presence of methaemoglobin the cyanide will dissociate from the enzyme and combine instead with the methaemoglobin. The cyanmethaemoglobin so formed will itself dissociate but recombination of cyanide with cytochrome C can be prevented by thiosulphate which reacts with the cyanide to produce the stable thiocyanate. In the treatment of cyanide poisoning, a very slow intravenous injection of sodium nitrite (about 500 mg) is followed by a very slow injection of a ten per cent solution of sodium thiosulphate. In recent years, another (and probably a better) antidote to cyanide has become available. This is cobalt edetate, a chelating agent (p. 796) that is given initially in doses of 300 to 600 mg by rapid intravenous injection. Cyanide poisoning produces a desperate situation and time lost in making up solutions would almost certainly prove fatal. If capsules of amyl nitrite are available, they can be administered by inhalation while sodium nitrite or cobalt edetate solutions are being prepared but in any situation where cyanide is used the antidotes should always be available in a form suitable for immediate use.

Amyl nitrite is an inflammable, volatile liquid with a characteristic and rather unpleasantly sweetish odour. It is taken only by inhalation and it is dispensed in the form of crushable glass capsules enclosed in a protecting fabric cover. The capsules (or 'perles') are crushed between the fingers and held to the nose and mouth. Amyl nitrite acts within 30 seconds of its being inhaled. Although the effect lasts for only about five minutes, this is long enough to cut short an acute anginal attack. Amyl nitrite is not nowadays very popular. The capsules are expensive, the flush is unpleasant and headache, nausea and vomiting commonly accompany their use. The means by which the drug is taken draws attention to the patient and makes the nature of his condition obvious even to the layman. Finally, even in patients who do not develop complete nitrite syncope, the fall of blood pressure is sometimes sufficiently great to reduce the blood flow through the heart and to make the ischaemia worse rather than better.

Octyl nitrite has similar properties to amyl nitrite. It is a highly volatile liquid which is used in an inhaler. Although it is less likely than amyl nitrite to produce side effects, its use is not widespread.

Glyceryl trinitrate (nitroglycerine) is an explosive liquid but it is, needless to say, quite safe in the tablet form in which it is normally presented. Nitroglycerine is well absorbed from the mouth and, as is indicated by one of its older proprietary names (Perglottal), the tablets are usually chewed or taken sublingually. The dose is one half to one milligram and the action of nitroglycerine, which appears within two to three minutes of its administration, lasts for up to 45 minutes. Like amyl nitrite, nitroglycerine sometimes causes a sufficiently severe hypotension to reduce the blood flow through the heart and injudicious doses have been known to precipate attacks of severe cardiac ischaemia. For this reason, the dose of nitroglycerine has to be carefully worked out for the individual patient. There is a remarkable unanimity of opinion that when this is done nitroglycerine is the best available drug for the treatment of anginal attacks. The wealth of proprietary preparations of nitroglycerine (Table 40.2) testifies to its popularity.

Nitroglycerine is absorbed through the skin and it is incorporated into an ointment (Nitrol), employed in the local treatment of conditions characterized by localized arterial spasms. One such condition is Raynaud's disease in which blood flow through one or more fingers or toes suddenly ceases, causing pallor or cyanosis and an incapacitating numbness in the affected digit. These attacks of vasoconstriction are often precipitated by exposure to cold and they have their origin in a localized increase in sympathetic activity. They are usually short lasting and though the condition is normally too trivial to merit the appellation 'disease', the temporary discomfort is often considerable so that drugs which relieve it are welcomed.

Preparations of nitroglycerine which release the drug slowly after oral administration have been developed. These preparations (Table 40.2) contain up to 30 mg of nitroglycerine and they should therefore provide protection for long periods of time. Opinion concerning their value is divided.

Other nitrites. All the other compounds listed in Table 40.2 have been developed as long acting vasodilators for the prophylaxis of angina. Their properties are, in general, similar but erythrityl tetranitrate and mannitol hexanitrate are the most effective and they can be taken sublingually in doses of up to 10 mg and 40 mg respectively. The other compounds are less useful and it is doubtful whether the effectiveness of any member of this group approaches that of nitroglycerine.

Mode of antianginal action of the nitrites

Healthy coronary arteries share in the generalized vasodilatation induced by the nitrites. Since this vasodilatation is achieved at the expense of no more than minor falls in blood pressure, the nitrites would be expected to increase the blood flow through the heart and for many years this action was assumed to underlie the therapeutic effectiveness of the nitrites. Recent studies have cast doubt on the validity of this explanation. Although the nitrites do increase blood flow through healthy hearts, there is more doubt concerning their effect on the diseased organ. Ischaemia itself causes coronary vasodilatation and it is thought by some that in subjects of anginal attacks, maximal vasodilatation has already occurred. It may be that the drugs produce a beneficial redistribution of blood in the coronary system without increasing total flow but against this possibility must be set the fact that glyceryl trinitrate does not relieve anginal attacks when it is given by direct injection into the coronary arteries of patients who are relieved by sublingual administration of the drug. The implication is that nitrites influence cardiac function by reason of their peripheral actions. It seems that the pooling of blood in the dilated vessels reduces the return of blood to the heart and hence the cardiac output. Energy demands on the heart are thereby reduced and a further contribution to this relief can be expected from the slight hypotensive action which will lighten the load against which the heart has to work. The reflex tachycardia caused by the initial hypotensive response partly, but not seriously, offsets the advantages conferred by the reduced stroke volume and the mild hypotension.

The fact that smaller smounts of blood are returned to the heart after taking the nitrites may have another beneficial consequence because the resulting fall in the tension to which the ventricular walls are exposed may allow a freer flow of blood through the coronary vessels. The heart is thus doubly favoured: it has less work to do and it is given more blood with which to do it.

Drugs that block adrenaline β receptors

In the previous edition of this book, propranolol was rather grudgingly allowed to occupy a few lines of text among a collection of miscellaneous drugs many of which, even then, were of dubious clinical value. It is a measure of the sway that the β-receptor blocking drugs have come to exert in therapeutics that they now have to be included as antianginal drugs of choice, occupying a position second only to glyceryl trinitrate itself.

The majority of patients with angina—about 70 per cent according to most authorities—benefit from continued treatment with a β-blocking agent. There are those who, knowing that the two drugs act synergistically, supplement the blocking agent with glyceryl trinitrate but the usual procedure is to use the latter drug only when an anginal attack threatens or when the circumstances are such as to demand extra protection, the blocking agent providing basal maintenance.

Since propranolol came into use as an antianginal drug, a whole range of congeners has appeared on the scene (Table 18.1, p. 303). Some of them might be expected, on superficial theoretical grounds, to hold more promise than propranolol as antianginal agents. Those with intrinsic sympathomimetic activity, for instance, might be able to prevent cardiac failure by providing sufficient sympathetic drive to ensure that the bradycardia induced by β blockade does not become excessive. There is, however, no evidence at all that drugs with intrinsic sympathomimetic activity are any more than marginally superior to those that lack it. Again, the cardioselective agents (acebutolol, atenolol and metoprolol) would be expected to have less widespread side effects than those that affect both types of β receptor. There is no evidence that this is so. The cardioselective agents are, of course, indicated in patients in whom coronary insufficiency and asthma coexist. Apart from this, the selection of a blocking agent for antianginal therapy is largely a matter of the physician's personal preference. At the time of writing, the blocking agents most frequently called into service for anginal prophylaxis are propranolol and oxprenolol.

Drugs that block β receptors prevent anginal attacks in susceptible subjects as a result of their ability to reduce myocardial energy requirements by slowing the heart and the velocity of cardiac contraction. They also inhibit the increased cardiac activity that otherwise accompanies the emotional stress that is so often a precipitant of an anginal attack. They do not increase coronary flow. Indeed some investigators have been able to demonstrate a coronary vasoconstriction after the administration of propranolol.

The properties and side effects of the drugs that block adrenaline β receptors are discussed in detail elsewhere (p. 302). Reviews of their antianginal value are provided by Prichard (1974) and by Sowton, Das Gupta and Baker (1975).

Other drugs

Over the years, claims that they possess useful antianginal activity have been made on behalf of many drugs; one survey (Charlier, 1971) discusses more than a hundred such agents. Few of them, apart from the nitrites and the β-blocking agents, merit serious consideration but from among the few we must make at least a passing mention of three.

PERHEXILENE MALEATE

Perhexilene (Pexid) is a piperidine compound (Fig. 40.7) that has been available in Britain since 1975 and on the continent of Europe for a rather longer period.

Perhexilene causes arteriolar dilatation but the resulting hypotension does not evoke the usual compensatory tachycardia because the drug also exerts a direct depressant action on the heart. Left ventricular work and, consequently, myocardial oxygen demand, fall but cardiac efficiency (the ratio of cardiac output to cardiac oxygen consumption) rises and this clearly explains the beneficial effect of perhexilene in cases of coronary insufficiency.

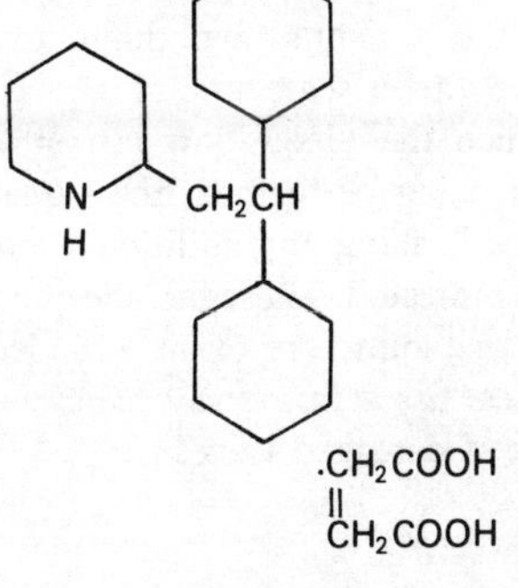

Perhexilene maleate

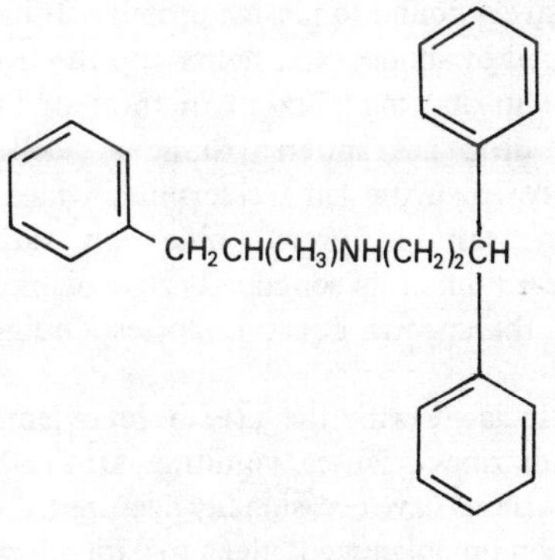

Prenylamine

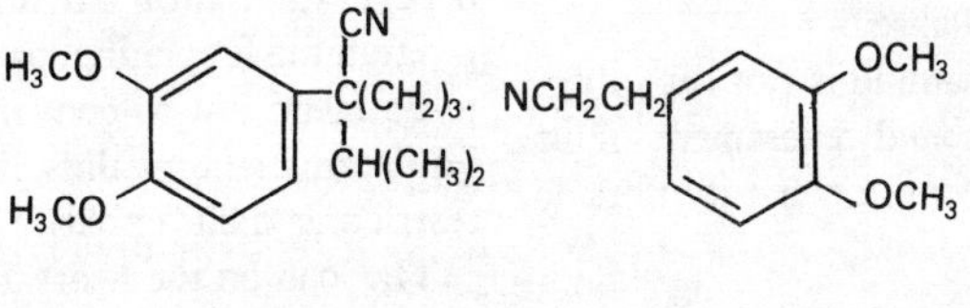

Verapamil

Fig. 40.7 Miscellaneous antianginal drugs.

Perhexilene is taken in twice daily oral doses each of 200 mgs. Mild side effects—dizziness and other autonomic disturbances, nausea and vomiting—are not infrequently experienced when the drug is first taken but these usually disappear completely within a week or so even if the dose is not reduced. It has, however, recently become evident that more serious side effects sometimes develop: liver damage, hypoglycaemia and a peripheral neuropathy head the list of these potentially more dangerous side effects.

Some individuals exhibit hypersensitivity to perhexilene and this constitutes an obvious signal to withdraw the drug. Other contraindications to its use are recent myocardial infarction and the presence of severe liver or kidney disease.

As a therapeutic agent, perhexilene does not seriously rival the older antianginal drugs.

PRENYLAMINE

Prenylamine (Synadrin, Segontin) causes some dilatation of blood vessels but its therapeutic effect stems principally from an action on myocardial metabolism. It prevents the incorporation of catecholamines into their storage sites in the myocardium (and, to a smaller degree, in other tissues) and it also hinders excitation-contraction coupling by blocking the calcium channels in the myocardial membrane. Sodium channels are not affected. As a consequence of these several actions, prenylamine causes bradycardia, a slight fall in blood pressure, and a reduction in the power of cardiac contraction. There is a fall in the demand of the myocardium for oxygen and cardiac efficiency improves.

Prenylamine is readily absorbed from the alimentary tract and is extensively bound to plasma proteins. It has a half life in the blood of about seven hours and the usual daily dose of 180 to 300 mg is taken in three or four instalments. The drug has antiarrhythmic as well as antianginal activity (p. 690). Like reserpine, which it resembles in some respects, prenylamine only slowly depletes the myocardium of its contained catecholamines and its maximal therapeutic effect is correspondingly delayed.

Side effects associated with the use of prenylamine include sedation, dizziness, nausea, vomiting, skin rashes and tremor. Convulsions have occasionally occurred. Care has to be taken when prenylamine is given to patients who are also receiving antihypertensive drugs or to those in heart failure lest too severe a depression of cardiovascular activity precipitate circulatory collapse.

Clinical experience with prenylamine is not yet sufficiently extensive to permit a reasoned assessment of its therapeutic value. Present indications are that it offers no special advantages.

VERAPAMIL

Like prenylamine, verapamil (Cordilox, Isoptin) has both antianginal and antiarrhythmic properties. It depresses myocardial activity by occluding calcium channels in a similar fashion to prenylamine and it also damps myocardial metabolism by lessening the utilization of the high energy phosphates through an inhibition of calcium-dependent ATPase.

Although the overt actions of verapamil on the heart recall those of propranolol, claims that the two drugs are equally efficaceous must be treated with caution until there is more solid evidence on which to base a judgment.

Verapamil is given in doses of 40 to 80 mg thrice daily, the usual care being needed in patients who are also receiving antihypertensive medication. Its antiarrhythmic action has been exploited by intravenous injection in cardiac emergencies. The principal side effects of verapamil are dizziness and nausea.

Surgical procedures

Over the past fifty years, many surgical measures aimed at correcting coronary insufficiency have been devised. Most of the earlier ones were as generally unsuccessful as they were dangerous but much more effective procedures are now available. Modern developments in cardiac surgery (with some contribution from prophylactic pharmacology) have virtually eliminated the risk of operative or immediately postoperative death while parallel advances in investigative techniques have made it possible to identify those who are likely to benefit from surgical interference. The day may be not far distant when the giving of antianginal drugs is relegated to the status of a reserve treatment.

It is no part of this book's task to describe surgical techniques but it is worth mentioning that the favoured operation for correcting inadequacies of coronary flow involves the grafting of lengths of saphenous vein, removed from the patient's own thigh, to provide bypass channels for those segments of the coronary arteries through which the blood flow is restricted. While the operation is being performed, the surgeon can take the opportunity of taking any additional remedial measures that may be indicated. These include endarterectomy (the removal of the solid core of an occluded major artery), removal of scar tissue from the ventricles and the repair or replacement of damaged valves.

General measures

As in cases of hypertension, general measures directed at reducing cardiac work and preventing further arterial degeneration form an important item in the treatment programme for anginal patients. At the same time, care has to be taken not to convert happily energetic individuals into permanent invalids, mental or physical, by needlessly restricting their activities.

The load on the heart can be reduced by correcting any obesity and by avoiding, as far as possible, heavy meals and situations that occasion stress. A mildly anxiolytic drug (p. 561) might be helpful.

Arterial degeneration is associated with elevated plasma

levels of cholesterol and triglycerides. The hyperlipoprot-einaemia can be reduced in severity by avoiding the consumption of animal fats. Drugs such as cholestyram-ine, flofibrate and nicotinic acid can be given when dietary measures alone do not suffice. Patients with coronary insufficiency should not smoke cigarettes: those who find it impossible to give them up completely should be encouraged to reduce their consumption of tobacco to a minimum and to take it in a pipe or in the form of cigars so as to reduce nicotine absorption by inhalation.

VASODILATOR DRUGS

The drugs discussed in the following paragraphs have vasodilator activity but they are not primarily employed in the treatment of either hypertension or angina pectoris.

Papaverine is an isoquinoline alkaloid found in opium, from which it was first isolated by Merck in 1848. It acts like the nitrites on smooth muscle throughout the body, causing vasodilatation and a general relaxation of smooth muscle tone. Its presence in opium is thought by some to explain why opium is less constipating than morphine.

Papaverine is a much more powerful coronary vasodila-tor than either amyl nitrite or nitroglycerine. It also depresses conduction and irritability in the heart and increases the refractory period of the myocardium, thus rendering it less sensitive to stimuli which might cause cardiac arrhythmias. Papaverine stimulates respiration by a similar mechanism to that by which nitrites exert their respiratory effect: in addition, it may increase the sensitiv-ity of the respiratory centre to carbon dioxide.

Although papaverine is a powerful coronary vasodilator, it is of little value in the treatment and prophylaxis of anginal attacks. It has been used in the treatment of such cardiac irregularities as extrasystoles when these arise in patients with coronary insufficiency. It is useful for the relief of arterial spasm during surgery or following the accidental injection into the artery of an irritant solution intended for intravenous use. Papaverine is also occasion-ally employed in the treatment of cerebral arteriosclerosis and spasm of the bile ducts, bronchi, ureters and intestine. It is of no great benefit in these conditions. Side effects of papaverine administration include sedation, sweating,

flushing, dyspnoea, dizziness, headache, nausea and loss of appetite. Heart block may also occur. Papaverine nitrite should combine the therapeutic effectiveness of both papaverine and the nitrites but in practice it does not seem to possess any advantages over papaverine alone.

Papaverine is useful in the laboratory as a reference compound, since it relaxes smooth muscle by a direct musculotrophic action and consequently it unselectively inhibits contractions of the intestine caused by acetylcho-line, histamine, 5-hydroxytryptamine and barium ions. If it is suspected that a substance which is being studied has a direct action on smooth muscle, it is useful to be able to compare its effects with those of papaverine. If, for instance, doses of papaverine and of the unknown antagon-ize acetylcholine-induced contractions of the guinea pig ileum to the same extent, they should be equally active as each other against contractions caused by other smooth muscle stimulants, if the substance under test has an exclusively musculotrophic action.

Papaverine's popularity in the past is reflected in the large number of proprietary names it enjoys. These include, among many other imaginative names, Cerebid, Dylate and Vasospan.

Papaverine should be distinguished from papaveretum (Omnopon, Pantopon) which is a mixture of the soluble salts of the morphine alkaloids. Papaveretum contains 50 per cent of morphine and only very small amounts of papaverine. It has no vasodilator or antispasmodic action.

Substances related to papaverine. Papaverine has mor-phine-like properties. This, and the further fact that it has a marked effect on coronary flow, encouraged the search for synthetic compounds of related structure with good vasodilator activity but no central action. A large number of such substances has been developed and tested but none

Ethaverine hydrochloride

has proved to be more effective or less toxic than the nitrites. Among the more successful are ethaverine (Ethaquin, Pavaspan, Perparin), the tetraethyl hom-ologue of papaverine and dioxyline phosphate (Paveril), an analogue of papaverine which is claimed to be as effective as, but less toxic than, papaverine. Neither of these compounds has found much favour.

Another papavarine derivative is verapamil, a drug that is more appropriately classified with the antianginal drugs proper. It is described on p. 704.

Papavérine

DIPYRIDAMOLE

Dipyridamole (Persantin) is a complex pyrimidine derivative with papaverine-like musculotrophic activity. It has a coronary vasodilator action but is less effective on other peripheral vascular beds. Adenosine is capable of causing coronary vasodilatation and increased amounts of adenosine occur in ischaemic heart muscle. It has been suggested that adenosine acts in heart muscle as a local regulator of blood flow. Dipyridamole inhibits adenosine deaminase and may exert part of its vasodilator action indirectly by raising the local concentration of adenosine in the heart. It also increases the concentration of adenosine triphosphate (ATP) in heart muscle damaged by lack of oxygen; ATP, like adenosine, causes coronary vasodilatation but its most important role in the heart as elsewhere is to act as a source of high energy phosphate. Although these considerations would suggest that dipyridamole should be a useful drug in the treatment of coronary insufficiency, it has proved disappointing in clinical use.

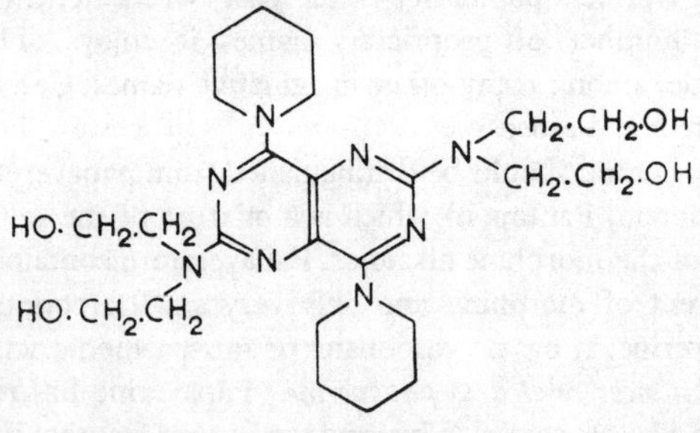

Dipyridamole

Dipyridamole inhibits platelet aggregation and it has occasionally been given to patients immobilized after surgery with the aim of reducing the incidence of thromboembolism.

CYCLANDELATE

Cyclandelate (trimethylcyclohexanyl mandelate, Cyclospasmol) is employed in the treatment of peripheral vascular disease (such as intermittent claudication, Raynaud's syndrome and cerebrovascular disease) and in

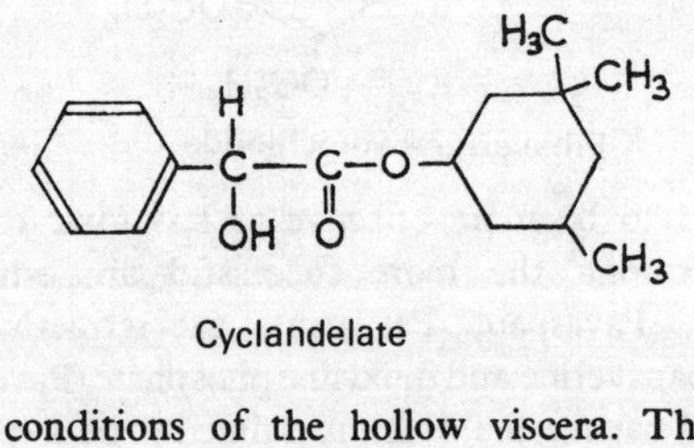

Cyclandelate

spastic conditions of the hollow viscera. The recommended oral dose is 200 to 400 mg three or four times daily. Gastrointestinal upsets sometimes occur in the course of treatment with cyclandelate. The drug should not be given to patients who have recently suffered myocardial infarction.

KHELLIN

Khellin is an obsolete drug whose chief claim to current fame is that a consideration of its chemical structure, pharmacological properties and clinical uses led to the synthesis of sodium cromoglycate (p. 410).

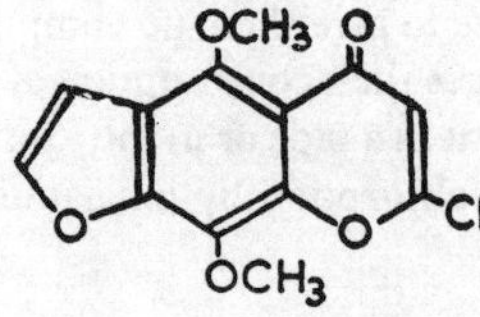

Khellin

Khellin was obtained from the fruits and seeds of an umbelliferous herb *Ammi visnaga* which grows in Egypt and was used there in folk medicine as an antispasmodic to relieve pain in renal colic and ureteral spasm. Khellin also causes relaxation of the bronchioles and the coronary arteries and has some blocking action on histamine H_1 receptors. At doses that cause marked coronary vasodilatation, khellin does not dilate the peripheral blood vessels nor does it cause hypotension. In its heyday, khellin was used in the treatment of angina pectoris, renal colic, asthma and whooping cough.

AMINOPHYLLINE

Although it is appropriate to consider the drug here, it should be noted that aminophylline is not primarily a vasodilator agent in the same sense as the drugs hitherto discussed. Its general antispasmodic effects are more marked than its vasodilator activity, it is a diuretic agent and it exerts a stimulant action on the central nervous system.

Aminophylline (theophylline ethylene diamine) is a solubilized form of theophylline and it possesses the pharmacological properties of that drug (p. 624). It dilates the blood vessels, including those of the coronary circulation and it has a stimulant action on the myocardium, increasing the cardiac output particularly when the output is depressed as in congestive cardiac failure. The central stimulant actions of aminophylline are most evident on the medullary centres: respiration is stimulated and excitation of the vagus centre sometimes causes bradycardia.

Uses of aminophylline. In left sided heart failure, blood accumulates in the pulmonary vessels, giving rise to cardiac asthma with dyspnoea and bronchospasm. Aminophylline dilates the bronchi and stimulates the respiratory centre and it produces an immediate relief of symptoms in attacks of cardiac asthma. It is also useful in the treatment of right sided heart failure, since it relieves the dyspnoea which may be a feature of the condition and it improves the cardiac output. It also controls oedema formation by reason of its diuretic action. Aminophylline is employed in the treatment of severe acute attacks of bronchial asthma and status asthmaticus but since it is most effective by the intravenous route it is less useful in chronic asthma, which demands continuous treatment. Aminophylline can be used to prevent or relieve the gastrointestinal spasm caused by morphine; combined with nikethamide (p. 515) it has been used as a respiratory stimulant in cases of respiratory failure.

When it is given by the intravenous route (as it must be in the acute conditions listed above), aminophylline is injected slowly (to prevent hypotension, syncope, headache or nausea) in doses of 100 to 500 mg. It is much less effective by mouth and high doses cannot be given by this route because of the frequency with which they cause nausea and vomiting. If aminophylline is used for the prolonged treatment of chronic conditions in the ambulant patient, suppositories are useful.

An elixir of theophylline (Elixophyllin) is absorbed more readily than aminophylline and is said to provide a more effective oral medicament than aminophylline itself.

Proprietary preparations of aminophylline include Cardophylin, Phyldrox, Phyllocontin and Theodrox.

The screening and clinical testing of vasodilator drugs

The detection of vasodilator and smooth muscle relaxant activity is simple but as has already been said it is much more difficult to predict whether a drug with coronary vasodilator activity in an isolated preparation will prove therapeutically useful.

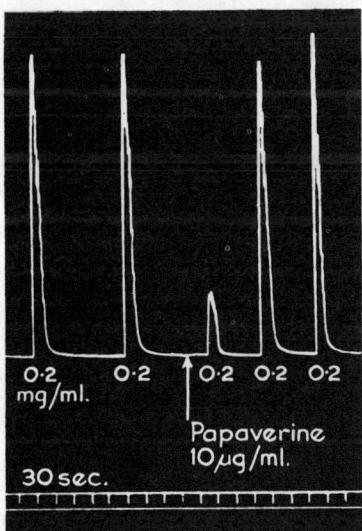

Fig. 40.8 Inhibition by papaverine of contractions of the guinea-pig ileum induced by barium chloride. All contractions are brought about by 0.2 mg/ml of barium chloride.

Papaverine-like musculotrophic activity can most easily be demonstrated by stimulating strips of isolated intestine with barium chloride and then showing that the drug being

tested reduces or prevents the contractions (Fig. 40.8). Barium chloride stimulates the muscle directly and independently of the specific receptors and it is therefore the most suitable spasmogen to use. When active compounds are found by the method, they should be subjected to the more detailed study described on p. 652 to determine

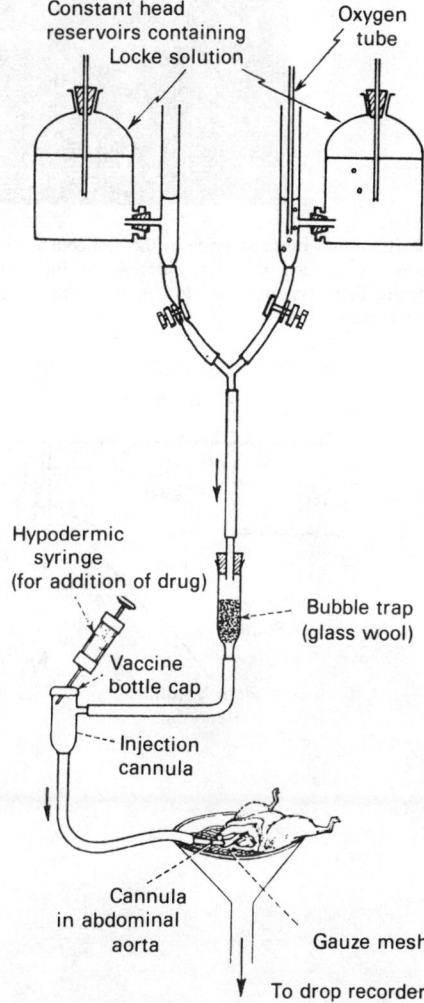

Fig. 40.9 Apparatus for perfusion of the rat hindquarters or rabbit ear. The drug is injected in a small volume into the perfusion fluid as shown. The use of two reservoirs allows the perfusion fluid to be changed to one containing noradrenaline in order to increase the tone of the vessels when potentially vasodilator substances are being studied. The oxygen delivery tube is placed in the reservoir in use.

whether they possess additional antispasmodic activity by virtue of their being also able to antagonize acetylcholine, histamine, 5-hydroxytryptamine or other humoral substances.

Action on blood vessels can be demonstrated by perfusing the isolated ear of a rabbit or the hindquarters of the

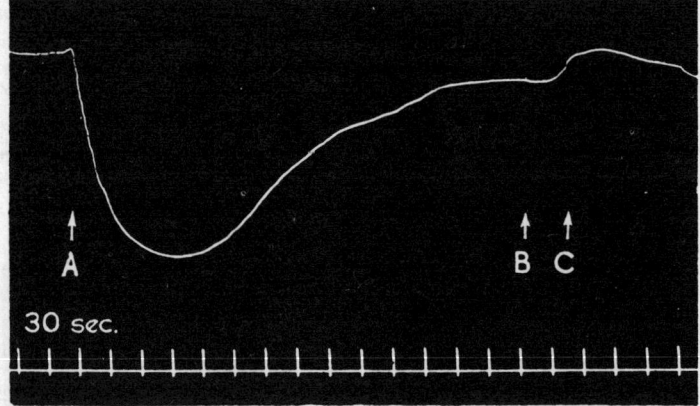

Fig. 40.10 Inhibition by papaverine of the vasoconstrictor action of barium chloride on the blood vessels of the rat's hindquarters. At A, 1 mg of barium chloride was injected into the cannula, at B, 0.2 mg of papaverine, and at C, 1 mg of barium chloride again. The apparatus used to obtain this record is shown in Figures 40.9 and 40.11. The hindquarters of other animals can also be used.

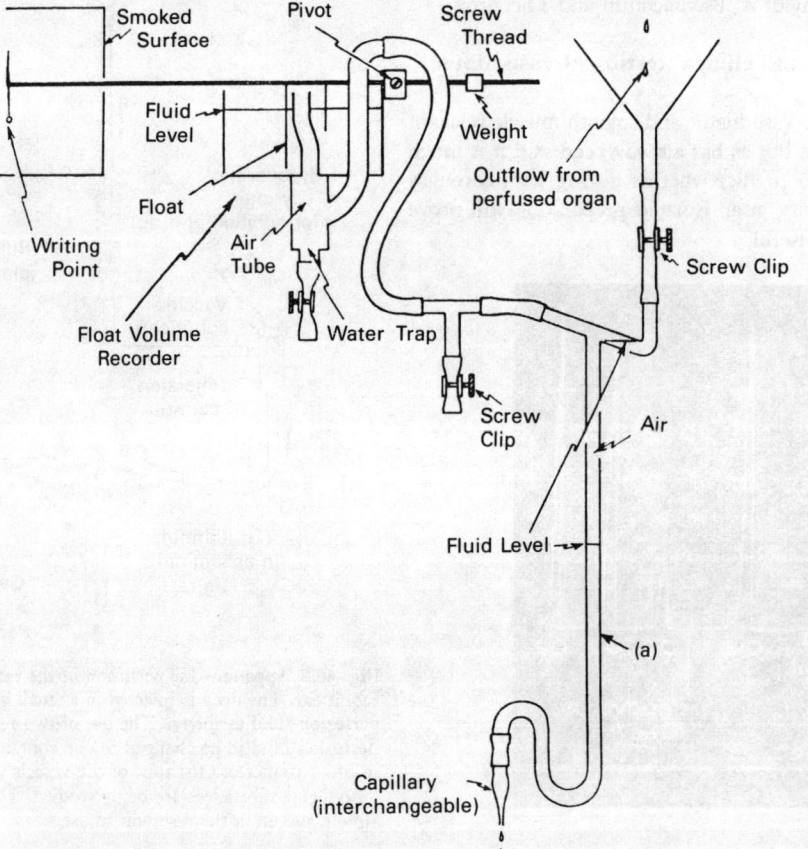

Fig. 40.11 Stephenson's outflow recorder. When using the apparatus a capillary is chosen whose length and bore are such that with a steady inflow the fluid level in tube (a) comes into equilibrium at approximately the position shown. If the inflow increases, the level in the tube rises until the increased hydrostatic pressure is sufficient to increase the flow through the capillary to a point when inflow and outflow are again equal. If inflow decreases, the fluid level sinks to a new equilibrium position. Changes in fluid level alter the volume of air in the system. The volume changes are recorded by the float recorder. (After Stephenson (1948) by permission of the editors of the *Journal of Physiology*.)

frog or rat with a solution containing noradrenaline, which constricts the vessels. Smooth muscle relaxants will overcome the vasoconstriction and increase the outflow from the preparation (Fig. 40.9 and 40.10). The outflow from the perfused organ can be measured either by means of Stephenson's recorder (Fig. 40.11) which can be made in any laboratory, or by one of the commercially available drop counters. The rabbit ear preparation is generally to be preferred to the hindquarters of the rat which become oedematous very rapidly. These preparations are used at room temperature, even when organs from homoiothermic animals are used, but it is also possible to perfuse limbs with blood at 37°C. For this purpose, dogs or cats are used and heparinized blood is pumped (using a Dale-Schuster pump) into the femoral artery of the isolated limb. Blood from the vein passes *via* an outflow recorder to an oxygenator whence it is returned to the leg of the pump. As much as possible of the tubing, which carries the blood, passes through a water bath maintained at 37°C. In refinements of this method, the blood is circulated at a constant rate and changes in vascular diameter are reflected in the changes of perfusion pressure required to maintain the constant perfusion rate. It should be remembered that in isolated organs or in the limbs of anaesthetized animals, vasodilatation is maximal or nearly so and the presence of vasodilator substances in injected material can only be demonstrated with certainty if the vessels are first constricted by an appropriate drug.

Coronary vasodilator activity can be assessed in isolated mammalian hearts by the Langendorff method described on page 698. Isolated rings of the coronary arteries can also be used, set up in a conventional organ bath.

A Langendorff preparation can also be used to measure the effect of drugs on coronary flow in the human heart if this is removed sufficiently soon after death. The use of this technique has shown that the reactivity of the vessels from hearts showing degeneration of the coronary arteries is frequently less than that of normal coronary vessels. The consequences of this finding have already been discussed.

In the intact human being, blood flow through the heart can be measured by a variety of techniques which measure the rate at which an identifiable substance is cleared from the heart after its injection into the venous blood or directly into the heart. If a radioactive substance is used (radioactive iodinated human albumin and radioactive rubidium have been employed), the passage of the material through the heart can be followed by counters placed on the chest wall. The application of these methods has been fully discussed by Charlier (1961) and Rowe (1966).

In the clinical testing of drugs which might be useful in the treatment of coronary vascular disease, it is very important to employ properly controlled double blind techniques. The only real criterion of effectiveness of these drugs is that the patient should be made free from pain. This state is a highly subjective one and it is important that the subjects of clinical tests should not be influenced in any way in their assessment of their condition. Many of the more recently developed antianginal agents were greeted enthusiastically by physicians, many of whom were convinced that the new drugs were better than the old. In almost every instance, later trials showed that the early enthusiasm had not been warranted and that the new drug was inferior to nitroglycerine.

VASOCONSTRICTOR AGENTS

The most important vasoconstrictor substances are the catecholamines, angiotensin and vasopressin. Their pharmacological properties and clinical uses are discussed in the chapters that deal specifically with these drugs in locations that can be traced by referring to the Index.

BIBLIOGRAPHY

Books, monographs and reviews

Butler, V.P. (1972) Assays of digitalis in the blood. *Prog. Cardiovasc. Dis.* **14**, 571-600.

Charlier, R. (1961) *Coronary Vasodilatation.* London: Pergamon Press.

Charlier, R. (1971). *Antianginal Drugs.* Heidelberg and New York: Springer-Verlag.

Dimond, E. G. (ed) (1957). *Digitalis.* Springfield, Ill.: Thomas.

Hodge, R.L. and Dornhorst, F. C. (1966). The clinical pharmacology of vasoconstrictors. *Clin. Pharmac. Ther.,* **7**, 639-647.

Julian, D. G. (ed) (1977). *Angina Pectoris,* Edinburgh and London: Churchill Livingstone.

Krikler, D. M. and Goodwin, J. F. (eds.) *Cardiac Arrhythmias.* London, Philadelphia and Toronto: W. B. Saunders Co.

Prichard, B. N. C. (1974) *β*-Adrenergic receptor blocking drugs in angina pectoris. *Drugs.* **7**, 55-84.

Repke, K. (1965) Effects of digitalis on membrane adenosine triphosphatase on cardiac muscle. In: *Proc. Second Int. Pharmac. Meeting.* New York: Pergamon Press

Rowe, G. G. (1966) Effects of drugs on the coronary circulation. *Clin. Pharmac. Ther.,* **7**, 547-557.

Singh, B. N. and Jewitt, D. F. (1974). *β*-Adrenergic receptor blocking drugs in cardiac arrhythmias. *Drugs,* **7**, 426-461.

Sowton, E., Das Gupta, D. S. and Baker, I. (1975). Comparative effects of beta-adrenergic blocking drugs. *Thorax,* **30**, 9-18.

Thorp, R. H. and Cobbin, L. B. (1967). *Cardiac Stimulant Substances.* New York and London: Academic Press

Vaughan Williams, E. M. (1975). Anti-dysrhythmic drugs— their mode of action. In: *Contraction and Relaxation of the Myocardium.* ed. Nayler, W. G., London: Academic Press.

Winbury, M. M. (1964). Experimental approaches to the development of anti-anginal drugs. In: *Advances in Pharmacology,* vol. 3, pp. 1-82, ed. Garattini, S. and Shore, P. A., *New York and London: Academic Press.*

Wright, S. E. (1960). *The Metabolism of the Cardiac Glycosides.* Oxford: Blackwell.

Original papers

Christiasen, N.J. B., Kolendorf, K., Siersback, K. and Molholm Hansen, J., (1973) Serum digoxin values following a dosage regimen based on body weight, sex, age and renal function. *Acta med. scand.,* **194,** 257-259.

Gillam, P. M. S. and Prichard, B. N. C. (1965). Use of propranolol in angina pectoris. *Br. med. J.,* **2,** 337-339.

Langer, G.A. (1970). The role of sodium ion in the regulation of myocardial contractility. *J. molec. cell. Cardiol.* **1,** 203- 207.

Nayler, W.G. (1973) An effect of ouabain on the superficially-located stores of calcium in cardiac muscle cells. *J. molec. cell. Cardiol.,* **5.,** 101-110.

Okita, G.T., Richardson F, and Roth-Schechter, B. F. (1973) Dissociation of the positive inotropic action of digitalis from inhibition of sodium and potassium activated adenosine triphosphatase. *J. Pharmac. exp. Ther.,* **185,** 1-11.

Richens, A. (1974) Drug estimation in the treatment of epilepsy. *Proc. R. Soc. Med.,* **67,** 1227-1229.

Soffer, A., Toribara, T., Moore-Jones, D. and Weber, D. (1960). Clinical application and untoward reaction of chelation in cardiac arrhythmias. *Archs intern. Med.,* **106,** 824-834.

Stephenson, R. P. (1948) An outflow recorder useful for detecting small amounts of vasopressin. *J. Physiol.,* **107,** 162-164.

Szekeres, L. and Vaughan Williams, E. M. (1962). Antifibrillatory action. *J. Physiol.,* **106,** 470-482.

Tanz, R.D. and Kerby, C.F. (1961). The inotropic action of certain steroids upon isolated cardiac tissue with comments on steroidal cardiotonic structure-activity relationships. *J. Pharmac. exp. Ther.,* 131, 55-64.

41.   Thyroid and antithyroid substances

The major portion of the thyroid gland is devoted to the production of thyroxine and triiodothyronine which we shall call the thyroid hormones. Though hallowed by long use this nomenclature is not completely satisfactory because the gland also produces *thyrocalcitonin,* a hormone that operates in concert with parathormone (the secretion of the parathyroids) to regulate calcium metabolism. Thyrocalcitonin is discussed in Chapter 46.

The thyroid hormones regulate energy metabolism at cellular and subcellular levels and they are therefore involved in the control of growth, tissue differentiation and development and in the regulation of the associated biochemical systems. The secretion of the thyroid hormones is under the supervision of the thyroid stimulating hormone (TSH or thyrotrophin) of the anterior pituitary and in this way its activity is integrated with that of related systems under hypothalamic control. The output of the thyroid stimulating hormone is also directly regulated by the concentration of thyroid hormone in the circulating blood. If the concentration changes, in the absence of any change in signals from the hypothalamus, the pituitary adjusts its output of thyroid stimulating hormone in such a direction as to restore the previous level of thyroid activity.

Production, release and metabolism of the thyroid hormones

The thyroid hormones are produced and stored in follicles which make up the bulk of the thyroid gland. Each follicle consists essentially of a closed spheroid of cubical or columnar cells one layer thick enclosing a cavity that is filled with a viscous, semifluid, yellowish colloid. The follicles vary in size, reaching diameters of up to about one millimetre so that they are visible to the naked eye in the intact gland. As would be expected of an organ whose secretions have to be distributed to virtually every cell in the body, the thyroid gland is highly vascular and profuse capillary networks embrace each follicle. In a quiescent gland the follicles are distended with colloid and the epithelial cells take on their cubical form. When the gland is very active, much of the colloid, which is being broken down more rapidly than it can be formed, disappears from the follicles and the epithelial cells revert to a columnar form (Fig. 41.1). The epithelial cells, as we shall see, are metabolically very active and they are equipped with the full range of cellular machinery described in Chapter 2.

Iodide from the diet is selectively taken up by the epithelial cells of the thyroid follicles where, under the influence of a peroxidase, it is oxidised to iodine. The follicular cells also synthesize a complex glycoprotein (*thyroglobulin*), one of those component amino acids is tyrosine. In the course of protein synthesis some of the tyrosine residues are iodinated to give 3-monoiodinated and 3,5- diiodinated compounds. Pairs of residues further unite to give triiodinated and tetraiodinated compounds. The resulting iodothyroglobulin is secreted into the follicles as the major component of the colloid. At the same time and at a rate determined by the rate of secretion of thyroid stimulating hormone, colloid is being taken up again by the epithelial cells and broken down to yield (in addition to its other component amino acids) 3- iodotyrosine, 3,5- diiodotyrosine, 3,5,3'- triiodothyronine and 3,5,3',5'- tetraiodothyronine (thyroxine). The two last named substances (often designated T_3 and T_4 respectively) are secreted into the blood as the thyroid hormones. The mono- and diiodinated compounds are degraded by a specific iodinase and the iodine so provided is available—to use contemporary jargon—for recycling.

When they reach the bloodstream, the thyroid hormones enter into a loose combination with plasma proteins. Three such proteins—albumin, an acid glycoprotein and a thyroxine-binding α -globulin—are capable of binding thyroid hormones and the amount of free hormone in the plasma is no more than 0.1 per cent of the blood's total complement.

The amount of protein bound iodine (often unnecessarily abbreviated to PBI) in the blood reflects the secretory

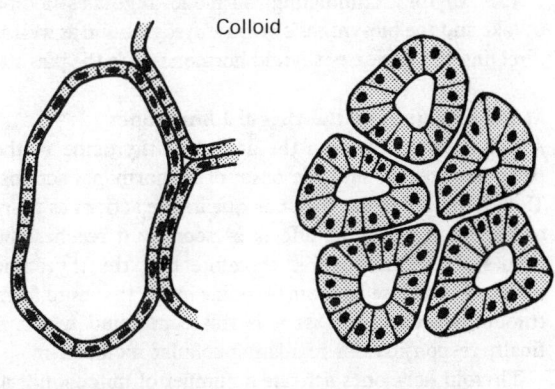

A   Quiescent gland   B   Active gland

Fig. 41.1 The thyroid gland.

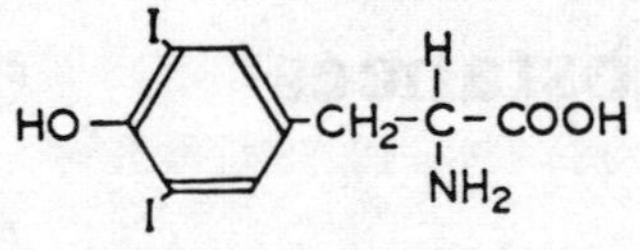

3,5-Diiodotyrosine

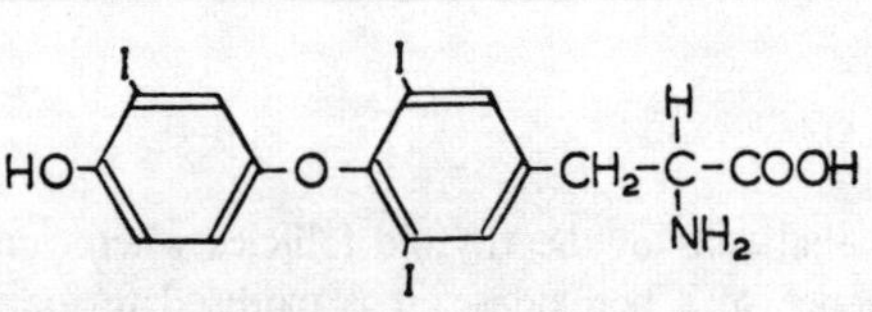

3,5,3'-triiodothyronine (T₃)

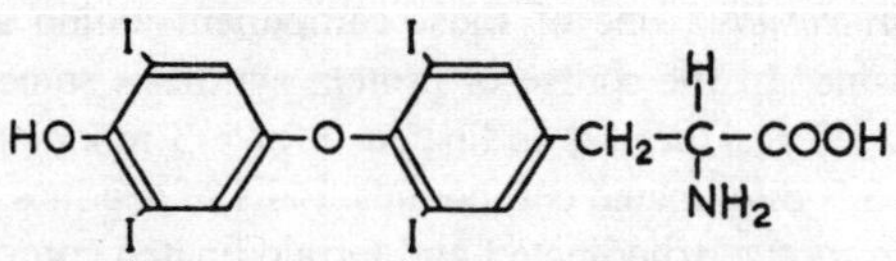

3,5,3',5'-tetraiodothyronine (thyroxine, T₄)

Fig. 41.2 Iodinated derivatives of tyrosine.

activity of the thyroid gland. It normally lies between about 4 and 7μ g per 100 ml of serum and is shared almost equally among the three species of binding protein. However, the thyroxine-binding α-globulin in some individuals has an abnormally high binding power and this results in the occurrence of high values of protein bound iodine (up to 15μ g per 100 ml) in the absence of any increase in thyroid activity. Conversely, a few otherwise normal subjects display abnormally low concentrations of protein bound iodine because they carry an α-globulin of inferior binding power. Both binding anomalies are of hereditary origin.

The thyroid hormones themselves are deiodinated in the liver, salivary glands and kidney. The iodine can be used again and the remainder of the molecules are disposed of, as conjugates, in the urine. Some of the deiodinated molecules undergo oxidative deamination before conjugation.

. The thyroid stimulating hormone regulates iodine uptake and the biosynthesis of iodothyroglobulin as well as directing the release of thyroid hormones into the plasma.

Mode of action of the thyroid hormones
A delay occurs between the arrival of thyroxine in the peripheral tissues and the onset of its hormonal actions. Triiodothyronine has the same qualitative actions as thyroxine but it exerts its effects as soon as it reaches the tissues. It seems possible therefore that the thyroxine molecule may lose an atom of iodine in the tissues to form triiodothyronine and that it is this compound which is finally responsible for regulating cellular metabolism.

Thyroid hormones activate a number of mitochondrial enzyme systems and thereby bring about a wide ranging stimulation of metabolic processes that is so characteristic

a feature of their physiological action. In high doses they uncouple oxidative phosphorylation (p. 31) so that heat production becomes excessive. This action may partly account for the hyperthermia, sweating and vasodilatation that form part of the clinical picture of hyperthyroidism (thyrotoxicosis, p. 714). The concurrent reduction in the supplies of ATP may well be a contributory cause of the muscle weakness that is often associated with thyrotoxicosis.

The thyroid hormones sensitize the tissues to adrenaline and noradrenaline and many of the signs of thyrotoxicosis—tremor, tachycardia, increased blood pressure, hyperglycaemia, increased heat production, etc.—are wholly or partly the consequence of this sensitization. Feelings of restlessness and anxiety accompany these peripheral signs of augmented sympathetic activity and it is sometimes difficult to make the differential diagnosis between thyrotoxicosis and an anxiety neurosis.

The sensitization induced by the thyroid hormones is the consequence of their being able to promote the synthesis of adenyl cyclase (p. 322) or (and this is perhaps the more likely in view of the special and specific relationship between the thyroid hormones and the catecholamines) to stimulate the production of additional catecholamine receptive moieties in the enzyme molecule. One important inhibitory action has to be noted among this welter of stimulating and sensitizing properties. The thyroid hormones (even in physiological amounts) restrain the synthesis of mucoprotein.

DISORDERS OF THYROID FUNCTION

In many patients with thyroid disease, the gland is enlarged and it produces an obvious swelling in the neck. An enlarged thyroid gland, however it is caused, is known as a *goitre* (French *goître* = neck). As will be seen, goitres may be associated with over-secretion, with under-secretion or with no change in the secretion of thyroid hormones. Goitres sometimes become large enough to cause serious pressure on adjacent structures (the trachea, the oesophagus and the laryngeal nerves) and in this event it may be necessary to remove some or all of the thyroid gland irrespective of whether the condition causing the goitre is one for which surgical treatment is normally indicated.

SIMPLE GOITRE
Simple goitre occurs when an essentially normal thyroid gland produces insufficient hormone to meet the body's demands. The gland hypertrophies in response to an increased secretion of thyroid stimulating hormone and this usually leads to a sufficiently increased production of thyroid hormones to maintain normal cellular metabolism. The increased demands made on the thyroid during

$$H_2C = C - HC \underset{H}{\overset{H_2C \text{———} NH}{\underset{O}{\bigg|}}} C = S$$

L-5-vinyl-2-thioxazolidine

puberty, menstruation and pregnancy are often sufficient to cause a small but obvious enlargement of the thyroid gland but the larger goitres are usually due to idoine lack, either because insufficient is provided in the diet or because its utilization is interfered with. It was once believed that iodine intake was more likely to be inadequate in those who, living far from the sea, ate food grown on soil which had not been exposed to the iodine vapour which was supposed to be borne on the sea breezes. Some credence was given to the idea by the observation that, in England, goitres were very common in Derbyshire although it was never explained why goitres appeared only in localized parts of the great land masses of the world. This view of the origin of simple goitre is now known to be untenable and it is clear that regional variations in the incidence of simple goitre are due to other factors: the presence of large amounts of calcium (or perhaps of other substances) in the drinking water, for instance, seems to interfere with the production of thyroid hormones. These factors will obviously operate to greater effect in those whose intake of iodine is only just above the minimal requirement. It is notable that, with improvement in the general standards of nutrition, 'Derbyshire necks'—the huge goitres which were not uncommon in the past in inhabitants of that county—are now rarely seen.

Simple goitre is sometimes due to ingestion of substances which prevent the synthesis of thyroxine. Goitres have been produced in rabbits by feeding them a diet consisting mainly of cabbage. Goitrogenic agents are also found in a number of other vegetable tissues including mustard seeds, turnips, swedes, linseed, kale and peanuts. The goitrogen in linseed and peanuts is a thiocyanate but the other plants mentioned all contain a glycoside together with an enzyme which is activated when the leaves or roots are broken during mastication. The enzyme causes the liberation of L-5-vinyl-2-thioxazolidine (goitrin) from the glycoside. It is doubtful whether even the most misguided devotee of the natural food cult eats enough raw cabbage or turnip to give himself a goitre. On the other hand, if dairy cattle eat large quantities of food containing a goitrogen, the latter may appear in harmful quantities in the milk. An interesting example of this occurred some years ago in Tasmania. Children were encouraged to drink increased amounts of milk but many of the cows which supplied the milk had been fed on kale. Even though the children's intake of iodine was more than adequate, many of them developed goitres.

It has already been mentioned that simple goitres usually represent a successful adaptation to a condition of sub-optimal iodide intake or utilization. The rational way of treating the condition is to give thyroxine, which reduces the output of thyroid stimulating hormone and hence the size of the gland. In order to ensure that the smaller gland produces adequate amounts of the thyroid hormones, sufficient iodide should be provided in the diet or supplied as a supplement. Potassium iodide is useful as a dietary supplement and in many countries (but not in Britain) iodide is compulsorily added to table salt. Fish is a good source of dietary iodide for those who are not attracted by seaweed.

CRETINISM

Cretinism is the consequence of severe hypothyroidism in infants. It is most often due to a congenital defect in thyroid development of function and it is usually not associated with a goitre since the gland cannot respond to the thyroid stimulating hormone.

In cretinism, growth is stunted, sexual development is arrested and the child is mentally retarded. The skin is coarse and thick and the tongue is enlarged so that it appears to be too large for the mouth. The basal metabolic rate is depressed. The rational treatment for cretinism is the provision of thyroxine. This stimulates growth and metabolism but the mental condition is less reponsive to thyroxine unless the disease is diagnosed and treated at a very early age.

The word cretin has the same origin as Christian: it implies that cretins do not have the intelligence (and, therefore, the guile) to indulge in any but purely innocent behaviour.

Cretinism is endemic in some regions of the world.

MYXOEDEMA

Myxoedema is a condition of hypothyroidism which usually appears in middle life though a condition of juvenile myxoedema is recognised. If thyrotoxicosis is to be called Graves' disease (p. 714), myxoedema should likewise be called Gull's disease but it only rarely attracts this eponym. Myxoedema may arise from no apparent cause ('spontaneous myxoedema') but it is now clear that many cases which would have been diagnosed in the past as spontaneous myxoedema are the consequence of lymphadenoid goitre (Hashimoto's disease). This condition is an autoimmune disease; the body manufactures antibodies to its own thyroid hormones which are thereby rendered ineffective. A goitre results but it does not remedy the hypothyroid state, for although more thyroid hormone may be manufactured it is immediately inactivated by the autoimmune reaction. In truly spontaneous myxoedema, goitre is unusual and the condition appears to be due to a simple atrophy of the thyroid gland which can no longer respond to the thyroid stimulating hormone. Other causes of myxoedema include pituitary deficiency, overdosage with antithyroid drugs and partial thyroidectomy with failure of the residual glandular tissue.

Drug effects and thyroid function

It is important to remember that a number of commonly-used drugs can depress thyroid function and the physician should be alert to the possibility that hypothyroidism may develop in patients receiving these drugs over a period of time. The list of suspect drugs includes, among others, lithium carbonate, phenylbutazone, ibuprofen, the sulphonylureas and *p* -aminosalicylic acid.

In myxoedema, the basal metabolic rate is reduced and there is a consequent reduction in all bodily activities. The skin is dry and coarse, the hair falls out and there is often an increase in weight. The amount of cholesterol in the blood increases and there is an increased risk of myocardial infarction. Mental symptoms may be severe enough to lead to a mistaken diagnosis of endogenous depression (p. 538). A characteristic feature of myxoedema and the one which gives its name to the disease (myxoedema = mucous swelling) is the accumulation in the subcutaneous tissues of a material consisting essentially of mucopolysaccharides combined with protein. The limbs and face are particularly affected and the puffy appearance of the face is similar to that which arises from the water retention of true oedema. However, since the myxoedematous swellings are not caused by fluid they do not 'pit' on pressure. Mucoprotein production increases in myxoedema because of relaxation of the restraint on its synthesis that is normally exerted by the thyroid hormones (p. 712).

Myxoedema, like cretinism, is treated with thyroxine.

THYROTOXICOSIS

In thyrotoxicosis, the thyroid gland secretes excessive quantities of hormone. The gland is usually enlarged but it does not reach the size of many simple goitres. The most important form of thyrotoxicosis is *Graves' disease* and for the purpose of this discussion thyrotoxicosis and Graves' disease will be regarded as synonymous.

For many years it was believed that Graves' disease was the result of an excessive stimulation of the thyroid by thyroid stimulating hormone, the secretion of which, it had to be assumed, was no longer subject to inhibitory feed back control by the circulating thyroid hormones. Although this hypothesis may explain the rare cases of thyrotoxicosis that are associated with pituitary tumours, there are compelling reasons for rejecting it in other cases: in thyrotoxicosis the concentration of thyrotrophin in the blood is not usually elevated (indeed, it is often depressed) and it is an easy matter to demonstrate that its secretion is still influenced by the circulating thyroid hormones. Moreover, Graves' disease has been known to occur in individuals who have undergone complete removal of the pituitary gland.

An alternative view of the origin of thyrotoxicosis was provided by the observation that the blood of patients with Graves' disease often carries a thyroid stimulating substance in addition to pituitary thyrotrophin and differing from it by reason of the fact that it provokes a long-lasting stimulating of the thyroid gland. Thus, whereas a single intravenous dose of pituitary thyrotrophin produces an effect that reaches its peak in some three hours and is complete within twenty-four, the response to the long acting compound climbs to a maximum in about twelve hours and persists for two or more days. What is now known as the *long acting thyroid stimulator* (inevitably and inelegantly abbreviated to LATS) was first detected by Adams and Purves in 1956 but it is only during the last few years that it has figured prominently in discussions concerning the aetiology of thyroid disease.

The long acting thyroid stimulator is a component of the immunoglobulin G fraction of the plasma proteins and many regard it as an autoantibody, thereby categorizing thyrotoxicosis like Hashimoto's disease as an autoimmune condition. It is not entirely clear how the immune system manages to produce autoantibodies that provoke hypothyroidism as well as others that cause hyperthyroidism but, as we saw in Chapter 24, its ways are complex and inscrutable. Some patients with Graves' disease later develop Hashimoto's disease, an indication perhaps that they have manufactured an abundance of thyroid autoantibodies.

The long acting thyroid stimulator is not found in all patients with Graves' disease and, among those in whose blood it does occur, there seems to be no very good correlation between the severity of the symptoms and the concentration of the stimulator. It is possible that it is not itself directly or entirely responsible for the augmented thyroid activity but that it merely signals in a rather inaccurate fashion the occurrence of more important changes taking place within the thyroid gland itself.

Because of the characteristic eye signs which frequently appear in Graves' disease, the condition is also called *exophthalmic goitre*. The eye signs include protrusion of the eyeballs (exophthalmos) and the retraction of the upper lids. These changes are brought about by the deposition of fat in the orbit which pushes the eye forward but they are probably not due directly to thyroid activity. It has been suggested that they are caused by an immunoglobulin related to, but distinct from, the long acting thyroid stimulator. An alternative supposition is that the pituitary gland secretes a factor that operates directly on the retrobulbar fat. Neither of these hypotheses is entirely satisfactory and the problem of exophthalmos awaits illumination from further informed reasearch.

Other features of thyrotoxicosis include an increased metabolic rate, loss of weight, nervousness, anxiety and a fine tremor of the fingers. As we have seen (p. 712), heat production is increased but the temperature regulating mechanisms cause widespread cutaneous vasodilatation and so prevent or minimise the hyperthermia that would otherwise be produced. The most serious consequences of thyrotoxicosis are seen in the heart. Atrial fibrillation or cardiac failure is likely to develop if thyrotoxicosis is not adequately treated. This may be partly a consequence of the long continued stimulation of the heart in response to metabolic needs but the heart also suffers directly from the effects of its continued exposure to excessive quantities of the thyroid hormones which, in addition to any direct toxic action they may exert, also sensitize the myocardium to the catecholamines to which it is exposed.

Some patients with Graves' disease display unsightly and irregular swellings on the legs. This condition is known as *pretibial myxoedema*. Although the designation is etymologically irreproachable (the swellings are produced by the accumulation of mucin) it is, perhaps, an unfortunate one because there is no suggestion of hypothyroidism in these patients.

Thyrotoxicosis is treated by partial thyroidectomy, by radioactive iodine or by antithyroid drugs. The indications for each of these therapeutic measures are mentioned later.

Thyroid crisis

This rare condition (also called *thyroid storm*) occurs when the blood stream is suddenly flooded with thyroid hormones. It may occur after thyroid surgery or in untreated thyrotoxic patients who suffer an infectious illness or other stress. It is characterized by hyperpyrexia and an exaggeration of the pre-existing signs of thyrotoxicosis.

The thyroid and muscle disease

A degree of weight loss and muscle wasting is a usual feature of thyrotoxicosis but many patients with this condition (or other thyroid disorders) also suffer from more definite disorders of muscle function. The most common of these thyroid linked diseases, according to the most authoritative work on the subject (Ramsay, 1974), are thyrotoxic myopathy and myasthenia gravis. The first named of these conditions is characterized by severe wasting and weakness of the limbs particularly in their proximal parts. The disorder arises in the muscles themselves (and not in the nerves that supply them) and may well be related to ATP deficiency. As we have already seen (p. 712) the production of ATP is likely to be hindered in thyrotoxicosis and the shortfall in supplies is accentuated by the increased demands for ATP that follow the increased activity of adenylcyclase. In addition, structural changes occur in the muscle fibres themselves.

The association of thyroid disease (both hypothyroidism and hyperthyroidism) with myasthenia gravis is probably a simple reflection of the fact that both these disorders are of autoimmune origin. In addition, many of the biochemical and morphological changes wrought by thyroid disease aggravate any existing myasthenic condition which may sometimes not make its presence felt until thyroid function is disturbed.

DRUGS USED IN THE TREATMENT OF THYROID DISEASE

IODIDES

Iodides increase thyroid secretion in cases of simple goitre, they inhibit secretion in hyperthyroidism and they have no effect in the normal (euthyroid) subject. In simple goitre, iodides clearly promote the synthesis of the thyroid hormones. If iodine deficiency is suspected, potassium iodide may be given in daily doses of 60 mg.

It is impossible to supply a convincing explanation for the ability of iodides to suppress secretion in patients with thyrotoxicosis. It has been suggested that they inactivate the thyroid stimulating hormone but if this is so it is difficult to see why no evidence of this effect is to be seen in the normal subject. Iodides certainly cause a dramatic remission of symptoms in patients with Graves' disease but the improvement is only maintained for a few weeks. Nevertheless, potassium iodide is a valuable drug for controlling thyroid activity in patients who are to undergo thyroidectomy. It is given during the two weeks immediately preceding operation. By its effect on the gland it reduces excitement, apprehension and cardiac output at the time when such an action is most necessary. Even if thiouracil derivatives are employed to suppress thyroid function in the weeks before operation, iodides still have to be given (p. 717). For the preoperative management of thyrotoxicosis, potassium iodide is given in doses of 60 mg three times daily. Until recently, Lugol's iodine (5 per cent of iodine in a 10 per cent solution of potassium iodide) was almost invariably used instead of potassium iodide but it offers no particular advantage over the simpler preparation.

Since the thyroid gland takes up most of the iodide supplied to the body, the radioactive isotope (^{131}I) can be used for the relief of thyrotoxicosis. It is concentrated in the gland and emits β-rays which effectively destroy some of the secretory tissue without affecting organs elsewhere in the body. Treatment with radioactive iodine is extraordinarily simple—the patient drinks a single glass of water containing the isotope, which is quite tasteless. The treatment may be repeated if the first dose does not produce sufficient depression of thyroid activity. This form of treatment is ideal for patients over the age of 45 (who usually do not respond to antithyroid drugs) or for those in whom concurrent conditions, such as heart failure, make surgery hazardous.

Because of the theoretical (but perhaps overemphasized) possibility of its causing thyroid carcinoma or chromosomal damage in the gonads, radioiodine should not be given to children or to adults in their reproductive years. Investigations are currently being conducted into the feasibility of replacing ^{131}I with the ^{125} isotope whose radiations are less penetrating and which should therefore be suitable for patients of all ages.

The only real danger that has to be guarded against in those receiving radioiodine is hypothyroidism although some patients develop *iodism* when they are given small doses of iodides. In this condition, there is an increased production of salivary nasal, lachrymal and bronchial secretions, skin rashes, gastric irritation, nausea and vomiting. The parotid and submaxillary glands may become painfully enlarged. The condition sometimes disappears if the administration of iodides is cautiously continued.

L-THYROXINE

This is the drug of choice for the treatment of simple goitre, cretinism and myxoedema. In the latter two conditions, relatively large doses of thyroxine may be required but hypothyroid patients are often very sensitive to the hormone and the dose should therefore be increased very slowly. Particularly in cretinism, the optimal dose is often only just below that which produces toxic symptoms (irritability, tachycardia, tremors, sweating and loss of weight) and it must therefore be carefully regulated. Because the thyroid deficiency is usually more severe in cretinism than in myxoedema, the optimal dose for children is of the same order (or slightly higher than) that for adults. It is usually 0.2-0.3 mg daily but initial doses should not exceed 0.05 mg.

TRIIODOTHYRONINE

Triiodothyronine is available under the name of liothyronine for the treatment of cretinism and myxoedema. It is more potent and it acts more quickly than thyroxine. On the other hand, its effects disappear very rapidly when treatment stops and relapses into the hypothyroid state are likely if the patient omits to take his daily dose. Liothyronine has no advantage over thyroxine in the routine treatment of hypothyroidism (indeed it can be positively dangerous) but it may be valuable in cases of coma due to myxoedema. This rare but grave condition occurs in severely myxoedematous patients who are not receiving adequate doses of thyroxine. It is precipitated by minor stresses (such as infection or injury) and the victim suffers acute heart failure, hypothermia and adrenal insufficiency as well as coma. The emergency may be desperate enough to justify the intravenous administration of liothyronine but it must be remembered that the drug is very active and that myxoedematous patients are often very sensitive to the thyroid hormone. Other forms of supportive treatment including the administration of cortisone must also be provided.

Liothyronine is also used in the diagnosis of thyrotoxicosis. The patient is given a small dose (100 μg) of liothyronine daily for a week and the uptake of radioiodine by his thyroid is measured. Liothyronine inhibits uptake of the labelled compound by the normal gland but has no effect on the uptake in thyrotoxic patients. On the rare occasions when liothyronine is indicated for the continuing treatment of hypothyroidism, it is given in daily doses of 50 to 250 μg.

THIOURACIL AND RELATED COMPOUNDS

The observation that a number of plants contain goitrogenic substances, stimulated a search for antithyroid activity in known drugs and in 1941 it was reported that sulphaguanidine (p. 817) caused hypothyroidism in laboratory rats. Shortly afterwards, phenylthiourea was found to posses a similar action. A number of other types of compound including nitrites and imidazolines inhibit the formation of thyroxine but most of those which have been used clinically are derivatives of thiourea. The names and formulae are given in Fig. 41.3. Although all of them have been used in the past, thiourea and thiouracil have now been largely abandoned. Of the remainder, only carbimazole (Carbazole; Neo-Mercazole) is extensively used today but if this drug is not well tolerated it can be replaced by methylthiouracil.

The precise mechanism by which these compounds inhibit the production of thyroid hormones is not known but they certainly prevent the incorporation of iodine into tyrosine. This may be so because, being reducing agents, they interfere with the oxidation of inorganic iodide. Alternatively, they may inhibit an enzyme which is involved in the oxidation process. In addition, they may prevent the conversion of the mono- and diiodotyrosines into the thyronines. They do not interfere with the action of the thyroid hormone on cellular metabolism.

Carbimazole is used in the treatment of thyrotoxicosis. It is given in daily oral doses of 30-60 mg until thyroid activity has been reduced to normal levels. Thereafter a maintenance dose of 10-20 mg is required but this may often be reduced further after a few more weeks.

The effects of carbimazole administration are not evident during the first one or two weeks because the thyroid gland continues to secrete the hormones manufactured

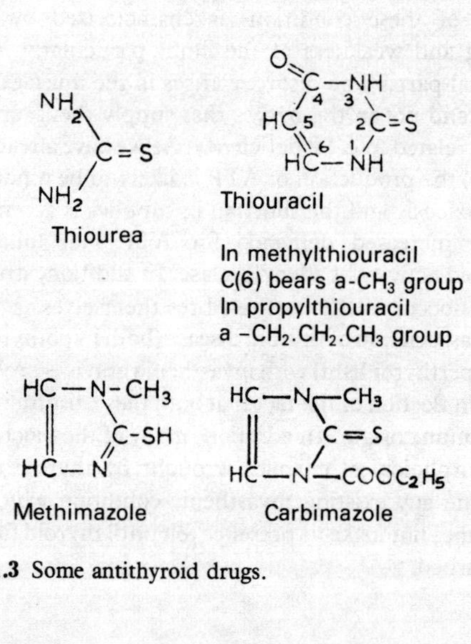

Fig. 41.3 Some antithyroid drugs.

before treatment began. After that, the benefits of treatment appear: the basal metabolic rate is reduced, nervousness and excitability diminish and the heart rate becomes slower. Exophthalmos may be unaffected, since it is probably not directly due to the thyroid hormone itself: this symptom is equally refractory to other forms of treatment. If excessive doses of antithyroid drug are given, the amount of thyroid hormone in the blood may reach levels low enough to provoke increased secretion of the stimulating hormone and the goitre will increase in size. Thus enlargement of the goitre is a useful warning sign of excessive dosage: it will usually be accompanied by the symptoms of incipient myxoedema.

Treatment with antithyroid drugs is usually continued for no more than one year. The drug is then withdrawn. In about 50 per cent of cases in the younger female patient, permanent cure will have been achieved. Results are usually much less satisfactory in the older female patient and in men of all ages. If a relapse occurs after withdrawal of the drug, partial thyroidectomy or treatment with radioiodine will be necessary. In either event (particularly when surgery is contemplated) a course of treatment with the antithyroid drugs is instituted in the months before operation or the administration of the isotope. For the two weeks immediately preceding surgery, iodine should be given instead of, or as well as, the antithyroid drug. The reason for this is that the thyroid of patients given antithyroid drugs becomes soft and vascular. Iodine makes the gland more firm and less vascular so that surgery is easier.

Although carbimazole is less toxic, in the doses commonly used, than the other thiouracil derivatives, its administration is not without risk to the patient. The most serious side effects of carbimazole treatment are allergic hypersensitivity reactions and agranulocytosis. Since treatment with carbimazole is necessarily protracted, a careful watch for signs of agranulocytosis must be maintained. If they appear, the drug must be immediately withdrawn and penicillin treatment must be instituted. Allergic reactions also necessitate the cessation of drug therapy. Less serious side effects include oedema of the legs and feet, enlargement of lymph nodes and salivary glands, conjunctivitis and skin rashes.

POTASSIUM PERCHLORATE

Potassium perchlorate inhibits the active transport processes that promote the uptake of iodide by the epithelial cells of the thyroid. By this means it prevents the biosynthesis of the thyroid hormones.

If its plasma concentration is sufficiently high, iodide can pass into the thyroid gland by simple diffusion in large enough quantities to obviate the need for the active transport mechanism. Thus iodine reverses or prevents the action of potassium perchlorate.

Potassium perchlorate has been used as an antithyroid drug but it is much less effective than the thiouracil derivatives and it is no less toxic. Blood disorders (particularly aplastic anaemia) and gastric irritation may be produced and the drug is of limited value, although it may have some place in the treatment of those who show hypersensitivity or other toxic reactions to carbimazole. In these circumstances, the daily dose is of the order of 1 gram. Potassium perchlorate should never be employed for the pre-operative treatment of thyrotoxicosis because the administration of potassium iodide (which is a necessary part of preoperative treatment) will reverse its antithyroid action and the patient will revert to the thyrotoxic state just at the time when a depressed thyroid activity is most necessary. Sodium thiocyanate has a similar action to potassium perchlorate but it is no longer used clinically.

BLOCKADE OF THE ADRENERGIC SYSTEM

As we have already emphasized, many of the signs and symptoms of thyrotoxicosis are at least partly a manifestation of increased sympathetic activity which arises because the thyroid hormones sensitize the tissues to catecholamines. It would therefore seem reasonable to expect therapeutic benefits from any procedure that reduced the impact of sympathetic activation or adrenaline release in thyrotoxic patients. This approach has only become widely known in recent years (it receives no mention at all in most textbooks of pharmacology or therapeutics more than five years old) but it is by no means a new form of treatment. As long ago as 1923, Bloch administered a high spinal anaesthetic to a delirious patient in the throes of a severe thyroid crisis and produced an immediate and dramatic improvement in her condition. Others later employed the same manoeuvre (which arrests the sympathetic outflow from the spinal cord) with equal success, not only when confronted with the actual emergency of a thyroid crisis but also when they wished to prevent its appearance during and after thyroid surgery. Crile (1938), another pioneer in this field, wishing to avoid the risk of inflicting permanent damage to the throats of professional singers with thyrotoxicosis, denervated their adrenal glands instead of performing thyroidectomy.

Drugs that antagonize activity in sympathetic neurones should also help to relieve thyrotoxicosis. The list of those that have been investigated includes reserpine, methyl dopa, guanethidine, phentolamine and propranolol among others. Not all of them have been successful (phentolamine indeed caused the patients' cardiac condition to deteriorate) but guanethidine and propranolol have earned a place for themselves as useful adjuncts to other forms of treatment. Their principal value lies in their being able to produce a rapid remission of symptoms while other antithyroid drugs are taking their effect or while the patient is awaiting surgery. Propranolol is the drug of choice for many patients (it is given three or four times a day in doses of 10 to 40 mg) because its ability to allay anxiety (p. 569) supplements its antiarrhythmic and other peripheral actions. Its quinidine-like properties add a further contribution to its usefulness. It is, however, contraindicated in patients with incipient or actual cardiac failure because it is liable to precipitate or aggravate cardiac failure, perhaps by preventing the operation of compensatory reflexes. Although guanethidine might be expected to have the same deleterious action, it is found in practice that this is not so and guanethidine becomes the blocking drug of choice when cardiac failure is present. The oral dose of guanethidine (given once daily) can be gradually increased to 1 mg per kilogram of body weight.

The mode of action of the blocking agents is discussed in detail elsewhere in this book while the whole topic of the relationship between thyroid activity and the autonomic nervous system is comprehensively reviewed by Leak (1970).

Taste and thyroid disease

Most people, asked to sample a very dilute solution (0.1–0.2M) of phenylthiourea, will agree that it has an extremely bitter taste but a few will be unable to detect any taste at all until the concentration of phenylthiourea has been increased at least tenfold. We can, therefore, divide the population into those who easily recognise (the 'tasters') and those who do not recognise (the 'non-tasters') a bitter taste in phenylthiourea. In Britain, Europe, Japan and most of the United States about 70 per cent of the population appear to be 'tasters' but the proportion is very much higher among Africans, American Indians and Mongoloid races. Some other compounds that contain the -NC= S grouping taste bitter to 'tasters' but not to 'non-tasters'. Among these substances are methylthiourea and propylthiourea, the antithyroid drugs we discussed previously. The inability to taste these compounds is carried on a recessive gene which is specific in the sense that 'non-tasters' can usually (though not always) readily detect the taste of quinine and other bitters that do not contain the -NC = S grouping.

Although there is no *a priori* reason why an inability to taste an antithyroid drug should go hand in hand with

Phenylthiourea

disturbances of thyroid function, a number of investigations during the past 25 years have established that the incidence of some forms of thyroid disorder (particularly cretinism and nodular goitre) is much higher in 'non-tasters' than it is in 'tasters' (Harris, Kalmus and Trotter, 1949; Fraser, 1961). The association seems to be a fortuitous one: presumably the gene that determines the inability to taste is also responsible for some of the aberrations of thyroid biochemistry that underlie thyroid disease. It is evidently not an entirely maleficent gene since it seems that tasters of phenylthiourea are much more likely than non-tasters to smoke more than 20 cigarettes a day!

BIBLIOGRAPHY

Books, monographs and reviews
Selected texts on general endocrinology
Ezrin, C., Godden, J. O., Volpe, R. and Wilson, R. (1973) (eds.) *Systematic Endocrinology.* Hagerstown: Harper and Row.
Hall, R., Anderson, J., Smart, G. A. and Besser, M. (1974). *Fundamentals of Clinical Endocrinology,* 2nd ed., London: Pitman.
Humphrey, J. H. and White, R. G. (1971). *Immunotherapy for Students of Medicine,* 3rd ed. Oxford: Blackwell.
Kutsky, R. J. (1973). *Handbook of Vitamins and Hormones.* New York: Van Nostrand Reinhold.
Tepperman, J. (1973). Metabolic and Endocrine Physiology, 3rd ed. Chicago: Year Book Medical Publishers.

Thyroid
Conference (1960). Modern concepts of thyroid physiology. *Ann. N. Y. Acad. Sci.,* **86,** 311-676.
Leak, D. (1970). *The Thyroid and the Autonomic Nervous System.* London: Heinemann.
Maloof, F. and Soodak, M. (1963). Intermediary metabolism of thyroid tissue and the action of drugs. *Pharmac. Rev.,* **15,** 43-95.
Means, J. H., DeGroot, L. J. and Stanbury, J. B. (1963). *The Thyroid and its Diseases,* 3rd ed. New York: McGraw Hill.
Ramsay, I. (1974). *Thyroid Disease and Muscle Function.* London: Heinemann.
Thomas, J. A. and Mawhinney, M. G. (1973). *Synopsis of Endocrine Physiology.* Baltimore: University Park Press.
Vanderlaan, W. P. and Storrie, V. M. (1955). A survey of the factors controlling thyroid function with especial reference to newer views on antithyroid substances. *Pharmac. Rev.,* **7,** 301-334.

Original papers
Fraser, G. R. (1961). Cretinism and taste sensitivity to phenylthiocarbamide. *Lancet,* (**i**) 964.
Harris, H., Kalmus, H. and Trotter, W. R. (1949). Taste sensitivity to phenylthiourea in goitre and diabetes. *Lancet,* (**ii**) 1038.

42. Insulin, glucagon and diabetes mellitus

Illness is as old as man himself, but the biochemical tests which help the modern physician to diagnose disease are of quite recent origin. Until they became available, the physician had to rely on simple observation of the patient's excretions and this led to the early recognition of a disease characterized by the passing of large amounts of very sweet or 'honeyed' urine. The name *diabetes*, which is derived from the Greek for syphon, was given to the disease by Aretaeus of Cappadocia (81–138 A.D.). The adjective *mellitus* which comes from the Latin for honey was added by the great Thomas Willis in 1674. Thus 'diabetes mellitus', notwithstanding its mixed parentage, succinctly describes two of the main signs of this disease and distinguishes it from *diabetes insipidus*, a quite different disorder (p. 637) which is characterized by the excretion of large quantities of tasteless (insipid) urine. Since diabetes mellitus is much more common than diabetes insipidus, the word diabetes standing alone is sometimes used to describe diabetes mellitus. The honeyed taste of the urine in diabetes mellitus results from the presence of glucose. The diuresis of diabetes mellitus is classified as an osmotic diuresis (p. 623) consequent on the large amounts of glucose and urea in the urine. Other prominent symptoms in this disease are thirst and wasting.

During the eighteenth century, several clinicians began to suspect that diabetes mellitus had its origin in a disorder of the pancreas and this fact was unequivocally established in 1889 by Minkowski and von Mering. These German physiologists removed the pancreas from dogs and noticed that the animals thereafter showed symptoms of diabetes and drank their own urine. This latter observation suggested that the dogs were thirsty and that the urine was potable as a dilute sweet urine would be. It was already known that islets of cells (called the islets of Langerhans, after their discoverer) were present throughout the glandular tissue proper of the pancreas and de Meyer in 1909 and Schäfer in 1916 independently suggested that the islets might secrete a hormone controlling carbohydrate metabolism. Because of its presumed origin, this hypothetical substance was called 'insuline', though it was not until 1922 that Banting and Best were able to produce convincing evidence that the hypothetical 'insuline' really existed: they prepared an extract of the pancreas of the foetal calf and showed that the extract was capable of reducing the blood sugar content of a diabetic dog. Previous attempts to prepare active 'insuline' had failed because the digestive juices in the pancreas destroyed the hormone during the extraction process. Foetal pancreas contains no proteolytic enzyme. In 1927 the active antidiabetic principle (now called *insulin*) was prepared in a crystalline form and in 1960 a landmark in the history of protein chemistry was reached when Sanger and his colleagues established the sequence of the 51 amino acid residues which make up the insulin molecule. Insulin was the first protein to be characterized in this way and it is appropriate that this should be so, for the whole history of insulin is a record of outstandingly original observations and deductions unsurpassed in any other field of medicine. Within the last decade, several groups of workers have independently achieved the remarkable feat of synthesizing insulin from its component aminoacids.

The human pancreas contains about a million islets of Langerhans, the cells of which can be grouped, on the basis of the size and number of their intracellular granules, into three principal types. The most numerous are designated β or B. They make up about 80 per cent of the total and they secrete insulin. The α or A cells account for about 15 per cent of the islet cell population and the δ or D cells the remaining 5 per cent. The α cells produce glucagon (which, as we shall see, operates in concert with insulin) while the δ cells, surprisingly enough, secrete gastrin (p. 641) and somatostatin (p. 770). Orci and Unger (1975) have shown, in a number of mammalian species, that some of the β cells and all the α cells are closely associated with δ cells. Pancreatic somatostatin can inhibit the secretion of both insulin and glucagon and Orci and Unger tentatively suggest that somatostatin mediates the rapid physiological variations that occur in insulin and glucagon production. A degree of reciprocal control may also be exerted by glucagon on the secretion of somatostatin. Most of the β cells are not associated with α and δ cells so that the steady background secretion of insulin, on which the acute secretory changes are superimposed, can proceed without interference from somatostatin. This interesting hypothesis warrants further study.

The δ cells have suffered from a confusing multiplicity of labels and they are still occasionally referred to as α_1 cells (what we have previously referred to as α cells then have to be designated α_2) or even as β_2 cells. On this latter classification the cells that produce insulin are labelled β_1.

The 51 amino acids in the insulin molecule form two chains, A and B, containing 21 and 30 residues respec-

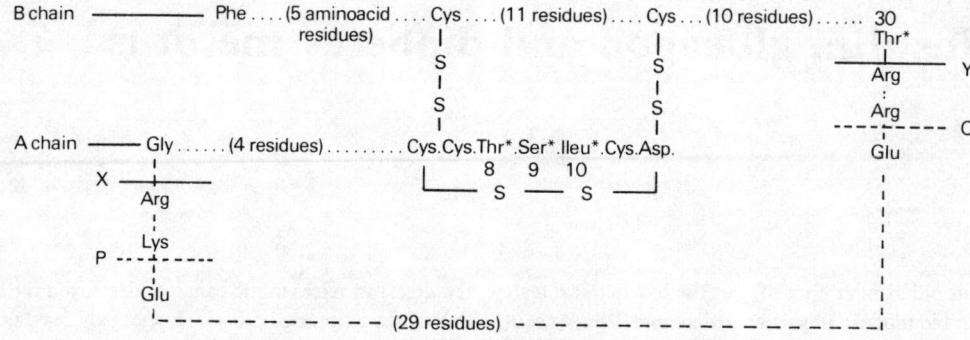

Residue number

	A. chain			B. chain
	8	9	10	30
Human	Thr	Ser	Ileu	Thr
Porcine	Thr	Ser	Ileu	Ala
Rabbit	Thr	Ser	Ileu	Ser
Beef	Ala	Ser	Val	Ala

(Thr – Threonine; Ser – Serine; Ileu – Isoleucine; Ala – Alanine; Val – Valine)

Fig. 42.1 The structure of human insulin (chains A and B), connecting peptide (between X and Y) and C-peptide (between P and Q). The whole molecule as shown here is proinsulin

tively, with a total molecular weight of 5807. The chains are connected by two disulphide linkages and a third disulphide bridge occurs within the shorter chain. The arrangement of the bridges in human insulin is shown in Figure 42.1. The integrity of the disulphide bridges is essential for biological activity but fragments of the rest of the molecule can be split off without loss of activity.

Although all mammalian insulins are made up of 51 aminoacid residues arranged in two chains they do differ very slightly from one another. The differences lie in the nature of one or more of the aminoacid residues in positions 8, 9 and 10 of the A chain and in position 30 of the B chain. These four residues are marked by asterisks in Figure 42.1 and the composition of the insulins of a few common species is indicated in the inset to the Figure. It will be noted that interspecies differences are minimal. All the insulins have the same type of activity as far as their effects on metabolic processes are concerned but the structural differences are sufficient for an animal to recognize as a foreign substance the insulin of another species. It is doubtful whether this ever creates a problem in the human being given pork or beef insulin. It is true that these insulins do induce the production of antibodies which may reduce their therapeutic effectiveness but this is largely a response to contaminating protein rather than to the insulin itself.

Insulin is derived from a precursor (proinsulin) which is

synthesized within the β cells of the islets. In proinsulin, a chain of aminoacid residues (35 in number in the human variety), known as the connecting peptide, links the terminal glycine of the insulin A chain to the terminal threonine of the B chain (Fig. 42.1). Proteolytic enzymes in the pancreas first split off the connecting peptide and then bring about the loss of the two terminal residues from each extremity of the chain. The truncated form of the connecting peptide is known as the C peptide. When insulin secretion is evoked, equivalent amounts of C peptide and a much smaller quantity of proinsulin appear in the blood. The proportion of proinsulin in the mixture is very much increased in patients with tumours affecting the islets of Langerhans.

The length and composition of the connecting peptide displays a considerable degree of interspecies variation. However, both the connecting and the C peptides are biologically inert and, as we have seen, all insulins behave in the same way. Consequently all proinsulins, notwithstanding their structural differences, exert biochemical effects that are qualitatively identical and indistinguishable from those of insulin itself.

Proinsulin was discovered some years ago by Steiner who has since reviewed the subject (Rubenstein and Steiner, 1971).

Insulin appears to be stored in the pancreas in a crystalline complex of six molecules of insulin and two atoms of zinc. Dorothy Hodgkin earned a Nobel prize for her work on the crystal structure of insulin as Sanger (also of Cambridge) had done some years earlier for elucidating the full aminoacid sequence in the molecule.

Before discussing the mode of action of insulin we must first remind the reader that when glucose appears in the urine (glycosuria) it is the result of the blood's glucose concentration having risen above the 'renal threshold' of about 180 mg per 100 ml of blood. At lower blood levels, all the glucose filtered into the glomeruli is reabsorbed by the kidney tubules. An increase in the blood glucose concentration (hyperglycaemia) sufficient to cause glycosuria is not, of itself, of serious import; it may occur transiently in normal people who have ingested large quantities of glucose or in emotional stress, when adrenaline release causes the liberation of glucose from liver glycogen (glycogenolysis). Glycosuria also results if tubular function is impaired. This occurs experimentally after the administration of phlorizin, a glycoside found in the root bark of some fruit trees. Biochemists sometimes speak of 'phlorizin diabetes' though this condition is not one of diabetes in the proper sense of the term. Phlorizin is only used, in animals, for experimental purposes. It has no clinical use.

A form of experimental diabetes that does resemble the clinical condition is that produced by the administration of alloxan (mesoxalyl urea) or streptozotocin. Both substances selectively destroy the β cells of islet tissue. In alloxan, streptozotocin and clinical diabetes alike the glucosuria is a consequence of the impaired utilization of glucose.

THE ACTIONS OF INSULIN

The most powerful stimulus to proinsulin synthesis and to the production and secretion of insulin is provided by the glucose in blood. Other substances that bring about the release of insulin include some aminoacids (arginine, leucine, lysine and phenylalanine) and three of the local hormones (gastrin, secretin and pancreozymin) that promote gastrointestinal activity during the digestion of food. These facts, together with the more immediate and obvious signs of diabetes mellitus (hyperglycaemia, tissue wasting and the breakdown of fat) make it clear that insulin is essentially an anabolic hormone, whose activity promotes the synthesis and prevents the unnecessary breakdown of glycogen, fat and protein.

For some time it was believed, following the suggestion of Cori, that insulin increased the activity of intracellular hexokinase, the enzyme which catalyzes the conversion of glucose to glucose-6-phosphate in the first stage of glucose metabolism. It is now known that the action of insulin is less specific than this and that it has a more general effect on the cell membrane. Even in the absence of glucose, insulin has an action on the erythrocyte, a cell which is incapable of synthesizing glycogen, fats and protein. It seems that the primary action of insulin is exerted at the cell surface where it regulates the redox-potential gradient and thus the energy available for glucose transport across the cell.

In the absence of insulin, a much higher concentration of blood glucose is required before it can cross the cell surface. Glucose is produced first from the glycogen reserves in the liver and the resulting hyperglycaemia can be regarded as a response directed towards increasing the extracellular-intracellular glucose gradient and hence the passage of glucose into the cells. The compensatory value of this mechanism is limited, for as soon as the renal threshold is reached glucose 'overflows' into the urine, preventing any further rise in blood sugar and leading to a depletion of the liver's stores of glycogen. Insulin inhibits the formation of cyclic AMP and hence the breakdown of glycogen (p. 321).

In the absence of insulin, protein breakdown, particularly in muscle, also supplies glucose. The amino acids so produced undergo transamination in the liver to pyruvic acid which is converted to glucose through the Embden-Meyerhof pathway (p. 26). This formation of glucose (gluconeogenesis) is accompanied by the production of urea derived from the amino nitrogen. In the normal individual, the amino acids produced by protein catabolism, or absorbed from the intestine, are not carried to the liver for transamination. Instead, under the influence of insulin, they are for the most part reconstituted into proteins, thus conserving the body's nitrogen supplies. This action of insulin seems to be independent of that on glucose metabolism.

Of the tissues that normally utilize glucose, fatty tissue is particularly sensitive to insulin lack. In this tissue, neutral fats (the triglycerides) break down into fatty acids but these are normally re-incorporated into triglycerides by esterification with glycerophosphate. This latter compound is itself produced by the breakdown of glucose (glycolysis) and in diabetic conditions the impaired utilization of glucose results in a deficiency of glycerophosphate. Fatty acids are, in consequence, released into the blood stream and some are taken up by the liver where they are resynthesized to neutral fat or converted into long-chain fatty acids. Those fatty acids not dealt with in this way are converted into ketone bodies (acetone, acetoacetic acid and β-hydroxybutyric acid) which can be metabolized by muscle. The ability of muscle to 'mop up' ketone bodies in this way is, however, not great and if their production increases a point is soon reached beyond which they can no longer be utilized. Ketosis then occurs. The production of long-chain fatty acids by the liver is impossible in the presence of ketone bodies so that, as soon as ketosis occurs, fat metabolism becomes even more deranged. Disturbances of protein and fat metabolism are responsible for most of the pathological changes of diabetes mellitus. There is accumulating evidence that insulin has another role, entirely unsuspected until quite recently and not allied in any way to its metabolic function. It seems likely that, in its passage through the liver, it exerts a protective action on the liver cells and also promotes the regeneration of atrophic liver tissue (see, for instance Starzo, Porter and Putnam, 1975). Well known facts such as the increased incidence of cirrhosis of the liver in diabetic patients find a ready explanation on this fascinating hypothesis.

GLUCAGON

Banting and Best noticed that their preparations of insulin produced a transient hyperglycaemia before hypoglycaemia set in. They attributed this hyperglycaemia to adrenaline release but Kimball and Murlin (1923) suggested that the insulin contained a hyperglycaemic contaminant to which they gave the name *glucagon*. This view was later shown to be correct and glucagon has now been isolated in a pure state. Its composition was established in 1957: it is a single-chain polypeptide of 29 aminoacids. Glucagon is secreted by the α cells of islet tissue (p. 719) but a substance very similar to glucagon *(enteroglucagon)* occurs in the mucosa of the small intestine distal to the duodenum. It now seems likely that, in addition, glucagon proper is produced in the stomach and duodenum where there are cells that are morphologically indistinguishable from pancreatic α cells.

Glucagon and insulin have opposite effects on the concentrations of glucose and free fatty acids in the blood. Like adrenaline, glucagon promotes glycogenolysis through the cyclic AMP-phosphorylase mechanism (p. 321) but unlike adrenaline (which operates on both liver and muscle) its action is restricted to the liver. It also brings about the production of glucose from aminoacids in the liver *(gluconeogenesis)* and it stimulates lipolysis.

Glucagon has a number of pharmacological actions that are not immediately related to its metabolic effects. Some of them have already been put to clinical use while the potentialities of others are still being explored. Thus it stimulates the release of adrenaline and of growth hormone and these responses form the basis of diagnostic tests for phaeochromocytomata (p. 274) and pituitary function respectively. Glucagon inhibits gastrointestinal movements and induces feelings of satiety though this last effect may represent a response to glucose release. These observations kindled the hope (which has not been realized) that the hormone might have a place in the treatment of obesity. It increases the rate and force of cardiac contraction. This response, like so many glucagon effects, resembles that exhibited by adrenaline and it probably has the same underlying cause—the activation of adenylcyclase. Glucagon has been employed in a few cases of cardiac failure refractory to other forms of treatment. Other pharmacological responses to glucagon administration include hypocalcaemia and insulin release. It is worth

adding that it was an investigation of glucagon action that led to the discovery of cyclic AMP by Sutherland (p. 321) and hence to an appreciation of the ubiquity and unique importance of this 'second messenger'.

Readers who wish to acquire more information concerning the actions of glucagon should begin with the authoritative work edited by Lefebvre and Unger (1972).

Glucagon secretion is stimulated by reductions in the glucose and free fatty acid contents of blood and by conditions associated with increased activity of the sympathetic nervous system. Starvation, hypoglycaemia and physical exercise are potent stimulants of glucagon secretion which, in these circumstances, clearly has the physiologically desirable effect of supplying much needed glucose. The reader who remembers that glucagon evokes insulin secretion might feel prompted to ask whether this effect does not operate too and blunt the desirable responses. In fact, the 'insulinotropic' action of glucagon is suppressed by the concomitant activity in the sympathetic nervous system and perhaps by metabolic consequences of the glucose lack. Consequently the direct metabolic actions of glucagon are allowed full play. Nevertheless there are some physiological circumstances in which glucagon release is followed by insulin secretion. Thus, during the digestion and absorption of a meal, a number of influences (local hormones and changes in the concentration of aminoacids and free fatty acids) provoke glucagon secretion which, because there is no enhanced activity in the sympathetic nervous system, stimulates insulin release. In these conditions it is, of course, entirely appropriate that insulin should be released. In its turn, insulin inhibits glucagon release. Thus the two hormones together form the complementary members of a balanced pair analogous to the many others that subserve homeostatic control mechanisms in the living organism. Since the effects of glucagon are similar to those of insulin lack it is perhaps natural to ask what part, if any, is played by glucagon in the aetiology of diabetes mellitus. Opinions on this presently controversial topic differ but, at one extreme, Unger and his colleagues have entered very convincing pleas on behalf of the hypothesis that glucagon is critically involved in the pathogenesis of diabetes (see, for instance, Unger and Orci, 1975). They maintain that a mere lack of insulin, however caused, will not induce hyperglycaemia unless glucagon is available. Their argument applies even when supplies of insulin are cut off by total pancreatectomy because glucagon is produced in the gut. Again, an injection of somatostatin (p. 770) which suppresses the secretion of both insulin and glucagon will not induce hyperglycaemia until glucagon is supplied from an external source. Similarly, somatostatin will moderate the hyperglycaemia in diabetic patients under treatment with insulin. Unger's concept of the parts played by the two hormones in diabetes is that insulin lack causes hyperglycaemia by preventing glucose utilization while glucagon does so by promoting gluconeogenesis. He also suggests that glucagon may be involved in the production of ketone bodies by the liver. Under experimental conditions, blood glucose level is more dependent on the concentration ratio of insulin to glucagon than on the absolute concentration of either hormone and this also argues for the view that the two hormones work together to maintain homeostasis. There is, however, no convincing evidence that an oversecretion of glucagon is ever the primary cause of idiopathic diabetes. Very occasionally, reports appear of patients with α cell tumours and symptoms of diabetes but the increased secretion of glucagon that undoubtedly occurs in idiopathic diabetes represents a compensatory response to insulin lack. It is probably still advisable, while keeping an open mind on the subject, to think of glucagon (operating in concert with small amounts of insulin) as exerting a fine control of glucose homeostasis leaving the major burden of blood sugar regulation to insulin. Indeed, and as we have already seen (p. 719) Unger himself has adduced histological evidence for such a view. It would be interesting to be able to study the actions and therapeutic potentiality of a substance that could selectively inhibit the secretion or activity of glucagon. Unfortunately no such substance exists.

OTHER SUBSTANCES THAT INFLUENCE THE AMOUNT OF GLUCOSE IN THE BLOOD

ADRENALINE
The actions of adrenaline resemble those of glucagon. In addition, both adrenaline and noradrenaline prevent insulin release by glucagon.

PITUITARY HORMONES
It is an old observation that the metabolic disturbances which follow pancreatectomy in the dog are partly alleviated if the animal is also hypophysectomised. This led to the suggestion that the pituitary gland secretes a diabetogenic hormone and that the blood sugar level is controlled by a balance of the mutually antagonist hormones, insulin and the diabetogenic factor. It is now clear that the diabetogenic action of pituitary extracts is due to their contained growth hormone since the continued administration of purified growth hormone to experimental animals produces a diabetic state. This arises partly from the action of the growth hormone itself and partly from a secondary exhaustion of the β-cells which become hyperactive in consequence of the increased blood glucose level. Over-production of growth hormone in human beings produces gigantism and acromegaly and diabetes is a common complication of these conditions. The pituitary gland also has an indirect effect on carbohydrate metabolism, since it stimulates the secretion of adrenal glucocorticoids which have themselves a diabetogenic action.

Although the actions of insulin and of pituitary growth hormones are antagonistic as far as their action on carbohydrate metabolism is concerned, insulin also has growth-promoting properties as a result of its facilitatory effect on protein and fat synthesis. It seems likely that growth hormone promotes the synthesis of protein largely by effecting insulin release.

OTHER HORMONES
Corticosteroids, aldosterone, oestrogen and the thyroid hormone all impair glucose tolerance and may aggravate the diabetic state.

DIABETES MELLITUS

Diabetes can occur as a consequence of recognizable pancreatic disease, it can accompany diseases of other organs (pituitary, adrenal cortex, thyroid, liver, kidney) or it can be precipitated by glucocorticoid therapy and, very occasionally, by other drugs particularly the thiazide diuretics. Most cases, however, are of idiopathic origin and it is usual and convenient to classify them into the so-called 'juvenile onset' and 'maturity onset' types. These two designations should not be taken too literally: 'juvenile onset' diabetes may first appear in adult life while young people occasionally develop diabetes of the 'maturity onset' type. The difference between the two types of diabetes is primarily one of degree and some diabetic patients cannot be allocated firmly to either category.

In 'juvenile onset' diabetes, a very severe deficiency of insulin typically declares itself in childhood or adolescence and causes disturbances of glucose, fat and protein metabolism that, if not corrected, lead to serious tissue wasting, an increased susceptibility to infection and degenerative diseases of the retina, nerves and arteries. These conditions constitute the real dangers to life in diabetic subjects. The incomplete oxidation of fat is reflected by the presence of intermediary metabolites in the blood (ketosis) and urine (ketonuria). The mechanism whereby a lack of insulin induces ketosis has already been mentioned (p. 721). If severe, ketosis produces coma. Nausea and vomiting, drowsiness or restlessness and giddiness occur with degrees of ketosis insufficient to cause coma. The acidic nature of the ketone bodies causes respiratory stimulation and diabetic patients who are discovered in hyperglycaemic coma sometimes appear, because of the accompanying hyperventilation ('air-hunger') to be suffering from a severe respiratory infection. The excretion of ketone bodies in the expired air, however, imparts a characteristic sweet smell to the breath which should enable the correct diagnosis to be made. Hyperglycaemic coma is treated by the intravenous injection of soluble insulin and the administration of saline solution to combat dehydration. Even in the patient whose insulin needs have been properly assessed and provided for, intercurrent infections, a missed or an incorrect dose of insulin, stress and other disturbances to the normal tenor of his life can cause unexpected alterations in the effectiveness of his treatment and he may experience sudden attacks of hypoglycaemia or hyperglycaemia even to the point of coma.

Juvenile diabetes sometimes appears with dramatic suddenness: a previously healthy young person may be found in a coma or may suddenly develop an intense and insatiable thirst and a heavy diuresis. On the other hand, the disease may arise quite insidiously with no more early warning signs than a loss of weight or the repeated occurrence of staphylococcal infections such as boils or carbuncles.

'Maturity onset' diabetes is more common in women than in men. In this condition the insulin deficiency is much less severe, the patient retaining a considerable number of functioning β cells. Ketosis does not occur and wasting is not a common feature. On the contrary, many patients are obese and there is an attractive hypothesis that attributes the diabetes to the obesity. This further emphasizes the evils of obesity and of the overindulgences that cause it. It is known that adipose tissue is less sensitive to

insulin than are other target tissues. Consequently the obese person has to secrete abnormally large amounts of insulin if her adipose tissue is to be prevented from disrupting homeostasis by refusing to take up glucose. This long term overstimulation of the β cells may lead to a partial exhaustion of their ability to produce insulin if the islet tissue was, for hereditary reasons, only marginally adequate in the first place. Thus this form of insulin deficiency is preceded by an excessive secretion of insulin and it is not uncommon for diabetes to be ushered in by episodes of hypoglycaemia. Many patients with 'maturity onset' diabetes are not obese and have never been so. Even their condition may be the result of a previously excessive stimulation of β cells consequent on their tissues being insulin resistant. The origin of this resistance is not firmly established but it is tempting to postulate the existence of a specific antagonist in blood. Alternatively the dissociation of insulin from the inactive form (bound to protein) in which it circulates may be deficient so that a large amount of protein bound hormone has to be secreted to provide adequate quantities of free insulin.

The reader will appreciate that there must be many

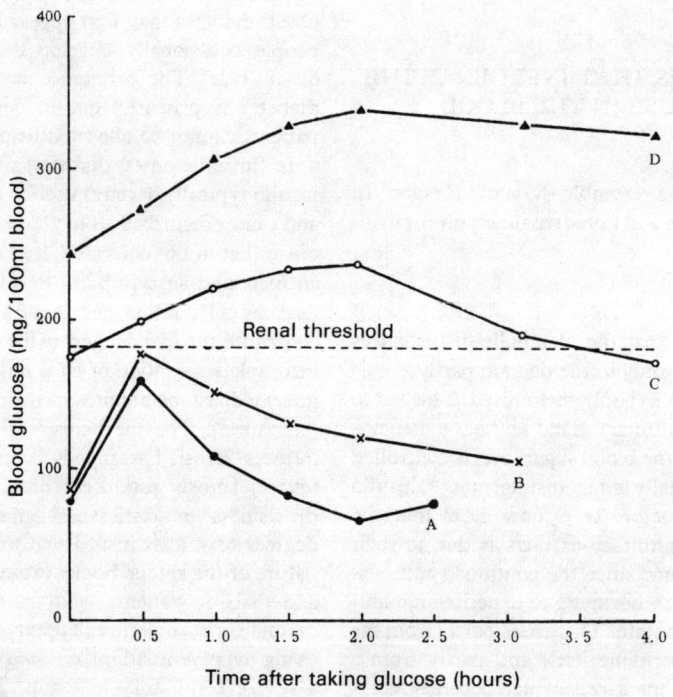

Fig. 42.2 Glucose tolerance curves.
A: normal subject. Blood glucose level has returned to fasting level within 1.5 hr
B: latent diabetes. Fasting blood glucose concentration is indistinguishable from that of the normal subject. After glucose ingestion the increase in blood glucose concentration is not excessive and glycosuria does not necessarily occur but fasting levels of blood glucose are not regained for several hours
C: Mild diabetes
D: Severe diabetes. There is glycosuria at all times and blood glucose concentrations of 300–400 mg per cent or more may be reached after glucose ingestion

potentially diabetic individuals who, by virtue of a modest food intake or other circumstances of their life style never expose their β cells to stresses that will exhaust them. Others (with so-called *latent diabetes*) display signs of impaired glucose tolerance only when they are exposed to such metabolic stresses as pregnancy or when they are given glucocorticoids. Frank diabetes may or may not appear in these patients later in life. Finally some patients must, on the basis of the usual tests, be classified as diabetic but they experience no, or only trivial symptoms of the disease.

Diabetes is a disease of affluence with a high incidence in well nourished populations. It has a strong familial tendency. Recent surveys suggest that overt or latent diabetes may be present in up to two per cent of the population.

GLUCOSE TOLERANCE CURVES

Determination of the patient's glucose tolerance curve is the most useful pathognomonic test of diabetes. The normal subject has a fasting blood glucose level of between 50 and 95 mg per 100 ml. If he now takes 50 g of glucose by mouth, the blood glucose rises rapidly for about a half to one hour but it soon begins to fall rapidly again and two to two-and-a-half hours after glucose ingestion it should be at or below the fasting level (Fig. 42.2). In the diabetic subject the fasting level and the peak glucose level are higher than in the normal subject and, most important of all, fall towards the fasting level much more slowly. The types of glucose tolerance curves exhibited by frank diabetics and those with mild and latent diabetes are also shown in Fig. 42.2: if blood glucose is higher than 110 mg per 100 ml two hours after the glucose meal, diabetes must be suspected. Although it has been usual to give glucose by mouth, its intravenous administration gives a more useful tolerance curve which is capable of detecting much milder degrees of diabetes than is possible with oral administration. The glucose tolerance test can be made even more sensitive if cortisone is given some nine and two hours before glucose. Cortisone inhibits the uptake of glucose by the liver and it thus serves to reveal deficiencies in the glucose utilization mechanisms in other tissues.

HYPOGLYCAEMIA

Low blood sugar occurs in diabetic patients if their insulin dosage is too high in relation to the amount of carbohydrate ingested. The low blood sugar calls forth a secretion of glucagon and adrenaline which promotes glycogenolysis and thus partly counters the hypoglycaemia. When the blood glucose content falls below about 70 mg per 100 ml of blood, hypoglycaemic symptoms occur. These are due partly to the glucose lack and partly to adrenaline release and they include, in moderate hypoglycaemia, a feeling of hunger, cold sweats, tremors, weakness and dizziness. Because the brain is almost entirely dependent on glucose as a source of energy, the effects of hypoglycaemia are most marked in this organ and convulsions can occur as a result

of severe hypoglycaemia. Insulin has been used in psychiatry for the purpose of causing therapeutic convulsions. Diabetic patients soon learn to recognize the onset of hypoglycaemia which can be rapidly corrected by taking glucose by mouth: diabetics usually carry tablets of glucose. Patients in hypoglycaemic coma are treated by the intravenous injection of a 5 per cent solution of glucose. Glucagon or adrenaline injections will also bring about a rapid return to consciousness, provided that liver glycogen reserves are not exhausted. Glucagon has the advantage of not producing the excessively high blood sugar levels that sometimes occur as a result of glucose administration.

It will be noted that the blood glucose concentration at which hypoglycaemic symptoms first occur falls within the range of fasting blood sugar levels in the normal subject so that mild hypoglycaemia is not an uncommon occurrence in non-diabetic individuals. For obvious reasons, it is particularly likely to occur before breakfast or after a period of exercise during which food has not been taken.

The treatment of diabetes mellitus

Patients with 'juvenile onset' diabetes need insulin. In the normal individual the secretion of insulin and its associated hormones is regulated by the blood glucose level but in the diabetic subject under insulin treatment the food intake has to be regulated in accordance with the predetermined dose of insulin. It is customary to insist on a fixed carbohydrate intake (this varies between 120 and 300 grams daily depending on the patient's age, sex and occupation) but not to restrict the intake of fat and protein though the wise physician will take the opportunity of instilling sensible dietary habits in his patient.

From what has already been said it will be clear that weight reduction is the overriding requirement in the obese patient with 'maturity onset' diabetes and this must be achieved as quickly as possible. Thereafter the patient can be prescribed a diet that is appropriate for all those with 'maturity onset' diabetes. It should be sufficient to ensure the maintenance of optimal weight but its carbohydrate content is restricted to about 150 grams daily and the patient must be urged not to take other than his daily allowances. If the diabetes fails to respond completely to dietary measures, oral hypoglycaemic agents (p. 728) are introduced into the attack, sulphonylurea derivatives being avoided in patients who are still obese. If these measures fail, insulin may be needed.

It will be appreciated that dietary regulation is the sheet anchor of treatment for all forms of diabetes whatever form of drug therapy is instituted.

Prospects for the future include the possibility of transplanting islet tissue.

INSULIN THERAPY

Insulin is destroyed in the gastrointestinal tract and it is therefore administered by subcutaneous injection, an operation that has to be performed by the patient himself. Even with a rigidly-controlled diet and the regular administration of the appropriate dose of insulin, his blood sugar may occasionally exhibit sharp changes and he has to be trained to recognize the signs of incipient hypo- or hyperglycaemia and the methods of dealing with these disturbances. Simple urine tests using sugar indicator papers enable him to check for himself that his insulin intake is adequate but it is clear that a good deal of intelligent cooperation is required on the part of the patient if his treatment is to be successful.

A number of different insulin preparations are available. They differ principally in the speed of onset and the duration of their hypoglycaemic action (Fig. 42.3).

Soluble insulin is an aqueous solution of crystalline insulin. It is the most rapidly acting form of the drug but it also has the shortest duration of effect. Its action begins in an hour or less after injection, its peak effect is reached in three or four hours and its total duration of action is about six hours. It is used for the stabilization of new cases, to treat patients who need large daily doses of insulin, for the rapid control of severe cases and for the treatment of hyperglycaemic coma.

Soluble insulin must be injected at least twice daily.

This is a disadvantage and, where possible, the longer acting preparations are now used. However, soluble insulin sometimes provides the only satisfactory means of controlling severe diabetes particularly in the early phases of treatment. A mixture of soluble insulin and a preparation with a more prolonged action taken twice daily before meals provides a steady background concentration of insulin with mealtime peaks that is very useful for patients ('brittle' diabetics) whose blood sugar concentration would fluctuate widely during the day if they received only morning and evening injections of soluble insulin.

Protamine zinc insulin is a suspension of an insulin-protamine complex containing a trace of zinc. It has a prolonged action and the effects of one dose may persist for up to 48 hours. Its hypoglycaemic effect is correspondingly slow to appear, taking from 6 to 12 hours. The slow onset of action and prolonged effect have certain disadvantages. It is not possible to give protamine zinc insulin just before a meal to prevent hyperglycaemia and the very prolonged action may cause hypoglycaemic reactions during the night or early hours of the morning. It is difficult to obtain a daily dose of protamine zinc insulin which will control the blood sugar level during the day without causing hypoglycaemia at night. Protamine zinc

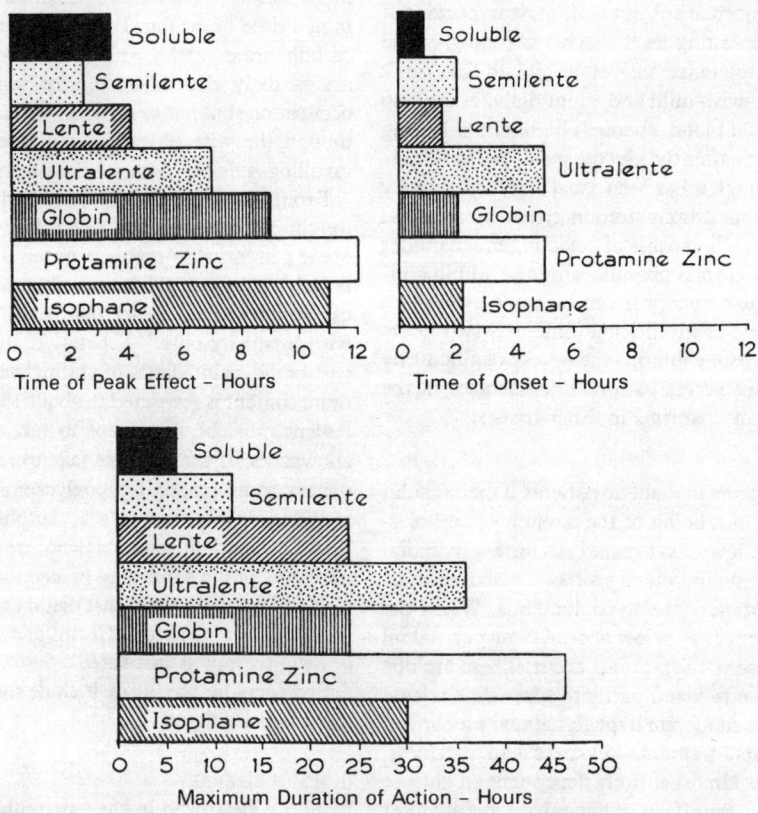

Fig. 42.3 The effects on the blood sugar level of different preparations of insulin

insulin was the first of the longer-acting insulins to be developed and the difficulties caused by its prolonged actions were often overcome by means of a combined therapy with soluble insulin. With the advent of the newer preparations described below, there is less need for this form of insulin.

Globin zinc insulin is a solution of an insulin-globin complex containing a trace of zinc. Unlike protamine zinc insulin, it acts fairly rapidly, being effective about two hours after injection. It shows a peak effect in from 6 to 12 hours and has a duration of effect which does not exceed 24 hours. It is therefore intermediate in effect between soluble insulin and protamine zinc insulin. It does not usually cause hypoglycaemia during the night but it may do so during the late afternoon. It is used mainly for those mild cases of diabetes mellitus which can be successfully controlled by one dose a day.

Isophane insulin is a modified protamine zinc insulin containing crystalline insulin, protamine and zinc in a buffered solution. The time relations of its action are similar to those of globin zinc insulin.

Insulin zinc suspensions also have a prolonged action. They consist of suspensions of zinc insulin in an acetate buffer of pH 7.2 to 7.5. The size of the particles or crystals in suspension determines the rate of solution and hence the duration of action. A suspension of the crystalline form of zinc insulin *(insulin ultralente)* has the longest action; a suspension of amorphous insulin *(insulin semilente)* has the shortest duration of action, while mixtures of the two forms *(insulin lente)* produce preparations with actions of intermediate length. Insulins lente and semilente, notwithstanding their prolonged action, begin to act within one to four hours of administration.

Since these preparations are buffered at the isoelectric point of insulin, they cannot be mixed with other types of insulin, though they can be mixed with one another. Insulin zinc suspensions are used for the same purpose as globin and isophane insulins.

Side effects of insulin administration
Some diabetic patients are tempted to make all their injections into one or two readily accessible sites and in so doing run the risk of developing tumours at the injection sites. The tumours are unsightly, they may be so large that they have to be excised and they hinder the absorption of insulin. An opposite effect is the production of a deep hollow in the region of the injection. It is caused by atrophy of the subcutaneous fat and since it can appear after a single injection it cannot be prevented by frequent changes of injection sites. Indeed, repeated injections in the affected area sometimes result in a reversal of the change, fatty tissue appearing in the areas of atrophy so that the affected limb regains a normal appearance. Protamine zinc insulin was prone to cause reactions (swelling, tenderness and pain) at the site of the injection and allergic

reactions to all forms of insulin are sometimes seen. Further attacks can be prevented by using a more highly purified preparation, changing the species of insulin or, as a last resort, by desensitization. Some elderly patients who have been taking insulin for many years become very resistant to insulin and need to inject perhaps hundreds of units of insulin daily to control their blood sugar levels. This resistance has an immunological basis and, like the allergic reactions referred to, it has been seen in an extreme form only very infrequently since the advent of highly purified insulins. These newer preparations are of porcine origin (in the past, bovine insulin was more common) and proprietary porcine preparations include Nuso and Actrapid (soluble insulins), Semitard (equivalent to a *semilente* preparation), Monotard *(lente)* and Rapitard, a biphasic preparation. It is a matter of some importance to realize that a hypoglycaemic crisis can be precipitated by a change from bovine to porcine insulin (or vice versa) since the new insulin when it is first injected will meet with no antibody or other acquired resistance to its action.

The assay and standardization of insulin
Two methods are available for the biological standardization of insulin. One relies on the fact that insulin causes convulsions in mice. It is suitable for the standardization of rapidly acting insulin. In the other method (recommended for the assay of protamine zinc insulin) the effect of insulin on the blood sugar of the rabbit is measured.

Insulin in plasma can now be determined in several ways and the application of these methods has greatly advanced our knowledge of diabetes and insulin action.

In one method of assay, the uptake of glucose by isolated rat diaphragm is measured in the presence of a sample of the plasma. Glucose uptake is stimulated by insulin. In a variant of this method the plasma under test is administered, by intraperitoneal injection, to the living rat. The animal is killed two and a half hours later and the glycogen content of its diaphragm is measured. In another method, the fat pad of the rat epididymis is incubated with 14-C labelled glucose. Insulin-containing plasma added to this system stimulates glucose metabolism and hence the output of labelled carbon dioxide. A specific and relatively simple *in vitro* method of insulin assay is a radioimmunological one based on the fact that human insulin can displace beef insulin from its combination with specific antibody. The beef insulin is labelled with 131-iodine and its displacement from the antigen-antibody complex can therefore be easily followed. This method permits the estimation of endogenous insulin in the presence of beef insulin in the plasma of diabetic patients being treated with the latter compound. It is also more specific than the other methods which are affected by the presence of insulin antagonists. If the apparent insulin content of a sample of diabetic plasma is assayed by the radio-immunological method and by the rat diaphragm method, it is possible to determine whether the insulin deficiency is due to a true lack of the hormone or to the presence of antagonists.

ORAL HYPOGLYCAEMIC AGENTS

The oral hypoglycaemic agents fall into two principal groups, the sulphonylureas and the biguanides.

The sulphonylureas

In 1942, Jambon was using the isoproyplthiadiazole derivative of para-aminobenzene sulphonamide (2254RP) for the treatment of typhoid fever and he noticed that some of his patients developed hypoglycaemia. Further work, by Loubatières, showed that 2254RP caused a progressive lowering of the blood sugar level in dogs. The hypoglycaemic action of the drug was only evident in the presence of functioning islet tissue and Loubatières concluded that 2254RP owed its effect to a stimulant action on the production and secretion of insulin. In 1955 Franke and Fuchs found that carbutamide, another sulphonamide drug then used clinically, produced hypoglycaemia. These observations led to the introduction of the sulphonylureas as hypoglycaemic agents. They are effective only in the presence of functional islet tissue and their principal action is to stimulate insulin secretion although glibenclamide, the newest sulphonylurea, appears to stimulate the synthesis as well as the release of insulin.

The sulphonylureas may also reduce the output of glucose from the liver by a mechanism (such as phosphorylase inhibition) independent of that which promotes insulin release. They do not potentiate the action of injected insulin so that they are only of value in patients who retain some islet function.

The names, formulae and recommended dose schedules of the sulphonylureas that have found clinical application are included in Table 42.1. Apart from the consequences of differences in their durations of action, they all have essentially the same properties and they are discussed as a group in the succeeding paragraphs.

Tolbutamide has a short half-life because it is rapidly metabolized by carboxylation of its methyl group. The other sulphonylureas are broken down more slowly into metabolites that retain some hypoglycaemic activity. This prolongation of action, which results in the drugs' having to be taken only once or twice daily, is not an entirely unmixed blessing because any unexpected response to their administration might also be correspondingly prolonged. In particular, the sulphonylureas occasionally bring about a profound and intractable hypoglycaemia which will obviously be the more dangerous the longer it lasts. Deaths from hypoglycaemia have been reported among patients taking chlorpropamide, a single dose of which will continue to promote the liberation of insulin during the night and at other times when none is needed.

The hypoglycaemic action of the sulphonylureas is potentiated by monoamine oxidase inhibitors, some antiinflammatory drugs such as aspirin and phenylbutazone and (not surprisingly, in view of their origin) some long acting sulphonamides.

Because the sulphonylureas and their metabolites are excreted in the urine they should be prescribed only with great circumspection for patients in renal failure. This caution applies particularly to the long acting compounds. Obese patients find it difficult to lose weight when they are taking a sulphonylurea alone and they should be prescribed a biguanide instead. It is, however, permissible to supplement the biguanide with small amounts of a sulphonylurea.

Apart from the possibility of their causing a severe hypoglycaemia if they are given in injudicious doses (and the disputed danger of inducing cardiovascular disease, to which reference is made on p. 730) the sulphonylureas are safe drugs, although they may produce a number of inconvenient side effects. They have a disulphiram-like action (p. 90) and patients sometimes experience nausea and uncomfortable flushes when they take alcoholic drinks during sulphonylurea treatment. This embarrassing side effect occurs in up to 20 per cent of those who take chlorpropamide but it is seen much less frequently with the other members of the group. Other minor side effects—skin rashes, gastrointestinal upsets, fatigue and a mild toxic hepatitis with jaundice—have been reported but they are not of common occurrence, they rarely incommode the patient and they disappear when the drug is withdrawn. Carbutamide can cause more serious liver damage and agranulocytosis but it is no longer used clinically.

The blood sugar response to an intravenous injection of tolbutamide (one gram) is employed as a diagnostic test for tumours of the pancreatic islet cells. The tumour cells manufacture insulin which is liberated by the tolbutamide to produce a much more profound hypoglycaemia than would occur if only the normal amount of islet tissue were available to respond to the tolbutamide challenge.

Chlorpropamide has recently been successfully applied to the treatment of diabetes insipidus. This development is discussed on p. 637.

The biguanides

Nearly 50 years ago, two guanidine derivatives (decamethylene diguanidine and dodecamethylene diguanidine) were found to have a hypoglycaemic action in diabetic patients. The drugs were, however, highly toxic and a number of fatalities led to their withdrawal from clinical use. The renewed upsurge of interest in oral hypoglycaemic agents revived interest in guanidine derivatives and led, in 1957, to the discovery of phenformin, a non-toxic biguanide. Another hypoglycaemic biguanide is metformin. Diguanides are compounds in which two guanidine molecules

Table 42.1 Oral hypoglycaemic agents

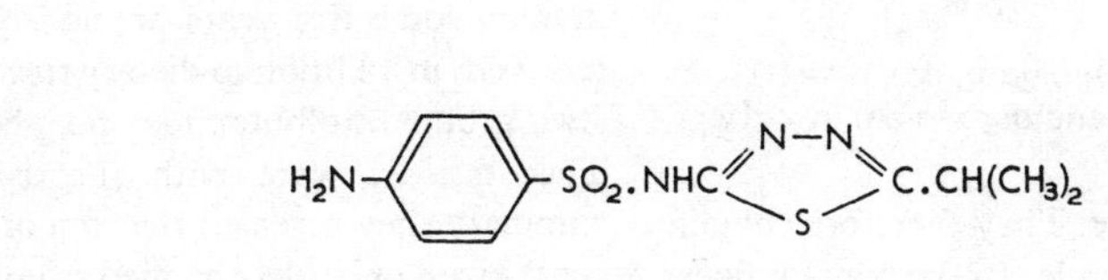

$$H_2N-\langle\text{benzene ring}\rangle-SO_2.NHC\overset{N-N}{\underset{S}{\diagdown}}C.CH(CH_3)_2$$

2254 RP

(paraaminobenzene sulphonamido isopropylthiadiozole)

The sulphonylureas

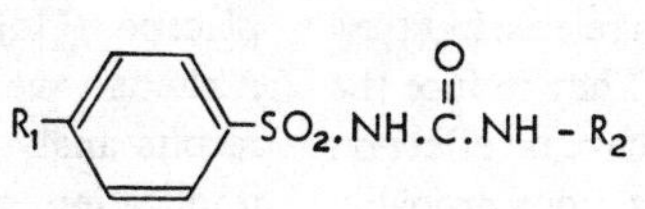

$$R_1-\langle\text{benzene ring}\rangle-SO_2.NH.\overset{O}{\overset{\|}{C}}.NH-R_2$$

Approved name	Proprietary name(s)	R_1	R_2	Approximate daily dose schedule
Tolbutamide	Artosin, Rastinon, Orinase, Pramidex	CH_3	$(CH_2)_3CH_2$	0.5–3 grams in 3 doses
Carbutamide	—	NH_2	$(CH_2)_3CH_3$	not used
Chlorpropamide	Diabinese, Melitase	Cl	$(CH_2)_2CH_3$	100–400 mg
Acetohexamide	Dimelor	CH_3CO	C_6H_{11}	0.5–1.5 grams
Tolazamide	Tolanase	CH_3	$-N\overset{(CH_2)_2CH_2}{\underset{(CH_2)_2CH_2}{\diagdown}}$	0.2–1 gram, in one or two doses daily
Glibenclamide	Daonil, Euglucon	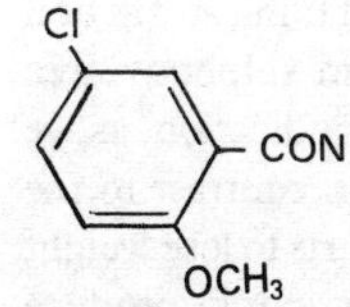 (chlorophenyl with CONH(CH₂)₂ and OCH₃)	C_6H_{11}	15–20 mg in one or two doses
Glymidine	Gondafon, Redul	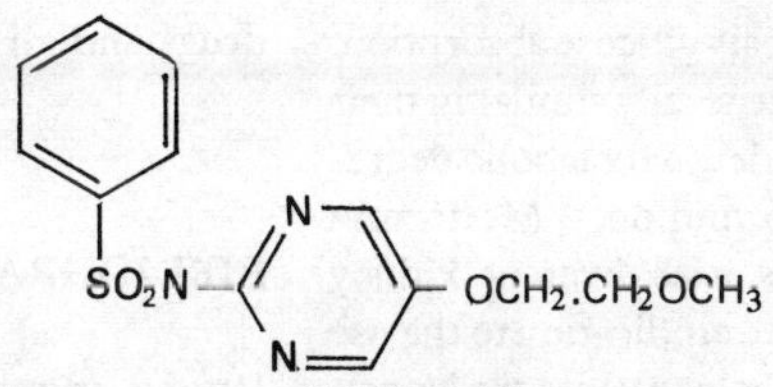 \multicolumn full formula		2 grams in one or two doses

Glymidine (full formula):

$$\langle\text{benzene}\rangle-SO_2N-\overset{N}{\underset{N}{\langle\text{pyrimidine}\rangle}}-OCH_2.CH_2OCH_3$$

(full formula)

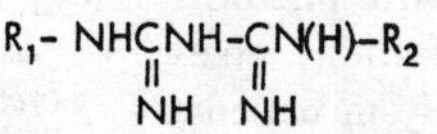

The biguanides

$$R_1-\underset{NH}{\overset{\|}{N}HC}NH-\underset{NH}{\overset{\|}{C}N}(H)-R_2$$

Approved name	Proprietary name(s)	R_1	R_2	Approximate daily dose schedule
Metformin	Glucophage, Metiguanide	H	$(CH_3)_2$	1.5–3 grams in 3 doses
Phenformin	Dibotin, Dipar, Meltrol	H	$(CH_2)_2\langle\text{phenyl}\rangle$ 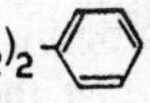	50–150 mg in 4 doses
Proguanil	Paludrine	$(CH_3)_2CH$	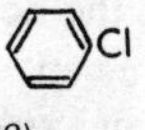 $\langle\text{phenyl}\rangle Cl$	

(Proguanil is an antimalarial drug; see p. 868)

$$H_2N-C-NH\ (CH_2)_n\ NH-C-NH_2$$
$$\|\qquad\qquad\qquad\qquad\|$$
$$NH\qquad\qquad\qquad\quad NH$$

In Synthalin A (decamethylene diguanide), n = 10
In Synthalin B (dodecamethylene diguanide), n = 12

are linked by a methylene bridge. They therefore contain six nitrogen atoms in their molecule. In the biguanidines, two guanidine derivatives are joined with the elimination of a molecule of ammonia and these compounds contain only five nitrogen atoms per molecule.

The biguanides do not stimulate insulin release but they are ineffective in the absence of insulin. They reduce the blood sugar level in diabetic subjects but have no effect on that of normal individuals. A number of actions probably contribute to the drugs' overall hypoglycaemic activity. These include a potentiation of the action of insulin on glucose transfer into the cell, inhibition of glucose absorption from the gut and inhibition of glucose formation by the liver.

Although they are not as dangerous as the diguanides, the biguanides produce more severe side-effects (gastrointestinal upsets, anorexia, nausea, vomiting and fatigue) than the sulphonylureas and they are not used in patients who respond to the sulphonylureas. They can, however, be used in diabetic patients of all kinds to reduce their insulin requirement, to augment the action of sulphonylureas in patients whose response to these drugs is failing and as oral hypoglycaemic agents in those for whom sulphonylurea treatment is contraindicated. One contraindication, as we have seen, is obesity. The biguanides, in contrast to the sulphonylureas, support the patient's efforts to lose weight largely because of the anorexia they commonly produce but also, perhaps, because they impair glucose absorption.

Phenformin and metformin are generally similar in their actions but metformin does not undergo metabolic degradation in the body whereas phenformin does. Metformin can therefore be given to patients with liver or kidney diseases that would constitute a contraindication to the use of phenformin. Metformin is less likely to cause the ketosis that is sometimes seen in patients treated with phenformin. Phenformin (but not, apparently, metformin) sometimes induces a lactic acidaemia particularly in patients with cardiac or renal disease. There is bicarbonate deficiency, acidosis and dehydration. Prolonged use of either biguanide may result in malabsorption of vitamin B_{12}.

In addition to the preparations named in Table 42.1 phenformin is available as Dibotin, a timed-release preparation. It should be added that the doses quoted in the table represent maximum requirements. Smaller amounts of drug will be needed if insulin or a sulphonylurea is also being taken.

Oral hypoglycaemic agents and cardiovascular disease
In 1970, an American group published the results of a prospective study (p. 111) in which more than a thousand then newly diagnosed diabetic patients had been randomly divided some five years previously into five groups who received, in addition to dietary treatment, placebo, insulin (two groups), tolbutamide and phenformin respectively. The statistics were both surprising and alarming: in summary they revealed that ten of the patients (14.9 per cent) given only placebo died from cardiovascular disease but in the tolbutamide and phenformin groups the figures were 26 (12.7 per cent) and 27 (13.2 per cent) respectively. The patients given insulin fared no worse than those given placebo (University Group Diabetes Program, 1970). Although the investigation was properly designed and the results analysed by impeccable statistical techniques the implication of the findings have not been universally accepted, particularly in Britain and Europe. In the years since 1970, other groups have produced their own more or less impressive reports which have done nothing but accentuate the differences between those who support and those who oppose the use of oral hypoglycaemic agents. To quote a commentary that is distinguished by a shrewd assessment of what exactly the published statistics do and do not tell us, 'the combatants are now obscured by increasingly heavy clouds of clinical, statistical and philosophical smoke' (Editorial, 1975). It seems likely that, within the lifetime of this book, knowledge will accumulate to an extent that will permit the physician to decide, on a weightier basis than that of preferring the look of one set of statistics to another, whether or not he should make use of the oral hypoglycaemic agents. In the meantime all that can be said is that the drugs should not be used unless there seems to be no other way of controlling the patient's condition. But that advice, of course, applies equally to all drugs and all conditions.

BIBLIOGRAPHY

Books, monographs and reviews

Best, C. H. (1959). Metabolic problems involving the pancreas, choline, insulin and glucagon. In *Significant Trends in Medical Research*, pp. 164-195. Ciba Foundation Symposium, ed. Wolstenholme, G. E. W., O'Connor, Cecilia M. and O'Connor, Maeve. London: Churchill.

Butterfield, W. J. H. and Mahler, R. F. (1962). Hypoglycaemic agents and diabetes mellitus. In *Recent Advances in Pharmacology*, pp. 179-213, ed. Robson, J. M. and Stacey, R. S. London: Churchill.

Karam, J. H., Matin, S. B. and Forsham, P. H. (1975) Antidiabetic drugs after the University Group Diabetes Program (UGDP). *A. Rev. pharmac.* **15**, 351-366

Krahl M. E. (1961). *The Action of Insulin on Cells*. New York: Academic Press.

Lefebvre, P. J. and Unger, R. H. (eds) (1972). *Glucagon*. Oxford: Pergamon

Marble, A. and Cahill, G. F. (1962). *The Chemistry and Chemotherapy of Diabetes Mellitus*. Springfield, Ill.: Thomas.

Oakley, W. G., Pyke, D. A. and Taylor K. W. (1975) *Diabetes and its Management*. 2nd Edn Oxford: Blackwell.

Rubenstein, A. H. and Steiner, D. F. (1971). Proinsulin. *A. Rev. med.*, **22**, 1-18.

Slater, J. D. H. (1961). Oral hypoglycaemic drugs. *Prog. med. Chem.*, **1**, 187-219.

Young, F. G., Broom, W. A. and Wolff, F. W. (1960). *The Mechanism of Action of Insulin*. Oxford: Blackwell.

See also the general texts listed on p. 718.

Original papers

Devrim, S. and Recant, Lillian (1966). Effect of glucagon on insulin release *in vitro*. *Lancet*, **2**, 1227-1228.

Dormandy, T. L. (1966). The mechanism of insulin action. The effect of insulin on the allosteric properties of intracellular haemoglobin. *J. Physiol.* **183**, 378-406.

Dormandy, T. L. and Zarday, Z. (1965). The mechanism of insulin action. The immediate electrochemical effects of insulin on red cell systems. *J. Physiol.*, **180**, 684-707.

Editorial (1975). Somatostatin and diabetes. *Lancet* **1**, 1323-1324.

Hunton, R. B., Wells, M. V. and Skipper, E. W. (1965). Hypothyroidism in diabetes treated with sulphonylurea. *Lancet*, **2**, 449-451.

Kimball, C. P. and Murlin, J. R. (1923). Aqueous extracts of pancreas-III. Some precipitation reactions of insulin. *J. biol. Chem.*, **58**, 337-346.

Orci, L. and Unger, R. H. (1975). Functional subdivision of islets of Langerhans and possible role of D cells. *Lancet* **2**, 1243-1244.

Sanger, F. (1960). Chemistry of insulin. *Br. med. Bull.*, **16**, 183-188.

Sterzi, T. E., Porter, K. A. and Putnam, C. W. (1975). Intraportal insulin protects from the liver injury of portacaval shunt in dogs. *Lancet* **2**, 1241-1242.

Unger, R. H. and Orci, L. (1975). The essential role of glucagon in the pathogenesis of diabetes mellitus. *Lancet* **1**, 14-16.

University Group Diabetes Program (1970). A study of the effects of hypoglycaemic agents on vascular complications in patients with adult-onset diabetes. *Diabetes*, **19**, Suppl. 2, 747-772.

43. The sex hormones

The sex hormones are divided into androgens, oestrogens and progestogens. All the naturally occurring hormones and most of the synthetic ones are steroids and are simple derivatives of the saturated tetracyclic hydrocarbon, cyclopentanoperhydrophenanthrene (Fig. 43.1).

ANDROGENS

The androgens or male sex hormones are responsible for the normal development, function and maintenance of the male sex organs and sexual characteristics. They also control spermatogenesis. Androgens are formed and secreted by the testes, the suprarenal cortex and the ovaries. Normally the amounts produced by the last named organs are small but some forms of ovarian tumour secrete large amounts of androgens and this may cause the development of male characteristics in women (virilism). Tumours or pathological overactivity of the adrenal cortex can also produce virilism but the secretions of the normal adrenal cortex are insufficient to prevent the complete cessation of sexual function in the castrated male animal. Given to immature male animals, the androgens cause premature development of the accessory sex organs and male characteristics and they will cause the appearance of these characteristics in males in whom normal sexual development has not occurred.

Androgens cause retention of water, nitrogen and a number of important inorganic substances (potassium, sodium, calcium, chloride, sulphate and phosphorus). They also increase protein metabolism and thus promote the laying down of new tissues. This *anabolic* effect of the androgens explains the spectacular growth which occurs in the male at puberty. The androgens also affect a number of enzyme systems, including kidney D-amino acid oxidase, alkaline and acid phosphatases, transaminases and arginase.

For the purpose of giving them systematic chemical names, the androgens are regarded as androstane derivatives. In the steroid compounds generally, the atom or groups on the carbon atoms may project above or below the plane of the steroid nucleus. In the former case, the bond is drawn as a solid line and the configuration is designated β. In the α configuration the bond projects below the plane of the nucleus and it is drawn as a dotted line. Among the naturally occurring steroids, the valencies

on C5 and C14 may take either the α or the β configuration though that on C14 is usually α. Those on the other carbon atoms always take the same form: α on C9 and β on C8 C10, C13 and C17. Among synthetic compounds variations from this arrangement are, of course, met with. In drawing the formulae of the steroids a valency bond is often represented with no radical or group attached to it. When this is done it can be assumed that a methyl ($-CH_3$) group is attached. The formula of the methyl group is omitted purely for convenience in drawing.

Testosterone is the natural male sex hormone. In the testis it is synthesized, under the influence of the luteinizing hormone (p. 771), by the interstitial (Leydig) cells. Its immediate precursor is androstenedione (Fig. 43.1) which is itself derived from cholesterol and pregnenolone by the same routes as those used in the adrenal cortex. These are depicted in Figure 44.3 (p. 756). Testosterone exerts its physiological activity through dihydrotestosterone (Fig. 43.2). Conversion of the inactive parent substance to the active metabolite takes place predominantly in the responding tissues but some transformation occurs in the blood stream en route to the target. Both compounds are transported to a large extent in the form of loose combinations with a specific binding globulin.

It will be appreciated by reference to its formula (Fig. 43.1) that the stereochemistry of the testosterone molecule at C5 does not need to be considered but its metabolic degradation involves reduction of the double bond and the principal product of metabolism occurs in both stereochemical forms (Fig. 43.1). Androsterone, which has the α configuration, retains androgenic activity; the β form (etiocholanolone) is physiologically inactive. Metabolism of testosterone also involves conversion of the hydroxyl group on C17 to a keto group. Androsterone and etiocholanolone are therefore components of the 17-oxosteroid fraction of the urinary metabolites although the total contribution they make is small, most of the urinary 17-oxosteroids being of adrenal origin (Chap. 44). For this reason, castration produces very little change in 17-oxosteroid excretion. Oxosteroids are sometimes known as ketosteroids.

Testosterone is converted into androstenedione before it is metabolized to androsterone and its stereoisomer. Thus androstenedione is both a precursor and a metabolite of testosterone.

If the testes are incapable of secreting testosterone the

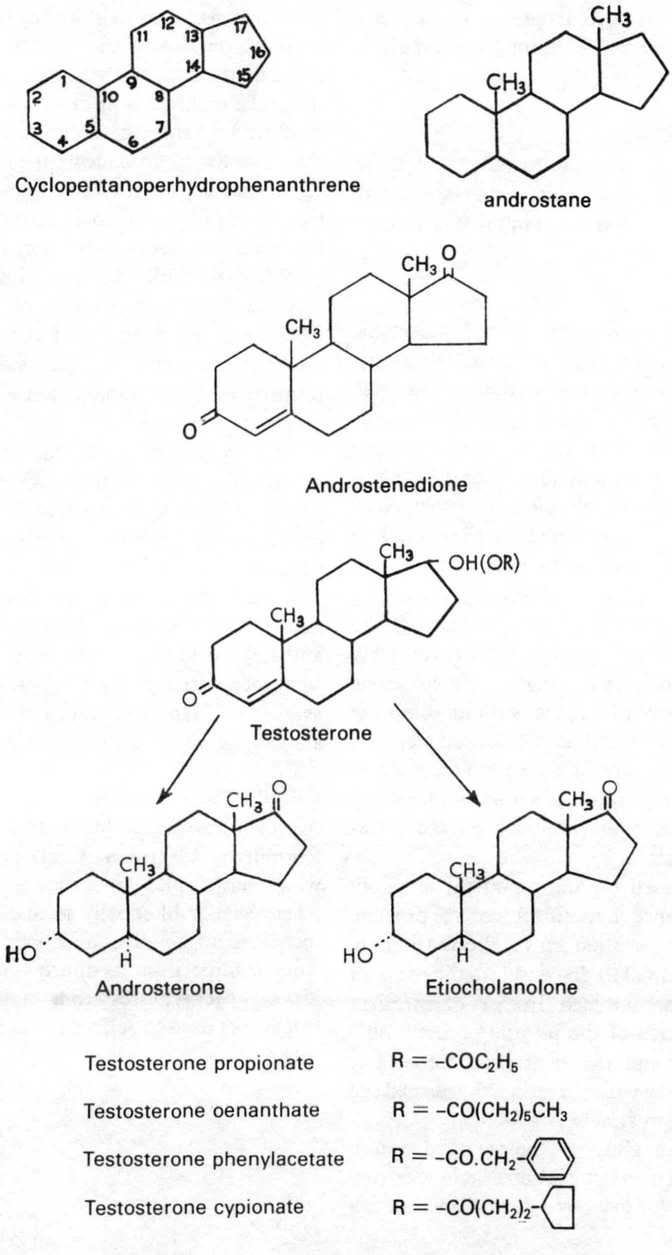

Fig. 43.1 Testosterone and related steroids

resulting condition is *eunuchism*. Partial deficiency causes *hypogonadism*. In both conditions the normal anatomical, sexual and psychological changes of puberty do not occur. The external genitalia retain their infantile appearance, the voice remains high pitched because the larynx fails to develop, muscle development is arrested and the body does not easily tan on exposure to sunlight. Fat may accumulate in the buttocks, hips and breast. The beard does not appear, hair does not grow in the axillae and the pubic hair, if it develops at all, takes on the female distribution, its upper boundary being concave. Union of the epiphyses which normally stops further growth in height is delayed, but eunuchs are not necessarily abnormally tall. Needless to say, sexual desire (*libido*) is not experienced and spermatozoa do not develop.

Castration may be needed for therapeutic reasons or testosterone secretion may fail after puberty. In these circumstances the irreversible changes which occurred at puberty (deepening of the voice, enlargement of the penis, etc.) are not affected but libido will disappear and spermatogenesis will cease.

Clinical use of the androgens

Androgens are used for their androgenic activity in replacement therapy, as anabolic agents to increase growth and the laying down of new tissues and in the treatment of some forms of cancer.

TESTOSTERONE

Replacement therapy. Testosterone is employed in the treatment of eunuchism and hypogonadism and to restore or maintain secondary sexual characteristics in those who have undergone surgical castration. It is usually given as the propionate or the oenanthate. All the esters are more active than testosterone itself and the oenanthate has a more prolonged action than the propionate. The cypionate, like the oenanthate, is long-acting: the phenylacetate has a similar duration of action to the propionate.

Testosterone propionate in oil is given by intramuscular injection in twice weekly doses of 25 to 50 mg. If the oenanthate is used, it need be given only at two-weekly intervals but the dose required is higher. Testosterone itself (Testoral) can be given in aqueous solution but the esters in oil are to be preferred. Once the desired response has been obtained, smaller amounts are used for maintenance therapy and for this purpose subcutaneous implants are utilized. New implants are required no more frequently than twice a year.

Testosterone is also used for the treatment of faulty spermatogenesis, impotence, hypertrophy of the prostate and cryptorchism. In the last named condition (literally 'hidden testes') the testes fail to descend into the scrotum and spermatogenesis is not initiated. In cases of dwarfism caused by lack of secretion of the pituitary growth hormone, thyroid hormone and a corticosteroid are used to promote growth. When the patient reaches the normal age of puberty, testosterone treatment is added.

Testosterone has been given to maintain or restore sexual function in ageing men but it is not clear how far any observed effect is really due to a physiological and not to a placebo response.

Application of anabolic activity It has already been pointed out that the androgens promote the laying down of tissue and attempts have been made to turn this anabolic property to good account by administering testosterone or related compounds to patients convalescing from wasting diseases. The anabolic activity of the androgens is associated with calcium retention and this is the rationale of the use of testosterone in the treatment of osteoporosis—a condition of rarefaction of bone seen particularly in the elderly. In the treatment of fractures in old people, the androgens ought to be doubly useful for they should accelerate the regeneration of the soft tissues by their general anabolic effect as well as aiding union of the broken bone by promoting the retention of calcium. Notwithstanding the apparently sound theoretical justification for using the androgens in this way, the therapeutic benefits conferred by their anabolic activity seem to be no more than marginal. An exception to this generalization may sometimes be provided when testosterone is used for the treatment of aplastic anaemia particularly in children. In this condition, testosterone may be successful when other methods fail (Fullerton and Girdwood, 1966).

Some of the side effects of corticosteroid therapy arise from the drugs' catabolic effect and there is some evidence that the incidence of these side effects is reduced if testosterone or an anabolic steroid (p. 735) is given with the corticosteroid.

Menstrual disorders. In the past, dysmenorrhoea, premenstrual tension, menopausal tension and some types of uterine bleeding were treated with testosterone. The oestrogens and progestogens are now preferred for this purpose.

Testosterone rejoices in a large number of proprietary names including, among others, Delatestryl (for the oenanthate), Andronate (the cypionate), Testoviron and Virormone (the propionate) while testosterone itself is available as Neo-Hombreol and Oreton. Testoral Sublings are sublingual tablets of testosterone.

METHYLTESTOSTERONE

Methyltestosterone (cavandrol-M, Neo-Hombreol-M, Perandren, Virormone-Oral) is a synthetic compound which has similar properties to testosterone. It is active when taken sublingually so that it can be used when it is inconvenient to give injections or to use implants. A suitable initial dose in eunuchism or hypogonadism is 75 to 150 mg. Methyltestosterone in daily doses of 25-35 mg is sometimes used to relieve the itching of obstructive jaundice.

Methyltestosterone

FLUOXYMESTERONE

As can be seen, (Fig. 43.2) fluoxymesterone (Halotestin, Oratestin, Ultandren) is the 9α-fluoro, 11β-hydroxy derivative of methyltestosterone. It is a much more potent agent than methyltestosterone itself. It has been used to replace the natural hormone after castration and in women it has been applied to the treatment of menstrual disorders and of inoperable carcinoma of the breast. Although fluoxy-

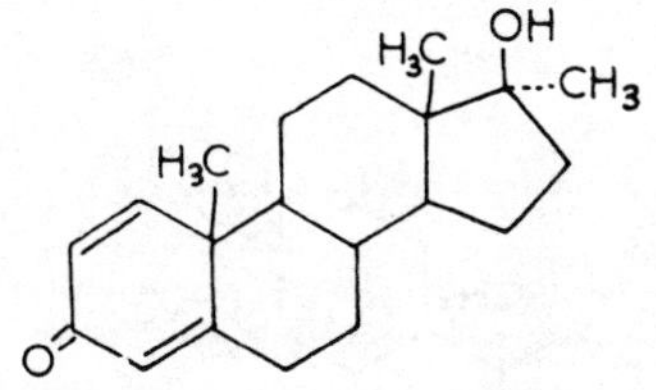

Methandienone (methandrosteno-
lone; Dianabol)
    Dose: 10-25 mg daily by mouth.

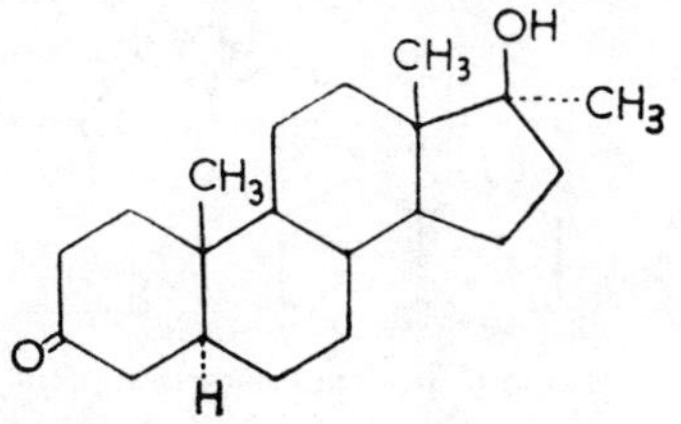

Mestanolone (methylandrostano
lone)

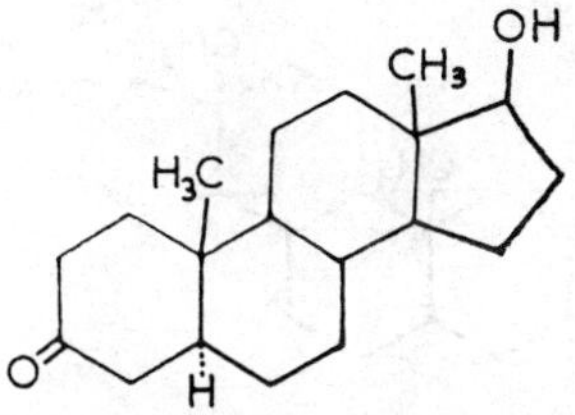

Stanolone (androstanolone, dihydrotestosterone, Anabolex
Dose: 150-75 mg daily,
sublingually

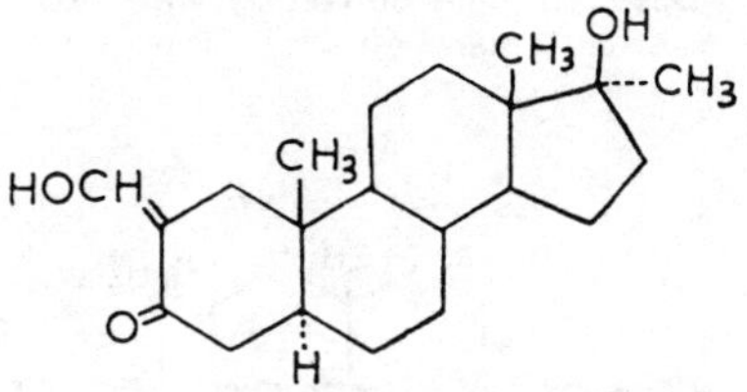

Oxymetholone (Anapolon Anadrol)
    Dose: 5-15 mg daily, by mouth.

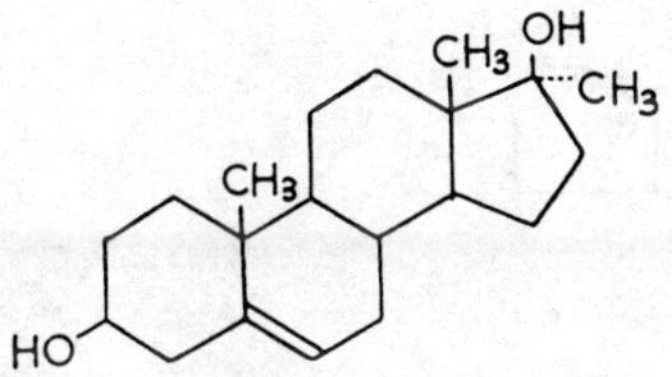

Methylandrostenediol (methandriol,
Stenediol)
Dose: 50-150 mg daily, by mouth

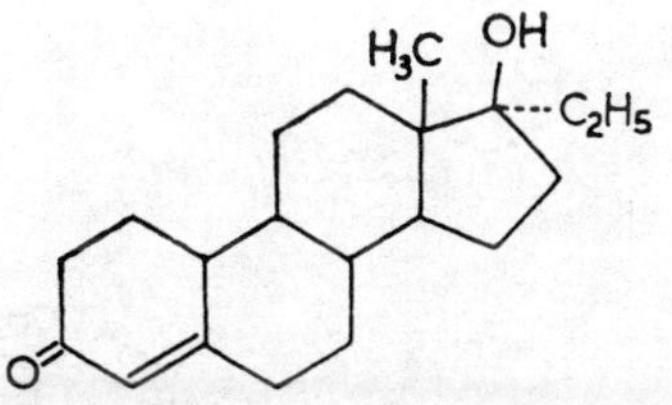

Norethandrolone
(17α-ethyl-19-nortestosterone; Nilevar)
Dose: 25-30 mg daily by mouth

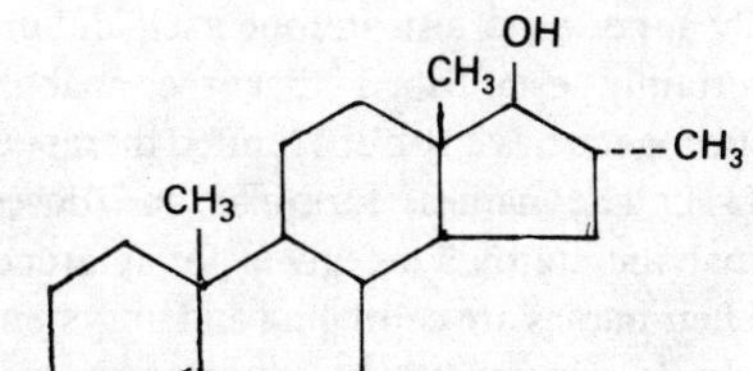

Oxymesterone (Oranabol)
Dose: 10-40 mg daily by mouth

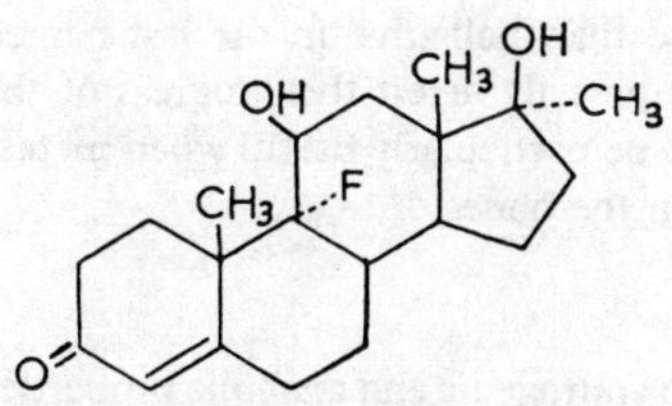

Fluoxymesterone (Ultandren)
Dose 2-20 mg daily by mouth

Fig. 43.2 Some anabolic steroids

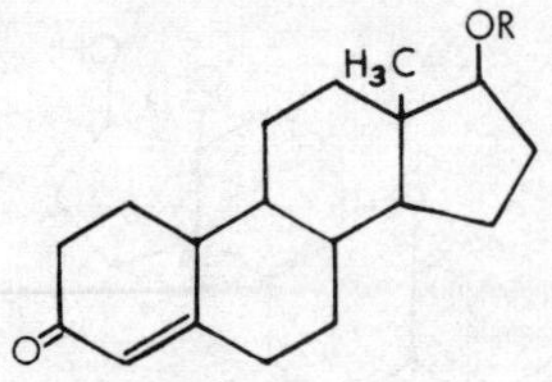

Nandrolone (19-nortestosterone), R = H

Nandrolone phenylpropionate (Durabolin)

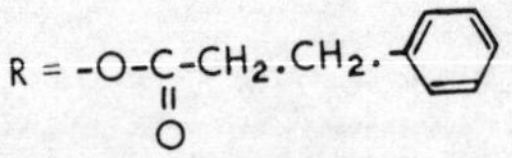

$$R = -O-\overset{\displaystyle O}{\underset{\displaystyle \|}{C}}-CH_2 \cdot CH_2 \cdot \bigcirc$$

Dose: 25 mg once weekly, intramuscular.

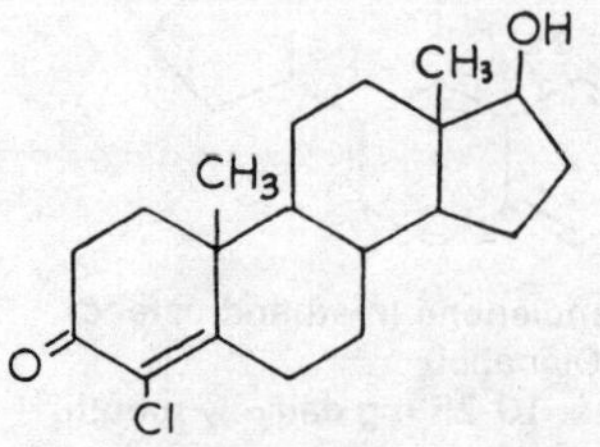

4-Chlorotestosterone

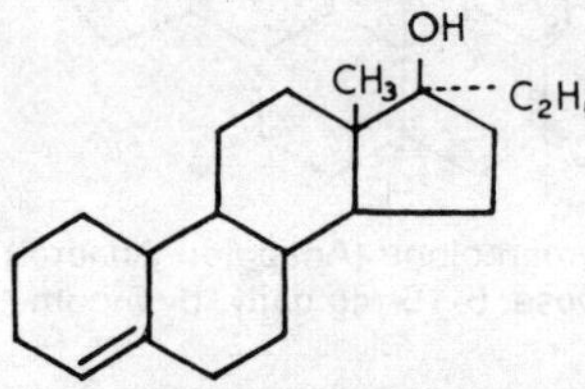

Ethyloestrenol (Orabolin)
Dose: 3 mg daily, by mouth.

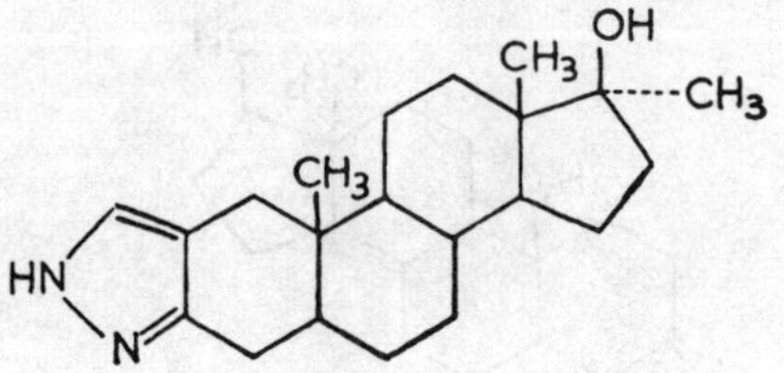

Stanozolol (methylstanazole, androstanazole, Stromba, Winstrol)
Dose: 5 mg daily, by mouth.

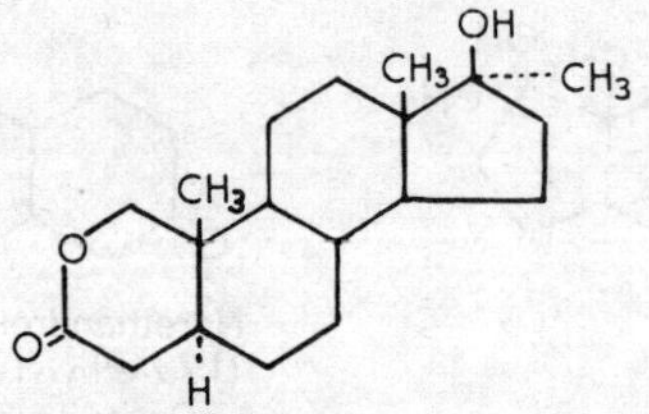

Oxandrolone (Anavar)
Dose: 2.5-10 mg daily, by mouth

Fig. 43.2 Some anabolic steroids—contd.

mesterone is no more than palliative in the last named condition, it may temporarily arrest the progress of the illness and it seems to be particularly useful when metastases have appeared in the bones.

ANABOLIC STEROIDS.

Testosterone has both androgenic and anabolic properties and attempts have been made to develop compounds with maximal anabolic and minimal androgenic activity. Such compounds could be used for their anabolic effects without causing virilism in women or premature sexual development in male children. Although a large number of compounds has been produced, none seems to be noticea-

bly superior to testosterone itself and in any event it is not certainly established that the anabolic action of the androgens has any but a limited therapeutic application (p. 734). The names, formulae and doses of some of the anabolic steroids are given for reference in Figure 43.2. Their names are confusing and unsystematic and no useful purpose is served by attempting to commit them to memory. Norethandrolone has progestational as well as anabolic properties. The corresponding ethynyl compound (p. 745) has even more powerful progestational properties and it is used as an oral contraceptive. Some of the anabolic steroids are active by mouth; the others are given by intramuscular injection.

Anabolic steroids and athletic training

Some few years ago the minds of British athletes were exercised at first by the suspicion and then by the conviction that some of their foreign rivals in endurance and heavyweight events were using anabolic steroids to develop the muscular strength that won them medals. Typically English epithets (the most popular was 'unsportsmanlike') were hurled against those who were believed to indulge in, to condone or to encourage this practice. Protests were of little avail and many an athlete lost his event, by a kind of reverse placebo effect, almost before he entered the stadium convinced as he was that his rivals would all be enjoying the benefits of a training programme that included the regular ingestion of anabolic steroids. It was not long before British athletes themselves took to the drugs, without, be it said, noticeably improving their performance in international competitions. It would be unfair to hazard a guess as to the proportion of athletes who take anabolic steroids and presumptuous for a mere pharmacologist to discuss the ethics of the situation. The effectiveness of this form of body building, however, is a proper and necessary topic for examination here.

Conclusions concerning this matter have only too often been based on prejudice, unreliably subjective impressions and indifferent experiments. Nevertheless, the literature does include reports of well designed and executed experiments, the best of which lead to the conclusion that body weight and muscle strength do increase to a greater extent in athletes who take anabolic steroids during training than in those who do not. Some authorities are of the opinion that the drugs might exert this effect indirectly by reducing fatigue and so permitting more prolonged and vigorous training (Hervey et al., 1976). It certainly seems to be true that athletes in training respond to anabolic steroids more readily and to a greater degree than do those who live a more sedentary life. Moreover even in the training athlete, muscles that are not exercised escape the beneficial effect of the drug (Freed and Banks, 1975). These facts may explain why anabolic steroids proved disappointing as aids to recuperation from debilitating diseases.

Methandienone seems to be the most popular anabolic steroid among athletes. It is sometimes taken in very large doses (300 mg daily has been mentioned) but it seems that smaller amounts (25 or 50 mg daily) are just as effective and are, presumably, less likely to produce side effects. The latter (which are detailed below) are occasionally severe enough to necessitate withdrawal of the drug but it seems that they occur less frequently and are probably less dangerous than has sometimes been supposed. Such adverse changes as are induced usually disappear rapidly when drug taking ceases. It has, however, to be added that, because anabolic steroids are taken surreptitiously (the practice is officially banned by British sports authorities and the drugs are not freely available) any assertions and conclusions concerning their possible adverse effects must necessarily be tentative.

Side effects of androgen therapy

When androgens are given to adult women, virilism (masculinization) may occur. These changes are progressive and they may become prominent in those requiring long term therapy. The voice deepens, hair grows on the face, the clitoris enlarges, the body becomes more muscular and baldness of the male type may develop.

In male children with normal testicular function, androgens cause premature development of the accessory sex organs and characteristics. Most authorities now agree that the androgens should not be employed to secure anabolic effects in young children of either sex.

Androgens promote retention of sodium so that oedema may occur in patients who have to take the drugs over a prolonged period.

Steroids with a methyl substituent in the α position on C17 are likely to cause liver damage (*cholestatic hepatitis*). In this condition, bile stagnates and accumulates in smaller ducts throughout the liver so that jaundice develops.

ANTIANDROGENS

Compounds capable of antagonizing androgen action fall into three principal categories.

a. Substances that compete with androgen for its receptor sites in the tissues. These are the true antagonists, the best known example being cyproterone.

b. Substances that inhibit the release of gonadotrophins. Oestrogens and progestogens have this ability but so has testosterone itself.

c. Substances whose pharmacological actions on the target tissues are the opposite of those exerted by the androgens. Oestrogens are obvious candidates for inclusion in this category. They antagonize androgen activity in doses too low to suppress gonadotrophin release.

Some of the antiandrogens have actions that permit their inclusion in more than one of these categories. Oestrogens provide a case in point as does cyproterone acetate. This compound is a true competitive antagonist but it also inhibits gonadotrophin release. Cyproterone itself does not depress the output of gonadotrophins. There are, indeed, some reports that the unesterified compound actually promotes release of the trophic hormones by reason of its ability to antagonize the action of testosterone on the hypothalamo-pituitary mechanisms so that the androgen can no longer exercise its feed-back inhibitory influence on gonadotrophin release. Chlormadinone (p. 744) also has a dual action similar to that of cyproterone acetate.

The antiandrogen activity of the oestrogens is exploited when they are applied to the treatment of carcinoma of the

CH₃
|
CO
|
CH₃
OCCH₃
‖
O

H₂C

CH₃

O

Cl

Cyproterone acetate

prostate (p. 741). Antiandrogens have been given to control behaviour in male sexual offenders (p. 741) but they have attracted most attention in relation to the possibility that they might be used as male contraceptives.

Most of the antiandrogens so far investigated can certainly inhibit sperm formation but at the same time they abolish sexual desire—surely the ultimate in contraceptive mechanisms. The major exception to this generalization is provided by testosterone itself. Given in sufficiently large doses, testosterone abolishes gonadotrophin release and hence both spermatogenesis and the synthesis of testosterone. Libido is not, however, affected because the administered testosterone takes the place of the missing androgen. Testosterone has to be given for some two months before spermatozoa finally disappear from the semen but the biggest obstacle to the adoption of testosterone as a contraceptive agent is the fact that it needs to be given by regular intramuscular injection. Only those who take their pleasures very seriously would willingly submit to so uncomfortable a contraceptive regime. The orally active androgens are, unfortunately, rather ineffective inhibitors of gonadotrophin release. Nevertheless, the possibility clearly remains that androgens will form the basis of the first successful oral contraceptive for males.

α-CHLOROHYDRIN AND COMPOUND CL88236
Although these substances are not antiandrogens it is relevant to mention them here in the context of male contraceptives. They prevent the maturation that spermatozoa normally undergo as they wend their way along the epididymis. α-Chlorohydrin itself has a toxic effect on the bone marrow but compound CL88236 seems to be less suspect in this respect (Coppola and Saldarini, 1974) and

CH₂Cl
|
CHOH
|
CH₂OH

α-Chlorohydrin

CH₂Cl
|
CHOH
|
CH₂NH₂

Compound CL88236

its structural simplicity encourages the hope that other glycerol derivatives might emerge as successful antifertility agents.

THE MENSTRUAL CYCLE

The course of a normal menstrual cycle is illustrated in Figure 43.3. Under the influence of the follicle stimulating and luteinizing hormones of the anterior pituitary, (which at this stage of the cycle are secreted in relatively small amounts) a Graafian follicle matures, one in each cycle. The maturing follicle secretes progressively increasing quantities of oestrogens which are responsible for causing an increase in thickness and vascularity of the endometrium. On about the 14th day of the cycle there is a sudden but short-lived increase in the rate of secretion of both trophic hormones. The cause of this surge of activity is not entirely clear: the increasing concentration of oestrogens in the blood might well trigger the release of the luteinizing hormone releasing factor from the hypothalamus but it would be expected at the same time to exert a feed back inhibition on the release of follicle stimulating hormone.

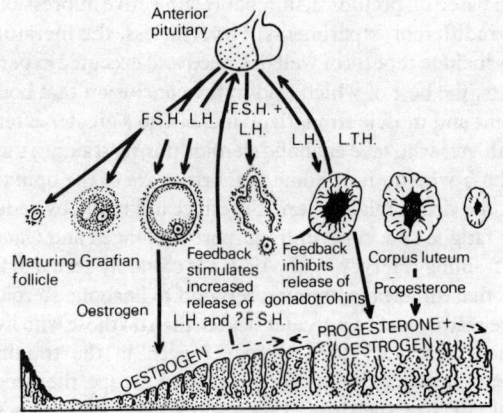

Fig. 43.3 The menstrual cycle. To show the influence upon the endometrium of secretions from the anterior pituitary gland, Graafian follicle and corpus luteum.
F.S.H. = Follicle stimulating hormone.
L.H. = Luteinizing hormone.

The luteinizing hormone, aided perhaps by the follicle stimulating hormone, causes the Graafian follicle to rupture and so to release its ovum, which begins its journey along the oviduct to the uterus. It also initiates the conversion of the empty follicle into a corpus luteum, which secretes progesterone and smaller amounts of oestrogens. Under the combined influence of oestrogens and progesterone, the endometrium develops further and enters its progestational phase in which the glands become elongated and tortuous and full of mucus. The other cells of the endometrium increase in size and number, the blood vessels become dilated and there is some exudation of fluid into the uterine cavity. In its progestational phase the endometrium is capable of receiving and imbedding a fertilized ovum and it enters this phase at about the time when the ovum reaches the uterus. The period between about the 14th and 21st day of a 28-day cycle is therefore the optimal time for fruitful sexual intercourse. If pregnancy does not occur, the corpus luteum degenerates on about the 26th day of the cycle, perhaps because it is exposed to the action of prostaglandin F2 α (p. 373), secreted by the endometrium. This withdrawal of oestrogens and progesterone causes the superficial layers of the endometrium to break down. On about the 28th day of the cycle menstruation occurs and over the next four or five days the shed endometrium leaves the body together with mucus and blood from the ruptured endometrial glands and blood vessels. Menstrual cycles vary considerably in length: they may be as short as 19 days or as long as 38 days in normal women. Whatever the length of the cycle, the interval between ovulation and menstruation is fairly constant at about 14 days.

In some animal species (but not in the human being), the proper functioning of the corpus luteum requires the presence of a third gonadotrophin, the luteotrophic hormone which is now known to be identical with prolactin (p. 776).

The follicle stimulating and luteinizing hormones are glycoproteins each with a molecular weight of about 30000.

Menstruation has been rather coyly described as the 'weeping of a disappointed uterus'. If the uterus is not disappointed, the corpus luteum persists and grows and continues to secrete progesterone so that the endometrium remains in a condition favourable to pregnancy. The continued secretion of progesterone suppresses secretion of the follicle stimulating hormone and thus prevents further ovulation during pregnancy. The corpus luteum of pregnancy persists until about the sixth month but its secretions are from an early date supplemented by those of the placenta. The placenta, in association with the developing foetus, is a veritable hormone factory. Its main products are progesterone, human chorionic gonadotrophin (HCG) and oestrogens but it also manufactures human placental lactogen, two thyrotrophins (one designated 'chorionic' and the other 'molar'), relaxin and a number of prostaglandins. These placental products are mentioned or discussed elsewhere in this volume. Further details concerning the less important members of the group can be found in current textbooks of endocrinology (see, for instance, Hall, et al. 1974).

The primitive placenta begins to secrete chorionic gonadotrophin as early as the third week of pregnancy. This hormone has actions similar to those of the luteinizing hormone so that the preservation of the corpus luteum is assured by the fertilized ovum whose own continued existence depends on the continuing activity of the corpus luteum. As the placenta develops its own capacity to secrete oestrogens and progesterone, the corpus luteum becomes less important. A major transfer of endocrine activity from corpus luteum to placenta occurs towards the end of the third month of pregnancy and it is during this change, when the continued retention of the foetus is in jeopardy, that spontaneous abortions are most likely to occur.

It has already been mentioned that chorionic gonadotrophin is produced very early in pregnancy and its presence in urine is diagnostic of that condition. This forms the basis of a number of tests the most sensitive of which is an immunological one. Specific antibodies are produced in the serum of rabbits by inoculating the animals with purified human chorionic gonadotrophin. Sheep erythrocytes coated with the hormone provide the other component of the system. The urine under test is mixed with antiserum and the coated erythrocytes are then added to the mixture. If chorionic gonadotrophin is present in the urine it will combine with the antibodies in the serum and no further reaction will occur when erythrocytes are added. If the urine comes from a woman who is not pregnant the serum will be unaffected and when the ethythrocytes are added agglutination will occur, the cells clumping together and being precipitated. Production of chorionic gonadotrophin reaches its peak in the ninth week of pregnancy but it can be detected in the urine soon after its manufacture begins, in the third week.

The newly fertilized ovum is surrounded by cells that constitute the *trophoblast*. Vascularized villi develop from this outer layer of tissue and penetrate into the endometrium to form the beginnings of the placenta. In the functioning placenta, exchanges of material between mother and foetus will take place across the villi. It sometimes happens that the villi undergo a pathological change in the early weeks of pregnancy, becoming changed into a large mass of vesicles or *hydatidiform mole*. In about 10 per cent of cases a malignant tumour (*choriocarcinoma*) develops in the wake of the mole. It secretes large amounts of chorionic gonadotrophin and measurement of the hormone in the urine provides a ready means of assessing the success of treatment. For this purpose the gonadotrophin is determined by radioimmunoassay.

The secretion of the gonadotrophic hormones is under the control of the hypothalamus and it is not therefore surprising that the menstrual cycle is very easily disturbed by emotional factors.

OESTROGENS

The naturally occurring oestrogens are three in number— oestradiol (17β-oestradiol), oestriol and oestrone—of which oestradiol is the most important. They are synthesized in the ovary along similar pathways to those used in

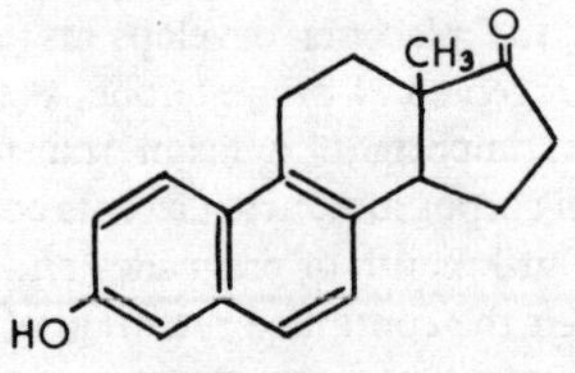

Equilenin

the adrenal cortex (Fig. 44.3). Oestradiol and oestrone are freely interconvertible. The liver is the principal site of interconversion but some takes place in the ovary and other tissues. The liver also converts oestrone to oestriol. All three oestrogens are excreted as sulphur esters and glucuronides. The ovary secretes small amounts of testosterone just as the testis secretes oestrogens. The adrenal cortex in both sexes produces small amounts of both androgens and oestrogens. It is an interesting fact that the stallion excretes more oestrogens in his urine than does the pregnant mare who is herself no mean performer in this respect. The principal oestrogen in mares' urine is equilenin.

The oestrogens can be regarded as derivatives of oestrane (Fig. 43.4). The resemblances between androstane, testosterone and androsterone on the one hand and oestrane, oestradiol and oestrone on the other will be evident by comparing the formulae in Figs. 43.1 and 43.4.

The oestrogens are responsible for the development and maintenance of the secondary sexual characteristics and accessory sex organs of the female. They stimulate (in association with adrenal androgens) the skeletal growth of immediately prepubertal girls but they also finally arrest the same process by ensuring closure of the epiphyses. They promote the deposition of subcutaneous fat in the appropriate areas of the body so moulding the characteristic female contours and they make a further contribution to

female beauty by preventing the action of androgens on sebaceous gland activity that so disfigures the skin of our adolescent sons. The anabolic actions of the oestrogens are less well marked than those of the androgens.

Clinical use of the oestrogens

The available oestrogens fall into three groups—the naturally-occurring, the semisynthetic and the synthetic agents. They have similar therapeutic uses which are first described without reference to particular compounds. The peculiar advantages of individual oestrogens are mentioned later.

Replacement therapy. Failure of the ovaries to develop is much less common than testicular failure. When it does occur, replacement therapy with the oestrogens is indicated in order to produce the physical changes of puberty. If menstrual cycles are to be initiated and maintained, large doses of oestrogen and progestogen have to be given for some three weeks. The hormones are then withheld until menstruation has occurred. Oestrogen treatment is more successful when the ovarian deficiency is caused by conditions in the ovary itself. Ovarian failure arising from pituitary defects demands the administration of other hormones to correct deficiencies in endocrine systems such as the thyroid and the adrenal cortex.

Treatment of menopausal symptoms. For many psychologically well-adjusted women the menopause is an event which arrives and passes almost unnoticed. Others suffer considerable discomfort, physical and mental, collectively known as the climacteric. There may be circulatory, autonomic and psychological changes that incluce hot flushes, headache, vertigo, dizziness, irritability, palpitations, fatigue, emotional instability, anxiety and melancholia. These effects appear to be attributable to both the

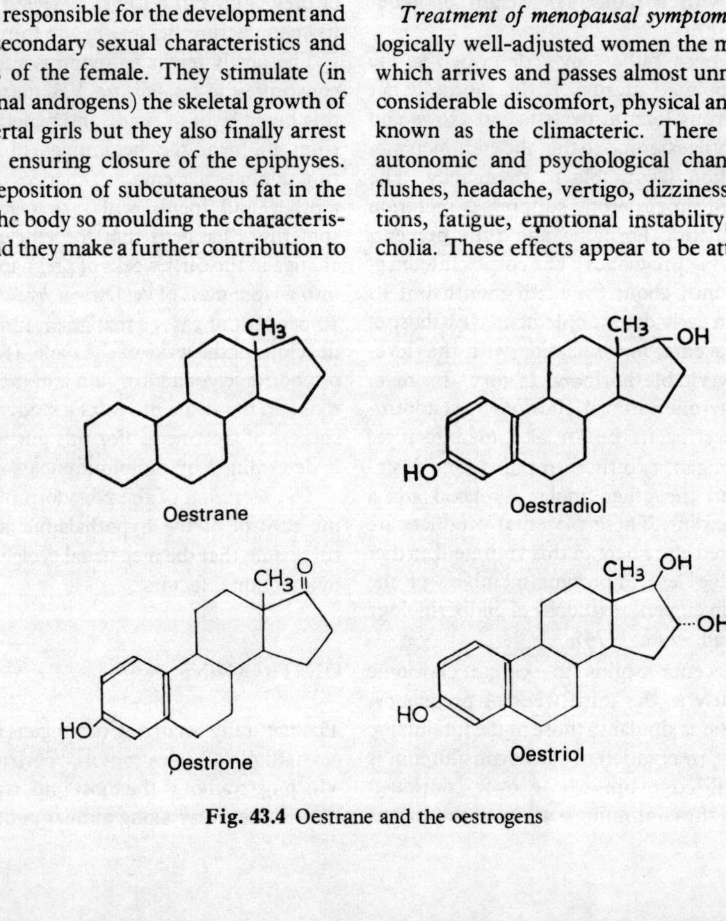

Oestrane

Oestradiol

Oestrone

Oestriol

Fig. 43.4 Oestrane and the oestrogens

deficiency of oestrogens and to the excess of pituitary gonadotrophins that arises naturally from the loss of oestrogens. Other effects of oestrogen deficiency include osteoporosis and a rise in the amount of cholesterol and fatty acids in the blood so that women are much more likely to develop cardiovascular disease after the menopause than they are before that event. Climacteric symptoms are relieved by treatment with oestrogens or with an oestrogen-progesterone mixture if they are associated with menstrual disturbances. A natural oestrogen such as piperazine oestrone sulphate (Harmogen) is to be preferred to synthetic or semisynthetic oestrogens such as mestranol or ethinyl oestradiol, the use of which is associated with a definite morbidity from thromboembolic disease (Report, 1977). Surgical removal of the ovaries during the period of reproductive life will precipitate an artificial menopause which is often more distressing than that which occurs naturally. In younger women, the osteoporosis and the increased concentration of plasma lipids constitute a threat to health which should be countered by oestrogen administration even if climacteric symptoms are absent.

There are those who advocate indefinite postponement of the menopause by giving oestrogens and progestogens on a cyclical basis as soon as endogenous hormone production begins to falter.

Menstrual disturbances. Dysmenorrhoea (painful menstruation) sometimes responds favourably to oestrogen treatment. The oestrogen is taken daily for two and a half weeks in each menstrual cycle, commencing on the fifth day. Menstruation usually occurs within a few days of oestrogen withdrawal. Oestrogens inhibit ovulation and this seems to be the origin of the relief they offer in dysmenorrhoea because they are ineffective if they are given after ovulation has occurred or if the dose used is too small to prevent ovulation. Not infrequently, menstruation is delayed for some days in patients receiving oestrogens. In itself, this is not of serious import but if ovulation takes place at the normal time in the next cycle it may already have occurred when oestrogen administration is recommenced on the fifth day. Regular oestrogen treatment may therefore result in freedom from pain only in alternate menstrual periods. If this happens, combined therapy with oestrogen and a progestogen is indicated. This will prevent the delay in menstruation and ensure that an equal degree of relief is obtained in every cycle. Sex hormone treatment of dysmenorrhoea amounts, of course, to giving an oral contraceptive (p. 750).

The actual cause of dysmenorrhoea is unknown. Oestrogens, progesterone, gonadotrophins, prostaglandins and other hormone as well as psychological and dietary factors and the state of the general health all play their part. Marriage often provides the best cure for dysmenorrhoea but some might consider this to be too drastic a form of treatment. The oestrogens are used for the treatment of other menstrual irregularities such as oligomenorrhoea (scanty periods) but they are not often successful in these conditions.

Cancer chemotherapy. The growth and activity of the prostate gland is dependent on the integrity of the testes and as many as 80 years ago castration was recommended as a form of treatment for prostatic cancer. The operation did not come into vogue until 1941 when Huggins and his collaborators re-introduced it. At the same time, they pointed out that the androgenic activity of the testes could be antagonized by oestrogens. Their suggestion that inoperable carcinoma of the prostate should be treated by orchidectomy (removal of the testes) combined with oestrogen administration was quickly adopted and it has been responsible for causing a significant prolongation of life in a large number of men. The treatment does not cure the cancer but the primary growth and secondary deposits regress, the patient feels better and he suffers less pain. Unfortunately, suppression of the primary growth is not permanent because of the development of cells resistant to the effects of the oestrogens. This suggests that the oestrogens operate directly on the prostatic cells but they may also act upon and through the suprarenal cortex and the anterior pituitary gland.

Oral contraceptives. The value of oestrogens as chemical contraceptives is discussed later (p. 746).

Other conditions The possible value of oestrogen therapy on a miscellany of other clinical conditions has been investigated. These include acne in the adolescent girl, excessive growth of facial and body hair in women (*hirsutism*) and osteoporosis. Oestrogens seem to be marginally effective in these conditions. Because arterial disease and coronary thomboses are rare in women, attempts have been made to prevent these conditions in men by administering regular doses of oestrogens, insufficient to provoke feminizing effects. There is little convincing evidence that this kind of attempted prophylactic treatment achieves the ends it seeks, but it is probably more successful in women who are exposed to the risk of coronary arterial disease by reason of their being in artificial menopause (see above). Oestrogens are sometimes given to accelerate closure of the epiphyses in prepubertal girls whose hereditary background threatens otherwise to make them abnormally tall. Like other antiandrogens (p. 737), the oestrogens can be made use of to reduce libido in males who fear that they may be driven to acts of sexual violence. Oestrogens have been used to arrest lactation after childbirth but better agents, such as bromocriptine (p. 777) have recently become available for suppressing milk secretion.

Individual oestrogens

A large number of compounds with oestrogenic activity are available for clinical use. In addition to the naturally occurring compounds (oestradiol, oestriol and oestrone) use is made of both semisynthetic oestrogens (ethinyloestradiol is an example) and of completely synthetic substances. As we have already indicated the natural oestrogens are less likely to cause venous thrombosis than are those of synthetic or semisynthetic origin. As a generalization, it can be said that the synthetic and semisynthetic compounds are more suitable for general use since they can be taken by mouth and their action is not as evanescent as that of the natural oestrogens. Stilboestrol has the added advantage of being cheap.

The properties of the natural oestrogens have already been discussed. In this section, details relevant to their clinical use are presented.

OESTRADIOL

Oestradiol is used as the alcohol itself (Ovocyclin), and as the monobenzoate (Benztrone, Ovocyclin M), dipropionate or valerate (Primogyn, Progynova). The esters have to be administered by parenteral (usually intramuscular) injection but oestradiol itself is effective when it is taken sublingually. It is also sometimes administered as a cream or ointment but it is extremely doubtful whether the hoped-for cosmetic results (removal of wrinkles, breast development) are achieved by the application of these expensive preparations. For the treatment of dysmenorrhoea or menstrual irregularities the daily requirement of oestradiol is about 2 mg in divided doses. Doses of 1 to 5 mg given at weekly intervals are suitable for the treatment of menopausal symptoms, pruritus vulvae or senile vaginitis. The esters should not be given for the treatment of menstrual irregularities. Quite apart from the fact that they have to be given by injection, they have the disadvantage that cessation of administration does not produce the sudden fall in the hormone concentration which is a prerequisite of successful menstruation.

OESTRIOL

The actions of oestriol (Ovestin) appear to be exerted primarily on the cervix and vagina immediately before parturition or menstruation. It has relatively little action on the endometrium. It has been used for the treatment of pruritus vulva (0.25 to 0.5 mg daily) and vulvitis and vaginitis (0.25 to 1 mg daily).

OESTRONE

Oestrone has similar properties and uses to oestradiol, over which it possesses no advantage.

ETHINYLOESTRADIOL

This semisynthetic compound is the most active available oestrogen. It can be taken by mouth. For replacement therapy in amenorrhoea, it is given for seventeen days in a daily dose of 0.05 to 0.1 mg. This is followed by a 10-day interval. The daily dose in dysmenorrhoea is 0.05 mg. Ethinyloestradiol is available under a number of proprietary names including Estigyn, Estinyl and Lynoral. The

Ethinyloestradiol

methyl ether is known as mestranol: mestranol and ethinyloestradiol itself are both constituents of several oral contraceptives (Table 43.1).

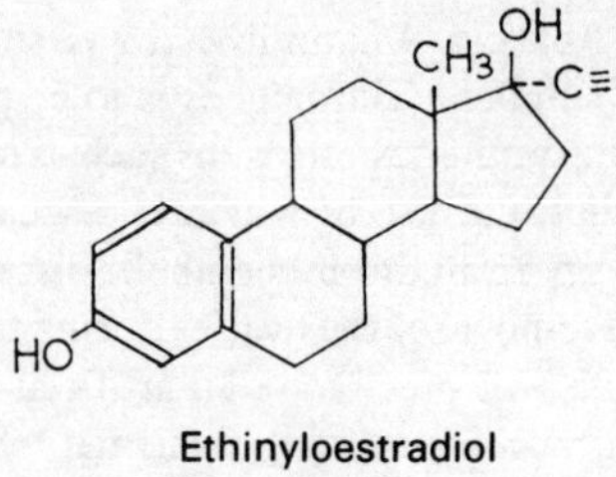

STILBOESTROL

Stilboestrol (sometimes known as diethylstilboestrol) is the most widely used of all oestrogenic preparations. It has only one-tenth of the potency of ethinyloestradiol but it is the cheapest available oestrogenic substance, even when account is taken of the necessity of giving relatively large doses of the drug. Stilboestrol is effective by mouth. Doses of up to 15 mg per day are needed for cancer chemotherapy. Menopausal symptoms are controlled by doses of 0.1 to 3 mg daily and disorders of the menstrual cyle by doses of 1 to 3 mg. Proprietary names include Clinestrol and Pabestrol. The diphosphate ester of stilboestrol is known as fosfestrol (Honvan). It is given in thrice daily doses of 100 mg in the treatment of carcinoma of the prostate.

OTHER SYNTHETIC OESTROGENS.

The names and formulae of some other synthetic oestrogens are presented in Fig. 43.5.

Side effects of oestrogen therapy

The oestrogens may cause nausea, vomiting and a painful swelling of the breasts but the incidence of these complica-

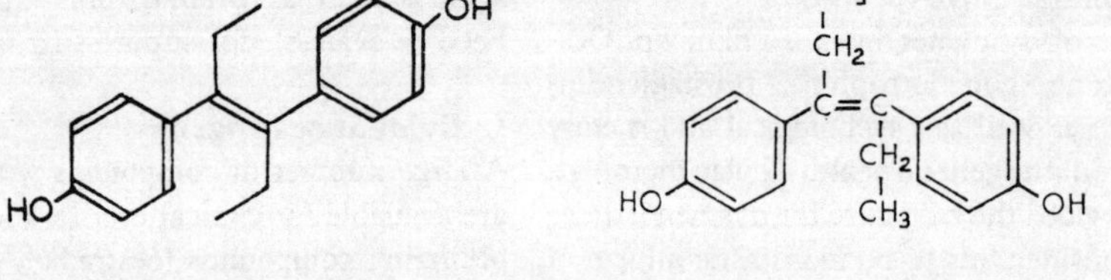

Stilboestrol

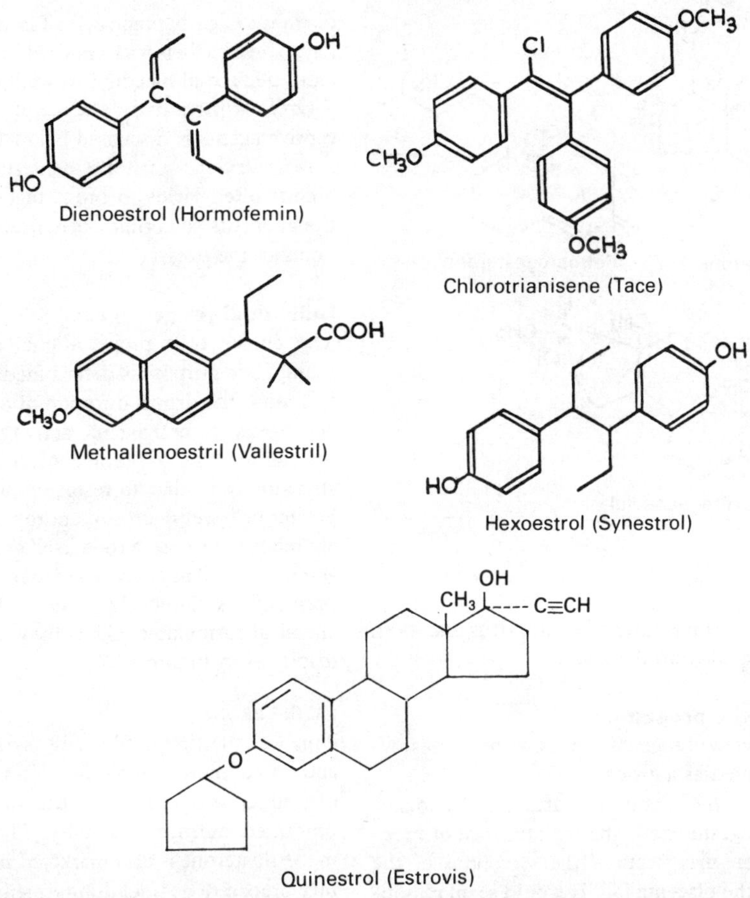

Dienoestrol (Hormofemin)

Chlorotrianisene (Tace)

Methallenoestril (Vallestril)

Hexoestrol (Synestrol)

Quinestrol (Estrovis)

Fig. 43.5 Some synthetic oestogens

tions is reduced if therapy is initiated with low doses of oestrogen, which are slowly increased until the desired effect is obtained. When oestrogens are given to male patients, an embarrassing growth of the breasts (*gynaeco-mastia*) may occur, but other signs of feminization are unusual. In patients who have secondary tumours in bone, sex hormone therapy may cause a noticeable rise in the calcium content of the plasma. If hypercalcaemia is of only a moderate degree, it may be countered by giving a chelating agent (p. 796) and ensuring a high fluid intake to prevent calcium deposition in the kidneys. In more severe degrees of the condition, hormone therapy may have to be stopped. Large doses of oestrogens cause retention of sodium and water. They are also prone to cause venous thrombosis, a complication that is discussed later in relation to the use of oral contraceptives (p. 749). The possibility that sex hormone therapy may actually acceler-ate the growth of tumours must always be borne in mind.

PROGESTOGENS (PROGESTINS)

The only naturally-occurring progestogen is progesterone, a substance whose functions have already been described (p. 739). The configuration of the biologically active form of progesterone and of its stereoisomer, known as retropro-gesterone, is shown in Figure 43.6. Progesterone itself is effective only when it is given by parenteral injection but a number of orally active progestogens have been produced during the past 20 years or so. This has greatly extended the scope of progestational therapy and has permitted the development of successful oral contraceptives.

Progesterone is rapidly metabolized in the body. In the urine, up to 30 per cent of an administered dose appears as a conjugate of glucuronic acid and pregnanediol (Fig. 43.6) and measurement of the urinary excretion of pregnanediol can be used to assess the rate at which progesterone is being secreted. The effects of progesterone on the target

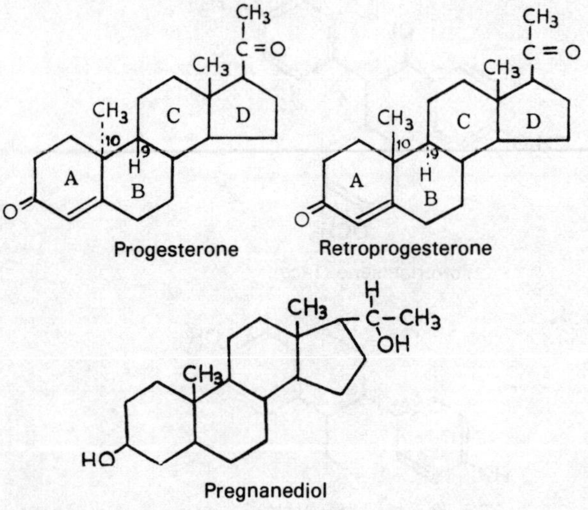

CH₃ ... (chemical structures)

Progesterone   Retroprogesterone

Pregnanediol

Fig. 43.6

tissues continue for some time after the drug has been completely eliminated from the body.

Clinical uses of the progestogens

From the point of view of their clinical uses, the progestogens can be considered as a group.

Habitual abortion. As its name indicates, the physiological function of progesterone is the maintenance of pregnancy and abortion may occur if the secretions of the corpus luteum or the placenta fail. It would seem reasonable, therefore, to provide progestogen treatment for women who, having suffered several abortions in the past, are anxious to carry a pregnancy through to a successful conclusion. In fact, progestogen treatment has not been so uniformly successful as was originally hoped (perhaps because abortion is not always caused by a hormone deficiency) but it always warrants a trial.

Functional uterine bleeding. This condition (which most commonly occurs at the two extremes of the reproductive life) is characterized by bouts of excessive and prolonged bleeding. It is the result of a lack of both oestrogens and progesterone but it can be successfuly treated with a progestogen such as norethynodrel which has some oestrogenic activity.

Dysmenorrhoea. In order to reproduce more closely the conditions which obtain in a normal menstrual cycle, oestrogens used in the treatment of dysmenorrhoea can be supplemented with progestogen during the last four or five days of each period of treatment. It has already been pointed out (p. 741) that the use of a progestational agent in this way prevents delay in menstruation and thereby permits the continued suppression of ovulation.

Pregnancy diagnosis. An oral progestogen together with an oestrogen (Pregornot, Primodos) can be used for the diagnosis of early pregnancy. The drugs are given for some days and are then withdrawn. If the patient is not pregnant, menstrual bleeding will follow within a few days.

Oral contraceptives. The use of progestogens as contraceptive agents is discussed below (p. 746).

Miscellaneous uses. Premenstrual discomfort in the breasts often yields to progestogen treatment. Progestational agents sometimes benefit advanced cases of carcinoma of the breast.

Individual progestogens

The choice of a progestational agent for a particular therapeutic purpose is determined by a number of factors including the drug's duration of action, its possession of androgenic or oestrogenic activity and its suitability for oral administration. Some of the synthetic agents are structurally similar to testosterone and therefore have a greater or lesser degree of androgenic activity. The others are related to progesterone itself and may have oestrogenic activity. It will be appreciated that many of the commercial preparations closely duplicate each other's activity. The chemical formulae of the substances mentioned here are displayed in Figure 43.7

ETHISTERONE

This was the first orally active synthetic progestogen. Its actions are more delayed in onset than those of progesterone itself and prolonged use may be associated with unwanted androgenic activity. The daily dose is 25 to 50 mg. Ethisterone is also marketed in a number of proprietary preparations (including Amenorone and Paralut) that also contain ethinyloestradiol. They are used in the treatment of amenorrhoea.

NORETHYNODREL AND NORETHISTERONE (NORETHINDRONE)

These isomers, which are derivatives of ethisterone, have structural features in common with both the oestrogens and the progestogens. They have oestrogenic and some androgenic activity. Both compounds are used in oral contraceptives.

MEGESTROL

Megestrol is a powerful oral progestational agent which is devoid of other hormonal actions, including androgenic activity. Mixed with an oestrogen, megestrol was once a popular contraceptive agent but it is no longer used for this purpose since the drug was found to increase the incidence of mammary tumours in dogs. When used for other purposes (including, oddly enough, the chemotherapy of malignant tumours of the breast and uterus) megestrol was given in daily doses of up to 40 mg.

CHLORMADINONE

This compound is closely related to megestrol. It has no oestrogenic or androgenic activity. It prevents ovulation

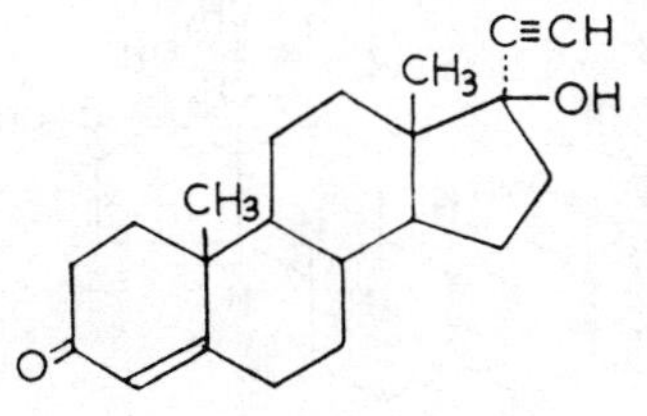

Fig. 43.7 Some synthetic progestational agents.

Ethisterone
(Gestone)

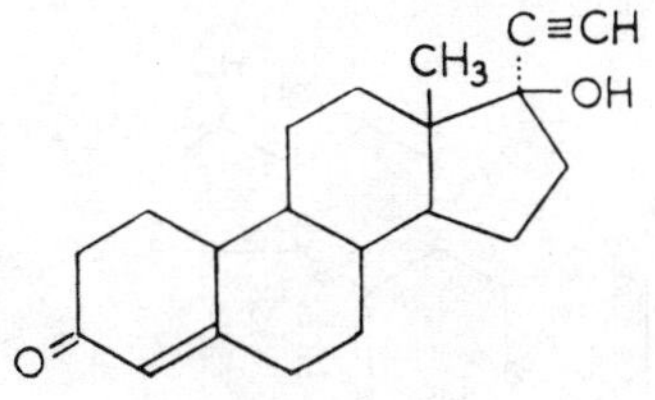

Norethisterone
(norethindrone, Norlutin, Primolut)

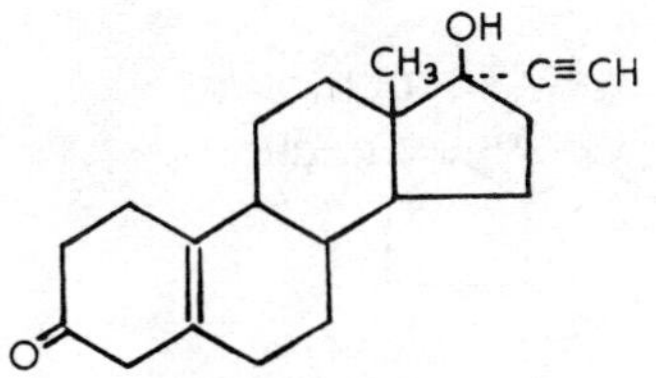

Norethynodrel

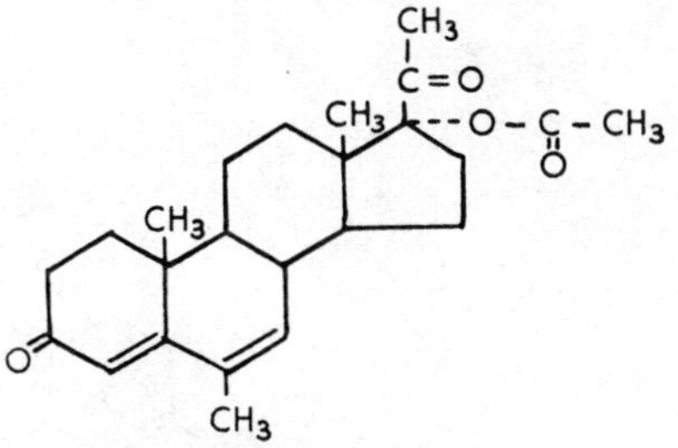

Megestrol acetate

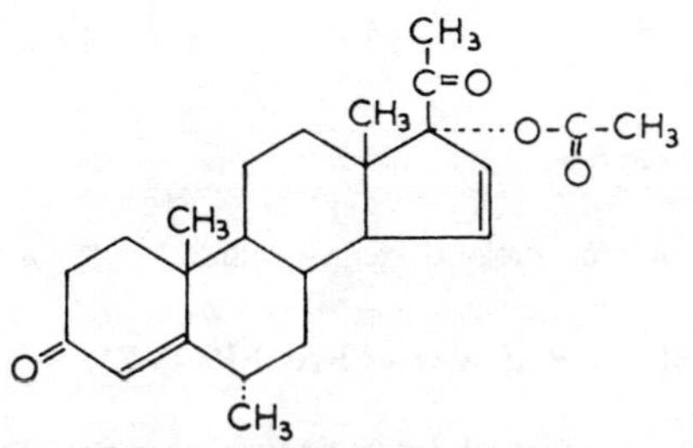

Medroxyprogesterone acetate
(Provera)

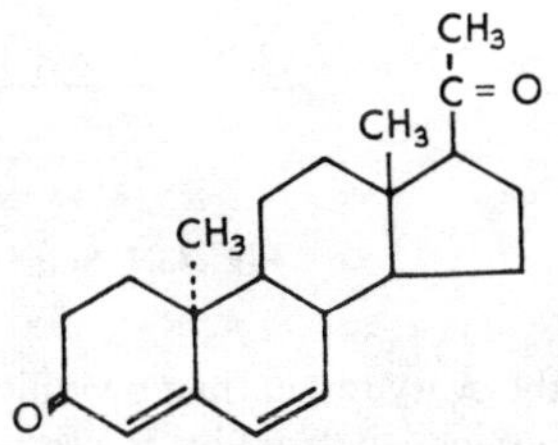

Dydrogesterone (dehydroprogesterone
Duphaston)

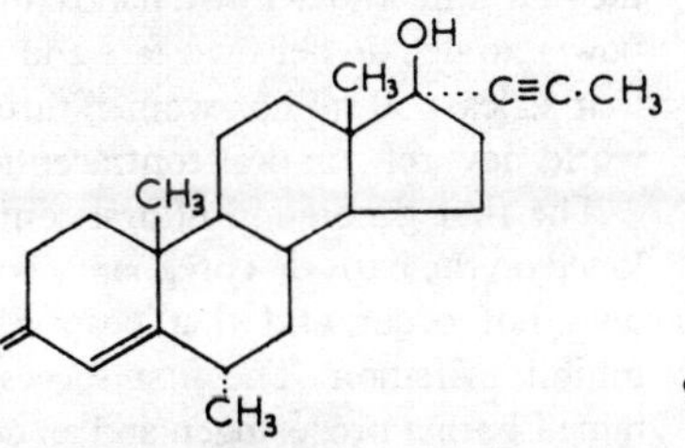

Dimethisterone
(Secrosteron)

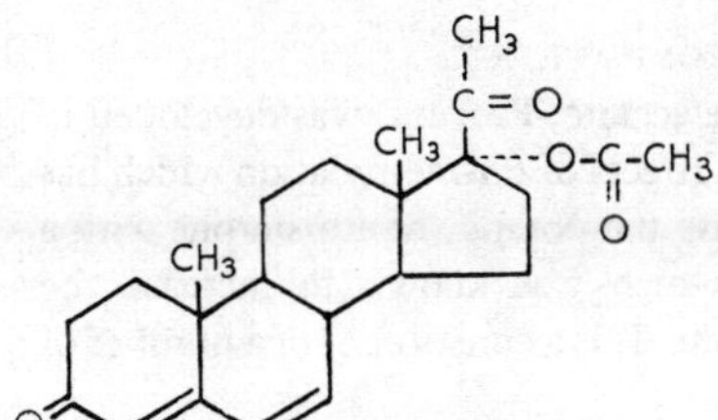

Chlormadinone acetate

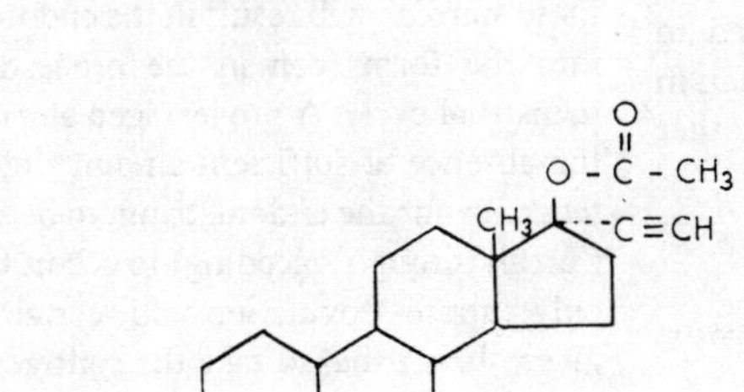

Ethynodiol diacetate

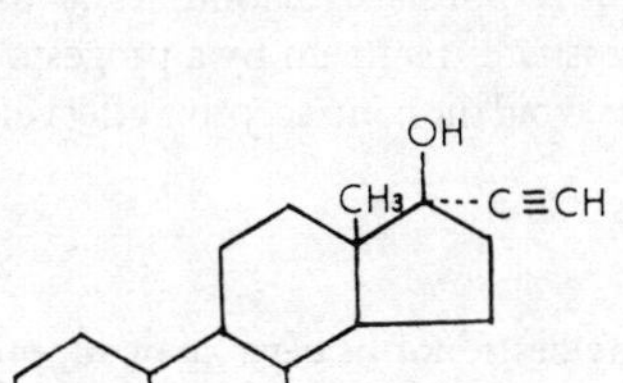

Lynoestrenol

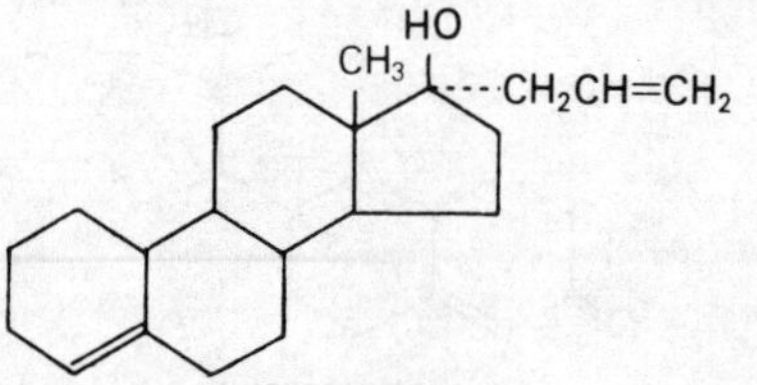

Allyloestranol (Gestanin)

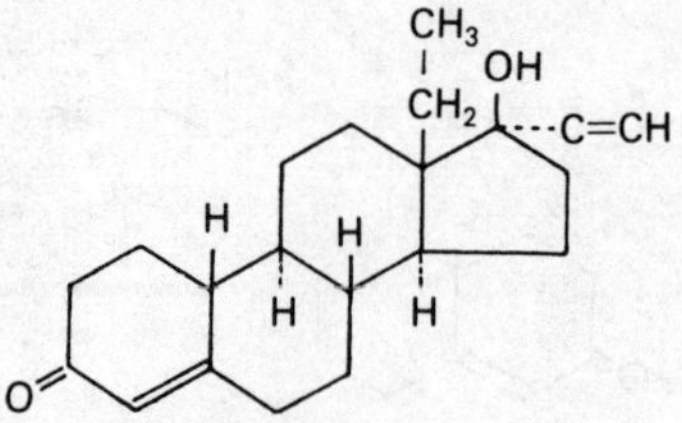

Norgestrel

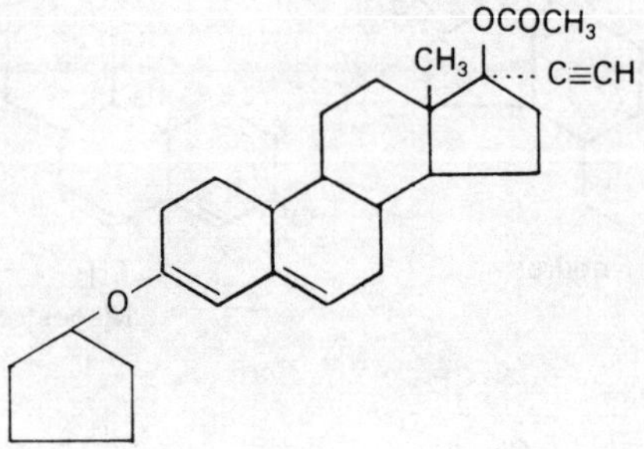

Quingestanol

Fig. 43.7 Some synthetic progestational agents—contd.

by a direct action on the ovary rather than by inhibition of the secretion of pituitary gonadotrophin. It also possesses some antioestrogenic activity. Like megestrol, chlormadinone is no longer used as a contraceptive agent.

MEDROXYPROGESTERONE ACETATE.

Medroxyprogesterone acetate (Provera) was developed in order to combine the effects of 6α-methylation which has been shown to increase the potency of ethisterone with a 17α-acetoxy group which was known to increase the potency of progesterone. It is a constituent of a number of oral contraceptives.

DYDROGESTERONE

Dydrogesterone (Duphaston) is a retroprogesterone (Fig. 43.1). It has no anabolic, androgenic or oestrogenic activity, and it does not suppress ovulation. It is used in conditions that necessitate treatment by a progestogen in patients who wish to avoid the contraceptive effect of other drugs.

LYNOESTRENOL

Lynoestrenol (ethinyloestrenol) is capable of suppressing ovulation for long periods of time.

DIMETHISTERONE

Dimethisterone was synthesized with the aim of increasing progestational activity by methylating C(6) and so protecting the compound from metabolic inactivation by hydroxylation. It is about as potent as norethisterone.

ORAL CONTRACEPTIVES

The oral contraceptive has proved to be one of the greatest liberating forces in the history of womankind, putting for the first time into her own hands (or rather her mouth) the power to decide her own fate and future. It is estimated that at least 50 million women throughout the developed world now rely on oral contraception.

The first generation of oral contraceptives were developed on the basis that pregnancy is impossible if ovulation does not occur and that oestrogens and progestogens inhibit ovulation. The first successful preparation contained both a progestogen and an oestrogen and *combined preparations* of this type are still very popular. Reference to Figure 43.3 will make it clear that the administration of these steroids will result in the endometrium's developing into the form seen in the progestational phase of the menstrual cycle. A progestogen alone achieves this but in the absence of sufficient amounts of oestrogen there is a tendency for the endometrium to be shed and for bleeding ('break through' bleeding) to occur. Oestrogens alone will only suppress ovulation with certainty if large doses are given. It is usual to take the contraceptive according to a dose schedule which will permit the maintenance of normal menstruation. The combined preparations are taken for 21 days, beginning on the fifth day of the menstrual cycle. Withdrawal of the drugs mimics the hormonal events that occur immediately before a natural menstruation and is followed after two or three days by

Table 43.1 Some oral contraceptive agents

Preparation	Oestrogen μg	Progestogen mg
COMBINED PREPARATIONS WITH HIGH DOSE OESTROGENS		
Conovid-E (Enavid-E)	Mestranol 100	Norethynordrel 2.5
Conovid (Enavid-S)	Mestranol 75	Norethynordrel 5
Ortho-Novin 2 mg	Mestranol 100	Norethisterone 2
Norinyl 2	Mestranol 100	Norethisterone 2
Ortho-Novin 1/80	Mestranol 80	Norethisterone 1
Demulen	Mestranol 100	Ethynodiol diacetate 0.5
Ovulen 1 mg	Mestranol 100	Ethynodiol diacetate 1
Metrulen	Mestranol 100	Ethynodiol diacetate 2
Lyndiol	Mestranol 75	Lynoestrenol 2.5
COMBINED PREPARATIONS WITH MEDIUM DOSE OESTROGENS		
Norinyl 1 (and 1/28)	Mestranol 50	Norethisterone acetate 1
Ortho-Novin 1/50	Mestranol 50	Norethisterone acetate 1
Anovlar 21	Ethinyloestradinol 50	Norethisterone acetate 4
Confer		Norethisterone acetate 1
Minovlar and Minovlar ED		Norethisterone acetate 1
Orlest 21		Norethisterone acetate 1
Gynovlar 21		Norethisterone acetate 3
Norlestrin		Norethisterone acetate 2.5
Demulen 50		Ethinynodiol diacetate 0.5
Ovulen 50		Ethinynodiol diacetate 1
Eugynon 50		DL-Norgestrel 0.5
Ovran		D-Norgestrel 0.25
Minilyn		Lynoestrenol 2.5
COMBINED PREPARATIONS WITH LOW DOSE OESTROGENS		
Microgynon 30	Ethinyloestradiol 30	D-Norgestrel 0.15
Ovranette	Ethinyloestradiol 30	D-Norgestrel 0.15
Eugynon 30	Ethinyloestradiol 30	DL-Norgestrel 0.5
Loestrin 20	Ethinyloestradiol 20	Norethisterone acetate 1
SEQUENTIAL PREPARATION		
Ovanon	Mestranol 80 (days 1–7) Mestranol 75 (days 8–22)	Lynoestrenol 2.5 (days 8–22)
PROGESTOGEN-ONLY PREPARATIONS ('MINI-PILLS')		
Micronor		Norethisterone 0.35
Micronovum		
Noriday	ZERO	
Nor Q.D.		
Femulen		Ethynodiol diacetate 0.5
Neogest		
Ovrette		DL-Norgestrel 0.75
Microlut		
Micro-30		D-Norgestrel 0.3
Microluton		
Turinal		Allylestrenol 0.5
Exluton		Lynoestrenol 0.5

menstrual bleeding. On the fifth day the drug taking cycle begins again. There seems, in fact, to be no real reason why the monthly cycle should be maintained except that if bleeding is allowed to occur at the traditional intervals the subject is assured that her normal functions have not been interfered with.

The first 'pills' contained mestranol (150 μg) and norethynodrel (10 mg). Mestranol is still used but in many combined preparations it has been replaced by ethinyloestradiol, an oestrogen that is twenty times more potent than mestranol. Similarly, the progestational element is supplied by one of number of the newer progestogens (Table 43.1), of which the most potent are ethynodiol diacetate and DL -norgestrel. A more important development has been the progressive reduction in the amount of each steroid in the preparation. This has been achieved without any loss of contraceptive effectiveness. The trend to low dose preparations accelerated after 1970 when it became evident that thromboembolic complications (p. 749) are more likely to occur in women whose daily intake of oestrogen is in excess of 50 μg. Many of the currently recommended combined preparations contain 50 μg of oestrogen but in a few even smaller amounts are present (Table 43.1).

Another way of achieving contraception involves a *sequential* dose schedule, intended to reproduce as nearly as possible the hormonal changes that occur during a normal menstrual cycle. The tablets to be taken for the first fifteen days of the cycle contain only oestrogen while those supplied for the next five days are made up of an oestrogen and a progestogen. Sequential type contraceptives are less reliable than combined preparations and they were never very popular, even in the days before their high content of oestrogen (75 or 80 μg per pill) aroused the suspicions concerning their safety that has led to their virtual disappearance from the contraceptive scene.

Progestogen-only contraceptives (sometimes known in these 'mini' days as mini-pills) are taken every day without the drug free interval that appears in the dose schedule of the combined and sequential type preparations. Although the preparation is taken daily, physiological mechanisms periodically re-assert themselves and uterine bleeding occurs at regular intervals which may be as inconveniently short as 10 days but which are more often of the order of three to five weeks. Mini-pills are not as reliable as combined preparations and, as we noted earlier, progestogens are likely to permit 'break through' bleeding. Moreover those containing chlormadinone acetate fell into disfavour on the suspicion (now dismissed) that they might cause carcinoma of the breast. Their only current use is in women who exhibit intolerance towards oestrogens.

The relative amounts of oestrogen and progestogen (as well as the absolute quantities of these substances) vary from one combined preparation to another and, as we shall see, there are sometimes reasons for switching from one preparation to another containing a different ratio of oestrogen to progestogen. Thus, side effects that are predominantly attributable to oestrogen action (fluid retention, premenstrual tension, discomfort in the breasts, etc) signal the desirability of changing to a preparation with a higher progestogen : oestrogen ratio. Effects such as acne, premenstrual depression and a dry vagina indicate that the reverse change should be made. These considerations do not imply that each one of the many available preparations has been developed to meet the needs of particular groups of patients. A glance at Table 43.1 will make it clear that many of the contraceptives listed there differ from one another only minimally if at all and they have clearly been developed in response to commercial rather than medical pressures. With millions of potential customers, each of whom might take up to 8000 contraceptive pills in her lifetime, the temptation to enter the market must be irresistible.

Side effects of oral contraceptive use

It is hardly surprising that a long list can be compiled of the extraneous effects that may accompany the taking of oral contraceptive agents. These drugs, after all, are taken by vast numbers of women in differing states of mental and physical health, they interfere with the natural hormonal balance of the organism and they intrude into the most personal and responsive areas of female physiology. Moreover, psychological factors can exert a strong influence on the systemic responses to oral contraceptives: some women experience feelings of well being as they lose the fear of an unwanted pregnancy but, even in these enlightened times, others experience adverse mental or physical symptoms from an underlying sense of guilt or even from an unacknowledged disappointment that the contraceptive method is so reliable that there is virtually no chance of their becoming pregnant by the 'accident' they subconsciously wish for, even while guarding against it. Pure hedonism, it seems, is not an easy state to acquire and accept. In view of all these circumstances, it is indeed remarkable that so few of those who take oral contraceptives suffer any adverse reaction at all.

The side effects of hormonal contraceptives can now be enumerated.

1. Oestrogens induce nausea, sometimes accompanied by vomiting and it has been estimated that between 10 and 25 per cent of women suffer in this way when they first begin to take oral contraceptives. The fact that the nausea is very similar to that experienced in early pregnancy adds a touch of piquant irony to the situation but the symptoms rarely persist for longer than the first three or four cycles of hormone administration. They are less likely to occur with combined preparations containing only small amounts of oestrogen.

2. The possibility that oral contraceptives may influence libido has excited much discussion particularly

among those (or the partners of those) who take them. It seems that, in most women, sex drive is not affected but that in a sizeable minority (this may amount to some 25 per cent of the total 'pill' taking population) there is at least a temporary sharpening or diminution of libido. In the light of what has already been said, the reader will appreciate that these changes are likely to have a psychological rather than an endocrinological origin, a view that is strongly supported by the results of an investigation in which women who did not mind becoming pregnant were given placebo preparations instead of the oral contraceptives they were expecting. More than half of the group complained of diminished libido, headache or nervousness (Aznar Ramos *et al.*, 1969). A depressed libido can sometimes be corrected by changing to a preparation whose progestogen component has marked androgenic properties. Norgestrel and norethisterone fall into this category.

3. A small proportion of women suffer severe migraine-like headaches during their drug free days. They may prove refractory to the usual analgesics and this may necessitate permanent withdrawal of the hormone preparations. There have been reports that the taking of oral contraceptives may have been a precipitating factor in a few fatal cases of subarachnoid haemorrhage.

4. Some five per cent of those who employ oral contraceptives complain of depression. Although it is reasonable to regard this as yet another 'psychological' side effect, at least one attempt has been made to explain the symptom on biochemical grounds. Oral contraceptives induce activity in hepatic microsomal enzymes (p. 80) including tryptophane pyrrolase and it has been suggested (though not very convincingly) that the enhanced activity of this enzyme leads to a loss of tryptophan, the precursor of 5-hydroxytryptamine, and hence to deficiency of a transmitter that is believed by some to be utilized by physiological systems that maintain mood (p. 546).

5. Women who adopt oral contraceptive methods should be told to watch their weight carefully. The unwanted gain in weight that might otherwise occur is often the simple result of an increased food intake consequent on relief from the worry of a possible pregnancy but other factors such as fluid retention caused by the oestrogen and the anabolic effect of 19-norsteroids may add their contribution.

6. Oral contraceptives exert a number of metabolic effects in addition to those already mentioned. They include an interference with carbohydrate metabolism so that glucose tolerance is impaired, sometimes to an extent that renders difficult the proper control of diabetic patients and a stimulation of immune mechanisms that may have a detrimental effect in patients with autoimmune disease. Induction of microsomal enzymes sometimes has adverse consequences. Thus, the synthesis of haem may be stimulated to give hepatic porphyria or the skin condition known as *porphyria cutanea tarda*. Another skin condition

sometimes seen is *chloasma*, a blotchy pigmentation of the skin. It is of endocrinological origin.

Bilirubin excretion is slowed by the oral contraceptive agents, sometimes to the point of causing cholestatic jaundice.

7. While oral contraceptives are being taken, negative feedback processes inhibit the output of the follicle stimulating and luteinizing hormones (p. 738). Withdrawal of the drugs is usually followed by release of the stimulating hormones and resumption of normal menstrual activity. It occasionally happens, however, that the trophic hormones do not make their expected reappearance and amenorrhoea, possibly accompanied by galactorrhoea (p. 776) follows in the wake of contraceptive withdrawal. This *over-suppression syndrome* can be the cause of considerable distress in the woman who wishes to become pregnant. It is treated with clomiphene (p. 776) or, oddly enough, by a weak oestrogen which can stimulate the release of the trophic hormones by a positive feedback mechanism that contrasts with the negative feed back processes initiated by the stronger oestrogens that suppressed hormone release in the first place.

8. The best known, most publicized and most dangerous side effects of oral contraceptive use are those that influence the vascular system. The danger of death from deep vein thrombosis and embolic accidents is seven times greater among those who take oral contraceptive agents than it is among women who do not. Even then the risk is minimal: deaths from vascular complications among women at risk amount to no more than 1.5 and 3.9 per 100 000 woman years in the age groups 20 to 34 and 35 to 44 respectively. Moreover even these figures give an exaggerated view of the position they were collected some time ago when contraceptive preparations containing 100 μg of oestrogen were still available. These are more than three times as likely to cause thrombosis than are those containing the smaller amounts of oestrogen that are favoured today. Finally it must be remembered that although the mortality directly associated with the use of some other methods of contraception (such as condoms and diaphragms) is zero, they are much more likely to fail and so expose the woman to the dangers of pregnancy or abortion. The mortality from pregnancy or labour is of the order of 20 and 60 per 100 000 pregnancies in the age groups 20 to 34 and 35 to 44 respectively. The risks associated with abortion are even higher and the arithmetic of the situation is such as to demonstrate that the safest form of contraceptive (vasectomy apart) is the low oestrogen combined preparation. Notwithstanding these reassuring statistics, prudence still dictates that oral contraceptive agents should be avoided by those with a history of thromboembolic disease and that the vascular health of those who do take them should be carefully monitored.

Very recently a number of reports have appeared that make it clear that deaths from myocardial infarction are more likely to occur in those who take oral contraceptives regularly than in those who use other methods of birth control. Women most at risk from this complication are those in the higher age groups (30 to 45), those who have been taking oral contraceptives for a number of years and, most particularly, those who smoke cigarettes. Although the absolute number of deaths from myocardial infarction among women of child bearing age is very small it is clear that they could and should be reduced even more by making sure that those who need to take oral contraceptives are warned of the danger of indulging in practices such as cigarette smoking that markedly increase the risk of a myocardial calamity.

The vascular side effects of oral contraceptives are attributable to increases in the stickiness of platelets and in the activity of several of the coagulation factors.

Some of those who take oral contraceptives suffer an increase in blood pressure, attributable to an increase in the amount of angiotensin in the plasma. That hypertension occurs relatively rarely is explained by the feed back inhibition of renin release evoked by the angiotensin.

BENEFICIAL EFFECTS OF ORAL CONTRACEPTIVES

Many women derive physical as well as psychological benefit from their oral contraceptives. The reader will have noted that the manoeuvres employed to secure contraception by the hormonal method are identical with those used in efforts to relieve dysmenorrhoea. Thus the woman who takes oral contraceptives may be pleasantly surprised to find that her dysmenorrhoea disappears and that to the peace of mind she expected there is added the unexpected bonus of freedom from menstrual pain. Premenstrual tension and discomfort may also improve. In addition, that same stimulation of immunological processes that exacerbates autoimmune diseases sometimes ameliorates the condition of patients with rheumatoid arthritis and may even offer some protection against cancer. And, although some women develop chloasma, many more note an improvement in their skin condition while they are taking the contraceptives.

DRUG INTERACTIONS INVOLVING ORAL CONTRACEPTIVES

During the course of their reproductive life, most women will suffer from one or more illnesses, however trivial, that demand drug treatment and it is important that those who prescribe these drugs should be aware of the possibility than an interaction might occur between the new drug and any oral contraceptive that might be being taken at the same time. It is easy for even the conscientious physician to forget that he might be exposing his patient to this risk particularly if she has been using oral contraceptives without complaint for many years.

As we have had occasion to remark earlier, oral contraceptives induce hepatic microsomal enzymes and so may accelerate the metabolism of any of the many drugs that are inactivated by processes dependent on these enzymes. Similarly, the new drug may stimulate the catabolism of the contraceptive. Thus each drug may jeopardize the effectiveness of the other. The risk of an incident of this kind is clearly greater with drugs that have to be taken over a relatively prolonged period. Rifampicin (p. 848) has already achieved some notoriety as a cause of contraceptive failure and ampicillin and some other antibiotics have also come under suspicion. Anticonvulsant drugs, particularly phenobarbitone and diphenylhydantoin, may also impair the effectiveness of, or may be rendered ineffective by, oral contraceptive agents. The reader will recall that oestrogens cause fluid retention and this may still further reduce the effectiveness of anticonvulsive agents in those taking oral contraceptives. Fluid retention and angiotensin production explain why an established and successful antihypertensive regime sometimes loses its grip on the blood pressure if the patient begins to take oral contraceptives. Our earlier discussions concerning the metabolic effects of the sex hormones should render it unnecessary to explain why the control of diabetes and of endogenous depression sometimes breaks down under the influence of oral contraceptives.

CONTRAINDICATIONS TO THE USE OF ORAL CONTRACEPTIVES

A history of thromboembolic disease or any suspicion of hepatic or renal malfunction constitutes an absolute contraindication to the use of oral contraceptives. For the time being, the contraceptives should also be banned in those with hormone dependent tumours such as carcinoma of the breast. This is a sensible precaution although there is no substantial evidence that oral contraceptives really do stimulate the growth of these tumours. Indeed there is some evidence that they may have the opposite effect.

The contraceptives may have to be forbidden to patients with hypertension or epilepsy if it seems that they are likely to reduce the effectiveness of the specific drug therapy in a way that cannot be overcome by adjusting drug dosage. Prudence would indicate the advisability of supplementing the oral contraceptives by mechanical methods of birth control if their effectiveness is threatened by the necessity of taking other drugs.

OTHER FORMS OF HORMONAL CONTRACEPTION

In recent years, the steroid hormones (and some other substances) have been used to secure contraception by giving them according to dose schedules different from those that apply to the longer established preparations. Many of these newer techniques are still in the early stages of development and several of them are certainly of principal interest to those who are concerned to provide effective birth control in underdeveloped nations condemned to perpetual misery and poverty unless their rates of population increase can be checked.

A long acting oestrogen combined with a short acting strong progestogen forms the basis of 'once-a-month' contraceptives. These are taken for the first time on day 22 of a normal menstrual cycle and every 28 days thereafter regardless of the point that the cycle has then reached. The usual components of the mixture are quinestrol (2 or 5 mg) and dydrogesterone (25 mg) or quingestanol (2.5 mg). Another preparation of the same type but given by intramuscular injection is Deladroxate. It contains oestradiol oenanthate (5 mg) and algestone (dihydroxyprogesterone) acetophenide (150 mg). It is given every 28 days beginning on day 5 of a normal menstrual cycle. Even longer periods of protection can be secured by giving large intramuscular doses of progestogen only. Suitable preparations and doses include medroxyprogesterone acetate (Depo-Provera, Depo-Clinovir 150) given in doses of 150 mg every three months, and norethisterone oenanthate in doses of 200 mg every nine weeks. The long term use of these methods of contraception is not, however, generally recommended. Megestrol acetate (115 mg) in small Silastic capsules has been deposited subcutaneously to provide effective contraception for periods of a year or longer but this drug is no longer used. Long term protection can also be secured by incorporating progestogen into Silastic rings or other devices implanted into the vagina or uterus. The possibility of achieving fertility control by immunising women against the luteinizing hormone or its releasing factor is now being actively explored. Other antigens that are involved in fertilization processes or in the maintenance of pregnancy and which might be susceptible to attack by antibodies include spermatozoal enzymes and components of the ovum or of the early placenta (Editorial, 1975).

The postcoital contraceptive (less delicately known as the 'morning-after pill') aims to prevent implantation of the ovum should it have been fertilized some hours previously. Norethisterone (Primolut N) in a single 5 mg dose or large doses of a strong oestrogen (stilboestrol 50 mg or ethinyloestradiol 5 mg) taken daily for 5 days have been used for this purpose. They induce endometrial changes inimical to implantation and the oestrogens also have a luteolytic action (p. 373). Postcoital contraceptives are intended only for emergency use. They can, for instance, be given to rape victims.

Some substances are capable of preventing the further development of the fertilized ovum even after implantation has occurred. They are known as interceptives although they would be more honestly described as abortifacients. The ergot alkaloids have some activity but the compounds that show most promise of developing into useful interceptives are the prostaglandins or their analogues.

The possibility that oral contraceptives for men will eventually make their appearance has been discussed earlier in this chapter (p. 738).

STANDARDIZATION AND ASSAY OF THE SEX HORMONES

A number of methods are available for the assay of the sex hormones.

Androgens
CAPON'S COMB METHOD
Male birds are castrated by the removal of both testes so that the comb does not grow in size. The length and height, or the area, of the comb are measured. The androgen is injected into the pectoral muscles and the final size of the comb is noted. The effect of the unknown is compared with that of the standard preparation. This can be done in two ways.

a. Several groups of five capons are used and a dose response curve is constructed by giving each group a different dose of androgen. The unknown is given to a group of five birds and its potency is calculated from the dose-response curve.

b. A comparison is made between the responses to two doses of the standard and two of the unknown. This enables the potency of the unknown to be calculated by a four-point assay technique (p. 134).

RAT SEMINAL VESICLE TEST
The response used is the increase in weight of the prostate glands and seminal vesicles of the young castrated rat. The assay is conducted in the same general fashion as that used in the capon's comb method.

ESTIMATION OF THE ANDROGENIC/ANABOLIC RATIO
The method usually employed is due to Hershberger and his colleagues. Two groups of male rats are castrated. The drug under investigation is injected into the animals of one group. The other group is used for control purposes. The prostate glands and levator ani muscles are removed from the animals in both groups. The increase in weight of the prostate glands in the drug-treated animals is an index of androgenic activity and the increase in weight of the levator ani muscles is an index of anabolic potency.

Oestrogens
Two standards are in use; these are oestrone and oestradiol monobenzoate. The international unit of each is the oestrus-inducing activity in 0.0001 mg of the standard preparation.

THE ALLEN-DOISEY TEST
This is also known as the vaginal smear or oestrus test. In spayed female rats or mice the vaginal smear contains numerous leucocytes, together with a few nucleated and some squamous (cornified) cells. Following treatment with oestrogens the vaginal smear consists predominantly of large, non-nucleated squamous cells but very few

leucocytes are present. Similar changes are seen during oestrus in the normal animal.

The test is carried out using a large group (40 or 50) of animals and the vaginal smears are examined for the presence of squamous cells and leucocytes. The dose of standard is varied and a dose-response curve is constructed in which the percentage of animals which go into oestrus is plotted against the dose administered. This method gives a measure of the potency of the unknown in terms of the standard but the results depend a great deal on the technique and criteria adopted by the individual worker.

METHOD OF BÜLBRING AND BURN

In castrated female rats the uterus does not develop but one injection of oestrogen will cause it to increase in size and weight and this is made the basis of the assay method.

Progestogens

The international unit of progestational activity is that which is contained in 1 mg of progesterone.

METHOD OF CLAUBERG AND McPHAIL

In this method, sexually immature female rabbits are used. Oestrus is induced by a course of injections of an oestrogen and the oestrogen-sensitized uterus is brought into the progestational phase by injections of the progestogen. Two groups of rabbits are used; one group receives the standard (progesterone), the other the unknown. Histological examination of the uteri of the members of each group shows the characteristic proliferative changes which take place in the endometrium. These are classified according to a scale and a comparison of the potencies of the two substances can then be made.

OTHER METHODS

a. Progestogens cause the carbonic anhydrase activity of the rabbit endometrium to rise. This can be used as a method of comparing the potency of synthetic progestogens.

b. If the ovaries are removed from pregnant rats, abortion follows. A method of assessing progestational activity in synthetic progestogens is to ovariectomize pregnant rats on the tenth day of pregnancy. The progestogen is then given until the twenty-first day and the extent to which the compound under test prevents abortion can be compared with that which results from administration of a progestogen of proved activity.

BIBLIOGRAPHY

Books, monographs and reviews

Briggs, M. H. and Briggs, Maxine (1976). *Biochemical Contraception. Prospects for Human Development.* London, New York, San Francisco: Academic Press.

Brotherton, J. (1976). *Sex Hormone Pharmacology.* London, New York, San Francisco: Academic Press.

Camerino, B. and Sala, G. (1960). Anabolic steroids. *Prog. Drug Res.,* **2,** 71-134.

Fullerton, H. W. and Girdwood, R. H. (1966). Disorders of the Blood. In *Textbook of Medical Treatment,* 10th ed., pp. 456-518. Ed. Dunlop, Sir D. and Alstead, S. Edinburgh: Livingstone.

Hempel, E. and Klinger, W. (1976). Drug stimulated biotransformation of hormonal steroid contraceptives: clinical implications. *Drugs,* **12,** 442-448.

Jackson, H. (1959). Antifertility substances, *Pharmac. Rev.,* **11,** 135-172.

Pincus, G. (1959). Progestational agents and the control of fertility. *Vitams Horm.,* **17,** 307-324.

Pincus, G. (1965). *The Control of Fertility.* New York and London: Academic Press.

Short, R. V. and Baird, D. T. (eds.) (1976). Discussion on contraceptives of the future. *Proc. R. Soc. Lond. B.* 1-224.

Thomson, J. A. (1976). *An Introduction to Clinical Endocrinology.* Edinburgh and London: Churchill Livingstone.

Tyler, E. T. (1967). Antifertility agents. *A Rev. Pharmac.,* **7,** 381-298.

Original papers

Aznar Ramos, R., Giner-Valasquez, J., Lara-Ricalde, R. and Martinez-Manau. J. (1969). Incidence of side effects with contraceptive placebo. *Am. J. Obstet. Gynec.,* **105,** 1144-1145.

Bolton, C. H., Hampton, J. R. and Mitchell, J. R. A. (1968). Effect of oral contraceptive agents on platelets and plasma-phospholipids. *Lancet,* **2,** 1336-1341.

Coppola, J. R. and Siadarini, R. J. (1974). A new orally active male anti-fertility agent. *Contraception.* **8,** 207-217.

Editorial (1975). Immunological control of fertility. *Lancet,* **1,** 1018-1019.

Freed, D. L. J. and Banks, A. J. (1975). A double-blind cross-over trial of Methandienone (Dianabol) in moderate dosage on highly trained experienced athletes. *Br. J. sports Med.* **9,** 78-81.

Hervey, G. R., Hutchinson, I., Knibbs, A. V., Burkinshaw, L., Jones, P. R. M., Norgan, H. G. and Levell, M. J. (1976). Anabolic effects of methandienone in men undergoing athletic training. *Lancet,* **2,** 699-702.

Medical Research Council (1967). Rise of thromboembolic disease in women taking oral contraceptives *Br. med. J.,* **2,** 355-359.

Report (1977). Natural and synthetic oestrogens in the female climacteric. *Practitioner.* **218,** 573-579.

Vessey, M. P. and Weatherall, Josephine (1968). Venous thromboembolic disease and the use of oral contraceptives. *Lancet,* **2,** 94-96.

44. The adrenocortical steroids

Unlike its medulla, the cortex of the adrenal gland is essential for life. Through hormonal secretions, it controls or influences a variety of vital activities including salt and water balance (and hence the control of blood volume and blood pressure) and the metabolism of carbohydrate, fat and protein. It is intimately involved in the operation of the processes that enable the body to resist infection and stress and it has some effect on sexual function. As a consequence of these multifarious activities the adrenal cortex has important interrelationships with many tissues and organs.

The hormones of the adrenal cortex are steroidal in nature. More than thirty steroids have been isolated from extracts of the mammalian cortex but (apart from the sex hormones) only three of these—hydrocortisone (cortisol), corticosterone and aldosterone—can be detected in physiologically active quantities in adrenal venous blood. These three corticosteroids are, therefore, the only ones which can justifiably be described as cortical hormones: the others are presumably precursors or breakdown products of the hormones proper. In man, cortisol is the most abundant adrenocortical hormone but the relative amounts of the three hormones varies widely among different mammalian species.

The adrenocortical steroids are, like all other steroids, based on the cyclopentanoperhydrophenanthrene ring (p.

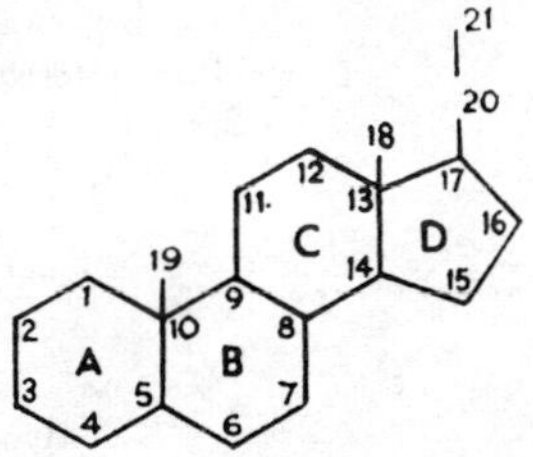

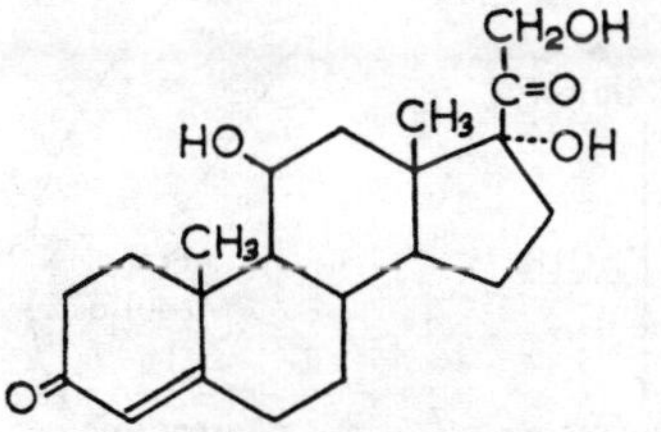

Hydrocortisone (cortisol, 17-hydroxycorticosterone)

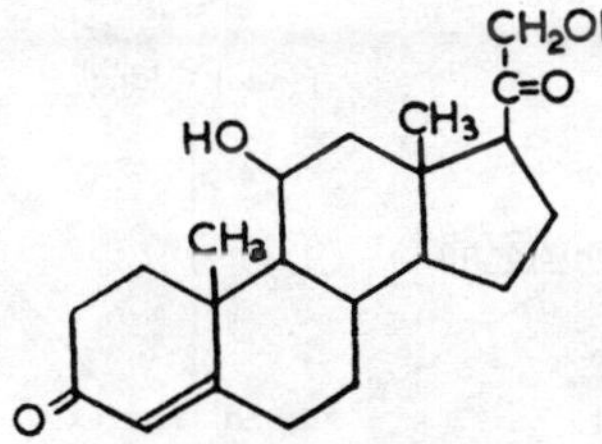

Corticosterone

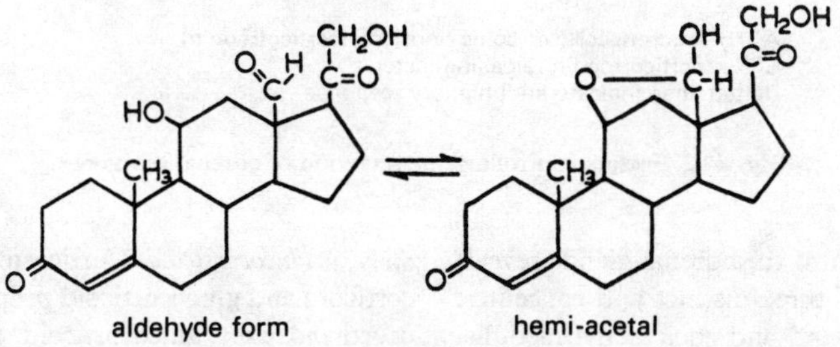

aldehyde form

hemi-acetal

Aldosterone

Fig. 44.1 The adrenocortical hormones.

753

733). All bear a two carbon side chain at position C17 (Fig. 44.1) so that they have 21 carbon atoms in their molecules in contrast to the oestrogens and androgens which possess 18 and 19 carbon atoms respectively. The side chain always includes a ketol grouping at position C20, which confers reducing properties on the molecule. A third characteristic feature of the adrenocortical steroids is the presence of an oxygen atom on carbon atom 3 and a double bond between C4 and C5: together these are described as the $\Delta^4$3-ketone grouping. The Δ symbol signifies a double bond.

Progesterone, androgens and oestrogens are produced in the adrenal cortex. Progesterone is a key intermediary in the synthesis of the adrenocortical hormones and the occurrence of the other sex hormones may be an incidental consequence of this. They are of no more than minor importance in the control of normal sexual functions although the adrenal androgens are said to regulate the growth of body hair in women and the oestrogens may be secreted in sufficient quantity to provoke the development, and maintain the growth, of carcinoma of the breast in women whose main source of oestrogens (the ovaries) has been removed. Overactivity of the adrenal cortex may also cause masculinization (virilism) in females and, less often, feminization in males.

adjoins the medulla is the *zona reticularis*. Aldosterone is elaborated only in the zona glomerulosa, the other two hormones are both formed in the other zones. Removal of the pituitary gland causes atrophy of the zonae fasciculata and reticularis but the zona glomerulosa is spared and aldosterone production is not interrupted. Thus the secretion of hydrocortisone and corticosterone is completely under pituitary control. This control is exerted by corticotrophin (the adrenocorticotrophic hormone, ACTH), which is secreted by the anterior pituitary gland (Fig. 44.2). Although the contrary view was held for many years, it is now known that corticotrophin influences aldosterone secretion (Ganong, Biglieri and Mulrow, 1966). but much the most important factor controlling aldosterone release is the renin-angiotensin system (p. 357).

The three adrenocortical hormones have some common properties and actions and as far as their physiological functions are concerned it is likely that they all participate to varying degrees in all the recognized actions of the adrenal cortex. Nevertheless, the control of salt and water metabolism is largely invested in aldosterone which is therefore called a *mineralocorticoid*. Cortisol is particularly concerned in the control of carbohydrate metabolism and other metabolic systems and it is called, not very appropri-

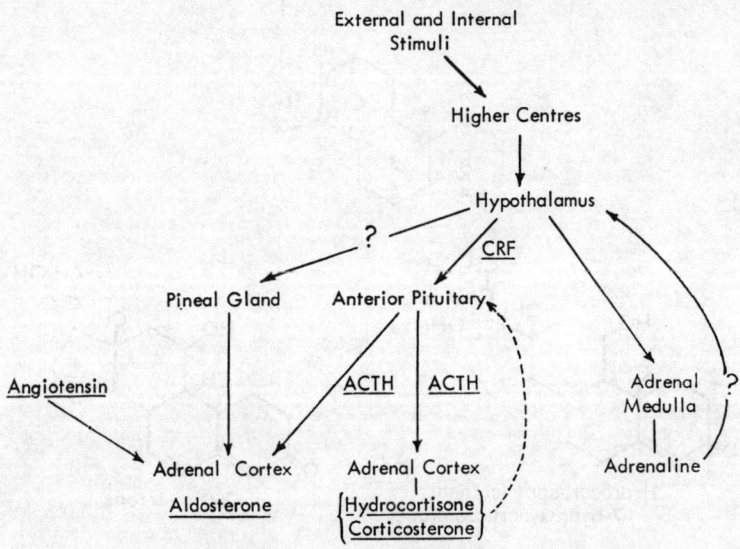

ACTH = adrenocorticotrophic hormone (corticotrophin)
CRF = corticotrophin releasing factor
Dotted lines indicate an inhibitory response

Fig. 44.2 Factors controlling the secretion of adrenal hormones.

Histological examination of the adrenal glands reveals that the cortex consists of three distinct and concentric cellular areas which surround and enclose the medulla. The outermost part of the cortex is the *zona glomerulosa*, the middle zone is the *zona fasciculata* and that which

ately, a *glucocorticoid*. Corticosterone has both mineralocorticoid and glucocorticoid properties. Because mineralocorticoid and glucocorticoid actions are fundamentally different, and to some extent antagonistic, a great deal of energy has been expended in efforts to achieve a complete separation of these activities in synthetic derivatives. The properties and uses of the individual synthetic compounds are detailed later.

PHARMACOLOGICAL ACTIONS OF THE GLUCOCORTICOIDS AND THE MINERALOCORTICOIDS

The following account relates to both the naturally occurring and the synthetic adrenocortical steroids. Some of these actions reproduce or caricature the physiological actions of the adrenal hormones but the others do not necessarily reflect any of the hormones' normal functions: they are only seen after the administration of large therapeutic doses of the steroids or in conditions in which the glands are over-active to a pathological degree.

The *glucocorticoids* have a number of actions. They

   a. promote gluconeogenesis (the formation of glucose from protein), increase the deposition of glycogen in the liver and inhibit the utilization of glucose, as a result of an anti-insulin action.

   b. increase the breakdown of protein. The amino acids so produced are available to support the accelerated gluconeogenesis already referred to.

   c. increase the mobilization of fat and stimulate its synthesis and storage.

   d. increase the glomerular filtration rate as a result of causing some increase in blood pressure. The urinary excretion of uric acid is increased but that of creatinine is unaffected. The effect on blood pressure is attributable partly to a sensitization of the arterioles to noradrenaline and partly to an increased production of angiotensinogen but the overall hypertensive action of the glucocorticoids is smaller than that of the mineralocorticoids.

   e. increase calcium excretion. This effect, together with the glucocorticoids' tendency to stimulate the breakdown of the protein matrix of bone may lead to osteoporosis.

   f. depress the production of eosinophils and lymphocytes but stimulate erythropoiesis and the production of polymorphonuclear leucocytes. They inhibit antibody formation and depress the response of the tissues to inflammation.

   g. stimulate the secretion of the several components of gastric juice.

   h. may have actions on the psyche: the production of a euphoric state is not unusual.

   i. suppress the output of corticotrophin by the pituitary gland. This is a reflection of the fact that the secretion of the pituitary hormone is reciprocally related to the concentration of the glucocorticoids in blood.

The variety of actions exhibited by these compounds explains the comment made earlier that the description 'glucocorticoid' is not entirely appropriate. It is nevertheless true that the principal effects of the glucocorticoids are those which influence carbohydrate metabolism. From the clinical point of view the antiinflammatory action of the glucocorticoids is of considerable importance. In some of the synthetic compounds high antiinflammatory potency

is associated with only moderate glucocorticoid activity, but there seems to be little doubt that the two types of activity are inseparable. The origin of the antiinflammatory activity of the glucocorticoids is discussed elsewhere (p. 453).

Mineralocorticoids. The actions of the mineralocorticoids are much more circumscribed than those of the glucocorticoids. They operate at the level of the cell membrane, stimulating the passage of sodium into, and of potassium out of, the cells. This is most evident in the kidney where ion exchange proceeds rapidly, but mineralocorticoids also reduce the loss of sodium in the saliva and sweat as well as in the urine. As a result of their causing sodium retention, physiological quantities of the mineralocorticoids maintain, and larger quantities elevate, the blood pressure.

STRESS AND THE ADRENAL CORTEX: THE GENERAL ADAPTATION SYNDROME

When an animal is exposed to stress (such as might be produced, for example, by physical injury, infection, irradiation or fatigue), it responds in a characteristic fashion. There is a specific local response at the site of stress (if this is localized) and a general non-specific response. The local response varies according to the nature of the stress but the generalized response is always the same. Selye has called the latter the *general adaptation syndrome,* which he sees as being divided into three successive phases—the 'alarm' (immediate) reaction, the stage of resistance and the stage of exhaustion. The last named stage only appears if the stress is sufficiently intense or prolonged to exhaust the physiological mechanisms responsible for initiating and maintaining the process of resistance.

In a stress situation, impulses from the stressed region reach the hypothalamus and call forth the secretion of the corticoids provide by their actions the means of resistance and they assist the body's return to its normal state. Failure of the adaptation syndrome is held to lead to *diseases of adaptation,* some of which are enumerated later (p. 767). As so often happens with new ideas, Selye's views were at first embraced too eagerly and indiscriminately, to their detriment, by many who now disown them. It remains a fact that, whatever their origin may prove to be, many of the so-called diseases of adaptation do respond, and some of them dramatically so, to treatment with glucocorticoids.

The place of adrenaline in supporting general adaptation responses is not clear. Some maintain that it facilitates the release of corticotrophin but this is disputed.

METABOLISM OF THE ADRENOCORTICAL HORMONES

The possible pathways of synthesis of the adrenocortical

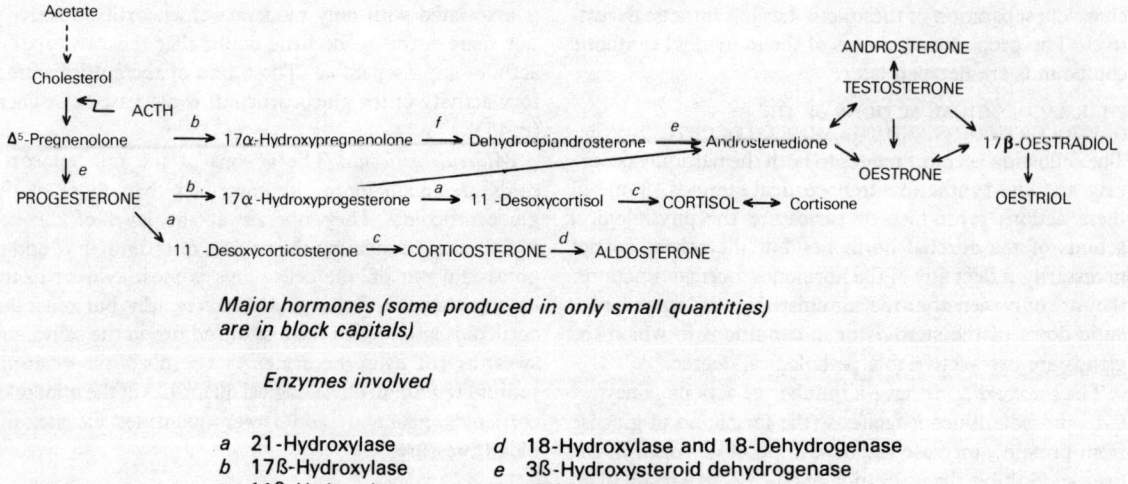

Acetate

Cholesterol

ACTH

Δ^5-Pregnenolone $\xrightarrow{\quad b \quad}$ 17α-Hydroxypregnenolone $\xrightarrow{\quad f \quad}$ Dehydroepiandrosterone $\xrightarrow{\quad e \quad}$ Androstenedione

PROGESTERONE $\xrightarrow{\quad b \quad}$ 17α-Hydroxyprogesterone $\xrightarrow{\quad a \quad}$ 11-Desoxycortisol $\xrightarrow{\quad c \quad}$ CORTISOL $\longleftrightarrow$ Cortisone

11-Desoxycorticosterone $\xrightarrow{\quad c \quad}$ CORTICOSTERONE $\xrightarrow{\quad d \quad}$ ALDOSTERONE

ANDROSTERONE
TESTOSTERONE
17β-OESTRADIOL
OESTRONE
OESTRIOL

Major hormones (some produced in only small quantities) are in block capitals)

Enzymes involved

a   21-Hydroxylase   d   18-Hydroxylase and 18-Dehydrogenase
b   17ß-Hydroxylase   e   3ß-Hydroxysteroid dehydrogenase
c   11ß-Hydroxylase   f   17,20-desmolase

Fig. 44.3 Hormone synthesis in the adrenal cortex.

hormones can be studied by adding potential precursors to the medium perfusing an isolated adrenal gland and identifying the steroids appearing in the gland and the perfusate. Of the synthetic pathways which have been so identified, those which seem to be the most important in the intact animal are indicated in Figure 44.3. By referring to the formula of progesterone (p. 744) and those of the adrenocortical and sex hormones given in this and the preceding chapter, the interested reader will be able to appreciate the nature of the intermediate steps in the synthesis. The important detail to remember is that, by whichever pathway the individual hormones are synthesized, the following changes in the progesterone molecule have to be brought about:

a. hydroxylation of the carbon atom C11.

b. hydroxylation of the terminal carbon atom C21 on the side chain.

These transformations produce corticosterone. The additional change required for the other two hormones is ß-hydroxylation at C17 (for hydrocortisone) or the attachment of an aldehyde (-CHO) group to C13 (for aldosterone).

The adrenal gland has no storage capacity, so that demands for additional supplies of adrenocortical hormones can only be met by an immediate increase in the rate of synthesis. Such demands are mediated by corticotrophin (ACTH) which itself stimulates synthesis by accelerating the conversion of cholesterol to progesterone. It may also act at other points in the synthetic pathway.

Up to 75 per cent of the cortisol released into the plasma is bound to a specific α-globulin (*cortisol binding globulin* or *transcortin*) and up to 25 per cent unites with albumin. Under normal circumstances, no more than 5 per cent is present in the free, physiologically active form. Aldoster-

one is bound to albumin to the extent of about 50 per cent of the total plasma content, the rest appearing in the unbound form.

Cortisol is metabolized principally in the liver where it suffers saturation of the double bond at C4-5 and conversion of the oxygen at C3 into an α-hydroxy group. Because these transformations involve the introduction of four hydrogen atoms into the molecule, the resulting metabolite is called tetrahydrocortisol. Cortisone, although it has some hormonal activities and occurs, in equilibrium with cortisol, in several tissues, can be regarded as a metabolite of cortisone. It, too, is degraded into a tetrahydro compound. Some of the tetrahydro compounds lose the two-carbon side chains on C17 and these are replaced by oxygen to give 17-oxosteroids.

A proportion of the cortisol and cortisone undergoes reduction at C20 (the carbonyl group is converted into >CHOH) before conversion to the tetrahydro derivatives. The compound finally produced in this way from cortisol is a cortol (because it carries an 11ß-hydroxy group) while that derived from cortisone (which has an 11-oxo group) is a cortolone. Very small amounts of cortisol are excreted in an unchanged form.

About 60 per cent of the cortisone that is secreted under normal circumstances appears in the urine as tetrahydrocortisol and tetrahydrocortisone, a further 25 per cent as the corresponding cortol and cortolone and 10 per cent as 17-oxosteroids. All these compounds are excreted as glucuronides, the conjugation occurring at position C3. The group of substances can be measured as a whole by a method (periodate oxidation) that results in the conversion of them all into 17-oxosteroids. The parent compounds are known as 17-oxogenic compounds.

An alternative way of assessing cortisol metabolism

makes use of the Porter-Silber reagent (phenylhydrazine in sulphuric acid) which reacts with the dihydroxyacetone side chain on the C17 atom of steroid molecules to give coloured compounds. However—and for obvious reasons—this method does not measure cortols and cortolones.

Nomenclature can become confused and confusing at this point and the reader should distinguish carefully (even if some authors do not) between the 17-oxosteroids (which have lost carbon atoms 20 and 21) and the 17-hydroxycorticosteroids. Only the latter group of substances (the *Porter-Silber chromogens*) are estimated by the Porter-Silber method.

In individuals whose adrenocortical activity is not grossly deranged, 17-oxogenic steroids are excreted at a rate that indicates the rate of cortisol secretion. However, if it is secreted in abnormally large quantities (as happens, for instance, in Cushing's syndrome) some of the hormone is metabolized along pathways that do not yield 17-oxogenic steroids. Under these circumstances, 17-oxosteroid excretion no longer reflects hormone secretion rates.

The amount of unchanged cortisol in the urine amounts to no more than one or two per cent of that of its metabolites but it changes in parallel with the unbound hormone in the plasma. Since only this free cortisol can exert a physiological action, measurement of 'urinary free cortisol' is a potentially valuable method of assessing adrenocortical secretion, particularly when this is high enough to result in saturation of the transcortin so that a higher than usual proportion of the secreted cortisol remains in the unbound state. The success of corticotrophin treatment can be evaluated in this way.

Like cortisol, aldosterone is metabolized principally to the tetrahydro derivative but only a small proportion of this (say 5 per cent) is further transformed into the 3-oxo compounds.

METYRAPONE

It has been pointed out that an essential step in the production of the adrenocortical hormones is the introduction of a hydroxyl group at position C11. This grouping, which is invariably orientated in the β position, is incorporated in the molecule under the influence of the enzyme 11β-hydroxylase (Fig. 44.3). This enzyme is inhibited by metyrapone (Metopirone, SU-4885) which therefore suppresses the synthesis of the hormones. Metyrapone has been used in a test for pituitary function. Since it prevents

Metyrapone

synthesis of the adrenocortical hormone, it should evoke an increased output of corticotrophin and hence lead to an accumulation of hormone precursors (11-desoxycorticosterone and 11-desoxycortisol, Fig. 44.3) and their metabolites in plasma and urine. Thus, if metyrapone administration is not followed by an increase in the urinary excretion of 17-oxogenic steroids it can be concluded that the pituitary is not responding to its normal physiological stimuli. It should hardly be necessary to add that the metyrapone test can only be applied to individuals whose adrenal cortex is known to be responsive to corticotrophin.

In the past metyrapone has been employed in the treatment of hyperaldosteronism but the drug is unpleasant to take (it frequently causes nausea) and is not devoid of toxicity so that it is now rarely used for therapeutic purposes and its popularity as a diagnostic tool is also waning.

DISORDERS OF ADRENOCORTICAL FUNCTION

A number of conditions caused by over- or underactivity of the adrenal cortex are recognized. They are briefly described here.

Disorders caused by impaired adrenocortical activity

The signs and symptoms of adrenocortical insufficiency in man serve to illustrate the physiological role of the cortical hormones by drawing attention to the consequences of their absence.

ADDISON'S DISEASE (PRIMARY HYPOADRENALISM)

In this condition, destructive or degenerative processes affect all zones of the cortex. Addison's disease may be the result of tuberculosis or a tumour but very often no obvious cause can be found: in many such instances particularly in women the disease is of autoimmune origin. In Addison's disease, there is weakness, loss of weight, vomiting and a dark brown pigmentation of the skin. Sodium excretion is increased but potassium is retained. The loss of sodium leads to dehydration with haemoconcentration, hypotension and an impairment of kidney function so that there is an accumulation of urea and nonprotein nitrogen in the blood. Patients suffering from Addison's disease are highly susceptible to the effects of infection, exertion and other forms of stress. The origin of the skin pigmentation is interesting. Lack of adrenocortical hormones evokes an increased secretion of corticotrophin. This cannot, of course, exert any action on an adrenal cortex whose function is lost but corticotrophin has structural resemblances to the melanocyte stimulating hormone of the anterior pituitary and it is possible that in the quantities in which it appears in Addison's disease, corticotrophin adds its own contribution to the skin darkening action of the melanocyte stimulating hormone. All the other findings in Addison's disease are attributable to a lack of the adrenocortical hormones.

Cases of Addison's disease of autoimmune origin may display the stigmata of other autoimmune conditions particularly thyroid disease, pernicious anaemia and diabetes mellitus.

ACUTE ADRENAL INSUFFICIENCY
If a subject whose adrenocortical activity is only marginally adequate is exposed to a sudden stress, there may be a complete failure of cortical function with the development of a state of shock. The same situation may arise if drugs are suddenly withdrawn from patients who have been treated with glucocorticoids for rheumatic or other conditions. These drugs suppress adrenocortical activity—because they inhibit the secretion of corticotrophin—and their withdrawal leaves the patient with no cortical hormone at all apart from aldosterone.

PITUITARY FAILURE
In this condition, corticotrophin output fails because of the breakdown in pituitary function. Aldosterone output is unaffected and the skin does not become pigmented. Otherwise the clinical picture is similar to that of Addison's disease with the added complication that there is failure of the other endocrine organs normally under pituitary control.

Disorders caused by overactivity of the adrenal cortex
The signs and symptoms of syndromes referable to adrenocortical overactivity serve to underline the pharmacological actions of the adrenocortical steroids.

CUSHING'S SYNDROME
Cushing's syndrome is the result of an excessive secretion of glucocorticoids. The adrenal overactivity is sometimes provoked by tumours within the substance of the cortex itself but in 80 per cent of cases it is the result of an excessively high rate of corticotrophin secretion engendered by tumours or other pathological changes in the pituitary gland or the hypothalamus. Occasionally, the corticotrophin emanates from tumours located in tissues other than those of the hypothalamo-pituitary axis. Cushing's syndrome is sometimes of iatrogenic origin, the result of overenthusiastic medication with adrenocortical hormones. In Cushing's syndrome carbohydrate metabolism is disturbed and this may lead to exhaustion of the body's supply of insulin and the development of diabetes. Protein breakdown (together with the loss of potassium caused by the mineralocorticoid activity of the glucocorticoid) causes the skeletal muscles (particularly those in the proximal parts of the limbs) to become weak and wasted but there is also obesity, the face and abdomen being particularly affected. The characteristically fattened features give rise to the description 'moon faced'. Loss of calcium from the bones and disappearance of the protein matrix leads to oesteoporosis. The thickness of the skin is much reduced and there is a tendency to spontaneous subcutaneous haemorrhages. Females may develop amenorrhoea and the increased secretion of adrenal androgens may cause excessive growth of body hair and other signs of virilism. Eosinophils and lymphocytes decrease in number, blood pressure and the erythrocyte count may increase.

ALDOSTERONISM (HYPERALDOSTERONISM)
An increased secretion of aldosterone may have its origin in the adrenal cortex itself (*primary aldosteronism*) or it may be associated with conditions such as cardiac failure or nephrosis, which indirectly stimulate secretion of the mineralocorticoid *(secondary aldosteronism)*. The pathognomonic feature of secondary aldosteronism is oedema: it is discussed in detail elsewhere (p. 621). In primary aldosteronism there is loss of potassium and retention of sodium. The blood pressure rises and the loss of potassium causes muscle weakness, though this is not as serious as it is in Cushing's syndrome since protein breakdown is not excessive.

ADRENAL VIRILISM
Adrenal tumours often result in an excessive secretion of all the adrenocortical hormones so that a classical Cushing's syndrome appears. Sometimes, however, the secretory overactivity is confined to the adrenal androgens (less often, the oestrogens) and the resulting condition is the *adrenogenital syndrome*. Adrogens have anabolic properties so that children who develop the adrenogenital syndrome grow rapidly and show a considerable degree of muscular development, earning them the description 'infant Hercules'. The voice deepens and in boys the secondary sex characteristics develop prematurely. The testes, however, remain undeveloped because secretion of pituitary gonadotrophin is prevented by reason of the high concentration of androgens in the blood. In girls, virilism occurs: the clitoris enlarges and the muscular body displays a male distribution of pubic hair. Similar effects are seen in adult women in whom, in addition, ovarian activity is suppressed. If oestrogen output is increased it may cause breast development in males.

CONGENITAL ADRENAL HYPERPLASIA
Congenital metabolic defects can afflict several of the enzymes that are involved in the synthesis of the adrenocortical hormones. The enzyme deficiencies result in adrenal hyperplasia but the enhanced activity of the adrenal cortex does not necessarily extend to its androgen synthesizing system. Whether it does (and, therefore, whether virilization occurs) is determined by the function of the specific enzyme whose deficiency occasioned the hyperplasia in the first place. The discussions elaborated in

the following paragraphs will be more intelligible if frequent references are made to Figure 44.3 (p. 756).

The most common variety of congenital adrenal hyperplasia is that resulting from loss of 21β-hydroxylase activity (Enzyme *a* in Fig. 44.3). The synthesis of cortisol is depressed and this provokes an increased secretion of corticotrophin. The adrenal cortex is thereby stimulated into increased synthetic activity, androgen production rises and virilism results. In some cases the increased drive exerted by corticotrophin stimulates the glucocorticoid synthesizing system to such good effect that the block imposed by the enzyme deficiency is overcome. In more severe cases, this does not occur and the picture is then one of androgen excess and cortisol deficiency. Aldosterone production also includes a 21-hydroxylating step and in severe cases of enzyme deficiency its synthesis becomes compromised to the extent of causing salt loss and hypotension. In less severe cases, aldosterone production, like that of cortisol, will be maintained, or even enhanced, by the concerted action of corticotrophin and plasma renin.

the discussions in the preceding paragraphs (these are summarized in Table 44.1) the interested reader should be able to decide for himself what will be the likely consequences of these rarer defects.

So far as sexual development is concerned, the effects of congenital adrenal hyperplasia with overproduction of androgens are similar to those of the adrenogenital syndrome. However, since the condition is of congenital origin, its effects are likely to make their appearance before birth and girls may be born with external genitalia so like those of a male child that they are mistaken for, and brought up as, boys.

INDIVIDUAL CORTICOSTEROIDS

The names and formulae of some of the naturally occurring and synthetic corticosteroids are set out in Table 44.2. It will be seen that most of the synthetic compounds are glucocorticoids with little or no mineralocorticoid activity.

Table 44.1 Congenital defects of adrenocortical hormone synthesis

Enzyme deficiency		Androgen synthesis	Cortisol synthesis	Aldosterone synthesis	Blood pressure
			[0 = no change; + = increase; − = decrease]		
21β-Hydroxylase	Compensated	+	0	0	0
	Uncompensated	+	−	−	−
17β-Hydroxylase	Compensated	0	0	+	+
	Uncompensated	−	−	+	+
11β-Hydroxylase	Compensated	+	0	0	0
	Uncompensated	+	−	−	+

If there is a deficiency of 17β-hydroxylase (Enzyme *b*) the synthesis of both androgens and cortisol will be threatened but the aldosterone synthesis pathway will remain clear. Corticotrophin output will rise and this may or may not be sufficient to restore androgen and glucocorticoid production. In either event, aldosterone synthesis will be boosted with hypertension as a likely consequence. It is clear that virilism will not occur.

A deficiency of 11β-hydroxylase (Enzyme *c*) inhibits the synthesis of both cortisol and aldosterone with the usual consequence for corticotrophin secretion. Androgen synthesis will be stimulated to the point of causing virilism and if the enzyme deficiency is not compensated for by the enhanced output of corticotrophin, desoxycorticosterone will accumulate. This may be sufficient to cause hypertension notwithstanding the lack of aldosterone.

Deficiencies of some of the other enzymes involved in the synthesis of the adrenocortical hormones (18-dehydrogenase and 3β-hydroxysteroid dehydrogenase; enzymes *d* and *e* respectively) occur rarely. In the light of

Most effort has been directed towards the production of this type of corticosteroid because it is glucocorticoid activity which is made use of in the non-specific treatment of the many so-called 'diseases of adaptation'. The drugs have to be given in large doses. As a result, those which possess even a small degree of mineralocorticoid activity are likely to cause retention of sodium and water and the production of an unwelcome hypertension.

As can be seen by reference to the formulae in Table 44.2, only minor structural differences exist among the different corticosteroids. These differences, and their consequences, are summarized in the course of the account which follows.

A double bond linking carbon atoms 4 and 5 and an oxygen atom on C3 are essential prerequisites for hormonal activity so that the tetrahydro derivatives discussed earlier (p. 756) are physiologically inactive. Cortisone differs from cortisol only in respect of the substituents on carbon atom 11: in cortisone it is an oxygen atom, in cortisol it is a hydroxyl group. The properties and uses of

Table 44.2 Some naturally occurring and synthetic corticosteroids

Compound	Formula	Proprietary name(s)	Remarks	Dose Equivalent (Dose needed to produce the same glucocorticoid effect as 50 mg of cortisone)
		ADRENAL HORMONES		
Aldosterone Electrocortin	see text (p. 753).	Aldocorten;	Mineralocorticoid	Not used clinically
Hydrocortisone (Cortisol)		Cobadex; Cortef; Cortifoam; Cortril; Ef-Cortelan; Genacort; Hydrocortistab; Hydro-Cortisyl; Hycortole; Hydrocortone; Pabracort.	Glucocorticoid	40 mg

(The sodium succinate is known as Corland and Solu-Cortef and the hydrochloride of the 21-diethylaminoacetate of hydrocortisone as Magnacort)

Corticosterone				Not used clinically

COMPOUNDS THAT OCCUR IN SMALL AMOUNTS IN ADRENAL VENOUS BLOOD

Cortisone (acetate)		Cortate; Cortelan; Cortistab; Cortisyl; Cortogen; Cortone;	Glucocorticoid; compound of choice for maintenance therapy in Addison's disease (Dose 25-35 mg)	50 mg
(11)-Desoxycorticosterone acetate (Deoxycortone)		Decortacetate; Decosterone; DOCA; Percorten	Mineralocorticoid	—

Table 44.2 Some naturally occurring and synthetic corticosteroids—contd.

Compound	Formula	Proprietary name(s)	Remarks	Dose Equivalent (Dose needed to produce the same glucocorticoid effect as 50 mg of cortisone)

SYNTHETIC COMPOUNDS

The ending '-onide' indicates that the compound is an acetonide. The hydrogen atom at C14 is indicated only when it takes the α configuration (p. 732).

Fludrocortisone		Florinef; F-cortef.	Some glucocorticoid activity but used only as a mineralocorticoid	—

CH$_2$OH
C=O
CH$_3$ ···OH
HO
CH$_3$
F
O

Halcinonide		Halciderm	Used locally in an 0.1 per cent cream for steroid-responsive dermatological conditions

CH$_2$Cl
CO
CH$_3$ ----OH
HO
----OH
CH$_3$
F
O

Prednisone (Δ'-Cortisone) Metacortandracin		DeCortisyl; Deltacortone Deltasone; Di-Adreson; Meticorten; Paracort; Ultracorten	Glucocorticoid with only small amounts of mineralocorticoid activity 10 mg

CH$_2$OH
C=O
CH$_3$ ···OH
O
CH$_3$
O

Chloroprednisone has a chlorine atom at C6. It is used topically

Prednisolone (Δ'-Cortisol) Metacortandrolone		Codelcortone; Delta Cortef; Deltacortril; Delta-Genacort; Delta-stab; Meticortelone; Metiderm; Paracortol; Pre Cortisyl; Sterane; Ultracorten-H	Glucocorticoid with only small amount of mineralocorticoid activity 10 mg

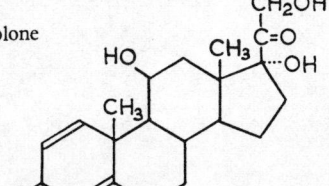

CH$_2$OH
C=O
CH$_3$ ···OH
HO
CH$_3$
O

(Prednisolone stearoylglycolate is known as Sintisone. Its dose equivalent is 13 mg)
(Prednisolone acetate is known as Prednelan or Sterane and the disodium phosphate as Hydeltrasol or Predsol.)

Table 44.2 Some naturally occurring and synthetic corticosteroids—contd.

Compound	Formula	Proprietary name(s)	Remarks	Dose Equivalent (Dose needed to produce the same glucocorticoid effect as 50 mg of cortisone)
Methylpredniso-lone		Medrol; Medrone	Glucocorticoid with minimal mineralocorticoid activity	8 mg
Fluprednisolone		Alphadrol	Glucocorticoid with minimal mineralocorticoid activity. May cause side effects	5 mg
Dexamethasone		Decadron; Dexameth; Deronil; Dexa-Cortisyl; Dextelan; Gammacorten; Hexadrol; Millicorten; Oradexon.	Glucocorticoid with minimal mineralocorticoid activity	1.5 mg
Betamethasone		Betnelan; Betnesol; Celestone; ß-Corlan.	Glucocorticoid with minimal mineralocorticoid activity	1.5 mg

(Betamethasone valerate is known as Betnovate.)

Table 44.2 Some naturally occurring and synthetic corticosteroids—contd.

Compound	Formula	Proprietary name(s)	Remarks	Dose Equivalent (Dose needed to produce the same glucocorticoid effect as 50 mg of cortisone)
Beclomethasone		Becotide Propaderm	Glucocorticoid administered by aerosol in metered doses of 50 μg in asthma and locally in an 0.025 per cent cream in dermatology.	
Flumethasone		Locorten	Used locally in an 0.02 per cent cream in dermatological conditions	
Paramethasone		Haldrate Holdrone Metilar	Glucocorticoid with minimal mineralocorticoid activity	4 mg
Triamcinolone (also available as the acetonide		Adcortyl; Aristocort; Kenacort; Ledercort.	Glucocorticoid with minimal mineralocorticoid activity. May cause side effects	8 mg

Table 44.2 Some naturally occurring and synthetic corticosteroids—contd.

Compound	Formula	Proprietary name(s)	Remarks	Dose Equivalent (Dose needed to produce the same glucocorticoid effect as 50 mg of cortisone)
Desonide (desfluoro-triamcinolone)		Tridesilon	Used locally in an 0.05 per cent cream for steroid-responsive dermatological conditions	—
Fluocinolone acetonide (Fluocinonide)		Metosyn Synalar Synandone Topsyn	Glucocorticoid with minimal mineralocorticoid activity. Used topically Also available as unmodified fluocinolone	—
Dichlorisone (acetate)		Diloderm	Glucocorticoid with some mineralocorticoid activity. Used topically	—
Fluorometholone		Oxylone	Glucocorticoid with some mineralocorticoid activity. Used topically	—

Table 44.2 Some naturally occurring and synthetic corticosteroids—contd.

Compound	Formula	Proprietary name(s)	Remarks	Dose Equivalent (Dose needed to produce the same glucocorticoid effect as 50 mg of cortisone)
Flurandrenolone	CH₂OH / CO / CH₃ / OH / OH / HO / CH₃ / O / F	Drenison; Haelan	Used topically in an 0.05 per cent cream	—
Fluocortolone	CH₂OH / CO / CH₃ / CH₃ / HO / CH₃ / O / F	Ficoid Ultralanum Ultraproct	Used topically in an 0.1 per cent cream	—
Fluclorolone	CH₂OH / CO / O–C–CH₃ / O–CH₃ / CH₃ / Cl / CH₃ / Cl / O / F	Topilar	Used topically in an 0.025 per cent cream	—
Difluocortolone	Nerisone / CH₂OH / CO / CH₃ / CH₃ / HO / CH₃ / F / O / F	Temetex Nerisone	Used topically in an 0.1 per cent cream	—

Table 44.2 Some naturally occurring and synthetic corticosteroids—contd.

Compound	Formula	Proprietary name(s)	Remarks	Dose Equivalent (Dose needed to produce the same glucocorticoid effect as 50 mg of cortisone)
Clobetasone		Molivate	Used topically in an 0.05 per cent cream	
Clobetasol		Dermovate	Used topically in an 0.05 per cent cream	

the two compounds are similar. Cortisone occurs in the adrenal cortex in small quantities and a little is liberated into the blood but the amounts are too small to have any physiological significance. Cortisone was the first corticosteroid to be used for the treatment of diseases other than adrenal insufficiency: its dramatic effects in rheumatoid arthritis and similar diseases stimulated a great deal of enthusiasm for the new 'miracle drug' when it was first used, in 1949. It was once known as compound E, a name derived from the early custom of lettering corticosteroids in sequence as they were discovered. The other compound found in small quantities in adrenal blood is desoxycorticosterone. It is a precursor of the corticoids (Fig. 44.3) but it also has mineralocorticoid activity in its own right and if abnormal quantities accumulate in the blood as a result of metabolic defects which prevent the final elaboration of the corticosteroids, salt retention with hypertension may occur.

All the naturally occurring corticosteroids and a majority of the synthetic analogues carry a hydroxyl group on the terminal carbon atom C21. Compounds that lack this feature retain a little glucocorticoid activity but they cannot induce sodium retention. High antiinflammatory

activity demands in addition an α-hydroxy group at C7 and a β-hydroxyl at C11.

Prednisone and prednisolone differ from cortisone and cortisol respectively only in their possession of an additional double bond at C1-2. This feature has the effect of increasing glucocorticoid and antiinflammatory activity and it is found in all the newer drugs. It may, however, lead to an increased tendency for the drugs to cause peptic ulcer. α-Methylation or fluorination at position C6, as in methyl prednisolone and fluprednisolone respectively, also leads to a potentiation of all types of cortical hormone activity. Fludrocortisone, which has very high mineralocorticoid activity, differs from cortisone in possessing a fluorine atom at C9. Halogenation always brings about an increase in both antiinflammatory and mineralocorticoid activity but the latter property can be reduced while retaining the antiinflammatory potency if halogenation is combined with hydroxylation or methylation at C16. Fluorine (at C9) and the hydroxyl group occur in triamcinolone which is otherwise similar to prednisolone. Dexamethasone has fluorine at C9 but a methyl group instead of hydroxyl at C16. Betamethasone is isomeric with dexamethasone but its methyl group takes the β instead of the α configuration.

Paramethasone is like dexamethasone except that its fluorine atom is on C6. Fluocinolone resembles triamcinolone save for an additional fluorine atom at C6. Both fluocinolone and triamcinolone are available as acetonides. In dichlorisone the hydroxyl group at C11 in prednisolone is replaced by chlorine and another chlorine atom is added on C9. Dichlorisone has no substituent on C16 and the compound therefore has mineralocorticoid as well as glucocorticoid properties.

THERAPEUTIC USES OF THE ADRENOCORTICAL STEROIDS

A recent textbook of therapeutics (Alstead and Girdwood, 1974) mentions more than 100 conditions which might respond to treatment with the corticosteroids. It is clearly not possible to do more than give a general indication here of the potentialities of these drugs.

REPLACEMENT THERAPY

In Addison's disease (or after surgical removal of both adrenal glands) it is necessary to provide both a glucocorticoid and a mineralocorticoid if a semblance of normal endocrine function is to be restored. The glucocorticoid of choice is cortisol which is given by mouth in daily doses of 25 to 50 mg. The best mineralocorticoid to use is fludrocortisone (0.05 to 2 mg daily): unlike its predecessor, desoxycorticosterone acetate, this drug can be taken by mouth. Although this regimen provides sufficient support so long as the patient is otherwise healthy, it may be totally inadequate in conditions such as an infectious disease or physical injury, which demand additional supplies of adrenocortical hormones. If these are not given as soon as the stress situation arises, the patient may pass into a state of acute adrenal insufficiency with hypotension, hypoglycaemia, vomiting and shock. The crisis is treated with intravenous infusions of glucose-saline and hydrocortisone sodium succinate (100 mg) combined with an intramuscular injection of desoxycorticosterone acetate (2 mg). It may be necessary to continue treatment by giving intramuscular injections of the corticosteroids three times daily until the patient can once more take drugs by mouth.

When pituitary failure causes the adrenals to be deprived of the drive normally supplied by corticotrophin, adrenocortical function can be restored by the administration of hydrocortisone alone. Fludrocortisone is not needed, since aldosterone secretion is maintained by extrapituitary mechanisms (p. 754).

Corticosteroids are of value in the treatment of congenital adrenal hyperplasia and those cases of adrenogenital syndrome which are not due to an adrenal tumour. The steroids suppress the secretion of corticotrophin and hence of the adrenal androgens. Prednisolone (10 to 20 mg daily) is a suitable drug for this purpose.

TREATMENT OF DISEASES OF ADAPTATION

Many of the conditions referred to in the preamble to this section can be loosely grouped together, following Selye and for want of a better descriptive classification, as diseases of adaptation. The very multiplicity of the diseases gathered under this head indicates that the effects of corticosteroid therapy are non-specific: the tissue reaction to the agent causing the disease is modified but the condition is not cured in the sense that the causative agent is eliminated or antagonized. Nevertheless, there can be no doubt that the drugs are valuable and often life saving therapeutic weapons. Diseases of adaptation include rheumatic fever, gout and rheumatoid arthritis (the treatment of which is discussed in detail elsewhere p. 453), the collagen diseases (disseminated lupus erythematosus, periarteritis nodosa, scleroderma, etc.), asthma and some other allergic conditions, blood disorders (such as aplastic anaemia, agranulocytosis and leukaemia) and infections of the eye. The effects of severe burns, shocks and serious systemic infections may also be mitigated by the steroids.

From what was said earlier, it will be appreciated that it is the glucocorticoids which are used in the treatment of these diseases. Because large doses have to be given, often for long periods, the development of toxic side effects referable to glucocorticoid excess must always be expected and guarded against, if necessary by discontinuing the drug. Among the more usual side effects are glaucoma, glycosuria, hypertension, dyspepsia or peptic ulcer and a 'moon face' similar to that seen in Cushing's syndrome. It must be remembered that since one effect of glucocorticoid administration is the elimination of pituitary control of adrenal activity, patients treated with these drugs are likely to be particularly susceptible to infection, especially if drug treatment is stopped suddenly.

Among the newer compounds, prednisolone seems to be particularly effective in the treatment of many conditions while betamethasone and fluocinolone acetonide constituted the vanguard of a long procession of compounds that are now available for local application in dermatological conditions. Many of these newer compounds are listed in Table 44.2. Another recent development has been the provision of aerosol inhalers that deliver metered doses of beclomethasone dipropionate (Table 44.1) for use by sufferers from asthma (p. 409). The use of other corticosteroids is determined to a large extent by personal preference and the availability and price of the preparations. Table 44.1 gives the potency, relative to that of cortisone, of each of the compounds used systemically for their glucocorticoid effects. The reference dose chosen (50 mg of cortisone) is the daily amount that was commonly given in cases of rheumatic disease.

PREVENTION OF TISSUE REJECTION

As even the layman now knows, one of the major hazards associated with kidney and heart transplantation is the possibility that the host tissues may reject the new organ. The attempts to prevent it involve suppression of the activities of the reticulo-endothelial system. A number of drugs, including mercaptopurine and antilymphocyte serum, can be used for this purpose. Prednisone which, because of its glucocorticoid action, suppresses lymphocyte formation, is also commonly employed.

TREATMENT OF CARCINOMA OF THE BREAST
It has been mentioned earlier that oestrogen secretion from the adrenals may be sufficient to maintain a carcinoma of the breast. In such instances an obvious therapeutic measure is to remove both adrenal glands but if this cannot be done recourse may be made to suppression of adrenocortical activity by administration of a glucocorticoid such as prednisolone.

USE OF ADRENOCORTICOIDS IN DIAGNOSIS
Administration of a glucocorticoid should suppress adrenocortical function and should therefore bring about a reduction in the excretion of urinary 17-oxosteroids. If it does not do so, the presence of a glucocorticoid secreting adrenal tumour should be suspected. A useful drug to employ in this test is dexamethasone given in a daily dose of 5 to 10 mg.

BIOLOGICAL ESTIMATION OF CORTICOSTEROID ACTIVITY

Glucocorticoid activity can be estimated by measuring the amount of glycogen deposited, under the influence of the agent being investigated, in the livers of bilaterally adrenalectomized rats. In these animals gluconeogenesis is depressed or abolished so that liver stores of glycogen are severely depleted.
Mineralocorticoid activity is determined by measuring the retention of sodium and the excretion of potassium in bilaterally adrenalectomized animals. The measurement of *antiinflammatory activity* is discussed elsewhere (p. 462).

Adrenal gland extracts, pure hormones or synthetic compounds can also be assayed on the basis of their ability to maintain life in animals which have undergone bilateral extirpation of the adrenal glands or which have been exposed to a stress such as low temperature.

A practical note may not be out of place here. Complete adrenalectomy is a very simple operation when performed on a rat or mouse. It may, however, happen that after operation the animals show extraordinarily few signs of adrenal insufficiency. Failure to achieve the desired result in these cases is usually the result of the operator's having neglected to strip off the kidney capsule under which may be left sufficient secretory cells to maintain life.

BIBLIOGRAPHY

Books, monographs and reviews
Alstead, S. and Girdwood, R. H. (eds) (1974) *Textbook of Medical Treatment*. Edinburgh and London: Churchill Livingstone.
Brandon, M. L. (1962). *Corticosteroids in Medical Practice*. Springfield: Thomas.
Brogden, R. N., Pinder, R. M., Sawyer, Phyllis R., Speight, T. M. and Avery, G. S. (1975). Beclomethasone dipropionate inhaler. *Drugs*, **10**, 166-217.
Currie, A. R., Symington, T. and Grant, J. K. (eds) (1962). *The Human Adrenal Cortex*. Edinburgh: Livingstone.
Ganong, W. F., Biglieri, E. G. and Mulrow, P. J. (1966). Mechanisms relating adrenalcortical secretion of aldosterone and glucocorticoids. *Recent Prog. Horm. Res.*, **22**, 381-430.
Leung, K. and Munck, A. (1975). Peripheral actions of glucocorticoids. *A. rev. Physiol.*, **37**, 245-272.
Myles, A. B. and Daly, J. R. (1974). *Corticosteroid and ACTH Treatment*. London: Edward Arnold.
Phillips, J. G. and Bellamy, D. (1963). Adrenocortical hormones. In *Comparative Endocrinology*. ed. von Euler, U. S. and Heller, H. **1**, 208-257. London: Academic Press.
Slater, J. D. H. (1965). The adrenal glands. In *Clinical Physiology*, 2nd ed. reprint. ed. Campbell, E. J. M., Dickinson, C. J. and Slater, J. D. H. Oxford: Blackwell.
Smelick, P. G. and Sawyer, C. H. (1962). Pharmacological control of adrenocortical and gonadal secretions. *Ann. Rev. Pharmac.*, **2**, 313-340.
Various Authors (1962). The adrenal cortex. *Br. med. Bull.*, **18**, 89-173.

45. The pituitary hormones

The pituitary gland (or hypophysis) is attached to the base of the brain by the pituitary (or hypophysial) stalk which is itself composed of pituitary tissue and which brings the gland into close anatomical and functional relationship with the hypothalamus.

The pituitary gland releases a number of hormones, some of which regulate the activity of other endocrine glands (that is, they have a *trophic* function) while the others have independent actions. Its ability to control other glands underlines the importance of its relationship with the hypothalamus. The hypothalamus controls the autonomic nervous system and it is involved in the initiation and modification of emotional states. It is itself influenced by activity in many other parts of the central nervous system and the hypothalamo-hypophysial link subserves the key function of integrating and coordinating the nervous and endocrine components of many of the organism's regulatory, reproductive and adaptive activities.

The importance of the pituitary gland has been appreciated for considerably less than a century. The ancients believed that it produced fluid to moisten the nose (*pituita* means phlegm) but in more modern times the pituitary was regarded, until about 1890, as a vestigial structure with no physiological function. 'Hypophysis' means a downgrowth.

The pituitary gland is made up of the *adenohypophysis* and the *neurohypophysis* which differ in origin, structure and function. The adenohypophysis develops as a diverticulum (Rathke's pouch) from the primitive mouth. It consists of three parts—the *pars tuberalis*, the *pars intermedia* and the *pars distalis*—but in man the pars tuberalis is usually missing and the pars intermedia is very small. When the pars tuberalis is present, it surrounds the infundibular stem (q.v.). Although the adenohypophysis develops from the oral cavity, it soon loses its connection with that organ and becomes associated with, and dependent upon, the hypothalamus.

The neurohypophysis appears as a downwards growing diverticulum from the developing third ventricle. It reaches a position immediately behind the adenohypophysis and in mammals the two structures unite to form the

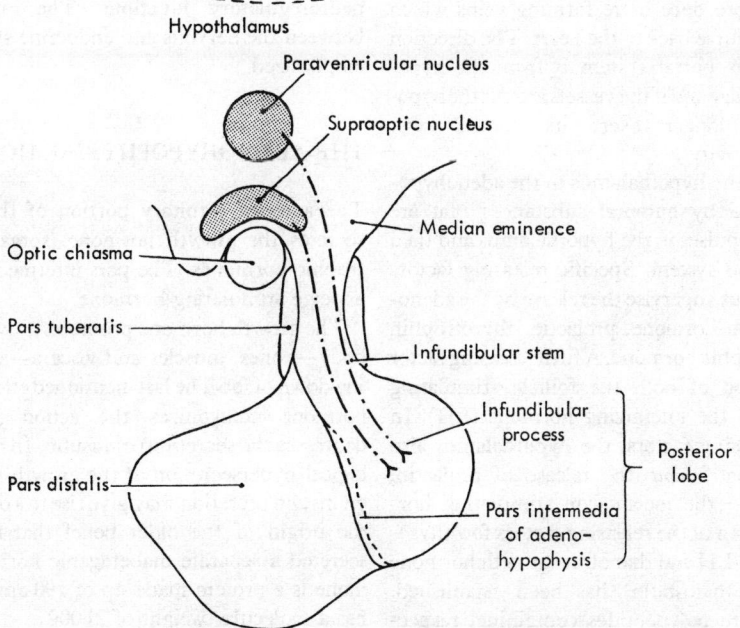

Fig. 45.1 Subdivisions of the pituitary gland

pituitary gland. The neurohypophysis also consists of three parts: the *median eminence* is contiguous with the hypothalamus; together with the *infundibular stem* it forms the pituitary stalk. The third part of the neurohypophysis is the *infundibular process* or *pas nervosa* (Fig. 45.1).

On dissection, the pituitary gland separates easily into anterior and posterior lobes. These do not correspond precisely to the functional divisions just referred to, because the natural line of division is a cleft which is the remnant of the original cavity of Rathke's pouch. Consequently, the anatomical anterior lobe is made up of the pars distalis and, where it exists, the pars tuberalis of the adenohypophysis. The anatomical posterior lobe consists of the pars nervosa of the neurohypophysis and the pars intermedia of the adenohypophysis. The remaining two parts of the neurohypophysis constitute, as we have seen, the pituitary stalk. The important division is the functional one but no great harm is done by the common practice of equating posterior and anterior lobe hormones with neurohypophysial and adenohypophysial hormones respectively, since the secretion of the pars intermedia is of minor importance. Nevertheless the several terms will be used in this chapter in their strict sense.

Nerve fibres from the supraoptic and the paraventricular nuclei of the hypothalamus constitute the hypothalamo-hypophysial tract which provides the means whereby the hypothalamus exerts its controlling influence over the pars nervosa of the posterior lobe. The connection between the hypothalamus and the adenohypophysis is a vascular one. Capillaries in the median eminence of the hypothalamus drain into veins that pass into the adenohypophysis (predominantly the pars distalis) where they break up into capillaries again before once more forming veins which then take a normal course back to the heart. The direction of blood flow in this portal system is from the hypothalamus to the pituitary and if the vessels are cut the hypothalamus can no longer exert its control over adenohypophysial activity.

Information from the hypothalamus to the adenohypophysis is transmitted by humoral substances that are liberated by nerve impulses in the hypothalamus and then enter the portal blood system. Specific releasing factors from the hypothalamus supervise the release by the adenohypophysis of growth hormone, prolactin, thyrotrophin and adrenocorticotrophic hormone. A fifth releasing factor controls the secretion of both the follicle stimulating hormone (FSH) and the luteinizing hormone (LH). In addition to the releasing factors, the hypothalamus also elaborates factors that *inhibit* the release of prolactin, growth hormone and the melanocyte stimulating hormone. The composition of the releasing factors for thyrotrophin and for FSH-LH and that of the growth hormone inhibitory factor (somatostatin) has been established. These compounds are polypeptides containing, respectively, three, ten and fourteen aminoacid residues. Most

authorities believed that the prolactin inhibitor would also prove to be a polypeptide until Schally and his colleagues obtained a purified preparation of the inhibitor (the source was hypothalmic tissue collected from 500 000 pigs!) and showed that it consisted largely of dopamine (Schally *et al.*, 1974; Takahara *et al.*, 1974). Dopamine receptors have been demonstrated in the adenohypophysis. When stimulated they inhibit prolactin release. It seems likely that the hypothalamus does produce a polypeptide with some ability to inhibit prolactin secretion but that it has but a minor physiological role. It does not activate the pituitary dopamine receptors but it may itself be under dopaminergic influences. These views are supported by the experimental observation that dopamine can inhibit prolactin release by direct actions on both the hypothalamus and the adenohypophysis.

The secretion of the trophic hormones is subject to feed back inhibition by the hormones whose output they have stimulated. Thus thyroid hormone in the plasma inhibits release of the thyrotrophic hormone. These inhibitory actions may be exerted at the pituitary or the hypothalamic level or at both sites. Which is the more important locus of action varies from one hormone to another.

The hormones of the neurohypophysis are elaborated in the hypothalamus itself. They are carried to the pars nervosa by way of the axons of the hypothalamo-hypophysial tract and they are held in the gland until they are released by nervous impulses that travel along the same nerve fibres as a result of stimulation of hypothalamic centres. Thus the hypothalamo-hypophysial tract and the hypothalamus are unique among nervous structures in that they have secretory as well as the more usual type of neuroregulatory functions. The intimate relationship between the nervous and endocrine systems is once more emphasized.

THE ADENOHYPOPHYSIAL HORMONES

The anterior pituitary portion of the adenohypophysis secretes the growth hormone (somatotrophin) and five trophic hormones. The pars intermedia secretes the melanocyte stimulating hormone.

The growth hormone promotes growth in all parts of the body—bones, muscles and viscera—and inhibits the laying down of fat. The last mentioned effect arises because the hormone antagonizes the action (and perhaps also depresses the secretion) of insulin. In conditions of pathological hypersecretion of the growth hormone, the effect on insulin secretion may give rise to a diabetic state. This is the origin of the older belief that the pituitary gland secreted a separate diabetogenic hormone. Growth hormone is a protein made up of 190 aminoacid residues. It has a molecular weight of 21 000.

The five trophic hormones whose existence has been

unequivocally established are corticotrophin, thyrotrophin, the follicle stimulating and luteinizing hormones and prolactin. The corticotrophin (adrenocorticotrophic hormone, ACTH) molecule is a polypeptide chain containing 39 amino acid residues. Among the corticotrophins so far isolated (those of pig, sheep and beef) differences in structure are restricted to the amino acid sequences in positions 25 to 33 of the chain. Corticotrophin regulates the release of the adrenal corticosteroids; its function is discussed elsewhere. Thyrotrophin (thyroid stimulating hormone, TSH) is a glycoprotein with a molecular weight of 28000; its action in relation to thyroid function is mentioned on page 711. The follicle stimulating (FSH) and the luteinizing (LH) hormones, both of which are glycoproteins with molecular weights of 30000, operate in concert to control the ovarian cycle and to maintain pregnancy. The luteinizing hormone also exerts a trophic action on the endocrine secretion of the testis and for this reason it is also known as the interstitial cell stimulating hormone (ICSH). The physiological functions of the gonadotrophic hormones are detailed in Chapter 43.

Prolactin (mammotrophin or the lactogenic hormone) is a protein hormone similar in composition, but distinct from, the growth hormone. It initiates and maintains lactation after parturition has taken place, but the maintenance of lactation is a complex process demanding the cooperative activity of a number of nervous and endocrine factors. Prolactin appears to exert actions on many tissues in addition to those of the breast. The variety of these actions justifies a separate discussion of prolactin physiology and this is done on p. 776.

The melanocyte (or melanophore) stimulating hormone (intermedin, melanotrophin, chromatophore exciting hormone) brings about the dispersion of the pigment granules in the melanocytes of amphibian skin. This scattering of the granules causes the skin to take on a darker appearance. Extracts of the pars intermedia of mammalian pituitary glands (including that of man) all have this effect in amphibia but they also have a more general effect on skin pigmentation even when, as in mammals, this is not dependent on the presence of melanocytes. This provides an explanation for the changes in skin colour that may be associated with disturbances of pituitary activity. In Addison's disease, for instance, the inability of the adrenal cortex to secrete its hormone leads to an increase in adenohypophysial activity and one of the characteristic features of Addison's disease is a darkening of the skin.

The melanophore stimulating hormone occurs in two forms. The α form , which never leaves the pituitary, has 13 amino acids arranged in the same sequence as those in positions 1 to 13 of corticotrophin. The β form, which appears in the bloodstream, has 22 amino acids seven of which (11 to 17) are identical with those occupying 4 to 10 in the corticotrophin molecule.

Some of the cells of the adenohypophysis (the chromo-phils) take up simple stains but the others (the chromophobes) do not The chromophils can be further subdivided into those that stain with acid dyes such as eosin (these are the acidophils or α cells) and those with an affinity for baser dyes, the basophils or β cells. The α-cells secrete growth hormone and prolactin while the β-cells secrete thyrotrophin and the follicle stimulating and luteinizing hormones. Corticotrophin and melanocyte stimulating hormone come, at least in part, from the chromophobes.

Electron microscope studies make it clear that the granules manufacturing each hormone are morphologically distinct, a finding that underlines the chemical individuality of the several hormones.

NEUROHYPOPHYSIAL HORMONES

Extracts of the neurohypophysis show three distinct pharmacological actions: they increase the blood pressure of anaesthetized animals, they abolish or prevent the diuresis otherwise produced by the ingestion of water and they cause contraction of the uterus. For many years it was believed that these effects were produced by separate hormones which were called vasopressin, the antidiuretic hormone and oxytocin respectively. It is now known that only two substances are involved, antidiuretic activity being vested in vasopressin. It is also now clear that oxytocin elicits contraction of smooth muscle in mammary glands as well as that of the uterus.

The structure of oxytocin and vasopressin was established and their synthesis was accomplished by Du Vigneaud and his colleagues in the course of a most impressive series of investigations that were completed in 1953. The arrangements of the amino acid residues in the two hormones are shown, in the form in which they are usually represented, in Figure 45.2 in which the formula of oxytocin is also drawn out in full. Both hormones are octapeptides linked in a cyclic disulphide form and the only difference between vasopressin and oxytocin is that in the latter, isoleucine and leucine replace phenylalanine and arginine respectively. Although the hormones are octapeptides the usual convention is followed in Figure 45.2, the aminoacid residues being numbered 1 to 9. This is because the two cysteine moieties that constitute the cystine molecule are represented separately.

The structures shown in Figure 45.2 relate to compounds isolated from beef pituitary but the beef hormones have the same composition as those secreted by most other mammals including man. The pig provides an exception: its vasopressin contains lysine instead of arginine. The two vasopressins are designated lysine-vasopressin and arginine-vasopressin. Some lower vertebrates contain a substance with the ring structure of oxytocin and the side chain of vasopressin. It is called arginine vasotocin and its

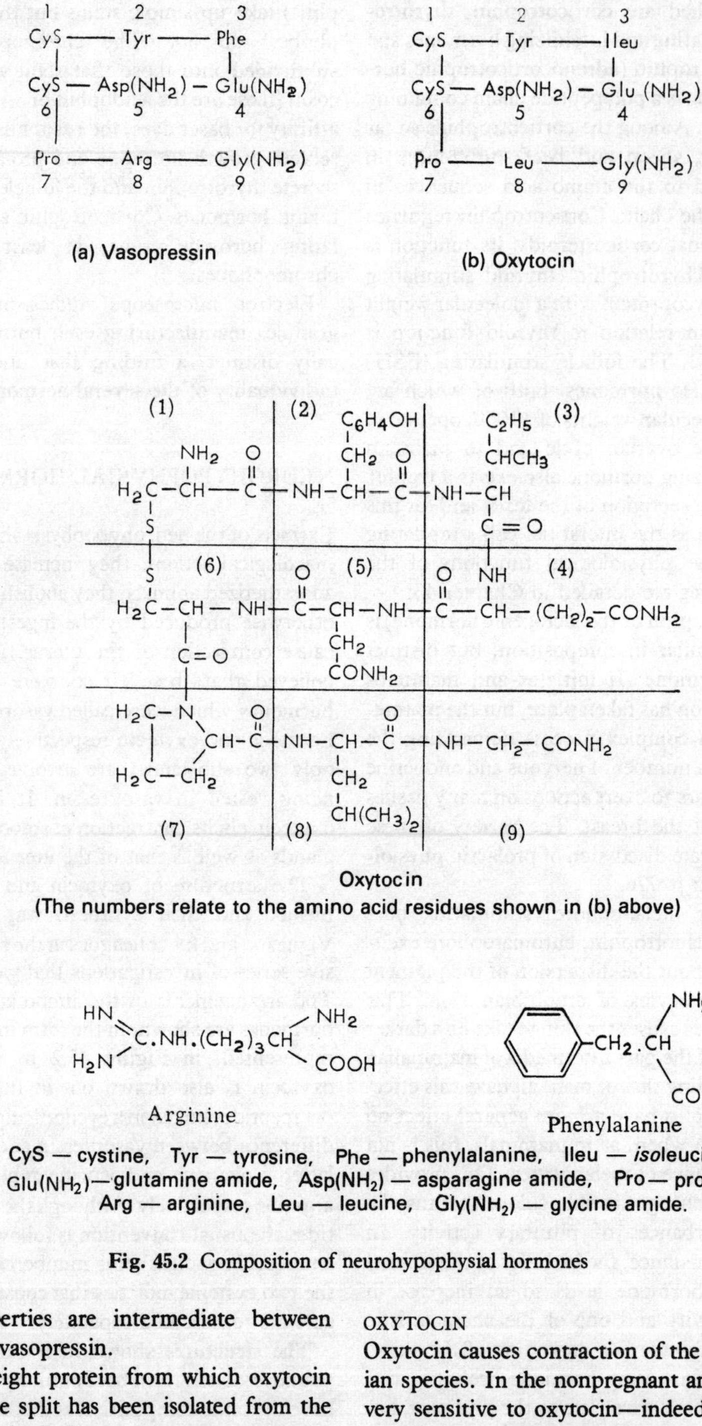

(a) Vasopressin

(b) Oxytocin

Oxytocin
(The numbers relate to the amino acid residues shown in (b) above)

Arginine

Phenylalanine

CyS — cystine,   Tyr — tyrosine,   Phe — phenylalanine,   Ileu — *isoleucine*,
Glu(NH₂)—glutamine amide,   Asp(NH₂) — asparagine amide,   Pro— proline,
Arg — arginine,   Leu — leucine,   Gly(NH₂) — glycine amide.

Fig. 45.2 Composition of neurohypophysial hormones

pharmacological properties are intermediate between those of oxytocin and vasopressin.

A low molecular weight protein from which oxytocin and vasopressin can be split has been isolated from the mammalian pituitary gland. It may represent a storage form of the neurohypophysial hormones from which the octapeptides are released in response to signals from the hypothalamus. Alternatively the protein itself may enter the blood stream, the hormones proper being liberated at the site of action.

OXYTOCIN

Oxytocin causes contraction of the uterus in all mammalian species. In the nonpregnant animal the uterus is not very sensitive to oxytocin—indeed, in the human being, contractions are more easily evoked by vasopressin—but in pregnancy its sensitivity progressively increases. At full term as little as 0.05 μg of the pure hormone is sufficient to induce labour and this extraordinarily high responsiveness persists throughout parturition. Mechanical stretching of the cervix of the uterus in a fashion simulating that occurring during labour causes the appearance in the blood of a substance with oxytocic activity. There is evidence, too, that the neurohypophysis is partly depleted of oxytocin during parturition. These observations suggest that the physiological function of oxytocin may be to maintain uterine contractility throughout labour. There is less evidence that it is involved in the *initiation* of labour but it is possible that oxytocin and the prostaglandins (p. 373) act together to achieve this end.

Vaginal stimulation during coitus brings about the release of oxytocin. In view of the relative insensitivity of the nonpregnant uterus, this response may be no more than a physiological curiosity. On the other hand, it may be sufficient to cause some uterine contraction and so to assist the progress of the spermatozoa into the uterine cavity and oviducts.

Oxytocin brings about milk ejection ('let down') from lactating mammary glands. It is reflexly released by the act of suckling and it causes contraction of the myoepithelial tissue around the mammary alveoli and the small lactiferous ducts. In this way the milk is passed into the larger ducts and the nipple.

Large doses of oxytocin may cause a fall followed by a rise of blood pressure in mammals. In birds (which are more sensitive) oxytocin has a depressor effect at all dose levels. This forms the basis of a method for the biological standardization of oxytocin. These cardiovascular responses are of no physiological significance and it is doubtful whether therapeutic doses of purified oxytocin ever affect blood pressure in the human subject.

Oxytocin-induced contractions of the isolated uterus are prevented by sodium thioglycollate, which reduces the disulphide linkage in the oxytocin molecule.

No function has yet been attributed to the oxytocin found in the neurohypophysis of male animals.

VASOPRESSIN

In experimental preparations this hormone has an antidiuretic action which reflects a physiological function and a pressor action which does not. It is, perhaps, a pity that the hormone should be widely (and officially) known as vasopressin (Pitressin). 'Antidiuretic hormone' is a more appropriate name and it is preferred by some authorities, particularly in physiological contexts. It has the disadvantage of being a more cumbersome term than vasopressin and this tempts writers to scatter yet another abbreviation (ADH) over their pages.

So far as its antidiuretic action is concerned, vasopressin operates by increasing the permeability of the kidney tubules to water. It is released from the neurohypophysis in response to stimulation of hypothalamic osmoreceptors. The details of this mechanism are discussed in more detail elsewhere (p. 618).

The pressor effect of vasopressin is the result of a direct action on the smooth muscle of the blood vessels. It is most evident in anaesthetized animals because the reactivity of the autonomic nervous system is depressed by anaesthetics. Compensatory depressor responses are therefore inhibited. Ganglion blocking agents have the same effect as anaesthetics. Even in anaesthetized animals, the dose of vasopressin needed to produce an obvious pressor response is several times greater than that needed to inhibit diuresis. The pressor response to a single injection of vasopressin is rather prolonged, persisting for up to a minute (Fig. 45.3).

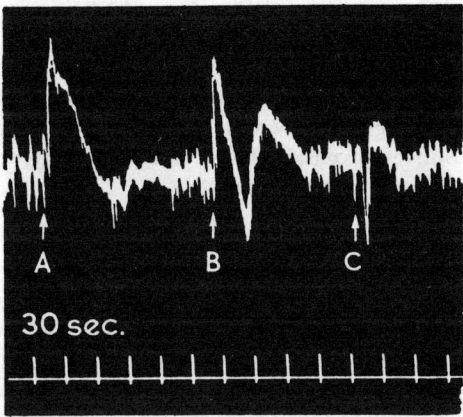

Fig. 45.3 The effects of 10 m units of vasopressin (A), 0.5 μg of adrenaline (B) and 10 m units of oxytocin (C) on the blood pressure of the rat.

Many a student of pharmacology, attempting to demonstrate the inhibition of diuresis by vasopressin in the anaesthetized or spinal animal, has been surprised to obtain a diuretic response. This arises because in this type of preparation the blood pressure tends to fall to a point where blood flow through the kidney becomes inadequate to maintain the normal rate of glomerular filtration. Vasopressin increases blood pressure, renal blood flow and urine formation and this more than offsets its antidiuretic action under these experimental conditions. This diuretic effect of vasopressin is of no physiological significance but it is sufficiently pronounced to have deceived the physiologists who first investigated the problem into the belief that the pituitary gland secreted a diuretic hormone.

There is no evidence that the vascular effects of vasopressin have any regulatory function in the intact animal under normal circumstances. Vasopressin is released in stress and it has been suggested that in haemorrhagic shock this may be sufficient to effect some restoration of blood pressure. In view of the insensitivity of the unanaesthetized human subject, it is doubtful whether usefully pressor amounts of vasopressin appear in the blood even in conditions of extreme stress. It is, however, certainly true that the doses of vasopressin employed in the treatment of diabetes insipidus (p. 637) are sufficient to affect blood pressure. The coronary arteries take part in the vasoconstrictor response and this is sufficient to provide a contraindication to the therapeutic use of vasopressin in patients with arterial disease.

Vasopressin causes contraction of smooth muscle in other organs. Large doses provoke peristalsis and induce uterine contractions. Thus the properties of vasopressin overlap to some extent with those of oxytocin. This is hardly surprising, in view of their similarities of structure.

DISORDERS OF PITUITARY FUNCTION

It is not usual for disease processes to affect both parts of the pituitary gland in the same individual and it is therefore justifiable to consider disorders of the adenohypophysis and neurohypophysis separately.

The adenohypophysis
UNDERSECRETION
In human beings, skeletal growth continues until the bony epiphyses unite at the time of adolescence. If the activity of the pituitary gland is depressed during the growing period, the growth rate is depressed and *pituitary dwarfism* results. Gonadotrophin secretion is usually depressed but thyrotrophin and corticotrophin secretion are likely to be adequate to maintain normal activity in their 'target organs'. Although pituitary dwarfs are small, they are normally proportioned and this serves to differentiate them from those whose stunted growth arises from other causes.

Unless it is artificially induced puberty is usually delayed in pituitary dwarfs. As a result, growth, though retarded, is not arrested as early as it is in normal children and almost normal heights may eventually be attained.

It is theoretically possible for secretion of one or more of the trophic hormones to be deficient in children whose output of growth hormone is not impaired but these conditions are rare.

When pituitary deficiency arises in adult life, it usually affects all the adenohypophysial secretions. This is the condition of *panhypopituitarism* or *Simmonds' disease*. There is atrophy of the sex glands, a depressed metabolism and a reduced ability to resist stress and the effects of surgery. Hypoglycaemia and an increased sensitivity to insulin occur as a result of the withdrawal of the antiinsulin action normally exerted by the growth hormone. It is even more unusual to encounter cases of isolated deficiency of a trophic hormone in adults than it is in children.

OVERSECRETION
Tumours of the α cells of the anterior pituitary result in the overproduction of growth hormone. If this occurs in early life *gigantism* results and heights of seven or eight feet may be attained before growth ceases. If α cell hyperactivity

develops in a previously normal pituitary gland in adults, *acromegaly* results. There is no increase in height but the spine becomes bowed and the extremities of the bones enlarge: the jaws thicken and the lower one becomes protuberant, the teeth separate and the hands and feet increase in size. Diabetes mellitus is likely to occur in consequence of the increased secretion of growth hormone. Sometimes diabetic symptoms appear in the absence of concomitant bony signs of acromegaly.

Oversecretion of individual trophic hormones (which are secreted by β cells) may occur. Some cases of thyrotoxicosis (p. 714) and of Cushing's syndrome (p. 758) are the result of oversecretion of the thyrotrophic and adrenocorticotrophic hormones respectively.

Overpigmentation of the skin as a consequence of hypersecretion of the melanophore stimulating hormone sometimes occurs in Cushing's syndrome and in Addison's disease (p. 757).

The neurohypophysis
UNDERSECRETION
Undersecretion of vasopressin produces diabetes insipidus, a condition that is discussed elsewhere (p. 637). Oxytocin deficiency may occur at the same time but this seems to be attended by no ill effect, even during labour.

OVERSECRETION
Disorders due to a primary overactivity of the neurohypophysial hormones have not been described. Continued stress, cerebral tumours and some forms of cardiovascular disease may be associated with an increased secretion of vasopressin so that water retention occurs.

CLINICAL USES OF THE PITUITARY HORMONES

GROWTH HORMONE
Limited amounts of purified human growth hormone are now available and almost normal adult heights have been produced in some of the dwarfs to whom it has been administered over a period of years. Some patients fail to respond, perhaps because their dwarfism is not primarily of pituitary origin. It may be the result of a neutralization of the growth hormone by antibodies.

Early clinical experiences with human growth hormone suggest doses of 5 to 10 mg twice weekly. It is given by subcutaneous or intramuscular injection and treatment is continued until the epiphyses finally unite. This may require several years of treatment. Growth hormone may have to be supplemented with other hormone preparations depending on the extent of pituitary involvement.

Because of its diabetogenic action, growth hormone should not be given to those whose stunted growth is not of pituitary origin.

THYROTROPHIN

Thyrotrophin (Thytropar) is used for diagnostic purposes to determine whether a myxoedematous condition is due to a primary thyroid deficiency or whether it is one of the rare cases that arise because of a failure of the pituitary to secrete thyrotrophin.

The patient receives a single dose (10 units) of thyrotrophin by intramuscular injection. Some time before, and one day after, the injection, he is also given a tracer of radioactive iodine (^{131}I). The uptake of labelled iodine by the thyroid gland is measured on both occasions. If the myxoedema is of pituitary origin, thyroid activity—and hence the uptake of labelled iodine—will be stimulated by the trophic hormone.

Thyrotrophin has also been employed to increase the concentration of radioactive iodine in thyroid tumours.

CORTICOTROPHIN

The adrenal corticosteroids are employed in the treatment of a wide variety of conditions (p. 767). Since corticotrophin regulates the secretory activity of the adrenal cortex, it might be expected to have a similar range of therapeutic utility as the adrenal hormones themselves except, of course, in conditions associated with depressed cortical function. Corticotrophin has indeed some advantages over the corticosteroids: it does not cause adrenal atrophy so that the glands can resume their normal activity when treatment ceases, it does not cause osteoporosis or muscle wasting and it is less likely to depress growth in children. On the other hand, it has an unselective action, stimulating the release of all the cortical hormones whereas some selectivity of action has been incorporated into the synthetic corticosteroids which can, therefore, be chosen in the light of the individual patient's clinical condition. Moreover, corticotrophin stimulates the synthesis of androgens and though this is sometimes an advantage it sometimes causes hypertension as well as effects such as acne, pigmentation of the skin and the growth of superfluous hair that are not especially welcomed by female patients. But the overwhelming disadvantage of corticotrophin is that it has to be given by intravenous or intramuscular injection. The synthetic corticosteroids are active when taken by mouth. Among the conditions for which corticotrophin is sometimes preferred we must include rheumatoid arthritis, asthma, Still's disease (an arthritic condition of childhood) and ulcerative colitis.

Corticotrophin has been used with some success for the treatment of some forms of infantile epilepsy (p. 529).

Corticotrophin is used to determine whether an adrenocortical insufficiency arises from failure of the cortex itself or from cessation of corticotrophin secretion by the pituitary gland. Corticotrophin is infused for several hours: if the adrenal cortex responds to this stimulus the concentration of corticosteroid metabolites in the urine will increase and it can be concluded that the adrenal insufficiency is secondary to pituitary failure.

Some authorities recommend that corticotrophin should be given to all patients receiving corticosteroid therapy. The reasoning behind this suggestion is that the administered corticosteroid may suppress the activity of the adrenal cortex and that the function of the cortex can be maintained, against the day when the corticosteroids are withdrawn, if it is subjected to continuous stimulation by the trophic hormone. Of course, the exogenous corticotrophin suppresses the release of the natural hormone but release is quickly re-established when the drug is withdrawn. Rational though it may seem, this practice of using corticotrophin as an adjunct to corticosteroid therapy has not been widely adopted.

Only 24 of corticotrophin's 39 aminoacid residues confer hormonal activity on the molecule. The remaining chain of 15 residues is responsible for antigenic activity. Compounds consisting of only the 24 active residues are available. They include tetracosactrin (Cortrosyn, Synacthen) and the longer acting tetracosactrin zinc (Cortrosyn-Depot, Synacthen-Depot). Their obvious value is in the treatment of patients who exhibit hypersensitivity reactions to corticotrophin itself. The complete molecule is available as Acthar. Longer acting preparations include Acthar Gel (corticotrophin gelatin injection), Cortrophin ZN (corticotrophin zinc hydroxide) and Cortico-Gel.

For the diagnostic test referred to earlier, tetracosactrin can be given in an intramuscular dose of 0.25 mg as an alternative to an infusion of corticotrophin itself. The depot preparations of tetracosactrin are given by twice weekly intramuscular injections each of 1 mg.

THE GONADOTROPHIC HORMONES

Although purified preparations of follicle stimulating hormone are prepared from human pituitary glands, the amounts available from this source are obviously very strictly limited. A more convenient and readily available source is the urine of postmenopausal women. Their blood lacks more than minimal amounts of oestrogen and this evokes an energetic secretion of follicle stimulating hormone. A commercial preparation of gonadtrophin of urinary origin is Pergonal. It contains some luteinizing hormone, as well as the follicle stimulating hormone, but this is no disadvantage. The urine of pregnant women provides a similarly rich source of human chorionic gonadtrophin (HCG) whose actions are similar to those of luteinizing hormone (p. 771). Proprietary preparations of human chorionic gonadtrophin from urinary sources include Gonadotraphon LH and Pregnyl. Gonadin is derived from the urine of pregnant mares: its actions are similar to those of Pergonal.

Follicle stimulating hormone has been successfully used to treat some cases of female sterility. Some of the patients apparently secreted normal amounts of gonadotrophin but the additional stimulus provided by the administered hormone provoked the ovulation that the unaided pituitary had failed to produce.

The dose for the treatment of sterility has not been well established but in one investigation 10 mg of purified hormone were given daily for ten days. It was supplemented by chorionic gonadotrophin, administration of which began after the course of pituitary hormone injections had ended.

The administration of gonadotrophin may cause the development of pelvic pain due to enlargement of the ovaries. In sensitive individuals, or after injudiciously chosen doses of the gonadotrophins, these changes may be exaggerated and accompanied by other changes such as thrombosis and pleural and abdominal effusions. The condition has occasionally proved fatal. Multiple pregnancy is another possible complication.

The gonadotrophins have also been applied to the treatment of male infertility.

CLOMIPHENE

The output of follicle stimulating hormone by the pituitary is normally restrained by the ovarian hormones. Clomiphene removes this restraint by reason of a gonadotrophin releasing action exerted directly on the hypothalamus so that its effects on the ovary are very similar to those of the gonadotrophic hormone itself. It has been very successfully employed to cure infertility and it is also of value in the treatment of menstrual irregularities and a number of other gynaecological disorders. When used to treat infertility, clomiphene is given in oral doses of 50 mg daily for one week. Side effects (abdominal pain and multiple pregnancies) are similar to those encountered in gonadotrophin therapy.

Clomiphene

It will be evident that clomiphene can only be effective if pituitary function is intact. Indeed, the drug can be given as a diagnostic test for hypopituitarism in which condition there will be no gonadotrophin response to clomiphene.

In some animal species, including the rat, clomiphene inhibits the secretion of gonadotrophins and induces sterility in both sexes.

OXYTOCIN

Oxytocin (Pitocin, Syntocinon) can be used to induce labour, to overcome uterine inertia during labour and to reduce discomfort in engorged breasts during lactation. For the induction of labour it is given by intravenous infusion in a solution containing one to five units of oxytocin per litre of 5 per cent dextrose. The drip rate is adjusted so that oxytocin is supplied at an initial rate of about 5 milliunits a minute. If signs of incipient labour do not appear within half an hour or so, the dose level is cautiously increased to about 20 milliunits a minute. The same regime is followed when oxytocin is given during labour but great care has to be exercised lest too powerful contractions—which might damage the uterus or obstruct the blood supply to the foetus—are induced. If this unfortunate contingency does arise, the patient must be anaesthetized so as to promote uterine relaxation.

For relieving engorgement of the breast, a convenient way of applying oxytocin is by nasal spray. Oxytocin can also be used to improve the supply of milk to the baby if the milk ejection mechanisms are responding only sluggishly to the stimulus of suckling.

After delivery of the baby and placenta, it is usual to give ergometrine or a related drug (p. 298) to encourage firm contraction of the uterus and thus to reduce the likelihood of post partum haemorrhage. Oxytocin can be used at this stage of labour if ergot alkaloids are contraindicated. It has also been used in early pregnancy to induce therapeutic abortions.

VASOPRESSIN

The therapeutic use of vasopressin is discussed elsewhere (p. 637).

GALACTORRHOEA AND THE PHYSIOLOGY OF PROLACTIN

Prolactin, as we have seen, is a pituitary hormone that initiates and helps to maintain lactation in response to the suckling of breasts prepared by pregnancy for this duty. The secretion of prolactin is under the control of hypothalamic factors, excitatory and inhibitory. Under normal conditions, the action of the inhibitory factors is dominant and the amount of prolactin in the blood, though subject to diurnal variation, does not rise beyond about 1 ng per ml. However, certain pathological conditions and a number of drugs provoke the release of prolactin which, as a result, sometimes attains plasma concentrations as high as 500 ng per ml. The increased amounts of prolactin may elicit a non-physiological secretion of the mammary glands (galactorrhoea) in the absence of suckling in women who are not, and may never have been, pregnant. It may even occur in men.

Tumours and other conditions of the hypothalamus and pituitary gland that result in the release of abnormally large amounts of hormones or their releasing factors can induce galactorrhoea which may therefore feature in the symptomatology of Cushing's syndrome and acromegaly. Indeed, galactorrhoea sometimes appears as the very first sign of acromegaly. The thyrotrophin releasing factor also evokes the release of prolactin so that galactorrhoea sometimes occurs in the course of hypothyroidism. In that condition the hypothalamus secretes the releasing factor in response to the low level of circulating thyroid hormone.

Damage to the chest wall or herpes zoster (shingles) affecting thoracic nerve segments is also sometimes associated with galactorrhoea, presumably because the irritation of sensory nerves activates the afferent pathways that in other circumstances are stimulated by suckling. Other less common causes of galactorrhoea are dealt with in the appropriate textbooks (see, for instance, Hall, Anderson, Smart and Besser, 1974) but the pharmacologist must be more concerned with the effects of drugs. Galactorrhoea can occur in the course of treatment with α-methyldopa, a number of psychotrophic drugs (reserpine, phenothiazines, haloperidol and some of the tricyclic antidepressant agents) and, very occasionally, oral contraceptives of the combined type. α-Methyldopa and the psychotropic drugs antagonize dopamine, the major hypothalamic prolactin inhibitor. It has been estimated that a degree of galactorrhoea exists in 50 per cent of women and 10 per cent of men who take phenothiazines. Hyperprolactinaemia suppresses gonadotrophin release so that galactorrhoea is usually accompanied by amenorrhoea in women and impotence in males.

Before turning to the treatment of galactorrhoea, mention has to be made of recent investigations (summarized by Horrobin 1973, 1974) that have made it clear that prolactin exerts a range of effects that are not obviously related to milk production. Some of these can only be demonstrated in response to amounts of prolactin in excess of those normally found in plasma but they may, nevertheless, mirror physiological effects of the hormone. This seems the more likely in the light of the interesting fact that, in experimental situations, prolactin is often more effective in small than in large doses.

The structure of human prolactin is similar to that of growth hormone and it is only recently that the chemical individuality of the two hormones has been unequivocally demonstrated. It is not surprising, then, that some of the effects of prolactin administration (stimulation of skeletal growth and protein synthesis, potassium retention, calcium mobilization, hyperglycaemia, etc.) resemble those produced by growth hormone. Other actions of prolactin include (among many others) stimulation of prostaglandin synthesis, a pressor effect attributable to both a direct action on the heart and a potentiating effect on endogenous vasoconstrictor substances, the promotion of sodium and potassium movements across cell membranes, stimulation of aldosterone secretion, fluid retention and the maintenance of mammary cancers and perhaps some other tumours. These findings imply a participation of prolactin in a large variety of fundamental physiological processes and its involvement in the aetiology of many clinical conditions.

Like so many other regulatory substances, prolactin appears to interact with the cylic AMP system.

It may well be asked why prolactin, of all hormones, should display such protean behaviour. Partly, of course, it is because the hormone has almost fortuitously attracted the attention of several groups of dedicated workers who might well have been able to demonstrate an equally wide spectrum of physiological activity in any other hormone they had chosen to study. On the other hand, milk secretion is dependent on the proper functioning of a number of basic physiological processes (blood flow, transfer of materials across membranes, etc.) and what prolactin does in the breast it can, presumably, do elsewhere. We have mentioned previously (p. 474) that many substances have actions on tissues other than their more obvious target organs.

BROMOCRYPTINE (PARLODEL)

It has been known since the middle of the seventeenth century that cessation of milk flow is one of the several possible consequences of ergot poisoning. This old observation can be said to have lain at the root of recent searches for an ergot alkaloid that would more specifically suppress lactation. This quest met with success in 1968 when Flückiger and Wagner demonstrated the actions of bromocryptine, the 2-bromo derivative of ergocryptine, itself an aminoacid alkaloid constituent of ergot (Fig. 18.4, p. 296). Bromocryptine is a potent inhibitor of prolactin secretion, a consequence of the fact that it stimulates dopamine receptors in the pituitary. In doses larger than those required to suppress lactation it produces effects attributable to stimulation of dopamine receptors elsewhere than in the pituitary. Thus, it induces vomiting, increases spontaneous motor activity and stereotyped movements in laboratory animals and it may be the cause of visual hallucinations.

It is convenient to summarize all the therapeutic uses of bromocryptine here although not all are referable to an interaction with pituitary mechanisms.

1. Bromocryptine, in doses of 2.5 mg, twice or thrice daily, is employed in the treatment of galactorrhoea from any cause and to suppress lactation in women who cannot, or are unwilling to, breast feed their new offspring.

As we have seen, amenorrhoea and impotence commonly accompany the galactorrhoea provoked by drugs or by abnormalities of pituitary function. It sometimes happens that hyperprolactinaemia arises from no obvious cause and though it may be insufficient to induce milk secretion it may nevertheless bring signs of hypogonadism in its train. It is often worthwhile to try the effect of bromocryptine in cases of amenorrhoea and other manifestations of hypogonadism, on the assumption that they may be the result of a hyperprolactinaemia.

2. Bromocryptine stimulates the output of growth hormone in endocrinologically normal subjects but, for no

very clear reason, it inhibits hormone release in those with acromegaly. It provides the only known form of drug treatment for this condition but daily doses of up to 60 mg have to be given to achieve any therapeutic effect. Bromocryptine reduces the amount of growth hormone in the plasma of the majority of those acromegalics who receive it but normal levels are not reached even in those who have responded well to treatment.

3. Because it stimulates dopamine receptors, bromocryptine has been applied to the treatment of Parkinson's disease (p. 592). It is not noticeably superior to L-dopa except perhaps in patients who suffer rapid swings in their response to L-dopa corresponding to fluctuations in its plasma concentration occasioned on the one hand by the twice daily ingestions of the drug and on the other by its rapid disappearance from the tissues. Bromocryptine has a longer half life than dopa in the plasma so that a steady concentration can be more easily maintained in the tissues. Bromocryptine can also be tried in those who are refractory to L-dopa although it is by no means certain that they will not prove to be just as resistant to bromocryptine.

Daily doses of up to 300 mg of bromocryptine have been given in the hope of alleviating the symptoms of Parkinson's disease.

4. Bromocryptine can be employed to prevent galactorrhoea in hypertensive patients receiving α-methyldopa. When this is done the antihypertensive action of α-methyldopa is seen to be potentiated and it has been suggested that bromocryptine might be used as an adjunct to α-methyldopa therapy, whether or not there is a threat of galactorrhoea. Changes brought about by bromocryptine that are probably related to its antihypertensive action include an increased excretion of salt and water and a reduction in the amount of angiotensin in the plasma. These changes lend some support to the idea that at least some of the actions of prolactin mentioned earlier do indeed reflect its physiological role.

Side effects of bromocryptine therapy. Side effects are more likely to appear in the course of treatment with the larger doses of drug such as those used in Parkinson's disease. Hallucinations are probably the most common unwanted response but nausea and vomiting, postural hypotension, constipation and dryness of the mouth also occur. Many of these effects are attributable to stimulation of dopamine receptors elsewhere than in the pituitary.

THE ASSAY AND STANDARDIZATION OF PITUITARY HORMONES

Polypeptide hormones can be assayed by radioimmunoassay, a technique that is described below. Although the method is exquisitely sensitive it is not always specific enough to distinguish between polypeptides with closely related structures and for this reason it is sometimes necessary to revert to the older technique of bioassay. Since bioassay will also be needed in laboratories that are not yet equipped to perform radioimmunoassay, descriptions of bioassay methods are retained in the account that follows.

Growth hormone can be assayed by measuring its effect on the growth of young hypophysectomized rats. Growth is assessed simply by weighing the animal or by removing the tibia, staining it and measuring the width of the epiphysial cartilage. The preparation to be assayed is given by subcutaneous injections that have to be repeated daily for at least one week if the animal is to be weighed or for four days if the tibia is to be inspected. The daily dose of growth hormone has to be not less than 10 μg so that the methods are of little value for determining the amount of hormone in blood: in the normal adult human being the growth hormone content of the serum reaches no more than 0.5 μg per ml and it may be much less. However, radioimmunoassay can deal satisfactorily with tiny amounts of growth hormone. In one method a small amount of growth hormone labelled with radioactive iodine (^{131}I) together with a small amount of growth hormone antibody are added to the solution to be assayed, or, when the method is being calibrated, to a series of standard solutions of growth hormone. The amount of labelled hormone that combines with the antibody depends upon the relative amounts of labelled and unlabelled hormone present in the solution. Thus, the growth hormone content of the solution under assay can be calculated from the amount of added labelled hormone that becomes bound to antibody. A convenient way of determining this is by electrophoresis: the unbound hormone does not move in the electrophoretic field. Further details of these methods are discussed by Berson and Yallow (1964).

Thyrotrophic hormone. Radioactive iodine (^{131}I) is readily taken up by the thyroid gland. The rate of release of radioactivity from the thyroid gland labelled in this way is determined by the physiological activity of the gland which is itself dependent on the stimulus received from the thyrotrophic hormone. This forms the basis of a very sensitive method for the bioassay of the hormone. Mice are used and the rate of appearance of radioactivity in the blood is measured following administration of the material being assayed.

Minnows can be used to measure the activity of the exophthalmos-producing factor (p. 714) to which the eyes of fish are very sensitive.

Even radioimmunoassay is not sensitive enough to detect the small amounts of thyroid stimulating hormones in the blood of endocrinologically normal individuals.

Corticotrophin. A method of biological standardization recommended by the British and other Pharmacopoeias makes use of the fact that corticotrophin reduces the ascorbic acid content of the adrenal gland. Hypophysectomized rats (kept in health by a saline supplement to their drinking fluid) are used. The operation is performed 18 to 36 hours before the assay so as to remove all endogenous sources of corticotrophin. The material to be standardized, or doses of a standard preparation, are given by subcutaneous or intravenous injection and the adrenal ascorbic acid is measured three hours after subcutaneous injection or one hour after intravenous injection. Although this method is simple and adequate for standardization purposes, it is too insensitive for physiological work. An alternative is to assess the adrenal response by measuring the corticosterone content of adrenal venous blood. By this method the corticotrophin of as little as 5 ml of blood can be measured.

The gonadotrophins. Gonadotrophin assay presents some difficulties. Pituitary extracts and blood plasma contain both hormones and the responses of sensitive tissues to one of the gonadotrophins are modified by the presence of the other. Luteinizing hormone can, however, be assayed by taking advantage of its action on male sex organs. Young, male, hypophysectomized rats are used and the effect of the hormone on the weight of the prostate gland is measured. In a more sensitive test, female rats are given large doses of urinary or chorionic gonadotrophin. Some days later the assay is performed, luteinizing activity being assessed by measuring the depletion of ascorbic acid from the ovaries. Follicle stimulating hormone does not interfere with this assay.

Preparations or extracts containing follicle stimulating hormone uncontaminated by luteinizing hormone are assayed on the basis of their ability to increase the weight of the ovaries of hypophysectomized rats. If luteinizing hormone is present, intact animals are employed. They are given a dose of chorionic gonadotrophin. This itself brings about an increase in ovarian weight but follicle stimulating hormone further augments the weight independently of the amount of luteinizing hormone contaminating the preparation.

It is sometimes sufficient or necessary to measure total gonadotrophic activity. For this purpose, the effect of the gonadotrophins on uterine weight in mice is utilized.

Radioimmunochemical assays for the gonadotrophins are very sensitive but not highly specific. In particular, some biologically inactive derivatives retain immunological reactivity and so are assayed as active hormones.

Oxytocin. One of the best methods of standardizing preparations of oxytocin makes use of the fact that the hormone has a hypotensive action in birds. This hypotensive action accurately reflects oxytocic activity. Young cockerels are anaesthetized with sodium barbitone which is given by intramuscular injection. The blood pressure is recorded from the popliteal artery. Drugs and standard solutions are administered intravenously. Another pharmacopoeial method uses the isolated uterus of non pregnant dioestrus rats and in experimental work oxytocin can

be measured on the basis of its ability to cause milk ejection from the mammary duct of the rabbit.

Oxytocin and vasopressin are small polypeptides and do not stimulate the production of antibodies. They cannot, therefore, be assayed by radioimmunological methods.

Vasopressin. For the biological *standardization* of vasopressin, blood pressure methods are used. Male rats are anaesthetized with urethane and are given hexamethonium (p. 252) or dibenamine (p. 299) to stabilize the blood pressure. The advantage of this method over the cat blood pressure assay previously favoured is that tachyphylaxis does not occur so that injections can be given at frequent intervals.

Although standardization is usually based on pressor activity, physiological experiments may demand measurement of the antidiuretic activity of serum or urine. For this purpose fasting male rats are water-loaded by stomach tube. They are anaesthetized with an aqueous solution of ethanol given by mouth. The jugular vein is cannulated and the bladder is catheterized. More water is then supplied, equal in volume to that voided up to the time of cannulation. At this stage the rat is put on to a balance pan and as urine is lost an equivalent weight of a 2.5 per cent solution of ethanol is given. This maintains the water load and the level of anaesthesia. When urine output becomes constant a dose of the material to be assayed is given by way of the venous cannula. Antidiuretic activity is shown by a reduction in urine flow.

An alternative method, which is favoured by some physiologists, makes use of conscious dogs trained to accept intravenous injections. It is very suitable in research laboratories but not for routine assays.

BIBLIOGRAPHY

Books, monographs and reviews

Astwood, E. B. and Beck, J. C. (eds) (1964). Proteins and polypeptides. *Metabolism*, **13**, 965-1296.

Bayliss, R. I. S., Turner, P. and Maclay, W. P. (eds) (1976). *Pharmacological and Clinical Aspects of Bromocryptine (Parlodel)*. Tunbridge Wells: MCS Consultants.

Caldeyro-Barcta, R. and Heller, H. (1961). *Oxytocin*. London: Pergamon.

Glick, S., Roth, J., Yallow, Rosalyn S. and Berson, S. A. (1965). The regulation of growth hormone secretion. *Recent Prog. Horm. Res.*, **21**, 241-283.

Hall, R., Anderson, J., Smart, G. A. and Besser, M. (1974). *Fundamentals of Clinical Endocrinology*, 2nd ed. London: Pitman Medical.

Harris, G. W. (1955). *Neural Control of the Pituitary Gland*. London: Arnold.

Hoffbrand, B. I., Maclay, W. P. and Turner, P. (eds) (1976). Ergot compounds - the changing scene. *Postgrad. med. J.*, **52**, Supp. (1), 7-86.

Horrobin, D. F. (1973) *Prolactin: Physiology and Clinical Significance*. Lancaster: Medical and Technical Publishing Co.

Horrobin, D. F. (1974). *Prolactin 1974*. Lancaster: Medical and Technical Publishing Co.

Kirkham, K. E. and Hunter, W. M. (1971). *Radioimmunoassay Methods.* Edinburgh and London: Churchill Livingstone.

Knobil, E. and Hitchkiss, J. (1964). Growth hormone. *A. rev. Physiol.*, **26**, 47-74.

Loraine, J. A. and Bell, E. T. (1971). *Hormone Assays and their Clinical Application.* Edinburgh and London: Churchill Livingstone.

Sawyer, W. H. (1961). Neurohypophysial hormones. *Pharmac. Rev.*, **13**, 225-277.

Wolstenholme, G. E. W. and Knight, J. (eds) (1972). *Lactogenic Hormones.* Edinburgh and London: Churchill Livingstone.

Yagi, K. and Koshida, S. (eds) (1973). *Neuroendocrine Control.* New York, Toronto and London: John Wiley.

Original papers

Berson, S. A. and Yallow, Rosalyn S. (1964). Immunoassay of protein hormones. In, Pincus. G., Thimann, K. V. and Astwood, E. B. (eds) *The Hormones,* Vol. IV, 557-629. New York: Academic Press.

Boissonnas, R. A., Guttman, St., Berde, B. and Konzett, H. (1961). Relationships between the chemical structures and the biological properties of the posterior pituitary hormones and their synthetic analogues. *Experientia (Basel),* **17**, 377-390.

Flückiger, E. and Wagner, H. R. (1968). 2-Br-α -ergokryptin: Beinflussing von Fertilität und Laktation bei der Ratte. *Experientia,* **24**, 1130-1131.

Schally, A. V., Arimura, A., Takahara, J., Redding, T. W. and Dupont, A. (1974). Inhibition of prolactin release *in vitro* and *in vivo* by catecholamines. *Fed. Proc.*, **33**, 237A.

Takahara, J., Arimura, A. and Schally, A. V. (1974). Suppression of prolactin release by a purified porcine PIF preparation and catecholamines infused into a rat hypophysial portal vessel. *Endocrinology,* **95**, 462-465.

46. Calcium, the parathyroid glands and calcitonin

Calcium is a metal of unique importance since it is required by the body in large quantities as an essential constituent of bone and teeth and in very much smaller quantities as a regulator of a number of vital processes. About ninety-seven per cent of the total calcium content of the human body is present in the bony skeleton which consists essentially of the phosphates and other salts of calcium deposited on an organic matrix. The rest of the calcium is found in connective tissue, the soft tissues, interstitial fluid and plasma. About one half of the calcium in plasma exists as calcium ions. The rest occurs in the form of a non-diffusible complex with protein. A minor fraction of the plasma's calcium is present in the form of diffusible but unionized complexes with organic acids. Only the calcium which is present as freely diffusible ions takes any part in the regulation of physiological processes. Thus in patients with a gross deficiency of plasma proteins, calcium dependent processes may be well maintained even if there is an overall deficiency of the metal.

The organic matrix of bone consists largely of collagen, a fibrous protein one of whose most important constituents is hydroxyproline.

Calcium ions have important regulatory actions on a number of vital processes. The permeability—and hence the excitability—of nerve and muscle membranes is inversely related to the calcium content of the fluid to which they are exposed but calcium ions play a more direct part in the initiation of muscle contraction. When a muscle is depolarized, calcium can pass into the fibre from the extracellular fluid but the excitatory process that provokes this depolarization of the boundary membrane of the fibre produces a similar change in the microsomal membrane and thereby permits the egress of calcium from the intracellular particles. The calcium thus made available induces, in concert with ATP, the shortening of the actomyosin filaments that constitutes muscle contraction.

Calcium is a mediator not only of excitation-contraction coupling in muscle but also of the analogous stimulus-secretion coupling which ensures the liberation of synaptic transmitter substances or of hormones in response to the stimulus provided, respectively, by nerve impulses or by trophic hormones. It seems that these stimuli permit the intracellular accumulation of calcium (derived, as before, partly from the extracellular fluid and partly from the mitochondria) and a consequent expulsion of transmitter or hormone from contractile tubules or vesicles.

As we have seen (p. 322) the hormones themselves operate, in many instances, by promoting the formation of cyclic AMP which activates the specific enzyme systems that support the hormone dependent metabolic processes. This activation can only take place in the presence of adequate amounts of calcium.

Calcium ions participate in the processes that culminate in the coagulation of blood (Chap. 39) and they are also necessary for the maintenance of some of the physical properties of cells, such as adhesiveness.

It would be wrong to think of the calcium in bone as being permanently sequestered there in a physiologically inactive and inaccessible form. The bony skeleton of the adult male contains about 1000 grams of calcium of which about 5 grams (that which has been most recently laid down) can be freely exchanged with the diffusible calcium of plasma. Some idea of the importance of this labile pool may be gleaned from the estimate that the total daily exchange of calcium between plasma and bone is 20 grams. Thus the contents of the pool are completely changed once in six hours. Movements of calcium into and out of the pool are determined simply by changes in the direction of the concentration gradient between pool and plasma: they are not under hormonal control but they will clearly help to maintain a steady level of plasma calcium.

The calcium content of plasma is of the order of 10 mg per 100 ml: individual values are kept remarkably constant. Calcium balance is achieved by the mutual interaction of a number of regulatory mechanisms. In addition to the plasma-bone exchange already referred to, these are as follows:

a. Variable proportions of the calcium ingested in the diet are absorbed into the blood. In addition, active secretory processes permit calcium to be excreted into the intestine. The total average daily calcium intake is one gram and about 900 mg are excreted in the faeces.

b. Diffusible calcium passes into the glomerular filtrate and variable amounts are reabsorbed by renal tubular mechanisms. The daily urinary excretion of calcium is usually about 100 mg.

c. In lactating women, calcium is lost in the milk.

d. Calcium can pass into plasma from the stable fraction in bone. This is the calcium in the mass of older bone which does not form part of the labile pool; it is mobilized by parathyroid hormone (see below).

In accordance with the general principles of homeostasis, changes in the loss or gain of calcium by one route are compensated, within the limits of the system, by reciprocal changes elsewhere. The calcium content of the plasma regulates the secretion of, and is in its turn controlled by, the parathyroid hormone.

THE PARATHYROID GLANDS

These glands, four in number, are in most species (including man) embedded in the thyroid gland. The glands synthesize a polypeptide 'prohormone' that is made up of 90 amino acid residues from which the hormone proper, which has 84 residues, is split off before release into the blood stream. The full sequences of amino acids in porcine and bovine hormones have now been established. It facilitates absorption of calcium from the intestinal tract, it increases the tubular reabsorption of calcium but promotes phosphate excretion, it reduces the calcium content of milk and it promotes the passage of calcium and phosphate into plasma from the stable fraction in bone. All these actions serve the same end—the maintenance of the level of plasma calcium required for vital physiological processes at the expense, if needs be, even of the body's own supporting skeleton or the well-being of its offspring. The presence of vitamin D (Chap. 47) is necessary before the parathyroid hormone can effectively perform any of its functions but, apart from promoting calcium absorption from the intestine (in which activity the vitamin is more important than the hormone), vitamin D alone cannot reproduce any of the actions of the parathyroid hormone.

Factors that influence the secretion of the parathyroid hormones operate directly on the glands themselves which (unlike so many endocrine organs) are not subject to pituitary control.

Bone is modelled, and the form of the fully developed structure is maintained, by the conjoint and coordinated activity of two types of cell: the *osteoblasts* which lay down the bone and the *osteoclasts* which remove it. The two processes operate simultaneously and so far as bone is concerned it seems that the parathyroid hormone owes its action to an ability to increase the number or the activity of the osteoclasts. The removal of bone by osteoclastic activity is referred to as *resorption*, an infelicitous word which unfortunately enjoys a wide currency. Parathyroid hormone also stimulates respiration and ion transport in mitochondrial preparations. This action presumably accounts for the hormone's ability to influence absorptive and secretory processes.

The actions of the parathyroid hormone on bone and kidney are mediated by cyclic AMP.

DISEASES DUE TO DISTURBANCES OF CALCIUM BALANCE

HYPOPARATHYROIDISM AND TETANY

Hypoparathyroidism is most often the result of the delib- erate removal of the parathyroid glands made necessary by a tumour in these organs or in the thyroid gland. Occasionally hypoparathyroidism arises in the absence of any obvious pathological process in the glands. The characteristic sign of hypoparathyroidism is *tetany*, a manifestation of a lack of ionized calcium. There are tingling sensations (*paraesthesiae*) in the limbs, an increased neuromuscular irritability with twitching and fibrillation of the skeletal muscles, laryngeal spasm (alternating spasm and relaxation of the laryngeal muscles may produce a characteristic 'crowing' sound) and finally convulsions. Two well known diagnostic signs of tetany, both providing evidence of the increased neuromuscular excitability, are *Chvostek's Sign* and *Trousseau's Sign*. To elicit the first, the facial nerve is tapped at its point of origin from the skull near the mastoid process. In tetany this results in a firm spasm of the muscles of the face. Trousseau's Sign (carpopedal spasm) is looked for by reducing, by means of a sphygmomanometer cuff, the blood supply to a limb. This has the effect of accentuating the already heightened neuromuscular excitability: if the arm is constricted the wrist and elbow are flexed but the fingers are firmly extended; if the test is applied to the lower limb, the feet will be drawn up with the toes flexed. Carpopedal spasm, affecting all four limbs, may occur spontaneously in severe tetany. In addition to tetany, hypoparathyroidism may also cause cataract (the parathyroid hormone prevents the deposition of calcium in the lens) and psychiatric disturbances.

Tetany is only rarely due to hypoparathyroidism; any condition which causes a sufficient depletion of ionized calcium in the plasma will produce tetany. The condition may be due to an inadequate intake of calcium or vitamin D or an impaired absorption of calcium consequent on some intestinal condition. Alkalosis, which reduces the ionization of calcium salts, is another likely cause of tetany. Alkalosis may arise as a result of excessive vomiting, overdosage with alkali or hyperventilation. Many students who have followed too enthusiastically instructions to overbreathe in the course of a practical class will themselves have experienced the symptoms (paraesthesia and twitching of the smaller muscles) of incipient tetany.

In clinical practice the aetiology of an individual case of tetany is rarely in doubt. If hypoparathyroidism is suspected the diagnosis can be confirmed by measuring the urinary excretion of the parathyroid hormone.

A possible explanation of the neuromuscular hyperexcitability seen in tetany is that calcium ions may be associated with some of the molecules that carry sodium ions across the nerve and muscle membrane. Deficiency of calcium ions would make more carrier molecules available for sodium transport so that depolarization of the excitable membranes would take place more readily. This increased excitability contrasts oddly with the failure of contraction which occurs when muscle is exposed to a solution which lacks calcium (for the action on the heart, see Fig. 40.6, p.

698) and with the known calcium dependence of acetylcholine release at the neuromuscular junction. Calcium deficiency of the grade met clinically does not proceed far enough seriously to affect the contractile processes of muscle and any neuromuscular blocking effect is more than offset by the increased excitability of the conducting and contractile tissues.

Acute attacks of tetany, whatever their origin, are treated by the intravenous injection of a calcium salt. The gluconate is usually employed: the dose (which can be repeated if the condition is not relieved) is 2 grams given very slowly in a 10 per cent solution. When the immediate objective of relieving convulsions, laryngeal spasm or carpopedal spasm has been achieved, attention can be directed towards remedying the underlying disorder. If this is nutritional, the provision of a diet containing adequate amounts of calcium, phosphate and vitamin D will usually be sufficient. Hypoparathyroidism raises more difficult problems. The sheet anchor of treatment in this condition is still dietary but in order to produce an internal environment similar to that created by parathyroid activity it is necessary to provide a diet which, though rich in calcium and vitamin D, is deficient in phosphate. Unfortunately, the necessity of avoiding phosphate involves restricting or forbidding some articles of diet—milk, cheese and eggs—which are the richest sources of calcium and adequate amounts of the metal can only be obtained by supplementing an already unattractive diet with calcium salts. Calcium lactate (6 grams daily) is cheap but unpleasant to take. Calcium gluconate is palatable but expensive as is calcium gluconogalactogluconate which is available in the form of effervescent tablets or a syrup. The daily dose is 750 mg to 3 grams.

The obvious therapeutic measure—administration of parathyroid extract (Parathorm) is often discouraged on the grounds that severe reactions may occur to the preparation (which is still only available in an impure form) and that patients rapidly develop a resistance to it. Nevertheless, parathyroid extract does have its place in treatment, particularly in the days following removal of a parathyroid tumour. There is some justification for attempting to use it over a longer period in individual cases, since not all patients become resistant to its effects. The onset of the hormone's action is slow and the initial doses may have to be given by the intravenous route. Later

they may be given by subcutaneous or intramuscular injection. Another substance which has been given in hypoparathyroidism is dihydrotachysterol (AT10; Hytakerol). Its actions appear to be similar to those of the parathyroid hormone. Among recent publications can be found statements that dihydrotachysterol does nothing that cannot be done more cheaply and effectively by vitamin D and assertions that it has considerable therapeutic potential which will ensure its more widespread use in future years. It seems justifiable to conclude that its value is in dispute.

HYPERPARATHYROIDISM

Hyperparathyroidism is usually due to a secreting tumour of the parathyroid glands but it may arise iatrogenically (p. 70) as a result of injudicious administration of parathyroid hormone. As would be expected, the bones tend to become decalcified. This may cause pain in the bones or joints or the condition may progress to a fully blown *von Recklinghausen's disease of bone.* In this disorder, which is also known as *osteitis fibrosa generalisata,* decalcification may progress so extensively that the bones become soft, bent and easily fractured. Long before this stage has been reached, however, the disease is likely to have drawn attention to itself by causing kidney or ureteric pain due to the deposition of calcium in the renal tubules or of stones in the ureter. Treatment is surgical.

CALCIUM DEFICIENCY DISEASES

Tetany occurs when there is a lack of calcium ions in the plasma. Because the free ions constitute but a minor fraction of the body's total supply of calcium, the occurrence of tetany does not necessarily betoken an overall deficiency of calcium. Conversely, since the parathyroid glands can maintain a normal concentration of calcium ions in the plasma in the face of considerable deficiencies elsewhere, tetany is only a feature of the most severe forms of calcium deficiency.

Calcium deficiency occurs if the dietary intake of calcium is very low or if its absorption is impeded by vitamin D deficiency or by diseases which cause *steatorrhoea*—the excretion of large quantities of undigested fat and their associated vitamins. In young children, severe calcium deficiency causes *rickets,* a disorder characterized by inadequate calcification of the bones which remain soft and become curved outwards. The deficiency may be severe enough to cause tetany, and both convulsions and laryngeal spasm are common in rickets. Calcium and vitamin D are synergistic in their actions and a deficiency of one may be compensated by an excess of the other. Underprivileged children are likely to be denied adequate amounts of both these items of diet but those fortunate enough to live in the sun will suffer less severely because the sunlight will produce vitamin D from endogenous precursors in the children's skin. Rickets was once widespread in the industrialized parts of Britain where nutrition

Dihydrotachysterol

was poor, the sun shone rarely and then through an industrial murk and where neither the weather nor the national *mores* permitted children to play naked and out of doors. With increasing affluence, parents have been able to provide foods which supply sufficient calcium and vitamin D to offset the unfavourable environmental and atmospheric conditions so that rickets is almost a disease of the past in Britain, although there are some recent reports which indicate that the disease may be re-emerging in some of the areas, where it was rife in the past. The rickety child with his bowed legs, decayed teeth and miserably vacant expression can be seen in any photograph of infant school children taken in the early years of the present century in the less salubrious areas of Britain. Rickets is, of course, still a problem in many underdeveloped countries.

Gross calcium deficiency in adults is more likely to be the result of some condition which prevents calcium absorption but it may develop in underprivileged women who have had many pregnancies to drain their calcium stores. The disease produced is *osteomalacia*, a condition in which there is a progressive weakening of the skeleton. It is still common among unemancipated women in India and elsewhere. *Osteoporosis* is a not dissimilar condition which most often occurs in postmenopausal women, though it is also seen in old men. It may develop in individuals who have not previously shown signs of calcium deficiency and its relatively frequent occurrence indicates that calcium requirements may increase in old age, perhaps because excretion is increased. Osteoporosis is treated by attention to the diet, sometimes supported by the administration of oestrogens or anabolic steroids. The treatment of rickets and osteomalacia is entirely nutritional, with corrective orthopoedic surgery when necessary. Rarefaction of the bones may also be a feature of some cases of Cushing's syndrome (Chap. 44). It arises because glucocorticoids increase calcium excretion.

HYPERCALCAEMIA

An increased concentration of calcium ions in the blood may arise, in the absence of a hyperparathyroid state, as a result of bone tumours or in patients who, having been immobilized for a long period of time, are suffering from disuse atrophy. Among the substances which have been used to treat this condition are mineralo-corticosteroids (Chap. 44), sodium sulphate, the chelating agent disodium edetate (Chap. 48), and calcitonin.

Paget's disease of bone In this not uncommon condition the turnover of calcium in bone is accelerated as a result of an increased activity in both the osteoblasts and the osteoclasts. The disease often gives rise to no symptoms at all but some victims suffer extreme pain in the affected bones. In advanced cases there may be limb deformities and spontensous fractures. The calcium content of the serum may be raised, particularly if the limbs are immobilized by the disease or it may be held within normal limits.

Its aetiology is obscure and the disease is difficult to treat although some therapeutic success has been claimed for calcitonin (p. 785).

CALCITONIN

In experiments that began as long ago as 1957, Copp infused a calcium salt into an experimental animal and showed that this caused the appearance in the blood stream of a substance capable of lowering the calcium content of the plasma. He came correctly to the conclusion that the hypocalcaemic factor was a hormone. He named it *calcitonin* and believed, not unnaturally, that the new hormone came from the parathyroid glands. However, the discovery of calcitonin in extracts of rat thyroid tissue (Hirsch, Ganthier & Munson, 1963) led to experiments that established its origin as the small so-called C cells that are irregularly distributed around and between the thyroid follicles. For this reason calcitonin was renamed thyrocalcitonin in some quarters but the most recent work has made it clear that the cell types that produce the hormone are not confined to the thyroid gland. It would seem that the original name was, after all, the better one. It is retained in this book.

It seems worthwhile to summarize some of the work that first clearly demonstrated the origin and the action of calcitonin. MacIntyre and his colleagues (Gudmundssohn, MacIntyre and Soliman, 1966; MacIntyre, 1968) devised some of the most elegantly simple of these early experiments. In one of these, the thyroid-parathyroid glands of dogs were perfused with blood to which calcium could be added as required. Whenever the calcium content of the perfusate was increased, blood deficient in calcium was infused into a suitable systemic vein. It should have been possible to ensure in this way that the calcium content of the blood as a whole did not change even when that of the blood circulating through the glands was increased. In fact this was not possible: the amount of calcium in the circulating blood fell whenever the glands were exposed to high concentrations of calcium. An obvious explanation of this finding was that the calcium had suppressed the secretion of parathyroid hormone, an action it is known to possess. However, surgical removal of the thyroid and parathyroid glands was followed by only a slow fall in the concentration of calcium in the blood in contrast to the brisk response to calcium perfusion in the intact animal. Thus it seemed more likely that either the thyroid or the parathyroid glands produced a hormone which was capable of actively reducing the calcium content of circulating blood. That this hormone came from the thyroid gland was demonstrated in experiments on goats. In the goat, the two superior parathyroid glands are not embedded in the substance of the thyroid gland as they are in many other species and it is therefore possible to remove the thyroid gland completely without interrupting parathyroid activity. When the parathyroid glands of thyroidectomized goats were exposed to an increased concentration of calcium, the systemic blood did not exhibit the rapid fall in its calcium content which characterizes the response of animals with intact thyroid glands. It was then demonstrated that the intravenous injection of an extract of the goats' excised thyroid tissue brought about a fall in the calcium content of their blood. The hormone has been detected in the thyroid glands of all mammalian species (including man) so far examined and all species are sensitive to its action.

Calcitonin is a polypeptide: the human variety (which has now been synthesized) has 32 amino acid residues arranged in a single chain with one disulphide linkage within the chain. The hormone reduces the phosphorus as well as the calcium content of blood but magnesium is unaffected. A hint to its site of action comes from the observation that calcitonin brings about a reduction in the urinary excretion of hydroxyproline. This finding suggests that calcitonin prevents the breakdown of bone, the source of most of the urinary hydroxyproline. To this extent, calcitonin can be regarded as an antagonist of the parathyroid hormone but the antagonism does not extend to the gut or kidney. In these organs calcium transport, which is facilitated by parathyroid hormone (p. 782), is unaffected by calcitonin.

Although the experimental evidence so far obtained is not inconsistent with the hypothesis that calcitonin is a component of the system which controls calcium homeostasis, its importance relative to the parathyroid hormone remains to be established. It is difficult to believe that a substance with so powerful an effect on the calcium content of the blood is without physiological significance and it is certainly true that hypercalcaemia stimulates both the synthesis and the release of calcitonin. Nevertheless, some findings are difficult to reconcile with the view that calcitonin plays a major physiological role. MacIntyre and his colleagues, for instance (Cunliffe et al., 1968), have reported finding a thyroid carcinoma which secreted enormous quantities of calcitonin. Yet the patient exhibited no sign of calcium deficiency and the parathyroid glands were not hyperplastic as would have been expected if normal calcium balance had been maintained by a compensatory secretion of its hormone to balance the hypocalcaemic action of calcitonin. Perhaps calcitonin is released only in the emergency situation of the amount of calcium in the blood's increasing to an extent or at a rate that cannot be immediately controlled by curtailing the supplies of parathyroid hormone.

A number of substances other than calcium will call forth the release of calcitonin. Among these is glucagon (p. 722) which is active in very low concentrations. The physiological significance of this observation is obscure.

THERAPEUTIC USE OF CALCITONIN

Clinical syndromes attributable to a deficient or an excessive secretion of calcitonin have not been clearly identified but the properties of the hormone are such as to suggest that it might be useful for treating conditions characterized by an increased mobilization of calcium from bone. These include hyperparathyroidism, Paget's disease of bone, osteoporosis, hypervitaminosis D and some bone tumours. Experience with this form of treatment is still extremely limited but the indications so far are that Paget's disease sometimes responds very well and osteoporosis not at all to calcitonin. Its value in the treatment of the other conditions mentioned is problematical.

The forms of calcitonin available for clinical use are derived from the pig (Calcitare) or the salmon (Calsynar). The latter is the more potent because it is only broken down very slowly in the mammal. Its chemical nature demands its administration by injection.

BIBLIOGRAPHY

Books, monographs and reviews

Copp, D. H. (1964). Parathyroids, calcitonin and control of plasma calcium. Recent Prog. Horm. Res., **20**, 59-88.

MacIntyre, I. (1968). Calcitonin. The Scientific Basis of Medicine, Annual Reviews, 1968, pp. 242-253.

MacIntyre, I. (ed). (1972). Clinics in Endocrinology and Metabolism. London: Saunders.

Nordin, B. E. C. (1973). Metabolic Bone and Stone Disease. Edinburgh and London: Churchill Livingstone.

Potts, J. T., Aurbach, G. D. and Sherwood, L. M. (1966). Parathyroid hormone: chemical properties and structural requirements for biological and immunological activity. Recent Prog. Horm. Res., **22**, 101-151.

Potts, J. T., Keutmann, H. T., Hall, H. D. and Tregear, G. W. (1971). The chemistry of parathyroid hormone and the calcitonins. Vitams. Horm., **29**, 41-93.

Rasmussen, H. (ed). (1970). International Encyclopedia of Pharmacology and Therapeutics Sect. 51, Vol. 1: Parathyroid Hormone, Thyrocalcitonin and Related Drugs, Oxford and London: Pergamon.

Talmage, R. V. and Belanger, L. F. (eds) (1968). Parathyroid Hormone and Thyrocalcitonin (Calcitonin). New York: Excerpta Medica.

Talmage, R. V., Cooper, C. W. and Park, H. Z. (1970). Regulation of calcium transport in bone by parathyroid hormone. Vitams. Horm. **28**, 103-140.

See also the texts on General Endocrinology listed on p. 718.

Original papers

Cunliffe, W. J., Black, M. M., Hall, R., Johnston, I. D. A., Hudgson, P., Shuster, S., Gudmundsson, T. V., Joplin, G. F., Williams, E. .D., Woodhouse, N. J. Y., Galante, L. and MacIntyre, I. (1968). A calcitonin-secreting thyroid carcinoma. Lancet, **2**, 63-65.

Gudmundsson, T. V., MacIntyre, I. and Soliman, H. A. (1966). The isolation of thyrocalcitonin and a study of its effects in the rat. Proc. R. Soc., B. **164**, 460-477.

Hirsch, P. F., Gauthier, G. F. and Munson, P. L. (1963). Thyroid hypocalcemic principle and recurrent laryngeal nerve injury as factors affecting the response to parathyroidectomy in rats. Endocrinology. **73**, 244-252.

47. The vitamins

Animals die if they are fed purified diets which provide only an adequate number of calories, a sufficiency of proteins, fats and carbohydrates and all the inorganic substances required by the body. This is because such diets lack *vitamins*—organic compounds which must be provided in minute amounts if the chemical processes which support growth and health are to be maintained. Because vitamins are only produced in the body in trivial amounts, if at all, they (or in some instances their precursors) must be supplied by the diet or administered in their pure form as dietary supplements.

In human beings, a reasonably varied diet should provide, except in infancy and pregnancy, all the vitamins needed but in undernourished populations and among those whose diet is inadequate for one of various reasons (poverty, ignorance, alcoholism, idiosyncratic beliefs, etc.) a serious deficiency of one or more vitamins is likely to occur. Vitamin deficiency diseases are responsible for much of the misery and ill health suffered by those who are denied a proper diet.

The name 'vitamine' was originally given to these accessory food factors because they were known to be vital for life and they were all believed to be amines. The terminal 'e' was dropped when it became clear that some were not amines.

Since vitamins are chemical substances which influence the activity of the body's normal mechanisms, they come properly within the pharmacologist's field of study. They are, however, of more immediate interest to the biochemist and the nutritionist and they are therefore considered only briefly in this book.

The vitamins are divided into 'fat soluble' and 'water soluble' groups. The individual members of each group are named in Figure 47.1. As they were discovered the vitamins were systematically identified by the letters A to E. This was a useful convention at a time when the chemical composition of the newly found substances was a mystery. But then it was realised that the material that had been named vitamin B was a mixture of chemically dissimilar substances with differing biological activities and it became necessary to label the several components separately. The addition of identifying subscripts to give vitamins B_1, B_2 and so on seemed sensible enough but, after a good start, chaos took over and numbers and letters were allocated in what now seems to be a completely undiscriminating, haphazard and illogical manner. As a result we have acquired a heterogeneous collection of confusing and largely uninformative identifying symbols for the several members of the vitamin B complex so that vitamins B_1 and B_2 rub uneasy shoulders with, among others, vitamins B_C, H and PP (Fig. 47.1). These designations have proved so inconvenient that most workers in the field identify the

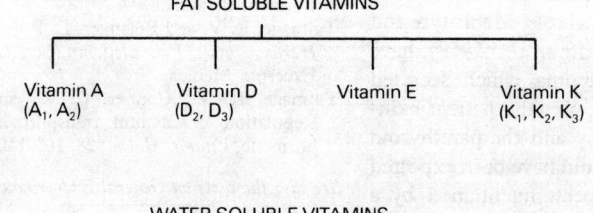

FAT SOLUBLE VITAMINS

Vitamin A (A_1, A_2) Vitamin D (D_2, D_3) Vitamin E Vitamin K (K_1, K_2, K_3)

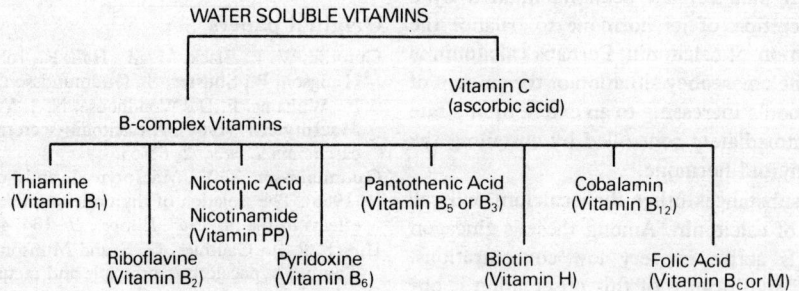

WATER SOLUBLE VITAMINS

Vitamin C (ascorbic acid)

B-complex Vitamins

Thiamine (Vitamin B_1) Nicotinic Acid / Nicotinamide (Vitamin PP) Pantothenic Acid (Vitamin B_5 or B_3) Cobalamin (Vitamin B_{12})

Riboflavine (Vitamin B_2) Pyridoxine (Vitamin B_6) Biotin (Vitamin H) Folic Acid (Vitamin B_C or M)

Fig. 47.1 Classification and nomenclature of the vitamins

members of the vitamin B complex by their chemical names. This practice is adopted in Figure 47.1 and throughout this book. It remains a matter of personal preference whether the reader adopts the same procedure in relation to the other vitamins or whether, as we have done here, he retains the original nomenclature. There is something to be said in support of both practices. It should, perhaps, be added that (unlike the situation represented by vitamin B) the substances labelled vitamins A_1 and A_2 are chemically similar and have identical biological functions. A similar remark applies to the D and K vitamins so that the use of identifying subscripts for the components of these vitamins is reasonable, helpful and logical.

Before the vitamins are discussed individually, one other general point should be made. Gross deficiency of vitamins gives rise to the specific disorders enumerated below and it can reasonably be expected that milder degrees of deficiency will cause less severe forms of the diseases. Thus, an individual whose intake of Vitamin A is slightly below the optimal level may be rather slow to adapt to the new conditions when he goes out into the night from a brightly lit room, although he cannot be said to be suffering from night blindness as he would be if his intake of Vitamin A was grossly inadequate. Moreover, it seems that a slight lack of some vitamins may be associated with suboptimal health and efficiency. Such minor deficiencies are probably rather more widespread, even in affluent communities, than is often believed but their existence should not be allowed to obscure the fact that there is no real evidence for the belief (which is not confined to the layman) that a whole host of minor complaints is the result of vitamin lack. These minor ailments can be neither cured nor prevented by the taking of vitamin preparations which serve merely as expensive placebos. In any event, adjustment of vitamin intake should come from the diet and not from a bottle.

FAT SOLUBLE VITAMINS

The chemical formulae of the fat soluble vitamins A, D and E are presented in Figure 47.2.

Vitamin A

Vitamin A occurs in two forms, A_1 or retinol and A_2 or dehydroretinol respectively. Vitamin A_1 has the more widespread occurrence. It can also be formed in the body from a number of dietary precursors (or provitamins). The most important of these are the α-, β-, and γ-carotenes and cryptoxanthine. The formula of β-carotene is given in Figure 47.2; the other compounds named have a closely similar structure.

Among the most valuable dietary sources of preformed Vitamin A are dairy produce, liver, kidney and vitamin-enriched margarines. The provitamins A, especially β-

carotene, are plentiful in carrots and green vegetables. Yellow corn contains cryptoxanthine.

In human subjects, vitamin A deficiency particularly affects the visual apparatus. Vision in dim light is mediated by the retinal rods. Rod pigment (rhodopsin or visual purple) absorbs light and initiates a series of chemical events that lead to excitation of fibres in the optic nerve. The rhodopsin is itself broken down in the process but in

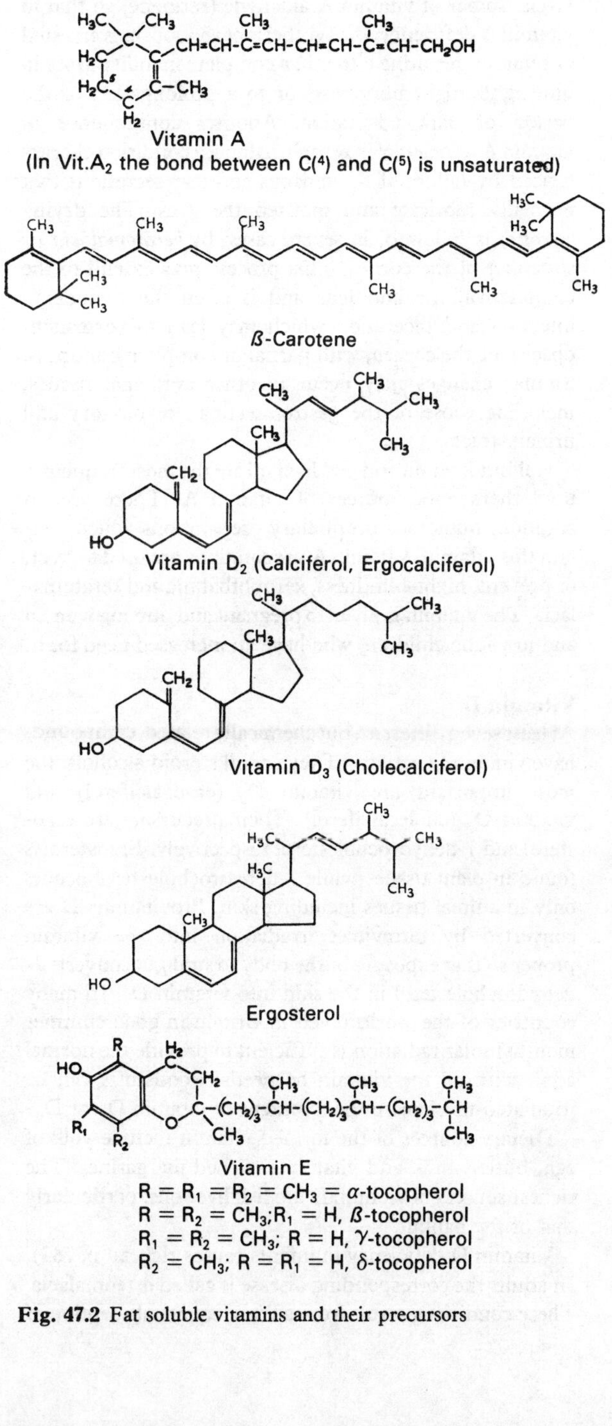

Vitamin A
(In Vit.A_2 the bond between $C(^4)$ and $C(^5)$ is unsaturated)

β-Carotene

Vitamin D_2 (Calciferol, Ergocalciferol)

Vitamin D_3 (Cholecalciferol)

Ergosterol

Vitamin E
$R = R_1 = R_2 = CH_3 = \alpha$-tocopherol
$R = R_2 = CH_3; R_1 = H$, ß-tocopherol
$R_1 = R_2 = CH_3; R = H$, γ-tocopherol
$R_2 = CH_3; R = R_1 = H$, δ-tocopherol

Fig. 47.2 Fat soluble vitamins and their precursors

dim light it is resynthesized sufficiently rapidly to ensure that supplies of the light sensitive pigment are maintained. Exposure of the eye to bright light (ordinary daylight or artificial light) brings about a complete breakdown of rhodopsin which cannot be resynthesized until the light dims again. This, of course, explains why a period of *dark adaptation* is needed when we move into the night from a well-lit room.

Rhodopsin is a combination of opsin (a protein) and the II-cis isomer of vitamin A aldehyde (retinene) so that in vitamin A deficiency, the synthesis of rhodopsin is arrested or retarded resulting either in a complete inability to see in dim light (night blindness) or to a prolongation of the period of dark adaptation. Another consequence of vitamin A deficiency is xerophthalmia, a condition characterized by failure of the mucous and tear secretions that normally lubricate and moisten the eyes. The drying (*xerosis*) is followed, in severe cases, by *keratomalacia* or softening of the cornea. This process may extend to the conjunctiva, iris and lens and is often the prelude to infection and ulceration which may lead to permanent opacity of the cornea, with partial or complete blindness. Similar changes may occur in other epithelial tissues, including those of the gastrointestinal, respiratory and urinary tracts.

Halibut liver oil and cod liver oil are the most frequently used therapeutic sources of vitamin A. There are, in addition, numerous proprietary preparations which contain this vitamin. Vitamin A preparations are used to treat, or prevent, night-blindness, xerophthalmia and keratomalacia. The vitamin is given to pregnant and nursing women and to young children, who have an increased need for it.

Vitamin D

At least seven different, but chemically related, compounds have vitamin D activity. They are all steroid alcohols: the most important are vitamin D_2 (ergocalciferol) and vitamin D_3 (cholecalciferol). Their precursors are ergosterol and 7-dehydrocholesterol respectively. Ergosterol is found in plant tissues while 7-dehydrocholesterol occurs only in animal tissues including skin. Provitamins D are converted by ultraviolet irradiation into the vitamin proper so that exposure of the body to sunlight converts 7-dehydrocholesterol in the skin into vitamin D_3. In many countries of the world (even in Britain in good summer months) solar radiation is sufficient to provide the normal adult with all the vitamin he needs. Foodstuffs can be irradiated to increase their content of vitamin D_2 or D_3.

Dietary sources of the formed vitamin include yolk of egg, butter, milk and vitamin-enriched margarines. The richest sources of vitamin D are fish liver oils, particularly that of the halibut.

Vitamin D deficiency in infants causes rickets (p. 783). In adults the corresponding disease is called osteomalacia. These conditions result from an inadequate absorption of calcium and phosphate from the intestine and an impaired uptake of the minerals by the bony tissues; consequently the matrix fails to calcify or ossify and the skeleton becomes deformed. If the diet contains large amounts of substances that form non-absorbable compounds with calcium, this may also lead to rickets or osteomalacia, despite an adequate dietary intake of vitamin D. Phytic acid, which is present in cereals and in cereal products, including wholemeal bread, can, for example, unless calcium is plentiful in the diet, reduce its absorption to inadequate levels. Rickets is associated not only with abnormalities of the skeleton, but with a low resistance to infection and with anaemia and generally poor health. The active forms of vitamins D_2 and D_3 are the 1,25-dihydroxy derivatives which probably influence the production of the proteins that serve as calcium carriers. Hydroxylation in position 25 occurs in the liver and the process is completed in the kidneys. The extent to which the monohydroxy derivatives is converted into the fully active forms is determined by the parathyroid hormone (p. 782).

For therapeutic purposes (the prevention or treatment of rickets and osteomalacia) vitamin D is administered in the form of cod liver oil, or halibut liver oil. Alternatively, calciferol tablets can be given. Because of its very high concentration of vitamin D, halibut liver oil need be given in very small doses which are much more acceptable than the larger doses of cod liver oil which are often nauseating to children. Halibut liver oil can also be presented in capsules.

Vitamin D is given prophylactically to pregnant women, nursing mothers and young children. There is no evidence that any useful purpose is served by adding vitamin D to the diet of other members of well-nourished communities except perhaps the elderly.

Vitamin D has been used in the treatment of tetany but dihydrotachysterol is usually preferred for this purpose.

Ergocalciferol has been used, apparently with some success, to supplement the effects of anticonvulsant drugs.

Hypervitaminosis A and D

Since the fat soluble vitamins are insoluble in water, they cannot be excreted in the urine. If they are taken in large quantities, they accumulate in the body and may have toxic actions. Hypervitaminosis A was first recognized as a toxic hazard by Arctic explorers who unwisely ate polar bear liver, an organ which contains astronomical quantities of vitamin A. Nowadays, hypervitaminoses A and D, when they occur, are most often seen in young children who have received a continued overdosage of the vitamins from over-conscientious mothers actuated by the misguided principle that the protection provided by vitamin preparations can be increased by increasing the dose.

The recommended prophylactic doses of vitamins A and D for infants up to one year of age are 1500 and 400 international units respectively. These doses have probably to be increased one hundred fold before toxic symptoms appear.

Hypervitaminosis A is characterized by headache, nausea, vomiting, drowsiness and the development of a dried and peeling skin. Softening of the bones and a tendency to bleeding may also occur but the condition is easily treated by reducing the vitamin intake to more realistic levels.

In hypervitaminosis D, the amount of calcium in the blood increases and, as a result, calcium phosphate is deposited in a variety of tissues, including the joints, kidneys, heart, arteries, intestine, skin and eyes. The bones are not uniformly more calcified than usual; although the growing parts of the bone may show dense calcification, osteoporosis (demineralization) occurs elsewhere and tends to affect the whole of the bone as the condition progresses.

Hypervitaminosis D is more serious the higher the intake of calcium. Unfortunately, children who are given excessive amounts of vitamin D usually receive a diet rich in calcium too.

Vitamin E

'Vitamin E is one of those embarrassing vitamins that have been identified, isolated and synthesized by physiologists and biochemists and then handed to the medical profession with a suggestion that a use be found for it, without any satisfactory evidence to show that human beings are ever deficient of it or even that it is a necessary nutrient for man' (Davidson and Passmore, 1963). This quotation should be borne in mind when reading the following account, since experimental vitamin E deficiency in animals produces a number of pathological changes reminiscent of some clinical conditions in man and not everyone has resisted the temptation to attribute these human disorders to vitamin E deficiency.

Vitamin E was discovered in the course of experiments in which rats were fed diets in which the fats were supplied by lard and butter. The diets were adequate in the then known vitamins but the male rats became sterile and pregnant females suffered abortions. The condition could be cured by adding vegetable oils to the diet and it was soon established that the antisterility factor (Vitamin E) in these oils was a mixture of tocopherols (Fig. 47.2) of which α-tocopherol is the most important.

Animals fed on diets deficient in vitamin E also develop a muscular dystrophy, necrosis of the liver, an increased tendency to intravascular haemolysis and discoloration of body fat.

In vitro, the tocopherols reduce the rate at which fats turn rancid. This is because they are antioxidants and it seems likely that all the effects of vitamin E deficiency result from the removal of a restraint which the vitamin normally imposes on oxidative processes. The oxygen consumption of vitamin E-deficient animals is certainly greater than that of normal animals.

The richest source of vitamin E is wheat germ oil, though it is also present in other vegetable fats and in eggs. Small quantities are found in a large number of other foodstuffs, including lettuce, grasses, some nuts and seeds and it seems inevitable that the intake of the vitamin will be adequate even in ill-nourished individuals and communities. The use of vitamin E to treat muscular dystrophy, sterility and the tendency to spontaneous abortions has, therefore, no rational basis and it is not surprising that it is of little therapeutic value. Very large doses of vitamin E (500 mg daily), which are far in excess of any that could conceivably be needed to correct a dietary deficiency (the daily requirement of the vitamin is no more than 20 mg) are sometimes resorted to for the treatment of Dupuytren's contracture and intermittent claudication. Dupuytren's contracture is a deformity of the hand attributable to degeneration and distortion of fibrous tissue; in intermittent claudication spasm of the limb vessels occurs during exercise but disappears at rest. The view that vitamin E offers a worthwhile treatment for these conditions has its adherents. A suitable proprietary preparation is Ephynal.

Vitamin K

Vitamin K is discussed in Chapter 39 (p. 673).

WATER-SOLUBLE VITAMINS

The water soluble vitamins include the members of the B-complex and ascorbic acid (vitamin C). Vitamin P is no longer recognized.

The B-complex vitamins

At least eight different vitamins make up the vitamin B complex (Figs. 47.1 and 47.3). Although they are chemically unrelated, it is not inappropriate to class these substances together, since they tend to occur together and some of them regulate different stages of the same metabolic processes. It should occasion no surprise therefore when a deficiency in one component of the complex produces similar effects to those induced by deficiency of another component. A much more worthy cause for comment is the fact that deficiency of individual members of the complex so often results in the production of recognisably different clinical syndromes.

THIAMINE

Thiamine (vitamin B_1) is, as its name indicates, a sulphur-containing amine. The discovery of the nutritional importance and biochemical significance of thiamine provides a story of great interest.

In 1890, Eijkman, a Dutch physician working in Java, noticed that domestic fowls developed weakness of the legs when they were fed on food left over from meals served to his own patients. The food consisted mainly of polished

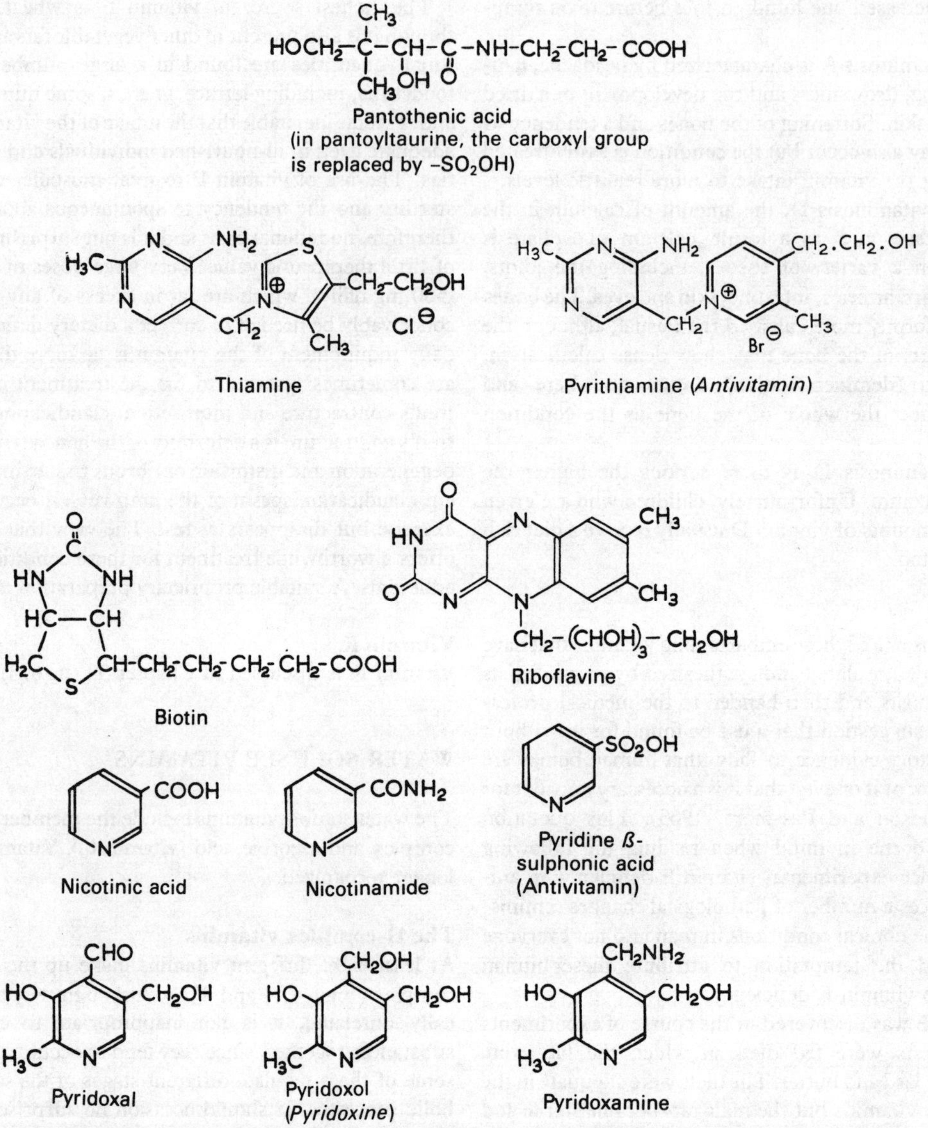

Fig. 47.3 Vitamins of the B-group and some of the corresponding antivitamins

rice (rice from which the husk had been removed) and when by chance it was replaced by unpolished rice the fowls' condition returned to normal. The appearance of the birds which had been fed the polished rice was similar to that of patients who were suffering from beriberi and Eijkman was soon able to report that the condition of his beriberi patients, as well as that of his fowls, improved when they were fed unpolished rice. This was not, in fact, the first demonstration that beriberi was caused by a nutritional deficiency: a few years earlier an ingenious large scale experiment carried out in the Japanese navy had established that beriberi did not occur in sailors whose diet contained barley instead of polished rice.

The anti-beriberi factor was not isolated in the pure state until 1926 and its chemical composition was not determined until 1936.

In 'wet' beriberi, cardiac failure and oedema are the predominant abnormalities. In 'dry' beriberi, progressive wasting of the muscles leads to severe incapacitation. In cerebral beriberi (*Wernicke's encephalopathy*) nervous and mental symptoms dominate the clinical picture. There may be vomiting and the pupillary reflexes disappear but the most prominent feature of the syndrome is a psychosis (*Korsakoff's psychosis*) that betrays itself in the victim's disorientation, delusions, abnormal or antisocial behaviour and stupor. Thiamine deficiency may also cause a peripheral polyneuritis which may appear alone or in association with Wernicke's encepholopathy. It should, perhaps, be added that neuritis of nutritional origin is not always attributable to a lack of thiamine and for this reason the vitamin is not now generally known by its once popular alternative name—aneurine—although 'aneurine hydrochloride' still appears in the B.P.

Some species of fish contain an enzyme (*thiaminase*) that destroys thiamine. It is fortunate that this antivitamin (p. 795) is destroyed by cooking but, in those parts of the world where raw fish is eaten, over indulgence in this undoubted delicacy may lead to thiamine deficiency. Deficiency may also occur in the course of conditions such as pregnancy and chronic alcoholism that increase the body's demands for thiamine: it may be severe enough, even in the apparently well nourished, to cause polyneuritis or Wernicke's encephalopathy. Even in the absence of an increased demand by the tissues, minor degrees of thiamine deficiency probably occur more frequently than is commonly supposed. They are particularly likely to occur in the elderly and the resulting fatigue, confusion, mental apathy and lack of initiative may be wrongly attributed to advancing years rather than to a simple and easily corrected vitamin deficiency.

The biochemical action of thiamine was elucidated as the culmination of an extensive series of researches by Peters who showed that thiamine pyrophosphate (diphosphothiamine) is the coenzyme of carboxylase (*cocarboxylase*), the enzyme which is responsible (in association with coenzyme A and nicotinamide adenine dinucleotide) for the oxidative decarboxylation of pyruvic and α-ketoglutaric acids. Thiamine thus has an important part to play in maintaining the operation of the citric acid cycle (p. 28). Moreover the oxidative decarboxylation of pyruvic acid yields acetylcoenzyme-A, the acetate donor in acetylcholine synthesis (p. 200). It is not difficult to understand why thiamine deficiency, with carbohydrate metabolism and acetylcholine synthesis both placed at risk, can wreak such havoc in the nervous system.

Diphosphothiamine is the coenzyme in the transketolase reaction. This additional pathway for glucose metabolism (the *hexose monophosphate shunt*) is important, since it results in the formation of ribose for nucleotide formation and it is a source of supply of reduced nicotinamide adenine dinucleotide phosphate (p. 792).

Thiamine is widely distributed in plant and animal tissues but the best sources are the bran and germ of cereals; wholemeal bread and bread made from white flour to which the vitamin has been added are therefore good dietary sources. Yeast is a particularly rich source and if it is necessary to supplement the normal diet with vitamin B_1, a yeast extract such as Marmite can be given. Other items of diet that provide useful quantities of the vitamin are beans, peas, green vegetables, fruit eggs and milk.

Benerva is a proprietary name for thiamine hydrochloride but the vitamin is also present, in company with other members of the B complex, in a number of other preparations (p. 792).

The possibility that thiamine has an action on peripheral nerves independently of its influence on carbohydrate metabolism is mentioned elsewhere (p. 472).

RIBOFLAVINE (VITAMIN B₂)

Soon after the discovery that beriberi was caused by deficiency of a dietary factor contained in the husk of rice grains, it was found that a water soluble substance was also needed for the proper growth of rats. It was at first thought that the two factors were identical but in 1920 it was shown that the anti-beriberi factor was more easily destroyed by heat than the growth factor. The latter was isolated in 1933 from milk (hence its present alternative name of lactoflavine) and identified as riboflavine. In the body, riboflavine is found largely in the form of a dinucleotide, flavine adenine dinucleotide or FAD (Fig. 47.4). A little is present as flavine mononucleotide (FMN). FAD and FMN form the prosthetic groups of a number of dehydrogenases whose biochemical functions are mentioned on page 63.

Like thiamine, riboflavine is present in large quantities in yeast and yeast extracts. Unlike thiamine, it also occurs in a high concentration in dairy produce but cereal grains provide a poor source of the vitamin.

Riboflavine deficiency, (*ariboflavinosis*) is, like beriberi, frequently complicated by the simultaneous presence of other dietary deficiencies. There is soreness and inflammation of the angles of the mouth (*angular stomatitis*), a sore, inflamed tongue (*glossitis*), inflamed pharynx (*pharyngitis*) and inflamed lips (*cheilosis*). In addition, there is dermatitis of the scrotum or vulva. These symptoms are collectively described as the 'orogenital syndrome' Characteristic changes also occur in the eyes. The normally avascular cornea is invaded by blood vessels along its whole circumference and may later develop opacities. Ariboflavinosis may also lead to neurological disorders.

Riboflavine (a proprietary preparation is Beflavit) is used to correct deficiencies of the vitamin in the diet. For no very good reason it has also found favour in some quarters for the treatment of migraine.

NICOTINIC ACID

Pellagra is usually remembered as the 'three D's' disease—the three D's representing dermatitis, diarrhoea and dementia. It has been known for at least 200 years among those peasant populations whose staple diet is maize. In Europe it has been particularly prevalent in Spain and Italy: the name pellagra itself (*pella* = skin, *agra* = rough) is of Italian origin. Although it had long been recognized that pellagra was caused by a dietary insufficiency, it was not until 1937 that the pellagra preventive factor was isolated from liver and identified as nicotinic acid (niacin). Like thiamine and riboflavine, nicotinic acid can be extracted from rice polishings and it is abundant in yeast

Flavine adenine dinucleotide (FAD)
Riboflavine-phosphate-phosphate-ribose-adenine
Flavine mononucleotide (FMN)
Riboflavine-phosphate

Coenzyme I: Nicotinamide adenine dinucleotide (NAD)

Nicotinamide — ribose — phosphate — phosphate — ribose —
adenine

Coenzyme II: Nicotinamide adenine dinucleotide phosphate (NADP)

Nicotinamide–ribose–phosphate–phosphate–ribose–phosphate
|
adenine

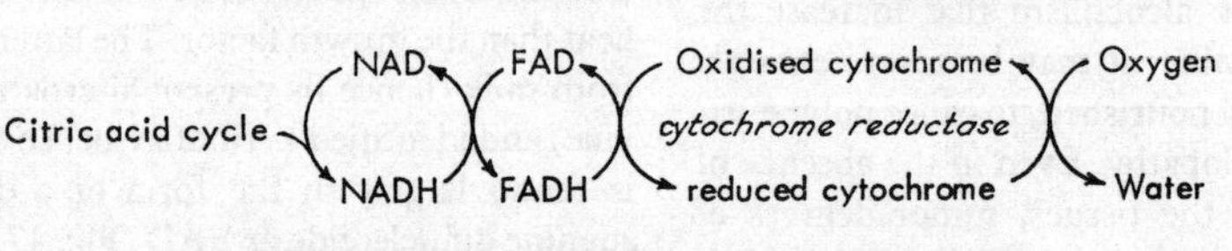

$$\text{Citric acid cycle} \underset{\text{NADH}}{\overset{\text{NAD}}{\bigg\langle}} \underset{\text{FADH}}{\overset{\text{FAD}}{\bigg\rangle}} \underset{\text{reduced cytochrome}}{\overset{\text{Oxidised cytochrome}}{\bigg\langle}} \underset{\text{Water}}{\overset{\text{Oxygen}}{\bigg\rangle}}$$

cytochrome reductase

Fig. 47.4 Derivatives of riboflavine and nicotinic acid

and yeast extracts. It is also present in kidney and meat. The ability of individual foodstuffs to prevent or precipitate pellagra is not strictly determined by their content of nicotinic acid. Thus milk has a low nicotinic acid content but it effectively prevents pellagra. This, it is now realised, is because milk contains much tryptophan which is converted in the body into nicotinic acid. On the other hand maize contains nicotinic acid in a form that cannot be absorbed from the gastrointestinal tract.

Nicotinic acid and nicotinamide are employed for the treatment and prevention of pellagra: since pellagra is probably the result of a multiple vitamin deficiency (the dementia is, for instance, very similar to that seen in Wernicke's encephalopathy) it is usual to employ a preparation which contains all the B-complex vitamins, such as a yeast extract. Proprietary preparations that include all or several of the B vitamins include Aluzyme, Becosym, Hemoplex and Hepacon-Plex. An even wider range of preparations includes all the B vitamins together with ascorbic acid and, often, other dietary requirements.

Nicotinic acid and some of its derivatives have also been employed as peripheral vasodilator agents.

In the body, nicotinic acid is present as the amide, nicotinamide (niacinamide) and it forms part of the molecules of coenzyme I (nicotinamide adenine dinucleotide, NAD) and coenzyme II (nicotinamide adenine dinucleotide phosphate, NADP) (Fig. 47.4). The nicotinamide moiety of coenzymes I and II acts as the hydrogen acceptor for dehydrogenase enzymes whose prosthetic groups are FAD or FMN. Thus riboflavine and nicotinamide, both members of the vitamin B group of enzymes, stand in an intimate functional relationship with one another. Moreover, as we saw earlier, the formation of the nucleotides of which they form a part is itself dependent on the presence of thiamine while the conversion of trypto-

phan into nicotinic acid is dependent on pyridoxal phosphate, a component of vitamin B_6. The functional interrelationship of NAD and FAD is best illustrated by reference to the oxidative processes mediated through the Krebs cycle (Fig. 47.4). Hydrogen liberated during the Krebs cycle is taken up by NAD which is thereby reduced to NADH. The hydrogen is immediately passed on to FAD which is itself reduced, to be immediately oxidized by cytochrome. The reduced cytochrome is oxidized by oxygen and water is formed. This is the chain of reactions which enables molecular oxygen to bring about an oxidative change without being directly involved in the events of the Krebs cycle. These reactions are discussed in more detail elsewhere (p. 27).

Flavine adenine dinucleotide is the prosthetic group of a number of enzymes (and flavine mononucleotide is present in a few others) which do not require coenzymes I or II.

PYRIDOXINE (VITAMIN B_6)

Vitamin B_6 is a mixture of an aldehyde (pyridoxal), an alcohol (pyridoxol) and an amine (pyridoxamine). The three components are interconvertible. Pyridoxol was previously known (and still is in some quarters) as pyridoxine but it is better to reserve this latter name for use as a synonym of vitamin B_6. Apart from the fact that 'pyridoxal' is easily confused with 'pyridoxol', particularly by careless proof readers, the newer terminology has much to recommend it. (Fig. 47.3). Vitamin B_6 is widely distributed in nature, where it is associated with the other members of the vitamin B complex. Thus it is particularly abundant in yeast, rice polishings and unmilled cereal grains. It is also found in egg yolk, liver, beans, peas and potatoes.

The existence of vitamin B_6 as a dietary factor different from those of the other members of the B group was recognized during the course of investigations into the pellagra preventing factor: rats being fed a diet thought to be deficient in this factor developed a dermatitis different from that seen in pellagra. The new vitamin thus discovered was isolated and identified in 1939. Other consequences of vitamin B_6 deficiency in experimental animals include anaemia and convulsions.

The most active constituent of vitamin B_6 is pyridoxal phosphate, which is the coenzyme of a large number of important enzymes including, among others, those that are involved in the biosynthesis of arichidonic acid, nicotinic acid, coenzyme-A and haemoglobin. Transaminations and aminoacid decarboxylations dependent on enzymes that contain pyridoxal phosphate include those that lead to the production of histamine, 5-hydroxytryptamine, the catecholamines and γ-aminobutyric acid, all substances that play important regulatory roles, particularly in the nervous system (Chap. 13). The coenzyme is especially important for the maintenance of supplies of γ-aminobutyric acid because it is involved in the reaction that provides the rate limiting step in the synthesis of this inhibitory substance. Failure of γ-aminobutyric acid production appears to be one of the most important consequences of vitamin B_6 deficiency: it would certainly seem to explain the tendency to convulsions which is so prominent a feature of the deficiency state in experimental animals. The relationship of γ-aminobutyric acid to convulsive activity is more fully discussed in Chapter 13 (p. 191).

Deficiency of vitamin B_6 does not arise as a result of dietary inadequacies but it can occur in patients receiving isoniazid since the drug combines with pyridoxal to form pyridoxal hydrazone which has no coenzyme activity. Peripheral neuritis, mental changes and epileptiform convulsions may all occur as complications of this form of tuberculosis therapy: they are all prevented or cured by vitamin B_6. Other drugs that reduce the effectiveness of pyridoxal phosphate include penicillamine (p. 455), hydrallazine (p. 311) and, perhaps, the steroid contraceptive agents.

Some cases of convulsions in infants have been traced to pyridoxine deficiency. In 1951, for instance, a large number of infants in various parts of the United States developed an illness in which convulsions were a prominent feature. The disorder was found to be caused by the destruction of vitamin B_6 during the processing of the milk preparation on which the infants were being fed. Other infantile seizures may arise because glutamic decarboxylase (which normally promotes the formation of γ-aminobutyric acid) is inactive by virtue of an inherited defect in the infant that prevents binding of pyridoxal phosphate to the apoenzyme.

Vitamin B_6 is sometimes useful in the treatment of forms of hypochromic anaemia resistant to other forms of therapy and it has also been extensively employed—on a completely empirical basis and with no firm evidence that it is of any value—for the relief of vomiting in pregnancy.

PANTOTHENIC ACID (VITAMIN B_5 OR B_3)

This substance is present in a wide variety of tissues and in all animal species (pantothenic is the Greek for 'everywhere'), where (as pantotheine, a sulphydryl derivative) it is a component of coenzyme-A (Co-acetylase). As its name implies this coenzyme is particularly important in reactions involving the transfer of acetyl groups so that it occupies a key role in the Krebs cycle, the synthesis of acetylcholine and steroid hormones and in fat metabolism. Some detoxication reactions also involve acetylation (p. 62). In rats, pantothenic acid deficiency causes arrest of growth, necrosis of the adrenal glands, greying of the hair (achromotrichia) and the deposition of porphyrins on the nose. In other animals fatty degeneration of the liver and degeneration of peripheral nerves have been observed.

Pantothenic acid deficiency in man is virtually unknown but the severe malnutrition suffered in Japanese prisoner of war camps led (among many other disorders) to the 'burning feet' syndrome which responded favourably to pantothenic acid but to no other vitamin. Pantothenic acid does not prevent or cure the greying of human hair.

BIOTIN (VITAMIN H)

Biotin is the coenzyme for a large number of metabolic reactions that involve the addition or transfer of carboxyl groups. It is widely distributed in nature and large amounts are also produced in the gut. The only practicable way of producing experimental biotin deficiency is to sterilize the intestine or to feed a diet in which the protein is supplied solely by raw egg white which contains avidin, a substance which combines with biotin.

Rats, pigs and other mammals with experimental biotin deficiency become wasted and develop a dermatitis that eventually covers the whole body. Poultry (particularly turkeys) are more susceptible than laboratory mammals to experimental biotin deficiency and, in these birds, disturbed bone formation is an additional feature of the biotin deficiency syndrome. Even in birds, biotin deficiency occurs only very rarely outside the laboratory. Broiler house chicks up to twenty days old are sometimes stricken with a sudden incapacitating paralysis which is associated with fatty changes in the liver and kidneys (the fatty liver and kidney syndrome). The condition rapidly responds to the addition of biotin supplements to the diet. Some forms of dermatitis in human infants also appear to be the result of a biotin deficiency. Oddly enough, one case of severe biotin deficiency in a human adult has been reported. It occurred in a man who lived on a bizarre diet of six dozen raw eggs and seven gallons of red wine a week. He developed a dermatitis which responded immediately to biotin treatment. It is unlikely that a similar case will be seen again and it hardly falsifies the statement that biotin deficiency does not occur in the adult human subject.

Biotin has been included in proprietary vitamin preparations. It adds a name on the package to impress the uninformed layman but it is difficult to believe that it is of any other value. Apart from the treatment of rare cases of biotin-deficiency dermatitis in infants, the vitamin has no therapeutic use.

COBALAMIN (VITAMIN B_{12}) AND FOLIC ACID (VITAMIN Bc)

These are discussed in detail in Chapter 39 (p. 676).

OTHER SUBSTANCES

Inositol, p-aminobenzoic acid and choline have all been included in the vitamin B group by some authorities but it is difficult to justify their classification as vitamins.

Vitamin C

Scurvy is a disease which has been known for centuries and everyone knows that the nickname 'limey' for the British sailor comes from the old practice, dating from the 18th century, of providing lemon or lime juice on Royal Navy ships to ward off the disease. Strangely enough, in the United States navy, attempts to prevent scurvy by supplying lime juice were not made until 1895.

The protective factor was isolated from lemon juice and in 1932 it was identified as 3-keto-L-gulofuranolactone. The trivial name—ascorbic acid—assigned to this compound recognizes its principal biological activity, *scorbutic* being an adjectival form of the word 'scurvy'. The laevorotatory isomer is the active form of ascorbic acid.

Ascorbic acid

Ascorbic acid is very easily oxidized (so that it is a useful reducing agent) first of all by removal of hydrogen from the two -OH groups in the ring. The resulting dehydroascorbic acid retains the biological activity of ascorbic acid itself but further oxidation results in loss of activity. In the human body, dehydroascorbic acid is metabolized to oxalic acid (the principal urinary representative of vitamin C) and 2,3-diketogulonic acid.

The symptoms of scurvy include weakness and fatigue, with muscle and joint pains, breathlessness and tachycardia. The gums bleed, become spongy and inflamed and the teeth loosen in their sockets. Haemorrhages then occur in the skin and elsewhere, with a consequent anaemia. Resistance to infection is much reduced, and this may be the cause of death.

Most animal species synthesize their own ascorbic acid but men and guinea pigs (laboratory managers should note this) cannot do so and must have it provided in the diet. The richest dietary sources of ascorbic acid are the citrus fruits (lime, lemon, grapefruit), oranges, blackcurrants, some green vegetables and tomatoes. Haws and rose hips contain up to one gram of ascorbic acid per 100 grams, a figure that should be compared with the modest 100 mg per cent yielded by broccoli and brussels sprouts and the 50 mg per cent of citrus fruits, the richest dietary sources of the vitamin. This statistic should not be interpreted as an injunction to return to nature: an orange is more delectable than a rose hip and the daily requirement of vitamin C for a healthy adult is no more than 50 mg. It is never necessary to become a crank in order to secure adequate nourishment. A proprietary name for ascorbic acid is Redoxon. Except in parts of the world where fruit is plentiful and cheap, most people obtain relatively little of their ascorbic acid from this source and in practice a large proportion of the daily intake comes from potatoes which do not contain a high concentration of the vitamin but which are consumed in large amounts. The importance of potatoes is underlined by the fact that, in the past, outbreaks of scurvy in Ireland coincided with the potato famines.

Since ascorbic acid is widely distributed, gross deficiencies of the vitamin are unlikely to occur in reasonably well fed individuals, although, because of the losses incurred in cooking, many people take amounts of vitamin C which probably border on the inadequate. More important than the losses which occur during the actual cooking process are those which take place when food is kept hot for long periods. Those—bachelors, widowers and students, for instance—who have to rely for their food on restaurants or residential institutions, suffer most from vitamin loss from this cause.

Ascorbic acid can be stored to a limited extent in many tissues in the body. When the tissues become saturated, any additional ascorbic acid intake is immediately excreted in the urine and this forms the basis of a test for determining the extent of tissue saturation. In this test, a large dose of ascorbic acid (11 mg per kilogram of body weight is usual) is taken by mouth and the urine which is excreted between the fourth and sixth hours thereafter is collected. If the tissues are saturated, at least 50 mg of ascorbic acid should be excreted during this period. Many people (particularly those denied the pleasures of home cooking) do not achieve this standard and some excrete no extra ascorbic acid at all after taking the loading dose. Thus while the present author (who takes an orange a day) excretes ascorbic acid all the time, the urine of most of his students remains resolutely devoid of vitamin activity even after a full loading dose of ascorbic acid. This is not to say that most people are necessarily suffering from even a marginal degree of vitamin deficiency, since their intake may be sufficient to supply their needs without being sufficient to add to the tissue stores. For this reason, many authorities pay little regard to the tissue saturation test. Nevertheless, it would seem that in those whose tissues do not hold a full complement of vitamin C, the standard of nutrition is not as high as it might and probably should be.

Vitamin C is used in the prevention and treatment of scurvy. Care should be taken to ensure that young children receive an adequate supply. As will have been appreciated from the discussion of vitamin C saturation, it is impossible to give too high a dose of the vitamin. The much canvassed view that high doses of vitamin C will prevent winter colds and other mild infections is still a controversial one. To the extent that ascorbic acid does prevent infection and that, as we have seen, many people do not fully fill their vitamin C stores, the taking of additional vitamin C during the winter months may have something to recommend it, particularly when we take into account the undoubted placebo effect that modern man derives from anything he takes out of a bottle. On the other hand, the person who is sensible enough to select a diet that keeps his tissues saturated with ascorbic acid would clearly achieve no useful object by dosing himself with tablets of vitamin C, the increased intake of which would be promptly countered by a corresponding increase in urinary excretion.

Since ascorbic acid is widely distributed in mammalian tissues, it is reasonable to assume that it exerts a regulatory action on fundamental cellular processes, although there is as yet relatively little precise knowledge concerning its mode of action. It seems to be involved in oxidation-reduction reactions and in the elaboration of intercellular cement, cartilage and collagen. It also takes part in the conversion of folic acid to folinic acid and in the oxidation of L-tyrosine. There is recent evidence that ascorbic acid is involved in the absorption of iron from the intestine and its transport to the bone marrow (p. 659). If this is so, the anaemia that develops in scorbutic patients may not be solely the consequences of the gingival and cutaneous haemorrhages.

Among individual organs, the adrenal cortex carries the highest concentration of ascorbic acid. Bodily injury or other forms of stress result in a depletion of adrenal ascorbic acid in response to an increased secretion of adrenocorticotrophic hormone by the pituitary gland. The significance of this response is obscure but it seems that the reduction in the concentration of ascorbic acid permits an accelerated production of the adrenal hormones required to meet the stress.

ANTIVITAMINS

Antivitamins are compounds which prevent the normal utilization of vitamins and in this way cause symptoms of a vitamin deficiency. As a rule the antivitamins are closely related chemically to the vitamins or growth factors which they antagonize. Examples include glucoascorbic acid and ascorbic acid; pantothenic acid and pantoyltaurine; pyrithiamine and thiamine; pyridoxine and deoxypyridoxine; nicotinic acid and pyridine-β-sulphonic acid. Some of these compounds are shown in Fig. 47.3. Most of these antivitamins are only of academic interest. Some of them, however, occur naturally and they may therefore reduce the effectiveness of a diet whose vitamin content would otherwise be adequate. A very good example of this type of antivitamin action is provided by dicoumarin, a constituent of spoiled sweet clover and an antagonist of vitamin K. Cattle fed on this clover develop a haemorrhagic disease because of an effective deficiency of vitamin K (p. 673). Thiaminase occurs in raw fish (p. 791) and folic acid antagonists find a place in cancer chemotherapy (p. 917).

ESSENTIAL FATTY ACIDS

The essential fatty acids include linoleic acid, linolenic acid and arachidonic acid. These compounds are sometimes referred to collectively as Vitamin F. They are essential for normal growth, development and reproduction in experimental animals. Vegetable oils that contain large amounts of these unsaturated fatty acids include corn oil, cotton seed oil, safflower oil and soya bean oil. The addition of these oils to the diet, particularly as a substitute for foodstuffs containing a high proportion of saturated fatty acids, lowers plasma cholesterol levels. The relationship between the essential fatty acids and the prostaglandins is discussed elsewhere (p. 367).

BIBLIOGRAPHY

Books, monographs and reviews

Arnstein, H. R. V. and Wrighton, R. J. (eds) (1971) *The Cobalamins* (Glaxo Symposium) Edinburgh and London: Churchill Livingstone.
Kutsky, R. J. (1973) *Handbook of Vitamins and Hormones.* New York and Toronto: Van Nostränd Reinhold
Lawson, D. E. M. (ed) (1978) *Vitamin D.* London and New York: Academic Press
Marks, J. (1975) *A Guide to the Vitamins.* Lancaster: MTP.
Sebrell, W. H. Jr. and Harris, R. S. (eds) (1971) *The Vitamins,* vols I to V. New York and London: Academic Press.
Sinclair, H. M. and Hollingsworth, Dorothy F. (1969) *Hutchinson's Food and the Principles of Nutrition.* 12th ed. London and New York: Academic Press.

48. Some metals of pharmacological and toxicological interest

A number of metals are essential, some in appreciable quantities and others in minute amounts, for the maintenance of normal body functions. Others are highly toxic. On both these counts, metals are of some interest to the pharmacologist.

A topic of some importance in pharmacology and medicine is chelation and this phenomenon is discussed before the individual metals are considered.

CHELATION

In 1935, Munz discovered the compound ethylene diamine tetraacetic acid (EDTA, edetic acid, Versene Acid, Edathamil, Sequestrene AA) and showed that it had a strong affinity for calcium ions with which it formed a complex containing unionized calcium. The nature of the reaction is shown in Figure 48.1. It is called *chelation* and the compound formed is a *chelate*. The words are pec16li-

arly appropriate. They are derived from the Greek 'chele' which means the crab's claw, and in a chelate compound the metal is surrounded by, and held firmly within, the rest of the molecule as the claw of a crab surrounds and seizes its victim. In chelates, the metal atom is held by a number of binding or *ligand* atoms usually of nitrogen, oxygen or sulphur. These bind the metal by coordinate bonds: an electron pair is shared between the metal and the ligand atoms. The bond is often indicated by an arrow with its head pointing away from the atoms (the ligands) which have donated the electron pair. If there are two co-ordinating groups present in a molecule and if they are in the correct spatial configuration, a chelate ring is formed. This can be seen in Figure 48.1: a large molecule containing several chelate groups may be able to form a series of rings which surround the metal atoms.

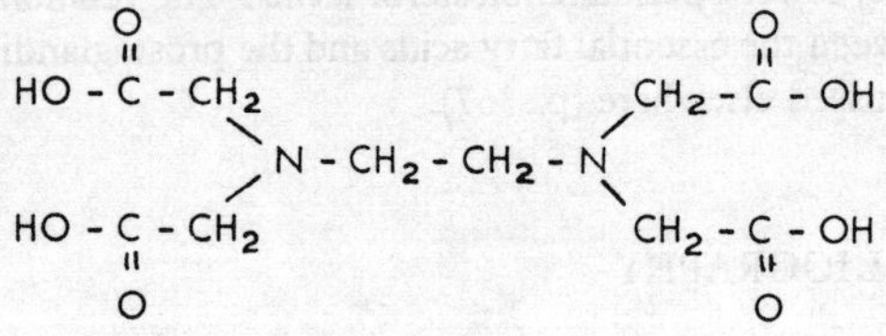

Munz applied his discovery to the textile industry. Because of its extremely high affinity for calcium, edetic acid was employed to remove calcium ions from the water used to wash the fibres. The first suspicion that chelates might be useful in medicine came in the early days of the Second World War when strenuous efforts were being made to develop antidotes to the poison gases to which, it was feared, troops and the civilian population were shortly to be exposed. Peters discovered that 2,3-dimercaptopropanol (dimercaprol, British anti-Lewisite or BAL) was an effective antidote to Lewisite. Dimercaprol owes its protective action to the formation of a chelate complex (Fig. 48.2). It was soon realized that nature had anticipated the discoveries of the chemists by several millenia because a number of naturally occurring compounds including haemoglobulin and cyanocobalamin (Fig. 48.6) are themselves chelates.

In the event, poison gas was not used in the war and the effectiveness of British anti-Lewisite was not put to the test in field conditions. However, in 1951 there occurred an event which gave the first real hint of the potentiality of

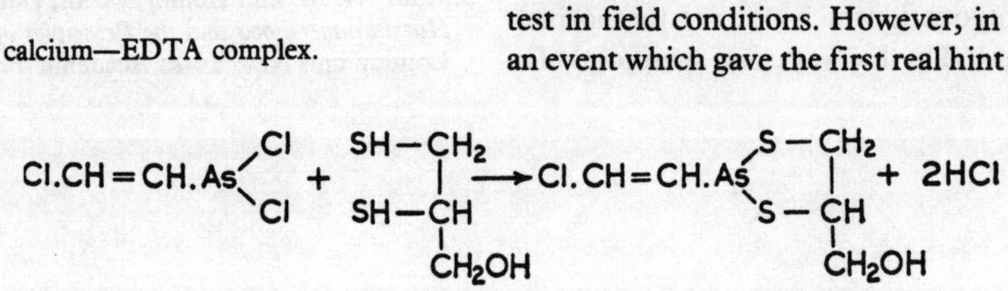

Ethylene diamine tetraacetic acid (EDTA)

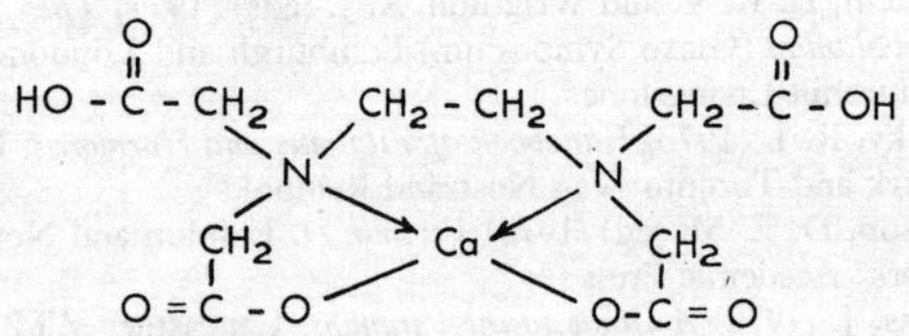

Calcium complex with EDTA

Fig 48.1 Formation of calcium—EDTA complex.

Lewisite   2,3, dimercapto-propanol   Stable Ring Compound

Fig 48.2 The reaction between Lewisite and 2,3-demercaptopropanol (dimercaprol) to give a stable, non-toxic ring compound.

chelate compounds. A young boy who was dying from lead poisoning was given repeated doses of disodium calcium edetate (Ledclair). Three days after treatment began, he had completely recovered and EDTA is now recognized as being the drug of choice for the treatment of lead poisoning. It will be appreciated that the disodium calcium edetate used in this first clinical trial is itself a chelate but the chelated calcium can be displaced by lead. There is an advantage in administering EDTA in this 'loaded' form. If edetic acid or sodium edetate itself were given, there would be the possibility that as the lead was cleared from the body, the calcium chelate would be produced and excreted and so cause calcium deficiency.

The value of EDTA in the treatment of lead poisoning lies in the fact that the lead-EDTA complex is non-toxic, soluble and rapidly excreted. This provides a most valuable combination of circumstances: the lead in the body is rendered harmless as soon as it comes into contact with the chelating agent, and then it is quickly disposed of. EDTA can be used to treat poisoning by other heavy metals such as plutonium; it has also been used (in the acid form, of course) for reducing the amount of calcium in the blood in hypercalcaemia, for dissolving renal calculi, for treating cardiac arrhythmias and digitalis poisoning (reducing the calcium content of the blood reduces the excitability of cardiac muscle) and for treating dermatitis caused by nickel or copper salts. Among other chelating agents, dimercaprol will remove gold, mercury, lead and arsenic from the body.

Wilson's disease is a condition affecting the liver and the brain, particularly the basal ganglia (p. 164). It is a hereditary condition associated with the deposition of copper in the affected tissues. Until recently, it was incurable and often fatal. The condition is now treated with chelating agents. Dimercaprol was used at first but better results are obtained with penicillamine (Cuprimine, Distamine). It is given by mouth in doses of 150 to 300 mg three times daily: the excretion of copper increases sharply. Clinical improvement is not noticeable for some weeks or months and its extent depends on the degree of irreversible change which has been produced in the nervous system before treatment starts. As in dimercaprol, the chelating effect of penicillamine is attributable to the — SH group.

$$H_3C - \underset{\underset{SH}{\overset{\overset{CH_3}{|}}{|}}{C} - \underset{\underset{NH_2}{|}}{CH} - COOH$$

Penicillamine

Desferrioxamine B is used for the treatment of iron poisoning. Another chelating agent is diethylene triamine pentaacetic acid (DTPA). It is similar in its actions and uses to EDTA except that it is more powerful and can also be used to treat iron poisoning. It is particularly valuable for the treatment of poisoning by radioactive elements.

It has been mentioned that iron is a toxic substance, yet relatively large amounts circulate in the plasma. The body uses its own chelate (iron-transferrin, p. 660) to protect itself from the toxic action of its own circulating iron. If an overdose of iron is taken (and young children are quite often tempted to eat ferrous sulphate tablets), the protective action of the transferrin chelating mechanism is overwhelmed and symptoms of iron poisoning appear.

$$\underset{HOOC - CH_2}{\overset{HOOC - CH_2}{\diagdown}} N - (CH_2)_2 - N - (CH_2)_2 - N \underset{CH_2 - COOH}{\overset{CH_2 - COOH}{\diagup}}$$

Diethylene triamine pentaacetic acid

In recent years several workers have pointed out that a large number of drugs, used to treat a variety of diseases, can form metal chelates and it has been suggested that these drugs may owe part at least of their action to chelate formation. It is clear that some investigators have been carried away by their enthusiasm for a new idea and caution has to be exercised when their claims are examined.

INDIVIDUAL METALS

It is convenient to divide the metals we shall discuss into essential and nonessential groups. Those in the latter category need concern us only because of their toxic actions or therapeutic potentiality but the metals essential for life are of additional interest because we have to consider not only their physiological actions but also the possible consequences of a deficient intake. As we shall see, some metals have been added only very recently to the list of essential elements so that statements concerning their biological significance are necessarily tentative.

Metals essential for life
Sodium, potassium and calcium occur in large quantities in the body and are of vital physiological importance. They are not further discussed in this chapter: calcium is dealt with separately in Chapter 46 (p. 781) but sodium and potassium are so ubiquitous that they have to be discussed in relation to the many functional systems in whose activity they participate and which form the subject of several other chapters in this book. Magnesium, the next most abundant element in the animal body, is considered but all the other essential metals mentioned in this section occur in only trace amounts. Iron is more appropriately discussed in connection with blood formation and this is done in Chapter 39 (p. 659).

CHROMIUM
Chromium has many industrial uses. The metal itself is

incorporated into a number of alloys and it is difficult to avoid chromium plating in our homes, our places of work and our cars. Chromium salts are employed as tanning agents and pigments: *chroma* is the Greek for colour. In the laboratory, radioactive chromium finds application as a label for erythrocytes and some chromium compounds are useful histological stains. Chromaffin tissue, as the name signifies, has a particular affinity for chromium salts.

Hitherto, chromium has not been a constituent of any therapeutic preparation, but the recent discovery that chromium is essential for life in man and the higher animals has prompted some enquiries into the possibility that its compounds might have a therapeutic role.

If rats are maintained on artificial diets that lack chromium, their glucose tolerance becomes disturbed and some authorities believe that the impaired glucose tolerance that is a feature of kwashiorkor is attributable to chromium lack. They have demonstrated their belief by adding chromium supplements, in the form of chromic chloride, to the diets of children with this disease. In some instances, glucose tolerance has improved within one day of initiating treatment. Similarly, glucose tolerance has been improved in elderly patients. The fact that the amount of chromium in the tissues decreases with advancing years provides some grounds for believing that chromium supplementation of the diet might be beneficial in the aged but it should be pointed out that not all investigators have been able to restore normal glucose tolerance with chromium in either old people or in children with kwashiorkor. Until further evidence is forthcoming, the question of chromium's value in these states must remain an open one. There can, however, be little doubt that the metal is a cofactor of insulin. It may also potentiate the action of insulin in other ways—for instance, by inhibiting its breakdown, stabilizing its structure or facilitating its binding to the tissues (Mertz, 1969).

Chromium facilitates the uptake of cholesterol and fatty acids by the liver and the cholesterol content of the blood of rats that have been given chromium supplemented diets over a long period of time is significantly lower than that of their untreated litter mates. There is some evidence that the same effect can be achieved in human beings given chromium acetate in doses of 2 mg daily. It seems that chromium also facilitates the utilization of glycine, serine and methionine.

Concern has sometimes been expressed in the past that chromium in toxic amounts might pass into the food from chromium plated or stainless steel cooking or storage vessels. The evidence is that only small and completely non toxic amounts of metal are dissolved in this way.

Salts of trivalent chromium are not very well absorbed from the gastrointestinal tract but substances containing the element in its hexavalent form or in organic compounds pass more readily into the blood where the chromium, after successful competition with iron, is attached to transferrin (p. 660) which transports it to the tissues. It is not evenly distributed throughout the body. Among the areas that contain high concentrations are the liver, the caudate nucleus and the hair. Determination of the amount of chromium in hair clippings is a useful way of assessing the adequacy of the dietary intake. Dietary sources of chromium include meat, condiments, thyme, cooked tomatoes. To this list must be added cigarette smoke!

Toxic effects of chromium that might appear in industrial workers exposed to it are skin lesions (dermatitis or ulcers), inflammation of the larynx, lesions of the nasal mucosa and respiratory disorders including carcinoma of the bronchus.

Ulcers produced by exposure to chromium salts have been treated with some success by the local application of a chelating agent such as BAL or sodium calcium edetate.

COBALT

Cobalt is a constituent of some of the fine alloys that are needed in the car, aircraft and electrical industries. The tool industry uses the metal for improving the cutting edge of its hard steel products and the quality of tungsten carbide tools. Some cobalt compounds are blue in colour and find application as pigments in the china industry. The radioactive isotope (cobalt 60) is used as a source of radiation in the treatment of cancers.

Cobalt is contained in vitamin B_{12}, as is indicated by the very names of the B_{12} components (cobalamin and hydroxocobalamin) and so is essential for life. It seems likely that cobalt also serves as a cofactor for other enzymes that are not immediately related to vitamin B_{12}.

Inorganic salts of cobalt stimulate red cell production probably because by inhibiting oxidative enzymes, they induce anoxia of the bone marrow and so promote the production of erythropoietin. This erythropoietic potentiality of cobalt (which is not shared by vitamin B_{12}) is of toxicological rather than therapeutic significance. Polycythaemia (p. 614) is a recognized sign of cobalt poisoning but attempts to relieve intractable anaemias by giving cobalt salts have not been very successful.

Both an excess and a deficiency of cobalt can inhibit thyroid activity. While cobalt deficiency probably does not occur in man, a number of diseases of livestock are caused by the animals' grazing on cobalt-poor land. One such condition (known as 'pine' or 'daising') is seen particularly in sheep. Symptoms include failure of proper growth, a poor coat or fleece, ataxia and muscular weakness. When confirmed, it is treated by means of drenches with cobalt chloride or cobalt sulphate. Minute amounts of cobalt will cure affected animals.

Cobalt poisoning is not a problem in industry. Occasional cases of allergic dermatitis and of gastrointestinal and respiratory upsets after exposure to cobalt have been reported but the incidence of these events is low. Most of the serious instances of cobalt poisoning have originated iatrogenically in anaemic patients treated injudiciously with cobalt salts, toxic responses to which include vomiting, diarrhoea, polycythaemia (and the associated symptoms of headache, tinnitus, dizziness and fatigue) and hypothyroidism. However, the most extraordinary cases of cobalt poisoning ever recorded had neither an industrial nor an iatrogenic origin.

Some ten years ago a serious form of cardiomyopathy (a disorder of cardiac muscle) appeared among the inhabitants of a localized area of Quebec. No fewer than twenty of the forty-eight reported cases had a fatal outcome but the origin of the affliction remained a mystery until it was realized that the disease only struck heavy drinkers of a particular brand of beer and that it was accompanied by polycythaemia and hypothyroidism, stigmata, we recall, of cobalt poisoning.

The advent of the newer generation of detergents brought gloom to beer drinkers who found that they were deprived of their froth. A film of detergent left in a beer glass after washing reduces the surface tension, and so destroys the froth, of the beer that next occupies the glass. One of the several measures that were introduced in order to restore froth to beer and joy to its drinkers was the addition of minute amounts of cobalt chloride to the brew. All the Quebec victims of cardiomyopathy had been drinking large amounts of the product of one particular brewery for many years. Epidemic outbreaks of cardiomyopathy were also reported from parts of Europe and the USA. In all instances, the culprit was beer from breweries that favoured the use of cobalt.

The practice of adding cobalt to beer has, it need hardly be said, been abandoned and it is even possible that some bartenders now preserve their customers' froth by the logical if drastic expedient of rinsing the beer glasses properly after washing.

Cobalt forms compounds with the usual chelating agents which can therefore be applied to the treatment of cobalt poisoning. At the same time, cobalt edetate is itself a valuable chelating agent. It is the preferred antidote in cyanide poisoning (p. 701).

COPPER

Copper is well known malleable and ductile metal. It is an extremely good conductor of heat and electricity, being inferior in this respect only to silver. It finds wide application in the electrical industry and in the construction of domestic cooking and other utensils. It is a contributor to a number of alloys and is the favoured material for gas and water pipes. Copper salts are used to kill algae in water reservoirs and as insecticides.

Copper is essential to life by virtue of its being a cofactor in a number of enzymes including, among others, caeruloplasmin, cytochrome-C oxidase, dopamine β-hydroxylase,

monoamine oxidase, tyrosinase and xanthine oxidase. It is also a component of a number of proteins whose functions have not yet been established but whose location in the tissues is indicated by their names—cerebrocuprein, erythrocuprein, haemocuprein, hepatocuprein and mitochondrocuprein. Haemoglobin production cannot proceed in the absence of copper, probably because globin synthesis is arrested. It may also be that copper brings about the release of iron from the liver and other storage sites.

Copper is so widespread in nature that an adequate intake can hardly be avoided by human beings who take enough food to sustain life although in kwashiorkor and severe malabsorption syndromes the amount reaching the tissues must be very close to the minimal compatible with normal enzyme function. In farm animals, on the other hand, copper deficiency is not very uncommon and it brings in its train such disorders as anaemia, defects in hair and fur pigmentation, myocardial fibrosis, rupture of the aorta and, most characteristically of all, swayback. The pigmentation defects are probably the result of impaired tyrosinase activity (tyrosine is a precursor of melanin) and the aortic rupture occurs because of thinning of the elastic coat of the vessel. This is a consequence of the fact that elastin formation from lysine is hindered by reason of a deficiency of the amine oxidase on which the synthesis depends. Swayback is a disease that affects lambs, which become ataxic as a result of demyelination of motor tracts in the spinal cord. It is associated with deficiency in a number of copper containing enzymes including cytochrome oxidase. The ingestion of molybdenum (for instance by cattle living on a soil rich in the element) can cause signs of copper deficiency which can be remedied by increasing the intake of copper.

Copper deficiency can apparently arise in both man and animals if they consume large quantities of a pea, *Larthyrus sativus*, which is grown in several poor countries in times of drought as an alternative to the more regular crops. The condition is called, predictably, lathyrism and the immediate cause of the copper deficiency is β-aminoproprionitrile. Symptoms of lathyrism include weakness, a spastic paralysis and skeletal deformities. Elastin production in the arteries is deficient.

Of the copper taken in the diet most is excreted in the faeces but a small amount is absorbed from the upper reaches of the small intestine. It is bound to plasma albumin for transport to the liver where it combines with a globulin to form caeruloplasmin, an enzyme whose possible function has been the subject of much so far unrewarded speculation. The enzyme is released into the circulation and about 95 per cent of the plasma's copper is present as caeruloplasmin. The remaining 5 per cent is associated with albumin. Some individuals are congenitally incapable of synthesizing caeruloplasmin so that uncombined copper is deposited in their tissues, particularly the liver, kidney, skin, ocular tissues and basal ganglia with the production of hepatolenticular degeneration (Wilson's disease). We have noted earlier in this chapter that the introduction of chelating agents into medicine has brought new hope to the previously doomed victims of this disease.

Metallic copper is a virtually non-toxic substance and it raises no problems among those who work with it. The salts, however, are poisonous and if taken by mouth they cause vomiting, severe abdominal pain, diarrhoea and prostration. The emesis and diarrhoea may be severe enough to save the victim's life by clearing the toxic material from the absorption sites. If they are absorbed into the circulation, copper salts may provoke renewed vomiting when they reach the vomiting centre. They also cause haematuria and convulsions. Survivors may show signs of kidney necrosis.

MAGNESIUM

Magnesium has many industrial uses but it does not constitute a hazard to the health of those exposed to it in their daily work. In medicine, magnesium compounds find employment as antacids and purgatives and magnesia is one of the more favoured compounds of the layman's self medication kit, particularly if his household contains young children.

Magnesium is essential to life, being a component of several enzyme systems especially those involved in the transfer of energy.

An intravenous injection of a soluble magnesium salt causes loss of consciousness. These effects are caused by the magnesium ion which in this respect is unique among metal ions.

The magnesium ion also has actions on the cardiovascular system causing vasodilatation and a fall in blood pressure and, if high blood levels are maintained, arrest of the heart beat. The depressor effect is due partly to the vasodilatation and partly to blockade of sympathetic ganglia. In the heart, magnesium ions cause slowing, prolong the PQ interval and widen the QRS complex. This may be the result of a direct effect on the myocardium, or of ganglion blockade. The actions of magnesium ions on the heart and elsewhere are antagonized by calcium ions, which can overcome a magnesium induced depression.

The effects of magnesium ions on neuromuscular transmission resemble those of tubocurarine and at concentrations which block transmission, the nerve and muscle remain excitable. Magnesium ions seem to reduce the sensitivity of the end plate to acetylcholine but magnesium, unlike curare, antagonizes the stimulant effects of potassium ions at the neuromuscular junction and on isolated tissues. In high doses magnesium has a direct depressant action on conduction in peripheral nerves.

Magnesium ions have a direct depressant action on all kinds of smooth muscle. Addition of magnesium ions to the bath fluid can be used to reduce spontaneous activity in preparations of isolated intestine. The magnesium ion penetrates cells very slowly and its actions appear to arise from an effect upon the cell surface.

The way in which magnesium ions exert the pharmacological effects outlined above is not understood, but it is possible that they prevent the synthesis of acetylcholine, inhibit the response of the effector cells to this substance, or exert both these effects.

Cattle that eat fodder lacking magnesium or containing it in a form that cannot be adequately assimilated, develop a condition known as 'grass staggers' when it affects adult cows and 'magnesium tetany' when it affects calves.

A number of circumstances can give rise to magnesium deficiency in human beings. These include prolonged diarrhoea and vomiting if no attempt is made to replace the magnesium that is being lost, severe malnutrition as in kwashiorkor, malabsorption syndromes, oversecretion of aldosterone or of the thyroid hormone and long continued treatment with certain diuritic agents. As might be expected from the description we have already given of the effects of magnesium administration, the sequelae of magnesium deficiency include tremor, hyperexcitability, uncontrolled and involuntary movements of the limbs, cardiac arrhythmias and, in man, such mental changes as agitation, confusion and hallucinations.

MANGANESE

Manganese is an essential trace element. It is found in highest concentration in the mitochondria and is a necessary component of a number of enzyme systems including, probably, those involved in the synthesis of mucopolysaccharides and cholesterol. In industry, the metal is mixed with steel to produce a high quality alloy and some of its salts find a range of applications. Potassium permanganate, a powerful oxidizing agent, has long been used as a disinfectant. Condy's fluid, which contains sodium permanganate, has similar uses.

Manganese salts are toxic and if taken by mouth they cause irritation of the gastrointestinal tract. Chronic poisoning may occur as a result of prolonged exposure to manganese dust. The central nervous system is particularly vulnerable to manganese which can cause hallucinations, restlessness, euphoria and emotional instability. However, to the pharmacologist, the most interesting manifestation of manganese toxicity is a disturbance of extrapyramidal function that produces a condition very similar, if not identical, to Parkinson's disease. Manganese can also cause cirrhosis of the liver, anaemia (manganese competes with iron for the transport system) and, occasionally, pneumonia.

Manganese deficiency in animals leads to arrested growth, skeletal deformities and abnormalities in their offspring. A deficiency of dietary origin has not been seen in man but some patients treated with hydrallazine (an anti-hypertensive agent, p. 311) have developed lupus erythematosus as a result of a manganese deficiency which results from the fact that hydrallazine has chelating properties. Both idiopathic and hydrallazine-induced lupus have responded favourably to treatment with manganese salts.

Manganese deficiency may also be an aetiological factor in the genesis of some other connective tissue diseases such as rheumatoid arthritis.

MOLYBDENUM

Molybdenum, a metal whose principal industrial value is as a hardener for steel and as a constituent of a number of high quality alloys, also finds applications in the glass, ceramics, dye and paint industries. Like the other essential trace metals it forms an integral part of a number of enzymes. Those dependent on molybdenum include xanthine oxidase and alcohol dehydrogenase. The actions of molybdenum are closely interwoven with those of copper and of iron. Thus the addition of molybdenum to the diet of animals whose intake of copper is only marginally adequate may induce signs of copper deficiency. On the other hand, molybdenum seems to exert a facilitatory effect on the absorption and utilization of iron.

Xanthine oxidase activity may be seriously depressed in sheep and cattle whose molybdenum intake has been inadequate by reason of their grazing pastures containing insufficient supplies of the metal. Animals so affected are likely to develop kidney stones. Experimentally induced molybdenum deficiency in laboratory chicks is associated with an increased excretion of xanthine, retarded growth and an increased mortality.

Molybdenum is usually present in adequate amounts in the normal human diet, peas, beans and cereals being particularly rich sources. Although deficiency does not produce a recognised clinical syndrome there is suggestive evidence that dental health is dependent on molybdenum. Thus the incidence of dental caries is high in children who live in areas such as Somerset in England where cattle exhibit signs of molybdenum deficiency. Moreover, in parts of the world where droughts, storms or other vagaries of the climate have led to a disappearance of much of the metal from the soil there may be even more serious manifestations of molybdenum deficiency. Some twenty years ago there was a considerable increase in the incidence of oesophageal cancer among the inhabitants of some native Bantu reserves in Africa. All the affected groups lived on land that had lost its fertility and its molybdenum some thirty years earlier.

Neither molybdenum nor its salts are toxic to man and molybdenum poisoning does not constitute an industrial hazard.

SELENIUM

Selenium has been a centre of controversy for many years. That it is a highly toxic substance is undeniable but the realization that it is also an essential trace element has dawned only slowly. It receives no mention in an otherwise authoritative text devoted to the essential metals and published as recently as 1972 (Davies, 1972). Few authorities yet seem disposed to admit that selenium has therapeutic possibilities largely, perhaps, because they are unaware of the results of recent studies that point in this direction.

The electrical and electronic industries use selenium in rectifiers and photoelectric cells and the metal is also found in some paints, metal coatings, glass, insecticides and (as the sulphide) in shampoos. Selenium sulphide has a long-standing reputation as an antiseborrhoeic agent (p. 810). Selenium poisoning, notwithstanding the element's toxicity, is not very common among industrial workers. Inorganic selenium compounds can cause dermatitis and some of them produce serious burns if they are spilled on the skin. Signs of chronic exposure include irritation of the upper respiratory and gastrointestinal tracts and a smell of garlic in the breath. Selenium poisoning is rather refractory to the usual forms of treatments including chelating agents. Selenium poisoning has occurred in South and East Africa in livestock that has consumed *Leucaena glauca* Benth. This plant extracts selenium from a selenium-rich soil and concentrates it in the seeds and elsewhere. Selenium poisoning of this kind can be chronic or acute and is called 'blind staggers' or 'alkali disease'. The former term is very descriptive of the symptoms—poor vision, blindness, ataxia and paralysis. Another prominent symptom of intoxication with selenium is loss of body hair.

Selenium is the prosthetic element in a number of enzymes that operate in conjunction with α-tocopherol (Vitamin E) to maintain the integrity of cellular and intracellular membranes and to synthesize immunoglobulins, some other proteins and ubiquinone. It is believed that, in physiological quantities, selenium facilitates the conversion of sulphydryl (-SH) into disulphide (-SS-) groups but in large amounts the selenite ion prevents the reformation of the sulphydryl groups and this action probably provides the reason for its toxicity.

Experimental selenium deficiency in animals is associated with hepatic and cardiovascular disorders, arthritis, degenerative muscle disorders, cataract, pancreatic lesions and loss of fur. Selenium is now sometimes added to animal feeding stuffs produced from grain grown on soils lacking selenium.

There is little acceptable evidence that states of selenium deficiency occur in human beings. Nevertheless there is evidence that selenium can improve the admittedly disputed benefit conferred by vitamin E (that other nutritional enigma) on patients with intermittent claudication, arthritis and some forms of heart disease (p. 789).

Although selenium is, as we have seen, a poisonous metal it can apparently confer a degree of protection against the toxic actions of some other heavy metals. It may also exert an anticancer action.

Readers who wish to extend their knowledge of selenium and its possibilities are referred to a recent review by Frost and Lish (1975).

ZINC

Iron that has a coating of zinc, deposited electrically, is known as galvanized iron and as such it and its industrial and domestic applications are very well known. Zinc is also a component of brass and other alloys and it has applications in the building and paint industries. Zinc salts have astringent and antiseptic properties that have led to their wide popularity as skin ointments and lotions.

Among workers in industry, 'brass founder's ague' (an influenza like condition) is attributable to their breathing the fumes of zinc oxide. In high concentration, zinc chloride fumes are also toxic and have caused some deaths from bronchopneumonia. Chronic zinc poisoning is seen only rarely.

As long ago as 1869, Raulin showed that zinc was essential for the growth of fungi but fifty years were to elapse before this finding was extended to animals. In 1940, carbonic anhydrase was isolated in a pure state and shown to contain zinc. Since then, zinc has been found in eight other enzymes (including alkaline phosphatase, carboxypeptidases and alcohol, lactate and glutamic dehydrogenases) while an even larger group of enzymes require zinc (and sometimes other trace metals) for optimal functioning. The synthesis of ribosenucleic acid can only proceed in the presence of zinc.

We have noted that alcohol dehydrogenase is a zinc dependent enzyme and in alcoholic cirrhosis the amount of zinc in the serum and the activity of the dehydrogenase are both depressed. Insulin in the islets of Langerhans is associated with zinc and it may be that the zinc-insulin complex serves as a store from which insulin is released on demand. Another possibility is that the zinc in some way contributes to the action of insulin, perhaps by exerting an insulin like action on its own account. Dithiazone, a zinc chelating agent, induces experimental diabetes in laboratory animals presumably because it inactivates the zinc-insulin complex. Patients with diabetes excrete more zinc in the urine than do nondiabetic subjects. Among the other physiological functions that seem to depend on the presence of adequate amounts of zinc are wound healing (some workers have been able to accelerate the healing of skin ulcers in human patients by applying zinc sulphate), the development of the gonads and spermatozoa and rod activity in the retina. There have been many reports concerning the possible relationship between zinc intake and the development of cancer but no definite conclusions concerning this association have yet emerged.

Zinc deficiency has been induced in laboratory animals and it sometimes occurs naturally in farm animals. Pigs suffer from dermatitis, diarrhoea and weight loss. This condition, which is often fatal, is known as *parakeratosis*. In laboratory animals (the rat has been most intensively studied), parakeratosis, testicular atrophy, impaired protein synthesis and skeletal deformities are seen. Experimental diets containing no zinc are markedly teratogenic.

Zinc deficiency is not commonly seen in human beings but reports have appeared of a few patients who exhibited iron deficiency anaemia in association with testicular atrophy and stunted growth and who responded remarkably well to zinc supplementation of their diet (Prasad, 1966).

These recent investigations into the significance of zinc in the animal organism clearly indicate that the therapeutic potentiality of this metal is greater than has hitherto been suspected.

Metals not essential for life

ALUMINIUM

Aluminium is widely used in industry and the home. It finds some applications in medicine: the hydroxide, glycinate and phosphate are employed as antacids and adsorbents in the treatment of peptic ulcer (p. 644) while alum and a number of other aluminium compounds have astringent and mildly caustic properties that render them useful for the local treatment of ulcers in the mouth and elsewhere and for arresting bleeding from minor cuts (p. 807).

Aluminium is present in small amounts in many items of diet, particularly fruits and vegetables and it is also present as aluminium dust in the atmosphere. About 50 to 100 mg of aluminium are ingested each day with the diet but only tiny amounts are absorbed from the gastrointestinal tract.

Ever since the end of the last century when the first aluminium cooking and storage vessels appeared, there have been sporadic outbreaks of anxiety and a number of official reports concerning the possibility that aluminium might be transferred from saucepans to food in sufficient quantities to constitute a hazard to health. These anxieties seem to have been misplaced. The amount of aluminium that passes into food during cooking in aluminium pans is increased if the contents of the vessel are acid or if baking soda (which contains aluminium) has been added. It is also increases if the vessels are stained or if they are made of soft aluminium instead of the more resistant variety that is more generally used nowadays. Even under the worst possible conditions (cooking acid foods with baking soda in stained old pans) the amount of additional aluminium that enters the food in cooking is no more than about 125 mg daily. Very little of this will be absorbed and there is no evidence that the trivial amounts of metal that gain access to the tissues are capable of exerting any toxic action at all. The larger amounts of aluminium that are deposited in the gut by those who take antacids containing the metal may cause loss of phosphate from the body but that is a different problem which is discussed elsewhere (p. 644).

Some industrial workers inhale considerable quantities of dusts containing aluminium or one of its compounds and much debate has centred on the possibility that they are thereby exposed to the risk of 'aluminosis' in the same way that those who inhale silica may develop silicosis. Clinical investigations and animal experiments alike have failed to provide clear cut evidence for the existence of any condition that could justifiably be described as aluminosis and the lungs of workers in the English pottery industry who are exposed in their daily work to alumina dust are remarkably free of fibrotic changes (pneumoconiosis) unless they have also been exposed to silica.

Far from inducing pathological changes in the lungs, aluminium is actually employed to prevent them in coal and gold miners and others who are at risk from silicosis. Aluminium powder is blown into the lungs in a stream of air. Usually each man is exposed to the powder for a period of some five minutes once weekly and in the course of a year he will receive more than 1500 mg of aluminium. Although this form of prophylactic treatment is neither used nor recommended in Great Britain it is much favoured in some other parts of the world whence some glowing reports concerning its efficacy have emanated. The rationale of the treatment is that the solubility and thus the toxicity of quartz in lung tissue will be reduced if the particles are coated with aluminium hydroxide that will be formed in the lungs. Other contributions to the beneficial effect may be provided by the increased size of the quartz particles consequent on their coating of aluminium and by the reported bronchodilator activity of the metal. It is unfortunate that the results of some investigations have failed to support the optimism of those who advocate this novel treatment and there is more than a suspicion that the successes attributed to it may be largely the consequences of placebo effects exerted both on those who give and those who receive the aluminium.

ANTIMONY

Several industrial processes involve the use of the chloride, oxides and sulphides of antimony as well as of antimony metal alloyed with copper, lead or tin. In medicine, compounds of trivalent antimony such as potassium antimony tartrate (tartar emetic) and of the pentavalent metal such as stibamine are employed in the treatment of schistosomiasis (p. 897) and leishmaniasis (p. 874) respectively.

Antimony is not a component of the diet but it does occur in some enamels and, in the past, cases of antimony poisoning arising as a result of preparing or storing acid foods or drinks in white enamelled vessels were occasionally seen. Antimony poisoning may also occur in those who mine or process stibnite or other antimony ores, in those who work with the metal and in typesetters.

Among the symptoms of antimony poisoning are vomiting, abdominal pains, gastrointestinal disturbances, fatigue and pain in the limbs, myocardial damage and, sometimes, skin rashes. These constitute a picture not dissimilar to that of chronic arsenic poisoning and the two conditions are treated in the same way (see below).

ARSENIC

Arsenic has no biological function but it is widely distributed in nature and small amounts are found in human tissues. In most contexts, 'arsenic' usually refers to the trioxide, the form in which the element is most commonly found. Arsenic trioxide is a constituent of some weedkillers and sheep dips and was used in the preparation of the once popular Fowler's solution which was used in the treatment of dermatological conditions until its carcinogenic nature became evident. The arsenates of lead and some other metals are employed as insecticides, potassium arsenite is a fungicide and copper compound (the arsenite and acetoarsenite) were much in vogue as wallpaper paints until it was realized that they were frequent causes of arsenic poisoning in the home. Organic compounds of arsenic still have a place in the treatment of amoebiasis, trichomoniasis and trypanosomiasis: they are discussed in the chapters that deal with these topics.

In both real life and detective fiction, arsenic (often obtained from weedkillers) has long been a favourite instrument of homicide and suicide but accidental poisoning is not common and it is becoming even more uncommon now that arsenic is less widely used and such hidden domestic menaces as poisonous wallpaper have been eliminated. Symptoms of acute arsenic poisoning include a burning mouth and lips, thirst, difficulty in swallowing, inflammation of the gums and mouth, abdominal pain, vomiting and diarrhoea. In severe poisoning there is cyanosis, weakness and prostration. The body temperature falls, the pulse is weak and rapid, loss of consciousness follows and death is due to circulatory failure. Arsenic may also cause nephritis, hepatitis, anaemia and various neurological distrubances.

The main signs of chronic arsenic poisoning are skin rashes, loss of hair and finger nails, malaise, weakness, loss of weight, sore and inflamed gums and mouth, vomiting, abdominal pain and diarrhoea or constipation. Nervous changes also occur and the breath has a characteristic odour of garlic. Arsenic poisoning is treated with dimercaprol (p. 796).

BERYLLIUM

Beryllium has no therapeutic applications but it is of considerable toxicological importance. It is used to manufacture special grades of metal alloy and pure rods of beryllium are used in atomic piles. It coats the tubes of fluorescent lights and X-ray tubes and it is present in some grades of porcelain. Compounds of beryllium are very toxic and inhalation of the dust causes symptoms of poisoning. These include conjunctivitis and facial dermatitis, irritation of the nasal passages and throat with nosebleeding, and swollen, congested mucous membranes.

Bronchitis and tracheitis may develop. The most serious toxic effect of beryllium compounds is acute pulmonary disease—usually an acute pneumonitis—which may be fatal. There is no specific treatment for beryllium poisoning but some amelioration of the condition can often be achieved by cortisone therapy.

CADMIUM

Cadmium has no therapeutic application but it is used in the metallurgical industries and in the manufacture of storage batteries and of pigments to resist high temperatures. If they are taken into the gastrointestinal tract, cadmium and its salts are powerful emetics but accidental cadmium poisoning in industry is usually the result of inhaling cadmium vapour or dust. In acute poisoning irritation of the eyes, nausea, giddiness, pain in the chest and dyspnoea are observed. The most serious complication is bronchopneumonia, which may be fatal. In chronic poisoning, pulmonary emphysema, chronic rhinitis and damage to the liver and kidneys dominate the clinical picture.

Chelating compounds will remove cadmium from the body but care has to be exercised in their use lest kidney damage is produced by the cadmium that enters the urine.

LEAD

This familiar metal has been in use for more than three millennia. From the very first, it was fashioned into water pipes and tanks (the modern tourist can still see the lead lining with which the Romans equipped their Pont du Gard, the famous French aqueduct) and lead is (or has been) extensively employed in the manufacture of shot, the plates of electric accumulators, pottery glazes and toys. It is a component of a number of alloys while lead oxides (litharge, red lead and white lead) and other compounds form the basis of some paints, varnishes, plastics, rubbers and insecticides. Organic compounds of lead are added to petrol as 'antiknock' agents: the threat to health posed by the discharge of lead into the atmosphere from our cars will be considered separately from the toxic actions of inorganic lead.

Over the centuries, lead poisoning has claimed many thousands of victims. The incidence of poisoning has fallen since employers have had to pay proper regard to the safety and welfare of their employees and now that other substances are replacing lead in water conduits, storage vessels and toys. Most cases of lead poisoning seen today are the result of accidental rather than occupational exposure. Inhalation of the fumes from burning lead can have dangerous sequelae and the use of old batteries for fuel has resulted in several cases of serious intoxication. Even though they no longer have lead soldiers to play with, young children still chew into painted wooden surfaces and can poison themselves in this way. It will be evident that acute poisoning is the more often seen but chronic lead poisoning does still occur.

Lead is not essential for life and no more than 10 per cent of any that is ingested is absorbed into the circulation. This ensures that the small amounts present in the diet will do no harm, but if more is added from other sources the concentration in the plasma soon reaches the toxic level of about 50 μg per 100 ml. Much of the lead that is absorbed is sequestered in the bones which carry about 90 per cent of the body's total complement of some 300 mg. Although uptake by bones provides useful protection, the lead can be released by any condition (such as leukaemia) that promotes osteolysis. Thus symptoms of lead poisoning may appear in people who have not been exposed to lead for many years.

The symptoms of acute lead poisoning include loss of appetite and sleep, severe abdominal pain, a feeling of weakness and pain in the joints and muscles. The central nervous system and the blood forming mechanisms are affected in cases of severe poisoning. Lead encephalopathy is characterized by headache, confusion, excitement, hallucinations and convulsions. Haematological changes include anaemia, haemolysis, punctate basophilia and impaired synthesis of haem. The gums frequently exhibit the blue 'lead line'.

As we have seen, lead poisoning is treated with calcium sodium edetate. The daily dose, by mouth or by infusion over five hours, is two grams. It is given in courses lasting five days with intervals of three days between successive courses.

The petrol peril

For the last half century, organic compounds of lead have been added to petrol to prevent uneven burning of the fuel ('knocking' or 'pinking') in the combustion chamber. Tetraethyl lead—$Pb(C_2H_5)_4$—was the first such additive but a number of other lead alkyls (the tetramethyl, methyltriethyl, ethyltrimethyl and dimethyldiethyl leads) are now in use. The actions of all of them are similar. The price we have had to pay for our fifty years of smoother motoring is a considerable increase in the amount of lead in the atmosphere. Thus, while the air above the open ocean contains only 0.001 μg of lead per cubic metre, that in the main streets of Los Angeles, where the automobile reigns supreme, has as much as 8 μg per cubic metre. Other cities lag behind Los Angeles: in New York, London and Edinburgh, the atmosphere contains about 4 μg, 3 μg and 0.2 μg per cubic metre respectively (Waldron and Stöfen, 1974). It is natural to enquire whether the lead in the atmosphere will eventually accumulate—or has already accumulated—to such an extent as to constitute a toxic hazard. Considerable differences of opinion exist concerning the answer to this question. Some authorities believe that lead is not dangerous until it reaches a threshold concentration in the plasma but others maintain that it is harmful even in amounts that do not produce overt signs of poisoning. There are disturbing reports that the exposure of young children to higher than average concentrations of atmospheric lead may retard both their physical growth and their intellectual development. It has even been suggested that the recent growth of juvenile crime in urban areas has its origin in the rising level of atmospheric lead.

In petrol, the 'antiknock' components are mixed with substances such as ethylene bromide that react in the combustion chambers with the decomposition products of the lead alkyls to produce inorganic compounds such as lead bromide which are themselves converted into carbonates and oxides when they come into contact with the atmosphere. Nevertheless, some unchanged lead alkyls escape into the air. They are much more toxic than inorganic lead compounds because they are lipid soluble and are taken up into nervous tissue instead of being safely deposited in bones. Thus the danger from car exhausts may be out of proportion to the actual amount of lead that they add to the atmosphere. Prudence would obviously dictate that the amount of lead in petrol should be curtailed to a point that prevents the accumulation of atmospheric lead beyond the upper limit of safety. Unfortunately, we do not yet known what the safety limit is. British and American workers have variously quoted, 2, 4 and 20 μg per cubic metre as the limit but the Russians (who perhaps love their motor cars less than we do) set the barrier at 0.7 μg per cubic metre.

The amount of lead taken up from the intestine (and some of the lead that is inhaled reaches the gut) is reduced if calcium is also present. This constitutes yet another excellent argument in favour of providing abundant quantities of cheap (or free) milk for infants and schoolchildren.

MERCURY

Metallic mercury is used in thermometers and barometers, in amalgams with copper, silver or gold and in the manufacture of artificial jewellery. Its salts find some industrial uses particularly and traditionally in the manufacture of felt hats while organic compounds of mercury are met in seed dressings and detonators. Mercury compounds have enjoyed a certain reputation as therapeutic agents but the only survivors are mercury diuretics (p. 627), ointments and disinfectants. Acute mercury poisoning is not seen very often: when it does occur it is characterized by kidney damage (causing albuminuria and haematuria), vomiting, acute gastric pain (if the offending compound has been taken by mouth) and respiratory embarrassment or frank pneumonia. Chronic mercury poisoning is rather more common and it brings a variety of disabilities in its train. A strange but characteristic form of neurosis (*erethism*) is sometimes seen in those who work with mercury. The principal features of erethism are feelings of intense embarrassment, anxious depression, irritability and an inability to concentrate. Other signs of chronic mercury poisoning are spongy and inflamed gums with loosening of the teeth, tremor, slurred speech, unsteady gait, peripheral neuritis and nephritis.

The toxic side effects that may accompany the administration of the mercurial diuretics are detailed elsewhere.

NICKEL

Nickel salts can cause dermatitis ('nickel itch') in those who work with them, but apart from this, the interest of toxicologists is confined, as far as this metal is concerned, to nickel carbonyl—$Ni(CO)_4$—the form in which nickel is extracted from its ores in the Mond process. It, or some substance formed from it, is carcinogenic and can cause cancer of the lung or nasal passages in those exposed to it. Acute nickel carbonyl poisoning is characterized by headache, dizziness and vomiting followed by signs of respiratory distress. Neither acute nor chronic poisoning is as common as it was in the early years of the century when the Mond process was first applied on an industrial scale. Indeed, acute poisoning is now so rare that it has not yet been possible to assess the value of chelating agents in its treatment. Experiments with animals, however, have not given encouraging results.

Nickel salts are no longer used medicinally.

SILVER

Silver nitrate (lunar caustic) is the only inorganic salt of silver used in therapeutics. It is a caustic and astringent used to treat warts and to cauterize ulcers and wounds. In solid form or as the strong solution, silver nitrate is an irritant and can cause tissue damage and scarring. More dilute solutions cause local redness and itching when applied to the skin. Symptoms of acute poisoning which follow ingestion of silver nitrate are similar to those which follow any corrosive poison. Silver compounds of various types have been used as antiseptics.

Chronic silver poisoning (Argyria) Prolonged absorption of small quantities of silver salts causes a dark bluish grey pigmentation resulting from the deposition of silver in the skin, mucous membranes and connective tissues. It may follow prolonged use of nasal drops which contain silver. It may also occur in workers in the photographic industry, in other industrial workers and in dentists who have worked for many years with silver amalgams. The skin and the eyes are likely to be particularly affected but deposition of silver in the kidneys may cause damage to these organs. Argyria is very difficult to treat, and as a rule pigmentation persists throughout life.

THALLIUM

Thallium is a soft and malleable metal, reminiscent of lead. It has a number of industrial uses particularly in the manufacture of lenses and imitation jewellery and as alloys with silver or lead. The metal itself is quite innocuous and those who work with it are not exposed to any industrial hazard on that account. The salts, on the other hand, are highly toxic and they have been the instruments of many a murder and suicide as well as being the cause of innumerable accidental deaths.

Thallium acetate (or the sulphate) was once a popular depilating agent but its use for this purpose was virtually abandoned once its high systemic toxicity became fully appreciated. The salts, however, still appear in insecticides and rat poisons that are freely available in some countries though not in Britain. Recently, thallous chloride incorporating radioactive thallium (T 201) has come into vogue as an agent for the radiographic scanning of the heart. It is given by intravenous injection for the detection of cardiac infarcts and the differential diagnosis of cardiac hypertrophy.

Thallium is readily absorbed from both the skin and the intestine. It is slowly excreted in the urine and faeces but this is a very slow process giving a serum half life of about one month. The likelihood of thallium cumulation (p. 68) is obviously a very real one.

Acute thallium poisoning affects principally the digestive and nervous systems giving, *inter alia*, restlessness, tremors, convulsions, paralysis, breathlessness and bloody diarrhoea. Thallium is taken up by many tissues but the principal sign of chronic thallium poisoning (as might be expected from its original therapeutic use) is loss of hair. The tissues of the eye may also be affected with a resulting keratitis, cataract and atrophy of the optic nerve.

Attempts to treat acute thallium poisoning by chelating agents such as diphenylthiocarbazone and dimercaprol have not been very successful largely because the thallium chelates are both toxic and lipid soluble so that they can cross the blood brain barrier and so interfere with nervous function. More success has attended the use of Prussian blue (potassium ferric cyanoferrate) given by mouth or intraduodenal tube. In the intestine, thallium exchanges with the potassium of Prussian blue. The thallium compound is not absorbed and is excreted in the faeces. Doses of up to 20 grams of Prussian blue may have to be given twice daily for two or three weeks to secure the complete clearing of a toxic dose of thallium from the body.

Tin. Metallic tin in powdered form and tin oxide have been used as anthelmintics in infestation with tapeworms. Tin has also been applied to the treatment of boils with no great success. It appears to be non-toxic; there is no evidence that storage of food in tin-plated containers is harmful but tin dust is responsible for the pneumoconiosis that is not infrequently seen in workers in the tin industry. The condition is not usually serious.

Organic compounds of tin such as the triethyl and diethyl tins, which have been used as fungicides and insecticides are much more toxic than the original salts. The dialkyl compounds are extremely irritant to the skin and they can also bring about inflammatory changes in the bile ducts. The trialkyl tins direct their main toxic attack against the central nervous system and cause tremors, weakness and paralysis of the limbs which may progress to a fatal end. An attempt to treat acne and boils with a preparation containing as it transpired, a misjudged dose of diethyl tin (which happened to be contaminated with the triethyl compound) had a catastrophic outcome some years ago in France. Some patients survived their treatment but no fewer than 102 died while another one hundred suffered permanent neurological damage.

URANIUM

Uranium has no therapeutic uses but it is used in connection with atomic energy plants and may thus be a hazard to health. Soluble compounds of uranium are toxic, exerting their effects upon the kidneys in which they are concentrated following absorption. A considerable amount of uranium is also concentrated in the bones, in which it replaces calcium. Death following uranium poisoning results from kidney failure

VANADIUM

Vanadium is used in the manufacture of hard alloy steels. It has no therapeutic uses but can cause poisoning. Symptoms arise from irritation of the tissues which come into contact with the vapour. It causes conjunctivitis, dermatitis and bronchitis. Bronchopneumonia may follow and this may be fatal. Workers who have been exposed to an undesirably high concentration of atmospheric vanadium often find that their tongues turn a greenish-black colour.

BIBLIOGRAPHY

Books, monographs and reviews

Albert, A. (1968). *Selective Toxicity*, 4th edn. London: Methuen.
Bidstrup, P. L. (1964). *Toxicity of Mercury and its Compounds.* Amsterdam: Elsevier.
Browning, Ethel (1969). *Toxicity of Industrial Metals*, 2nd edn. London: Butterworths.
Buchanan, W. (1962). *Toxicity of Arsenic Compounds* Amsterdam: Elsevier.
Davies, E. J. T. (1972). *The Clinical Significance of the Essential Biological Metals.* London: Heinemann.
Frost, D. V. and Lish, P. M. (1975). Selenium in biology. *A. rev. Pharmac*, **15**, 259-284.
Mertz, W. (1969). Chromium Occurrence and Function in Biological Systems. *Physiol. Rev.*, **49**, 163-239.
Passow, H. Rothstein, A. and Clarkson, T. W. (1961). The general pharmacology of the heavy metals. *Pharmac. Rev.*, **13**, 185-224.
Prasad, A. S. (1966) *Zinc Metabolism.* Springfield: Thomas.
Schubert, J. (1966). Chelation in medicine. *Scient. Am.* (May issue), **214**, 40-50.
Ussing, H. H. (1960). The alkali metal ions in isolated systems and tissues. *Handb. exp. Pharmak.*, **13**, 1-195.
Waldron, H. A. and Stofen, D. (1974). *Subclinical Lead Poisoning.* London and New York: Academic Press.

Original papers

Anonymous (1974). Thallium. *Lancet* (ii), 564-565.
Morin, Y. L., Foley, A. R., Martineau, G. and Roussel, J. (1967). Quebec beer-drinkers' cardiomyopathy. *Can. med. Ass. J.*, **97**, 881-885.
Sullivan, J. F., George, R., Bluvas, R. and Egan, J. D. (1969). Myocardiopathy of beer-drinkers: subsequent course. *Ann. intern. Med.*, **70**, 277-282.

49. Drugs used mainly in dermatology

The skin is more than a mere integument. It is the boundary between man and his external environment, a fact which is reflected in the skin's rich supply of sensory nerve endings, blood vessels and sweat glands. It is a matter of common experience that the skin is frequently the site of local eruptions and minor injuries, often accompanied by pain and itch. However, it is also affected by general as well as local conditions and many skin disorders demand systemic treatment rather than the topical application of medicaments. Moreover, the fact that portions of the skin are normally exposed to view adds a strong psychogenic element which may influence the course of dermatological conditions. The presence of a rash or other skin blemish may be the cause of considerable embarrassment and unhappiness. On the other hand, the circumstance that lesions of the skin are visible for all to see sometimes provides the patient with a subconscious wish (and the psychosomatic mechanism) to delay his recovery. So long as he has a visible lesion he can be *seen* to be ill and this may well provide him with the means of escaping from a difficult personal situation without incurring the charge of malingering.

Skin eruptions constitute the most common of all adverse drug reactions. They take various forms and are attributable to the independent or conjoint operation of a number of different mechanisms but many of them can be classified as hypersensitivity reactions and, as such, they are discussed in some detail in Chapter 24. Idiosyncratic reactions to ingested foodstuffs and to chemical substances with which the body has been in simple contact fall into the same category.

Large sums of money are spent every day on cosmetic preparations. Some of these are pleasantly decorative (provided that they do not evoke an allergic skin reaction) and some serve a truly cosmetic purpose by obscuring unsightly blemishes but expensive concoctions that purport to 'nourish' the skin (whatever that may mean), remove wrinkles, provide schoolgirl complexions for aging matrons and perform other dermatological miracles are not of sufficient value to warrant the attention of the serious pharmacologist. The substances described in this chapter are those which have some therapeutic effect when they are applied to the skin. Some of them are equally effective when they are taken systemically and some, indeed, are better taken in this way. Others, on the other hand, are dangerous if they are absorbed into the body and

their use is precluded when the skin is damaged or severely eczematous. Healthy, unbroken skin is not easily penetrated by chemical substances. This is a hardly surprising consequence of its boundary function.

Figure 49.1 should serve to remind the reader of the nature and disposition of the several components of the skin to which reference is made in this (and other) chapters.

ASTRINGENTS, KERATOLYTICS, EMOLLIENTS AND ANTIPRURITIC AGENTS

Astringents are protein precipitants. When they are applied to the skin and mucous membranes, only the proteins on the surface are precipitated so the cells are not killed. Many metallic salts have astringent properties. Among those that have been used in dermatology are alum, aluminium acetate and aluminium chloride. Alum sticks are used to stop bleeding from minor cuts. Solutions of copper sulphate, zinc sulphate and zinc chloride have both astringent and antiseptic properties: zinc sulphate is used in mouth washes while zinc oxide and calamine (zinc oxide with 2 per cent ferric oxide) are employed in the treatment of minor skin conditions. They are present in many proprietary creams and ointments; their astringent properties help to reduce itching. Lead salts were once popular but, because of the danger of poisoning, they should be avoided.

Iron salts have astringent properties. They are liable to produce staining if used for long periods on damaged skin, but a solution of ferric chloride provides a very good protection against poison ivy. This plant, *Rhus toxidendron*, which is common in North America, produces a violent reaction if it comes into even momentary contact with skin and it can provide a considerable hazard for the country walker. The active agent in poison ivy is ivy oil (urushiol or toxidendrol), a mixture of catechol derivatives with side chains based on fifteen carbon atoms.

Among organic substances, tannic acid is the best known astringent, though its therapeutic usefulness is limited. It is a mixture of the digallic esters of D(+)glucose and it precipitates, as tannates, certain alkaloids and the salts of some heavy metals. For many years tannic acid was used to treat burns, the precipitated proteins forming a protective layer on the damaged skin. It is no longer

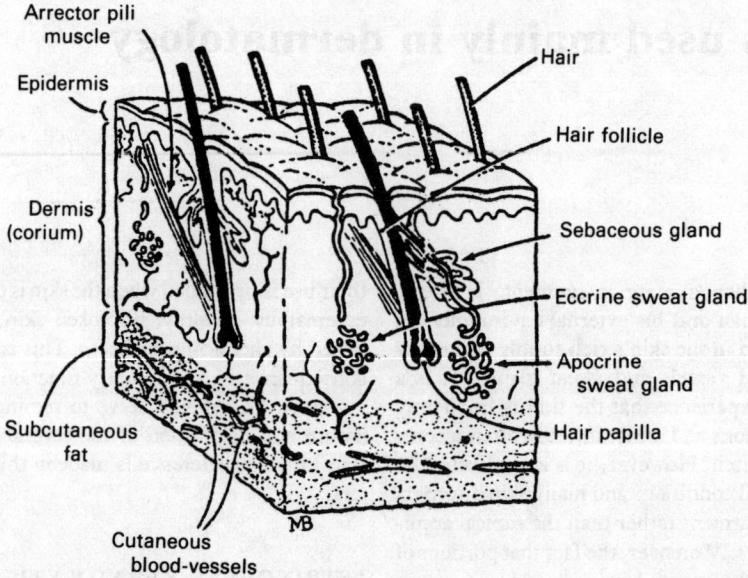

Fig. 49.1 Low power view of the structures found in hairy skin. (Reproduced by kind permission of the authors and publishers, from Bell, Enslie-Smith and Paterson (1976) '*Textbook of physiology and biochemistry*' 9th ed. Edinburgh: Churchill Livingstone)

employed for this purpose: antibiotics and other antibacterial substances are more effective and tannic acid absorbed from raw surfaces is now known to cause liver damage. Strong tea (which contains tannic acid) is a traditional antidote to poisoning by heavy metals and alkaloids. Though it can be used in an emergency, it is important to realise that gastric lavage must be carried out as soon as possible since tannates gradually dissolve in both acid and alkaline solutions of the strength found in the gastrointestinal tract. If this happens the poison is absorbed. Moreover, tannic acid does not precipitate the salts of some heavy metals (mercury is an example) nor some alkaloids (atropine and morphine are examples).

Keratolytics soften the horny layer (*stratum corneum*) of the skin so that it is more easily removed. Dilute solutions are used to remove scales in psoriasis or to remove portions of the stratum corneum affected by fungi. They are also used in the treatment of dandruff; more concentrated solutions are utilized as corn removers. Substances in this group include dithranol (1,8-dihydroxyanthranol), resorcinol and salicylic acid.

The more powerful keratolytics are known as *caustics:* they destroy the tissues with which they come into contact. *Escharotic agents,* though caustic, also produce an exudate which is organized into a protective scale. Caustics are used for the treatment of such blemishes as warts and moles; they are of some use in fungal infections. Podophyllum (a resin obtained from the dried roots of the May apple or American mandrake, *Podophyllum peltatum*) is a caustic commonly used as a wart remover. Formalin (5 per cent) and salicylic acid (50 per cent) will also remove warts but

the best agent (though not the one most readily available) is liquid nitrogen.

Emollients are substances used to protect the skin from irritation, to soothe irritated areas and to render the skin more supple and flexible. Emollients are also used as ointment bases though they do not promote the passage of drugs into the skin. A very large number of substances has been used as emollients. They include vegetable oils (olive oil, etc.), animal fats (wool fat, etc.), hydrocarbons (paraffin, etc.) and waxes. They are of pharmaceutical interest but their pharmacological importance is negligible.

Antipruritics. Itching (*pruritus*) is a common and distressing feature of many skin conditions and some systemic diseases. Those who itch are tempted to scratch: scratching causes skin damage which produces more itching and leads to further scratching. Thus scratching prevents or retards the healing of the original condition and may make it worse by introducing infection into the skin or by exposing it to infection from other extraneous sources. Not infrequently, itching is intensified by psychogenic factors. Indeed, pruritus (particularly when it involves the anus, the vulva or the scalp) is sometimes completely psychological in origin and may then be totally refractory to the usual antipruritic agents. By the same token, of course, some patients whose pruritus has a large psychogenic component respond in a gratifyingly dramatic manner to the placebo effect of the treatment they are given or that of the physician who gives it. Substances that have been used to treat itch include the antihistamines (Chap. 21), the corticosteroids and some of the astringents and caustics (calamine and phenol, for instance) which, by their action

CH₃ ... (chemical structure)

$$CH_3$$

Crotamiton

on the superficial layers of the skin, impair the activity of the fine sensory nerve terminals and thus act as local anaesthetics. They may also reduce the sensitivity of the skin and so reduce the liberation of itch-producing substances. Crotamiton (crotonyl-N-ethyl-*o*-toluidide; Eurax) is a potent nonspecific antipruritic agent which has some antibacterial activity. It is used, in the form of a cream or lotion, to provide rapid relief from severe itching in pruritus ani, pruritus vulvae, senile pruritus, eczema, dermatitis, psoriasis, etc. It is also useful in the control of itching accompanying scabies, since it kills the itch mite. Although they may be effective when applied locally, antihistamines should not be given in this way because of the real possibility of their provoking a hypersensitivity reaction which would add the insult of a drug eruption to the injury of the original dermatological condition. For a similar reason, the skin should not be exposed to preparations containing local anaesthetics although they may be effective antipruritic agents. Antihistamines can be safely taken by mouth.

The pharmacology of itch is discussed in Chapter 25.

THE TREATMENT OF DERMATOLOGICAL CONDITIONS

Substances of the types discussed in the preceding pages are incorporated in a variety of medicaments: ointments, creams, lotions, dressings and dusting powders. Zinc oxide is a very common constituent of these preparations. They are used to provide symptomatic relief of minor skin conditions but more effective medicaments are available for the more serious diseases. These include benzyl benzoate (p. 905) whose value in scabies has been recognized for many years, a number of specific drugs that are given locally or systemically to relieve fungal infections of the skin (Chap. 60) and immunosuppressive drugs such as methotrexate and azathioprine (p. 917) which have a place in the treatment of cases of psoriasis that have failed to respond to less drastic remedies. However, the real revolution in dermatology came about with the introduction of corticosteroid therapy. Many skin disorders (particularly those that are partly or wholly of allergic origin) respond extremely well to the corticosteroids. The drugs are sometimes administered systemically, especially in emergencies, and in these circumstances prednisone is usually chosen. In *pemphigus*, for instance, large oral doses of prednisone (up to 120 mg daily) can be life saving although in resistant cases it may be necessary to give ACTH intravenously instead. Pemphigus is a disease characterized by the widespread occurrence of fluid-filled bullae (blisters); if untreated it may prove fatal, particularly in the newly born.

The first corticosteroid to be made available for local application was hydrocortisone. It is usually applied as a one per cent ointment. Although more powerful compounds are now extensively used, hydrocortisone, as we shall see, still has much to recommend it.

A complete catalogue of the corticosteroids that are available for dermatological use, together with their formulae and proprietary names can be found in Chapter 44 (pp. 761-766); here it is only necessary to say that, at present, the most extensively used are betamethasone (Betnovate), beclomethasone (Propaderm) and fluocinolone (Synalar) and that some of the more recently-introduced compounds such as fluocinocide (Metosyn) and fluclorolone (Topilar) may be even more effective. For topical application, betamethasone and beclomethasone are presented as a 1 in 5 or a 1 in 10 dilution in a Cetomacrogol cream. This reduces the extent to which the drugs are absorbed into the deeper layers of the skin or into the systemic circulation. The necessary penetration into the superficial layers can be promoted by covering the treated area with polyethylene film or some other form of occlusive dressing.

Other agents can be incorporated in the corticosteroid ointments: the suffixes A, C and N (as in Betnovate A, etc.) indicate the addition of chlortetracycline, clioquinol and neomycin respectively.

Complications of corticosteroid therapy

The remarkable effectiveness of the corticosteroids and the natural demand of patients to be rid of embarrassing skin lesions as quickly as possible has led to an extensive use of the more powerful corticosteroids, often for quite trivial conditions which would be better left alone or treated with simpler remedies. Conditions of the skin often require prolonged treatment and it is unfortunate that those who prescribe the corticosteroids are not always fully aware of the extent to which the drugs can produce unpleasant and irreversible changes in the skin.

The first adverse change that may be produced by the continued application of corticosteroids is atrophy of the epidermis so that the skin takes on a thin, transparent, waxy appearance as it does in old age. The collagen fibres in the dermis may also undergo partial atrophy and, having lost some of their elasticity, they stretch and produce unsightly striations in the skin. These streaks are at first purple in colour, as, indeed, is the atrophied epidermis. Although normal skin colour is eventually restored, the scars remain.

Some conditions of the skin are associated with telangiectasis (areas in which the small vessels are dilated) and the epidermal atrophy consequent on corticosteroid therapy allows the telangiectatic areas to show through the now transparent skin. This is very unsightly if it occurs on the face, a part of the body to which the corticosteroid preparation is likely, of course, to have been most assiduously applied. The face may also develop an acne like rash after some weeks' exposure to corticosteroids.

Apart from the rash, which never appears before puberty, the changes described in the preceding paragraphs are particularly likely to occur in children and adolescents in the body folds such as the groin and armpits (in these locations, two treated areas of skin are likely to be in opposition and the rubbing that occurs on movement, together with the sweat produced in these regions, encourages absorption), in patients in whom absorption has been encouraged by covering the treated part with an occlusive dressing and in areas of skin that are wet (such as a baby's buttocks that are in continued contact with saturated diapers) or exposed to sunlight (Sneddon, 1974).

There is the theoretical possibility that sufficient corticosteroid will be absorbed from the skin into the systemic circulation to reduce the production of endogenous hormone. In practice, this does not occur in adults but it is not unknown in children, particularly in cases of severe eczema where the raw surface facilitates drug absorption.

The incidence of these unfortunate sequelae of corticosteroid therapy can be minimised by restricting the prolonged use of the more powerful drugs to the most serious skin conditions, by keeping a careful watch for evidence of incipient skin atrophy and, best of all perhaps, by using hydrocortisone instead of the more powerful compounds whenever this is practicable. Prolonged and repeated applications of hydrocortisone are only rarely attended by untoward consequences.

When corticosteroids are given systemically the usual precautions (p. 767) must be observed when the drugs are withdrawn.

Barrier creams are used to protect the skin from contact with substances likely to be injurious. Substances coming into prolonged contact with the skin may have a direct toxic action by virtue of their irritant or other properties, or they may give rise to allergic-sensitization reactions. The skin lesion so produced is a *dermatitis* (literally inflammation of the skin), a term used to refer to the large number of skin conditions that arise as a reaction to irritant substances or agencies. Almost every type of substance used in industry, and many of those found in the home, can produce dermatitis.

The skin is normally protected by its stratum corneum whose flexibility is maintained by the secretions of the sebaceous glands and even, to some extent, by the sweat. Many of the substances causing dermatitis remove the sebum and they may also act as keratolytics. The function of a barrier cream is to penetrate the stratum corneum and reinforce its protective action. Barrier creams are also

employed to protect the skin from the effects of discharges from drainage tubes, varicose ulcers, fistulae and colostomies and to assist in the treatment of excessive perspiration and salivation. They can be used to protect the skin against ultraviolet rays and in the prevention of diaper rash in infants.

Some barrier creams contain silicones which have water-repellent properties. They may also contain antibacterial agents and emollients. Before the introduction of silicones, a large number of pastes, creams and ointments were used as barrier preparations. A common constituent was the ubiquitous zinc oxide. Many of these preparations still find favour in the home.

SUBSTANCES AFFECTING SEBACEOUS AND SWEAT GLANDS

Selenium sulphide (which is contained in such preparations as Selsun) is a potent antiseborrhoeic. It is used in a 2.5 per cent concentration for the treatment of seborrhoeic dermatitis *(pityriasis circinata)*, an inflammatory condition affecting the hair follicles and sebaceous glands. Overactivity of the sebaceous glands promotes an oily scalp and skin which is a predisposing condition. Cadmium sulphide has similar properties. Both compounds are extremely toxic if taken internally or if they are absorbed from damaged skin. They affect the liver and kidney and need to be used with care.

Overactivity of the sweat glands can cause discomfort and embarrassment. Most of the preparations intended to reduce excessive sweating *(the deodorant anhydrotics)* contain zinc sulphate.

AGENTS THAT AFFECT SKIN PIGMENTATION

Melanin, the pigment in the skin, performs the valuable function of absorbing ultraviolet radiation and protecting the body against the otherwise harmful effects of exposure to sunlight. Some individuals lack pigment and they are consequently extremely sensitive to natural light; they may only be able to venture out of doors if the whole of their skin is completely covered. Others suffer from excessive skin pigmentation. This may take the form of the familiar and not unattractive freckles but it often appears as large patches which may be very disfiguring. Overpigmentation is a feature of Addison's disease (p. 757) and it may occur during pregnancy, but it most often arises from no detectable cause. Conditions in which skin pigmentation is deficient or excessive are described, respectively, as *vitiliginous* and *lentiginous*. Drugs are now available for treating each of these conditions.

A number of substances which themselves absorb light

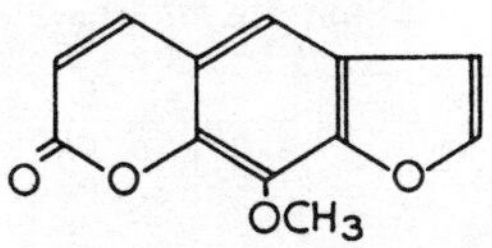

Methoxsalen

can be applied to vitiliginous skin. Hydroquinone and *p*-aminobenzoic acid have been used for this purpose. Methoxsalen, however, actually promotes the production of melanin. It is given in the form of a 1 per cent lotion no more than once a week. It is followed by a one-minute exposure to ultraviolet light which causes an inflammatory reaction, thickening of the stratum corneum and the deposition of melanin. The use of methoxsalen has to be very carefully supervised if violent skin reactions are to be avoided. It can cause liver damage and it is advisable not to administer methoxsalen orally, though it is effective by this route.

The formation of melanin is closely related to that of noradrenaline. An early stage in the biosynthesis of both is the conversion of tyrosine to dihydroxyphenylalanine (DOPA). Monobenzone, which is used in the production of rubber, has been shown to inhibit tyrosinase and hence the formation of DOPA and melanin. When applied to the skin several times a day in a 5 per cent lotion, monoben-

Monobenzone

zone reduces pigmentation. It is not toxic but care has to be exercised in its use, since over-enthusiastic application may simply result in the conversion of patches of pigmentation into equally unsightly patches of pallor.

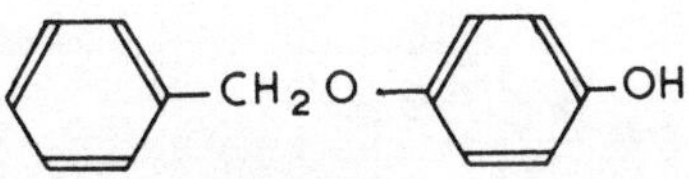

BIBLIOGRAPHY

Books

Andrews, G. C. and Domonkos, A. N. (1963). *Diseases of the Skin*, 5th ed. Philadelphia and London: Saunders.
Bruinsma, W. (1973). *A Guide to Drug Eruptions*. Amsterdam: Excerpta Medica.
Carruthers, C. (1962). *Biochemistry of the Skin in Health and Disease*. Springfield, Ill.: Thomas.
Hall-Smith, P., Cairns, R. J. and Beare R. L. B. (1973) *Dermatology*, 2nd edn. London: Crosby Lockwood Staples.
Levene, G. M. and Calnan, C. D. (1974) *A Colour Atlas of Dermatology*. London: Wolfe.
Marshall, J. (1960). *Diseases of the Skin*. Edinburgh: Livingstone.
Montagna, W. and Parakkal, P. F. (1974). *The Structure and Function of Skin*. New York: Academic Press.
Montagna, W., Van Scott, E. J. and Stoughton, R. B. (eds.), (1972). *Pharmacology and the Skin* (Advances in Biology of Skin, Vol. 12). New York: Appleton-Century-Croft.

Original papers

Fitzpatrick, T. B., Seijic, M. and McGugan, A. D. (1961). Melanin pigmentation. *New Engl. J. Med.*, **265**, 328-332, 374-378, 430-434.
Herxheimer, A. (1961). The action of drugs on the skin. *A. Rev. Pharmac.*, **1**, 351-368.
Sneddon, E. B. (1974). The dangers of the indiscriminate use of topical corticosteroids. *Prescriber's Journal*, **14**, 1-6.

PART IV

CHEMOTHERAPY

50. The chemotherapy of bacterial infections

Three quarters of the drugs prescribed today could not have been supplied forty years ago. This is the measure of the therapeutic revolution which has transformed medical treatment. Its most spectacular success has certainly been in the treatment of bacterial infections and many diseases which were a menace to life as recently as the early thirties have now been conquered.

Modern chemotherapy began with the work of Paul Ehrlich (1854–1915) who successfully used atoxyl in the treatment of sleeping sickness. He achieved an even more remarkable success in his search for a drug which would cure syphilis, then a major scourge of Europe. He synthesized a large number of organic arsenicals all of which proved to be useless until he reached number 606 in his

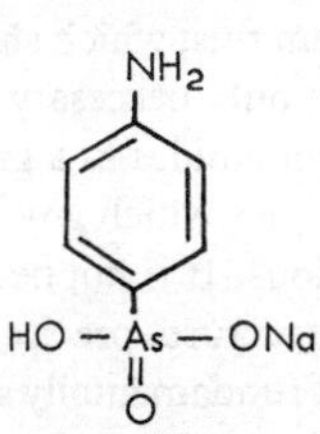

Atoxyl

series. This compound (Salvarsan) was found to be capable of curing syphilis and relapsing fever.

Sleeping sickness is caused by trypanosome infection, while syphilis and relapsing fever are caused by spirochaetes. These are relatively large organisms and the arsenicals were of no value in the treatment of diseases attributable to bacteria proper. The sulphonamides (introduced in the mid nineteen thirties) were the first successful antibacterial drugs and because they were active against a large range of pathogenic bacteria their impact on medicine was much greater than that of the arsenicals had been. The sulphonamides have now to a large extent been superseded by the antibiotics, a group of substances whose arrival on the medical scene caused almost as great a stir as had the appearance of the sulphonamides a few years earlier, not least because they became available at a time when sulphonamide resistant organisms were beginning to appear. The viruses, the smallest of all pathogenic organisms, have proved to be the most resistant to attack by chemical agents, but some progress has been made towards the development of successful antiviral drugs. These are discussed in Chap. 51 (p. 856).

THE SULPHONAMIDES

Sulphanilamide was synthesized in Germany as a dye-stuffs intermediate in 1908 and it was later incorporated into the molecules of a number of azo dyes including sulphonamido-chrysoidine (Prontosil Red). Nearly thirty years after sulphanilamide was first synthesized, Domagk (1935) was studying the phagocytosis of streptococci by the Kupffer cells of the liver. He wished to find a substance with which he could treat the streptococci in order to reduce their pathogenic effect when they were injected into his experimental mice. He already knew, from the work of Ehrlich and others, that certain dyestuffs were selectively absorbed by bacteria and it is perhaps not

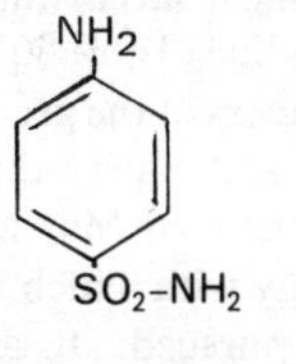

Sulphanilamide

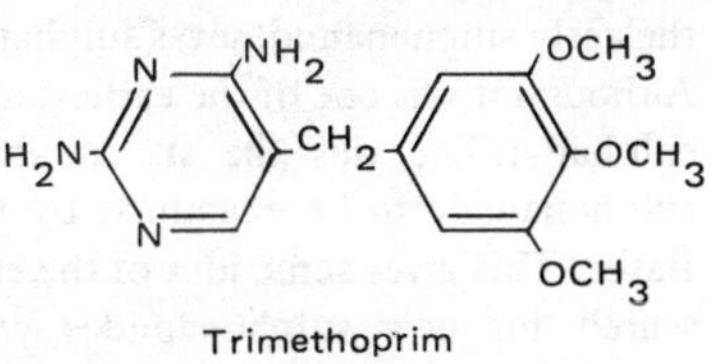

Trimethoprim

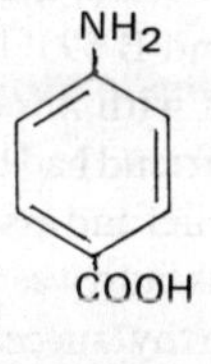

Aminobenzoic acid

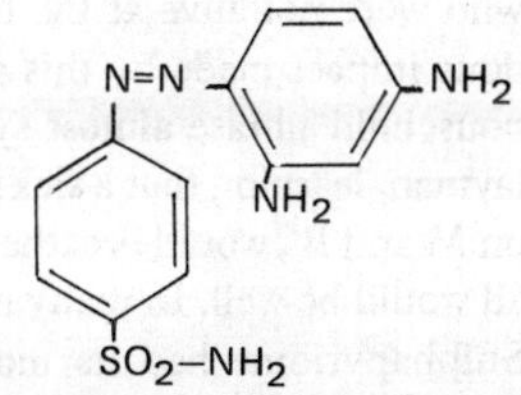

Prontosil Red

surprising that he included Prontosil among the compounds he tested. His choice was most fortunate, for his animals survived the injection of streptococci treated with the dye so well that Domagk decided to see whether Prontosil was capable of curing established streptococcal infections in mice. It was. Mice infected with a large dose of haemolytic streptococci died unless they were also given Prontosil. The first clinical trial of the drug was surely the most dramatic in medical history. Domagk's own daughter was at the brink of death from streptococcal septicaemia contracted as a result of a trivial accident—the puncturing of her hand with a knitting needle. Knowing only that Prontosil was effective against experimentally induced streptococcal infections in mice, Domagk gave some to his daughter. She recovered and bacterial chemotherapy was with us. In the next few years Prontosil was successfully used in the treatment of puerperal sepsis, a disease which until then had been responsible for the deaths of large numbers of women after childbirth. It was equally effective against other types of streptococcal infection. The story of these early clinical experiences may serve to illustrate not only the effectiveness of the new chemotherapeutic agent but also the extent of the threat to life presented, until then, by bacterial infections which could strike so swiftly and without warning.

It was soon realized that Prontosil was inactive *in vitro*. By 1937, Tréfouch and his colleagues in France and Fuller in England had shown that it was broken down in the body to release its contained sulphanilamide and that the latter substance was the active antibacterial agent. Sulphanilamide was found to have an activity similar to that of Prontosil. In addition, it proved to be effective in the treatment of gonorrhoea and meningococcal meningitis. The recognition that antibacterial activity resided in the simpler substance led to the replacement of Prontosil by sulphanilamide and to the development of a very large number of related compounds which are known collectively as the *sulphonamides*. One of the most successful of the early sulphonamides was sulphapyridine (Table 50.1). Although it was one of the earliest members of the group, sulphapyridine was the six hundred and ninety-third sulphonamide to be examined by the firm of May and Baker. This gives some idea of the energy with which the search for new sulphonamides was pursued. It also explains the name—M and B 693—by which sulphapyridine was universally known. It is very difficult for those who were not alive at the time to appreciate the tremendous impact made by this drug. 'M and B 693' became a household phrase almost synonymous with miracle. The layman, learning that a sick relative or friend had been 'put on M and B', would breathe a sigh of relief and assume that all would be well. In many instances his faith was justified. Sulphapyridine had its most noteworthy success in the treatment of pneumococcal pneumonia.

Sulphonamides continued to be produced at an ever-increasing rate and sulphapyridine was soon replaced by sulphathiazole, sulphadiazine, sulphamethazine and sulphamerazine (Table 50.1), all of which were more potent and less toxic than sulphapyridine.

It has been estimated that no fewer than 5000 different sulphonamides have been synthesized. About one hundred of these have found their way into clinical practice. Although most of them were developed before the advent of the antibiotics, some (particularly the longer-acting sulphonamides) are of more recent origin. Toxic reactions to the longer-acting drugs are, however, not uncommon and, to the extent that sulphonamides are used at all, there has been some tendency to revert to the use of the compounds with a less prolonged action. Table 50.1

provides the names and formulae of the only sulphonamides that need to be considered for their historical, pharmacological or current therapeutic interest. The oral doses and the principal characteristics of those which still have some use in therapeutics are also mentioned in the table.

Individual sulphonamides show no selectivity in their antibacterial actions. In other words, if a member of the group is active against a particular bacterial species, it can be assumed that it will be equally active against all other sulphonamide-susceptible organisms. Sulphonamides do, however, differ from one another in solubility, in the extent to which they are bound to protein and converted into acetylated derivatives and in their rates of absorption and excretion. As will be seen later, these factors influence the distribution of individual drugs among the blood, tissues, cerebrospinal fluid and urine and so help to determine the choice of sulphonamide for particular therapeutic purposes. Even when this has been said, however, it remains true that there is still a superfluity of useful sulphonamides, many of which differ from one another only in trivial detail. When an organism is resistant to one sulphonamide, it is resistant to them all and the multiplicity of these agents cannot be justified on the grounds that if one fails to achieve the desired therapeutic end another can be tried. The lesson from this, which should not be lost on the reader, is that it is only necessary to understand the properties of the sulphonamides as a group and to appreciate the general principles which govern their choice for specific clinical conditions. It is not necessary to learn the minutiae of chemical structure, precise solubilities and so on of a large number of fundamentally similar compounds and Table 50.1 should be used for reference purposes only.

The sulphonamides shown in Table 50.1 have been derived from sulphanilamide by substitution in the amido ($-SO_2NH_2$) group. In a few instances substitution has also been made in the amino group ($-NH_2$). The presence of a free amino group is essential for antibacterial activity and compounds in which this group carries substituents are, like Prontosil, broken down in the body to produce substances bearing the amino group. Substitution in the amido group of sulphanilamide increases antibacterial activity; 5- and 6-membered heterocyclic groups are particularly useful substituents in this respect.

CO-TRIMOXAZOLE

Trimethoprim (p. 815) was originally brought into therapeutics as an antimalarial drug but it also has bacteriostatic properties with a spectrum of activity similar to that of the sulphonamides. Co-trimoxazole (Bactrim, Septrin, Septra) is a mixture of trimethoprim and sulphamethoxazole (Table 50.1) which can be used to advantage in almost all the conditions for which a sulphonamide alone might otherwise be prescribed. The two components of the mixture exert mutually synergistic antibacterial effects so that the drug is effective in relatively small and nontoxic

Table 50.1 Sulphonamides of historical or current medicinal interest

Core structure: benzene ring with NHR_1 (para) and SO_2NHR_2.

Approved name(s)	Proprietary name(s)	R_1	R_2	Dose of recommended drugs	Remarks
The early sulphonamides					
Sulphacetamide	Albucid Sulamyd	H	–COH	—	Still used in ophthalmology
Sulphadiazine Sulphapyrimidine	Adiazine Cremodiazine Microsulfon Pyrimal	H	pyrimidine ring	Up to 4 g daily	Slowly absorbed and excreted; relatively low degree of protein binding. Sometimes used in meningitis but liable to cause crystalluria
Sulphadimidine Sulphamezathine	Diazil	H	4,6-dimethylpyrimidine ring (CH_3)	Initial dose: 2-3 g. Then 1 g six hourly	Highly soluble. Low toxicity
Sulphapyridine	M & B 693	H	pyridine ring	—	Toxic: not now used except as sulpha-salazine
Sulphathiazole	Thiazamide; Cibazol; M & B 760	H	thiazole ring	—	Toxic; not recommended
LOW SOLUBILITY COMPOUNDS					
Sulphaguanidine		H	$-C(=NH)NH_2$	3-6 g six hourly	Now little used
Succinylsulphathiazole	Sulphasuxidine	$-CO(CH_2)_2-$ $-COOH$	thiazole ring	5-10 g daily	Used in intestinal disinfection
Phthalysulphathiazole	Sulphathalidine Thalazole	benzene–CO	thiazole ring	10-20 g daily	Used in intestinal disinfection
More recent sulphonamides					
SHORT ACTING COMPOUNDS					
Sulphafurazole Sulfisoxazole	Gantrisin	H	$H_3C-C=C-CH_3$ isoxazole ring ($-C-O-N$)	Initial dose: 3 g. Then 1.5 g six hourly	Rapidly excreted so useful for urinary infections. Low toxicity
Sulphamethizole	Sulfurine Thiosulfin Ultrasul Urolucosil	H	thiadiazole ring ($-CH_3$)	0.25-0.5 g every four to six hours	Rapidly excreted, largely (90%) in free form. Useful for urinary infections
Sulphasomidine	Aristamid Elkosin	H	2,6-dimethylpyrimidine ring (CH_3)	Initial dose: 3 g. Then 1.5 g six hourly	Useful general purpose drug. Low toxicity. Rapid excretion

Table 50.1 (contd)

Approved name(s)	Proprietary name(s)	R_1	R_2	Dose of recommended drugs	Remarks
INTERMEDIATE ACTING COMPOUNDS					
Sulphamethoxazole	Gantanol	H		Initial dose: 1-2 g. Then 0.5-1 g every twelve hours	
Sulphasomizole	Bidizole	H		Initial dose: 1-2 g. Then 0.5-1 g every twelve hours	Sodium salt gives a neutral solution; useful for parenteral administration.
LONG ACTING COMPOUNDS					
Sulphadimethoxine	Madribon	H		Initial dose: 1 g. Then 0.5 g every 24 hours.	High degree (95%) of protein binding. Excreted as highly soluble glucuronide. Effective against staphylococci. May cause nausea and vomiting
Sulphamethoxydiazine	Durenate	H		Initial dose: 1 g. Then 0.5 g every 24 hours	Low degree of acetylation; smaller degree of protein binding than with others in the group
Sulphamethoxy-pyridazine	Lederkyn Midicel	H		Initial dose: 1 g. Then 0.5 g every 24 hours	Drug reactions and headache rather frequent
Sulphaphenazole	Orisulf	H		Initial dose: 1 g. Then 0.5 g every 24 hours	
ULTRA-LONG ACTING COMPOUNDS					
Sulfametopyrazine Sulfalene	Kelfizine	H		Initial dose: 0.8 g. Then 0.2 g every 24 hr or 2 g once weekly	Has been used for single dose treatment of acute infection
Sulfadoxine Sulphormethoxine	Fanasil	H		Initial dose: 0.5 g. Then 0.1 g every 24 hr or 1 g once weekly	As for sulpha-metopyrazine
Sulphasalazine Salicylazo-sulfapyridine (USA)	Salazopyrin Azulfidine (USA)		(full formula)	0.5 g four times daily	Used in the treatment of ulcerative colitis

doses. Drug resistance to co-trimoxazole develop less rapidly than it does to the sulphonamides proper and some sulphonamide-resistant organisms still succumb to co-trimoxazole.

Sulphamethoxazole rather than any other sulphonamide was chosen to partner trimethoprim in the combined preparation because the two drugs have similar pharmacokinetic characteristics. Consequently, when both are taken together, they arrive simultaneously in the tissues where they maintain, until they leave, a constant and therapeutically optimum concentration ratio of the one to the other.

Tablets and capsules of co-trimoxazole for oral administration contain 80 mg of trimethoprim and 400 mg of sulphamethoxazole. The usual adult dose is two tablets every twelve hours. Infants and young children need no more than a quarter of this dose. Side effects (nausea, vomiting, skin rashes) are generally similar to those seen with other sulphonamides but an additional possible complication, attributable to the trimethoprim moiety of the mixture, is folic acid deficiency with its associated blood dyscrasia (p. 677). This possibility is taken up again in a later paragraph.

Co-trimoxazole is rapidly absorbed from the alimentary tract and its components attain their maximum plasma concentrations within four hours. They are excreted, largely unchanged, by both glomerular filtration and tubular secretion. They have plasma half-lives of the order of ten hours.

The indications for co-trimoxazole therapy and other aspects of its actions and properties are discussed in later paragraphs along with those of the sulphonamides.

Trimethoprim acts synergistically with the polymyxins (p. 844) just as it does with the sulphonamides. Some clinical investigators have used mixtures of trimethoprim, sulphamethoxazole and colistin to treat infections caused by highly resistant strains of Gram-negative organisms.

Although the sulphonamides are discussed at length in most text books of pharmacology (including this one), their days as useful therapeutic agents are numbered. Sulphonamide-resistant strains of previously susceptible organisms are emerging in greater numbers and many of the sulphonamides produce unwelcome, or even dangerously toxic, side effects. The antibiotics are more potent and less toxic. It is probably true to say, indeed, that the sulphonamides would already have disappeared as useful therapeutic agents had it not been for the introduction of the very antibiotics that are replacing them! This paradoxical state of affairs arises because the use of antibiotics to treat conditions which would otherwise have been treated exclusively by a sulphonamide has delayed the development of sulphonamide-resistant organisms. The introduction of co-trimoxazole has also somewhat prolonged the life of at least one sulphonamide.

Current indications for sulphonamide therapy are discussed later.

Mode of action of the sulphonamides

For the most part, sulphonamides are bacteriostatic substances: that is, they arrest the growth and reproduction of bacteria but do not kill established organisms. However, when high tissue concentrations of the drugs are maintained some true bactericidal activity can often be demonstrated.

Sulphonamides are active against a wide range of bacteria so that it is easier to list those against which they are *ineffective.* These include *Mycobacterium tuberculosis* and the typhoid and paratyphoid bacilli.

The most widely held theory concerning the mode of action of sulphonamides is that put forward in 1940 independently by Fildes and by Woods. Both these workers showed that the antibacterial action of sulphanilamide was inhibited by very low concentrations of p-aminobenzoic acid. Fildes and Wood suggested that p-aminobenzoic acid was required by bacteria for their growth and development and that sulphanilamide competed with p-aminobenzoic acid for occupancy of an essential enzyme site. The fact that the antibacterial action of sulphanilamide could be reversed by extremely small amounts of p-aminobenzoic acid indicated that the acid had much the greater affinity for the enzyme and it emphasized the necessity of maintaining a high concentration of drug in the tissue of patients receiving sulphonamide therapy. This was an important practical point and those who ignored it found that sulphonamide treatment not only failed to cure their patients but sometimes made the infection more virulent since the more active bacteria grew and reproduced at the expense of the more susceptible organisms.

The obvious structural similarity between p-aminobenzoic acid and the sulphonamides makes the Fildes-Wood hypothesis an inherently reasonable one and there is other evidence to support it; p-aminobenzoic acid is synthesized by bacteria, it is demonstrably a growth factor in some species and some organisms which have developed sulphonamide-resistance are characterized by having a higher content of p-aminobenzoic acid than have the sensitive strains.

Folic acid contains a p-aminobenzoic acid residue and we now know that sulphonamides prevent the synthesis of folic acid by preventing the incorporation of p-aminobenzoic acid. Mammalian cells also require folic acid. However, unlike bacterial cells, they possess transport mechanisms that enable them to absorb folic acid in the preformed state from dietary sources. They do not, therefore, need to synthesize the compound—indeed they are incapable of so doing, so that their growth is not affected by inhibitors of folic acid synthesis.

The enzyme that is competitively inhibited by the sulphonamides is tetrahydropteroic acid synthetase, which promotes the union of p-aminobenzoic acid with the pteridine compound.

In bacterial and animal cells alike, folic acid is reduced to

HOOC-CH$_2$-CH$_2$-CH(COOH)NH┼OC—⟨ ⟩—NH┼CH$_2$ [pteridine ring structure] OH

glutamic acid residue   *p*-amino benzoic   pteridine residue
                         acid residue

Pteroyl glutamic acid: folic acid

folinic (tetrahydrofolic) acid under the influence of folic acid (dihydrofolic acid) reductase. In this form, folate promotes the incorporation of thymidine into DNA. Trimethoprim inhibits folic acid reductase and so prevents the synthesis of DNA.

The synergistic action of sulphonamides and trimethoprim is the consequence of their acting on successive stages of the process by which folinic acid is produced. It is easy to see, too, why resistance to co-trimoxazole develope less rapidly than it does to either component of the drug. Spontaneous mutations lead to the emergence of organisms which are resistant to either the sulphonamides or to trimethoprim by virtue of a reduced susceptibility to inhibition of their tetrahydropteroic synthetase or folic acid reductase respectively. The likelihood that both enzymes will be modified in the same way in the same organism is, of course, very low.

Since the enzymatic conversion of folic acid to its reduced form is as essential a process in animals as it is in microorganisms, it might be thought that trimethoprim would be as toxic to infected cells as it is to their invaders. That it is not, is a reflection of the fact that the bacterial enzyme is much more susceptible to trimethoprim (by a factor of several thousands) than is the mammalian version. It should, nevertheless, be withheld from patients who exhibit disorders of folate metabolism or who are threatened with folate deficiency from other causes.

The mutual antagonism of sulphonamides and *p*-aminobenzoic acid forms the basis of the usual test for sulphonamide activity. Sensitive organisms are grown in the presence of known amounts of *p*-aminobenzoic acid and the concentration of sulphonamide required to bring about bacteriostasis is measured. The ratio of the concentrations of sulphonamide and *p*-aminobenzoic acid constitutes the *antibacterial index* for the particular organism and sulphonamide. It is of value for the comparison of the activities of different sulphonamides *in vitro*.

Other substances that antagonize the actions of the sulphonamides include methionine, certain purines and pyrimidines, peptone and unidentified material present in pus. The inhibitors in pus are sufficiently powerful to render sulphonamides inactive in its presence. It should also be noted that, unlike *p*-aminobenzoic acid, methionine inhibits sulphonamides non-competitively.

General pharmacology of the sulphonamides
Many sulphonamides are only sparingly soluble in water.

Their acetylated derivatives are even less soluble and since sulphonamides are, for the most part, excreted partly unchanged and partly as the acetylated compounds, the possibility of crystallization in the kidney tubules has always to be considered. Crystalluria gives rise to pain, haematuria and, in severe cases, a complete arrest of urine excretion. Solubility is increased in alkaline urine and if it is necessary to use a relatively insoluble sulphonamide a high fluid intake should be maintained and sodium bicarbonate and sodium citrate should be given to ensure that an adequate volume of alkaline urine is produced. Sulphasomidine, sulphafurazole and sulphamethizole are more soluble and although the acetyl derivative of sulphasomidine is of low solubility, little of the drug is excreted in this form. Renal complications are, therefore, unlikely to accompany the use of these compounds. The solubility of a sulphonamide is not materially reduced by the presence of other sulphonamides in the solution and in the days before the more soluble members of the group became available it was a fairly common practice to prescribe a mixture of three sulphonamides. One such triad (which is still available) contained sulphadiazine, sulphathiazole and sulphamerazine. It permitted the use of adequately bacteriostatic concentrations of total sulphonamide without the risk of crystalluria.

Sulphonamides are usually given by mouth as those intended for systemic use are generally well absorbed from the stomach and (particularly) the small intestine. Intravenous injection is difficult because of the drugs' generally low solubility. The sodium salts of some sulphonamides are quite soluble and can be given intravenously, but apart from sodium sulphasomizole and sodium sulphadimidine they give alkaline solutions which are not suitable for intramuscular administration. Sulphonamides attain peak concentrations in the plasma (50–100 μg per ml) some three hours after ingestion. The plasma half life of the more rapidly excreted members of the group is two to three hours.

Sulphaguanidine, succinylsulphathiazole and phthalylsulphathiazole are not absorbed from the intestine and they have been used for the treatment of bacterial infections of the intestine. Although sulphaguanidine (the first of the unabsorbable group to be discovered) was very successfully used to treat bacillary dysentery in troops stationed in the Middle and Far East during the Second World War, it is now clear that sulphonamides that are not absorbed at all are not entirely suitable for the treatment of intestinal infections since antibacterial action is required within the tissues of the gut. The unabsorbable sulphonamides are more useful in the prevention of infection.

After absorption, a variable amount of the sulphonamide is bound to plasma protein and to the erythrocytes. The amount bound ranges from about 10 per cent with sulphanilamide to 80 per cent or more with sulphadimidine and with many of the recently introduced long-acting compounds. Protein binding is a factor that determines the distribution of sulphonamides in the tissues. For example, protein bound sulphonamide cannot pass into the cerebrospinal fluid.

Substances that bind to plasma protein compete with one another for available binding sites and we have already seen (p. 71) that sulphonamides, by displacing bilirubin, have caused fatal kernicterus in premature infants who have received the drugs in a misguided attempt to protect them from infection during the dangerous days of the early neonatal period. In this connection it should also be noted that sulphonamides pass the placental barrier. They persist in the foetus for quite long periods (sometimes for several weeks) and they should clearly not be given to pregnant women if there is any possibility that an unexpectedly early birth might lead to a premature infant's being born with a sulphonamide in its blood.

Drugs such as phenylbutazone can, of course, displace sulphonamides from their union with plasma protein (p. 78) but this is not likely to constitute a serious hazard.

It has already been mentioned that most of the sulphonamides are partly excreted as acetyl derivatives. The amount acetylated varies among different members of the group. It is normally about 20 per cent but sulphadimidine is acetylated to the extent of about 50 per cent in blood and 70 per cent in the urine. Sulphonamide in the glomerular filtrate is partly reabsorbed in the tubules but the acetylated derivative is less readily absorbed than the free drug. For this reason, the proportion of the acetylated compound in the urine is always greater than that in blood. Acetylated sulphonamides are more toxic than the parent compounds. Sulphasomidine and sulphamethizole are acetylated to a smaller extent than other sulphonamides and this fact partly explains their generally low toxicity.

Acetylation occurs in the liver (the formula of an acetylated sulphonamide appears on p. 67) but some individuals effect a more complete transformation of administered drug than do others. This genetically determined difference in acetylating activity is also reflected in the way in which other drugs (notably izoniazid) are handled. This topic is further discussed in Chapter 6 (p. 73).

Active acetylators convert up to 90 per cent of an administered sylphonamide into the acetylated form but the rest of the population dispose of no more than half their dose in this way.

Not all of the drug administered is excreted in the unchanged or acetylated form. Some is oxidized and the oxidized product may itself be excreted as the glucuronide. Sulphadimethoxine is unusual in that 80 per cent of the drug is excreted as the glucuronide. Both the sulphonamide and its glucuronide are very soluble. Like the acetylated compounds, the oxidation products are more toxic than the parent substances.

A drug which is rapidly excreted will reach a high concentration in the urine while slow excretion will permit the prolonged maintenance of a high plasma concentration. The long-acting compounds listed in Table 50.1 are all slowly excreted partly because they all undergo a high degree of protein binding and partly because they are to some extent reabsorbed by the renal tubules.

Soon after the sulphonamides were brought into general use it was observed that some patients developed a metabolic acidosis. This was found to be caused by carbonic anhydrase inhibition and, as a direct result of this observation, sulphonamide-like compounds came to be used as diuretics, operating by inhibiting the carbonic anhydrase of the renal tubule cells. The enzyme is involved in the regulation of a number of physiological activities which are discussed in more detail, as are the diuretic actions of its inhibitors, in Chap. 36 (p. 631). In hens, carbonic anhydrase is involved in egg shell formation and when hens were given sulphanilamide they laid eggs with very thin, or no, shells. Only those sulphonamides which possess an unsubstituted sulphonamido group, or which can form one by hydrolysis *in vivo*, are capable of inhibiting carbonic anhydrase.

Toxic effects of the sulphonamides

The earliest sulphonamides, particularly sulphapyridine and sulphathiazole, were prone to cause toxic side reactions, some of them serious. The later ones were less toxic and it was hoped that the most recently introduced drugs would be free of all toxic actions. This hope has not been realized, for although some of them do not produce the same type of toxic side effects as the earlier sulphonamides, they are particularly likely to cause sensitization reactions, headaches and general malaise.

The toxic effects which may arise during sulphonamide therapy can be enumerated as follows:

(i) Crystalluria and renal complications resulting therefrom. This aspect of sulphonamide toxicity has already been discussed. It can be avoided by choosing a soluble sulphonamide. If a compound likely to cause crystalluria (such as sulphadiazine) has to be used, a high urinary volume should be maintained and the urine should be kept alkaline.

(ii) Cyanosis. This complication, which was common when sulphapyridine was in use, is now rare. It reflected the formation of methaemoglobin and sulphaemoglobin.

(iii) Nausea, vomiting and other gastrointestinal upsets. These toxic reactions are unfortunately as likely to occur with the newer sulphonamides as with the older established members of the group. Sulphadimethoxine and sulphamethoxydiazine are frequent offenders in this respect.

(iv) Agranulocytosis and anaemia. Agranulocytosis is the most serious complication of sulphonamide therapy. Though rare, it carries a high mortality rate. An acute haemolytic anaemia sometimes appears in the course of sulphonamide therapy. It is often associated with a deficiency of glucose-6-phosphate dehydrogenase in the erythrocytes and so is more likely to occur in Negroes than in members of white-skinned races (p. 74). Blood dyscrasias can occur in the course of treatment with any of the sulphonamides but most of the recorded cases have appeared after long-term treatment which is less often resorted to at the present time.

(v) Headache, dizziness, mental depression and other signs of central nervous system involvement.

(vi) Sensitivity reactions. Fever and a rash (which may be of an urticarial variety) may occur after some days of treatment with sulphonamides or at the very beginning of a second or later course of treatment. These reactions are of an allergic nature, the allergen presumably being the sulphonamide-plasma protein complex. Allergic reactions can occur to any sulphonamide by whatever route it is given: they arose so frequently after the application of sulphonamides to the skin that this mode of administration is no longer employed.

(vii) Pulmonary fibrosis and fibrosing alveolitis are sometimes seen in patients who are taking sulphasalazine, the sulphonamide without antibacterial activity (p. 823). The occurrence of these complications demands the immediate withdrawal of the drug.

(viii) Hepatitis is a rare but potentially dangerous complication of sulphonamide therapy.

Resistance to sulphonamides

Bacteria are prone to acquire resistance to the sulphonamides particularly in individuals who have been treated with inadequate doses of the drugs or in those who have received prolonged treatment. As has already been mentioned, the development of resistance is associated in some bacterial species with an increased ability to produce *p*-aminobenzoic acid. Some organisms, however, seem to acquire resistance even when their ability to synthesize *p*-aminobenzoic acid is not stimulated. In these instances, it has to be assumed that the resistant bacteria are using metabolic pathways that by-pass those involving *p*-aminobenzoic acid. It may be that the resistant strains convert the sulphonamide into a utilizable metabolite. The general topic of bacterial resistance is taken up again later (p. 851).

Therapeutic uses of the sulphonamides and cotrimoxazole

Between 1936 and 1944, the sulphonamides were the only drugs capable of curing bacterial diseases. The enthusiasm with which they were prescribed is understandable but the lack of discrimination and the ignorance of the basic facts of sulphonamide action which accompanied this enthusiasm are less excusable. Inevitably, drug resistant microorganisms were quick to make their appearance. The antibiotics appeared just in time to save the situation but they, too, were prescribed with more enthusiasm than discretion. When, in its turn, penicillin resistance arose, there was some move back towards the sulphonamides which enjoyed, for a time, a new burst of popularity. This is now declining and the sulphonamides now occupy a very lowly position in the list of favoured antibacterial agents.

The following are the principal contemporary indications for sulphonamide therapy:

(i) *Urinary tract infections.* Infections by *Escherichia coli* and *Proteus mirabilis* usually respond to sulphonamides which are at least as effective as antibiotics. Sulphonamide resistance does, however, occur in both these species and some other organisms which are commonly responsible for urinary tract infections (*Streptococcus faecalis* and *Klebsiella aerogenęs*) are only sensitive to antibiotics. Care has therefore to be taken in selecting cases for treatment with sulphonamides. Some of those encountered in domiciliary practice will respond to sulphonamides alone but cotrimoxazole is likely to be more useful in hospital patients.

If infection is restricted to the renal tubules, a high urinary concentration of drug is required and for this purpose a rapidly excreted sulphonamide which undergoes little acetylation is indicated. Sulphafurazole, sulphasomidine and sulphamethizole meet these requirements and they have all been successfully used in the treatment of urinary tract infections. On the other hand, if the substance of the kidney is also infected, a high concentration of sulphonamide must be attained in all the renal cells. As has already been pointed out, a high tissue concentration is incompatible with rapid excretion and if the kidney parenchyma is affected a slowly excreted sulphonamide must be used. Drugs in the 'long-acting' group are useful for this purpose.

Uncomplicated urinary tract infections by sensitive organisms constitute (apart from the rather exceptional case of the sulphasalazine treatment of ulcerative colitis) the only conditions for which sulphonamides can now be regarded as the drugs of first choice.

(ii) Some infections caused by *Haemophilus influenzae* (otitis media, pharyngitis, etc.) respond well to combined sulphonamide and antibiotic (erythromycin) therapy. Cotrimoxazole is a preferable alternative to the antibiotic-sulphonamide mixture but ampicillin (p. 829) provides the best treatment of all.

(iii) *Intestinal disinfection.* It was mentioned earlier that those sulphonamides which cannot be absorbed from the intestine can be used to prevent intestinal infection. They are also sometimes used for sterilizing the large intestine before operations on this organ. Antibiotics such as neomycin may be needed in addition if complete sterilization is to be achieved.

(iv) *Meningococcal meningitis.* The sulphonamides can no longer be regarded as first choice drugs for the treatment of meningococcal meningitis but they retain some utility when infection is caused by sensitive organisms. The two best sulphonamides for this purpose are sulphadiazine and sulphadimidine. The latter has the advantage of low toxicity and high solubility. On the other hand, it is easier to maintain high blood and cerebrospinal fluid concentrations with sulphadiazine. Co-trimoxazole is as useful as the sulphonamides in meningococcal meningitis.

(v) *Eye infections.* Although sulphonamides should not be applied to the skin, lest they provoke hypersensitivity reactions, this prohibition does not extend to the eye and solutions of sodium sulphacetamide are still sometimes employed for the treatment of conjunctivitis. It is permissible to instil solutions as concentrated as 30 per cent for this purpose. Sulphasomidine has occasionally been used instead of sulphacetamide.

(vi) *Ulcerative colitis.* Sulphasalazine has a role in the treatment of ulcerative colitis, a condition of chronic ulceration of the colonic mucosa. In the course of the disease there are attacks of acute diarrhoea, with blood and large quantities of mucus appearing in the stools. Sulphasalazine does not always relieve these acute attacks but it does much to reduce their incidence.

Sulphasalazine is broken down by bacterial action in the large intestine to yield sulphapyridine and 5-aminosalicylic acid. For many years, it was generally believed that the undoubtedly beneficial effect of sulphasalazine was attributable to its sulphapyridine component operating otherwise than as an antibacterial drug. Very recently, however, evidence has appeared to support the view that 5-aminosalicylic acid is the active moiety (Azad Khan, Piris and Truelove, 1977). If this proves to be so it should be possible to devise an even more satisfactory medicament by combining 5-aminosalicylic acid with a less toxic carrier than sulphapyridine. The active substance cannot be taken on its own (except presumably by the rectal route) as it would suffer almost complete absorption in the small intestine.

The therapeutic dose of sulphasalazine is 500 mg taken four times daily by mouth or (in suitable cases) by rectum.

(vii) *Other conditions.* A number of conditions can be satisfactorily treated by co-trimoxazole but not by sulphonamides alone. These include infections of the prostate, typhoid and paratyphoid fevers, salmonellosis, gonorrhoea, toxoplasmosis, brucellosis and nocardiosis. In none of these conditions, apart from the first mentioned, is co-trimoxazole to be regarded as a first choice drug.

In appropriate cases, sulphonamides have some advantages over the antibiotics. They are cheap, simple to administer and their use is not attended by the danger of candidiasis (p. 907) which sometimes complicates prolonged treatment with antibiotics.

THE PENICILLINS

The observation that led to the next phase of the therapeutic revolution is probably as well known to the layman as that which inspired Newton to formulate the theory of gravity. Both provide classical illustrations of the momentum that can be imparted to scientific progress on the rare occasions when a chance event happens to be noticed by an individual possessed of sufficient serendipity to appreciate its significance.

In 1928 Alexander Fleming found that a plate culture of staphylococci in his laboratory had become contaminated with spores of the common green mould, *Penicillium notatum.* He noted that the bacterial colonies in the immediate neighbourhood of the spores were showing signs of lysis. The significance of this observation, with the hint that the mould was producing a material toxic to pathogenic bacteria, was not lost on Fleming who later attempted to use filtrates of the medium in which the mould had grown to promote the healing of infected wounds. Penicillin, as the active material had become called, did not, however, come into its own until after 1940 when Florey and Chain and their colleagues isolated it and described its properties in detail.

Florey's work came at a most propitious time: it indicated that penicillin was potent, non-toxic and active in the presence of pus in which environment the sulphonamides are ineffective. Europe was embroiled in war and penicillin seemed to offer just what would be needed in field hospitals. At first penicillin was so rare that, after administration to patients, it had to be recovered from their urine so that it could be used again.

These early experiences were extremely encouraging and the large-scale production of penicillin began when it became obvious that it was going to fulfil all the hopes that its discovery had raised.

Thus, within a few years of the appearance of 'M and B', another miracle drug had entered the scene. It was the first of the antibiotics and, although it was followed by many more during the next quarter of a century, it is still in many ways the best. 'Some of its properties are unique and it is nothing short of a miracle that so astonishing a substance should have been the first of its kind to be discovered' (Garrod, Lambert and O'Grady, 1973). The extraordinary value of the penicillins is illustrated by the fact that several of the newer antibiotics, introduced into clinical practice because they were active against strains of organisms resistant to penicillin, have themselves been supplanted by new penicillins which have a wider range of usefulness than the original members of the group.

The word antibiotic is, perhaps, unfortunate. Etymologically it suggests merely something that kills living organisms although 'antibiosis' was originally coined (in 1889) to describe the condition of one creature's being in absolute opposition to life of another. Some modern antibiotics are not derived from living organisms.

As we have seen, *Penicillium notatum* provided the source of the first penicillin but it was soon replaced by *P. chrysogenum*. The antibiotic as it was first produced proved to be a mixture of four closely related substances (Table 50.2) which were designated F, G, X and K by American investigators or I, II, III and IV respectively in the original English nomenclature. It was later found that individual penicillins could be produced, to the virtual exclusion of the others, by suitably modifying the culture medium. Penicillin G (benzylpenicillin) is the most satisfactory of the four compounds and for many years it has been the only component of the original mixture to be manufactured in quantity. It is obtained by growing *P. chrysogenum* in a medium to which phenylacetic acid has been added. Nearly forty years after its introduction into clinical medicine, benzylpenicillin is still widely used although it has had to yield to ampicillin the distinction of being the most popular of all antibiotics. Ampicillin is one of the large number of semisynthetic penicillins the nature and properties of which are described later.

All the penicillins are dipeptides and they are all derivatives of ß-lactam thiazolidine, a structure which was first discovered in the penicillins.

The properties of benzylpenicillin will be described in detail. Mention will then be made of the other penicillins currently available for clinical use and of the ways in which they differ from benzylpenicillin. Finally, the therapeutic uses of the group as a whole will be considered. When reference is made to 'penicillin' without naming the actual compound, it can be assumed that the remarks apply to all members of the penicillin group of antibiotics.

Benzylpenicillin

Benzylpenicillin (penicillin G) is an unstable acid but its sodium or potassium salt ('soluble' or 'crystalline' penicillin) is stable when dry. It is readily soluble in water but the solution is unstable, its activity being slowly lost even at 4°C. Deterioration occurs much more rapidly at higher temperatures.

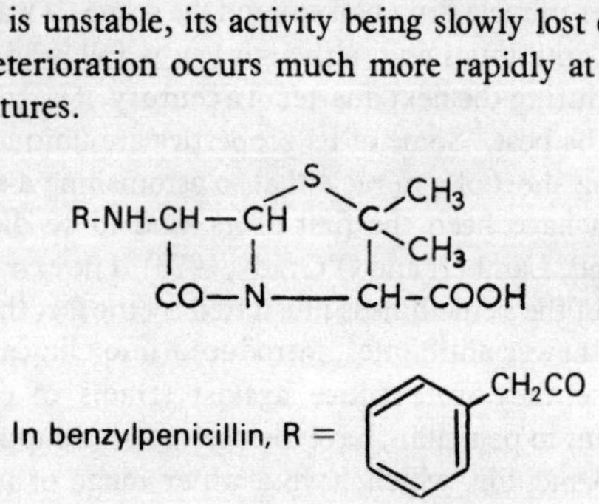

R-NH-CH—S—C—CH₃ ... CO—N—CH-COOH

In benzylpenicillin, R =   CH₂CO

Fig. 50.1 General formula of the penicillins

Antimicrobial activity. Because of its almost complete lack of toxicity in patients who show no hypersensitivity to it (see below), penicillin can usually be given, if necessary, in very large doses. Consequently, it can be employed for the treatment of infections caused by organisms that exhibit widely differing sensitivities to the drug. It is active against sensitive strains of almost all the Gram-positive organisms. Gram-negative cocci also succumb to penicillin but Gram-negative bacilli are not affected. Sensitive bacteria include the streptococci, staphylococci, gonococci, pneumococci, meningococci, the spirochaetes, the actinomyces and the large viruses. In clinical terms this means that the range of conditions likely to respond to penicillin therapy includes wound sepsis, cellulitis, puerperal sepsis, bacterial endocarditis, meningococcal meningitis, pneumonia, syphilis, gonorrhoea and some infections of the skin, the eye and the throat. Penicillin can also be used to provide an antibiotic umbrella to prevent the accumulation of microorganisms in the blood (*bacteraemia*) following the removal of infected teeth or tonsils from patients with valvular heart disease. Harmless in most people, a bacteraemia might lead to a fatal endocarditis in these patients.

Some strains of some of the bacterial species listed as penicillin sensitive are resistant to the drug and their numbers have increased with the years. This is particularly true of *Staphylococcus aureus*. In the early days of antibiotic chemotherapy, infections by this microorganism almost invariably responded to penicillin. Today, almost all the strains found in hospital, and at least twenty per cent of those encountered outside, are resistant to penicillin. Many resistant strains of gonococcus have also appeared.

General properties. Benzylpenicillin is active when taken by mouth but no more than one-third of the amount ingested reaches the blood stream and absorption is still further reduced if food is present in the stomach or duodenum. The unabsorbed penicillin is excreted in the faeces. Benzylpenicillin is unstable in acid and some destruction takes place in the stomach.

Benzylpenicillin is absorbed largely from the duodenum. It is excreted by secretion into the renal tubules. Consequently it is very rapidly eliminated from the body and large and frequently-repeated doses have to be given if an effective concentration of the antibiotic is to be maintained in the blood and tissues. Intramuscular injection provides the most useful mode of administration.

Some penicillin is broken down in the body but at least sixty per cent of a parenterally administered dose appears in the urine in an unchanged form.

Enzymatic inactivation. An enzyme, penicillinase, splits penicillin to give penicilloic acid (Fig. 50.2). The ability to produce penicillinase is one of the reasons why an organism may not be sensitive to penicillin—the tubercle bacillus and resistant strains of *Staph. aureus,* for example, are penicillinase producers. Mixed infection by a number of

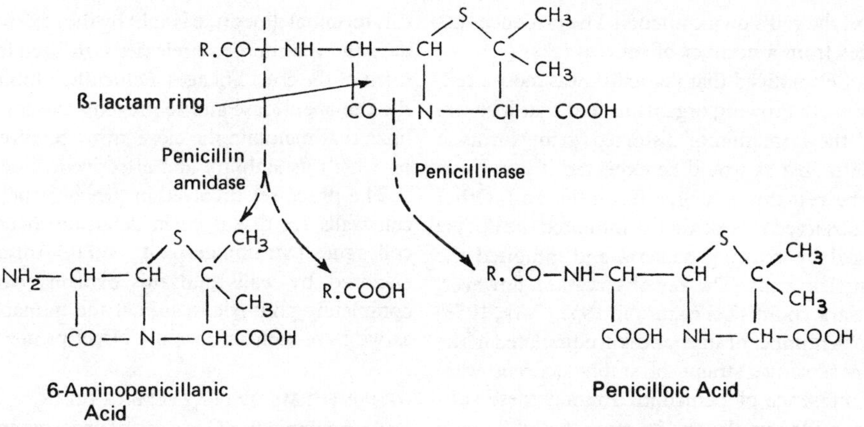

Fig. 50.2 Cleavage of penicillin by penicillinase and by penicillin amidase

bacterial species, only one of which produces penicillinase, may be completely resistant to penicillin because the enzyme released by the one species protects all the others.

Penicillin amidase (which is also produced by some microorganisms) splits penicillin to give 6-aminopenicillanic acid (Fig. 50.2).

Hypersensitivity reactions to penicillin. Early investigators were struck by penicillin's apparently complete lack of toxicity even when high doses had been given. Later experience has revealed that a few individuals react very violently indeed to penicillin, even when it is given by mouth. The reaction is an anaphylactic one with urticaria, laryngeal oedema and a precipitous fall in blood pressure. It demands emergency treatment of the kind that is detailed elsewhere (p. 409) but this does not always prevent a fatal outcome. Indeed, it is said that penicillin now claims more victims than do sera. The total number of fatalities—it is probably of the order of 1 in 50 000 of those who receive penicillin—is, of course, tiny in comparison with the vast number of lives which have been saved by the drug.

Milder forms of allergic response are seen. Sometimes they are benign versions of the fatal type of anaphylactic collapse and they can occur at any time from half an hour to two days after penicillin administration. Skin rashes, whose appearance may be even more delayed, are other manifestations of penicillin sensitivity.

It has been variously estimated that between 5 and 10 per cent of those who are given penicillin exhibit an allergic sensitivity to the drug.

Penicillin reactions can occur even in those who are apparently being exposed to the drug for the first time. In these instances, it has to be assumed that the patient has become sensitized as a result of a previous contact of which he was unaware. He may, for instance, have drunk milk from an animal that had itself received penicillin.

Those who, in any capacity, handle penicillin also run the risk of becoming sensitized to it.

The offending substance in cases of hypersensitivity to penicillin is sometimes penicillin itself and sometimes a breakdown product linked, in both instances of course, to an appropriate protein (p. 396).

It is not easy to predict that a particular patient will exhibit sensitivity to penicillin. Skin testing has been recommended but some authorities claim that this method does not adequately identify hypersensitive individuals. Moreover, a few instances are known of patients in whom the skin testing procedure has itself precipitated a fatal anaphylaxis. Before prescribing penicillin the physician should enquire whether his patient has ever had a serious allergic condition such as asthma or whether he has ever suffered an untoward reaction to drugs, injections or foodstuffs. He should enquire of those patients known to have handled the drug in the past whether they ever experienced skin rashes that could be attributed to penicillin. If he suspects that a reaction to penicillin may occur, the physician should, of course, prescribe an antibiotic less likely to provoke an anaphylactic response.

Notwithstanding their serious nature, anaphylactic responses represent an idiosyncratic reaction attributable more to the patient than to the drug. The vast majority of people do not exhibit hypersensitivity reactions and for them penicillin is completely harmless. It has been said that, hypersensitivity reactions apart, no dose of penicillin, however large, will harm anyone whose kidneys are functioning normally. This is not entirely true since a few reports have appeared of neurotoxic and nephrotoxic effects among patients who have received large doses of penicillin over a long period of time.

The mode of action of penicillin. High osmotic pressures develop in bacterial cells. The ingress of water, with consequent lysis, is prevented by the cell wall, a substantial structure which forms up to one-fifth of the dry weight of the cell. Penicillin interferes with the formation of the cell wall of the developing microorganism and thus exposes it to the lytic action of any solution whose osmotic pressure is less than that of the cell's own contents. The evidence that this is so comes from a number of sources.

Fleming himself noticed that penicillin was most effective against actively growing organisms and that it sometimes induced the formation of distorted 'giant' forms of sensitive bacteria just as would be expected if water was passing into the cell through breaches in its wall. Other early workers observed that penicillin inhibited the uptake of glutamic acid by growing bacteria and inhibited the synthesis of nucleic acids. The key observation, however, was made by Park and his colleagues in 1957 (Park, 1958) who found that a number of substances accumulated in the medium when sensitive strains of staphylococcus were grown in the presence of penicillin. Among these substances was a peptide complex and its components— L-and D-alanine, D-glutamic acid, L-lysine, uridine-5'-pyrosphosphate and N-acetylmuramic acid which was already known to be an integral part of the cell wall structure. The unique importance of muramic acid in the cell wall is indicated by its very name. Later, direct confirmation was obtained that penicillin inhibits the synthesis of the cell wall (so that precursors accumulate in the medium) without affecting protein synthesis in the bacterial cell itself (Rogers and Jeljaszewickz, 1961). Defects in the cell wall may nevertheless impair bacterial protein synthesis in an indirect way by deranging the processes that normally ensure the balanced transport of amino acids across the wall.

The bacterial cell wall consists essentially of elongated strands of carbohydrate that carry tetrapeptide side chains that are themselves linked by chains of five glycine residues. These glycine pentapeptides connect adjacent side chains on the same carbohydrate strand as well as forming cross linkages with neighbouring strands. This arrangement (which is illustrated schematically in Fig. 50.3) bestows stability, rigidity and water impermeability on the cell wall. It will be appreciated that this arrangement of side chains and linking peptides is such that it can lead to the production of very large molecules. In most Gram-positive organisms, indeed, the entire wall is composed of a single *mucopeptide* molecule of this kind. In Gram-negative bacteria the wall is thicker and is composed of alternating layers of mucopeptide and lipoprotein.

The carbohydrate skeleton of the mucopeptide molecule appears as the result of the union (by way of their hydroxyl groups) of alternating molecules of N-acetylglucosamine and N-acetylmuramic acid (Fig. 50.3). The tetrapeptide side chains usually take the form L-alanine-D-glutamic acid-L-lysine-D-alanine and they are attached to the -O.CH(CH₃)COOH (lactate) side chain of N-acetylmuramic acid. The glycine pentapeptide links connect the terminal D-alanine of one side chain with the L-lysine of another.

The tetrapeptide side chain begins life as a pentapeptide with a pair of D-alanine residues instead of the single one found in the finished product. During the building process

this terminal dipeptide is split by the action of a transpeptidase and the energy so released is utilized for the establishment of the cross linkages. Penicillin inhibits the activity of the transpeptidase and so prevents the construction of the links that maintain the close knit structure of the cell wall on which its stability and effectiveness depends.

The processes involved in the construction of bacterial cell walls are discussed in detail by Strominger and his colleagues (Strominger et al. 1971). Animal cells are not enclosed by walls and this explains why penicillin is completely nontoxic to animal and human subjects since, as we have seen, it does not affect protein synthesis.

OTHER FORMS OF BENZYLPENICILLIN

Procaine penicillin G is a salt of procaine and benzylpenicillin, which is sparingly soluble in water. It is usually presented as a suspension in oil, with aluminium monostearate added as a water repellent. It has a number of proprietary names—Avloprocin, Crysticillin, Lenticillin, Pro-Stabillin and PAM—and it can be injected together with penicillin itself. In this way the high blood level can be achieved rapidly and maintained without the necessity of frequent injections. A dose of 300 000 units given twice daily by intramuscular injection is sufficient to ensure this. Other salts which have a low solubility and hence a delayed and prolonged action are benzathine penicillin (Bicillin, Dibencil, Neolin, Penidural, Permapen) and benethamide penicillin.

Other penicillins

The names, formulae and principal characteristics of a number of other penicillins are set out in Table 50.2. Some general points concerning their production, properties and uses follow.

Phenoxymethylpenicillin (Penicillin V) is a natural penicillin in the sense that it is produced by adding a suitable side-chain precursor (phenoxyacetic acid) to the *Penicillium* culture medium. The other penicillins are described as 'synthetic'. They are obtained by adding the appropriate side chain, by purely chemical means, to 6-aminopenicillanic acid. The acid can be synthesized chemically but this method is not adopted on the commercial scale. Instead, *P. chrysogenum* is cultivated in a medium which lacks side-chain precursor. Alternatively, penicillin amidase, obtained from growing bacteria, is used to produce 6-aminopenicillanic acid from penicillin (Fig. 50.2). Since both these methods of production are essentially biological in nature, the description 'synthetic' for the newer penicillins is something of a misnomer.

The penicillins listed in Table 50.2 differ from benzylpenicillin in one or more of four ways—acid sensitivity, susceptibility to inactivation by penicillinase, antibiotic potency and spectrum of antibacterial activity.

The acid stable penicillins are not destroyed by gastric acid and they can therefore be taken by mouth. As a matter

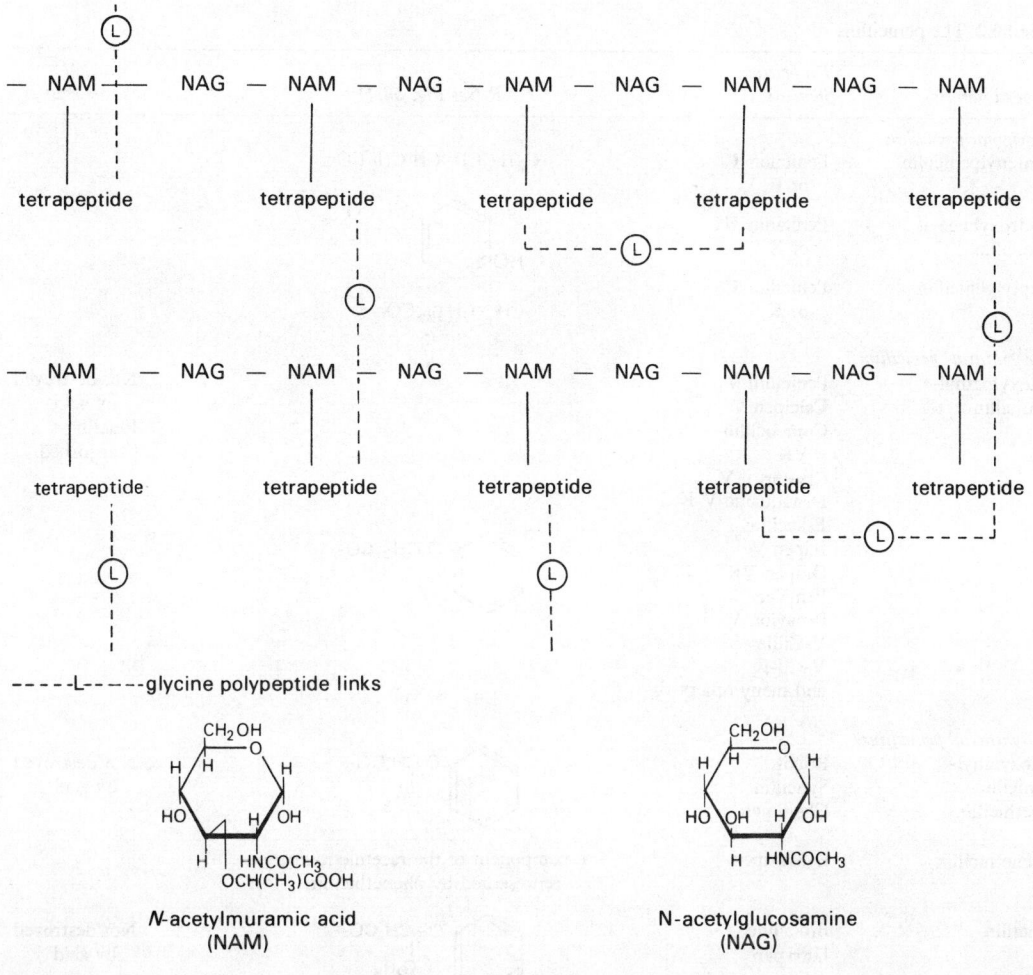

---- L ----glycine polypeptide links

N-acetylmuramic acid
(NAM)

N-acetylglucosamine
(NAG)

NAM and NAG molecules are joined by oxygen links resulting from the union of OH groups and the elimination of water, thus:

Fig. 50.3 Schematic representation of the structure of the bacterial cell wall

of fact, only small amounts of these penicillins appear in the blood stream after oral administration but their absorption is more regular than that of benzylpenicillin. Phenoxymethylpenicillin is the most readily absorbed of the acid stable penicillins although it is also the least active. The potassium (and sodium) salts are more easily absorbed than the free acids: the reader will note that several of the proprietary preparations of phenoxymethylpenicillin include the designation 'K' in their trade names (Table 50.2). The acid resistant penicillins are less active agents, weight for weight, then benzylpenicillin.

The penicillinase resistant penicillins are not inactivated by the enzyme produced by *Staph. aureus* and they are

therefore employed to treat infections caused by resistant strains of this organism. They are not equally resistant to the penicillinase elaborated by other organisms such as the tubercle bacillus and they are not used in tuberculosis therapy. It should also be noted that penicillin resistance, even among staphylococci, is not always the result of penicillinase production. The penicillinase resistant penicillins have a generally lower activity than benzylpenicillin against organisms that do not produce penicillinase.

Ampicillin is active against several Gram-negative organisms that are not attacked by the other penicillins. It is particularly valuable for the treatment of respiratory infections by mixed organisms that include *Haemophilus*

Table 50.2 The penicillins

Approved name(s)	Proprietary names(s)	R (see Fig. 50.1)	Principal characteristics
The original penicillins			
2-Pentenylpenicillin	Penicillin I or F	$C_2H_5.CH=CH.CH_2CO-$	
p-Hydroxybenzyl-penicillin	Penicillin III or X	HO—⬡—CH_2CO-	
n-Heptylpenicillin	Penicillin IV or K	$CH_3(CH_2)_6CO-$	
Other 'natural' penicillin			
Phenoxymethyl-penicillin	Penicillin V Calcipen V Compocillin VK Crystapen V Distaquaine V-K Eskacillin Icipen V Orapen VK Pen Vee Penavlon V V-Cillin V-Cil-K and many others	⬡—$O.CH_2.CO-$	Not destroyed by acid Readily absorbed
The 'synthetic' penicillins			
Phenoxyethyl-penicillin Phenethicillin	Broxil Syncillin Chemipen	⬡—$O.CH.CO-$ | CH_3	Not destroyed by acid
L-Phenethicillin	L-Maxipen	L-component of the racemic mixture represented by phenethicillin	
Propicillin	Brocilline Ultrapen	⬡—$O-CH.CO-$ | C_2H_5	Not destroyed by acid
Phenbenicillin	Penspek	⬡—$O.CH.CO-$ | ⬡	Not destroyed by acid. No longer man-ufactured
Methicillin	Celbenin Dimocillin Staphcillin	OCH_3 / ⬡—$CO-$ / OCH_3	Not destroyed by peni-cillinase
The isoxazoyl penicillins			
Oxacillin	Bactocill Prostaphlin Resistopen	As cloxacillin without chlorine atom	Not destroyed by penicillinase or acid
Cloxacillin	Orbenin Tegopen	Cl / ⬡—$C-C-CO-$ N O CH_3	As for oxacillin

Table 50.2 (contd)

Approved name(s)	Proprietary names(s)	R (see Fig. 50.1)	Principal characteristics
Dicloxacillin	Dynapen Pathocil Veracillin	As cloxacillin but with an additional Cl atom at*	As for cloxacillin
Flucloxacillin	Floxapen	As cloxacillin but with an F atom at*	As for cloxacillin
Nafcillin	Unipen	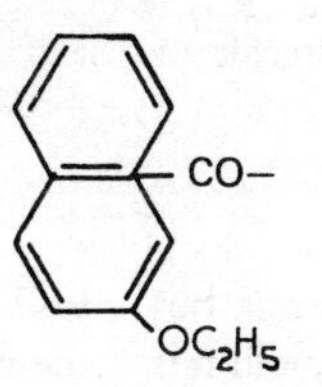	Not destroyed by penicillinase

Broad spectrum penicillins

Ampicillin	Penbritin Polycillin	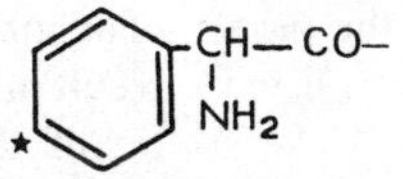	Not destroyed by acid but susceptible to inactivation by penicillinase
Talampicillin	Talpen	Talampicillin is the phthalidyl- 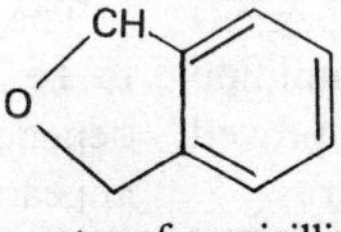 ester of ampicillin	As for ampicillin but more readily absorbed from alimentary tract. Releases ampicillin after absorption

Other compounds that release ampicillin in the tissues include hetacillin (Penplenum, Versapen) and pivampicillin (Alphacillin, Berocillin, Maxifen, Pondocillin).

Amoxycillin Amoxicillin (USA)	Amoxil Imacillin Larotid Polymox	As ampicillin but with an OH group at*	As for ampicillin
Carbenicillin	Fugacillin Geopen Pyopen	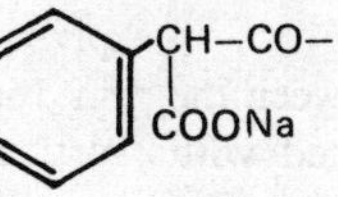 Carbenicillin is a disodium salt. The other Na replaces the acid hydrogen in the penicillinic acid moiety as in most other penicillin preparations	Unlike other penicillins, it is active against *Pseudomonas aeruginosa*. Useful in urinary tract infections. Not destroyed by penicillinase. Not absorbed from gastrointestinal tract
Carfecillin	Uticillin (Note that Uticillin VK is a proprietary name for phenoxy-methylpenicillin)	Carfecillin is the phenol ester of carbenicillin	Can be taken orally. After absorption releases carbenicillin but gives only low blood levels.

Table 50.2 (contd)

Approved name(s)	Proprietary names(s)	R (see Fig. 50.1)	Principal characteristics
The amidinopenicillins			

In mecillinam (Selexid), R is H
In pivmecillinam hydrochloride (Selexid), R is $CH_2OCOC(CH_3)_3.HCl$.

(For details, see text)

influenzae. Ampicillin is active against *Escherichia coli,* but this organism develops resistance rapidly and ampicillin is now recommended for the treatment of urinary infections with noticeably less enthusiasm than it was in the past. Similar remarks apply to the ampicillin derivatives listed in Table 50.2.

The amidinopenicillins

Mecillinam and pivmecillinam hydrochloride are the first serviceable representatives of an entirely new class of antibiotic agents. Strictly speaking they are not penicillins—true penicillins are acylamino derivatives of penicillanic acid, whereas the new compounds are amidino derivatives—and this fact is emphasized by their approved names, which do not end in the traditional 'icillin'.

Pivmecillinam hydrochloride is the pivaloyloxymethyl hydrochloride ester of mecillinam. It is readily absorbed from the alimentary tract and releases the parent compound into the circulation (*cf.* pivampicillin) so that it is suitable for oral administration. Mecillinam itself is given parenterally. Both compounds are marketed as Selexid. In the account that follows, 'mecillinam' can be taken to include pivmecillinam hydrochloride.

The relatively minor structural difference between the acylamino and amidino compounds is associated with surprisingly large differences in antibacterial activity. The outstanding feature of mecillinam is that it is much more active against a range of Gram-negative bacilli then it is against Gram-positive cocci. In this respect, its spectrum of activity is the precise opposite of penicillins.

Gram-negative bacilli that are highly sensitive to mecillinam include *Escherichia coli,* klebsiella species, the enterobacteriaceae, salmonellae and shingellae. Some species of proteus (*mirabilis* and *vulgaris*) are killed by mecillinam but others (*morgani* and *rettergi*) are resistant. Pseudomonas is totally resistant to mecillinam.

Mecillinam has some activity against some species of streptococci by virtue of its being able, like the penicillins, to interfere with the proper synthesis of the bacterial cell wall. It owes its lethal effect on Gram-negative bacilli to the operation of a unique mechanism. Organisms exposed to mecillinam take on a spherical shape, the result perhaps of an inhibition of the cell division processes that normally result in the production of the elongated form characteristic of the bacillus. Susceptible organisms need to be exposed to mecillinam over several generations before they succumb completely.

It is interesting to note that, although both ampicillin and mecillinam kill *E. coli,* they utilize different means to achieve this end.

The amidinopenicillins are new drugs and it is difficult to be dogmatic about their clinical future. Much will depend on the rate at which resistant organisms make their appearance. Currently they are being successfully applied to the treatment of both sufferers from and carriers of the enteric (typhoid and paratyphoid) fevers, urinary and respiratory tract infections and septicaemia caused by susceptible organisms. Useful synergism with ampicillin and the other broad spectrum penicillins has been demonstrated.

The usual daily dose of mecillinam (in the form of pivmecillinam hydrochloride) ranges from 0.8 to 2.4 grams in four instalments. Nausea, vomiting, diarrhoea and urticarial skin rashes have occurred in a few patients taking mecillinam. Anaphylactic reactions must be expected but none seems yet to have been reported.

THERAPEUTIC USES OF THE PENICILLINS

The conditions which yield to penicillin treatment have been indicated in the foregoing paragraphs and only a few general points need to be made here.

Benzylpenicillin and phenoxymethylpenicillin are still in many ways the best penicillins and they should be employed whenever there is no positive indication, of the kind mentioned in the previous paragraphs or implied by the entries in Table 50.2, for preferring another. There is no point in choosing a particular penicillin in the hope that it will prove less likely than another to precipitate a hypersensitivity reaction: those who show allergic or anaphylactic responses to one species of penicillin will do so to all others and these patients should avoid penicillins altogether.

The activity of the natural penicillins is expressed in International units. One unit is now the specific antibiotic activity contained in 0.6 μg of a standard preparation. The synthetic penicillins are prepared in a pure form. For the treatment of acute infections, benzylpenicillin is given in intramuscular doses of up to one million units (one mega unit) which may have to be repeated at three-hourly intervals. The total daily dose of the synthetic penicillins is of the order of one gram. For reasons that have already been discussed, the quoted doses are by no means critical.

Because of its high rate of elimination by the kidneys, penicillin has to be given in high and frequent doses. Excretion can be slowed by giving probenecid (p. 459) or carinamide. These substances compete with penicillin for the transport mechanism in the renal tubules. They have sometimes been given, with penicillin, to patients with subacute bacterial endocarditis, a condition whose treatment demands the maintenance of high concentrations of penicillin in the blood. In general it is preferable to increase the dose of penicillin to achieve this end.

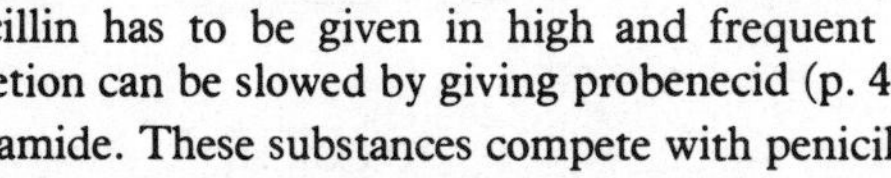

Carinamide

Hypersensitivity reactions apart, the only side effect of penicillin therapy seen with any frequency is candidiasis (p. 907).

The cephalosporins

In 1948, Brotzu found a mould of the *Cephalosporum* genus in the sea off Sardinia close to a sewage outlet. The mould, it was eventually discovered, produced three antibiotics which were named the cephalosporins N, C and P. It has transpired that cephalosporin N is a penicillin (adicillin) and that cephalosporin C is a derivative of 7-aminocephalosporanic acid (Fig. 50.4). Cephalosporin P is steroidal in nature.

Cephalosporin C made only a minimal contribution to the overall activity of the original antibiotic mixture and for this reason it was the last member of the trio to declare

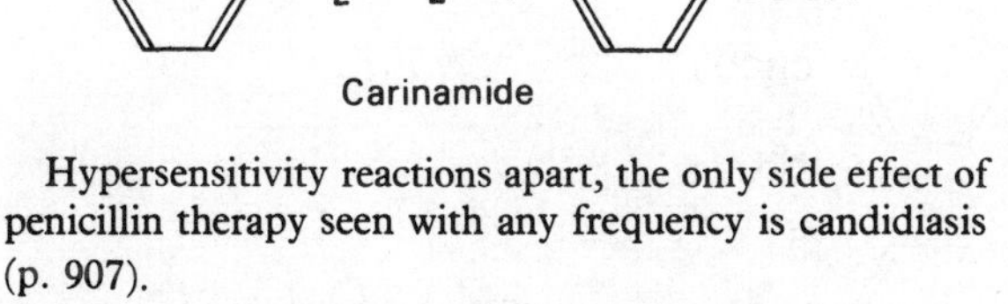

Fig. 50.4 The structure of cephalosporins N and C. In cephalosporin N, R is 6-aminopenicillanic acid (p. 825). In cephalosporin C, R is 7-aminocephalosporanic acid (formula shown)

its individual presence. Even then a good deal of effort and ingenuity had still to be expended in order to obtain enough material for detailed analysis. This labour was, however, well rewarded because cephalosporin C proved to be much the most valuable member of the group by virtue of its being unaffected by the penicillinases. Semi-synthetic cephalorsporins, obtained by attaching side chains to 7-aminocephalosporanic acid just as penicillins are made from 6-aminopenicillanic acid, were quick to make their appearance (Table 50.3). Two of these derivatives, cephaloridine and cephalothin will be described.

A compound structurally similar to cephalosporin P is fusidic acid, an antibiotic produced by the mould *Fusidium coccineum*. The sodium salt of this acid is fucidin. Although this substance is neither a penicillin nor a cephalosporin, it is convenient to include it here in view of the fact that it is related to cephalosporin P.

The mechanism of action of the cephalosporin antibiotics is similar to that of the penicillins.

CEPHALORIDINE

Cephaloridine has a wide spectrum of activity. It is bactericidal for a large number of pathogenic Gram-positive and Gram-negative microorganisms including those that secrete penicillinase although recent observations have made it clear that this antibiotic is more susceptible to the action of this enzyme than had originally been supposed. Nor is it necessarily effective against strains whose resistance arises from factors other than the presence of penicillinase and it has been reported that infections of the urinary tract by penicillin resistant strains of coliform organisms will not respond to cephaloridine. Bacterial species that are wholly or partially resistant to cephaloridine include *Pseudomonas aeruginosa*, *Proteus mirabilis*, *Streptococcus faccalis* and *Haemophilus influenzae*.

Cephaloridine is destroyed by acid and it is but poorly absorbed from the intestine. It is therefore given by intramuscular injection or, in cases of pneumococcal or meningococcal meningitis, by intrathecal injection.

Cephaloridine is used principally as an alternative to penicillin for the treatment of severe streptococcal and staphylococcal infections, if the patient is sensitive, or the organism is resistant to penicillin. It is excreted rapidly in an unchanged form and so reaches a high concentration in the urine. For this reason, it is particularly useful in cases of staphylococcal infections of the urinary tract. Cephaloridine is also a valuable drug for the treatment of severe septicaemia caused by gram-negative organisms such as *Eschericia coli* and *Proteus mirabilis* that are not attacked by penicillin.

The dose of cephaloridine is 500 mg every six hours or 50 mg for intrathecal injection. Reported side effects include hypersensitivity reactions, ranging from simple skin rashes to acute serum sickness. Serious kidney damage (proximal tubular necrosis) is a potential hazard in

Table 50.3 Semisynthetic cephalosporins

Approved name	Proprietary name(s)	R_1	R_2
Cephaloridine	Ceporin; Ceporan Keflodin	thiophene-CH₂CO–	$-N^+$ pyridinium
Cephalothin	Keflin	thiophene-CH₂CO–	–O.CO.CH₃
Cephalexin	Ceporex; Keflex	C₆H₅–CHCO– NH₂	CH₃–
Cephadrine		cyclohexadienyl–CHCO– NH₂	CH₃–
Cephaloglycin	Kafocin	C₆H₅=CHCO– NH₂	–CH₂.O.CO.CH₃
Cephazolin		tetrazolyl–CH₂CO–	thiadiazolyl –CH₂S– CH₃
Cephapirin		pyridyl–SCH₂CO–	–CH₂.O.CO.CH₃
Cephacetrile		N = C.CH₂.CO–	–CH₂.O.CO.CH₃
Cefoxitin		thiophene-CH₂CO.HN–(7) OCH₃	(3) CH₂OCONH₂

patients who have received high doses of cephaloridine. The danger is accentuated in the presence of impaired renal function and in those taking powerful diuretics such as ethacrynic acid or frusemide. Cephaloride should not be given in association with gentamicin or kanamycin since these aminoglycosides are also potentially nephrotoxic. Serious anaphylactic reactions to cephaloridine do not occur.

Drowsiness may be experienced by patients who have received cephaloridine by the intrathecal route.

CEPHALOTHIN
Cephaloridine is used in Britain but cephalothin is favoured in the United States. Unlike cephaloridine, cephalothin is completely unaffected by penicillinase and it seems to be rather less toxic than cephaloridine at high dose levels. These circumstances certainly confer some advantages on cephalothin but cephaloridine injections are less painful and less likely to cause tissue necrosis at the site of injection. These considerations apart, the actions and uses of the two drugs are in every way similar.

Cephalothin can be given in intramuscular injections of up to 5 g at six hourly intervals. The intravenous route can also be used. As with cephaloridine, skin rashes may appear in those taking cephalothin.

CEPHALEXIN
Cephalexin was the first orally active cephalosporin to be developed. Its spectrum of antibacterial activity is similar to that of cephalothin but it is a generally less potent antibiotic. Cephalexin has found a niche for itself in the treatment of infections of the urinary and, more particularly, the respiratory tract. Streptococcal sore throats, especially in children, also respond well to the drug.

Cephalexin is given in six hourly doses within the range of 250 mg to one gram, the actual dose being determined by the severity of the infection. It is not to be given parenterally. Skin rashes may appear in sensitive subjects during treatment with cephalexin. Candidiasis (p. 907) is another possible complication as it is with other antibiotics that are taken by mouth.

The most effective cephalospirins are those that gain access to the body by the parenteral route.

CEPHADRINE
Cephadrine has a structure very similar to that of cephalexin (see Table 50.3) but it can be given by either oral or parenteral routes. Actions, uses and side effects otherwise duplicate those of cephalexin.

OTHER CEPHALOSPORINS
Cephaloglycin is used in the United States for the treatment of urinary tract infections. Although it is usually taken orally cephaloglycin is not very well absorbed from the gastrointestinal tract.

Cephazolin is indistinguishable from cephaloridine in most respects but it has only minimal nephrotoxicity.

Similar claims are made for *cephapirin* and *cephacetrile*. Cephapirin has the additional merit of causing less discomfort than do the other cephalosporins when it is injected into muscle.

CEPHAMYCINS
The cephamycins are naturally produced compounds analogous in structure to the cephalosporins. Three principal members of the group have been identified and labelled A, B and C. Semisynthetic derivatives of the cephamycins have recently been produced and some of them show considerable promise as chemotherapeutic agents.

Cefoxitin is a semisynthetic derivative of cephamycin C and reports of its clinical effectiveness are already beginning to appear. It is to be hoped that the use of an Anglicized form (cephoxitin) will soon be permissible for those who prefer to adopt a unified spelling convention throughout the range of the cephalosporins and related compounds.

Cephamycins differ from cephalosporins in carrying a carbamoyl group in position 3 and a methoxy group in position 7 of their nucleus (Table 50.3). These features confer on the antibiotics and properties, respectively, of stability and resistance to the β lactamases. They are retained in cefoxitin but the semisynthetic compound also carries a thienylacetyl side chain that confers an activity against Gram-positive bacteria that is lacking in cephamycin C. Cephamycin C is analogous to cephalosporin C and cefoxitin is analogous to cephalothin.

Cefoxitin, then, is a broad spectrum antibiotic that is totally unaffected by the β lactamases that bestow resistance to penicillins and cephalosporins on many Gram-negative organisms. Organisms that do not succumb to cefoxitin include *Pseudomonas aeruginosa, Streptococcus faecalis* and the enterobacteriaceae.

Cefoxitin has more favourable pharmacokinetic properties than cephalothin, its cephalosporin rival. It reaches higher plasma concentrations that are better maintained and its plasma half life is twice that of cephalothin. The drug is excreted unchanged in the urine.

Cefoxitin has been successfully employed in the treatment of pyelonephritis, respiratory infections, septicaemic infections of the abdominal and pelvic cavities and osteomyelitis. Side effects are minimal, although thrombophlebitis and local reactions at the site of injection have occasionally been seen.

FUCIDIN
Fucidin is active against a range of Gram-positive organisms, most particularly *Staph. aureus*. It is not affected by gastric acid and it is rapidly absorbed from the gastrointestinal tract. Excretion is in the bile (with some reabsorption from the small intestine) and faeces. Very little, if any, appears in the urine and there is some tendency for the drug to accumulate in the blood and tissues. It is slowly

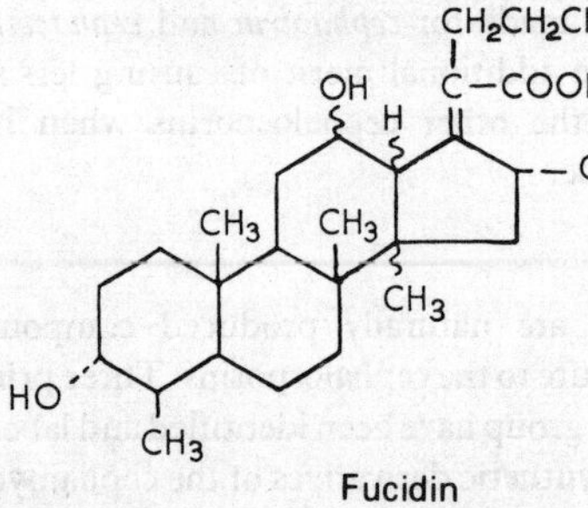

Fucidin

broken down and lost from the body when treatment ceases.

Fucidin and benzylpenicillin show an interesting type of synergistic action. If staphylococci that produce penicillinase are exposed to a mixture of benzylpenicillin and fucidin, the latter may inhibit the growth of the organisms so that penicillinase production is minimal. In these circumstances the penicillin is able to destroy the staphylococci.

Fucidin is capable of promoting recovery from staphylococcal infections—carbuncles, infected wounds, lung abscesses, etc—with remarkable rapidity. Unfortunately, resistance to the antibiotic develops rapidly and most authorities recommend that fucidin should be reserved for the treatment of severe staphylococcal infections in patients who are likely to be hypersensitive to the penicillins.

The dose for adults is 500 mg thrice daily. Side effects appear to be minimal.

THE STREPTOMYCIN GROUP OF ANTIBIOTICS (THE AMINOGLYCOSIDES)

The early success achieved with penicillin, coupled with the need for a drug that would attack a wider range of Gram-negative bacteria, stimulated the search for other organisms capable of producing antibacterial substances. One such search was that conducted by Wacksman and his colleagues. It began in 1939 and it culminated, five years later and after more than ten thousand organisms had been examined, in the discovery of streptomycin, an antibiotic produced by *Streptomyces griseus,* a soil-dwelling actinomycete.

Streptomycin has a more complex molecule than penicillin: in it, the base streptidine is linked to streptobiosamine a disaccharide composed of *N*-methylglucosamine and streptose (Fig. 50.5). The three basic amino groups in streptomycin can be used for salt formation. The activity of streptomycin is maximal at pH 7.8, falling off sharply in more acid media.

Dihydrostreptomycin was obtained by reduction of the aldehyde group in the streptose residue of streptomycin but it is now known that some species of *Streptomyces* produce the compound naturally.

Streptomycin was found to be lethal to a range of both Gram-negative and Gram-positive organisms (especially the former) but over the years, resistance to streptomycin has become widespread so that relatively few bacterial species now succumb to the antibiotic. Moreover, even members of still susceptible species rapidly develop resistance on exposure to streptomycin. This may happen after only a few days' exposure. Some strains may actually become dependent on streptomycin and can only multiply in its presence. It is usual to give streptomycin in combination with at least one other antibacterial drug which can attack any resistant strains that may be present or that develop during the course of treatment. It may, of course, happen that the infection is caused entirely by resistant organisms and tests for streptomycin sensitivity should be made on the bacteria isolated from individual cases before

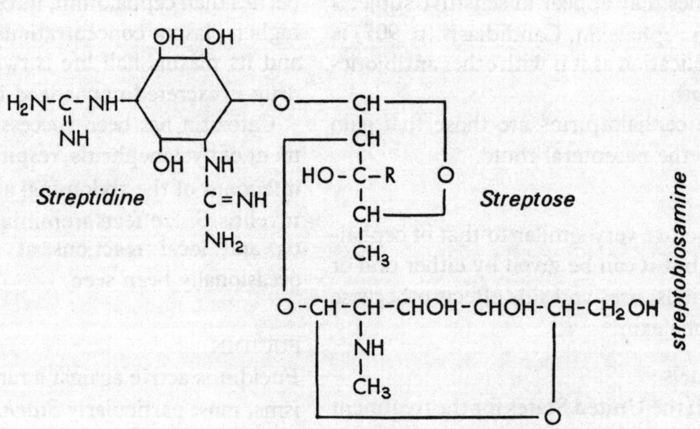

In Streptomycin R = CHO
In Dihydrostreptomycin R = CH$_2$OH

Fig. 50.5 Streptomycin and dihydrostreptomycin

treatment is instituted. This is particularly necessary with urinary infections.

In spite of these limitations, streptomycin retains its therapeutic importance by virtue of its activity against *Mycobacterium tuberculosis*. Fortunately, the tubercle bacillus does not lose its sensitivity to streptomycin until it has been exposed to the drug for a few weeks. The role of streptomycin in tuberculosis therapy is discussed later (p. 845). It is also of value, in association with tetracycline, in the treatment of brucellosis, plague and tularaemia. The last named condition is a fever which may occur in those who work with animals—butchers, poultry men and laboratory workers—particularly in the United States and Japan. Meningitis caused by *Haemophilus influenzae* and urinary infections by coliform organisms resistant to other agents may also respond to streptomycin.

Streptomycin is badly absorbed from the gastrointestinal tract. Except when it is being used to treat intestinal infections it is usually given by intramuscular injection although this may lead to the development of pain at the injection site. Subarachinoid injection is permissible (though probably no more effective than a parenteral administration) in cases of meningitis. Streptomycin is very readily excreted by the kidney. Unlike penicillin it is excreted into the glomerular filtrate so that the concurrent administration of probenecid will not lead to any reduction in its rate of excretion. In acute infections, the dose of streptomycin is 0.5 to 1 gram two to four times daily.

Streptomycin is bound to plasma proteins to the extent of some 30 per cent. Its half life in plasma is two and a half hours.

Side effects of streptomycin administration. The most characteristic toxic actions of streptomycin are the result of damage to the vestibular division of the eighth cranial nerve: loss of balance and a feeling of dizziness are common complaints among those (particularly the elderly) who have taken the drug.

Dihydrostreptomycin is even more likely to cause damage to the eighth nerve but in this instance it is the acoustic division which is more likely to be affected. The risk of producing permanent deafness has led to the disappearance of dihydrostreptomycin as a therapeutic agent.

Hypersensitivity reactions are common sequelae of streptomycin administration. They are also likely to occur in those who do not wear protective gloves when handling the drug. They take the form of rashes which usually yield to histamine H_1 antagonists. Fatal anaphylaxis such as is sometimes precipitated by penicillin does not occur.

Depression of the bone marrow leading to aplastic anaemia or agranulocytosis is another possible side effect.

Streptomycin exerts a weak though not insignificant curare-like effect at the skeletal neuromuscular junction. This action can constitute a hazard in patients with myasthenia gravis or in those undergoing surgery under conditions involving the use of neuromuscular blocking

agents and the administration at the end of the operation of large prophylactic doses of streptomycin.

Mode of action of streptomycin. Streptomycin appears to inhibit protein synthesis in the bacterial cell by becoming bound to ribosomes which, as a result, can no longer react with messenger RNA. It is suggested that streptomycin cannot combine with the ribosomes of highly resistant organisms as a result of a mutation that results in a change in the composition of one of the ribosomal proteins. Moderately resistant organisms acquire their immunity to streptomycin by developing less permeable cell walls. Resistance of this type can be overcome or prevented by giving penicillin with the streptomycin. Streptomycin-resistance in organisms that have not previously been exposed to the drug ('wild' strains) is attributable to their acquiring, by transfer from resistant organisms, genetic material that confers an ability to synthesize enzymes (streptomycin phosphotransferase and streptomycin adenylyl synthetase) that break down the antibiotic. The mode of action of streptomycin in relation to that of other antibiotic agents is discussed in more detail later (p. 854).

In the account that follows, other aminoglycosides are described in the order in which they were discovered.

NEOMYCIN

The next aminoglycoside to be discovered was neomycin.

Like streptomycin itself, it was discovered by Wacksman and his group who isolated it in 1949 from cultures of a soil dwelling actinomycete *Streptomyces fradiae*. The original antibiotic was early shown to be a mixture of three compounds (neomycins A, B and C) but neomycin A is now known to be a breakdown product of the other two compounds. Commercial neomycin (Mycifradin, Myciguent, Neomin, Nivemycin) consists of neomycin B with a small admixture of neomycin C. The two substances are isomeric compounds.

The properties and antibacterial activity of neomycin are qualitatively similar to those of streptomycin. Organisms do not become resistant to neomycin quite so rapidly as they do to streptomycin but this advantage is offset by neomycin's greater oto- and nephrotoxicity which considerably reduces its range of usefulness. Neomycin is used for local application (in a 0.5 per cent solution) to infected wounds, burns and other skin infections and (by those who believe the procedure to be worthwhile) for clearing the intestine of bacteria in patients who are about to undergo intestinal surgery. Intestinal sterilization is also one of a repertoire of therapeutic manoeuvres that are available for the management of hepatic coma. Neomycin can be used for this purpose too. When neomycin is given by mouth, little is absorbed so that systemic toxic effects do not appear. Neomycin is sometimes effective in dysentery. Intestinal candidiasis (p. 907) and atrophic changes in the intestinal mucosa are possible sequels to the prolonged administration of neomycin by the oral route.

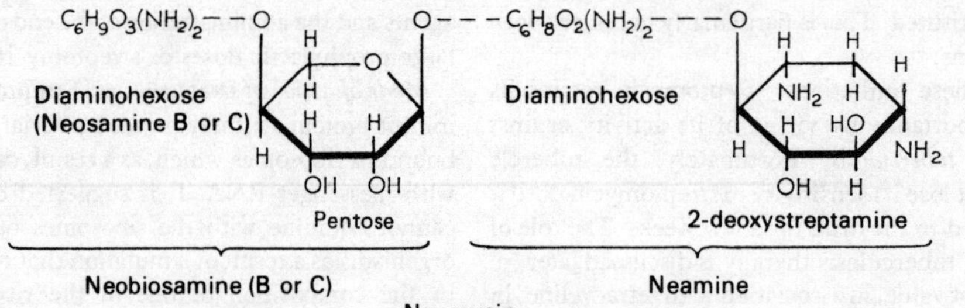

$C_6H_9O_3(NH_2)_2$– – O   O – – –$C_6H_8O_2(NH_2)_2$– – – O

Diaminohexose
(Neosamine B or C)

Diaminohexose

Pentose

2-deoxystreptamine

Neobiosamine (B or C)   Neamine

Neomycin

The potential toxicity of neomycin is so high as to constitute a firm contraindication to its administration by systemic routes.

When neomycin is employed it is usual to give another antibacterial agent—bacitracin, polymyxin or chlorhexidine, for example—at the same time, to eliminate microorganisms that may be, or may become, resistant to neomycin.

The pre-operative dose of neomycin is 4 grams (given in divided doses over a period of four hours) followed by one gram six times daily for two or three days.

Organisms that become resistant to neomycin will also resist streptomycin but streptomycin resistant organisms may still succumb to neomycin.

FRAMYCETIN

This antibiotic (Framygen, Soframycin) which is obtained from *Streptomyces decaris* is now known to be identical with neomycin B. It is so similar to neomycin that any further description of the drug would be quite superfluous. It is not widely used.

KANAMYCIN

Kanamycin (which was isolated in 1957 from a species of *Streptomyces*) has properties and actions similar to streptomycin and neomycin. Though more toxic than strep-

2-deoxystreptamine

CH_2NH_2

H_2N

OH

H_2N

CH_2OH

OH

OH NH_2

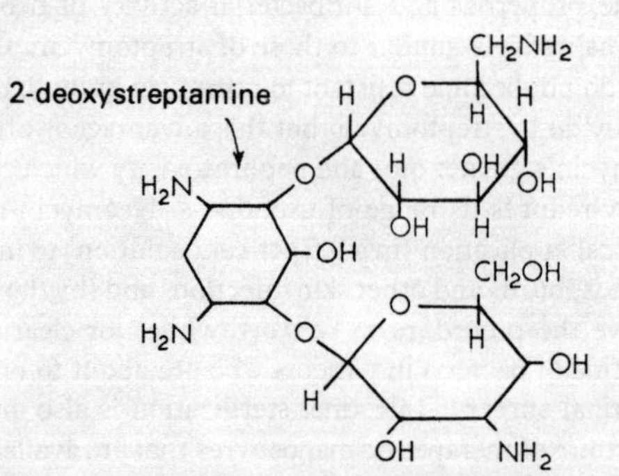

Kanamycin

(For purposes of illustration, the formulae of streptomycin, neomycin and kanamycin have been drawn according to different conventions. Careful comparison of the formulae will reveal a closer structural similarity than might at first sight appear. For instance, kanamycin, like neomycin, contains the 2-deoxystreptamine moiety.)

tomycin, it is less so than neomycin and it may be administered, with caution, by parenteral routes. Its antibacterial activity is such as to suggest that its range of therapeutic uses should be the same as those of streptomycin and neomycin. It should, however, be reserved for treating the most acutely serious infections with Gram-negative organisms, particularly those affecting the urinary tract. Like neomycin, it has also been given by the oral route to sterilize the bowel before surgery or in hepatic coma. It is still listed as an alternative to streptomycin for tuberculosis therapy but it now occupies a lowly position on that list. After intramuscular injection, kanamycin attains a peak serum concentration in about one and a half hours. It has a serum half life of about four hours and an effective concentration is maintained there for some six hours. Kanamycin is excreted unchanged by glomerular filtration but this process is not completely mature during the first three months of life and care must be exercised when kanamycin is given to very young children lest a dangerous accumulation of the drug occurs. Signals for extreme caution in adult patients include the existence of renal disease, hepatic failure or partial deafness. Unless contraindicated by any of these circumstances, the dose of kanamycin is 250 mg every six hours. Proprietary names include Kannasyn and Kantrex.

The side effects of kanamycin treatment are in every way similar to those that might result from the administration of streptomycin including a light blockade of the skeletal neuromuscular junction.

GENTAMICIN

Gentamicin is an antibiotic of recent (1963) origin. It is obtained from *Micromonospora purpurea* and this explains the apparent inconsistency in the spelling of the drug's name: the termination '-ycin' is reserved for antibiotic agents obtained from *Streptomyces* sp. It is a pity that this convention was unknown to (or ignored by) those who further confounded the confusion by deciding that Garamycin was a suitable proprietary name for a new drug.

Notwithstanding its origin, the chemical structure of gentamicin is very similar to that of the aminoglycosides obtained from *Streptomyces*. Even a superficial comparison of the formula of gentamicin with those of, say, kanamycin and tobramycin will illustrate this point.

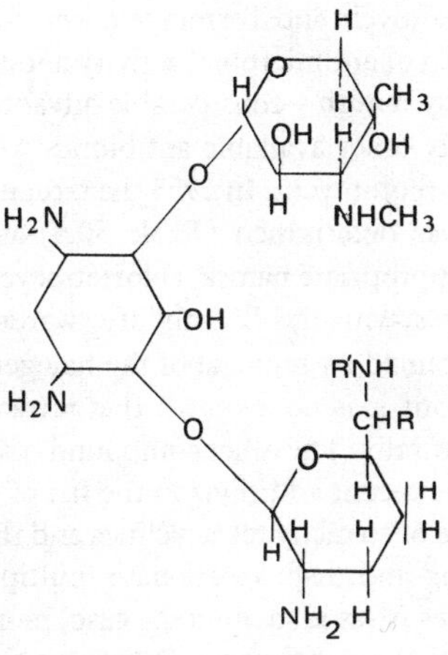

	R	R'
Gentamicin C$_1$	CH$_3$	CH$_3$
Gentamicin C$_2$	CH$_3$	H
Gentamicin Cl$_q$ (C3)	H	H

Fig. 50.6 The gentamicins

Gentamicin is a mixture of three closely related compounds (Fig. 50.6). Its spectrum of antibacterial activity is similar to that of the other aminoglycosides but it is much the most active member of the whole group. It is particularly lethal to *Pseudomonas aeruginosa*. Its high antibacterial activity is not, fortunately, accompanied by a proportionate increase in toxicity. While it is certainly true that gentamicin can cause eighth nerve damage (affecting particularly the vestibular division of the nerve) it is unlikely to damage the kidneys of normal individuals.

Gentamicin is used by local application and parenteral injection. In the plasma it is bound, to a total extent of about 40 per cent, to proteins and the erythrocytes. It has a serum half life of about four hours but, as with the other aminoglycosides, is considerably prolonged in the very young. It is excreted unchanged largely by glomerular filtration.

Gentamicin has a similar mode of action to its fellow aminohexose antibiotics: it inhibits the synthesis of ribosome proteins. Its particular point of intervention is in the process whereby phenylalanine is incorporated into peptides.

Gentamicin's high potency and relatively low toxicity coupled (until recently) with a virtual absence of resistant strains of susceptible organisms combined to give an antibiotic of high popularity and wide usefulness. It was first used only by topical application. Applied as a cream containing 0.1 per cent of the antibiotic, gentamicin is of proved efficacy for the treatment of severe burns particularly when infection with staphylococci or pseudomonas has occurred or threatens. Gentamicin has saved the lives of many burn victims who would otherwise have died.

The other major use of gentamicin is in the treatment of serious infections with Gram-negative organisms (especially *Pseudomonas aeruginosa*) particularly when these involve the urinary tract. A combination of penicillin and gentamicin has proved to be particularly valuable in the control of enterococcal endocarditis.

Now that resistant strains of previously susceptible organisms are emerging, it is prudent to combine gentamicin with other antibiotic agents when treating cases of grave septicaemia that demand the rapid and complete elimination of the infecting bacteria if life is to be saved. Cephaloridine and carbenicillin (as well as penicillin as mentioned above) form suitable partners for gentamicin. Gentamicin and carbenicillin interact in infusion fluids to the detriment of gentamicin's antibacterial activity but this interaction can be avoided by giving gentamicin by rapid intravenous injection before carbenicillin is introduced into the infusion.

By the usual intramuscular route, the daily dose of gentamicin currently recommended for adults with normal kidney function is 3 to 5 mg per kilogram of body weight.

Proprietary names for gentamicin, in addition to the one previously mentioned, include Genticin and Cidomycin.

PAROMOMYCIN

Paromomycin (Humatin), which appeared in 1959, is similar to neomycin except that it is very active against *Entamoeba histolytica*. It also, surprisingly, has anthelmintic properties. It has been employed, in daily oral doses of two grams, in the treatment of amoebic dysentery and in a

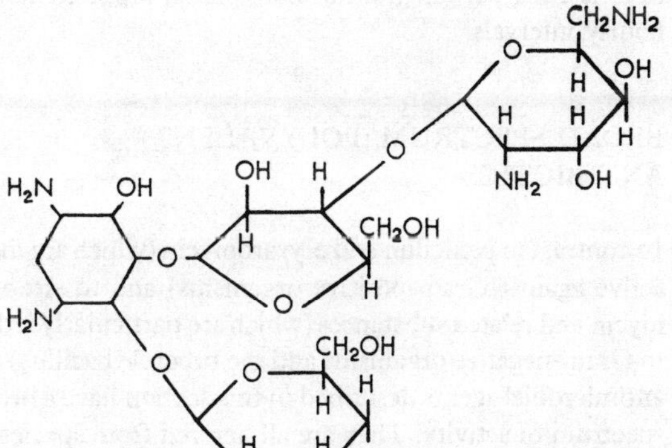

Paromomycin

single dose of four grams for the elimination of tapeworms from the body. Its use in the conditions treated by the other aminoglycosides has been minimal.

TOBRAMYCIN

With tobramycin (which first appeared in 1967) we return to antibiotics obtained from streptomyces—*Streptomyces tenebrarius* in this instance. In many ways, tobramycin closely resembles gentamicin. Even such pharmacokinetic variables as plasma half lives, time to peak concentration and extent of plasma protein binding are similar for the two drugs. However, tobramycin is very effective against *Pseudomonas aeruginosa* including strains that have become resistant to gentamicin. It is also rather less toxic than gentamicin.

Tobramycin

As might be expected, the conditions that respond to tobramycin are precisely the same as those that are indicated for gentamicin.

The adult dose of tobramycin, by intramuscular injection, is 1 mg per kilogram of body mass, repeated at six-hourly intervals.

BROAD SPECTRUM (POLYVALENT) ANTIBIOTICS

In contrast to penicillin and erythromycin (which are most active against Gram-positive organisms) and to streptomycin and related substances (which are particularly lethal to Gram-negative organisms and the tubercle bacillus) the antimicrobial agents described in this section have a broad spectrum of activity. They are all derived from species of *Streptomyces*.

The tetracyclines
Like streptomycin, the tetracyclines were discovered as a result of a deliberate search for a new antibiotic. The first member of the group was found, by Duggar, in 1948. The name of the organism (*Streptomyces aureofaciens*) which produces it and the original (now a proprietary) name of the antibiotic itself (Aureomycin) recognize the fact that both have a golden yellow colour. Two years later another tetracycline (Terramycin) was isolated, this time from *S.*

rimosus. Aureomycin and Terramycin were found to have a wide spectrum of antimicrobial activity and to be effective when taken by mouth—considerable advantages at a time when the only other available antibiotics were benzylpenicillin and streptomycin. In 1953 the structure of the new antibiotics was determined (Table 50.4) and they were given more appropriate names, chlortetracycline and oxytetracycline respectively. Shortly afterwards tetracycline itself was obtained by removal of the halogen from chlortetracycline but it is now known that tetracycline is also produced naturally. The other compounds named in Table 50.4 are more recent additions to the list of tetracyclines. The existence of so many tetracyclines and the embarrassing, confusing and disproportionate multiplicity of proprietary names is (as is so often the case) more a reflection of commercial competitiveness and acquisitiveness than it is a response to clinical demand. As we shall see, one or two of the individual compounds have special features that give them some therapeutic advantage over their congeners in particular situations but, with these exceptions, there is little to choose between one tetracycline and another.

The tetracyclines are weak bases, insoluble in water but soluble in organic solvents. In solution they are stable at an acid *p*H. Apart from rolitetracycline (which is given parenterally) the tetracyclines are usually taken by mouth although they are not completely absorbed from the gastrointestinal tract. After normal doses, they appear in the faeces in concentrations of up to 1 mg per gram. Tetracyclines are also excreted in the bile and urine. Biliary excretion accounts for the fact that they can be found in the faeces even after intravenous administration: some of the drug carried into the intestine by the bile is excreted and the rest is reabsorbed. Urinary excretion is by way of the glomeruli. About 20 per cent of an oral dose and 50 per cent of an intravenous dose is excreted in this way.

Most tetracyclines do not undergo an appreciable degree of metabolic degradation after absorption but chlortetracycline and doxycycline provide exceptions to this generalization. They are metabolized by hepatic microsomal enzymes and the possibility that less than effective doses of these antibiotics are being prescribed, because of the simultaneous administration of other drugs that may enhance enzyme activity (p. 80), must always be borne in mind.

Tetracyclines are absorbed from all parts of the gastrointestinal tract from the stomach onwards. They reach their maximum concentration in the plasma some 2 hr after being taken by mouth and this concentration is then maintained for some hours as a result of continuing absorption, release from binding to plasma proteins and recycling in the bile.

Tetracycline, oxytetracycline and chlortetracycline need to be taken every six hours but the newer compounds are less readily disposed of and can be taken at longer intervals—24 hr in the case of doxycycline.

Table 50.4 The tetracyclines

General Formula of the tetracyclines

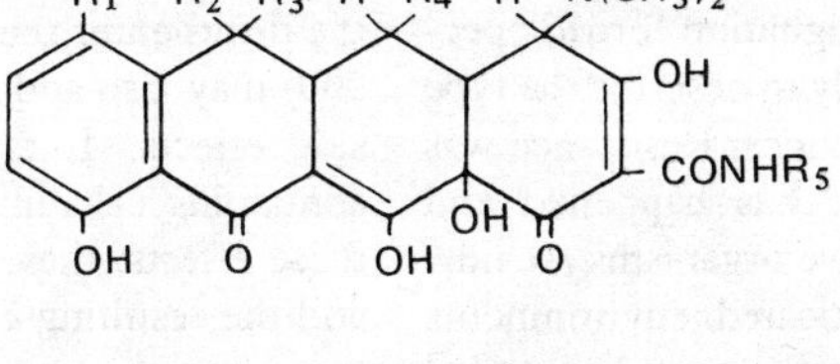

R_1 R_2 R_3 H R_4 H $N(CH_3)_2$

OH

$CONHR_5$

OH O OH O (with OH groups)

Approved name(s)	Proprietary name(s)	Substituents				
		R_1	R_2	R_3	R_4	R_5
Chlortetracycline	Aureomycin	Cl	CH_3	OH	H	H
Oxytetracycline	Terramycin Imperacin	H	CH_3	OH	OH	H
Tetracycline	Anchromycin Ambramycin Steclin Tetracyn Totomycin	H	CH_3	OH	H	H
Demethylchlor-tetracycline Demeclocycline	Declomycin Ledermycin	Cl	H	OH	H	H
Pyrrolidinomethyl-tetracycline Rolitetracycline	Reverin Synetrin Velocycline	H	CH_3	OH	H	(1) below
Methacycline 6-Methylene oxytetracycline	Rondomycin	H		CH_2	OH	H
Lymecycline Tetracycline L-methylene lysine	Tetralysal	H	CH_3	OH	H	(2) below
Sancycline	Bonomycin	H	H	H	H	H
Minocycline	Klinomycin Minocin Minomycin Vectrin	$N(CH_3)_2$	H	H	H	H
Doxycycline	Vibramycin	H	CH_3	H	OH	H
Clomocycline	Megaclor	Cl	CH_3	OH	H	CH_2OH

(1) is $-CH_2.N$ ⟨pyrrolidine ring⟩

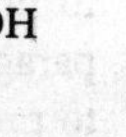

(2) is $-CH_2.NH(CH_2)_4\,CH.COOH$
with NH_2

Therapeutic uses of the tetracyclines

When they were first discovered, the tetracyclines were found to possess a remarkably extensive range of antimicrobial activity, being capable of inhibiting the growth of almost all known pathogenic bacteria as well as that of some bigger organisms such as the rickettsiae (p. 000) and some of the larger viruses. The designation 'broad spectrum' was, indeed, coined specifically to describe the type of activity displayed by the tetracyclines. Resistance was slow to appear but the inevitable has happened and resistant strains of nominally sensitive organisms are now commonplace in medically sophisticated environments such as are found in hospitals in the affluent and advanced nations of the world where the tetracyclines' spectrum of usefulness is considerably narrower than it was a few years ago.

Except when they are the result of infection with resistant strains of the responsible organisms, the principal conditions for which tetracyclines provide a satisfactory treatment are as follows:

a. infections of the respiratory tract, particularly pneumonia caused by *Mycoplasma pneumoniae* and attacks of acute bronchitis occurring in the course of a chronic bronchitis,

b. diseases such as actinomycosis, anthrax, syphilis and gonorrhoea which would normally be treated with penicillin but which have been caused by penicillin resistant strains of the responsible organisms or have occurred in individuals known to be hypersensitive to penicillin.

c. conditions caused by sensitive rickettsiae and viruses. These include lymphogranuloma venerum, psittacosis, trachoma, typhus and bubonic plague.

d. non-gonococcal urethritis,

e. acne vulgaris.

The use of tetracyclines in such relatively trivial conditions as tonsillitis is to be deprecated.

With one exception, cross resistance among the several tetracyclines is absolute: when an organism develops resistance to one tetracycline it is equally resistant to all the others. The exceptional drug is minocycline, the newest of the group which is active against many bacterial strains that have acquired resistance to the other tetracyclines. Tetracycline resistance seems to develop because the wall of the bacterial cell becomes impermeable to the drugs but minocycline can, apparently, still penetrate the cell wall even when other tetracyclines are refused admittance. Minor points of difference among the individual drugs relate to the rate of onset and the duration of action (and hence the frequency of dosage), potency and the tendency to produce the side effects enumerated in the following paragraphs. These considerations apart, there is no reason to prefer one tetracycline to another.

Side effects of tetracycline administration. Hypersensitivity reactions of the kind seen with penicillin are unusual after tetracycline administration but skin eruptions, angioedema and even severe anaphylactic responses have been reported. Much the most common side effects, however, involve the gastrointestinal tract. Nausea, vomiting and diarrhoea may be due to a direct irritant action of the drugs on the gastric mucosa and this may occur even in patients who have received tetracyclines parenterally since the drugs enter the intestine with the bile. Candidiasis (p. 000) may also add its contribution to the gastrointestinal side effects. It is important not to give preparations containing calcium or aluminium in an effort to obtund these effects: these ions are chelated by the tetracyclines and the resulting complex is not easily absorbed. For the same reason, patients taking tetracyclines should be warned against self medication with 'tonics' or other preparations containing iron (see also p. 77).

While some diarrhoea is not unusual in patients receiving the tetracyclines, the onset of severe diarrhoea may signal the development of a serious enteritis which may be fatal. It is the result of infection by a tetracycline-resistant strain of *Staph. aureus* which, freed of competition from other organisms, multiplies in the intestine causing extensive destruction of the intestinal mucosa, an incapacitating diarrhoea and circulatory collapse. Infection of this kind is more likely to occur in hospitals (which harbour the resistant strains of staphylococcus) than in private practice and patients who have undergone abdominal surgery are especially susceptible. The appearance of *Staph. aureus* in the faeces should be taken as a warning that tetracycline therapy should be stopped. Because of their ability to chelate calcium ions, tetracyclines become incorporated into growing bony tissues and the milk teeth of children who have been given the drugs in early infancy may develop a yellow, brown or greenish brown discolouration, the precise hue varying with the tetracycline. Staining of the teeth is sometimes seen in the newly erupted teeth of infants whose mothers have received tetracyclines in the second half of pregnancy. It is, of course, a much more unfortunate occurrence if the permanent teeth suffer an ugly discolouration and tetracyclines should not be given to children between six months and six years of age (when the permanent teeth are acquiring their mineral structure) except in situations of dire necessity or unless it is clear that the therapeutic goal can be reached by giving a low total dose of the chosen drug. There is some evidence that tetracyclines may actually induce structural defects in teeth. Oxytetracycline and doxycycline are rather less likely than the other tetracyclines to produce dental side effects.

In patients with renal failure, the tetracyclines not uncommonly have a nephrotoxic action which may result in a further serious impairment of renal function. This occurs partly as a result of the drugs' inhibiting protein synthesis so that the kidneys have to carry the extra burden of excreting aminoacids that would otherwise have been incorporated into tissue protein. In addition, tetracyclines may exert a direct toxic action on the kidneys. Doxycycline, which undergoes metabolic transformation in the liver (p. 838) does not accumulate in the body if renal function is impaired so that, unlike the other tetracyclines it can be given to patients with renal disease. Chlortetracycline is also metabolized in the liver but this does not prevent its having a nephrotoxic action.

Patients who have received large doses of demethyl-chlortetracycline may become photosensitive so that they suffer severe burning if they are exposed to very bright sunlight. Giddiness or dizziness, sometimes of an incapacitating severity, can occur in people taking minocycline.

Large doses of any tetracycline can cause liver damage particularly if the drug is given intravenously to pregnant subjects.

Mode of action of the tetracyclines
The tetracyclines inhibit bacterial protein synthesis by interfering with the formation of peptide linkages. Organisms that develop resistance to the tetracyclines probably do so by becoming less permeable to the drugs. The mode of action of the tetracyclines is considered again later in this chapter (p. 854).

Chloramphenicol
Chloramphenicol (Chloromycetin) was originally isolated (in 1947) from the soil dwelling organism *Streptomyces venezuelae* but it is now produced by chemical synthesis. It is a crystalline compound which, though insoluble in water, is readily absorbed when taken by mouth. Excretion is slow and high blood concentrations can be maintained by giving doses at intervals of six, eight or twelve hours. Peak concentrations are attained within two to three hours of commencing treatment. Chloramphenicol is excreted in the urine, largely as a pharmacologically inactive glucuronide. It penetrates the blood-brain barrier more readily than does any other antibiotic.

Chloramphenicol has a spectrum of antimicrobial activity very similar to that of the tetracyclines except that it is considerably less active against some Gram-positive organisms. Because of the possibility of its producing seriously toxic side effects, chloramphenicol is now less widely used than it was some years ago. It is, however, still the drug of choice for the treatment of typhoid and paratyphoid fever. It is also valuable for the treatment of

NO$_2$

CHOH
CH-NH-CO-CH-Cl$_2$
CH$_2$OH

Chloramphenicol

meningitis and pneumonia produced by *Haemophilus influenzae* in infants, particularly if the infecting organism is resistant to ampicillin. It has also been extensively employed as a remedy for chronic bronchitis but it is being replaced for this purpose by the tetracyclines. It may have to be employed for the treatment of infections caused by strains of *Staph. aureus* resistant to other antibiotics. Resistance to the tetracyclines, however, is likely to be associated with some degree of resistance to chloramphenicol.

Chloramphenicol itself has a very bitter taste but the palmitate and the cinnamate are tasteless compounds.

Chloramphenicol is usually given by mouth in total daily doses of up to 3 grams. For intravenous injection the succinate is used.

Side effects of chloramphenicol administration
The most serious toxic effect of chloramphenicol, and the one that explains the drug's waning popularity, is aplastic anaemia caused by depression of the bone marrow. This condition, which is usually ascribed to the nitrobenzene moiety of the chloramphenicol molecule, affects all the formed elements of the blood (including the platelets) and usually has a fatal outcome. It is generally agreed that this particular complication is a rare one but authorities differ in their assessment of the risk which attends administration of the drug in moderate doses, with careful and regular inspection of the blood picture to detect aplastic changes at a stage when they might still be reversible. Prudence would obviously dictate that chloramphenicol should be given only when it is the only preparation likely to save the patient's life.

A somewhat bizarre event in the history of chloramphenicol (the *grey syndrome* episode) is recorded on p. 71.

Gastrointestinal upsets, similar to, but less serious than, those produced by the tetracyclines, may also occur in patients receiving chloramphenicol.

Mode of action of chloramphenicol
Chloramphenicol blocks protein synthesis by preventing the transfer of amino acids into the ribosomes. This is essentially a non-selective action, multiplying microorganisms only being more susceptible than the host tissues because of their need for new protein. It also explains why chloramphenicol attacks the bone marrow and why the toxic effects of the drug are dose dependent (see also p. 854).

THE PENICILLIN SUBSTITUTES

These antibiotics have a spectrum of antibacterial activity similar to that of the penicillins. They are brought into service for the treatment of infections caused by penicillin resistant organisms or of patients who may suffer hypersensitivity reactions if given penicillin. They are not affected by penicillinase but organisms may develop resistance to them by other means. Moreover, some of the newer penicillins are resistant to penicillinase. These circumstances have had the effect of somewhat reducing the range of usefulness of the penicillin substitutes.

Erythromycin and other macrolides

ERYTHROMYCIN

Erythromycin is yet another antibiotic produced by a species of *Streptomyces*. It was first obtained in 1952 by McGuire and his associates who isolated it from *S. erytheus*, a soil dwelling organism first collected in the Philippines. It is a *macrolide;* the name (= macrocyclic lactone) is given to large ring lactones. Lactones are organic anhydrides formed from a hydroxy acid by the loss of water. The macrolides prevent protein synthesis by arresting the translocation movements that permit the sequential linking of aminoacids to produce the ribosomal protein. This process is discussed in more detail later (p. 854).

Erythromycin (Erythrocyn, Ilotycin) is active when taken by mouth but it is destroyed by acid and it has to be protected against hydrochloric acid in the stomach by presenting it in capsules, as enteric coated tablets or as a stearate (Bristamycin, Ethrilk) or estolate (Ilosone). The last named compound may cause liver damage. The glucoheptonate and the lactobionate are soluble in water and thus suitable for parenteral administration but intramuscular injection is very painful and the preferred parenteral route is the intravenous one.

Erythromycin is excreted to a large extent in the bile and faeces. It is a relatively non-toxic drug but it sometimes causes nausea, vomiting and other forms of gastrointestinal upset. Jaundice sometimes occurs in patients who have taken the estolate for more than two weeks. The total daily oral dose of erythromycin is 0.5 to 2 grams divided into four doses. For parenteral routes a generally similar dose schedule can be followed.

Among the conditions that respond well to erythromycin are middle ear infections and bronchopneumonia when these result from a mixed attack by Gram-positive cocci and *Haemophilus influenzae*. In this situation, indeed, erythromycin should be regarded as being preferable to penicillin. Otherwise, and as we have already noted, it is employed as an alternative to penicillin for the treatment of conditions attributable to infection by Gram-positive organisms.

OLEANDOMYCIN AND TRIACETYLOLEANDOMYCIN

Oleandomycin (Matromycin) is a compound of similar structure to erythromycin (Fig. 50.7). It is produced by *Streptomyces antibioticus*. It offers no particular advantage over erythromycin. Triacetyloleandomycin (troleandomycin, Cyclamycin, Tae) is obtained by esterification of oleandomycin. It is stable in acid and this permits the drug to be given by mouth without protection by enteric coating. Unfortunately, its administration over periods of longer than two weeks may result in liver damage similar to that caused by erythromycin estolate. This is a pity because these compounds (which liberate the parent compound after absorption) are absorbed much more readily and regularly than the unesterified bases.

SPIRAMYCIN

Spiramycin (Rovamycin) is less active than erythromycin or the oleandomycins but some authorities recommend its use in particular circumstances on the ground of its prolonged persistence in the tissues. Garrod, Lambert and O'Grady (1973), for example, note the value of this property in the prevention of sepsis following prostatec-

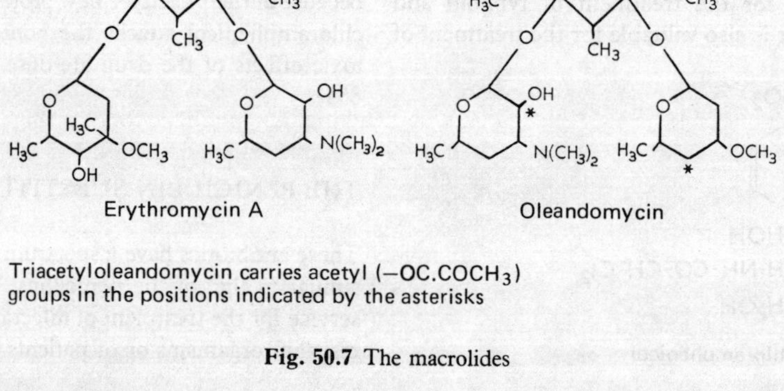

Erythromycin A

Oleandomycin

Triacetyloleandomycin carries acetyl (—OC.COCH₃) groups in the positions indicated by the asterisks

Fig. 50.7 The macrolides

tomy. Otherwise, spiramycin is in no way preferable (or inferior) to the other macrolides.

Other penicillin substitutes

Some other compounds have antibacterial activity similar to that of the penicillins and the erythromycins. All except lincomycin are much more toxic than the other antibiotics so far discussed and the number of occasions on which they can be justifiably used is very limited. They probably all inhibit bacterial cell wall synthesis.

VANCOMYCIN

Vancomycin (Vancocin) is an antibiotic, of so far undetermined structure, elaborated by *Streptomyces orientalis*. It has to be given by intravenous injection (250 to 500 mg four times daily) and it is excreted in the urine. Toxic side effects include allergic skin reactions, nerve deafness, kidney damage and phlebitis at the site of injection.

Vancomycin finds a use, and the only justification for its continued existence, in the treatment of serious infections caused by staphylococci resistant to other agents. It is especially useful in refractory cases of staphylococcal endocarditis. Resort to the drug may also have to be made in patients who are infected with resistant varieties of some streptococci (particularly the enterococci) or who are hypersensitive to the penicillins.

In some cases of staphylococcal enterocolitis, vancomycin has been given, with success, by mouth and it can also be applied locally in serious infections of the gums.

NOVOBIOCIN AND RISTOCETIN

Novobiocin (Albamycin, Biotexin, Cathomycin) and ristocetin (Riston, Spontin) were obtained from species of

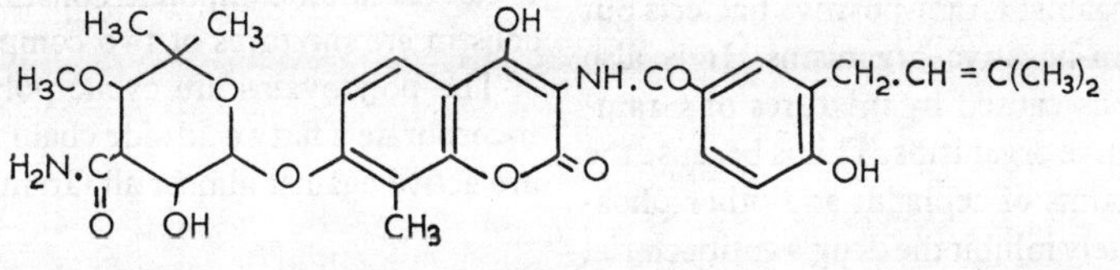

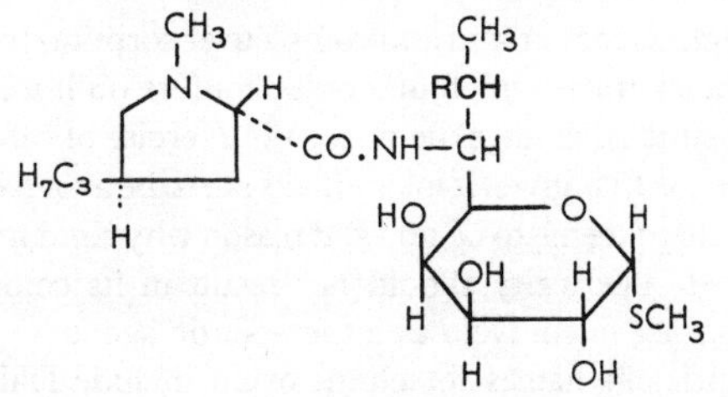

Fig. 50.8 Lincomycin (R is –OH) and clindamycin (R is –Cl)

faeces. Much of the faecal drug comes from the bile which is an important channel of excretion but the rest is derived by transfer through the intestinal wall.

The half life of lincomycin in the plasma is five hours but this increases considerably in patients whose liver function is depressed. The oral dose of the drug is 500 mg three or four times daily. The presence of food in the alimentary tract inhibits the absorption of lincomycin which should, therefore, be taken between meals.

A unique property of lincomycin (Fig. 50.8) is its ability to penetrate into bone and this has established for it a place in the therapy of bone and joint conditions (particularly osteomyelitis) arising from infection by penicillin resistant strains of *Staph. aureus*. It is also valuable in infections caused by bacteroides (the small bacilli that form the largest group of dwellers in the faeces) which may afflict many regions of the body.

Lincomycin is a less innocent drug than was at one time supposed. About one in five of those who receive it complain of diarrhoea which is sometimes so severe that the drug has to be withdrawn. Occasionally a much more severe colitis develops and this has been the cause of a

Novobiocin

Streptomyces and *Actinomyces* respectively. They are no longer used and none need mourn their departure from the antibiotic scene.

LINCOMYCIN AND CLINDAMYCIN

Lincomycin (Lincocin, Mycivin), which is obtained from *Streptomyces lincolnensis* (found in Lincoln, Nebraska) resembles the erythromycins in its mode of action and spectrum of antibacterial activity. However, lincomycin does not attack organisms of the *Haemophilus* and *Neisseria* groups although these are sensitive to erythromycin, while *Mycoplasma hominis* responds to lincomycin but not to the macrolide. Lincomycin can be taken by mouth and is only partly excreted in the urine. Even after intramuscular or intravenous injection, lincomycin appears largely in the

number of fatalities. Skin rashes, urticaria, itching and a variety of minor gastrointestinal upsets have also been reported from time to time.

Lincomycin first appeared in 1963 and clindamycin, a synthetic derivative, was introduced some four years later. Clindamycin is the more readily absorbed from the gastrointestinal tract and its antibacterial activity is much greater than that of lincomycin. It is given orally in doses of 150 mg three times daily not necessarily between meals. Its plasma half life (about 2.5 hr) is shorter than that of lincomycin, the drug being metabolized to a considerable extent. The principal urinary metabolites (which are also found in the bile) are N-demethylated and sulphoxide derivatives.

Clindamycin is no less (or more) toxic than its parent

although its more rapid and complete absorption from the alimentary tract (which otherwise confers on it a distinct therapeutic advantage) demands the exercise of care when the drug is first given if toxic effects are to be avoided. This apart, there seems to be no valid reason why clindamycin's manifest superiority should not result in its completely supplanting lincomycin as a therapeutic agent.

Proprietary names for clindamycin include Dalacin C and Clinimycin.

POLYPEPTIDES

In respect of their biological origin (which is from bacteria and not moulds) and chemical structure, the polypeptide antibiotics form a homogeneous group. The individual members, however, have different antibacterial activities and modes of action.

TYROTHRICIN

This substance is included here largely out of historical respect for an antibiotic that was in clinical use as long ago as 1940. Its success was one of the factors that redirected attention to the therapeutic potentialities of penicillin, then a substance of no more than academic interest notwithstanding Fleming's early attempts to exploit its properties to promote the healing of infected wounds.

Tyrothricin was isolated in 1939 by Dubos from a soil dwelling organism *Bacillus brevis*. It is a mixture of gramicidin and tyrocidine. Gramicidin itself is made up of at least four components. In structure, the gramicidins and tyrocidine are cyclic decapeptides. The structure of one of the gramicidins is shown in Fig. 50.9.

Tyrothricin is active against Gram-positive bacteria but it does not affect Gram-negative organisms. It is also inactive against infections caused by mixtures of Gram-positive and Gram-negative organisms. This is because the latter secrete small amounts of cephalin and other phospholipids which completely inhibit the drug's antibacterial activity.

Tyrocidine lyses the bacterial cell membrane because it acts as a detergent. Gramicidin interferes with bacterial growth processes by preventing the phosphorylation of carbohydrates. Thus tyrothricin as a whole is a bacteriostatic substance.

Tyrothricin is a toxic substance which may cause liver

and kidney damage if it is administered systemically. Its only current therapeutic use is for local application to the skin or body cavities. Its proprietary names include Solutricine, Tyordac and Tyroderm. Gramicidin (Gramidin) can be used in place of tyrothricin itself.

BACITRACIN

This antibiotic was discovered in 1945 by Meleney who found that road dirt contaminating a wound harboured an organism (later identified as *Bacillus licheniformis*) which produced a powerful antibiotic. The wounded patient was a girl called Tracey and the antibiotic was therefore named bacitracin.

Bacitracin (Baciguent) is a mixture of at least three similar polypeptides of which bacitracin A (Fig. 50.10) is the most abundant. Its antibacterial activity is directed largely against Gram-positive organisms. Its mode of action is similar to that of penicillin.

Bacitracin, like tyrothricin, can cause serious necrosis of the kidney tubules if it is given systemically, particularly by the intravenous route. It is occasionally employed, by topical application, for the treatment of burns, ulcers, wounds and abscesses infected with mixed organisms. Its sole advantage is that it hardly ever causes hypersensitivity reactions.

THE POLYMYXINS

The polymyxins, which were first isolated in 1947, are obtained from *Bacillus aerosporus* (hence the original—now a proprietary—name, Aerosporin) and from *B. polymyxa*. At least five polymyxins (designated by the letters A to E) are known but only polymyxin B and polymyxin E are suitable for clinical use. To prevent confusion it is usual to call the latter compound colistin. Both polymyxin B and colistin are mixtures of two components (Fig. 50.11).

The polymyxins are cyclic polypeptides but they also incorporate a fatty acid side chain in their molecules. They are active against almost all Gram-negative bacilli (except

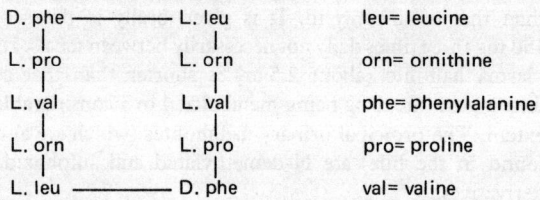

Fig. 50.9 The structure of gramicidin S

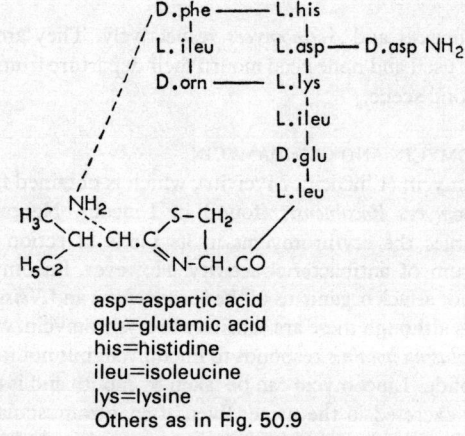

Fig. 50.10 Proposed structure for bacitracin A

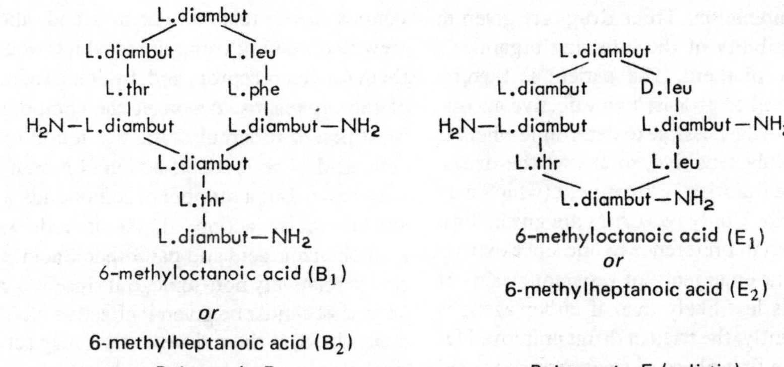

```
                    L.diambut
                    |
        L.diambut   L.leu
        |           |
        L.thr       L.phe
        |           |
H₂N—L.diambut       L.diambut—NH₂
        |
        L.diambut
        |
        L.thr
        |
        L.diambut—NH₂
        |
    6-methyloctanoic acid (B₁)

            or

    6-methylheptanoic acid (B₂)
        Polymyxin B
```

```
                    L.diambut
                    |
        L.diambut   D.leu
        |           |
H₂N—L.diambut       L.diambut—NH₂
        |           |
        L.thr       L.leu
        |
        L.diambut—NH₂
        |
    6-methyloctanoic acid (E₁)
            or
    6-methylheptanoic acid (E₂)

    Polymyxin E (colistin)
```

diambut=diaminobutyric acid; thr=threonine. Others as in Fig. 50.9)

Fig. 50.11 Structures of polymyxins B and E.

the *Proteus* group) but Gram-negative cocci and all Gram-positive microorganisms are not affected. The polymyxins (like tyrothricin and many disinfectants) exhibit surface activity which results in their being able to disrupt cell membranes. The phospholipid content of susceptible organisms is higher than that of resistant bacteria so that they take up the polymyxins more readily.

Polymyxin (Aerosporin) is highly toxic. Like the other polypeptides it may damage the renal tubules but it also exerts a variety of effects on the central nervous system so that the patient may complain of dizziness, ataxia and paraesthesiae affecting particularly the hands and feet. These effects are sufficiently common and serious to militate against the parenteral administration of the drug except in circumstances of dire necessity. These include severe infections of the urinary tract or meninges by Gram-negative organisms (particularly *Pseudomonas*) that are resistant to any other available antibiotic agent or that occur in patients known to react badly to what otherwise would be the first choice drug. Polymyxin B (as the sulphate) is given by intramuscular injection when the urinary tract is infected and by the intrathecal route in meningitis. Intramuscular injection causes considerable pain. Polymyxin can be taken by mouth if intestinal infections have to be treated since it is only poorly absorbed from the gut. It can also be applied topically to infected burns and sores. For this purpose it is sometimes mixed with bacitracin or neomycin.

The toxicity of polymyxin B is such as to demand a very close surveillance of those receiving the drug lest the kidneys be damaged.

Colistin (Colomycin, Coly-Mycin) is much less toxic than polymyxin and it can be given (as the sulphate or the sodium methanesulphonate) by painless intramuscular injection. It is of considerable value for the treatment of meningeal, urinary tract and generalized infections produced by strains of Gram-negative bacilli resistant to other antibiotics, in particular the *Pseudomonas* group. The intramuscular dose of colistin is 75 to 150 mg twice daily. The sulphate (but not the sodium methanesulphonate) can be given intravenously.

OTHER ANTIBIOTICS

Some other antibiotics which are used largely or exclusively for the treatment of tuberculosis are described in the following sections.

THE CHEMOTHERAPY OF TUBERCULOSIS

Until relatively recent years, no really effective anti-tuberculosis drug was available and treatment of the disease was directed towards fortifying the patient's own powers of resistance to the invading organism. This necessitated prolonged sanatorium treatment, the imposition of long periods of complete mental and physical rest in isolation from the patient's family and, frequently, extensive surgery to remove affected areas of the lungs. The advent of effective chemotherapeutic agents has completely changed this picture. The period of hospital treatment has been drastically reduced so that, although treatment is still prolonged, the patient need not be separated from his family for long periods and for most of the time it is usually possible for him to stay at work. Apart from streptomycin, which is usually only given in the early stages of treatment, the effective drugs are all active by mouth so that self medication is a simple matter. The psychological effects associated with a form of treatment which enables the patient to follow a more or less normal life cannot be exaggerated. They cannot but assist the curative processes initiated by the drugs.

There is general agreement concerning the chemotherapeutic regime which must be instituted in the treatment of tuberculosis. For the first three months or so, three drugs are given in combination. Three drugs are given to guard against the possibility of the infecting organism's being resistant to one of them. The patient is thereby assured of being exposed to at least two effective agents. During this period it will be possible to determine whether he is resistant, or unduly sensitive, to any of the drugs. Thereafter, and for the duration of treatment (which may last for two or more years), only two drugs are given. Two effective drugs are given in preference to one since experience has shown that the emergence of resistant strains of the tubercle bacillus is less likely than if either agent is given alone. Until recently, the triad of drugs employed (at least in Britain) for the first phase of treatment consisted almost invariably of streptomycin, p-aminosalicylic acid and isoniazid with the two last-named members of the trio providing the necessary pair of drugs for the remainder of the treatment period. If the infecting organism was resistant to one of the pair, the ineffective agent was replaced by streptomycin. This regimen is still followed in appropriate cases but the range of useful drugs has increased in recent years. The most valuable of the newer agents are ethambutol and rifampicin. Either can be used instead of p-aminosalicylic acid and with a smaller risk of causing unpleasant side effects or they can be used together to provide the drug combination needed for the second phase of treatment. Other new drugs, which have a place in the treatment of infections caused by organisms that are resistant to one or more of the more usual agents, include capreomycin, cycloserine, ethionamide, pyrazinamide and viomycin. Thiacetazone also falls into this category but its particular value is seen in those poor countries where tuberculosis is still widespread. It has the great advantage of being cheap.

All forms of the disease—pulmonary tuberculosis, tuberculous meningitis, genito-urinary and acute miliary tuberculosis—yield to combined drug therapy of the kind outlined.

STREPTOMYCIN
The properties and uses of streptomycin have already been described (p. 834).

PARA-AMINOSALICYLIC ACID
In 1940, Bernheim noted that the oxygen uptake of the tubercle bacillus was increased by salicylates and benzoates. It seemed likely that the organism was using them as metabolites. Lehman later investigated the effect on the metabolism of the tubercle bacillus of a number of compounds closely related to benzoic and salicylic acids with a view to obtaining compounds which would compete with them for cell receptors and, by doing so, inhibit the growth of the organisms. Amongst the compounds studied, the most potent tuberculostatic was found to be p-aminosalicylic acid. The mode of action of p-aminosalicylic acid is not known, but a number of compounds will antagonize its antitubercular action. These include salicylic acid, p-aminobenzoic acid and pantothenic acid. p-Aminosalicylic acid is relatively non-toxic, but since it is rapidly excreted, large doses must be given if effective blood levels are to be maintained; at these dose levels it may act as a gastrointestinal irritant and cause diarrhoea, nausea, vomiting and loss of appetite. There may also be sensitization reactions. These most commonly take the form of itchy rashes but more serious reactions sometimes occur and there have been reports of deaths from acute liver failure in patients who have taken the drug.

p-Aminosalicylic acid has an antithyroid action and, although the condition is a very rare complication, symptoms of hypothyroidism must be carefully looked for in patients undergoing long-term treatment with the drug. The hypothyroidism yields easily to thyroxine. Resistance to p-aminosalicylic acid may develop but the risk of this occurring is a good deal less than with streptomycin. The free acid is not well tolerated in the large doses which must be given and the sodium and calcium salts are usually used. The total daily dosage of the sodium salt is 10-15 g divided into three or four doses. It is sometimes presented in cachets made of rice paper which are dipped in water and then immediately swallowed. We have seen that, at least until recently, the preferred drug combination for the second phase of tuberculosis therapy has been p-aminosalicylic acid and isoniazid. It is essential that one drug should not be taken without the other and in order to ensure this, cachets containing both drugs are available. Their proprietary names include Pycasix, Pasinan and Inapasade. They need to be taken twice daily but Inapasade S.Q contains a daily dose (12 g of p-aminosalicylic acid and 300 mg of isoniazid) in a single packet. It seems that satisfactory plasma levels of the two drugs are maintained round the clock if Inapasade S.Q. is taken once daily.

The days of p-aminosalicylic acid as a preferred agent for the treatment of tuberculosis are numbered, at least in developed countries.

ISONIAZID
In 1952, workers in America and in Germany showed independently that isoniazid (isonicotinic acid hydrazide) inhibited the growth of the tubercle bacillus *in vitro* and had powerful antitubercular activity when used to treat experimental tuberculosis in laboratory animals. Chemically isoniazid bears some resemblance to thiacetazone (see below) and to the hydrazide of p-aminosalicylic acid but it probably acts as an antimetabolite and by so doing inhibits

COOH

OH

NH_2

Para-amino
salicylic acid

$$O$$
$$\overset{\parallel}{C}-NH-NH_2$$

Isoniazid

the functioning of essential enzyme systems in the bacteria. It is known that very low concentrations of isoniazid inhibit mycolase synthetase, an enzyme that is specific to mycobacteria and which is involved in the synthesis of mycolic acid, itself an essential component of *Mycobacterium tuberculosis* (Takayama, Wang and David, 1972). However the antimetabolic action of isoniazid extends to other enzyme systems and its therapeutic effectiveness is not necessarily entirely attributable to its being able to inhibit mycolase synthetase (McDonald, 1974).

Isoniazid is probably the most potent antitubercular compound available. Mycobacteria resistant to isoniazid are occasionally encountered in previously untreated patients living in poorly developed areas of the world but primary resistance of this type is extremely rare in more affluent regions where the cases of isoniazid resistance that do occur have usually to be classified as 'secondary' or 'acquired' and are the result of exposure to an inappropriate concentration of the drug. There is no cross resistance between isoniazid, *p*-aminosalicylic acid and streptomycin.

Isopropylisoniazid (iproniazid) was also used for a time as an antituberculosis drug but it had to be discarded because of its tendency to induce behavioural excitement. It is now known only as an antidepressant drug (p. 578).

The total daily dose of isoniazid is normally 300 mg but the treatment of very ill patients sometimes demands higher doses than this.

In the second phase of the tuberculosis treatment programme, two drugs have to be taken for periods of up to two years or more. Many patients, through forgetfulness, indolence or a careless disregard of their own welfare, fail to adhere to a treatment regimen that demands their having to take drugs once or twice daily. Recently some attention has been given to the practicability of intermittent treatment schedules that require drugs to be taken only twice or even once weekly. So far as isoniazid is concerned the recommended dose for intermittent therapy is 30 mg per kilogram once weekly or half that amount taken twice weekly. The position is complicated by the fact that the potential patient population is divided into two groups. the slow and the rapid inactivators of isoniazid (p. 73). If isoniazid is given only once weekly it is difficult to sustain an effectively antibacterial concentration of drug in the blood of rapid acetylators and this encourages the development of drug resistance in the infecting organisms. On the other hand, toxic reactions may be precipitated in slow inactivators. Intermittent therapy will probably not be completely successful until more adequate slow-release preparations have been developed but even then it will be difficult to escape the obligation to determine, before intermittent chemotherapy is embarked on, whether the patient is a slow or a rapid inactivator of isoniazid. The rate of inactivation does not appear to influence the clinical effectiveness of isoniazid given once or twice daily. It seems almost superfluous to add that there is little point in attempting to give one drug at infrequent intervals unless its chosen partner can be given in the same way.

Isoniazid is given alone, in daily doses of 5-10 mg per kilogram as a prophylactic against tuberculosis in subjects at risk. Treatment has to be continued for one year.

Isoniazid is rapidly absorbed from the gastrointestinal tract but antacids like aluminium hydroxide gell interfere with the absorption processes and should not be taken during the one hour period following the ingestion of isoniazid.

Isoniazid is excreted in the urine as the free compound, an acetylated derivative and hydrazones. Slow and rapid inactivators differ only in the effectiveness of their acetylation processes. The most common side effects of isoniazid therapy are a peripheral neuropathy, mental changes and hepatitis.

The first two complications are particularly likely to occur in slow inactivators. Toxic actions on the peripheral nerves result in sensations of burning, pricking or numbness in the limbs—'burning feet' is a very common complaint. The peripheral neuropathy is probably due to a deficiency of pyridoxine (vitamin B_6) since isoniazid treatment increases the urinary excretion of the vitamin. The administration of vitamin B_6 will prevent the development of toxic changes in the nerves but since it antagonizes the action of isoniazid, minimal doses must be given: 6 mg per day appears to be adequate (Fox, 1965). Other components of the vitamin B complex (pantothenic acid and aneurin) and glutamic acid have also been used in attempts to prevent or cure the peripheral neuropathy but they have not been particularly successful. The cerebral side effects of isoniazid therapy include major epileptiform seizures and toxic psychoses. They too yield to small doses of pyridoxine. The relationship of isoniazid seizures to γ-aminobutyric acid in the brain is discussed elsewhere (p. 191).

Liver damage is a less rare complication of isoniazid therapy than was at one time believed. It apparently occurs in about one per cent of those who receive the drug (Black 1974) but the incidence is greater than this in those over 35 and in regular drinkers. Isoniazid treatment should be discontinued at once if overt signs of hepatitis appear.

In laboratory animals, isoniazid is carcinogenic. It can cause lung cancer and stimulate the growth of implanted tumours. These rather alarming findings do not yet seem to have caused anxiety among the users of isoniazid.

Isoniazid and rifampicin (below) are available in combined preparations (Rifinah, Rimactazid) analogous to the mixtures of isoniazid and *p*-aminosalicylic acid to which reference has already been made (p. 846). Isoniazid itself is marketed under a number of proprietary names which include Nydrazid, Pycazide, Rimifon, and Vazadrine.

RIFAMPICIN

Rifampicin (rifampin, rifaldazine) is the most successful of a series of semi-synthetic derivatives (500 in all!) of a new antibiotic (rifamycin) obtained from *Streptomyces mediterranei*. It is active against a range of bacteria but it has achieved its greatest therapeutic success as an antituberculosis drug. Rifampicin in association with isoniazid (with, of course, a third drug—streptomycin or ethambutol—in the early phase of treatment) is now highly favoured in those countries that can afford this still expensive substance.

The usual daily oral dose of rifampicin is 600 mg (10 mg per kilogram for children) given in one to three instalments but twice-weekly doses, each of 900 mg, are equally effective. Attempts to institute intermittent treatment programmes in which the drug was given at even more widely spaced intervals proved unsuccessful by reason of the side effects induced by the larger single doses that these schedules demanded.

Rifampicin is readily absorbed from the gastrointestinal tract and much of it is deacetylated in the liver. The metabolite, which retains a considerable amount of antibacterial activity is excreted in the bile into the intestine. Some of it is reabsorbed to appear again in the bile. The amounts of metabolite that escape reabsorption in successive turns of the bile cycle represent a total of 60 to 65 per cent of the initial dose. They appear in the faeces. The remainder of the metabolite (and some unchanged rifampicin) is excreted in the urine. Rifampicin is extensively bound (about 80 per cent of a normal dose) to plasma proteins.

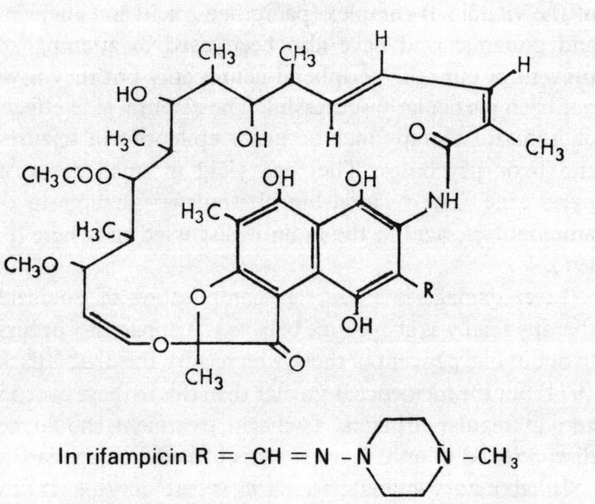

Provided that the recommended doses are adhered to, rifampicin is a safe drug and reports of adverse side effects have usually related only to one or two cases. Moreover it is generally agreed that some of the toxic responses in those taking rifampicin may well have to be attributed to the other member of the pair of drugs to which the patients have been exposed. Isoniazid in particular is a less innocuous drug than was once believed (p. 847). On the other hand, it must be remembered that rifampicin is still a relatively new drug and a more realistic appraisal of its safety waits on more extensive clinical experience. The side effects that have been reported include a thrombocytopenia of immunological origin (this was the major complication seen in patients given high doses of rifampicin in a once-weekly treatment programme), liver damage, acute but reversible renal failure and rashes. High doses of rifampicin (100 mg per kilogram) are teratogenic in rats and mice and pregnancy constitutes a contraindication to the use of the drug.

Rifampicin inhibits the synthesis of RNA by bacteria. It does not have this effect in man because of the lower sensitivity of the human version of the enzyme (RNA polymerase) that is affected by rifampicin.

Rifampicin has also been used in the treatment of leprosy and some infections by straphylococci resistant to the more usual antibiotics. Rifamide (Rifocin; Fig. 50.12) has no place in tuberculosis therapy: it is employed in the treatment of cholecystitis. Proprietary names for rifampicin include Rifadin and Rimactane. The drug is also available in a combined preparation with isoniazid.

ETHAMBUTOL

One of the newest antituberculosis drugs, ethambutol (Myambutol, Mynah) was first discovered in 1961 but it has only recently won popularity. It was found in the course of a screening programme in which a variety of synthetic compounds was tested for possible antituberculosis activity. It is a highly specific antibiotic, its only antibacterial activity being that exhibited towards mycobacteria which are extremely susceptible to it.

Like rifampicin, ethambutol can substitute for *p*-aminosalicylic acid and it is increasingly being employed for this purpose. As we have already noted (p. 846), rifampicin and

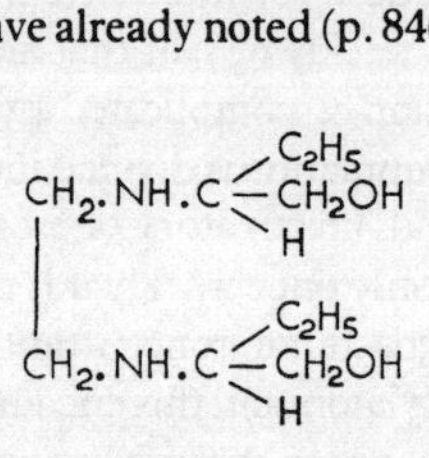

In rifampicin R = -CH = N - N⟨   ⟩N -CH₃

In rifamide R = -O.CH₂.CON(C₂H₅)₂

Fig. 50.12 Some rifamycin derivatives

Ethambutol

ethambutol are rapidly acquiring the status of the most favoured pair of drugs for tuberculosis therapy.

Ethambutol is active when taken by mouth and it is given (together with one or two other drugs according to the customary procedure) in daily doses of 1.5 g (15 mg per kilogram of body mass) reducing, after two months, to one g. Some recent clinical investigators have reported favourably on the results of giving the drug once weekly in amounts that approach four times the normal daily dose.

Ethambutol is rapidly excreted in the urine, 80 per cent of it in the unchanged form.

Ethambutol is a safe drug provided that recommended dose schedules are followed. Retrobulbar neuritis (an inflammation of the optic nerve) may occur with high doses. The main symptoms of the condition are blurred vision and a red-green colour blindness which usually does not persist provided that drug administration is stopped as soon as the symptoms appear. It is wise to instruct patients to report at once any ocular symptom they experience. A less common side effect (which is likewise associated with too high an intake of ethambutol) is peripheral neuritis. Very occasionally, sodium urate accumulates in the blood during treatment with ethambutol.

Ethambutol is probably an antimetabolite that inhibits the synthesis of bacterial RNA.

THI(O)ACETAZONE

This compound (which is also known as amithiozone) is a thiosemicarbazone which is chemically related to some of the heterocyclic sulphonamides as will be made clear by reference to Fig 50.13.

Thiacetazone has had a somewhat chequered history. In 1947, Domagk (of sulphonamide fame) found that thiacetazone was very active against the tubercle bacillus. It was introduced into clinical practice but because of toxic side effects the drug was soon abandoned. More recently, thiacetazone has been reintroduced and a number of thorough therapeutic trials have been carried out in Africa and India. It has now been established that thiacetazone is as effective and can be as safe a drug as *p*-aminosalicylic acid. It has proved to be a boon in many poor countries with a need for large quantities of cheap drugs. In more

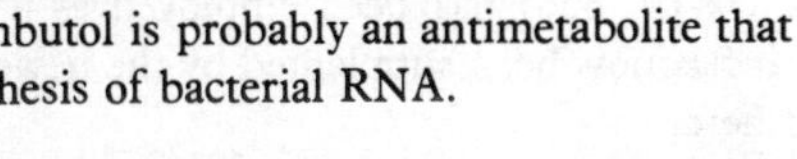

Thiacetazone

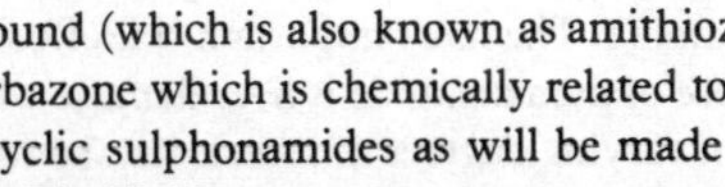

Sulphathiazole

Fig. 50.13 Structural similarities between thiacetazone and sulphathiazole

economically healthy communities, its use is generally restricted to the treatment of cases that have proved resistant to the more usual range of drugs.

Toxic side effects of thiacetazone treatment include nausea, vomiting, agranulocytosis and hepatitis. In addition, ototoxicity (which manifests itself as dizziness, tinnitus and perhaps deafness) is sometimes seen. Moreover, thiacetazone can potentiate streptomycin ototoxicity and it is important to remember the heightened possibility of eighth nerve damage when the two drugs are given together. Rashes can constitute a further complication but the incidence of this side effect varies from country to country. It is, fortunately, rare in Africa and India (where the drug has to be widely used) but its incidence among the Chinese is sufficiently high to preclude its administration to members of this race. These differences may have an environmental rather than a genetic basis so that a Chinese patient living in Africa might be no more likely than a native African to develop a drug rash in response to thiacetazone treatment.

It is easy to give a toxic overdose of thiacetazone (and of the other drugs described in this section) because many patients in Africa are very small. It is, therefore, better to quote the daily dose of thiacetazone in terms of body weight (2 to 2.5 mg per kilogram) although, as is pointed out elsewhere (p. 72), this way of expressing dosage is, for patients in affluent countries usually less precise than might appear at first sight.

Proprietary names for thiacetazone include Berculon A, Conteben, Neustab, Seroden, Thioparamizone, TBI and Tibione.

OTHER DRUGS

The substances to be described in the following paragraphs occupy only a lowly place in the hierarchy of antituberculosis drugs, being generally less effective and much more toxic than the first-line drugs that have been our concern up to this point. As reserve drugs, they are conscripted only to fight infections by organisms that exhibit primary or secondary resistance (p. 851) towards the more favoured chemotherapeutic agents. Primarily resistant strains of mycobacteria are most frequently encountered in the developing countries where the reserve drugs find their principal field of application.

Capreomycin. Capreomycin (which was first isolated in 1960 from *Streptomyces capreolus*) is a mixture of four cyclic polypeptides. Its antibacterial activity is directed against mycobacteria alone so that in this respect capreomycin resembles ethambutol. Like streptomycin, it has to be given by intramuscular injection and this constitutes an obvious disadvantage in a drug that has to be given over a long period of time. The initial dose is about one gram daily reducing, in the second phase of treatment, to one gram twice weekly. The drug is excreted in the urine, to a large extent in an unchanged form. The most serious side effects of capreomycin treatment are kidney damage and ototoxicity and blood dyscrasias have also been reported.

Capreomycin has been used in combination with ethionamide or ethambutol. It is supplied in the form of its sulphate as Capastat.

Cycloserine. Cycloserine (Oxamycin, Seromycin) is synthesized by *Streptomyces orchidaceous* and *S. garyphalus*. The oral dose range is from a half to one gram daily. Cycloserine has also been used for the treatment of urinary tract infections; it is one of the best available drugs for the treatment of *Escherichia coli* infections of the kidney. When employed for this purpose it is given in only half the dose that is considered appropriate for the treatment of tuberculosis and adverse reactions to it are less likely to occur.

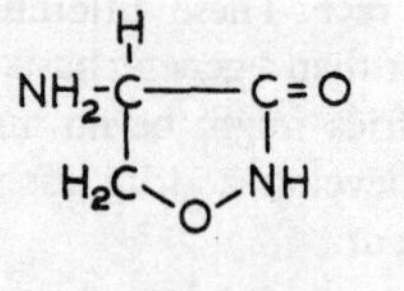

Cycloserine

Side effects may be serious and appear to be due mainly to effects upon the central nervous system. They include drowsiness, excitement, depression, mental confusion and epileptiform attacks. Skin rashes have also been seen. Patients with impaired kidney function or a history of epilepsy or mental illness are not suitable for therapy with cycloserine. Side effects are much reduced if the daily dose is divided and well spaced out and if the concentration of cycloserine in the blood is maintained below 25 μg per millilitre.

Cycloserine inhibits the synthesis of bacterial cell walls by a mechanism different from that which underlies the antibacterial action of the penicillins.

Ethionamide and prothionamide. Ethionamide (Trecator, Trescatyl, Trescazide) is a synthetic compound. It possesses twice the potency of streptomycin but it is less effective than isoniazid with which it has some structural affinity. It is active in daily oral doses of a half to one gram but adverse side effects occur frequently. The gastrointestinal tract is most commonly affected and it has been said that a degree of nausea, vomiting and diarrhoea occur in

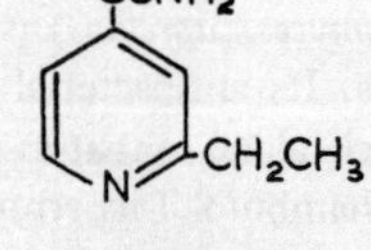

Ethionamide

the majority of those who receive ethionamide (Schwartz, 1966). Liver damage, peripheral neuritis and a variety of mental changes similar to those induced by high doses of cycloserine have also been reported. High doses of ethion-

amide are teratogenic in animals and pregnancy is a contraindication to its use.

In prothionamide (Trevintix) the ethyl group ($-CH_2.CH_3$) of ethionamide is replaced by the *n*-propyl radical ($-CH_2.CH_2.CH_3$). The actions, properties and uses of prothionamide and ethionamide are in every way similar except that prothionamide has a slightly lower toxicity.

Isoxyl. This drug has not achieved the popularity that was expected and it is now rarely used. The daily dose is 6 grams.

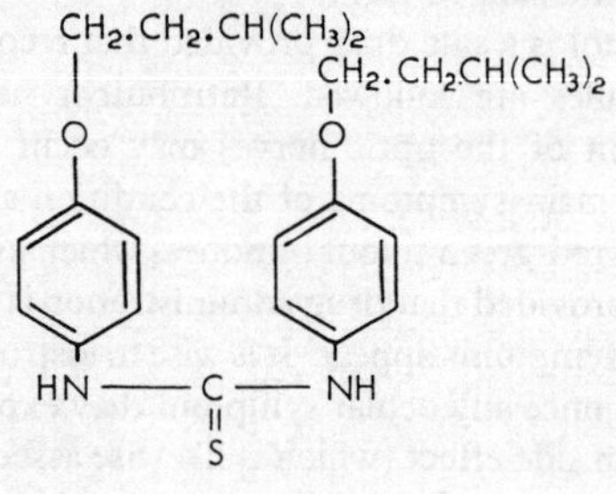

Isoxyl

Kanamycin (p. 836) has been employed as a reserve drug but it has now been supplanted by the newer drugs described here.

Pyrazinamide This is another compound closely related to nicotinamide. The most important side effect associated with the use of pyrazinamide is liver damage which causes jaundice of varying degrees of severity in about 10 per cent of patients. The possible occurrence of liver damage poses a serious problem when the drug is used in under-developed countries in which facilities for detecting liver damage (such as by estimating the activity of serum glutamic-oxaloacetic transaminase) may not be available. The dose of pyrazinamide is one gram twice daily. It can also be given, with no increase in toxicity, in once-weekly doses of 6 grams (90 mg per kilogram body mass).

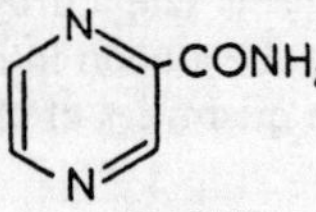

Pyrazinamide

Pyrazinamide is a drug of relatively low potency and resistance to it develops rapidly. Its proprietary names are Aldinamide and Zinamide.

Viomycin. Viomycin is obtained from a number of species of *Streptomyces*. Toxic effects include damage to the eighth cranial nerve, kidney damage and allergic reactions. The daily dose of viomycin is one gram. It is given by intramuscular injection, but its high toxicity precludes its being used in all but the most exceptional circumstances.

OTHER ANTIBACTERIAL SUBSTANCES

A large number of other substances are capable of destroying pathogenic microorganisms (including viruses) although they do not necessarily eliminate bacterial spores. Many of them find employment as *disinfectants*—substances which remove bacterial contaminants from objects (such as dishes and bed pans) used in sick rooms or from infected buildings and equipment in farms or other places where there has been contagious disease among animals. Some of these antibacterial substances can also be applied to the skin, to surface wounds or to the mucous surface of the gastrointestinal tract while those which are readily excreted by the kidney may also, if they have a low systemic toxicity, be administered with the aim of clearing the urinary tract of an infecting organism. Antibacterial substances applied to the living body in these ways are usually described as *antiseptics*.

Disinfectants and antiseptics as such are of minimal interest to pharmacologists but some of them are of service in the treatment of diseases caused by several types of non-bacterial organisms. Those used as intestinal or urinary antiseptics also merit a brief mention.

In the first-named category are included the furan derivatives (nitrofurazone, nitrofurantoin and furazolidone) and propamidine. Their clinical applications are discussed elsewhere in this book.

Nalidixic acid

Methenamine mandelate

Urinary antiseptics include mandelic acid and the mandelates such as methenamine (hexamine) mandelate (Mandelamine, Mandelurine), hexylresorcinol, nalidixic acid (NegGram, Wintomylon) and nitrofurantoin. Chlorhexidine (Hibitane) can be given with neomycin to rid the intestine of microorganisms before surgery and for application to surface wounds.

SOME GENERAL ASPECTS OF ANTIMICROBIAL ACTIVITY

In the course of this chapter we have had occasion to make repeated mention of two topics that relate to all the groups of drugs that have appeared for discussion. These two topics are bacterial resistance and the mode of action of antimicrobial agents and it seems appropriate that the disparate comments that have been made on these matters should now be brought together, co-ordinated and discussed in rather more detail with the aim of providing the reader with a cohesive summary of these important aspects of antimicrobial action.

Bacterial resistance

Bacteria are the most adaptable of organisms, a feature that ensures that a species will survive the hostile environment created by the presence of an antibiotic agent even though many individual members of the species have to perish before the line is safely reestablished. From the point of view of those who seek to conquer bacterial disease in man and animals, this adaptation appears as drug resistance and much of the history of the development of antibiotic drugs is the story of a struggle to produce new agents before their predecessors have been rendered useless by the appearance of resistance in their erstwhile victims.

The development of resistance to antibacterial agents has been hastened by such iatrogenic factors as the over-zealous use of the drugs (so that bacteria have been provided more often than they need have been with the conditions that encourage the proliferation of resistant forms) and the resort to unsatisfactory dosage schedules that fail to deliver the necessary 'overkill' that would ensure the elimination of all the sensitive organisms in the target area. Organisms that are permitted to escape such an ineffective attack are ripe for the acquisition of resistance. Although these facts are undeniable, it is important that the reader should appreciate at the outset that populations of bacteria that have never previously been exposed to a particular antibacterial agent are likely to contain some resistant individuals. In at least some instances, the appearance of resistance to a drug has predated the discovery of the drug itself. We can be sure, for example, that penicillin resistant organisms lay in wait for the new antibiotic. They were able, when the necessity arose, to father populations of resistant bacteria and this would have happened (albeit later than it did) even if the antibiotic had been used with the care that prudence should have dictated.

Although there is experimental evidence for the view that bacterial cells can acquire resistance by simple adaptation to the presence of a drug in their enviroment, most authorities would agree that bacteria usually develop resistance as a result of random mutations. Mutations are, of course, rare events in the sense that they occur no more often than once every million cell divisions. Nevertheless, these rare events operating among the teeming millions of a rapidly growing population of bacterial cells can soon produce a considerable number of mutants some of which will be drug resistant.

Organisms that have acquired a resistance to agents to which they have never been exposed are generally among the less successful members of their community since they are burdened by the necessity of maintaining mechanisms that serve no useful purpose. They only come into their own in the presence of the drug that is attacking their sensitive fellows but to which they themselves are immune.

Drug resistant mutants can, of course, give rise to resistant offspring by the normal process of cell division but they can also transmit their resistance to previously sensitive cells by the processes of transduction, conjugation and, perhaps, transcription. The existence of these mechanisms clearly extends the cell's opportunities for spreading its resistance.

Transduction

Bacteriophages (more often called phages) are virus-like particles that infect bacteria and in so doing may incorporate into their own substance part of the host's genetic material. The modified phage reproduces itself and its offspring escape from the now dead host to infect other bacteria. The new hosts receive the genetic material derived from the organism that was infected in the first place. The modified phages are less virulent than their parents and they do not necessarily kill the bacteria they infect. If the material they transfer contains genes that determine drug resistance the infected cells (and their offspring) will also acquire resistance.

The material transferred by the transduction process is occasionally derived from chromosomes but more usually it takes the form of *plasmids*. Plasmids are extrachromosomal particles of genetic material (DNA).

Phage transduction can occur in both Gram-negative and Gram-positive organisms. Plasmids containing genes that determine drug resistance are found particularly in *Staphylococcus aureus* in relation to resistance to penicillin, chloramphenicol, tetracyclines and erythromycin. They have also been detected in some streptococci.

The rapid development of resistant staphylococci in the hospital environment is probably the result of phage transduction.

Conjugation

Some Gram-negative bacteria can conjugate with other members of the same or a related species by a process that is reminiscent of sexual union. The 'male' member of each pair carries a hair-like projection known as the *sex pilus* which comes into contact with its partner, which lacks a pilus. The conjugation bridge so formed permits the passage of plasmid DNA from the 'male' to the 'female' cell. Plasmids that can be transferred in this way are described as *transmissible*. They are of several closely similar types: fertility (F) plasmids convert 'female' into 'male' cells so that they in their turn can transfer material

into other 'female' cells; colicinogenic plasmids confer on bacteria the ability to produce bactericidal substances known as *bacteriocins* while drug resistance plasmids (the so-called R factors) direct the production of resistant organisms.

Not all plasmids can be transferred by conjugation. In particular, Gram-positive organisms cannot form conjugal pairs and the drug resistance plasmids carried, for instance, by resistant strains of *Staph. aureus* and which, as we have seen, are carried from cell to cell by phage transduction, are said to be non-transmissible.

Transfer of drug resistance by conjugation occurs in many members of the Enterobacteriaceae family (*Escherichia, Klebsiella, Salmonella, Shingella, Pseudomonas*, etc.) and leads to the development of bacterial strains resistant to sulphonamides, penicillin, chloramphenicol, streptomycin, tetracyclines and a number of other antibiotic agents.

Transformation

Under experimental conditions it is possible, with certain bacterial species, to transfer the special properties of the members of one group of organisms to others of the same species that lack these properties. The transfer vehicle is purified DNA extracted from the donor cells and the classical example of this procedure is the conversion of 'rough' noncapsulated pneumococci into 'smooth' capsulated forms. This transformation also occurs naturally in populations of infecting pneumococci and there is no theoretical reason why a similar process should not lead to the transformation of sensitive into resistant bacteria particularly since this change can be effected in the laboratory. As yet, however, there is no solid experimental evidence that this mechanism—which would in any event be a most inefficient one—operates to produce resistant strains in populations of infecting organisms exposed to antibiotic drugs.

THE MECHANISMS OF DRUG RESISTANCE

Having surveyed the means whereby drug resistance can be disseminated among populations of previously sensitive organisms, we can now enquire into the nature of the changes that enable resistant organisms to withstand an onslaught by antimicrobial drugs. The reader will not be surprised to learn that a number of mechanisms operate, that some are more widely used than others and that bacterial species differ from one another in the number and nature of the mechanisms they make use of. Franklin and Snow (1971), following Davis, have enumerated seven possible mechanisms of drug resistance. These will emerge in the course of the following discussion.

1. Some resistant organisms elaborate enzymes that inactivate the antimicrobial drug. The best known example of this mechanism is provided by penicillin-resistant organisms which, as we have already noted (p. 824),

produce penicillinase (ß-lactamase), an enzyme that opens the ß-lactam ring. Other resistant organisms may produce penicillin amidase (p. 825).

Penicillin resistance arises in *Staph. aureus* and *E. coli*, among many other bacterial species. As we have already noted, that in the staphylococci is determined by genetic material in non-transmissible plasmids whereas that in *E. coli* is associated with a transmissible R-factor. Nevertheless, the resistance of both species is attributable to penicillinase.

Other examples of enzyme dependent resistance include the acetylation of chloramphenicol (by chloramphenicol acetyltransferase) and the inactivation of aminoglycoside antibiotics by a number of enzymes that develop in resistant organisms. The reactions involved include phosphorylation, adenylation and acetylation. There is no evidence that any aminoglycoside resistant bacterium makes use of more than one of these enzyme systems.

2. An alternative to destroying an antimicrobial agent is to deny it access to its site of action. This can be done by reducing the permeability of the organism to the drug. The walls of Gram-negative bacteria have an external lipoprotein coat which is not found in Gram-positive organisms. This reduces the sensitivity of Gram-negative organisms in general to antimicrobial drugs and it is easy to see that an increase in the thickness, or a change in the composition, of the external layer could easily convert a sensitive bacterium into a resistant one. It seems that changes of this kind account for the development of ampicillin resistance in *E. coli* and in *Salmonella typhimurium* and of streptomycin and erythromycin resistance in pneumococci.

Some antimicrobial agents gain access to the bacterial cell by making use of the transport systems provided for the transfer of essential nutrients into the cell. Interference with these systems could lead to the exclusion from the cell of the drugs that use them. The resistance of *E. coli* to cycloserine and of *E. coli*, *Staph. aureus* and other organisms to the tetracyclines probably arises in this way.

3. Even if an antimicrobial drug does penetrate into the bacterial cell, its mission can still be thwarted if the site at which it should act undergoes structural changes that prevent the proper apposition of drug and target. Streptomycin and other aminoglycoside antibiotics have ribosomal sites of action (p. 854) and trivial changes in the composition of the ribosomal proteins are sufficient to confer immunity to antibiotic attack. This kind of adaptation certainly underlies the resistance of many organisms to this group of antibiotics. A somewhat similar situation arises with the sulphonamides. In sensitive organisms these drugs, as we have seen (p. 819), compete with *p*-aminobenzoic acid for tetrahydropteroic acid synthetase. In resistant organisms, structural changes in the enzyme have reduced its affinity for sulphonamides while leaving it with an unchanged affinity for the physiological substrate.

4. The remaining putative mechanisms of drug resistance are much less important than those we have just considered. They can be dismissed briefly.

a. Some organisms that have become resistant to sulphonamides are able to acquire larger concentrations of *p*-aminobenzoic acid which therefore compete more effectively with the drugs for tetrahydropteroic acid synthetase.

b. A similar end could be achieved by elaborating more enzyme rather than more substrate and this seems to be one of the manoeuvres adopted by cells that become resistant to amethopterin (p. 000). Some resistant species have developed the ability to synthesize dihydrofolate reductase far more effectively than their sensitive brethren.

c. An organism may be able to produce such vital substances as the nucleic acids along more than one synthetic pathway. One of these pathways will normally be dominant while the other (or others) will serve in a reserve capacity. If an antibiotic agent relies for its efficacy on an ability to interrupt the normally dominant pathway, organisms exposed to it may be able to achieve resistance by opening up a reserve pathway.

Mode of action of antibacterial agents

Chemotherapeutic agents should, ideally, destroy or immobilize invading organisms and yet leave the host completely unharmed. This will happen if the drugs act on mechanisms that are represented in bacteria but not in their mammalian hosts. This state of affairs exists, as we have seen, with the sulphonamides and the penicillins. The former inhibit a unique bacterial process—the synthesis of folic acid—and the latter prevent the production of a unique bacterial structure, the cell wall. The toxic effects of the drugs in man are attributable to actions that are not related to their special properties.

We have already discussed (p. 827) the nature of the bacterial cell wall and the effect on it of the penicillins and the cephalosporins. Other antibiotics that prevent the proper construction of the cell wall include cycloserine, bacitracin and vancomycin. They all operate at an earlier stage in the building process than does penicillin.

Synthesis of glycan strands begins with the conversion of L -alanine into the dextrorotatory isomer and the union of pairs of the newly formed amino-acids to form dipeptides. Both these processes are inhibited by cycloserine.

Each pair of dipeptides is linked with three more aminoacids to form the pentapeptides that are originally attached to acetylmuramic acid (p. 827). The new complex is united with acetylglucosamine and the five-glycine chain. The whole is then transported by a phospholipid carrier to the site where it is needed. The complex is liberated and the carrier re-forms so that it can return for a further load of the complex from which the glycan strands will be assembled. Vancomycin prevents the release of the complex from its carrier while bacitracin interferes with the regeneration of the carrier itself.

The final stage in the construction of the complete mucopeptide molecule involves the establishment of cross linkages with the aid of energy released by the conversion of the original pentapeptide side chains into tetrapeptides. It is this conversion that is prevented by penicillin and the cephalosporins.

A number of antibiotic agents influence the permeability of the cell *membrane* without affecting the structure of the wall. The membrane is found inside the wall and it is not, of course, a structure unique to bacterial cells. Antibiotics that owe their therapeutic action to a more or less specific effect on the bacterial cell membrane include polymyxin B, tyrothricin, nystatin, colistin and novobiocin. Their concentration at the bacterial rather than the host's cell membrane is attributable to differences in chemical composition among membranes in different species. Some antibiotics, however, are less selective in their choice of targets and for this reason they cannot be used clinically.

The folic acid of bacterial cells is destined (as it is in other organisms) for conversion into cofactors necessary for the synthesis of nucleic acids and antimicrobial agents may intervene in the chain of events initiated by folic acid, even if they do not inhibit its synthesis. Trimethoprim prevents the conversion of folic into folinic acid, nalidixic acid arrests the replication of DNA and the rifamycins operate similarly against RNA. None of the three last mentioned processes is unique to the bacterial cell. Nevertheless, the drugs that interfere with them are not particularly toxic to man. This is a consequence of the fact that the bacterial enzymes involved are much more susceptible to the drugs than are the corresponding enzymes in the mammalian hosts.

Protein synthesis is the most important of all the metabolic processes carried out in the cell. It is conducted under the joint aegis of the three types of RNA and it follows a course described in detail in an earlier chapter (p. 21). The reprise provided here is intended merely to refresh the memory as a prologue to an enumeration of the loci of action of those antibacterial agents that inhibit protein synthesis.

Bacterial ribosomes are formed, under the influence of ribosomal RNA (r-RNA) by the attachment of a 30S and a 50S ribosomal fragment (or subunit) to the end of a thread of messenger RNA (m-RNA). Each ribosome carries two binding sites and the nature of the region of the m-RNA to which the ribosome is attached determines which aminoacid shall be attached to the first binding site. Each aminoacid is borne to its destination by a specific transfer RNA (t-RNA). When the appropriate aminoacid has been attached, the ribosome moves along the m-RNA thread (the process of translocation) and the attached aminoacid is transferred to the other binding site (the so-called donor site) leaving the original site free to receive a second aminoacid, the identity of which is determined by the codon on the part of the thread to which the ribosome has now moved. The first aminoacid is detached from the donor site and is linked with the second to form a dipeptide. In its turn, the dipeptide is shifted to the donor site, the ribosome takes another step along the thread of m-RNA and a third aminoacid arrives for incorporation into the dipeptide. So the molecule grows.

Streptomycin binds to, and inhibits the attachment of, the 30S subunit to the m-RNA. In high concentrations it also distorts protein synthesis by causing the incorporation into the polypeptide chain of an aminoacid different from that ordered by the m-RNA. Streptomycin cannot bind to 30S subunits from organisms that are resistant to the antibiotic. The other aminoglycosides operate in a similar (if not identical) fashion.

The tetracyclines also bind to the 30S subunits but they do not prevent their becoming attached to the m-RNA molecule. Instead, they arrest protein synthesis by preventing the approach and access of the aminoacids to the ribosomes.

Chloramphenicol attaches itself to the 50S subunit and prevents the transfer process whereby the stripling polypeptide is moved from the donor site to become attached to the newly arrived aminoacid.

Finally, erythromycin (and the other macrolides), fusidic acid and lincomycin all halt protein synthesis by preventing translocation.

It remains a mystery as to why interference with protein synthesis has sometimes a bactericidal and sometimes a bacteriostatic effect depending on the point at which the synthetic process is interrupted.

BIBLIOGRAPHY

Books, monographs and reviews

Anonymous (1964). Today's drugs—the sulphonamides. *Br. med. J.*, **1**, 419-421 and 483-486.

Ball, A.P., Gray, J.A. and Murdoch, J.McC. (1975a). Antibacterial drugs today: 1, *Drugs*, **10**, 1-55.

Idem (1975b). Antibacterial drugs today: 2, *Drugs*, **10**, 81-111.

Brogden, R.N., Pinder, R.M., Sawyer, Phyllis R. and Speight, T.M. (1976). Tobramycin: a review of its antibacterial and pharmacokinetic properties and therapeutic use. *Drugs*, **12**, 166-200.

Brogden, R.N., Speight, T.M. and Avery, G.S. (1975). Minocycline: a review of its antibacterial and pharmacokinetic properties and therapeutic use. *Drugs*, **9**, 251-291.

Burchall, J., Ferone, R. and Hitchings, G., (1965). Antibacterial chemotherapy. *Ann. rev. Pharmac.*, **5**, 53-76.

Fleming, A. (1946). History and development of penicillin. In *Penicillin* (A. Fleming, ed.). Philadelphia: Blakiston.

Fox, W. (1965). Recent advances in the chemotherapy of tuberculosis. In *Advances in Chemotherapy*. (A. Goldin, F. Hawking and R.J. Schnitzer, eds.) Vol. 2. pp. 197-268 New York and London: Academic Press.

Franklin, T.J. and Snow, G.A. (1971). *Biochemistry of Antimicrobial Action.* 2nd edn. London: Chapman and Hall.

Gale, E.F. (1963). Mechanisms of antibiotic action. *Pharmac. Rev.,* **15,** 481-530.

Garrod, L.P., Lambert, H.P. and O'Grady, F. (1973). *Antibiotic and Chemotherapy.* 4th edn. Edinburgh: Churchill Livingstone.

Kucers, A. and Bennett, N. McK. (1975). *The use of Antibiotics,* 2nd edn. London: Heinemann.

McDonald, H.M. (1974). Antibiotics, antiseptics and tubercle bacilli. *Med. J. Aust.,* **2,** 41-45.

Park, J.T. (1958). *Strategy of Chemotherapy.* Cambridge: University Press.

Pratt, W.B. (1973). *Fundamentals of Chemotherapy.* New York and London: Oxford University Press.

Rinehart, K.L. (1964). *The Neomycins and related antibiotics.* New York: Wiley.

Rollo, I.M. (1966). Antibacterial chemotherapy. *Ann. rev. Pharmac.,* **6,** 209-230.

Salton, M.R.G. and Tomasz, A. (eds) (1974). Mode of action of antibiotics on microbial walls and membranes. *Ann. N.Y. Acad. Sci.,* **235,** 1-620.

Schwartz, W.S. (1966). Comparison of ethioamide with isoniazid in original treatment cases of pulmonary tuberculosis. *Am. Rev. resp. Dis.,* **93,** 685-692.

Smith, H. (1977). *Antibiotics in Clinical Practice,* 3rd edn. London: Pitman Medical.

Waksman, S.A. (1958), (ed). *Neomycin, its nature and practical application.* Baltimore: Williams & Wilkins.

Woods, D.D. (1962). The biochemical mode of action of the sulphonamide drugs. *J. gen. Microbiol.,* **29,** 687-702.

Original papers

Azad Khan, A.K., Piris, J. and Truelove, S.C. (1977). An experiment to determine the active therapeutic moiety of sulphasalazine. *Lancet,* **ii,** 892-895.

Black, M. (1974). Isoniazid and the liver. *Am. R. Resp. D.,* **110,** 1-3.

Collins, J.F. and Richmond, M.H. (1962). A structural similarity between N-acetylmuramic acid and penicillin as a basis for antibiotic action. *Nature (Lond.),* **195,** 142-143.

Domagk, G. (1935). Ein Beitrag zur Chemotherapie der bakterellen Infektionem. *Dr. med. Wschr.,* **61,** 250-253.

Kodmidis, J., Hamilton-Miller, J.M.T., Gilchrist, J.N.G., Kerry, D.W. and Brumfitt, W. (1973). Cefoxitin, a new semisynthetic cephamycin: an *in vitro* and *in vivo* comparison with cephalothin. *Br. med. J.,* **4,** 653-655.

Rogers, H.J. and Jeljaszewicz, J. (1961). Inhibition of the biosynthesis of cell wall mucopeptides by the penicillins. A study of penicillin sensitive and penicillin resistant strains of *Straphylococcus aureus. Biochem. J.,* **81,** 576-584.

Strominger, J.L., Blumberg, P.M., Suginaka, H., Umbreit, J. and Wickus, G.G. (1971). How penicillin kills bacteria: progress and problems. *Proc. R. Soc. Lond. B.,* **179,** 369- 383.

Takayama, K., Want, L. and David, H.L. (1972). Effect of isoniazid on the *in vivo* mycolic acid synthesis, cell growth and viability of Mycobacterium tuberculosis. *Antimicrob. Ag. Chemother.* **2,** 29-35.

Williams, J.D., Andrews, J., Mitchard, M. and Kendall, M.J. (1976). Bacteriology and pharmacokinetics of the new amidinopenicillin—mecillinam. *J. Antimicrob. Chemother.,* **2,** 61-69.

51. The chemotherapy of virus diseases

Viruses are obligatory intracellular parasites. They represent indeed the ultimate in parasites since their growth and reproduction are totally dependent on the metabolism of the host cell, which provides not only the actual material required for development but also the energy-supplying processes and the biochemical systems which enable this material to be incorporated into the substance of the virus. For this reason, it was at first believed that the only means of preventing the growth and multiplication of viruses would be by the use of agents which, by their very nature, would have to be toxic to the tissues of the host. This situation contrasts with that obtaining with bacteria which have self-contained biosynthetic systems.

Later advances in our knowledge of virus biochemistry made it plain that the earlier assumptions were too pessimistic and that virus growth does involve some specific biochemical processes which can be inhibited without prejudice to the continued functioning of the host cell. The realization that this was so stimulated a search for effective antiviral agents. The largest viruses (which give rise to diseases such as lymphogranuloma venereum, psittacosis and ornithosis) are sensitive to the sulphonamides and to antibiotics but this chapter is more particularly concerned with the prophylaxis and treatment of diseases caused by the smaller viruses, which are responsible for a large proportion of the infectious diseases that affect man. They include the common cold, poliomyelitis, influenza, smallpox, rabies and yellow fever, to name but a few. Several potentially useful compounds have been shown to inhibit virus growth in experimental animals and in tissue cultures and a few have been introduced into clinical practice. More will doubtless follow.

Viruses consist of nucleic acid (either DNA or RNA) enclosed in a 'shell' of protein known as the *capsid*. The capsid is often spherical but other shapes are seen and it is sometimes clear that the capsid is made up of a number of subunits (*capsomeres*). In the herpes virus, for instance, twenty capsomeres in the form of equilateral triangles are arranged so that the capsid itself is a regular icosahedron. The viruses that cause influenza and mumps have spirally organized capsids and the smallpox virus is brick shaped. The structure of some viruses is completed by an encircling membrane (the *envelope*) but in other viruses the capsid is naked. The complete virus particle is sometimes referred to as a *virion*. Reactive sites on the capsid become attached to receptors on the host cell and once this intimacy has been established, nucleic acid passes into the host cell. The nucleic acid sometimes loses its capsid covering before it penetrates the host cell but it more often happens that it is uncovered within the cell. That in some of the RNA-containing viruses is capable of acting as 'messenger RNA'. In other viruses, messenger RNA is synthesized from the RNA or DNA contained in the virus: in either event, it directs the synthesis of new virus protein and the production of more nucleic acid. Nucleic acid and capsid protein are synthesized in different parts of the host cell and the several subunits have then to be brought together for assembling into new virions. The new particles accumulate in the cells in large numbers until they kill it. They are then released from the lysed cell. Some viruses induce the formation of toxic substances that add to their pathogenicity. Others, on the other hand, live innocently enough for many years in the cells that produced them and only cause ill effects if some event triggers a new burst of reproductive activity. As we note below, herpes simplex provides a good example of a virus that, once established in the body, only occasionally announces its presence to its host.

The smallest viruses have a diameter of no more than 20 nm while the largest attain dimensions of up to 300 nm which is about one third that of a staphylococcus.

The properties of the more common viruses (particularly those that are specifically mentioned in this chapter) and the diseases they cause can be summarized as follows.

DNA VIRUSES

The *pox viruses* are large, brick shaped, DNA viruses. They have envelopes, they are the largest viruses and they are the causative agents of smallpox (variola) and cowpox.

The *herpes viruses* are also large, enveloped viruses and they are of icosahedral shape. They cause herpes simplex and chickenpox. The virus of herpes simplex is of very common occurrence and most of us were infected early in life. The primary infection may pass unnoticed, it may cause only fever or the fever may be accompanied by an eruption of herpetic vesicles in the mouth or on the skin or conjunctiva. In more serious cases encephalitis or a fatal generalized infection may supervene. The herpes virus acquired in the early years often lies dormant for life but it may also give rise to recurrent outbreaks of so called cold sores on the lips or nostrils or of herpetic vesicles on the eyes or the mucous membrane of the genital tract. Factors that goad the dormant virus into renewed activity include the common cold or other minor infections, changes in environmental temperature and menstruation. The virus that causes chickenpox is varicella. In adults it may cause herpes zoster ('shingles'), a condition characterized by a herpetic eruption and severe pain in the area of skin supplied by one or more sensory nerves.

The *adenoviruses* are small viruses of icosahedral shape without an envelope. They cause infections of the pharynx and the upper respiratory tract.

RNA VIRUSES

The *myxoviruses* are medium sized viruses (diameter 75–150 nm) with an outer envelope that bears minute projections. They produce such conditions as influenza, parainfluenza, mumps and measles. One species of influenza virus infects pigs and was probably responsible for the notorious influenza epidemic in 1918 which killed more people than did the war that had just ended. Since that epidemic, human beings have not been infected on a large scale by the pig virus but there are recent disturbing reports that this long period of immunity may be ending.

Very small viruses containing RNA are grouped together as the *picornaviruses*. 'Picornavirus' is a semantic delight, a pronounceable word having been formed from pico (very small), RNA and virus. Among the picornaviruses are those that are responsible for poliomyelitis, foot and mouth disease and rubella (German measles) as well as the groups of echoviruses and rhinoviruses. 'Echovirus' is another example of the wordmaker's art, echo being derived from the initial letters of enteric cytopathogenic human orphan. In this context, 'orphan' implies that when they were first discovered the viruses were not related to any known human disease but it is now clear that they can produce infections of the meninges and the gastrointestinal and respiratory tracts. The rhinoviruses include a large group of picornaviruses all the members of which, as their generic name implies, can produce the common cold (*coryza*).

The *arboviruses* (arbo = arthropod borne) are small viruses transmitted by such arthropods as mosquitoes, ticks and sand flies. They particularly infect animals and birds but some of them produce serious diseases in man. These include yellow fever and sand fly fever.

ANTIVIRAL DRUGS

Before describing the individual drugs two general points should be made. The first is that, with the agents currently available, the development of resistant strains of virus occurs quite readily. The other is the generalization that substances that are effective against viruses which contain RNA are usually inactive against those which contain DNA. The converse is also true.

IDOXURIDINE

Idoxuridine (5-iodo-2'-deoxyuridine) has been successfully used in the treatment of some conditions caused by the herpes simplex virus, particularly herpetic keratitis. This represents a notable achievement for the first antiviral agent to be used in clinical practice, because herpetic keratitis is otherwise extremely difficult to treat and, if not cured, it can lead to serious impairment of vision. In the early stages of treatment, idoxuridine is applied to the eye in a one per cent solution, hourly during the day and every two hours during the night. As the lesions heal, it is given less frequently. 5-Bromo-2'-deoxyuridine has a similar action to the iodinated compound but the fluoro derivative is ineffective. Some success has also attended the use of idoxuridine in cases of herpes zoster. In this condition the drug is applied to the affected skin in a 40 per cent solution in dimethylsulphoxide. The vehicle facilitates absorption of the drug and it appears in addition to have some slight therapeutic action in its own right.

Idoxuridine is too toxic a substance for systemic use except in the emergency presented by herpetic encephalitis. The benefits of any treatment in this often fatal condition are difficult to assess but there are some well authenticated claims for the effectiveness of idoxuridine in at least a few series of cases. In viral encephalitis the drug is given by intravenous infusion or sometimes, more heroically, by the intracarotid arterial route.

Thymidine

Idoxuridine (5-iodo-2'-deoxyuridine)

As can be seen from the formulae, idoxuridine is chemically very similar to thymidine, a compound which in the normal cell is phosphorylated and then incorporated into the DNA molecule. When idoxuridine is given, it replaces thymidine and is itself taken into DNA. The distorted molecule thus produced differs from the virus's normal DNA in a number of ways but its most important deficiency, from the point of view of preventing viral replication, would seem to be that, while not preventing the synthesis of the subunits it cannot direct their assembly into viral particles.

The question naturally arises as to why idoxuridine affects the virus but not the host cells. The most likely explanation appears to be that of Tamm and Eggers (1965) who point out that the synthesis of viral DNA proceeds continuously and at a high rate whereas in the host cell it is more discontinuous. Consequently the idoxuridine has a much greater opportunity of becoming incorporated in the viral DNA. Nevertheless some effect on the host DNA does occur which could become serious after prolonged treatment. Moreover, idoxuridine may cause other untoward reactions in the host. In experimental preparations, it increases the mutation rate and it may also affect those enzyme reactions in the host cells which are regulated by deoxythymidine-5-triphosphate, some of which will be replaced by phosphorylated idoxuridine. Since idoxuridine is usually given topically, serious ill effects rarely attend its use, but itching, photophobia and oedema of the ṣkin around the eyes are irritatingly inconvenient minor side effects. Depression of the bone marrow, manifested as leucopenia and thrombocytopenia, has sometimes followed its systemic administration and it is clear that only an emergency situation can justify its use in this way.

CYTOSINE ARABINOSIDE

Cytosine arabinoside (cytarabine) is employed principally as an antineoplastic drug and, as such, its mode of action and detailed properties are more properly discussed elsewhere (p. 920). It is sometimes used to treat herpetic keratitis but, because of its greater local toxicity, it should

Cytosine arabinoside (cytarabine)

be reserved for cases that are resistant to idoxuridine. It has also been given systemically (in daily intravenous doses of up to 100 mg per square metre of body surface) to patients with serious herpes infections.

AMANTADINE

Amantadine (L-adamantanamine; Symmetrel) is active against some of the myxoviruses including those of influenza A, A_1 and A_2, rubella (German measles) and parainfluenza 1 (the Sendai virus) but its only therapeutic application is in the prophylaxis of influenza A_2 ('Asian flu') in the ill, the elderly and others who might not be able to withstand an attack of the disease.

Amantadine prevents penetration of the host cell by the virus and this explains its prophylactic action. It might be expected that it would have no curative value in established cases of influenza since there is no apparent reason why it should prevent the multiplication of viruses that

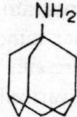

Amantadine

have already entered the tissues of the host. Nevertheless there is some evidence to suggest that, in addition to having a prophylactic action, amantadine can also ameliorate established symptoms. This additional property, if confirmed, will constitute an added recommendation for the drug since it will enable amantadine to diminish the effect of any virus that penetrates the protective barrier it has erected as its primary action.

Amantadine is given in twice daily oral doses each of 100 mg. Treatment is continued for as long as the threat of infection persists. Side effects of the drug include a medley of symptoms originating in the central nervous system (depression, nervous excitability, tremors, ataxia, lethargy, insomnia) and, occasionally, gastrointestinal disturbances and skin rashes. It is contraindicated in those with epilepsy, cerebral arteriosclerosis or mental illness requiring treatment with antidepressant drugs.

Although amantadine can induce tremors it can also abolish them and the other symptoms of Parkinsonism, as was first fortuitously noticed some eight years ago in a patient with Parkinson's disease who was also, by chance, taking amantadine because of an epidemic of influenza. This quite unexpected and inexplicable effect of amantadine led to its regular use for the treatment of Parkinson's disease (p. 591).

RIMANTADINE

Rimantadine is the α-methyl derivative of amantadine and it has similar actions and use. The twice daily dose is 150–200 mg by mouth. Nightmares, hallucinations and vomiting have been reported as side effects.

METHISAZONE

As we read elsewhere (p. 849) Domagk discovered that some derivatives of benzaldehyde thiosemicarbazone protected laboratory animals against tuberculosis. This observation led to an extensive investigation of the thiosemicarbazones and it soon became evident that some of them possessed more activity against some large viruses than they did against the tubercle bacillus. The only one of

N-methylisatin-β-thiosemicarbazone
(methisazone, Marboran)

the antiviral thiosemicarbazones in use today, however, is the N-methylisatin derivative which is known as methisazone or Marboran.

Methisazone prevents the pox viruses and some of the adenoviruses from reproducing themselves but its therapeutic application has been restricted to the prevention of smallpox in those who have been in contact with the disease and to the prevention and treatment of complications following smallpox vaccination in patients who are receiving immunosuppressive drugs or in children with a history of eczema who might otherwise develop generalized vaccination eczema or worse. The results of a number of well designed trials testify to the efficacy of methisazone as a prophylactic agent. In one such trial, in India, only six out of 2192 treated contacts developed smallpox. By contrast, 114 cases of the disease were reported among 2589 contacts who did not receive methisazone. The drug was effective even if it was given after infection had actually occurred but before signs of smallpox had appeared. Vaccination confers no protection if it is given during this incubation period but in other respects it is superior to methisazone as a prophylactic measure. Fortunately the past few years have witnessed the complete elimination of smallpox from every corner of the earth and it is unlikely that mass vaccinations on the scale seen in the quite recent past will be needed in the foreseeable future.

The prophylactic dose of methisazone, taken twice daily, is three grams. Treatment is usually for about one week. Vomiting (sometimes associated with diarrhoea) is often troublesome. Methisazone is contraindicated in pregnancy and in patients with liver or kidney disease.

In the presence of methisazone, pox viruses produce messenger RNA quite normally during the first three hours or so after gaining entry into the host cells but thereafter they lose much of their ability to induce the synthesis of the 'late' viral protein.

INTERFERONS

When a cell is infected with a living virus or is exposed to an inactivated one, it and its neighbours may become resistant to infection with other species of virus. This phenomenon has been described as *virus interference* and it occurs because when they are synthesizing virus material, cells also produce substances that reduce their susceptibility to other viruses. These substances, which diffuse readily from their site of production and so can protect cells that were not infected by the inducing virus, are known as *interferons* and they are highly specific in the sense that each animal species produces its own characteristic interferon which is effective only in that or a closely related species. In another sense, however, the interferons are quite unspecific because that produced in a particular species confers a degree of protection against a wide range of viruses irrespective of the nature of the inducing virus. Not all viruses are equally effective in provoking the synthesis of interferon (or its liberation if, as some think, it is preformed) and not all viruses are equally sensitive to the action of interferon. It should be added that some bacteria and protozoa have some ability to induce interferon production and are themselves less effective in the presence of interferon. Interferon production is presumably one of the components of the defence system erected by the animal organism against invasion by pathogenic organisms.

Interferons are small proteins that also contain carbohydrate. Their molecular weights range from about 20 000 to about 150 000. They are not antibodies as is evident from their lack of specificity and the fact that they appear very soon (sometimes within seconds) after viral invasion.

The interferons are not toxic (except to viruses), they have no antigenic activity and they are active in extremely low concentrations. These qualities are all desirable attributes of a successful therapeutic substance. To them we can add their lack of selectivity which would point to their potential value in the prophylaxis of conditions such as the common cold which are caused by a variable miscellany of viruses. It is virtually impossible to prepare a common cold vaccine that will provide protection in all outbreaks of the disease but interferon therapy should be effective at all times. Unfortunately it has not yet proved possible to harness this potential for the common good. To be of utility in human disease the interferon will have to be obtained from human subjects (or, at best, from some other primate animal) and this immediately raises so far insuperable problems concerning both the production and the purification of interferon for therapeutic use. The difficulties are accentuated by the fact that interferon is rapidly distributed and excreted so that it has an almost evanescently brief survival in the body: its serum half life amounts to no more than ten minutes in human subjects. Consequently, vast amounts of purified material would be required, their high potency notwithstanding, if interferon therapy were to be generally available. Nevertheless, sufficient interferon has been produced to permit the completion of promising clinical trials in several parts of the world. In most of these studies, interferon has been obtained from monkey kidney cells exposed to an influenza virus.

An alternative way of utilizing the activity of interferon would be deliberately to introduce a virus infection and so promote endogenous interferon production in patients needing protection from other more virulent viruses. Unfortunately the production of antibodies against the inducing virus would probably destroy the effectiveness of this manoeuvre. Another possibility is to exploit the fact that some relatively simple compounds can induce the production of interferon. It seems likely that interferon is formed in response to instructions from double stranded RNA (p. 21) which is present in a few viruses but is otherwise presumably produced in host cells when viruses (even those of the DNA category) are multiplying. A complex of polyinosinic and polycytidylic acids, known as poly–IC, is a synthetic analogue of double stranded RNA and is a potent inducer of interferon. It is non toxic on local application and in clinical trials it has been able to prevent coryza when instilled into the nose and conjunctival sacs. However, its clinical future is not bright because it can cause autoimmune disease (p. 395) if it is given systemically and large doses are also teratogenic. The principal dividend from the work with poly–IC will no doubt prove to be the renewed incentive to search for interferon inducers with low systemic toxicity.

It is perhaps worth concluding our discussion of antiviral agents with a reminder that the best prophylactic agents are vaccines because they are much more certain and long lasting in their effects than the alternatives we have mentioned whose application is, or will be, limited to conditions for which specific vaccines are not available or to patients for whom vaccines are contraindicated.

BIBLIOGRAPHY

Books, monographs and reviews

Becker, Y. (1976). *Mode of Action and Chemotherapy of Viral Infections in Man (Monographs in Virology: Vol. XI)* Chichester: Wiley.

Bucknall, R.A. (1973). The continuing search for antiviral drugs. *Adv. Pharmac. Chemother.*, **11**, 295–320.

Eggers, H.J. and Tamm, I. (1966). Antiviral Chemotherapy. *Ann. Rev. Pharmac.*, **6**, 231–250.

Herrman, E.C., Jr. (1961). The detection, assay and evaluation of antiviral drugs. *Progr. med. Virol.*, **3**, 158–192.

Ho, M. and Armstrong, J.A. (1975). Interferon. *A. rev. microbiol.*, **29**, 131–162.

Isaacs, A. (1961). Nature and function of interferon. In *Perspectives in Virology*, vol. II, pp. 117–125. ed. Pollard, M. Minneapolis: Burgess.

Knight, C.A. (1963). Chemistry of viruses. *Protoplasmatologia*, **4** (2), 1–117.

Symposium (1962). Basic mechanisms in animal virus biology. *Cold Spr. Harb. Symp. quant. Biol.*, **27**.

Tamm, I. and Eggers, H.J. (1965). Selective inhibition of viral replication. In *Viral and Rickettsial Infections of Man*, pp. 305–338, ed. Horsfall, F.L., Jr. and Tamm, I. Philadelphia: Lippincott.

Thompson, R.L. (1964). Viral diseases. *Adv. in Chemother.*, **1**, 85–131.

Various authors (1967). Aspects of medical virology. *Br. med. Bull.*, **23**, 105–197.

Original papers

Bauer, D.J. (1965). Clinical experience with the antiviral drug Marboran (1-methylisatin 3-thiosemicarbazone). *Ann. N.Y. Acad. Sci.*, **130**, 110–117.

Bauer, D.J., St. Vincent, L., Kempe, C.H. and Downie, A.W. (1963). Prophylactic treatment of smallpox contacts with N-methylisatin ß-thiosemicarbazone (compound 33T57, marboran). *Lancet*, **2**, 494–496.

Galbraith, A.W., Oxford, J.S., Schild, G.C. and Watson, G.I. (1969) Protective effect of 1-adamantanamine hydrochloride on influenza A2 infections in the family environment. *Lancet*, **2**, 1026–1028.

Renis, H.E. & Buthala, D.A. (1965). Development of resistance to antiviral drugs. *Ann. N.Y. Acad. Sci.*, **130**, 343–354.

Tamm, I. and Eggers, H.J. (1965). Biochemistry of virus reproduction, *Am. J. Med.*, **38**, 678–698.

52. The chemotherapy of the treponematoses

The treponemas are motile, non-flagellated organisms with a characteristic spiral conformation. They have affinities with both bacteria and protozoa. They give rise to a variety of diseases of which the most common are venereal and endemic syphilis (caused by *Treponema pallidum*) and yaws or framboesia (caused by *T. pertenue*). Less common are bejel, dichuchiva (conditions identical with or very closely related to endemic syphilis) and pinta. The causative organism of pinta is *T. carateum*. Other diseases, classed with the treponematoses and attributable to infection by treponema like organisms, are Vincent's angina (caused by *Borrelia vincentii*), relapsing fever (caused by *B. recurrentis*), rat-bite fever (caused by *Spirillum minus*) and Weil's disease or infectious jaundice, which follows infection by *Leptospira ictero-haemorrhagiae*. The treponemas, borreliae and leptospirae are collectively known as spirochaetes.

Venereal syphilis is transmitted by close sexual contact and has a world wide distribution. Endemic syphilis, bejel and dichuchiva are not of venereal origin; they occur in the

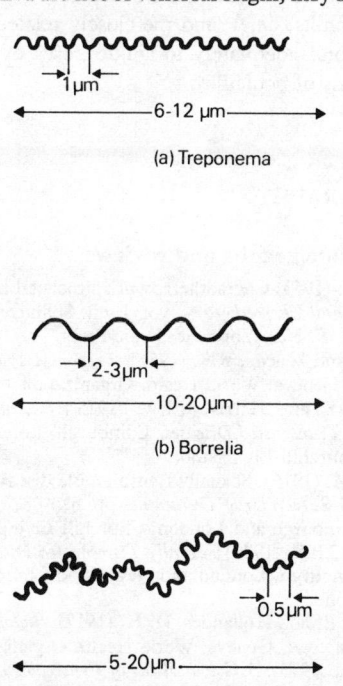

Fig. 52.1 The three genera of pathogenic spirochaetes

underprivileged communities of Asia and the Middle East. Yaws occurs in the tropical areas of Africa, South America and Asia. The disease particularly affects dark skinned peoples and is characterized by fever, bone and joint pains and a discharging skin rash. Vincent's angina is a form of acute tonsillitis which is often confined to one tonsil. It is of worldwide distribution, as are the rest of the diseases mentioned.

Except for relapsing fever, which is transmitted by lice, the treponematoses need no intermediate host for their propagation. Organisms are passed directly or indirectly from one person to another by way of cups and other vessels, kitchen utensils and direct bodily contact. Rat-bite fever and Weil's disease are carried by rats.

The treatment of all the treponematoses is essentially the same with a few exceptions to be mentioned.

Arsenic

We have seen elsewhere (p. 815) that the introduction of arsenic-containing compounds by Ehrlich and his colleagues for the treatment of relapsing fever and syphilis was one of the early events in the chemotherapeutic revolution which has transformed the treatment of infectious diseases during the present century.

The first effective synthetic antisyphilitic agent was arsphenamine. It cured early cases and prevented later cases from deteriorating. Arsphenamine has, however, a relatively high toxicity and its administration was painful to the patient, who had to endure a long course of intravenous injections. There was a high relapse rate, arsphenamine was of variable composition and special precautions had to be taken to prevent its chemical decomposition during storage. Some of these disadvantages were removed by the later introduction of neoarsphenamine ('914') and then of oxophenarsine. Bismuth was used with arsenic therapy to prevent relapses. The organoarsenicals are now virtually obsolete.

Penicillin

The treponema are highly susceptible to penicillin, which has been widely used in the treatment of all the treponematoses. Fortunately, treponema resistant to penicillin have not yet appeared, although there has been a recent increase in the incidence of syphilis in Great Britain, a country from which the disease had been almost eradicated.

To be effective in syphilis and other treponematoses,

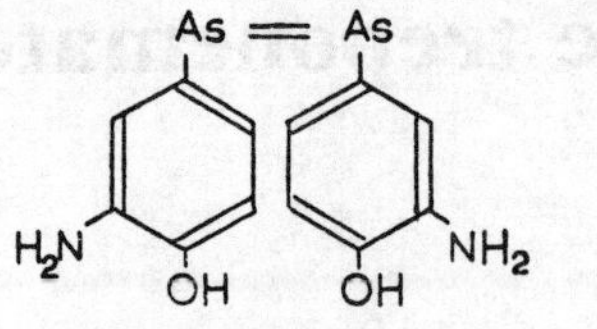

Arsphenamine

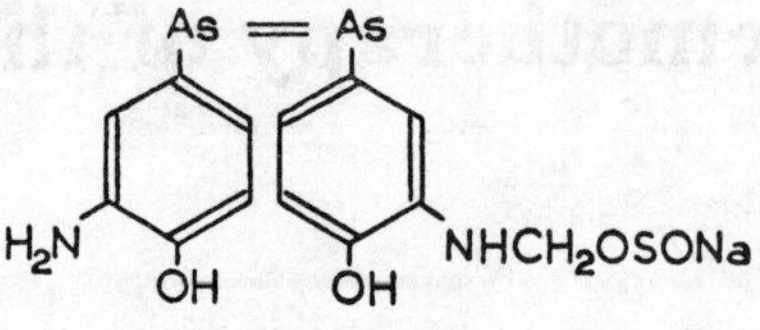

Neoarsphenamine

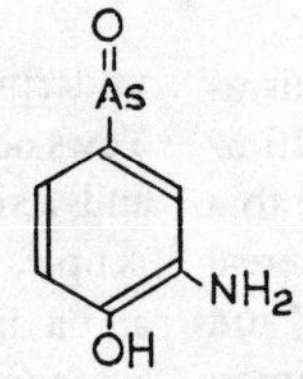

Oxophenarsine

high blood concentrations of penicillin (0.03 units per ml) must be attained. Moreover because penicillin only attacks actively dividing organisms and treponemas divide only slowly, this high concentration must be maintained for periods of up to 15 days to ensure that all the organisms have been killed and to prevent relapses. In syphilis, penicillin is best given in daily intramuscular doses of 600 000 to one million units of procaine penicillin G. Alternatively a long acting preparation such as benethamine or benzathine penicillin G can be given as a single injection containing 2.5 million units. This method of attack has some advantages. It certainly ensures that the action of the antibiotic will persist long enough to render the patient non-infectious even if he absconds after his first visit to the clinic. It also avoids the risk of the allergy that sometimes develops in patients who receive repeated injections of penicillin. The disadvantage of the method is that it is rarely completely curative and it is preferable to give penicillin daily if it is known that the patient will not default.

Soon after receiving their first injection of penicillin, patients in the early stages of syphilis (and those suffering from other spirochaete infections) frequently exhibit a more or less violent reaction compounded of sweating, high fever, headache and a temporary worsening of their condition. This *Jarisch-Herxheimer reaction* is not a consequence of the penicillin administration *per se* because it was also seen in the days when syphilis was treated with arsenic. It is evidently a response to the presence of dead organisms and it may be that there is a massive post mortem release of endotoxins. Alternatively the reaction may represent a simple allergic response to proteins liberated from the defunct spirochaetes.

The Jarisch-Herxheimer reaction (which usually persists for only a day or two) is rarely serious. When it is of unusual violence it can be controlled by a corticosteroid such as prednisolone.

Other antibiotics, notably the tetracyclines, are also effective in the prophylaxis and treatment of treponematoses and if the patient is sensitive to penicillin a tetracycline is given. Other useful antibiotics in these conditions are erythromycin and cephaloridine although individuals who exhibit adverse reactions to penicillin are likely to be equally sensitive to cephaloridine. In infection with *L. icterohaemorrhagiae*, good results are obtained with penicillin in large doses, provided that treatment starts early in the course of the disease. In *B. recurrentis* infections, the tetracyclines are effective, and they are to be preferred to penicillin in the treatment of rat-bite fever due to *S. minus*. Unlike syphilis, bejel (and the closely related pinta) and yaws respond adequately to single doses of long acting preparations of penicillin.

BIBLIOGRAPHY

Books, monographs and reviews

Doak, G.O. (1963) Chemotherapy of spirochetal infections. In: *Experimental Chemotherapy*, vol. 1, ed. Schnitzer, R.J. and Hawking, F. New York: Academic Press.

Guthe, T. and Wilcox, R.R. (1954). *Treponematoses. A World Problem*. Geneva: World Health Organization.

Morton, R.S. and Harris, J.R.W. (1975). *Recent Advances in Sexually Transmitted Diseases*. Edinburgh, London & New York: Churchill Livingstone.

Platts, W.M. (1976). Sexually transmissible diseases. In: Avery, G.S. (ed) *Drug Treatment*. pp. 875-887. Sydney: Adis; Edinburgh and London: Churchill Livingstone

Schofield, C.B.S. (1979) *Sexually Transmitted Diseases*, 3rd edn. Edinburgh, London and New York: Churchill Livingstone.

Turner, T. B. and Hollander, D. H. (1957). *Biology of the Trepanematoses*. Geneva: World Health Organization.

Wisdom, A. (1973). *A Colour Atlas of Venereology*. London: Wolfe Medical Books.

53. The chemotherapy of protozoal disease: malaria

Malaria is primarily a disease of the tropics and sub-tropics but its distribution is widespread and it extends to the warm temperate regions. Its incidence is highest in warm, wet and marshy regions.

Malaria is caused by infection with protozoan parasites of the genus *Plasmodium*. Four species infect man; these are *Plasmodium vivax*, *P. falciparum*, *P. ovale* and *P. malariae*. They are transmitted by the bite of an infected female anopheles mosquito. It has been estimated that each year some 300 million people become infected and that three million die from the disease.

The life cycle of the malaria parasite

The female anopheles mosquito is a bloodsucking insect. When it takes blood from an infected host it ingests erythrocytes carrying plasmodia in different stages of development. Some of them (see below) are still dividing by asexual division but others have differentiated into male and female gametocytes. The asexual forms of the parasite are digested and destroyed in the mosquito's stomach, but the gametocytes undergo rapid changes. The nucleus of

the male gametocyte divides to form about eight daughter nuclei which migrate to the periphery of the cell. Flagellae are extruded from each nucleus, the rest of the gametocyte disintegrates and the motile flagellated nucleated organisms, the *microgametes*, or male gametes are set free. The process is known as *exflagellation*.

The female gametocyte, by a process of maturation division, changes into the female gamete (or *macrogamete*). The male gamete swims towards and fuses with the female and conjugation takes place with subsequent fusion of the nuclei to form the *zygote*. The zygote alters in shape and becomes worm-shaped and motile. It is now called the *ookinete* (or *travelling vermicule*). It enters the tissues of the stomach wall of the mosquito and forms a rounded cyst (the *oocyst*) on the outer surface. The oocyst enlarges and undergoes nuclear division to form thousands of motile *sporozoites* which, when the enlarged oocyst bursts, are liberated into the body cavity of the mosquito. They migrate into various parts of the body and reach the salivary glands, entering the host's blood stream in the saliva when the mosquito bites. The cycle of sexual

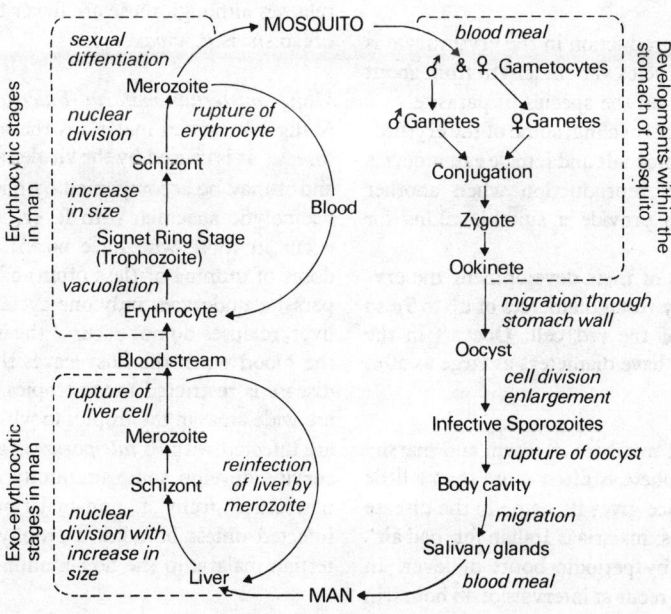

Fig. 53.1 The life cycle of the malaria parasite in man and mosquito

reproduction in the mosquito is known as *sporogony*. It occupies a period of seven to eleven days, being shorter the higher the environmental temperature.

In man, the malaria parasite continues its life cycle at first outside and then within the red blood cells.

The exoerythrocyte phase

The sporozoites enter the parenchyma cells of the host's liver, where they grow and undergo repeated nuclear divisions to form *schizonts*. Each schizont becomes surrounded by a layer of protoplasm and grows until the liver cell is many times its original size. It finally bursts and the parasites (now known as *merozoites*) enter the circulation and pass into the erythrocytes. Some invade fresh liver cells and repeat the exoerythrocytic cycle. This reinvasion is responsible for the late relapses of vivax malaria. Only *P. ovale*, *P. vivax* and *P. malariae* are repeatedly recycled through the liver in this way.

The erythrocyte phase

Inside the erythrocytes, the merozoites continue to grow. They form rounded, vacuolated cells or *trophozoites*. The vacuole enlarges and the nucleus is displaced to one side—this is the *signet ring form* of the parasite. Growth continues and nuclear division takes place resulting in the production of daughter cells which, like the cells formed in the liver, are called schizonts. Each schizont divides to give up to thirty offspring which acquire coatings of cytoplasm to become merozoites, again as in the liver. These are liberated by the rupture of the erythrocytes and enter fresh erythrocytes. The process of asexual multiplication is repeated in this way until large numbers of red corpuscles are parasitized.

The cycle of asexual reproduction in the erythrocyte is known as *schizogony:* the cycles vary in length from about 48 to 72 hours depending on the species of parasite.

After some days of asexual cycling, some of the erythrocytic merozoites develop into male and female gametocytes in preparation for sexual reproduction when another mosquito comes along to provide a suitable nidus for sporogony.

During the later stages of their development the erythrocytic trophozoites may reach diameters of up to 5μ so that they occupy most of the red cell. Oocysts in the mosquito's stomach often have diameters as large as 50μ.

Malaria

Mosquitoes live in largest numbers in warm and marshy country where the atmosphere is often more than a little noisome. This circumstance gives its name to the disease transmitted by mosquitoes: malaria is Italian for 'bad air'. Malaria is characterised by periodic bouts of fever. In tertian malaria the attacks recur at intervals of 48 hours; in the quartan form of the disease the periodicity of the attacks is 72 hours. These differences correspond to

differences in the length of the life cycle of the infecting parasites. The symptoms of malaria are caused by the parasitaemia and the recrudescences of fever take place when the erythrocytes rupture to liberate the merozoites. *P. malariae* causes quartan fever while the other plasmodia precipitate tertian malaria.

Devotees of novels set in the days of England's colonial adventuring will be familiar with over dramatized descriptions of the sufferings of malaria victims during their bouts of fever. These typically progress from a cold to a hot and then to a sweating stage. In the cold stage, the patient experiences chilling, shivering and rigors. The temperature then rises, sometimes to very high levels and the feeling of coldness gives way to one of heat. Resolution of the fever is accompanied by profuse sweating. The continuing destruction of erythrocytes causes a hypochromic anaemia, the spleen and liver are enlarged and pathological changes may also develop in the brain and kidneys.

Benign tertian malaria

Benign tertian malaria (vivax malaria) is a chronic form of the disease. It is the result of infection with *P. vivax,* an organism which is widely distributed north and south of the equator, extending from the tropics to the temperate zones. The exoerythrocyte forms of *P. vivax* persist in the liver for up to two years so that relapses are very frequent in this form of malaria.

Tertian malaria of a milder type and less prone to relapse is caused by *P. ovale*. Malaria due to this organism has a restricted distribution, being found only in tropical Africa and the western Pacific. *P. ovale* passes through an exoerythrocyte phase in the liver and these may cause late relapses although these are fewer than when the causative organism is *P. vivax*.

Malignant tertian malaria (Falciparum malaria)

Malignant tertian malaria is the most severe form of the disease. It is caused by the virulent pathogen *P. falciparum* and it may be accompanied by blackwater fever, a severe haemolytic anaemia, with fever, which is more likely to occur in those who have taken irregular or inadequate doses of quinine or (less often) of chloroquine. Since the parasite undergoes only one cycle of development in the liver, relapses do not occur if the infection is cleared from the blood when the host leaves the malarious zone. The disease is restricted to the tropics and sub-tropics. There are wide areas in the tropics in which all of the inhabitants are infected with *P. falciparum* at an early age. Those who survive develop some immunity to the infection, but a newcomer from a non-malarious zone is inevitably infected unless he takes a prophylactic drug. Malignant tertian malaria in the non-immune is often fatal.

Quartan malaria

Quartan malaria is caused by infection with *P. malariae*; it is the mildest but most persistent form of the disease and relapses may take place years after infection. The parasite's geographical distribution is similar to that of *P. falciparum*.

CHEMOTHERAPY

The drugs to be discussed in the following pages are used to treat malaria in those who have contacted the disease and to prevent it in those who have been bitten by an infected mosquito or who are exposed to the possibility of being so bitten. The control and eradication of the disease demand measures, at both the personal and the community level, that go beyond mere chemotherapy. These measures must be ignored here since they relate, in the main, to areas of study that lie outside the scope of this book except to the extent that one of the most important control measures is the use of insecticides. It is indeed not unreasonable to assert that the most valuable of all antimalarial drugs are dichlorodiphenyltrichloroethane (DDT) and benzene hexachloride (p. 901). Those who need reliable summaries of the control techniques actually applied in the field are referred to specialized texts such as, for instance, that by Nnochiri (1975). However vigorously these techniques are applied in some quarters, the realities of the malaria situation and of the world's sense (or lack of it) of economic priorities are such that we are a long way from abolishing the disease and the chemotherapeutic agents to be discussed here seem destined to remain in the textbooks for many years to come.

Some of the drugs available for treating malaria are capable of destroying plasmodial merozoites. These so-called *schizonticides* can provide a clinical cure in patients who are first seen when attacks of malarial fever have already begun. Other drugs are not lethal to the parasite but can inhibit their growth (the reader will be reminded of the difference between a bacteriocidal and a bacteriostatic drug) and are employed in *suppressive treatment*. Suppressive treatment is called for in individuals who have been exposed to infection but who are not displaying any overt sign of clinical malaria. It also provides the only form of prophylactic measure that can be offered to those about to enter a malaria ridden area because it is impossible to prevent the entry of merozoites into the blood of those bitten by infected mosquitoes. For personal prophylaxis, suppressive treatment has to be initiated some days before entering a malarious area and has to be continued for at least one month after leaving it.

Individuals who have not taken prophylactic measures during their sojourn in a malarious area may develop the disease some time after they have left the area. When that happens, the opportunity can be taken of achieving a *radical cure* of their condition by giving a combination of drugs that will kill the parasites actually responsible for the attack of malarial fever and will also completely eliminate those still developing in the erythrocytes and other tissue cells. No useful purpose is served by attempting to achieve radical cures in patients who remain in malarious areas.

The traditional drug for treating malarial fever is, of course, quinine. Although quinine is much less extensively used since the advent of the synthetic antimalarials, it still has a place, if a limited one, in antimalarial therapy. The extensive use of the synthetic antimalarials is leading to drug resistance, particularly among strains of *P. falciparum*. Quinine may be the only drug capable of relieving malarial fever caused by infection by these resistant organisms. Moreover, it is cheap and this fact alone may well dictate its use in those economically poor countries where malaria is rife. Of the synthetic drugs, the 4-aminoquinolines are recommended for the clinical cure of malaria (Table 53.1). These drugs could also be employed as suppressive agents but in practice their use for this purpose is avoided because of the danger of their needlessly accelerating the development of resistant organisms. Pyrimethamine and proguanil are used instead. So far as radical cure is concerned, the 8-aminoquinolines (which are particularly effective against the erythrocyte phase of

Table 53.1 Antimalarial drugs

Purpose	Drugs of first choice	Reserve drugs
Clinical cure	4-aminoquinolines (particularly chloroquine and amodiaquine)	Quinine Mepacrine
Suppressive treatment and personal prophylaxis	Pyrimethamine	Proguanil Quinine
Radical cure	Combined treatment with 4-aminoquinolines (as above) and 8-aminoquinolines (particularly primaquine and quinocide)	

plasmodial development) provide the required supplement to the schizonticidal activity of the 4–aminoquinolines.

Some of those who have lived for long periods of time in malarious areas develop a degree of immunity to the disease so that, even if they do succumb, they need more modest doses of antimalarial drugs than are prescribed for those who have not previously had the disease.

Quinoline derivatives

These compounds can be conveniently divided into three groups:

(a) the alkaloids of cinchona bark
(b) the 4-aminoquinolines
(c) the 8-aminoquinolines

QUININE

Quinine is the most important alkaloid of cinchona bark. It exerts its actions on the erythrocytic forms of the malaria parasite, and it also attacks the gametocytes of *P. vivax, P. ovale and P. malariae* but not those of *P. falciparum.* It is very effective in destroying the asexual forms in the erythrocytes and when used alone it is, therefore, a very effective suppressant.

Therapeutic dose levels of quinine do not cause serious side effects but *cinchonism* with ringing in the ears, blurred vision, headache, nausea and dizziness may occur when treatment is begun. Damage to the optic and auditory nerves is sometimes sufficiently severe to cause blindness or deafness. These complications are more likely to arise as a result of overdosage particularly in hypersensitive individuals. Very occasionally, patients display typical allergic symptoms such as asthma, urticarial skin rashes or oedema.

In addition to its antimalarial action, quinine and its congeners exhibit a variety of other pharmacological properties, some of which have found therapeutic applications.

Quinine affects all types of muscle. It has a curare-like action at the skeletal neuromuscular junction and this has led to its use as a diagnostic test for myasthenia gravis (p. 245) and as a therapeutic agent in certain rare muscular disorders such as dystrophia myotonica. In doubtful cases of myasthenia gravis, an oral dose of 600 mg of quinine will precipitate obvious signs of the disease. If these are reversed by neostigmine the diagnosis can be regarded as established. In dystrophia myotonica, efforts to produce voluntary contraction of the muscle cause muscle spasm. Oral doses of quinine (500 mg once or twice daily) relieve the spasm. Quinine has also been used to relieve nocturnal cramps in elderly patients. The pregnant uterus is stimulated to contract by quinine but the drug is not now used in obstetric practice. Among the laity it has a not entirely unjustified (or unexploited) reputation as an abortifacient. It can cause contraction of other smooth muscle too;

contraction of the bronchial muscle by quinine itself (rather than by material liberated as a result of an allergic reaction) may partly explain the asthma-like attacks seen in hypersensitive individuals. Vascular smooth muscle, however, is relaxed by quinine and rapid intravenous injections may cause a considerable fall of blood pressure. Retinal vessels apparently constrict when large doses of quinine are given and this may be partly responsible for the disturbances of vision which are experienced in cinchonism. On the other hand, the vascular response may be the consequence of a pathological condition of the retina induced by quinine rather than a direct action of the drug itself. On cardiac muscle, quinine has the same actions as quinidine (the isomer of quinine). These are described elsewhere (p. 685).

Quinine has local anaesthetic, antipyretic and analgesic activity. Strangely enough, chloroquine, another antimalarial drug, also has analgesic and anti-inflammatory properties (p. 456). Quinine inhibits the activity of a number of enzymes, including cholinesterase.

Quinine has a characteristic taste and it has often been used (often mixed with strychnine) as bitter (p. 640). It is a constituent of tonic water.

THE 4-AMINOQUINOLINES

The most important members of this group of drugs are chloroquine (Aralen, Nivaquine) and amodiaquine (Camoquin). Both drugs are very active against the asexual erythrocytic forms of all species of *Plasmodium* and they are therefore valuable agents for the rapid control of acute

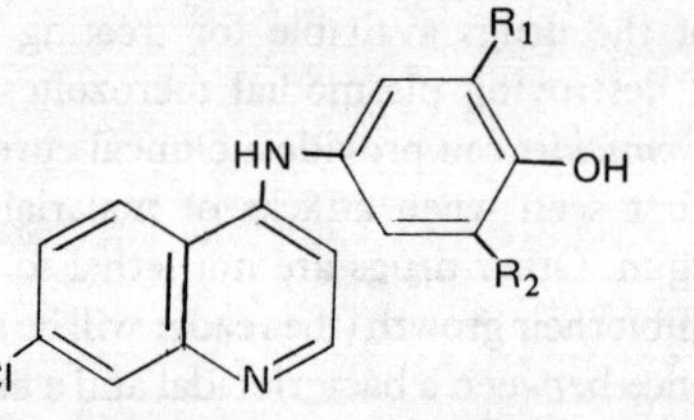

	R_1	R_2
Amodiaquine	$-CH_2N(C_2H_5)_2$	H
Amopyroquine	$-CH_2N(CH_2)_4$	H
Cycloquine	$-CH_2N(C_2H_5)_2$	$-CH_2N(C_2H_5)_2$

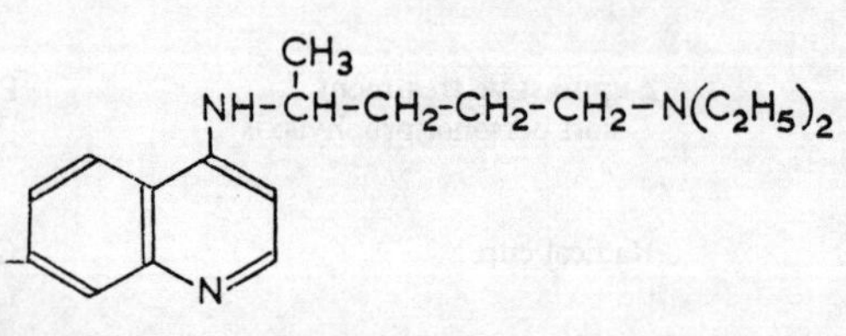

Chloroquine

Fig. 53.2 The 4-aminoquinolines

attacks of malaria. They were also, at one time, extensively employed as suppressant drugs because they are able to kill parasites leaving the liver but, as we have already noted (p. 865) their use for this purpose is now frowned upon. Neither drug has any action against the gametocytes of *P. falciparum* and malaria caused by this organism may therefore still be transmitted by the mosquito from patients who have themselves been cured by these drugs.

The 4–aminoquinolines are readily absorbed from the gastrointestinal tract and are extensively bound to plasma and tissue proteins from which they are only slowly released. Consequently, the usual dosage regime involves the administration of an initial 'loading' dose (800 mg and 600 mg respectively for chloroquine sulphate and amodiaquine hydrochloride) followed by a smaller maintenance dose for 3 to 5 days. For both drugs the once daily dose is 400 mg. Maintenance doses are not needed by patients who have acquired some immunity to the disease.

As with all drugs that leave the body slowly, prolonged or overenthusiastic medication with chloroquine or amodiaquine carries the danger of the drugs' accumulating in the body. If this occurs, such seriously toxic changes as corneal opacities and nerve deafness may supervene. The damage is not necessarily arrested if the drugs are completely withdrawn. Less severe degrees of poisoning are signalled by such symptoms as blurred vision, headache, gastric upsets, itching and dermatitis. It has been reported that amodiaquine, in addition, may cause a greyish purple discoloration of the nails if it is taken over long periods. Chloroquine has some teratogenic activity and, unless no other suitable drug is available, it should not be given to women in the early months of pregnancy.

In emergencies, chloroquine can be given by intramuscular or intravenous injection. A suitable preparation for intravenous use is Nivaquine. Combined preparations with pyrimethamine or chlorproguanil are available as Darachlor and Lapaquin respectively. Chloroquine (which was introduced during the Second World War) is more extensively used than amodiaquine.

The 4–aminoquinolines owe their effectiveness to the fact that they are taken up avidly by the erythrocytes where they inhibit nucleic acid and protein synthesis in the malarial parasite.

Chloroquine is also used in the treatment of amoebiasis (p. 871) and clonorchiasis (p. 892). It also has analgesic and antiinflammatory actions and it has enjoyed some success in the treatment of rheumatoid arthritis (p. 456). To be effective in this condition, chloroquine has to be given in larger doses and over a longer period of time than when it is used as an antimalarial drug and in these circumstances toxic side effects may become troublesome. Chloroquine inhibits anaphylactic responses (p. 393) in some species and it has been applied to the treatment of some allergies. Chloroquine has a quinidine-like action on the heart.

Mepacrine (Quinacrine)

Mepacrine was the first synthetic antimalarial to find widespread clinical application. It is most active against the asexual erythrocytic form of all the *Plasmodia* species and it was a popular suppressant drug. The chemical structure of mepacrine is similar to that of chloroquine except for the extra ring in mepacrine. Mepacrine can therefore legitimately be classified with chloroquine as a 4–aminoquinoline.

Mepacrine is now much less widely used than formerly because of its tendency to produce serious side effects. These include abdominal pain, nausea, vomiting, diarrhoea, dermatitis and mental disturbances. Though usually mild, the side effects (particularly those referable to the nervous system) are sometimes very severe or fatal. In addition, mepacrine is a yellow dyestuff and its prolonged administration causes an unpleasant yellowing of the skin and the conjunctivae.

Mepacrine

Other compounds

Other 4–aminoquinolines that have achieved some popularity include amopyroquine (Propoquine) and cycloquine (Haloquine). Their properties, uses and side effects are similar to those of chloroquine. Cycloquine has been extensively used in Russia.

THE 8-AMINOQUINOLINES

The first synthetic antimalarial was pamaquin: it was introduced into clinical practice in 1926. Later, primaquine, pentaquine and isopentaquine were synthesized but only primaquine (which is less toxic than the other compounds) is used now.

Primaquine attacks the exoerythrocytic forms of the malarial parasite and this explains its ability to produce, in conjunction with a drug such as chloroquine, a radical cure of malaria. For this purpose, primaquine phosphate is given in daily doses of 15 mg for fourteen days during the first three of which chloroquine has also to be taken.

Primaquine is rapidly absorbed and rapidly excreted. It is not bound extensively to proteins so that problems of accumulation do not normally arise.

Primaquine is a relatively non-toxic drug but large doses may cause haemolytic anaemia, haemoglobinuria, methaemoglobinaemia, nausea, vomiting, headache and epigastric pain. The toxic symptoms are likely to be more severe, and to appear at lower dose levels in those with a genetically determined deficiency of glucose-6-phosphate dehydrogenase in their erythrocytes (p. 74). Severe toxic

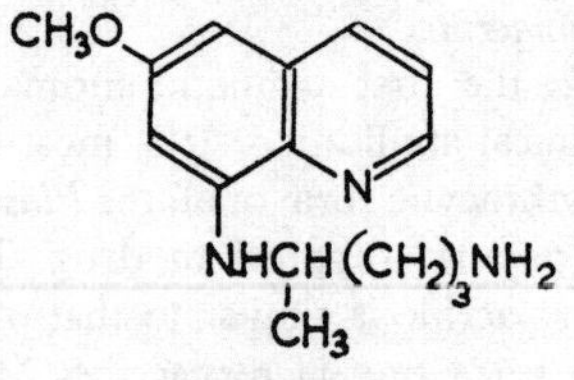

Primaquine

symptoms may also appear as a result of interactions between primaquine and certain other drugs (including mepacrine and proguanil) that inhibit its metabolic degradation.

Primaquine lacks the versatility of quinine and apart from its schizonticidal activity it exerts no pharmacological action of note. So far as its therapeutic activity is concerned, its mode of action is similar to that of chloroquine.

Quinocide

Quinocide is a structural isomer of primaquine and the two drugs have generally similar actions, uses and side effects, although quinocide is said to be the rather less effective member of the pair. The daily dose of quinocide is 50 mg.

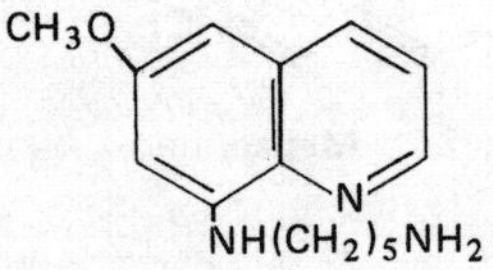

Quinocide

Biguanides

PROGUANIL

Proguanil (chloroguanide, Paludrine) was first synthesized, in Britain, in 1945. It destroys the asexual erythrocytic forms of all species of human malaria parasites but its action is slow and it is better to use another drug to treat an acute attack of malaria. Proguanil is active against the exoerythrocytic forms of *P. falciparum* and it therefore provides a radical cure in cases of malaria caused by this organism. For malaria attributable to other species, proguanil is an effective suppressive agent, although pyrimethamine is the drug of first choice. Continued suppressive treatment with proguanil of those who have left malarious areas will eventually rid them of all their malarial parasites.

Proguanil is probably the least toxic of all the currently available antimalarial drugs but it may cause gastric upsets

with reduced secretion of hydrochloric acid, nausea, vomiting and diarrhoea. The malaria parasite develops resistance to proguanil with relative ease and the drug may be useless in areas where resistant strains are appearing in large numbers.

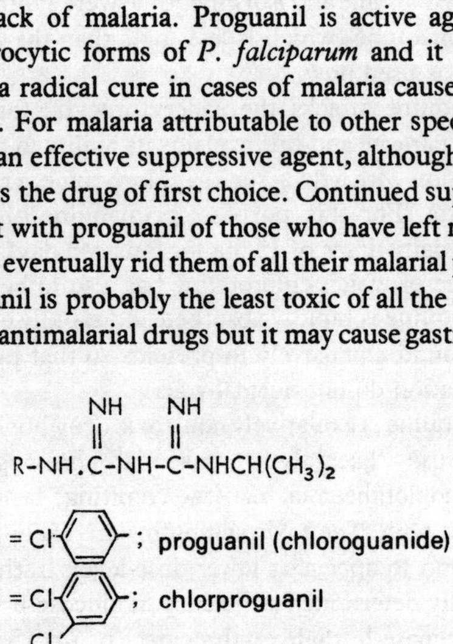

Proguanil is metabolized *in vivo* to a dihydrotriazine (cycloguanil) which, as can be seen, has some structural resemblances to pyrimethamine. The metabolite is probably responsible for the antimalarial activity of proguanil. Proguanil and pyrimethamine have very similar antimalarial properties as might be expected and cross resistance to the two drugs sometimes occurs. Both drugs probably owe their antimalarial activity to their being able to prevent the utilization of folic acid by the parasite. Their potency is enhanced by sulphadiazine, an effect which makes it likely that the drugs inhibit nucleic acid synthesis.

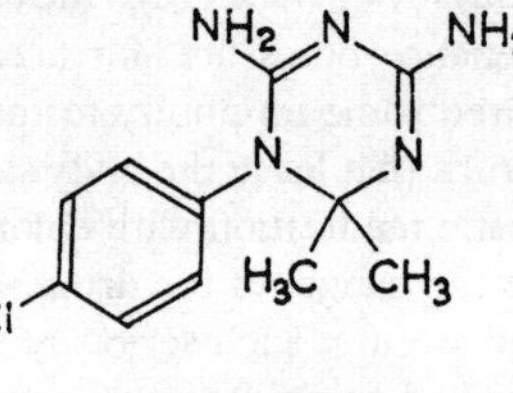

Cycloguanil

In the form of its embonate, cycloguanil has been used for antimalarial prophylaxis: a single dose, suspended in oil and given by the intramuscular route, confers protection for several months. The suppressive dose of proguanil is 250 mg daily. As we have already noted, proguanil interacts with primaquine and the two drugs should not be taken together.

CHLORPROGUANIL

Chlorproguanil (Lapudrine) has properties and uses similar to those of proguanil. A single dose (20 mg) taken as a prophylactic provides protection for at least one week.

2, 4-Diaminopyrimidines

PYRIMETHAMINE

Pyrimethamine (Daraprim) is active against the exoerythrocytic forms of all species of *Plasmodium*. Otherwise its properties and uses are similar to those of proguanil: it is the drug of choice for the suppressive treatment of malaria, particularly the malignant tertian form. Prolonged use of high doses of pyrimethamine may cause a macrocytic anaemia due perhaps to its action on folic acid metabolism

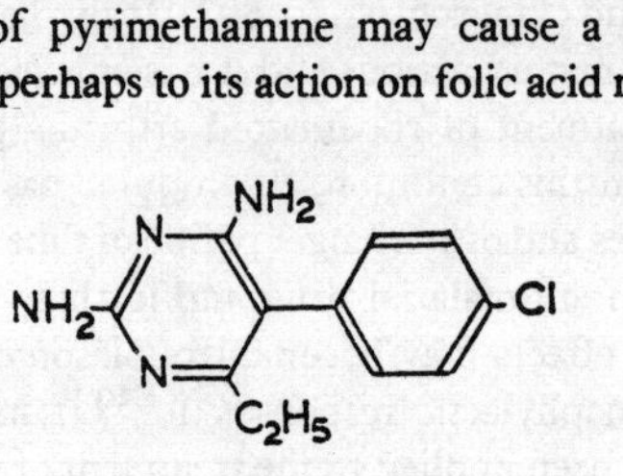

Pyrimethamine

but its toxicity is, in general, very low. Drug resistance to pyrimethamine does occur.

For prophylactic purposes, pyrimethamine is taken once weekly in doses of 50 mg.

LABORATORY EVALUATION OF ANTIMALARIAL ACTIVITY

A number of strains of plasmodia are known which infect laboratory animals (canaries, chicks, mice and monkeys). Laboratory strains of these organisms are not difficult to maintain and, although they differ from the species that parasitize man, their use has led to the discovery of some of the more valuable synthetic drugs including mepacrine, pamaquin and pyrimethamine.

BIBLIOGRAPHY

Books, monographs and reviews

Chemotherapy of Malaria. *Wld Hlth Org. techn. Rep. Ser.*, No. 226 (1961).

Covell, G., Coatrey, G.R., Field, J.W. and Singh, J. (1955). *Chemotherapy of Malaria.* Wld Hlth Org. Monogr. Ser., No. 27.

Davey, D.G. (1963). Chemotherapy of malaria. Part I, Biological basis of testing methods. In *Experimental Chemotherapy.* Ed. Schnitzer, R.J. and Hawking, F. New York: Academic Press.

Elsager, E.F. (1974). New perspectives on the chemotherapy of malaria, filariasis and leprosy. *Prog. drug Res.*, **18**, 99-172.

Expert Committee on Malaria. *Wld Hlth Org. techn. Rep. Ser.*, No. 8 (1950); No. 39 (1951); No. 80 (1954); No. 123 (1957); No. 162 (1959); No. 205 (1961); No. 243 (1962).

Findlay, G.M. (1951). In *Recent Advances in Chemotherapy*, Vol. II. London: Churchill.

Hill, J. (1963). Chemotherapy of malaria. Part II, the antimalarial drugs. In *Experimental Chemotherapy.* Ed. Schnitzer, R.J. and Hawking, F. New York: Academic Press.

Malaria Conference in Equatorial Africa. *Wld Hlth Org. techn. Rep. Ser.*, No. 38 (1951).

Malaria Conference of the Western Pacific and South-east Asia Regions. *Wld Hlth Org. techn. Rep. Ser.*, No. 103 (1956).

Malaria Conference for the Eastern Mediterranean and European Region. *Wld Hlth Org. techn. Rep. Ser.*, No. 132 (1957).

Marshall, E.K. Jr (1942). Chemotherapy of avian malaria. *Physiol. Rev.*, **22**, 190-204.

Nnochiri, E. (1975). *Medical Parasitology in the Tropics.* London: Oxford University Press.

Pampana, E. (1963). *A Textbook of Malaria Eradication.* London: Oxford University Press.

Rollo, I.M. (1964). Chemotherapy of malaria. In *Biochemistry and physiology of protozoa*, Vol. III. Ed Hutner, S.H. New York: Academic Press.

World Health Organization (1954). Malaria control. *Bull. Wld Hlth Org.*, **11**, 509-890.

54. The chemotherapy of protozoal disease: amoebiasis

Amoebiasis is caused by infection with the protozoan parasite, *Entamoeba histolytica*. Infection occurs in many regions of the world and it has been estimated that at least 5 to 10 per cent of the population of the USA and of Britain harbour the parasite. The majority of those who carry the parasite are symptom free, only cysts appearing in their stools. If amoebae develop and multiply, however, infective illnesses supervene. These include amoebic dysentery and amoebic hepatitis. Rarely, amoebic abscesses develop in the lungs and the brain. In mild cases of amoebiasis there may be no more than slight gastrointestinal upset but in severe amoebic dysentery the intestinal ulceration may be sufficiently severe to produce perforation, haemorrhage and death.

Life cycle
Infection is caused by the ingestion of viable cysts following contamination of food, drink or hands with infected faeces. Motile amoebae are digested by the juices of the stomach and are not infective. The infective cysts contain four nuclei which divide once to form eight. The cyst hatches in the small intestine and liberates eight trophozoites which grow into mature amoebae in the large intestine.

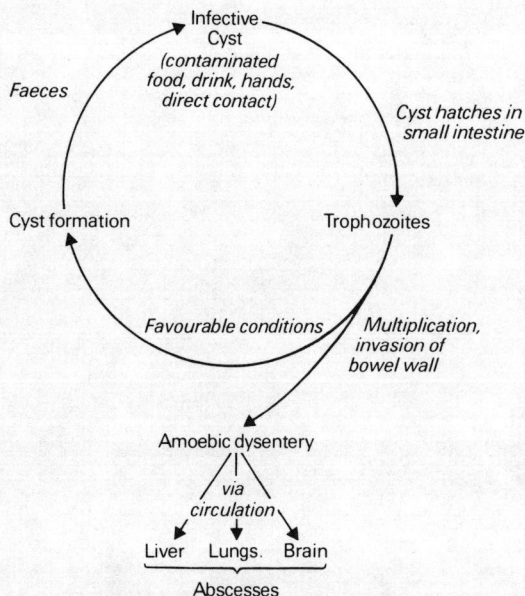

Fig. 54.1 The life cycle of *Entamoeba histolytica*

The mature motile amoebae undergo multiplication by simple fission. They normally live on bacteria but may invade the intestinal wall and cause areas of ulceration which then become infected with bacteria. Some of the amoebae enter the portal circulation and reach the liver where they may cause abscess formation whilst others may reach the brain or the lungs (Fig. 54.1). In acute cases of amoebic dysentery encystment does not take place. Cysts are formed when conditions in the lumen of the large intestine are favourable for survival. This occurs when there is plenty of food and when the bowel movement is placid and well ordered. Cyst formation enables the amoeba to survive the hardships encountered during the passage from one host to another. Cysts are not found in amoebic abscesses or ulcers.

AMOEBICIDAL DRUGS
For most of this century, emetine was the drug of choice for the treatment of amoebiasis but it has recently had to yield pride of place to metronidazole. Both substances are effective in all forms of the disease. Within the lifetime of emetine, the tetracyclines and paromomycin have enjoyed a few years of glory but they are now falling into disrepute as amoebicides. Other drugs of long standing that are still used often enough to justify their being accorded at least a passing mention are diloxanide furoate, the iodinated hydroxyquinoline compounds and the organic arsenicals. Chloroquine can be used for the treatment of liver abscess but not for other forms of amoebiasis.

METRONIDAZOLE
This drug (which is active against several species of protozoa) is fully described elsewhere (p. 882).

EMETINE
Emetine is an alkaloid obtained from the dried roots of *Cephaëlis ipecacuanha,* a shrub which grows in Brazil. It is the most potent amoebicide available. It is given by subcutaneous or intramuscular injection in the form of emetine hydrochloride and by mouth in enteric coated capsules as emetine bismuth iodide. When given by injection emetine is concentrated by the liver, to a smaller extent by the lungs, spleen and kidneys but not at all by the intestine or smooth or striated muscles.

The main value of emetine is in the treatment of amoebic

abscess of the liver and other organs. In amoebic dysentery it is reserved for the treatment of acute cases but it is of no value in the treatment of carriers and should not be used when symptoms are mild or prolonged. Emetine does not bring about a radical cure in more than a small proportion of cases, but it does suppress the symptoms of the disease. Treatment is completed with emetine bismuth iodide or other suitable drugs. It has a direct toxic action upon the amoebae, but does not destroy cysts. This is not a serious disadvantage because if the motile forms are all destroyed no more cysts will appear. Nevertheless, after a period of time cysts may appear again in the faeces so that the patient becomes a carrier or might even suffer a recurrence of the disease in its acute form. The dose of emetine usually employed is 30 mg given twice daily for not longer then ten to twelve days. Children are given smaller doses. The period of treatment with emetine can often be considerably shortened and the risk of toxic side effects lessened if it is given in conjunction with another amoebicidal agent. After the first two or three days of treatment with emetine, the acute symptoms will have subsided and the remaining amoebae can be dealt with by the other drug.

Emetine is a toxic substance and toxic side effects occur even at therapeutic dose levels. For this reason, cases for emetine treatment should be carefully selected and close medical supervision is required throughout the period of treatment. As the name implies, emetine causes vomiting. Associated with the vomiting—which is caused by a direct irritative action on the gut as well, perhaps, as through stimulation of the chemoceptive trigger zone (p. 599)—there is abdominal pain, diarrhoea and fever. Oedema, purpura, urticaria muscle pain and weakness have also been reported but the most dangerously toxic action of emetine is exerted on the myocardium and this may result in hypotension, precordial pain, tachycardia and dyspnoea.

Emetine is excreted very slowly and the consequent accumulation of the drug in the tissues may result in the appearance of toxic symptoms in response to the repeated administration of what at first seem to be safe doses of the drug.

Emetine

The mode of action of emetine is uncertain but it may inhibit the synthesis of RNA.

In small doses, extracts of ipecacuanha have long been employed as expectorants.

EMETINE BISMUTH IODIDE
Emetine bismuth iodide is used for the oral treatment of amoebiasis in which dysentery has been controlled with injections of emetine hydrochloride. When given at a dose level of 200 mg daily for ten days it effectively destroys the intestinal infection in over ninety per cent of cases. Although its activity resides primarily in its content of emetine, emetine bismuth iodide is a more potent amoebicide than parenteral emetine. It is insoluble in the stomach contents and the alkaloid is not liberated until it reaches the alkaline intestinal juices. Toxic side effects are similar to those associated with parenteral emetine. Nausea, vomiting and diarrhoea are frequent but not serious if the drug is given before sleeping and together with a sedative.

DEHYDROEMETINE
Dehydroemetine (Mebadin) is a recently introduced derivative of emetine which has been used successfully to treat acute intestinal amoebiasis and hepatic amoebiasis. It is eliminated more rapidly than the older compound and, perhaps because of this, it is much less toxic, particularly to the myocardium. When toxic effects do appear they are qualitatively similar to those seen with emetine.

The dose of dehydroemetine—given according to the same schedule as that recommended for emetine—is 30 mg. There seems to be no reason in view of its higher toxicity, why emetine should ever be preferred to dehydroemetine.

Synthetic halogenated quinoline derivatives

CHLOROQUINE
Chloroquine (Avloclor, Bemasulph, Nivaquine, Resochin) is used for the treatment of hepatic amoebiasis and because of its lower toxicity it is preferred to emetine. Its specificity against E. histolytica in the liver is attributable to the fact that it is concentrated in this organ. The oral dose is 300 mg given three times a day for four days followed by 300 mg once daily for fourteen to twenty-one days. Chloroquine is of little value in intestinal amoebiasis and in hepatic amoebiasis it is used in combination with another drug (such as carbarsone or chiniofon) which is active on the intestinal forms. Side effects are not serious provided that treatment is not prolonged: those which may be encountered include headache, visual disturbances, gastric upset and pruritus. The related drug, amodiaquine is used for the same purpose as chloroquine. The antimalarial actions of both drugs are discussed elsewhere (p. 866).

THE IODINATED 8-HYDROXYQUINOLINES
The three compounds shown in Fig 54.2 have all been applied to the management of chronic intestinal amoebia-

sis but chiniofon (Avlochin, Quinoxyl, Yatren), once the most popular member of the group, is now rarely used. Iodochlorhydroxyquinoline (clioquinol, Barquinol, Vioform) has suffered the same fate so far as its employment as a systemic amoebicide is concerned but it is retained for local application in impetigo and other skin infections.

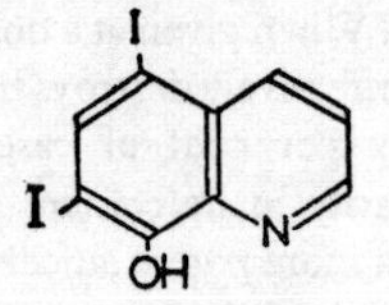

Di-iodohydroxyquinoline 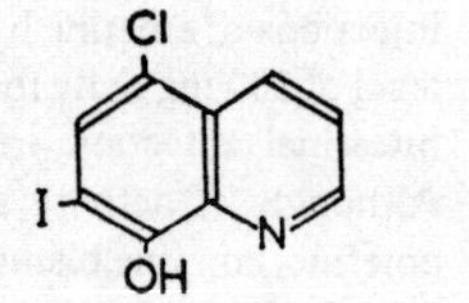   Iodochlorhydroxyquinoline

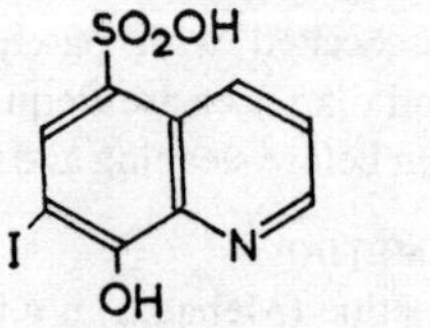

Chiniofon

Fig. 54.2 Iodinated 8-hydroxyquinolines with amoebicidal activity

Travellers will also recognise the drug, through its best known proprietary name, as a popular prophylactic against traveller's diarrhoea but its efficacy in this respect is doubtful since so few cases of this condition are of amoebic origin. The drug has been withdrawn in Japan because of the high incidence of optic nerve degeneration in patients who had taken it systemically. There is little profit to be gained by taking a potentially dangerous drug merely as an expensive placebo.

DI-IODOHYDROXYQUINOLINE
Di-iodohydroxyquinoline (Diodoquin, Embequin) is used to treat symptom-free carriers and cases of chronic intestinal amoebiasis. In acute amoebiasis the use of emetine or carbarsone is combined with that of di-iodohydroxyquinoline. It is ineffective in amoebic abscess of the liver or of other organs because it is not absorbed to any extent from the intestine. The dose employed is from 300 to 600 mg three or four times a day for up to twenty-one days. Di-iodohydroxyquinoline causes few toxic side effects and because of this it has been employed for the large-scale treatment of ambulant patients. It does not invariably give a complete cure. Side effects include gastrointestinal upset, headache and pruritus. Optic neuritis has also been reported thus raising the suspicion that di-iodohydroxyquinoline may sometimes be as dangerous a drug as clioquinol. Although di-iodohydroxyquinoline contains 62 to 64 per cent of iodine it seems that amoebicidal activity is due not to this but to the possession of the 8-hydroxyquinoline nucleus. The iodine may serve to reduce

solubility and hence to slow absorption from the intestine and increase the local effectiveness of the drug. Di-iodohydroxyquinoline should be used cautiously in cases of hypersensitivity to iodine or in cases of thyroid dysfunction and is contraindicated in the presence of liver disease.

Diloxanide furoate
Diloxanide furoate (Furamide) is one of the newer amoebicidal agents. Its main value lies in the treatment of chronic amoebiasis. It has a specific action upon the cysts of *E. histolytica* but is less effective against the trophozoites. The effective adult dose in chronic amoebiasis is 500 mg three times daily for a minimum period of ten days. The toxicity of this compound is low and it has the advantage of being cheap and relatively free from side effects.

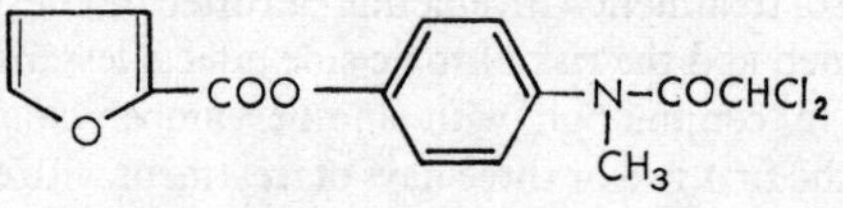

Diloxanide furoate

Organic arsenicals
The organic arsenicals are usually prescribed, for the management of both acute and chronic intestinal amoebiasis, in conjunction with emetine, di-iodohydroxyquinoline or another amoebicide. Compounds containing pentavalent arsenic are preferred to those with the trivalent ion. Though rather less effective they are much less toxic.

CARBARSONE
Carbarsone is particularly used in the treatment of chronic intestinal amoebiasis and to treat symptom-free carriers; the dose level employed is 250 mg two or three times daily for a total of twenty doses (seven to ten days). After a rest period of ten days the same treatment may be repeated. Carbarsone is of no value in amoebic hepatitis or in amoebic abscesses of other organs. It may owe its effectiveness to an inhibitor action upon thiol-enzymes. Side effects include nausea, vomiting, diarrhoea, skin rashes and liver and kidney damage.

GLYCOBIARSOL
Glycobiarsol (Milibis) has the same uses as carbarsone. The dose recommended is 500 mg three times a day for seven days. Glycobiarsol has been employed together with

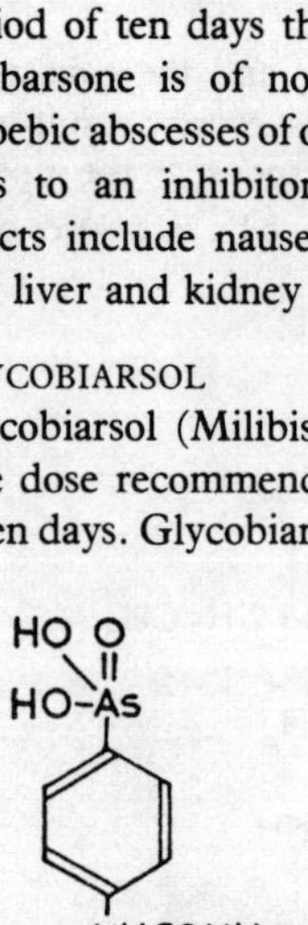

Carbarsone 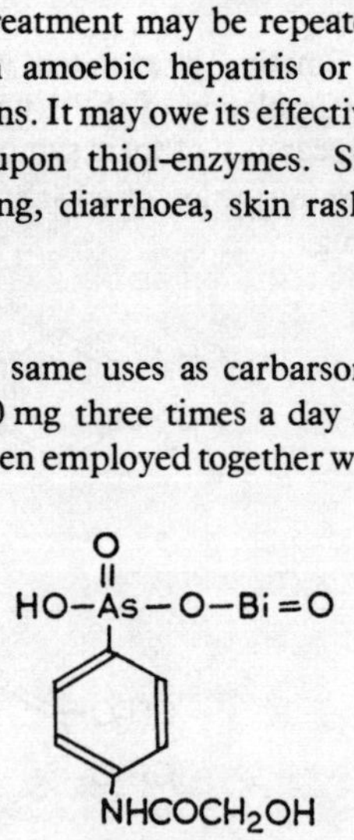   Glycobiarsol

chloroquine in the successful mass treatment of intestinal amoebiasis in mental institutions.

Antibiotics

Antibiotics, particularly the tetracyclines and paromomycin, have been used for treating amoebiasis on the grounds that they destroy the bacterial flora that produce the metabolites essential for the establishment and growth of *E. histolytica* but this form of medication is not now generally recommended.

LABORATORY EVALUATION OF AMOEBICIDES

Provided that special culture media are used, human strains of *E. histolytica* can be cultured and maintained in the laboratory.

A screening method routinely employed for the *in vitro* evaluation of amoebicides consists of preparing a range of dilutions of the compound under test in the culture medium and then inoculating these with a rich culture of the test organism. The tubes containing the drugs plus the culture are incubated at 37°C and samples are removed from time to time for microscopic examination. The results are compared with those obtained from controls that do not contain the drug.

Tests may also be made using monkeys, young rats or guinea pigs infected, naturally or artificially, with *E. histolytica*. In the artificial infection of experimental animals the culture of amoebae may be injected into the caecum after laparotomy or it may be given *per rectum*. Drug treatment is commenced before infection and, after a sufficient period of time, the animal is killed and the large intestine examined for ulceration, motile amoebae and cysts.

BIBLIOGRAPHY

Reviews

Anderson, H.H. and Hansen, E.L. (1950). The chemotherapy of amoebiasis. *Pharmac. Rev.*, **2**, 399-434.

Balamuth, W. and Thompson, P.E. (1955). Comparative studies on amoebae and amoebicides. In *Biochemistry and Physiology of Protozoa*, vol. II, ed. Hutner, S.H. and Lwoff, A. New York: Academic Press.

Findlay, G.M. (1950). *Recent Advances in Chemotherapy*, pp. 191-233. London: Churchill.

Nnochiri, E. (1975). *Medical Parasitology in the Tropics*. London: Oxford University Press.

Powell, S.J. (1969). Amebiasis. In *Current Therapy*. ed. Conn, H.F. Philadelphia: Saunders.

Symposium (1960). Amoebiasis and other intestinal infections, Lucknow, 1959. *Ann. Biochem.*, **20**, Supplement.

Woolfe, G. (1963). Chemotherapy of amoebiasis. In *Experimental Chemotherapy*, vol. I, ed. Schnitzer, R.J. and Hawking, F. New York: Academic Press.

55. The chemotherapy of protozoal disease: leishmaniasis

Three forms of leishmaniasis are recognised. These are visceral leishmaniasis (kala azar), mucocutaneous leishmaniasis (espundia) and dermal or cutaneous leishmaniasis (oriental sore, Baghdad button, Delhi boil). The causative organisms are *Leishmania donovani*, *L. braziliensis* and *L. tropica* respectively. The best method of detecting the organisms is by means of Leishman's stain: the originator of this stain (Sir William Leishman) discovered the organisms that now bear his name. As stained in the tissues, the protozoa take the form of spherical or ovoid bodies, some 2.5 to 5 μm in diameter (the Leishman–Donovan bodies). On culture at room temperature, they become larger and each develops a flagellum.

Kala azar is a disease found in India, China, East Africa and South East Asia. It is characterized by enlargement of the spleen and liver, severe anaemia, wasting and prolonged fever. It may be complicated by dysentery. Protozoa can be detected in the blood and the organs of the reticulo-endothelial system of infected patients. Infection is transmitted by the bites of sand flies that have themselves become infected after biting dogs, the principal vertebrate reservoir.

The other two forms of leishmaniasis occur in scattered areas of South America as well as in Africa and the East. Infection is transmitted to man by the sand fly from dogs, cats and rodents.

The *Leishmania* form a genus of the *Trypanosomidae*.

CHEMOTHERAPY OF KALA AZAR

Compounds of antimony

Organic antimonials containing pentavalent antimony remain the most widely used and most effective drugs for the treatment of kala azar. A large number of these compounds has been synthesized and tested. Some are of simple chemical composition but others are complex and in some instances different batches of the same preparation vary in composition. Since these variations in composition may affect both toxicity and therapeutic potency, it is necessary to exercise careful biological control of each new batch of these drugs.

Many of the pentavalent antimonials are derivatives of *p*-aminophenylstibonic acid. The simplest is stibamine, the sodium salt of the acid. More complex compounds include ethylstibamine (a complex derivative of *p*-amino-

phenylstibonic acid, *p*-acetylaminophenyl stibonic acid and diethylamine), urea stibamine (a mixture of derivatives of phenylstibonic acid), stibamine glucoside and sodium stibogluconate. Among the more recently introduced derivatives are Glucantime (*N*-methylglucamine antimonate) and Pentastib (the *N*-methylglucamine salt of *p*-aminophenylstibonic acid). The most useful of these compounds are urea stibamine, sodium stibogluconate and ethylstibamine.

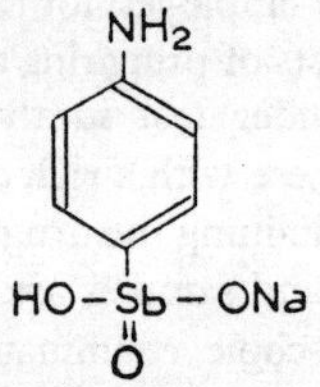

Sodium p-aminophenylstiboate (stibamin)

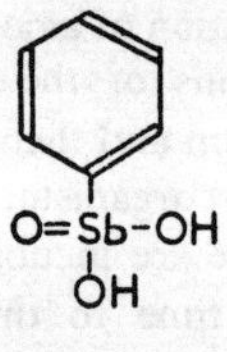

Phenyl stibonic acid

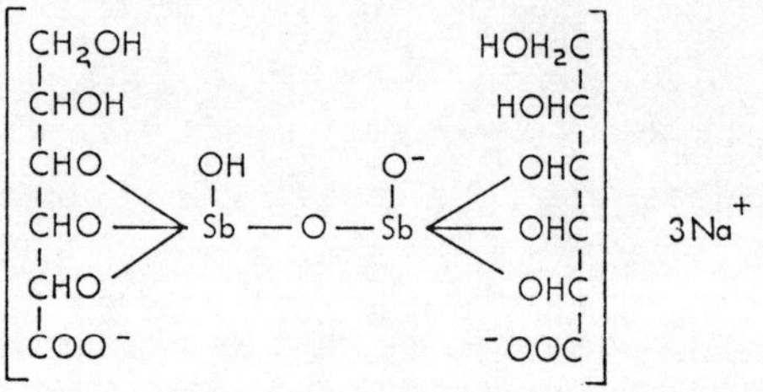

Sodium stibogluconate

Urea stibamine (Carbostibamide, Stiburea, Ureastibol) is given by intravenous injection. A total dose of 2.5 to 3 g given over a 2 to 4 weekly period is usually adequate to effect a cure of Indian kala azar. The African and Sudanese forms of the disease are more refractory and more than one course of treatment with urea stibamine may be necessary. Sodium stibogluconate (Pentostam, Solustibosam), the drug of choice, is given in a daily dose of 500 mgs for ten days but the course of treatment may have to be repeated once or twice at 14-day intervals. It is usually more effective than the other organic arsenicals for the treatment of the Sudanese variety of kala azar. Ethylstibamine (Neostibosam, Stibosamine, Astril) is given in daily doses of 250 mg by intramuscular or intravenous injection until 3 g have been given. The dose schedule for glucantime (protostib) is a similar one.

The organic pentavalent antimonials may produce toxic

side effects including nausea, vomiting, headache, diarrhoea, dizziness, skin rashes and hypotension. Agranulocytosis has occasionally occurred during the treatment of kala azar and large doses of urea stibamine may cause retinal and cerebral haemorrhages. All the compounds are hepatotoxic and should, if possible, be avoided in patients with pre-existing kidney, heart or liver disease.

They owe their therapeutic effectiveness to their ability to prevent the anaerobic metabolism of glucose by *L. donovani*.

Aromatic diamidines

A number of aromatic diamidines are effective against *Leishmania*. The most active are stilbamidine and pentamidine but the toxicity of stilbamidine is so high that its employment is no longer justified. Pentamidine is much less toxic and it is a useful drug for the treatment of cases of kala azar resistant to the organic compounds of antimony. It is given by intramuscular injection as the ethionate in daily doses of 2 to 4 mg per kilogram until temperature and spleen size are reduced. Pentamidine is also employed in the treatment of trypanosomiasis and its pharmacology is discussed in more detail in relation to other trypanocidal drugs on p. 878.

cases of espundia which have not responded to other drugs. Success has also attended the use of cycloguanil pamoate (p. 868). It is given in single intramuscular injections of 350 mg. The dose may have to be repeated.

Dermal leishmaniasis responds to dehydroemetine (p. 871) and metronidazole (p. 882) while both the dermal and mucocutaneous forms of the disease sometimes yield to mepacrine (p. 867) or melarsen (p. 877). Oriental sore can be prevented by inoculating live leishmania into the skin of a part of the body normally hidden by clothing. A small sore is produced but it confers immunity so that the risk of developing a disfiguring ulcer on the face is removed. Other preventive measures against leishmaniasis include the use of insecticides to eliminate the sand fly and, in areas where kala azar is rife, the slaughter of dogs.

BIOLOGICAL EVALUATION OF LEISHMANICIDAL DRUGS

Hamsters can be infected with *Leishmania donovani* and the effectiveness of new drugs can be assessed by their action upon experimental infections. The drug effect is estimated by taking liver or spleen biopsies, counting the

Dihydroxystilbamidine isethionate

Dihydroxystilbamidine isethionate is much less toxic than stilbamidine itself and it has had some success in the treatment of otherwise resistant cases of kala azar. It is given in daily doses of 250 mg for 10 days. The course of treatment can be repeated once or twice if necessary at fortnightly intervals. Like the other diamidines, dihydroxystilbamidine causes histamine release but the resulting itching and headache can be mitigated by antihistamines.

CHEMOTHERAPY OF ESPUNDIA AND ORIENTAL SORE

Drugs used for the treatment of kala azar ought also to be effective in the other forms of leishmaniasis but in practice espundia and oriental sore respond less readily to these agents. Amphotericin B (p. 908) is sometimes of benefit in

number of parasites, and comparing this figure with the values obtained before drug treatment.

BIBLIOGRAPHY

Reviews

Beveridge, E. (1963). Chemotherapy of leishmaniasis. In *Experimental Chemotherapy*, vol. 1, ed. Schnitzer, R.J. and Hawking, F. New York: Academic Press.

Findlay, G.M. (1950). *Recent Advances in Chemotherapy*, vol. 1, pp. 289-358. London: Churchill.

Goodwin, L.G. and Rollo, I.M. (1955). The chemotherapy of malaria, piroplasmosis, trypanosomiasis and leishmaniasis. In *Biochemistry and Physiology of Protozoa*, pp. 225-276, ed. Hutner, S.H. and Lwoff, A. New York: Academic Press.

Nnochiri, E. (1975) *Medical Parasitology in the Tropics*. London: Oxford University Press.

56. The chemotherapy of protozoal disease: trypanosomiasis

Trypanosomes are motile, flagellate protozoa, parasitic on vertebrates including man and on invertebrates, particularly insects. The order *Trypanosomidae* includes the leishmanias (p. 874) as well as the trypanosomes.

Some trypanosomes have a single vertebrate or invertebrate host; others require two hosts, one invertebrate (usually an insect), the other a vertebrate.

Although some trypanosomes are non-pathogenic and live within the tissues of the host without causing ill-health, the pathogenic species produce serious disease in man and in domestic animals, creating immense medical, social and economic problems in tropical Africa and in some parts of South and Central America. It has been estimated that trypanosomiasis has made one half of the total land surface of Africa unsuitable for the rearing of animals.

The organisms which cause disease in animals (nagana) include *T. congolense* and *T. vivax* in cattle and *T. evansi* and *T. equiperdum* in horses. In man, the trypanosomes *T. gambiense* and *T. rhodesiense* cause sleeping sickness in Africa. *T. cruzi* is responsible for *Chagas' disease* in South America.

Chagas' disease is transmitted by the reduviid bugs (assassin or kissing bugs) which defaecate as they suck the blood of their human victims. The bite (usually on the face) causes itching and the victim scratches, rubbing infected faeces into the wounds. *T. cruzi* principally infects muscle, particularly that of the heart and alimentary tract. Chagas' disease which is essentially a disease of poverty, does not usually respond to the drugs that can control African trypanosomiasis and it is very often fatal. However, recent investigations have provided some

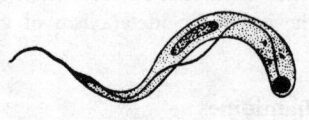

Fig. 56.1 T cruzi

grounds for believing that nitrofurazone (p. 879) and metronidazole (p. 882) might be able to succeed where other drugs have failed. Steck (1972) has surveyed and evaluated the many other drugs that have from time to time been applied to the treatment of Chagas' disease. None achieved more than a limited success.

Sleeping sickness is transmitted by the bite of the tsetse fly. The symptoms of the disease signal the presence of trypanosomes in the central nervous system. Patients are drowsy, lethargic and apathetic; they sleep for long periods and become weak and emaciated. Unlike Chagas' disease, sleeping sickness does respond to drugs, some of which can also be used to prevent the disease.

Trypanosomiasis can also be attacked by destroying insects and their breeding places and by destruction of game which can act as reservoirs of pathogenic trypanosomes. Gamma benzene hexachloride and dieldrin (p. 901) are widely used in the campaign to eliminate insect vectors. Improved housing and hygenic conditions will also help to reduce contact between man and fly.

CHEMOTHERAPY OF TRYPANOSOMIASIS IN MAN

Compounds of arsenic
A large number of arsenic compounds have been used in

Table 56.1 Drugs used in the treatment of trypanosomiasis in man

	Prophylaxis	*Treatment*	
American trypanosomiasis (Chagas' disease)		? nitrofurazone ? metronidazole	
African trypanosomiasis		*Early cases*	*Late cases*
West African type (caused by *T. gambiense*)	pentamidine suramin	pentamidine	melarsoprol tryparsamide (rarely) nitrofurazone (rarely)
East African type (caused by *T. rhodesiense*)	Prophylaxis not recommended	suramin	melarsoprol nitrofurazone (rarely)

the past in the chemotherapy of trypanosomiasis. Their margin of safety is generally low and with the development of other drugs, most of them are now obsolescent. The only survivors are tryparsamide and melarsoprol.

TRYPARSAMIDE

Tryparsamide contains about 25 per cent of pentavalent arsenic in organic combination. In the body it is reduced to the pharmacologically active trivalent form.

Tryparsamide is effective in the treatment of the more advanced cases of sleeping sickness because of its ability to cross the blood brain barrier and render the cerebrospinal fluid trypanocidal. It is frequently used with suramin or pentamidine. Treatment with tryparsamide usually involves weekly injections, a course lasting from 6 to 15 weeks. The adult dose in advanced cases is 0.06 g per kg of body mass. Treatment may be followed by a relapse. Many strains of trypanosome are now resistant to tryparsamide and this severely limits the drug's usefulness.

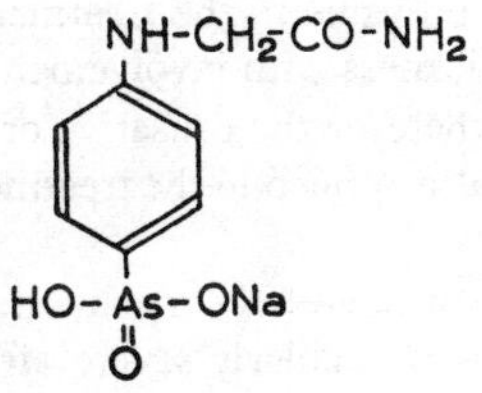

Tryparsamide

Tryparsamide causes some toxic side-effects which are aggravated by the debility, malnutrition and disease that afflict so many African communities. The most important toxic effect is optic nerve atrophy, which may be severe enough to cause permanent impairment of the vision or even blindness. Tryparsamide may also cause skin rashes, fever and diarrhoea. The toxic side-effects of tryparsamide can be prevented or partially reversed, by dimercaprol (p. 796).

MELARSOPROL

This substance (also known as mel B) is a compound of melarsen oxide with dimercaprol. It contains trivalent arsenic. Although melarsoprol is effective in all stages of sleeping sickness, it is not without danger and its use is therefore restricted to the hospital treatment of advanced cases which show severe involvement of the central nervous system and will not respond to other drugs. In these circumstances it is an extremely valuable therapeutic agent. It is usually given by slow intravenous injection in daily doses of 3.6 mg per kilogram of body mass for three days. The course can be repeated after two to three weeks if necessary. East African patients are often more sensitive to the drugs than their West African counterparts and it may be necessary to initiate their treatment with only small amounts of melarsoprol which are slowly increased until an effective dose level is reached.

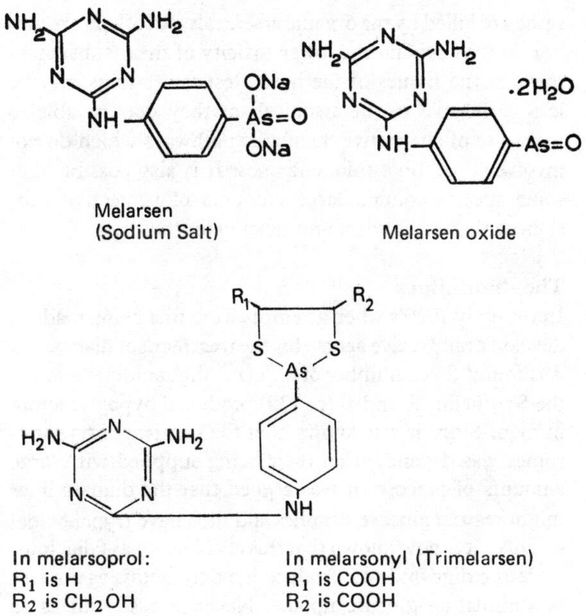

In melarsoprol: In melarsonyl (Trimelarsen)
R_1 is H R_1 is COOH
R_2 is CH_2OH R_2 is COOH

Fig. 56.2 Melarsen and related compounds

On the very rare occasions when, because of intolerance to other drugs, early cases of sleeping sickness have to be treated with melarsoprol only a single injection is given.

Side-effects are frequent and include abdominal pain, dermatitis, agranulocytosis, allergic reactions to the dead trypanosomes (the Jarisch-Herxheimer reaction), reactive encephalopathy and damage to the heart.

Mode of action of the organic arsenicals
Trypanosomes sensitive to arsenic are able to remove it from the medium in which they are suspended, bind it firmly and transport it into the interior of their bodies. The organic arsenicals (after conversion, where relevant, into a trivalent compound) are believed to combine with and inactivate vital enzymes by reacting with free thiol groups. Trypanosomes have a very high metabolic rate and oxidize large amounts of glucose. It may be that the arsenicals inhibit hexokinase which catalyzes the conversion of glucose to glucose-6-phosphate. Many other enzymes involved in glycolysis and the tricarboxylic acid cycle possess essential thiol groups.

An earlier hypothesis concerning the mode of action of the arsenical trypanocides, due to Voegtlin and his co-workers, was that the drugs combine with the thiol compounds glutathione and cysteine and perhaps others. This would inhibit cellular oxidation-reduction systems and cause the death of the cell. Glutathione, cysteine and dimercaprol have all been shown to protect trypanosomes (and their human hosts) against the toxic effects of the organic arsenicals, a point in favour of this hypothesis. Neither hypothesis explains why some species of trypanosome are killed by the organic arsenicals and others are not, nor do they explain the lower toxicity of these substances towards the tissues of the host. Resistant strains may be less permeable to the arsenicals or they may be able to make use of alternative metabolic pathways which do not involve susceptible thiol enzymes. It is also possible that some species contain large amounts of protective substances that react with, and inactivate, the drug.

The diamidines

In the early 1920's when attempts were first being made to develop orally active agents for the treatment of diabetes, it was found that a number of aliphatic diguanidines such as the Synthalins A and B (p. 730) produced hypoglycaemia in man. Since it was known that the survival of trypanosomes was dependent on their being supplied with large amounts of glucose, it was argued that the diguanidines might restrict glucose supplies and thus have trypanocidal activity. It is now known that this argument was fallacious, since the diguanidines produce hypoglycaemia as a result of stimulating glucose uptake. Nevertheless—and as so often happens in pharmacology—the prediction, though

$$H_2N \diagup C-NH \cdot (CH_2)_n-NH-C \diagdown NH_2$$
$$HN \qquad\qquad\qquad\qquad NH$$

$n=10=$decamethylene diguanidine

$$H_2N \diagup C-(CH_2)_{11}-C \diagdown NH_2$$
$$HN \qquad\qquad\qquad NH$$

Undecane diamidine

Propamidine

Pentamidine

Stilbamidine

based on a false premise, was fulfilled. Work with these substances led to the synthesis of related compounds—first the aliphatic diamidines such as undecane diamidine and then the aromatic diamidines, propamidine, pentamidine and stilbamidine. The last named compounds have all been used in the treatment of trypanosomiasis but pentamidine is much the least toxic of the three and it is, consequently, the most widely used.

PENTAMIDINE

Pentamidine is used in both the treatment and mass prophylaxis of sleeping sickness. It has already provided protection for whole populations in Africa. Unfortunately, mass prophylaxis of this type carries with it the danger that resistant organisms will develop and proliferate. This is already happening with pentamidine which is no longer recommended for the prevention of infection by *T. rhodesiense*, the East African trypanosome.

Pentamidine is usually given by intramuscular or intravenous injection. It is used as the dimethyl sulphonate (Lomidine) or diisethionate. The prophylactic dose is 3 to 4 mg of base per kg of body mass every six months. The average dose for the treatment of early cases of sleeping sickness caused by *T. gambiense* is 1.5 to 4 mg of base per kg of body mass for six to ten days. Many strains of *T. rhodesiense*, as we have already seen, are resistant to pentamidine and an alternative drug such as suramin is needed to control early infections with this organism. Moreover, pentamidine is of no value in the treatment of advanced cases of sleeping sickness with involvement of the central nervous system, whatever the causative organism.

Pentamidine is also applied to the treatment of kala azar (p. 874).

The most common side-effect of pentamidine treatment is itching, which is particularly severe after intravenous administration of the drug. It is probably caused by histamine release (p. 342). Among unsophisticated populations, the itching is often taken as a welcome sign of the drug's effectiveness. Other side-effects include diarrhoea, vomiting, headache, faintness and (after intravenous injection) a sudden fall in blood pressure.

Mode of action of pentamidine

The origin of pentamidine's trypanocidal activity is not precisely known but in *in vitro* experiments it has been shown to inhibit no fewer than 20 enzyme systems (Newton, 1964a). Its inhibitory action on the growth and reproduction of trypanosomes should therefore occasion no surprise.

Other compounds

SURAMIN

In the early years of this century a number of dyestuffs were shown to be capable of curing experimental trypanosome infections in mice. Trypan red, trypan blue and afridol violet were among the first chemotherapeutic agents to be discovered. They were not effective, however, in the treatment of trypanosomiasis in man. It was soon realized that there was no need for trypanocidal compounds to be coloured and that colourless compounds based upon the structure of active dyestuffs were just as likely to be effective. One of these compounds was suramin (Antryptol; Germanin; Moranyl) a complex derivative of urea.

Suramin is effective in early African trypanosomiasis but, because of the large size of its molecule, it does not penetrate nervous tissue so that it is of no value in treating advanced forms of the disease. It has a very prolonged action and it is therefore a useful prophylactic drug. Binding to plasma and tissue proteins and reabsorption by the tubular epithelium of the kidneys account for its prolonged action although the strong negative charge on the molecule may also be important. The trypanosomes themselves bind the drug and this is probably the first step in its lethal action. The mode of action of suramin is not known, but it has been suggested that it inhibits anaerobic glycolysis and also that it sensitizes the organisms to phagocytes which then destroy them.

Retention of suramin by the kidneys not infrequently gives rise to albuminuria but signs of more serious renal damage sometimes appear and the drug is contraindicated in patients with inadequate kidney function. A small minority of people suffer anaphylactic like reactions to suramin and it is wise to give a preliminary test dose of the drug to patients for whom treatment with suramin is contemplated.

Other side effects associated with the use of suramin include nausea, vomiting, diarrhoea, skin rashes, fever, headache, paraesthesiae and collapse. In undernourished communities, side effects are more common and more severe.

When used prophylactically, suramin is given in intravenous doses of one gram at two-weekly intervals. Prophylactic treatment should be restricted to those exposed to the possibility of infection with *T. gambiense*.

Early cases of sleeping sickness are given one gram of suramin intravenously at weekly intervals until five doses have been given. An alternative schedule is to give the drug on days 1, 4, 7, 14 and 21. Suramin is particularly useful for treating infections with *T. rhodesiense,* an organism that is often resistant to pentamidine. Suramin also finds a place in the therapy of onchocerciasis (p. 893).

NITROFURAZONE

We have already mentioned nitrofurazone (Furacin) in connection with Chagas' disease. It is also employed in late cases of African trypanosomiasis but its high toxicity precludes it from consideration as anything more than a reserve drug in this condition, to be tried only when all else fails. Side effects include haemolytic anaemia and polyneuritis. The polyneuritis appears to be associated with the drug's ability to antagonize thiamine. Haemolytic anaemia occurs only in susceptible patients but, unfortunately, the cause of their susceptibility—a deficiency of glucose-6-

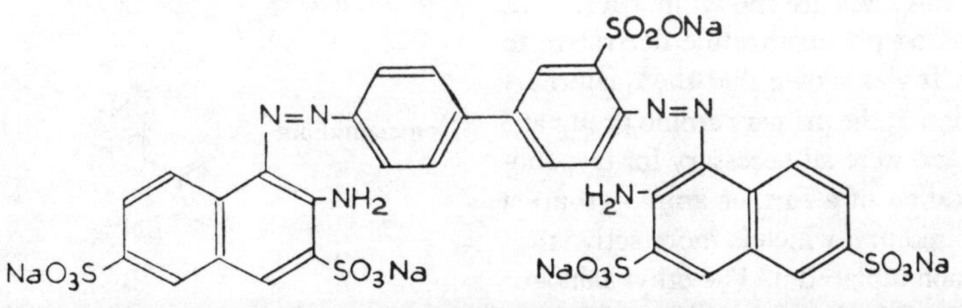

Trypan Red

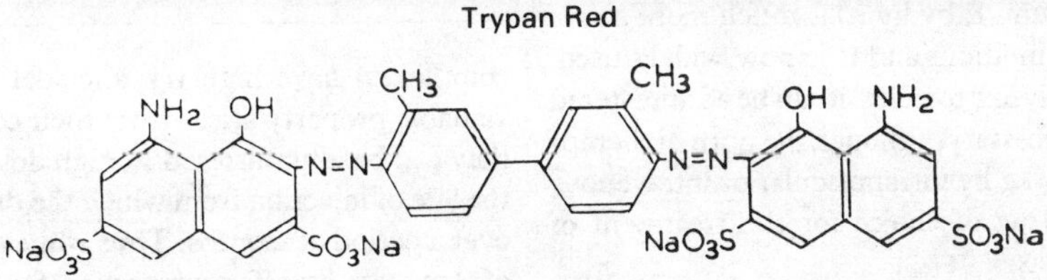

Trypan Blue

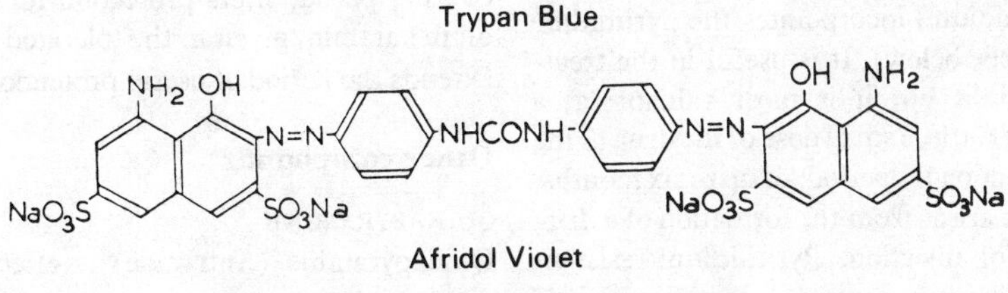

Afridol Violet

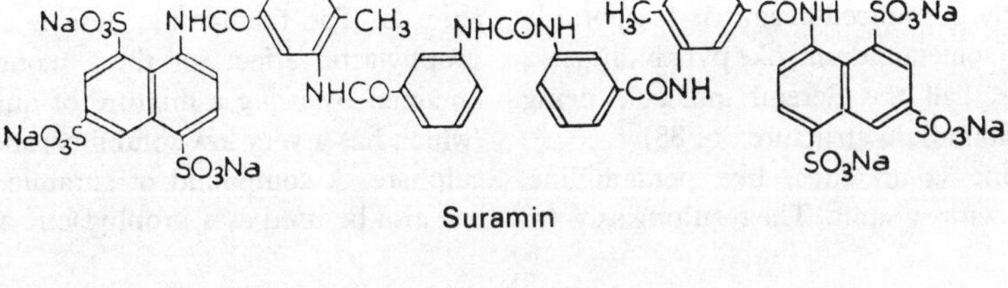

Suramin

Nitrofurazone

phosphate dehydrogenase in the erythrocytes—occurs most often in dark-skinned people, particularly men (p. 74). These are the very people who will form the greater number of those most in need of the drug.

CHEMOTHERAPY OF TRYPANOSOMIASIS IN DOMESTIC ANIMALS

In terms of food productivity, standard of living and ultimately the health of the population, trypanosomiasis in cattle has been a more serious menace in Africa than has the human disease. Recent advances in chemotherapy have greatly improved the situation but the emergence of resistant strains to individual drugs necessitates the continued development of new substances for the prophylaxis and treatment of trypanosome infections. Attempts to destroy the trypanosome breeding grounds thus become of considerable importance.

Phenanthridine derivatives
Useful compounds in this class are shown in Table 56.2.

Phenidium was the first phenanthridine derivative to undergo clinical trials. It was shown that the quaternary nitrogen atom at position 5, the primary amino group at 8 and the phenyl group at 6 were all necessary for trypanocidal activity. The addition of a further amino group at position 3 produced dimidium, which is more active than phenidium and very soon replaced it. The ethyl analogue of dimidium (homidium, Ethydium) is much more active and less toxic than dimidium and it is now widely used. Because of its relatively low toxicity, it can be administered in high doses when necessary, although the normal therapeutic dose is 2 mg per kg by intramuscular or intravenous injection. It is the drug of choice for the treatment of bovine trypanosomiasis.

Pyrithidium (Prothidium) incorporates the pyrimidine ring of quinapyrine (see below). It is useful in the treatment of trypanosomiasis but it is most valuable as a prophylactic agent. In cattle, a small dose of the drug (2 mg per kg) provides protection for periods of up to six months. This prolonged action arises from the formation of a drug depot at this point of injection. Pyrithidium-resistant strains of trypanosomes are appearing but isometamidium, a more recently introduced drug, has temporarily solved this problem. Isometamidium, like pyrithidium is a 'combined' molecule, half the Berenil molecule being incorporated in the homidium structure (p. 88).

The phenanthridine compounds, like pentamidine, have been combined with suramin. The resulting salts (or

Table 56.2 Some useful phenanthridine derivatives

	R_1	R_2	R_3	R_4
Phenidium	H	-	CH_3	NH_2
Dimidium	H	NH_2	CH_3	-
Homidium (*Ethydium*)	H	NH_2	C_2H_5	-
Pyrithidium (*Prothidium*)			NH_2	CH_3
Isometamidium			NH_2	C_2H_5

complexes) have high trypanocidal activity. Their most valuable property arises from their colloidal structure, for they can be administered in high doses to form a depot at the site of injection from which the drug is released slowly over a period of months. Thus while pyrithidium in a dose of 2 mg per kg offers protection for six months, pyrithidium suramin, given in the tolerated dose of 10 mg per kg extends the period of useful protection to almost one year.

Other compounds

QUINAPYRAMINE
Quinapyramine (Antrycide) is effective against a wide range of the trypanosomes that cause disease in domestic animals. The therapeutic dose is about 5 mg per kg. A prophylactic effect for three months or longer can be obtained by using a mixture of quinapyramine chloride (which has a very low solubility) and the soluble methylsulphate. A compound of suramin with quinapyramine can also be used as a prophylactic agent.

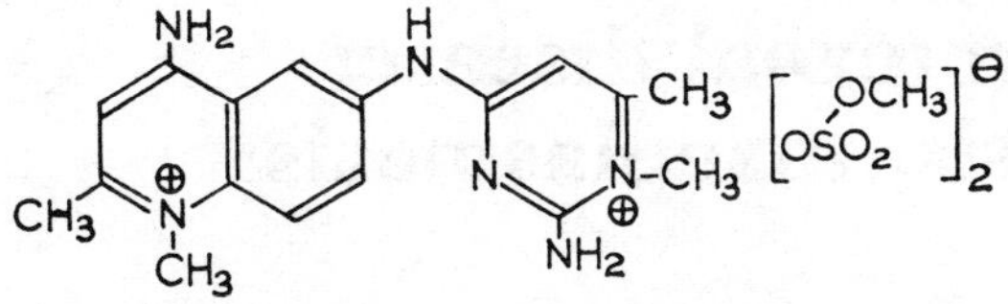

Quinapyramine

DIMINAZENE

Some diamidines possess trypanocidal activity. The most important of these is diminazene (Berenil) which is used successfully to treat infections in cattle. Diminazene has no prophylactic uses.

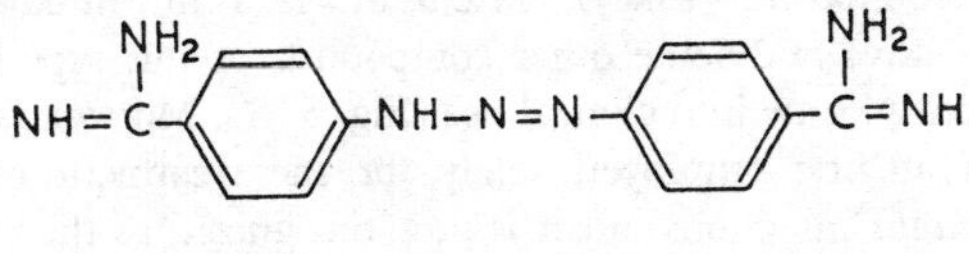

Diminazene
(Berenil)

Mode of action of the phenanthridine derivatives and related compounds

As the work of Newton and others has shown, the phenanthridine derivatives interfere with the synthesis of nucleic acids and protein. Quinapyramine has a similar action and the other trypanocides also seem to block vital enzyme reactions. The question then arises as to why the host, as well as the parasite, is not killed by the drug. A large number of possible explanations has been put forward: they are summarized and examined by Newton (1964b). They include the possibility that only the parasite has the appropriate drug binding sites or that it may be more permeable to the drug. The parasite may not be able to resynthesize essential cellular components as quickly as the host. Some trypanosomes (unlike their hosts) cannot synthesize the purine ring, so inhibition of adenine incorporation would be fatal.

EVALUATION OF DRUGS FOR TRYPANOCIDAL ACTIVITY

In essence, the methods used consist of infecting mice with trypanosomes, waiting until the blood shows that trypanosomes are present in the circulation and then injecting the drug under test. The organisms employed experimentally are *T. brucei*, *T. equiperdum* and *T. rhodesiense*. Normally the infected mice will die in about six days. An active drug will prolong life by eliminating or reducing the numbers of trypanosomes in the tissues. New drugs are compared with compounds of known potency and against non-drug treated controls.

For studying the mode of action of trypanocides, trypanosome-like organisms such as *Crithidia oncopelti*, found in some insects, can be cultured *in vitro*. Trypanosomes themselves have not, as yet, been satisfactorily cultured.

BIBLIOGRAPHY

Reviews and monographs

Brener, Z. (1975). Chemotherapy of *Trypansoma cruzi*. *Adv. Pharmac. Chemother.*, **13**, 1-44.
CIBA Symposium No. 20 (1974). *Trypanosomiasis and Leishmaniasis with Special Reference to Chagas' Disease.* Amsterdam: Associated Scientific Publishers.
Findlay, F.M. (1950). *Recent Advances in Chemotherapy*, vol. 1, pp. 359-576. London: Churchill.
Goodwin, L.G. and Goss, I.M. (1955). The chemotherapy of malaria, piroplasmosis, trypanosomiasis and leishmaniasis. In *Biochemistry and Physiology of Protozoa*, vol. 2, ed. Hutner, S.H. and Lwoff, A. New York: Academic Press.
Newton, B.A. (1964a). Trypanocidal Agents. In *Metabolic Inhibitors*, vol. 2, pp. 285-310, ed. Quastel, J.H. and Hochster, R.M. New York: Academic Press.
Newton, B.A. (1964b). Mechanism of action of phenanthridine and aminoqualdine trypanocides. In *Advances in Chemotherapy*, vol. 1, p. 35-83, ed. Golden, A. and Hawkins, F. New York: Academic Press.
Nnochiri, E. (1975). *Medical Parasitology in the Tropics*. London: Oxford University Press.
Noble, E.R. (1955). The morphology and life cycles of trypanosomes. *Q. Rev. Biol.*, **30**, 1-28.
Steck, E.A. (1972). *The Chemotherapy of Protozoan Diseases.* Washington D.C: Walter Reed Army Institute.
Walls, L.P. (1963). The chemotherapy of trypanosomiasis. *Prog. med. Chem.*, **3**, 52-88.
World Health Organization (1960). Chagas' disease. *Tech. Rep. Ser. Wld Hlth Org.* No. 202.
World Health Organization (1962). Expert committee on trypanosomiasis. *Tech. Rep. Ser. Wld Hlth Org.* No. 247.

57. The chemotherapy of protozoal disease: trichomoniasis, piroplasmosis, toxoplasmosis and coccidiosis

The miscellaneous group of conditions discussed here are all caused by protozoan parasites. Some of them are treated with drugs which, since they are also useful in the treatment of other diseases, are more appropriately considered elsewhere. In this chapter, attention is directed towards drugs which are more specifically employed in the treatment of the conditions named.

TRICHOMONIASIS

The trichomonads are unicellular, oval or pear-shaped organisms some 12–25 μm long with three or four flagella emerging from the wider end. Parasitic species are found in many vertebrate and invertebrate hosts but most of them are not pathogenic. Among those which do cause disease are *Trichomonas vaginalis* in man, *T. foetus* in cattle and *T. columbae* in pigeons.

T. vaginalis causes vaginitis in the female and urethritis in the male. In the male, trichomonal urethritis is frequently symptomless and infection and reinfection of the female by her sexual partner, unaware that he is harbouring the parasite, is common. For this reason, it is advisable to treat both parties, even when treatment is sought only by the woman. Trichomonal vaginitis causes a vaginal discharge (in which the organism can be identified) and an intense pruritus.

Susceptibility to infection in the female varies with her age and the period of the menstrual cycle. Multiplication of trichomonads and other infecting organisms is prevented by acid conditions in the vagina. The vaginal contents are almost neutral in reaction before puberty, after the menopause, after parturition and during and immediately after menstruation. At these times, susceptibility to trichomonal infection is high. At other times the vaginal secretions are acid because Döderlein's bacilli,

normal commensals in the vagina, form lactic acid from glycogen.

METRONIDAZOLE
Metronidazole (Flagyl, Trichazol) is a nitroimidazole derivative and some other compounds of this type have recently come into clinical use (Fig. 57.1). Metronidazole was at first employed solely for the treatment of *T. vaginalis* infections but it is now recognized as the treatment of choice for all forms of amoebiasis. It has also been used with considerable success in Vincent's angina (p. 861) and it is rapidly establishing a reputation as the best available drug for dracunculiasis (p. 885), giardiasis and balantidiasis. The two last named diseases are protozoal infections of the gastrointestinal tract. Metronidazole has occasionally been applied to the treatment of alcoholism (see below), exophthalmos (p. 714) and haemorrhoids but there can be few occasions when it is necessary or desirable to resort to such an unlikely treatment for these conditions. Metronidazole is active by mouth and it is therefore suitable for the treatment of trichomonal infections in both male and female patients to whom it is given in doses of 250 mg twice or thrice daily. A single course of treatment usually lasts for 7 to 10 days. Alternatively, a dose of two grams can be given on a single occasion: this one-dose regime seems to be as effective as the more prolonged treatment programme. In amoebiasis, the dose of metronidazole is 800 mg given thrice daily for five days but in the more chronic forms of the disease is it sometimes preferable to halve the daily dose and to continue drug administration for ten days. Side effects, whose incidence is not high, include gastric upsets, a metallic taste in the mouth, skin rashes, pruritus and disturbances of the central nervous system manifested by dizziness, paraesthesiae, ataxia and muscular inco-ordination. People receiving metronidazole may experience nausea, headache and vom-

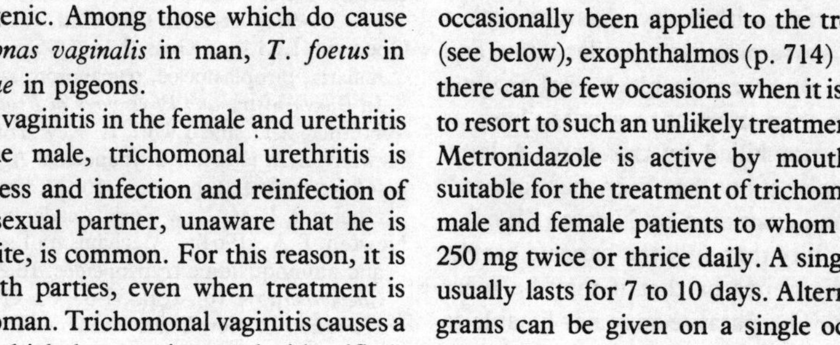

	R_1	R_2
metronidazole	CH_3	CH_2CH_2OH
nimorazole	H	CH_2CH_2N (morpholine ring with O)
tinidazole	CH_3	$CH_2CH_2SO_2C_2H_5$

Fig. 57.1 Some nitroimidazole derivatives

iting if they also take alcohol. The occurrence of this disulphiram like response (p. 89) led to the introduction of metronidazole aversion therapy in alcoholism (Lal, 1969) but the value of this treatment is dubious. Acute psychotic changes have been seen in alcoholic subjects who have been given disulphiram and metronidazole together (Rothstein and Chancy, 1969).

Moniliasis (p. 907) may sometimes occur in patients receiving metronidazole and it is a wise precaution to give nystatin or topical amphotericin B to these patients if by reason, for instance, of pregnancy or diabetes, they are particularly exposed to the risk of moniliasis, with metronidazole. Treatment with metronidazole should be stopped if symptoms of central nervous system involvement appear. The drug is capable of causing leucopenia but few serious cases directly attributable to the drug have been reported.

Metronidazole is contra-indicated in patients with blood dyscrasias but there is no convincing reason for withholding the drug in early pregancy. There is no evidence that it has a teratogenic action but there is ample evidence that trichomonal vaginitis, if left untreated, increases the likelihood of premature labour.

The mode of action of metronidazole is unknown.

NIMORAZOLE AND TINIDAZOLE

Nimorazole (nitrimidazine, Naxogin, Nulogyl) has a spectrum of activity and a range of therapeutic applications similar in every way to those of metronidazole. Even the effective dose (250 mg thrice daily) is the same. Tinidazole is similar to the other two nitroimidazoles although it is rather more potent (probably because it is more resistant to metabolic degradation) and is effective at a dose level of 125 mg.

PIMARICIN AND HACHIMYCIN

These polyene antibiotics (p. 908) are employed in the treatment of vaginal candidiasis but they also possess some trichomonacidal activity, a fortunate circumstance in view of the frequency with which candidiasis and trichomoniasis coexist in the same patient.

ACETARSOL

Acetarsol is used in the form of vaginal pessaries (SVC) each containing 250 mg of the drug. Acetarsol is frequently used with lactose which acts as a substrate for the Döderleins bacilli. Boric acid, to increase vaginal acidity,

may also be incorporated in the pessaries and treatment with acetarsol may be supplemented with oestrogens to stimulate the deposition of glycogen in the cells of the vaginal epithelium. Before administration of the drug, the vagina is douched with normal saline to remove cellular debris and viscous secretions and thus enable the drug to operate more effectively. Although acetarsol is often effective in cases of vaginal trichomoniasis, the complex nature of the treatment indicates the difficulty of controlling the infection by local application of drugs in contrast to the simplicity of metronidazole therapy. Side effects of acetarsol treatment include skin rashes and vaginal irritation.

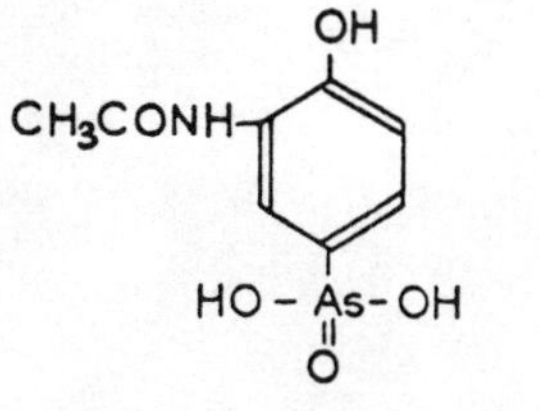

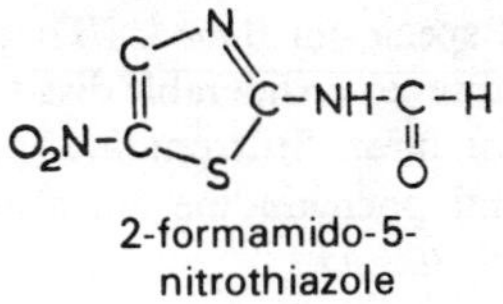

2-formamido-5-
nitrothiazole

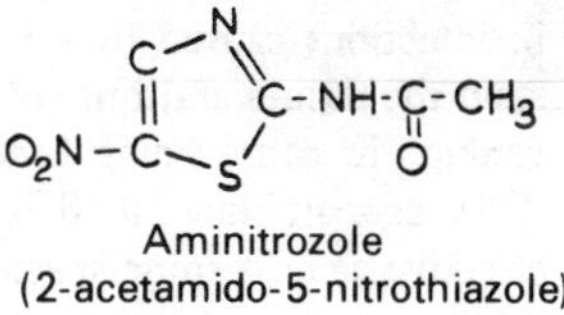

Aminitrozole
(2-acetamido-5-nitrothiazole)

AMINITROZOLE

A number of nitrothiazoles are effective in the prevention and treatment of trichomonal disease in poultry. Two of these, 2-formamido-5-nitrothiazole and 2-acetamido-5-nitrothiazole (aminitrozole) have also been used for the therapy of trichomonal vaginitis but they are of very limited value in human beings.

PIROPLASMOSIS

Piroplasmosis is essentially a disease of tame and domestic animals which are susceptible to many members of the *Babesia, Theileria* and *Anaplasma* species. These protozoa infect the red blood corpuscles. Infection is spread by the bite of infected ticks and the disease is sometimes called 'tick fever'. Piroplasmosis is widespread throughout the world and it is responsible for much loss of value livestock. Very rarely, piroplasmosis occurs in man: a fatal case of human infection by *B. bovis,* the organism which causes European red water in cattle, has been reported from Yugoslavia.

QUINURONIUM METHYL SULPHATE

Quinuronium methyl sulphate (Ludobal) is effective against many species of *Babesia* and is the best available drug for the treatment of this type of infection in horses and cattle. It is less effective against *Theileria* and *Anaplasma* infections although it has been used with some

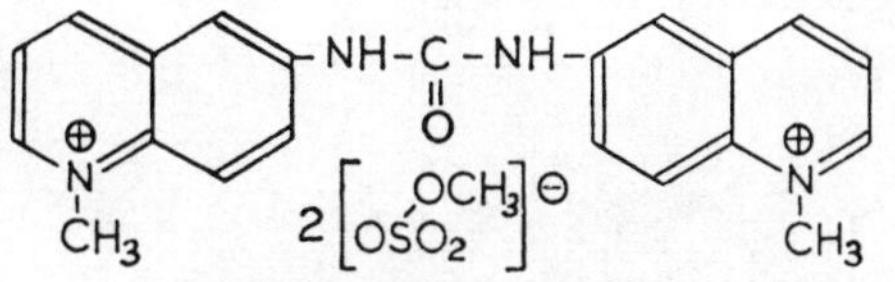

Acetarsol

Quinuronium methyl sulphate

success in these conditions. Quinuronium has some acetyl-choline-like activity which is the source of most of the drug's side effects.

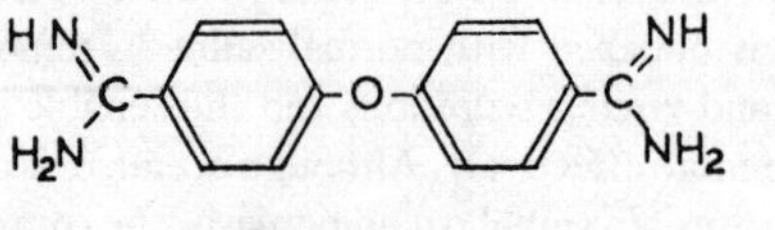

Phenamidine

OTHER COMPOUNDS
These include the dyes trypan blue and euflavine. Given by intravenous or subcutaneous injection, they are useful in infections caused by several species of *Babesia*. They stain the tissues and this constitutes a considerable disadvantage in cattle being bred for meat. Stilbamidine (p. 878), propamidine (p. 878) and phenamidine are also effective against some species of *Babesia*.

OTHER PROTOZOAL DISEASES

Toxoplasmosis is the result of infection by species of *Toxoplasma* which can become parasitic on both man and animals. The most usual infecting organism is *T. gondi,* a small, non-motile, oval shaped protozoon, some 5 μm long and 2 μm wide, first obtained from the gondi, an African rodent. Large numbers of human beings throughout the world carry the parasite which dwells within the cells of the nervous system and heart and the macrophages of the reticuloendothelial system. Overt signs of disease are rare but a fatal hydrocephalus or encephalitis may afflict infants who have acquired the infection, before birth, from their mothers. In older subjects, toxoplasmosis sometimes gives rise to a condition resembling infectious mononucleosis ('glandular fever'). When it is not of congenital origin, toxoplasmosis is probably transmitted from domestic animals. The cat has developed something of a reputation as a reservoir of *T. gondi*. The drug of choice for the treatment of toxoplasmosis is pyrimethamine (p. 868), with sulphadiazine. *Balantidium coli* may cause dysentery in man. As we have already seen (p. 882), balantidiasis is now treated by metronidazole.

Histomonas meleagridis causes enterohepatitis ('black-head disease') in turkeys. The liver and caecum are infected and the disease can cause serious losses to poultry breeders. Drugs used for the prevention or treatment of

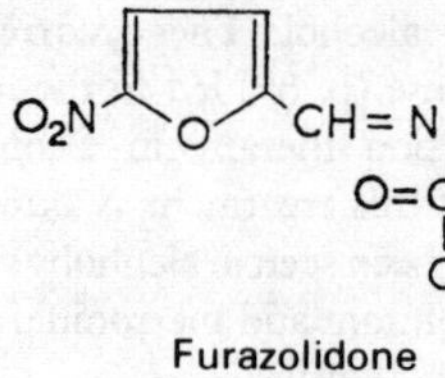

Furazolidone

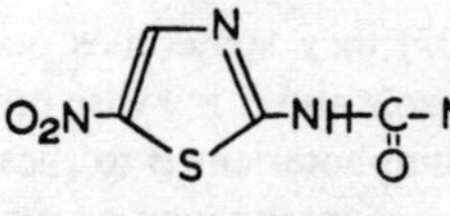

Nithiazide

enterohepatitis include the 8-hydroxyquinolines, organic arsenicals (acetarsol, tryparsamide and carbarsone), the nitrothiazoles, furazolidone and nithiazide.

Infection with species of *Eimeria* causes coccidiosis in chickens, rabbits, dogs, cattle, sheep and pigs. Coccidiosis is rare in man. The most effective drugs in this condition are furazolidone and nitrofurazone (p. 879). They are added to the food.

BIBLIOGRAPHY

Books, monographs and reviews
Conference (1956). Some protozoan diseases of man and animals: anaplasmosis, babesiosis and toxoplasmosis. *Ann. N.Y. Acad. Sci.,* **64,** 25-277.
Conference (1959). The vagina. *Ann. N.Y. Acad. Sci.,* **83,** 77-358.
Sawyer, Phyllis R., Brogden, R.N., Pinder, R.M., Speight, T.M. and Avery, G.S. (1976). Tinidazole: a review of its antiprotozoal activity and therapeutic efficacy. *Drugs.* **11,** 423-440.
Schnitzer, R.J. and Hawking, F. (1963). *Experimental Chemotherapy,* Vol. 1. New York: Academic Press.
Trussell, R.E. (1947). *Trichomonas Vaginalis and Trichomoniasis.* Oxford: Blackwell.

Original papers
Lal, S. (1969). Metronidazole in the treatment of alcoholism. A clinical trial and review of the literature. *Q. Jl. Stud. Alc.* **28,** 544-546.
Lehmann, H.E. and Ban, T.A. (1967). Chemical reduction of compulsion to drink with metronidazole: new treatment modality in therapeutic program of alcoholics. *Current Therap. Research.* **9,** 419-428.
Rothstein, E. and Clancy, D.D. (1969). Toxicity of disulfiram combined with metronidazole. *New Engl. J. Med.* **280,** 1006-1007.

58. The chemotherapy of helminthiasis

Infestation with parasitic worms (*helminthiasis*) and its control by means of drugs and social and educational measures is an urgent problem in many tropical and subtropical countries.

Drugs that are employed to destroy and eliminate parasitic worms are known as *anthelmintics*. Drugs that kill worms are also called *vermicides*, those which expel them from the body are called *vermifuges*.

The poorer the community, the greater the extent of worm infestation. This fact has made it imperative to develop cheap, non-toxic, effective drugs that can be given by mouth.

Helminthiasis rarely causes death directly but in some communities it takes a very serious toll of health, leading to lowered efficiency, reduced resistance to disease and retardation of growth. Infestation with several species of parasite is not uncommon and helminthiasis is frequently superimposed upon other diseases, including malaria and trypanosomiasis.

The extent of worm infestation throughout the world is indicated by the figures quoted by Watkins (1958) who estimated that one species alone—the roundworm, *Ascaris lumbricoides*—infects 600 million people. Victims of infestation by other species are numbered in tens or hundreds of millions.

In this chapter the more common types of parasitic worm (classified as in Fig. 58.1) and the diseases they cause are briefly described in the text. The individual drugs used in the treatment of helminthiasis are then considered. The information provided in the text is summarized, with some additional notes (intended only for reference) in Tables 58.1 to 58.5.

TYPES OF WORM INFESTATION

Conditions caused by roundworms

FILARIASIS

Filariasis (which also includes the related conditions onchocerciasis and dracontiasis) is a major social and economic problem in the tropics.

Filarial worms that cause disease in man include: *Wuchereria bancrofti, Brugia malayi, Loa loa, Onchocerca volvulus* and *Dracunculus medinensis*.

Some other filarial worms also infest man but they do no more than cause minor allergic reactions. *Litomosoides*

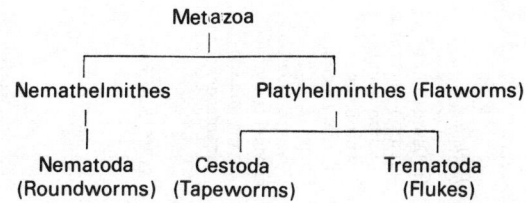

Fig. 58.1 Classification of parasitic worms, some of which infest man and domestic animals

carinii is parasitic to the cotton rat and is used in the laboratory evaluation of antifilarial drugs.

The life cycle of filarial worms that infest man is presented schematically in Fig. 58.2 and the main types of filariasis are summarized in Table 58.1.

Adult filaria are long, thin, round worms which are whitish in colour. Their size varies from species to species but the female is always longer than the male. The length of a typical female of *W. bancrofti* is about 10 cm and that of the male 5 cm. The microfilariae are motile thread-like organisms of about 250 μ in length. The female of *Dracunculus medinensis* may reach a length of 100 cm or more. The adult worms of some species live in the subcutaneous tissues but those of *W. bancrofti* and *B. malayi* are found in lymph vessels. If they obstruct the flow of lymph they cause *elephantiasis*, a condition characterized by a massive enlargement of the scrotum and of one or both legs.

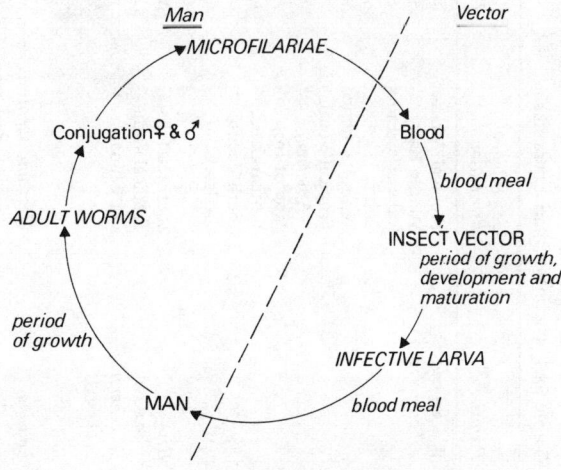

Fig. 58.2 The life cycle of a filarial worm

Table 58.1 The major filarial parasites

Parasite	Geographical distribution	Definitive host	Intermediate host (vector)	Method of transmission	Pathology	Treatment
Wuchereria bancrofti	Tropical Africa, Middle East, Indonesia, India, China, Central America, Tropical South America, Parts of tropical Australasia. South Pacific Islands.	Man *Adults* Lymph ducts, Lymph glands. *Microfilariae* Lymph ducts, Lymph glands, Blood.	Various species of mosquito.	Bite of infected mosquito.	Inflammation of lymph ducts and lymph glands with fever. Allergic reactions Blockage of lymph ducts causing hydrocoele and elephantiasis.	Diethylcarbamazine (kills microfilariae and some adults). Surgery (hydrocoele; elephantiasis).
Brugia malayi (Wuchereria malayi)	South-east Asia, Tropical India and China.	Man *Adults* as *W. bancrofti*. *Microfilariae* as *W. bancrofti*.	Various species of mosquito.	Bite of infected mosquito	As *W. bancrofti*.	As *W. bancrofti*.
Loa loa	West and Central Africa (Regions 10° north and south of the Equator).	Man *Adults* Subcutaneous tissues (Calabar swellings). *Microfilariae* Blood.	Red mangrove fly (*Chrysops sp.*).	Bite of infected fly	Subcutaneous (Calabar) swellings. Allergic itching. Anaemia.	As *W. bancrofti* but may kill all adult worms
Onchocerca volvulus	Central America, Southern Mexico, Tropical Africa (mainly in regions 10° north or south of the Equator).	Man *Adults* Subcutaneous tissues. *Microfilariae* Skin, eyes.	Buffalo gnat (*Simulium sp.*).	Bite of infected gnat.	Subcutaneous nodules that contain adults. Allergic itching, urticaria. Injury to the eyes (including blindness).	Diethylcarbamazine followed by suramin Adults removed surgically. Antihistamines. Cortisone.
Dracunculus medinensis (Guinea worm)	Middle East, India, West Indies. Tropical West and Central Africa.	Man *Adults* Subcutaneous tissues. Deeper connective tissues. *Larvae* Fresh water.	Fresh water crustacean (*Cyclops*)	Drinking water containing infected *Cyclops*.	Allergic reactions including; Urticaria, erythema, nausea, vomiting and diarrhoea. Secondary infection of worm track.	Thiabendazole Niridazole Removal of mature worm by surgery or gentle traction.

The prevention and treatment of filarial infestations is carried out by the following methods:

1. The use of insecticides and other measures to destroy the vectors and of insect repellants to prevent insect bites.

2. If practicable, the surgical removal of adult worms. Native populations have for many years used their own method of removing adult filariae present in subcutaneous tissue. When a worm emerges on the surface of the body it is attached to a small piece of wood round which it is wound, a little each day until the whole worm is withdrawn. The surgeon achieves the same end (but without the danger of causing severe infection along the worm track) by incising the skin over the length of the worm and removing it whole. The operation is simple and can be carried out under a local anaesthetic.

3. The use of drugs to kill the microfilariae, to kill or sterilize the adult worms and to prevent or reduce allergic symptoms due to dead worms. The systemic response to dead worms is often quite violent particularly in patients with onchocerciasis. There is fever, oedema, intense itching, swelling and tenderness of the lymph nodes and headache. The symptoms may persist for up to a week and may need treatment by cortisone and antihistamines.

4. The education of native populations and the improvement of hygiene and water supplies.

INFESTATION BY OTHER NEMATODES

Other nematodes that infect man include *Ascaris lumbricoides,* hookworms and the threadworm or pinworm *Enterobius vermicularis.* They all differ from the filariae in that infection is transmitted without the intervention of an intermediate host. *A. lumbricoides,* for instance, normally lives in the intestine. Its eggs are voided with the faeces and may then infect food. The larvae thus find themselves in the intestine but before they develop into adult worms they penetrate the intestinal wall and take a tour *via* the blood, liver, heart, lungs and trachea to the oesophagus whence they return to the intestine. Hookworm eggs live in the soil, penetrate the victim's skin and take a similar course from the bloodstream to the intestine.

The threadworm causes perianal itching, particularly at night and may cause considerable discomfort, sleeplessness and irritability in young children. The other worms cause a variety of symptoms ranging from itching, allergic symptoms and simple anaemia to severe vomiting and diarrhoea, pneumonia and heart failure (Table 58.2).

Conditions caused by tapeworms (cestodes)

Tapeworms that use man as their definitive host include *Diphyllobothrium latum* (the fish tapeworm), *Hymenolepis nana* (the dwarf tapeworm), *H. diminuta, Taenia saginata* (the beef tapeworm) and *T. solium* (the pork tapeworm). The larval forms of *T. solium* may infect man to give rise to cysticercosis cellulosae. In man the larval forms of the dog tapeworm, *T. echinococcus (Echinococcus granulosus)* cause

Tissue flukes	Intestinal	Fasciolopsis (*F. buski*) Gastrodiscoides (*G. hominis*) Heterophyes (*H. heterophyes*) Metagonimus (*M. yokogawai*)
	Pulmonary	Paragonimus (*P. westermanii*)
	Biliary	Clonorchis (*C. sinensis*) Fasciola (*F. hepatica*) Opisthorchis (*O. felineus*)
Blood flukes (Schistosomes)	Vesical	Schistosoma (*S. haematobium*)
	Intestinal	*S. mansoni* *S. japonicum*

Fig. 58.3 Classification of the pathogenic trematode worms with important members of each group

hydatid disease. A cysticercus (or bladder worm) consists of a larva of *T. solium* contained in a white, fluid filled sac that approaches 1 cm in diameter. In cysticercus cellulosae, tissues such as subcutaneous tissue, muscle, bone and brain are invaded by larvae which develop into cysticerci often in sufficient numbers to give rise to an obvious mass. In the brain, cysticerci are prone to precipitate grand mal epileptic seizures. In hydatid disease (echinococcosis) cysts containing many larvae form in one or more tissues particularly the lungs and liver. The cysts grow slowly but continuously so that they may eventually produce pressure symptoms from their sheer bulk or they may rupture and cause a severe anaphylactic shock as well as disseminating the disease to other tissues. With the exception of *H. nana* tapeworms need at least one intermediate host. *D. latum* requires two intermediate hosts.

The symptoms of infestation by these organisms are summarized in Table 58.3. Tapeworm infection is uncommon in Britain but *T. saginata* still presents a potential hazard since if it infects cattle it is unlikely (because of the popularity of underdone beef) to be destroyed in the cooking process.

There is no drug available at present for the treatment of hydatid disease or cysticercosis cellulosae. Hydatid disease is treated surgically where this is possible and epilepsy caused by cysticercosis is treated by means of anticonvulsant drugs.

Adult tapeworms are removed from the gastrointestinal tract by the use of appropriate anthelmintics, the most important of which are described below and listed in Table 58.3.

Conditions causes by trematodes (flukes)

Like the tapeworms, the trematodes are flat worms. Almost all the pathogenic trematodes (which are classified in Fig. 58.3) use the snail as intermediate host. Many of those that infect man pass through two intermediate hosts but the schistosomes require only one. Typical life cycles are illustrated in Figs. 58.4 and 58.5.

Trematode infestation poses serious medical and social

Table 58.2 Nematodes that infest man

Parasite	Geographical distribution	Host	Source of infestation	Symptoms	Treatment
Enterobius vermicularis (Oxyuris vermicularis) Threadworm, pinworm, seatworm	Worldwide	Man Ileum, caecum, colon	Ingestion of eggs (faecal contamination of hands, clothes, bedding, food)	Enterobiasis. Oxyuriasis Perianal itching, especially at night and causing loss of sleep. Children may become easily tired and irritable	Pyrantel pamoate Piperazine Viprynium
Hookworm (Ancylostoma duodenale and Necator americanus)	Tropical and subtropical regions Ancylostoma (the Old World hookworm) in Europe and Middle East; Necator (the New World species) in tropical Africa and the Americas.	Man Small intestine	As S. stercoralis	Causes chronic debility with anaemia from blood loss Larvae: Allergic reactions with itching, urticaria and dermatitis at points of entry. Heavy infestation with adults in intestine Cough, severe anaemia, abdominal pain, debility, weakness, prostration, vomiting, diarrhoea	Piperazine Pyrantel pamoate Bephenium hydroxy-naphthoate Thiabendazole Tetrachloro-ethylene
The roundworm (Ascaris lumbricoides)	Tropical and subtropical regions	Man Small intestine	Ingestion of eggs (faecal contamination of soil)	Ascariasis Mild: Gastrointestinal upset, pain and discomfort, cough, dyspnoea. Allergic reactions Severe: Pneumonia, pleurisy. Intestinal obstruction	Piperazine Thiabendazole Bephenium hydroxy-naphthoate Diethylcarbamazine

Table 58.2 (contd)

Parasite	Geo-graphical distribution	Host	Source of infestation	Symptoms	Treatment
Strongyloides stercoralis (the dwarf thread worm)	Tropical and sub-tropical regions	*Man, cat, dog* Small intestine	Contact with soil which contains larvae (faecal contamination) Ingestion of larvae (contamination of hands or food with infected faeces)	*Larvae:* Allergic reactions at site of penetration and secondary infection. Itching *Heavy infestation with:* *Adults in intestine* Diarrhoea, abdominal pain, urticaria, anaemia, debility *Adults in lungs* Cough, pneumonia, pneumonitis *Migrating larvae* Inflammation and haemorrhage in the brain. Urticaria	Thiabendazole Viprynium
Trichinella spiralis	Europe, America, India, Middle East	*Man, rat, pig* *Adult worm* Small intestine *Larvae* Skeletal muscles	Consumption of raw or under-cooked infected pork	*Heavy infestations:* *Adult worms* Nausea, vomiting, diarrhoea *Migrating larvae* Pyrexia, urticaria, tachycardia, tachypnoea, pain in limbs and muscles, facial oedema, haemorrages under finger nails *In very severe cases* Pneumonia and coma, heart failure	*Adult worms* Thiabendazole Methyridine Piperazine *Larvae* Manifestations of the disease treated symptomatically Cortisone may give considerable symptomatic relief
Whipworm (*Trichuris trichiura*)	World-wide	*Man* Caecum and colon	Food contaminated with faeces which contain eggs	*Heavy infestations* Diarrhoea, abdominal pain, weight loss, anaemia	Mebendazole Thiabendazole Bephenium hydroxy-naphthoate Hexylresorcinol

Table 58.3 Tapeworms that infest man

Tapeworm	Geographical distribution	Definitive hosts	First intermediate hosts	Second intermediate hosts	Cause of infestation in man	Symptoms of infestation	Treatment
Diphyllobothrium latum (Fish tapeworm, broad tapeworm)	Central, Southern and Eastern Europe Baltic States, Middle and Far East, U.S.A., Canada	*Man, dog, cat, pig* Ileum	Crustaceans *Cyclops sp. Diaptomus sp.*	Freshwater fish, including pike, perch, trout, salmon, eel	Consumption of raw or inadequately cooked infected fish	Macrocytic anaemia (cyanocobalamin deficiency) Digestive upsets Abdominal discomfort	Paromomycin Niclosamide Dichlorophen
Hymenolepis nana (Dwarf tapeworm)	World-wide	*Man, rodents* Ileum	None	Insects	Faecal contamination of food	Anaemia Digestive upsets Allergic reactions	As *D. latum*
Hymenolepis diminuta	World-wide	*Man (rare), rodents* Small intestine	Rat and mouse fleas	None	Ingestion of infected flea	As *H. nana*	As *D. latum*
Taenia echinococcus (syn. Echinococcus granulosus)	World-wide	*Dog* Small intestine	Man (accidental) to cause hydatid cysts Cattle, horses, pigs, sheep	None	Ingestion of eggs (contact with infected dogs)	*Hydatid disease in man* Symptoms from presence of cysts in brain, lungs, bones, liver and kidneys Allergic or anaphylactic symptoms from release of hydatid fluid	Surgery In *dogs*, worms removed by arecoline Bunamidine
Taenia satinata (Beef tapeworm)	World-wide	*Man* Jejunum	Ox, camel (*Cysticercus bovis*)	None	Consumption of inadequately cooked infected beef	Anaemia Digestive upset	As *D. latum*
Taenia solium (Pork tapeworm)	World-wide	*Man*	Pig Man (*Cysticercosis cellulosae*)	None	Consumption of inadequately cooked infected pork	Digestive upset, diarrhoea, constipation *Cysticercosis cellulosae* Symptoms from presence of cysticerci in brain (epilepsy, paraesthesia, aphasia, etc.)	As *D. latum* Anticonvulsants in epilepsy

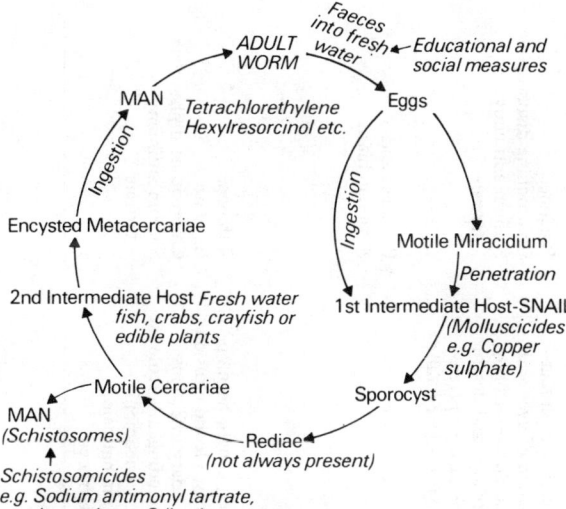

Fig. 58.4 An example of the life cycle of a trematode worm. The diagram shows the points at which drugs act and the various other measures which may be taken to break the life cycle.

problems in countries of the Middle and Far East and in parts of Africa, India and Eastern Europe, where infestation of the intestine, lungs and liver with flukes may be superimposed upon other types of infection and infestation. Symptoms are more severe in undernourished communities and are rendered more serious by the simultaneous presence of other diseases.

Measures to combat fluke infestation may be taken at different stages in the organism's complex life cycle. They include:

1. Educational measures designed to prevent people from eating, or feeding animals with, uncooked fresh water fish, crabs, crayfish or edible water plants which may bear metacercariae

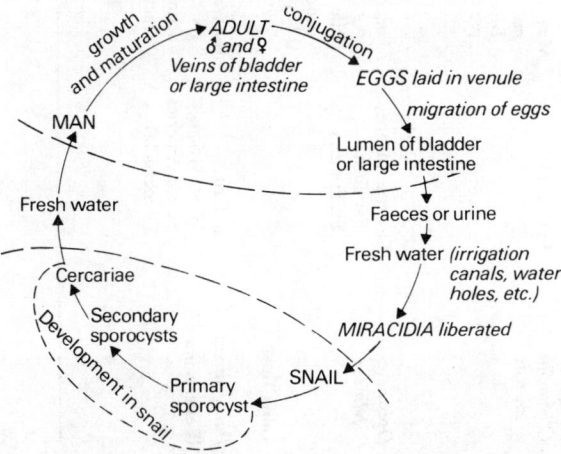

Fig. 58.5 The life cycle of a schistosome

2. Measures aimed at the prevention of contamination of water with faeces

3. Elimination of snails by means of molluscicides

4. Therapeutic measures. The drugs employed are listed in Table 58.4 and are briefly described later in the text.

The main features of diseases caused by intestinal, liver and lung flukes are also summarized in Table 58.4. It will be seen that the lung flukes cause fever, cough and haemoptysis (spitting of blood) while infection with intestinal and liver flukes is signalled by abdominal symptoms.

SCHISTOSOMIASIS (BILHARZIASIS)

The schistosomes differ from the other pathogenic trematodes in that the sexes are separate. The adult female is worm-like and cylindrical, while the male is elongated and leaf-like. The male is folded along its longitudinal axis to form a groove (*the gynaecophoric canal*) in which the female lies. The males are 10–20 mm in length and are slightly shorter than the females. The species which most commonly infect man are *Schistosoma haematobium*, *S. mansoni* and *S. japonicum*. The adult forms of *S. haematobium* are found in the veins of the bladder, while the other two inhabit the mesenteric and intestinal veins. The eggs pass into the bladder or intestine and are voided with the urine or faeces. They hatch in water to liberate a motile larval form (*the miracidium*) which is then taken up by snails. The cercariae which develop in the intermediate host are liberated into water. When they meet the definite host, they penetrate his skin and pass into the circulation by way of the lymphatic vessels. They mature in the portal veins and then pass to the bladder and intestine. The eggs are laid in the venules of these organs and then pass into their lumina. The symptoms of schistosomiasis are summarized in Table 58.5. They are caused mainly by the movements of the eggs through the tissues although the cercariae set up areas of irritation and itching at the points of penetration while the presence of the immature schistosomes in the blood vessels of the lungs and liver sometimes causes fever, allergic sensitization reactions and enlargement of the spleen and liver. In haematobium schistosomiasis symptoms are caused by the passage of the eggs from the venules of the bladder into the lumen. In mansoni and japonicum schistosomiasis they are caused by their passage into the large intestine. In some cases eggs are deposited in other organs such as the lungs, heart and brain and may cause serious disturbances.

Schistosomiasis is a major social and medical problem in the tropics and in some countries more than 75 per cent of the population harbour schistosomes. The disease is more serious in undernourished communities and although it may not be directly responsible for many deaths it causes ill health and inefficiency and reduces resistance to other diseases.

Table 58.4 Tissue flukes pathogenic to man

Fluke	Geographical distribution	Definitive host	First intermediate host	Second intermediate host	Symptoms	Treatment
Intestinal flukes						
Fasciolopsis buski	Phillipines, India and Far East	*Man, dog, pig* Small intestine	Aquatic snail	Water plant	Local inflammation, abdominal pain and tenderness, diarrhoea	Hexylresorcinol Tetrachloroethylene,
Gastrodiscoides hominis	India and Malaya	*Man, pig* Large intestine	Probably aquatic snail	Probably a water plant	Diarrhoea	Hexylresorcinol Tetrachloroethylene,
Heterophyes heterophyes	Middle East, Far East	*Man, cat, dog* Small Intestine	Aquatic snail	Freshwater fish	Diarrhoea, abdominal pain and tenderness	Hexylresorcinol Tetrachloroethylene,
Metagonimus yokogawai	Far East, Eastern U.S.S.R.	*Man, cat, dog, pig* Small intestine	Aquatic snail	Freshwater fish	Diarrhoea, abdominal pain and tenderness	Hexylresorcinol Tetrachloroethylene,
Liver flukes						
Clonorchis sinensis	Far East	*Man, cat, dog, pig* Bile and pancreatic ducts	Aquatic snail	Freshwater fish	*Clonorchiasis*—inflammation of liver and bile ducts—atrophy, cirrhosis and destruction of liver parenchyma—liver failure	Emetine Chloroquine disphosphate Sodium antimony tartrate
Opisthorchis felineus	Eastern Europe, Far East, Philippines	*Man, cat, dog, pig* Bile and pancreatic ducts	Aquatic snail	Freshwater fish	*As clonorchiasis*	Bithionol and as clonorchiasis
Lung fluke						
Paragonimus Westermanii	Far East, West Africa, South America (Venezuela)	*Man, cat, dog, goat, pig, etc.* Lungs, intestinal tract, brain	Aquatic snail	Freshwater crabs, crayfish	Fever, cough, haemoptysis, pleural effusion Secondary infections including tuberculosis, and pneumonia Abdominal pain, diarrhoea	Bithionol Emetine Chloroquine diphosphate Sodium antimony tartrate

Table 58.5 Schistosomes pathogenic to man

Schistosome sp.	Geographical distribution	Definitive host and region infested	Intermediate host	Pathological changes (Schistosomiasis = bilharziasis)	Treatment
Schistosoma haematobium	Africa, Middle East	Man Adults found in veins of bladder	Aquatic snails	Haematobium schistosomiasis Pain and frequency of urination. Haematuria, cystitis, fever, headache, backache, ulcers and papillomata of bladder General debility.	Molluscicides, niridazole, hycanthone, metriphonate, sodium (or potassium) antimony tartrate, stibocaptate, stibophen Surgery if indicated. All drugs are least effective against S. japonicum.
Schistosoma japonicum	Far East (China, Japan etc.) Pacific (Formosa, Philippines)	Man, rodents, domestic animals Adults found in veins of large and small intestine	Amphibious snails	Japonicum schistosomiasis Dysentery, enlarged spleen and liver. Cirrhosis. Damage by eggs to central nervous system. Anaemia, debility.	
Schistosoma mansoni	South and Central America, Africa, Middle East	Man and monkeys Adults found in veins of large intestine	Aquatic snails	Mansoni shcistosomiasis Abdominal pain, frequent bloody stools, ulceration of rectum. Enlarged spleen and liver. Weakness, anaemia, debility. Damage to lungs.	

DRUGS USED IN THE TREATMENT OF HELMINTHIASIS

In the accounts that follow, drugs are described in the order in which they are named in Tables 58.1 to 58.5.

Drugs particularly active against filariae

DIETHYLCARBAMAZINE
Diethylcarbamazine is the most effective antifilarial drug at present available in infestations with W. bancrofti, B. malayi and L. loa. It does not destroy the microfilariae in vitro but when it is injected, the organisms are removed from the blood by macrophages in the sinusoids of the liver, spleen and bone marrow and are destroyed by phagocytosis. The drug appears to sensitize the microfilariae to the actions of the phagocytes. In W. bancrofti, B. malayi and L. loa the majority of adults are killed or sterilized. In cases of O. volvulus infestation diethylcarbamazine is given to kill the microfilariae but the adult worms escape and have to be dealt with by a subsequent course of suramin treatment.

Diethylcarbamazine

The toxicity of diethylcarbamazine is very low. Most of the toxic reactions which follow its use are responses to the products liberated by decomposition of the dead worms (p. 887).

Diethylcarbamazine is used in the form of the dihydrogen citrate, under the names Banocide, Hetrazan and Notezine. It is given by mouth and is well absorbed. Peak blood levels are attained in about three to four hours. The dose for adults is 4 mg per kilogram body mass thrice daily but it is usual to begin treatment with lower amounts than this and to reach the full dose over a period of some 3 to 4 days. A course of treatment lasts for 3 to 4 weeks.

SURAMIN
This compound was originally introduced as a trypanocide and as such it is described elsewhere (p. 878). When used in the treatment of onchocerciasis, suramin (Antrypol) is given by intravenous injection in doses of 1 g at once-weekly intervals for no more than six weeks, although in view of the possibility of its evoking adverse responses it is advisable to give a small test dose of the drug (200 mg) before embarking on a full course of treatment. Suramin administration should begin ten days after completion of diethylcarbamazine treatment. Suramin may cause nausea, vomiting, fainting, blood dyscrasias and skin eruptions. In addition to these side effects, allergic responses to the dead parasites may appear during suramin treatment.

THIABENDAZOLE
Originally employed only in the treatment of nematode infestation in domestic animals, thiabendazole (Mintezol) now occupies a valuable place in human medicine. It is a

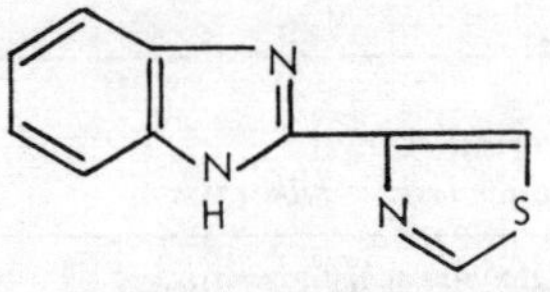

Thiabendazole

drug of first choice in cases of stronglyloidosis, dracontiasis and trichuriasis (Tables 58.1 and 58.2) but it is lethal to a wide variety of roundworms (perhaps because it interferes with the activity of an essential enzyme) and it can also be applied to the treatment of infestations by hookworms and *Trichinella*.

Thiabendazole is given in doses of 25 mg per kilogram of body mass on two or three successive days. It is rapidly absorbed after oral administration and is largely excreted within 24 hours. Side effects are frequent and varied and may be temporarily incapacitating but they are short lived. They chiefly involve the gastrointestinal tract (vomiting, diarrhoea, abdominal pain), the central nervous system (dizziness, drowsiness, headache) and the skin (flushes and rashes). Signs of hepatotoxicity (changes in serum enzyme activity) are sometimes seen and the drug must be given circumspectly to those with existing evidence of liver disease.

NIRIDAZOLE
Although this substance is usefully employed in the treatment of dracontiasis (Table 58.1), it is primarily an antischistosomial agent and as such it is described elsewhere (p. 899).

Drugs particularly active against other forms of roundworm

PIPERAZINE
Piperazine is employed as the adipate, citrate, phosphate or tartrate. It is a vermifuge but not a vermicide, the worms being paralysed and expelled alive. This has the advantage that it avoids the reactions to dead worms retained in the body that often follow the use of vermicides. Piperazine causes paralysis of the worms by antagonizing the action of the intrinsic acetylcholine on which neuromuscular activity depends. It has recently been suggested (Phillips, Sturman & West, 1976) that piperazine promotes the uptake of histamine by the worm from the gastrointestinal tract of its host. It may be that histamine is the inhibitory transmitter at the worm's neuromuscular junction and if so the effectiveness of piperazine may reside in its ability both

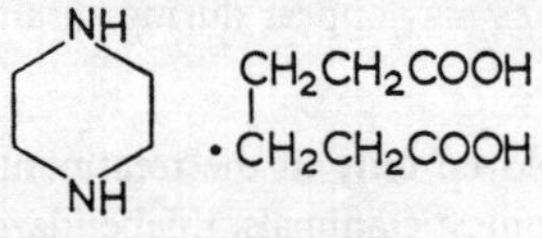

to antagonize excitatory processes and to potentiate inhibitory activity. It is used mainly to treat infestation with *E. vermicularis* and *A. lumbricoides,* in which it is very effective. For enterobiasis the adult dose of the adipate is 0.6 g three times a day for seven days. Children over six years receive a similar dose, younger children being given proportionally less. In ascariasis a single dose of 3 to 4.5 g of adipate is usually adequate. For children the effective dose is 2.5 to 3.5 g according to age and body weight. The toxicity of piperazine is low but side effects occasionally occur in adults and children. These include nausea and vomiting, blurred vision, headache and dizziness. Convulsions have occasionally been reported in children. Piperazine is marketed under a variety of trade names. These include Antepar, Entacyl, Helmezine, Parazine, Piperate and Pipizan.

PYRANTEL PAMOATE
Pyrantel (Antiminth, Combantrin) is gaining popularity as an anthelmintic agent. It is particularly useful for the treatment of infestation by threadworms, roundworms and hookworms: it is said to be as valuable as bephenium at least as far as countering hookworm attacks is concerned.

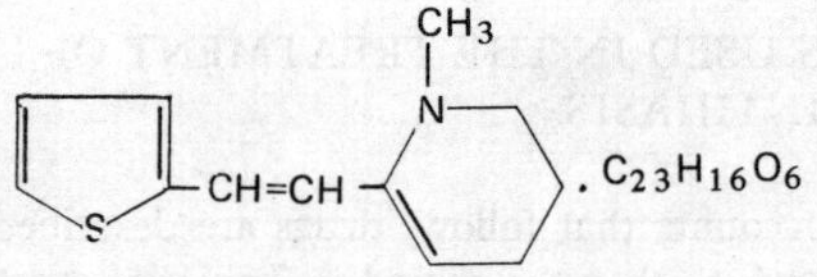

pyrantel pamoate

The usual dose of pyrantel is 11 mg per milogram of body mass. It is given by mouth. Depending on the nature of the infesting agent (and perhaps on the predilection of the therapist) this dose is repeated once or twice after the lapse of one day (*Necator* attacks) or two weeks (*Ancylostoma* attacks).

Pyrantel is a depolarizing neuromuscular blocking agent and, in accordance with this property, it causes a spastic paralysis of worms exposed to it. In this respect it provides an interesting contrast to piperazine which is a competitive antagonist of acetylcholine and so causes a flaccid paralysis of the worm.

VIPRYNIUM (PYRVINIUM)
Viprynium embonate or pyrvinium pamoate (Vanquin, Pamovin) is used to treat infestations with *E. vermicularis* (threadworm) and *S. stercoralis*. The dose for a child is

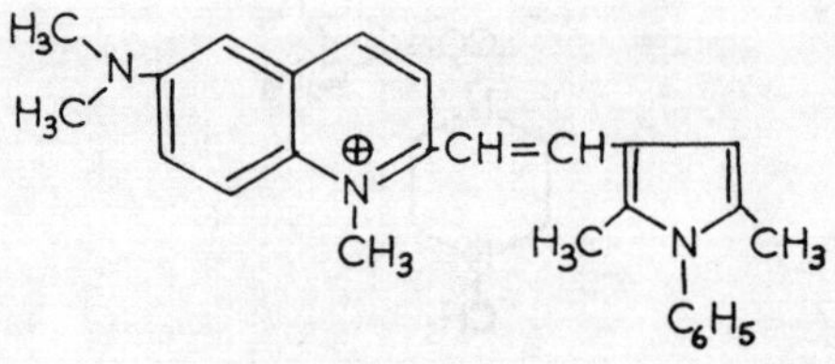

Piperazine adipate

Viprynium (Pyrvinium)

5 mg per kg as a single dose. Viprynium embonate appears to be virtually free from toxicity but it is a red dyestuff and the child and its parents should be warned that the drug will impart a vividly red colour to the faeces. Viprynium embonate is also employed in veterinary medicine.

TETRACHLOROETHYLENE

Tetrachloroethylene ($Cl_2C = CCl_2$) is very effective in the treatment of hookworm infestation. Its toxicity is low but it may cause epigastric burning, nausea and dizziness. Tetrachloroethylene is chemically related to chloroform and inhalation of the vapour can result in anaesthesia; patients who have been treated with tetrachlorethylene sometimes complain that they feel drunk. The absorption of tetrachloroethylene—and hence the possibility of systemic side effects—is increased if fat is present in the intestine and before treatment patients should take only a light, fat-free meal. The dose for adults is 5 ml. Children receive 0.3 ml per year of age. The drug is given in a capsule or as an emulsion. In the past, saline purges were given together with the tetrachloroethylene but this is no longer regarded as being necessary. Tetrachloroethylene is also effective against nematode infection in domestic animals.

HEXYLRESORCINOL

Hexylresorcinol has a broad spectrum of anthelmintic activity and it may be employed to treat infestation with tapeworms (D. latum, H. nana and T. saginata) as well as nematodes (A. lumbricoides, A. duodenale, N. americanus, E. vermicularis and T. trichiura). The drug is a vermicide and the worms, killed in situ, have to be removed by means of a saline purge. Hexylresorcinol is supplied in enteric-coated pills which, to avoid irritation of the mouth, are swallowed and not chewed. The gastric, as well as the buccal, mucosa is also sensitive to hexylresorcinol which is to be avoided in patients with gastric ulcers. In the treatment of infestation with nematodes, food, but not water, is withheld for 5 hours before giving the drug. A cleansing enema is given shortly after the drug is taken followed one hour later by a retention enema of a solution of hexylresorcinol. This is retained for from 15 to 20 minutes. For the treatment of tapeworm infestation the drug is given in the morning on an empty stomach. About two hours after the drug has been administered a saline purgative is given to remove the dead worms, food being withheld until treatment is completed. The adult dose of hexylresorcinol and that for children over 12 years is 1 g.

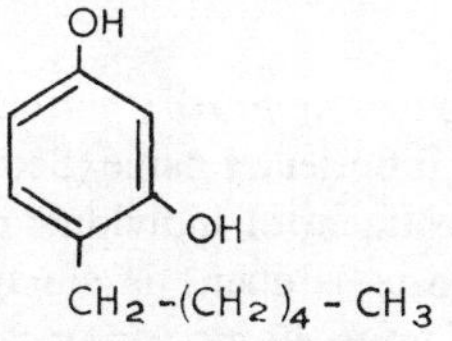

Hexylresorcinol

For children aged 6 to 8 years, 600 mg are given and for ages 8 to 12 the dose is 800 mg. Hexylresorcinol can also be given in the form of an enema in the treatment of whipworm infestation.

BEPHENIUM HYDROXYNAPHTHOATE

Bephenium hydroxynaphthoate (Alcopar) is the drug of choice for the treatment of infections by the hookworm, A. duodenale. It is also active against roundworms and whipworms. This is a useful circumstance since ancylostomiasis and ascariasis frequently coexist in the same patient. Bephenium is rather less effective against infections with the hookworm N. americanus. The drug has a very low toxicity. The daily dose for an adult is five grams. Rare side effects include nausea, vomiting and diarrhoea.

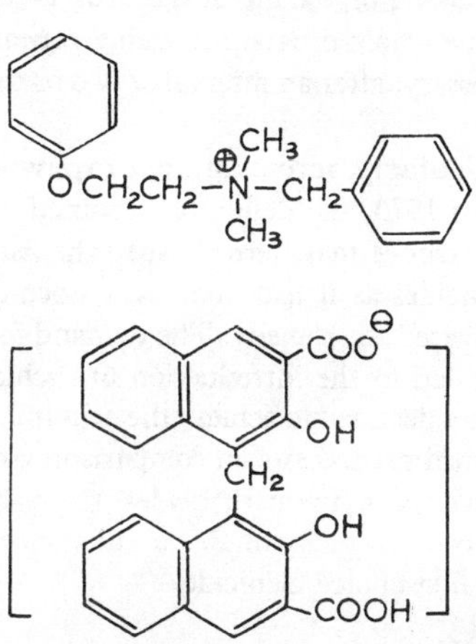

Bephenium hydroxynaphthoate

METHYRIDINE

Methyridine (Mintic, Promintic) is a vermifuge that is used primarily in veterinary practice for the treatment of roundworm infestation.

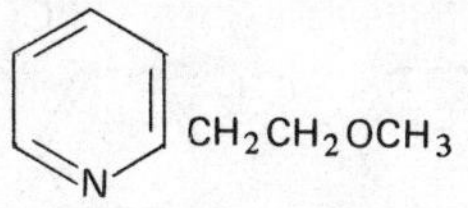

Methyridine

MEBENDAZOLE

Mebendazole (Vermox) is a useful drug. Its anthelmintic activity is exerted against whipworms, roundworms, threadworms and hookworms as well as the tapeworms T. saginata and T. solium. It is the agent of choice for the treatment of whipworm infections but its wide spectrum of activity also makes it particularly valuable in the not uncommon cases of mixed nematode infections.

Mebendazole

No more than 10 per cent of an oral dose of mebendazole is absorbed from the intestine and this circumstance certainly contributes to the drug's safety. Apart from allergic skin rashes, systemic side effects are seen only rarely during treatment with mebendazole. Nevertheless it should be withheld during pregnancy.

The usual course of treatment with mebendazole involves the taking of 100 mg of the drug twice daily for three days, the whole programme being repeated, if it is thought necessary, after an interval of two or three weeks.

Drugs particularly active against tapeworms

As recently as 1970, the delightfully named oleoresin of aspidium (extract of male fern) headed the list of recommended taenicides as it had done ever since the ancient Greeks discovered the remedy. The demand for less toxic medicaments led to the introduction of dichlorophen, a drug that is not destined to achieve the near immortality of its distinguished predecessor in comparison with which it is less effective and not remarkably less toxic. It is already being displaced by niclosamide, a substance that now ranks as the first choice taenicide.

DICHLOROPHEN

Dichlorophen (Anthiphen) had been employed as a taenicide in veterinary medicine for a number of years before it was introduced for the treatment of *T. saginata* infestation in man. It appears to kill the worm *in situ* and the dead parasite disintegrates and may be partly digested by the host. In *T. solium* infestation this may increase the risk of cysticercosis. Dichlorophen is not without value in cases of infestation with other tapeworms (Table 58.3).

Dichlorophen

Side effects of dichlorophen treatment include mild abdominal pain, diarrhoea, and, in rare instances, jaundice. With the older drugs, it was usual to seek visual confirmation of the effectiveness of the treatment by looking for the worm in the faeces voided in response to a saline purgative taken immediately after the taenicidal agent. Since dichlorophen has some purgative action in its own right it is not necessary to give it in association with a separate purgative drug although this makes it less easy to confirm the success of the taenicidal operation by demonstrating the presence of the head in the faeces, particularly since the worm will have been partially digested. Consequently a search for segments and eggs has to be made if the patient reports the reappearance of symptoms. The recommended dose of dichlorophen for an adult is 2 g taken every eight hours for two or three successive days.

NICLOSAMIDE

Niclosamide (Cestocide, Yomesan) is effective in tapeworm infestation in man and animals. It is almost totally unabsorbed from the gut, a circumstance that explains its lack of systemic toxicity. Although it is active against all species of tapeworm, the possibility of its causing cysticercosis cannot be excluded if it is applied to the elimination of *T. solium,* the ova of which are immune to attack by the drug. The danger can be largely avoided if a purgative is given after the worm has been killed but vigorous purging should be avoided in debilitated patients.

Niclosamide

Niclosamide inhibits the oxidative metabolism of tapeworms and, like dichlorophen, it also renders them more susceptible to attack by the proteolytic enzymes of the gastrointestinal secretions so that it may be difficult to recognize expelled worm segments in the faeces.

The normal adult dose of niclosamide is two grams. It is sometimes given in two equal doses, the second following the first after an interval of one hour.

ARECOLINE

Arecoline hydrobromide, a cholinomimetic substance whose pharmacology is more fully considered elsewhere (p. 204) is as ancient a vermifuge as extract of male fern. It is still used routinely as a taenicide in dogs in countries where there is a high incidence of hydatid disease caused by the larval form of *T. echinococcus* and where the mass treatment of animals is necessary. The deworming dose is 2 mg per kg of body mass. Arecoline causes the worms to relax their grip on the tissues of the intestine and the worms are then expelled by the drug's purgative action.

BUNAMIDINE

Bunamidine is a new veterinary vermifuge which rejoices in a descriptive proprietary name (Scolaban) and which is used for the treatment of individual cats and dogs. The hydroxynaphthoate (Buban) is suitable for sheep and goats. Doses of up to 40 mg per kg can be given, usually with impunity.

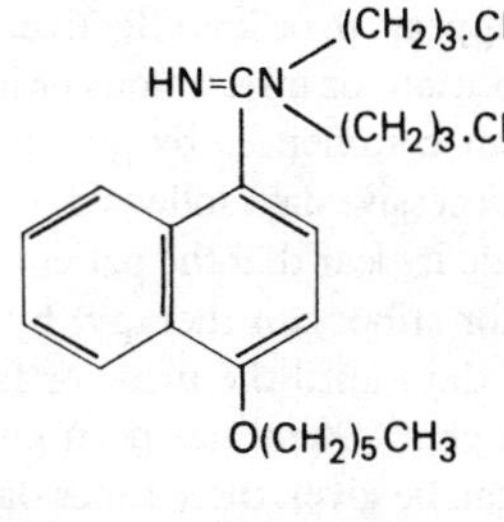

HN=CN
(CH₂)₃.CH₃
(CH₂)₃.CH₃

O(CH₂)₅CH₃

Bunamidine

PAROMOMYCIN

This drug is an antibiotic and is more appropriately discussed with the other members of the streptomycin group of chemotherapeutic agents (p. 834).

Drugs particularly active against tissue flukes

BITHIONOL

Bithionol (Actamer, Bitin) is particularly useful for the treatment of infections by the lung fluke *P. westermanii* but it also is active against liver flukes. It is given by mouth in divided doses of about 50 mg per kg of body mass which are repeated on alternate days for up to five days. Patients given bithional may suffer urticaria, photosensitivity reactions or gastrointestinal upsets.

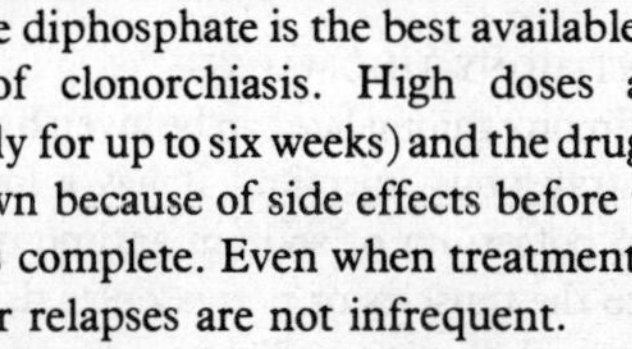

OH S OH
Cl Cl

Cl Cl

Bithionol

CHLOROQUINE

Chloroquine diphosphate is the best available drug for the treatment of clonorchiasis. High doses are required (750 mg daily for up to six weeks) and the drug may have to be withdrawn because of side effects before the course of treatment is complete. Even when treatment is not interrupted, later relapses are not infrequent.

Chloroquine has other therapeutic uses and it is discussed in more detail in the chapter that collects together all the antimalarial drugs (p. 866).

EMETINE

This drug is also used (though to a much smaller extent than previously) for the treatment of amoebiasis and its general properties are described in the chapter devoted to the amoebicides (p. 870).

As far as its use as an anthelmintic is concerned, there is general agreement that emetine is a drug of choice for the treatment of infestation by *Fasciola hepatica*, the sheep liver fluke. Although fascioliasis most commonly affects sheep, cattle and horses, outbreaks in human populations do occur and are treated by daily subcutaneous injections of emetine. The usual daily dose is 65 mg (1 mg per kilogram body mass) and a course of treatment lasts for ten days. An alternative drug is bithionol.

OTHER DRUGS

Other substances applied to the therapy of tissue flukes are described elsewhere in this chapter. They include potassium antimony tartrate (below), hexylresorcinol (p. 895) and tetrachloroethylene (p. 893).

Drugs particularly active against blood flukes (schistosomes)

Prevention is always better than cure and the eradication of schistosomiasis from areas plagued with the disease is primarily the concern of the civil engineer, the ecologist and the public health experts working together to prevent contamination of water supplies either by snails or by human excreta (Nnochiri, 1975). If snails are already established in reservoirs and irrigation systems they will have to be eliminated by molluscicides added to the water at a time when the snails are beginning to multiply. The traditional molluscicide is copper sulphate but it is being supplanted by the much more active copper pentachlorophenate which is toxic to snails when it is present in water to the extent of no more than one part in a million. Cheaper but effective agents include calcium oxide (unslaked lime) and calcium cyanamide.

While preventative measures are taking effect, cases of established schistosomiasis will continue to need treatment. Indeed, the elimination of flukes from large numbers of people living in infected areas is as much a prophylactic as it is a curative measure. The drugs listed below are those currently used to treat schistosomiasis in man. Antimony compounds are discussed first because for many years they have been the most favoured antischistosomial agents. Newer compounds are beginning to challenge their supremacy except in cases of infection by *S. japonicum*, a fluke that resists all but the most powerful schistosomicides.

SODIUM (AND POTASSIUM) ANTIMONY TARTRATE

The use of potassium antimony tartrate in the treatment of schistosomiasis was the outcome of observations made during the treatment of kala azar and venereal disease when it was noted that the symptoms of concurrent schistosomiasis improved.

Both sodium antimony tartrate and potassium antimony

$$
\begin{array}{l}
COO - Sb = O \\
| \\
CHOH \\
| \qquad\qquad \cdot \tfrac{1}{2}\,H_2O \\
CHOH \\
| \\
COOK
\end{array}
$$

Potassium antimony
tartrate (*Tartar Emetic*)

tartrate (tartar emetic) effectively kill adult schistosomes. They cause toxic side reactions during injection and later, but have the advantage of being cheap. Both compounds can be given by the slow intravenous injection of a solution in glucose-saline. The sodium compound is the less toxic and is the one preferred in several countries. Side effects during injection include coughing, vomiting, salivation and collapse. Following the injection, they include haematuria, skin rashes, urticaria and liver damage. There may also be a toxic effect on the heart. The side effects are more severe when the drug is being used in poorly nourished communities who should, when possible, be given less toxic compounds. This will not generally be possible, as we have already indicated, when *S. japonicum* is the infesting organism. Its elimination necessitates very slow injections of an antimony tartrate in doses of about 150 mg every two or three days until 2.5g have been given. It is prudent to preface this treatment by a few test doses beginning at 50 mg and increasing by increments of 25 mg on alternate days. Patients who display unexpectedly severe reactions before the full daily dose of 150 mg is reached should be transferred to a different drug. The tartrates inhibit glycolysis in schistosomes. This effect upon carbohydrate metabolism arises from inhibition of phosphofructokinase, the enzyme which catalyses the formation of fructose-1, 6-diphosphate from fructose-6-phosphate. This is presumably the site of their toxic action upon the organisms.

POTASSIUM ANTIMONY DIMERCAPTOSUCCINATE

This compound (stibocaptate, Astiban) and the corresponding sodium derivative are given by intravenous or intramuscular injection. They are rather less toxic than the older antimonials. The total dose for adults is about 3 g given in five instalments once or twice weekly. Side effects (fatigue, skin rashes, nausea and vomiting) are not uncommon and if severe may necessitate temporary or permanent withdrawal of the drug. The drug is contraindicated in the presence of liver, kidney or cardiovascular disease and in patients weakened by reason of extensive worm infestation.

Potassium antimony dimercaptosuccinate

S. japonicum responds less readily to stibocaptate than do the other blood flukes.

STIBOPHEN

Stibophen (sodium antimony pyrocatechol disulphate; Fuadin) is less toxic than sodium or potassium antimony

tartrate but it also appears to be less effective. It is supplied as a 6.3 per cent solution for intravenous or intramuscular injection. Treatment commences by giving doses of 1.5, 3.5 and 5.0 ml on successive days followed (unless the early injections have made it clear that the patient is an unsatisfactory candidate for stibophen therapy) by 5.0 ml doses every two or three days until the urine or faeces are free from eggs or until about 90 ml has been given. Alternatively a 4 ml dose can be given three times daily for one or two weeks but the incidence of uncomfortable side effects is greater with this régime. Relapses may occur, so that follow-up examinations are essential.

Stibophen

Side effects of and contraindications to treatment with stibophen are similar to those detailed for stibocaptate.

SODIUM ANTIMONYL GLUCONATE

Sodium antimonyl gluconate (sodium stibogluconate; Pentostam, Solubistam, Triostam) is less toxic than sodium or potassium antimony tartrate. It is also used in the management of leishmaniasis and its chemical formula will be found on p. 874 among those of other leishmanicidal agents. So far as the treatment of schistosomal infections are concerned, a total dose of 1.5 g given in divided doses by intravenous injection over six days may be adequate to destroy the adult flukes.

Sodium antimonyl gluconate is supplied as a dry powder which contains 30 per cent of trivalent antimony and is dissolved in water immediately before use.

LITHIUM ANTIMONY THIOMALATE

Lithium antimony thiomalate can be given by intramuscular or by intravenous injection; it has a lower systemic toxicity than potassium or sodium antimony tartrate and injection into the muscles or perivascular tissues does not cause pain or inflammation. This compound contains 16 per cent of trivalent antimony (tartar emetic and its sodium analogue contain about 40 per cent) and is administered in the form of a 6 per cent solution. The initial dose is 0.5 to 1.0 ml increasing by 1 ml increments to 4 ml, the drug being given every second or third day. Treatment is continued until the urine or faeces no longer contain eggs

Lithium antimony thiomalate

or until a maximum of about 16 injections have been given. Lithium antimony thiomalate is somewhat less effective and more expensive than sodium or potassium antimony tartrate but its lower toxicity may make it more suitable for use in communities in which schistosomiasis is endemic and the population is already weakened by disease.

NIRIDAZOLE

Niridazole (Ambilhar) first appeared in 1964 and has now established itself as the drug of first choice for the treatment of infections by *S. haematobium*. It is often useful too when the infecting agent is *S. mansoni* (provided that the victim's hepatic function is not seriously disturbed) or the guinea worm, *Dracunculus medinensis*. Although niridazole has amoebicidal activity, its relatively high toxicity has militated against its general use in amoebiasis.

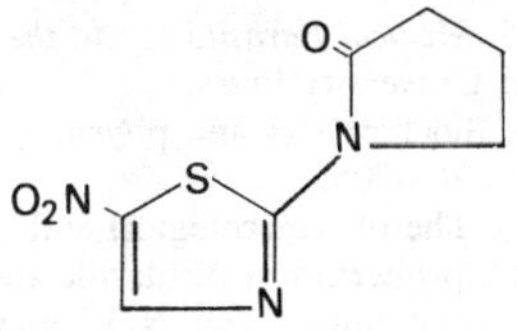

Niridazole

Niridazole exerts its primary effect on the vitellogenic gland of the female schistosome so that egg shell formation ceases and viable fertile eggs no longer reach the uterus. It may also be that spermatogenesis is arrested in sensitive males.

Niridazole is given by mouth in daily doses of 25 mg per kg for 5 to 10 days. It sometimes causes nausea, vomiting or other types of gastrointestinal upset as well as more general symptoms such as skin rashes but its more characteristic toxic effects are exerted on the heart (an apparently benign flattening of the T-wave of the electrocardiogram) or on the psyche with insomnia, agitation, hallucinations or convulsions.

Niridazole is absorbed only slowly from the gut and it is metabolized to a considerable extent during its first passage through the liver so that the blood in the portal vein, where the adult schistosomes congregate will, fortunately, carry the highest concentration of drug. Its hepatic function is impaired as a result of the infection (and this, as we have seen, is particularly likely to occur with *S. mansoni*) the resulting sluggish metabolism of niridazole may cause unacceptability toxic responses to the drug. Niridazole is contraindicated in pregnancy (it might be teratogenic) and haemolysis is to be expected in patients with an inborn deficiency of glucose-6-phosphate dehydrogenase (p. 74).

LUCANTHONE AND HYCANTHONE

Just before the Second World War, Mauss prepared a series of xanthenones and thioxanthenones. Four of them described as the Miracils, were investigated in detail after the war and they were shown to be lethal to *S. mansoni* and

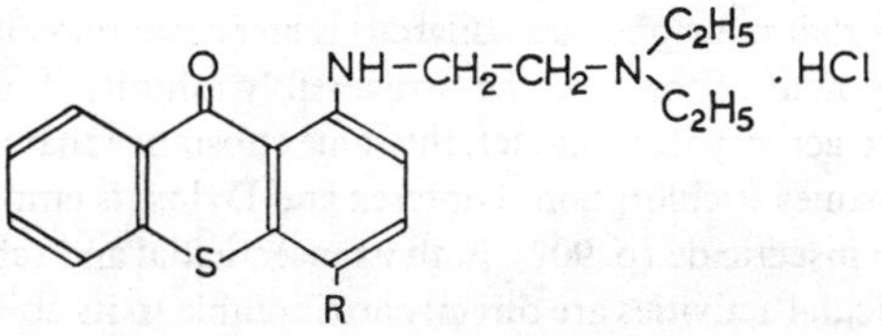

Fig. 58.6 Schistosomicidal thioxanthenones. In lucanthone, R is CH_3; in hycanthone, R is CH_2OH

to be active when taken by mouth. The most active (Miracil D) was a thioxanthenone (the sulphur-containing compounds are more active than the xanthenones) and it entered the therapeutic ring as lucanthone (Fig. 58.6). Derivatives of lucanthone were not slow to appear and one of them, hycanthone (Etrenol) is preferred to lucanthone in some countries.

Lucanthone is given by mouth and at dose levels of about 20 mg per kg twice daily for up to six days. Repeat courses may be necessary one month after the completion of the initial treatment. Successful results have been obtained in the treatment of *S. haematobium* (although niridazole is to be preferred) and *S. mansoni* infestation but *S. japonicum* is resistant to lucanthone.

Lucanthone possesses some obvious advantages over the trivalent antimonials; it can be given by mouth, it is less toxic and treatment need not be so prolonged. On the other hand, like the antimonials, it does not destroy the immature schistosomes and it often causes side effects which include headaches, dizziness and irritation of the gastrointestinal tract with pain, loss of appetite, nausea and vomiting—a decided disadvantage in the field when the co-operation of the indigenous population is essential if treatment is to be successful.

Lucanthone, like niridazole, is quickly destroyed in the liver but some of the metabolites (including hycanthone) are as active as the parent compound. Lucanthone is contraindicated in pregnancy and in patients with liver disease.

The indications, contraindications, advantages and disadvantages of hycanthone are similar to those of lucanthone except that it is usual to give the drug in a single intramuscular injection of 3 mg per kg of body mass.

Lucanthone and hycanthone, like alkylating agents (p. 914), interpose themselves between matching bases in the DNA molecule so that egg laying and cell replication are prevented. In addition, they prevent uptake of 5-hydroxytryptamine by the flukes' nervous apparatus (although uptake by the fluke as a whole is increased) and this may constitute the real basis of the drugs' activity. Neurohumoral substances are no less important in these relatively humble creatures than they are in man.

METRIPHONATE

Those who have read the chapter that discusses the anticholinesterases will recognise from its chemical formula that metriphonate (Bilarcil) is an organophosphorus compound of the type that irreversibly inhibits cholinesterase activity. It is, in fact, the same substance that under the names trichlorphon, Dipterex and Dylox, is employed as an insecticide (p. 902). Both its insecticidal and schistosomicidal activities are directly attributable to its ability to inhibit cholinesterase and it further underlines the point made earlier that the wellbeing of worms is as dependent on the proper functioning of neurohumoral processes as is the health of man.

$$CH_3O \diagdown \underset{\displaystyle CH_3O \diagup}{\overset{\displaystyle O}{P}} \diagup \underset{CHOH}{\overset{CCl_3}{}}$$

Metriphonate

When metriphonate is used therapeutically, the dose has to be very carefully regulated because the host's own cholinesterase is as vulnerable as that of his parasite and even a small overdose of drug might precipitate disaster (p. 221). In spite of this, metriphonate has in practice not emerged as a particularly toxic substance. It is recommended chiefly for cases of haematobial schistosomiasis, for which purpose it is given in doses of 5 to 15 mg per kg. The actual dose is determined by the frequency of the drug's administration which is, in its turn, influenced by the nature of infesting organism.

BIBLIOGRAPHY

Books, monographs and reviews

Brown, H.W. (1968). Anthelmintics new and old. *Clin. Pharmac. Ther.* **10**, 5-21.

Craig, J.C. and Tate, M.E. (1961). Structure-activity relationships in certain anthelmintics. *Prog. Drug. Res.,* **3**, 75-150.

Hawking, F. (1963). Chemotherapy of filariasis. In *Experimental Chemotherapy,* vol. I, pp. 893-912. Ed. Schnitzer, R.J and Hawking, F. New York: Academic Press.

Keeling, J.E.D. (1968). The chemotherapy of cestode infections. *Adv. Chemother,* **3**, 109-152.

Lämmler, G. (1968). The chemotherapy of trematode infections. *Adv. Chemother.,* **3**, 153-251.

Mansour, T.E. (1964). The pharmacology and biochemistry of parasitic helminths. In *Advances in Pharmacology,* vol. 3, pp. 129-165. Ed. Garattini, S. and Shore, P.A. New York and London: Academic Press.

Nnochiri, E. (1975) *Medical Parasitology in the Tropics.* London: Oxford University Press.

Read, C.P. (1963). Biochemistry and physiology of tapeworms. *Physiol. Rev.,* **43**, 263-305.

Symposium (1969). The pharmacological and chemotherapeutic properties of niridazole and other antischistosomal compounds. *Ann. N.Y. Acad. Sci.* **160**, 423-946.

Original papers

Phillips, Jean L., Sturman, Gillian and West, G.B. (1976) The interaction between anthelminitic drugs and histamine in *Ascaris suum. Br. J. Pharmac.* **57**, 417-420.

59. Insecticides

As we have emphasized in the preceding chapter, the final elimination of many parasitic diseases will depend on the destruction of insect vectors. Insecticides have thus become an important weapon in the therapeutic armoury. By their very nature, some insecticides are highly toxic to man as well as to animals. Since they are applied as sprays or dusts to prevent insect attack on food crops, they come into contact with man and they may also cause accidental contamination of his foodstuffs. Some knowledge of the chemical nature, the pharmacological properties and the toxic effects of the insecticides is therefore desirable. In this chapter this information is briefly presented for a few of the more important insecticides. They are grouped according to their chemical structure under the following heads:

(a) chlorinated hydrocarbons
(b) organophosphorus derivatives
(c) the pyrethrins and the pyrethroids
(d) rotenone and the rotenoids
(e) a large group of miscellaneous compounds of varied structure

Chlorinated hydrocarbons

A large number of chlorinated hydrocarbons have been employed as *contact poisons* — substances that exert their lethal action after they have passed through the insect cuticle. The names and formulae of some of the more important contact poisons in this group are presented in Fig. 59.1. The insecticidal and toxicological properties of all the active chlorinated compounds are qualitatively similar. As far as their insecticidal effects are concerned, the chlorinated hydrocarbons act primarily on the nervous system. Dicophane (D.D.T.), for instance, at first increases the muscular activity of insects with which it comes into contact. Then it disorganizes the insect's reflex activity and causes ataxia, tremor, neuromuscular paralysis and death. The chlorinated hydrocarbons are toxic to man and animals (although they can be safely used as dusting powders for the elimination of body lice) and they should be kept well away from foodstuffs and animal feed. In areas where these compounds are widely used, it is almost inevitable that small amounts will be ingested by a large proportion of the population. They are taken up by, and sequestered safely in, the fatty tissues of the body but there is a limit to the extent of the protection that can be offered in this way and the use of the chlorinated hydrocarbons needs to be carefully controlled.

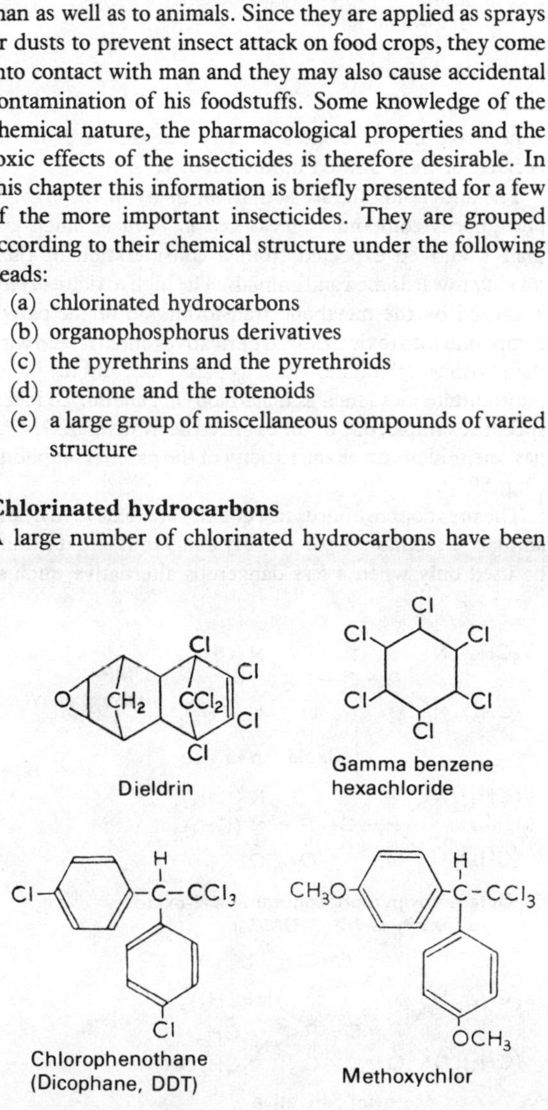

Certain substituents on the benzene rings (C_2H_5-, CH_3O-, C_2H_5O-, -F, -Cl and -Br) increase the potency of these insecticides either by increasing the lipid solubility of the compounds or by improving the fit on the receptor surface. Other substituents (C_4H_9-, C_6H_5-, NH_2-, NO_2-, -OH and -COOH) reduce the potency. All the active compounds are very soluble in lipids and their molecular weights lie within the range 270 to 450. Thus the overall bulk of the molecule as reflected by the molecular weight, the presence or position of 'fixing' or 'hindering' groups, lipid solubility and molecular flexibility all play a part in determining the potency of this group of insecticides.

Some chemically simpler chlorinated hydrocarbons such as chloroform, paradichlorbenzene, carbon tetrachloride and trichloroethylene also have insecticidal activity. They are used as *fumigants*—substances that are applied in gaseous form or as an aerosol in enclosed spaces such as rooms, cupboards or the holds of ships. These chlorinated hydrocarbons are highly dangerous to man and they must be used with care.

Two of the chlorinated hydrocarbons are used for therapeutic purposes in man.

Dieldrin

Gamma benzene hexachloride

Chlorophenothane (Dicophane, DDT)

Methoxychlor

Fig. 59.1 Some chlorinated hydrocarbons used as contact poisons

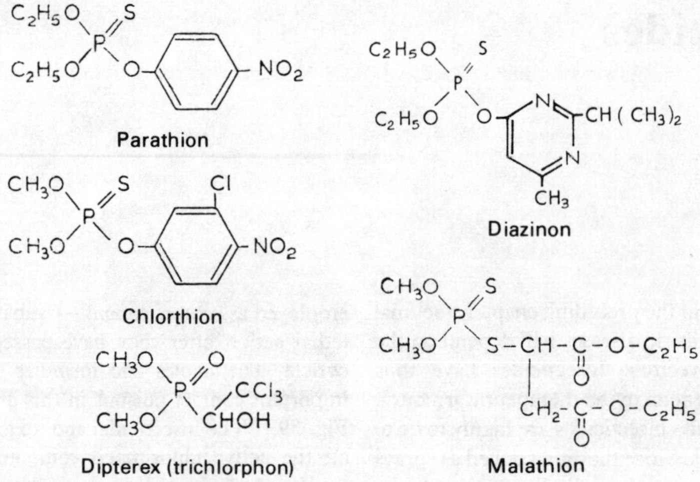

Parathion

C_2H_5O, C_2H_5O — P(=S)—O—(benzene ring)—NO_2

Chlorthion

CH_3O, CH_3O — P(=S)—O—(benzene ring with Cl)—NO_2

Dipterex (trichlorphon)

CH_3O, CH_3O — P(=O)—CHOH—CCl_3

Diazinon

C_2H_5O, C_2H_5O — P(=S)—O—(pyrimidine ring with CH_3)—$CH(CH_3)_2$

Malathion

CH_3O, CH_3O — P(=S)—S—CH(—C(=O)—O—C_2H_5)—CH_2—C(=O)—O—C_2H_5

Fig. 59.2 Some organophosphorus insecticides

GAMMA BENZENE HEXACHLORIDE (QUELLADA)
This compound is used to destroy head lice. For this purpose about 30 ml of an 0.1 per cent emulsion is rubbed into the infested scalp and is left to act for 24 hours. It is also used in the treatment of scabies.

DICOPHANE
Dicophane is also employed for the eradication of head lice. It is applied as a 2 per cent emulsion or as a dusting powder in a 10 per cent dilution with calcium carbonate and kaolin.

Organophosphorus derivatives
Members of this group of insecticides include (among many others) tetraethylpyrophosphate (TEPP), parathion, chlorthion, diazinon, trichlorphon (dipterex) and octamethylpyrophosphoramide (OMPA). The formula of TEPP will be found on p. 217, those of the other organophosphorus compounds are presented in Figs. 59.2 and 59.3.

The organophosphorus compounds are used both as contact poisons and as systemic poisons. A *systemic poison* is one that is ingested by the insect and distributed from the alimentary tract throughout its tissues. Systemic poisons are applied to plants liable to attack by insects.

The organophosphorus insecticides form stable compounds with a number of esterases including cholinesterase; their general actions are discussed together with those of the other anticholinesterases elsewhere (p. 213). The acetylcholine-cholinesterase system is necessary for the normal functioning of many insect species—the head of the house fly, for instance, synthesizes acetylcholine at a rate which is phenomenal in comparison with that attained by mammalian brain tissue—and the insecticidal action of the organophosphorus compounds is likely to be attributable, partly at least, to their inhibiting cholinesterase. Some anticholinesterases, such as eserine and neostigmine, have no insecticidal activity but this is probably because of their limited lipid solubility.

The anticholinesterase activity of many of the organophosphorus compounds measured *in vitro* is much less than would be expected from a consideration of their toxicity towards men and animals. The high toxicity *in vivo* is caused by the metabolic transformation of the parent compound into toxic oxidized derivatives and it is seen with the phosphorothionates (such as parathion) and the phosphorodithionates (such as malathion) in general. To take a specific example, one of the oxidized derivatives of OMPA has one million times the toxicity of the parent compound (Fig. 59.3).

The organophosphorus insecticides are toxic to man and animals. Parathion is particularly dangerous and it should be used only when a less dangerous alternative, such as

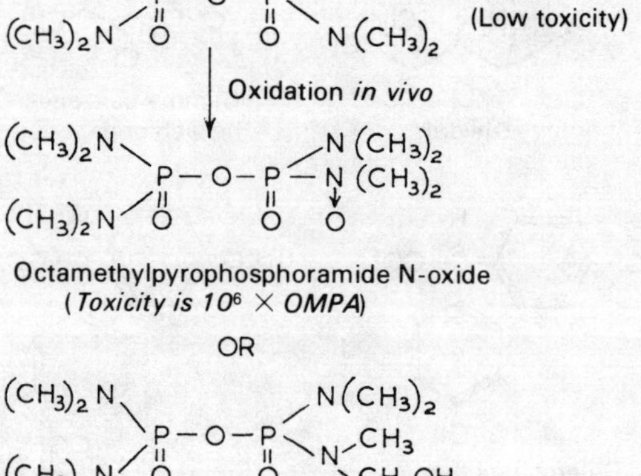

$(CH_3)_2N$, $(CH_3)_2N$ — P(=O)—O—P(=O)— $N(CH_3)_2$, $N(CH_3)_2$ OMPA (Low toxicity)

Oxidation *in vivo* ↓

$(CH_3)_2N$, $(CH_3)_2N$ — P(=O)—O—P(=O)— N(→O)$(CH_3)_2$... $N(CH_3)_2$

Octamethylpyrophosphoramide N-oxide (*Toxicity is $10^6 \times$ OMPA*)

OR

$(CH_3)_2N$, $(CH_3)_2N$ — P(=O)—O—P(=O)— $N(CH_3)_2$, $N(CH_3)$—CH_2OH

Methylol derivative

Fig. 59.3 OMPA and its toxic derivatives

malathion, is not available. Whichever organophosphorus insecticide is used, extreme care must be taken to prevent its coming into contact with the skin of, or being inhaled or ingested by, those who handle it. Gloves, protective clothing and a suitable respirator must be worn. It is hardly necessary to add that the greatest care should be taken to avoid contamination of food or food containers. The toxic effects of the anticholinesterase drugs and the treatment of poisoning by these agents is discussed elsewhere (p. 221).

The simultaneous presence of two or more organophosphorus compounds may cause a marked potentiation of toxicity. Malathion and tri-o-tolylphosphate show this type of potentiation and a number of other examples are known. The potentiation appears to be caused by one compound's inhibiting the enzyme that metabolizes the other.

Although the organophosphorus compounds are dangerous to those who handle them carelessly, their actual use as insecticides seems to have no adverse consequences in man. They are being successfully employed in regions in which insects have developed resistance to the chlorinated hydrocarbons. Malathion (Carbofos; Prioderm) is extensively used as a dusting powder in cases of infestation with body lice: a 1 per cent malathion powder is as effective in this respect as one containing 10 per cent of dicophane.

Pyrethrins and the pyrethroids

The insecticidal activity of pyrethrum arises from four esters, the pyrethrins I and II and the cinerins I and II. They are complex esters of chrysanthemum carboxylic acid (Compounds I) and the monomethyl ester of chrysanthemum dicarboxylic acid (Compounds II) with pyrethrolones and cinerolones (Fig. 59.4). They are obtained from the flower heads of several species of chrysanthemum. The pyrethroids (or rethroids) are synthetic compounds of a similar structure of the pyrethrins themselves. The most important pyrethroids are allethrin, furethrin and cyclethrin (Fig. 59.5).

The naturally occurring compounds can exist in several isomeric forms. In pyrethrin I, for example, there are two optically active centres. In addition, there is a double bond and a cyclopropane ring, both able to show geometric isomerism.

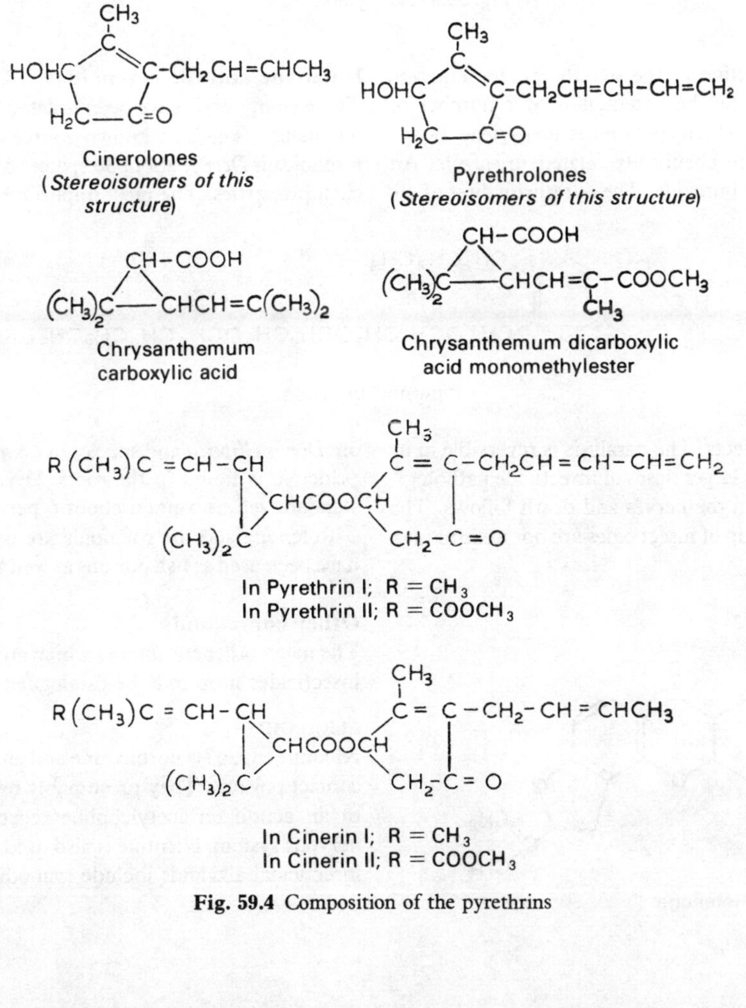

Fig. 59.4 Composition of the pyrethrins

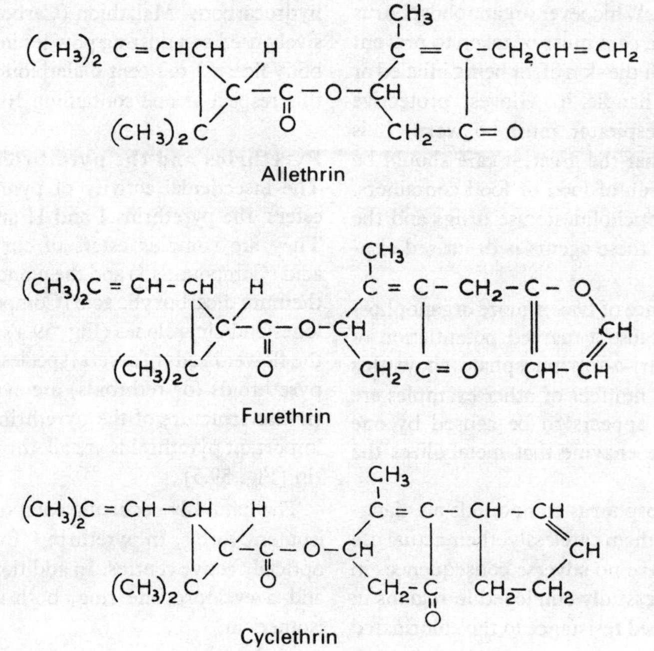

$(CH_3)_2\ C = CHCH$ ... Allethrin

$(CH_3)_2C = CH - CH$ ... Furethrin

$(CH_3)_2C = CH - CH$ ... Cyclethrin

Fig. 59.5 The pyrethroids

The insecticidal action of the pyrethrins, the cinerins and the pyrethroids can be potentiated by a number of compounds, most of which contain the methylene dioxyphenyl group and are chemically related to safrole. An example is piperonyl butoxide. The pyrethrins first of all

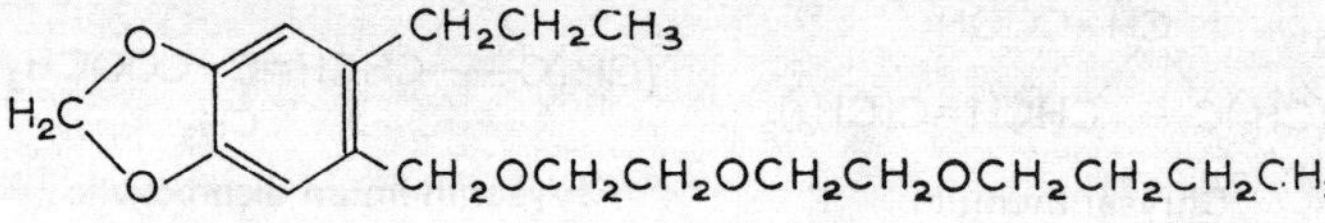

Piperonyl butoxide

cause paralysis in insects. The paralysis is reversible in its early stages but with larger doses of insecticide pathological changes appear in the nerves and death follows. The members of this group of insecticides are not toxic to man or to animals.

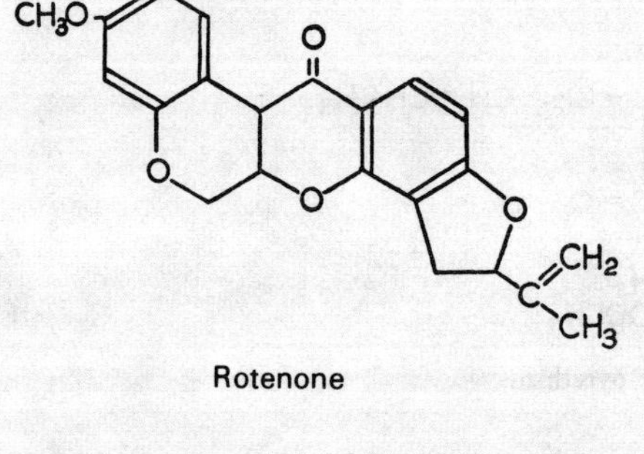

Rotenone

Rotenone and the rotenoids

These compounds have been isolated from many leguminous plants. The best known source of rotenone and the rotenoids is *Derris,* about 30 species of which have insecticidal properties. The most important commercial sources are *Derris elliptica* and species of *Lonchocarpus.* The active principle is found in the roots. Derris powder is usually standardized to contain about 6 per cent of rotenone.

Rotenone and the rotenoids are contact poisons. They have been used as fish poisons as well as insecticides.

Other compounds

The many other substances which are or have been used as insecticides need only be catalogued.

ALKALOIDS
Nicotine (p. 205), nornicotine and anabasine are powerful contact poisons. They presumably owe their effectiveness to an action on acetylcholine receptors in the insect's nervous system. Nicotine is also used as a fumigant. Other insecticidal alkaloids include ryanodine and veratrine (p. 310).

INORGANIC INSECTICIDES

Inorganic compounds of arsenic (such as copper arsenite and lead arsenate), selenium (sodium selenite) and fluorine (sodium fluoride, sodium fluosilicate) all have insecticidal activity. Simple organic compounds of selenium or fluorine (sodium fluoracetate) are also used. Sodium fluoracetate is lethal to man and animals as well as to insects: it inhibits many of the enzyme systems upon which cellular respiration depends. It is a useful laboratory tool for the study of enzyme activity *in vitro*. Other inorganic insecticides include sulphur dioxide and hydrogen cyanide, both of which are used as fumigants.

MISCELLANEOUS COMPOUNDS

These include naphthalene, reduced thiadiazines, ethylene dichloride, chloropicrin (CCl_3NO_2), the nitrophenols and some nitriles.

SCABIES

Scabies ('the itch') is the result of infestation of the keratinized layers of the skin by the scabies or itch mite, *Sarcoptes scabiei var hominis*.

It is occasionally caused by other species of mite which infect domestic and tame animals. The disease is very highly contagious and is readily transmitted (especially in institutions) by contaminated blankets or clothing or by carriers. The symptoms of scabies are caused by the burrowing of the female mite in the skin and include severe itching at the site of the burrows especially at night.

Burrows are most commonly formed in the sides and backs of the fingers, the wrists, palms of the hands and soles of the feet, glans penis, prepuce, buttocks, nipples and umbilical region. These sites may become infected following scratching, causing boils and abscesses and there may be severe skin irritation as a result of sensitization reactions.

Chemotherapy of scabies

SULPHUR

Sulphur is the traditional and ancient remedy for scabies. Sulphur itself can be used as an ointment. It is not a very convenient preparation: for the successful treatment of scabies, the whole of the body has to be covered with a layer of the ointment because scabies mites may lurk even in areas where there is no itching or skin eruption. The ointment is greasy, it soils clothes and bed linen, it has an unpleasant smell and it may give rise to a dermatitis. Other preparations of inorganic sulphur include solutions containing calcium or potassium polysulphides. Another way of using sulphur is to precipitate it on to the skin by making use of the reaction which takes place between dilute hydrochloric acid and sodium thiosulphate. All these preparations are as likely to cause dermatitis as is sulphur

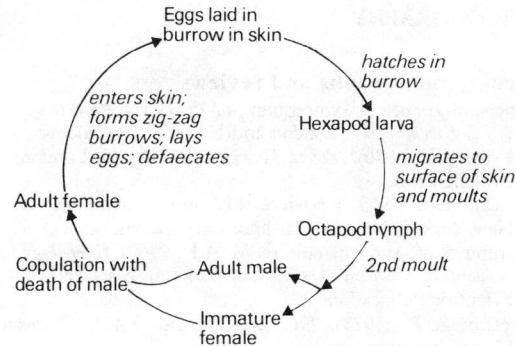

Fig. 59.6 The life cycle of the scabies mite (*Sarcoptes scabiei*)

ointment and they have the same offensive smell. Tetraethylthiuram monosulphide, an organic sulphur compound, is as effective as sulphur, it is clean to use and it rarely causes dermatitis. It is used as a soap containing 5 per cent of the active substance or as a 25 per cent solution in alcohol which is diluted before use. Tetraethylthiuram monosulphide is also used in the prophylaxis of mange, a condition caused by the scabies mite, in dogs, cats, horses, pigs and cattle.

$$C_2H_5 \atop C_2H_5 \hspace{-0.5em}>\hspace{-0.5em}N-\underset{S}{\overset{\|}{C}}-S-\underset{S}{\overset{\|}{C}}-N\hspace{-0.5em}<\hspace{-0.5em}{C_2H_5 \atop C_2H_5}$$

Tetraethylthiuram
monosulphide

BENZYL BENZOATE

Benzyl benzoate is present in Balsam of Peru, a preparation which has been used for many years for the treatment of scabies. It is an extremely effective sarcopticide. It is applied as an emulsion and two or three applications separated by intervals of 12 hours are usually sufficient to effect a complete cure.

Benzyl benzoate

OTHER COMPOUNDS

Gamma benzene hexachloride (p. 901) and other insecticides have also been used for the prevention and treatment of scabies in man and animals.

After the skin has been cleared of the scabies mite, itching is likely to continue for some time. An antipruritic agent such as calomel should therefore be applied for a few weeks after cure has been effected. Crotamiton (crotonyl-N-ethyl-*o*-toluidide) has the advantage of possessing both sarcopticidal and antipruritic actions. It is applied as a cream containing 10 per cent of the agent.

BIBLIOGRAPHY

Books, monographs and reviews

Biochemical Society Symposium no. 25 (1965). *Aspects of Insect Biochemistry*. London and New York: Academic Press.

Busvine, J.R. (1976). *Insects, Hygiene and History,* London: Athlone Press.

De Ong, E.R. (1960). *Chemical and Natural Control of Pests.* New York: Reinhold Publishing Corporation.

Gordon, R.M. and Lavoipierre, M.M.J. (1962). *Etomology for Students of Medicine.* Oxford and London: Blackwell's Scientific Publications

Greenberg, B. (1973). *Flies and Disease,* vol. 2. Princeton: University Press.

Gunther, F.A. and Jeppson, L.R. (1960). *Modern Insecticides and World Food Production.* London: Chapman and Hall.

Heath, D.F. (1961). *Organophosphorus Poisons.* London: Pergamon.

Jager, K.W. (1970). *Aldrin, Dieldrin, Endrin and Telodrin.* Amsterdam, London and New York: Elsevier.

Snow, K.R. (1974). *Insects and Disease,* London: Routledge and Kegan Paul.

Tschirly, F.H. (1973). Pesticides—relation to environmental quality. *J. Am. med. Ass.,* **224,** 1157-1159.

Winteringham. F.P.W. and Lewis, S.E. (1959). On the mode of action of insecticides. *Ann. Rev. Entomol.,* **4,** 303-318.

60. The chemotherapy of diseases caused by fungi and actinomycetes

Fungi come in a variety of shapes and sizes. Some (like toadstools and mushrooms) are large but the others are minute parasitic and saprophytic cells such as the familiar yeasts, moulds, mildews and similar growths. Many of the saprophytes are useful scavengers of vegetable matter but some fungi have had a much more elevated role thrust upon them, for where would modern man be without his bread and wine, not to say his antibiotics?

We live in contact with and surrounded by fungal organisms with most of which we establish a harmonious relationship but some fungi are pathogenic to man and are responsible for disorders ranging in severity from the trivial to the seriously life threatening.

Actinomyces is a genus of anaerobic organisms that grow as thin branching filaments and are parasitic to man and animals. Together with similar genera, such as *Nocardia*, these organisms are known as the 'higher bacteria' or actinomycetes but are often, as here, grouped with the fungi.

Actinomycosis infects cattle and man. The pathogenic organism in man is *A. israeli* which enters the body by a wound or by way of the respiratory passages. Actinomycosis affects the lungs, causing a widespread suppurating pneumonia.

The yeasts proper include yeasts, yeast-like fungi, filamentous and dimorphic fungi.

Yeasts are spheroidal cells, some 20 μ in diameter, that reproduce by budding. The yeast of particular relevance in the context of this chapter is *Cryptococcus neoformans*. It causes cryptococcosis (torulosis), a rare but extremely serious infection. Although torulosis can attack any part of the body it most frequently gives rise to abscesses in the brain or lungs or to a meningitis that is almost invariably fatal if it is not promptly treated.

Yeast-like fungi sometimes take the same form as the yeast themselves but sometimes they grow in chains of elongated cells. One such organism is *Candida albicans*. It was formerly known as *Monilia albicans* and the terms used to describe the infections it causes—moniliasis and candidiasis—can be used interchangeably. The organism is a normal commensal in the mouth, anus and vagina of healthy adults from which it is transferred to the infant's mouth at birth or shortly afterwards. The suppression of the growth of other organisms in patients receiving long term treatment with broad-spectrum antibiotics permits the proliferation of *C. albicans*. In infants, thrush may result. Thrush (monilial stomatitis) is an infection of the mouth and oesophagus. In adults pruritus vulvae, pruritus ani, a thrush-like condition in the mouth, ophthalmic candidiasis or generalized moniliasis may occur. Moniliasis may also occur in diseased portions of the lung of tuberculosis patients who have received antibiotic treatment. Localized candidiasis can be irritating, embarrassing and exhausting by its very persistence but when the infection becomes generalized the sequelae are much more serious. Candidial endocarditis or meningitis are particularly grave conditions.

Although most cases of candidiasis today arise as a consequence of therapy with broad spectrum antibiotics, other circumstances favour the overgrowth of *Candida*. These include undernutrition in infants and, in adults, the taking of oral contraceptives which, by altering the acidity of the vaginal secretions, predispose to the development of a local candidiasis. Candidiasis may also complicate corticosteroid therapy.

Filamentous fungi appear as long filaments (*hyphae*) arranged in irregular tangles (*mycelia*). Members of this very large group of fungi include *Microsporum*, *Trichophyton* and other genera that together form the dermatophytes, *Aspergillus* and the famous *Penicillium* moulds. The dermatophytes cause ringworm (tinea). Ringworm infections occur in the scalp (tinea capitis), the skin (tinea circinata), the feet (tinea pedis or athlete's foot), the groin (tinea cruris) and the nails (onychomycosis). Not all organisms are equally active at all these sites so that a particular drug may relieve one form of tinea but be useless for the treatment of another form.

Infection by species of *Aspergillus* (aspergillosis) most frequently affects the lungs (particularly when these are already diseased). The fungal mycelium may be so large as to constitute a tumour (aspergilloma) that demands surgical removal. Aspergillosis may also be associated with a severe and distressing asthma-like state as well as general reactions to the fungal attack.

Dimorphic fungi, as the name implies, exist in two forms: in the body they are yeast-like in appearance but outside the body they grow as filaments. Among them are included *Histoplasma*, *Sporotrichum* and *Blastomyces*, fungi that produce extremely serious infections. Histoplasmosis, which occurs in either a pulmonary or a systemic form, is virtually unknown in Britain but it occurs in some parts of the United States and some other parts of the world.

Blastomycosis occurs in a North American and a South American version. The disease may occur in a generalized form or it may be localized to the skin.

Other fungal diseases are very rare. The interested reader can obtain details of these diseases and the fungi which cause them from the sources quoted in the bibliography to this chapter.

Fungal diseases generally are called *mycoses* though in compound words 'mycosis' is often shortened to 'osis' as in histoplasmosis and aspergillosis.

ANTIMYCOTIC AGENTS

Antibiotics

Many antibiotics are derived from fungi and it is not surprising that few antibiotics can be applied to the treatment of fungal disease. Dog does not eat dog even in the fungal world.

PENICILLIN, TETRACYCLINES AND RIFAMPICIN

Penicillin is useful in the treatment of actinomycosis but penicillin-resistant strains of *A. israeli* are not uncommon. Tetracyclines are used in infections caused by these resistant strains. Tetracyclines and rifampicin, which normally have no fungicidal action, attack some fungal species in the presence of amphotericin B.

AMPHOTERICIN

Amphotericin is a mixture of two compounds, amphotericins A and B, formed by a soil dwelling streptomycete *Streptomyces nodosus*. As their name implies, the amphotericins are amphoteric substances. Compounds containing unsaturated carbon rings or chains ($-CH=CH-CH=$ etc.) are known as *polyenes*. The amphotericins are haptaenes. Amphotericin B (Fungizone) is the more potent compound and although it has a narrower spectrum of antifungal activity it is now used instead of the mixture. Until recently it was the only drug that offered any hope of cure in torulosis and systemic candidiasis and it retains an important therapeutic role in these conditions notwithstanding the advent of less toxic drugs. It is also the drug of choice for the treatment of serious varieties of some of the rarer mycoses such as histoplasmosis, blastomycosis and sporotrichosis.

Amphotericin B is poorly absorbed from the gastrointestinal tract and it is best administered by slow intravenous infusion in a five per cent glucose solution. Doses of up to 5 mg of the drug are given over a period of six hours. This is repeated on alternate days, increasing the dose until a total of three grams has been given (Simpson, 1966). The drug has also been given by intrathecal and intraventricular injection in severe cases of cryptococcal meningitis. Nausea, vomiting and thrombophlebitis may occur as side effects of amphotericin treatment but these are relatively unimportant when it is the only effective drug for the treatment of an infection which might otherwise prove fatal. Amphotericin B is toxic to the kidneys and it is said that all patients display at least minor degrees of kidney malfunction when they are receiving the drug. These toxic effects usually disappear when treatment ends but if signs of more serious renal failure develop during the treatment period it will be necessary to reduce the dose of, or to temporarily withdraw, the drug. Concurrent administration of heparin reduces the incidence of thrombophlebitis and hydrocortisone, aspirin and antihistamines can be given in the hope of minimizing headache, nausea and vomiting.

Amphotericin B can be applied topically to treat oral and vaginal candidiasis. The proprietary name of the drug, when it is in the form of lozenges and cream, is Fungilin.

The amphotericins owe their antifungal activity to an ability to increase the permeability of the outer fungal membrane. Their selectivity is attributable to the fact that they bind to a sterol found only in fungi (Kinsky, 1962, 1970).

NYSTATIN

Nystatin (Mycostatin), so called because it was discovered by workers in New York State, is another polyene (tetraene) antibiotic. Its mode of action is similar to that of the amphotericins but it is so insoluble that its only practicable use is for the local treatment of oral, vaginal and gastrointestinal candidiasis and fungal infections of the cornea. Given in an aerosol it has also been employed to treat pulmonary aspergillosis.

The practice of giving nystatin (or amphotericin B) with the tetracyclines in the hope of preventing the moniliasis that is so often precipitated by the tetracyclines is of doubtful efficacy.

OTHER POLYENE ANTIBIOTICS

Among the other polyene antibiotics that have found their way into the pharmacopoeias are natamycin (pimaricin, Pimafucin), hachimycin (Trichomycin), candicidin (Candeptin) and hamycin. The most widely used of these agents has been natamycin. In its actions and uses it is virtually indistinguishable from nystatin. Hachimycin (as its proprietary name indicates) is effective against trichomonal (p. 882) as well as candidial infections of the vagina. Candicihin is another polyene used topically in vaginal candidiasis. Hamycin is active when taken by mouth but it is quite toxic.

PECILOCIN

This newly introduced antibiotic is active against dermatophytes and has been used successfully to treat ringworm infections of the scalp, groin and feet. It is applied topically as an ointment (Variotin). Leofungine and Supral are European proprietary names.

5-Fluorocytosine

5-Fluorocytosine (flucytosine, Ancobon) began life in 1957

as a cytosine antimetabolite that did not fulfil the expectation that it might prove to be a useful anticancer drug. It was nearly ten years before its antifungal properties were discovered and its therapeutic role established.

Flucytosine has a restricted spectrum of antifungal activity but it is very effective against yeasts and yeast-like fungi. It is readily absorbed from the gastrointestinal tract and it penetrates with ease into the cerebrospinal fluid. It is principally applied to the treatment of serious cryptococcal and systemic candidial infections. It can be taken by mouth but its outstanding advantages over amphotericin B is its very low toxicity. Unfortunately, organisms rapidly become resistant and may do so even in the course of treatment, necessitating replacement of flucytosine by amphotericin B. In the absence of contraindications to the use of amphotericin, there is some merit in initiating combined therapy with amphotericin and flucytosine: the drugs show some synergy in their combined action and resistance to flucytosine develops less rapidly in the presence of the antibiotic.

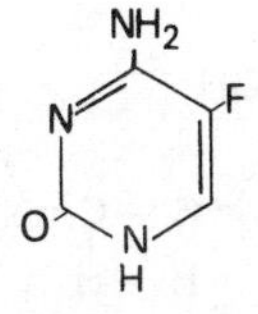

5- Fluorocytosine

Flucytosine is excreted by the kidney, to a large extent in an unchanged form. In the fungal organism, however, it is transformed into 5–fluorouracil (p. 919) where it probably prevents nucleic acid synthesis.

Because it is excreted entirely by glomerular filtration some care is needed if flucytosine is given to patients in renal failure. Liver function should also be monitored during exposure to the drug. One or two authenticated cases of aplastic anaemia attributable to flucytosine have been reported but these few indications of toxicity should excite fewer comments than the fact that there are so few reports of untoward responses among patients receiving the drug.

The daily oral dose of flucytosine is 120 to 150 mg per kg taken in four instalments. It can be given intravenously but, because of the ease with which it induces the emergence of resistant organisms, it is never applied topically.

Imidazole derivatives

Imidazole derivatives have been employed as anthelmintics (Chap. 58) for at least a quarter of a century. Others are active against some protozoa and bacteria but their antifungal properties, though long recognized, have only been exploited in the last few years so that much of what is said in the following paragraphs is necessarily tentative.

The two imidazole derivatives at present in vogue are clotrimazole and miconazole which appeared on the therapeutic scene almost simultaneously though from different sources.

CLOTRIMAZOLE

Clotrimazole (Canesten, Lotrimin) exhibits activity against a wide range of fungi but it is at present principally employed, by topical application, in the treatment of mycotic infection of the eye, vaginal candidiasis and candidial and ringworm infections of the skin particularly in cases where the infecting organisms have become resistant to the polyene antibiotics. Clotrimazole can be given by mouth, alone or to supplement its local effects but the frequency with which it causes disturbances of central nervous activity as well as nausea, vomiting and diarrhoea, constitutes a discouragement to a more extensive adoption of this route of administration.

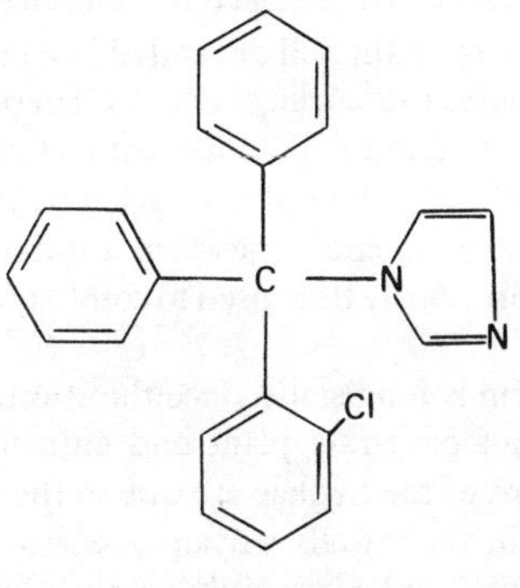

Clotrimazole

Clotrimazole, like the polyene antibiotics, damages the fungal cell membrane but, unlike the antibiotics, it does not attach itself to the specific membrane sterol. There is also evidence that it strengthens the patient's ability to attack the invading fungus. Myeloperoxidase is an enzyme that enables leucocytes to destroy the organisms they have ingested. The enzyme's activity is enhanced by clotrimazole (Renz et al., 1974).

MICONAZOLE

Miconazole (Brentan, Daktarin, Dermonistat, Monistat) has similar actions and uses not dissimilar to those of clotrimazole except that it is possible to administer the

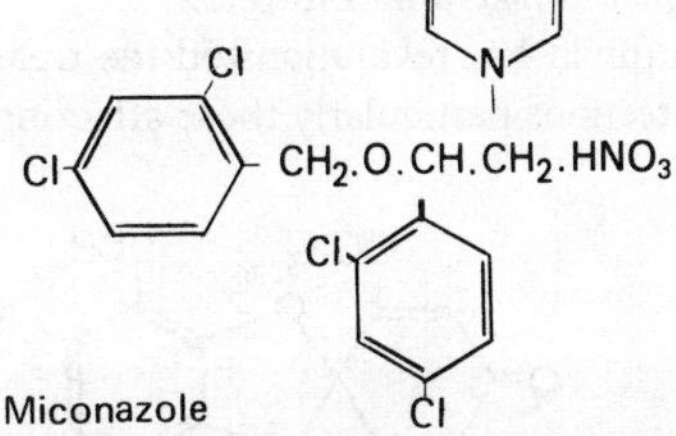

Miconazole

drug intravenously and oral administration is not attended by serious gastrointestinal or central nervous disturbances. This implies that, unlike clotrimazole, it might be applied to the treatment of systemic fungal infections and early reports of its use for this purpose have been encouraging.

ECONAZOLE

Econazole is a new imidazole derivative with antifungal activity. It is similar in structure to miconazole and appears to have much the same potential value but little information is yet forthcoming concerning its clinical effectiveness.

Griseofulvin

Griseofulvin was isolated as long ago as 1939 (Oxford, Raistrick and Simonart, 1939) from *Penicillium griseoful-vum* but other varieties of the mould also produce it: griseofulvin has, for example, been identified as the culprit responsible for the stunted growth of conifer trees in an area of Dorset. It damaged the soil dwelling fungi on which the health of the soil depended in a fashion that led to its being called the 'curling factor'. Griseofulvin was not introduced into clinical practice until after the work of Gentles (1958), who showed that, given by mouth, griseo-fulvin cured experimental ringworm infestations in guinea pigs. It had previously been used to combat fungal diseases in lettuce.

Griseofulvin is fungistatic since the stunted and curled hyphae cannot penetrate plant and animal tissues. The malformations of the hyphae are due to the production of weak spots in their walls perhaps because nucleic acid synthesis is inhibited. Griseofulvin only affects fungi with chitinous cell walls; those with cellulose walls are not attacked. It is a stable compound and although only slightly soluble in water it is adequately absorbed from the intestine. After absorption it is concentrated in the skin and nails which are thereby protected from further attacks by griseofulvin sensitive fungi. Fungi already established in the cells are not affected and the ringworm is not cured until new nails or skin replace the infected tissue. The oral dose of griseofulvin is 0.5 to 1 g daily; it is ineffective when applied locally but if necessary it can be used in connection with a topically applied fungicide. Griseofulvin is inacti-vated by demethylation in the liver. The responsible microsomal enzyme is susceptible to induction by barbitu-rates (p. 80) and it may be necessary to increase the dose of griseofulvin if the treated patient has also, for any reason, also to take a barbiturate.

Griseofulvin has revolutionized the treatment of ring-worm infections particularly those affecting the scalp and

finger nails. It is remarkably non-toxic though transient leucopenia, headache, gastric upsets, diarrhoea and skin rashes have occasionally been reported in patients receiv-ing the drug. It should be avoided in pregnancy and, since it interferes with porphyrin metabolism, it should be used with circumspection in patients with porphyria.

FATTY ACIDS

Sweat contains propionic and caprylic acids and the observation that sweat had antifungal properties led to the introduction of mixtures of sodium or calcium propionate and propionic acid for the treatment of moniliasis and ringworm. Undecylenic acid and zinc undecylenate are used in the treatment of ringworm and monilial vaginitis. They are applied in the form of an ointment, lotion or dusting powder, and they have been widely used in the treatment of athlete's foot and onychomycosis. As with all locally applied antifungal agents it is essential that dead skin be removed before the drugs are applied so that they can reach the infected tissue. Keratolytics (p. 808) may usefully be used in conjunction with locally applied agents.

Hydroxystilbamidine isethionate

Amidines

Stilbamidine and hydroxystilbamidine have proved to be very useful in the treatment of North American blastomy-cosis and in systemic moniliasis. They have also been used to treat cryptococcosis and actinomycosis.

Other compounds

Ringworm of the scalp and feet and monilial infections of the mouth and vagina, cause considerable irritation and embarrassment and they may prove difficult to treat. A large number of compounds other than those already described has been used in the treatment of these condi-tions and some of them still have a place in the treatment of the less severe fungal diseases. Diiodohydroxyquinoline and gentian violet may be useful in the treatment of local infections due to *C. albicans*. For the topical treatment of ringworm, diamthazole (Asterol), iodine, iodochlorhy-

Griseofulvin

Diamthazole

droxyquinoline, phenylmercuric nitrate and Whitfield's ointment have been used. Whitfield's ointment contains salicylic acid and benzoic acid and it is useful in the treatment of the more chronic types of the disease. Iodine and iodides have also been tried in cases of actinomycosis and North American blastomycosis

Tolnaftate

Tolnaftate (Tinaderm, Tinactin) is a new antifungal agent with much the same actions and range of usefulness as pecilocin.

Tolnaftate

BIBLIOGRAPHY

Books, monographs and reviews

Ainsworth, G.C. (1951). *Medical Mycology*. London: Pitman.

Dalldorf, G. (1962). *Fungi and Fungous Diseases*. Springfield: Thomas.

Haffbrand, B.I. (ed.) (1974) Clotrimazole. *Postgrad. med. J.* (Supp. 1) 1-108.

Riddle, R.W. and Stewart, G.T. (1958). *Fungous Diseases and Their Treatment*. London: Butterworth.

Sawyer, Phyllis R., Brogden, R.N., Pinder, R.M., Speight, T.M. and Avery, G.S. (1975). (i) Miconazole: a review of its antifungal activity and therapeutic efficacy. *Drugs*, **9**, 406-423. (ii) Clotrimazole: a review of its antifungal activity and therapeutic efficacy. *Drugs*, **9**, 424-447.

Original papers

Gentles, J.C. (1958). Experimental ringworm in guinea pigs: oral treatment with griseofulvin. *Nature, Lond.*, **182**, 476-477.

Kinsky, S.C. (1962). Nystatin binding by protoplasts and a particulate fraction of *Neurospora crassa* and a basis for the selective toxicity of polyene fungal antibiotics. *Proc. natn. Acad. Sci. USA*, **48**, 2049-2056.

Kinsky, S.C. (1970). Antibiotic interactions with model membranes. *A. Rev. Pharmac.* **10**, 119-142.

Oxford, A.E., Raistrick, H. and Simonart, P. (1939). Studies on the biochemistry of micro-organisms. LX. Griseofulvin. *Biochem. J.*, **33**, 240-248.

Renz, M. Farquar, J.W., Cohen, M. and Harkness, R.A. (1974). Elevation of myeloperoxidase activity in infants with oral candidiasis treated with clotrimazole. *Postgrad. med. J.* **50**, (Suppl. 1) 30-34.

Simpson, J.A. (1966). In *Textbook of Medical Treatment*, p. 875, ed Dunlop, D. and Alstead, S. Edinburgh: Livingstone.

61. The chemotherapy of neoplastic diseases

A malignant *neoplasm* (loosely, a cancer) or new growth is a proliferation of cells which is no longer under the control of the organism which harbours it and which can, therefore, grow without restriction, invade other tissues and (by splitting off cells which are then transported in the lymphatic or vascular systems) cause secondary growths (*mestases*) in the bones and soft tissues. The unregulated growth of the neoplasm makes overwhelming demands on the body's supply of food material and metabolic energy (even when the actual new growth is itself quite small) so that the patient becomes progressively weaker and more emaciated. The invasion by the new growth, or its metastases, of blood vessels or other vital structures is another factor contributing to malignancy.

The type of neoplastic cell varies with the tissue in which it develops and the new growth is named accordingly. A *carcinoma* is a malignant new growth that affects epithelial tissue and a *sarcoma* is one that affects connective tissue. A large number of different types of tumour are included within the last named category: thus, a lymphosarcoma is a malignant growth of the lymph nodes, a melanoma is a malignant black tumour arising from the choroid coat of the eye or from pigmented blemishes in the skin. Malignant tumours (teratoma and chorion-epithelioma) may arise from the germinal epithelium.

The word 'cancer' is sometimes loosely used to describe any form of malignant tumour. It is not inappropriate (the word is Latin for 'crab') for it suggests the slow but inexorable spread of the neoplasm, clawing its way to other locations in the body.

Connective, epithelial and germinal cells may also give rise, in addition, to benign tumours. They grow slowly, they are not disseminated to other tissues and they make few demands on the host's economy. They can become dangerous if their growth causes them to exert pressure on neighbouring structures and, if left, they may become malignant. Usually they can be treated by simple excision.

THE PLACE OF DRUGS IN THE TREATMENT OF MALIGNANT DISEASE

Surgery and X-ray therapy still provide the most important means of attacking malignant disease. In recent years, however, a number of useful anticancer agents have become available. They are used alone or in combination with one or both of the traditional methods of treatment. Among the factors that determine the value of chemother-apy in a particular instance are the nature of the tumour, its response to X-ray therapy and its accessibility to the surgeon. The conditions in which chemotherapeutic agents may be used can be summarized and assessed as follows:

1. *Conditions completely curable by chemotherapy.* Only a very few malignant neoplasms fall into this category. The most important is chorioepithelioma, a tumour that develops in early pregnancy. The epithelial cells of the chorionic villi (the means whereby the developing embryo obtains nourishment from the mother) undergo a rapid and malignant proliferation. The uterus enlarges rapidly and haemorrhages occur but in many instances chemotherapy alone will effect a complete cure. A tumour of lymphoid tissue, the Burkitt lymphoma, which is found in the tropics, may also respond to chemotherapy alone.

2. *Conditions for which chemotherapy, though not curative, produces longer remissions than do other forms of treatment.* The leukaemias and polycythaemia rubra vera (p. 917) together with some other neoplastic conditions of the bone marrow fall into this category.

3. *Conditions for which chemotherapy forms an additional, or an alternative, treatment to surgery or to X-ray therapy.* Many patients do not report their symptoms until a neoplastic process has advanced beyond the reach of surgery or X-irradiation. In some of these neoplasms (Hodgkin's disease, some other tumours of the reticulo-endothelial system, carcinoma of the ovary and a number of sarcomas, for example) chemotherapy, with or without X-irradiation, may make the patient's symptoms less obtrusive and his life more tolerable. Chemotherapy can also be employed to treat patients with these conditions who, previously sensitive, become resistant to X-rays.

A special form of chemotherapy which should be considered in this category is that represented by the use of sex hormones as adjuncts to the surgical treatment of carcinoma of the breast and prostate (p. 741).

4. *Other conditions.* In most other neoplastic conditions drug therapy has no established value. On the other hand, in otherwise intractable cases, chemotherapy tried as a last resort can do no more harm than the disease process itself and it occasionally secures useful remissions. Carcinoma of the breast, bronchus, and urinary tract, brain metastases and malignant melanomas are all conditions which have been known to respond favourably to chemotherapeutic agents when all else had failed.

It should be noted that none of the chemotherapeutic

agents in clinical use exerts any *specific* effect on neoplastic cells. All are toxic to host and tumour cells alike but because the latter are dividing more rapidly they more readily succumb to the cytotoxic action of the drugs. The so-called anticancer drugs are therefore potentially dangerous to normal tissues and the dose regime has to be adjusted with extreme care for each patient. In the account that follows the doses of many of the chemotherapeutic agents are expressed in terms of drug weight per unit of body mass per square metre of body surface. This reflects the necessity of adjusting the dose carefully.

Because of the highly toxic nature of most of the agents used, the chemotherapy of malignant conditions can only be undertaken when laboratory facilities enable a careful watch to be maintained on the response of the patient's tissues so that the intensity and duration of treatment can be appropriately adjusted.

The drugs used in the treatment of malignant diseases can be conveniently grouped as follows:

1. Alkylating agents
2. Antimetabolites
3. The nitrosoureas and related compounds
4. Plant alkaloids and their derivatives
5. Antibiotics
6. Enzymes
7. Hormones
8. Radioactive isotopes.

The drugs to be discussed in this chapter — like the antibacterial agents featured in Chap. 50—owe their effectiveness to actions on cell growth and division and the reader may need to revise his knowledge of these processes as set out on pp. 16-23 in order properly to understand the mode of action of the neoplastic drugs.

ALKYLATING AGENTS

These substances affect cells (both normal and malignant) in much the same way as does irradiation with ionizing rays. For this reason they have, in the past, been called *radiomimetic* drugs. They transfer alkyl groups to the proteins and nucleic acids of living cells. The attachment of the alkyl groups takes place through the medium of nitrogen, sulphur or oxygen and all the biological alkylating agents possess at least one such alkylating atom.

THE SULPHUR AND NITROGEN MUSTARDS

In 1917, German forces launched a gas attack on unprepared Allied troops. This was the first act of chemical warfare in history and the substance used was sulphur mustard (mustard gas; Fig. 61.2). Sulphur mustard is a volatile liquid which causes severe blistering of the skin, serious damage to the eyes and an extensive necrosis of cells lining the respiratory tracts. Gas attack victims who did not succumb to these immediate effects, or to secondary infections to which these infections exposed them, suffered a delayed and generalized systemic poisoning which put them in a state of chronic ill health for the rest of their lives. Both the immediate and the delayed effects of mustard gas poisoning are quite irreversible but minor degrees of poisoning are not incompatible with life and a few of the victims of the first gas attack at Ypres are still alive today.

The delayed effects of mustard gas poisoning produce headache, vomiting, diarrhoea, loss of appetite, epigastric pain, shock and prostration. There is salivation, bradycardia and hypotension, indicating an increased activity of the parasympathetic nervous system. The haemopoietic tissues are very sensitive to the effects of mustard gas and the leucocyte count is especially depressed.

The nitrogen mustards, the general formula of which is shown in Fig. 61.2, were also developed originally as war gases. Their toxic actions are the same as those of the sulphur mustards.

The irreversible effect of the mustards on proliferating tissues is the origin of the compounds' use in the treatment of neoplastic diseases, particularly those which affect blood forming tissues. Some of the compounds which have

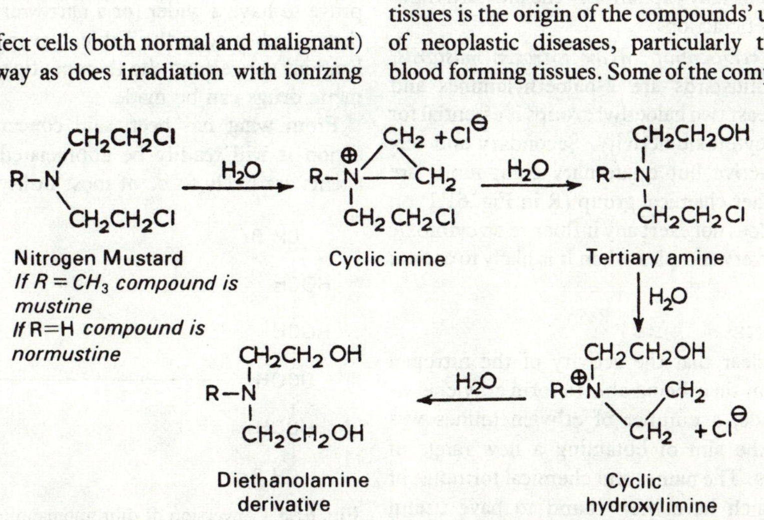

Nitrogen Mustard
If R = CH₃ compound is mustine
If R=H compound is normustine

Cyclic imine

Tertiary amine

Diethanolamine derivative

Cyclic hydroxylimine

Fig. 61.1 Formation of active cyclic intermediates from nitrogen mustard

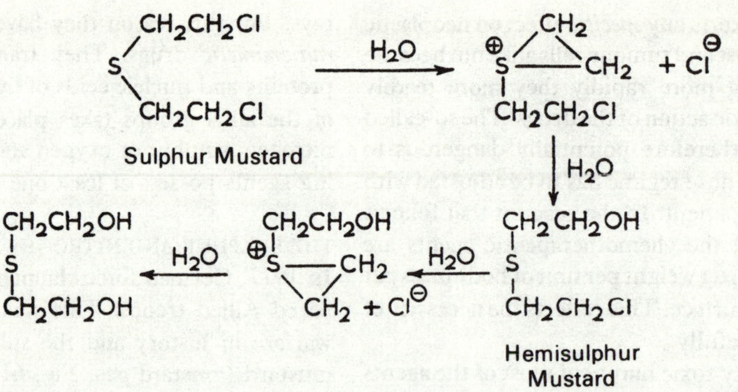

Fig. 61.2 Formation of active cyclic sulphonium intermediates from sulphur mustard

found clinical application are shown in Table 61.1 and the therapeutic uses of the alkylating agents in general are considered in more detail below.

Mode of action of the mustards. When the nitrogen or sulphur mustards come into contact with an aqueous medium, a series of chemical reactions takes place leading to the formation of the reactive cyclic ethyleneimmonium or ethylenesulphonium intermediates respectively (Figs. 61.1 and 61.2). These intermediates can react with negatively charged (nucleophilic) chemical groupings in the tissue proteins. They are, therefore, likely to interfere with the activity of enzymes, co-enzymes and other substances that regulate cellular activity. However, the most significant reaction is that which takes place between the mustards and the nucleic acids of the chromosomes. Biological alkylating agents alkylate the guanine moiety of DNA and this leads to cross linking between these moieties in adjacent chains. Consequently the DNA strands cannot separate and replication is prevented.

The cyclic ethyleneimmonium and ethylenesulphonium intermediates bear a resemblance to the quaternary choline esters and this may explain why the mustards have parasympathomimetic actions.

Structure-action relationship in the nitrogen mustards. All the nitrogen mustards are 2-haloethylamines and the presence of at least two haloethyl groups is essential for the characteristic cytotoxic activity. Secondary and tertiary amines are active but quaternary compounds are ineffective. The other chemical group (R in Fig. 61.1) on the nitrogen atom does not exert any influence on cytotoxic activity unless it is very complex when it is likely to cause a loss of potency.

THE ETHYLENEIMINES

When it became clear that the activity of the nitrogen mustards arose from their being able to form ethyleneimmonium compounds, a number of ethyleneimines was synthesized with the aim of obtaining a new range of radiomimetic drugs. The names and chemical formulae of some of those which have been found to have useful chemotherapeutic activity are set out in Table 61.1.

Triethylene melamine (Tretamine) may be taken as a typical member of the group.

OTHER COMPOUNDS

Many other groups of compounds have biological alkylating activity and a few members of some of the groups have useful clinical activity. Thus ethoglucid is a diepoxide, busulphan is a di-(methanesulphonyloxy) alkane and dibromomannitol is a halogenated sugar. Dibromomannitol owes its activity, at least partly, to its conversion into its diepoxide (Fig. 61.3). The nitrosoureas (p. 920) and dacarbazine (p. 919) also show a degree of alkylating activity.

Therapeutic uses of the alkylating agents

Some of the conditions which have been treated, with some degree of success, by the individual alkylating agents are listed in Table 61.1. The reader should not assume that the usefulness of each drug is restricted to the conditions named: the entries in Table 61.1 record the results of what in several instances were relatively limited clinical investigations. It may well be that some drugs may eventually prove to have a wider (or a narrower) field of application than is indicated in the Table. Nevertheless, some generalizations concerning the therapeutic value of the radiomimetic drugs can be made.

From what has been said concerning their mode of action it will readily be appreciated that the alkylating agents are likely to be of most utility in the treatment of

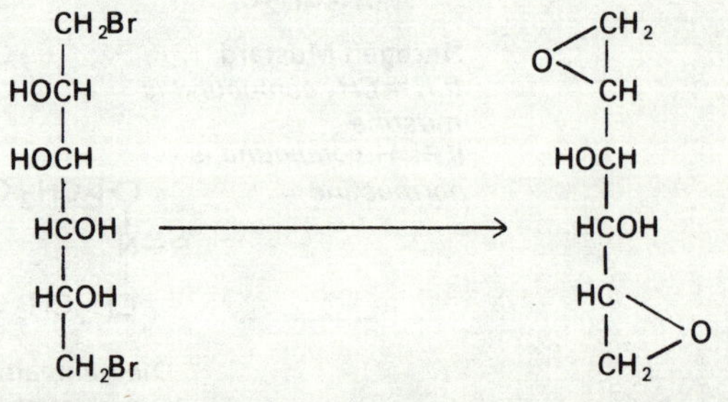

Fig. 61.3 Conversion of dibromomannitol into an alkylating diepoxide

Table 61.1 Names, formulae and therapeutic uses of some alkylating drugs

Approved name(s)	Proprietary name(s)	Formula	Possible therapeutic uses	Approximate dose

THE NITROGEN MUSTARDS

Approved name(s)	Proprietary name(s)	Formula	Possible therapeutic uses	Approximate dose
Nitrogen mustard Mustine HN2 Mechlorethamine	Mustargen	See text (Fig. 61.1)	Hodgkin's disease Other lymphomas Polycythaemia rubra vera Chronic lymphatic leukaemia Mycosis fungoides (by topical application)	250 μg/kg (15 mg/m^2) for 4 days intravenously
Trimustine	Trillekamin Leukamin	N⟨ CH$_2$CH$_2$Cl / CH$_2$CH$_2$Cl / CH$_2$CH$_2$Cl	Indications and dosage as for mustine. Rarely used.	
Uramustine Uracil mustard		(structure) N⟨CH$_2$CH$_2$Cl / CH$_2$CH$_2$Cl	Chronic lymphatic leukaemia Malignant lymphomas	50-70 μg/kg daily by mouth for 3 weeks, followed by 1 week free of drug. Repeat for up to 3 months
Mannomustine	Degranol	H$_2$C-NH-CH$_2$-CH$_2$-Cl HO-C-H HO-C-H H-C-OH 2HCl H-C-OH H$_2$C-NH-CH$_2$-CH$_2$-Cl	Hodgkin's disease Other lymphomas Chronic lymphatic leukaemia Pleural tumours (by intrapleural injection)	Initially: 100 mg daily, or less often
Chlorambucil	Leukeran	Cl CH$_2$CH$_2$ ⟩N- (ring) -CH$_2$CH$_2$CH$_2$COOH Cl CH$_2$CH$_2$	Lymphatic leukaemia Lymphomas Ovarian and mammary carcinoma Hodgkin's disease	Initially: up to 4-8 mg/m^2 daily. Maintenance: 1-2 mg/m^2 daily. Active by mouth
Cyclophosphamide	Cytoxan; Endoxan(a); Enduxan; Genoxal; Procytox; Sendoxan	(structure) N⟨CH$_2$.CH$_2$.Cl / CH$_2$.CH$_2$.Cl	Hodgkin's disease Other lymphomas Burkitt's tumour Lymphatic leukaemias Ovarian and lung tumours	Single intravenous doses of 30-40 mg/ kg (1 gram/m^2) every 3 weeks. Can also be given by mouth in daily doses of 2 mg/kg (100 mg/m^2)
Melphalan	Alkeran	HOOC - C - CH$_2$- (ring) -N⟨CH$_2$ CH$_2$ Cl / CH$_2$ CH$_2$ Cl with H and NH$_2$	Multiple myelomata Macroglobulinaemia Mammary and ovarian tumours	Up to 1 mg/kg (40 mg/m^2) given over 3 to 7 days. Dose repeated at 6-weekly intervals. Active by mouth
Mitoclomine		Cl CH$_2$CH$_2$ ⟩N- (quinoline ring) -OCH$_3$ Cl CH$_2$CH$_2$ CH$_3$	Lymphatic leukaemia	100 mg daily. Active by mouth

Table 61.1 (contd)

Approved name(s)	Proprietary name(s)	Formula	Possible thera-peutic uses	Approximate dose

THE ETHYLENEIMINES

General formula:

Triethylene-melamine Tretamine TEM			Hodgkin's disease Lymphosarcoma Chronic leukaemias	50-100 μg/kg by mouth once weekly for 4 weeks. Not widely used
Triethylenethio-phosphoramide; ThioTEPA			Chronic myeloid leukaemia Carcinoma of the ovary, breast and brain Particularly employed for injection into body cavities and instillation into the bladder.	0.2 mg/kg (7 mg/m²) daily for four successive days each month.
Diethylene-iminobenzo-quinone Inproquone			Not now used	

THE DIEPOXIDES

General formula:

Ethoglucid	Epodyl	R is HO(CH$_2$CH$_2$O)$_3$ CH$_2$CH	Not now used	
Dibromo-mannitol Mitobronitol	Myelobromol	See Fig. 61.3	Chronic myeloid leukaemia Polycythaemia rubra vera	1.5 mg/kg initially; Maintenance: 0.2 mg/k Active by mouth

THE DI-(METHANESULPHONYLOXY) ALKANES

General formula: CH$_3$SO$_2$O-(CH$_2$)$_n$-O.SO$_2$.CH$_3$

Busulphan	Myleran	n = 4	Chronic myeloid leukaemia Polycythaemia rubra vera	Initially: 3 mg/m² daily. Maintenance: 1 mg/m or less, daily. Active by mouth

OTHER COMPOUNDS

The nitrosoureas (p. 920) and dacarbazine (p. 919) also have some alkylating activity.

conditions associated with overactivity of the blood-forming tissues. These disorders can be divided into two groups: the *myeloproliferative diseases* and the *reticuloses.* In the former group of diseases the activity of the bone marrow is increased so that excessive numbers of red or white cells appear in the blood giving the conditions of *polycythaemia rubra vera* and the various *leukaemias* respectively. The adjective *vera* is attached to the first named disease to make it clear that the increase in the number of red cells is a true one and is not merely an apparent elevation of the red cell count caused by haemoconcentration.

The reticuloses arise as a result of the proliferation of the reticular cells of the reticulo-endothelial system in the spleen, liver, bone marrow, lymph nodes and other situations. The most common reticulosis is *Hodgkin's disease,* a disorder characterized by progressive enlargement of the lymph nodes, liver and spleen with attendant systemic complications (anaemia, pyrexia and jaundice) which, if not treated, may have a rapidly fatal outcome.

Of the alkylating agents, busulphan is particularly active against the bone marrow and it consequently finds its principal application in the treatment of myeloproliferative disorders. The other alkylating agents (particularly cyclophosphamide and chlorambucil) are used in the treatment of Hodgkin's disease and the chronic myeloid and lymphatic leukaemias. For this purpose they are usually administered in conjunction with other chemotherapeutic agents such as vinblastine (see below, p. 922). Cyclophosphamide depresses the formation of platelets from megakaryocytes to a much smaller extent than does chlorambucil and it is therefore to be preferred whenever it is desirable to avoid too severe a reduction in the platelet count (*thrombocytopenia*) with its attendant danger of haemorrhages.

Other conditions that sometimes respond to the alkylating agents include tumours of the ovary, bronchus, liver and urinary tract.

Chlorambucil and busulphan are usually given by mouth while mustine is given by dilute intravenous infusion over a period of several days. The other alkylating agents can be given by either of these routes depending on the circumstances of the individual case. Other modes of administration are available such as direct injection into the tumour or into the pericardial, peritoneal, pleural and meningeal cavities. Sometimes a tumour is perfused with blood from a source outside the body. The alkylating agent is added to the blood in this extracorporeal circulation and in this way minimal damage is done to normal tissues although the tumour itself is exposed to the full effects of the drug. A similar advantage attends injection into the serous cavities. Among the alkylating agents, mannomustine, melphalan and thioTEPA have been favoured for intracavity injections and for administration by way of an extracorporeal circuit. It should be noted that cyclophosphamide is not effective by either of these routes because it is devoid of alkylating activity until its nitrogen-phosphorus bond has been broken. This occurs as a result of enzyme action in the liver.

In the treatment of Hodgkin's disease, the alkylating agent is given until the clinical condition improves or until it is clear that none will occur. This may necessitate the administration of chlorambucil or cyclophosphamide for up to six weeks. Bone pain, pyrexia and pruritus diminish, the lymphoid organs are reduced in size and the patient feels better. The remission may last for some months but further courses of treatment will then be required and the periods of remission tend to become progressively shorter until finally the disease becomes resistant to the drug. The use of mustine and trimustine is reserved for the more seriously ill patients. Treatment is interrupted every two or three days in order to assess the severity of any toxic effects.

The other conditions mentioned are treated in a similar fashion to Hodgkin's disease except that it is usual to administer small maintenance doses of the radiomimetic drug when the initial remission has been obtained. Particularly when treating leukaemia, a close watch must be kept on the leucocyte count.

The side effects likely to be encountered during treatment with the alkylating agent are those inseparable from the cytotoxic effects of the compounds that form the basis of the therapeutic action. These have already been listed (p. 913).

In addition to the side effects seen with all the alkylating agents, a few peculiar to one or a small number of drugs are seen: cyclophosphamide often causes loss of hair while busulphan treatment may lead to amenorrhoea and to a pigmentation of the skin similar to that which occurs in Addison's disease (p. 757).

ANTIMETABOLITES

In the present context, antimetabolites are substances that are structurally similar to compounds needed for the synthesis of nucleic acids and which, because of this, compete with the metabolites proper for enzymes involved in the synthetic processes. For obvious reasons they are sometimes referred to as *metabolite analogues.*

Folic acid analogues

Folic acid deficiency (p. 677) depresses the formation of white cells. This observation led, long before the precise role of folic acid was known, to the suggestion that antimetabolites to folic acid should be synthesized with the object of obtaining drugs which might inhibit malignant hyperactivity of the leucocyte forming tissues. The first antimetabolite to be synthesized (in 1948) was aminopterin. It had some therapeutic success but it has now been largely replaced by methotrexate (Amethopterin) which is a less toxic compound.

METHOTREXATE

Under the influence of dihydrofolic reductase, folic acid is converted into tetrahydrofolic acid. Tetrahydrofolic acid takes up single-carbon (formyl) residues generated by various metabolic processes to form coenzymes (the formyltetrahydrofolic acids) that provide the formyl and methyl groups that are required for the synthesis of the thymidine and purine components of the nucleic acids. Methotrexate combines, virtually irreversibly, with the reductase and so prevents the synthesis of nucleic acids. It also directly inhibits thymidyl synthetase (p. 920) thus further hindering the synthesis of DNA. Inhibition of nucleic acid production leads to unregulated and unbalanced cell growth and so to cell death.

Because the combination with the enzyme is tight an overdosage with methotrexate cannot be corrected by giving folic acid. Folinic acid, (5-formyltetrahydrofolic

R=H=Aminopterin;   R=CH$_3$=Amethopterin (Methotrexate)

acid) however, can be used as an antidote if one is needed. Folinic acid is freely convertible into the other formyltetrahydrofolic acids.

Methotrexate is used in the treatment of acute lymphatic leukaemia, particularly in children. Although it has been used as the sole therapeutic agent in this condition, it is now more usual to reserve methotrexate for the maintenance of remissions induced by other drugs. For this purpose it is given in intramuscular doses of 20-30 mg per square metre of body surface, twice weekly.

Methotrexate is one of the drugs that are capable of effecting a complete cure of choriocarcinoma. In adult women, daily oral doses of up to 25 mg of the drug are given for five consecutive days at one- or two-weekly intervals. The course of treatment is repeated until the urinary excretion of chorionic gonadotrophin is permanently depressed to normal levels. This may necessitate treatment over a period of up to eighteen months and resistance to the drug may develop before the therapeutic goal is attained. The development of resistance is less likely if mercaptopurine (see below) is given along with the methotrexate.

Methotrexate has also been applied, with some success, to the chemotherapy of some other tumours including carcinoma of the breast, testes and tongue. These cases

usually demand combined therapy with other cytotoxic agents.

Suppression of platelet formation may lead to subcutaneous haemorrhages, bleeding gums and effusion of blood into the joint cavities of patients who receive methotrexate. Anaemia and leucopenia are other possible complications, as are disorders of liver and sex gland function.

Purine analogues

MERCAPTOPURINE

The best known purine antagonist is 6-mercaptopurine (Puri-Nethol).

The first stage in the formation of the nucleic acids is the transformation of hypoxanthine to its ribonucleotide (inosinic acid). The enzyme (a pyrophosphorlyase) responsible for bringing about this change also converts mercaptopurine into its ribonucleotide. Consequently, when the drug is administered, much of the hypoxanthine nucleotide is replaced by the 'fraudulent metabolite' as it has been called. This interferes, in a number of ways, with the proper formation of adenylic and guanylic acids and hence of the nucleic acids.

Mercaptopurine has had most of its success in the treatment of acute lymphatic leukaemia. It is relatively ineffective in acute myeloid leukaemia except in children, in whom it sometimes induces remissions lasting for several months. The chronic form of myeloid leukaemia is rather more susceptible to the drug. Mercaptopurine is also of value (particularly when it is given with methotrexate) in the treatment of choriocarcinoma.

In adenine,
R = NH$_2$
In hypoxanthine,
R = OH
In mercaptopurine,
R = SH

The dose of mercaptopurine has to be carefully adjusted. It is usual to commence treatment with oral doses of 2.5 mg per kilogram of body weight daily. This is reduced when signs of clinical improvement appear or is increased if no remission occurs after some weeks of treatment.

Mercaptopurine is broken down by xanthine oxidase and the effective dose of the drug is no more than one third of that quoted above if allopurinol (an inhibitor of xanthine oxidase, p. 460) is given at the same time.

Mercaptopurine has a low systemic toxicity but it may cause anorexia, nausea, vomiting and diarrhoea. Its main toxic actions are exerted on the bone marrow and on the epithelium of the gastrointestinal tract and it causes a marked reduction in the number of granulocytes, platelets and reticulocytes in the blood.

THIOGUANINE

Thioguanine (Lanvis) is structurally similar to mercaptopurine but it is said to be less toxic. It is employed in conjunction with cytosine arabinoside, in the treatment of

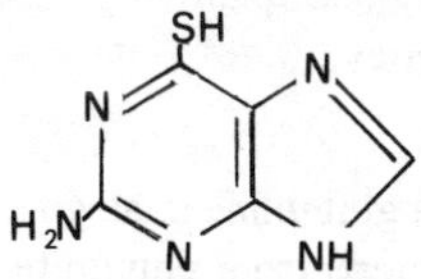

Thioguanine

myeloid leukaemia, in daily oral doses of 2 to 3 mg per kg of body mass. Its immunosuppressive properties have also been exploited.

AZATHIOPRINE

Mercaptopurine is fairly unstable *in vivo* owing to the ease with which the sulphydryl (–SH) group is oxidized. Azathioprine (Imuran) is one of several mercaptopurine derivatives which were synthesized with the aim of replacing the sulphydryl group by one less likely to be oxidized before reaching its intended destination in the body. Mercaptopurine is slowly released from azathioprine *in vivo*.

In spite of the expectations aroused by its apparently favourable structure, azathioprine offers no advantage over mercaptopurine for the treatment of leukaemia and other malignant conditions. Its real success has been as an immunosuppressive agent, employed to prevent the rejection from the body of newly transplanted organs.

Tissue rejection is an immune reaction which is dependent on the activity of the lymphocytic system and the immunosuppressive effect of azathioprine is a reflection of the fact which has already been noted, that mercaptopurine and its derivatives exert their main action on the development of this type of cell.

For the purpose of preventing tissue rejection, azathioprine is usually given in combination with one or more other immunosuppressive agents such as mercaptopurine itself, actinomycin D, prednisone or azaserine. Apart from these drugs, a specific serum (antilymphocytic serum) has proved to be an immunosuppressive agent of considerable value.

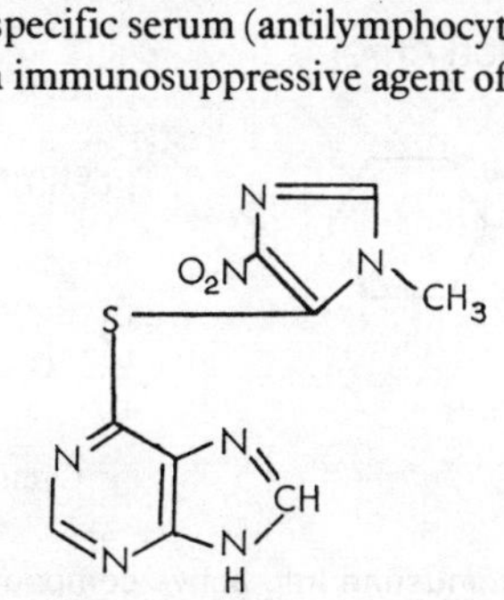

Azathioprine

Azathioprine has also been used, with varying degrees of success, in the treatment of a wide range of autoimmune diseases.

Azathioprine and the other purine antagonists have teratogenic actions and are therefore contraindicated in pregnancy. Other kinds of tumour development have also been linked with azathioprine therapy and the drug must clearly be used with circumspection.

The daily dose of azathioprine is 2 mg per kg of body weight by intravenous injection. As with mercaptopurine a lower dose is needed if allopurinol is given at the same time.

IMIDAZOLCARBOXAMIDE

Although it is included here with the purine antimetabolites, imidazolcarboxamide (dacarbazine) could equally well have appeared among the alkylating agents since the drug apparently functions in both capacities. Structurally, however, it is certainly a purine analogue.

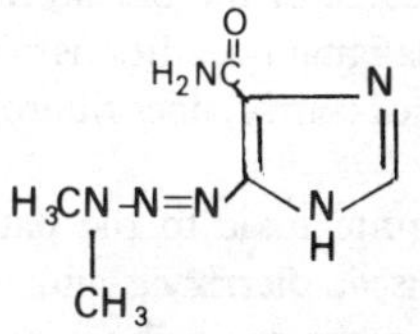

Imidazolcarboxamide (dacarbazine)

Hitherto, dacarbazine has been employed almost exclusively for the treatment of malignant melanomas and a few soft tissue sarcomas but it is a new drug and it may well prove to have a wider range of applications than it presently enjoys.

Dacarbazine is one of the least toxic of antineoplastic agents but it sometimes causes nausea and vomiting and there may be a delayed depression of bone marrow, with the usual haematological sequelae, among those who have received the drug. Some patients develop a short-lived pyrexial illness reminiscent of influenza.

Dacarbazine is given in intravenous doses of 250 mg per square metre of body surface for five successive days each month.

Pyrimidine analogues

A number of pyrimidine antagonists have antitumour activity. Although these substances have considerable activity, they are also highly toxic, affecting particularly the bone marrow, the mouth and the gastrointestinal tract.

5-FLUOROURACIL

Fluorouracil must be converted into its phosphorylated nucleotide before it can exert any cytotoxic action. This 'lethal synthesis' is accomplished in two stages that involve successively the enzymes nucleoside phosphorylase and nucleoside kinase. The resulting nucleotide acts as a 'fraudulent metabolite' which attaches itself firmly to thymidylate synthetase, the enzyme that promotes the conversion of thymine to thymidine. 'Thymineless death' follows. The absence of thymidine prevents DNA synthesis while general cell growth and RNA production continue unabated. The imbalance of growth activities thus imposed on the cell is generally accepted as the cause of fluorouracil's cytotoxic action. The reader will recall that methotrexate operates partly through a similar mechanism (p. 918).

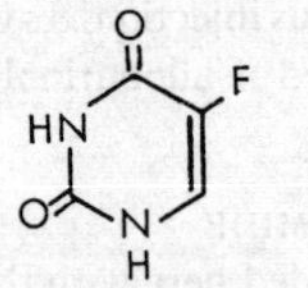

5-Fluorouracil

Fluorouracil is usually given by intravenous injection since its absorption from the gastrointestinal tract is irregular. Tumours that have responded favourably to the drug include carcinoma of the breast, intestine, prostate and pancreas and malignant conditions of the skin. In none of these conditions, of course, does fluorouracil offer more than palliation.

Fluorouracil is quite toxic to the patient. Toxic side effects include nausea, diarrhoea and ulceration of the mouth. Reduction in the red cell, white cell and platelet counts result from a depressant action on the bone marrow. Hair is sometimes lost.

The daily dose of fluorouracil (which has to be carefully adjusted at a level that prevents the appearance of toxic effects) is 6 to 12 mg per kg of body mass.

Proprietary preparations of fluorouracil, for topical application to skin tumours, include Efudex and Fluoroplex.

FLOXURIDINE (FLUORODEOXYURIDINE)

Floxuridine is formed as the first step in the conversion of fluorouracil into the active cytotoxic agent. It is given in similar doses and for similar purposes as fluorouracil.

CYTOSINE ARABINOSIDE

Cytosine arabinoside (cytarabine, Cytosar) has to be converted into its di- and triphosphates before it can exert any cytotoxic activity. The phosphorylated compounds interfere with DNA synthesis by inhibiting both DNA polymerase and the reductase that promotes the conversion of cytidine diphosphate into its deoxy derivatives and DNA. In addition, the phosphorylated molecule can disturb nucleic acid function by being incorporated into both DNA and RNA.

Cytosine arabinoside is used in the treatment of Burkitt's tumour and both myeloid and lymphatic leukaemia. It can be given either in weekly intravenous injections of 15 mg per kg or as twice daily infusions each of 1 to 1.5 mg per kg of body mass.

Cytosine also has antiviral properties that have led to its

being used in the treatment of herpes zoster (shingles). Its chemical formula will be found on p. 858.

The toxic effects of cytosine arabinoside are exerted principally on the bone marrow but nerve damage and renal dysfunction have also been reported. It is contraindicated in the early months of pregnancy.

Aminoacid analogues

AZASERINE

Azaserine (Azur) is a glutamine analogue. It prevents the transfer of amino groups from glutamine to nucleic acid intermediates. It has immunosuppressor as well as antineoplastic activity but it is rarely used clinically.

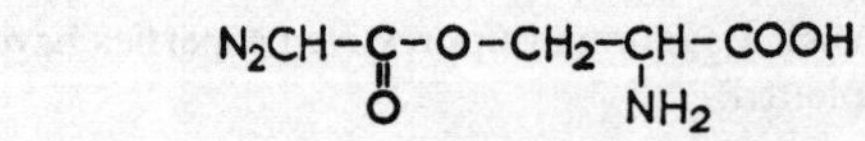

Azaserine

The nitrosoureas and related substances

Like the antimetabolites, all the compounds included within this category interfere with nucleic acid production.

THE NITROSOUREAS

The nitrosoureas were originally classified with the alky-

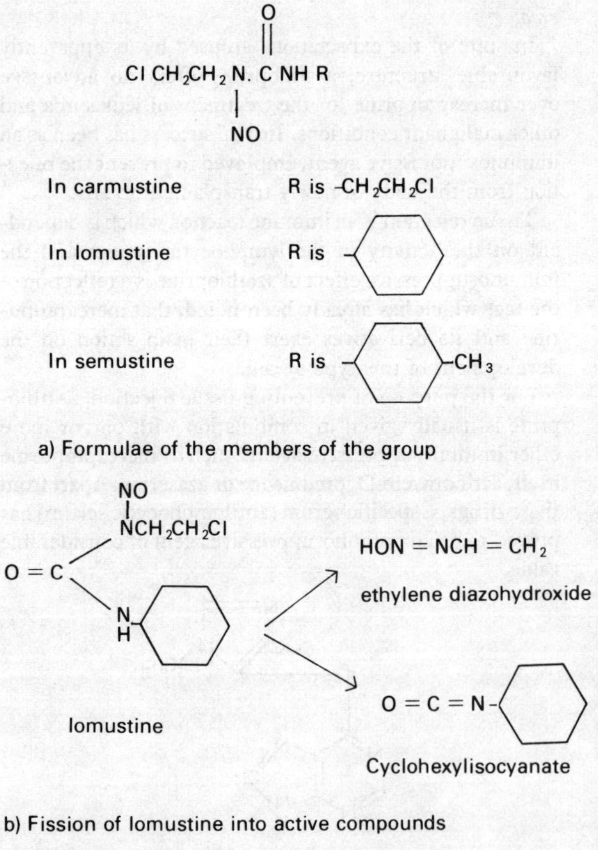

a) Formulae of the members of the group

b) Fission of lomustine into active compounds

Fig. 61.4 The nitrosoureas

lating agents but lomustine and semustine only possess one alkylating side chain in their molecules and so, unlike the alkylating agents, they cannot form cross links between the strands of DNA. The molecule of carmustine does carry two alkylating side chains but its primary mode of action seems, nevertheless, to be similar to that of the other nitrosoureas.

The nitrosoureas owe their cytotoxic activity to active compounds produced from the parent molecule *in vivo*. Thus lomustine gives ethylene diazohydroxide and cyclohexylisocyanate (Fig. 61.4b). The first named of these compounds binds to base residues in nucleic acids and proteins while cyclohexylisocyanate binds to aminoacid residues in the proteins. In addition, the active compounds operate at several other points in the sequence of events that leads to the production of nucleic acids.

The nitrosoureas pass the blood brain barrier and they are employed in the chemotherapy of brain tumours and of leukaemia involving the central nervous system. Other conditions for which they have been used include Hodgkin's disease, cancer of the lung and tumours (adenocarcinomas) of the gastrointestinal tract. The principal side effects of treatment are nausea, vomiting and a delayed depression of the bone marrow. Carmustine is more likely to produce serious side effects than are the other members of the group. Amounts of the drugs of the order of 100 to 150 mg per square metre of body surface are given in single doses at intervals of approximately six weeks. Carmustine is usually given by intravenous injection but the other two members of the group can be taken by mouth.

STREPTOZOTOCIN

Streptozotocin (or streptozocin) is an antibiotic but its chemical structure demands its inclusion among the nitrosoureas. It inhibits nucleic acid synthesis but, perhaps because of its glucosamine residue, it displays a particular affinity for the β cells of the pancreas. It has been used in the treatment of islet cell carcinoma of the pancreas, the Zollinger-Ellison syndrome (p. 354) and malignant carcinoid (p. 329).

Streptozotocin

The therapeutic dose of streptozotocin is of the order of 1 to 1.5 g per square metre of body surface in single weekly injections but the drug is very toxic and the dose has to be very carefully adjusted to the requirements of the individual patient. The kidney is the principal victim of this toxicity but the liver and gastrointestinal tract are sometimes affected too. There may be hyperglycaemia.

Streptozotocin is also used to produce experimental diabetes in laboratory animals.

HYDROXYUREA

Hydroxyurea (Hydrea) is more selective in its action than the nitrosoureas: it inhibits the synthesis of DNA without noticeably affecting that of RNA or protein. It achieves this by preventing the action of ribonucleotide reductase, the enzyme that converts cytidine phosphate into the deoxy compounds. It is most often employed in the treatment of myeloid leukaemia that no longer responds to busulphan but some cases of melanoma and other skin cancers have also responded favourably to the drug. In association with methotrexate, hydroxyurea also finds a place in the treatment of psoriasis.

Hydroxyurea

Hydroxyurea has a brief half life and for that reason it is usually given twice daily in doses of up to one gram per square metre of body surface. Side effects include skin rashes, alopecia and a delayed depression of the bone marrow manifested by anaemia and thrombocytopenia. Withdrawal of the drug rapidly arrests these changes.

PROCARBAZINE

Procarbazine (Matulane, Natulan) is not a nitrosourea but it does inhibit nucleic acid and protein synthesis by a number of actions. Through its metabolites it inhibits nucleic acid polymerase, it methylates the guanine residues in the nucleic acids and it degrades DNA. In these respects the consequences of its administration are similar to those of irradiation. Procarbazine is employed for the treatment of Hodgkin's disease, often in association with mustine, vinblastine and prednisolone. This combination of cytotoxic agents has proved to be particularly successful. Other conditions that have yielded to procarbazine include non-Hodgkin lymphomas, myeloma, melanoma and lung cancer.

Procarbazine is a substituted hydrazine and it is not, therefore, surprising to find that it inhibits monoamine oxidase (p. 578). Indeed, the cytotoxic action of procarbazine and its congeners was discovered in the course of investigations into their psychotropic activity. Procarbazine is not a very powerful enzyme inhibitor but those who receive the drug may experience hypertensive crises if they succumb to the temptation to partake of any of the

Procarbazine

traditionally forbidden foods and drinks (p. 79). On the other hand, the drug does not inhibit monoamine oxidase to the extent of inducing an antidepressant effect. Indeed, it so markedly potentiates the depressant effect of the phenothiazine drugs that this combination of agents has to be listed among those likely to produce undesirable interactions. Procarbazine also has a disulphiram like action (p. 89) and patients receiving it should be warned of the inadvisability of taking alcohol.

Nausea, vomiting and depression of the bone marrow have also to be included among the side effects of procarbazine administration.

Procarbazine is given in daily oral doses of 100 to 200 mg per square metre of body surface. It is contraindicated in pregnancy.

PLANT ALKALOIDS

THE VINCA ALKALOIDS

Some twenty years ago, Johnson and his associates discovered that extracts of the periwinkle plant (*Vinca rosea*) possessed antitumour activity, thus supporting an ancient belief that this particular plant had miraculous healing powers. Noble, working independently of, but concurrently with, Johnson isolated an active alkaloid from the plant in 1958. He called this vincaleukoblastine but later work showed that it was a mixture of four separate alkaloids—vinblastine, vincristine, vinleurosine and vinrosidine. The two first named have been studied in detail and are now recognized as effective anticancer drugs.

Vinblastine and vincristine are closely similar compounds, their complex molecules differing from one another by only one small radical. Nevertheless the two

In vinblastine, R = CH₃; in vincristine, R = CHO

In vinglycinate the -OCOCH₃ group of vinblastine is replaced by

$$-OCOCH_2N\begin{array}{l}C_2H_5\\C_2H_5\end{array}$$

drugs differ markedly in their actions, therapeutic uses and toxicities. Their differences are underlined by the fact that a patient who has received one of the drugs may become resistant to it while retaining his sensitivity to the other.

Both alkaloids arrest cell division in the metaphase of the mitotic process, vincristine being more active than vinblastine in this respect. They achieve their end by combining with a precursor of the mitotic spindle. The precursor is, of course, protein in nature and it has other functions in the cell so that the cytotoxic effect of these compounds is not as specific as it might at first appear. The actions of the alkaloids (particularly vinblastine) are reversed by glutamic acid, suggesting the possibility that vinblastine, at least, is a glutamic acid antagonist.

Vinblastine. Vinblastine (Velbe, Velban) is used for the treatment of Hodgkin's disease and other lymphomas and for cases of choriocarcinoma which have not yielded to treatment with other drugs. In the treatment of Hodgkin's disease it is often given, as we have seen (p. 921) in association with other drugs. Other tumours that have yielded to vinblastine include cancers of the breast, testis, lung, kidney and bladder and some neoplasms of bone.

Vinblastine has a severely depressant action on the bone marrow and the resulting anaemia, leucopenia or thrombocytopenia represents the major toxic effects of the drug. It may also exert adverse effects on the central nervous system. These are similar to, but much less severe than, those which sometimes result from vincristine administration. Pain in the jaws is another possible complication. Nausea, vomiting and other gastrointestinal disturbances may occur as with all cytotoxic drugs.

Vinblastine is given intravenously in a dose of 0.1 to 0.15 mg per kg of body weight at weekly intervals.

Vincristine Vincristine (Oncovin) is less effective than vinblastine for the treatment of Hodgkin's disease. On the other hand, it produces remissions in acute leukaemia in children as effectively as does mercaptopurine. Like the latter drug, vincristine is given in association with prednisolone for this purpose. It appears, also, that vincristine is superior to vinblastine as a chemotherapeutic agent against lymphocytic lymphosarcoma. This is a condition which arises in the lymph nodes or spleen and then spreads to the bone marrow. A wide range of other tumours (neuroblastoma, Wilms' tumour of the kidney, and cancers of the brain, breast, testis and ovary) have also been successfully treated with vincristine, often in association with other chemotherapeutic agents.

Vincristine depresses the bone marrow to a much less severe degree than does vinblastine. On the other hand, it has more marked actions on the nervous system. Toxic effects referable to this facet of its activity include paraesthesiae, neuritic pains, convulsions, muscle weakness, hoarseness or loss of voice and double vision or other visual disturbances. Vincristine is more prone than vinblastine to cause loss of hair.

The treatment regime for vincristine is similar to that already described for vinblastine but dose levels are no more than one quarter of those recommended for the latter drug. Orally active preparations of both alkaloids are available but their absorption from the gastrointestinal tract is irregular.

COLCHICINE DERIVATIVES

Demecolcine (Colcemid) has been used to treat chronic myeloid leukaemia but its value is limited. Colchicine and its derivatives arrest mitosis in metaphase but the mechanism of action appears to be different from that of the vinca alkaloids.

Demecolcine

ANTIBIOTICS

Several antibiotics, isolated from species of *Streptomyces* (and a few related organisms) inhibit the growth of tumours. They do this by interfering with the action of DNA.

THE ACTINOMYCINS

The actinomycins are a large group of closely related red-coloured antibiotics obtained from several species of *Streptomyces*.

The actinomycins do not prevent the synthesis of DNA but they do distort the molecule once formed, being bound by alkylation to the guanine bases. As a result, the synthesis of RNA is interfered with. The tricyclic moiety in the actinomycin molecule (actinocin; Fig. 61.5) is responsible for the antibiotic's characteristic colour and it also provides the means whereby attachment is made to the guanine in the DNA molecule.

Of the several actinomycins, that designated 'D' (actinomycin D, dactomycin or Cosmegen) is the least toxic and it has been used with some success in the treatment of cancer of the uterus and testis, Wilms' tumour, neuroblastoma and a variety of solid tumours particularly in children. For all these purposes it is usually used in conjunction with other drugs or with deep X-ray therapy.

The actinomycins have powerful antimicrobial activity and they also inhibit the production of some types of virus but their toxicity precludes the therapeutic exploitation of these properties.

Toxic side effects of actinomycin administration include nausea, vomiting, diarrhoea, ulceration of the mouth and tongue, damage to the spleen and depression of the bone marrow. In addition, skin eruptions, similar to those produced by X-irradiation, are likely to occur.

For cancer chemotherapy, actinomycin D is given intravenously in amounts of 15 μg per kilogram of body weight. This dose is given either once weekly or on five successive days every four weeks.

MITHRAMYCIN

Like actinomycin, mithramycin (Mithracin) attaches itself to DNA and so prevents the production of RNA. It is obtained from several species of *Streptomyces*. A tricyclic chromophore (Fig. 61.5) confers a yellow colour on the antibiotic.

Mithramycin is a very toxic substance but it has proved useful in the chemotherapy of malignant and inoperable testicular tumours of embryonic cell origin. It also appears to have a specific effect on the bone cells which results in its bringing about a lowering of the plasma calcium concentration and a depression of alkaline phosphatase activity. This property has led to its being employed to treat the hypercalcaemia associated with some malignant tumours. It shows promise too as a drug for the treatment of Paget's disease of bone, a non-malignant condition characterized by the development, in many bones, of patchy areas of increased bone formation alternating with areas of rarefaction.

Mithramycin is given by intravenous infusion in doses of 1.0 to 1.5 mg per square metre of body surface on alternate days until signs of toxicity appear. The treatment can be repeated at monthly intervals. For the treatment of hypercalcaemia and Paget's disease smaller doses (not more than 0.5 mg per square metre) are recommended.

The most potentially dangerous side effect of mithramycin therapy is haemorrhage: depression of the bone marrow causes thrombocytopenia, the possible consequences of which are aggravated by a hepatotoxicity that impairs the synthesis of clotting factors. Other side effects include skin rashes, disturbances of kidney function and a general systemic upset presenting as malaise, fever, nausea and vomiting.

The toxic consequences of mithramycin administration are not commonly seen in patients who have received the modest doses of the drug prescribed for hypercalcaemia and Paget's disease.

DAUNORUBICIN

Daunorubicin (daunomycin, Cerubidin, Rubidomycin) is obtained from *Streptomyces peucetius*. The tetracyclic chromophore indicated in Fig. 61.5 confers an orange red colour on the drug. Daunorubicin appears to owe its cytotoxicity to daunorubicinol, a metabolite formed by enzymatic reduction of the keto group at C13. This compound intercalates itself between adjacent base pairs of the DNA molecule which becomes partly untwisted so that further synthesis of DNA, and hence of RNA, is interfered with.

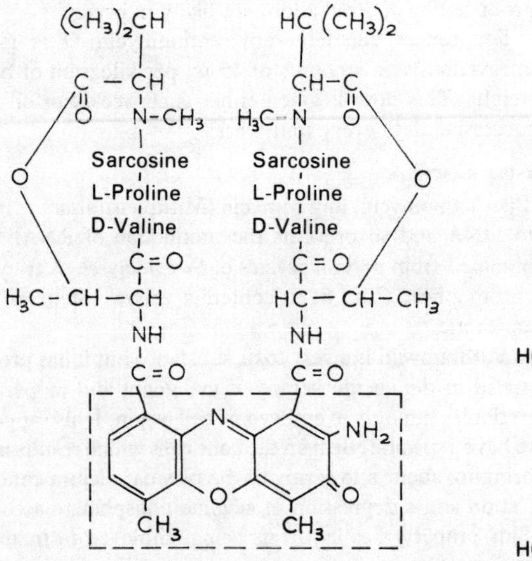

Actinomycin D

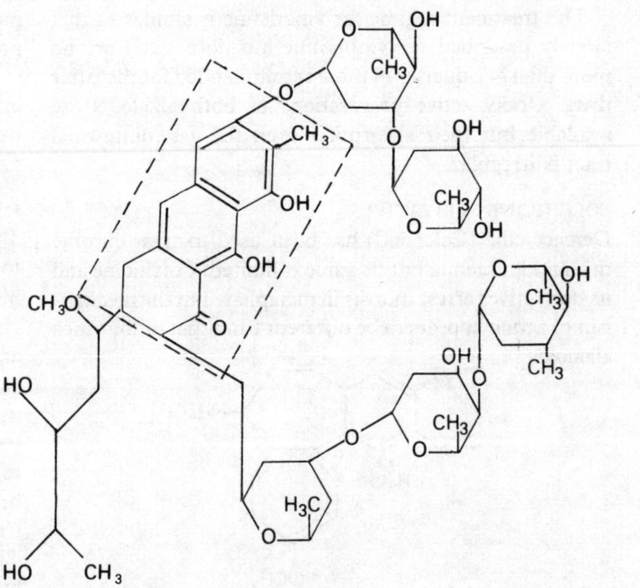

Mithramycin

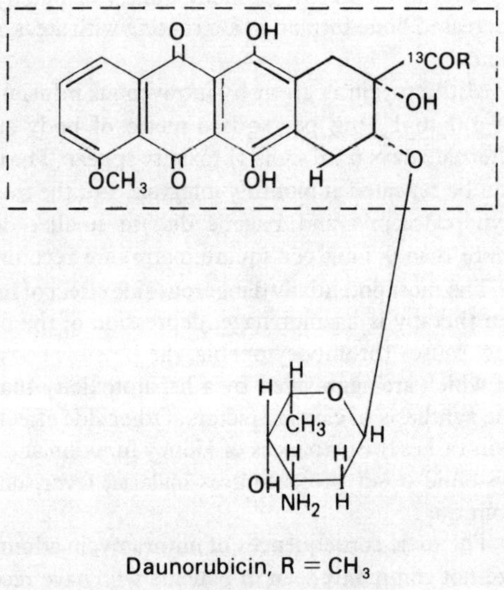

Daunorubicin, R = CH₃

Doxorubicin,   R = CH₂OH

Portions of the molecule surrounded by broken lines indicate the chromophore moieties

Fig. 61.5 Some antibiotic drugs with antineoplastic activity

Daunorubicin's principal value is in the treatment of acute lymphatic and myeloid leukaemia: leucocytes are rich in the reductase that converts the parent molecule into daunorubicinol. While it has been used as the sole medication in leukaemia, it is more usual to give daunorubicin in association with other cytotoxic drugs such as prednisone, vincristine and cytarabine.

Daunorubicin is administered by fast intravenous infusion twice weekly in doses of 10 to 30 mg per square metre of body surface, but the total amount given to any one patient should not exceed 750 mg per square metre. Daunorubicin seems to have a particular affinity for DNA in the myocardium and too high a dose can precipitate an irreversible cardiac failure. The appearance of tachycardia during treatment with daunorubicin should be read as a danger signal and the drug is contraindicated in those with heart disease. Other side effects include anaemia, thrombocytopenia, alopecia, arthritis and phlebitis.

DOXORUBICIN

Doxorubicin (Adriamycin, Adriblastina) like daunorubicin, is extracted from a strain of *Streptomyces peucetius,* its chemical structure differing in only one trivial detail from that of daunorubicin (Fig. 61.5) and like the latter drug, it seems to owe its cytotoxic action to a reduction product (doxorubicinol) that intercalates itself into the DNA molecule. Yet doxorubicin displays cytotoxic activity against a much wider range of neoplasms than does daunorubicin. The reason for this difference in activity between such closely related compounds is obscure but it may be that doxorubicin can contribute cytotoxic metabolites additional to doxorubicinol itself.

Doxorubicin has been applied to the chemotherapy of a number of solid tumours (including Hodgkin's disease and other lymphomas, Wilms' tumour, carcinoma of the breast, bladder, lung, thyroid and ovary and osteogenic sarcoma) but it also retains the antileukaemia activity of daunorubicin.

Dose schedules and side effects are similar to those recorded for daunorubicin.

BLEOMYCIN

Bleomycin (Blenoxane) is a mixture of several glycopeptide antibiotics of complex structure. Originally extracted from *Streptomyces verticillus,* the components of the mixture can now be synthesized. Bleomycin is used in the treatment of lymphomas (including Hodgkin's disease) and a variety of other malignant growths.

Bleomycin is given in twice weekly intravenous (occasionally intramuscular) doses of 10 mg per square metre of body surface. It is a radiomimetic drug and cutaneous side effects (blistering, itch, rash and alopecia) are not uncommon. Other toxic reactions include anorexia, fever, headache and vomiting but depression of the bone marrow is minimal.

ENZYMES

L-Asparagine is an aminoacid that is normally synthesized in the cells from glutamine and aspartic acid. Some types of malignant cell, particularly those of lymphoid origin, are, however, devoid of the enzyme (asparagine synthetase) under whose aegis this synthesis is brought about and they have therefore to rely on the arrival of supplies of the aminoacid from extraneous sources. If these supplies were to be cut off, synthetase deficient malignant cells would be denied an essential nutrient and would, consequently, die. *L. Asparaginase* (colaspase, Crasnitin), an enzyme obtained from *E. coli,* brings about this interruption of supplies because it promotes the cleavage of L-asparagine into aspartic acid and ammonia.

It was at one time believed that lack of asparagine synthetase was a feature exclusive to malignant cells and L-asparaginase was hailed as the first specifically antineoplastic drug. It promised to attack malignant cells while ignoring normal tissue. These early hopes have not, alas, been realised. Some normal cells demand external supplies of L-asparagine and treatment with L-asparaginase is no less likely to be attended by toxic effects than is the administration of other cytotoxic agents.

L-Asparaginase is used primarily in the treatment of acute lymphatic leukaemia although it is occasionally given to patients with myeloid leukaemia, lymphosarcomas or other tumours.

Treatment with L-asparaginase usually begins with daily slow infusions of the enzyme in amounts of 200 units per kg of body mass. The dose can be progressively increased until it reaches 1000 units per kg. The most pure specimens of the enzyme contain about 250 units per mg of drug.

A range of systemic side effects has been reported among patients receiving L-asparaginase. These include functional disturbances of the liver and of pancreatic islet tissue, severe depression of the bone marrow (fatal cases of haemorrhage and of leucopenia have occurred), mental confusion and depression. L-Asparaginase has teratogenic activity and it is, consequently, contraindicated in pregnancy.

Glutaminase, which brings about the hydrolysis of glutamine and so hinders the synthesis of asparagine has sometimes been employed in association with L-asparaginase further to reduce supplies of asparagine particularly when treating tumours that show evidence of being resistant to L-asparaginase.

It is unfortunately true to say that L-asparaginase has not lived up to its early promise.

HORMONES

The use of the oestrogens, the adrenocorticosteroids and corticotrophin in the chemotherapy of neoplastic diseases is discussed elsewhere (pp. 741, 768, and 775 respectively). Here it is only necessary to attempt an evaluation of the hormones in relation to the other chemotherapeutic agents discussed in this chapter.

The value of oestrogens in the treatment of carcinoma of the prostate is now well established: they are unsurpassed for this purpose by any chemotherapeutic agent. They also have a place in the treatment of cancer of the breast. Corticotrophin and the corticosteroids (particularly prednisone) may induce remissions in cases of acute leukaemia and Hodgkin's disease when all else fails. They can be combined with other drugs, either from the beginning of treatment or when resistance to the other agents has begun to appear. Their utility as immunosuppressive agents has already been mentioned.

ESTRAMUSTINE PHOSPHATE

Estramustine phosphate (Estracyt) is a compound of normustine (Fig. 61.1, p. 913) and oestradiol with a particular affinity for prostatic tissue. It is particularly useful in the treatment of cases of advanced prostatic carcinoma that are (or have become) resistant to the oestrogens. It seems to have more than a merely palliative effect since bony metastases have been seen to regress during treatment with estramustine.

Estramustine is broken down in the prostate gland (and in the liver) into its component molecules but the fact that it is active in oestrogen resistant patients indicates that its cytotoxic action owes more to normustine than to oestradiol. Its oestrogenic activity is, in any event, low: gynaecomastia, for instance, is rarely seen in patients who have received the drug.

Estramustine can be taken by mouth: treatment is initiated with total daily oral doses of 560 mg divided into fractions taken with meals. The daily dose can be cautiously increased to a maximum of 840 mg but it should be reduced to a maintenance level of 280 mg as soon as possible. The doses quoted here take into account the fact that the drug is supplied in capsules in 140 mg quantities.

Side effects of estramustine treatment include gastrointestinal upsets, transient disturbances of liver function, anginal attacks and allergic reactions. The drug is contraindicated in patients with peptic ulceration, liver disease or cardiovascular complaints.

RADIOACTIVE ISOTOPES

Radioactive isotopes emit three types of ray: α particles, β particles and γ rays. Alpha particles are identical with the nuclei of helium atoms, β particles are electrons and γ rays are short wave electromagnetic radiations. Certain organs selectively absorb particular elements: if these elements can be made radioactive they will, on administration, provide an intense local irradiation of the organs that take them up.

In the tissues, α and β particles are slowed down because they collide with the atoms and molecules of the tissue substances. These collisions cause the displacement of electrons from the atomic nuclei so that ionization takes place. For this reason, the emitted α and β particles are often referred to as *ionizing radiations* and it seems certain that the ionization effect is the basis of their cytotoxic action.

The γ rays possess no mass and they are not, therefore, absorbed or slowed down by the tissues. On the other hand, they have considerable penetrative power so that the uptake of a γ-radiating substance by a particular organ can be assessed by means of a counter placed on the body surface near the organ even when the administered dose of radioactivity is low.

The effects just described form the basis of the use of radioactive elements both to irradiate tumours and for investigatory purposes.

RADIOACTIVE IODINE
Radioactive iodine has an atomic weight of 131. It is used in the form of sodium radioiodide ($Na^{131}I$), a compound with a half-life of eight days. On injection it is concentrated in the thyroid gland. Small doses of radioiodide are employed for the diagnosis of disorders of the gland, larger amounts are needed for the treatment of diffuse toxic goitre and still larger doses are given for the chemotherapy of cancers of the thyroid involving cells that concentrate iodine (follicular cell carcinomas).

For diagnostic purposes, the uptake of iodine by the thyroid gland is measured. The glands of normal individuals take up some 30 per cent of the administered iodide but those of patients suffering from toxic goitre may absorb up to 70 per cent. Very little is taken up by the glands of hypothyroid patients. Determinations of uptake can be supplemented with estimations of the amount of radioactivity eliminated in the urine; the greater the retention by the gland the smaller the loss in the urine.

When larger doses of radioiodide are given for therapeutic purposes, the β irradiation to which the gland is exposed is sufficiently intense to destroy the glandular tissue.

RADIOACTIVE PHOSPHORUS
Radioactive phosphorus has an atomic weight of 32 and a half-life of 14.3 days. It emits only β particles and the cytotoxic effect of a dose of radiophosphorus is therefore localized to the organs that concentrate it. These are bone, liver, lymph nodes and spleen. Rapidly proliferating cells take up more phosphorus than do quiescent tissues, presumably because of the higher rate of nucleic acid turnover. The isotope is, therefore, concentrated to a somewhat greater degree in cancer cells than it is in normal tissues.

When radioactive phosphorus leaves soft tissues which have taken it up, much passes into bone so that finally the largest amounts of radioactivity are found there.

Radioactive phosphorus in the form of sodium dihydrogen phosphate ($NaH_2{}^{32}PO_4$) or disodium hydrogen phosphate ($Na_2H^{32}PO_4$) has been used in the treatment of polycythaemia rubra vera and chronic myeloid leukaemia; its value in cases of chronic lymphocytic leukaemia is dubious and in acute leukaemia it is negligible.

When it is used for the treatment of polycythaemia, a single oral or intravenous dose of radioactive sodium phosphate is often sufficient to produce a remission lasting for several years after which the treatment may be repeated as necessary. Regular haematological examinations must be performed in order to assess the effect of the isotope on the formation of the white cells. Some have suggested that radioactive phosphorus may predispose to the development of leukaemia in patients with polycythaemia rubra vera.

A colloidal suspension of radioactive chromic phosphate ($Cr^{32}PO_4$) is sometimes used in the treatment of pleural or intraabdominal effusions which have arisen as secondary complications of neoplasms of the thoracic or abdominal viscera.

RADIOACTIVE GOLD
Radioactive gold (^{198}Au) has a half-life of 2.7 days and it emits β particles and γ rays. It has been used to treat abdominal and pleural effusions due to cancer but it offers no advantages over other chemotherapeutic agents.

RESISTANCE TO ANTINEOPLASTIC DRUGS

Many tumour cells, like bacteria, readily develop resistance to some chemotherapeutic agents so that a patient needing extended treatment may require changes of medication with the passage of time. In addition to this 'secondary' form of drug resistance, consequent on exposure to the drug, a 'primary' form is recognised. In primary resistance, tumour cells do not respond to an antineoplastic agent to which they should be sensitive, even on their first exposure to the drug.

The several causes of resistance, primary or secondary, can be briefly summarized as follows.

a. Some agents (particularly the purine and pyrimidine analogues) only acquire cytotoxicity after they have been converted into nucleotides. This conversion is brought about enzymatically and cells are sometimes resistant because they lack the enzymes necessary for achieving this lethal conversion.

b. Methotrexate combines, virtually irreversibly, with dihydrofolate reductase and so prevents the formation of tetrahydrofolic and folinic acids. Continued exposure of malignant cells to the cytotoxic agent is likely to be followed by the production of additional supplies of the enzyme which can thereby break through the inhibition previously imposed by methotrexate.

c. In response to the continuing presence of particular cytotoxic agents, some tumour cells can elaborate additional supplies of enzymes that break down the drugs. In this way the amount of the drug to which the target tumour cells are exposed may be reduced below an effective level. This provides one of the ways by which resistance develops to the alkylating agents.

d. Tumour cells may be (or may become) impermeable to the antineoplastic drugs to which they would otherwise be sensitive or they might lose the ability to bind the drugs to the appropriate intracellular molecules. Resistance to vinblastine, vincristine, actinomycin D and the alkylating agents probably arises, partly at least, from the operation of this mechanism.

e. Some tumour cells defeat an attacking cytotoxic agent by accelerating repair processes to such an extent that they can keep pace with the destructive efforts of the drug.

THE SCREENING OF DRUGS FOR ANTICANCER ACTIVITY

The usual method of testing for anticancer activity involves the use of tumours maintained in culture, portions of which are transplanted into experimental animals. Mice and rats are usually employed for this purpose and a number of different tumours are available for transplantation in this way. They are usually implanted subcutaneously and when they have become properly established, their rate of growth in animals which have received the agent under test is compared with that in untreated animals. Since the tumours are located subcutaneously, it is relatively easy to determine their size by palpation and the use of callipers. In some cases it is better to use the animals' survival time, rather than the size of the tumour, as the criterion of activity. The drug is usually given by intraperitoneal injection, the first dose being delayed until the neoplasm is well established.

When these screening tests are performed, it is necessary also to assess the effect of the new drug on the animal as well as on the tumour. By their very nature, all anticancer agents are likely to damage normal tissues and some attempt should be made to assess the overall toxic effect of new drugs in relation to their ability to retard tumour growth.

The tumours used in animal experiments are not identical with those which afflict human beings and it is quite surprising that the activity of so many substances of undoubted therapeutic value in human beings should have been identified as a result of animal experiments. Attempts to maintain human tumours in tissue culture and to transfer them to experimental animals have so far met with little success.

The possibility of developing *in vitro* methods for the screening of anticancer drugs is now being studied. It is not sufficient simply to add the substance under test to a tumour maintained in culture because the situation is too far removed from that obtaining *in vivo*. However, when more is known of the metabolic processes which specifically sustain the growth of neoplasms, it should be possible to discover new anticancer drugs by studying the nature of substances which modify these basic metabolic processes. In other words, significant new advances in the field of cancer chemotherapy can be expected only when more basic biochemical and physiological information is available—a conclusion which echoes in one particular field the generalization concerning pharmacology as a whole which was expressed in the opening pages of this book.

BIBLIOGRAPHY

Books, monographs and reviews

Brodsky, I. and Kahn, S.B. (eds) (1972). *Cancer Chemotherapy II*. New York: Grune and Stratton.

Brulé, G., Eckhardt, S.J., Hall, T.C. and Winklev, A. (1973). *Drug Therapy of Cancer*. Geneva: World Health Organization.

Busch, H. (1962). *An Introduction to the Biochemistry of the Cancer Cell*. New York: Academic Press.

Chabner, B.A., Myers, C.E., Coleman, C.N. and Johns, D.G. (1975). The clinical pharmacology of antineoplastic agents. *New Engl. J. Med.*, **292**, 1107-1113; 1159-1168.

Clark, R.L. (1961). *Cancer Chemotherapy*. Springfield: Thomas.

Clarysse, A., Kenis, Y. and Mathé, G. (1976). *Cancer Chemotherapy*. Berlin, Heidelberg, New York: Springer-Verlag.

Delmonte, L. and Jukes, T.H. (1962). Folic acid antagonists in ·cancer chemotherapy. *Pharmac. Rev.*, **14**, 91-135.

Dustin, J., Jr., (1963). New aspects of the pharmacology of antimitotic agents. *Pharmac. Rev.*, **15**, 449-480.

Elias, E.G. and Evans, J.T. (1972). Mithramycin in the treatment of Paget's disease of bone. *J. Bone Jt. Surg.*, **54A**, 1730-1736.

Elson, L.A. (1963). *Radiation and Radiomimetic Chemicals.* London: Butterworth.

Galton, D.A.G. (1966). Trends in the therapy of leukaemia. In, Deeley, T.J. and Wood, C.A.P. (Eds.) *Modern Trends in Radiotherapy.* London: Butterworth.

Galton, D.A.G. (1967). The chemotherapy of malignant disease. In, Fulton, W.F.M. (Ed.) *Modern Trends in Pharmacology and Therapeutics,* vol. 1. London: Butterworth.

Harris, R.J.C. (1961). *Biological Approaches to Cancer Chemotherapy.* New York: Academic Press.

Heidelberger, C. (1967). Cancer chemotherapy with purine and pyrimidine analogues. *Ann. rev. Pharmac.,* **7,** 101-124.

Holland, J.F. and Frei, E. (eds) (1973). *Cancer Medicine.* Philadelphia: Lea and Febiger.

Pratt, W.B. (1973). *Fundamentals of Chemotherapy.* New York, London and Toronto: Oxford University Press.

Sartorelli, A.C. and Johns, D.G. (eds) (1975). *Antineoplastic and Immunosuppressive Agents.* Berlin: Springer-Verlag.

Stoll, B.A. (ed) (1972). *Endocrine Therapy in Malignant Disease.* Philadelphia: W.B. Saunders.

Symposium (1963). Chemotherapy of cancer. *Proc. R. Soc. Med.,* **56,** 629-670.

Wheeler, G.P. (1962). Studies related to the mechanisms of action of cytotoxic alkylating agents: a review. *Cancer Research,* **22,** 651-688.

Index

In the index, proprietary names are *italicized:* against each such entry is placed the corresponding approved name. The proprietary names for a particular drug can be found in the text itself, where they are given capital initial letters.

chromium *(cont.)*
 sources and toxicity, 797-8
chromium salts:
 acetate, 798
 phosphate, 926
chromodacryorrhesis, 226
chromone-2-carboxylic acid, 409
chromosomes, 13
chronic toxicity tests, 141-3
chronotropic action, 263
chrysanthemum carboxylic acid esters, 903
chrysotherapy, 454
Chvostek's sign, 782
chymotrypsin, 217
Ciatyl – clopenthixol
Cibazol – sulphathiazole
Cidomycin – gentamycin
cigarette smoking, 206-7
 as a means of absorbing drugs, 34
ciliary ganglion, 159
ciliary muscle, 225
cimetidine, 344, 346, 353-4, 382
cinanserin, 575
cinchocaine, 468, 471
cinchona, 640
cinchona alkaloids, 866
cinchonism, 866
cinchophen, 457
cinerins, 903-4
cingulate gyrus, 167-8
cingulectomy, 168
cinnarazine, 604
circus movement, 681
cirrhosis of the liver, 622, 656, 673, 722, 800, 893
cis – aconitic acid, 29
cisterna magna, 37
Citanest – prilocaine
citrated calcium carbimide, 90
citrates, 611, 665
citrate synthetase, 27
citric acid, 611, 612
citric acid cycle – *see* Krebs cycle
citrovorum factor, 679
citrus fruits as vitamin sources, 794
clam heart preparation, 208, 333
Clark, Alfred J., 6, 97
clathrate fromation, 494
Clauberg and McPhail assay, 752
clearance value, 619
clemizole, 350, 352
clindamycin, 843-4
Clinestrol – stilboestrol
clinical trials, 143-6
Clinimycin – clindamycin
clioquinol – *see* iodochlorhydroxy quinoline
Clistin – carbinoxamine
clobetasol, 766
clobetasone, 766
clofibrate, 671, 705
clomiphene, 749, 776
clomipramine, 546, 581, 582
clomocycline, 839
clonal selection hypothesis, 398
clonazepam, 527, 530, 574
clonic convulsions, 512

clonidine, 299, 310-1, 316, 481
 rebound, 311
clonixin, 446, 447
Clonodin – clonazepam
clonorchiasis, 892
clopamide, 634
clopenthixol, 564
clorazepate, 572
Clorexan – chlorphenoxamine
clorexolone, 634
close arterial injection, 172
closed method of anaesthetic administration, 499
clothiapine, 566
clotrimazole, 909
clotting – *see* coagulation
clotting time, 663
cloxacillin, 828
clozapine, 552, 565, 566
coagulants, 672-4
coagulation of blood, 661-3
cobalamin, *see* cyanocobalamin
Cobalin – cyanocobalamin
cobalt
 physiological significance, dietary sources and toxicity, 798-9
 production of experimental epilepsy, 798
cobalt compounds:
 chloride, 798
 edetate, 701, 799
 sulphate, 798
Cobadex – hydrocortisone
cobra venom, 665
cocaine
 and the 'two sympathins' hypothesis, 171-2
 and morphine receptors, 330
 central actions, 467
 dependence, 85, 91
 effects on sympathetic system, 269
 local anaesthetic action, 466-7
 prevention of noradrenaline uptake, 269
 toxicity, 467
cocarboxylase, 791
coccidiosis, 884
cockerel blood pressure assay, 779
codeine, 429, 652
 antitussive action, 609
 histamine liberating action, 342
Codelcortone – prednisolone
cod liver oil, 788
Codone – hydrocodone
codons, 20
coefficient of variation, 116
coeliac disease, 647
coeliac ganglion, 160
coenzyme I – *see* nicotinamide adenine dinucleotide
coenzyme II – *see* nicotinamide adenine dinucleotide phosphate
coenzyme A, 25, 65, 793
coenzyme Q, 24, 25, 30
Cogentin – benztropine
cohort surveys, 111
coitus, oxytocin in, 773
 prostaglandins in, 374

Colace – dioctyl sodium sulphosuccinate
colaspace – *see* asparaginase
colbenemid, 459
Colcemid – demecolcine
colchicine
 in gout, 457-8
 in leukaemia, 923
 malabsorption caused by, 78
cold compress, 672
colistin, 814, 839-40, 849
collagen diseases, 455
 synthesis, 386
colloidal aluminium hydroxide, 644
colloidal purgatives, 649
colocynth, 650
Colofac – mebeverine
Colomycin – colistin
colour vision defects, 579
Coly-Mycin – colistin
Combantrin – pyrantel pamoate
Committee on Safety of Medicines, 141, 143
common cold
 and antiviral agents, 857, 859
 and vitamin C, 795
Compazine – prochlorperazine
competitive antagonists, 100-104, 237-43
complement fixation test, 399
complement system, 398-9, 400
complete heart block, 683
compliance of lung, 616
Compocillin VK – phenoxymethylpenicillin
compound CL88236, 738
compound 3113CT, 213
compound E – *see* cortisone
compound SQ20881, 314
compound 33T57 – *see* methisazone
compound 48/80, 342, 410
COMT – *see* catechol-*O*-methyltransferase
conditioning, 594
Condon's manometer, 150
Condy's fluid, 800
Confer – ethinyloestradiol + norethisterone acetate
confidence limits, 117-8
congenital adrenal hyperplasia, 758-9, 767
congestive cardiac failure, 693
conjugation as detoxication mechanism, 52, 58, 60-62
 change with age, 70-1
 in bacteria, 852
connective tissue diseases, 440
Conovid, 747
Conovid E, 747
constipation, 427
constrictor pupillae muscle, 224
contact dermatitis, 401
contact poisons, 901
Conteben – thiacetazone
contingency tables, 112-3
contraception, 373, 730, 746-51
contracture, 208
contrast media, 657-8
control experiments, 110-111

nornicotine, 206, 904
Norpace – disopyramide
norpethidine, 431
norphenylephrine, 270
Norpramin – desipramine
Nor Q.D. – ethynodiol diacetate
norsynephrine – *see* octopamine
19-nortestosterone – *see* nandrolone
nortriptyline, 581, 582
noscapine – *see* narcotine
Nospan – tybamate
Nostyn – ectyl urea
Notensil – acepromazine
notezine, 893
Nothiazine – mepazine
Novatrin – homotropine
Noveril – dibenzepin
novobiocin, 843, 854
Novocaine – procaine
Novurit – mercurophyllin
Nozinan – methotrimeprazine
NSD-1055 – *see* 4-bromo-3-
    hydroxybenzyloxyamine
nuclear envelope, 9
nuclear pores, 9
nucleolus, 8, 11
nucleoside kinase, 919
nucleoside phosphorylase, 919
nucleotides, 18-20
nucleus, 8-9
Nulacin (antacid) 644
null hypothesis, 110
Nulogyl – nimorazole
Numorphan –oxymorphine
Nuncital – emylcamate
Nupercaine – cinchocaine
Nuso – soluble insulin
nutmeg, 93, 369, 382
nutritional macrocytic anaemia, 678
nutritional oedema, 621
nux vomica, 621
Nydrazid – isoniazid
nylidrin, 271
nystagmus, 524, 526
nystatin, 854, 883, 908
    in testing antiinflammatory agents,
    463

obesity, 281-5, 573, 724, 749
obidoxine chloride, 222
obligatory excretion of water, 618
obligatory reabsorption of water, 618
Oblivon – methylparafynol
obsessional neuroses, 537
obstructive jaundice, 734
octamethylpyrophosphoramide, 902
Octin – 2-methylaminoheptane
octoclothepine, 565, 566
octopamine, 189, 259, 319
octopus sting, 420
octylamine, 342
octyl nitrite, 700, 701, 702
oculomotor nerve, 159
oculomucocutaneous syndrome, 302
oedema, 376-7, 450, 463, 622, 635
oestradiol, 739-40, 742, 925
oestrane, 740

oestriol, 738, 742
Oestroform – oestradiol
oestrogens, 739-43, 784
    and cyclic GMP, 328
    and glucose tolerance, 723
    antiandrogen effect, 737
    assay, 751
    occurrence, 740, 754
    therapeutic uses, 740-2, 749, 883
oestrone, 739-40, 742
oestrus test, 751
oil of mustard – *see* allyl isothiocyanate
oil of turpentine, 422, 611
oil of wintergreen – *see* methyl salicylate
oil-water partition coefficient, 40, 494
old age, drugs in, 71
oleandomycin, 842
oligomenorrhoea, 741
oligomycin, 31
olive oil, 808
O-methylation of catecholamines, 260-1
O-methylisoprenaline, 272
Omnopan – papaveretum
OMPA – *see*
    octamethylpyrophosphoramide
Onazine – chlorpromazine
onchocerca volvulus, 885
onchocerciasis, 885, 888
Oncovin – vincristine
onychomycosis, 907, 910
open drop method of anaesthesia, 499
open field tests, 594
operant conditioning, 594
opiate receptors, 436-8
Operidine – phenoperidine
Opilon – thymoxamine
opipramol, 581
opisthotonus, 514
opium, 426-7, 428, 652
    dependence, 86
Oppazone – phenylbutazone
opsonins, 400
opsonization, 400
optic nerve, 455, 676
opticrom, 410
Orabolin – ethyloestranol
Oradexon – dexamethasone
oral administration of drugs, 33-4
oral contraceptives, 746-50, 907
Orap – pimozide
Orapen VK – phenoxymethylpenicillin
oral hypoglycaemic agents, 728-30
    and cardiovascular disease, 730
Oranabol – oxymesterone
Oratestin – fluoxymesterone
Oratrol – dichlorphenamide
Orbenin – cloxacillin
Orbinamon – thiothixene
orchidectomy, 741
orciprenaline, 270, 272
Oreton – testosterone propionate
organelles in cell, 7-14
organic psychoses, 537, 538
organoarsenical agents, 861
organomercurial diuretics, 627-9
organophosphorus compounds, 215-8,
    902-3
oriental sore, 874, 875

Orinase – tolbutamide
oripavines, 430
Orisulf – sulphaphenazole
Orlest – ethinyloestradiol +
    norethisterone acetate (p.747)
orogenital syndrome, 791
orphenadrine, 596
Orpidan – chlorazanil
Ortal –hexethal
orthocaine, 468
Orthoform – orthocaine
Ortho-Novin – mestranol +
    norethisterone (p.747)
Orthoxine – methoxphenamine
Orudis – ketoprofen
osmoreceptors, 618
osmotic diuretics, 623
Ospolot – sulthiame
osteitis fibrosa generalisita, 783
Ostensin – trimethidinium
osteoarthritis, 386, 440, 451, 452
osteoblasts, 782
osteoclasts, 387, 782
osteomalacia, 525, 784, 788
osteomyelitis, 843
osteoporosis, 453, 666, 734, 741, 754,
    784, 785, 789
Othello, 4
otitis media, 822
otolith organs, 601, 602
ototoxicity, 630
ouabagenin, 491-2
ouabain, 42, 691, 697
ouabain-sensitive ATPase, 44
Ovanon – mestranol + lynoestrenol
    (p.747)
ovarian failure, 740
ovarian tumour, 732, 912, 915, 916,
    922, 924
overbreathing in diagnosis of epilepsy,
    520
overpigmentation, 544, 771, 774, 810-1
over-suppression syndrome, 749
Overton-Meyer rule of anaesthesia, 494
Ovestin – oestriol
Ovocyclin – oestradiol
Ovocyclin M – oestradiol monobenzoate
Ovran – ethinyloestradiol + norgestrel
    (p.747)
Ovranette – ethinyloestradiol +
    norgestrel (p.747)
Ovrette – norgestrel
ovulation, 738, 741
Ovulen – ethinyloestradiol (or
    mestranol) + ethynodiol acetate
    (p.747)
oxacillin, 828
oxaloacetic acid, 27, 28, 29
oxalosuccinic acid, 28-9
oxamides, 213, 215
Oxamycin – cycloserine
oxandrolone, 736
7-oxaprostanoic acid, 370
7-oxa-13-prostynoic acid, 370
oxazepam, 527, 572, 574
oxazolidinediones, 528
oxedrine – *see* synephrine
oxeladin, 610